AAOS

Intermediate
Emergency
Care and Transportation of the Sick and Injured

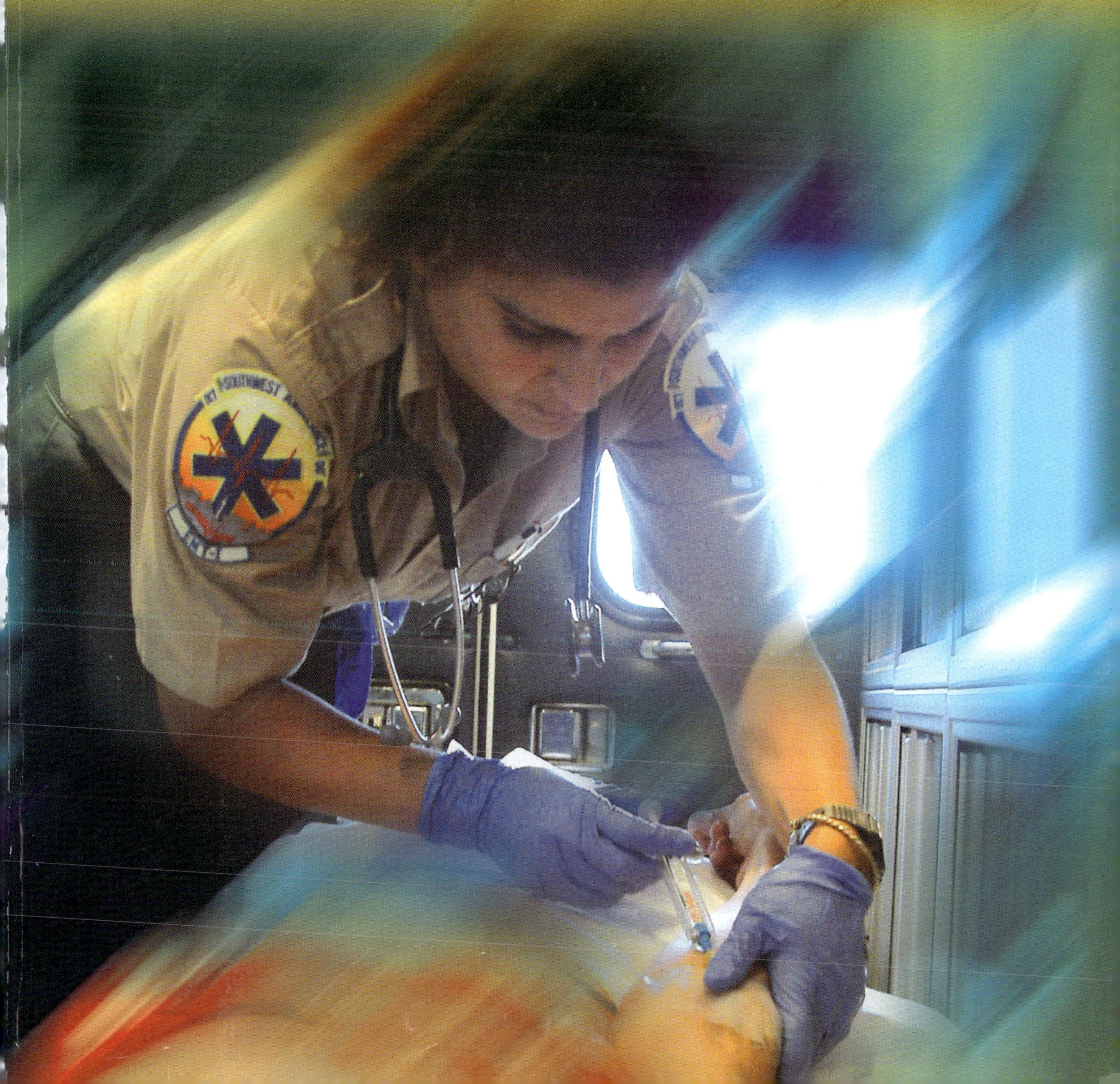

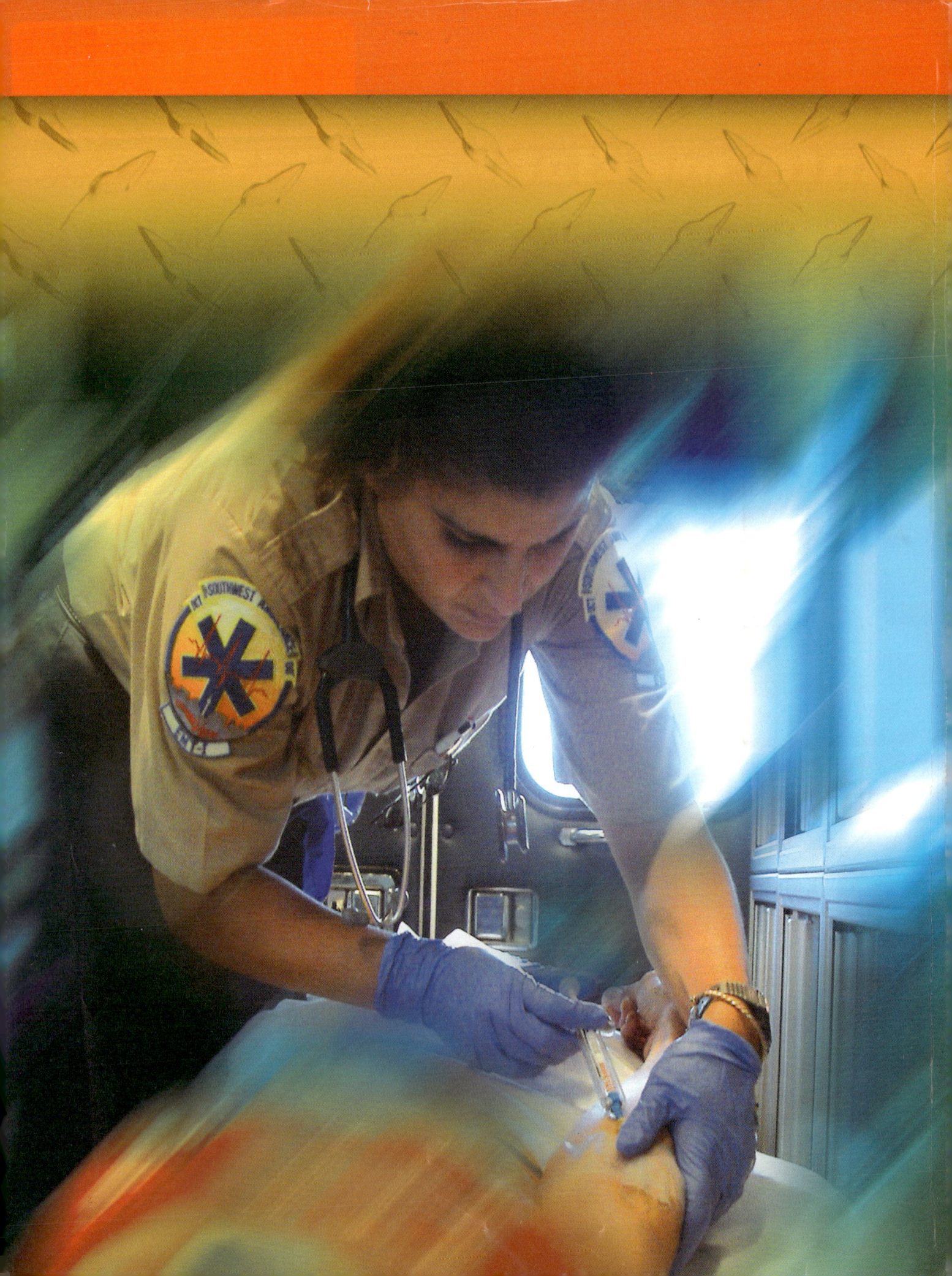

AAOS

Intermediate Emergency
Care and Transportation of the Sick and Injured

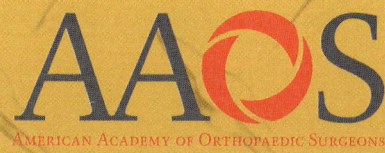
AMERICAN ACADEMY OF ORTHOPAEDIC SURGEONS

Author:
Rhonda J. Beck, NREMT-P
Editor:
Stephen J. Rahm, NREMT-P
Series Editor:
Andrew N. Pollak, MD, FAAOS

JONES AND BARTLETT PUBLISHERS
Sudbury, Massachusetts
BOSTON   TORONTO   LONDON   SINGAPORE

Jones and Bartlett Publishers

World Headquarters
Jones and Bartlett Publishers
40 Tall Pine Drive, Sudbury, MA 01776
978-443-5000
info@jbpub.com
www.EMSzone.com

Jones and Bartlett Publishers Canada
6339 Ormindale Way
Mississauga, ON L5V 1J2
Canada

Jones and Bartlett Publishers International
Barb House, Barb Mews
London W6 7PA
United Kingdom

Production Credits
Chief Executive Officer: Clayton Jones
Chief Operating Officer: Donald W. Jones, Jr.
President, Higher Education and Professional Publishing: Robert Holland
V.P., Sales and Marketing: William J. Kane
V.P., Production and Design: Anne Spencer
V.P., Manufacturing and Inventory Control: Therese Bräuer
Publisher, Public Safety: Kim Brophy
Publisher, Emergency Care: Lawrence D. Newell
Managing Editor: Carol E. Brewer
Associate Managing Editor: Jennifer Reed
Production Editors: Scarlett Stoppa, Susan Schultz
Text Design: Anne Spencer, Kristin Ohlin
Composition: Graphic World
Illustrations: Imagineering, Graphic World
Cover Design: Kristin Ohlin
Cover Photograph: © Eddie Sperling
Photo Research: Scarlett Stoppa, Kimberly Potvin, Kristin Ohlin
Printing and Binding: Replika Press Pvt. Ltd.

AAOS
American Academy of Orthopaedic Surgeons

Editorial Credits
Chief Education Officer: Mark W. Wieting
Director, Department of Publications: Marilyn L. Fox, PhD
Managing Editor: Lynne Roby Shindoll
Managing Editor: Barbara A. Scotese

Board of Directors 2004
Robert W. Bucholz, MD, *President*
Stuart L. Weinstein, MD
Richard F. Kyle, MD
Edward A. Toriello, MD
James H. Herndon, MD
Vernon T. Tolo, MD
Frederick M. Azar, MD
Frances A. Farley, MD
Oheneba Boachie-Adjei, MD
Laura L. Tosi, MD
Peter J. Mandell, MD
Frank B. Kelly, MD
Dwight W. Burney, III, MD
Glenn B. Pfeffer, MD
Mark C. Gebhardt, MD
Andrew N. Pollak, MD
Leslie L. Altick
Karen L. Hackett, FACHE, CAE, *Ex-Officio*

Copyright © 2005 by Jones and Bartlett Publishers, LLC and American Academy of Orthopaedic Surgeons
All rights reserved. No part of the material protected by this copyright notice may be reproduced or utilized in any form, electronic or mechanical, including photocopying, recording, or by any information storage and retrieval system, without written permission from the copyright owner.

The procedures and protocols in this book are based on the most current recommendations of responsible medical sources. The American Academy of Orthopaedic Surgeons and the publisher, however, make no guarantee as to, and assume no responsibility for, the correctness, sufficiency, or completeness of such information or recommendations. Other or additional safety measures may be required under particular circumstances.

This textbook is intended solely as a guide to the appropriate procedures to be employed when rendering emergency care to the sick and injured. It is not intended as a statement of the standards of care required in any particular situation, because circumstances and the patient's physical condition can vary widely from one emergency to another. Nor is it intended that this textbook shall in any way advise emergency personnel concerning legal authority to perform the activities or procedures discussed. Such local determinations should be made only with the aid of legal council.

Library of Congress Cataloging-in-Publication Data
Intermediate emergency care and transportation of the sick and injured /
American Academy of Orthopaedic Surgeons ; editors, Rhonda J. Beck, Andrew N. Pollak, Stephen J. Rahm.
  p. ; cm.
 Includes index.
 ISBN 0-7637-2244-8 (pbk. : alk. paper)
 1. Medical emergencies. 2. Transport of sick and wounded. 3. Emergency medical technicians.
 [DNLM: 1. Emergency Medical Services--methods--Handbooks. 2. Emergency Medical Technicians--education--Handbooks. 3. Transportation of Patients--methods--Handbooks. WX 39 I61 2005] I. Beck, Rhonda J. II. Pollak, Andrew N. III. Rahm, Stephen J. IV. American Academy of Orthopaedic Surgeons. V. Title.

RC86.7.I563 2005
616.02'5--dc22
                                        2004020315
6048

ISBN-13: 978-0-7637-9589-4

Additional illustrations and photo credits appear on page 1598, which constitutes a continuation of the copyright page.
Printed in India
14 13 12 11 10   10 9 8 7 6 5 4

Brief Contents

Section 1 — Preparing to be an EMT-I
- Chapter 1 Introduction to Emergency Medical Care ... 2
- Chapter 2 The Well-Being of the EMT-I 24
- Chapter 3 Medical, Legal, and Ethical Issues 74
- Chapter 4 Medical Terminology 96
- Chapter 5 The Human Body 114

Section 2 — Pharmacology and Intravenous Therapy
- Chapter 6 Pharmacology 242
- Chapter 7 Intravenous Access 284
- Chapter 8 Medication Administration............. 326

Section 3 — Airway
- Chapter 9 Airway Management and Ventilation..... 362

Section 4 — Patient Assessment
- Chapter 10 Patient Assessment................... 488
- Chapter 11 Communications and Documentation 576

Section 5 — Trauma
- Chapter 12 Trauma Systems and Mechanism of Injury . 616
- Chapter 13 Hemorrhage and Shock 642
- Chapter 14 Burns and Soft-Tissue Injuries 674
- Chapter 15 Thoracic Trauma 712
- Chapter 16 Abdomen and Genitalia Injuries 742
- Chapter 17 Head and Spine Injuries 758
- Chapter 18 Musculoskeletal Care 798

Section 6 — Medical Emergencies
- Chapter 19 Respiratory Emergencies 848
- Chapter 20 Cardiovascular Emergencies 880
- Chapter 21 Diabetic Emergencies 984
- Chapter 22 Allergic Reactions and Envenomations .. 1004
- Chapter 23 Poisonings and Overdose Emergencies .. 1032
- Chapter 24 Neurologic Emergencies.............. 1058
- Chapter 25 Nontraumatic Abdominal Emergencies .. 1082
- Chapter 26 Environmental Emergencies........... 1098
- Chapter 27 Behavioral Emergencies 1130
- Chapter 28 Gynecologic Emergencies............. 1150

Section 7 — Special Considerations
- Chapter 29 Obstetric Emergencies 1166
- Chapter 30 Neonatal Resuscitation 1200
- Chapter 31 Pediatric Emergencies 1228
- Chapter 32 Geriatric Emergencies 1336

Section 8 — Operations
- Chapter 33 Ambulance Operations 1372
- Chapter 34 Lifting and Moving 1402
- Chapter 35 Gaining Access 1444
- Chapter 36 Special Operations 1460
- Chapter 37 Response to Terrorism and Weapons of Mass Destruction 1490

Section 9 — Enrichment
- Chapter 38 Assessment-Based Management 1524
- Chapter 39 BLS Review 1544

Index 1578

Additional Credits 1596

Contents

Section 1 Preparing to be an EMT-I

1 Introduction to Emergency Medical Care 2

Introduction to Emergency Medical Care 6
Course Description 6
EMT-Intermediate Training: Focus and Requirements 7
Certification Requirements 8
Overview of the Emergency Medical Services System 9
    History of EMS 9
Levels of Training 10
    Public Basic Life Support and Immediate Aid 11
    First Responders 11
    EMT-Basic 11
    EMT-Intermediate 12
    EMT-Paramedic 12
Components of the EMS System 12
    Access 12
    Administration and Policy 13
    Medical Direction and Control 13
    Quality Control and Improvement 14
    Other Physician Input 15
    Regulation 15
    Equipment 15
    The Ambulance 15
    Transport to Specialty Centers 15
    Interfacility Transports 16
    Working With Hospital Staff 16
    Working With Public Safety Agencies 16
    Training 17
    Providing a Coordinated Continuum of Care 17
Roles and Responsibilities of the EMT-I 18
    Professional Attributes 18
Continuing Education 19
Prep Kit 21

2 The Well-Being of the EMT-I 24

The Well-Being of the EMT-I 26
Emotional Aspects of Emergency Care 26
Death and Dying 26
    Physical Signs of Death 27
    Medical Examiner Cases 28
    The Grieving Process 28
    What Can the EMT-I Do? 29
    Dealing With the Patient and Family Members ... 29
Initial Care of the Dying, Critically Ill, or Injured Patient ... 30
    Anxiety 30
    Pain and Fear 30
    Anger and Hostility 30
    Depression 30
    Dependency 30
    Guilt 31
    Mental Health Problems 31
    Receiving Unrelated Bad News 31
Caring for Critically Ill and Injured Patients 31
    Avoid Sad and Grim Comments 31
    Orient the Patient 31
    Be Honest 32
    Acknowledge the Seriousness of the Condition .. 32
    Allow for Hope 32
    Locate and Notify Family Members 32
Injured and Critically Ill Children 32
    Dealing With the Death of a Child 32
    Helping the Family 33
Stressful Situations 33
    Uncertain Situations 34
Stress Warning Signs and the Work Environment 34
    Stress and Nutrition 36
    Stress Management 37
    Critical Incident Stress Debriefing 40
Workplace Issues 41
    Cultural Diversity on the Job 41
    Your Effectiveness as an EMT-I 42
    Avoiding Sexual Harassment 42
    Substance Abuse 43
Scene Safety and Personal Protection 44
Communicable Diseases 45
    Routes of Transmission 45
Risk Reduction and Prevention 45
    Universal Precautions and Body Substance
        Isolation 45
    Employer Responsibilities 50
    Exposure Control Plan 51
Immunity 52
    Immunizations 52
Duty to Act 53
Some Diseases of Special Concern 54
    HIV Infection 54
    Hepatitis 55
    Meningitis 56
    Tuberculosis 56
    Other Diseases of Concern 57
General Postexposure Management 57
Establishing an Infection Control Routine 58
Illness and Injury Prevention 59
    Prevention Strategies 59
Scene Hazards 60
    Hazardous Materials 60
    Electricity 61
    Fire 62
Protective Clothing: Preventing Injury 63
    Cold Weather Clothing 63
    Turnout Gear 63
    Gloves 64
    Helmets 64
    Boots 64
    Eye Protection 65
    Ear Protection 65
    Skin Protection 65
    Body Armor 65

| Violent Situations 65
| Behavioral Emergencies 66
| Prep Kit 69

3   Medical, Legal, and Ethical Issues   74

Medical, Legal, and Ethical Issues 78
Scope of Practice 78
Standards of Care 78
   Standards Imposed by Local Custom 78
   Standards Imposed by Law 79
   Professional and Institutional Standards 79
   Standards Imposed by States 80
Laws 81
   Legislative, Administrative, and Common 81
   Criminal Law 81
   Civil (Tort) Law 81
Duty to Act 81
Negligence 81
Abandonment 82
Consent 82
   Expressed Consent 83
   Implied Consent 83
   Minors and Consent 83
   Mentally Incompetent Adults 84
   Forcible Restraint 84
Assault and Battery 84
The Right to Refuse Treatment 85
Good Samaritan Laws and Immunity 85
Advance Directives 86
Ethical Responsibilities 87
Confidentiality 88
   HIPAA 88
Records and Reports 88
Special Reporting Requirements 89
   Abuse of Children, Elderly People, and Others . . . 89
   Injury During the Commission of a Felony 89
   Drug-Related Injuries 89
   Childbirth 89
   Other Reporting Requirements 89
   Scene of a Crime 90
   The Deceased 90
Special Situations 90
   Organ Donors 90
   Medical Identification Insignia 91
Prep Kit 92

4   Medical Terminology   96

Medical Terminology 98
Prefixes 98
Suffixes 101
Root Words 101
Abbreviations 104
Prep Kit 112

5   The Human Body   114

Introduction 118
The Structure of the Human Body 118
   Cells 118
   Tissues 118
   Organs 118
   Organ Systems 118
   Homeostasis 118
Anatomic Terminology 119
   The Anatomic Position 119
   Anatomic Planes 120
   Directional Terms 122
   Abdominal Quadrants 123
   Anatomic Positions 123
   Movement and Positions 123
Cellular Transport Mechanisms 126
   Permeability of the Cell Membrane 126
   Cellular Metabolism 128
   Cellular Respiration 128
Tissues 129
   Epithelial Tissue and Glands 129
   Connective Tissue 129
   Muscle Tissue 130
   Nerve Tissue 130
Integumentary System 130
   Functions of the Skin 131
   Anatomy of the Skin 132
Skeletal System 133
   The Skull 134
   The Neck 138
   The Spine 139
   The Thorax 141
   The Abdomen 143
   The Appendicular Skeleton 145
   The Pelvic Girdle 148
   The Lower Extremity 149
   Cartilage, Tendons, and Ligaments 152
   Bones: Their Growth and Organization 152
   Joints 156
The Musculoskeletal System 158
   Skeletal Muscle 158
   Smooth Muscle 160
   Cardiac Muscle 160
The Nervous System 160
   The Central Nervous System 162
   The Peripheral Nervous System 168
   The Autonomic Nervous System 171
The Endocrine System 173
   The Pituitary Gland and Hypothalamus 174
   The Thyroid Gland 175
   The Parathyroid Glands 176
   The Pancreas 176
   The Adrenal Glands 177
   The Reproductive Glands and Hormones 178
Blood and Its Components 178
   Plasma and Formed Elements (Cells) 178
The Heart 181

Location and Major Structures of the Heart 181
Valves of the Heart 182
Blood Flow Within the Heart 182
Electrical Properties of the Heart and Conduction System 184
The Cardiac Cycle 187

The Vascular System 188
The General Scheme of Blood Circulation 188
Circulation to the Heart 188
The Pulmonary Circulation 189
Systemic Arterial Circulation 189
The Systemic Venous Circulation 194

Physiology of the Circulatory System 196
Normal Circulation in Adults 197
Inadequate Circulation in Adults 198

The Lymphatic System 198
Lymphatic Vessels 198
Lymph Organs 200

The Respiratory System 201
The Upper Airway 201
The Lower Airway 202
Respiratory Physiology 204

The Digestive System 207
How Digestion Works 207
Anatomy of the Digestive System 208

The Urinary System 209
The Genital System 210
The Male Reproductive System and Organs 210
The Female Reproductive System and Organs 210
Fluids and Electrolytes 212
Body Fluid Balance 212
Acid-Base Balance 213
Buffer Systems 213
Prep Kit 216

Section 2 Pharmacology and Intravenous Therapy

6 Pharmacology 242

Pharmacology 244
How Medications Work 244
Medication Names 245
Methods of Drug Classification 246
Standardization of Drugs 246
The Scope of Practice 247
Nervous System Divisions 247
Drug Properties 250
Drug Forms 250
Solid Drugs 250
Liquid Drugs 251
Metered-Dose Inhalers 252
Topical Medications 252
Transcutaneous Medications 252
Gels 253
Gases 254

Overview of the Routes of Drug Administration 254
Mechanism of Action 255
Pharmacokinetics: Movement of Drugs Through the Body 257
Drug Absorption 257
Drug Distribution 258
Biotransformation 258
Drug Elimination 258

Pharmacodynamics: Drug Actions 259
Drug-response Relationship 259
Predictable Responses 259
Iatrogenic Responses 259
Unpredictable Adverse Responses 259

Factors Influencing Drug Interactions 260
Drug Storage and Security of Controlled Substances 262
Activated Charcoal 262
General Steps in Administering Medication 263
Prep Kit 280

7 Intravenous Access 284

Intravenous Access 286
Basic Cell Physiology 286
Electrolytes 286
Fluid and Electrolyte Movement 287
Fluid Compartments 289
Fluid Balance 290

Principles of Fluid Balance 291
Internal Environment of the Cell 291
Body Fluid Composition 292
IV Fluid Composition 293
Types of IV Solutions 293

IV Techniques and Administration 296
Assembling Your Equipment 296
Choosing an IV Solution 297
Choosing an Administration Set 297
Choosing an IV Site 298
Choosing a Catheter 301
Inserting the IV Catheter 303
Drawing Blood 304
Securing the Line 305
Discontinuing the IV Line 306
Alternative IV Sites and Techniques 306
Dimensional Analysis 312
Drip Rates 312
Drops per Minute 313

Possible Complications of IV Therapy 313
Local IV Site Reactions 313
Systemic Complications 316

Troubleshooting 318
Pediatric Considerations 318
Catheters 318
Volutrol IV Sets 318
IV Locations 318

Geriatric Considerations 319
Catheters 319

IV Sets 319
  Locations 319
Prep Kit 321

8 Medication Administration 326

Medication Administration 328
Mathematical Principles Used in Pharmacology 328
  The Metric System 328
Weight and Volume Conversion 329
  Weight Conversion 329
  Volume Conversion 330
Converting Pounds to Kilograms 330
The Apothecary System 331
Fahrenheit and Celsius Scales 331
Calculating Medication Doses 331
  Desired Dose 331
  Drug Concentrations 332
  Volume to be Administered 332
Weight-Based Drug Doses 333
Calculating the Dose and Rate for a Medication Infusion .. 333
Pediatric Doses 334
Medical Direction 334
Principles of Medication Administration 335
Medications Administered by the Inhalation Route 336
Enteral Medication Administration 337
  Oral Administration 337
  Rectal Administration 338
Parenteral Administration of Medications 340
  Equipment 340
  Packaging of Parenteral Medications 340
Administration of Medication by the Subcutaneous Route . 343
Administration of Medication Via the
  Intramuscular Route 347
Administration of Medication Via Intravenous Bolus 349
Administration of Medication Via the IO Route 351
Administering Medications Via the Sublingual Route 352
Prep Kit 357

Section 3 Airway

9 Airway Management and Ventilation 362

Airway 368
Anatomy of the Upper Airway 368
  Nasopharynx 368
  Oropharynx 369
  Larynx 369
Anatomy of the Lower Airway 370
Lung and Respiratory Volumes 370
Ventilation 372
  Inspiration 372
  Expiration 372
  Respiration 372
Causes of Decreased Oxygen Concentrations
  in the Blood 373
  Carbon Dioxide in the Blood 373
  The Measurement of Gases 373
Respiratory Rate 374
  Neural Control 374
  Chemical Stimuli 374
  Control of Respiration by Other Factors 375
Airway Evaluation 376
  Essential Parameters 376
  Recognition of Airway Problems 376
Acid-Base Balance 378
  Defining the Acidity of a Solution 378
  Ion Shifts 378
  Buffers 378
  Compensatory Mechanisms 380
  Clinical Presentations 380
Maintaining the Airway 383
Airway Management 384
  Manual Maneuvers 385
Airway Obstructions 388
  Possible Causes of Airway Obstruction 389
  Recognition 391
  Emergency Medical Care for Foreign Body Airway
    Obstruction 392
Suctioning 397
  Suctioning Equipment 398
  Techniques of Suctioning 398
  Airway Adjuncts 402
  Nasal Airway 405
Supplemental Oxygen 406
  Liquid Oxygen 408
  Pin-Indexing System 408
  Regulators 409
  Flowmeters 409
Operating Procedures 410
  Hazards of Supplemental Oxygen 411
Supplemental Oxygen-Delivery Devices 412
  Nonrebreathing Mask 412
  Nasal Cannula 412
  Simple Face Mask 413
  Partial Rebreathing Mask 413
  Venturi Mask 413
  Small Volume Nebulizer 413
  Oxygen Humidifiers 413
Assisted and Artificial Ventilation 414
  Mouth-to-Mouth, Mouth-to-Nose, and Mouth-to-
    Mask Ventilation 414
  One-Person BVM Device 415
  Two-Person BVM Ventilation Method 417
  Three-Person BVM Ventilation 418
  Technique 418
  Flow-Restricted, Oxygen-Powered Ventilation
    Devices 420
  Automatic Transport Ventilators 422
  Cricoid Pressure/Sellick Maneuver 422

Gastric Distention 423
    Gastric Tubes 423
    Dental Appliances 428
    Facial Bleeding 430
Multilumen Airways 430
    Advantages and Disadvantages of
        Multilumen Airways 431
    Indications for Multilumen Airways 431
    Contraindications for Multilumen Airways 431
    Complications of Multilumen Airways 431
    Equipment for Multilumen Airways 431
    Technique for Multilumen Airway Insertion 436
Advanced Airway Management 438
    Endotracheal Intubation 438
    Orotracheal Intubation by Direct Laryngoscopy .. 440
    Tracheobronchial Suctioning 451
    Pediatric Endotracheal Intubation 453
    Intubation Technique 456
    Esophageal Obturator Airway (EOA) 461
    The Laryngeal Mask Airway 463
Tracheostomy, Stoma, and Tracheostomy Tubes 466
    Ventilation of Stoma Patients 467
Special Patient Considerations 471
Prep Kit 477

Section 4 Patient Assessment

10 Patient Assessment — 488

About This Chapter 495
    Patient Assessment 495
Scene Size-up 497
Body Substance Isolation 497
Scene Safety 497
    Personal Protection 497
    Making the Unsafe Scene Safe 498
**Determine the Mechanism of Injury or Nature
of the Illness** 498
    Mechanism of Injury 499
    Nature of the Illness 501
    Determine the Number of Patients 502
Initial Assessment 505
Form a General Impression of the Patient's Condition ... 505
Distinguishing Between Medical and Trauma Patients 506
Approach to the Assessment Process 508
Assess Mental Status 508
Assess the Airway 509
    Responsive Patients 510
    Unresponsive Patients 511
Assess Breathing 511
Assess Circulation 512
    Assess the Pulse 512
    Assess and Control External Bleeding 512
    Evaluate Skin Color, Temperature,
        and Condition 513

Identify Priority Patients 514
Focused History and Physical Exam: Trauma Patients ... 517
    Goals of the Focused History and Physical Exam 517
    Reconsider the MOI 518
    Significant Mechanisms of Injury 518
    Infant and Child Considerations 518
    Hidden Injuries 518
Trauma Patients With a Significant MOI 520
Rapid Trauma Assessment 520
    Head, Neck, and Cervical Spine 520
    Chest 521
    Abdomen 524
    Pelvis 524
    Extremities 524
    Back 524
    Baseline Vital Signs and SAMPLE History 525
    Transport 526
Trauma Patients With No Significant MOI 526
    Focused Assessment: Chief Complaint 526
    Baseline Vital Signs and SAMPLE History 528
    Transport 528
    Documentation 528
    Other Considerations 529
Focused History and Physical Exam: Medical Patients ... 531
    Evaluate Responsiveness 531
    History of Present Illness 531
    OPQRST-I 532
    The SAMPLE History 534
    The Focused Physical Exam 535
    Baseline Vital Signs 536
    Reevaluate the Transport Decision 536
    Documentation 536
Evaluating the Unresponsive Patient 536
    Rapid Medical Assessment 537
    Baseline Vital Signs 537
    History of Present Illness/
        SAMPLE History 537
    Reevaluate the Transport Decision 538
    Documentation 538
Detailed Physical Exam 541
Steps of the Detailed Physical Exam 542
    Head, Neck, and Cervical Spine 543
    Chest 546
    Chest: Chest Wall 546
    Chest: Breath Sounds 547
    Chest: Heart Sounds 548
    Abdomen 548
    Pelvis 549
    Extremities 549
    Cranial Nerve Assessment 550
    Back 550
    Cardiovascular System 550
    Baseline Vital Signs 551
    Mental Status 551
Ongoing Assessment 553
    Steps of the Ongoing Assessment 553
    Repeat the Initial Assessment 554
    Reassess Vital Signs 554
    Repeat the Focused Assessment 554

Check Interventions 555	Communicating With Non-English-Speaking
Transportation Considerations 555	Patients 600

Clinical Decision Making 557
The Prehospital Environment 557
The Spectrum of Prehospital Patients 558
   Levels of Patient Acuity 558
Protocols, Standing Orders, and Algorithms 559
Critical Thinking and the EMT-I 559
   Concept Formation 559
   Data Interpretation 560
   Application of Principles 560
   Evaluation 560
   Reflection on Action 560
Fundamental Elements of Critical Thinking 561
Field Application of Assessment-Based Management 561
   The Spectrum of Patient Acuity 561
   Thinking Under Pressure 561
   Mental Checklist for Thinking Under Pressure . . 562
   Facilitating Behaviors 562
   Situational Awareness 562
Putting It All Together: "The Six Rs" 563
   Read the Patient 563
   Read the Scene 564
   React 564
   Reevaluate 564
   Revise the Management Plan 564
   Review Performance at the Run Critique 564
Prep Kit 568

11 Communications and Documentation   576

Communications and Documentation 580
Communications Systems and Equipment 580
   Base Station Radios 580
   Mobile and Portable Radios 581
   Repeater-Based Systems 582
   Digital Equipment 582
   Cellular Telephones 583
   Other Communications Equipment 584
Components of the Local Dispatch Communications System and Function 584
Radio Communications 586
   Responding to the Scene 586
   Communicating With Medical Control and
      Hospitals 588
   Standard Procedures and Protocols 591
   Reporting Requirements 591
   Maintenance of Radio Equipment 591
Verbal Communications 593
   Communicating With Other Health Care
      Professionals 593
   Communicating With Patients 594
   Communicating With Older Patients 596
   Communicating With Children 597
   Communicating With Hearing-Impaired
      Patients 598
   Communicating With Visually Impaired
      Patients 598
   Communicating With Non-English-Speaking
      Patients 600
Written Communications and Documentation 600
   Minimum Data Set 600
   Prehospital Care Report 600
   Types of Forms 602
   General Considerations 603
   Elements of a Properly Written EMS Document . 603
   Reporting Errors 604
   Documenting Refusal of Care 604
   Systems of Narrative Writing 604
   Data Collection 606
   Special Reporting Situations 606
   Consequences of Errors, Omissions, and
      Inappropriate Documentation 606
Prep Kit 610

Section 5   Trauma

12 Trauma Systems and Mechanism of Injury   616

Kinematics of Trauma 618
Trauma Systems 618
   Components 618
   Trauma Centers 619
   Transport Considerations 619
Energy and Trauma 620
   Energy Exchange 622
Blunt and Penetrating Trauma 622
Mechanism of Injury Profiles 623
Blunt Trauma 623
   Blunt Trauma: Vehicular Collisions 623
   Frontal Collisions 626
   Rear-End Collisions 630
   Lateral Collisions 630
   Rollover Crashes 631
   Rotational Impacts 632
Restraints 633
   Lap Belts 633
   Shoulder Restraints 633
   Air Bags 633
   Child Safety Seats 634
Motorcycle Collisions 634
Pedestrian Versus Motor Vehicle 635
Falls 635
Penetrating Trauma 636
Blast Injuries 638
Prep Kit 640

13 Hemorrhage and Shock   642

Hemorrhage and Shock 646
Physiology and Perfusion 646
Hemorrhage 648
   The Significance of Bleeding 648

Physiologic Response to Hemorrhage 649
　　　　Assessment 651
　　　　Management 651
　　　　Bleeding from the Nose, Ears, and Mouth 658
　Shock 659
　　　Pathophysiology of Shock 659
　　　Compensation for Decreased Perfusion 660
　　　Stages of Shock 661
　　　Etiologic Classifications 663
　　　Differential Shock Assessment Findings 666
　　　Management 666
　Prep Kit 670

14 Burns and Soft-Tissue Injuries — 674

Burns and Soft-Tissue Injuries 678
The Anatomy and Function of the Skin 678
　　Anatomy of the Skin 678
　　Functions of the Skin 679
Types of Soft-Tissue Injuries 679
Closed Injuries 680
　　Emergency Medical Care 681
Open Injuries 681
　　Emergency Medical Care 684
Chest Wounds 686
Abdominal Wounds 688
Impaled Objects 689
Amputations 690
Neck Injuries 690
Burns 691
　　Pathophysiology 691
　　Management 692
　　Burn Severity 692
　　Mechanisms of Burn Injuries 694
　　Signs and Symptoms of Burn Injuries 694
　　Emergency Medical Care 695
　　Inhalation Burns 698
　　Chemical Burns 699
　　Electrical Burns 702
　　Radiation Exposure 705
Dressing and Bandaging 707
　　Sterile Dressings 707
　　Bandages 707
Prep Kit 709

15 Thoracic Trauma — 712

Thoracic Injuries 716
Anatomy and Physiology Review of the Thorax 716
　　Anatomy 716
　　Physiology 718
Injuries of the Chest 719
　　Pathophysiology of Thoracic Trauma 720
　　Management 722
Chest Wall Injuries 723
　　Rib Fractures 723
　　Flail Chest 724
　　Sternal Fracture 725
Injury to the Lung 725
　　Simple Pneumothorax 725
　　Open Pneumothorax 726
　　Tension Pneumothorax 727
　　Hemothorax 730
　　Pulmonary Contusion 731
Myocardial Injuries 732
　　Pericardial Tamponade 732
　　Myocardial Contusion 733
Vascular Injuries 733
　　Aortic Dissection and Rupture 733
　　Penetrating Wounds of the Great Vessels 733
Other Thoracic Injuries 734
　　Diaphragmatic Injury 734
　　Esophageal Injury 734
　　Tracheobronchial Injuries 734
　　Traumatic Asphyxia 734
Management of Thoracic Injuries 735
Prep Kit 739

16 Abdomen and Genitalia Injuries — 742

Abdomen and Genitalia Injuries 744
Anatomy of the Abdomen 744
Injuries to the Abdomen 745
　　Signs and Symptoms 746
　　Evaluating Abdominal Injuries 746
Types of Abdominal Injuries 747
　　Blunt Abdominal Wounds 747
　　Injuries From Seat Belts and Airbags 748
　　Penetrating Abdominal Injuries 749
　　Abdominal Evisceration 750
Management of Abdominal Injuries 751
Anatomy of the Genitourinary System 751
Injuries to the Genitourinary System 751
　　Injuries to the Kidney 751
　　Injuries to the Urinary Bladder 753
　　Injuries to the External Male Genitalia 754
　　Injuries to the Female Genitalia 754
Prep Kit 756

17 Head and Spine Injuries — 758

Head and Spine Injuries 762
Anatomy and Physiology of the Nervous System 762
　　Central Nervous System 762
　　Protective Coverings 762
　　Peripheral Nervous System 764
　　How the Nervous System Works 765
Anatomy and Physiology of the Skeletal System 766
Injuries of the Spine 767
　　Assessment of Spinal Injuries 767
　　Emergency Medical Care 769

Preparation for Transport 771
   Supine Patients 771
   Sitting Patients 773
   Standing Patients 774
Head Injuries 775
   Scalp Lacerations 775
   Skull Fracture 777
   Brain Injuries 779
   Other Brain Injuries 780
   Complications of Head Injury 781
Assessing Head Injuries 781
   Types of Head Injuries 781
   Signs and Symptoms of Head Injury 782
   Emergency Medical Care 783
   Immobilization Devices 785
Helmet Removal 788
   Preferred Method 789
   Alternative Method 789
Prep Kit 794

18 Musculoskeletal Care   798

Musculoskeletal Care 800
Anatomy and Physiology of the Musculoskeletal System .. 800
   Muscles 800
   The Skeleton 801
Musculoskeletal Injuries 802
   Mechanism of Injury 804
   Fractures 804
   Dislocations 807
   Sprains 807
Assessing Musculoskeletal Injuries 808
   Assessing Pulse, Motor, and Sensory Function .. 809
   Assessing the Severity of Injury 812
Emergency Medical Care 812
   Splinting 813
   Transportation 824
Specific Musculoskeletal Injuries 824
   Injuries of the Clavicle and Scapula 824
   Dislocation of the Shoulder 826
   Fracture of the Humerus 827
   Elbow Injuries 829
   Fractures of the Forearm 830
   Injuries of the Wrist and Hand 830
   Fractures of the Pelvis 831
   Dislocation of the Hip 834
   Fractures of the Proximal Femur 834
   Femoral Shaft Fractures 836
   Injuries of Knee Ligaments 836
   Dislocation of the Knee 836
   Fractures About the Knee 837
   Dislocation of the Patella 838
   Injuries of the Tibia and Fibula 838
   Ankle Injuries 839
   Foot Injuries 839
Prep Kit 842

Section 6 Medical Emergencies

19 Respiratory Emergencies   848

Respiratory Emergencies 850
Anatomy and Function of the Lungs 851
Causes of Dyspnea 854
   Upper or Lower Airway Infection 854
   Acute Pulmonary Edema 854
   Obstructive Airway Disease 858
   Assessment Findings 861
   Spontaneous Pneumothorax 862
   Pneumonia 863
   Pleural Effusions 863
   Mechanical Obstruction of the Airway 863
   Pulmonary Thromboembolism 864
   Hyperventilation Syndrome 865
Emergency Care of Respiratory Emergencies 866
   Scene Size-Up and Initial Assessment 867
   Approach to the Patient in Respiratory Distress . 868
   Prescribed Inhalers 871
Prep Kit 876

20 Cardiovascular Emergencies   880

Cardiovascular Emergencies 884
Cardiovascular Anatomy and Physiology 884
   The Heart 884
   Valves of the Heart 885
   Blood Flow Within the Heart 885
Electrical Properties of the Heart and the
  Conduction System 888
   Pacemaker Function 888
   Pacemaker Settings 888
   The SA Node 889
   The Internodal Pathways 889
   The AV Node 889
   The Bundle of His 890
   The Left Bundle Branch (LBB) 890
   The Right Bundle Branch (RBB) 890
   The LAF 891
   The LPF 891
   The Purkinje System 891
   Special Electrical Properties of Cardiac Cells 891
   Regulation of Heart Function 891
   Electrolytes (Ions) and the Heart 892
   The Electrical Potential 892
   Depolarization and Cardiac Contraction 892
   Repolarization 893
The Cardiac Cycle 895
The Blood Vessels 896
   The General Scheme of Blood Circulation 896
   Circulation to the Heart 897

    The Pulmonary Circulation 898
    Systemic Arterial Circulation 898
    Venous Return 899
    Atherosclerosis 899
    Angina Pectoris 900
Acute Myocardial Infarction 901
    Initial Assessment Findings 901
    Consequences of AMI 902
    Hypertensive Emergencies 906
    Initial Cardiovascular Assessment 907
Cardiac Surgery and Pacemakers 912
    Automatic Implantable Cardiac Defibrillators ... 913
Cardiac Arrest 915
    Termination of Resuscitation 915
    Automated External Defibrillation 916
ECG Monitoring 925
    Introduction to Basic Components 926
    Wave Nomenclature 927
Individual Components of the ECG Complex 928
    The P Wave 928
    The Tp Wave 928
    The P-R Segment 929
    The P-R Interval 929
    The QRS Complex 929
    The ST Segment 930
    The T Wave 931
    The Q-T Interval 931
    The U Wave 932
    Additional Intervals 932
Boxes and Sizes 933
ECG Tools 934
    Calipers: The Clinician's Best Friend 934
    ECG Rulers 935
    Straight Edge 935
The Rate 936
    Establishing the Rate 936
Artifact 937
Major Concepts: Interpreting a Cardiac Rhythm 938
    General 939
    P Waves 939
    QRS Complexes 939
Individual Rhythms 940
    Supraventricular Rhythms 940
    Junctional Rhythms 944
    Ventricular Rhythms 945
    Heart Blocks 949
Premature Complexes 951
    An Arrhythmia vs an Event 951
Escape Complexes and Rhythms 952
Ectopic Foci and Their Morphologic Features 952
    Ectopic Foci in the Ventricles 955
Aberrancy 956
Premature Junctional Contraction 957
    PAC With Aberrancy vs PJC With Aberrancy ... 958
Premature Ventricular Contraction 960
    Coupling Interval 960
    R-on-T Phenomenon 960
    End-diastolic PVC 960

    Compensatory vs Noncompensatory Pauses 961
    Unifocal vs Multifocal PVCs 961
    Bigeminy, Trigeminy, and More 962
    Couplets, Triplets, and Salvos 962
    Interpolated PVC 963
Bundle Branch Blocks 963
    What Happens If One Side Is Blocked? 964
Electrical Interventions 965
    Defibrillation 965
    Transcutaneous Pacing 967
Management 967
    Chest Pain and Stroke 967
    Tachycardias 969
    Bradycardias 970
    V-fib and Pulseless V-tach 971
Prep Kit 975

21 Diabetic Emergencies   984

Diabetic Emergencies 986
Diabetes 986
    Defining Diabetes 986
    Types of Diabetes 986
    The Role of Glucose and Insulin 987
    Hyperglycemia 989
    Hyperglycemia and Hypoglycemia 990
    Emergency Medical Care 992
    Giving Oral Glucose 993
    Administering 50% Dextrose 996
Complications of Diabetes 996
    Seizures 997
    Altered Mental Status 998
    Alcoholism 998
    Relationship to Airway Management 998
Prep Kit 1000

22 Allergic Reactions and Envenomations   1004

Allergic Reactions and Envenomations 1006
Allergic Reactions 1006
    Insect Stings 1008
    Anaphylactic Reaction to Stings 1010
Patient Assessment 1010
Emergency Medical Care 1011
Specific Bites and Envenomations 1017
    Spider Bites 1017
    Snake Bites 1018
    Scorpion Stings 1022
    Tick Bites 1023
    Dog Bites and Rabies 1024
    Human Bites 1024
    Injuries From Marine Animals 1025
Prep Kit 1028

23 Poisonings and Overdose Emergencies   1032

Substance Abuse and Poisoning 1034
Identifying the Patient and the Poison 1035

How Poisons Get Into the Body 1037
    Ingested Poisons 1037
    Inhaled Poisons 1038
    Injected Poisons 1039
    Absorbed (Surface Contact) Poisons 1039
Emergency Medical Care 1040
Geography-specific Toxic Emergencies 1041
Specific Poisons 1041
Grouping Toxicologically Similar Agents 1041
    Alcohol 1041
    Narcotics and Opiates 1042
    Sedative-Hypnotic Drugs 1043
    Psychiatric Medications 1044
    Abused Inhalants 1044
    Carbon Monoxide 1045
    Sympathomimetics 1045
    Marijuana 1046
    Hallucinogens 1046
    Anticholinergic Agents 1047
    Cholinergic Agents 1048
    Miscellaneous Drugs 1048
Food Poisoning 1049
Plant Poisoning 1050
Prep Kit 1054

24 Neurologic Emergencies 1058

Neurologic Emergencies 1060
Brain Structure and Function 1060
Common Causes of Brain Disorders 1061
    Stroke 1061
    Seizures 1064
    Altered Mental Status 1066
Signs and Symptoms of Brain Disorders 1068
    Stroke 1068
    Other Conditions 1069
Assessing the Patient 1069
    Stroke 1069
    Seizures 1072
    Syncopal Episodes 1073
    Altered Mental Status 1073
Emergency Medical Care 1074
    Stroke 1074
    Seizures 1075
Prep Kit 1078

25 Nontraumatic Abdominal Emergencies 1082

Nontraumatic Abdominal Emergencies 1084
Physiology of the Acute Abdomen 1084
Signs and Symptoms of Acute Abdomen 1084
Causes of Abdominal Pain 1088
    Gastrointestinal and Urinary Tract 1088
    Uterus and Ovaries 1089
    Other Organ Systems 1090
Emergency Medical Care 1091
Prep Kit 1094

26 Environmental Emergencies 1098

Environmental Emergencies 1102
Cold Exposure 1102
    Hypothermia 1103
    Advanced Cardiac Life Support Considerations 1107
    Management of Cold Exposure in a Sick or
       Injured Person 1107
    Local Cold Injuries 1108
    Cold Exposure and You 1110
Heat Exposure 1111
    Heat Cramps 1111
    Heat Exhaustion 1113
    Heatstroke 1115
Lightning Injuries 1116
    Emergency Medical Care 1117
Drowning and Near Drowning 1117
    Emergency Medical Care 1118
    Spinal Injuries in Submersion Incidents 1120
    Recovery Techniques 1120
    Resuscitation Efforts 1122
Diving Emergencies 1122
    Descent Emergencies 1122
    Emergencies at the Bottom 1123
    Ascent Emergencies 1123
Other Water Hazards 1124
Prevention 1125
Prep Kit 1127

27 Behavioral Emergencies 1130

Behavioral Emergencies 1132
Myth and Reality 1132
Defining Behavioral Emergencies 1132
The Magnitude of Mental Health Problems 1133
    Pathology: Causes of Behavioral Emergencies .. 1134
    Safe Approach to a Behavioral Emergency 1134
Assessing a Behavioral Emergency 1134
    Initial Assessment 1137
    Focused History and Physical Exam 1138
Suicide 1138
Management Considerations 1139
Medicolegal Considerations 1140
    Consent 1141
    Limited Legal Authority 1141
    Restraint 1141
The Potentially Violent Patient 1143
Prep Kit 1146

28 Gynecologic Emergencies 1150

Gynecologic Emergencies 1152
Anatomy of the Female Reproductive System 1152
Normal Physiology 1153
General Assessment 1154
    Obstetric History 1154

History of Gynecologic Problems 1155
Physical Exam 1156
General Management 1156
Specific Gynecologic Emergencies 1157
Pelvic Inflammatory Disease 1157
Ruptured Ovarian Cyst 1158
Ectopic Pregnancy 1158
Vaginal Bleeding 1158
Traumatic Abdominal Pain 1159
Sexual Assault 1159
Prep Kit 1161

Section 7 Special Considerations

29 Obstetric Emergencies 1166
Introduction 1168
Obstetric Emergencies 1168
The Female Reproductive System 1168
The Ovaries 1168
The Fallopian Tubes 1168
The Uterus 1168
The Vagina 1169
The External Genitalia 1170
The Mammary Glands 1170
Gestation 1170
Normal Gestation 1170
Trimesters of Pregnancy 1173
Normal Maternal Changes of Pregnancy 1173
Emergencies Prior to Delivery 1175
Abortion 1175
Ectopic Pregnancy 1175
Hypertension 1176
Supine Hypotensive Syndrome 1177
Gestational Diabetes 1177
Late Pregnancy Complications 1177
Stages of Labor 1179
Preparing for Delivery 1180
Delivering the Infant 1182
Delivering the Head 1184
Delivering the Body 1186
Postdelivery Care 1186
Delivery of the Placenta 1188
Abnormal or Complicated Delivery Emergencies 1189
Breech Delivery 1189
Limb Presentations 1189
Prolapsed Cord Presentation 1190
Prolapsed Uterus 1191
Prep Kit 1194

30 Neonatal Emergencies 1200
Neonatal Emergencies 1204
Neonatal Pathophysiology 1204
Fetal Oxygenation In Utero 1204
Fetal Transition 1204

Fetal Distress 1205
Newborn Bradycardia 1206
Anticipating the Need for Resuscitation 1206
Resuscitation Equipment 1207
Basic Equipment 1207
Advanced Life Support Equipment 1207
Interventions Immediately Following Delivery 1208
Assessment of the Newborn 1208
Depressed Newborn Resuscitation 1208
The Initial Steps of Resuscitation 1209
Essential Parameters 1210
Assess Respiratory Effort 1211
Assess Heart Rate 1212
Assess Color 1213
Advanced Life Support Interventions 1214
Orogastric Tube Insertion 1214
Endotracheal Intubation 1216
Venous Access 1217
Medication Therapy 1217
Special Considerations 1219
Meconium Staining and Aspiration 1219
Hypothermia 1220
Diaphragmatic Hernia 1220
Twins 1220
Delivering a Newborn of an Addicted Mother . . 1221
Premature Newborn 1221
Fetal Death 1222
Prep Kit 1224

31 Pediatric Emergencies 1228
Unique Needs of Children 1234
Epidemiology 1234
Pediatric Trauma 1234
Pediatric Illness 1234
Injury and Illness Prevention 1234
Continuing Education 1235
Growth and Development 1235
The Infant 1236
The Toddler 1236
The Preschool-Age Child 1237
The School-Age Child 1237
The Adolescent 1237
Anatomy and Physiology 1238
The Head 1238
The Airway 1238
Chest and Lungs 1239
The Abdomen 1240
The Extremities 1240
Skin and Body Surface Area 1240
The Respiratory System 1240
Cardiovascular System 1241
The Nervous System 1241
Metabolic Differences 1242
Pediatric Assessment 1242
General Considerations 1242
Scene Size-up 1242
Initial Assessment 1244

Pediatric Assessment Triangle 1244
Vital Functions 1246
Pediatric Vital Signs 1248
Transport Decision 1250
Transition Phase 1250
Focused History and Physical Exam 1251
Focused History 1251
Physical Exam 1251
Ongoing Assessment 1252
Pediatric Airway Management 1252
Manual Airway Positioning 1252
Foreign Body Upper Airway Obstruction 1252
Partial Upper Airway Obstruction 1254
Complete Upper Airway Obstruction 1254
Removal of an Airway Obstruction With Magill
Forceps 1257
Suctioning 1258
Airway Adjuncts 1259
Oropharyngeal Airway 1259
Nasopharyngeal Airway 1260
Oxygenation 1263
Oxygen Delivery Devices 1263
Ventilation 1264
BVM Device 1264
Cricoid Pressure 1265
Endotracheal Intubation 1266
Equipment for Endotracheal Intubation 1267
Preparation for Endotracheal Intubation 1268
Gastric Decompression 1272
Preparation of Equipment 1272
NG Tube Insertion 1273
OG Tube Insertion 1273
Complications of NG or OG Tube Insertion . . . 1273
Circulation 1273
Cardiopulmonary Resuscitation 1274
Intravenous Access 1276
IO Infusion 1278
Fluid Resuscitation 1279
Medication Therapy 1280
Manual Defibrillation 1280
Transport Considerations 1284
Pediatric Medical Emergencies 1284
Respiratory Compromise 1285
Phases of Respiratory Compromise 1285
Emergency Medical Care 1286
Upper Airway Diseases 1286
Croup 1286
Epiglottitis 1287
Lower Airway Diseases 1288
Asthma 1288
Bronchiolitis 1290
Pneumonia 1290
Foreign Body Lower Airway Obstruction 1291
Shock 1291
Classifications of Shock 1292
General Shock Management 1292
Etiologies of Shock 1294

Hypovolemic Shock 1294
Distributive Shock 1294
Cardiogenic Shock 1296
Cardiac Dysrhythmias 1296
Tachydysrhythmias 1296
Bradydysrhythmias 1297
Absent Rhythms 1297
Other Medical Emergencies 1299
Seizures 1299
Altered Level of Consciousness 1301
Poisoning 1302
Fever 1303
Meningitis 1303
Dehydration 1304
Hypoglycemia 1305
Hyperglycemia 1306
Sudden Infant Death Syndrome 1307
Assessment and Management 1307
Communication and Support of the Family . . . 1308
Scene Assessment 1308
Apparent Life-Threatening Event 1308
Death of a Child 1309
Pediatric Trauma Emergencies 1310
Anatomic Differences 1310
Injury Patterns 1311
Physical Differences 1311
Psychological Differences 1312
Child Safety Seats 1312
Automobile Collisions 1312
Sports Activities 1313
Special Considerations 1313
Airway Control 1313
Immobilization 1314
Fluid Management 1314
Traumatic Brain Injury 1314
Injuries to Specific Body Systems 1315
Head Injuries 1315
Chest Injuries 1316
Abdominal Injuries 1316
Injuries of the Extremities 1316
Burns 1316
Submersion Injury 1318
Emergency Medical Care 1318
Airway 1319
Breathing 1319
Immobilization 1320
Child Abuse 1321
Signs of Abuse 1321
Symptoms and Other Indicators of Abuse 1324
Emergency Medical Care 1324
Sexual Abuse 1324
EMS Response to Pediatric Emergencies 1325
Prep Kit 1327

32 Geriatric Emergencies 1336

Geriatric Assessment 1338
The GEMS Diamond 1338

The Economic Impact of Aging 1340
Independent and Dependent Living 1341
Leading Causes of Death 1342
Physiologic Changes That Accompany Age 1342
Skin 1343
Senses 1343
Respiratory System 1344
Cardiovascular System 1344
Renal System 1345
Nervous System 1345
Musculoskeletal System 1346
Gastrointestinal System 1346
Immune System 1346
Advance Directives 1346
Patient Assessment 1348
Scene Size-up 1348
Initial Assessment 1348
Most Common Geriatric Complaints 1349
Focused History and Physical Exam 1352
Response to Nursing and Skilled Care Facilities 1356
Trauma 1356
Mechanism of Injury 1356
Systemic Impact of Aging and Trauma 1357
Falls and Trauma 1357
Cardiovascular Emergencies 1358
Syncope 1358
Myocardial Infarction 1358
The Acute Abdomen 1358
Altered Mental Status 1360
Elder Abuse 1360
Assessment of Elder Abuse 1361
Signs of Physical Abuse 1362
Prep Kit 1365

Section 8 Operations

33 Ambulance Operations 1372
Ambulance Operations 1374
Emergency Vehicle Design 1374
Phases of an Ambulance Call 1375
The Preparation Phase 1376
The Dispatch Phase 1384
En Route to the Scene 1384
Arrival at the Scene 1391
The Transfer Phase 1392
The Transport Phase 1393
The Delivery Phase 1393
En Route to the Station 1394
The Postrun Phase 1394
Air Medical Operations 1395
Safety Precautions Around Helicopters 1396
Landing Sites 1396
Prep Kit 1399

34 Lifting and Moving 1402
Lifting and Moving Patients 1404
Body Mechanics 1404
Anatomy Review 1404
Weight and Distribution 1408
Directions and Commands 1414
Additional Lifting and Carrying Guidelines 1415
Principles of Safe Reaching and Pulling 1417
General Considerations 1419
Emergency Moves 1419
Urgent Moves 1421
Rapid Extrication Technique 1421
Nonurgent Moves 1426
Direct Ground Lift 1426
Extremity Lift 1427
Transfer Moves 1427
Patient-Moving Equipment 1430
The Wheeled Ambulance Stretcher 1430
Portable/Folding Stretchers 1435
Flexible Stretchers 1435
Backboards 1436
Basket Stretchers 1437
Scoop Stretcher 1437
Stair Chairs 1437
Moving and Positioning the Patient 1438
Prep Kit 1441

35 Gaining Access 1444
Gaining Access 1446
Fundamentals of Extrication 1446
Scene Size-Up 1447
Patient and Bystander Safety 1448
Gaining Access to the Patient 1449
Patient Care During Entrapment and
 Extrication 1450
Preparation for Removal 1450
Removal 1451
Specialized Rescue Situations 1451
Prep Kit 1456

36 Special Operations 1460
Special Operations 1462
Incident Command Systems 1462
Components and Structure of an Incident
 Command System 1462
Introduction to Hazardous Materials 1465
Identifying Hazardous Materials 1467
Caring for Patients at a Hazardous Materials
 Incident 1469
Resources 1471
Mass-Casualty Incidents 1473
Triage 1473
Disaster Management 1477
Clandestine Drug Laboratories 1478
Location of Illegal Drug Laboratories 1479

Recognizing Illegal Drug Laboratories 1479		Recognizing Patterns and Obtaining a Field Impression 1529

Recognizing Illegal Drug Laboratories 1479
Hazards Associated with Clandestine Drug Labs . 1481
Emergency Scene Operations 1481
EMS Operations 1482
Fire Suppression Operations 1482
Positive-Pressure Ventilation 1483
Monitoring Personnel Working in the Hot Zone . 1483
Interacting with a Methamphetamine User 1484
Prep Kit 1486

37 Response to Terrorism and Weapons of Mass Destruction   1490

Introduction 1492
What Is Terrorism? 1492
Weapons of Mass Destruction (WMD) 1493
What Are WMDs? 1493
Chemical Warfare/Terrorism 1493
Biological Terrorism/Warfare 1494
Nuclear/Radiological Terrorism 1494
EMT-I Response to Terrorism 1494
Recognizing a Terrorist Event (Indicators) 1494
Response Actions 1495
Chemical Agents 1498
Vesicants (Blister Agents) 1498
Pulmonary Agents (Choking Agents) 1499
Nerve Agents 1500
Industrial Chemicals/Insecticides 1503
Biological Agents 1505
Viruses 1505
Bacteria 1506
Neurotoxins 1508
Other EMT-I Roles During a Biological Event .. 1509
Radiological/Nuclear Devices 1511
What Is Radiation? 1511
Sources of Radiological Material 1511
Radiological Dispersal Devices (RDD) 1513
Nuclear Energy 1513
Nuclear Weapons 1513
Symptomology 1513
Medical Management 1513
Protective Measures 1514
Prep Kit 1517

Section 9 Enrichment

38 Assessment-Based Management   1524

Assessment-Based Management 1528
Effective Patient Assessment 1528
Gathering Information 1528
The Importance of History 1528
Physical Assessment 1529

Recognizing Patterns and Obtaining a Field
  Impression 1529
BLS/ALS Treatment 1529
Choreographing Assessment and Management 1530
Team Leader 1530
Patient Care Person(s) 1530
The Right Stuff 1531
Optional "Take In" Equipment 1531
Aspects of Assessment and Decision Making 1532
Uncooperative Patients 1532
Distracting Injuries 1532
The Environment, Patient Compliance, and
  Manpower Considerations 1533
General Approach 1533
The Initial Assessment 1533
The Role of Experience 1534
Transferring the Patient 1534
Drills for Common Prehospital Complaints 1535
Prep Kit 1540

39 BLS Review   1544

BLS Review 1546
Elements of BLS 1546
Automated External Defibrillation 1548
Assessing the Need for BLS 1549
When to Start and Stop BLS 1549
Positioning the Patient 1551
Opening the Airway in Adults 1552
Head Tilt–Chin Lift Maneuver 1553
Jaw-Thrust Maneuver 1554
Foreign Body Airway Obstruction in Adults 1554
Recognizing Foreign Body Obstruction 1554
Removing a Foreign Body Obstruction in Patients
  Over 1 Year of Age...................... 1555
Foreign Body Obstruction in Infants and Children 1557
Removing a Foreign Body Airway Obstruction . 1557
Rescue Breathing in Adults 1558
Ventilation 1559
Ventilation Through a Stoma 1560
Gastric Distention 1561
Recovery Position 1561
Adult CPR   1562
External Chest Compression 1562
One-Rescuer Adult CPR 1564
Two-Rescuer Adult CPR 1565
Switching Positions 1567
Infant and Child CPR 1569
External Chest Compression 1569
Proper Hand Position and Compression
  Technique 1570
Interrupting CPR 1572
Prep Kit 1574

Index 1578
Photo Credits................................ 1596

EMT-I Skill Drills

1985 and 1999 Skill Drills

Section 1 Preparing to be an EMT-I

Chapter 2
- 2-1 Proper Glove Removal 48

Section 2 Pharmacology and Intravenous Therapy

Chapter 7
- 7-1 Spiking the Bag 299
- 7-2 IV Therapy 307
- 7-4 Determining if an IV is Viable 315

Section 3 Airway

Chapter 9
- 9-1 Placing a Patient in the Recovery Position 383
- 9-2 Positioning an Unresponsive Patient 384
- 9-3 Head Tilt–Chin Lift Maneuver 386
- 9-4 Jaw-Thrust Maneuver 388
- 9-5 Jaw-Thrust Maneuver With Head Tilt 389
- 9-6 Tongue–Jaw Lift Maneuver 390
- 9-7 Managing Complete Airway Obstruction in an Unconscious Adult 393
- 9-8 Managing Complete Airway Obstruction in an Unconscious Child 394
- 9-9 Managing Complete Airway Obstruction in an Unconscious Infant 395
- 9-10 Managing Complete Airway Obstruction or Incomplete Airway Obstruction With Poor Air Exchange in a Conscious Adult or Child 396
- 9-12 Suctioning a Patient's Airway 401
- 9-13 Inserting an Oral Airway 403
- 9-14 Inserting an Oral Airway With a 90° Rotation 404
- 9-15 Inserting a Nasal Airway 406
- 9-16 Placing an Oxygen Cylinder Into Service 411
- 9-17 Mouth-to-Mask Ventilation 416
- 9-18 Manual Gastric Decompression 424
- 9-21 Insertion of the PtL 432
- 9-22 Insertion of the Combitube 434
- 9-30 LMA Insertion 468
- 9-31 Mouth-to-Stoma Ventilation (Using a Resuscitation Mask) 470
- 9-32 BVM to Stoma Ventilation 471
- 9-33 Suctioning of a Stoma 473

Section 4 Patient Assessment

Chapter 10
- 10-1 Performing a Rapid Trauma Assessment 522
- 10-2 Performing a Rapid Medical Assessment: Unresponsive Patient 538
- 10-3 Performing the Detailed Physical Exam 544

Section 5 Trauma

Chapter 13
- 13-1 Controlling External Bleeding 652
- 13-2 Applying a Pneumatic Antishock Garment (PASG) 655
- 13-3 Applying a Tourniquet 657
- 13-4 Treating Shock 667

Chapter 14
- 14-1 Controlling Bleeding From an Extremity Soft-Tissue Injury 686
- 14-2 Sealing a Sucking Chest Wound 687
- 14-3 Stabilizing an Impaled Object 689
- 14-4 Caring for Burns 696

Chapter 17
- 17-1 Performing Manual In-Line Stabilization 770
- 17-2 Immobilizing a Patient to a Long Backboard 772
- 17-3 Immobilizing a Patient Found in a Sitting Position 776
- 17-4 Immobilizing a Patient Found in a Standing Position 778
- 17-5 Application of a Cervical Collar 786
- 17-6 Removing a Helmet 790

Chapter 18
- 18-1 Assessing Neurovascular Pulse 810
- 18-2 Caring for Musculoskeletal Injuries 813
- 18-3 Applying a Rigid Splint 816
- 18-4 Applying a Zippered Air Splint 817
- 18-5 Applying an Unzippered Air Splint 818
- 18-6 Applying a Vacuum Splint 819
- 18-7 Applying a Hare Traction Splint 820
- 18-8 Applying a Sager Traction Splint 822
- 18-9 Splinting the Hand and Wrist 832

Section 6 Medical Emergencies

Chapter 19
- 19-1 Assisting a Patient With a Metered-Dose Inhaler 873

Chapter 20
- 20-1 Treating Cardiogenic Shock 904
- 20-2 Treating CHF 906
- 20-3 Treating a Conscious Patient for Chest Discomfort 910
- 20-4 AED and CPR 920

Chapter 21
- 21-1 Administering Glucose 994
- 21-2 Administration of D_{50} 997

Chapter 22
- 22-1 Using an Auto-Injector 1013
- 22-2 Using an AnaKit 1014

Chapter 26
- 26-1 Treating for Heat Exhaustion 1114
- 26-2 Stabilizing a Suspected Spinal Injury in the Water 1121

Section 7 Special Considerations

Chapter 29
- 29-1 Delivering the Infant 1185

Chapter 30
- 30-1 Giving Chest Compressions to a Newborn 1213

Chapter 31
- 31-1 Positioning the Airway in a Child 1253
- 31-2 Removing a Foreign Body Airway Obstruction in an Unresponsive Child 1256
- 31-3 Inserting an Oropharyngeal Airway in a Child 1261
- 31-4 Inserting a Nasopharyngeal Airway in a Child 1262
- 31-5 One-Person BVM Ventilation on a Child 1266
- 31-7 Performing Infant Chest Compressions 1275
- 31-8 Performing Chest Compressions on a Child 1276
- 31-10 General Shock Management 1293
- 31-11 Immobilizing a Child 1322
- 31-12 Immobilizing an Infant 1323

Section 8 Operations

Chapter 34
- 34-1 Performing the Power Lift 1407
- 34-2 Performing the Diamond Carry 1410
- 34-3 Performing the One-Handed Carrying Technique . . . 1411
- 34-4 Carrying a Patient on Stairs 1413
- 34-5 Using a Stair Chair 1416
- 34-6 Performing Rapid Extrication Technique 1424
- 34-7 Extremity Lift 1428
- 34-8 Using a Scoop Stretcher 1430
- 34-9 Loading a Cot into an Ambulance 1434

Section 9 Enrichment

Chapter 39
- 39-1 Positioning the Patient 1552
- 39-2 Performing Chest Compressions 1565
- 39-3 Performing One-Rescuer Adult CPR 1568
- 39-4 Performing Two-Rescuer Adult CPR 1570

1999 Skill Drills

Section 2 Pharmacology and Intravenous Therapy

Chapter 7
- 7-3 Pediatric Intraosseous Infusion 310

Chapter 8
- 8-1 Administering Medication Via Small-Volume Nebulizer 337
- 8-2 Drawing Medication From an Ampule 342
- 8-3 Drawing Medication From a Vial 344
- 8-4 Administering Medication Via the Subcutaneous Route 346
- 8-5 Administering Medication Via the Intramuscular Route 348
- 8-6 Administering Medication Via the Intravenous Bolus Route 350
- 8-7 Administering Medication Via the IO Route 353
- 8-8 Administering Medication Via the Sublingual Route . . 354

Section 3 Airway

Chapter 9
- 9-11 Removal of an Upper Airway Obstruction With Magill Forceps 397
- 9-19 Nasogastric Tube Insertion in a Conscious Patient . . . 426
- 9-20 OG Tube Insertion 428
- 9-23 Intubation of the Trachea Using Direct Laryngoscopy . 446
- 9-24 Performing End-tidal Carbon Dioxide Detection 448
- 9-25 Securing an Endotracheal Tube With Tape 450
- 9-26 Securing an Endotracheal Tube With a Commercial Device 452
- 9-27 Performing Extubation 454
- 9-28 Performing Pediatric Endotracheal Intubation 458
- 9-29 Securing an Endotracheal Tube 460
- 9-34 Replacing a Dislodged Tracheostomy Tube 474

Section 5 Trauma

Chapter 15
- 15-1 Decompression of a Tension Pneumothorax 728

Section 6 Medical Emergencies

Chapter 20
- 20-5 Using Paddles for Cardiac Monitoring 927
- 20-6 Defibrillation 966
- 20-7 Transcutaneous Pacing 968

Section 7 Special Considerations

Chapter 30
- 30-2 Inserting an Orogastric Tube in the Newborn 1215

Chapter 31
- 31-6 Performing Pediatric Endotracheal Intubation 1270
- 31-9 Pediatric IO Infusion 1280

Resource Preview

The American Academy of Orthopaedic Surgeons is pleased to bring you *Intermediate: Emergency Care and Transportation of the Sick and Injured*, a modern integrated teaching and learning system. It combines current content with dynamic features, interactive technology, and both instructor and student resources.

Intermediate: Emergency Care and Transportation of the Sick and Injured addresses the objectives in both the 1985 and 1999 DOT EMT-Intermediate National Standard Curricula. It bridges the gap between the two curricula while still keeping them separate, making it user friendly for instructors and students. Material that is specific to the 1999 curriculum is identified with a 1999 icon. Users of the 1985 curriculum skip over the 1999 content, or incorporate it at the instructor's discretion for further study.

Chapter Resources

The text is the core of the teaching and learning system with features that will reinforce and expand on the essential information and make information retrieval a snap. These features include:

Chapter Objectives

1999 and 1985 National Standard Curriculum objectives and additional noncurriculum objectives are provided for each chapter with corresponding page references.

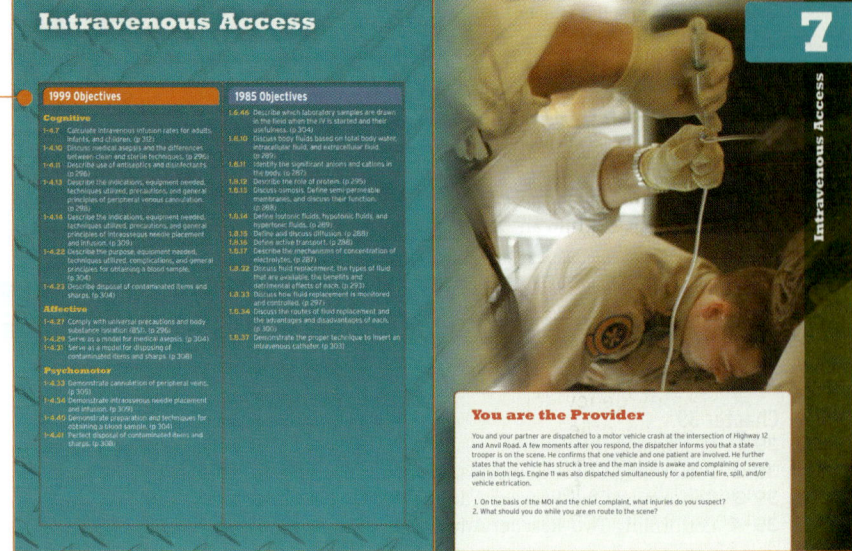

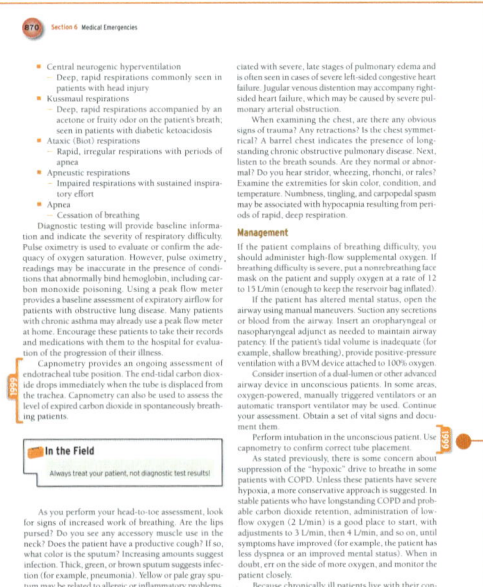

1999 Icon

A bar is used to flag content that applies only to students of the 1999 National Standard Curriculum. Students of the 1985 National Standard Curriculum should skip over the content marked by the 1999 icon, or incorporate it at the instructor's discretion for further study.

Resource Preview

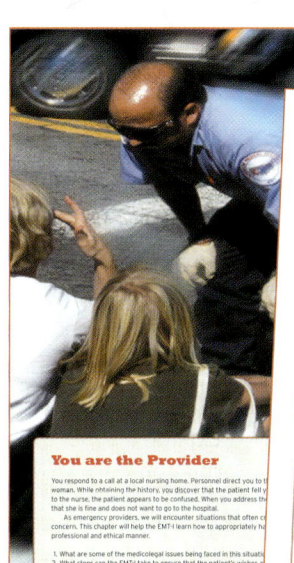

You are the Provider

Each chapter contains a progressive case study to make students start thinking about what they might do if they encountered a similar case in the field. The case study introduces patients and follows their progress from dispatch to delivery at the emergency department. The case becomes progressively more detailed as new material is presented. This feature is a valuable learning tool that encourages critical thinking skills. Answers and rationales for the case study appear at the end of the chapter.

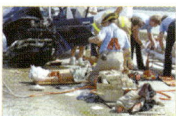

Technology Toolbar

Found at the beginning of each chapter, the technology toolbar will guide you through the resources available for that chapter at www.EMSzone.com/EMTI.

Resource Preview

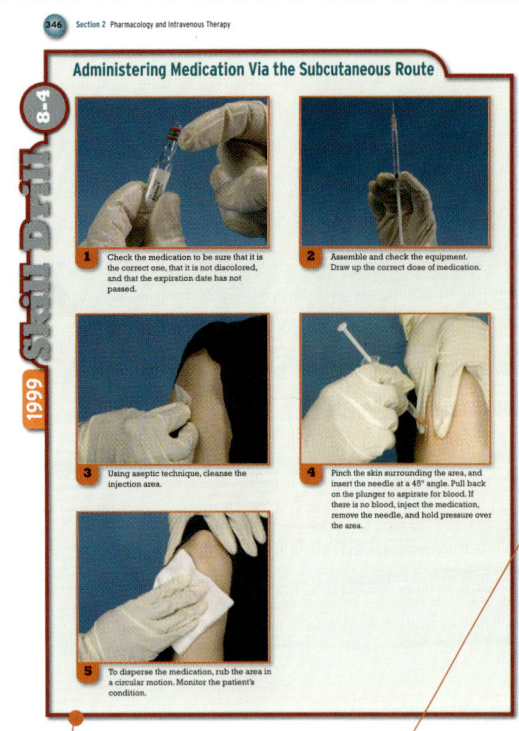

Skill Drills

Skill Drills provide written step-by-step explanations and visual summaries of important skills and procedures. Those skills that apply only to the 1999 National Standard Curriculum are labeled with the 1999 icon.

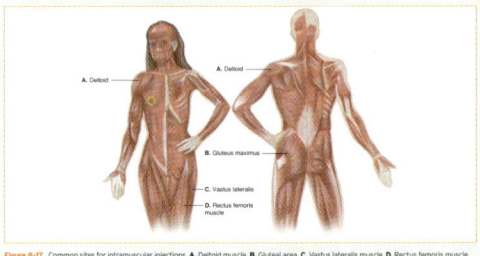

Terminology Tips and Vital Vocabulary

Terminology Tips discuss how to remember the meaning of medical terms by using root words, prefixes, and suffixes. Vital Vocabulary is easily identified and defines key terms students must know in the field.

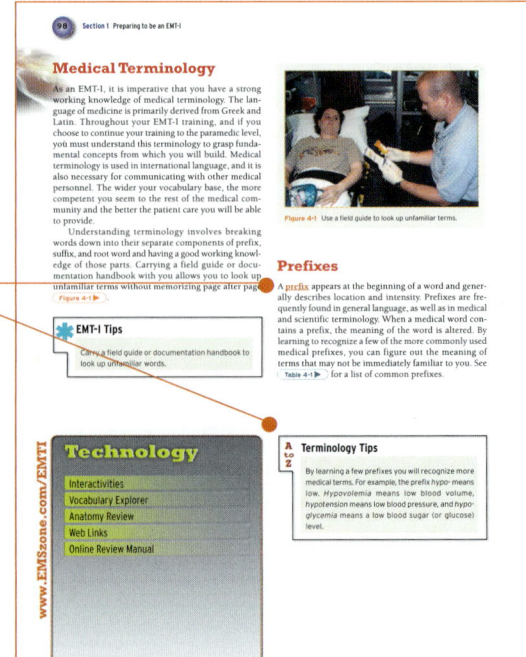

Resource Preview

EMT-I Tips
Provide advice from masters of the trade.

EMT-I Safety
Reinforces safety concerns for both the EMT-I and the patient.

In the Field
Discusses practical applications of material for use in the field.

Documentation Tips
Provide advice on how to document patient care and highlight situations where documentation is especially crucial.

Resource Preview

Chapter 19 Respiratory Emergencies 867

Geriatric Needs

Normal aging processes alter the respiratory system and the ability to exchange oxygen and carbon dioxide. If the patient is a smoker, the disease processes of emphysema or chronic bronchitis can exacerbate these age-related changes.

Several changes occur as we age. The chest wall, including the muscles and ribs, become less resilient. In addition, the bronchi and bronchioles lose their muscle mass or tone, and the air sacs (alveoli) become stiffer and less able to recoil (relax and empty) during exhalation. If the chest wall, including muscles and ribs, is weaker or less flexible, the chest cavity cannot expand as easily, and the total amount of air that is allowed into the lungs will be reduced. With decreased recoil of the lungs, alveoli can become distended with air trapped inside. If you are required to ventilate an apneic (nonbreathing) geriatric patient, you will notice that it is more difficult because of increased resistance of the chest and airways and reduced compliance of the lungs.

The geriatric patient is at an increased risk of pneumonia or a worsening of asthma or COPD if the airways have lost muscle mass or tone. Secretions might not be expelled from the airways, allowing pneumonia to develop.

The results of normal changes with aging include a reduction of the total amount of air the lungs can hold, air becoming trapped in overstretched alveoli, and increased resistance to air flow into and out of the lungs. Ultimately, these changes cause decreased oxygen and carbon dioxide exchange in the respiratory system with reduced oxygen delivery to the cells. Consider changes in aging that affect the respiratory system, and provide adequate ventilation and oxygenation according to the patient's needs. Geriatric patients may need ventilatory support for conditions that, in younger adults, are easily accommodated by the respiratory system.

patients with COPD. Slowing of respirations after oxygen administration does not necessarily mean that the patient's condition is improving; it may be deteriorating. If respirations slow after oxygen administration, simply assist breathing with a bag-valve-mask (BVM) device.

Scene Size-Up and Initial Assessment

Pulmonary complaints may be associated with exposure to a wide variety of toxins, including carbon monoxide, toxic products of combustion, or environments that have deficient ambient oxygen (such as silos and enclosed storage spaces). It is critical to assure a safe environment

You are the Provider — Part 4

You apply a nonrebreathing mask at 15 L/min and prepare to transport the patient. Your partner brings the stretcher in, and together you lift the patient onto it.

Vital Signs	Recording Time: 3 Minutes After Patient Contact
Respirations	30 breaths/min, shallow
Pulse	124 beats/min, regular
Blood pressure	150/100 mm Hg
Level of consciousness	Becoming lethargic, but still alert and oriented
SaO$_2$	87%

7. In what position should you transport the patient?
8. Why do you think the patient's condition is not improving?
9. How should you adjust your treatment?

---

874 Section 6 Medical Emergencies

Pediatric Needs

Asthma is a common childhood illness. When assessing a pediatric patient, look for retraction of the skin above the sternum and between the ribs. Retractions are typically easier to see in children than in adults. Cyanosis is a late finding in children. Keep in mind that a cough may not be a symptom of a cold; it could signal pneumonia or asthma. Even if you do not hear much wheezing, the presence of a cough can indicate some degree of reactive airway disease (for example, asthma or bronchiolitis).

The emergency care of a child with shortness of breath is the same as it is for an adult, including the use of supplemental oxygen. However, many small children will not tolerate (or may refuse to wear) a face mask. Rather than fighting with the child, hold the oxygen mask in front of the child's face or ask the parent to hold the mask (**Figure 19-15**). Many children with asthma also will have prescribed hand-held metered-dose inhalers. Assist with the use of these inhalers just as you would with an adult.

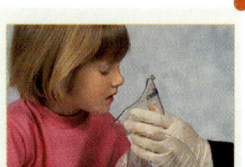

Figure 19-15 Because children may refuse to wear an oxygen mask, you may have to hold the mask in front of the child's face. If the child still refuses, enlist the parents' help.

12. **Instruct the patient** to hold his or her breath for as long as he or she comfortably can to help the lungs absorb the medication (**Step 3**).
13. **Replace the oxygen mask.**
14. **Allow the patient** to breathe a few times, then give the second dose per direction from medical control or according to local protocol (**Step 4**).

In the Field

While one EMT-I is getting oxygen ready, the second EMT-I should try to coach the patient with asthma or COPD to use pursed-lip breathing. This further opens the bronchioles to help air to escape.

You are the Provider — Part 6

The patient's color and mental status improve with the BVM ventilation, and his spontaneous respirations become deeper. You are able to reapply the nonrebreathing mask as your partner drives to the hospital.

Vital Signs	Recording Time: 7 Minutes After Patient Contact
Respirations	22 breaths/min, regular, good tidal volume
Pulse	110 beats/min, regular
Blood pressure	148/88 mm Hg
Level of consciousness	Alert and oriented to person, place, and time
SaO$_2$	94% with oxygen via nonrebreathing mask

12. What should you do en route to the hospital?
13. Would a Combitube be appropriate for this patient?

Pediatric Needs and Geriatric Needs

Highlight specific concerns and procedures for special populations.

Resource Preview xxvii

Prep Kit

End-of-chapter activities reinforce important concepts and improve student comprehension.

Vital Vocabulary provides key terms and definitions from the chapter. Vocabulary Explorer on www.EMSzone.com/EMTI provides interactivities.

Ready for Review thoroughly summarizes chapter content. An interactive Ready for Review is provided on www.EMSzone.com/EMTI to help students prepare for exams.

Points to Ponder tackles cultural, social, ethical, and legal issues through case studies.

Assessment in Action promotes critical thinking through the use of case studies and provides you with discussion points for your classroom presentation.

Instructor Resources

A complete teaching and learning system developed by educators with an intimate knowledge of the obstacles you face each day supports *Intermediate: Emergency Care and Transportation of the Sick and Injured*. The supplements provide practical, hands-on, time-saving tools like PowerPoint presentations, customizable test banks, and web-based distance learning resources to better support you and your students.

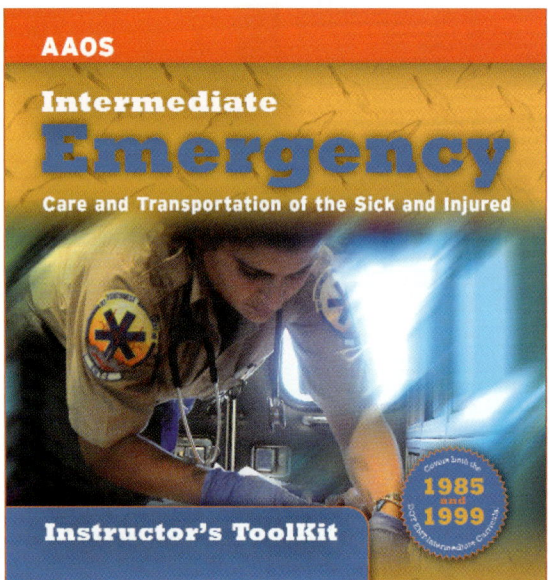

Instructor's ToolKit CD-ROM
ISBN: 0-7637-2670-2
Preparing for class is easy with the resources found on this CD-ROM, including:

- PowerPoint Presentations, providing you with a powerful way to make presentations that are both educational and engaging to your students. Separated into two folders, 1999 presentations and 1985 presentations, the slides can be modified and edited to meet your needs.
- Lecture Outlines, providing you with complete, ready-to-use lesson plans that outline all of the topics covered in the text. Separated into two folders, 1999 outlines and 1985 outlines, the lesson plans can be modified and edited to fit your course.
- Electronic Test Bank, containing multiple-choice and scenario-based questions, allows you to originate tailor-made classroom tests and quizzes quickly and easily by selecting, editing, organizing, and printing a test along with an answer key, that includes page references to the text. All test questions are separated into 1999 questions and 1985 questions.
- Image and Table Bank, providing you with many of the images and tables found in the text. You can use them to incorporate more images into the PowerPoint presentations, make handouts, or enlarge a specific image for further discussion.

The resources found on the Instructor's ToolKit CD-ROM have been formatted so that you can seamlessly integrate them into the most popular course administration tools. Please contact Jones and Bartlett Publishers technical support at any time with questions.

Instructor Resources

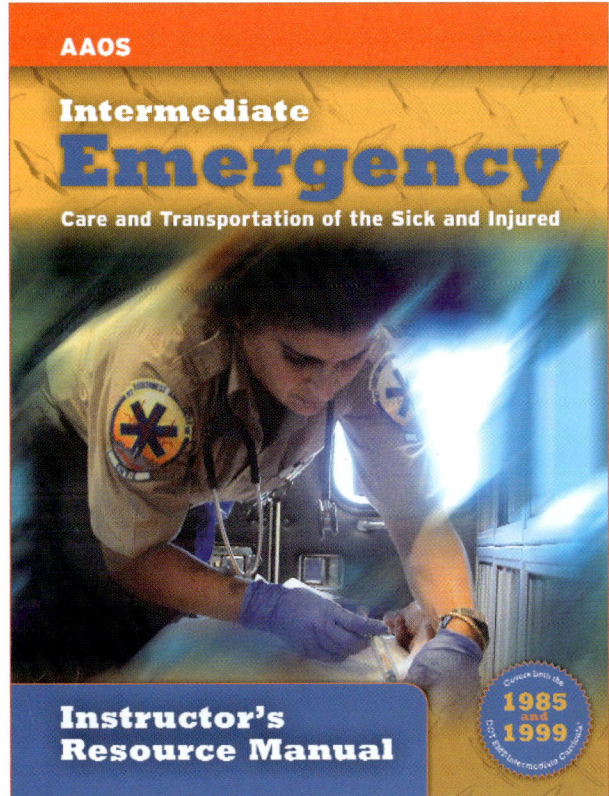

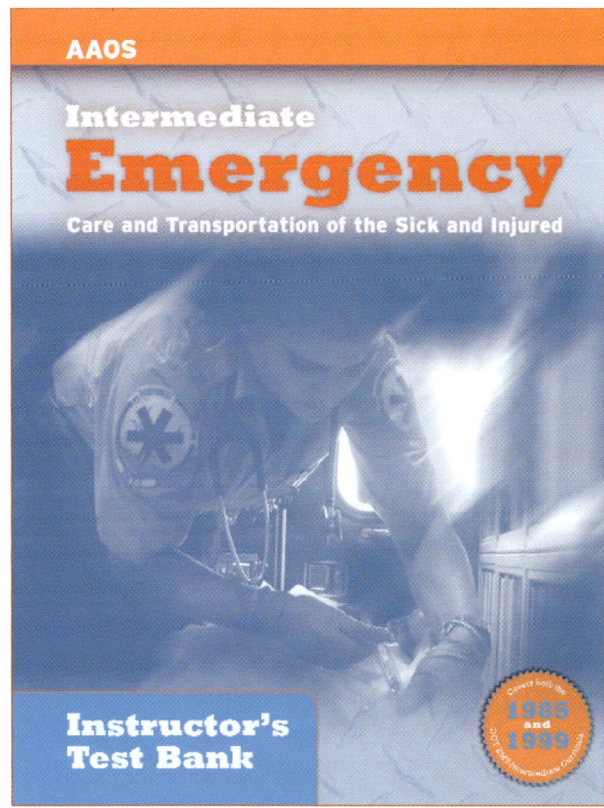

Instructor's Resource Manual
ISBN: 0-7637-2668-0
The Instructor's Resource Manual is your guide to the entire teaching and learning system. This indispensable manual contains:
- Detailed lesson plans that are keyed to the PowerPoint presentations with sample lectures, lesson quizzes, and teaching strategies.
- Teaching tips and ideas to enhance your classroom presentation.
- Answers to all end-of-chapter student questions found in the text.
- Skill Drill evaluation sheets.

Instructor's Test Bank (print)
ISBN: 0-7637-2740-7
This is the printed version of the Test Bank available on the Instructor's ToolKit CD-ROM. It contains multiple-choice questions with page references.

Student Resources

To help students retain the most important information and to assist them in preparing for exams, we have developed the following resources:

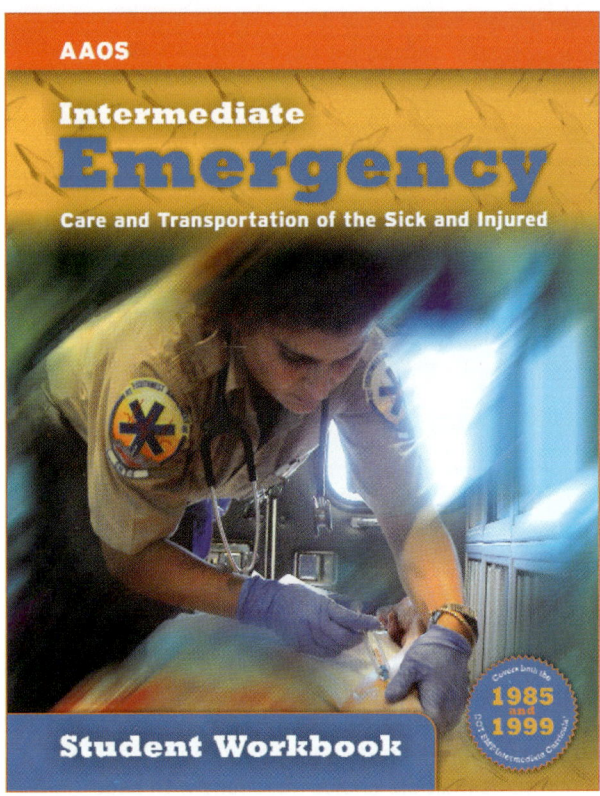

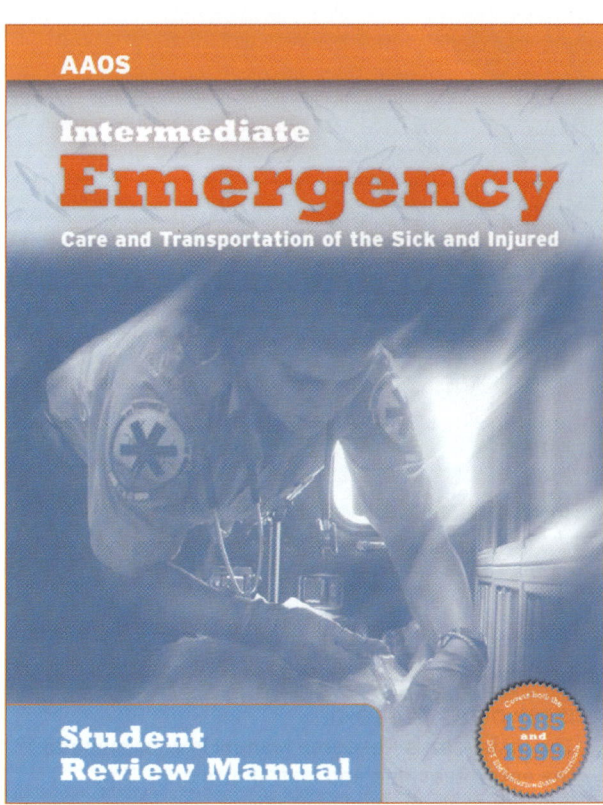

Student Workbook
ISBN: 0-7637-2669-9
This resource is designed to encourage critical thinking and aid comprehension of the course material through:
- Case studies and corresponding questions
- Skill drill activities
- Figure labeling exercises
- Crossword puzzles
- Matching, fill-in-the-blank, short answer, and multiple-choice questions

Student Review Manual
Print - ISBN: 0-7637-3084-X
CD-ROM - ISBN: 0-7637-3466-7
Online - ISBN: 0-7637-3467-5
This Review Manual has been designed to prepare students for exams by including the same type of questions that they are likely to see on classroom and national examinations. The manual contains multiple-choice question exams with an answer key and page references. It is available in print, on CD-ROM, and online.

Technology Resources

A key component to the teaching and learning system are interactivities and simulations to help students become great providers.

www.EMSzone.com/EMTI

Make full use of today's teaching and learning technology with www.EMSzone.com/EMTI. This site has been specifically designed to compliment *Intermediate: Emergency Care and Transportation of the Sick and Injured* and is regularly updated. Some of the resources available include:

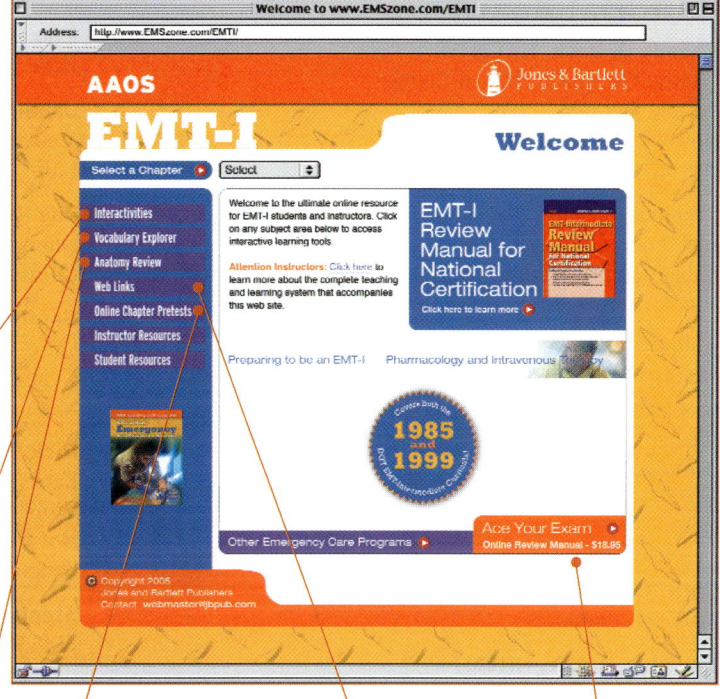

Interactivities allow your students to experiment with the most important skills and procedures in the safety of a virtual environment.

Vocabulary Explorer is your virtual dictionary. Here, students can review key terms, test their knowledge of key terms through quizzes and flashcards, and complete crossword puzzles.

Anatomy Review provides an interactive anatomical figure labeling exercise to reinforce student's knowledge of human anatomy.

Web Links present current information including trends in health care, the EMS community, and new equipment.

Chapter Pretests to prepare students for training. Each chapter has a pretests and provides instant results, feedback on incorrect answers, and page references for further study.

Review Manual allows students to prepare for classroom and national examinations providing instant results, feedback, and page references.

Acknowledgments

Editorial Board

Rhonda J. Beck, NREMT-P
Central Georgia Technical College
Macon, Georgia
Houston Healthcare EMS
Warner Robins, Georgia

Stephen J. Rahm, NREMT-P
EMS Professions Educator
Bulverde-Spring Branch EMS
Spring Branch, Texas

Andrew N. Pollak, MD, FAAOS
Medical Director, Baltimore County Fire Department
Associate Professor, University of Maryland
  School of Medicine
Baltimore, Maryland

Contributors

Christopher M. Andolsek
Aurora, Colorado

Daniel A. Batsie, NREMT-P
Yarmouth Fire/Rescue
Yarmouth, Maine

Rhonda J. Beck, NREMT-P
Central Georgia Technical College
Macon, Georgia
Houston Healthcare EMS
Warner Robins, Georgia

Christopher Bell, BA, NREMT-P, FP-C
Columbus State Community College
Columbus, Ohio

Julie F. Chase, BS, BM, NREMT-P
Seattle, Washington

Alice (Twink) Dalton, RN, NREMT-P, MS
Pridemark Paramedic Services
Boulder, Colorado

Tomas B. Garcia, MD, FACEP
University of Miami
Miami, Florida

Donell Harvin
Effort, Pennsylvania

Rick Hilinski, BA, EMT-P
Public Safety Institute
Community College of Allegheny County
Pittsburgh, Pennsylvania

Sara Houston, BS, AS, NREMT-P
Durham Technical Community College
Durham County, EMS
Durham, North Carolina

Mary Ellen Hurban, RN, EMT-P
Lake Hospital System
Painesville, Ohio

Janelle Johnson, NREMT-P
Metropolitan Emergency Medical Services
Little Rock, Arkansas

Jay Keefauver, BS, EMT-P, CEMSI
National Emergency Resource Center
Columbus, Nebraska

Geoffrey T. Miller, NREMT-P
University of Miami School of Medicine
Center for Research in Medical Education
Miami, Florida

Rick Petrie, EMT-P
Kennebec Valley EMS
Winslow, Maine
Northeastern Maine EMS
Bangor, Maine

Stephen J. Rahm, NREMT-P
EMS Professions Educator
Bulverde-Spring Branch EMS
Spring Branch, Texas

Jose V. Salazar, MPH, NREMT-P
Loudoun County Department Fire-Rescue
Leesburg, Virginia

Jana Szostek, MS, EMT-P
STREETWISE, INC.
Crown Point, Indiana

David S. Teeter, PharmD
Wishard Hospital Pharmacy
Indianapolis, Indiana

Reviewers

Pamela M. Armentrout, NREMT-P
Southwest Healthcare Services
Bowman, North Dakota

Richard W. Campbell, AS, NREMT-P, PI
Lowcountry Regional EMS Council
North Charleston, South Carolina

Wesley Carter, NREMT-P
Lenoir County EMS, Lenoir Community College
Kinston, North Carolina

Jon S. Cooper, NREMT-P
Baltimore City Fire Academy EMS Training Division
Baltimore, Maryland

Rick Criste, BHS, NREMT-P
Fayetteville Technical Community College
Fayetteville, North Carolina

Scott A. Culp, Firefighter/EMT
Cheyenne Fire & Rescue
Cheyenne, Wyoming

Alton W. Fowler, Jr, EMT-P
Central Georgia Technical College
Macon, Georgia

Mark E. Franzese, EMT-I, EMS-I
Campion Ambulance Service, Inc.
Waterbury, Connecticut

Jon Hallum
Fort Gibson, Oklahoma

Randy Hardick, BA, NREMT-P
Saddleback College, South Orange County Community
   College District
Mission Viejo, California

Clint Harper, MA
Pipers Gap Rescue Squad
Carroll County EMS
Galax, Virginia

Adele C. Hill, PhD(c), APRN, BC, EMT-P
Westover Air Reserve Base
Chicopee, Massachusetts
Riverbend Medical Group
Springfield, Massachusetts

Larry J. Hill, EMT-P
Memorial Health University Medical Center
Savannah, Georgia

Bill J. Hufford, REMT-P, PI
FMH Emergency Training Academy
Connersville, Indiana

Edward Kalinowski MEd, DrPH
University of Hawaii
Honolulu, Hawaii

William R. Kerney, MA, EMTP-A
Community College of Southern Nevada
Las Vegas, Nevada

Robin Kinsella, EMT-I, NECEMS I/C
Mad River Valley Ambulance Service
Waitsfield, Vermont

Gregory R. LaMay, BS, NREMT-P
Madison Area Technical College
Reedsburg, Wisconsin

Jay Lovelady, RN, BSN, CEN, NREMT-P
John Randolph Medical Center
Hopewell, Virginia

Barry L. McCammon, EMT-P
Richland Community College
Decatur, Illinois

Tamara L. Meyers, NREMT-P, EMSI
Southeast Community College
Lincoln, Nebraska

William R. Montrie, EMT-P
Owens Community College
Toledo, Ohio

Robert B. Morris, EMT-I
Clackamas Community College
Oregon City, Oregon

Scott Nelson, EMT-P
Medical Resource Consultation
Aurora, Colorado

Kenneth A. Noel, AS, NREMT-I
StarFire EMS
Manchester, New Hampshire

Dennis Patterson
College of Southern Idaho
Twin Falls, Idaho

Jose V. Salazar, MPH, NREMT-P
Loudoun County Department Fire-Rescue
Leesburg, Virginia

Howard A. Shaw, Jr., Paramedic
Wayne County EMS
Wayne Community College
Goldsboro, North Carolina

Helen Yurong, NREMT-P, MSN
Naval Medical Clinic Pearl Harbor
Pearl Harbor, Hawaii

Mark S. Zinn, NREMT-P
Baltimore City Fire Academy
Baltimore, Maryland

Jeff Zuckernick, BS, MBA, NREMT-P
Kapi`olani Community College
University of Hawai`i
Honolulu, Hawaii

The American Academy of Orthopaedic Surgeons would like to acknowledge the contributors and reviewers of *Emergency Care and Transportation of the Sick and Injured, Eighth Edition.*

Photographic Contributors

Rhonda J. Beck, NREMT-P
Central Georgia Technical College
Macon, Georgia
Houston Healthcare EMS
Warner Robins, Georgia

Department of Public Information and Media Services
Maryland Institute for Emergency
   Medical Services Systems
Baltimore, Maryland

Loudoun County Department Fire Rescue
Leesburg, Virginia

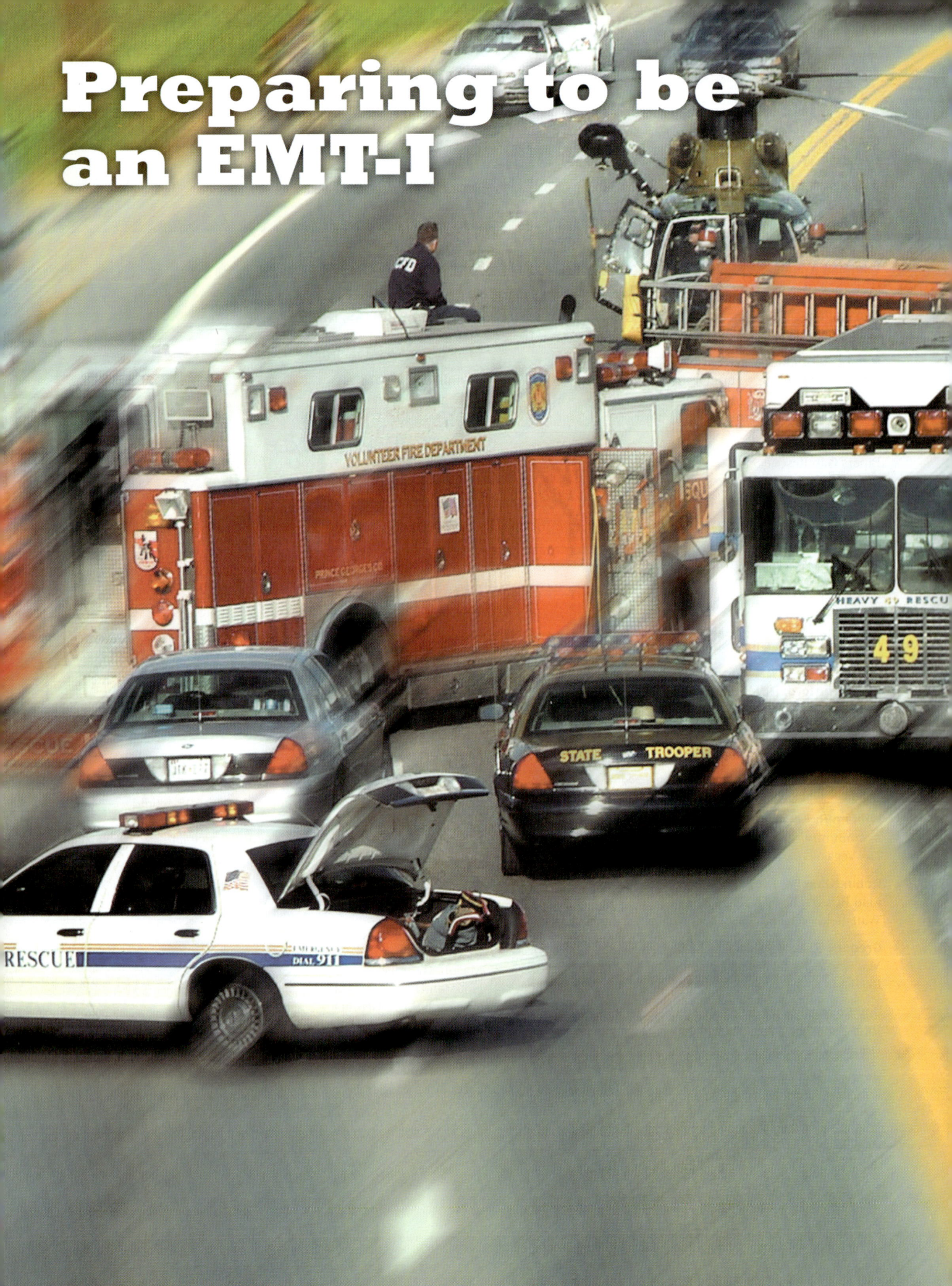

Preparing to be an EMT-I

Section 1

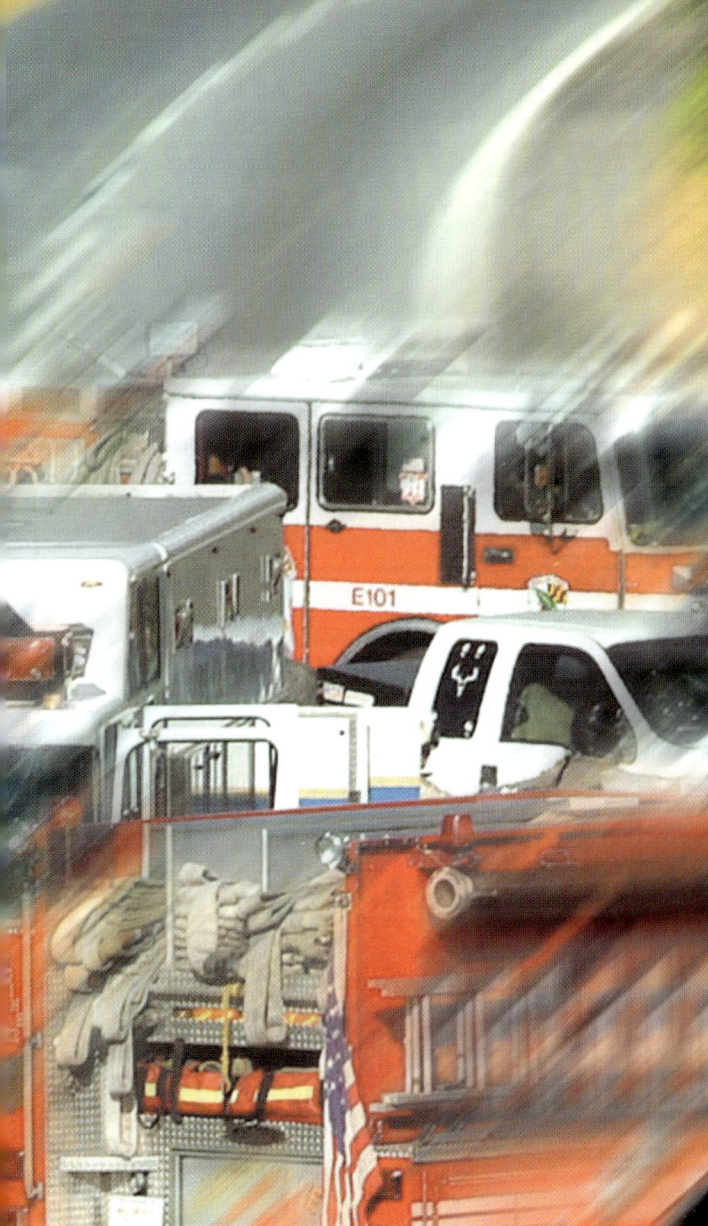

1	Introduction to Emergency Medical Care	2
2	The Well-Being of the EMT-I	24
3	Medical, Legal, and Ethical Issues	74
4	Medical Terminology	96
5	The Human Body	114

Introduction to Emergency Medical Care

1999 Objectives

Cognitive

1-1.1 Define the following terms: EMS systems, certification, registration, profession, professionalism, health care professional, ethics, medical direction, and protocols. (p 6)

1-1.2 Describe the attributes of an EMT-Intermediate as a health care professional. (p 6)

1-1.3 Explain EMT-Intermediate licensure/certification, registration, and reciprocity requirements in his or her state. (p 6)

1-1.4 Describe the benefits of EMT-Intermediate continuing education. (p 15)

1-1.5 List current state requirements for EMT-Intermediate education in his/her state. (p 8)

1-1.6 Describe examples of professional behaviors in the following areas: integrity, empathy, self-motivation, appearance and personal hygiene, self confidence, communications, time management, teamwork and diplomacy, respect, patient advocacy, and careful delivery of service. (p 18)

1-1.7 Provide examples of activities that constitute appropriate professional behavior for an EMT-Intermediate. (p 18)

1-1.8 Describe how professionalism applies to the EMT-Intermediate while on and off duty. (p 19)

1-1.9 List and explain the primary and additional roles and responsibilities of the EMT-Intermediate. (p 6)

1-1.10 Describe the importance and benefits of quality EMS research to the future of EMS. (p 9)

1-1.11 Describe the role of the EMS physician in providing medical direction. (p 15)

1-1.12 Describe the benefits of medical direction, both on-line and off-line. (p 13)

1-1.13 Describe the relationship between a physician on the scene, the EMT-Intermediate on the scene, and the EMS physician providing on-line medical direction. (p 19)

1-1.14 Describe the components of continuous quality improvement. (p 14)

Affective

1-1.49 Serve as a role model for others relative to professionalism in EMS. (p 19)

1-1.50 Value the need to serve as the patient advocate inclusive of those with special needs, alternative life styles, and cultural diversity. (p 18)

1-1.51 Defend the importance of continuing medical education and skills retention. (p 19)

1-1.52 Advocate the need for supporting and participating in research efforts aimed at improving EMS systems. (p 15)

1-1.53 Assess personal attitudes and demeanor that may distract from professionalism. (p 19)

1-1.55 Exhibit professional behaviors in the following areas: integrity, empathy, self-motivation, appearance and personal hygiene, self-confidence, communications, time management, teamwork and diplomacy, respect, patient advocacy, and careful delivery of service. (p 18)

1-1.61 Assess his/her own prejudices related to the various aspects of cultural diversity. (p 18)

Psychomotor

None

1

1985 Objectives

1.1.1 Identify and describe those activities performed by an EMT-Intermediate in the field. (p 13)

1.1.2 Define the role of an EMT-Intermediate. (p 18)

1.1.3 Describe and contrast the difference between an EMT-Ambulance and EMT-Intermediate training program. (p 8)

1.1.4 Define the term "ethics" and "professionalism." (p 14)

1.1.9 Define the term "professional." (p 17)

1.1.10 Define the term "health care professional." (p 15)

1.1.11 Identify whether a particular activity is professional or unprofessional given certain patient care situations. (p 13)

1.1.12 State certain activities that are most appropriate to professional behavior. (p 13)

1.1.13 List current State requirements for EMT-Intermediate continuing education. (p 13)

1.1.14 Define and discuss at least three reasons why continuing education is important for the EMT-Intermediate. (p 14)

1.1.15 Define the terms certification/licensure/registration. (p 14)

1.1.16 Name and describe current state legislation outlining the scope of prehospital advanced life support. (p 6)

1.1.17 State the reason it is important to keep one's EMT-Intermediate certification current. (p 19)

1.1.18 State the major purposes of a national association. (p 19)

1.1.19 State the major purposes of a national registration agency. (p 8)

1.1.20 State the major benefits of subscribing to professional journals. (p 19)

1.1.21 State the benefits of EMT-Intermediates teaching in their community. (p 18)

1.2.1 Discuss citizen access and the various mechanisms of obtaining it. (p 12)

1.2.2 Discuss prehospital care as an extension of hospital care. (p 15)

1.2.4 Define and describe medical control. (p 13)

1.2.5 Describe physician responsibility for Medical Control. (p 13)

1.2.6 Describe the relationship between the physician on the scene, the EMT-I, and the physician on the radio. (p 13)

1.2.7 Describe the benefits of EMT-I follow up on patient condition. (p 13)

1.2.10 Define the national standard levels of prehospital provider as defined by curriculum, respectively. (p 7)

1.2.11 Discuss the medical community role in overseeing prehospital care. (p 13)

1.2.12 Define protocols and standing orders. (p 13)

1.2.13 Describe the development of protocols. (p 15)

1.2.14 Define local training standards. (p 6)

1.2.15 Describe the legislation in the EMT-I's state as regards prehospital care. (p 15)

1.2.16 Describe integration of prehospital care into the continuum of total patient care with the emergency department phase of hospital care. (p 18)

1.2.19 Describe the relationship between the physician on radio and the EMT-I at the scene. (p 13)

1.2.21 Describe the transition of patient care from the EMT-I, including, A) transfer of responsibility (legal and medical), B) reporting of patient status to physician or nurse. (p 18)

1.2.23 Describe retrospective evaluation of patient care, including run report review, continuing education, skill practice, and skill deterioration. (p 19)

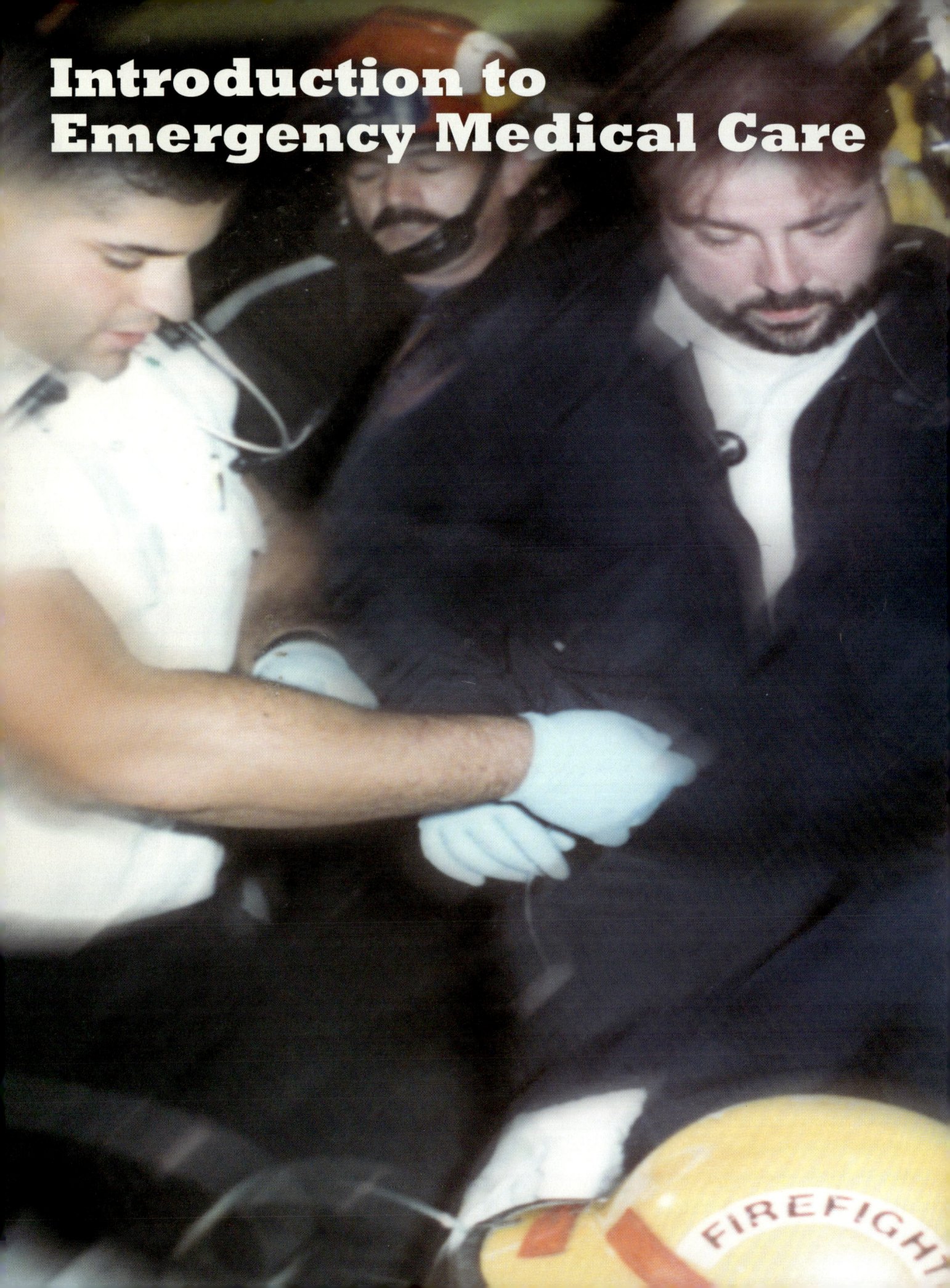

Introduction to Emergency Medical Care

1
Introduction to Emergency Medical Care

You are the Provider

You are responding to your first call as an EMT-Intermediate. Dispatch advises you that a patient is reported to be lying unresponsive on the ground.

You mentally review your protocols while en route. Since your partner is an EMT-Basic, you will be in charge of the call.

This chapter will help you to understand the roles and responsibilities of an EMT-Intermediate.

1. What role does medical direction play in the EMT-Intermediate's delivery of prehospital care?
2. What is the distinction between off-line and online medical control?

Introduction to Emergency Medical Care

This book has been designed to serve as the text and primary resource for the emergency medical technician intermediate (EMT-Intermediate) course. This chapter describes the content and objectives of the EMT-Intermediate course. It also discusses what will be expected of you during the course and what other requirements you will have to meet to be licensed or certified as an EMT-Intermediate in most states. The differences between basic first aid training, a Department of Transportation (DOT) First Responder training course, and the training for the EMT-Basic, EMT-Intermediate, and EMT-Paramedic are described.

Emergency medical services (EMS) is a system. The key components of this system and how they influence and affect the EMT-Intermediate and his or her delivery of emergency care are carefully discussed. Next, the administration, medical direction, quality control, and regulation of EMS services are presented. The chapter ends with a detailed discussion of the roles and responsibilities of the EMT-Intermediate as a health care professional.

Course Description

Emergency medical services (EMS) consists of a team of health care professionals who, in each area or jurisdiction, are responsible for and provide prehospital emergency care and transportation to the sick and injured (Figure 1-1). Each emergency medical service is part of a local or regional EMS system that provides the prehospital components required for the delivery of proper emergency medical care. The standards for prehospital emergency care and the individuals who provide it are governed by the laws in each state and are typically regulated by a state office of EMS.

The individuals who provide the emergency care in the field are trained and, except for licensed physicians, must be state-licensed or certified emergency medical technicians (EMTs). EMTs are categorized into three training and licensure levels: EMT-Basic, EMT-Intermediate, and EMT-Paramedic. An EMT-Basic (EMT-B) has training in basic emergency care skills, including automated external defibrillation, use of basic airway adjuncts, and assisting patients with certain medications. An EMT-Intermediate (EMT-I) has advanced training in specific aspects of advanced life support, such as intravenous (IV) therapy, advanced airway management, and cardiac monitoring. An EMT-Paramedic (EMT-P) has extensive training in advanced life support, including IV therapy, pharmacology, cardiac monitoring, and other advanced assessment and treatment skills. The EMT-Ambulance (EMT-A) certification used previously was comparable to the EMT-B, but is now obsolete.

Although the specific training and licensure requirements vary from one state to another, the training that is required in almost every state meets or exceeds the guidelines that are recommended in the current US DOT National Standard Curriculum for each level of EMS provider.

After you have successfully completed the Basic Life Support/Cardiopulmonary Resuscitation (BLS/CPR) course for health care providers and met the other prerequisites, which may include EMT-B, you are ready to take the EMT-I course. Like any continuing course, the

Technology

- Interactivities
- Vocabulary Explorer
- Anatomy Review
- Web Links
- Online Review Manual

www.EMSzone.com/EMTI

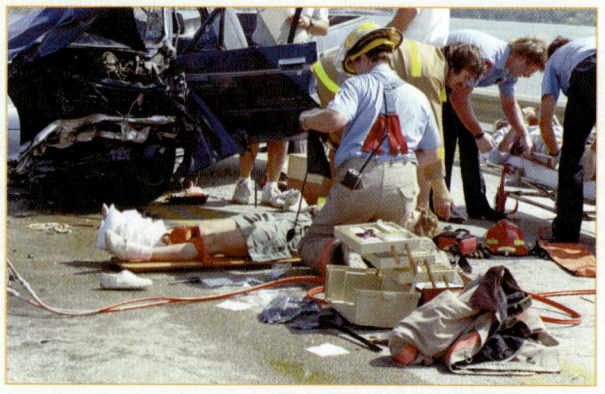

Figure 1-1 As an EMT-I, you will be part of a larger team that responds to a variety of calls and provides a wide range of prehospital emergency care.

EMT-I course covers a great deal of information and introduces many skills. Everything you learn in the course will be important in your ability to provide high-quality emergency care once you are certified and ready to practice. In addition, the knowledge, understanding, and skills that you acquire in the EMT-I course will serve as a foundation for the additional knowledge and training that you will receive in future years.

Once you have passed your state's requirements you are then certified to work for an EMS service to provide care within your level of training. You are issued a certification, which is a legal document that indicates you have successfully completed a prescribed course of training and have met certain standards. You may also be registered with a certifying agency such as the National Registry of Emergency Medical Technicians. EMTs do not receive a licensure, which grants permission to perform professional actions in various fields. Even with an EMT certification, you will still work under the license of your medical director.

This textbook covers the knowledge objectives that are identified in the US DOT 1985 and 1999 EMT-Intermediate National Standard Curriculum and in the 1994 National EMS Education and Practice Blueprint. In addition to the required core content, it includes additional information that will help you to understand and apply the material and skills that are included in the EMT-I level. Your instructor will furnish you with reading assignments. It is important that you complete the assigned reading before each class.

In class, the instructor will review the key parts of the reading assignment and clarify and expand on them Figure 1-2 ▼. The instructor will also answer any questions that you have and will clarify any points that you or others find confusing. Unless you have carefully read the assignment and made notes before coming to class, you may not fully understand or benefit from the classroom presentation and discussions. You will also need to take additional notes during class (Table 1-1 ▼).

The EMT-I course will include four types of learning activities:

1. **Reading assignments** from the textbook and presentations and discussions held in class will provide you with the necessary knowledge base.
2. **Step-by-step demonstrations** will teach you hands-on skills that you then need to practice repeatedly in supervised small group workshops.
3. **Summary skills sheets** will help you to memorize the sequence of steps in complex skills that contain a large number of steps or variations so that you can perform the skill with no errors or omissions.
4. **Case presentations and scenarios** used in class will help you learn how to apply the knowledge and skills acquired in classroom situations to those you will find in the field.

EMT-Intermediate Training: Focus and Requirements

EMT-I training is divided into three main categories. The first and most important category focuses on the care of life-threatening or potentially life-threatening conditions. To deal with these, you will learn how to do the following:

- Size up the scene and situation.
- Ensure that the scene is safe.
- Perform an initial assessment of the patient.
- Obtain a history of this episode and a pertinent past medical history.
- Identify life-threatening injuries or conditions.
- Establish and maintain an open airway.
- Provide adequate ventilation.

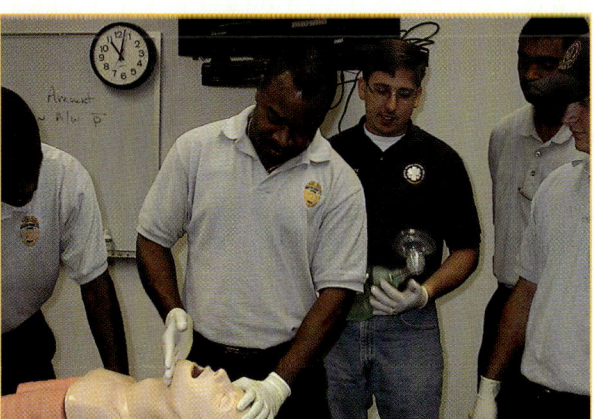

Figure 1-2 In the classroom, you will learn both didactic and practical skills to prepare you for various types of calls.

TABLE 1-1	Study Tips for Using This Textbook

- **Complete each assignment** diligently and carefully.
- **Read the textbook** like a textbook, not like a newspaper, magazine, or novel.
- **Read each chapter** several times and underline key points. Take notes!
- **Ask your instructor** to clarify any questions you note in your reading or in class.
- **Take additional notes** when the assigned material is expanded upon in class.
- **Remember:** The only absurd question is the one that a student has and fails to ask.

- Manage conditions that prevent proper ventilation.
- Provide high-flow supplemental oxygen.
- Perform cardiopulmonary resuscitation (CPR).
- Perform automated or semiautomated external defibrillation (with an AED).
- Control external bleeding.
- Recognize and treat shock.
- Care for patients in an acute life-threatening medical emergency.
- Assist patients in taking certain medications that they carry and that their physician has prescribed for an acute episode.
- Identify and rapidly prepare, or "package," patients (by positioning, covering, and securing them) for rapid initiation of transport when necessary.

The second category of training covers conditions that, although not life-threatening, are key components of emergency care or are necessary to prevent further harm before the patient is moved. You will learn to do the following:

- Identify patients for whom spinal precautions should be taken and immobilize them properly.
- Dress and bandage wounds.
- Splint injured extremities.
- Care for burns.
- Care for cases of poisoning.
- Deliver a baby.
- Assess and care for a newborn.
- Manage patients with behavioral or psychological problems.
- Cope with the psychological stresses on patients, families, your fellow EMT-Is, and yourself.

The third category covers important issues that are related to your ability to provide emergency care. You will develop the following related skills:

- Understanding the role and responsibilities of the EMT-I
- Following your service's protocols and orders from medical direction
- Understanding ethical and medicolegal problems
- Driving the emergency vehicle and defensive driving
- Using equipment carried on the ambulance
- Checking and stocking the ambulance
- Communicating with patients and others at the scene
- Using the radio and communicating with the dispatcher
- Giving a precise radio report about the patient and obtaining direct medical direction
- Giving a full verbal report when transferring the patient's care at the hospital
- Preparing proper documentation and completing the patient care report
- Working with other responders at an emergency scene
- Cooperating with operations at special rescue, mass-casualty, and hazardous materials incidents

Certification Requirements

To be recognized and to perform as an EMT-I, you must meet certain training and other requirements. The specific requirements differ from state to state. You should ask your instructor or contact your state EMS office to find out about the requirements in your state. Generally, the criteria will include the following:

- High school diploma or equivalent
- Proof of immunization against certain communicable diseases
- Valid driver's license
- Successful completion of a recognized health care provider's BLS/CPR course
- Successful completion of a state-approved EMT-I course
- Successful completion of a state-approved written certification examination
- Successful completion of a state-approved practical certification examination
- Demonstration that you can meet the psychological and physical criteria necessary to be able to safely and properly perform all the tasks and functions described in the defined role of an EMT-I
- Compliance with other state and local provisions

The state-recognized written and practical examination may be the National Registry Exam based on the individual state. The National Registry of Emergency Medical Technicians (NREMT) was established to certify and register EMS professionals through a valid and uniform process that assesses their knowledge and skills to ensure competent practice. The NREMT requires a reregistration process every 2 years to assure continued competence. Since most states now recognize the NREMT certification, it is easy for an EMT-I to move to another state and continue to work without the process of attending another course and taking another certification test for that area. If you decide to transfer to a different state, you may be allowed to apply for reciprocity rather than starting your training all over or taking that state's certification exam. **Reciprocity** is the recognition by one state of another state's certification, allowing a health care professional from another state to practice in the new state.

The Americans With Disabilities Act (ADA) of 1990 protects individuals who have a disability from being denied access to programs and services that are provided by state or local governments and prohibits employers from failing to provide full and equal employment to the disabled. To obtain further information about the ADA and employment as an EMT-I, you should contact your state EMS office.

In most states, individuals who have been convicted of driving while under the influence of alcohol or other drugs or have been convicted of certain felonies may be denied certification as an EMT-I.

States may exclude from certification persons with a history of a health problem that could make their performance of EMT-I tasks dangerous to themselves or others.

Overview of the Emergency Medical Services System

History of EMS

As an EMT-I, you will be joining a long tradition of people who have provided emergency medical care to their fellow human beings. With the early use of motor vehicles in warfare, volunteer ambulance squads were organized and went overseas to provide care for the wounded in World War I. In World War II, the military trained special corpsmen to provide care in the field and bring the casualties to aid stations staffed by nurses and physicians. In the Korean conflict, the care system evolved to the field medic and rapid helicopter evacuation to nearby Mobile Army Surgical Hospital units, where immediate surgical intervention was provided. Many advances in the immediate care of trauma patients resulted from the casualty experiences in the Korean and Vietnam conflicts.

Unfortunately, emergency care of the injured and ill at home had not progressed to a similar level. As late as the early 1960s, emergency ambulance service and care across the United States varied widely. In some places, care was provided by well-trained advanced first aid squads

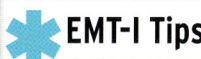

EMT-I Tips

As an EMT-I, you will be continuing a long tradition of people who have provided emergency medical care to their fellow human beings.

that had well-equipped modern ambulances. In a few urban areas, it was provided by hospital-based ambulance services that were staffed with interns and early forms of medics. In many places, the only emergency care and ambulance service was provided by the local funeral home using a hearse that could be converted to carry a cot and serve as an ambulance. In other places, the police or fire department used a station wagon that carried a cot and a first aid kit. In most cases, both of these were staffed by a driver and an attendant who had some intermediate first aid training. In the few areas where a commercial ambulance was available to transport the ill, it was usually similarly staffed and served primarily as a means to transport the patient to the hospital.

Many communities had no formal provision for prehospital emergency care or transportation. Injured persons were given intermediate first aid by police or fire personnel at the scene and were transported to the hospital in a police or fire officer's car. Customarily, patients with an acute illness were transported to the hospital by a relative or neighbor and were met by their family physician or an on-call hospital physician who assessed them and then summoned any specialists and operating room staff that were needed. Except in large urban centers, most hospitals did not have the staffed emergency departments to which we are accustomed today.

The EMS system as we know it today had its origins in 1966 with the publication of Accidental Death and Disability: The Neglected Disease of Modern Society. This report, prepared jointly by the Committees on Trauma and Shock of the National Academy of Sciences/National Research Council, revealed to the public and Congress the serious inadequacy of prehospital emergency care and transportation in many areas.

You are the Provider Part 2

When arriving on scene, you note an elderly man lying on the front lawn. You and your partner get out of your vehicle to begin patient care.

3. What is the first step in caring for this patient?
4. What precautions, if any, should you consider?

A number of key items were recommended in the report, some of which follow:

- Development of national courses of instruction for prehospital emergency care and transportation by fire, police, rescue, and ambulance personnel
- Development of nationally accepted textbooks and training aids for these courses
- Development of federal guidelines for the design of ambulances and the equipment they carry
- Development and adoption of general policies and regulations pertaining to ambulance services and qualification and supervision of ambulance personnel in each state
- Adoption by each municipality (or district or county) of means to supply the necessary proper prehospital emergency care and transport within its jurisdiction
- Establishment of hospital emergency departments with staffing by physicians, nurses, and other personnel who are trained in resuscitation and the immediate care of the seriously injured and ill

As a result, Congress mandated that two federal agencies address these issues. The National Highway Traffic Safety Administration (NHTSA) of the DOT, through the Highway Safety Act of 1966, and the Department of Health and Human Services, through the Emergency Medical Act of 1973, created funding sources and programs to develop improved systems of prehospital emergency care.

In the early 1970s, the DOT developed and published the first National Standard Curriculum to serve as the guideline for the training of EMT-Bs. To support the EMT course, the American Academy of Orthopaedic Surgeons prepared and published the first EMT textbook—*Emergency Care and Transportation of the Sick and Injured*—in 1971. The textbook you are reading is the first edition of that publication at the EMT-I level. Through the 1970s, following the recommended guidelines, each state developed the necessary legislation, and the EMS system was developed throughout the United States. During the same period, emergency medicine became a recognized medical specialty, and the fully staffed emergency departments that we know today became the accepted standard of care.

In the late 1970s and early 1980s, the DOT developed a recommended National Standard Curriculum for the training of paramedics and identified a part of the course to serve as training for EMT-Is.

By 1980, EMS had been established throughout the nation. The system was based on the following two key changes:

- The introduction of legislation that made it the responsibility of each municipality, township, or county to provide proper prehospital emergency care and transportation within its boundaries
- The establishment of recognized and regulated standards for the training of ambulance personnel and equipment required on each ambulance

These changes ensured that, regardless of where an individual became injured or acutely ill, he or she would receive timely, proper emergency care and transport to the hospital. During the 1980s, many areas enhanced the EMT National Standard Curriculum by adding EMTs with higher levels of training who could provide key components of **advanced life support (ALS)** care (advanced lifesaving procedures). The availability of paramedics (EMT-Ps) on calls that require or benefit from advanced care has grown steadily in recent years. In addition, with the evolution in training and technology, the EMT-B and EMT-I can now perform a number of important advanced skills in the field that were formerly reserved for the EMT-P.

The way EMS systems work may differ depending on the geographic area and population served. Regardless of the area, however, the NHTSA is available to evaluate EMS systems, based on the following 10 categories of criteria in their Technical Assistance Program Assessment Standards:

1. Regulation and policy
2. Resource management
3. Human resources and training
4. Transportation equipment and system
5. Medical and support facilities
6. Communications system
7. Public information and education
8. Medical direction
9. Trauma system and development
10. Evaluation

Levels of Training

Certification of EMT-Is is a state function, subject to the laws and regulations of the state in which the EMT-I practices. For this reason there is some variation from state to state on the scope of EMT-I practice, as well as training and recertification requirements.

There are some national guidelines, however. The DOT National Standard Curriculum serves as the basis for the development of state curricula. The EMT-B, EMT-I, and EMT-P curricula can be downloaded from the National Highway Traffic Safety Administration's (NHTSA's) website. In addition, the National Registry of Emergency Medical Technicians is a nongovernmental agency that provides a national standard for EMT-I testing and certification throughout the United States. Many states utilize the National Registry testing process in certifying their EMT-Is, and grant licensing reciprocity to Nationally Registered EMT-Is. It is important to remember, however, that EMS is regulated entirely by the state in which you are certified.

Public Basic Life Support and Immediate Aid

With the development of EMS and increased awareness of the need for immediate emergency care, millions of laypeople have been trained in BLS/CPR. In addition to CPR, many individuals have taken short basic first aid courses that include control of bleeding and other simple skills that may be required to provide immediate essential care. These courses are designed to train individuals so that those in the workplace, teachers, coaches, baby-sitters, and the like, can provide the necessary critical care in the minutes before EMTs or other responders arrive at the scene.

In addition, many individuals, such as those who regularly accompany groups on camping trips or are in other situations in which the arrival of EMS may be delayed because of remote location, are trained in advanced first aid. This course includes basic life support and the essential additional care and packaging that may be necessary until the help of rescuers and EMTs can be obtained at a remote location.

One of the most dramatic recent developments in prehospital emergency care is the use of an **automated external defibrillator (AED)**. These remarkable devices, some no larger than a cellular phone, detect treatable life-threatening cardiac arrhythmias (ventricular fibrillation and ventricular tachycardia) and deliver the appropriate electrical shock to the patient. Designed to be used by the untrained layperson, they are now included at every level of prehospital emergency training.

First Responders

Because the presence of a person who is trained and able to initiate basic life support and other urgent care cannot be ensured, the EMS system includes immediate care by **first responders**, such as law enforcement officers, fire fighters, park rangers, ski patrollers, or other organized rescuers who often arrive at the scene before the ambulance and EMTs (Figure 1-3 ▶). The DOT has established a First Responder Curriculum to provide these individuals with the training necessary to initiate immediate care and then assist the EMTs on their arrival. The course focuses on providing immedi-

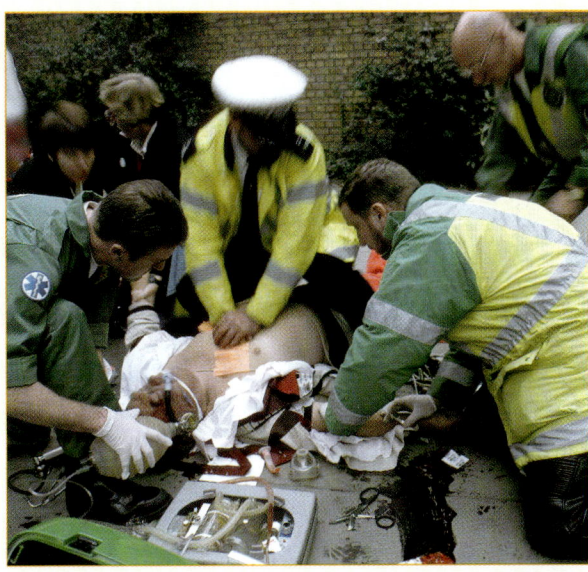

Figure 1-3 First responders, such as law enforcement officers, are trained to provide immediate basic life support until EMTs arrive on the scene.

ate intermediate life support and urgent care with limited equipment. It also familiarizes the student with the additional procedures, equipment, and packaging techniques that EMTs may use and with which the first responder may be called upon to assist.

In addition to professional first responders, EMT-Is often encounter a variety of people on scene eager to help. You will encounter Good Samaritans trained in first aid and CPR, physicians and nurses, and other well-meaning individuals with or without prior training and experience. Identified and utilized properly, these individuals can provide valuable assistance when you are short-handed. At other times, they can interfere with operations and even create problems or danger to themselves or others. It will be your task in your initial scene size up to identify the various persons on the scene and orchestrate well-meaning attempts to assist.

EMT-Basic

The EMT-B course requires a minimum of 110 hours (more in some states) and includes essential knowledge and skills required to provide basic emergency care in the field. The course serves as the foundation upon which additional knowledge and skills are built in advanced EMT training. On arrival at the scene, you and the other EMTs who have responded with the ambulance should assume responsibility for the assessment and care of the patient, followed by proper packaging and transport of the patient to the emergency department.

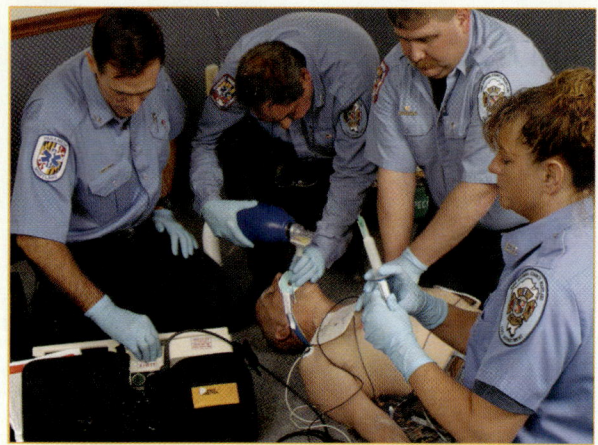

Figure 1-4 EMT-Is have EMT-B training and various advanced skills such as arrhythmia recognition.

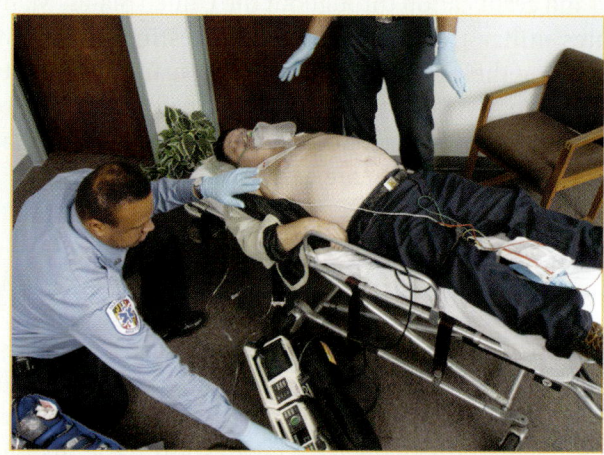

Figure 1-5 EMT-P training includes advanced skills such as cardioversion.

EMT-Intermediate

The EMT-I course and training is designed to provide additional knowledge and skills in specific aspects of advanced life support to individuals who have been trained and have experience in providing emergency care as an EMT-B. These additional skills include IV therapy, interpretation of cardiac rhythms and defibrillation, orotracheal intubation, and, in many states, the knowledge and skills necessary to administer medications (Figure 1-4 ▲). Keep in mind that you must follow guidelines specific for your area.

EMT-Paramedic

The EMT-P has completed an extensive course of training that significantly increases knowledge and mastery of intermediate skills and covers a wide range of ALS skills (Figure 1-5 ▶). These skills include the following:

- Electrocardiogram monitoring and interpretation of cardiac rhythms
- Advanced cardiac life support (ACLS) protocols and skills
- Manual defibrillation, synchronized cardioversion, and external cardiac pacing
- Orotracheal and nasotracheal intubation
- Needle cricothyroidotomy
- Needle decompression for tension pneumothorax
- Intravenous therapy
- Advanced pharmacology: drug calculations and medication administration (IV, IV infusion, intraosseous [IO], endotracheal [ET], and injections)

Components of the EMS System

Access

Easy access to the help needed in an emergency is essential. In most of the country, an emergency communications center that dispatches fire, police, rescue, and EMS units can be reached by dialing 9-1-1. At the communication center, trained dispatchers obtain the necessary information from the caller and, following dispatch protocols, dispatch the ambulance crew and other equipment and responders that might be needed (Figure 1-6 ▼).

In an enhanced 9-1-1 system, the address of the telephone from which the call is made is displayed on a

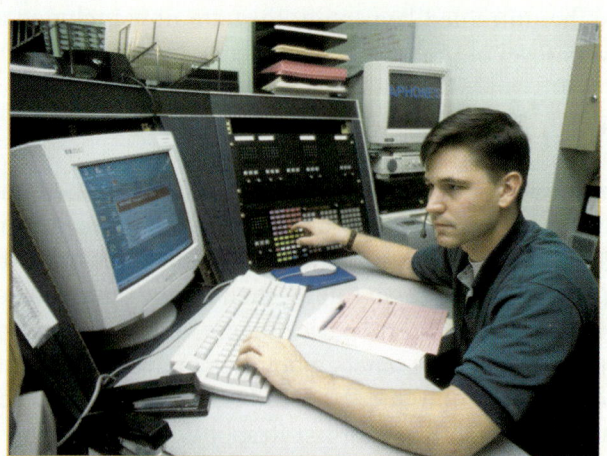

Figure 1-6 Trained dispatchers obtain information about the call and then send responders to the scene as needed.

screen. The connection is frozen until the dispatcher releases it so that if the caller is unable to speak, his or her location remains displayed. Most emergency communications centers also include special equipment so that individuals with speech or hearing disabilities can communicate with the dispatcher via a keyboard and printed messages. In some areas, rather than 9-1-1, a different special published emergency number may be used to call for EMS. Training the public in how to summon an EMS unit is an important part of the public education responsibility of each EMS service.

Enhanced 9-1-1 systems for cellular phones are now becoming available that identify not only the cellular phone number from which an emergency call is being placed, but also the exact geographic coordinates of the phone at the time the call is made. Such systems utilize GPS (global positioning satellite) technology. Because cellular phones capable of transmitting a GPS signal and a system capable of receiving that signal are both required, the technology will require many years to implement.

A system called **Emergency Medical Dispatch (EMD)** has been developed to assist dispatchers in providing callers with vital instructions to help them deal with a medical emergency until the arrival of EMS crews. Dispatchers are provided with training and scripts to help them relay relevant instructions to the callers. The system also helps dispatchers select appropriately resourced units to respond to a request for assistance. It is the dispatcher's duty to relay all relevant and available information to the responding crews in a timely manner. Keep in mind, however, that current technology doesn't allow the dispatcher to "see" what is actually going on at the scene, and that it is not uncommon for you to find the reality of the call quite different from the dispatch information.

In many municipalities, EMS is a part of the fire department. In others, it is a part of the police department or is an independent public or private safety service. In some areas, a contractor may provide either BLS or ALS service. In some areas, ALS is provided by paramedics who are based at a hospital or who may cover a number of towns in a region.

New technologies are constantly being developed that can assist responders in locating their patients. As previously described, cellular telephones can be linked to GPS units to display their location. Rescue squads can transmit their position to dispatch and dispatch can transmit the location of a call to a moving digital map in the squad, complete with turn-by-turn directions. Medical databases can be queried and patient information directly downloaded to the EMT-I's computer, or uploaded from the EMT-I's laptop to the database. The pace of technological developments in communications makes the latest device soon obsolete, so constant training and education are required to keep the EMT-I's knowledge up to date.

Administration and Policy

Each EMS service operates in a designated **primary service area (PSA)** in which it is responsible for the provision of prehospital emergency care and the transportation of the sick and injured to the hospital.

The EMS services are usually administered by a senior EMS official. Daily operational and overall direction of the service is provided by an appointed chief executive officer and several other officers who serve under him or her. When the EMS service is a part of a fire or police department, the department chief will usually delegate the responsibility for directing EMS to an assistant chief or other officer whose sole responsibility is to manage the EMS activities of the department. To provide clear guidelines, most services have written operating procedures and policies. When you join a service, you will be expected to learn and follow them.

The chief executive of the service is in charge of both the necessary administrative tasks (such as scheduling, personnel, budgets, purchasing, and vehicle maintenance) and the daily operations of the ambulances and crews. Except for medical matters, he or she operates as the chief (similar to a fire chief or police chief) of EMS for the service and the PSA that it covers.

Medical Direction and Control

Each EMS system has a physician **medical director** who authorizes the EMTs in the service to provide medical care in the field. The appropriate care for each injury, condition, or illness that you will encounter in the field is determined by the medical director and is described in a set of written standing orders and protocols. Protocols are described in a comprehensive guide delineating the EMT-I's scope of practice. Standing orders are part of protocols, and designate what the EMT-I is required to do for a specific complaint or condition.

The medical director provides the ongoing working liaison between the medical community, hospitals, and the EMT-Is in the service. If treatment problems arise or different procedures should be considered, these are referred to the medical director for his or her decision and action. To ensure that the proper training standards are met, the medical director determines and approves the continuing education and training that are

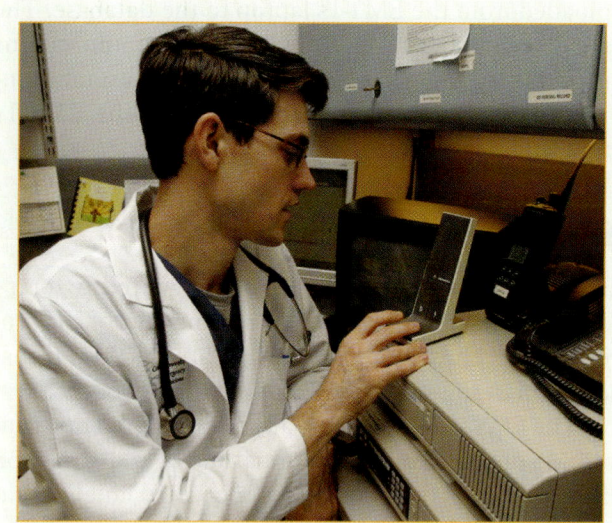

Figure 1-7 Online or direct medical control is provided by a physician.

required of each EMT-I in the service and approves any that individuals obtain elsewhere.

Medical control is either off-line (indirect) or online (direct), as authorized by the medical director. Online medical control consists of direction given over the phone or radio directly from the medical director or designated physician. The medical direction can be transferred by the physician's designee; it does not have to be transferred by the physician himself or herself. Off-line medical control consists of standing orders, training, and supervision authorized by the medical director. Each EMT-I must know and follow the protocols developed by his or her medical director.

The service's protocols will also identify an EMS physician who can be reached by radio or telephone for medical control during a call (Figure 1-7▲). This is a type of direct online medical control. On some calls, once the squad has initiated any immediate urgent care and given its radio report, the online medical control physician may confirm or modify the proposed treatment plan or may prescribe any additional special orders that the EMT-Is are to follow for that patient. The point at which the EMT-Is should give their radio report or obtain online medical direction will vary.

 EMT-I Tips

Each EMS system has a physician medical director who authorizes the EMT-Is in the service to provide medical care in the field.

The medical director is the ongoing working liaison among the medical community, hospitals, and the EMTs in the service. If treatment problems arise or different procedures should be considered, these are referred to the medical director for decision and action. To ensure that the proper training standards are met, the medical director determines and approves the continuing education and training that are required of each EMT in the service and approves any that individuals obtain elsewhere.

Quality Control and Improvement

The medical director is responsible for maintaining quality control to ensure that all staff members who are involved in caring for patients meet appropriate medical care standards on each call. To provide the necessary quality control, the medical director and other involved staff review patient care reports.

Continuous quality improvement (CQI), which may also be known as quality assurance (QA), is a circular system of continuous internal and external reviews and audits of all aspects of an EMS call. To provide CQI, periodic run review meetings are held in which all those who are involved in patient care review the run reports and discuss any areas of care that seem to need change or improvement. Positive feedback is also discussed. If a problem seems to be repeated by a single EMT-I or crew, the medical director will discuss the details with the individuals involved and, if necessary, assign remedial training or some other development activity. The medical director is also responsible for ensuring that appropriate continuing education and training are available.

Information and skills in emergency medical care change constantly. You need refresher training or continuing education as new modalities of care, equipment, and understanding of critical illnesses and trauma develop. In addition, when you have not done a particular procedure for some time, skill decay may occur. Therefore, your medical director might establish a CQI process to correct the deficit. For example, an emergency department physician noted that despite their assessments, many EMT-Is were missing a high number of closed long bone fractures, resulting in inadequate prehospital care. A subsequent audit of calls led to a review and retraining session for assessment and care of fractures. This same process can apply to CPR or any other type of skill that you do not use often. You may also choose to follow up on specific patients delivered to the hospital. By doing so, you have the opportunity to critique your prehospital care and, in turn, improve any weak areas. Ensuring that your skills and knowledge are current is one of the ongoing commitments of being an EMT-I.

Other Physician Input

EMS is an extension of the emergency medical care provided in the emergency department by the physicians and other specialists who provide definitive care in the hospital. Besides the direction that the medical director and direct online medical control physicians provide, your training and practices are based on input from many specialty professional associations at the national, state, and local levels.

As an EMT-I, you are part of the professional continuum of care provided to patients who often have life-threatening conditions. Many physician experts from the specialties of emergency medicine, traumatology, orthopaedics, cardiology, anesthesiology, radiology, and other medical disciplines participate in the ongoing work of EMS. The efforts of these groups—often through professional associations such as the American Academy of Orthopaedic Surgeons, the American College of Emergency Physicians, the American College of Surgeons, and the National Association of EMS Physicians—include research, the establishment of standards for quality assurance, continuing education, and publications. Constant research and quality improvement are the cornerstones of advances in emergency medicine and the future of EMS.

Regulation

Although each EMS system, medical director, and training program has vast latitude, their training, protocols, and practices must conform to the EMS legislation, rules, regulations, and guidelines adopted by each state. Medical directors, along with EMS supervisors and others, develop protocols for individual service areas based on the training levels of the EMS providers in that area. The state EMS office is responsible for authorizing, auditing, and regulating all EMS services, training institutions, courses, instructors, and providers within the state. In most states, the state EMS office obtains input from an advisory committee made up of representatives of the services, service medical directors, medical associations, hospitals, training programs, instructors' associations, EMT associations, and the public.

Equipment

As an EMT-I, you will use a wide range of different emergency equipment. During the EMT-I course, you will be introduced to, and learn how to use, a variety of the different appliances and devices that you may need to use on a call. You will also learn when the use of each is indicated and when it is contraindicated because it will

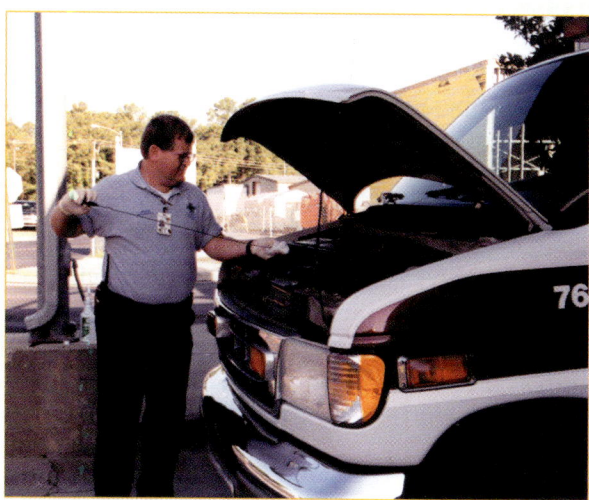

Figure 1-8 Making sure the ambulance is in good working condition is your responsibility as an EMT-I.

not be of benefit or may cause harm. Although the use of different models and brands of a given device will follow the same generic principles and methods, some variations and peculiarities exist from one model to another. When you join a service, you should check each key piece of equipment before going on duty to ensure that it is in its assigned place, that it is working properly, and that you are familiar with the specific model carried on your ambulance.

The Ambulance

Each EMT-I may be called upon to drive the ambulance. Therefore, you must familiarize yourself with the roads in your PSA or sector. Before going on duty, you should check all the equipment and supplies and communication equipment that the ambulance carries and make sure that it is fully fueled, that it has sufficient oil and other key fluids, and that the tires are in good condition and properly inflated (**Figure 1-8 ▲**). You should also test each of the driver's controls and each built-in unit and control in the patient compartment. If you have not driven the specific ambulance before, it is a good idea to take it out and become familiar with it before you respond to a call. Maintenance and safe driving of the ambulance are discussed in detail in Chapter 33.

Transport to Specialty Centers

In addition to hospital emergency departments, many EMS systems include specialty centers that focus on specific types of care (such as trauma, burns, poisoning, or psychiatric conditions) or specific types of patients (for example, children). Specialty centers require in-house staffs of surgeons and other specialists; other facilities must page operating teams, surgeons, or other specialists from outside the hospital. Typically, only a few hospitals in a region are designated as specialty centers. Transport time to a specialty center may be slightly longer than that to an emergency department, but patients will receive definitive care more quickly at a specialty center. You must know the location of the centers in your area and when, according to your protocol, you must transport the patient directly to one. Sometimes, air medical transport will be necessary. Local, regional, and state protocols will guide your decision in these instances.

Interfacility Transports

Many EMS services provide interfacility transportation for nonambulatory patients or patients with acute and chronic medical conditions requiring medical monitoring (Figure 1-9). This transportation may include transferring patients to and from hospitals, skilled nursing facilities, board and care homes, or even their home residence.

During ambulance transportation, the health and well-being of the patient is the EMT-I's responsibility. The EMT-I should obtain the patient's medical history, chief complaint, and latest vital signs and provide ongoing patient assessment. In certain circumstances, depending on local protocols, a nurse, physician, respiratory therapist, or medical team will accompany the patient. This is especially true when the patient requires care that extends beyond the EMT-I's scope of practice.

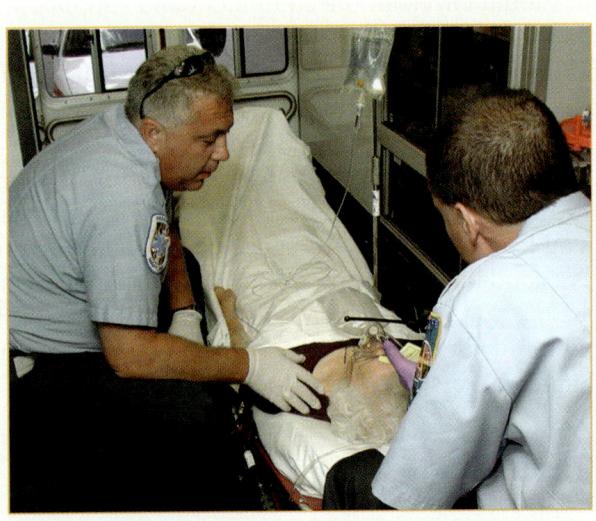

Figure 1-9 As an EMT-I, part of your job will be transporting patients to other facilities.

Working With Hospital Staff

You should become familiar with the hospital by observing hospital equipment and how it is used, the functions of staff members, and the policies and procedures in all emergency areas of the hospital. You will also learn about advances in emergency care and how to interact with hospital personnel. This experience will help you to understand how your care influences the patient's recovery and will emphasize the importance and benefits of proper prehospital care. It will also show you the consequences of delay, inadequate care, or poor judgment.

Physicians are not likely to be in the field with you to provide personal, on-the-spot instructions. However, you may consult with appropriate medical staff by using the radio through established medical control procedures.

In the emergency department, hospital staff may train you by showing you assessment and treatment techniques on patients. A physician or nurse may serve as an instructor for medical subjects in your training program. Through these experiences, you will become more comfortable using medical terms, interpreting patient signs and symptoms, and developing patient management skills.

Hospital staff members are usually willing to help you improve your skills and efficiency throughout your career. Some physicians and nurses may have completed the EMT curriculum as part of their formal medical training. The best patient care occurs when all emergency care providers have close rapport. This allows you and hospital staff the opportunity to discuss mutual problems and to benefit from each other's experiences.

Working With Public Safety Agencies

Some public safety workers have EMS training. As an EMT-I, you must become familiar with all the roles and responsibilities of these agencies. Personnel from certain agencies are better prepared than you to perform certain functions. For example, employees of a utility company are better equipped to control downed power lines than you or your partner. Law enforcement personnel are better able to handle violent scenes and traffic control, while you and your partner are better able to provide emergency medical care (Figure 1-10). If you work together and recognize that each person has special training and a job to do at the scene, effective scene and patient management will result. Remember that the best, most efficient patient care is achieved through cooperation among agencies.

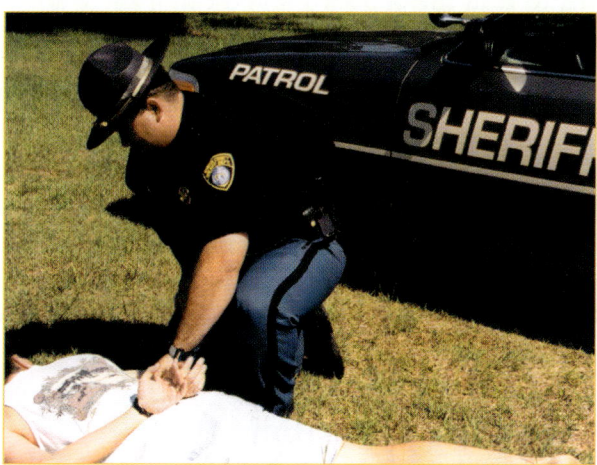

Figure 1-10 As an EMT-I, you will work with law enforcement personnel when dealing with violent patients.

Training

Your training will be conducted by many knowledgeable EMS educators. In most states, the instructors who are responsible for coordinating and teaching the EMT-I course and continuing education courses are approved and certified by the state EMS office or agency. To be certified in some states, an instructor must have extensive medical and educational training and teach for a designated period while being observed and supervised by an experienced instructor.

Most ALS training is provided in a college or hospital setting. In most states, educational programs that provide ALS training must be approved by the state and have their own medical director. In these courses, many of the lectures and small group sessions will be presented by the medical director or other physicians and nurses. In clinical sessions in which supervised practice is obtained in the emergency department or other in-hospital settings, students are also supervised directly by physicians and other medical staff.

The quality of care that you will provide depends on your ability and the quality of your training. Therefore, your instructor and the many others who developed and participated in your training program are key members of the emergency care team.

Providing a Coordinated Continuum of Care

The emergency care of patients occurs in three progressive phases:

1. **The first phase** consists of patient assessment, initial prehospital care, proper packaging, and safe transport to the hospital.
2. **In the second phase**, the patient receives continued assessment and stabilization in the hospital emergency department.
3. **In the third phase**, the patient receives the necessary definitive specialized care.

These three phases must be provided in a coordinated continuum of care to maximize survival and reduce patient suffering and lasting adverse effects. The EMS system is designed to produce such a coordinated effort among the local EMS services, emergency department staff, and the medical staff who provide definitive care.

You are the Provider — Part 3

You perform your initial assessment and determine the following:

Initial Assessment	Recording Time: Zero Minutes
Appearance	Motionless on the ground
Level of consciousness	No response
Airway	Open and clear
Breathing	Absent
Circulation	No pulse

5. What is your next step in caring for this patient?
6. What information should you provide to receiving emergency department personnel?

Roles and Responsibilities of the EMT-I

As an EMT-I, you will be the first health care professional to assess and treat the patient; as such, you have certain roles and responsibilities (Table 1-2). Often, patient outcomes are determined by the care that you provide in the field and your identification of patients who need prompt transport.

Educating patients in the field is also an important role the EMT-I must assume. Frequently patients are rushed through a physician's office and given a prescription that is filled by a pharmacist with the instructions to read the paperwork and call if there are any questions. Quite often the EMS provider is the only health care professional to recognize that the patient is noncompliant with medications because of a lack of knowledge. By simply explaining to the patient and his or her family how to eat properly and take the appropriate amount of the medication, trips to the emergency room may be reduced drastically. This is especially true for people with diabetes. Taking the extra time to educate the patient and family members may save money and reduce the unnecessary use of resources.

Professional Attributes

As an EMT-I, whether you are paid or a volunteer, you are a health care professional. A **professional** is skilled and trained for work by extended study or practice. Part of your responsibility is to make sure that patient care is given a high priority without endangering your own safety or the safety of others. Another part of your responsibility to yourself, other EMTs, the patient, and other health care professionals is to maintain a professional appearance and manner at all times. Your attitude and behavior must reflect that you are knowledgeable, proficient, and sincerely dedicated to serving anyone who is injured or experiencing an acute medical emergency. This includes ethical responsibilities as well. **Ethics** are moral principles or standards governing conduct.

As a professional, you must take pride in your appearance, grooming, and hygiene (Figure 1-11). You must look the part to be respected as an efficient, knowledgeable provider. A professional appearance and manner help to build confidence and ease the patient's anxiety. You will be expected to perform under pressure with composure and self-confidence. Patients and families who are under stress need to be treated with understanding, respect, and compassion.

Most patients will treat you with respect and appreciation, but some will not. Some patients are uncooperative, demanding, unpleasant, ungrateful, and verbally abusive. You must be nonjudgmental and overcome your instincts to react poorly to such behavior. Remember that when individuals are hurt, ill, under stress, frightened, despondent, under the influence of alcohol or drugs, or feel threatened, they will often react with inappropriate behavior, even toward those who are trying to help and care for them. Every patient, regardless of his or her attitude or beliefs, is entitled to compassion, respect, and the best care that you can provide. This includes patients with special needs, alternative lifestyles, and culturally diverse backgrounds. Personal prejudices should not interfere with appropriate medical care.

TABLE 1-2 Roles and Responsibilities of the EMT-I

- Ensuring your own safety and the safety of your fellow EMT-Is, the patient, and others at the scene
- Locating and safely driving to the scene
- Sizing up the scene and situation
- Rapidly assessing the patient's gross neurologic, respiratory, and circulatory status
- Providing any essential immediate intervention
- Performing a thorough, accurate patient assessment
- Obtaining an expanded SAMPLE history
- Reaching a clinical impression and providing prompt, efficient, prioritized patient care based on your assessment
- Communicating effectively with the patient and advising him or her of any procedures you will perform
- Properly interacting and communicating with fire, rescue, and law enforcement responders at the scene
- Identifying patients who require rapid packaging, and initiating transport without delay
- Identifying patients who do not need emergency care and will benefit from further detailed assessment and care before they are moved and transported
- Properly packaging the patient
- Safely lifting and moving the patient to the ambulance and loading the patient into it
- Providing safe, appropriate transport to the hospital emergency department or other designated facility
- Giving the necessary radio report to the medical control center or to the receiving hospital emergency department
- Providing any additional assessment or treatment while en route
- Monitoring the patient and checking vital signs while en route
- Documenting all findings and care on the patient care report
- Unloading the patient safely and, after giving a proper verbal report, transferring the patient's care to the emergency department staff
- Safeguarding the patient's rights

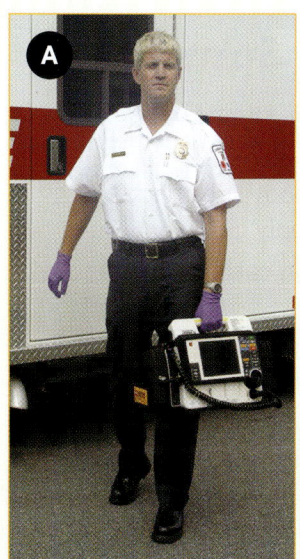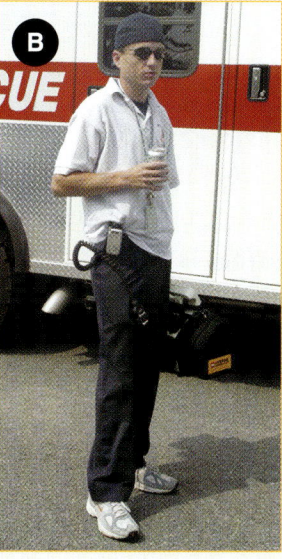

Figure 1-11 **A.** A professional appearance and manner help to build confidence and ease patient anxiety. **B.** An unprofessional appearance may promote distrust.

Most people can obtain proper routine medical care when they are ill and are surrounded by relatives and friends who will help to take care of them. However, when you are called to a home for a medical problem that is clearly not an emergency, remember that for some individuals, calling an ambulance and being transported to the emergency department is their only way to obtain medical care. You may find yourself in the role of patient advocate in these cases. The issue may arise from lack of funds, special needs, or other problems. If there is an issue that is not addressed, your job as a professional is to bring it to the attention of the individuals who are designated to find assistance for patients in need. It may be as simple as providing transportation or as complex as investigating a possible abuse or neglect case.

As a new EMT-I, you will be given a lot of advice and training from the more experienced EMT-Is with whom you serve. Some may voice a callous disregard for some patients. You should not be influenced by the unprofessional attitude of these individuals, regardless of how experienced or skilled they seem.

As a health care professional and an extension of physician care, you are bound by patient confidentiality. You should not discuss your findings or any disclosures made by the patient with anyone but those who are treating the patient or, as required by law, the police or other social agencies. If you must discuss a call with other providers, you should be careful to avoid any information that might disclose the name or identity of patients you have treated. Be careful not to gossip about calls and patients with others, even in your own home.

Continuing Education

Once you no longer have the structured learning environment that is provided in your initial training course, you must assume the responsibility for directing your own study and learning. As an EMT-I, you will be required to attend a certain number of hours of continuing education approved for EMT-Is each year to maintain, update, and expand your knowledge and skills. In many services, the training officer and medical director provide the required number of hours. In addition, most EMS education programs and hospitals offer a number of regular continuing education opportunities in each region. You may also attend state and national EMS conferences to help keep you up-to-date regarding local, state, and national issues affecting EMS. Some professional journals, such as the *Journal of Emergency Medical Services* (*JEMS*) and *EMS Magazine*, offer distance learning through continuing education articles and evaluations as well. Aside from continuing education credits, conferences and professional journals also introduce new procedures, medications, and other advances to keep providers up-to-date on changes in emergency medicine.

Since there are many levels of certification, you should ensure that the continuing education you receive is approved for the EMT-I. Whether you take advantage of these opportunities depends on you. Whether you decide to remain an EMT-I or achieve a higher level of training and certification, you should always strive for personal improvement. The key to being a good EMT-I and providing high-quality care is your commitment to continual learning and ever-increasing knowledge and skills.

EMT-Is possess special knowledge and skills that are directed to the care of patients in emergency situations. The authority that is delegated to you to care for patients is a very special one. Time management is yet another professional attribute. Maintaining your knowledge and skills is a substantial responsibility. This means making the time to stay current and proficient with training and skills that you have already learned, as well as those that are new in the field. Knowledge and skills that are learned in any profession decay and weaken when they are not used on a continual basis. Consider CPR skills. If you have not used these skills since your original training, it is likely that you will perform CPR in a way that is less than desirable. Continuing education and refresher courses are one way that you can maintain your skills and knowledge.

You are the Provider — Summary

1. What role does medical direction play in the EMT-I's delivery of prehospital care?

The medical director, under the auspice of his or her medical license, authorizes the EMT-I to provide medical care in the prehospital setting.

2. What is the distinction between off-line and online medical control?

Off-line medical control involves the use of written orders, which are to be followed in the event the patient's condition requires immediate lifesaving intervention or direct communication with the physician fails. Online medical direction refers to direct verbal orders provided by the physician, via two-way radio or cellular phone.

3. What is the first step in caring for this patient?

The first step is to ensure that the scene is safe.

4. What precautions, if any, should you consider?

The EMT-I should consider body substance isolation precautions and apply gloves.

5. What is your next step in caring for this patient?

The next step is to begin immediate care including ventilations and chest compressions.

6. What information should you provide to the receiving emergency department (ED) personnel?

ED personnel need to be notified of the EMT-I's assessment findings, treatment modalities, and the patient's response to treatment so they can take steps to prepare to receive the patient.

Prep Kit

Ready for Review

- EMS is the system that provides the emergency medical care that is needed by people who have been injured or have an acute medical emergency.
- When the dispatcher at the 9-1-1 emergency communications center receives a call for emergency care, he or she dispatches to the scene the designated EMS ambulance squad and any fire, rescue, or police units that may be needed.
- The EMS ambulance is staffed by EMTs who have been trained to the EMT-B, EMT-I, or EMT-P level according to recommended national standards and have been certified or licensed by the state.
- After the EMTs size up the scene and assess the patient, they provide the emergency care that is indicated by their findings and ordered by their medical director, in the service's standing order protocols, or the physician who is providing online medical direction. The EMTs then package the patient and provide transport to the nearby hospital or designated specialized care facility (for example, trauma center, pediatric hospital) for further evaluation and stabilization in the emergency department and, after admission, definitive surgical or medical care.
- The EMT-I course that you are now taking will present the information and skills that you will need to pass the required examinations for licensure certification and start as an EMT-I in the field. This course will provide you with the training that you need to function as an EMT-I and will serve as the essential foundation upon which you can advance your training and expertise.
- The following are the essential keys to being a good EMT-I:
  - Compassion and motivation to reduce suffering, pain, and death in people who are injured or acutely ill
  - Desire to provide each patient with the best possible care
  - Commitment to obtain the knowledge and skills that this requires
  - The drive to continually increase your knowledge, skills, and ability
- Once you have successfully completed this course and have been certified as an EMT-I, you will enter the next key phase of your training. With your new level of certification, your first task will be to learn the medical protocols and operating procedures of the squad pertinent to the EMT-I level. You will also have to learn where each piece of equipment is kept on the ambulance and become familiar with how the equipment works.
- From your experience and the guidance provided by your crew chief and the other experienced EMT-Is you work with, you will gain increased mastery of the skills that you learned in the course and learn how to apply your knowledge and skills in the diverse situations that are actually encountered in the field.
- Once you have completed the course, you must assume responsibility for directing your own study through continuing education provided by your service's training officer and medical director or through other opportunities available to you. Your commitment to continued learning is the key to being a good EMT-I.

Vital Vocabulary

advanced life support (ALS) Advanced lifesaving procedures, some of which are now being provided by the EMT-I.

Americans With Disabilities Act (ADA) Comprehensive legislation that is designed to protect individuals with disabilities against discrimination.

automated external defibrillator (AED) A device that detects treatable life-threatening cardiac arrhythmias (ventricular fibrillation and ventricular tachycardia) and delivers the appropriate electrical shock to the patient.

Technology

- Interactivities
- Vocabulary Explorer
- Anatomy Review
- Web Links
- Online Review Manual

Prep Kit continued...

continuous quality improvement (CQI) A system of internal and external reviews and audits of all aspects of an EMS system.

emergency medical dispatch (EMD) A system that assists dispatchers in selecting appropriate units to respond to a particular call for assistance and in providing callers with vital instructions until the arrival of EMS crews.

emergency medical services (EMS) A multidisciplinary system that represents the combined efforts of several professionals and agencies to provide prehospital emergency care to the sick and injured.

emergency medical technician (EMT) An EMS professional who is trained and licensed by the state to provide emergency medical care in the field.

EMT-Basic (EMT-B) An EMT who has training in basic emergency care skills, including automated external defibrillation, use of a definitive airway adjunct, and assisting patients with certain medications.

EMT-Intermediate (EMT-I) An EMT who has training in specific aspects of advanced life support, such as IV (intravenous) therapy, interpretation of cardiac rhythms, defibrillation, and orotracheal intubation.

EMT-Paramedic (EMT-P) An EMT who has extensive training in advanced life support, including IV (intravenous) therapy, pharmacology, cardiac monitoring, and other advanced assessment and treatment skills.

ethics Moral principles or standards governing conduct.

first responder The first trained individual, such as a police officer, fire fighter, or other rescuer, to arrive at the scene of an emergency to provide initial medical assistance.

medical control Physician instructions that are given directly by radio (online or direct) or indirectly by protocols or guidelines (off-line or indirect), as authorized by the medical director of the service program.

medical director The physician who authorizes or delegates to the EMT the authority to perform medical care in the field.

primary service area (PSA) The designated area in which the EMS service is responsible for the provision of prehospital emergency care and transportation to the hospital.

professional One who is skilled and trained for work by extended study or practice.

quality control The responsibility of the medical director to ensure that the appropriate medical care standards are met by EMT-Is on each call.

reciprocity The recognition by one state of another state's certification, allowing a health care professional from another state to practice in the new state.

Points to Ponder

You are asked to represent your agency at the local city council meeting. Apparently there have been discussions concerning the cost and effect of providing ALS service to the local community. Several council members feel that since they paid for AEDs to be placed on the city's fire engines, there is not much need for ALS personnel when EMT-Bs could perform almost the same care.

What is your immediate reaction to this? How would you explain the need for ALS in the city, even with the addition of AEDs on fire engines? What skills does an EMT-I provide beyond the EMT-B level that could justify the need?

Issues: Professionalism, Advocating for the Patient, Personal Attitudes, Demeanor, Roles and Responsibilities

Assessment in Action

You are on your way to becoming an EMT-I, an advanced life support provider. In this course, you will learn new terms, theories, and techniques as they relate to advanced life support. These advanced concepts and principles serve as the basis for the skills and knowledge you are about to obtain.

You have been an EMT-B for a couple of years now and you enjoy your job. However, you wish to enhance your skills and knowledge by advancing to the next level of certification. You also know this will help your career. You enjoy this field and have the desire and ethics needed to continue. You know that the EMT-I is one of the levels recognized nationally. You are prepared to garner the skills and knowledge needed to function as an EMT-I. You also look forward for the opportunity to work closer with your medical director.

1. The term *ethics* is defined as:
    A. skills and training for work by extended study or practice.
    B. moral principles or standards governing conduct.
    C. documenting all findings and care on the patient transport report.
    D. safeguarding the patient's rights.

2. The main purpose of the National Registry of EMTs is to:
    A. ensure compliance with state and local provisions.
    B. recognize each state's EMS certification.
    C. assess minimum competency through standardized testing.
    D. facilitate testing within each state's paramedic course.

3. Which of the following is the EMT-I's primary role in an out-of-hospital setting?
    A. Scene security
    B. Make decisions on behalf of the medical director
    C. Dispense medications ordered by a patient's doctor
    D. Identify and care for life-threatening conditions

4. The EMS system as we know it today had its origins with the publishing of the:
    A. American With Disabilities Act.
    B. EMS Act of 1973.
    C. EMT national standard curriculum.
    D. Accidental Death and Disability: The Neglected Disease of Modern Society.

5. The individual who authorizes the EMT-I to provide medical care in the field is the:
    A. medical director.
    B. senior EMS official.
    C. state EMS director.
    D. state EMS training coordinator.

6. The level of training that includes training in basic emergency care skills such as automated external defibrillation, use of basic airway adjuncts, and assisting patients with certain medications is the:
    A. first responder.
    B. EMT-B.
    C. EMT-I.
    D. EMT-P.

7. The importance and benefits of quality EMS research to the future of EMS includes:
    A. providing a mechanism for disciplinary action against an EMT-I.
    B. staying current on information and skills in emergency medical care, which change constantly.
    C. justification for billing insurance companies.
    D. preventing any legal action against the agency or provider.

8. A team of health care professionals who, in each area or jurisdiction, is responsible for and provides prehospital emergency care to the sick and injured best describes:
    A. emergency medical service providers.
    B. hospital administrations.
    C. quick response teams.
    D. community emergency response teams.

www.EMSzone.com/EMTI

The Well-Being of the EMT-I

1999 Objectives

Cognitive

- **1-1.14** Explain the components of wellness for the EMS provider. (p 26)
- **1-1.15** Discuss the importance of universal precautions and body substance isolation practices and develop strategies to prevent the transmission of diseases. (p 45)
- **1-1.16** Describe the steps to take for personal protection from airborne and blood borne pathogens. (p 47)
- **1-1.17** Explain what is meant by an exposure and describe principles for management. (p 46)
- **1-1.18** Describe the incidence, morbidity, and mortality of preventable injury and illness. (p 26)
- **1-1.19** Identify the human, environmental, and socioeconomic impact of preventable injury and illness. (p 59)
- **1-1.20** Describe the feasibility of EMS involvement in illness and injury prevention. (p 59)
- **1-1.21** Develop strategies for the implementation of EMS related illness and injury prevention programs in the community. (p 59)
- **1-1.22** Identify health hazards and potential crime areas within the community. (p 60)
- **1-1.23** Identify local municipal and community resources available for physical and socioeconomic crises. (p 59)
- **1-1.24** Identify the role of EMS in local municipal and community prevention programs. (p 59)

Affective

- **1-1.54** Advocate the need for injury prevention, including abusive situations. (p 59)
- **1-1.56** Advocate the benefits of working toward the goal of total personal wellness. (p 36)
- **1-1.57** Serve as a role model for other EMS providers in regard to a total wellness lifestyle. (p 36)
- **1-1.58** Value the need to assess his/her own lifestyle. (p 38)
- **1-1.59** Challenge him/herself to teach wellness concept in his/her role as an EMT-Intermediate. (p 38)
- **1-1.60** Defend the need to treat each patient as an individual, with respect and dignity. (p 41)
- **1-1.62** Improve personal physical well-being through achieving and maintaining proper body weight, regular exercise, and proper nutrition. (p 38)
- **1-1.63** Defend the need to respect the emotional needs of dying patients and their families. (p 29)
- **1-1.64** Advocate and practice the use of personal safety precautions in all scene situations. (p 44)
- **1-1.65** Advocate and serve as a role model for other EMS providers relative to body substance isolation practices. (p 47)
- **1-1.66** Value and defend tenets of prevention for patients and communities being served. (p 59)
- **1-1.67** Value personal commitment to success of prevention programs. (p 59)

Psychomotor

- **1-1.74** Demonstrate the proper procedures to take for personal protection from disease. (p 47)

1985 Objectives

There are no 1985 objectives for this chapter.

2

The Well-Being of the EMT-I

You are the Provider

You and your partner respond to a motor vehicle crash. Upon arrival you determine that the scene is safe. Your scene size-up reveals that there is one vehicle that hit a bridge guardrail. There is one victim in the car.

This chapter will discuss the importance of body substance isolation and how the EMT-I can be an injury prevention advocate for the community.

1. What are some of the potential exposure concerns that the EMT-I should consider with this call?
2. What steps should be taken to protect emergency personnel from infectious disease exposure?

The Well-Being of the EMT-I

There is an ancient proverb, "Physician, heal thyself." As providers of health care, doctors need to look after themselves—in all respects—so that they can minister to others. Ill physicians are in no position to provide care as they were trained to do. That dictum applies to all health care providers and goes well beyond just physical issues. In caring for the critically ill and injured, there are many factors and situations that can interfere with the ability of the EMT-I to treat the patient.

The personal health, safety, and well-being of all EMT-Is are vital to an EMS operation. As a part of your training, you will learn how to recognize possible hazards and protect yourself from them. These hazards vary greatly, ranging from personal neglect to environmental and human-made threats to your health and safety. You will also learn about the mental and physical stress that you must cope with as a result of caring for the sick and injured. Death and dying challenge you to deal with the realities of human weaknesses and the emotions of the survivors.

It is important to remain calm in order to perform effectively when you are confronted with horrifying events, life-threatening illness, or injury. A special kind of self-control is needed to respond efficiently and effectively to the suffering of others. This self-control is developed through the following:

- Proper training
- Ongoing experience in dealing with all types of physical and mental distress
- A dedication to serve humanity

Emotional Aspects of Emergency Care

At times, even the most experienced health care providers have difficulty overcoming personal reactions and proceeding without hesitation. Patients need to be removed from life-threatening situations. Life support measures need to be given to patients who are severely injured. You may also be called on to recover human remains from highway accidents, aircraft disasters, or explosions (Figure 2-1 ▼). In all of these situations, you must be calm and act responsibly as a member of the emergency medical care team. You should also realize that even though your personal emotions must be kept under control, your own reactions to the situation are normal feelings. Every EMT-I who must deal with such situations has these feelings. The struggle to remain calm in the face of horrible circumstances contributes to the emotional stress of the job.

Death and Dying

Today, life expectancy has dramatically increased; nearly two thirds of all deaths occur among people age 65 years and older. Of all deaths today, 60% are attributed to heart disease. From the age of 1 year to the age of 34 years, trauma is the leading cause of death. Death today is likely to occur quite suddenly or after a prolonged terminal illness. The setting of death may be somewhere other than the home—such as in the hospital, in a convalescent home, at work, or on the highway. For this

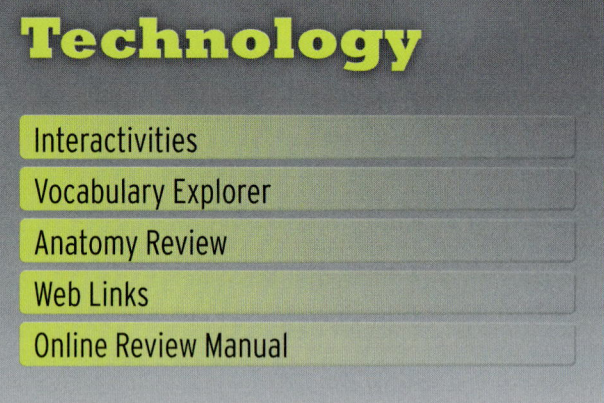

Technology

- Interactivities
- Vocabulary Explorer
- Anatomy Review
- Web Links
- Online Review Manual

www.EMSzone.com/EMTI

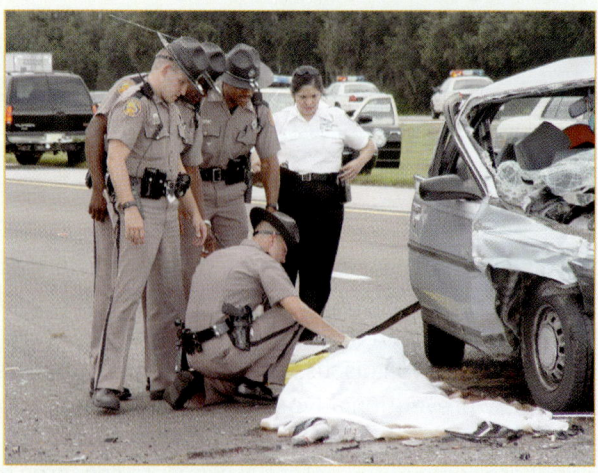

Figure 2-1 As an EMT-I, you may have to deal with removal of the deceased.

reason, we are less familiar with death than our ancestors were. We tend to deny death in America. Illness can be much more drawn out and removed from daily life. Life support systems and impersonal care remove the whole experience of death from most people's awareness. The mobility of families also makes it less likely that there will be extended family support when death occurs.

Death was once an expected and accepted fact in earlier American history. Life expectancy was brief (compared with today's), mortality rates (the ratio of number of deaths to a given population size) were high, and childbirth was hazardous, often resulting in the death of the mother and the baby. Hardships of the times, both natural and human-made, were great. Children and adults died from disease, injuries, and the traumas of war. Most people experienced the death of someone close to them. There were no funeral homes; mourning occurred at home in the family setting. The presence of a dead body was a natural event.

No matter what the frequency of response to emergency calls, death is something that every EMT-I will face. For some of you, it may be infrequent. Others, especially in urban settings, may see death many times in responding to motor vehicle crashes, drug overdoses, suicides, or homicides. Some EMS providers may have to deal with the mass-casualty incident of an airplane crash or a hazardous materials accident. In all of these cases, coming to grips with your thoughts, understandings, and adjustment to death is not only important personally, but also a function of providing emergency medical care.

Physical Signs of Death

Determination of the cause of death is the medical responsibility of a physician. There are definitive and presumptive signs of death. In many states, death is defined as the absence of circulatory and respiratory function. Many states have also adopted "brain death" provisions; these provisions refer to irreversible cessation of all functions of the brain and brain stem. Questions often arise as to whether to begin basic life support. In the absence of physician orders such as do not resuscitate (also called DNR) orders, the general rule is as follows: If the body is still warm and intact, initiate emergency medical care. An exception to this rule is cold temperature (hypothermia) emergencies. Hypothermia is a general cooling of the body in which the core body temperature becomes abnormally low: 95°F (35°C). It is a serious condition and is often fatal. At 86°F (30°C), the brain can survive without perfusion for about 10 minutes. When the core temperature drops to 82.4°F (28°C), the patient is in grave danger; however, people have survived a hypothermia accident with a body temperature of 64.4°F (18°C). In cases of hypothermia, the patient should not be considered dead until he or she is warm and dead.

> **EMT-I Tips**
>
> *Clinical death* is the absence of respirations and a pulse. *Biological death* begins within 4 to 6 minutes of clinical death, as cells start to die.

Presumptive Signs of Death

Most medicolegal authorities consider the presumptive signs of death that are listed in Table 2-1 adequate, particularly when they follow a severe trauma or occur at the end stages of a long-term illness such as cancer or other prolonged diseases. These signs alone may not be adequate in cases of sudden death due to hypothermia, acute poisoning, or cardiac arrest. Usually in these cases, all of the signs plus evidence of irreversibility are necessary.

Definitive Signs of Death

Definitive or conclusive signs of death that are obvious and clear to even nonmedical persons include the following:

- Obvious mortal damage, such as dismemberment at the neck or waist (decapitation)
- Dependent lividity: blood settling to the lowest point of the body, causing discoloration of the skin.
- Rigor mortis, the stiffening of body muscles caused by chemical changes within muscle

TABLE 2-1	Presumptive Signs of Death
■ Unresponsiveness to painful stimuli
■ Lack of a pulse or heartbeat
■ Absence of breath sounds
■ No deep tendon or corneal reflexes
■ Absence of eye movement
■ No blood pressure
■ Profound cyanosis
■ Lowered or decreased body temperature

tissue. It develops first in the face and jaw, gradually extending downward until the body is in full rigor. The rate of onset is affected by the body's ability to lose heat to its surroundings. A thin body loses heat faster than a fat body. A body on a tile floor loses heat faster than a body wrapped up in a blanket in a bed. Rigor mortis occurs sometime between 2 and 12 hours after death.
- <u>Putrefaction</u> (decomposition of body tissues). Depending on temperature conditions, this occurs sometime between 40 and 96 hours after death.

> ### EMT-I Tips
>
> Definitive Signs of Death
> - Obvious mortal damage
> - Dependent lividity
> - Rigor mortis
> - Putrefaction

Medical Examiner Cases

Involvement of the medical examiner, or the coroner in some states, depends on the nature and scene of the death. In most states, when trauma is a factor or the death involves suspected criminal or unusual situations such as hanging or poisoning, the medical examiner must be notified (Figure 2-2). When the medical examiner or coroner assumes responsibility for the scene, that responsibility supersedes all others at the scene, including the family's. The following are considered medical examiner's cases:
- When the person is dead at the scene
- Death without previous medical care or when the physician is unable to state the cause of death
- Suicide (self-destruction)
- Violent death
- Poisoning, known or suspected
- Death resulting from accidents
- Suspicion of a criminal act

If emergency medical care has been initiated, keep thorough notes of what was done or found. These records may be important during a subsequent investigation. These records should include the position the patient was found in; any weapons, pill bottles, or other important objects; and anything else witnessed by the EMT-I relating to the scene.

The Grieving Process

The death of a human being is one of the most difficult events for another human being to accept. If the survivor is a relative or close friend of the deceased, it is even more difficult. Emotional responses to the loss of a loved one or friend are appropriate and should be expected. In fact, it is expected that you will feel emotional about the death of a patient. Feelings and emotions are part of the grieving process. All of us experience these feelings after a stressful situation that causes us personal pain.

In 1969, Dr Elisabeth Kubler-Ross published research revealing that people go through several stages of grieving. The stages of grieving are as follows:

1. **Denial.** Refusal to accept diagnosis or care, unrealistic demands for miracles, or persistent failure to understand why there is no improvement.
2. **Anger, hostility.** Projection of bad news onto the environment and commonly in all directions, at times almost at random. The person lashes out. Someone must be blamed, and those who are responsible must be punished. This is typically an unpleasant phase.
3. **Bargaining.** An attempt to secure a prize for good behavior or promise to change lifestyle. "I promise to be a 'perfect patient' if only I can live until 'x' event."
4. **Depression.** Open expression of grief, internalized anger, hopelessness, or the desire to die. It sometimes involves suicidal threats, complete withdrawal, or giving up long before the illness seems terminal. The patient is usually silent.

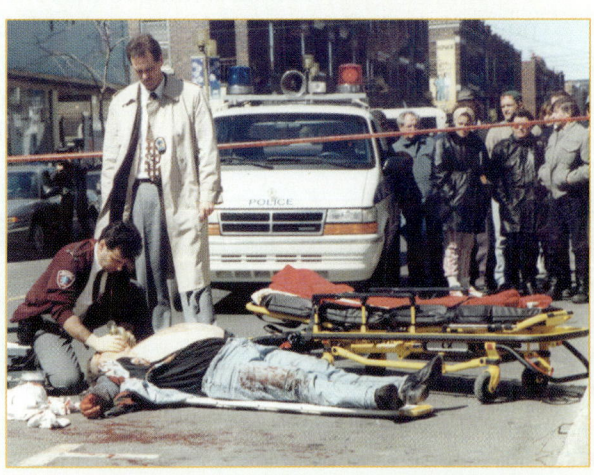

Figure 2-2 When trauma is a factor or the death involves a suspected criminal situation, the medical examiner is required.

5. Acceptance. The simple "yes." Acceptance grows out of a person's conviction that all has been done and the person is ready to die. While the acceptance phase is usually the most peaceful for the patient, it is often the most traumatic for the family.

Stages may follow one another or occur simultaneously. They may last for different spans of time. Family members may experience similar phases.

Even though the event (death) has not yet happened, the patient knows that it will happen. The patient has no control over this process. The patient will die whether or not he or she is ready. Furthermore, being ready to die does not mean that the patient will be happy about dying. You may encounter situations in which the patient is close to death, and you may need to provide reassurance and emotional care.

What Can the EMT-I Do?

Do helpful things, and make simple suggestions. Ask whether there is anything that you can do that will be of help, such as calling a relative or religious advisor. Provide gentle and caring support. Reinforcing the reality of the situation is important. This can be accomplished by merely saying to a grieving person, "I am so sorry for your loss." It is not important that you have a well-rehearsed script, for it is not likely that your exact words or consolations will be remembered. Being yourself and sincere are important. Sometimes it is better to say nothing at all and let the grieving person talk about the deceased. It can be a comfort for them to remember the positive times.

Some statements tend to be trite, and some suggest a kind of silver lining behind the clouds. Although they may be intended to make the person feel better about a situation, they also can be viewed as an attempt to diminish the person's grief. The grieving person needs to grieve. Statements like these can also indicate our inability to comprehend the profound sadness of grief because we have not experienced that kind of loss.

Attempts to take grief away too quickly are not good. If you do not know how the person really feels, you should not say that you do. People may be offended by responses that give advice or explanations about the death (Table 2-2). Statements such as "Oh, you shouldn't feel that way" are judgmental. If you judge what the grieving person is feeling, it is likely that he or she will stop talking with you. There is no reason why grieving people should not feel what they are feeling. Remember that anger is a stage of grieving. The anger may be directed at you. The anger seems irrational to everyone but the person grieving. A professional attitude is a necessity, and you must not take this anger as a personal attack.

Statements and comments that suggest action on your part are generally helpful. These statements imply a sense of understanding; they focus on the grieving person's feelings. It is not necessary to go into an extensive discussion. All you need to do is be sincere and say, "I am so sorry. I just want you to know that I am thinking about you." What people really appreciate is somebody who will listen to them. Simply ask, "Would you like to talk about how or what you are now feeling?" Then accept the response.

Dealing With the Patient and Family Members

There is no right or wrong way to grieve. Each person will experience grief and respond to it in his or her own way. Family members may express rage, anger, and despair. Many people will be rational and cooperative. Their concerns will usually be relieved by your calm, efficient manner. Your actions and words, even a simple touch, can communicate caring. While you must treat all patients with respect and dignity, use special care with dying patients and their families. Be concerned about their privacy and their wishes, and let them know that you take their concerns seriously. However, it is best to be honest with patients and their families; do not give them false hope.

TABLE 2-2	Responding to Grief
Don't Say...	
Give it time. Things will get better.	
You should not question God's will.	
You have to get on with your life.	
You have to keep on going.	
You can always have another child.	
You're not the only one who suffers.	
The living must go on.	
I know how you feel.	
Try Instead...	
I'm sorry.	
It is okay to be angry.	
It must be hard to accept.	
That must be painful for you.	
Tell me how you are feeling.	
If you want to cry, it's okay.	
People really cared for...	

Initial Care of the Dying, Critically Ill, or Injured Patient

People who are in the process of dying as a result of trauma, an acute medical condition, or a terminal disease will feel threatened. That threat may be related to their concern about survival. These concerns may involve feelings of helplessness, disability, pain, and separation. They are related to the person's sense of self and understanding of death (Table 2-3).

Anxiety

Anxiety is a response to the anticipation of danger. The source of the anxiety is often unknown, but in the case of seriously injured or ill patients, the source is usually recognizable. What may increase the anxiety are the unknowns of the current situation. Patients may ask the following:

- What will happen to me?
- What are you doing?
- Will I make it?
- What will my disabilities be?

Patients who are anxious may have the following signs and symptoms:

- Emotionally upset
- Sweaty and cool (diaphoretic)
- Rapid breathing (hyperventilation)
- Fast pulse (tachycardia)
- Restlessness
- Tense
- Fearful
- Shaky (tremulous)

For the anxious patient, time seems to be extended; seconds seem like minutes, and minutes seem like hours.

TABLE 2-3	Ways the Dying, Critically Ill, or Injured Patient May Express Concern About Survival

- Anxiety
- Pain and fear
- Anger and hostility
- Depression
- Dependency
- Guilt
- Mental health problems

Pain and Fear

Pain and fear are interrelated. Pain often is associated with illness or trauma. Fear is generally thought of in relation to the oncoming pain and the outcome of the damage. It is often helpful to encourage patients to express their pains and fears, since expression of them begins the process of adjustment to the pain and acceptance of the emergency medical care that may be necessary. Some people have difficulty openly admitting their fear. The fear may be expressed as bad dreams, withdrawal, tension, restlessness, "butterflies" in the stomach, or nervousness. In some cases, it may be expressed as anger.

Anger and Hostility

Anger may be expressed by very demanding and complaining behavior. Often this may be related to the fear and anxiety of the emergency itself or the medical care that is being given. Sometimes the fear is so acute that the patient may want to express anger toward you or others but is unable to do so because of the dependency factor. If you find that you are the target of the patient's anger, make sure that you are safe; do not take the anger or insults personally. Be tolerant, and do not become defensive.

The anger may also be expressed physically, and you may be the target of the displaced aggression. If the patient or a relative becomes so emotionally upset that you are physically assaulted or you believe that this could happen, retreat from the situation. Such hostility must be contained. If emergency medical care is not possible under these circumstances, law enforcement intervention is required.

Depression

Depression is a natural physiological and psychological response to illness, especially if the illness is prolonged, debilitating, or terminal. Whether the depression is a temporary sadness, or clinical depression that is long-term, there is, of course, little the EMT-I can do to alleviate the pain of depression during the brief time the patient is being treated and transported. The best one can do in treating and transporting a patient experiencing depression is to be compassionate, supportive, and nonjudgmental.

Dependency

Dependency usually takes longer to develop than during the very brief relationships developed in EMS. When medical care is given to any individual, a sense of dependency may develop. Individuals who are placed in this position may feel helpless and become resentful. The resentfulness may arouse feelings of inferiority, shame, or weakness.

Guilt

Many patients who are dying, their families, or the caregivers of the patients may feel guilty about what has happened. Occasionally family members and long-term caregivers may feel a degree of relief when an extended illness is finally over. That relief may later turn into guilt. Most of the time, however, no one can explain these feelings. The magnitude of the guilt may be great. Sometimes, feelings of guilt can result in a delay in seeking emergency medical care.

Mental Health Problems

Mental health problems such as disorientation, confusion, or delusions may develop in the dying patient. In these instances, the patient may display behavior inconsistent with normal patterns of thinking, feeling, or acting. Common characteristics of such behavior may include the following:

- Loss of contact with reality
- Distortion of perception
- Regression
- Diminished control of basic impulses and desires
- Abnormal mental content, including delusions and hallucinations

In some long-term situations, generalized personality deterioration may occur.

Receiving Unrelated Bad News

A patient who is in critical condition or is dying may not want to hear unrelated bad news, such as the death of a close relative or friend. Such news may depress the patient or cause the patient to give up hope.

Caring for Critically Ill and Injured Patients

Patients need to know who you are and what you are doing. Let the patient know that you are attending to his or her immediate needs and that these are your primary concerns at that particular moment (Figure 2-3). As soon as possible, explain to the patient what is going on. Confusion, anxiety, and other feelings of helplessness will be decreased if you keep the patient consistently informed.

Avoid Sad and Grim Comments

EMT-Is, other safety personnel, family, and bystanders must avoid grim comments about a patient's condition. Remarks such as "This is a bad one," or "The leg is badly damaged, and I think he will lose it," are inappropriate. These remarks may upset or increase anxiety in the patient and compromise possible recovery outcomes. This is especially true for the patient who may be able to hear but not respond.

Orient the Patient

You should expect a patient to be disoriented in an emergency situation. The aura of the emergency situation—lights, sirens, smells, and strangers—is intense. The impact and effect of injuries or acute illness may cause the patient to be confused or unsettled. It is important to orient the patient to the surroundings (Figure 2-4). Use brief, concise statements such as "Mr. Smith, you have had an accident, and I am now splinting your arm. I am John Foxworth of the New Britain EMS; I will be caring for you."

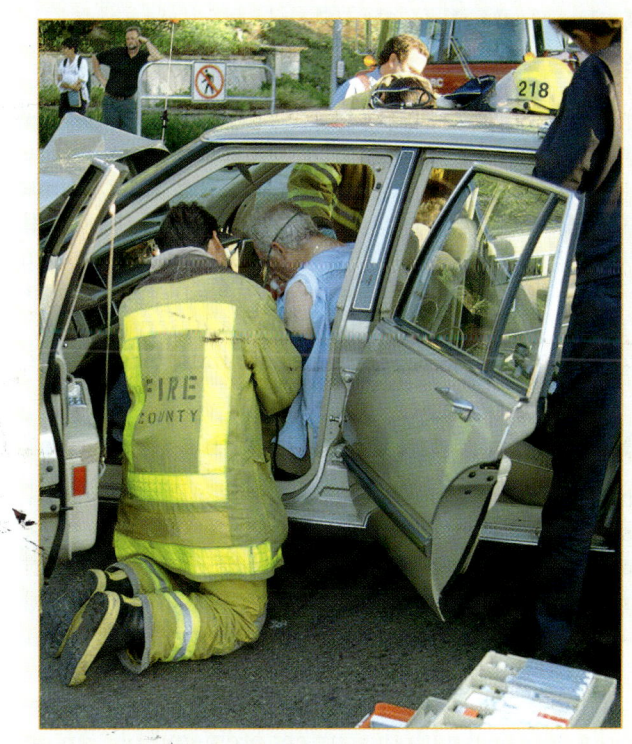

Figure 2-3 Let the patient know immediately that you are there to help.

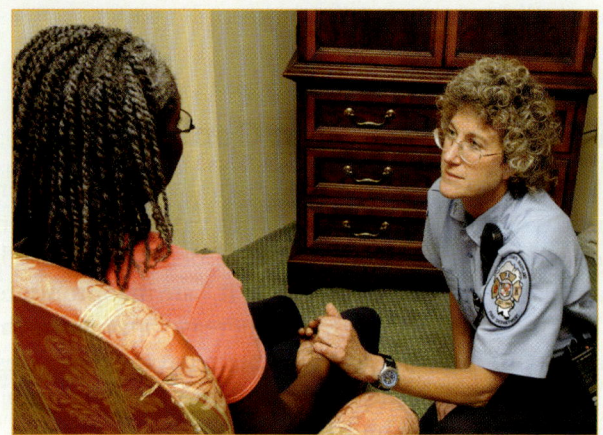

Figure 2-4 The aura of an emergency situation can be confusing and frightening to the patient. Make sure you explain to the patient what has happened and what you are doing.

Be Honest

When approaching any patient, you must determine the patient's ability to understand and accept. You should be honest without additionally shocking the patient or giving information that is unnecessary or that may not be understood. Simply explain what you are doing and allow the patient to be part of the care being given; this can relieve feelings of helplessness and some of the fear.

Acknowledge the Seriousness of the Condition

There may be occasions when a patient may refuse emergency medical care and insist that you do nothing and leave him or her alone. In these cases, it is important to impress upon the patient the seriousness of the condition without causing undue alarm. Saying, "Everything will be okay," when it is obvious that they will not be makes you appear dishonest. Generally, seriously ill or injured patients know that they are in trouble.

Allow for Hope

In trauma and acute medical conditions, patients may ask whether they are going to die. You may feel at a loss for words. You may also know, on the basis of experience or in view of the seriousness of the present situation, that the prognosis is poor. But it is not your responsibility to tell the patient that he or she is dying. Statements such as "I don't know when you are going to die; let's deal with the current problem," or "I'm not going to give up on you, so don't give up on yourself,"

are helpful. These statements transmit a sense of trust and hope, and they let the patient know that you are doing everything possible to save his or her life. If there is the slightest chance of hope remaining, you want that message transmitted in your attitude and in the statements you make to the patient.

Locate and Notify Family Members

Many patients will be concerned and ask you to notify their family or others close to them. The patient may or may not be able to assist you in doing this. You should ensure that an appropriate and responsible person makes an effort to locate the desired persons. Assuring the patient that someone is going to do this is a significant part of the patient's care.

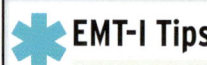

EMT-I Tips

When transporting an elderly patient who lives with a spouse or other elderly relative or friend, try to transport that person along with the patient if time permits. Many elderly people cannot drive and are left at home while the patient dies alone at the hospital.

Injured and Critically Ill Children

Children who are critically ill or injured should be cared for as any patient would be, insofar as an assessment of airway, breathing, and circulation (the ABCs) and immediate life threats are concerned. Due regard should be given to variations in height, weight, and size in providing emergency medical care. Because of the increased excitement and extraordinary nature of the emergency scene for a child, it is important that a relative or responsible adult accompany the child, to relieve anxiety and assist in care as appropriate.

Dealing With the Death of a Child

The death of a child is a tragic and dreaded event. It is not unusual to think about the fact that the dead or dying child has a lot more to do and should have many more years to live. In our society, we assume that only elderly people are supposed to die. Children die less frequently now than they did in earlier times, so most people are unprepared for what they will feel when a child dies. You may think about your own children and those whom you know: nephews, nieces, grandchildren, and children of close friends. And you may think, "Why should this child, who is only 5 years old, die?"

Answering the difficult questions of your own mortality will be of help when dealing with the death of a child. Still, the death of a child will not be an easy subject to discuss. This will be especially true for the family. And as an EMT-I involved in a call that involves the death of a child, you will also likely experience stress.

One of your responsibilities is to help the family through the initial period after the death (Figure 2-5 ▼). As an EMT-I, until more definitive and professional help can be available, you may be in the best position to help the family begin to cope with their loss. How a family initially deals with the death of a child will affect their stability and endurance. You can help a family through its initial period of grief and alert them to the follow-up counseling and support services that are available.

Helping the Family

If the child is dead, acknowledging the fact of the death is important. This should be done in a private place, even if that is inside an ambulance. Often, the parents cannot believe that the death is real, even if they have been preparing for it, as in the case of a child with a terminal illness. Reactions vary, but shock, disbelief, and denial are common. Some parents show little emotion at the initial news.

Sometimes cultural or religious practice will dictate that the parents avoid viewing the dead body. Be respectful of these issues. If appropriate, find a place where the mother and father can hold the child. This is important in the parents' grieving process; it helps to lessen the sense of disbelief and makes the death real. Even if the parents do not ask, you should tell them that they can see the child. Your decision in permitting the parents to see the child may need some discretion. For example, in the case of a traumatic death in which there is significant disfigurement, that decision might have to be delayed. The delay may involve having support services available or contacting the family physician or others who can help the parents through this difficult situation. This may involve preparing the parents for what they will see and the changes brought on by rigor mortis, asphyxiation, and so forth. Also remember that if the death is suspicious, no one should be allowed into the scene or to touch the body until proper law enforcement authorities can be notified and an investigation has been completed. In cases such as this, you should follow your local protocols and adhere to any state laws.

Sometimes you do not need to say much. In fact, sometimes silence is more comforting than words. You can express your own sorrow. Do not overload grieving parents with a lot of information; at this point, they cannot handle it. Nonverbal communication, such as holding a hand or touching a shoulder, may also be valuable. Let the family's actions be your guide regarding what is appropriate. It is important to encourage parents to talk about their feelings.

Stressful Situations

Many situations such as mass-casualty scenes; serious automobile crashes; excavation cave-ins; house fires; infant and child trauma; amputations; abuse of an infant, child, spouse, or elderly person; or death of a coworker or other public safety personnel will be stressful for everyone involved. During these situations, you must exercise extreme caution in your words and your actions. Present a professional demeanor in your words and actions at the scene. Words that do not seem important or that are said jokingly may hurt someone. Conversations at the scene must be professional. You should not say, "Everything will be all right," or "There is nothing to worry about." A person who is trapped in a wrecked car, hurting from head to foot, and worrying about a loved one knows that all is not well. Your calm and caring approach to the emergency situation will reassure the patient. Briefly explain your plan of action to assist the patient in the crisis. Inform the patient that you

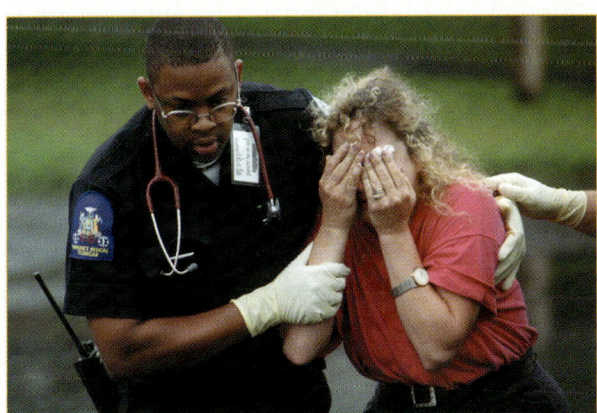

Figure 2-5 One of your responsibilities is to help the family through the initial period after the death.

need his or her help and the assistance of family members or bystanders to carry out the plan of action.

How a patient reacts to injury or illness may be influenced by certain personality traits. Some patients may become highly emotional over what may seem to be a minor problem. Others may show little or no emotion, even after serious injury or illness. Many other factors influence how a patient reacts to the stress of an emergency incident. Among these factors are the following:

- Socioeconomic background
- Fear of health care personnel
- Alcohol or substance abuse
- History of chronic disease
- Psychological disorders
- Reaction to medication
- Age
- Nutritional status
- Feelings of guilt

You are not expected to always know why a patient is having a particular emotional response. However, you can quickly and calmly assess the actions of the patient, family members, and bystanders. This assessment will help you to gain the confidence and cooperation of everyone at the scene. In addition, you should use a professional tone of voice and show courtesy, along with sincere concern and efficient action. These simple considerations will go far to relieve worry, fear, and insecurity. Calm reassurance will inspire confidence and cooperation. Compassion is important, but you must be careful. Your professional judgment takes priority over compassion. For example, suppose a screaming, frightened child with no obvious life-threatening injuries is covered with another patient's blood. This frightened child appeals to your compassion and, thus, gets your attention. In the meantime, an unconscious, non-breathing adult nearby could die because of lack of care.

Patients must be given the opportunity to express their fears and concerns. You can easily relieve many of these concerns at the scene. Usually patients are concerned about the safety or well-being of others who are involved in the accident and about the damage or loss of personal property. Your responses must be discreet and diplomatic, giving reassurance when appropriate. If a loved one has been killed or critically injured, you should wait, if possible, until clergy or emergency department staff can inform the patient. They can then provide the psychological support the patient may need.

Some patients, especially children and elderly people, may be terrified or feel rejected when separated from family members by the uniformed EMS provider team. Other patients may not want family members to share their stress, see their injury, or witness their pain. It is usually best if parents go with their children and relatives accompany elderly patients.

Religious customs or needs of the patient must also be respected. Some people will cling to religious medals or charms, especially if any attempt is made to remove them. Others will express a strong desire for religious counsel, baptism, or last rites if death is near. You must try to accommodate these requests if it is practical. Some people have religious convictions that strongly oppose the use of drugs and blood products. If you obtain such information, it is imperative that you report it to personnel responsible for the next level of care.

In the event of a death, you must handle the body with respect and dignity. It must be exposed as little as possible. Learn your local regulations and protocols about moving the body or changing its position, especially if you are at a possible crime scene. Even in these situations, cardiopulmonary resuscitation (CPR) and appropriate treatment must be given unless there are obvious signs of death.

Uncertain Situations

There will be times when you are unsure whether a true medical emergency exists. *If you are unsure, contact medical control about the need to transport.* If you cannot reach medical control, it is always best to err on the side of caution and transport the patient. For ethical and medicolegal reasons, a physician must examine all patients who are transported and determine the degree of medical need.

Many minor signs or symptoms may be early indicators of severe illness or injury. Symptoms of many illnesses can be similar to those of substance abuse, hysteria, or other conditions. You must accept the patient's complaints and provide appropriate care until you are able to transfer care of the patient to a higher level (such as a paramedic, nurse, or physician). Your local protocols will direct your actions in these situations. When in doubt, err on the side of caution, and acquire the patient's consent and transport to the medical facility.

Stress Warning Signs and the Work Environment

Working in EMS is a high-stress job. Understanding the causes of stress and knowing how to deal with them are critical to your job performance, health, and interpersonal relationships. To prevent stress from affecting your life negatively, you need to understand what stress is, its physiologic effects, what you can do to minimize these effects, and how to deal with stress on an emotional level.

Stress is the impact of stressors on your physical and mental well-being. Stressors include emotional, physical, and environmental situations or conditions that may cause a variety of physiologic, physical, and psychological responses. The body's response to stress begins with an alarm response, followed by a stage of reaction and resistance, and then recovery or, if the stress is prolonged, exhaustion. This three-stage response is referred to as the general adaptation syndrome Table 2-4.

The physiologic responses involve the interaction of the endocrine and nervous systems, resulting in chemical and physical responses. This is commonly known as the fight-or-flight response. You will cover this response more in-depth in later chapters. Positive stressors, such as exercise, and negative stressors, such as shift work, long hours, or the frustration of losing a patient, all result in the same physiologic manifestations. These include the following:

- Increased respirations and heart rate
- Increased blood pressure
- Dilated venous vessels near the skin surface (causes cool, clammy skin)
- Dilated pupils
- Muscle tension
- Increased blood glucose levels
- Perspiration
- Decreased blood flow to the gastrointestinal tract

Stress may also have physical symptoms such as fatigue, changes in appetite, gastrointestinal problems, or headaches. Stress may cause insomnia or hypersomnia, irritability, inability to concentrate, and hyperactivity or underactivity. In addition, stress may manifest itself in psychological reactions such as fear, dull or non-responsive behavior, depression, oversensitivity, anger, irritability, and frustration. Often, today's fast-paced lifestyles compound these effects by not allowing a person to rest and recover after periods of stress. Prolonged or excessive stress has been proven to be a strong contributor to heart disease, hypertension, cancer, alcoholism, and depression.

Many people are subject to cumulative stress, whereby insignificant stressors accumulate and lead to a larger stress-related problem. In the emergency services environment (EMS personnel, police, firefighters), stressors may also be sudden and severe. Some events are unusually stressful or emotional, even by emergency services standards. These acute severe stressors result in what is referred to as critical incident stress. Events that can trigger critical incident stress include the following:

- Mass-casualty incidents
- Serious injury or traumatic death of a child
- Crash with injuries caused by an emergency services provider while responding to or from a call
- Death or serious injury of a coworker in the line of duty

Posttraumatic stress disorder (PTSD) may develop after a person has experienced a psychologically distressing event. PTSD is characterized by reexperiencing the event and over-responding to stimuli that recall the event. Sometimes PTSD is referred to as "Vietnam veteran's disease" because of its classification as a mental disorder after the Vietnam conflict. Stressful events in EMS are sometimes psychologically overwhelming. Some of the symptoms include depression, startle reactions, flashback phenomena, and dissociative episodes (such as amnesia of the event).

A process called critical incident stress management (CISM) was developed to address acute stress situations and potentially decrease the likelihood that PTSD will develop after such an incident Figure 2-6. This process theoretically confronts the responses to critical incidents and defuses them, directing the emergency

TABLE 2-4	Response to Stress

General Adaptation Syndrome
- Alarm response
- Reaction and resistance
- Recovery or exhaustion

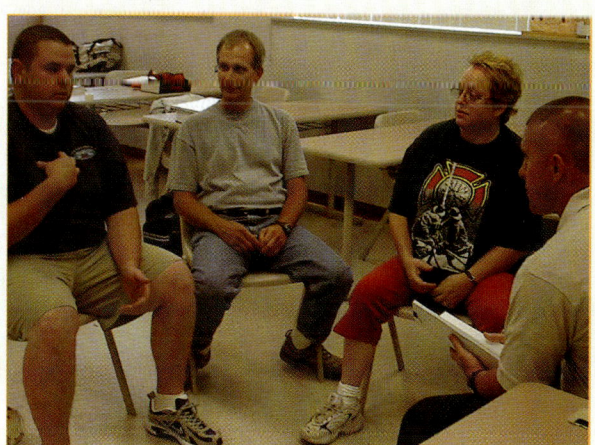

Figure 2-6 Critical incident stress management is sometimes used to help providers to relieve stress.

services personnel toward physical and emotional equilibrium. CISM can occur formally, as a debriefing for those who were at the scene. Trained CISM teams of peers and mental health professionals may facilitate this. In addition, CISM can occur at an ongoing scene in the following circumstances:

- When personnel are assessed for signs and symptoms of distress while resting
- Before reentering the scene
- During a scene demobilization in which personnel are educated about the signs of critical incident stress and given a buffer period to collect themselves before leaving

The most common form of CISM is peer defusing, when a group informally discusses events that they experienced together.

In the Field

Coworkers often notice a change in behavior or attitude before a supervisor does. This is especially true in EMS, where close relationships develop between people who work together and share rooms, meals, and social interaction. This may allow you to help someone before job performance is negatively affected.

Stress and Nutrition

Anyone can respond to a sudden physical stress for a short time. If stress is prolonged, especially if physical action is not a permitted response, the body can quickly be drained of its reserves. This can leave it depleted of key nutrients, weakened, and more susceptible to illness.

Your body's three sources of fuel—carbohydrates, fat, and protein—are consumed in increased quantities during stress, particularly if physical activity is involved. The quickest source of energy is glucose, taken from stored glycogen in the liver. However, this supply will last less than a day. Protein, drawn primarily from muscle, is a long-term source of glucose. Tissues can use fat for energy. The body also conserves water during periods of stress. To do so, it retains sodium by exchanging and losing potassium from the kidneys. Other nutrients that are susceptible to depletion are the vitamins and minerals that are not stored by the body in substantial quantities. These include water-soluble B and C vitamins and most minerals.

As EMS providers, we do not have control of what stressors we will face on any given day. Consequently, stress in one form or another is an unavoidable part of our lives. As one would study for a test, dress properly for a day of snow skiing, or train for a sporting event, we should physically prepare our bodies for stress. Physical conditioning and proper nutrition are the two variables over which we have absolute control. Muscles will grow and retain protein only with sufficient activity.

You are the Provider — Part 2

After gaining access to the patient, you direct your partner to manually stabilize the patient's C-spine. You perform an initial assessment, which reveals the following:

Initial Assessment	Recording Time: Zero Minutes
Appearance	Motionless, slumped forward in the driver's seat of the vehicle
Level of Consciousness	No response to verbal stimuli
Airway	Open
Breathing	Respirations, noisy, rapid, and shallow
Circulation	Pulses, weak and thready; skin, cool and clammy

3. What is your next step in the treatment of this patient?
4. What else should you consider when treating this patient?

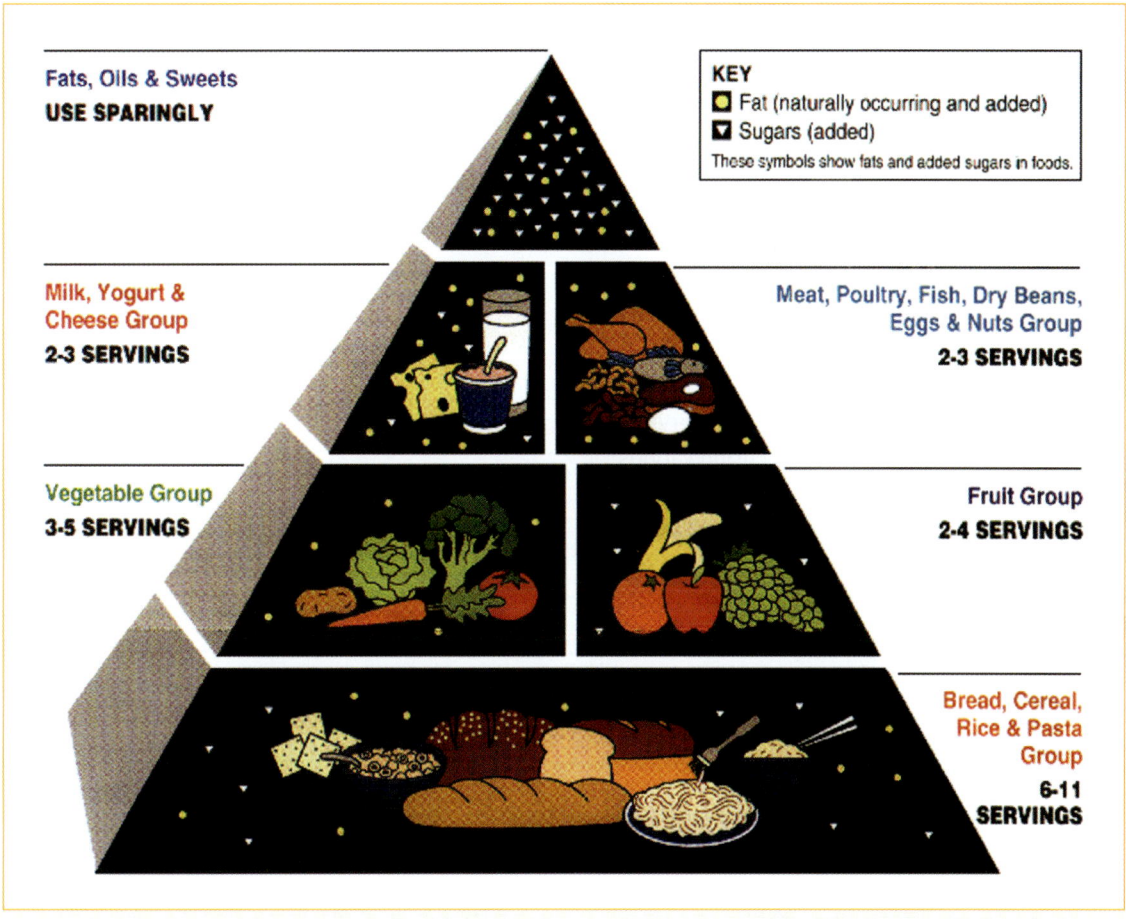

Figure 2-7 A healthy diet is illustrated by the US Department of Agriculture Food Guide Pyramid.

Bones will not passively accumulate calcium. In response to the physical stress of exercise, bones store calcium and become denser and stronger. Regular, well-balanced meals are essential to provide the nutrients that are necessary to keep your body fueled Figure 2-7 ▲ . Vitamin-mineral preparations that provide a balanced mix of all the nutrients may be necessary to supplement a less than perfectly balanced diet.

Stress Management

There are many methods of handling stress. Some are positive and healthy; others are harmful or destructive. Americans consume more than 20 tons of aspirin per day, and doctors prescribe muscle relaxants, tranquilizers, and sedatives more than 90 million times per year to patients in the United States. Although these medications have legitimate uses, they do nothing to combat the stress that may cause the medical problems previously described.

The term "stress management" refers to the tactics that have been shown to alleviate or eliminate stress reactions. These may involve changing a few habits, changing your attitude, and perseverance Table 2-5 ▶ .

A clue to the management of stress comes from the fact that it is not the event itself but the person's reaction to it that determines how much it will tax the body's resources. Remember that stress results from anything that you perceive as a threat to your equilibrium. Stress is an undeniable and unavoidable part of our everyday life. By understanding how it affects you physiologically, physically, and psychologically, can help you manage it more successfully.

TABLE 2-5	Strategies to Manage Stress

Identify, change, or eliminate stressors.
Change partners to avoid a negative or hostile personality.
Change work hours.
Cut back on overtime.
Change your attitude about the stressor.
Do not obsess over frustrating situations such as relapsing alcoholics and nursing home transfers. Focus on delivering high quality care.
Try to adopt a more relaxed, philosophical outlook.
Expand your social support system apart from your coworkers.
Sustain friends and interests outside emergency services.
Minimize the physical response to stress by using various techniques, including:
- A deep breath to settle an anger response
- Periodic stretching
- Slow, deep breathing
- Regular physical exercise
- Progressive muscle relaxation

Supporting patients in emergency situations is difficult. It is stressful for them and also for you. You are vulnerable to all the stresses that go with your profession. It is critical that you recognize the signs of stress so that it does not interfere with your work and your personal life. The signs and symptoms of chronic stress may not be obvious at first. Rather, they may be subtle and not present all the time (Table 2-6).

The following sections provide some suggestions about how to cope with stress. Some of them may be useful in helping you prevent problems from developing. Others may help you to solve problems should they develop.

Lifestyle Changes

Your well-being is a crucial factor for providing safe and effective patient care. The effectiveness and efficiency with which you do your job depends on your ability to stay in shape and avoid the risk of personal injury. **Burnout** is a condition of chronic fatigue and frustration that results from mounting stress over time. To avoid burnout, you need to be in good physical and mental health. Be aware of the potential hazards in rescue and emergency medical care. You must also learn how to avoid or prevent personal injury or illness.

Nutrition

To perform efficiently, you must eat nutritious food. Food is the fuel that makes the body run. The physical exertion and stress that are a part of your job require a high-energy output. If you do not have a readily available source of fuel, your performance may be less than optimum. This can be dangerous for you, your partner, and your patient. Therefore, it is important for you to learn about and follow the rules of good nutrition.

Candy and soft drinks contain sugar. These foods are quickly absorbed and converted to fuel by the body. But simple sugars also stimulate the body's production of insulin, which reduces blood glucose levels. For some people, eating a lot of sugar can actually result in lower energy levels.

Complex carbohydrates rank next to simple sugars in their ability to produce energy. Complex carbohydrates such as pasta, rice, and vegetables are among the safest, most reliable sources for long-term energy production (Figure 2-8). However, some carbohydrates take hours to be converted into usable body fuel.

Fats are also easily converted to energy, but eating too much fat can lead to obesity, cardiac disease, and other long-term health problems. The proteins in meat, fish, chicken, beans, and cheese take several hours to convert to energy.

Carry an individual supply of high-energy food to help you maintain your energy levels. Try eating several small meals throughout the day in order to keep your energy resources at consistent levels, thus allowing you to function. Remember, however, that overeating may reduce your physical and mental performance. After a large meal, the blood that is needed for the digestive process is not available for other activities.

TABLE 2-6	Warning Signs of Stress

Irritability toward coworkers, family, and friends
Inability to concentrate
Difficulty sleeping, increased sleeping, or nightmares
Anxiety
Indecisiveness
Guilt
Loss of appetite (gastrointestinal disturbances)
Loss of interest in sexual activities
Isolation
Loss of interest in work
Increased use of alcohol
Recreational drug use

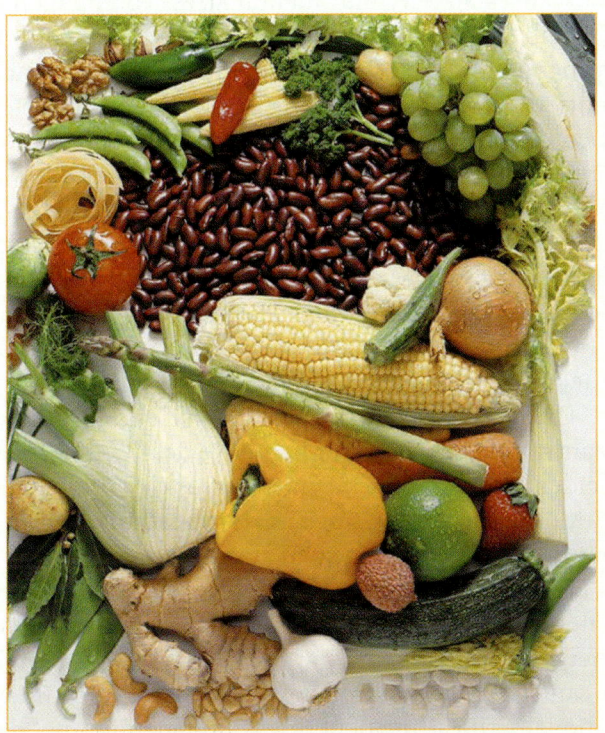

Figure 2-8 Complex carbohydrates are a good source of long-term energy.

You must also make sure that you maintain an adequate fluid intake (Figure 2-9 ▼). Hydration is important for proper functioning. Fluids can be easily replenished by drinking any nonalcoholic, noncaffeinated fluid. Water is generally the best fluid available. The body absorbs it faster than any other fluid. Avoid fluids that contain high levels of sugar. These can actually slow the rate of fluid absorption by the body. They can also cause abdominal discomfort. One indication of adequate hydration is frequent urination. Infrequent urination or urine that is dark yellow indicates dehydration.

Exercise and Relaxation

A regular program of exercise will enhance the benefits of maintaining good nutrition and adequate hydration. When you are in good physical condition, you can handle job stress more effectively. A regular program of exercise will increase your strength and endurance (Figure 2-10 ▼). You may want to practice relaxation techniques, meditation, and visual imagery.

Balancing Work, Family, and Health

As an EMT-I, you will often be called to assist the sick and injured any time of the day or night. Unfortunately, there is no rhyme or reason to the timing of illness, injury, or interfacility transfers. Volunteer EMT-Is may often be called away from family or friends during social activities. Shift workers may be required to be apart from loved ones for long periods. You should never let the job interfere excessively with your own needs. Find a balance between work and family; you owe it to yourself and to

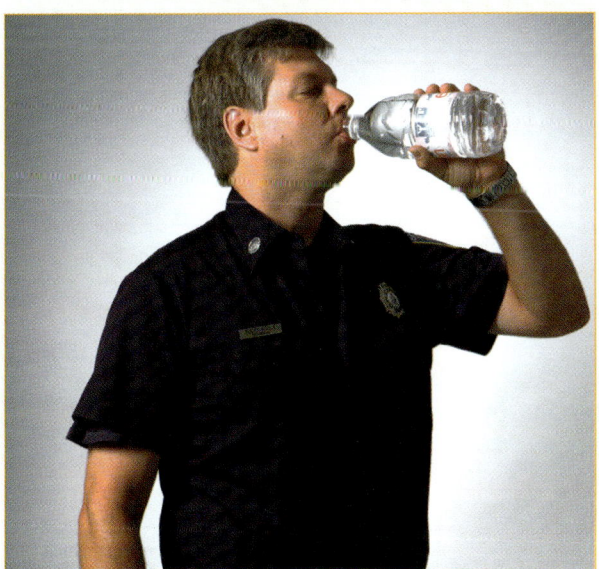

Figure 2-9 Maintain an adequate fluid intake by drinking plenty of water or other nonalcoholic, caffeine-free fluids.

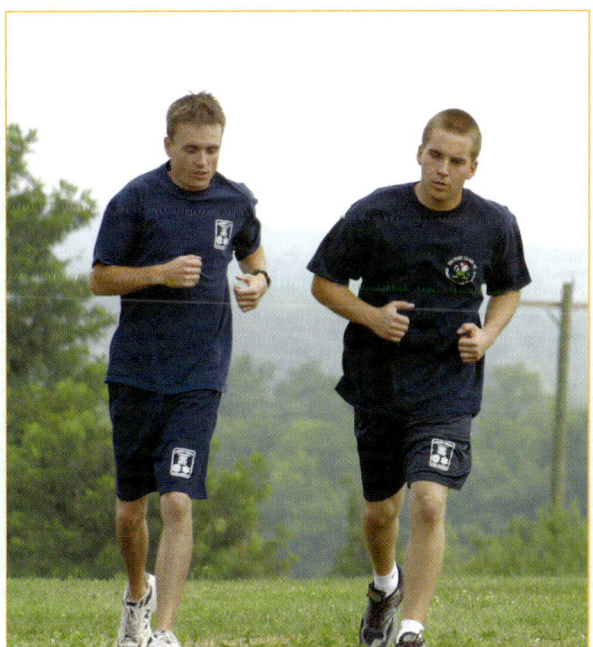

Figure 2-10 A regular program of exercise will increase strength and endurance.

them. It is important to make sure that you have the time that you need to relax with family and friends.

It is also important to realize that coworkers, family, and friends often may not understand the stress caused by responding to EMS calls. As a result of a "bad call," you might not feel like going out to a movie or attending a family event that has been planned for some time. In these situations, help from a critical incident stress debriefing team or information sessions conducted by the EMS unit's employee assistance program may assist you in resolving these problems.

When possible, rotate your schedule to give yourself time off. If your EMS system allows you to move from station to station, rotate to reduce or vary your call volume. Take vacations to provide for your good health so that you will be able to respond the next time you are needed. If at any point you feel that the stress of work is more than you can handle, seek help. You may want to discuss your stress informally with your family or coworkers. Help from more experienced team members can be invaluable. You may also want to get help from peer counselors or other professionals. Seeking this help does not make you weak in the eyes of others. Rather, it shows that you are in control of your life.

Critical Incident Stress Debriefing

You may be called to a situation so horrible that you find it difficult to respond as you were trained. You may have an immediate or a delayed negative response to the incident. Do not be ashamed of such feelings; almost all responders have had the same reaction at one time or another. If you feel overwhelmed, step back and call additional resources. Sometimes simply knowing that help is on the way can help you overcome your fear or anxiety and enable you to respond effectively to the situation. Remember that if you have these feelings from time to time, your partner and other members of the team may have them, too. Keep an eye on other members of your team. Confirm that they are under control and act appropriately during a major disaster. If a team member is behaving ineffectively, help the person to focus on the needs of the emergency situation.

After a stressful call or a disaster, there may be an emotional letdown, which is often overlooked. However, it may be more important to deal with than the initial contact response. A critical incident is any event that causes anxiety and mental stress to emergency workers. Critical incident stress debriefing (CISD) is a program in which severely stressful job-related incidents are discussed. These discussions are conducted in confidence with other emergency workers who are trained in CISD (Figure 2-11 ▼). The purpose of CISD is to relieve personal and group anxieties and stress. Although utilized extensively now for many years, CISD has never been demonstrated to be effective. In fact, several recent studies indicate that CISD may actually *increase* rescuer distress and result in worse outcomes.

CISD teams consist of peer counselors and mental health professionals who help you deal with critical incident stress. The CISD meetings are typically held within 24 to 72 hours of a major incident, and they may also have to be repeated at a later time.

CISD programs are located throughout the United States. Teams can usually be found by calling telephone directory assistance in your area and asking for CISD or can be requested through your employer. The International Critical Incident Stress Foundation, Inc. has an emergency access number: (410) 313-2473. For general information, call (410) 750-9600, or contact the foundation by e-mail at info@icisf.org.

A comprehensive CISM system includes the following 10 components:
- Preincident stress education
- On-scene peer support
- One-on-one support

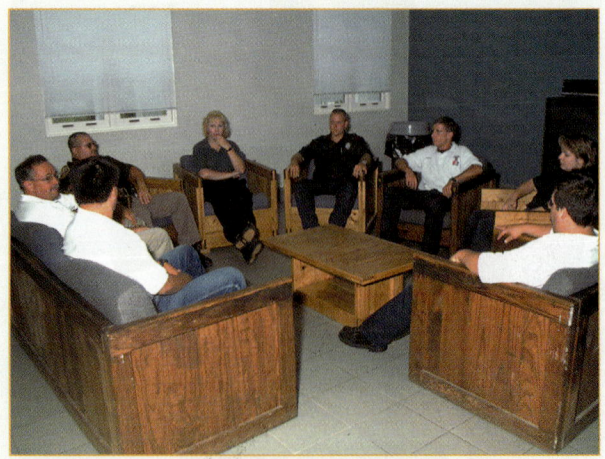

Figure 2-11 CISD sessions are conducted in confidence with other emergency workers who are trained in CISD.

- Disaster support services
- Defusing meetings
- CISD
- Follow-up services
- Spouse and family support
- Community outreach programs
- Other health and welfare programs

Workplace Issues

As our society continues to grow more culturally diverse, some groups that may have been satisfied in the past to accept and participate in American cultural traditions may seek instead to assert, preserve, and nurture their differences. As our society grows more culturally diverse, so do EMS workplaces. There will be challenges as these changes continue to occur. With the greater involvement of people of different backgrounds, EMS has the opportunity to serve people with more sensitivity to cultural variances.

Cultural Diversity on the Job

Each person is different, and you should communicate with coworkers and patients in a way that is sensitive to everyone's needs (Figure 2-12). Look at cultural diversity as a resource, and make the most of the differences among people in EMS, thus allowing them to provide optimum patient care. As the public safety workplace becomes more culturally diverse, changes may occur that could be considered disruptive. It is possible to build the strength of your workgroup through the use of diversity.

For many years, EMS and public safety has primarily consisted of caucasian males, though to a lesser extent than police and fire departments because of the traditional involvement of female nurses in EMS. This trend continues to decline; more women and minorities are working in public safety. The proactive EMT-I understands the benefits of using cultural diversity to improve patient care and expects to work alongside workers with different backgrounds and to accept their cultural differences.

As an arm of public safety, EMS has not been in existence for as long as law enforcement and fire departments. Therefore, there may be less resistance to cultural diversity in EMS than in other areas of public safety. Depending on your work experience, you may or may not have worked with people of varying backgrounds, attitudes, beliefs, and values.

Compared with traditional workplaces, EMS might seem like chaos. People who work in an office or a manufacturing facility can reasonably expect to go to work every day, see the same people, and perform basically the same tasks. In EMS and public safety work, you are exposed to people in crisis. This exposure brings out the traits and qualities that your partners and coworkers use to manage their stress. Coworkers in traditional workplaces may not be willing to show this side of themselves to others. Debriefing after the call will help in this process.

Cultural diversity in EMS allows EMT-Is to enjoy the benefits of accentuating the skills of a broad range of people. When you accept coworkers as individuals, the need to fit them into rigid roles is eliminated. To be more sensitive to cultural diversity issues, you must first be aware of your own cultural background. Ask yourself, "What are my own issues relative to race, color, religion, and ethnicity?" Since culture is not restricted to different nationalities, you should also consider age, handicap, gender, sexual orientation, marital status, work experience, and education.

In sports, you play to your team's strengths. For example, in football, offensive lines have a fast side and a strong side, and they run plays toward either side depending on the situation. As part of an effective EMS team, you can make it part of your team culture to play to your group's strengths. This may be difficult to do, but once you begin the process, the benefits in improved patient care are immeasurable.

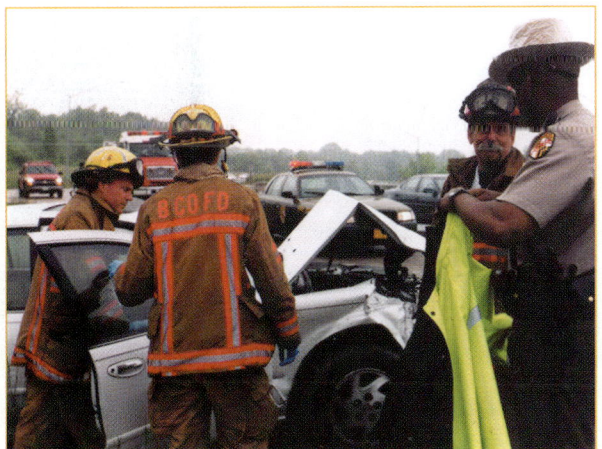

Figure 2-12 Communicate with coworkers in a way that is sensitive and respectful of individual differences.

Your Effectiveness as an EMT-I

To be an effective EMT-I, you need to discover the diverse cultural needs of your coworkers, as well as those of your patients and their families. Although it is unrealistic to expect EMT-Is to become cross-cultural experts with knowledge about all ethnicities, you should learn how to relate effectively.

Teamwork is essential in public safety and EMS. To work effectively as a team, you must be able to communicate in order to effectively deal with cultural diversity issues.

As a health care professional, you should try to be a role model for new EMT-Is by showing them the value of diversity. If you are working with a coworker or patient from a particular cultural group, be careful about any opinion you may have formed about that group. Do not assume that there is a language barrier, and do not seem patronizing by saying, "Some of my best friends are…." There are legitimate differences in how various cultures respond to stress. For example, you should be prepared to accept that people of different cultures might respond differently to the death of a loved one.

When you are working with patients or calling the hospital on the radio, other EMT-Is may be sensitive to how you treat patients from their cultural group. Therefore, when referring to patients, you should use the appropriate terminology. Avoid using terms such as "crippled," "deformed," "deaf," "dumb," "crazy," and "retarded" when referring to patients. Instead, use the term "disabled," and describe the specific disability.

You might want to consider taking multilingual training classes (Figure 2-13 ▶). This not only will be useful in communicating with your coworkers, it will also help to improve communication with your patients and accustom you to the cultural richness of the people who are using the language.

Even the perception of discrimination can weaken morale and motivation and negatively affect the goal of EMS. Therefore, to achieve the benefits of cultural diversity in the EMS workplace, EMT-Is must understand how to communicate effectively with coworkers from various backgrounds.

Avoiding Sexual Harassment

The number of sexual harassment lawsuits skyrocketed during the 1990s because of increased media attention to the problem. Furthermore, guilty verdicts encouraged others to bring suit concerning conduct that would have previously gone unchallenged.

Sexual harassment is any unwelcome sexual advance, unwelcome request for sexual favors, or other unwelcome verbal or physical conduct of a sexual nature when submitting is a condition of employment, submitting or rejecting is a basis for an employment decision, or such conduct substantially interferes with performance and/or creates a hostile or offensive work environment.

There are two types of sexual harassment: quid pro quo (the harasser requests sexual favors in exchange for something else, such as a promotion) and hostile work environment (jokes, touching, leering requests for a date, talking about body parts). Seventy percent of sexual harassment today is considered hostile work environment. Remember, it does not matter what the intent or who the harasser was. What matters are the other person's perceptions and what impact the behavior had on that person. For many years, it was not uncommon to walk into a fire station and see sexually suggestive posters, calendars, or cartoons and to hear sexual jokes or comments. With the increase of women working in EMS and public safety, it is becoming more apparent that this behavior is not appropriate in the work force.

Because EMT-Is and other public safety professionals depend on each other for their own safety, it is especially important to try to develop nonadversarial relationships with coworkers. Most EMS facilities and fire stations make arrangements for different bunkrooms for men and women. If this is not the case at your facil-

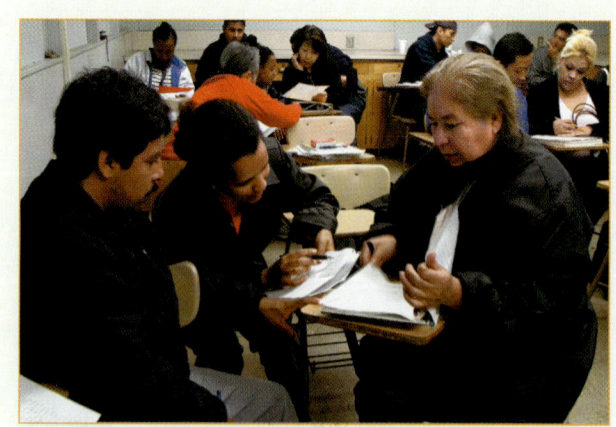

Figure 2-13 Taking a multilingual training class can help improve communication with coworkers.

ity, you should discuss this with your supervisor and talk openly with coworkers of the opposite gender to allow for their privacy.

If you are concerned about a particular behavior, it may be helpful to ask yourself these questions: "Would I do or say this in front of my spouse, significant other, or parents?" "Would I want my family members to be exposed to this behavior?" "Would I want my behavior videotaped and shown on the evening news?"

If you have been harassed, you should report it to your supervisor immediately and keep factual documentation of what happened and what was said. You should confront the harasser only if you feel comfortable doing so. If you are asked for a date, say, "I'm not interested." If remarks or touching offends you, say, "Please don't say/do that to me; it offends me."

Substance Abuse

In the past, part of the fire service ritual was to go back to the fire station after the fire, clean and maintain the equipment, and discuss the call. At some locations, having a few beers was not uncommon. Today, EMS is very different from the ambulance service in which one of your parents may have participated years ago.

The use of drugs and alcohol in the workplace causes an increase in accidents and tension among workers, but most important, it can lead to poor treatment decisions. The EMS personnel who abuse substances such as alcohol or marijuana are more likely to have problems with their work habits, and their drivers' licenses may be revoked as a result. They may be absent from work more often than other workers. If the abuse has occurred within hours before the start of their shift, their ability to provide safe and effective emergency medical care may be lessened because of mental or physical impairment. Because of the seriousness of substance abuse, many EMS systems now require their personnel to undergo periodic random tests for illegal drug use. Since public safety workers depend so much on coworkers for their own safety, it is even more important that ways be found to manage this problem.

As an EMT-I, you will witness firsthand the tremendous effects of violence, trauma, and disease. It is important to understand that the problem behavior will usually get worse before it gets better. Unfortunately, the stereotypical image of the alcoholic or addict lying in the gutter in an urban area often blinds EMS personnel to the existence of a coworker's drug or alcohol problem. People with substance abuse problems often do not fit that description.

As a member of the EMS team, you are responsible for responding to the community's emergency medical needs. Hazards in the EMS workplace are many. If you or one of the members of your team has an alcohol or other drug problem, these risks increase significantly. Furthermore, drug use that occurs off the job does not necessarily decrease the risk. Although laws and rules vary from state to state, a drug- or alcohol-related arrest may result in the revocation of some or all driving privileges and even loss of EMS certification. Because of the tremendous risk potential, it is critical that EMT-Is seek help or find a way to confront their partner or coworker even though there will be great pressure to allow the behavior to continue. People with drug addiction or alcoholism develop great skill at covering their behavior; you might even decide not to bother your coworker because you believe that he or she has run too many emotionally trying calls lately and needs to blow off some steam. Do not let this happen. You have to find a way to confront a person with a substance abuse problem. Because of the tremendous hazard to patients, the public, and other team members, you have a legitimate right to confront coworkers with drug and alcohol problems.

When confronting a coworker with a potential drug or alcohol problem, make it clear to the worker that if the problem is personal, it is the worker's responsibility to take care of it. You have the ability to assist this person. In many workplaces, coworkers are often in a position to notice a change in a coworker's behavior or attitude before a supervisor does. This is even more the case in EMS because of the close relationship that develops between people who work in an ambulance for so many hours, share rooms and meals, and socially interact while waiting for the next call. This may allow you to help someone before his or her job performance and subsequent patient care are negatively affected.

To help reduce the potential for drug and alcohol use in the EMS workplace, EMT-Is can learn about alcohol and other drugs. Beyond following company policy, EMT-Is can agree among themselves what constitutes unacceptable behavior. The best time to confront these issues is usually after a call. Management sets the tone on these issues, but senior EMT-Is can also emphasize to new personnel that drug and alcohol abuse will not be tolerated.

In a manufacturing or office environment, supervisors refer employees with problems to employee assistance programs (also called EAPs). The EMS operations might not lend themselves easily to employee assistance programs. Operations may be geographically spread out with minimal supervision and irregular work hours. Calls may range from a relatively simple 5-minute call to complex mass-casualty incidents that last several hours. Your partners may change regularly. And since you depend so much on each other for your safety, there will be pressure not to rock the boat. You are not "turning someone in." You may be saving his or her life. Your coworker may be a great EMT-I, but if this person has unresolved substance abuse issues, the risk to coworkers and patients is too great. If a substance abuse–related incident occurs during a call, it may dramatically increase the workload for other emergency responders when they respond to assist you. Early intervention is the best bet to ensure a safe, alcohol- and drug-free workplace.

> ### EMT-I Safety
>
> Substance abuse does not just reduce an EMS responder's ability to provide safe and effective patient care. It also compromises the safety of that responder and other members of the team. Ignoring a substance abuse problem puts you and those you work with at increased risk.

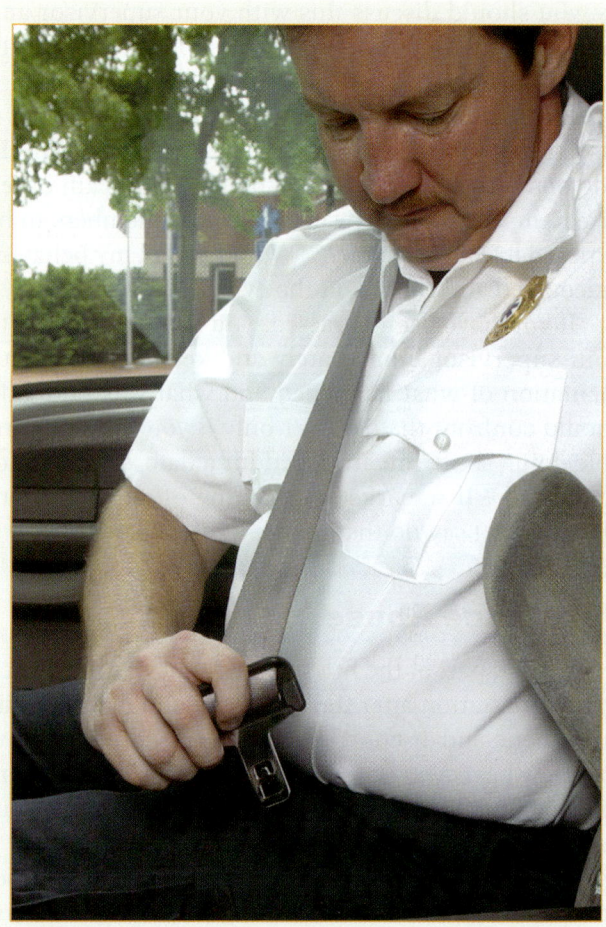

Figure 2-14 Wear seat belts and shoulder harnesses en route to the scene.

Scene Safety and Personal Protection

The personal safety of all people involved in an emergency situation is very important. In fact, it is so important that the steps you take to preserve personal safety must become automatic. A second accident at the scene or an injury to you or your partner creates more problems, delays emergency medical care for patients, increases the burden on the other EMT-Is, and may result in unnecessary injury or death.

You should begin protecting yourself as soon as you are dispatched. Before you leave for the scene, begin preparing yourself both mentally and physically. Make sure you wear seat belts and shoulder harnesses en route to the scene. Wear seat belts and shoulder harnesses at all times unless patient care makes it impossible (Figure 2-14). Many EMS units have mandatory seat belt policies for the driver at all times, for all EMT-Is during transit to the scene, and for anyone who is riding in the patient compartment.

Protecting yourself at the scene is also very important. A second accident may damage the ambulance and may result in injury to you or your partner or additional injury to the patient. Crash scenes must be well marked (Figure 2-15). If law enforcement has not already done so, you should make sure that proper warning devices are placed at a sufficient distance from the scene. This will alert motorists coming from both directions that a crash has occurred. You should park the ambulance at a safe but convenient distance from the scene. Before attempting to access patients trapped in a vehicle, check the vehicle's stability. Then take any necessary measures to secure it. Do not rock or push on a vehicle to find out whether it will move. This can overturn the vehicle or send it crashing into a ditch.

When working at night, you must have plenty of light. Poor lighting increases the risk of further injury to you and the patient. It also results in poor emergency medical care. Reflective emblems or clothing helps to make you more visible at night and decreases your risk of injury (Figure 2-16).

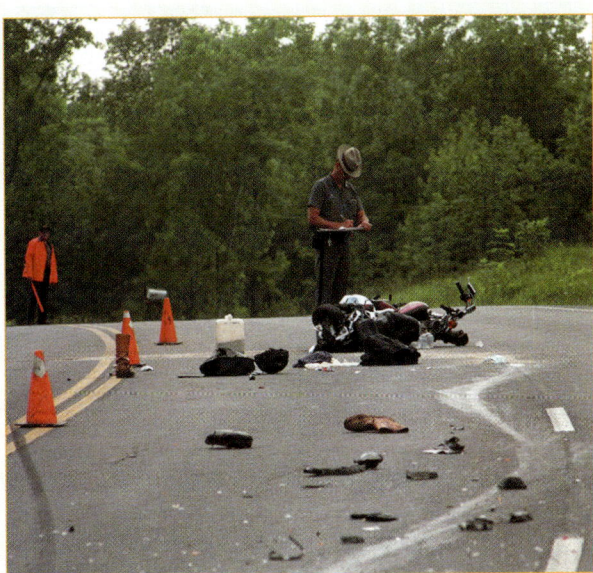

Figure 2-15 Make sure the crash scene is well marked to prevent a second crash that may damage the ambulance or result in injury to you, your partner, or the patient.

Communicable Diseases

As an EMT-I, you will be called upon to treat and transport patients with a variety of communicable or infectious diseases. Most of these diseases are much harder to contract than is commonly believed. In addition, there are many immunizations, protective techniques, and devices that can minimize the health care provider's risk of infection. When these protective measures are used, the risk of the health care provider contracting a serious communicable disease is minimized.

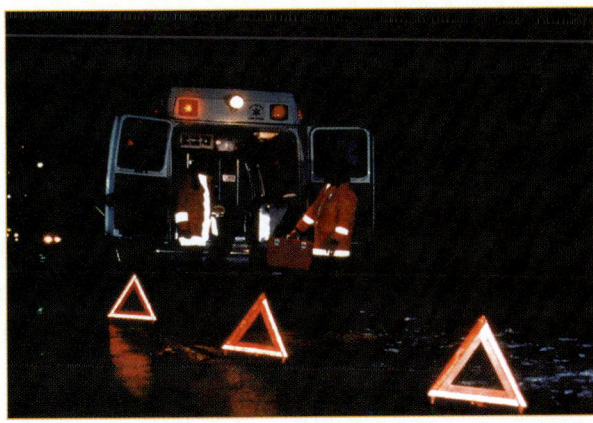

Figure 2-16 Wear reflective emblems or clothing to help make you more visible at night and improve your safety in the dark.

Routes of Transmission

While all infections result from an invasion of body spaces and tissues by germs, different germs use different means of attack. These means are known as the mechanisms of transmission. <u>Transmission</u> is the way an infectious agent is spread. There are four mechanisms: direct transmission, vehicle-borne, vector-borne, and airborne . In this context, "vehicle" means an inanimate object, while "vector" means a living object.

> ### EMT-I Tips
>
> **Infectious, contagious, or communicable**
> Many people confuse the terms "infectious" and "contagious." In fact, all contagious diseases are infectious, but only some infectious diseases are contagious. For example, pneumonia caused by pneumococcus bacteria is an infectious process, but it is not contagious. In other words, it will not be transmitted from one person to another. However, other infectious agents, such as the hepatitis B virus, are contagious because they can be transmitted from one person to another. An <u>infection</u> is an abnormal invasion of a host or host tissue by organisms such as bacteria, viruses, or parasites. A <u>pathogen</u> is a microorganism that is capable of causing disease in a host. A <u>host</u> is simply the person invaded by the pathogen. An <u>infectious disease</u>, then, is a disease that is caused by an infection. For example, Lyme disease is an infectious disease caused by the *Borrelia burgdorferi* bacterium, which lives in deer ticks. However, Lyme disease is not contagious. Again, a <u>contagious</u> or <u>communicable disease</u> can be transmitted from one person to another. The only way to get Lyme disease is to be bitten by a deer tick.

Risk Reduction and Prevention

Universal Precautions and Body Substance Isolation

The <u>Occupational Safety and Health Administration (OSHA)</u> develops and publishes guidelines concerning reducing risk in the workplace. It is also responsible for

| TABLE 2-7 | Mechanisms of Transmission of Infectious Diseases |||

In this table, the routes of transmission and some examples are outlined. Remember, while some germs frequently cause disease after transmission, transmission to a susceptible host is much more likely to cause asymptomatic infection and colonization.

Route	Descriptions	Source	Examples
UNIVERSAL PRECAUTIONS REQUIRED			
Direct	Contact directly with the person or with droplets sprayed (for example, by sneezing or coughing)	Ordinary contact	Measles, mumps, chickenpox, bacterial meningitis, influenza, diphtheria, herpes simplex
		Sexual contact	Syphilis, gonorrhea, HIV infection, hepatitis B, herpes simplex
Indirect			
Vehicle-borne	Spread by inanimate objects (for example, food, needles, clothing, transfused blood)	Food or water	Hepatitis A, B, C; *Salmonella*; *Shigella*; poliomyelitis
		Blood or other bodily fluid	HIV infection
		Other	Measles, tetanus
Vector-borne			
Mechanical	Simple carriage by insects; vector simply carries the germs	Houseflies	*Shigella*
Biological	Transmission by insect in which the germ lives and grows	Ticks	Lyme disease, Rocky Mountain spotted fever
		Mosquitoes	Malaria, equine encephalitis
AIRBORNE DISEASE PRECAUTIONS REQUIRED			
Airborne Droplet nuclei	Residues after partial evaporation of droplets; germs may remain viable, and the droplets may remain suspended for long periods.		*Mycobacterium tuberculosis*, chickenpox
Dust	Small particles of dust from the soil may carry fungal spores and remain airborne for long periods.		Histoplasmosis, Coccidioides, Mycobacterium avium intracellulare

HIV = human immunodeficiency virus.

Data from Benenson AS (ed): *Control of Communicable Diseases in Man*, ed 15. Washington, DC, American Public Health Association, 1990

enforcing these guidelines. All EMS providers are required by OSHA to be trained in the handling of bloodborne pathogens and in approaching the patient who may have a communicable or infectious disease. Training must also be provided for issues including blood and body fluid precautions and contamination procedures.

Because health care workers are exposed to so many different kinds of infections, the Centers for Disease Control and Prevention (CDC) developed a set of <u>universal precautions</u> for health care workers to use when providing patient care. These protective measures are designed to prevent workers from coming in direct contact with germs carried by patients. <u>Direct contact</u> is the exposure or transmission of a communicable disease from one person to another by direct physical contact. Gonorrhea, a sexually transmitted disease (also called STD), is an example of a disease transmitted by direct contact. <u>Exposure</u> is contact with blood, body fluids, tissues, or airborne droplets by direct or indirect contact. <u>Indirect contact</u> is exposure or transmission of a disease from one person to another by contact with a contaminated object. Common colds are typically spread in this manner.

The goal of universal precautions is to interrupt the transmission of germs by decreasing the chance that you will come into contact with them. Universal precautions are not universal in the sense that they will help to protect you against all infectious diseases. Instead, the word "universal" is meant to remind you to apply precautions in all situations in which you have direct patient contact. It is impossible to tell whether a person is free of a communicable disease, even if he or she appears healthy. For this reason, it is safest to assume that all patients are infected and use the appropriate precautions.

You can also reduce your risk of exposure by following <u>body substance isolation (BSI)</u> precautions. BSI is the preferred infection control concept for fire and EMS personnel. BSI differs from universal precautions in that it is designed to approach all body fluids as being potentially infectious. To provide maximum safety, EMS follows the BSI concept rather than relying on universal precautions.

Modes of transmission for infectious diseases include the following:
- Blood or body fluid splash
- Surface contamination
- Needlestick exposure
- Oral contamination due to lack of or improper handwashing

> **EMT-I Tips**
>
> One of the most effective ways to control disease transmission is by washing your hands thoroughly with soap and water after any patient contact.

Proper Handwashing

Proper handwashing is perhaps one of the simplest yet most effective ways of controlling disease transmission. You should always wash your hands before and after contact with a patient, regardless of whether you wore gloves. The longer the germs remain with you, the greater their chance of getting through your barriers. Although soap and water are not protective in all cases, in certain cases their use provides excellent protection against further transmission from your skin to others (cross-contamination).

If no running water is available, you may use waterless handwashing substitutes Figure 2-17. If you use a waterless substitute in the field, make sure that you wash your hands as soon as possible. The proper procedure for handwashing is as follows:

1. Use soap and warm water.
2. Rub your hands together for at least 10 to 15 seconds to work up a lather.

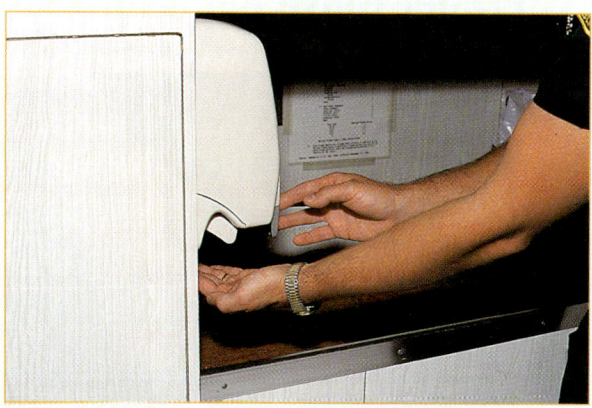

Figure 2-17 Use a waterless handwashing solution if there is no running water available. Be sure to wash your hands with soap once you arrive at the hospital.

3. Rinse your hands, and dry them with a paper towel.
4. Use the paper towel to turn off the faucet.

Gloves and Eye Protection

Gloves and eye protection are the minimum standard for all EMS personnel. Both vinyl and latex gloves provide adequate protection. Your department may prefer one type of glove over the other, or you may choose the glove. You should evaluate each situation and choose the glove that works best. Some people are allergic to latex. If you suspect that you are, consult your supervisor for options. Vinyl gloves may be best for routine procedures, and latex gloves may be best for invasive procedures. Never use vinyl or latex gloves for cleaning. Change latex gloves if they have been exposed to motor oil, gasoline, or any petroleum-based product. Do not perform tasks such as using a radio, driving, writing a patient care report, or using any monitoring device such as a cardiac monitor or pulse oximeter when wearing contaminated gloves. Wear double gloves if there is substantial bleeding. You may also wear double gloves if you will be exposed to large volumes of other body fluids. Be sure to change gloves as you move from one patient to another. For cleaning and disinfecting the unit, you should use heavy-duty utility gloves Figure 2-18. *You should never use lightweight latex or vinyl gloves for cleaning.*

Removing used latex or vinyl gloves requires a methodical technique to avoid contaminating yourself with the materials from which the gloves have protected you Skill Drill 2-1.

1. **Begin by partially removing one glove.** With the other gloved hand, pinch the first glove at the

Proper Glove Removal Technique

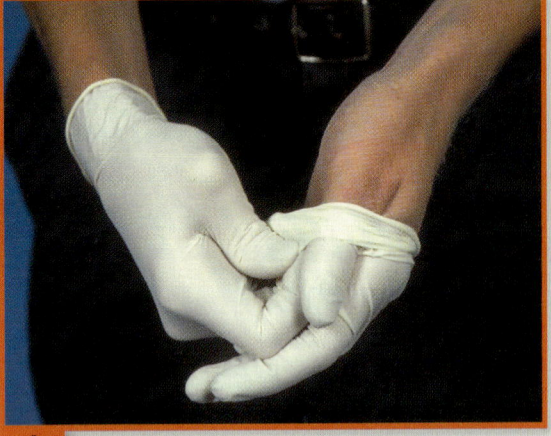

1. Partially remove the first glove by pinching at the wrist. Be careful to touch only the outside of the glove.

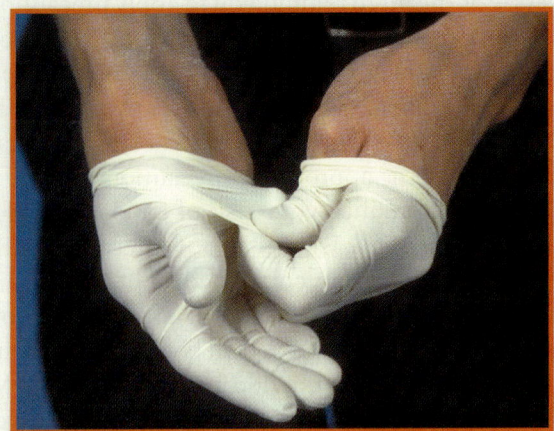

2. Remove the second glove by pinching the exterior with the partially gloved hand.

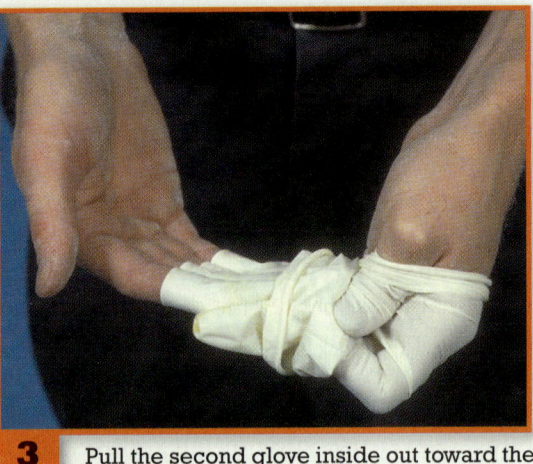

3. Pull the second glove inside out toward the fingertips.

4. Grasp both gloves with your free hand touching only the clean, interior surfaces.

wrist—being certain to touch only the outside of the first glove—and start to roll it back off the hand, inside out. Leave the exterior of the fingers on the first glove exposed (**Step 1**).

2. **Use the still-gloved fingers** of the first hand to pinch the wrist of the second glove and begin to pull it off, rolling it inside-out toward the fingertips as you did with the first glove (**Step 2**).
3. **Continue pulling the second glove off** until you can pull the second hand free (**Step 3**).
4. **With your now-ungloved second hand**, grasp the exposed inside of the first glove and pull it free of your first hand and over the now-loose second glove. Be sure that you touch only clean, interior surfaces with your ungloved hand (**Step 4**).

Gloves are the most common type of <u>personal protective equipment (PPE)</u>. In many EMS rescue operations, you must also protect your hands and wrists from injury. You may wear puncture-proof leather gloves, with latex gloves underneath. This combination will allow you free use of your hands with added protection from blood and body fluids. Remember that latex or vinyl gloves are considered medical waste and must be disposed of properly. Leather gloves must be treated as contaminated material until they can be properly decontaminated.

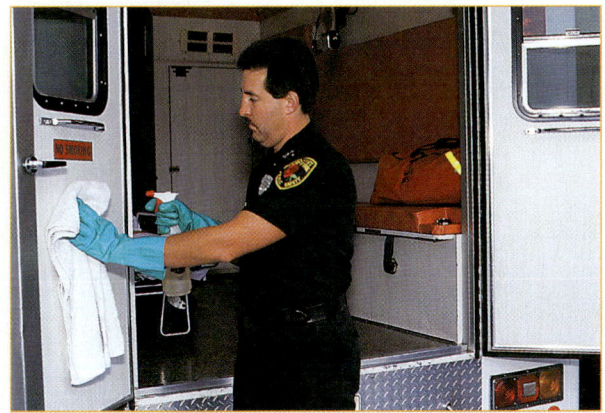

Figure 2-18 Use heavy-duty utility gloves to clean the unit. You should never use lightweight latex or vinyl gloves for cleaning.

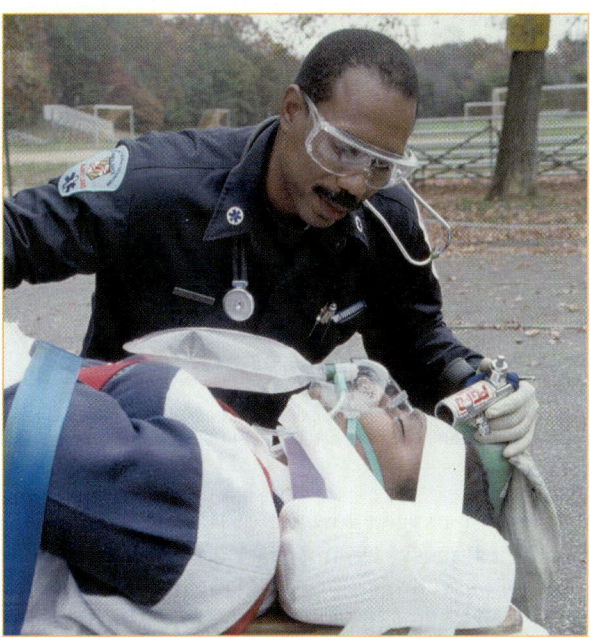

Figure 2-19 Wear eye protection to prevent blood from splattering into your eyes.

> **EMT-I Tips**
>
> **Personal protective equipment** is protective equipment that blocks entry of an organism into the body.
>
> **Body substance isolation** is the use of PPE and the assumption that all body fluids are potentially infectious.

Eye protection is important in case blood splatters toward your eyes 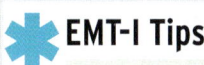 Figure 2-19 . If this is a possibility, wearing goggles is your best protection. Prescription glasses are acceptable as eye protection; however, you must add removable side shields when on duty. This will ensure that your eyes are shielded from all angles.

Gowns and Masks

Occasionally, you may need to wear a mask and gown. A mask and gown provide protection from extensive blood splatter. Gowns may be worn in situations such as field delivery of a baby or major trauma. However, wearing a gown may not be practical in many situations. In fact, in some instances, a gown may pose a risk for injury. Your department will likely have a policy regarding gowns. Be sure you know your local policy. There are times when a change of uniform is preferred because trying to clean off contaminants is difficult and sometimes impossible without professional cleaning and disinfection or disposing of the uniform entirely.

Masks, Respirators, and Barrier Devices

The use of masks is a complex issue, especially in light of OSHA and CDC requirements regarding protection from tuberculosis. You should wear a standard surgical mask if blood or body fluid splatter is a possibility. If you suspect that a patient has an airborne disease, you should place a surgical mask on the patient. However, if you suspect that the patient has tuberculosis, place a surgical mask on the patient and a high-efficiency particulate air (HEPA) respirator on yourself Figure 2-20 . If the patient needs oxygen, apply a nonrebreathing

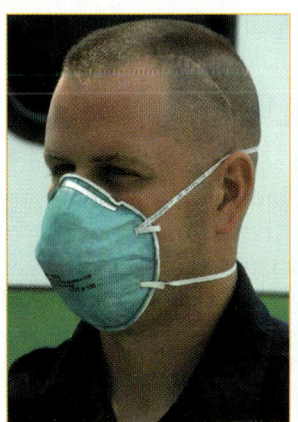 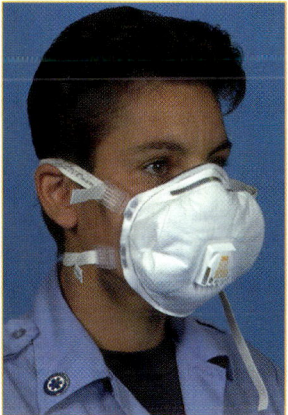

Figure 2-20 Wear a HEPA respirator if you treat a patient whom you suspect has tuberculosis.

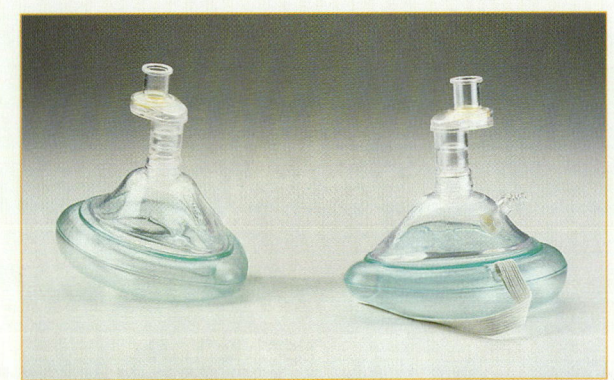

Figure 2-21 Barrier devices such as a pocket mask are necessary when providing artificial ventilations.

mask with an oxygen flow rate of 10 to 15 L/min instead of a surgical mask. Do not place a HEPA respirator on the patient; it is unnecessary and uncomfortable. A simple surgical mask will reduce the risk of transmission of germs from the patient into the air. Use of a HEPA respirator should comply with OSHA standards, which state that facial hair, such as long sideburns or a mustache, will prevent a proper fit.

Although there are no documented cases of disease transmission to rescuers as a result of performing unprotected mouth-to-mouth resuscitation on a patient with an infection, you should use a pocket mask with the one-way valve or bag-valve-mask device (Figure 2-21). Mouth-to-mouth resuscitation is discouraged.

Remember that the outside surfaces of these items are considered contaminated after they have been exposed to the patient. You must ensure that gloves, masks, gowns, and all other items that have been exposed to infectious processes or blood are properly disposed of according to local guidelines. If you are stuck by a needle, get blood or other body fluid in your eye, or have contact with any body fluid from the patient, seek medical care as soon as it is feasible and report the incident to your supervisor.

Proper Disposal of Sharps

Be careful when handling needles, scalpels, and other sharp items. The spread of human immunodeficiency virus (HIV) and hepatitis in the health care setting can usually be traced to careless handling of sharps.

- Do not recap, break, or bend needles. Even the most careful people may stick themselves accidentally.
- Dispose of all sharp items that have been in contact with human secretions in approved, closed, puncture-proof containers. Such containers are typically red and are labeled with a biohazard insignia (Figure 2-22).

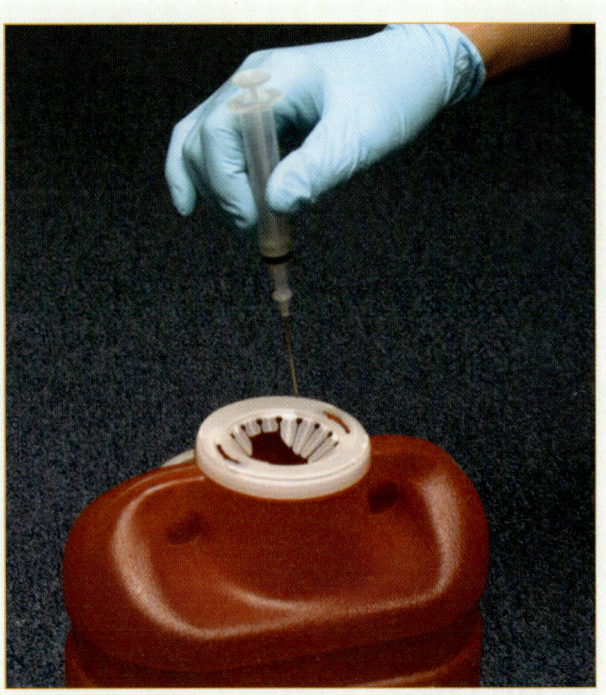

Figure 2-22 Properly dispose of sharps in a closed, rigid, marked container.

Employer Responsibilities

Your employer cannot guarantee a 100% risk-free environment. Taking the risk of exposure to a communicable disease is a part of your job. You have a right to know about diseases that may pose a risk to you. Remember, though, that your risk for infection is not high; however, OSHA regulations, especially for private and federal agencies, require that all employees be offered a workplace environment that *reduces* the risk for exposure. Note that in some states that have their own OSHA plans, state and municipal employees must also be covered.

In addition to OSHA guidelines, other national guidelines and standards, including those from the CDC and National Fire Protection Association Infection Control Standard 1581, address reducing the risk for exposure to bloodborne pathogens (disease-causing organisms) and airborne diseases. The standards set by these agencies provide for a standard of care for all fire and EMS personnel and apply whether you are a full-time paid employee or a volunteer.

Personal Protective Equipment

PPE is equipment that blocks entry of an organism into the body. OSHA requires that the following PPE be made available to you:

- Vinyl and latex gloves
- Heavy-duty gloves for cleaning

- Protective eyewear
- Masks (including a HEPA respirator)
- Cover gowns
- Devices for respiratory assistance (ie, pocket mask with one-way valve)

The proper PPE for each task is selected according to the way in which a communicable disease is transmitted. For example, wearing a mask can block transmission of an airborne disease.

Wear protective eyewear such as goggles or a face shield whenever there is a possibility that blood or another body fluid will splatter into your eyes. If you wear prescription eyeglasses, you can add removable side shields to your glasses while you are on duty.

Because some cover gowns are not practical in the field, your department will decide whether your uniform will serve as PPE. If so, the department's exposure control plan should outline how and where contaminated uniforms are to be laundered.

The recommendations for PPE use should be followed; however, OSHA recognizes that there are times when these procedures cannot be performed. There is an exception statement in the OSHA regulation that states that when you believe that taking the time to use PPE will delay provision of care to the patient or will pose a risk to your personal safety, you may choose not to use PPE. Risk to personal safety refers to the likelihood of being attacked by a person or an animal, not to concern about acquiring a communicable disease. If you choose not to use PPE, you may have to justify this action, as an inquiry will follow.

Exposure Control Plan

Another way to reduce risk of exposure is by following your department's *exposure control plan*, which is a comprehensive plan that incorporates CDC guidelines, OSHA regulations, National Fire Protection Association Infection Control Standard 1581, and other applicable state and local regulations (Table 2-8).

TABLE 2-8 Components of an Exposure Control Plan

Determination of Exposure
- Determines who is at risk for ongoing contact with blood and other body fluids
- Creates a list of tasks that pose a risk for contact with blood or other body fluids
- Includes PPE required by OSHA

Education and Training
- Explains why a qualified person is required to answer questions about communicable diseases and infection control, rather than relying on packaged training materials
- Includes availability of an instructor able to train EMT-Is regarding bloodborne and airborne pathogens, such as hepatitis B and C viruses, HIV, and the bacteria that cause diseases such as syphilis and tuberculosis
- Ensures that the instructor provides appropriate education, which is the best means for correcting many myths surrounding these issues

Hepatitis B Vaccine Program
- Spells out the vaccine offered, its safety and efficacy, record keeping, and tracking
- Addresses the need for postvaccine antibody titers to identify people who do not respond to the initial three-dose vaccination series

Personal Protective Equipment
- Lists the PPE offered and why it was selected
- Lists how much equipment is available and where to obtain additional PPE
- States when each type of PPE is to be used for each risk procedure

Cleaning and Disinfection Practices
- Describes how to care for and maintain vehicles and equipment
- Identifies where and when cleaning should be performed, how it is to be done, what PPE is to be used, and what cleaning solution is to be used
- Addresses medical waste collection, storage, and disposal

Tuberculin Skin Testing and HEPA Mask Fit Testing
- Addresses how often employees should undergo tuberculin skin testing (purified protein derivative or PPD)
- Addresses how often fit testing should be done to determine the proper size HEPA mask to protect the EMT-I from tuberculosis
- Addresses all issues dealing with HEPA respirator masks

Postexposure Management
- Identifies whom to notify when exposure may have occurred, forms to be filled out, where to go for treatment, and what treatment is to be given

Compliance Monitoring
- Addresses how the service or department evaluates employee compliance with each aspect of the plan
- Ensures that employees understand what they are to do and why it is important
- States that noncompliance should be documented
- Indicates what disciplinary action should be taken in the face of noncompliance

Record Keeping
- Outlines all records that will be kept, how confidentiality will be maintained, and how records can be assessed and by whom

Immunity

Even if germs do reach you, they may not infect you. For example, you may be immune, or resistant, to those particular germs. Immunity is a major factor in determining which hosts become ill from which germs (Table 2-9). One way to gain immunity from many diseases today is to be immunized, or vaccinated, against them. Vaccinations have almost eliminated some childhood diseases, such as measles and polio.

Another way in which the body becomes immune to a disease is to recover from an infection from that germ. Afterward, the body recognizes and repels that germ when it shows up again. Once exposed, healthy people will develop lifelong immunity to many common pathogens. For example, a person who contracts and becomes infected with the hepatitis A virus may be ill for several weeks, but because immunity will develop, he or she will not have to worry about getting the illness again. Sometimes, however, the immunity is only partial. Partial immunity protects against new infections, but germs that remain in the body from the first illness may still be able to cause the same disease again when the body is stressed or has some impairment in its immune system. For example, tuberculosis can cause a mild, unnoticeable infection before the body builds up a partial immunity. If the infection is never treated, it may be reactivated when immunity is weakened; however, people with partial immunity are protected against a new infection from another person.

Humans seem unable to mount an effective immune response to some infections, such as HIV infection, which is infection with the human immunodeficiency virus that can progress to acquired immunodeficiency syndrome (AIDS).

Although OSHA does not require hepatitis A immunization, you may want to be vaccinated as a preventive measure. Hepatitis A vaccination is not necessary if you have had hepatitis A in the past. All these vaccines are effective and rarely cause side effects. Many EMS systems require you to show proof that you are up-to-date with your immunizations.

Remember, germs that cause no symptoms in one person may cause serious illness in another.

Immunizations

As an EMT-I, you are at risk for acquiring an infectious or communicable disease. Using basic protective measures can minimize the risk. You are responsible for protecting yourself.

TABLE 2-9 Immunity to Infectious Diseases

Type of Immunity	Characteristics	Examples	Comments
Lifelong	The illness will not recur.	Measles Mumps Polio Rubella Hepatitis A Hepatitis B	Infection or vaccination provides long-term immunity to new infection. A live vaccine is required for measles only.
Partial	The person who has recovered from a first infection is unlikely to get a new infection from another person, but may develop illness from germs that lie dormant from the initial infection.	Chickenpox Tuberculosis	Infection provides lifelong immunity to the patient from acquiring a new infection, but the original illness may recur, or it may recur in a different way. In the case of chickenpox, which is caused by the varicella virus, an infection may recur years later in the form of shingles.
None	Exposure confers no protection from reinfection. The infection may wear down the patient's resistance.	Gonorrhea Syphilis HIV infection	No vaccine is available. Repeated infections are common. For example, there is effective immediate treatment for gonorrhea, and the germs may be eradicated; however, reinfection is likely if the high-risk practices (eg, unprotected sex) continue. For syphilis and HIV infection, the lack of immunity allows the germs to continue to cause damage within the host.

Prevention begins by maintaining your personal health. EMS personnel should receive annual health examinations. A history of all your childhood infectious diseases should be recorded and kept on file. Childhood infectious diseases include chickenpox, mumps, measles, rubella, and whooping cough. If you have not had one of these diseases, you must be immunized.

The CDC and OSHA have developed requirements for protection from bloodborne pathogens such as the hepatitis B virus. An immunization program should be in place in your EMS system. Immunizations should be kept up-to-date and recorded in your file. Recommended immunizations include the following:

- Tetanus-diphtheria boosters (every 10 years)
- Measles, mumps, rubella (MMR) vaccine
- Influenza vaccine (yearly)
- Hepatitis B vaccine

You should also have a skin test for tuberculosis before you begin working as an EMT-I. The purpose of the test is to identify anyone who has been exposed to tuberculosis in the past. Testing should be repeated every year. It is important to know that testing positive for a tuberculosis skin test does not mean that you have the disease; it indicates that you have been exposed. Additional follow-up will be needed to determine whether the disease is active.

If you know that you will be transporting a patient who has a communicable disease, you have a definite advantage. This is when your health record will be valuable. If you have already had the disease or been vaccinated, you are at minimal risk. However, you will not always know whether a patient has a communicable disease. Therefore, you should always follow BSI precautions when caring for any patient.

Duty to Act

You cannot deny care to a patient you suspect has a communicable disease, even if you believe that the patient poses a health risk to you. To deny care to such a patient is considered abandonment, which is illegal and unethical and can result in civil and criminal actions against you. By always wearing PPE when caring for any patient, you minimize your risk. It can also be considered a breach of duty (a situation in which the EMT-I does not act within an expected and reasonable standard of care). In addition to breach of duty, if the following factors are present, you may be considered negligent in your duties:

- **Duty to act**—Having a duty to respond
- **Breach of duty**—Failure to respond

You are the Provider   Part 3

The patient is quickly removed from his vehicle, and care is initiated immediately to support airway, breathing, and circulation. After performing a rapid head-to-toe assessment, you obtain the following set of vital signs:

Vital Signs	Recording Time: 2 Minutes After Patient Contact
Respirations	8 breaths/min, shallow (ventilations are being assisted)
Pulse	132 beats/min, weak and thready
Skin	Pale, cool, and clammy
Blood pressure	72/48 mm Hg
SaO_2	95% (ventilations assisted with 100% oxygen)

After fully immobilizing the patient's spine, you load him into the ambulance and begin transport to a local trauma center. Additional interventions are performed en route.

5. How can the EMT-I help reduce the occurrence of traumatic injuries, such as those sustained by this patient?
6. What measures can the EMT-I take to help prevent the spread of potentially infectious diseases?

- **Injury**—An injury has occurred
- **Proximate cause**—Injury was caused by your actions or inactions

Denying care to a patient you suspect has a communicable disease can also be considered discrimination according to the Americans with Disabilities Act (also called ADA), especially when a public department or agency such as EMS is involved.

Some Diseases of Special Concern

HIV Infection

Exposure to the virus that causes AIDS is the most feared infection risk for EMS providers. It is this prospect that led to the development of universal precautions and BSI precautions. There is no vaccine to protect against HIV infection, and despite great progress in drug treatments, AIDS is still fatal. Fortunately, it is not easily transmitted in your work setting. For example, it is far less contagious than hepatitis B. HIV infection is a potential hazard only when deposited on a mucous membrane or directly into the bloodstream. Exposure can take place in the following ways:

- The patient's blood is splashed or sprayed into your eyes, nose, or mouth or into an open sore or cut, however tiny; even a microscopic opening in the skin is an invitation for infection with the virus.
- You have blood from the infected patient on your hands and then touch your own eyes, nose, mouth, or an open sore or cut.
- A needle used to inject the patient breaks your skin. The risk to you from a single injection, even with a hollow-bore needle, is small, probably less than 1 in 1,000. However, this is the most common route of transmission.
- Broken glass at a motor vehicle crash or other incident may penetrate your glove (and skin), which may have already been covered with blood from an infected patient.

Many patients who are infected with HIV do not show any symptoms. This is why health care workers should wear certain types of gloves any time they are likely to come into contact with secretions or blood from any patient. You should always put on the proper

TABLE 2-10	Characteristics of Hepatitis		
Type	**Route of Infection**	**Incubation Period** (time before clinical signs and **symptoms** appear but infection may still be transmitted)	**Acute Disease** (when patient usually appears sick)
Viral (infectious)			
Hepatitis A	Fecal-oral, infected food	2 to 6 weeks	Early symptoms of all viral hepatitis include loss of appetite, vomiting, fever, fatigue, sore throat, cough, and muscle and joint pain.
Hepatitis B	Blood, saliva, urine, sexual contact, breast milk	4 to 12 weeks	Several weeks later, jaundice (yellow eyes and skin) and right upper quadrant abdominal pain develop.
Hepatitis C	Blood, sexual contact	2 to 10 weeks	
Hepatitis D	Blood, sexual contact	4 to 12 weeks	
Toxin-Induced			
Medication, Drugs, Alcohol	Inhalation, skin exposure, oral ingestion, exposure or IV administration	Within hours to days following exposure	Severity of disease depends on amount of agent absorbed and duration of exposure.

type of gloves before leaving the ambulance to care for a patient. In addition, you must take great care in handling and disposing of needles and scalpels so that others are not inadvertently exposed to them. Finally, you should cover any open wounds that you have whenever you are on the job.

If you have any reason to think that a patient's blood or secretions may have entered your system, especially through inoculation with the patient's blood, you should seek medical advice as soon as possible. If you know that the patient is infected with HIV, your physician may suggest immediate treatment to try to prevent you from becoming infected. However, if the patient seems an unlikely candidate for HIV infection, your physician may recommend that both you and the patient be tested before you undergo prophylactic therapy. As scientists learn more about HIV infection, testing and treatment recommendations will change. So, it is important that you immediately see your doctor (or your program's designated doctor) any time you are potentially exposed to a communicable disease. Know the policy for your system and consider now what you would do in the event of exposure.

Hepatitis

The term **hepatitis** refers to an inflammation (and often infection) of the liver. Hepatitis causes fever, loss of appetite, jaundice, and fatigue. It can be caused by a number of different viruses and toxins. There is no definitive way to determine which patients with hepatitis have a contagious form of the disease and which do not.

Table 2-10 ▼ shows the characteristics of different types of hepatitis, from which you can assess your risk of exposure. Hepatitis A can be transmitted only from a patient who has an acute infection, while hepatitis B and hepatitis C can also be transmitted from long-term carriers who have no signs of active illness. A **carrier** is a person (or animal) in whom an infectious organism has taken up permanent residence and who may or may not transmit any active disease. Carriers may never know that they harbor the organism; however, they can infect other people.

Hepatitis A is transmitted through oral or fecal contamination. This means that, generally, you must eat or drink something that is contaminated with the virus. **Contamination** is the presence of an infectious organism on or in an object. The organisms that cause

Chronic Infection (patient may no longer have signs of the relevant illness)	Vaccine Available?	Treatment	Comments
Chronic condition does not exist.	Yes	None	Mild illness; approximately 2% of patients die. After acute infection, patient has lifelong immunity.
Chronic infection affects up to 10% of patients; up to 90% of newborns who have the disease.	Yes	Yes, but poor results	Up to 30% of patients may become chronic carriers. Patients are asymptomatic and without signs of liver disease, but they may infect others. Approximately 1% to 2% of patients die.
Chronic infection affects 90% of patients.	No	Yes, but poor results	Cirrhosis of the liver develops in 50% of patients with chronic hepatitis C; chronic infection increases the risk of cancer of the liver.
Chronic infection is very common.	No	None	Occurs only in patients with active hepatitis B infection. Fulminant disease may develop in 20% of patients.
Some chemicals may initiate an inflammatory response that continues to cause liver damage long after the chemical is out of the body.	No	Stop exposure. In patients with overdose of acetaminophen, certain drugs may subdue liver injury if given early enough.	This type of hepatitis is not contagious. Patients with toxin-induced hepatitis may have signs of liver damage, such as jaundice. Not every exposure to a toxin will cause liver damage.

hepatitis B and C are transmitted through vehicles other than food or water. For example, these organisms may enter the body through a transfusion or needlestick with infected blood, which puts health care workers at high risk for contracting hepatitis B, the more contagious and virulent form. <u>Virulence</u> is the strength or ability of a pathogen to produce disease. Hepatitis B is far more contagious than HIV. For this reason, vaccination with hepatitis B vaccine is highly recommended for EMS providers. Unfortunately, not everyone who is vaccinated develops immediate immunity to the virus. Occasionally, an additional dose will be required to achieve immunity. You should be tested (titer) after vaccination to determine your immune status.

If you are stuck with a needle or injured in some other way while caring for a patient who might have hepatitis, you should seek medical care as soon as possible and report the incident to your supervisor.

Meningitis

<u>Meningitis</u> is an inflammation of the meningeal coverings of the brain and spinal cord. Patients with meningitis will have signs and symptoms such as fever, headache, stiff neck (nuchal rigidity), and altered mental status. It is an uncommon but frightening infectious disease. Viruses and bacteria, most of which are not contagious, can cause meningitis. However, one form, meningococcal meningitis, is highly contagious. The meningococcal bacterium colonizes in the human nose and throat and only rarely causes an acute infection. When it does, the infection can be lethal. Patients with this kind of infection often have red blotches on their skin. This sign can also be seen in patients with other noncontagious forms of meningitis.

Because laboratory analysis is required to identify the strain of meningitis, you should use universal precautions and follow BSI precautions with any patient who is suspected of having meningitis. Gloves and a mask will go a long way to prevent the patient's secretions from getting into your nose and mouth. Again, the risk of infection is small, even if the organism is transmitted. For this reason, vaccines, which are available for most types of meningococcus, are rarely used. There are no effective treatments for the disease.

After treating a patient with meningitis, you should contact your employer health representative.

Tuberculosis

Most patients who are infected with *Mycobacterium tuberculosis* (the tubercle bacillus) are well most of the time. Tuberculosis that involves the bone or kidneys is only slightly contagious. In the United States, however, <u>tuberculosis</u> is a chronic bacterial disease that usually affects the lungs. Disease that occurs shortly after infection is called primary tuberculosis. Except in infants, this infection is not usually serious. After the primary infection, the tubercle bacillus is rendered dormant by the patient's immune system. However, even after decades of lying dormant, this germ can reactivate. Reactive tuberculosis is common and can be much more difficult to treat, especially because an increasing number of tuberculosis strains have grown resistant to most antibiotics.

Although tuberculosis is often hard to distinguish from other diseases, patients who pose the highest risk almost invariably have a cough. Therefore, for your safety, you should consider respiratory tuberculosis to be the most contagious form, as it is the only one that is spread by airborne transmission. The droplets that are produced by coughing are not the real problem. The real problem is the droplet nuclei, which are what remains of droplets after excess water has evaporated. These particles are tiny enough to be totally invisible and can remain suspended in the air for a long time. In fact, as long as they are shielded from ultraviolet light, they can remain alive for decades. So you may be at risk by simply entering a closed room that the patient left long ago. Routine surgical masks do not stop particles of that size. Inhaled, they are carried directly to the alveoli of the lungs, where the bacteria may begin to grow.

> **EMT-I Tips**
>
> Place a surgical mask on the patient suspected of having tuberculosis and a HEPA mask on yourself.

Why is tuberculosis not more common than it is? After all, absolute protection from infection with the tubercle bacillus does not exist. Everyone who breathes is at risk. And the vaccine for tuberculosis, called BCG, is only rarely used in the United States. Under normal circumstances, however, the mechanism of transmission used by *M tuberculosis* is not very efficient. Infected air is easily diluted with uninfected air, and *M tuberculosis* is one of the germs that typically does not cause illness in a new host. In fact, many patients with tuberculosis do not even transmit the infection to family members. In crowded environments with poor ventilation, however, the disease spreads relatively easily.

If you are exposed to a patient who is found to have pulmonary tuberculosis, you will be given a tuberculin skin test. This simple skin test determines whether a person has been exposed to *M tuberculosis*. A positive result means that exposure has occurred; it does not mean that the person has active tuberculosis. It takes at least 6 weeks for the bacteria to show up in the laboratory test. So if you have the test within a few weeks of the exposure and results are positive, this means that you had already acquired the infection from somebody else. You will probably never identify the source. Most transmissions occur silently. This is why health care workers have tuberculin skin tests regularly. If the infection is found before the person becomes ill, preventive therapy is almost 100% effective. Usually, a daily dose of isoniazid (INH) will result in a cure.

> **Geriatric Needs**
>
> Everyone has defenses against illness, but the aging process can pose a threat to our natural defense mechanisms against invading microorganisms. Our physical defenses weaken or are eliminated as we age. The skin's thinning and loss of supportive collagen, along with a reduction in the number of blood vessels, can allow bacteria or viruses to enter the body with less resistance. The respiratory system cannot trap and eliminate bacteria or viruses in the airways as it once did. Finally, the gastrointestinal system allows an easier entry for bacteria or viruses through the intestines. Not only do our physical barriers to entry weaken, but our immune system deteriorates, and invading organisms are not as easily identified as abnormal. Infectious agents can take hold in elderly patients much more easily because of reduced defenses.
>
> When transporting an elderly patient, protect the patient from the environment, since extremes in heat or cold can further reduce the body's defenses. If you have a cold or the flu, use respiratory precautions, including a face mask for yourself so that the patient is not exposed to your illness. If your patient has a cold or the flu, protect yourself. However, remember that your defense system is probably much stronger than that of the patient.

Other Diseases of Concern

Syphilis

Although syphilis is commonly thought of as a sexually transmitted disease, it is also a bloodborne disease. There is a small risk for transmission through a contaminated needlestick injury or direct blood-to-blood contact.

Whooping Cough

Whooping cough, also called pertussis, is an airborne disease caused by bacteria that mostly affects children younger than 6 years. Signs and symptoms include fever and a "whoop" sound that occurs when the patient tries to inhale after a coughing attack.

The best way to prevent exposure is to try to place a mask on the patient and on yourself.

Newly Recognized Diseases

Newly recognized diseases, such as those caused by Hantavirus or enteropathogenic *Escherichia coli* (also called *E coli*), are being reported. These diseases are not transmitted from person to person directly; rather, they are carried by a vehicle, such as food, or a vector, such as rodents. Although not a newly discovered illness, West Nile Virus has caused some concern recently. This virus' vector is the mosquito, and also affects birds. The virus is actually tracked by tests done on birds suspected of being killed by the virus. These diseases are not communicable and do not pose a risk to you during patient care.

Another virus that has caused significant concern of late is best known as <u>SARS</u>, or severe acute respiratory syndrome. SARS is a serious, potentially life-threatening viral infection caused by a recently discovered family of viruses best known as the second most common cause of the common cold. SARS usually starts with flu-like symptoms, which may progress to pneumonia, respiratory failure, and, in some cases, death. The SARS virus strain probably spread from in Guangdong province in southern China to Hong Kong, Singapore, and Taiwan. Canada has had a significant outbreak in the Toronto area. SARS is thought to be primarily transmitted by close person-to-person contact. Most cases have involved persons who lived with or cared for a person with SARS or who had exposure to contaminated secretions from a SARS patient.

Multiple antibiotic-resistant organisms have recently been the subject of media scrutiny. These organisms should be viewed as no more or less contagious than other less resistant organisms of the same type. The same precautions apply.

General Postexposure Management

In many instances, you will not know that a patient has an airborne or bloodborne disease, and you could be exposed without knowing it. The Ryan White Law requires that the hospital notify your department's <u>designated officer</u>, the person in the department who is charged with the responsibility of managing exposures and infection control issues, within 48 hours of the time the hospital identifies the patient's disease. In the event of possible exposure, there should be a protocol in place to obtain information from your local hospital or other medical resource. You should be screened and given information about the necessity of medical follow-up. Treatment depends on the disease. Your designated officer will assist you with the necessary information.

If you experience a needlestick injury or some other unprotected exposure to blood, you must notify your department's designated officer as soon as possible and complete an incident report. The designated officer can contact the hospital for information; the hospital has 48 hours to report back to the designated officer. Depending on your state laws and whether it is possible, patient testing should be done, followed by baseline testing on you.

Because there are many diseases for which there are no outward signs of infection, your protection lies in the use of PPE and prompt reporting of exposure. Be familiar with the postexposure protocols outlined in your department's exposure control plan.

> **Documentation Tips**
>
> The ability of your EMS system to support you in case of exposure to a communicable disease depends on your understanding of how exposure can occur and your immediate report of exposure to potentially infectious materials. Document the event as soon as possible to ensure that you remember all pertinent information, and report immediately after the exposure, following your service's guidelines.

Establishing an Infection Control Routine

Infection control, or the use of procedures to reduce infection in patients and health care personnel, should be an important part of your daily routine. Take the following steps when dealing with potential exposure situations:

1. **En route to the scene**, make sure that all equipment is out and available.
2. **Upon arrival**, make sure the scene is safe to enter, and then do a quick visual assessment of the patient, noting whether any blood is present.
3. **Select the proper PPE** according to the tasks you are likely to perform.
4. **Change gloves and wash hands** between patients; do not unnecessarily delay treatment for use of PPE, thereby potentially putting patients at risk. Remove gloves and other gear after contact with the patient, unless you are in the patient compartment of the ambulance. *Remember that good handwashing is the most effective way of preventing the spread of disease.*
5. **Limit the number of people** who are involved in patient care if there are multiple injuries and a substantial amount of blood at the scene.
6. **If you or your partner are exposed** while providing care, try to relieve one another as soon as possible so that you can seek care. Notify the designated officer and report the incident. This will also help to maintain confidentiality.

Be sure to routinely clean the ambulance after each run and on a daily basis. Cleaning is an essential part of the prevention and control of communicable diseases and will remove surface organisms that may remain in the unit.

You should clean your unit as quickly as possible so that it can be returned to service. Address the high-contact areas, including surfaces that were in direct contact with the patient's blood or body fluids or surfaces that you touched while caring for the patient after having contact with the patient's blood or body fluids.

Whenever possible, cleaning should be done at the hospital. If you clean the unit back at the station, make sure you have a designated area with good ventilation and a floor drain.

Bag any medical waste and dispose of it in a red bag at the hospital whenever possible. Any contaminated equipment that is left with the patient at the hospital should be cleaned by hospital staff or bagged for transport and cleaning at the station.

You can use a solution of bleach and water at a 1:10 dilution to clean the unit. A hospital-approved disinfectant that is effective against *M tuberculosis* can also be used. Use the cleaning solution in a bucket or pistol-handled spray container. Do not use alcohol or aerosol spray products to clean the unit.

Remove contaminated linen, and place it into an appropriate bag for handling. Each hospital may have a different system for handling contaminated linen; you should learn hospital protocols Figure 2-23 ▶.

Learn the regulations defining medical waste in your area. The procedures for disposal of infectious waste such as needles and heavily soiled dressings may vary from hospital to hospital and from state to state.

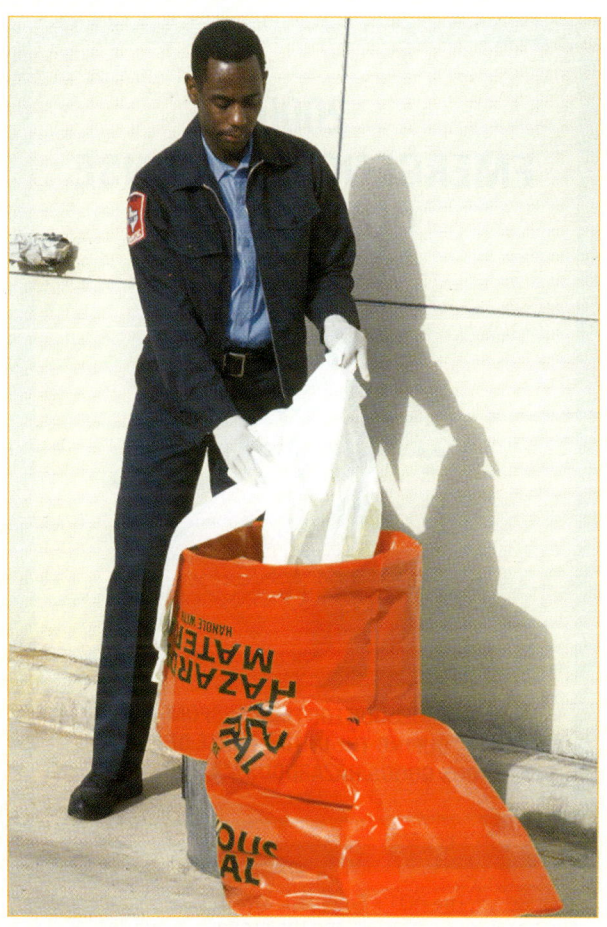

Figure 2-23 Contaminated linen should be bagged appropriately and disposed of according to your local protocols.

Illness and Injury Prevention

In the United States, injury has surpassed stroke as the third leading cause of death. For each injury-related death that occurs, there are an estimated additional 19 hospitalizations and 254 emergency department visits, and the estimated lifetime cost of injuries is greater than $114 billion. It is important that you as an EMS provider educate the public on ways to prevent injuries through the use of protective equipment and education.

Another factor to consider is the early release of patients from hospitals. Whether the reason is insurance restrictions or physician discretion, the outcome is the same—an increased number of at risk patients for EMS providers to manage.

In most areas, EMS providers are considered high-profile role models. They generally reflect the composition of the community and, in a rural setting, may be the most medically educated people. EMS providers are often considered advocates of the injured or ill and, as such, are welcomed into schools and other environments. They are considered authorities on injury and prevention.

> **A to Z Terminology Tips**
>
> **Primary injury prevention**—Preventing an injury from occurring
>
> **Secondary and tertiary prevention**—Care and rehabilitation activities, respectively, that prevent further problems as a result of an event that has already occurred
>
> **Teachable moment**—The time after an injury has occurred when the patient and observers remain acutely aware of what has happened and may be more receptive to teaching about how the event or illness could have been prevented

Prevention Strategies

There are many prevention strategies that may be implemented simply by recognizing signs and symptoms related to specific illnesses or injuries. Patient care considerations include recognizing signs and symptoms of suspected abuse and abusive situations and taking the necessary steps to resolve the conflict without the use of violence. This may involve leaving a patient temporarily until your suspicions can be reported to local law enforcement or other appropriate authorities.

Other situations include recognizing signs and symptoms of exposure to hazardous materials, temperature extremes, vectors, communicable diseases, assault and battery, and structural risks. *Remember, personal safety first!* Each of these situations may be detrimental to the EMT-I and must be considered as such. Always ensure safety before entering the scene, and take necessary BSI precautions.

Public education by way of objective, nonjudgmental, and effective communications with consideration of ethnic, religious, and social diversity is important. It is essential to recognize recurrent problems or sense the potential for recurrences and to inform people about how they can prevent recurrence through knowledge of the situation or use of protective devices. Resources for further assistance should be provided. These may include child protective services; shelters for sexual, spousal, or elder abuse; food; clothing; counseling; alternative sources of health care such as free clinics; grief support; and numerous others. Keeping a list of resources or a few pamphlets from a local shelter in your ambulance can be very beneficial in a time of crisis.

Scene Hazards

During your career, you will be exposed to many hazards. Some situations will be life threatening. In these cases, you must be properly protected, or you must avoid the hazard completely.

Hazardous Materials

Your safety is the most important consideration at a hazardous materials incident. Upon your arrival, you should first try to read labels and identification numbers. All hazardous materials should be marked with safety placards. These placards are marked with colored diamond-shaped labels (Figure 2-24). Although it is important for you to obtain information from the placards, you should never approach any object marked with a placard until the substance has been identified as not being a threat to you.

It is useful to carry binoculars in the ambulance so that you can read placards from a safe distance. A specially trained and equipped hazardous materials team will be called to handle disposal of materials and removal of patients. You should not begin caring for patients until they have been moved away from the scene or the scene is safe for you to enter.

The *Emergency Response Guidebook* from the Department of Transportation (DOT) is an important resource (Figure 2-25). It lists most hazardous materials and the proper procedures for scene control and emergency care of patients. Several similar resources are available. Some state and local government agencies may also have information about the hazardous materials in their areas. A copy of the guidebook and other information relevant to your area should be available in your unit or at the dispatch center. Thus, you should be able to begin proper emergency management as soon as the hazardous material is identified. Again, do not go into an area and risk exposure to yourself. Do not enter the area unless you are absolutely sure that no hazardous spill has occurred.

Hazardous materials are substances that may cause personal injury or property damage, and are classified according to toxicity levels, which dictate the level of protection required. The toxicity levels, which are listed on a scale of 0 to 4, measure the risk the substance poses to a person. The higher the number, the greater the toxicity and the greater the protection needed (Table 2-11). It is important to remember that you are at great risk in hazardous materials situations. *Do not enter the scene unless it is safe.*

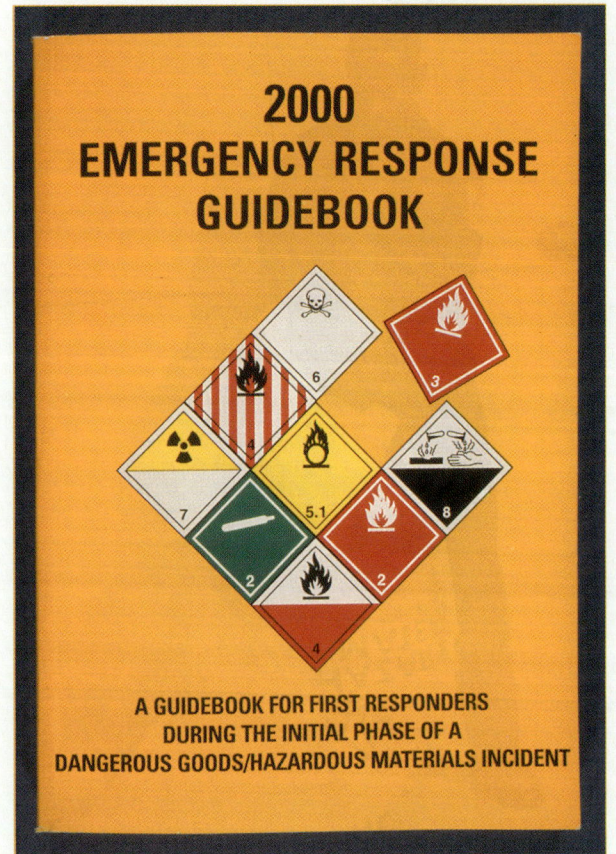

Figure 2-25 The DOT's *Emergency Response Guidebook* lists many hazardous materials and the proper procedures for scene control and emergency care of patients.

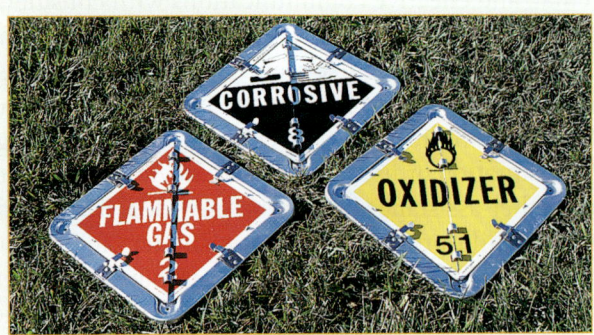

Figure 2-24 Hazardous materials safety placards are marked with colored diamond-shaped labels.

> ### EMT-I Safety
>
> EMT-Is should be aware of the potential hazards that may be present when responding to the scene. At times, these situations may be dangerous to you and your crew. The best protection when hazards are present is early recognition that a hazard may exist.

TABLE 2-11	Toxicity Levels of Hazardous Materials	
Level	Hazard*	Protection Needed
0	Little to no hazard	None
1	Slightly hazardous	Self-contained breathing apparatus only (level C suit)
2	Slightly hazardous	Self-contained breathing apparatus only (level C suit)
3	Extremely hazardous	Full protection, with no exposed skin (level A or B suit)
4	Minimal exposure causes death	Special HazMat gear (level A suit)

*Protection for levels 1 and 2 is the same, but there are differences in the toxicity level of the materials in these two categories. For more information on classification of hazardous materials, see Table 36-1.

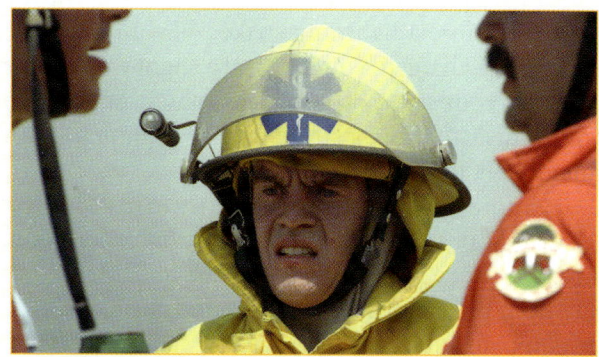

Figure 2-26 Wear a helmet made of a certified electrical non-conductor material, making sure that the chin strap is fastened securely.

Electricity

Electrical shock can be produced by human-made sources (power lines) or natural sources (lightning). No matter what the source, you must evaluate the risk to you and to the patient before you begin patient care.

Power Lines

The amount of current that is involved greatly affects the level of risk for injury. Your local power company can help you by providing training to evaluate the risks in electrical emergencies. Its staff can also teach you how to deal with power lines once the risks have been determined. You should not touch downed power lines. Dealing with power lines is beyond the scope of EMT-I training. However, you should mark off a danger zone around the downed lines.

Energized, or "live" power lines, especially high-voltage lines, behave in unpredictable ways. You need in-depth training to be able to handle the equipment that is used in an electrical emergency. The equipment also has specific storage needs and requires careful cleaning. Dirt or other contaminants can make this equipment useless or dangerous.

At the scene of a motor vehicle crash, above-ground and below-ground power lines may become hazards. Disrupted overhead wires may or may not be a visible hazard. You must be careful even if you do not see sparks coming from the lines. Visible sparks are not always present in charged wires. The area around downed power lines is always a danger zone. This danger zone extends well beyond the immediate accident scene.

Use the utility poles as landmarks for establishing the perimeter of the danger zone. The danger zone must be a restricted area. Only emergency personnel, equipment, and vehicles are allowed inside this area.

If you must enter this type of situation, be sure to wear the proper protective equipment according to the type of incident. A helmet and turnout gear Figure 2-26 are typically indicated, although you cannot count on this equipment for complete protection from electrical hazards. Other protective equipment may be needed. The "Protective Clothing" section in this chapter covers turnouts and helmets more in depth.

Lightning

Lightning is a complex natural phenomenon. You are unwise to think "lightning never strikes in the same place twice." If the right conditions remain, a repeated strike can occur in the same area.

Lightning is a threat in two ways: through a direct hit and through ground current. After the lightning bolt strikes, the current drains along the earth, following the most conductive pathway. To avoid being injured by a ground current, stay away from drainage ditches, moist areas, small depressions, and wet ropes. If you are involved in a rescue operation, you may need to delay

 EMT-I Tips

Recognize the warning signs before a lightning strike. You may feel a tingling sensation on your skin, or your hair may stand on end. Move immediately to a low-lying area. If caught in an open area, make yourself the smallest possible target.

it until the storm has passed. Recognize the warning signs just before a lightning strike. As your surroundings become charged, you may feel a slight tingling sensation on your skin, or your hair may even stand on end. In this situation, a strike may be imminent. Move immediately to the lowest possible area.

If you are caught in an open area, try to make yourself the smallest possible target for a direct hit or for ground current. To keep from being hit by the initial strike, stay away from projections from the ground, such as a single tree. Drop all equipment, particularly metal objects that project above your body. Avoid fences and other metal objects. These can transmit current from the initial strike over a long distance. Position yourself in a low crouch. This position exposes only your feet to the ground current. If you sit, both your feet and your buttocks are exposed. Place an object made of nonconductive material, such as a blanket, under your feet. Get inside a car or your unit, if possible, as vehicles will protect you from lightning.

Fire

You will often be called to the scene of a fire to care for victims or to stand by in anticipation of possible injuries to fire personnel on the scene. Therefore, you should understand some basic information about fire. There are five common hazards in a fire:

1. Smoke
2. Oxygen deficiency
3. High ambient temperatures
4. Toxic gases
5. Building collapse

Smoke is made up of particles of tar and carbon. These particles irritate the respiratory system on contact. Most smoke particles are trapped in the upper respiratory system, but many smaller particles enter the lungs. In addition to airway irritation, some smoke particles may be deadly. You must be trained in the use of appropriate airway protection, such as a self-contained breathing apparatus or a disposable short-term device, and have it available at all fire scenes (Figure 2-27).

Fire consumes oxygen, particularly in an enclosed space, and will make breathing difficult for anyone in that space. The high ambient temperatures in a fire can result in thermal burns and damage to the respiratory system. Breathing air that is heated to more than 120°F (49°C) can damage the respiratory system.

A typical building fire emits a number of toxic gases, including carbon monoxide and carbon dioxide. Carbon monoxide is a colorless, odorless gas that is responsible for more fire deaths each year than any

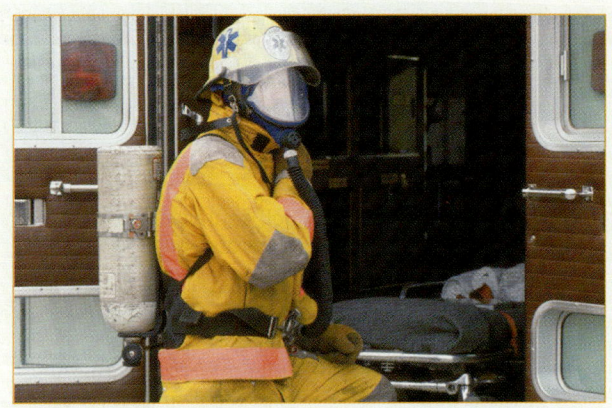

Figure 2-27 You should be trained in the use of a self-contained breathing apparatus and have it available if you may be working near fire scenes.

other by-product of combustion. Carbon monoxide has an affinity for hemoglobin that is 200 times greater than that of oxygen. It blocks the ability of the hemoglobin to transport oxygen to your body tissues. Carbon dioxide is also a colorless, odorless gas. Exposure causes increased respirations, dizziness, and sweating. Breathing concentrations of carbon dioxide that are higher than 10% to 12% will result in death within a few minutes.

During and after a fire, there is always a possibility that all or part of the burned structure will collapse. Therefore, you should never run into a burning building. Your hasty entry into a burning structure may result in serious injury and possibly death. Once inside the burning building, you are subject to an uncontrolled, hostile environment. Fires are not selective about their victims. You must be extremely cautious whenever you are near a burning structure or one in which a fire has just been put out. Fire suppression crews will be at the scene, and EMT-Is should follow their directions.

Fuel and fuel systems of vehicles that have been involved in crashes are also a hazard. A car leaking fuel may ignite under the right conditions. If you see or smell a fuel leak or if people are trapped in the vehicle, you must coordinate appropriate fire protection.

Make sure that you are properly protected if there is or has been a fire in the vehicle. Wear appropriate respiratory protection and thermal protection, as the smoke from a vehicle fire contains many toxic by-products. The use of appropriate protective gear at a crash scene can reduce your risk of injury. Avoid using oxygen in or near a vehicle that is smoking, smoldering, or leaking fuel.

Protective Clothing: Preventing Injury

Wearing protective clothing and other appropriate gear is critical to your personal safety. Become familiar with the protective equipment that is available to you. Then you will know what clothing and gear are needed for the job. You will also be able to adapt or change items as the situation and environment change. Remember that protective clothing and gear are safe only when they are in good condition. It is your responsibility to inspect your clothing and gear. Learn to recognize how wear and tear can make your equipment unsafe. Be sure to inspect equipment before you use it, even if you must do so at the scene.

Clothing that is worn for rescue must be appropriate for the activity and the environmental conditions in which the activity will take place. For example, bunker gear that is worn for firefighting may be too restrictive for working in a confined space. In every situation involving blood or other body fluids, be sure to follow BSI precautions. You must protect yourself and the patient by wearing gloves and eye protection and any additional protective clothing that may be needed.

Cold Weather Clothing

When dressing for cold weather, you should wear several layers of clothing. Multiple layers provide much better protection than a single thick cover. You have more flexibility to control your body temperature by adding or removing a layer. Cold weather protection should consist of at least the following three layers:

1. **A thin inner layer** (sometimes called the transport layer) next to your skin. This layer pulls moisture away from your skin, keeping you dry and warm. Underwear made of polypropylene or polyester material works well.
2. **A thermal middle layer** of bulkier material for insulation. Wool has been the material of choice for warmth, but newer materials, such as polyester pile, are also commonly used.
3. **An outer layer** that will resist chilling winds and wet conditions, such as rain, sleet, or snow. The two top layers should have zippers to allow you to vent some body heat if you become too warm.

When choosing clothing to protect yourself from the weather, pay attention to the type of material used. Cotton should be avoided in cold, wet environments. Cotton tends to absorb moisture, causing chilling from wetness. For example, if you wear cotton trousers and walk through wet grass, the cotton soaks up the moisture from the grass. However, cotton is appropriate in warm, dry weather because it absorbs moisture and pulls heat away from the body.

As an outer layer in cold weather, you might consider plastic-coated nylon, as it provides good waterproof protection. However, it can also hold in body heat and perspiration. Newer, less airtight materials allow perspiration and some heat to escape while the material retains its water resistance. Avoid flammable or meltable synthetic material anytime there is a possibility of fire.

Turnout Gear

Turnout or bunker gear is a fire service term for protective clothing designed for use in firefighting environments Figure 2-28. Turnout gear provides head-to-toe protection. It uses different layers of fabric or other material to provide protection from the heat of fire, to reduce trauma from impact or cuts, and to keep water away from the body. Like most protective clothing, turnout gear adds weight and reduces range of motion to some degree.

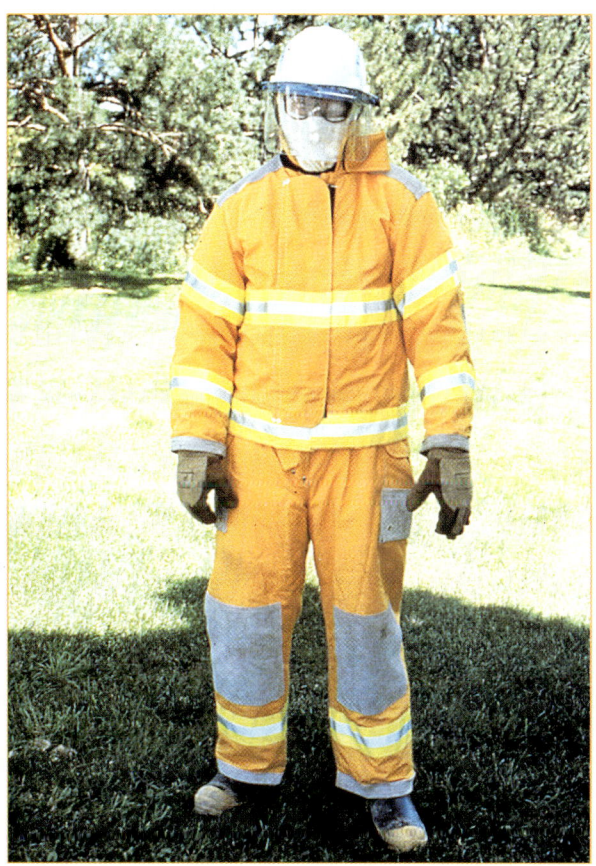

Figure 2-28 Turnout or bunker gear provides complete head-to-toe protection.

The exterior fabrics provide increased protection from cuts and abrasions. They also act as a barrier to high external temperatures. In cold weather, an insulated thermal inner layer of material that helps to retain body heat is recommended.

Turnout gear or a bunker jacket provides minimal protection from electrical shock. But it does protect you from heat, fire, possible flashover, and flying sparks. The front opening of the jacket should be fastened, and the jacket should be worn with the collar up and closed in front to protect your neck and upper chest. Proper fit is important so that you can move freely while still being protected.

Gloves

Firefighting gloves will provide the best protection from heat, cold, and cuts Figure 2-29 ▼, but these gloves reduce manual dexterity. In addition, firefighting gloves will not protect you from electrical hazards. In rescue situations, you must be able to use your hands freely to operate rescue tools, provide patient care, and perform other duties. Puncture-proof leather gloves, with latex gloves underneath, will permit free use of your hands with added protection from injury and body fluids. The "Communicable Diseases" section in this chapter discusses the use of latex gloves for infectious exposure prevention.

Helmets

You should wear a helmet any time you are working in a fall zone. A fall zone is an area where you are likely to encounter falling objects. The helmet should provide top and side impact protection. It should also have a secure chin strap Figure 2-30 ▶. Objects will often fall one after another. If the strap is not secure, the first

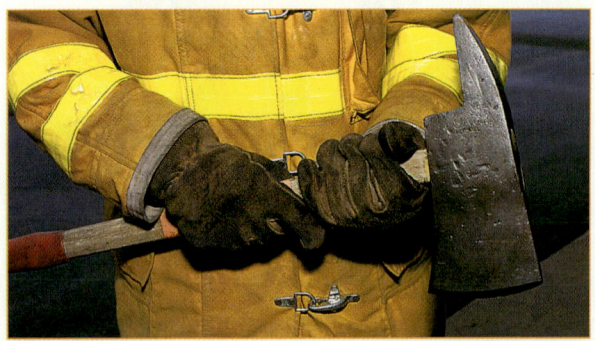

Figure 2-29 Firefighting gloves protect your hands and wrists from heat, cold, and injury.

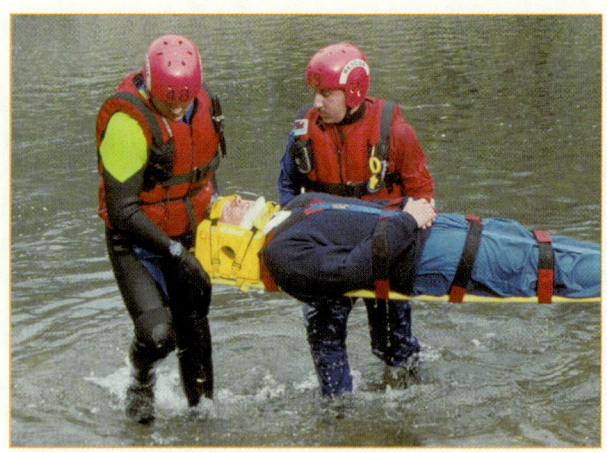

Figure 2-30 A helmet with side impact protection and a chin strap will not dislodge if struck by an object.

falling object may knock off your helmet. This leaves your head unprotected as the remaining objects fall.

Construction-type helmets are not well suited for rescue situations. They offer minimal impact protection and have inadequate chin straps. Modern fire helmets afford the best impact protection. In cold weather, you can lose significant body heat if you are not wearing a hat or helmet. An insulated hat made from wool or a synthetic material can be pulled down over the face and the base of the skull to reduce heat loss in extremely cold weather.

In situations that may involve electrical hazard, you should always wear a helmet with chin strap and face shield (see Figure 2-26). The shell of the helmet should be made of a certified electrical nonconductor. The chin strap should not stretch. In fact, it should fasten securely so that the helmet stays in place if you are knocked down or a power line hits your head. You should also be able to lock the face shield on the helmet. This will protect your face and eyes from power lines and flying sparks. A standard fire turnout helmet should meet all of these needs.

Boots

Boots should be water resistant, well-fitting, and flexible so that you can walk long distances comfortably. If you will be working outdoors, you should choose boots that cover and protect your ankles, keeping out stones, debris, and snow. Steel-toed boots are preferred Figure 2-31 ▶. In cold weather, your boots must also protect you from the cold. Leather is one of the best materials for boots. However, other materials, such as Gore-Tex® water-repellent fabric, are also very good.

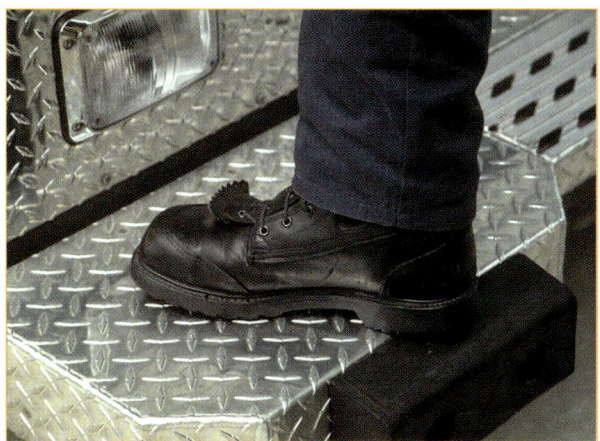

Figure 2-31 Boots should cover and protect your ankles, keeping out stones, debris, and snow. Steel-toed boots are preferred.

The soles of your boots must provide traction. Lug-type soles may grip well in snow, but they become very slippery when caked with mud.

The fit of boots and shoes is extremely important because a minor annoyance can develop into a disabling injury. You may develop painful blisters if your feet slip around inside your boots. However, make sure you have enough room to wiggle your toes.

Boots should be puncture-resistant, protect the toes, and provide foot and ankle support. It may be difficult to obtain a good fit with firefighting boots; shoe inserts or sock layering may be needed for a comfortable fit. Make sure the tops of your boots are sealed off to prevent entry of rain, snow, glass, or other materials.

Socks will keep your feet warm and provide some cushioning for you as you walk. In cold weather, two pairs of socks are generally preferable to one thick pair. A thin sock next to the foot helps to wick perspiration away to a thicker, outer sock. This tends to keep your feet warmer, drier, and generally more comfortable. When you purchase new shoes or boots, keep these points in mind.

Eye Protection

The human eye is fragile, and permanent loss of sight can occur from very minor injuries. You need to protect your eyes from blood and other body fluids, foreign objects, plants, insects, and debris from extrication. You may wear eyeglasses with side shields during routine patient care. (The "Communicable Diseases" section in this chapter covers eye protection against splattering body fluids.)

When tools are being used during extrication, you should wear a face shield or goggles. In these instances, prescription eyeglasses do not provide adequate protection. In snow or white sand, particularly at higher altitudes, you must protect your eyes from ultraviolet exposure. Specially designed glasses or goggles can provide this protection. In addition, your eye protection must be adaptable to the weather and the physical demands of the task. It is critical that you have clear vision at all times.

Ear Protection

Exposure to loud noises for long periods can cause permanent hearing loss. Certain equipment, such as helicopters, some extrication tools, and sirens, produce high levels of noise. Wearing soft foam industrial-type earplugs usually provides adequate protection.

Skin Protection

Your skin needs protection against sunburn while you are working outdoors. Long-term exposure to the sun increases the possibility of skin cancer. It might be considered an annoyance, but sunburn is a type of thermal burn. In reflective areas such as sand, water, and snow, your risk of sunburn increases. Protect your skin by applying a sunscreen with a minimum SPF (sun protection factor) rating of 15.

Body Armor

Although policy and common sense direct avoidance of situations that may involve shootings, EMS responders in some areas wear body armor (bulletproof or flak vests) for personal protection. Several types of body armor are available. They range from extremely lightweight and flexible to heavy and bulky. The lighter vests do not stop large-caliber bullets. However, they offer more flexibility and are preferred by most law enforcement personnel. Lighter vests are commonly worn under a uniform shirt or jacket. The larger, heavier vests are worn on the outside of your uniform.

Violent Situations

The safety of you and your team is of primary concern. Civil disturbances, domestic disputes, and crime scenes, especially those involving gangs, can create many hazards for EMS personnel. Large gatherings of hostile or potentially hostile people pose an even greater threat. Several agencies will respond to large civil disturbances. In these instances, it is important for you to know who is in

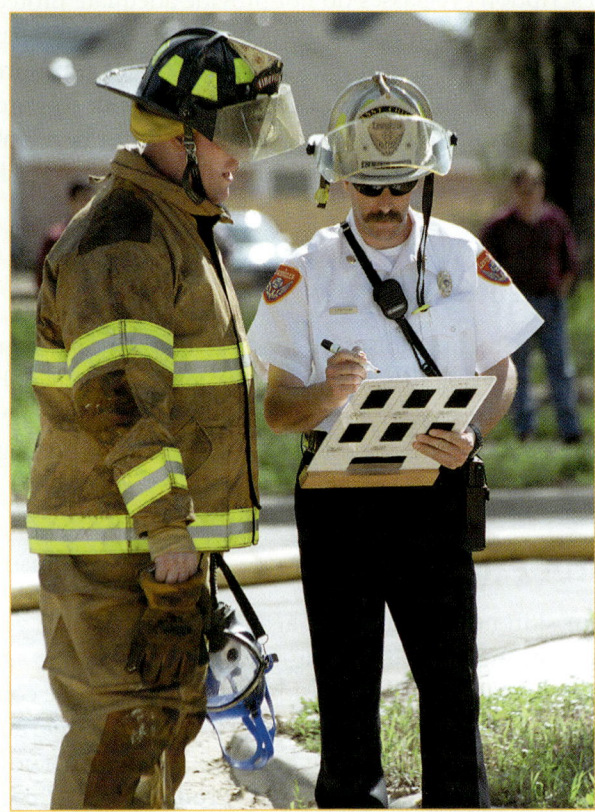

Figure 2-32 Several agencies may respond to large disturbances. It is important for you to know who is in command and will be issuing orders.

nel. A perpetrator who is still at the scene could reappear and threaten you and your partner or attempt to further injure the patient you are treating. Bystanders who are trying to be helpful may interfere with your emergency medical care. Family members may be distraught and not understand what you are doing when you attempt to splint an injured extremity and the patient cries out in pain. Be sure that you have adequate assistance from the appropriate public safety agency in these cases.

Sometimes EMT-Is are at a scene where a dangerous situation is underway, such as a hostage situation or riot. In these instances, it may be necessary for EMS personnel to be protected from projectiles such as bullets, bottles, and rocks. Law enforcement personnel will ordinarily provide for <u>concealment</u> or cover of personnel who are involved in the response to the incident. <u>Cover</u> involves the tactical use of an impenetrable barrier for protection. Concealment involves hiding behind objects such as shrubs or bushes to limit a person's visibility of you. EMT-Is should not be placed in a position that will endanger their lives or safety during such incidents.

Remember that your personal safety is of utmost importance. You must thoroughly understand the risks of each environment you enter. Whenever you are in doubt about your safety, do not put yourself at risk. Never enter an unstable environment, such as a shooting, a brawl, a hostage situation, or a riot. Therefore, as part of sizing up the scene, evaluate it for the potential for violence. If possible, call for additional resources. Failure to do so may put you and your partner at serious risk. Rely on the advice of law enforcement personnel, as they have more experience and expertise in handling these situations.

If you believe that an event is a crime scene, you must attempt to maintain the chain of evidence by disturbing the scene as little as possible. Remember however, that patient care takes priority.

command and will be issuing orders Figure 2-32 . However, you and your partner may be on your own when a group of people grows larger and becomes increasingly hostile. In these cases, you should call law enforcement immediately if they are not already at the scene. You may need to remove yourself from the scene and wait for law enforcement to arrive before you can begin treatment.

Remember that you and your partner must be protected from the dangers at the scene before you can provide patient care. Law enforcement must make sure the scene is safe before you and your partner enter. A crime scene often poses potential problems for EMS person-

Behavioral Emergencies

Although Chapter 27 goes into greater depth about behavioral emergencies, consider these questions as you evaluate the patient in terms of a behavioral or psychiatric emergency that may lead to a violent patient reaction:

- How does this patient relate to you? Are your questions answered appropriately? Are the patient's vocabulary and expressions what you would expect under the circumstances?

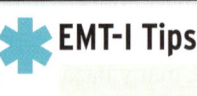

EMT-I Tips

Law enforcement must make sure the scene is safe before you and your partner enter.

- Is the patient withdrawn or detached? Is the patient hostile or friendly?
- Does the patient understand why you are present?
- How is the patient dressed? Is the dress appropriate for the time of the year and occasion? Are the clothes clean? Dirty?
- Does the patient appear relaxed, stiff, or guarded? Are the patient's movements coordinated? Does the patient make sudden movements? Is the patient hyperactive?
- Are the patient's movements purposeful, for example, in putting his or her clothes on? Are the actions aimless, such as sitting and rocking back and forth in a chair?
- Has the patient harmed himself or herself? Is there damage to the surroundings?
- Does the patient appear physically rigid, or is there waxy flexibility?
- What are the patient's facial expressions? Are they bland or flat, or are they expressive? Does the patient show joy, fear, or anger to appropriate stimuli? If so, to what degree?

It might not be possible for you to obtain answers to all of these questions. Sometimes a patient who is experiencing a behavioral emergency will not respond at all. In those cases, the patient's facial expressions, pulse and respirations, tears, sweating, and blushing may be significant indicators of his or her emotional state.

The following principal determinants of violence, although not intended to be all-inclusive, are of value to the EMT-I:

- **History.** Has the patient previously exhibited hostile, overly aggressive, or violent behavior? This information should be solicited by EMS personnel at the scene or requested from law enforcement personnel, family, or previous EMS records.
- **Posture.** How is the patient sitting or standing? Does the patient appear to be tense or rigid, or is the patient sitting on the edge of the bed, chair, or wherever he or she is positioned? The observation of increased tension as shown by physical posture is often a warning signal of hostile behavior.
- **Vocal activity.** What is the nature of the speech the patient is using? Loud, obscene, erratic, and bizarre speech patterns usually indicate emotional distress. The patient who is conversing in quiet, ordered speech is not as likely to strike out against others as is the patient who is yelling and screaming.
- **Physical activity.** Perhaps one of the most demonstrative factors to look for is the motor activity of a person who is undergoing a behavioral crisis. The patient who is pacing, cannot sit still, or is displaying protection of his or her boundaries of personal space needs careful watching. Agitation is a prognostic sign to be observed with great care and scrutiny.

Other factors to take into consideration for potential violence include the following:

- Poor impulse control
- The behavior triad of truancy, fighting, and uncontrollable temper
- Instability of family structure
- Inability to keep a steady job
- Tattoos, such as those with gang identification or statements like "born to kill" or "born to lose"
- Substance abuse
- Functional disorder (If the patient says that he or she is hearing voices that say to kill, believe it!)
- Depression, which accounts for 20% of violent attacks

You are the Provider / Summary

1. What are some of the potential exposure concerns that the EMT-I should consider with this call?

It is prudent for EMS personnel to assume that all patients are a potential exposure threat; therefore, the appropriate precautions should be taken.

2. What steps can be taken to protect emergency personnel from infectious disease exposure?

Body substance isolation precautions are necessary, including eye and facial protection and gloves. These measures are designed to prevent emergency personnel from coming into contact with potentially communicable diseases. The goal is to interrupt the transmission of germs by decreasing the chance of contact.

3. What is your next step in the treatment of this patient?

While protecting the patient's C-spine, you must quickly remove him from his car and begin care aimed at supporting airway, breathing, and circulation.

4. What else should you consider when treating this patient?

The mechanism of injury is an important consideration in helping to predict potentially life-threatening injuries. This, along with careful observation of the scene, will facilitate the most effective care, both at the scene and in the emergency department.

5. How can the EMT-I help reduce the occurrence of traumatic injuries?

By observing certain behavior patterns of the driver (eg, not using seatbelts, driving with excessive speed) that contribute to injury severity, the EMT-I can help implement community education programs that would help decrease the potential for serious injury or death.

6. What measures can the EMT-I take to help prevent the spread of potentially infectious diseases?

According to the Centers for Disease Control and Prevention (CDC), frequent and thorough handwashing, especially between patients, is the single most effective way to prevent the spread of potentially infectious diseases.

Prep Kit

Ready for Review

- EMT-Is will encounter death, dying patients, and the families and friends of those who have died. Death will be no stranger to EMS personnel. Therefore, coming to grips with death and dying and understanding the concerns of the dying patient, assisting a family following the death of a loved one, and dealing with one's own feelings about death are personally and professionally important.

- When signs of stress such as fatigue; anxiety; anger; feelings of hopelessness, worthlessness, or guilt; and other such indicators manifest themselves, behavioral problems can develop. Recognizing the signs of stress is important for all EMT-Is.

- Posttraumatic stress disorder is a syndrome with onset following a traumatic, usually life-threatening event.

- As an EMT-I, you will arrive at scenes where potential danger to you is easily apparent. Every patient encounter should be considered potentially dangerous. Therefore, it is essential that you take all available precautions to minimize exposure and risk. Potential risks include scene hazards and infectious and communicable diseases.

- Infectious diseases can be transmitted in one of four ways: direct transmission, vehicle-borne, vector-borne, and airborne. Even if you are exposed to an infectious disease, your risk of becoming ill is minimal. Whether an acute infection occurs depends on several factors, including the amount and type of infectious organisms and your resistance to the infection caused by those organisms. Most germs colonize the human body without causing any disease.

- You can take several steps to protect yourself against exposure to infectious diseases, including remaining up-to-date with recommended vaccinations, using universal and BSI precautions at all times, and handling all needles and other sharp objects with great care. Sharp items should be disposed of in closed, rigid, puncture-proof containers.

- Because it is often impossible to tell which patients have infectious diseases, you should avoid direct contact with the blood and body fluids of all patients. Use special caution if you have any open sores or cuts, no matter how small. If you think you may have been exposed to an infectious disease, see your physician (or your employer's designated infection control officer) immediately.

- Five infectious diseases of special concern are HIV infection, hepatitis B, meningitis, tuberculosis, and SARS. Of these, meningitis, tuberculosis, and SARS are transmitted through the air. The tubercle bacillus that causes tuberculosis can remain dormant for decades without causing disease.

- Because medical therapy is almost always effective if you have not already become ill, you should get a tuberculosis test on an annual basis. Hepatitis B is by far the most common threat to health care workers. It is highly contagious and usually transmitted by needlestick. Vaccination against hepatitis B vaccine is highly recommended.

- Meningitis is rare; your risk of disease, even if you are exposed, is very small. Using a mask and gloves will go a long way to protect you against meningitis.

- You should know what to do if you are exposed to an airborne or bloodborne disease. Your department's designated officer will be able to help you follow the protocol set up in your area.

- Infection control should be an important part of your daily routine. Be sure to follow the proper steps when dealing with potential exposure situations.

- During your career, you will be exposed to many hazards. Some situations will be life-threatening. In these cases you should be properly protected, or you must avoid the situation altogether.

- Scene hazards include potential exposure to hazardous materials, electricity, and fire. At a hazardous materials incident, your safety is the most important consideration. Never approach an object labeled with a hazardous materials placard. Use binoculars to read the placards from a safe distance.

Technology

- Interactivities
- Vocabulary Explorer
- Anatomy Review
- Web Links
- Online Review Manual

Prep Kit continued...

- Do not begin caring for patients until they have been moved away from the scene by the hazardous materials team and properly decontaminated or the scene has been made safe for you to enter.

- Electrical shock can be produced by power lines or by lightning. If you encounter a downed power line, do not touch it. Mark off a danger zone around the downed lines and contact the power company. To protect yourself from lightning, recognize the warning signs just before a lightning strike. Move immediately to the lowest area possible. If you are in an open area, make yourself the smallest target by dropping all equipment and getting into a low crouch. If possible, get inside a car or your unit.

- There are five common hazards in a fire: smoke, oxygen deficiency, high ambient temperatures, toxic gases, and building collapse. You must be trained in the use of appropriate protective equipment and have it available at all scenes. Do not rush into a burning building to retrieve a patient. This is a function of the fire department.

- Violent situations such as civil disturbances, domestic disputes, and crime scenes can create many hazards for EMS personnel. Whenever you are in doubt about your safety, do not put yourself at risk. If you see the potential for violence when you are sizing up the scene, call for the appropriate resources. Rely on the advice of law enforcement.

- Remember, your personal safety is of the utmost importance.

Vital Vocabulary

body substance isolation (BSI) An infection control concept and practice that assumes that all body fluids are potentially infectious.

burnout A condition of chronic fatigue and frustration that results from mounting stress over time.

carrier An animal or person who may transmit an infectious disease but may be asymptomatic.

communicable disease Any disease that can be spread from person to person or from animal to person.

concealment The use of objects such as shrubs or bushes to limit a person's visibility of you.

contagious The capability of transmitting an infectious disease from one person to another.

contamination The presence of infectious organisms on or in objects such as dressings, water, food, needles, wounds, or a patient's body.

cover The tactical use of an impenetrable barrier to conceal EMS personnel and protect them from projectiles (for example, bullets, bottles, and rocks).

critical incident stress debriefing (CISD) A confidential group discussion of a severely stressful incident that usually occurs within 24 to 72 hours following the incident.

critical incident stress management (CISM) A process that confronts responses to critical incidents and defuses them.

dependent lividity Blood settling to the lowest point of the body, causing discoloration of the skin.

designated officer The person in the department who is charged with the responsibility of managing exposures and infection control issues.

direct contact Exposure to or transmission of a communicable disease from one person to another by physical contact.

exposure A situation in which a person has had contact with blood, body fluids, tissues, or airborne particles that increases the risk of disease transmission.

exposure control plan A comprehensive plan that helps employees reduce their risk of exposure to or acquisition of communicable diseases.

general adaptation syndrome The body's three-stage response to stress. First, stress causes the body to trigger an alarm response, followed by a stage of reaction and resistance, and then recovery, or if the stress is prolonged, exhaustion.

hepatitis Inflammation of the liver, usually caused by a virus, that causes fever, loss of appetite, jaundice, fatigue, and altered liver function.

HIV infection Infection with the human immunodeficiency virus (HIV) that can progress to acquired immunodeficiency syndrome (AIDS).

host The organism or person attacked by the infecting agent.

indirect contact Exposure or transmission of disease from one person to another by contact with a contaminated object.

infection The invasion of a host or host tissues by organisms such as bacteria, viruses, or parasites, with or without signs or symptoms of disease.

infection control Procedures to reduce transmission of infection among patients and health care personnel.

infectious disease A disease that is caused by infection or one that is capable of being transmitted with or without direct contact.

meningitis An inflammation of the meningeal coverings of the brain; it is usually caused by a virus or a bacterium.

Occupational Safety and Health Administration (OSHA) The federal regulatory compliance agency that develops, publishes, and enforces guidelines concerning safety in the workplace.

pathogen A microorganism that is capable of causing disease in a susceptible host.

personal protective equipment (PPE) Protective equipment that the Occupational Safety and Health Administration (OSHA) requires to be made available to EMS providers. In the case of infection risk, PPE blocks entry of an organism into the body.

posttraumatic stress disorder (PTSD) A delayed stress reaction to a previous incident. This delayed reaction is the result of one or more unresolved issues concerning the incident.

putrefaction Decomposition of body tissues.

rigor mortis Stiffening of the body, which is a definitive sign of death.

SARS (severe acute respiratory syndrome) Potentially life-threatening viral infection that usually starts with flu-like symptoms.

stress Any demand that is placed on the body, either physical or psychological.

stressors Include emotional, physical, and environmental conditions that may cause a variety of physiologic, physical, and psychologic responses.

transmission The way in which an infectious agent is spread: contact, airborne, by vehicles (for example, food or needles), or by vectors.

tuberculosis A chronic bacterial disease caused by *Mycobacterium tuberculosis* that usually affects the lungs but also can affect other organs such as the brain or kidneys.

universal precautions Protective measures developed by the Centers for Disease Control and Prevention (CDC) for use in dealing with objects, blood, body fluids, or other potential exposure risks of communicable disease.

virulence The strength or ability of a pathogen to produce disease.

Assessment in Action

You and your partner have been asked to participate in the department's health and wellness committee. You have been asked to prepare a list of issues to bring to a meeting.

After reviewing the health and safety records of the department, you notice that several issues need to be addressed. There is a need to update the exposure control plan. You also notice that there is no wellness program in place. You feel that a wellness program will not only help your department, but will also help providers teach and follow important health and safety aspects during public education events. You want to find out what providers currently know about safety and wellness.

1. All of the following are considered components of a wellness program for the EMS provider, except:
   A. safety.
   B. compensation.
   C. health.
   D. well-being.

2. The difference between BSI precautions and universal precautions is:
   A. universal precautions are designed to approach all body fluids as being potentially infectious.
   B. BSI precautions are designed to approach all body fluids as being potentially infectious.
   C. BSI is not a concept that applies to fire and EMS personnel.
   D. universal precautions were developed by OSHA and BSI precautions were developed by the CDC.

3. Contact with blood, other body fluids, tissues, or airborne droplets by direct or indirect contact is called:
   A. BSI.
   B. a pathogen.
   C. an infection.
   D. an exposure.

4. One of the reasons that EMS providers may become involved in illness and injury prevention programs in the community is because:
   A. they have significant down time to work on prevention.
   B. insurance companies pay for injury prevention services done by EMS providers.
   C. patients are more likely to listen to an EMS provider.
   D. EMS providers are considered role models within the community.

5. As an EMS provider, you may have to care for injured people at a fire scene or be on standby in case someone is injured. Of the following, which is not a common hazard of fire?
   A. Oxygen deficiency
   B. Toxic gases
   C. Low ambient temperature
   D. Building collapse

6. When EMS providers are called to a potential hazardous materials incident, the resource that all responding units should have is:
   A. a DMV driver's manual.
   B. an Emergency Response Guidebook.
   C. a Medical Care of Hazardous Materials manual.
   D. an NIOSH manual.

Points to Ponder

Your department has decided to take a proactive stance on establishing a fitness program for all providers. You are asked to take the lead in advocating this program to all personnel. You believe it is a good idea and you are in full support of this initiative. When you start talking to some of your colleagues about this idea, they get very defensive and do not understand why the department is getting involved in dictating their lifestyle outside of work. How could you defend this program and present it as an important and valuable initiative for the wellness of all providers?

Issues: Serving as a Role Model for Other EMS Providers, Valuing the Need to Assess Lifestyle, Challenging Oneself to Teach Wellness, Improving Personal Physical Well-being

Medical, Legal, and Ethical Issues

1999 Objectives

Cognitive

1-1.25 Review legal and ethical responsibilities. (p 78)
1-1.26 Identify and explain the importance of laws pertinent to the EMT-Intermediate. (p 78)
1-1.27 Differentiate between licensure and certification as they apply to the EMT-Intermediate. (p 80)
1-1.28 List the specific problems or conditions encountered while providing care that an EMT-Intermediate is required to report, and identify each instance to whom the report is to be made. (p 88)
1-1.29 Review the following terms: abandonment, advance directives, assault, battery, breach of duty, confidentiality, consent (expressed, implied, informed, involuntary), do not resuscitate (DNR) orders, duty to act, emancipated minor, false imprisonment, immunity, liability, libel, minor, negligence, proximate cause, scope of practice, slander, standard of care, and tort. (p 78)
1-1.30 Differentiate between the scope of practice and the standard of care for EMT-Intermediate practice. (p 78)
1-1.31 Discuss the concept of medical direction and its relationship to the standard of care of an EMT-Intermediate. (p 80)
1-1.32 Review the four elements that must be present in order to prove negligence. (p 81)
1-1.33 Given a scenario in which a patient is injured while an EMT-Intermediate is providing care, determine whether the four components of negligence are present. (p 81)
1-1.34 Given a scenario, demonstrate patient care behaviors that would protect the EMT-Intermediate from claims of negligence. (p 82)
1-1.35 Explain the concept of liability as it might apply to EMT-Intermediate practice, including physicians providing medical direction and EMT-Intermediate supervision of other care providers. (p 79)
1-1.36 Review the legal concept of immunity, including Good Samaritan statutes and government immunity, as it applies to the EMT-Intermediate. (p 85)
1-1.37 Review the importance and necessity of patient confidentiality and the standards for maintaining patient confidentiality which apply to the EMT-Intermediate. (p 88)
1-1.38 Review the steps to take if a patient refuses care. (p 85)
1-1.39 Identify legal issues involved in the decision not to transport a patient, or to reduce the level of care being provided during transportation. (p 85)
1-1.40 Review the conditions under which use of force, including restraint, is acceptable. (p 84)
1-1.41 Explain the purpose of advance directives relative to patient care and how the EMT-Intermediate should care for a patient who is covered by an advance directive. (p 86)
1-1.42 Discuss the responsibilities of the EMT-Intermediate relative to resuscitation efforts for patients who are potential organ donors. (p 90)
1-1.43 Review the importance of providing accurate documentation (oral and written) in substantiating an incident. (p 89)
1-1.44 Review the characteristics of a patient care report required to make it an effective legal document. (p 89)
1-1.45 Review the premise that should underlie the EMT-Intermediate's ethical decisions in out-of-hospital care. (p 87)
1-1.46 Review the relationship between the law and ethics in EMS. (p 87)
1-1.47 Identify the issues surrounding the use of advance directives in making an out-of-hospital resuscitation decision. (p 87)
1-1.48 Describe the criteria necessary to honor an advance directive in your state. (p 87)

Affective

1-1.68 Advocate the need to show respect for the rights and feelings of the patient. (p 87)
1-1.69 Assess his/her personal commitment to protecting patient confidentiality. (p 88)
1-1.70 Defend personal beliefs about withholding or stopping patient care. (p 85)
1-1.71 Defend the value of advance medical directives. (p 86)
1-1.72 Reinforce the patient's autonomy in the decision-making process. (p 82)
1-1.73 Given a scenario, defend an EMT-Intermediate's actions in a situation where a physician orders therapy the EMT-Intermediate feels to be detrimental to the patient's best interests. (p 78)

Psychomotor

None

3

1985 Objectives

1.1.5 Describe the differences between ethical behavior and legal requirements. (p 78)

1.1.6 State specific activities that are most appropriate to ethical behavior. (p 82)

1.1.7 Identify whether a particular activity is unethical and/or illegal, given certain patient care situations. (p 81)

1.1.8 Identify whether a particular activity is ethical or unethical given certain patient care situations. (p 82)

1.2.22 Describe the ability of physician run critique based on documentation. (p 89)

1.3.1 Discuss the significance and scope of the following in relationship to EMT practice: State Medical Practice Act, Good Samaritan Act/Civil Immunity, state EMS statutes, state motor vehicle codes, and state and local guidelines for "Do Not Resuscitate." (p 80)

1.3.2 Define the following: negligence, medical liability, tort, duty to act, battery, slander, informed consent, expressed consent, implied consent, abandonment, libel, assault, and false imprisonment. (p 81)

1.3.3 Describe the significance of accurate documentation and record keeping in substantiating an incident. (p 81)

1.3.4 Identify those situations that require the EMT-I to report those incidents to appropriate authorities. (p 89)

1.3.5 Describe the four elements to prove medical liability. (p 81)

1.3.6 Describe the significance of obtaining expressed consent. (p 83)

1.3.7 Describe the extent to which force and restraint may be used to protect the EMT, the patient, and the third party. (p 84)

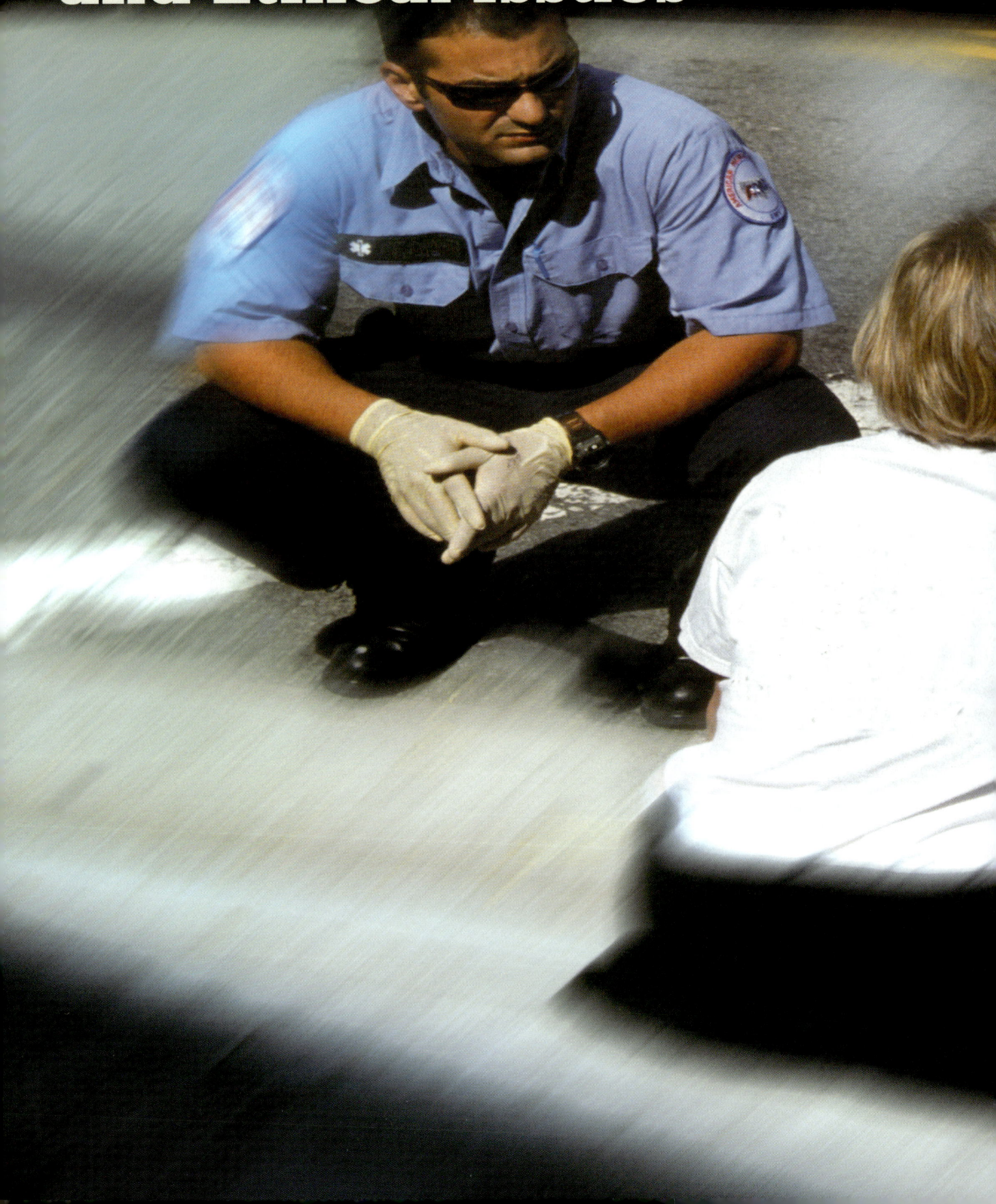

Medical, Legal, and Ethical Issues

3

Medical, Legal, and Ethical Issues

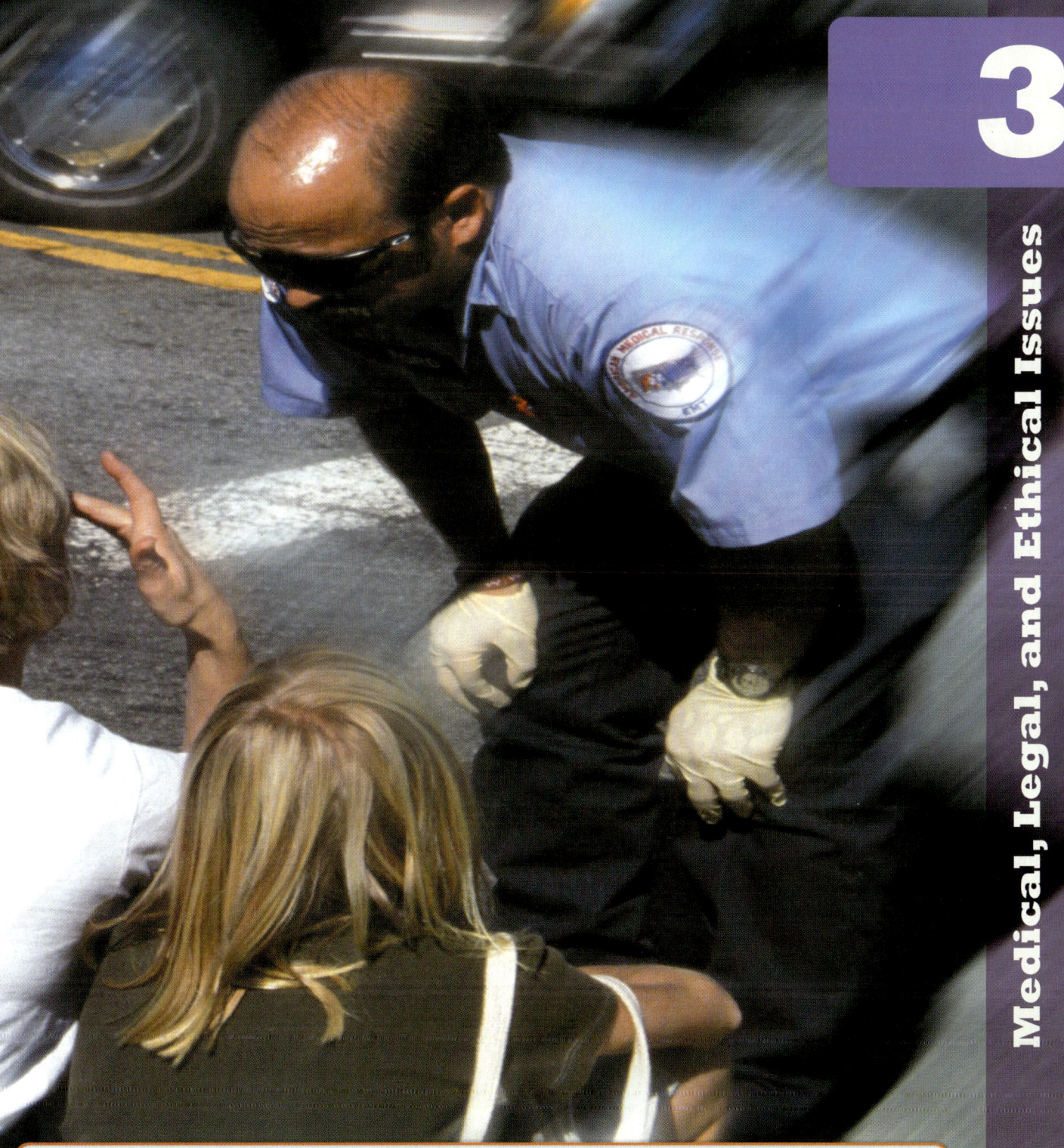

You are the Provider

You respond to a call at a local nursing home. Personnel direct you to the room of an elderly woman. While obtaining the history, you discover that the patient fell yesterday and, according to the nurse, the patient appears to be confused. When you address the patient, she tells you that she is fine and does not want to go to the hospital.

As emergency providers, we will encounter situations that often create frustration and concern. This chapter will help the EMT-I learn how to appropriately handle these situations in a professional and ethical manner.

1. What are some of the medicolegal issues being faced in this situation?
2. What steps can the EMT-I take to ensure that the patient's wishes and needs are met?

Medical, Legal, and Ethical Issues

A basic principle of emergency care is to do no further harm. Any health care provider who acts in good faith and according to an appropriate standard of care usually avoids legal exposure. Providing emergency medical care in an organized system is a recent phenomenon. <u>Emergency medical care</u>, or immediate care or treatment, is often provided by an EMT, who may be the first link in the chain of prehospital care. As the scope and nature of emergency medical care become more complex and EMS becomes more widely available, litigation involving participants in EMS systems will no doubt increase. Providing competent emergency medical care that conforms with the standard of care taught to you will help you to avoid civil and criminal actions. Consider the following situations:

- You are transporting a patient, and while the stretcher is being loaded into the ambulance, your partner slips, the stretcher crashes to the ground, and the patient is injured.
- You are about to begin treating a child, and the father commands you to stop.

What should you do? Even when emergency medical care is properly given, there are times when you may be sued by a patient who seeks to obtain relief, often in the form of a monetary award, for economic damages or pain and suffering. Or administrative action, such as suspension of your state license or EMT-I certificate, may be brought against you for failure to abide by the regulations of your state EMS agency. For this reason, you must understand the various legal aspects of emergency medical care.

You must also consider ethical issues. As an EMT-I, should you stop and treat patients who were involved in an automobile crash while you are en route to another emergency call? Should you begin cardiopulmonary resuscitation (CPR) on a patient who, according to the family, has terminal cancer? Should patient information be released to a patient's attorney on the telephone?

Scope of Practice

The scope of practice, which is most commonly defined by state law, outlines the boundaries for the care you are permitted to provide for the patient. This care is based on generally accepted standards. Your medical director further defines the scope of practice by developing <u>protocols</u> and <u>standing orders</u>. The medical director gives you the legal authorization to provide patient care through telephone or radio communication (online) or standing orders and protocols (off-line).

You and other EMS personnel have a legal responsibility to provide proper, consistent patient care and to report problems, such as possible liability or exposure to airborne or bloodborne pathogens or infectious disease, to your medical director immediately.

Standards of Care

The law requires you to act or behave toward other individuals in a certain, definable way, regardless of the activity involved. Under given circumstances, you have a duty to act or not. Generally speaking, you must be concerned about the safety and welfare of others when your behavior or activities have the potential for causing others injury or harm Figure 3-1▶. The manner in which you are required to act or behave is called a <u>standard of care</u>.

The standard of care is established in many ways, among them published medical research, local custom, statutes, ordinances, administrative regulations, and case law. In addition, professional and institutional standards have a bearing on determining the adequacy of your conduct.

Standards Imposed by Local Custom

The care that you provide is compared with the care a reasonably prudent person with similar training and experience would provide under similar circumstances.

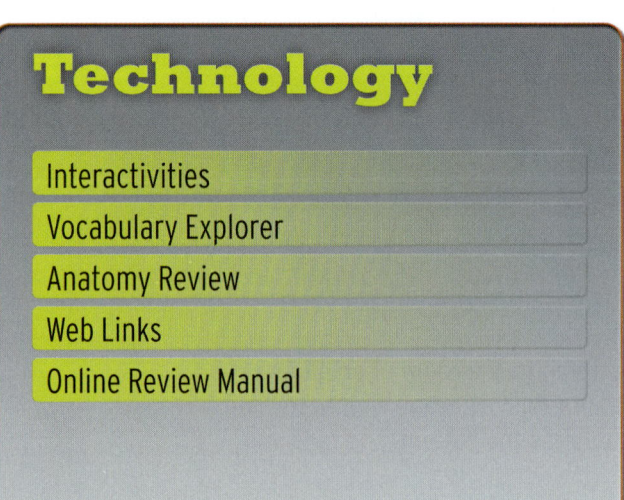

www.EMSzone.com/EMTI

Technology
- Interactivities
- Vocabulary Explorer
- Anatomy Review
- Web Links
- Online Review Manual

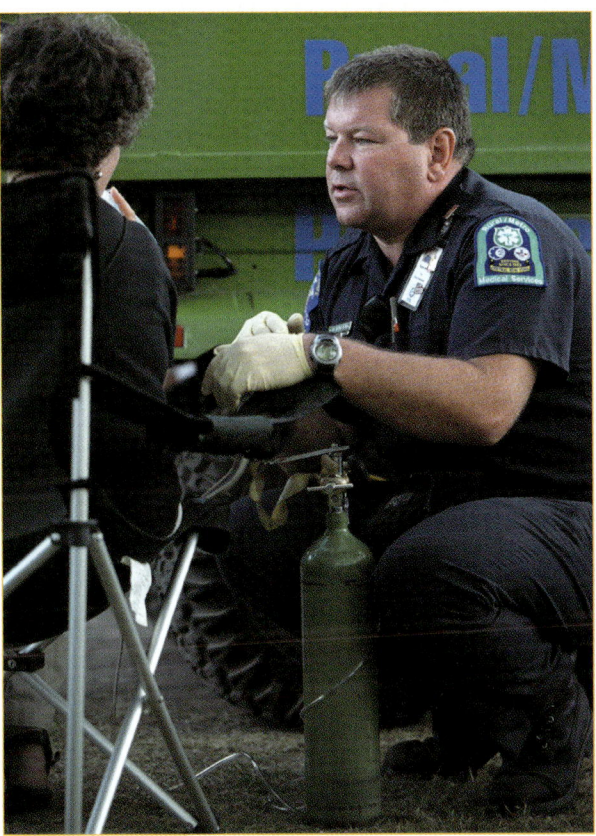

Figure 3-1 Act or behave toward others in a way that shows your concern for their safety and welfare.

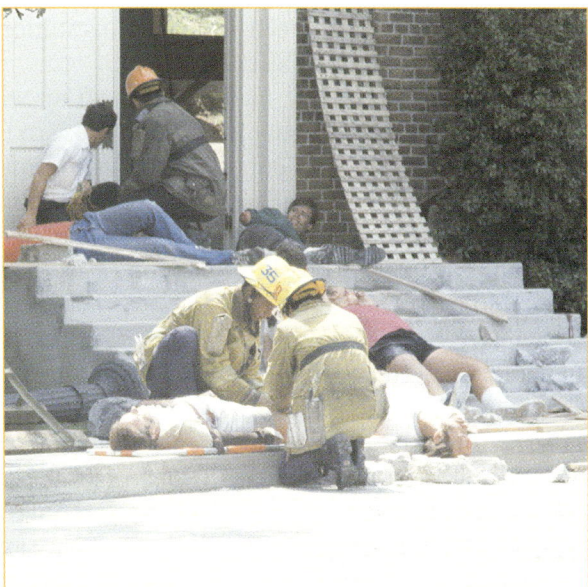

Figure 3-2 An emergency is a serious situation that arises suddenly, threatens the life or welfare of one or more people, and requires immediate intervention.

For example, the conduct of an EMT-I who is employed by an ambulance service is to be judged in comparison with the expected conduct of other EMT-Is from comparable ambulance services. These standards are often based on locally accepted protocols.

As an EMT-I, you will not be held to the same standard of care as physicians or other more highly trained professionals. In addition, your conduct must be judged in the light of the given emergency situation, taking into consideration the following factors:

- The atmosphere at the scene of the emergency, such as a state of general confusion
- The needs of other patients
- The type of equipment available

In this context, an <u>emergency</u> is a serious situation, such as injury or illness that arises suddenly, threatens the life or welfare of a person or group of people, and requires immediate intervention (Figure 3-2).

The prevailing custom of the community is an important element in determining the standard of emergency care required.

Standards Imposed by Law

In addition to local customs, standards of emergency medical care may be imposed by statutes, ordinances, administrative regulation, or case law. In many jurisdictions, violating one of these standards is said to create *presumptive negligence*. Therefore, you must become familiar with the particular legal standards that may exist in your state. In many states, the standards may take the form of treatment protocols published by a state agency.

Professional and Institutional Standards

In addition to standards imposed by law, professional and institutional standards may be used as evidence in determining the adequacy of an EMS provider's conduct. Professional standards include recommendations published by organizations and societies that are involved in emergency medical care. Institutional standards include specific rules and procedures of the EMS service, ambulance service, or other organization to which you belong.

Two notes of caution: First, you must be familiar with the standards of your organization. Second, the standards formulated for a particular agency should be reasonable and realistic so that they do not impose an unreasonable burden on EMS providers. Providing the best emergency medical care should be every EMS provider's goal, but it is not realistic to have institutional standards that *demand* the best care.

Many standards of care may be imposed on you. State health department regulations usually govern the scope and level of training. Court decisions have resulted in case law that defines standards of care. Professional standards are also imposed, such as the American Heart Association's standard for basic life support (also known as BLS) and CPR Figure 3-3 ▼.

Ordinary care is a minimum standard of care. In general, it is expected that anyone who offers assistance will exercise reasonable care and act prudently. If you act reasonably, according to the accepted standard, the risk of losing in a civil suit may be decreased. If you apply the standard practices you have been trained to use, you can likely avoid liability. For example, various organizations have defined standards for performing CPR. If you deviate from these standards, you may be liable for civil action and possibly criminal prosecution. In addition, state regulatory agencies that oversee EMS operations can sanction EMS personnel for deviating from the standard of care.

Standards Imposed by States

Medical Practices Act

In most states, EMS personnel are exempt from the licensure requirements of the Medical Practices Act because an EMT-I is regarded as a nonlicensed professional. As an EMT-I, you work directly under the license of your individual medical director. The physician medical director may also be directly involved in critiquing run reports as a means of ensuring proper care for every patient.

The practice of medicine is defined as the diagnosis and treatment of disease or illness. EMT-Is and others in the prehospital care chain assess the need for life support and begin care. Therefore, the standard of care must be maintained within the scope of your state's provisions and licensing requirements.

When unsure of proper care you should contact medical control for orders. Any order that is unclear or seems inappropriate should be questioned. Do not blindly follow an order that does not make sense to you. The physician may have misunderstood or may have missed part of the report. In that case, he or she may not be able to respond appropriately to the patient's needs.

Certification and Licensure

Some states provide certification or licensure of people who perform emergency medical care. Certification is the process by which an individual, institution, or program is evaluated and recognized as meeting certain predetermined standards to ensure safe and ethical patient care. Once certified, you are obliged to conform to the standards that are generally recognized nationally by various registry groups and provide an important link in nationwide EMS. Licensure is the process by which a governmental agency, such as a state medical board, grants permission to an individual who meets established qualifications to engage in the profession or occupation. Be familiar with the laws of your own state regarding licensure or certification requirements for EMT-I.

Licensure, certification, or both may be required by state or local authorities to practice as an EMT-I. You must also ensure that your certification or licensure remains current; skills competency must remain current.

Some organizations have recently changed their concept of certification. The American Heart Association, for example, now acknowledges only the successful completion of a CPR course. Certification has specific legal meaning and is generally restricted to licensing agencies.

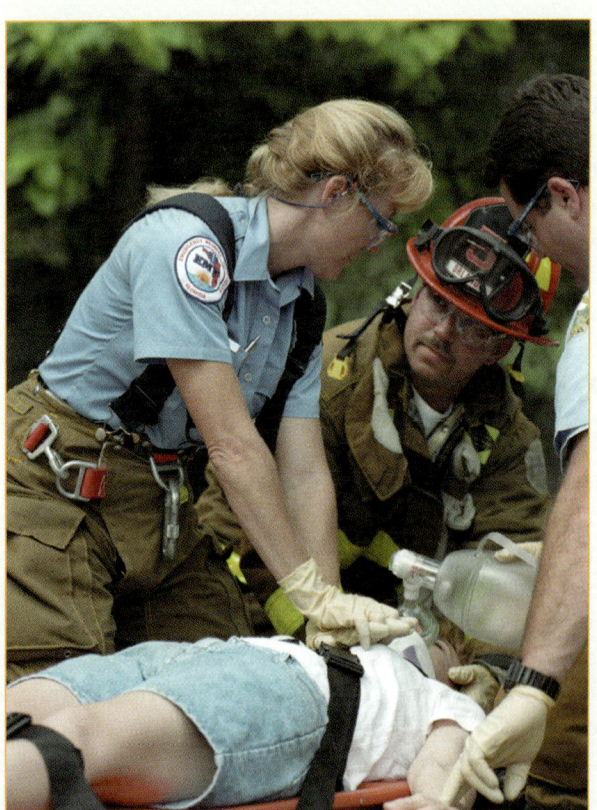

Figure 3-3 Many standards of care are imposed on you, such as those for performing CPR.

State EMS Legislation

Each state is legally required to provide for the practice of emergency care. One purpose of state statutes is to define the scope of practice for that particular area. The statutes also set forth the requirements for licensure, regulations, and certification within the state's boundaries. Regulations regarding medical control, protocols, and communications also are usually included in state legislation.

Motor vehicle laws fall under state legislation as well. These vary considerably from state to state. It is mandatory for the EMT-I to be familiar with appropriate state statutes regarding operation of emergency vehicles.

Laws

Legislative, Administrative, and Common

Laws are enacted at federal, state, and local levels by legislative branches of government. They are products of Congress, city councils, district boards, and general assemblies. Administrative laws or regulations are developed by governmental agencies that have the authority to enforce legislation. Common law is "case" or "judge-made" law. It is derived from society's and the legal system's acceptance of customs or norms over time.

Criminal Law

Criminal law is an area of law in which the federal, state, or local government prosecutes individuals on behalf of society for violating laws designed to safeguard society. Violation of these laws may be punishable by fine, imprisonment, or both. Examples of violation of criminal laws include robbery, rape, murder, and kidnapping.

Civil (Tort) Law

Civil (tort) law is an area of law dealing with private complaints brought by a plaintiff against a defendant for a wrongful act or wrongdoing (tort). It is enforced by bringing about a civil lawsuit in which the plaintiff requests that a court award damages, which are usually monetary. Examples of civil cases include those involving wrongful death, malpractice, and negligence.

In some cases, prosecution based on violation of a criminal law can also lead to a civil suit. For example, a person can be charged in a criminal court for murder and be found not guilty. Families of the victim can then sue the defendant in a civil court for wrongful death. In this case, the defendant can be found "responsible" and be ordered to pay for damages, despite the outcome of the criminal trial.

Duty to Act

Duty to act is a person's responsibility to provide patient care. Responsibility comes from statute or function. A bystander is under no obligation to assist a stranger in distress; there is no legal duty to act. There may be a duty to act in certain instances, including the following:
- You are charged with emergency medical response.
- Your service or department's policy states that you must assist in any emergency.

Once your ambulance responds to a call or treatment is initiated, you have a legal duty to act. If you are off duty and come upon a crash, you are not legally obligated to stop and assist patients. However, you do have a moral and ethical duty to act because of your special training and expertise.

Negligence

Negligence is the failure to provide the same care that a person with similar training would provide. It is deviation from the accepted standard of care that may result in further injury to the patient. Determination of negligence is based on the following four factors:

1. **Duty to Act.** It is the EMT-I's responsibility to act reasonably within the standards of his or her training.
2. **Breach of Duty.** There is a breach of duty when the EMT-I does not act within an expected and reasonable standard of care.
3. **Damages.** There are damages when a patient is physically or psychologically harmed in some noticeable way.
4. **Proximate Cause.** The EMT-I is directly responsible for the patient's injury. There must be a reasonable cause and effect. An example is dropping the patient during lifting, causing a fracture of the patient's leg. Inaction may also cause damage. If a person has a duty and abuses it, resulting in harm to another individual, the EMT-I, EMS agency, and/or medical director may be sued for negligence.

All four elements must be present for the legal doctrine of negligence to apply. In some cases, negligence

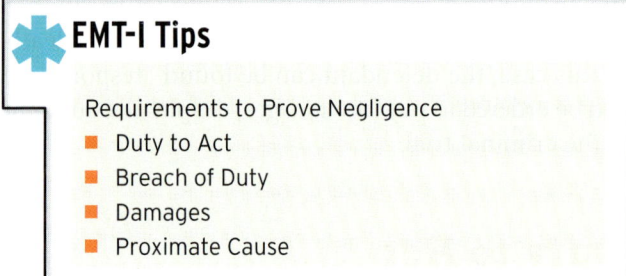

EMT-I Tips

Requirements to Prove Negligence
- Duty to Act
- Breach of Duty
- Damages
- Proximate Cause

may be so obvious that it does not require extensive proof. *Res ipsa loquitur* is Latin for "the thing speaks for itself." The injury could only have been caused by negligence. An example would be a patient who had surgery and then developed peritonitis (inflammation in a membrane in the abdominal cavity) because a piece of sponge or gauze was left in the abdominal cavity when the incision was closed.

The best protection against claims of negligence includes the following:
- Appropriate education and training and continuing education
- Appropriate medical direction, online and off-line
- Accurate, thorough documentation
- Professional attitude and demeanor

Abandonment

Abandonment is the unilateral termination of care by the EMT-I without the patient's consent and without making any provisions for continuing care by a medical professional with skills at the same or a higher level.

Once you have started care, you have assumed a duty that must not stop until an equally competent person with an equal or higher level of training assumes responsibility (that is, a paramedic, nurse, or physician). Not fulfilling that duty exposes the patient to harm and is a basis for a negligence suit. Abandonment is a legally and ethically serious matter that can result in civil and criminal actions against an EMT-I.

For example, suppose you arrive at the scene of a single-car accident and begin the care of two injured patients. A passerby tells you of a two-car accident further down the road in which five people are injured. You turn care of the two injured patients from the first accident over to the passerby and leave to go to the other accident. Abandonment has occurred because you did not turn care of the patients over to a person with a level of training equal or higher to yours. Consider the following general questions when you are faced with making a decision such as this one:
- What problems may develop from your actions?
- Are you neglecting your duty to your patient?
- Are you abandoning the patient if you leave the scene?
- Are you violating a standard of care?
- Are you acting prudently?

Consent

Under most circumstances, consent is required from every conscious, mentally competent adult before care can be started. A person receiving care must give permission, or consent, for treatment. If a person is in control of his or her actions, even though injured, and

You are the Provider — Part 2

Your patient consents to be examined. Your initial assessment reveals the following:

Initial Assessment	Recording Time: Zero Minutes
Appearance	Calm, sitting in a chair, and in no obvious distress
Level of consciousness	Oriented to person and place
Airway	Open and clear
Breathing	Respiratory rate appears normal.
Circulation	Strong radial pulses; skin, pale, warm, and dry

3. What other pertinent information should be obtained?
4. Does this patient have the right to refuse transport?

refuses care, you may not legally care for the patient. In fact, doing so may be grounds for criminal and civil action such as a charge of assault and battery or false imprisonment. Consent can be actual or implied. Consent may also be involuntary, such as an incidence where a patient who is under arrest by law enforcement is refusing care. If the patient is under arrest, he or she cannot refuse the orders given by the law enforcement officer. Similarly, if a parent gives consent for treatment of a young child, the child cannot refuse.

> **EMT-I Tips**
>
> Under most circumstances, consent is required from every conscious, mentally competent adult before care can be started.

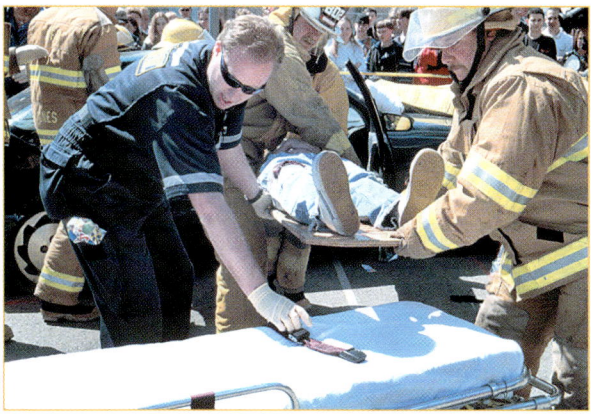

Figure 3-4 When a serious threat to life exists and the patient is unconscious or otherwise unable to give consent, the law assumes that the patient would give consent to care and transport to the hospital.

Expressed Consent

Expressed consent (or actual consent) is the type of consent in which the patient expressly authorizes you to provide care or transport. It must be informed consent, which means that the patient has been told of the potential risks, benefits, and alternatives to treatment and has given consent to treatment. The legal basis for this doctrine rests on the assumption that the patient has a right to determine what is to be done with his or her body. The patient must be of legal age (18 years in most states) and able to make a rational decision.

A patient might agree to certain emergency medical care but not to other care. For example, a patient might agree to receive oxygen and transport but refuse insertion of an intravenous line. An injured person might agree to emergency care at home but refuse to be transported to a medical facility. Informed consent is valid if given orally; however, it may be difficult to prove. Having the patient sign a consent form does not eliminate your responsibility to fully inform the patient.

Implied Consent

When a seriously ill or injured person is unconscious and unable to give consent, the law assumes that the patient would consent to care and transport to a medical facility 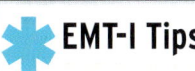. This is called implied consent. Implied consent is limited to true emergency situations and is appropriate when the patient is unconscious, delusional, unresponsive as a result of drug or alcohol use, or otherwise physically unable to give expressed consent. However, many things may be unclear about what represents a "serious threat to life." Legal proceedings would likely revolve around that question. This becomes a medicolegal judgment, which should be supported by the EMT-I's best efforts to obtain consent. Medicolegal is a term that relates to medical jurisprudence (law) or forensic medicine. In most instances, the law allows the spouse, a close relative, or next of kin to give consent for an injured person who is unable to give consent. Refusal of your offer to provide emergency care may also be implied. For example, a patient's action in pulling his or her arm from your splint may be an indication of refusal of consent.

Minors and Consent

Because a minor might not have the wisdom, maturity, or judgment to give valid consent, the law requires that a parent or legal guardian give consent for treatment or transport Figure 3-5 . However, in some states, a minor can give valid consent to receive medical care, depending on the minor's age and maturity. Many states also allow emancipated, married, or pregnant minors to be treated as adults for the purposes of consenting to medical treatment. An emancipated minor is one who is living independently of his or her parents and is self-sufficient, a member of the armed services, married, or a parent. You should obtain consent from a parent or legal guardian whenever possible; however, if a true emergency exists and the parent or legal guardian is not available, the consent to treat the minor is implied, just as with an adult. You must never withhold lifesaving care.

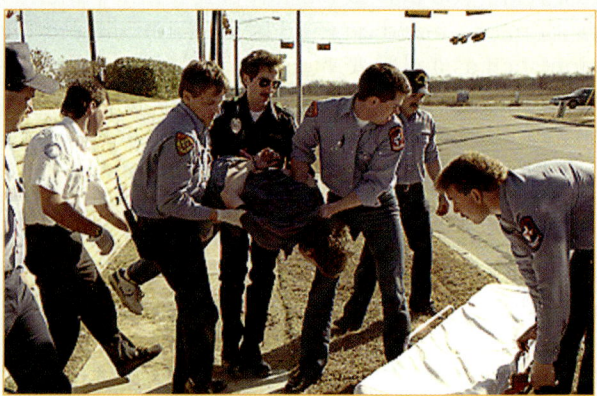

Figure 3-6 Be sure that you know the local laws about forcible restraint of a patient. In some states, only a law enforcement officer has the authority to restrain a patient.

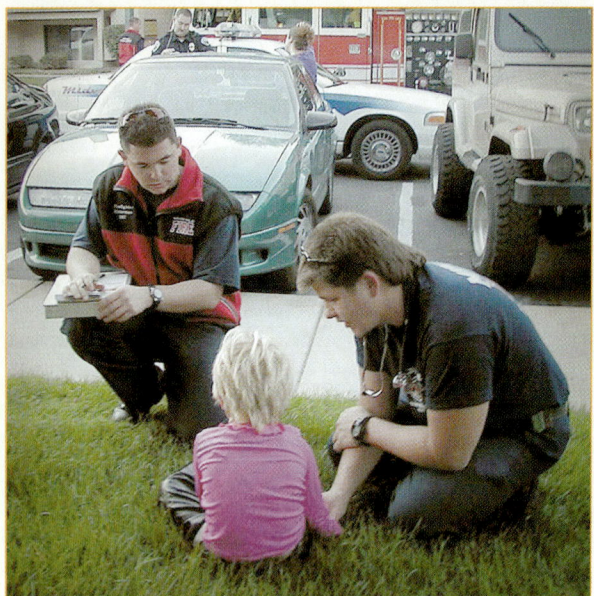

Figure 3-5 The law requires that a parent or legal guardian give consent for treatment or transport of a minor. However, you must never withhold lifesaving care.

Mentally Incompetent Adults

Assisting patients who are mentally ill, in behavioral (psychological) crisis, under the influence of drugs or alcohol, or developmentally delayed is complicated. An adult patient who is mentally incompetent is not able to give informed consent. From a legal perspective, this situation is similar to situations involving minors. Consent for emergency care should be obtained from someone who is legally responsible, such as a guardian or conservator. In many cases, however, such permission will not be readily obtainable. Many states have protective custody statutes allowing such a person to be taken, under law enforcement authority, to a medical facility. Know the provisions in your area. Remember that when a true emergency exists, you can assume that implied consent exists.

Forcible Restraint

<u>Forcible restraint</u> of a patient is the act of physically preventing the patient from a mental or physical action. This may help to prevent the patient from harming himself or herself or the EMT-I. Forcible restraint of a mentally disturbed individual may be required before emergency care can be given. If you believe that a patient will injure himself, herself, or others, you can legally restrain the patient. However, you must consult medical control, online or off-line depending on local protocol, for authorization to restrain, or contact law enforcement personnel who have authority to restrain people. In some states, only a law enforcement officer may forcibly restrain a person (Figure 3-6). You should clearly understand local laws. Restraint without authority exposes you to civil and criminal penalties. Restraint may be used only in circumstances of risk to the patient, yourself, or others.

Your service should have clearly defined protocols pertaining to situations involving restraint. After restraints are applied, they must not be removed en route even if the patient promises to act calmly. It is also important to closely monitor the restrained patient for any signs of breathing difficulty. It is possible to suffocate the patient if he or she is face down, creating positional asphyxia, or if a mask placed over the patient's face occludes airflow.

Remember that if the patient is responsive and the situation is not urgent, consent is required. Adults who appear to be in control of their senses cannot be forced to submit to care or transportation.

Assault and Battery

<u>Assault</u> is defined as threatening, attempting, or causing a person fear of immediate bodily harm without the person's consent. <u>Battery</u> is unlawfully touching a person; this includes providing emergency care without consent. Serious legal problems may arise in situations in which a patient has not given consent for treatment. Battery could be charged if you apply a splint to a suspected fracture of the lower leg or use a prefilled epi-

nephrine syringe (for example, an EpiPen) on a patient without the patient's consent. The patient may have grounds to sue you for assault, battery, or both. To protect yourself from these charges, make sure that you obtain expressed consent or that the situation allows for implied consent. Consult your medical director if you have questions or doubts about a specific situation.

The Right to Refuse Treatment

Mentally competent adults have the right to refuse treatment or withdraw from treatment at any time. If they do, you are faced with a dilemma. Should you provide care against their will and risk being accused of battery? Should you leave them alone? If you leave patients alone, you risk being accused of negligence or abandonment if their condition becomes worse.

If a patient refuses treatment or transport, you must make sure that he or she understands, or is informed about, the potential risks, benefits, treatments, and alternatives to treatment. You must also fully inform the patient about the consequences of refusing treatment and encourage the patient to ask questions. Remember that competent adults who refuse specific kinds of treatment for any reason, including religious reasons, have a legal right to do so.

When a patient refuses treatment, you must assess whether the patient's mental condition is impaired. If the patient refusing treatment is delusional or confused, you cannot assume that the refusal is an informed refusal. When in doubt, it is always best to proceed with treatment. This is the best course of action because providing treatment is a much more defensible position than failing to treat a patient. Failure to treat a patient can be considered negligence.

You may also be faced with a situation in which a parent refuses to permit treatment of an ill or injured child. In this situation, you must consider the emotional impact of the emergency on the parent's judgment. In this and virtually all cases of refusal, you can usually resolve the situation with patience and calm persuasion. You may also need the help of others, such as your supervisor or law enforcement officials. In most states, consent to treat a minor is required from only one parent.

There will be times when you are not able to persuade the patient, guardian, conservator, or parent of a minor or mentally incompetent patient to proceed with treatment. In this case, you must obtain the signature of the person who is refusing treatment on an official release form that acknowledges refusal. You must be sure to document any assessment findings and any emergency care that you provided. You must also obtain a signature from a witness to the refusal. You should then keep the release form with the patient care report. In addition to the release form itself, you should write a note about the refusal on the patient care report. If the patient refuses to sign the release form, the best you can do is inform your medical director and thoroughly document the situation and the refusal. Report to medical control, and follow your local protocols with regard to this situation.

> **Documentation Tips**
>
> When a patient, parent, or guardian refuses treatment or transport, protect yourself with a thorough patient care report and an official refusal form. Have the patient or other refusing party sign the form, document in the patient care report what you have done to ensure an informed refusal, and note the involvement of medical control in the situation. Be sure to submit the refusal form with your patient care report.

Good Samaritan Laws and Immunity

Most states have adopted Good Samaritan laws, which are based on the common law principle that when you reasonably help another person, you should not be liable for errors and omissions that are made in giving good faith emergency care. However, Good Samaritan laws do not protect you from a lawsuit. Only a few statutory provisions provide immunity from a lawsuit, and those usually are reserved for governments. Good Samaritan laws provide an affirmative defense if you are sued for providing care, but they do not protect you from liability if you have not provided proper care, nor do they pertain to acts outside your scope of care. These laws do not protect anyone from wanton, gross, or willful negligence (for example, the failure to exercise due care), or if care is provided for remuneration.

Another group of laws grants immunity from liability to official emergency medical care providers, such as EMT-Is. These laws, which vary from state to state, do not provide immunity when injury or damage is caused by gross negligence or willful misconduct.

The statute of limitations, which limits the number of years after an incident during which a lawsuit can be filed, may also aid in protecting EMT-Is from litigation. It is set by law, may differ for cases involving adults and children, and varies from state to state.

Most states have also adopted specific laws granting special privileges to EMS personnel, authorizing them to perform certain medical procedures. Many states also grant partial immunity to EMS providers, physicians, and nurses who give emergency instructions to EMS personnel via radio or other forms of communication. Consult your medical director for more information about the laws in your area.

A plaintiff may be found liable of contributory negligence, which means that he or she is found to have contributed to his or her own injury. In cases such as this, damages awarded may be reduced or eliminated based on the plaintiff's own contribution to the injury.

Another form of protection EMT-Is may want is liability insurance. Most EMS services provide liability insurance that covers EMT-Is while on duty. Purchasing a personal policy may provide additional coverage. Insurance coverage does not prevent you from being sued, but it can offer financial protection or legal representation in the event you are sued. Be sure to understand your insurance coverage requirements.

Advance Directives

Occasionally, you and your partner may respond to a call in which a patient is dying of an illness. When you arrive at the scene, you may find that family members do not want you to try to resuscitate the patient. Without valid written documentation, such as an advance directive, living will, or <u>DNR (do not resuscitate) order</u> (also known as a "Do Not Attempt Resuscitation" order), this type of request places you in a very difficult position. An <u>advance directive</u> is a written document that specifies medical treatment for a <u>competent</u> patient, should he or she become unable to make decisions. In this situation, a competent patient is able to make rational decisions about his or her well-being. An advance directive is also commonly called a living will. DNR orders give you permission not to attempt resuscitation. Although laws might differ from state to state, generally speaking, to be valid, DNR orders must meet the following requirements:

- Clearly state the patient's medical problem(s)
- Be signed by the patient or legal guardian
- Be signed by one or more physicians
- Be dated in the preceding 12 months

However, even in the presence of a DNR order, you are still obligated to provide supportive measures (oxygen, pain relief, and comfort) to a patient who is not in

You are the Provider   Part 3

You are able to determine that the patient is not normally oriented to time. She appears to answer your questions appropriately. She does not remember falling; however, she does acknowledge having a headache.

Vital Signs	Recording Time: 2 Minutes After Patient Contact
Respirations	14 breaths/min, good air movement
Pulse	88 beats/min, irregular
Skin	Pale, warm, and dry
Blood pressure	182/68 mm Hg
Sao$_2$	92% on room air

5. What are some of the concerns that you might have regarding this patient's medical condition?
6. What are your care and transport options for this patient?

cardiac arrest, whenever possible. Each ambulance service, in consultation with its medical director and legal counsel, must develop a protocol to follow in these circumstances.

> 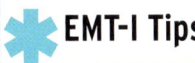**EMT-I Tips**
>
> An **advance directive** specifically states what type of care the patient wishes to receive in a given situation. This may include the desire to have basic life support performed, but no advance procedures or life support equipment.
>
> **DNR orders** typically state that if the patient is apneic and pulseless, no resuscitative measures are to be taken.

TABLE 3-1	Ethical Decision Making

1. Consider all options available to you and the consequence of each option.
2. What decisions have been made regarding a similar situation? Is this a type of problem that reflects a rule or policy? Can an existing policy or rule be applied? *This uses the concept of "precedence."*
3. How would this action affect you if you were in your patient's or patient's family's position? *This is a form of the "Golden Rule."*
4. Would you feel comfortable having all prehospital care providers apply this action in all similar circumstances? *This is an application of Kant's "Categorical Imperative."*
5. Can you justify your action(s) to
   - Your peers?
   - The public?
   - Your supervisor?
   - Your medical director?
6. Will the treatment you provide yield the greatest benefit in comparison to all of the alternatives? *This is the test of "utility."*
7. What is in the patient's best interest?

Because of terminal nursing home placement, hospice, and home health programs, you may often be faced with this situation. Specific guidelines vary from state to state, but the following four statements may be considered general guidelines:

1. **Patients have the right to refuse treatment**, including resuscitative efforts, provided that they are able to communicate their wishes in a competent manner. Patients also have the right to withdraw a DNR for themselves and request emergency care.
2. **A written order from a physician is required** for DNR orders to be valid in a health care facility.
3. **You should periodically review** state and local protocols and legislation regarding advance directives.
4. **When you are in doubt** or the written orders are not present, begin basic life support and contact medical control for guidance.

Ethical Responsibilities

In addition to legal duties, EMS providers have certain ethical responsibilities as health care providers. These responsibilities are to themselves, their coworkers, the public, and the patient. Ethics are related to action, conduct, motive, and character and how they relate to the EMS provider's responsibilities. Ethics are principles that identify conduct deemed morally desirable. From an EMS standpoint, ethics are associated with what the EMS profession deems right or fitting conduct. Treating a patient ethically means doing so in a manner that conforms to professional standards of conduct.

How can you make sure that you are acting ethically, especially with all the decisions you have to make in the field (Table 3-1)?

You must meet your legal and ethical responsibilities while caring for your patients' physical and emotional needs. Patient needs vary depending on the situation. This also includes supervising care given by first responders and others on scene to ensure that the patient is receiving proper attention.

An unquestionable responsibility is honest reporting. Absolute honesty in reporting is essential. You must provide a complete account of the events and the details of all patient care and professional duties. Accurate records are also important for quality improvement activities.

To provide the best level of care, it is necessary to maintain mastery of skills. Participating in continuing education and refresher training not only provides updates on changes and new procedures in EMS, but also keeps you current in the areas that are dealt with infrequently such as obstetrics and pediatrics. As an EMT-I, you have a moral obligation to make sure that you are knowledgeable in all areas of emergency care and to care for patients to the best of your ability. Critically reviewing your performance and seeking improvement are ethical concerns.

Failing to live up to legal or ethical standards may result in the EMT-I being charged civilly, criminally, or both. The best legal protection is performing an appropriate assessment and providing care that is safe, effective, and competent, coupled with accurate and complete documentation. Laws differ from state to state and area to area, so be sure to seek legal advice if needed. By staying up-to-date on skills and information and treating patients with the same consideration and respect that you would give one of your close family members, you may limit possible complications that can have legal ramifications.

Confidentiality

Communication between you and the patient is considered confidential and generally cannot be disclosed without permission from the patient or a court order. Confidential information includes the patient history, assessment findings, and treatment provided. You cannot disclose information regarding a patient's diagnosis, treatment, or mental or physical condition without consent; if you do, you may find yourself liable for breach of confidentiality.

In certain situations, you may release confidential information to designated individuals. In most states, records may be released when a legal subpoena is presented or the patient signs a written release. The patient must be mentally competent and fully understand the nature of the release.

Another means for disclosing information is through automatic release, which does not require a written form. This type of release allows you to share information with other health care providers so that they may continue the patient's care.

In many states, you do not need a written release to report information about cases of rape or abuse to proper authorities. Third-party payment billing forms may also be completed without written consent.

Improper release of information or release of inaccurate information can result in liability. Invasion of privacy is the release, without legal justification, of information about a patient's private life that might reasonably expose the patient to ridicule, notoriety, or embarrassment. The fact that the information is true is not a defense. <u>Libel</u> (making false statements in writing) and <u>slander</u> (making false verbal statements) fall under the category of defamation of character. <u>Defamation</u> is making an untrue statement about someone's character or reputation without legal privilege or consent of the individual. These statements, whether verbal or written, are made with malicious intent or reckless disregard for the veracity of the statements.

To protect yourself, be sure to document only objective findings and omit personal opinions. Do not give information to anyone other than other health care professionals directly involved in the patient's continuing care. Briefly, but politely, explain to others such as family members and concerned friends that you cannot give out information regarding the patient's condition. Instead, suggest that they follow up with immediate family members once the patient has been seen in the emergency department.

HIPAA

HIPAA is the acronym for the Health Insurance Portability and Accountability Act of 1996. Although this act had many aims, including improving the portability and continuity of health insurance coverage and combating waste and fraud in health insurance and the provision of health care, the section of the act that most affects EMS relates to patient privacy. The aim of this section was to strengthen laws for the protection of the privacy of health care information and to safeguard patient confidentiality. As such, it provides guidance on what types of information is protected, the responsibility of health care providers regarding that protection, and penalties for breaching that protection.

The law has the effect of dramatically limiting the ability of EMS providers to obtain follow-up information about patients they treat, including information that would serve to improve their knowledge of medical conditions or help them understand the degree to which they may have been exposed to a communicable disease as a result of a patient encounter.

Most personal health information is protected and should not be released without the patient's permission. If you are not sure, do not give any information to anyone other than those directly involved in the care of the patient. For specific policies, each EMS service is required to have a manual and a compliance officer who can answer questions. You can expect to receive further training on how this act impacts your specific response agency and resource hospital.

Records and Reports

Certain people and agencies, such as the EMS system, are in a position to obtain information about diseases, injuries, and emergency events, and they may be required by statute or regulation to compile the information and report it to regulatory or accreditation agencies. Even if there is no such requirement, you should compile a complete and accurate record of all incidents in which you come into contact with sick or injured patients. Most medical and legal experts believe that a complete and accurate record of an emergency medical incident is an important safeguard against legal action. The absence of a record or a substantially incomplete record may mean that you have to testify about the events, your findings, and your actions by relying on memory alone, which can prove to be inadequate and embarrassing in the face of aggressive cross-examination.

The courts often consider the following two rules of thumb regarding reports and records:
- **If an action or procedure** is not recorded on the written report, it was not performed.
- **An incomplete or untidy report** is evidence of incomplete or inexpert emergency medical care.

You can avoid both of these potentially dangerous presumptions by compiling and maintaining accurate reports and records of all events and patients.

Patient care reports also help the EMS system evaluate individual and service provider performance. These reports are an integral part of most quality assurance programs.

> **Documentation Tips**
>
> Remember: If you did not document it, you did not do it! Make sure your documentation is accurate and thorough.

Special Reporting Requirements

Abuse of Children, Elderly People, and Others

All states and the District of Columbia have enacted laws to protect abused children, and some have added other protected groups such as elderly and "at-risk" adults. Most states have a reporting obligation for certain individuals, ranging from physicians to any person. You must be aware of the requirements of law in your state. Such statutes frequently grant immunity from liability for libel, slander, or defamation of character to the person who is obligated to report, even if the reports are subsequently shown to be unfounded, as long as the reports are made in good faith.

> **EMT-I Tips**
>
> When taking a history from a patient you suspect has been abused, you may get more accurate information if your partner interviews the parents or other caregivers separately. Abused patients are usually reluctant to speak openly in front of their abusers.

Injury During the Commission of a Felony

Many states have laws requiring the reporting of any injury that is likely to have occurred during the commission of a crime, such as gunshot wounds, knife wounds, or poisonings. Again, you must be familiar with the legal requirements of your state.

Drug-Related Injuries

In some instances, drug-related injuries must be reported. These requirements may affect the EMT-I. However, it should be stressed that the US Supreme Court has maintained that drug addiction, in contrast with drug possession or sale, is an illness and not a crime. Hence, an injury as a result of a drug overdose may not be within the definition of an injury resulting from a crime.

Some states, by statute, specifically establish confidentiality and excuse certain specified individuals from reporting drug cases, either to a government agency or to a minor's parents, if, in the opinion of those individuals, withholding reporting is necessary for the proper treatment of the patient. Once again, you must be familiar with the legal requirements of your state.

Childbirth

Many states require that anyone who attends a live birth in any place other than a licensed medical facility report the birth. You must be familiar with state requirements.

Other Reporting Requirements

Other reporting requirements may include attempted suicides, dog bites, certain communicable diseases, assaults, and rapes.

Most EMS agencies require that all exposures to infectious diseases be reported. You may be asked to transport certain patients in restraints, which may also need to be reported. Each of these situations can present significant legal problems. You should learn your local protocols regarding these situations.

Scene of a Crime

If there is evidence at an emergency scene that a crime may have been committed, you must notify the dispatcher immediately so that law enforcement authorities can be informed. Such circumstances should not stop you from providing necessary emergency medical care to the patient; however, your safety is a priority, so you must ensure that the scene is safe to enter. If the patient shows signs of obvious death (such as dependent lividity or decapitation), take necessary precautions not to disturb the crime scene because this may interfere with the subsequent investigation.

At times, you may have to transport the patient to the hospital before the authorities arrive. While emergency medical care is being provided, you must be careful not to disturb the scene of the crime any more than absolutely necessary. Notes and drawings should be made of the position of the patient and of the presence and position of any weapon or other objects that may be valuable to the investigating officers. If possible, do not cut through holes in clothing from weapon or gunshot wounds. You should confer periodically with local authorities and be aware of the actions they want you to take at the scene of the crime. It is best if these guidelines can be established by protocol.

The Deceased

In most states, EMT-Is do not have the authority to pronounce a patient dead. If there is any chance that life exists or that the patient can be resuscitated, you must initiate resuscitative efforts at the scene and during transport. However, at times death is obvious, such as in the following circumstances:
- Rigor mortis (stiffening of the body) has set in.
- Mortal injury, such as decapitation.
- Dependent lividity (discoloration of the body as a result of pooling of the blood) is present Figure 3-7 ▶.
- The body is decomposed.

In such instances, there is no urgent reason to move the body. The only immediate action that is required of you is to cover the body and prevent its disturbance. Local protocol will determine your ultimate action in these instances.

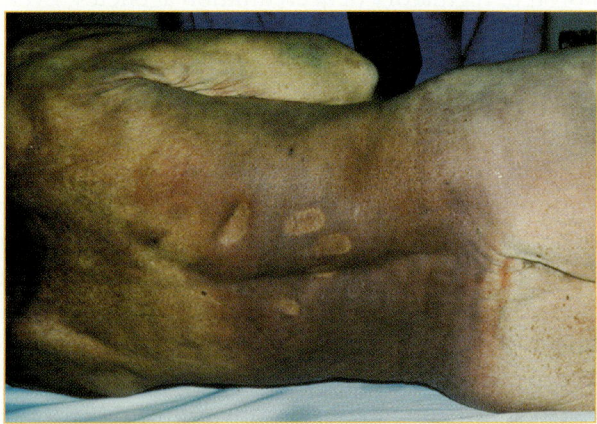

Figure 3-7 Dependent lividity is an obvious sign of death that is caused by discoloration of the body by pooling of the blood in the lowermost parts of the body.

Special Situations

Organ Donors

You may be called to a scene involving a potential organ donor. A person who has expressed a wish to donate organs is a potential organ donor. Consent to organ donation is voluntary and informed. Consent is evidenced by a donor card or a driver's license indicating that the person wants to be a donor Figure 3-8 ▼. You may need to consult with medical control when faced with this situation.

You should treat a potential organ donor in the same way that you would any other patient needing treatment. The fact that a patient is a possible donor does not mean that you should not use all means necessary to keep that patient alive. Organs that are donated, such as a kidney, heart, or liver, need oxygen at all times; you must give the possible donor oxygen, or the organs will be damaged and become useless.

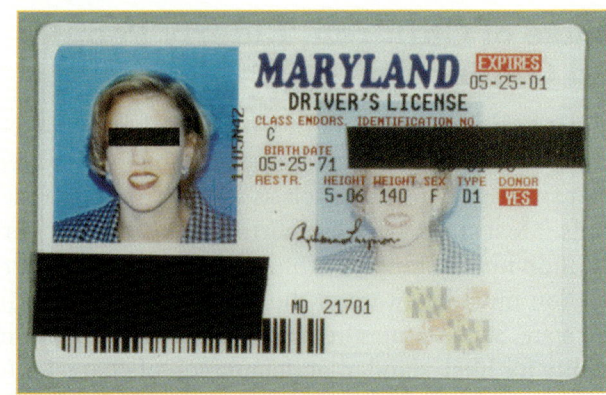

Figure 3-8 The patient may be carrying a donor card or driver's license indicating that he or she wishes to be an organ donor.

Remember that your priority is to save the patient's life. You may encounter potential organ donor situations at a multiple-casualty incident. The potential organ donor should be triaged with other patients and assigned a category; the potential organ donor may require a lower priority than other less severely injured patients.

Be sure to learn the specific protocols in your area for these situations.

Medical Identification Insignia

Many patients will carry important medical identification and information, often in the form of a bracelet, necklace, or card that will identify whether the patient has allergies, diabetes, epilepsy, or some other serious condition (Figure 3-9 ▶). This information is helpful to you in assessing and treating the patient.

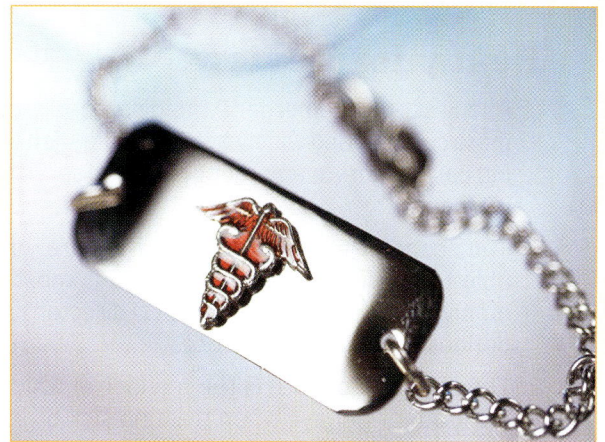

Figure 3-9 The patient may be carrying a medical identification card or wearing a bracelet or necklace that may indicate a serious medical condition.

You are the Provider — Summary

1. What are some of the medicolegal issues being faced in this situation?

The medicolegal issue here is the patient's refusal to be treated and transported to the hospital. Competent, oriented, alert patients have the right to determine whether or not they will receive medical care and transport to the hospital.

2. What steps can the EMT-I take to ensure that the patient's wishes and needs are met?

The EMT-I needs to perform a thorough, accurate assessment to determine the patient's level of consciousness and orientation. This will help the provider determine the patient's ability to make an informed decision. In addition, the provider needs to be familiar with state and local laws pertaining to these circumstances. The EMT-I has a legal responsibility to provide proper care that is consistent with the standard of care.

3. What other pertinent information should be obtained?

The patient's medical history and medication intake need to be noted, which can help direct the appropriate care.

4. Does this patient have the right to refuse transport?

Yes. Mentally competent adults have the right to refuse treatment and/or transport. If a patient refuses treatment or transport, you must make sure that he or she clearly understands the potential risks of refusing treatment. You must also fully inform the patient about the benefits and risks of treatment and transport, should he or she elect to accept it.

5. What are some of the concerns that you might have regarding this patient's medical condition?

This patient is not completely oriented and has no recollection of the events that led staff to call 9-1-1. Her complaint of a headache is concerning because it can be indicative of a potentially serious underlying problem.

6. What are your care and transport options for this patient?

Remember, competent adults have a legal right to refuse treatment or transport. The EMT-I can also contact and consult with medical control when these difficult situations arise. If the provider has any doubt as to the mental condition of the patient, it is always best to proceed with treatment. This is the best course of action because providing treatment is a much more defensible position than failing to treat a patient. Failure to treat a patient could lead to allegations of negligence and/or abandonment.

Prep Kit

Ready for Review

- As the scope of emergency medical care becomes more complex and widely available, litigation involving participants in emergency medical services will increase.

- The scope of practice outlines the care you are able to provide to the patient and is most commonly defined by law; the medical director further defines the scope of practice.

- The standard of care is the manner in which you must act or behave when treating sick or injured patients. Some standards are imposed by local custom, the law, or institutions.

- A duty to act is the responsibility of an individual to provide patient care. If you are off duty or out of your jurisdiction, you may not have a legal duty to act; however, you do have a moral and ethical duty to act because of your training and expertise.

- Negligence is the failure to provide the same care that a person of similar training would provide in a similar situation. Determination of negligence is based on duty, breach of duty, damages, and proximate cause.

- Abandonment is the termination of care without the patient's consent and without making provisions for the transfer of care to a health care professional with skills at the same or a higher level than yours. Abandonment is a legally and ethically serious act.

- You must receive consent from a patient before beginning care. A conscious adult patient who can make a rational decision will be able to give you expressed consent. Expressed consent must also be informed.

- When a patient is unconscious and unable to give consent, the law assumes implied consent, therefore treatment should proceed.

- You should try to obtain consent from a parent or guardian of a minor whenever possible. You should never withhold lifesaving care.

- Assault is defined as unlawfully placing a person in fear of immediate harm without the person's consent.

- Battery is unlawfully touching a person; this includes providing emergency care without consent.

- To protect yourself from charges, be sure to obtain expressed consent whenever possible.

- Mentally competent patients have the right to refuse treatment. In these instances, be sure to have the patient sign a refusal form, and make sure your department keeps a copy.

- Many states have adopted Good Samaritan laws and other laws that provide immunity to EMS personnel, provided that injury to the patient was not the result of gross negligence or willful misconduct on the part of the EMT-I, and that treatment was not provided for remuneration.

- An advance directive is a written document that specifies medical treatment in case a mentally competent patient becomes unable to make decisions.

- A DNR order gives you permission to not attempt resuscitation in the event of cardiac arrest. Your ambulance service should have protocols to follow when you are faced with an advance directive or a DNR order.

- Communication between you and the patient is confidential and should not be disclosed without permission from the patient or a court order.

- Records and reports are important; make sure that you compile a complete and accurate record of each incident in which you come in contact with sick or injured patients. You may need to testify some day, and the courts consider an action or procedure that was not recorded on the written report as not having been performed, and an incomplete or untidy report can be considered evidence of incomplete or inexpert medical care.

- You should know the special reporting requirements about abuse of children, elderly people, and others; injuries related to crimes; drug-related injuries; and childbirth. Be sure to note whether patients are carrying some type of medical identification information. If you fail to take this information into account, you may harm the patient.

Technology

- Interactivities
- Vocabulary Explorer
- Anatomy Review
- Web Links
- Online Review Manual

Vital Vocabulary

abandonment Unilateral termination of care by the EMT-I without the patient's consent and without making provisions for transferring care to another health care professional with skills at the same level or higher.

advance directive Written documentation that specifies medical treatment for a competent patient should he or she become unable to make decisions; also called a living will.

assault Unlawfully placing a patient in fear of bodily harm.

battery Touching a patient or providing emergency care without consent.

certification A process in which a person, an institution, or a program is evaluated and recognized as meeting certain predetermined standards to provide safe and ethical care.

civil (tort) law Area of law dealing with private complaints brought by a plaintiff against a defendant for a wrongful act or wrongdoing.

competent Able to make rational decisions about personal well-being.

consent Permission from a patient or guardian to provide care.

criminal law Area of law in which the federal, state, or local government prosecutes individuals on behalf of society for violating laws designed to safeguard the public.

defamation Making an untrue statement about someone's character or reputation without legal privilege or consent of the individual.

DNR (do not resuscitate) order Written documentation giving permission to medical personnel not to attempt resuscitation in the event of cardiac arrest.

duty to act A medicolegal term relating to certain personnel who by statute or by function have a responsibility to provide care.

emergency A serious situation, such as injury or illness that threatens the life or welfare of a person or group of people and requires immediate intervention.

emergency medical care Immediate care or treatment.

ethics Principles that identify conduct deemed morally desirable.

expressed consent A type of consent in which a patient gives express authorization for provision of care or transport.

forcible restraint The act of physically preventing a person from taking physical action.

Good Samaritan laws Statutory provisions enacted by many states to protect citizens from liability for errors and omissions when giving good faith emergency medical care, unless there is wanton, gross, or willful negligence or acceptance of remuneration.

implied consent A type of consent in which a patient who is unable to give consent is given treatment under the legal assumption that he or she would want treatment.

informed consent Permission for treatment given by a competent patient after the potential risks, benefits, and alternatives to treatment have been explained.

libel False statements about a person made in writing or through the mass media.

licensure The process by which a governmental agency, such as a state medical board, grants permission to an individual who meets established qualifications to engage in the profession or occupation.

medicolegal A term relating to medical jurisprudence (law) or forensic medicine.

negligence Failure to provide the same care that a person with similar training would provide under similar circumstances.

protocols Precise and detailed plans for a regimen of therapy (for example, advanced cardiac life support [or ACLS] algorithms).

slander False verbal statements about a person.

standard of care Accepted levels of medical care expected by reason of training and profession; determined by legal or professional peer organizations so that patients are not exposed to unnecessary risk or harm.

standing orders Local protocols, usually pertaining to a particular service or area.

Assessment in Action

You are dispatched to an "unconscious male" at a private residence. You arrive at the scene 5 minutes after being dispatched. You ring the doorbell and knock loudly several times but there is no response.

While you are tempted to go in, you remember that your training did not include forcible entry. Police arrive on the scene, gain access into the house, and summon you inside. You enter the house and see a man lying on the floor. Your partner starts to assess his level of consciousness. The patient begins to wake up and tells you to go away.

1. The process by which an individual, institution, or program is evaluated and recognized as meeting certain predetermined standards to ensure safe and ethical patient care is called:
   A. licensure.
   B. certification.
   C. standard of care.
   D. authorization.

2. Unlawfully touching a person even while attempting to provide care is called:
   A. battery.
   B. assault.
   C. slander.
   D. libel.

3. All of the following are required to prove negligence against an EMT-I, except:
   A. breech of duty.
   B. duty to act.
   C. consent.
   D. proximate cause.

4. A type of consent in which the patient has been told of the potential risks, benefits, and alternatives to treatment and has given consent to treatment is:
   A. expressed consent.
   B. implied consent.
   C. informed consent.
   D. actual consent.

5. The act of physically restraining a patient from a mental or physical action is called:
   A. malfeasance.
   B. forcible restraint.
   C. assault.
   D. battery.

6. A written document that specifies medical treatment for a competent patient should he or she become unable to make decisions is called:
   A. do not resuscitate order.
   B. advance directive.
   C. standard of care.
   D. standing order.

7. The law dealing with private complaints brought by a plaintiff against a defendant for an illegal act or wrong doing is called:
   A. criminal law.
   B. tort law.
   C. administrative law.
   D. common law.

8. Which of the following is true regarding consent of a minor?
   A. Parents or legal guardians may not give consent if the patient is competent.
   B. In some states, emancipated minors may consent for medical treatment.
   C. You can always provide care under implied consent to a minor.
   D. If you do not have proper consent, you must withhold lifesaving care.

9. If the EMT-I is on the scene of a potential organ donor, the EMT-I should:
   A. not attempt any resuscitation.
   B. wait for law enforcement to authorize any treatment.
   C. treat the patient the same way that you would any other patient needing treatment.
   D. not supply oxygen because it will damage potential organs.

10. Good Samaritan laws that exist in many states are designed to:
    A. prevent anyone from bringing a lawsuit against you.
    B. avoid liability for errors or omissions that are made in giving good faith emergency care.
    C. grant complete immunity from liability.
    D. apply only to compensated providers who are part of a municipality.

Points to Ponder

You are dispatched to a home of a 70-year-old woman in severe respiratory distress. Upon arrival you are met by her son who states that she is very sick and prepared to die. Her religious beliefs do not allow for any type of resuscitative measures. You ask the family member if they have a DNR order for the patient. The son states that she has a living will and that he has power of attorney. Your state does not recognize living wills in the prehospital setting. While you examine this patient, you notice that she is deteriorating rapidly. You are providing care to her when the patient experiences cardiac arrest. You direct your BLS crew to initiate CPR. As you prepare to call medical control and talk to the son about the current situation, a neighbor who happens to be a doctor comes in and begins to order you to initiate ALS interventions or he will do it himself. What do you do?

Issues: Advocating for Respect of Patient Rights and Feelings, Defending Personal Beliefs About Withholding or Stopping Patient Care, Defending Values of Medical Directives, Defending EMT-I Actions

Medical Terminology

1999 Objectives

There are no 1999 objectives for this chapter.

1985 Objectives

Cognitive

1.4.1 Define and contrast medical terms. (p 98)
1.4.2 Identify various medical terms given one or more anatomical parts of the body. (p 101)
1.4.3 Identify common medical abbreviations. (p 105)
1.4.4 Identify common root words and determine their meaning. (p 101)
1.4.5 Identify and define common prefixes and suffixes. (p 98)
1.4.6 Locate one or more medical terms in a medical dictionary. (p 112)

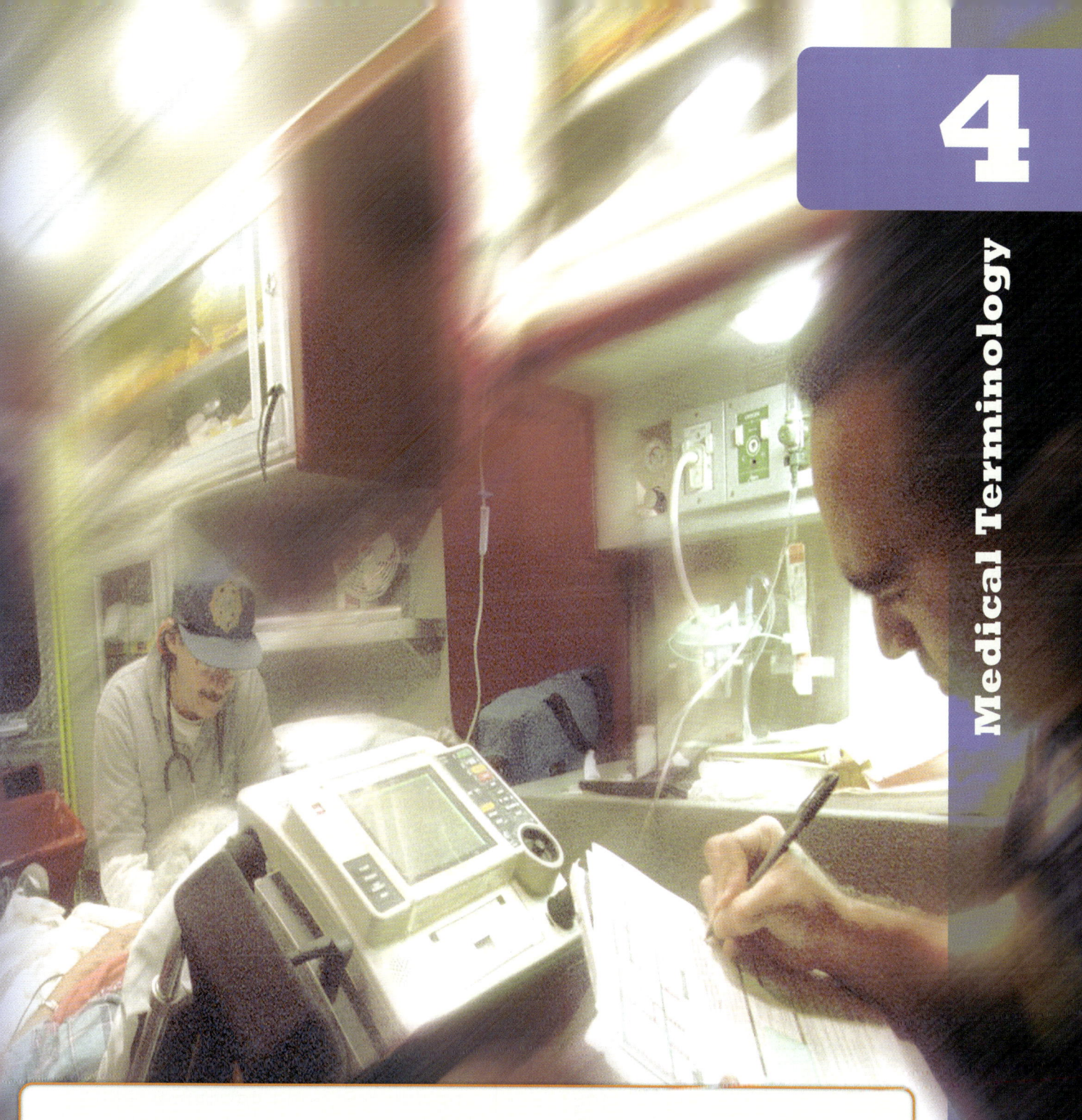

4

Medical Terminology

You are the Provider

You are dispatched for an unknown medical call. Upon arrival at the scene, you find an elderly man who tells you that he is having difficulty breathing. He describes a history of chronic obstructive pulmonary disease (COPD). You call the emergency department and report that you are en route with a patient complaining of dysphagia.

This chapter will help the EMT-I learn the language of medicine. Proper use of medical terminology will lend credibility to the EMS provider's report.

1. What is the medical term that describes difficulty breathing?
2. Can patient care be affected by using incorrect medical terminology?

Medical Terminology

As an EMT-I, it is imperative that you have a strong working knowledge of medical terminology. The language of medicine is primarily derived from Greek and Latin. Throughout your EMT-I training, and if you choose to continue your training to the paramedic level, you must understand this terminology to grasp fundamental concepts from which you will build. Medical terminology is used in international language, and it is also necessary for communicating with other medical personnel. The wider your vocabulary base, the more competent you seem to the rest of the medical community and the better the patient care you will be able to provide.

Understanding terminology involves breaking words down into their separate components of prefix, suffix, and root word and having a good working knowledge of those parts. Carrying a field guide or documentation handbook with you allows you to look up unfamiliar terms without memorizing page after page 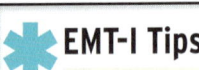.

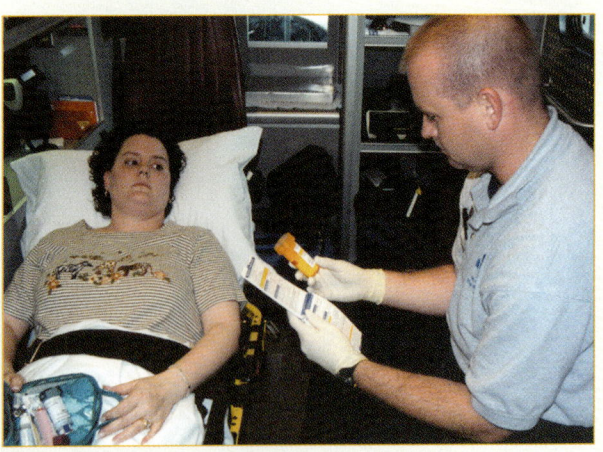

Figure 4-1 Use a field guide to look up unfamiliar terms.

EMT-I Tips

Carry a field guide or documentation handbook to look up unfamiliar words.

Prefixes

A **prefix** appears at the beginning of a word and generally describes location and intensity. Prefixes are frequently found in general language, as well as in medical and scientific terminology. When a medical word contains a prefix, the meaning of the word is altered. By learning to recognize a few of the more commonly used medical prefixes, you can figure out the meaning of terms that may not be immediately familiar to you. See Table 4-1 for a list of common prefixes.

A to Z Terminology Tips

By learning a few prefixes you will recognize more medical terms. For example, the prefix *hypo-* means low. *Hypovolemia* means low blood volume, *hypotension* means low blood pressure, and *hypoglycemia* means a low blood sugar (or glucose) level.

Technology

- Interactivities
- Vocabulary Explorer
- Anatomy Review
- Web Links
- Online Review Manual

www.EMSzone.com/EMTI

TABLE 4-1	Common Prefixes		
Prefix	**Meaning**	**Prefix**	**Meaning**
a-	without, lack of	cyst(o)-	pertaining to the bladder or any fluid-containing sac
ab-	away from	cyt(o)-	pertaining to a cell
abdomi(n)-	abdomen	dermat(o)-	pertaining to the skin
acr(o)-	pertaining to an extremity	di-	twice, double
ad-	to, toward	dia-	through, completely
aden(o)-	pertaining to a gland	dys-	difficult, painful, abnormal
an-	without, lack of	ect(o)-	out from
ana-	up, back, again	electro-	pertaining to electricity
angio-	vessel	end(o)-	within
ante-	before, forward	enter(o)-	pertaining to the intestines
anti-	against, opposed to	epi-	upon, on
arteri(o)-	artery	erythr(o)-	pertaining to red or to erythrocytes (red blood cells)
arthro-	pertaining to a joint	eu-	easy, good, normal
auto-	self	ex(o)-	outside
bi-	two	extra-	outside, in addition
bi(o)-	pertaining to life	gastr(o)-	pertaining to the stomach
blast(o)-	germ or cell	glyc(o)-	sugar
blephar(o)-	pertaining to an eyelid	gynec(o)-	pertaining to females or the female reproductive organs
brady-	slow	hemat(o)-	pertaining to blood
calc-	stone; also heel	hemi-	half
cardi(o)-	pertaining to the heart	hem(o)-	pertaining to blood
cephal(o)-	pertaining to the head	hepat(o)-	pertaining to the liver
cerebr(o)-	pertaining to the cerebrum, a part of the brain	hydr(o)-	water
cervic(o)-	pertaining to the neck or the uterine opening (cervix)	hyper-	over, excessive
		hypo-	under, deficient
chole-	pertaining to bile	hyster(o)-	pertaining to the uterus
chondr(o)-	pertaining to cartilage	infra-	below
circum-	around, about	inter-	between
contra-	against, opposite	intra-	within
cost(o)-	pertaining to a rib		
cyan(o)-	blue		

Continued

TABLE 4-1	Common Prefixes—cont'd		
Prefix	**Meaning**	**Prefix**	**Meaning**
iso-	equal	phag(o)-	pertaining to eating, ingesting, or engulfing
latero-	side	pharyng(o)-	pertaining to the throat or pharynx
leuk(o)-	pertaining to anything white or to leukocytes (white blood cells)	phleb(o)-	pertaining to a vein
lith(o)-	pertaining to a stone	pneum(o)-	pertaining to respiration, the lungs, or air
macro-	large	poly-	many
mal-	bad or abnormal	post-	after, behind
mening(o)-	pertaining to a membrane, particularly the meninges	pre-	before
micro-	small	pro-	before, in front of
mono-	one	proct(o)-	pertaining to the rectum
myel(o)-	pertaining to the spinal cord, the bone marrow, or myelin	pseud(o)-	false
my(o)-	pertaining to muscle	psych(o)-	pertaining to the mind
nas(o)-	pertaining to the nose	pulm(o)-	pertaining to the lung
ne(o)-	new	pyel(o)-	pertaining to kidney pelvis
nephr(o)-	pertaining to the kidney	py(o)-	pertaining to pus
neur(o)-	pertaining to a nerve or the nervous system	quadr(i)-	four
noct-	night	retr(o)-	backward or behind
olig(o)-	little, deficient, or minimal	rhin(o)-	pertaining to the nose
oophor(o)-	pertaining to the ovary	salping(o)-	pertaining to a tube
ophthalm(o)-	pertaining to the eye	scler(o)-	hard; also means pertaining to the sclera
orchid(o)-	pertaining to the testicles	semi-	half or partial
orchi(o)-	pertaining to the testicles	sub-	under, moderately
ortho-	straight or normal	super-	high, excessive, or more than normal
oste(o)-	pertaining to bone	supra-	above
ot(o)-	pertaining to the ear	tachy-	fast
para-	by the side of	thorac(o)-	pertaining to the chest
path(o)-	pertaining to disease	trans-	across
per-	through	tri-	three
peri-	around	uni-	one
		vas(o)-	vessel

TABLE 4-2 Common Suffixes

Suffix	Meaning	Suffix	Meaning
-algia	pertaining to pain	-ostomy	surgical creation of an opening
-asthen(o)	weakness	-pathy	disease or a system for treating disease
-blast	immature cell		
-cele	pertaining to a tumor or swelling	-phagia	pertaining to eating or swallowing
-centesis	pertaining to a procedure in which an organ or body cavity is punctured, often to drain excess fluid or obtain a sample for analysis	-phasia	pertaining to speech
		-phobia	pertaining to an irrational fear
		-plasty	reconstruction
-cyte	cell	-plegia	paralysis
-ectomy	surgical removal of	-pnea	pertaining to breathing
-emia	pertaining to the presence of a substance in the blood	-ptosis	drooping
		-rrhage	abnormal or excessive flow or discharge
-esthesi(o)-	pertaining to sensation or perception	-rrhagia	abnormal or excessive flow or discharge
-genic	causing		
-gram	record	-rrhaphy	suture of; repair of
-graph	a record or the instrument used to create the record	-rrhea	flow or discharge
-itis	inflammation	-scope	instrument for examination
-lysis	decline, disintegration, or destruction	-scopy	examination with an instrument
-megaly	enlargement of	-sis	a process, action, or condition
-ology	science of	-taxis	order, arrangement of
-oma	tumor	-trophic	pertaining to nutrition
-osis	pertaining to a disease process (see also -sis)	-uria	pertaining to a substance in the urine or the condition so indicated

Suffixes

Suffixes are placed at the end of words to change the meaning. In medical terminology, a suffix usually indicates a procedure, condition, disease, or part of speech. A commonly used suffix is *-itis*, which means "inflammation." When this suffix is paired with the prefix *arthro-*, meaning joint, the resulting word is *arthritis*, an inflammation of the joints. Sometimes it is necessary to change the last letter or letters of the root word or prefix when a suffix is added to aid in pronunciation. See Table 4-2 for a list of common suffixes.

Root Words

The main part or stem of a word is called a root word. A root word conveys the essential meaning of the word and frequently indicates a body part. It may be combined with another root word, a prefix, or a suffix to describe a particular structure or condition. A frequently used term in EMS is CPR, which stands for cardiopulmonary resuscitation. When we break it down, *cardio* is a root word meaning "heart," and *pulmonary* is a root word meaning "lungs." By performing CPR we introduce air into the lungs and circulate blood by compressing the heart to resuscitate the patient. Some root words may also be used as prefixes or suffixes. See Table 4-3 for a list of common root words.

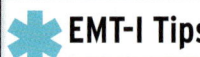

EMT-I Tips

When documenting, use only abbreviations that are commonly accepted.

TABLE 4-3 Common Root Words

Root Word	Meaning	Root Word	Meaning
abdomin-	abdomen	carotid	great arteries of the neck
acou-	hear	carp-	wrist
aden-	gland	cent-	a fraction in the metric system; one hundredth or 100
adip-	fat		
alb-	white	cente-	to puncture (a body cavity)
alges-	pain	cephal-	head
andr-	male	cervic-	neck
angi-	vessel	chol-	bile
aorta	large artery exiting from the left ventricle of the heart	chondr-	cartilage
		cili-	eyelid
aqua-	water	cleid(o)-	clavicle
arteri-	artery	cubitus	elbow
arthr-	joint	cyan-	blue
asphyxia	lack of oxygen or excess of carbon dioxide in the body that results in unconsciousness	cycl-	circle or cycle
		cyst-	bladder
		cyt-	cell
asthen-	weak	derm(at)-	skin
audi-	to hear	digit	finger or toe
bi-	life; also two	ede-	swelling
bronch-	windpipe	enter-	intestine
bucc-	cheek	erythr-	red
bursa	pouch or sac	esthe-	sensation or perception
callus	hard, thick skin; also a meshwork of connective tissue that forms during the healing process after a fracture	febr-	fever
		-flex-	bend
carcin-	cancer	foramen	opening
cardi-	heart		

TABLE 4-3 Common Root Words—cont'd

Root Word	Meaning	Root Word	Meaning
fract-	break	ot-	ear
gastr-	stomach	ov-	egg
gest-	carry, produce, congestion	palpate	to examine by touch
glyc(y)-	sweet	path-	disease
gno-	know	ped-	child or foot
-gram	something written or recorded	percuss	to examine by striking
graph-	write, record	phag-	eat
gyn(ec)-	female	pharyng-	throat
hem(at)-	blood	photo-	light
hepat(ic)-	liver	pleur-	rib, side
heter-	other, different	pneum(at)-	breath
hom-	the same	pneumo(n)-	lung
humerus	the bone in the upper arm	pod-	foot
hydr-	water	pseud-	false
idi-	separate, distinct	psych-	mind
iod(o)-	iodine	pto-	fall
lact-	milk	ptyal-	saliva
leuk-	white	pur-, py-	pus
lingu-	tongue	pyr-	fire
mal-	abnormal	quadr, quar-, quat-	four
medi-	middle	radius	the forearm bone on the thumb side; also a line from the center of a circle or sphere to the edge
mega-	large		
melan-	black		
men-	month	ren-	kidney
mening-	membrane, usually refers to the meninges	retina	inner nerve-containing layer of the eye
		rhin-	nose
myel-	marrow or spinal cord	sangui(n)-	blood
my-	muscle	scler-	hard
nephr-	kidney	sebum	a fatty secretion of the sebaceous glands
neur-	nerve	sect-	cut
ocul-	eye	sepsis	the presence of microorganisms or their toxins in the blood; also the toxic condition caused by such presence
ophthalm-	eye		
ost(e)-	bone	sept-	wall, divider; also seven

Continued

TABLE 4-3 Common Root Words—cont'd

Root Word	Meaning	Root Word	Meaning
serum	the clear portion of body fluids, including blood	thorac-	chest
		tom-	cut
sinus	cavity, channel or hollow space	toxic	poisonous
som(a)-	body	trich-	hair
spir-	coil	ur-	urine
stasis	slowing or stopping of the normal flow of a fluid, such as blood	varic-	varicose vein
stature	height	vas-	vessel
stern(o)-	sternum (breastbone)	vertigo	a disordered sensation in which one's own body or the surroundings are perceived as moving or spinning
stoma	any small opening on the surface of the body, such as a pore; also, the opening created in the abdominal wall for the passage of urine or feces	viscer-	internal organs
		viscous	sticky
tach(y)-	rapid	xen-	foreign (material)
tact-	touch	xer-	dry
tetra-	four		

Abbreviations

Abbreviations take the place of words to shorten notes or documentation. When using abbreviations on patient care reports, remember to use only standard, accepted abbreviations to avoid confusion and errors. See Table 4-4 for a list of commonly used abbreviations. This list is intended to help you decipher documents written by other health care professionals. Before using any abbreviations in your own reports, be familiar with accepted use of abbreviations in your local jurisdiction or service area.

You are the Provider — Part 2

You have completed your assessment. You have initiated 100% oxygen via nonrebreathing mask.

Vital Signs	Recording Time: 2 Minutes After Patient Contact
Respirations	32 breaths/min, shallow
Pulse	128 beats/min, irregular
Skin	Pale, warm, and dry
Blood pressure	182/68 mm Hg
Sao_2	88% on 100% oxygen

Your patient is only able to speak in one- or two-word sentences. When you arrive at the emergency department, you discover that they are not prepared to receive a patient in respiratory distress.

3. What responsibility does the EMT-I have regarding medical terminology?
4. What potential affects can incorrect medical terms have on both the patient and the provider?

TABLE 4-4 Common Abbreviations*

Abbreviation	Meaning
A & P	anatomy and physiology
ā	before
aa	of each (used in writing prescriptions)
abd	abdomen
ABG	arterial blood gas
ac	before meals
ACLS	advanced cardiac life support
ADL	activity of daily living
ad lib	as much as desired
AED	automated external defibrillator
AF	atrial fibrillation
AIDS	acquired immunodeficiency syndrome
AK	above the knee
AKA	above the knee amputation
A-line	arterial line
AMA	against medical advice
amb	ambulatory
AMI	acute myocardial infarction
AMS	altered mental status
ant	anterior
AO × 4	alert and oriented to person, place, time, and self
AP	anteroposterior, front-to-back, action potential, angina pectoris, anterior pituitary, arterial pressure
APC	atrial premature complex, activated protein C, aspirin-phenacetin-caffeine
Aq	water
ARDS	adult respiratory distress syndrome
ASA	aspirin (acetylsalicylic acid)
ASAP	as soon as possible
ASHD	arteriosclerotic or atherosclerotic heart disease
AV, A-V	atrioventricular, arteriovenous
BBB	bundle branch block
bid	twice daily
BKA	below the knee amputation
BM	bowel movement
BP	blood pressure
BS	blood sugar, breath sounds, bowel sounds, bachelor of science (degree)
BSA	body surface area
BVM	bag-valve-mask (ventilation device)
bx	biopsy
c̄	with
°C	degrees Celsius (centigrade)
Ca	calcium
CA	cancer, cardiac arrest, chronological age, coronary artery, cold agglutinin
CABG	coronary artery bypass graft
CAD	coronary artery disease
CBC	complete blood count
cc	cubic centimeter
CC or C/C	chief complaint
CCU	coronary care unit
CHF	congestive heart failure
Cl$^-$	chloride
cm	centimeter
cm^3	cubic centimeter
CNS	central nervous system

*Sometimes abbreviations are written with periods (for example, abd. and a.c.), and sometimes different capitalization might be used and might convey a different meaning. Not all possible meanings for the abbreviations in this table are given here. Unless you are certain about the meaning, ask the person who used the abbreviation.

Continued

TABLE 4-4 Common Abbreviations—cont'd

Abbreviation	Meaning	Abbreviation	Meaning
c/o	complaining of	DVT	deep venous thrombosis
CO	cardiac output, carbon monoxide	D_5W	dextrose 5% in water
CO_2	carbon dioxide	Dx	diagnosis
COLD	chronic obstructive lung disease	ECG	electrocardiogram
COPD	chronic obstructive pulmonary disease	ED	emergency department
CP	chest pain, chemically pure, cerebral palsy	EDC	estimated date of confinement
		EEG	electroencephalogram
CPR	cardiopulmonary resuscitation	eg	for example
CRNA	certified registered nurse anesthetist	EKG	electrocardiogram
CRT	capillary refill time, cathode-ray tube	ENT	ears, nose, and throat
CSF	cerebrospinal fluid	ER	emergency room
CSM	carotid sinus massage, cerebrospinal meningitis	ET	endotracheal tube, endotracheal
CVA	cerebrovascular accident	ETA	estimated time of arrival
CVP	central venous pressure	ETOH	ethyl alcohol
CXR	chest x-ray	ETT	endotracheal tube
D & C	dilatation and curettage	°F	degrees Fahrenheit
D/C	discontinue	F_{IO_2}	fraction of inspired oxygen
diff	differential	FBS	fasting blood sugar
dig	digoxin	Fe	iron
DM	diabetes mellitus	FHR	fetal heart rate
DOA	dead on arrival	FHT	fetal heart tones
DOE	dyspnea on exertion	FHx	family history
DON	director of nursing	fL	femtoliter
DOS	dead on scene	fl or fld	fluid
DPT	diphtheria and tetanus toxoids and pertussis vaccine	FSH	follicle-stimulating hormone
		fx	fracture
DSD	dry sterile dressing	g	gram
DtaP	diphtheria and tetanus toxoids and acellular pertussis vaccine	GB	gallbladder
DTP	diphtheria and tetanus toxoids and pertussis vaccine	GI	gastrointestinal
		gm	gram
DTs	delirium tremens		

Abbreviation	Meaning
gr	grain
GSW	gunshot wound
gtt	drop(s)
GTT	glucose tolerance test
GU	genitourinary
gyn	gynecology
h	hour
H, (H)	hypodermic
H & H	hemoglobin and hematocrit
H & P	history and physical
H/A	headache
Hb, Hgb	hemoglobin
Hct	hematocrit
Hg	mercury
HH	hiatal hernia
HIV	human immunodeficiency virus
H_2O	water
H_2O_2	hydrogen peroxide
HPI	history of present illness
hr	hour
hs	at bedtime
HTN	hypertension
Hx	history
Hz	hertz
I & O	intake and output
IC	intracardiac, inspiratory capacity, irritable colon
ICP	intracranial pressure
ICU	intensive care unit
IDDM	insulin-dependent diabetes mellitus
IM	intramuscular
IO	intraosseous
IPPB	intermittent positive pressure breathing
IUD	intrauterine (contraceptive) device
IV	intravenous
JVD	jugular venous distention
K^+	potassium
KCL	potassium chloride
kg	kilogram
KUB	kidneys, ureters, and bladder
KVO	keep vein open
L	liter
LAC	laceration, laparoscopic-assisted colectomy
lb	pound
LE	lower extremity, left eye, lupus erythematosus
LLL	left lower lobe of the lung
LLQ	left lower quadrant of the abdomen
L/M	liters per minute
LMP	last menstrual period
LOC	level of consciousness, loss of consciousness
LPM	liters per minute
LPN	licensed practical nurse
LR	lactated Ringer's
LSD	lysergic acid diethylamide
LUL	left upper lobe of the lung
LUQ	left upper quadrant of the abdomen
LVN	licensed vocational nurse
m	meter
MAE	moves all extremities
MAEW	moves all extremities well

Continued

TABLE 4-4 Common Abbreviations—cont'd

Abbreviation	Meaning	Abbreviation	Meaning
MAP	mean arterial pressure	NSR	normal sinus rhythm
mcg	microgram	NTG	nitroglycerin
MCL	midclavicular line, modified chest lead	N/V	nausea and vomiting
mEq	milliequivalent	N/V/D	nausea, vomiting, and diarrhea
mg	milligram (mgm is a former symbol)	NVD	neck vein distention
MI	myocardial infarction	O_2	oxygen
MICU	mobile intensive care unit; medical intensive care unit	OB	obstetrics
		OBS	organic brain syndrome
min	minute	OD	overdose, right eye, optical density, outside diameter, doctor of optometry
mL	milliliter		
mm	millimeter	OP	outpatient
mm Hg	millimeters of mercury	OPA	oropharyngeal airway
MRI	magnetic resonance imaging	OR	operating room
MS	morphine sulfate, multiple sclerosis	OS	left eye
MSO_4	morphine sulfate	OU	both eyes
MVA	motor vehicle accident	oz	ounce
MVC	motor vehicle crash	$\bar{p}$	after
MVP	mitral valve prolapse	pc	after meals
Na	sodium	pco_2	partial pressure of carbon dioxide
NA, N/A	not applicable	PDR	Physician's Desk Reference
NaCl	sodium chloride	PE	pulmonary embolism, physical examination
NAD	no apparent distress, no appreciable disease		
		PEA	pulseless electrical activity
$NaHCO_3$	sodium bicarbonate	PEARL or PERL	pupils equal and reactive to light
NC	nasal cannula		
NG	nasogastric	ped or peds	Pediatric
NICU	neonatal intensive care unit	PEEP	positive end-expiratory pressure
NIDDM	non-insulin-dependent diabetes mellitus	PERRL	pupils equal, round, and reactive to light
NKA	no known allergies	pH	hydrogen ion concentration
NKDA	no known drug allergies	PID	pelvic inflammatory disease
NPA	nasopharyngeal airway	PND	paroxysmal nocturnal dyspnea
NPO	nil per os (nothing by mouth)	po	per os (by mouth)
NS	normal saline	PO	postoperative, "post op"
		po_2	partial pressure of oxygen

Abbreviation	Meaning
PRN	pro re nata (as needed)
psi	pounds per square inch
PSVT	paroxysmal supraventricular tachycardia
pt	patient
PT	physical therapy
PTA	prior to admission, plasma thromboplastin antecedent
PTT	partial thromboplastin time
PVC	premature ventricular complex, polyvinyl chloride
PVD	peripheral vascular disease
q	every
qd	every day
qh	every hour
qid	four times a day
qod	every other day
RA	rheumatoid arthritis, right atrium
RAD	reactive airway disease, right axis deviation
RBC	red blood cell
Rh	Rhesus blood factor, rhodium
RHD	rheumatic heart disease
RL	Ringer's lactate
RLL	right lower lobe of the lung
RLQ	right lower quadrant of the abdomen
RN	registered nurse
R/O	rule out
ROM	range of motion, rupture of membranes
RUL	right upper lobe of the lung
RUQ	right upper quadrant of the abdomen
Rx	prescription
s̄	without
SC	subcutaneous, secretory component
SICU	surgical intensive care unit
SIDS	sudden infant death syndrome
SL	sublingual
SOB	shortness of breath
SQ	subcutaneous
ss	half
S/S	signs and symptoms
stat	immediately
STD	sexually transmitted disease
Sub Q	subcutaneous
SVT	supraventricular tachycardia
sym or Sx	symptoms
tab	tablet
TB	tuberculosis
TBA	to be admitted, to be announced
tbsp	tablespoon
tech	technician, technologist
TIA	transient ischemic attack
tid	three times a day
TKO	to keep open
TPR	temperature, pulse, respiration
tsp	teaspoon
Tx	treatment
U	unit
UA	urinalysis
UE	upper extremity
URI	upper respiratory infection
USP	United States Pharmacopeia
UTI	urinary tract infection
VD	venereal disease
vol	volume
VS	vital signs
W/	with

Continued

TABLE 4-4 Common Abbreviations—cont'd

Abbreviation	Meaning	Abbreviation	Meaning
WBC	white blood cell	β	beta
WNL	within normal limits	≅	approximately
wt	weight	o	normal
yo	year old	×2	times two
x̄	except	/	per
1°	first, first degree, primary	≠	not equal
2°	secondary, second degree	>	greater than
↑	increased	<	less than
↓	decreased	?	questionable, possible
∅	none	Δ	change
Ⓡ	right	-	negative
Ⓛ	left	♀	female
μ	micro	♂	male
α	alpha		

You are the Provider　　　　　　　　Summary

1. What is the medical term that describes difficulty breathing?

Dyspnea.

2. Can patient care be affected by using incorrect medical terminology?

Inaccurate communication regarding patient complaints and care can have potentially adverse affects on the smooth transfer of care to emergency department personnel.

3. What responsibility does the EMT-I have regarding medical terminology?

An understanding of correct medical terminology is necessary for communicating with other medical personnel. The use of proper medical terms adds to the credibility of the provider and provides a more accurate description of the patient's condition.

4. What potential effects can incorrect medical terms have on both the patient and the provider?

Misuse of medical terms can create confusion and interfere with the delivery of patient care.

Prep Kit

Ready For Review

- By learning some of the most common root words, prefixes, and suffixes, and by using a medical dictionary, you will gain a good working knowledge of medical terminology. This will help in your career as an EMT-I and aid in communication with patients, hospital personnel, and coworkers.
- Learning abbreviations will assist you in documentation and decrease the length of your reports. Remember to only use standard, accepted, and approved abbreviations when completing your trip reports and medical documentation.
- The terms listed in this chapter are but a select few of the most commonly used prefixes, suffixes, and root words. As you continue throughout this text and throughout your career, you will continuously add to your medical vocabulary.

Vital Vocabulary

prefix Appears at the beginning of a word and generally describes location and intensity.

root word The main part or stem of a word that conveys the essential meaning of the word and frequently indicates a body part.

suffix Placed at the end of a word to change the meaning and usually indicates a procedure, condition, disease, or part of speech.

Points to Ponder

You are caring for a patient who is experiencing a diabetic emergency. He has a low blood glucose level that you are able to treat. En route to the hospital, the patient begins to experience an altered level of consciousness. You ask your driver to relay to the hospital that you are coming in with a patient who is experiencing hypoperfusion. The hospital directs you to bring the patient into Trauma Bay 1.

Upon arrival to the hospital, you give your hospital report. The staff was expecting a patient in shock, based on what your driver relayed in his radio report. Your driver actually should have used the term hypoglycemia to describe the patient's condition.

Issues: Importance of Knowing Correct Terminology, Understanding Benefits of Plain English, Being Aware of the Effect of One's Own Actions on Others

Technology

- Interactivities
- Vocabulary Explorer
- Anatomy Review
- Web Links
- Online Review Manual

www.EMSzone.com/EMTI

Assessment in Action

You are dispatched to care for a person with "chest pain" in a rural part of your jurisdiction. Your travel time is approximately 17 minutes, so you request that the local volunteer fire department be dispatched to respond with you.

Upon your arrival, one of the volunteers meets you at the ambulance and informs you that the patient is a 64-year-old man with an extensive medical history. He hands you the paperwork from the patient's most recent hospitalization. You walk inside and begin sorting through the chart as your partner assesses the patient's level of responsiveness and vital signs.

1. You note a history of hyperglycemia and NIDDM in the chart. You know that the prefix *hyper-* means:

   A. up.
   B. down.
   C. high.
   D. low.

2. You check your field guide to find that *NIDDM* is an abbreviation for:

   A. no inherent drug dose maximum.
   B. non-insulin-dependent diabetes mellitus.
   C. non-insulin diabetes drug maintenance.
   D. not in dry dose manner.

3. You continue reading and find a list of medications including K^+. This is the abbreviation for:

   A. potassium.
   B. chloride.
   C. sodium.
   D. calcium.

4. Your partner requests your assistance while filling out the trip report after the call. He tells you the patient has a history of high blood pressure. How will you abbreviate it?

   A. Hyperten
   B. Hprtn
   C. HBP
   D. HTN

The Human Body

1999 Objectives

Cognitive

1-2.1 Define anatomy, physiology, and pathophysiology. (p 118)

1-2.2 Name the levels of organization of the body from simplest to most complex, and explain each. (p 118)

1-2.3 Define homeostasis. (p 118)

1-2.4 State the anatomical terms for the parts of the body. (p 119)

1-2.5 Identify terminology to describe the location of body parts with respect to one another. (p 119)

1-2.6 Review the body cavities and the major organs within each. (p 141)

1-2.7 Identify the anatomical planes. (p 120)

1-2.8 Identify areas of the abdomen and underlying organs. (p 123)

1-2.9 Define each of the cellular transport mechanisms and give an example of the role of each in the body: diffusion, osmosis, facilitated diffusion, active transport. (p 126)

1-2.10 Define metabolism, anabolism, catabolism. (p 128)

1-2.11 Describe how glucose is converted to energy during cellular respiration. (p 128)

1-2.12 Describe the general characteristics of each of the four major categories of tissues. (p 129)

1-2.13 Name the three major layers of the skin. (p 132)

1-2.14 Describe the functions of the skeleton. (p 133)

1-2.15 Explain how bones are classified. (p 133)

1-2.16 Explain how joints are classified. (p 156)

1-2.17 Describe the structure and function of muscles. (p 158)

1-2.18 List the three types of muscles. (p 159)

1-2.19 State the functions of the nervous system. (p 160)

1-2.20 Name the divisions of the nervous system. (p 160)

1-2.21 Explain the structure of neurons. (p 160)

1-2.22 Describe the types of nerves. (p 161)

1-2.23 Describe the role of polarization, depolarization, repolarization in nerve impulse transmission. (p 892-894)

1-2.24 Identify the components of the central nervous system. (p 162)

1-2.25 State the function of the meninges and cerebrospinal fluid. (p 165)

1-2.26 Identify the divisions of the autonomic nervous system and define their functions. (p 171)

1-2.27 Discuss the regulator processes of hormonal secretion. (p 173)

1-2.28 State the functions of hormones. (p 173)

1-2.29 State the function of the hormones of the pancreas. (p 176)

1-2.30 State the functions of epinephrine and norepinephrine and explain their relationship to the sympathetic division of the autonomic nervous system. (p 177)

1-2.31 Describe the characteristics of blood and its composition. (p 178)

1-2.32 Explain the function of red blood cells, white blood cells, and platelets. (p 179)

1-2.33 State the importance of blood clotting. (p 180)

1-2.34 Describe the location of the heart. (p 181)

1-2.35 Describe the function of the pericardium. (p 181)

1-2.36 Identify the major vessels and chambers of the heart. (p 182)

1-2.37 Identify the valves of the heart, and explain their functions. (p 182)

1-2.38 Describe coronary circulation, and explain its purpose. (p 182)

1-2.39 Describe the cardiac cycle. (p 182)

1-2.40 Explain how heart sounds are created. (p 183)

1-2.41 Name the parts of the cardiac conduction pathway. (p 184)

1-2.42 Explain the relationship between stroke volume, heart rate, and cardiac output. (p 187)

1-2.43 Explain how the nervous system regulates heart rate and force of contraction. (p 187)

1-2.44 Describe the structure of arteries and veins, and relate their structure to function. (p 188)

1-2.45 Describe the structure of capillaries, and explain the exchange processes that take place in capillaries. (p 188)

1-2.46 Describe the pathway and purpose of pulmonary circulation. (p 189)

1-2.47 Describe the pathway and purpose of systemic circulation. (p 189)

5

1-2.48 Define blood pressure. (p 197)
1-2.49 Explain the factors that maintain and regulate blood pressure. (p 197)
1-2.50 Describe the functions of the lymphatic system. (p 198)
1-2.51 Describe the immune response. (p 200)
1-2.52 State the function of the respiratory system. (p 201)
1-2.53 Describe the structure and functions of the components of the respiratory system. (p 201)
1-2.54 Describe normal inhalation and exhalation. (p 201)
1-2.55 Differentiate between ventilation and respiration. (p 205)
1-2.56 Explain the diffusion of gases across the alveolar-capillary junction. (p 205)
1-2.57 Describe how oxygen and carbon dioxide are transported in the blood. (p 204)
1-2.58 Explain the nervous and chemical mechanisms that regulate respiration. (p 163)
1-2.59 Describe the functions of the digestive system, and name its major divisions. (p 207)
1-2.60 Describe the water compartments and the name for the fluid in each. (p 212)
1-2.61 Explain how water moves between compartments. (p 212)
1-2.62 Explain the regulation of the intake and output of water. (p 212)
1-2.63 Describe the three buffer systems in body fluids. (p 214)
1-2.64 Explain why the respiratory system has an effect on pH, and describe respiratory compensating mechanisms. (p 213)
1-2.65 Explain the renal mechanisms for pH regulation of extracellular fluid. (p 213)
1-2.66 Describe the effects of acidosis and alkalosis. (p 213)

Affective

1-2.67 Appreciate how anatomy and physiology are the foundation of medicine. (p 118)

Psychomotor

None

1985 Objectives

There are no 1985 objectives for this chapter.

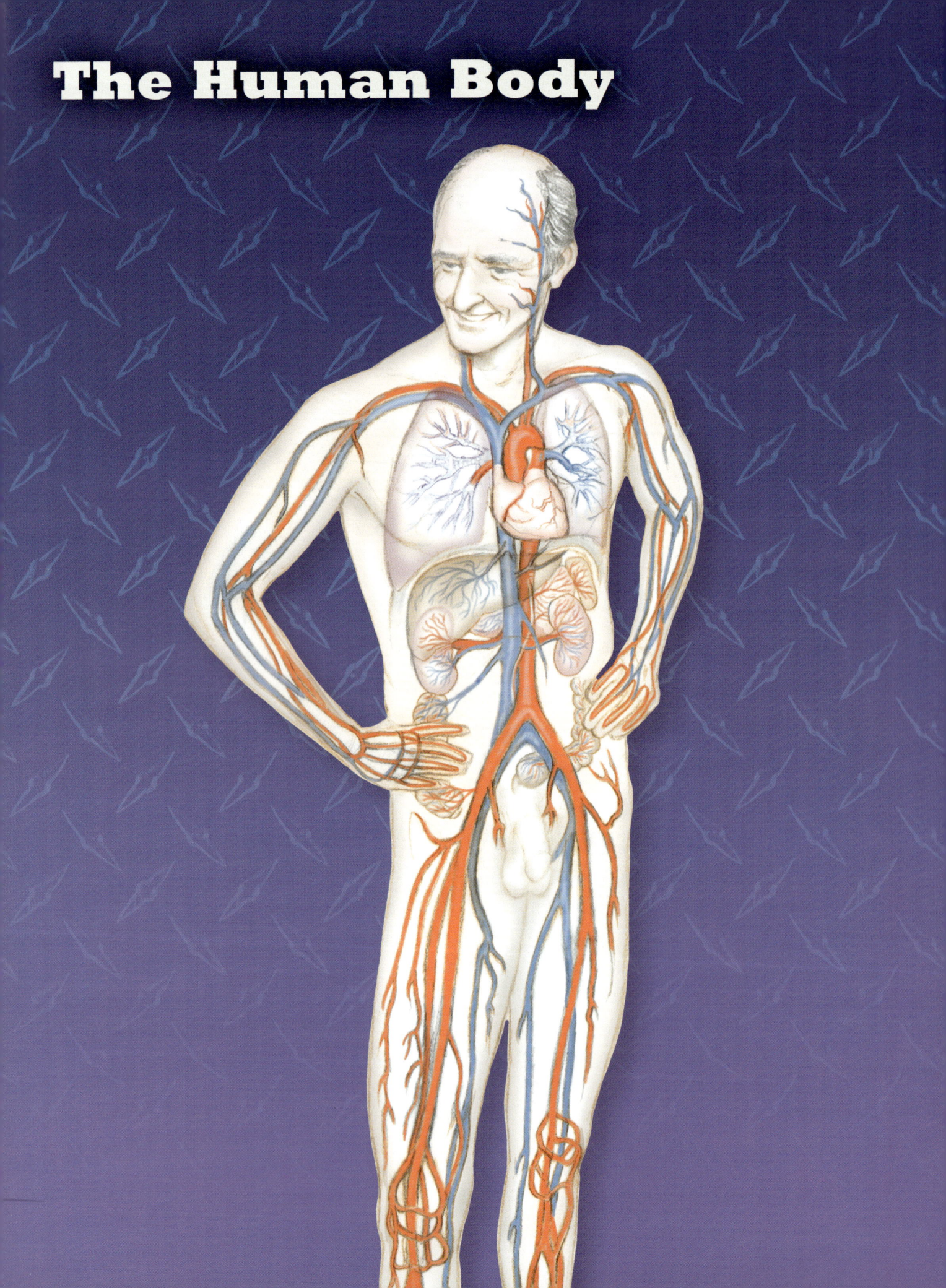

The Human Body

5

The Human Body

You are the Provider

You and your partner are on duty when a call comes in for an MVC involving a minivan and a passenger vehicle. Initial reports from law enforcement on scene state that there are possibly four injured people.

This chapter provides essential information about the basic workings of the human body and will also help you answer the following questions:

1. How does each body system respond when another body system is damaged from illness or injury?
2. What are anatomy, physiology, and pathophysiology?

Introduction

The study of anatomy is concerned with the structure of an organism and the components that make up the organism, in this case, the human body. Gross anatomy includes body parts that are generally visible to the naked eye—the bones, the muscles, and the organs. Microscopic anatomy involves components of the body that are small, often visible only through a microscope. Physiology examines the body functions of the living organism. Pathophysiology is the study of the body functions of a living organism in an abnormal state, such as a disease. With general knowledge of the structures and function of the body's systems, you will be able to better assess a patient as well as predict potential complications resulting from occult injuries (those not visible to the eye). In addition, all EMT-Is must be familiar with the language of topographic anatomy. By using the proper medical terms, you will be able to communicate correct information with the least possible confusion.

The Structure of the Human Body

The body comprises building blocks, from the minute cells and their internal structures to the tissues, organs with special functions, and organ systems, which work together to accomplish essential functions of the body. The building blocks of the body work closely together to provide a normal environment so that the cells, tissues, organs, and organ systems can live and function properly.

Technology

- Interactivities
- Vocabulary Explorer
- Anatomy Review
- Web Links
- Online Review Manual

www.EMSzone.com/EMTI

Cells

Cells are the most basic component of an organism. Some organisms, such as bacteria, are made up of only one cell. More complex organisms, such as the human body, contain numerous cells that may be specialized to perform a particular function. The human body contains about 100 trillion cells, which are specialized to fulfill particular roles in the body.

Tissues

Tissue refers to a group of similar cells working together to perform a common function. Tissues are classified as one of the following four types: epithelial, connective, muscle, and nerve.

Organs

Organs comprise different types of tissues working together to perform a particular function. For example, muscle, nerves, and fibrous connective tissue all coexist in the heart. Together, these components serve to pump blood throughout the arteries and veins of the circulatory system. The skin contains all four types of tissues and is the largest organ in the body. It preserves heat, prevents fluid loss (dehydration), functions as a sensory organ, and protects against invasion of the body's surface by infection-causing bacteria. Other organs include the liver, spleen, digestive organs, reproductive organs, and the organs of special sense.

Organ Systems

While organs are made of different types of tissue working together, an organ system is a group of organs that work together. Organ systems may be located near each other, or may be located far from each other, in different parts of the body. Combined, the various organ systems form an organism, any living thing considered as a whole (ie, the human body). The human organism is very complex, consisting of mutually dependent organs and organ systems. Organ systems inside the body carry out vital functions. The organ systems of the human body include musculoskeletal, circulatory, respiratory, nervous, gastrointestinal, urinary (excretory), reproductive, immune, endocrine, lymphatic, integumentary, and special sensory systems.

Homeostasis

Maintenance of the internal environment of the cell is regulated by elaborate systems of checks and balances. As systems in the body become imbalanced and begin to shift, feedback systems create an appropriate response to return the internal environment to normal. This normally balanced condition is referred to as <u>homeostasis</u>, or the resistance to change. These checks and balances can be seen in the way that the body regulates blood glucose: too little circulating blood glucose and the feedback system responds to create glucose; too much circulating blood glucose and the feedback system responds to store the excess glucose.

Anatomic Terminology

Using topographic anatomy is like using a road map. The terms that are introduced in this chapter will help you to identify the topographic (on the surface) landmarks of the body. These landmarks are used as guides to locate the internal structures that lie beneath them. These terms also refer to the names of the major regions of the body and the way in which the locations of these regions are described in relation to one another.

The Anatomic Position

<u>Topographic anatomy</u>, also called regional anatomy, refers to terms that uniformly describe the position and movement of the body. The universal position from which all body positions and movements are described is referred to as the <u>anatomic position</u> (Figure 5-1 ▶). In the anatomic position, the subject is standing upright, facing the observer. The arms are straightened, with the palms of the hands forward.

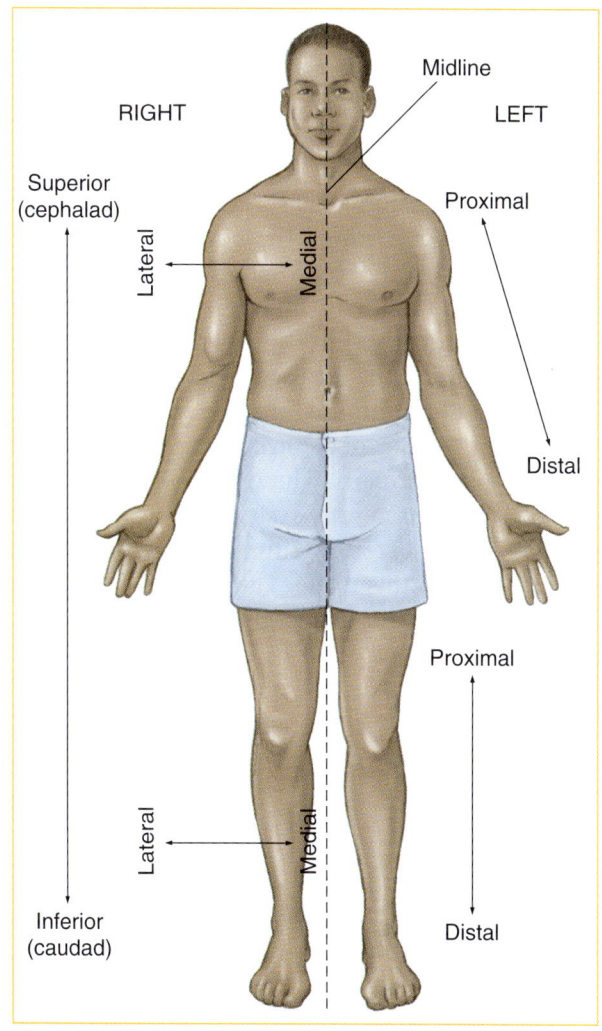

Figure 5-1 The anatomic position. Directional terms indicate the distance and direction from the midline.

You are the Provider Part 2

Ample additional personnel and vehicles have responded to the scene. Your first victim, the unrestrained driver of the minivan, is conscious and complaining of difficulty breathing. You note the following:

Initial Assessment	Recording Time: Zero Minutes
Appearance	Respiratory distress; pale
Level of consciousness	Conscious and alert
Airway	Open and clear
Breathing	Increased and labored
Circulation	Radial pulse, rapid; skin, cool and pale

3. How can knowledge of medical terminology help the EMT-I care for this patient?

Directional terms pertain to the patient, not the observer; therefore, right or left refers to the patient's right or left.

Anatomic Planes

In the anatomic position, flat surfaces, or planes, can be imagined to pass through the body Figure 5-2. These are the frontal (coronal), transverse (cross-horizontal), and median (midsagittal) planes. These planes describe distinct three-dimensional frames of reference from which the location of various organs and their relation to one another may be specified.

The frontal plane, or coronal plane, divides the body into front and back parts. These parts may be equal or unequal. The terms anterior (situated toward the front of the body) and posterior (situated toward the back of the body) refer to this plane. The transverse plane, or cross-horizontal plane, divides the body into the cranial or cephalad (upper, toward the head) and caudad (lower, toward the feet) parts. This plane is perpendicular to the long axis of the body. The median plane, also called the midsagittal plane or midline, passes longitudinally through the middle of the body and divides the body into left and right halves. The terms medial and lateral refer to the median plane and describe how close (medial) or far away (lateral) locations are on the body compared to the median plane. A sagittal plane is any vertical plane that is parallel to the median plane and divides the body into unequal left and right parts.

Terms that describe locations based on the division of the body by the frontal, transverse, or median planes are universally used. These terms include anterior, posterior, ventral, dorsal, superior, inferior, medial, and lateral. The terms anterior and ventral refer to the front of a part, organ, or structure. Posterior and dorsal refer to the back. Cranial (or cephalad) and superior refer to a structures that are closer to the head or higher than

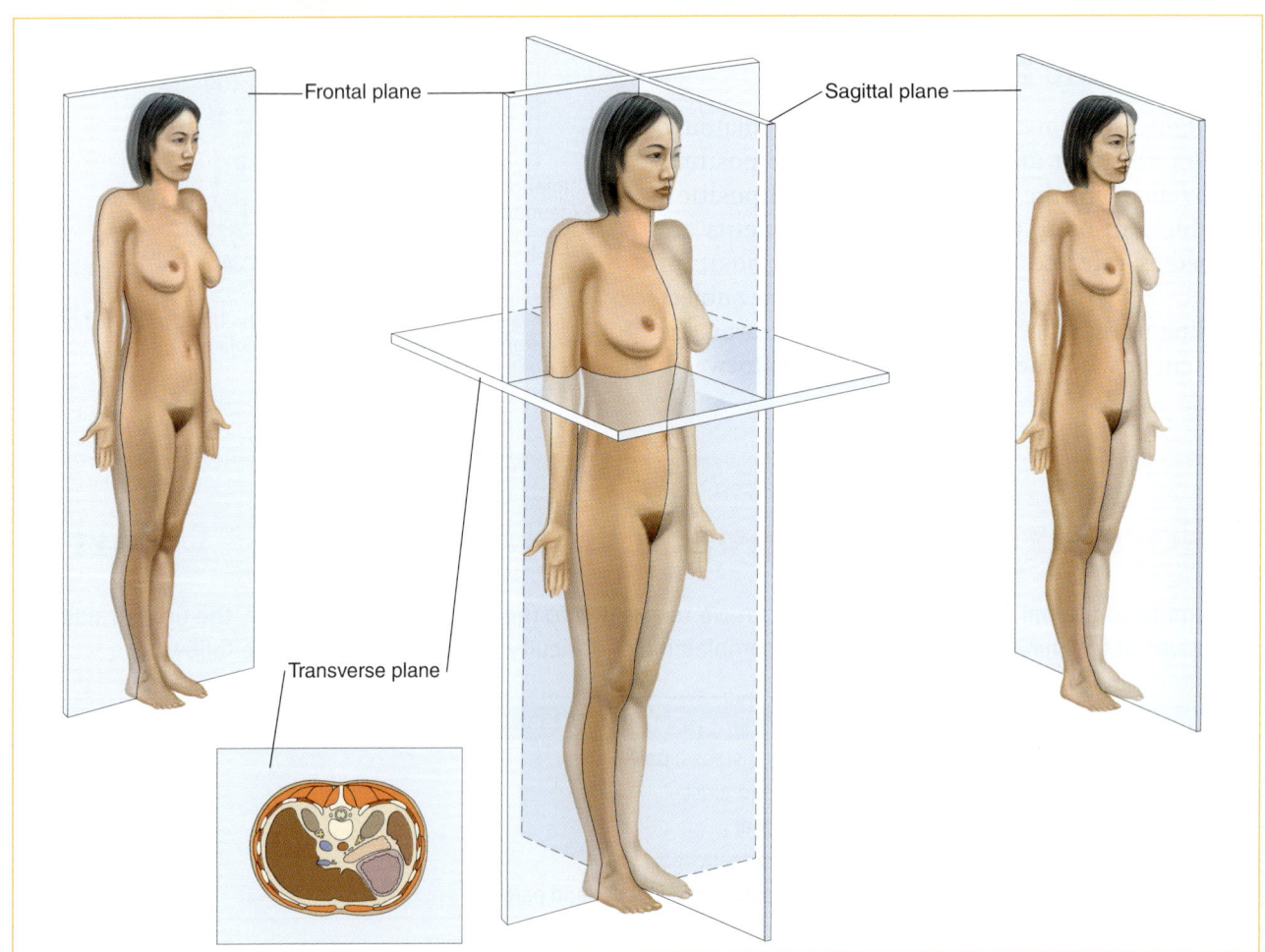

Figure 5-2 The anatomic planes of the body.

another structure. Caudad and inferior refer to structures that are closer to the feet or lower than another structure. Medial means situated toward the midline or central portion of a structure or organ, whereas lateral means situated away from the midline. Proximal and distal describe the relationship of any two structures on an extremity; proximal means nearer to or toward the trunk of the body and distal means farther from the trunk and toward the free end of an extremity. For example, the knee is proximal to the ankle, and the wrist is proximal to the fingers; the toe is distal to the ankle, and the wrist is distal to the elbow.

The frontal plane runs through the body from head to toe, dividing it into anterior (or ventral) and posterior (or dorsal) sections. For example, pain in the breast area would be described as being located on the anterior, or ventral, portion of the chest wall. An injury near the buttocks, on the other hand, would be specified as being located on the posterior, or dorsal, portion of the body.

The transverse plane runs through the body parallel to the horizon. There is no specified area of the body through which this plane must pass. A body part that is closer to the head than another part in the transverse plane is described as being superior (or cephalad) to the other part. Any body part closer to the feet than another part in the transverse plane is described as being inferior (or caudad) to the other part. An injury to the breast area would be described as being located superior to the navel (a possible transverse plane), whereas pain in the foot may be described as being inferior to it.

The median plane, also referred to as the midline, runs through the body in line with the umbilicus (navel). It is perpendicular to the frontal plane and divides the body into right and left halves. As discussed earlier, structures that are closer to the midline are specified as being medial to those situated farther to the side. On the other hand, areas closer to a side are specified as lateral to those nearer the midline.

A number of "imaginary lines" can also be used to help describe the location of an injury or landmark on the body Figure 5-3 ▼. The midaxillary line is an imaginary vertical line drawn through the axilla (armpit) to the waist. A parallel line drawn just an inch or so in front of the midaxillary line would be the anterior axillary line; a parallel line drawn an inch or so behind the midaxillary line would be the posterior axillary line. An imaginary line drawn vertically through the middle portion of the clavicle (collarbone) and parallel to the midline would be the midclavicular line.

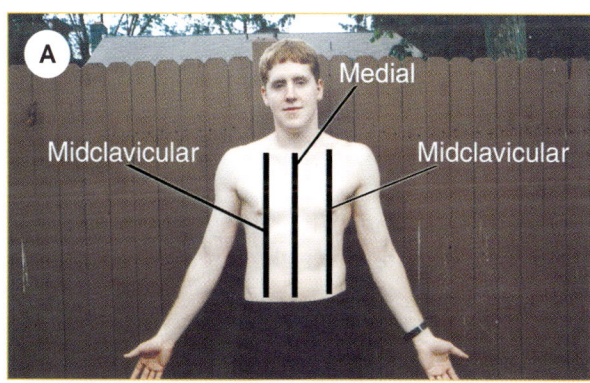

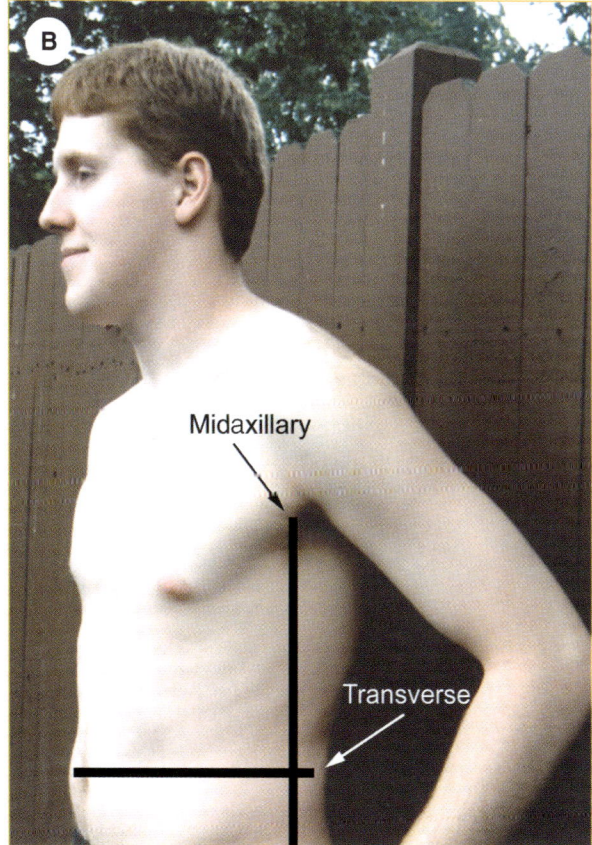

Figure 5-3 Imaginary lines can be used to describe the location of an injury or a landmark on the body. **A.** The midclavicular lines. **B.** The midaxillary lines.

> ✱ **EMT-I Tips**
>
> When a patient experiences an injury, the anatomic planes, body surfaces, and imaginary lines are often used to describe the location of the injury. For example, the patient may have received a laceration to the medial aspect of the right forearm.

EMT-I Tips

Often the lungs are auscultated for the presence of air movement in the location where the anterior axillary line intercepts the nipple level. An understanding of the imaginary lines helps the EMT-I decide exactly where to place the diaphragm of the stethoscope.

Directional Terms

In this section, terms that indicate direction are introduced. These terms indicate distance and direction from the midline (Table 5-1 ▼).

Right and Left

The terms "right" and "left" refer to the patient's right and left sides, not to your right and left sides.

TABLE 5-1	Directional Terms
Term	**Definition**
Anterior	Toward the front of the body
Posterior	Toward the back of the body
Right	The patient's right
Left	The patient's left
Lateral	Away from the midline of the body
Medial	Toward the midline of the body
Superior (cephalad)	Toward the head; structure that is situated higher than another
Inferior (caudad)	Toward the feet; structure that is situated lower than another
Proximal	Nearer to or toward the trunk of the body
Distal	Located away from the trunk of the body and toward the free end of an extremity
Dorsal	The posterior surface of the body (including the back of the hand)
Ventral	The anterior surface of the body
Palmar (volar)	The front region of the hand
Plantar	The bottom of the foot

Superior and Inferior

The superior (cephalad) part of the body, or any body part, is the portion nearer to the head. The part nearer to the feet is the inferior (caudad) portion. These terms are also used to describe the relationship of one structure to another. For example, the nose is superior to the mouth and inferior to the forehead.

Superficial and Deep

Superficial means closer to or on the skin. Deep means farther inside the body and away from the skin.

Ventral and Dorsal

Ventral refers to the anterior surface of the body. Dorsal refers to the posterior surface of the body, including the back of the hand.

Palmar and Plantar

The front region of the hand is referred to as the palm or palmar (volar) surface. The bottom of the foot is referred to as the plantar surface.

Apex

The apex (plural: apices) is the tip or the uppermost portion of a structure. For example, the tips of the shoulders are the apices of the shoulder. The most superior portions of the lungs are the apices of the lungs. An exception to this is the apex of the heart, which is the most inferior (lower) portion due to its inverted position within the chest cavity.

Other Directional Terms

Many structures of the body occur bilaterally. A bilateral structure is a body part that appears on both sides of the midline. For example, the eyes, ears, hands, and feet are bilateral structures. This is also true for structures inside the body, such as the lungs and kidneys.

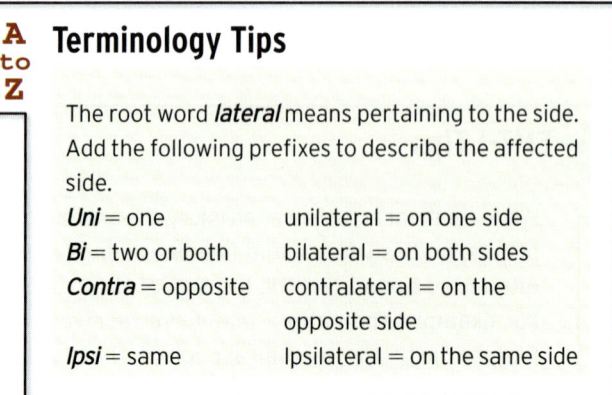

Terminology Tips

The root word *lateral* means pertaining to the side. Add the following prefixes to describe the affected side.

Uni = one	unilateral = on one side
Bi = two or both	bilateral = on both sides
Contra = opposite	contralateral = on the opposite side
Ipsi = same	Ipsilateral = on the same side

Structures that are on only one side of the body are said to be unilateral. For example, the spleen is on the left side of the body only, and the liver is on the right side. Contralateral refers to the opposite side of the body. For example, a right hemispheric stroke causes weakness on the contralateral, or opposite, side of the body. Ipsilateral refers to the same side of the body. A right hemispheric stroke, for example, affects the right side (ipsilateral) of the face.

Abdominal Quadrants

The abdomen is another area where imaginary lines are used. An imaginary vertical line drawn from the inferior tip of the sternum (breastbone) to the genital area and a horizontal line drawn from the iliac crest straight across the umbilicus (navel) identify the four distinct abdominal quadrants: the right upper quadrant, left upper quadrant, right lower quadrant, and left lower quadrant. Specific organs are located in each of the four quadrants, and pain or injury is often described as being in a specific quadrant Figure 5-4.

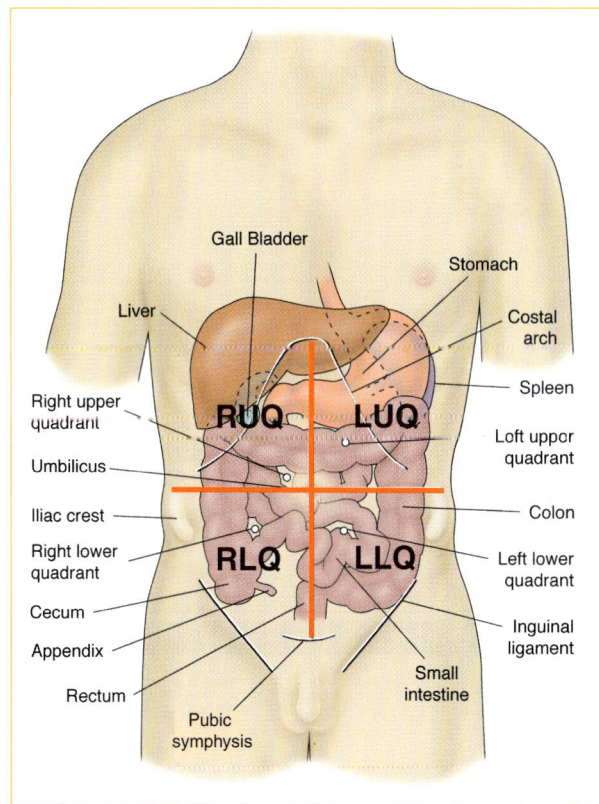

Figure 5-4 The abdomen is divided into quadrants.

Anatomic Positions

You will use these terms to describe the position of the patient as you find him or her or as you eventually transport the patient to the emergency department. These various anatomic positions are illustrated in Figure 5-5.

Prone, Supine, and Lateral Recumbent

The terms prone, supine, and lateral recumbent describe the position of the body. The body is in the prone position when lying face down; the body is in the supine position when lying face up. The body is lying on the side in the lateral recumbent position (or lateral decubitus position). If the patient is lying on his or her left side, it is called the left lateral recumbent position—also known as the recovery position.

Fowler's Position and Semi-Fowler's Position

A patient who is sitting up at a 45° angle with the knees bent is in semi-Fowler's position. A patient sitting up at a 90° angle is in a Fowler's position.

Trendelenburg's Position

In Trendelenburg's position, the body is supine with the head down and the lower extremities elevated approximately 12″ to help increase blood flow to the torso and brain.

Shock Position

In the shock position, or modified Trendelenburg's position, the head and torso (the trunk without the head and limbs) are supine, and the lower extremities are elevated 6″ to 12″. This helps to increase blood flow to the brain.

Movement and Positions

All movements of the body, from the simplest grasp to the most complicated ballet maneuver, can be broken down into a series of simple components and described with specific terms. As with the terms for anatomic positions, an accepted set of terms describes body movements. These are particularly useful in describing how an injury occurred.

Range of motion (ROM) is the full distance that a joint can be moved. In the anatomic position, moving a distal point of an extremity toward to the trunk is usually called flexion. Flexion of the elbow brings the hand closer to the shoulder, flexion of the knee brings the foot up to the buttocks, and flexion of the fingers

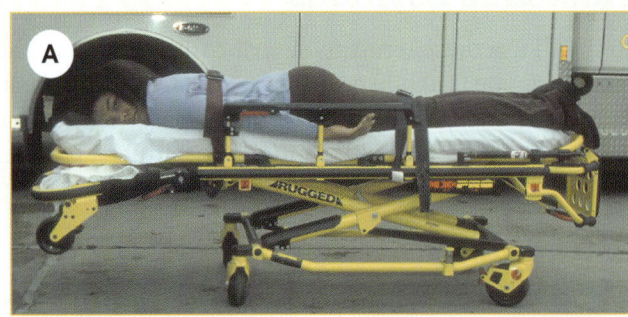
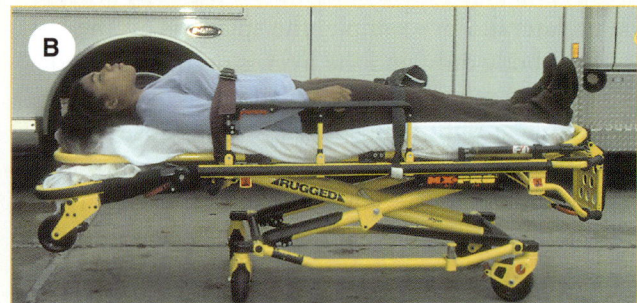
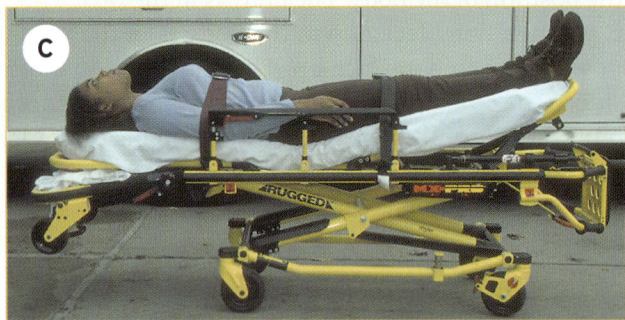
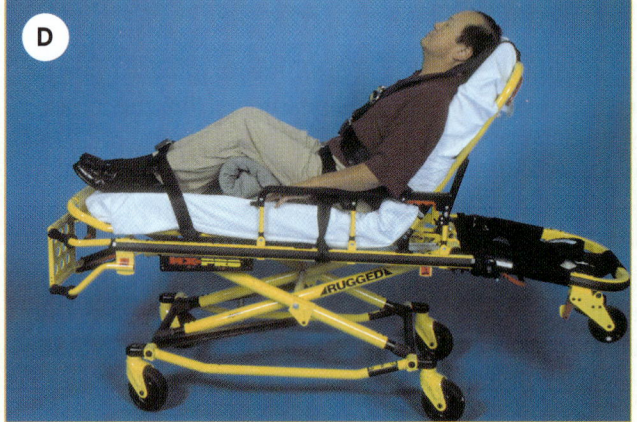
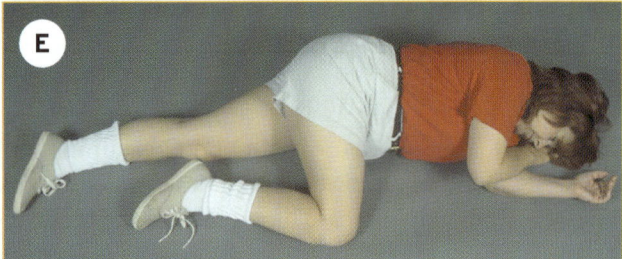

Figure 5-5 Positions in which patients may be found or transported. **A.** Prone. **B.** Supine. **C.** Trendelenburg's. **D.** Semi-Fowler's. **E.** Lateral recumbent.

You are the Provider — Part 3

Your continued assessment of Patient 1 reveals the following:

Vital Signs	Recording Time: 2 Minutes After Patient Contact
Respirations	28 breaths/min, labored
Pulse	114 beats/min, irregular
Blood pressure	90/60 mm Hg
Sao_2	95% on supplemental oxygen

4. How can knowledge of anatomy and physiology help the EMT-I care for patients?

forms the hand into a fist. Extension is the motion associated with the return of a body part from a flexed position to the anatomic position. In the anatomic position, all extremities are in extension. A patient's neck can be in one of several positions when the patient is found in the supine position (Figure 5-6 ▼).

The prefix hyper often is added to the terms flexion or extension to indicate a mechanism of injury. "Hyper" implies that the normal range of motion for the particular movement was maximized or even exceeded, potentially resulting in injury. This prefix is used commonly in clinical literature, as well as in written and verbal communication among health care providers. The term hyperflexion refers to a body part that was flexed to the maximum level or even beyond the normal ROM. Hyperextension refers to a body part that was extended to the maximum level or even beyond the normal ROM. A hyperextension injury occurs when an individual falls on an outstretched hand, resulting in a distal radius fracture (Figure 5-7 ▼). A hyperflexion injury to the back can occur while bending. Wrist injuries can also be described using the terms supination and pronation. Turning the palms upward constitutes supination of the forearm. Turning the palms downward is described as pronation of the forearm.

Internal rotation describes turning an extremity medially toward the midline. The lower extremity is internally rotated when the toes are turned inward. External rotation describes turning an extremity away from the midline. Often, when an injured extremity is compared to the uninjured extremity, rotational deformities are noted. A hip can be dislocated anteriorly or posteriorly. In an anterior hip dislocation, the foot is externally

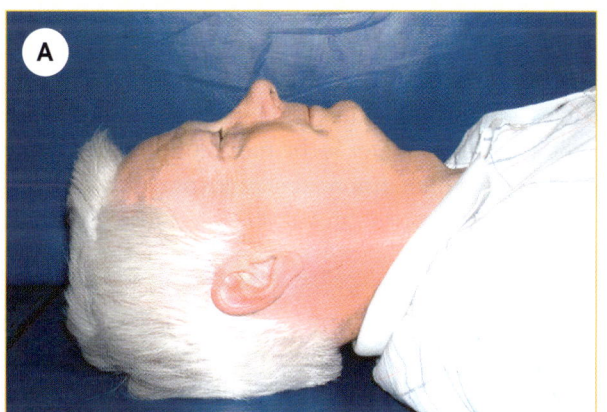
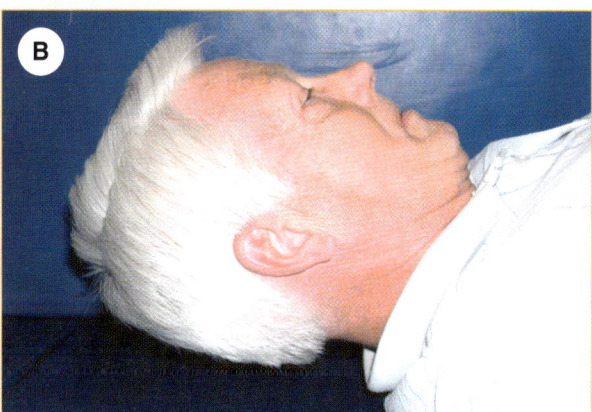
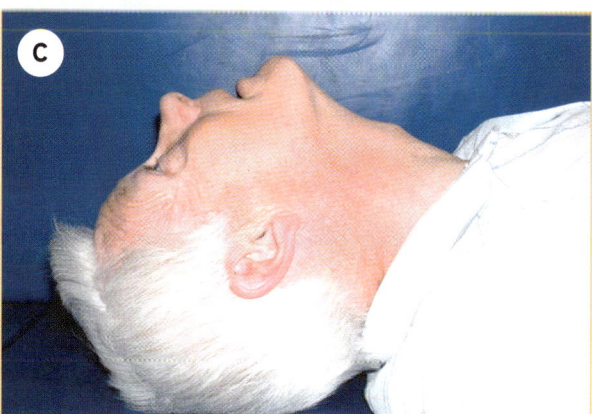

Figure 5-6 Positions of the neck in a patient found in a supine position. **A.** Neutral. **B.** Flexed. **C.** Extended.

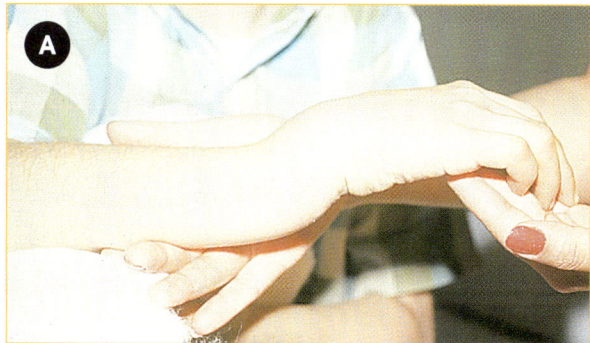
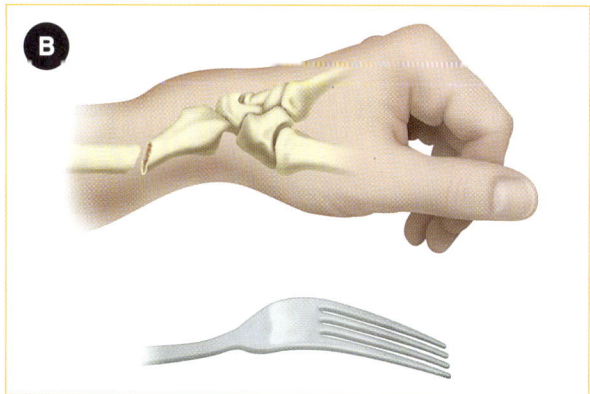

Figure 5-7 A. Exceeding the range of motion of an extremity can result in a fracture. **B.** Fractures of the distal radius produce a characteristic silver fork deformity and can result from hyperextension at the wrist secondary to falling on an outstretched hand.

rotated and the head of the femur is palpable in the inguinal area. In the more common posterior hip dislocation, the knee and foot usually are flexed and internally rotated. The term rotation also can be applied to the spine. The spine is rotated when it twists on its axis. Placing the chin on the shoulder rotates the cervical spine.

Abduction of an extremity moves it away from the midline. Adduction moves the extremity toward the midline.

Cellular Transport Mechanisms

Permeability of the Cell Membrane

The cell membrane (the cell wall) is described as being selectively permeable, which means that it allows some substances to pass through it, but not others Figure 5-8 ▼.

Selective permeability allows normal differences in concentrations between intracellular and extracellular environments to be maintained. The separation of the extracellular and intracellular areas by a selectively permeable membrane helps to maintain homeostasis, the maintenance of a stable internal physiologic environment including a stable temperature, fluid balance, and pH balance. Various enzymes, sugar molecules, and electrolytes freely pass in and out of the cell. Electrolytes are chemicals that are dissolved in the blood and are made up of salt or acid substances that become ionic conductors when dissolved in a solvent such as water.

Several mechanisms, such as diffusion, osmosis, facilitated diffusion, active transport, endocytosis, and exocytosis, allow material to pass through the cell wall Figure 5-9 ▶.

Diffusion

Particles such as molecules and ions live in water, which creates a solution. Water is the most common solvent or substance, in which other substances or solutes will dissolve. Diffusion is the movement of solutes, particles such as salts that are dissolved in a solvent, from an area of high concentration to one of low concentration, to produce an even distribution of particles in the space available. The degree of diffusion across a membrane depends on the permeability of the membrane to that substance and the concentration gradient, which is the

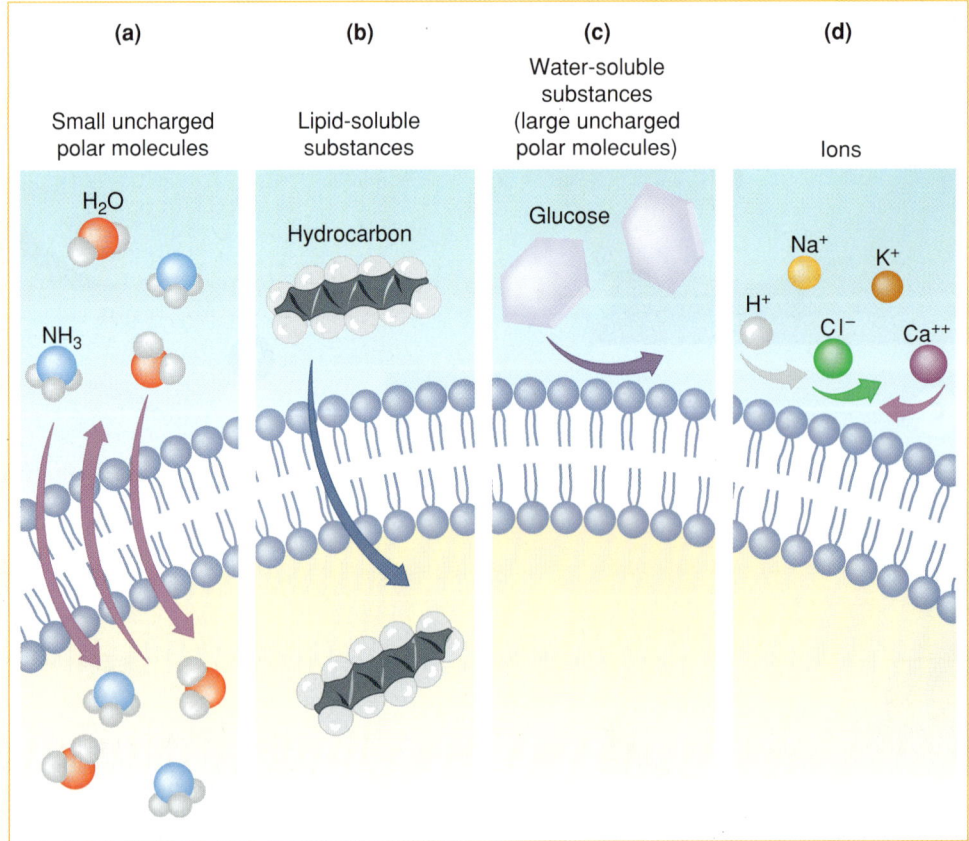

Figure 5-8 A selectively permeable membrane maintains homeostasis by allowing some molecules to pass through while others may not.

difference in concentrations of the substance on either side of the membrane. Small molecules diffuse more easily than large ones. Watery solutions diffuse more rapidly than thicker, viscous solutions. Many of the cell's nutrients, such as oxygen, enter the cell by diffusion.

Osmosis

Osmosis is the movement of a solvent, such as water, from an area of low solute concentration to one of high concentration through a selectively permeable membrane. The membrane is permeable to the solvent but not to the solute. Movement generally continues until the concentrations of the solute equalize on both sides of the membrane.

Osmotic pressure is a measure of the tendency of water to move by osmosis across a membrane. If too much water moves out of a cell, the cell shrinks abnormally, a process known as crenation. If too much water enters a cell, it will swell and burst, a process known as lysis.

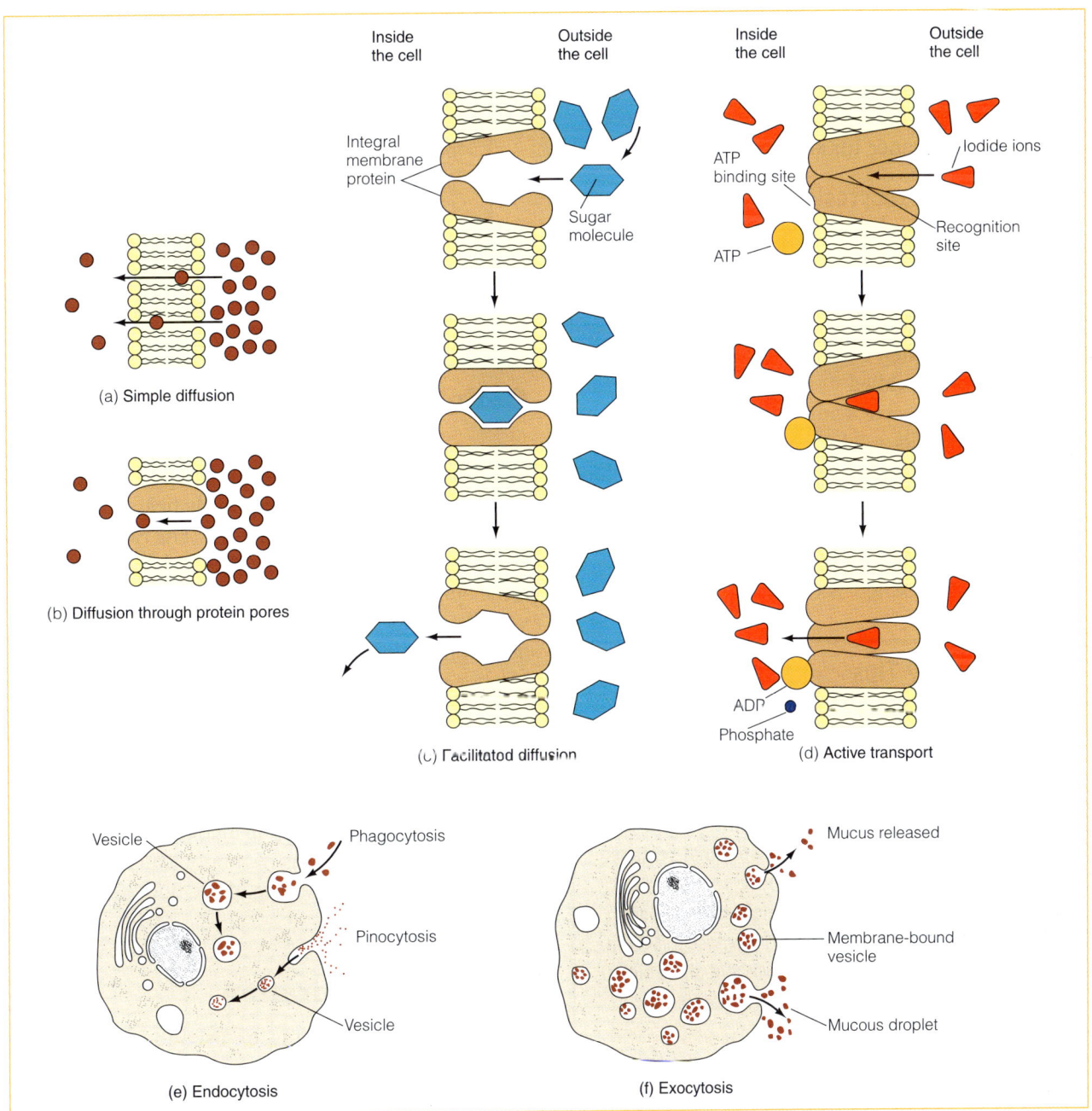

Figure 5-9 Methods of material transport through the cell wall. **A.** Simple diffusion. **B.** Diffusion through protein pores. **C.** Facilitated diffusion. **D.** Active transport. **E.** Endocytosis. **F.** Exocytosis.

Facilitated Diffusion

Facilitated diffusion is the process in which a carrier molecule moves substances in or out of cells from areas of high concentration to areas of lower concentration (see Figure 5-9). Energy is not required; the number of molecules transported is directly proportional to the amount of concentration.

Active Transport

Active transport is the movement of a substance against a concentration or gradient such as the cell membrane (see Figure 5-9). Active transport requires energy as well as some type of carrier mechanism and is a movement opposite that of the normal movement of diffusion. Both glucose and amino acids are absorbed via active transport. At times, the active transport mechanism may exchange one substance for another.

Endocytosis and Exocytosis

Endocytosis is the uptake of material through the cell membrane by a membrane-bound droplet or vesicle that forms within the protoplasm of the cell. The cell membrane surrounds the material, engulfing it within the cell (see Figure 5-9). When endocytosis involves solid particles, the process is called phagocytosis, which means "cell eating." A phagocyte is any cell that ingests microorganisms or other cells and foreign particles. Phagocytosis occurs commonly when infection-fighting white blood cells consume bacteria and foreign particles. In certain disease states, these cells lose their ability to phagocytize, resulting in life-threatening infections. Endocytosis of liquids, or "cell drinking," is called pinocytosis.

> **A to Z Terminology Tips**
>
> Osmolality refers to the number of osmotically active particles in a kilogram of solvent. The term serum osmolality refers to the number of osmotically active particles in a liter of serum, the clear straw-colored, liquid portion of the plasma that remains after the solid elements have been separated out. Abnormal elevations of blood glucose and sodium concentrations may result in an increase in serum osmolality. When this occurs, movement of the blood is impeded and tissue oxygenation decreases. A condition known as hyperosmolar hyperglycemic nonketotic coma (HHNC) may result. HHNC is a diabetic emergency that occurs when a relative insulin deficiency results in marked hyperglycemia in the absence of ketones and acidosis.

Exocytosis is the release of secretions from the cells. These secretions accumulate within vesicles, which then move to the cell membrane (see Figure 5-9). The vesicles bond or fuse to the membrane, and the content of the vesicle is eliminated from the cell. Examples of exocytosis include secretion of digestive enzymes from the pancreas, mucous secretion from the salivary glands, and secretion of milk from the mammary glands.

> **EMT-I Tips**
>
> The transport of glucose in and out of most cells occurs by facilitated diffusion. If glucose accumulates within the cell to a concentration that is as high as the concentration outside the cell, the process would stop. Thus, when it enters the cell, glucose is rapidly converted to other molecules. If the cell's ability to convert glucose is hindered, such as in severe shock, low glucose concentrations or hypoglycemia will occur within the cell.

Cellular Metabolism

Metabolism is the sum of all the physical and chemical processes that produce and maintain the body. It includes growth, generation of energy, body heat, elimination of wastes, and other body functions. The two components of metabolism are anabolism and catabolism. Anabolism is the building phase, in which smaller molecules are converted to larger molecules. Catabolism is the breakdown phase, in which larger molecules are converted to smaller molecules. These are sometimes referred to as the constructive phase and destructive phase.

The body's sources of "fuel" or energy are carbohydrates (mostly as glucose), fats, and proteins. Ultimately, glucose serves as the main cell "food," whether taken orally, parenterally, or made from conversion of stored fats and proteins. A major cause of and contributor to disease is failure of the body to make sufficient energy.

Cellular Respiration

Glucose, fat, and proteins are used to generate energy in a process called cellular respiration, not to be confused with respiration that occurs by breathing. Cellular respiration creates energy in the form of adenosine triphosphate (ATP) molecules that fuel all of the body's functions. Cellular respiration is a biochemical process that takes place in the cell within the mitochondria. In the mitochondria, foodstuffs are metabolized to ATP, carbon dioxide, and water through the Krebs cycle and oxidative phosphorylation. For each molecule of glucose metabolized, these chemical processes produce almost 40 molecules of energy-rich ATP, as well as CO_2 and H_2O. More than 40 molecules of ATP are yielded per fat molecule through this process. Cellular respiration produces the majority of the body's ATP (Figure 5-10 ▼). Another intracellular process, glycolysis, also contributes to ATP stores, but to a lesser extent.

> **A to Z Terminology Tips**
>
> Oxidative phosphorylation is the production of ATP, which takes place in the mitochondria during cellular respiration.

Cellular respiration is called normal aerobic metabolism because it normally occurs in the presence of oxygen. However, when oxygen levels are low, the reactions described previously do not occur and the cell reverts to anaerobic metabolism. Anaerobic metabolism produces less energy than does aerobic metabolism, and produces lactate acid waste products.

Tissues

Epithelial Tissue and Glands

Epithelium is a type of tissue that covers all of the external surfaces of the body and forms the secreting portions of glands. Epithelial tissue also lines hollow organs within the body, such as the intestines and bronchial tubes. In addition to providing a protective barrier, epithelial tissues function in the absorption of nutrients in the intestines and the secretion of various body substances, such as in the sweat glands.

Connective Tissue

Connective tissue, as the name implies, connects other types of tissue together. Extracellular matrix is a nonliving substance consisting of protein fibers, nonfibrous protein, or fluid that separates connective tissue cells from each other. Bone and cartilage are subtypes of connective tissue. Adipose tissue is a special type of connective tissue that contains large amounts of lipids (fat). Other types of connective tissues aid in the formation of blood vessels and participate in the body's defense system against disease-causing agents. Scar tissue is an example of connective tissue that can develop in almost any part of the body to help repair or replace damaged areas.

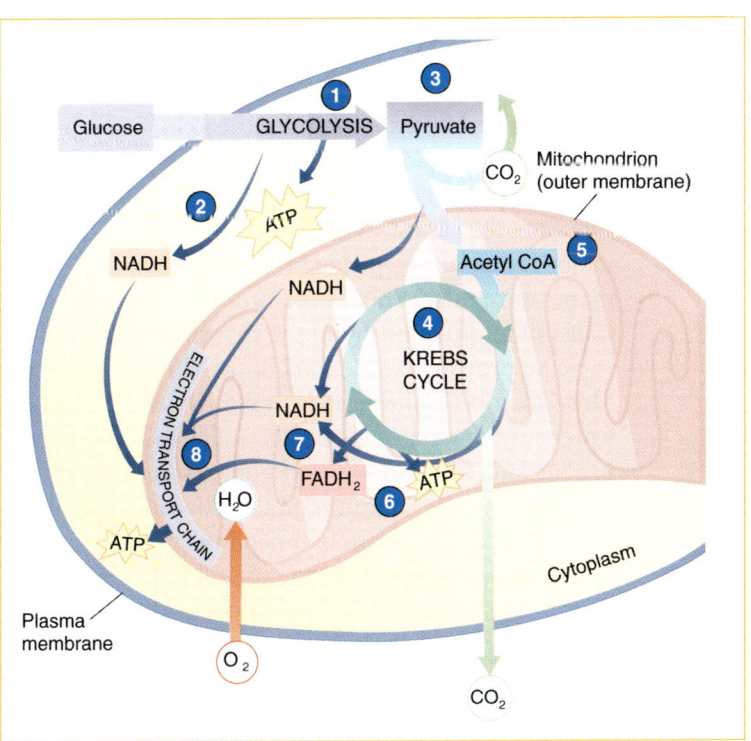

Figure 5-10 Summary of cellular respiration.

Muscle Tissue

Muscle tissue is located within the substance of the body and is invariably enclosed by connective tissue. Muscles overlie the framework of the skeleton and are classified by both structure and function. Structurally, muscle tissue is either <u>striated</u>, in which microscopic bands or striations can be seen, or <u>nonstriated</u> (smooth).

Functionally, muscle is either <u>voluntary</u> (consciously controlled) or <u>involuntary</u> (not normally under conscious control). The three types of muscle are skeletal muscle (striated voluntary), cardiac muscle (striated involuntary), and smooth muscle (nonstriated involuntary) (Figure 5-11 ▼). Most of the muscles used in day-to-day activities are skeletal muscles. The heart consists of <u>cardiac muscle</u>. We have no conscious control over the beating of this muscle. Smooth muscle lines most glands and digestive organs. Smooth muscle also is responsible for constriction and widening of the pupil of the eye when it is exposed to light or dark. Typically, we have no conscious control over the function of smooth muscle.

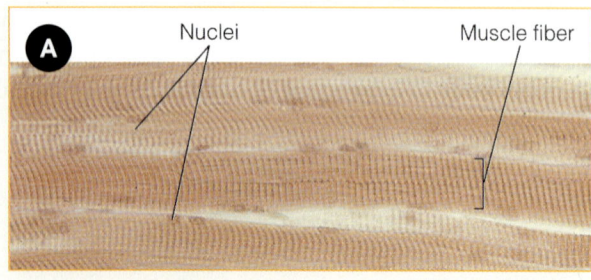
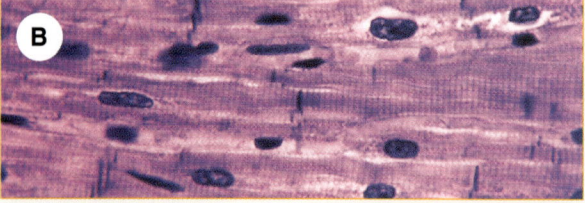
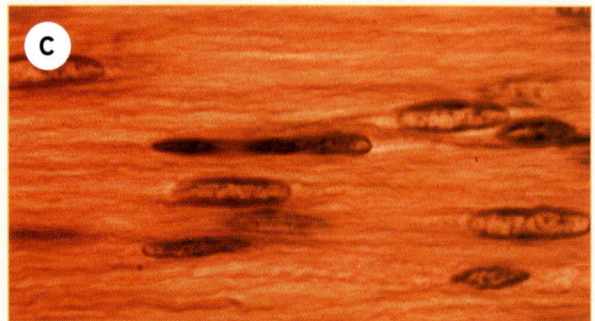

Figure 5-11 Light micrograph of the types of muscle tissue. **A.** Skeletal. **B.** Cardiac. **C.** Smooth.

Nerve Tissue

The brain, spinal cord, and peripheral nerves are examples of nerve tissue. <u>Peripheral nerves</u> include all of the nerves that extend from the brain and spinal cord, exiting from between the vertebrae to various parts of the body. <u>Neurons</u> are the main conducting cells of nerve tissue. The cell body of the neuron includes the nucleus and is the site of most cellular functions.

Two projections typically extend from nerve cells: dendrites and axons. <u>Dendrites</u> receive electrical impulses from the axons of other nerve cells and conduct them toward the cell body. <u>Axons</u> typically conduct electrical impulses away from the cell body. Each neuron has only one axon but may have several dendrites. The connective and supporting tissues of nerve tissue are collectively referred to as <u>neuroglia</u> (Figure 5-12).

> **✳ EMT-I Tips**
>
> The details of cellular metabolism are well beyond the intended scope of this text. The key core concepts are simple: When we breathe, we take in oxygen. Through various metabolic processes, oxygen is metabolized to energy in the form of adenosine triphosphate (ATP) and heat. Water and carbon dioxide are also formed as by-products.

Integumentary System

The <u>integumentary system</u> is essentially the outer surface of the body. It includes the skin, nails, hair, and sweat and oil glands. The integumentary system (or integument) accounts for about 15% of body weight. The skin, the largest single organ in the body, serves three major functions: to protect the body from the environment, to regulate the temperature of the body, and to transmit information about the environment to the brain.

The protective functions of the skin are numerous. More than 60% of the body is composed of water. The water contains a delicate balance of chemical substances in solution. The skin is watertight and serves to keep this balanced internal solution intact. The skin also protects the body from invasion by infectious organisms: bacteria, viruses, and fungi. These organisms are everywhere and are routinely found lying on the skin surface and deep in its grooves and glands. However, they do not penetrate the skin unless it is broken by injury; thus, the skin provides constant protection against outside invaders.

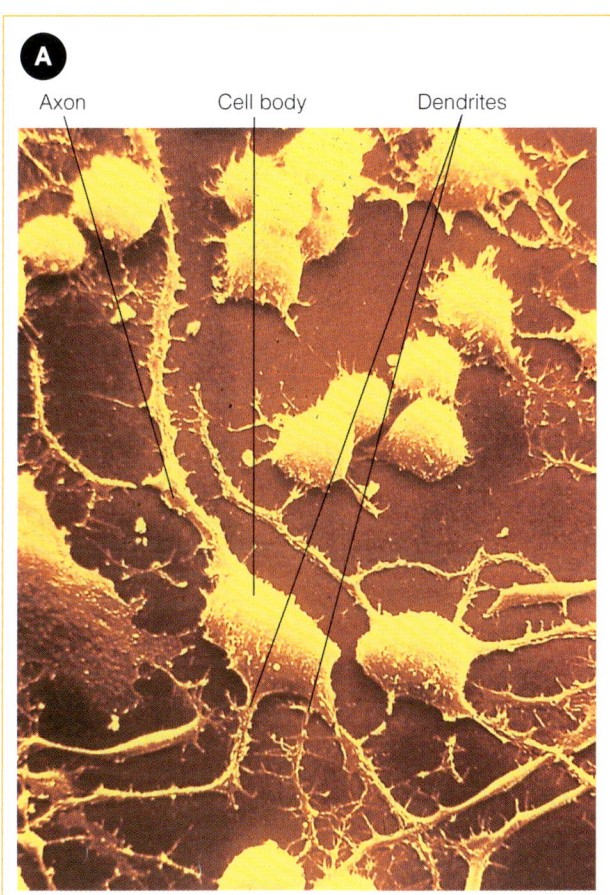

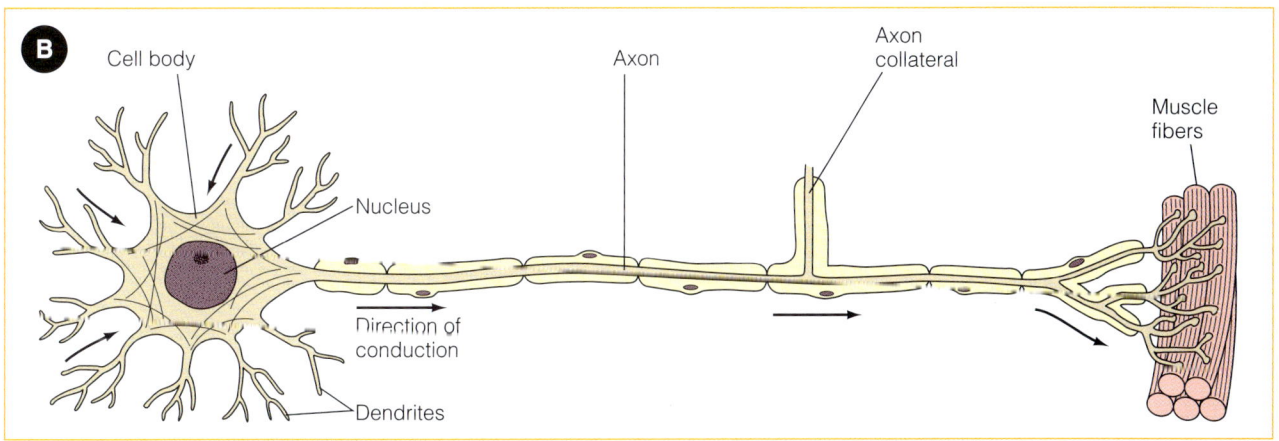

Figure 5-12 The neuron. **A.** A scanning electron micrograph of the cell body and dendrites of a multipolar neuron, which resides in the central nervous system. **B.** Collateral branches may occur along the length of the axon. When the axon terminates, it branches many times, ending on individual muscle fibers.

Functions of the Skin

The major organ for regulation of body temperature is the skin. Blood vessels in the skin constrict when the body is in a cold environment and dilate when the body is in a warm environment. In a cold environment, constriction of the blood vessels diverts the blood away from the skin to decrease the amount of heat radiated from the body surface. When the outside environment is hot, the vessels in the skin dilate, the skin becomes flushed or red, and heat radiates from the body surface.

Also, in the hot environment, sweat is secreted to the skin surface from the sweat glands. Evaporation of the sweat requires energy. This energy, as body heat, is taken from the body during the evaporation process, which causes the body temperature to fall. Sweating alone will not reduce body temperature; evaporation of the sweat must also occur.

Regulation of body temperature is a critical function of the skin. The energy of the body is derived from metabolism (chemical reactions) that must take place within a very narrow temperature range. If the body temperature is too low, these reactions cannot proceed, metabolism ceases, and the body dies. If the temperature becomes too high, the rate of metabolism increases. Dangerously high temperatures producing a metabolic rate that is too high can result in permanent tissue damage and death.

Information about the environment is carried to the brain through a rich supply of sensory nerves that originate in the skin. Nerve endings that lie in the skin are adapted to perceive and transmit information about heat, cold, external pressure, pain, and the position of the body in space. The skin thus recognizes any changes in the environment. The skin also reacts to pleasurable stimuli.

Anatomy of the Skin

The skin is divided into two parts: the superficial epidermis, which is composed of several layers of cells, and the deeper dermis, which contains the specialized skin structures. Below the skin lies the subcutaneous tissue layer Figure 5-13 ▶. The cells of the epidermis are sealed to form a watertight protective covering for the body.

The epidermis is actually composed of several layers of cells. At the base of the epidermis is the germinal layer, which continuously produces new cells that gradually rise to the surface. On the way to the surface, these cells die and form the watertight covering. The epidermal cells are held together securely by an oily substance called sebum, which is secreted by the sebaceous glands of the dermis. The outermost cells of the epidermis are constantly rubbed away and then replaced by new cells produced by the germinal layer. The deeper cells in the germinal layer also contain pigment (melanin) granules that (along with the blood vessels lying in the dermis) produce skin color.

The epidermis varies in thickness in different areas of the body. On the soles of the feet, the back, and the scalp, it is quite thick, but in some areas of the body, the epidermis is only two or three cell layers thick. The watertight seal provided by the epidermis prevents the invasion of bacteria and other organisms.

The deeper part of skin, the dermis, is separated from the epidermis by the layer of germinal cells. Within the dermis lie many of the special structures of the skin: sweat glands, sebaceous (oil) glands, hair follicles, blood vessels, and specialized nerve endings.

Sweat glands produce sweat for cooling the body. The sweat is discharged onto the surface of the skin through small pores, or ducts, that pass through the epidermis onto the skin surface. The sebaceous glands produce sebum, the oily material that seals the surface epidermal cells. The sebaceous glands lie next to hair follicles and secrete sebum along the hair follicle to the skin surface. In addition to providing waterproofing for the skin, sebum keeps the skin supple so that it does not crack.

You are the Provider — Part 4

Your second victim was the front seat passenger in the minivan. She was restrained and is complaining of pain in her right shoulder and abdomen from her seatbelt. You note the following:

Initial Assessment	Recording Time: Zero Minutes
Appearance	In pain
Level of consciousness	Conscious and alert
Airway	Open and clear
Breathing	Respirations, normal rate and unlabored
Circulation	Skin, warm and dry to touch; pulse, present and normal

5. What is the function of the skeletal system?
6. What is the musculoskeletal system designed to do?

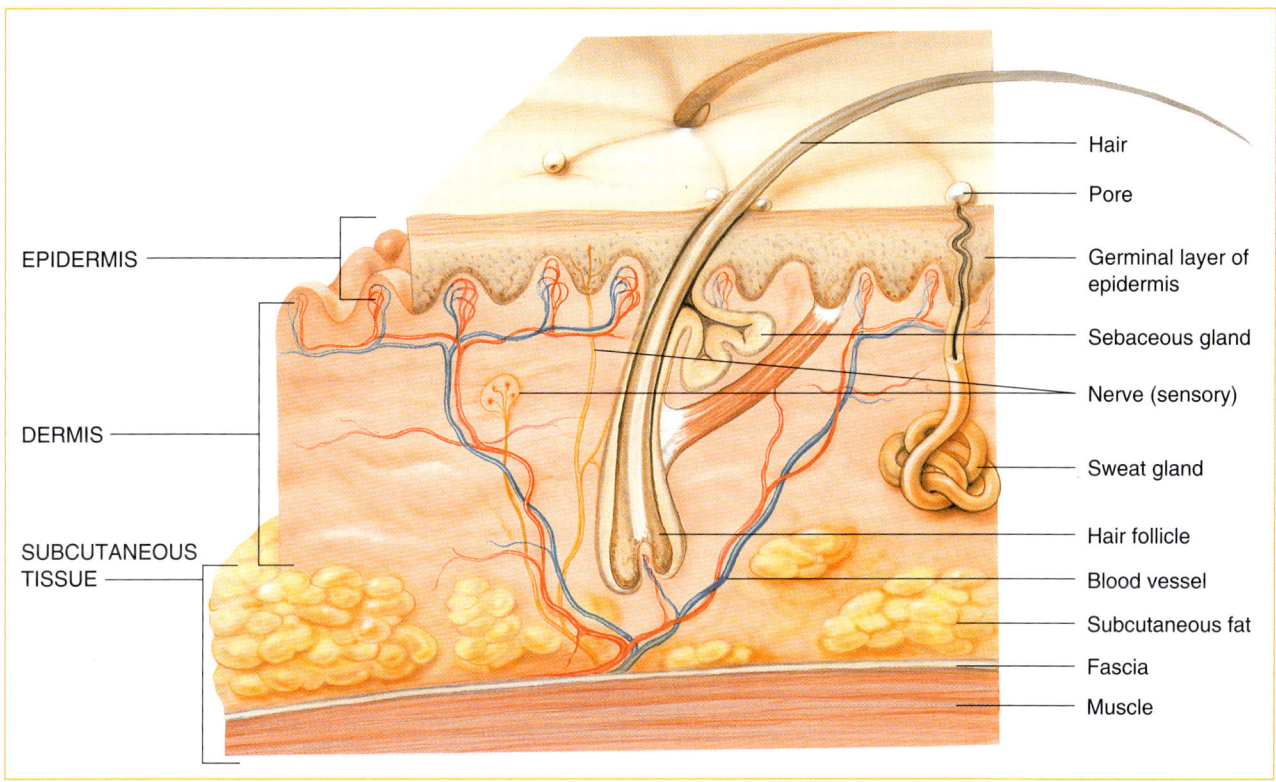

Figure 5-13 The skin has two principal layers: the epidermis and the dermis. Below the skin is a layer of subcutaneous tissue.

Hair follicles are the small organs that produce hair. There is one follicle for each hair connected with a sebaceous gland and also with a tiny muscle. This muscle, the erector pili, pulls the hair into an erect position when the individual is cold or frightened. All hair grows continuously and is either cut off or worn away by clothing.

Blood vessels provide nutrients and oxygen to the skin. The blood vessels lie in the dermis. Small branches extend up to the germinal layer. There are no blood vessels in the epidermis. A complex array of nerve endings also lies in the dermis. These specialized nerve endings are sensitive to environmental stimuli; they respond to these stimuli and send impulses along the nerves to the brain.

Beneath the skin, immediately under the dermis and attached to it, lies the subcutaneous tissue. The subcutaneous tissue is composed largely of fat. The fat serves as an insulator for the body and as a reservoir to store energy. The amount of subcutaneous tissue varies greatly from individual to individual. Beneath the subcutaneous tissue lie the muscles and the skeleton.

The skin covers the entire external surface of the body. The various orifices (openings to the body)—including the mouth, nose, anus, and vagina—are not covered by skin. Orifices are lined with mucous membranes. Mucous membranes are quite similar to skin in that they provide a protective barrier against bacterial invasion. Mucous membranes differ from skin in that they secrete mucus, a watery substance that lubricates the openings. Thus, mucous membranes are moist, whereas the skin is dry. A mucous membrane lines the entire gastrointestinal tract from the mouth to the anus.

Skeletal System

The skeleton gives us our recognizable human form and protects our vital internal organs Figure 5-14 ▶. The skeleton has two major components: the axial skeleton and the appendicular skeleton. The axial skeleton forms the upright part or axis of the body. It consists of the hyoid, skull, vertebral column, ribs, and sternum. The appendicular skeleton is attached to the axis as appendages. It consists of the shoulder and pelvic girdles and the upper and lower extremities.

The 206 bones of the skeleton provide a framework for the attachment of muscles. The skeleton is also designed to allow motion of the body. The body's support framework consists of bones and their associated connective tissues: cartilage, tendons, and ligaments. Virtually every muscle in the body attaches to bones. Muscle contraction results in the movement of the bones at joints. Bony structures provide protection for the most vital organs of the body such as the skull, which encases the brain, and the rib cage, which surrounds the heart, lungs, and mediastinum. Finally, the skeletal system serves several vital metabolic functions such as the production of blood cells, platelets, and regulation of serum levels of the essential mineral calcium. Bones come into contact with one another at joints where, with the help of muscles, the body is able to bend and move.

The Skull

At the top of the axial skeleton is the skull, which consists of 28 bones in three anatomic groups: the auditory ossicles, the cranium, and the face. The six auditory ossicles function in hearing and are located, three on each side of the head, deep within cavities of the temporal bone. The remaining 22 bones comprise the cranium and the face.

The cranial vault consists of the eight bones that encase and protect the brain: the parietal, temporal, frontal, occipital, sphenoid, and ethmoid bones. The brain and the spinal cord are connected through a large opening at the base of the skull called the foramen magnum.

The bones of the skull are connected together at special joints known as sutures (Figure 5-15 ▼). The paired parietal bones join together at the sagittal suture. The parietal bones abut the frontal bone at the coronal suture. The occipital bone attaches to the parietal bones at the lambdoid suture. Fibrous tissues called fontanelles, which soften and expand during childbirth, link the sutures. The tissue felt through the fontanels are layers of the scalp and thick membranes overlying the brain. Under normal conditions, the brain may not be felt through the fontanels. By the time a child reaches age 2 years, the sutures should have solidified and the fontanels closed.

At the base of the temporal bone is a cone-shaped section of bone known as the mastoid process. This area

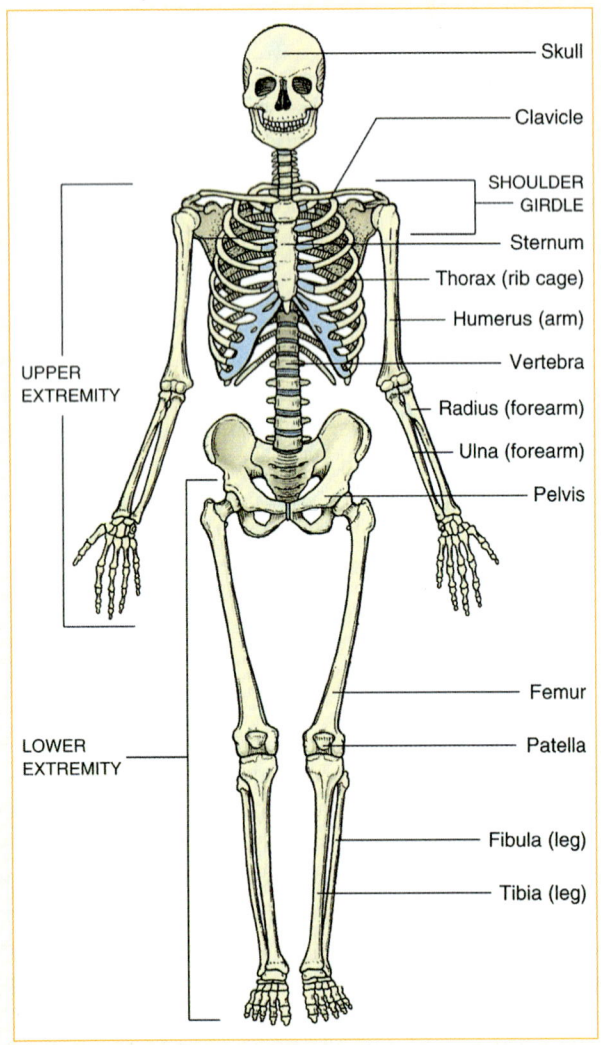

Figure 5-14 The 206 bones of the skeleton give us our form, protect our vital organs, and allow us to move.

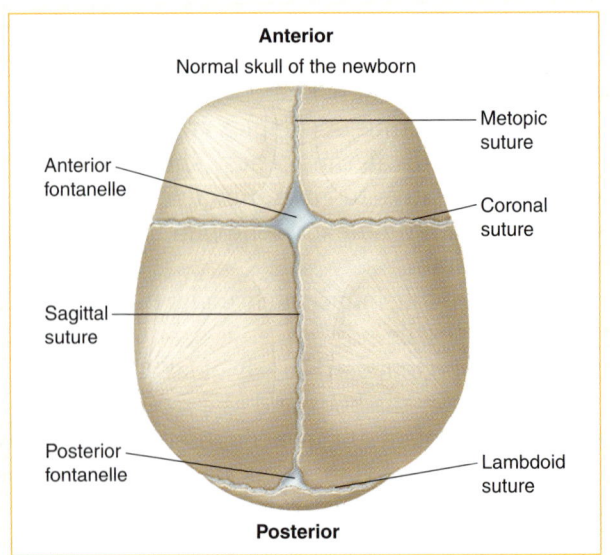

Figure 5-15 The sutures of the skull.

is an important site for attachment of various muscles. In addition, a portion of the mastoid process contains hollow mastoid air cells Figure 5-16 .

Superior and anterior to the mastoid process is the external auditory meatus, which is an opening in the temporal bone that leads to the ossicles (the three small bones in the middle ear: the malleus, incus, and stapes) and the inner ear structures of hearing deep within the bone. Below the meatus is a bony protuberance, the styloid process, made up of several long, slender, and pointed bones that project downward and forward from the temporal bone. The facial nerve supplies sensory and motor nerve functions to the face and jaw and runs through the styloid process.

The Floor of the Cranial Vault

Viewed from above, the floor of the interior of the skull, or cranial vault, is divided into three compartments: the anterior fossa, middle fossa, and posterior fossa Figure 5-17 .

The crista galli forms a prominent bony ridge in the center of the anterior fossa and is the point of attachment of the meninges, the three layers of membranes—the dura mater, arachnoid, and pia mater—that surround the brain. On either side of the crista galli is the cribriform plate of the ethmoid bone, the horizontal bone that is perforated with numerous openings (foramina) for the passage of the olfactory nerve filaments from the nasal cavity. The olfactory bulb, the cranial nerve for smell, sends projections through the foramina in the cribriform plate and into the nasal cavity, the chamber inside the nose that lies between the floor of the cranium and the roof of the mouth.

The sella turcica is a saddle-shaped depression in the middle of the sphenoid bone, between the anterior and posterior fossae. The pituitary gland, which is an endocrine gland that directly or indirectly affects all body functions, resides in this area. The foramen magnum is located behind the sella turcica, in the posterior fossa. Numerous other foramina are located in the base of the skull. Their names often are derived from the structure that passes through them. For example, the carotid foramen in the temporal bone contains the carotid artery.

> **EMT-I Tips**
>
> Fractures of the cribriform plate result in leakage of cerebrospinal fluid (CSF) from the nose. CSF is the fluid that bathes and provides hydraulic cushioning to the brain and spinal cord. Leakage of clear, watery fluid from the nose following head trauma suggests leakage of CSF.

The Base of the Skull

When the mandible is removed, the base of the skull appears amazingly complex, with numerous visible foramina Figure 5-18 . The occipital condyles on the occipital bone, which are the points of articulation between the skull and the vertebral column, lie on either

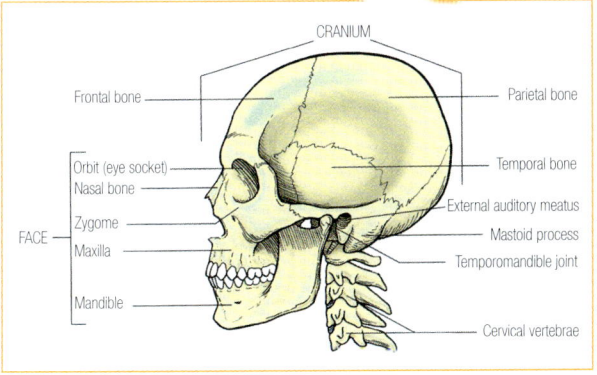

Figure 5-16 The mastoid air cells are located in the mastoid process. Just anterior to the mastoid is the external auditory meatus, which is associated with the ear canal.

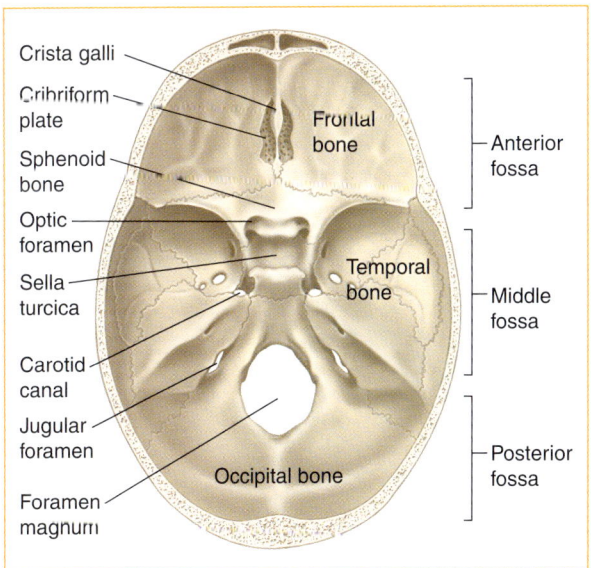

Figure 5-17 The floor of the cranial vault and its anatomy.

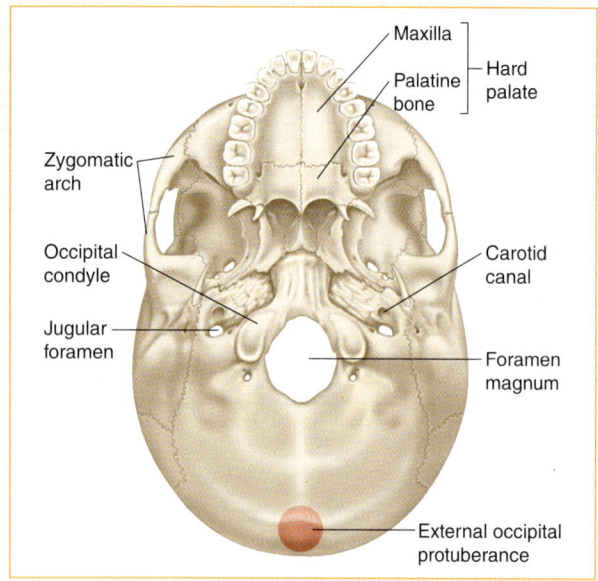

Figure 5-18 The base of the skull from below.

The Facial Bones

The frontal and ethmoid bones are part of both the cranial vault and the face. The 14 facial bones form the structure of the face, without contributing to the cranial vault. These bones include the <u>maxillae</u>, mandible, zygoma, palatine, nasal, lacrimal, vomer, and inferior nasal concha bones Figure 5-19 .

The facial bones protect the eyes, nose, and tongue and provide attachment points for the muscles that allow chewing. The zygomatic process of the temporal bone and the temporal process of the zygomatic bone form the zygomatic arch Figure 5-20 . The zygomatic arch lends shape to the cheeks.

Bones of the Orbit

The <u>orbits</u> are cone-shaped fossae that enclose and protect the eyes. In addition to the eyeball and muscles that move it, the orbit contains blood vessels, nerves, and fat. The frontal, sphenoid, zygomatic, maxilla, lacrimal, ethmoid, and palatine bones each form portions of the orbits.

A blow to the eye may result in fracture of the floor of the orbit. This bone is extremely thin and breaks easily. The result is transmission of forces away from the eyeball itself to the bone. Blood and fat then leak into the maxillary sinus below. This type of fracture is called a <u>blowout fracture</u> Figure 5-21 .

side of the foramen magnum. Portions of the maxilla and the <u>palatine bone</u>, the irregularly shaped bone in the posterior nasal cavity, form the <u>hard palate</u>, which is the bony anterior part of the palate, or the roof of the mouth. The <u>zygomatic arch</u>, the bone that extends along the front of the skull below the orbit, also is visible in this view.

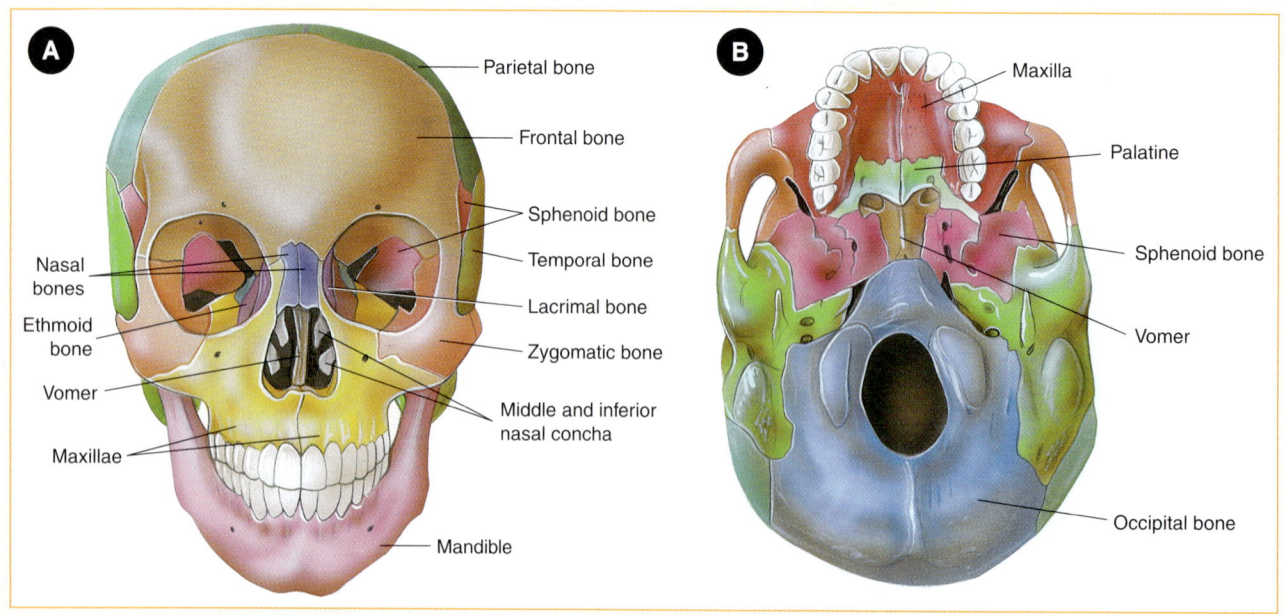

Figure 5-19 The skull and its components. **A.** Front view. **B.** Bottom view.

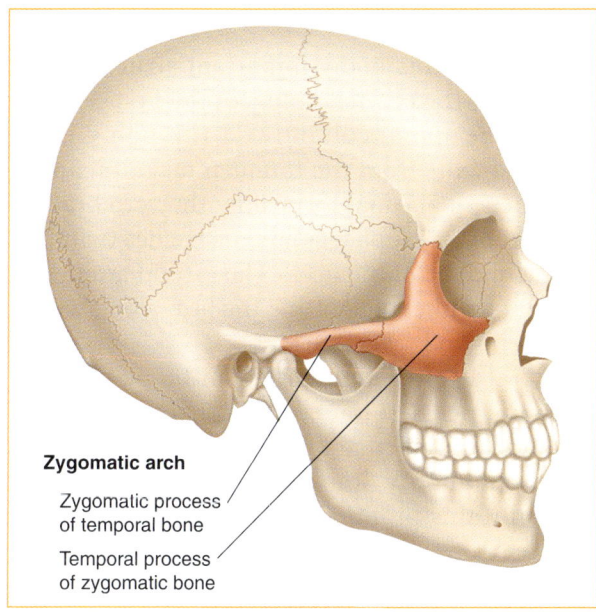

Figure 5-20 The zygomatic arch.

of the skull as well as provide resonance for the voice. The contents of the sinuses drain into the nasal cavity.

The Mandible and Temporomandibular Joint

The mandible is the large movable bone comprising the lower jaw and containing the lower teeth. The horizontal curved portion is the body of the mandible; two perpendicular rami join the body at nearly right angles. At the top of each ramus are the anterior coronoid process and the posterior condyle, which are separated by the mandibular notch. Numerous muscles of chewing attach to the mandible and its rami. The posterior condyle of the mandible articulates with the temporal bone at the temporomandibular joint (TMJ), allowing movement of the mandible (see Figure 5-16).

The Hyoid Bone

The hyoid bone "floats" in the superior aspect of the neck just below the mandible. It is not actually part of the skull, but it supports the tongue and serves as a point of attachment for many important neck and tongue muscles.

Bones of the Nose

The nasal cavity comprises portions of several of the facial bones, including the frontal, nasal, sphenoid, ethmoid, inferior nasal concha, maxilla, palatine, and vomer bones. The nasal septum is the separation between the nostrils and is located in the midline. Often, it bulges slightly to one side or the other. The external portion of the nose is formed mostly of cartilage.

Several of the bones associated with the nose contain cavities known as the paranasal sinuses, or sinuses (Figure 5-22▶). These hollowed sections of bone are lined with mucous membrane and decrease the weight

> **✴ EMT-I Tips**
>
> Sinusitis is an inflammation of the paranasal sinuses that is relatively common. Sinusitis may range in severity from a simple upper respiratory tract infection consisting of headache and nasal drainage to a potentially life-threatening brain infection, depending on the extent of the infection and which sinuses are affected.

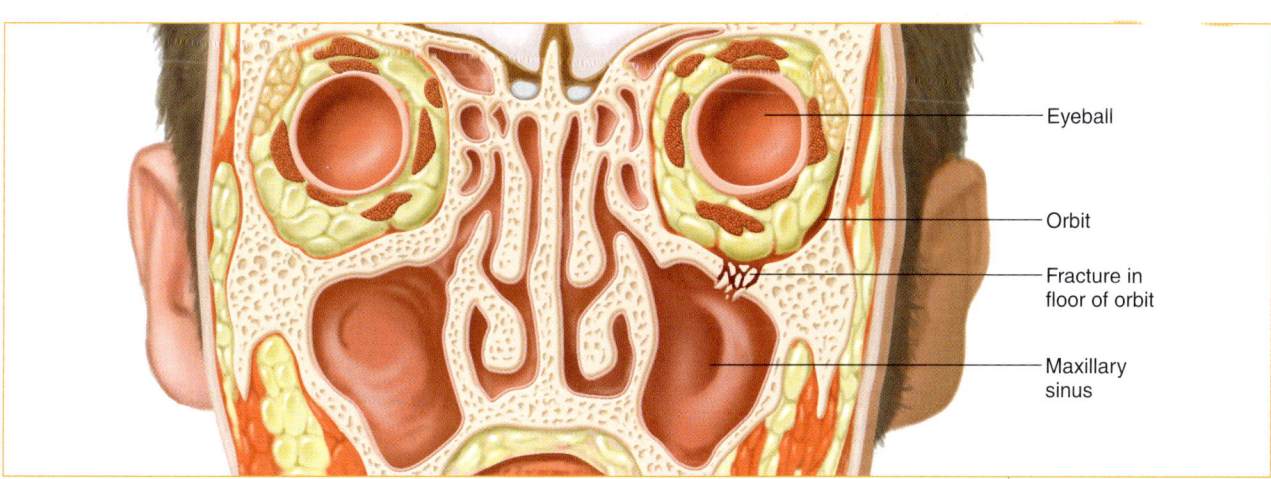

Figure 5-21 A blowout fracture of the left orbit.

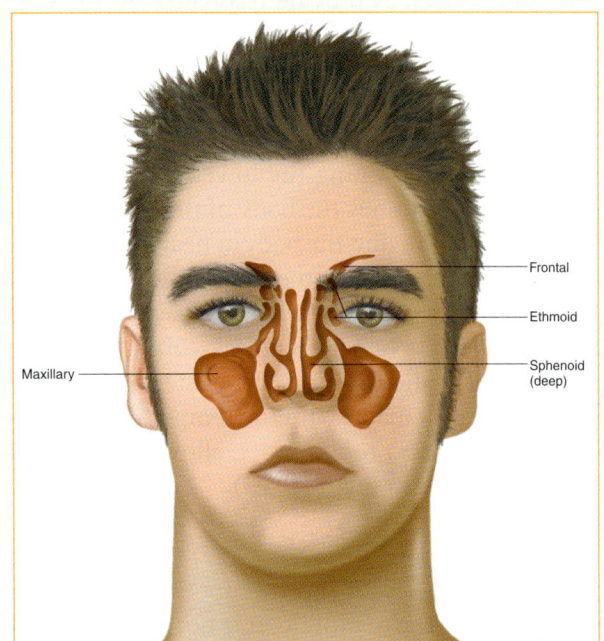

Figure 5-22 The paranasal sinuses.

> ### EMT-I Tips
>
> TMJ syndrome is an abnormal condition characterized by pain in the jaw and difficulty chewing and talking. Although dental malocclusion is regarded as the primary cause of TMJ syndrome, multiple factors, including head trauma, systemic disease, and stress, also may cause the syndrome. A genetic or acquired predisposition to TMJ syndrome may result in underlying alterations of the bones and soft tissues of the joint.
>
> Patients with TMJ syndrome report pain in and around the joint itself, although it also may radiate to the back and shoulders. Often, the pain is severe, resulting in headaches, and there may be clicking and popping of the joint, a grinding sensation (crepitus), or spasm in the muscles of chewing (trismus) that result in difficulty talking and chewing. Problems such as ringing in the ears (tinnitus) and dizziness also may occur. No single treatment method appears to be uniformly successful. Physical therapy is helpful, especially in patients who have sustained trauma. Intraoral appliances to adjust malocclusion and prevent bruxism (grinding together of the upper and lower teeth) help many patients, along with stress management techniques. Surgery is a last resort.

The Neck

The neck contains many important structures. It is supported by the cervical spine, or the first seven vertebrae in the spinal column (C1 through C7). The spinal cord exits from the foramen magnum and lies within the spinal canal formed by the vertebrae. The upper part of the esophagus and the trachea (windpipe) lie in the midline of the neck. The carotid arteries may be found on either side of the trachea, along with the jugular veins and several nerves.

Several useful landmarks can be palpated and seen in the neck (Figure 5-23 ▶). The most obvious is the firm prominence in the center of the anterior surface commonly known as the Adam's apple. Specifically, this prominence is the upper part of the thyroid cartilage. It is more prominent in men than in women. The other, lower portion is the cricoid cartilage, a firm ridge of cartilage inferior to the thyroid cartilage, which is somewhat more difficult to palpate. Between the thyroid cartilage and the cricoid cartilage in the midline of the neck is a soft depression, the cricothyroid membrane. This is a thin sheet of connective tissue (fascia) that joins the two cartilages. The cricothyroid membrane is covered at this point only by skin.

Inferior to the larynx, several additional firm ridges are palpable in the anterior midline. These ridges are the cartilage rings of the trachea. The trachea connects the larynx with the main air passages of the lungs (the bronchi). On either side of the lower larynx and the upper trachea lies the thyroid gland. Unless it is enlarged, this gland is usually not palpable.

Pulsations of the carotid arteries are easily palpable in a groove about half an inch lateral to the larynx. Lying immediately adjacent to these arteries, but not palpable, are the internal jugular veins and several important nerves. Lateral to these vessels and nerves lay the sternocleidomastoid muscles, which allow movement of the head. These muscles originate from the mastoid process of the cranium and insert into the medial border of each collarbone and the sternum (breastbone) at the base of the neck.

A series of bony prominences lie posteriorly, in the midline of the neck. They are the spines of the cervical vertebrae. The lower cervical spines are more prominent than the upper ones, and they are more easily palpable when the neck is flexed. At the base of the neck posteriorly, the most prominent spine is the seventh cervical vertebra (Figure 5-24 ▶).

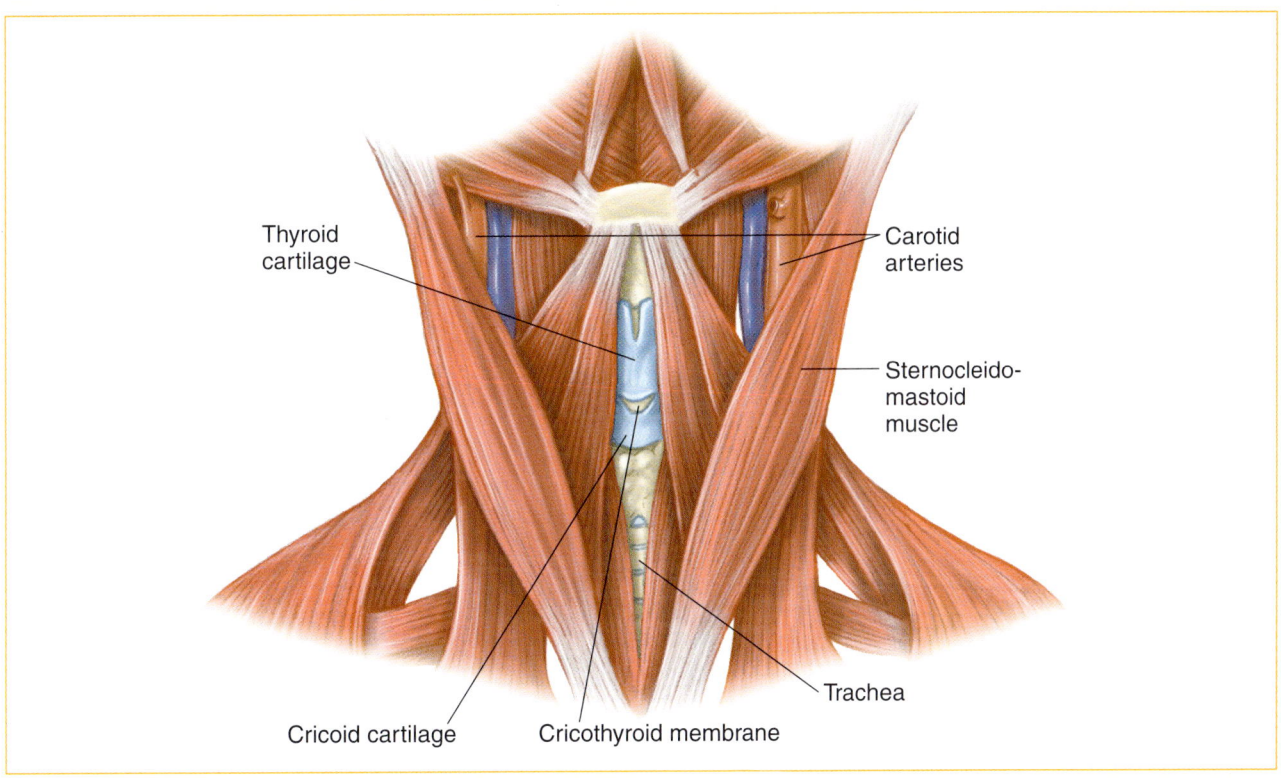

Figure 5-23 The principal structures of the neck include the trachea, along with many blood vessels, muscles, and nerves.

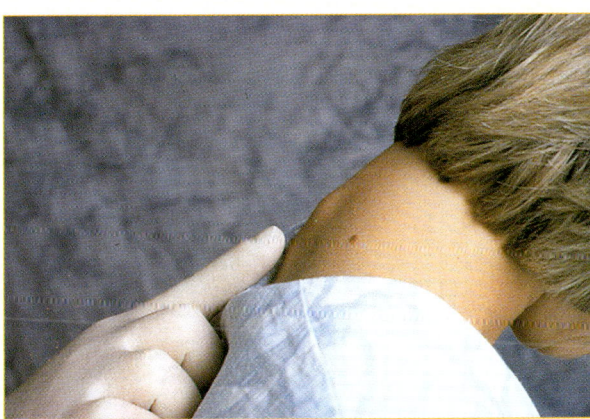

Figure 5-24 The most prominent of the cervical vertebrae is the spine of C7.

The Spine

The spine, or <u>vertebral column</u>, serves as a primary support structure for the body and houses the spinal cord and peripheral nerves. The spinal column is the central supporting structure of the body and is composed of 33 bones, each called a vertebra, which protect the spinal cord, provide a site for muscle attachment, and permit movement of the head and trunk. The <u>vertebrae</u> are named according to the section of the spine in which they lie and are numbered from top to bottom **Figure 5-25** ▶. From the top down, the spine is divided into five sections:

- <u>Cervical spine</u>. The first seven vertebrae (C1 through C7), which lie in the neck, form the cervical spine. The skull rests on the first cervical vertebra (the atlas) and articulates with it.
- <u>Thoracic spine</u>. The next 12 vertebrae make up the thoracic spine. One pair of ribs is attached to each of the thoracic vertebrae.
- <u>Lumbar spine</u>. The next five vertebrae form the lumbar or dorsal spine.
- <u>Sacrum</u>. The five sacral vertebrae are fused together to form one bone called the sacrum. The sacrum is joined to the iliac bones of the pelvis with strong ligaments at the sacroiliac joints to form the pelvis.
- <u>Coccyx</u>. The last four vertebrae form the coccyx or tailbone.

Seven cervical vertebrae are located in the neck. The first cervical vertebra (C1) is called the <u>atlas</u>. The atlas

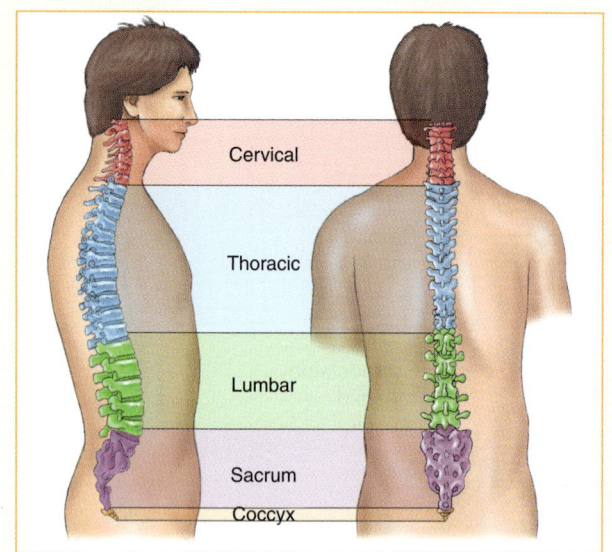

Figure 5-25 The spinal column is composed of 33 bones divided into five sections.

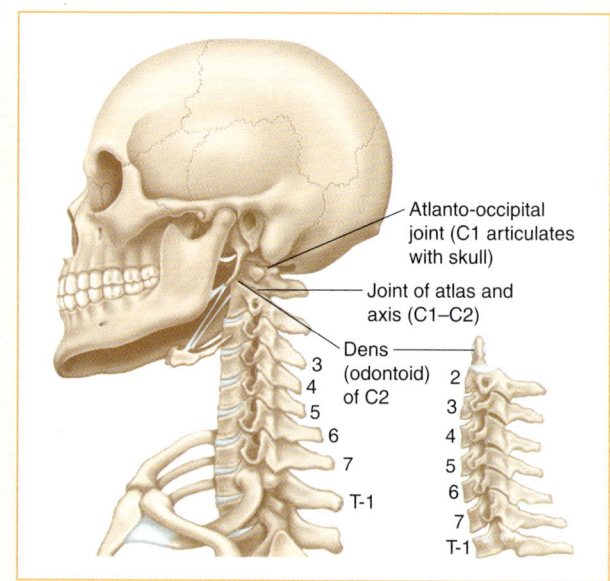

Figure 5-26 The cervical vertebrae.

is located directly beneath the skull and provides support for the head. The atlas articulates with the occipital condyles at the base of the skull at the <u>atlanto-occipital joint</u>. The only motions of this joint are flexion and extension and lateral bending.

The second cervical vertebra (C2) is known as the <u>axis</u> and is the point at which the head rotates, such as in a "no" motion. A large offshoot of C2 is the dens, or odontoid process, which fits into the enlarged vertebral foramen of the atlas. The atlas rotates around the axis at the dens. The cervical vertebrae numbered C3 through C6 form the cervical curve. C7, called the vertebra prominens, is different. It has a large spinous process that may be seen and felt at the base of the neck (Figure 5-26 ▶).

The spinal cord is an extension of the brain, composed of virtually all the nerves that carry messages between the brain and the rest of the body. It exits through a large hole in the base of the skull called the foramen magnum and is contained within and protected by the vertebrae of the spinal column. The spinal column is virtually surrounded by muscles. However, the posterior spinous process of each vertebra can be felt as it lies just under the skin in the midline of the back.

The anterior part of each vertebra consists of a round, solid block of bone called the body. The posterior part of each vertebra forms a bony arch. This series of arches from one vertebra to the next forms a tunnel that runs the length of the spine called the spinal canal. The bones of the spinal canal encase and protect the spinal cord (Figure 5-27 ▼). Nerves branch from the spinal cord and exit from the spinal canal between each two vertebrae to form the motor and sensory nerves of the body.

The vertebrae are connected by ligaments, and between each vertebra is a cushion called the intervertebral disk. These ligaments and disks allow some motion

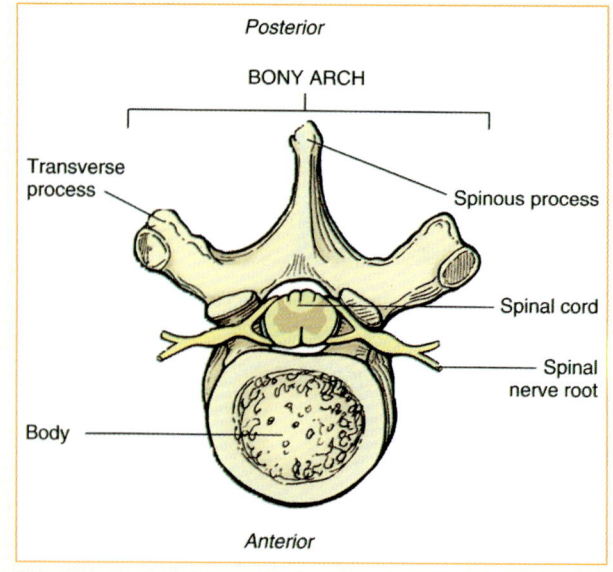

Figure 5-27 The bones of the spinal column encase and protect the spinal cord.

so that the trunk can bend forward and back. However, they also limit motion of the vertebrae so that the spinal cord will not be injured. An injury to the spine may damage part of the spinal cord and its nerves that may not be protected by the vertebrae. Therefore, until the injury is stabilized, you must use extreme caution in caring for the patient to prevent injury to the spinal cord.

The Thorax

The thorax (chest) is the cavity that contains the heart, lungs, esophagus, and great vessels (the aorta and two venae cavae). It is formed by the 12 thoracic vertebrae (T1 through T12) and their 12 pairs of ribs. The clavicle (collarbone) overlies the superior boundaries of the thorax in front and articulates posteriorly with the scapula (shoulder blade), which lies in the muscular tissue of the thoracic wall. The inferior boundary of the thorax is the diaphragm, which separates the thorax from the abdomen.

Anterior Aspects

The dimensions of the thorax are defined by the thoracic cage (bony rib cage) and its attachments Figure 5-28A ▼. Anteriorly, in the midline of the chest is the sternum. The superior border of the sternum forms the easily palpable jugular notch. The sternum has three components: the manubrium, the body, and the xiphoid process. The upper quarter of the sternum is called the manubrium. The body comprises the rest of the sternum except for a narrow, cartilaginous tip inferiorly, which is called the xiphoid process. The junction of the manubrium and the body forms a very prominent ridge on the sternum, called the angle of Louis. The angle of Louis lies at the level where the second rib is attached to the sternum; it provides a constant and reliable bony landmark on the anterior chest wall.

In the midline of the upper back, the spines of the 12 thoracic vertebrae can be palpated. Twelve ribs on each side form small joints with their respective thoracic vertebrae and extend around to the front to create the

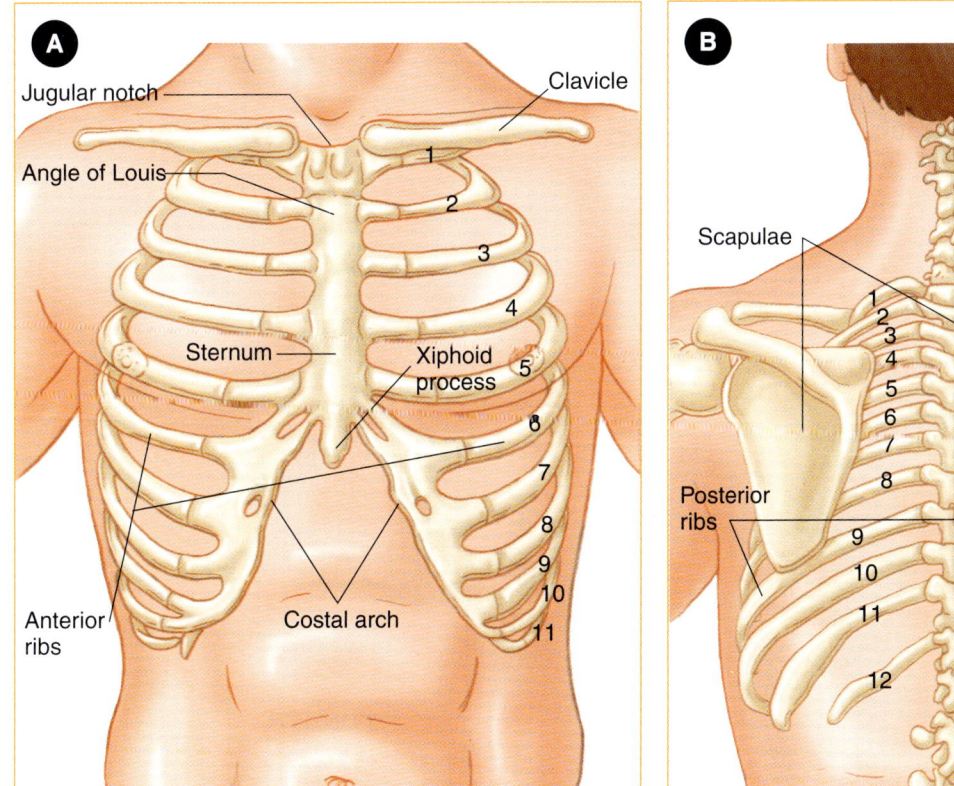
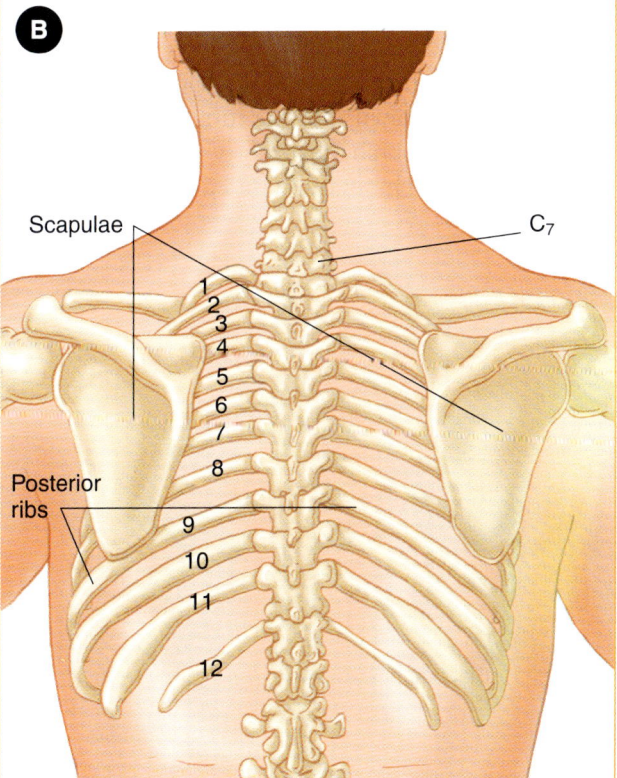

Figure 5-28 **A.** The anterior aspect of the thorax includes the following bony landmarks: the clavicle, the sternum, the xiphoid process, the angle of Louis, and the anterior ribs. **B.** The posterior aspect of the thorax includes the following bony landmarks: the scapulae, the thoracic vertebrae, and the posterior ribs.

walls of the thoracic cage. The upper five ribs connect to the sternum through a short bridge of cartilage. The sixth through tenth ribs insert into the costal arch. The costal arch is a bridge of cartilage that connects the ends of the sixth through tenth ribs with the lower portion of the sternum. The eleventh and twelfth ribs are called floating ribs, because they do not attach to the sternum through the costal arch. The costal arch is easily palpable and represents the boundary between the lower border of the thorax and the upper border of the abdomen.

Posterior Aspects

On the posterior chest wall, the scapulae overlie the thoracic wall and are surrounded by large muscles Figure 5-28B◀. When the patient is standing or sitting erect, the two scapulae should lie at approximately the same level, with their inferior tips at about the level of the seventh thoracic vertebra. In the lower part of the thorax on each side, the junction of the spine and the tenth rib forms an angle called the costovertebral angle. The kidneys lie deep to (beneath) the back muscles in the costovertebral angle.

Diaphragm

The diaphragm is a muscular dome that forms the inferior boundary of the thorax, separating the chest from the abdominal cavity Figure 5-29▼. Its contraction, along with that of the chest wall muscles, assists with allowing air to be drawn into the lungs. Anteriorly, it attaches to the costal arch; posteriorly, it attaches to the lumbar vertebrae. The diaphragm cannot be seen or palpated.

Organs and Vascular Structures

Within the thoracic cage, the largest structures are the heart, lungs, and great vessels Figure 5-30▼. The heart lies immediately behind the sternum (retrosternal). It extends from the second to the sixth ribs anteriorly and from the fifth to the eighth thoracic vertebrae posteriorly. The inferior border of the heart extends into the left side of the chest. Diseased hearts may be larger or smaller. The major blood vessels that travel to and from the heart also lie in the chest cavity. On the right side of the spinal column, the superior and inferior venae cavae carry blood to the heart.

Just beneath the manubrium of the sternum, the arch of the aorta and the pulmonary artery exit the heart. The arch of the aorta passes to the left and lies along the left side of the spinal column as it descends into the abdomen. The esophagus lies behind the great vessels and directly on the anterior aspect of the spinal column as it passes through the chest into the abdominal cavity.

All space within the chest that is not occupied by the heart, great vessels, and esophagus is occupied by

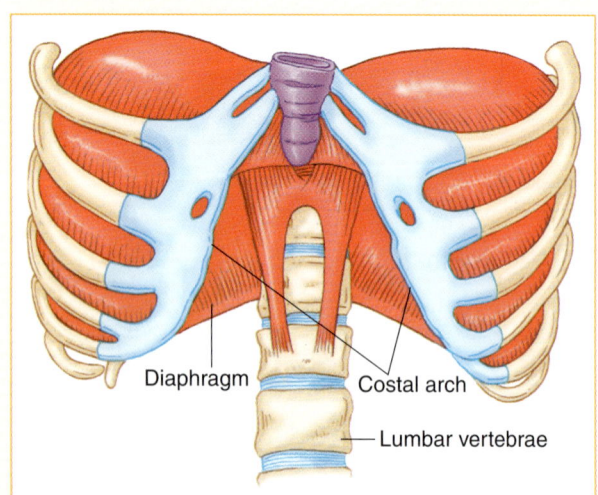

Figure 5-29 The diaphragm forms the undersurface of the thorax, separating the chest from the abdominal cavity.

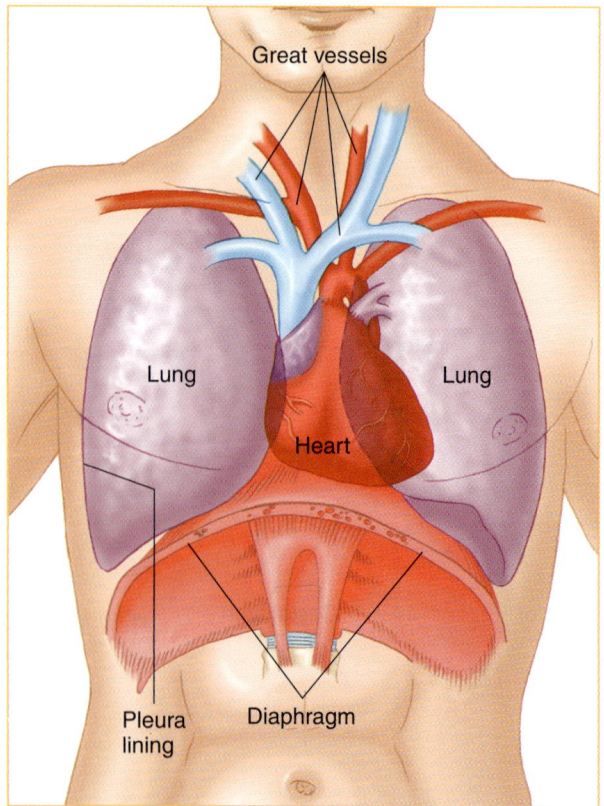

Figure 5-30 The anterior aspect of the thorax shows the relative positions of the principal organs beneath the surface.

the lungs. Anteriorly, the lungs extend down to the surface of the diaphragm at the level of the xiphoid process. Posteriorly, the lungs extend farther inferiorly to the surface of the diaphragm at the level of the twelfth thoracic vertebra.

Anatomic Landmarks

The major palpable landmarks in the chest are the ribs. Most of them can be easily felt except for the first, which is hidden under and behind the clavicle. Between each rib is an intercostal space. You can locate these spaces by palpating the jugular notch and moving laterally (the first intercostal space). Counting the successive spaces between the ribs gives us the second, third, etc. Both clavicles and the sternum can be easily palpated. The jugular notch is the top portion of the sternum. Lateral to that is the first intercostal space. Inferiorly, the costal arch is readily palpable on both sides of the anterior chest wall. In the midline, the tip of the xiphoid process is a tender and easily palpated landmark.

The Abdomen

The <u>abdomen</u> is the second major body cavity; it contains the major organs of digestion and excretion. The diaphragm separates the thoracic cavity from the abdominal cavity. Anteriorly and posteriorly, thick muscular abdominal walls create the boundaries of this space. Inferiorly, the abdomen is separated from the pelvis by an imaginary plane that extends from the pubic symphysis through the sacrum (Figure 5-31 ▶). Many organs lie in both the abdomen and the pelvis, depending on the posture of the patient.

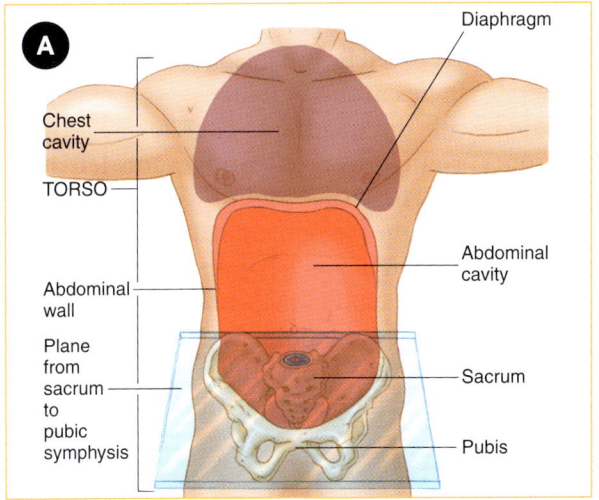
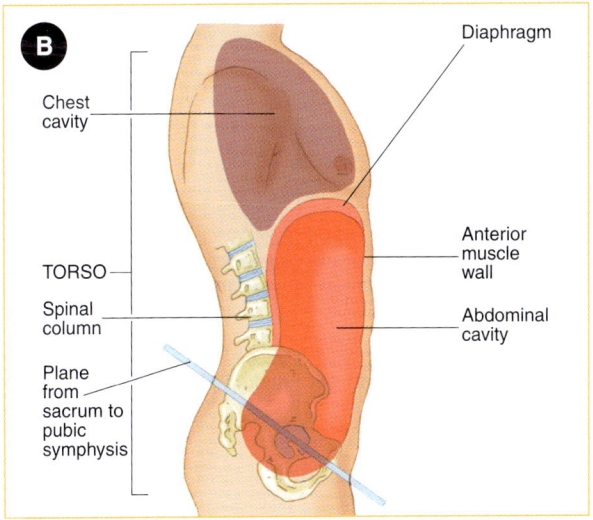

Figure 5-31 The boundaries of the abdomen are the anterior and posterior abdominal cavity walls, the diaphragm, and an imaginary plane from the pubic symphysis to the sacrum. **A.** Anterior view. **B.** Lateral view.

You are the Provider   Part 5

Your continued assessment of Patient 2 reveals the following:

Vital Signs	Recording Time: 2 Minutes After Patient Contact
Respirations	18 breaths/min, unlabored
Pulse	88 beats/min, strong and regular
Blood pressure	120/60 mm Hg
Sao_2	98% on supplemental oxygen

7. What is the most common method used to describe the abdomen?
8. Why is it important for the EMT-I to use these designations?

The simplest and most common method of describing the portions of the abdomen is by quadrants, the four equal areas formed by two imaginary lines that intersect at right angles at the umbilicus. On the anterior abdominal wall, the quadrants thus formed are the right upper, right lower, left upper, and left lower Figure 5-32 ▼). The terms "right quadrant" and "left quadrant" refer to the patient's right and left as you face them, not to your right and left sides. Pain or injury in a given quadrant usually arises from or involves the organs that lie in that quadrant. This simple means of designation will allow you to identify injured or diseased organs that require emergency attention.

Organs and Vascular Structures

In the right upper quadrant (RUQ), the major organs are the liver, the gallbladder, and a portion of the colon and small intestine. Most of the liver lies in this quadrant, almost entirely under the protection of the eighth to twelfth ribs. The liver fills the entire anteroposterior depth of the abdomen in this quadrant. Therefore, injuries in this area are frequently associated with injuries of the liver.

In the left upper quadrant (LUQ), the principal organs are the stomach, the spleen, and a portion of the colon and small intestine. The spleen is almost entirely under the protection of the left rib cage, whereas the stomach may sag well down into the left lower quadrant when full. The spleen lies in the lateral and posterior portion of this quadrant, under the diaphragm and immediately in front of the ninth to eleventh ribs. The spleen is frequently injured, especially when these ribs are fractured.

The right lower quadrant (RLQ) contains two portions of the large intestine: the <u>cecum</u>, the first portion into which the small intestine (ileum) opens, and the ascending colon. The <u>appendix</u> is a small tubular structure that is attached to the lower border of the cecum. Appendicitis is the most frequent cause of tenderness and pain in this region. In the left lower quadrant (LLQ) lie the descending and the sigmoid portions of the colon.

Several organs lie in more than one quadrant. The small intestine, for example, occupies the central part of the abdomen around the umbilicus, and parts of it lie in all four quadrants. The pancreas lies just behind the abdominal cavity on the posterior abdominal wall in both upper quadrants. The large intestine also traverses the abdomen, beginning in the RLQ and ending in the LLQ as it passes through all four quadrants. The urinary bladder lies just behind the pubic symphysis in the middle of the abdomen and therefore lies in both lower quadrants and also in the pelvis.

The kidneys are called <u>retroperitoneal</u> organs because they lie behind the abdominal cavity Figure 5-33 ▶). They are above the level of the umbilicus, extending from the eleventh rib to the third lumbar vertebra on each side. They are approximately 5″ long and lie just anterior to the costovertebral angle.

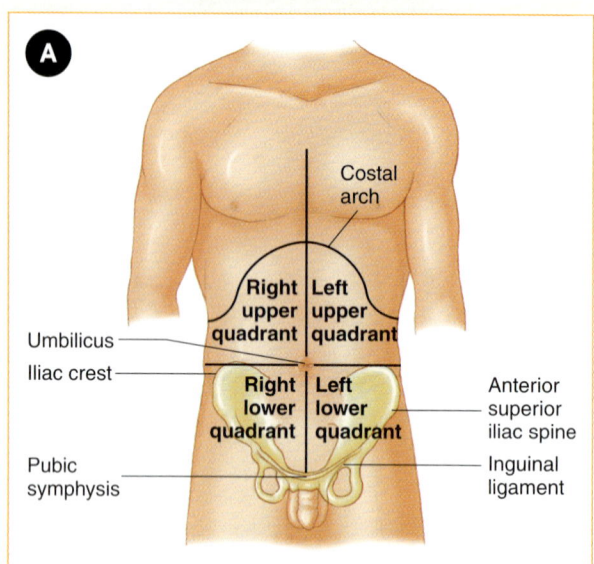

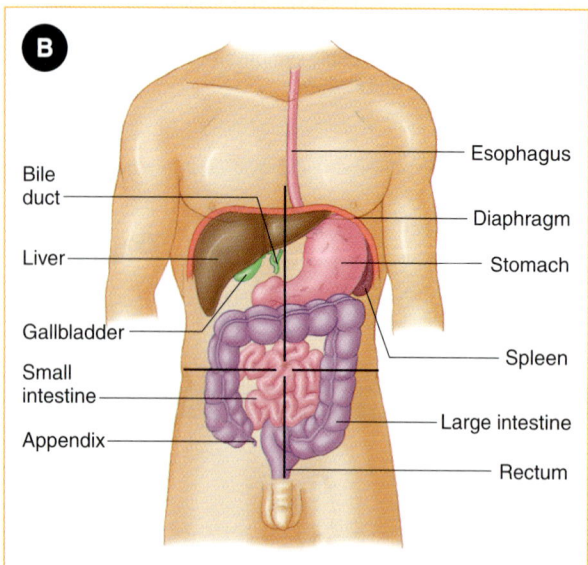

Figure 5-32 A. In the abdomen, quadrants are the easiest system for identifying areas. Major bony landmarks are also shown. **B.** Many of the organs in the abdomen lie in more than one quadrant.

A to Z Terminology Tips

Retro means back or behind and *peritoneal* refers to the peritoneal cavity surrounding the abdominal organs. Therefore, *retroperitoneal* means "behind the peritoneal cavity."

Chapter 5 The Human Body

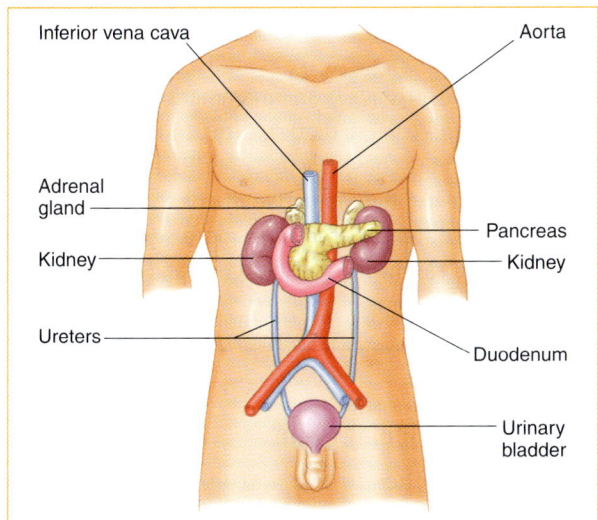

Figure 5-33 The major organs of the retroperitoneal space lie behind the abdominal cavity, above the level of the umbilicus, and extend from the eleventh rib to the third lumbar vertebra. Note that the bladder, inferior vena cava, and aorta also lie in this plane.

Posteriorly, you do not usually refer to abdominal quadrants. The posterior portion of the iliac crest can be palpated, as can the spines of the five lumbar vertebrae (Ll through L5) in the midline.

The Appendicular Skeleton

The Shoulder Girdle

The shoulder girdle attaches the upper extremity to the body. The two components of the shoulder girdle are the triangular shaped scapula (shoulder blade) and the clavicle (collarbone). Prominent features of the scapula include the acromion process (the tip of the shoulder), the coracoid process, the scapular spine, the glenoid fossa, the supraspinous fossa, and the infraspinous fossa.

The acromion process protects the shoulder joint and provides a site of attachment for both the clavicle and various shoulder muscles (Figure 5-34A ▼). The clavicle

Anatomic Landmarks

The chief landmarks in the abdomen are the costal arch, the umbilicus, the anterior superior iliac spines, the iliac crest, and the pubic symphysis. The costal arch, as was noted earlier, is the fused cartilages of the sixth through the tenth ribs. It forms the superior arching boundary of the abdomen. The umbilicus, a constant structure, is in the same horizontal plane as the fourth lumbar vertebra and the superior edge of the iliac crest, the rim of the pelvic bone. The anterior superior iliac spines are the bony prominences of the pelvis (ilium) at the front on each side of the lower abdomen just below the plane of the umbilicus. In the midline in the lowermost portion of the abdomen is another hard bony prominence, the pubic symphysis. Between the lateral edge of the pubic symphysis and the anterosuperior spine on each side, you can palpate the tough inguinal ligament, which stretches between these two structures. Below the ligament lie the femoral vessels.

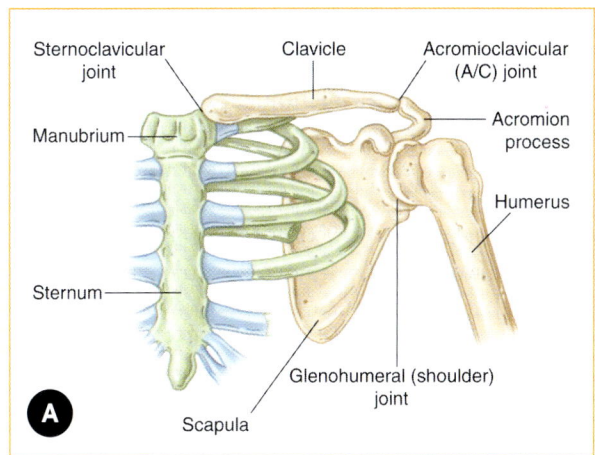

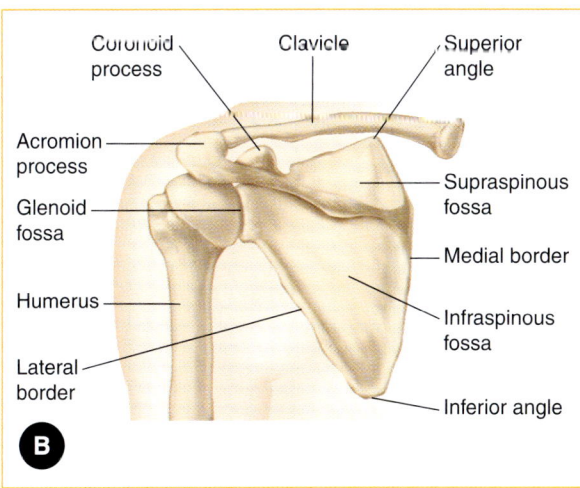

Figure 5-34 **A.** Anterior view of the shoulder girdle, including the clavicle. **B.** Posterior view of the shoulder girdle, including the scapula.

> **A to Z Terminology Tips**
>
> Pay close attention to spelling to prevent misunderstandings. Even though *ilium* and *ileum* are pronounced the same, they refer to two different parts of the body.
> **Ilium** = the bony prominences of the pelvis
> **Ileum** = the lower 3/5 of the small intestine

and shoulder muscles also attach to the coracoid process of the scapula. The scapular spine divides the posterior surface of the scapula into the supraspinous fossa, which is above the spine, and the infraspinous fossa, which is below the spine (Figure 5-34B). Important muscles of the shoulder, including those of the rotator cuff, originate here.

The clavicle is an S-shaped bone that is easily felt on either side of the jugular notch. The lateral end of the clavicle articulates with the acromion and the medial end with the manubrium.

The Shoulder Joint

The shoulder joint is a ball-and-socket joint in which the head of the humerus articulates with the glenoid fossa, which is part of the scapula (Figure 5-35). The hip and shoulder are typical ball-and-socket joints (Figure 5-36). Possible motions at a ball-and-socket joint include flexion, extension, abduction, adduction, rotation, and circumduction.

The four ligaments that attach the humeral head to the glenoid fossa include the glenohumeral, transverse humeral, coracohumeral, and coracoacromial ligaments. A fibrocartilage ring, the glenoid labrum, surrounds the glenoid rim and provides a point of attachment for the capsule, which is made up of fibrous connective tissue. A bursa is a fluid-filled sac situated between a tendon and a bone that cushions and protects joints such as the shoulder, hip, or knee. The subscapular bursa and the subacromial bursa are the two bursae located in the shoulder joint.

> 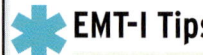 **EMT-I Tips**
>
> Costochondritis is an inflammation of the costocartilage (rib cartilage), often in the anterior portion of the chest. Costochondritis is a relatively common and benign cause of chest pain, but it must be differentiated from more severe conditions such as myocardial infarction and pulmonary embolism.

The Acromioclavicular Joint

The clavicle attaches to the acromion process at the acromioclavicular (AC) joint, where it is held in place by the acromioclavicular, coracoacromial, trapezoid, and conoid ligaments. The trapezoid and conoid ligaments sometimes are jointly referred to as the coracoclavicular ligament.

The Upper Extremity

The upper extremity consists of the arm (more commonly thought of as the upper arm), forearm, wrist, hand, and fingers.

The humerus is the bone of the upper arm (Figure 5-37A). It articulates proximally with the glenoid fossa and distally with the radius and ulna at the elbow joint. The elbow joint is a hinge joint, permitting motion in one plane only. Several ligaments connect the humerus, radius, and ulna at the elbow joint, and a fluid-filled bursa cushions and protects the joint posteriorly (Figure 5-38).

The Forearm and Wrist

The forearm extends from the elbow to the wrist. The forearm contains two bones, the radius and ulna (see Figure 5-37A). The radius is the bone located on the lateral side (the thumb side) of the forearm when the forearm is in the anatomic position, and the ulna is located on the little finger side. The proximal portion of the radius is called the radial head. The distal portion contains a small bony protrusion, the styloid process, to which ligaments of the wrist are attached.

The proximal portion of the ulna consists of the hooked olecranon process and the coronoid process; both articulate with the distal humerus at the elbow. At the distal end, the head of the ulna also contains a styloid process that serves the same function as its counterpart at the distal radius. A band of connective tissue,

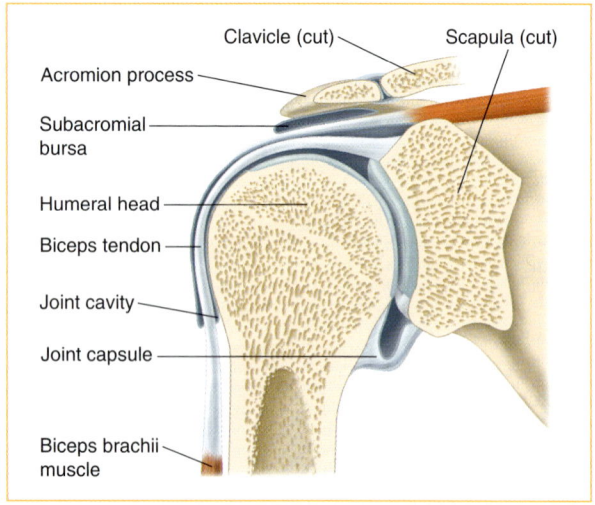

Figure 5-35 Anterior view of the shoulder joint.

Chapter 5 The Human Body 147

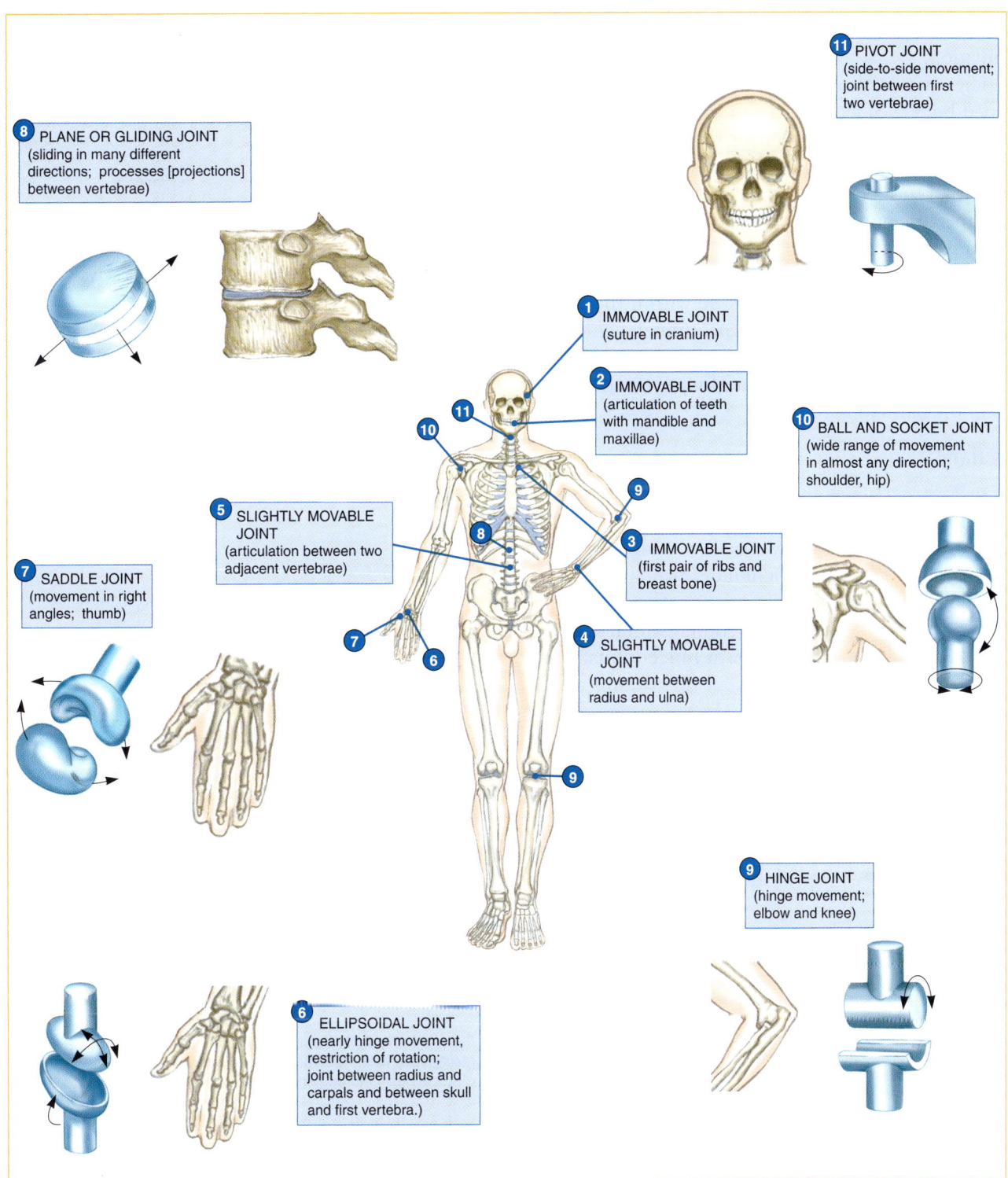

Figure 5-36 Joints in the body.

the interosseous membrane, connects the radius and the ulna and permits movements such as pronation and supination.

The wrist is made of a group of eight irregularly shaped bones, called the carpals. The carpals include the triquetrum, pisiform, capitate, lunate, hamate, trapezoid, trapezium, and scaphoid (carpal navicular) bones. The carpal tunnel is formed by the space bounded by the trapezium and hamate dorsally and the flexor retinaculum, a sheath of tough connective tissue that forms the roof of the carpal tunnel, on the palmar side. Tendons, nerves, and blood vessels lie within the carpal tunnel. Structures within the carpal tunnel include the long flexor tendon to the fingers and the median nerve, which supplies sensory and motor function to the radial half of the palm of the hand.

The Hand

The metacarpal bones are the bones that form the hand. The phalanges is a series of small bones that exist in each finger. Often, one or two small, rounded sesamoid bones are present at the junction of the phalanges and the metacarpals, at the metacarpophalangeal (MCP) joint. Sesamoid bones are formed entirely within tendons. The phalanges in the fingers form hinge joints. Each finger has three phalanges, except the thumb, which has only two (Figure 5-37B ▶). The carpometacarpal joint of the thumb is a saddle joint, consisting of two saddle-shaped articulating surfaces that are oriented at right angles to one another so that the complementary surfaces articulate with each other. Movement in these joints can occur in two planes. Arthritis commonly affects the carpometacarpal joint, resulting in stiffness and deformity.

> ### ✴ EMT-I Tips
>
> Acromioclavicular separation (AC separation), also called a separated shoulder, occurs when any of the four ligaments of the AC joint are partially or completely torn. In partial tears, no deformity is noted unless the patient attempts to hold a weight with the arm directed downward. In this case, the weakened joint is transiently widened, a finding visible on radiographs. In cases of complete separation, in which all four ligaments are severely damaged, the clavicle essentially lies above the acromion, causing a visible deformity in the patient's shoulder area.

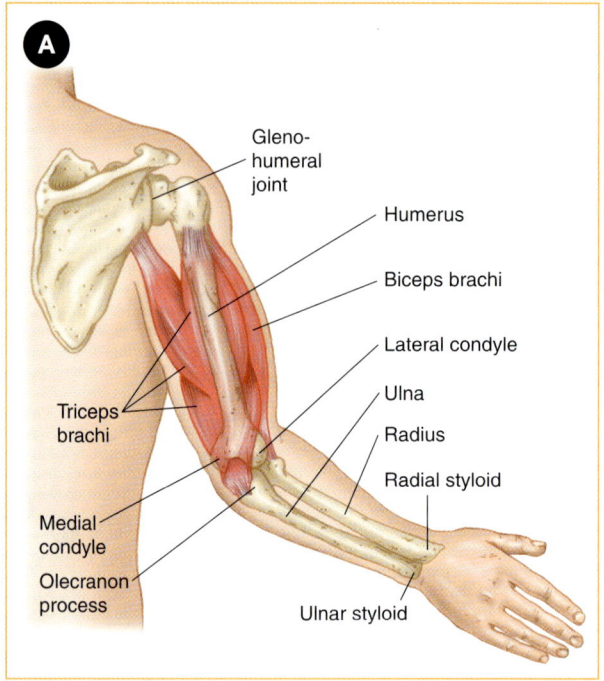

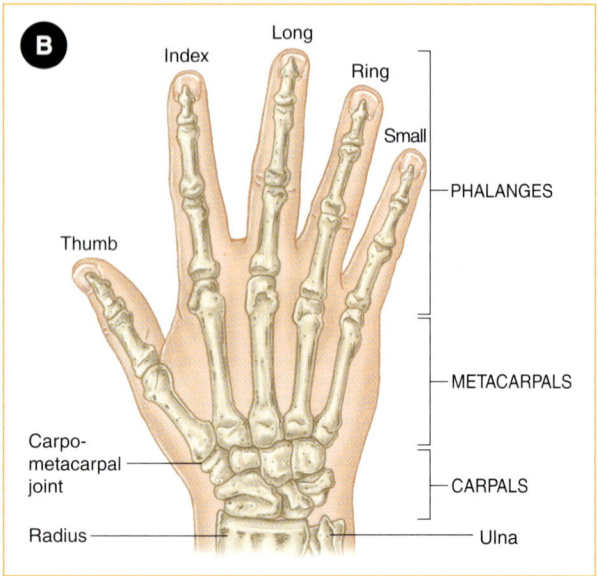

Figure 5-37 **A.** The upper arm contains the humerus; the forearm contains the radius and ulna. **B.** The carpals, metacarpals, and phalanges form the hand.

The Pelvic Girdle

The pelvis, or pelvic girdle, is where the lower extremity attaches to the body (Figure 5-39 ▶). The pelvis contains a ring of bones formed by the sacrum and the coxal, or pelvic bones; the sacrum is posterior and the coxal bones are on each side. Each coxa consists of three fused bones: the ilium, ischium, and pubis. The pelvis contains three joints: the two posterior sacroiliac joints and the

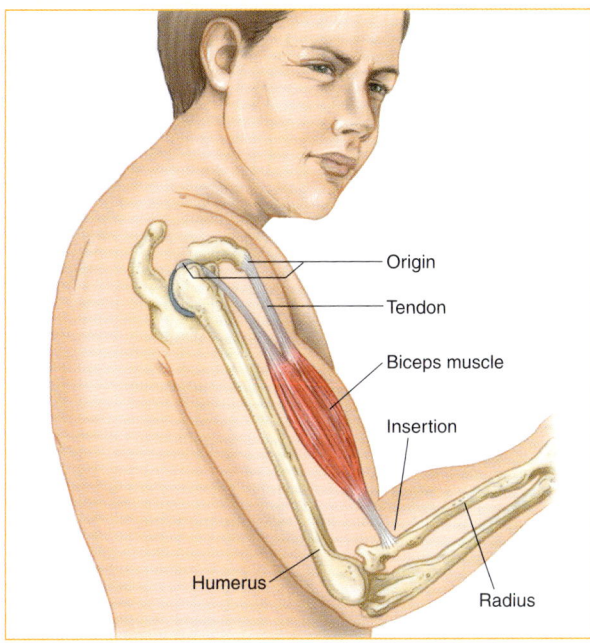

Figure 5-38 Ligaments connect the humerus, radius, ulna. A fluid-filled bursa cushions and protects the joint.

and pubis that contains several important nerves and muscles. The pelvic girdle supports the body weight and protects the internal organs. In a pregnant woman, the bones protect the developing fetus and provide a passageway through which the infant passes during delivery.

The Lower Extremity

The lower extremity is made of the hip, thigh, knee, leg, ankle, foot, and toes. The acetabulum is the socket of the ball-and-socket joint that connects the pelvic girdle with the lower extremity (Figure 5-40 ▼). The thigh is the part of the lower extremity that extends from the hip to the knee and contains the femur, which is the longest and strongest bone in the body. The uppermost portion of the femur, the femoral head, articulates with the pelvic girdle at the acetabulum. In addition to the femoral head, the proximal femur consists of the neck, greater trochanter, and lesser trochanter. The intertrochanteric

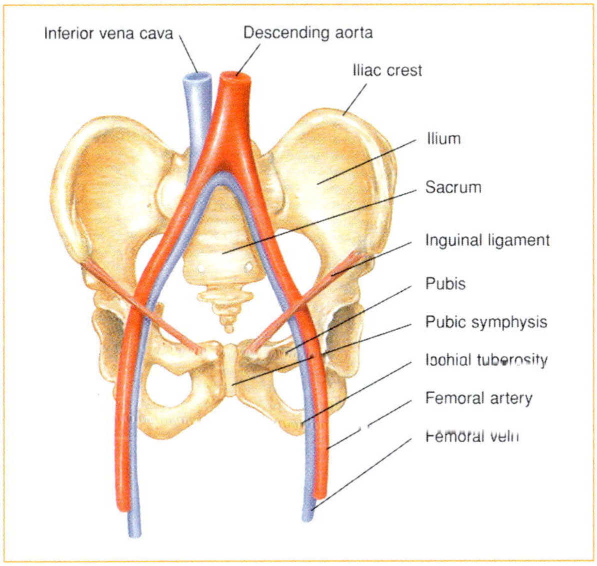

Figure 5-39 The pelvic girdle.

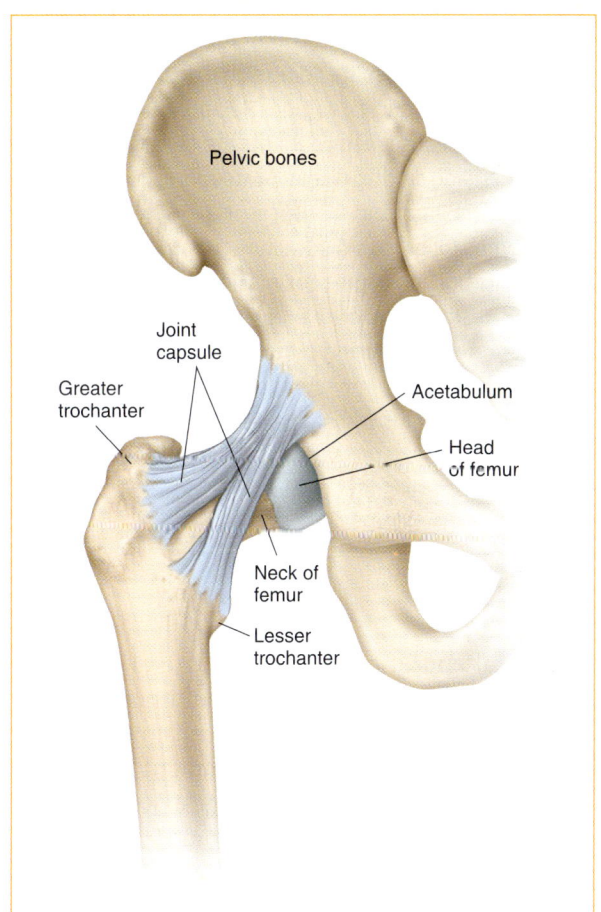

Figure 5-40 The hip joint and its surrounding structures.

interior midline pubic symphysis. The location where the ilium connects with the sacrum is the sacroiliac joint. The pubic symphysis is the lower midportion of the pelvic ring where the left and right sides fuse together. The superior portion of the ilium is the iliac crest. The obturator foramen is an opening between the ischium line runs between the greater and the lesser trochanter. The greater trochanter arises lateral to the juncture of the neck and shaft and is clinically considered as part of the hip. Several ligaments and muscle tendons provide integrity to the hip joint. The articular capsule is supported by three ligaments and is quite strong. In fact, the iliofemoral, pubofemoral, and ischiofemoral ligaments support much of the body's weight.

> ### ✱ EMT-I Tips
>
> Hip fractures actually are fractures of the proximal portion of the femur near or at the site of articulation with the acetabulum. These fractures are classified based on the structures of the femur involved. Fractures between the femoral head and the trochanteric region are termed femoral neck fractures. These include subcapital, mid-cervical and basi-cervical variants. Fractures between trochanters are described as intertrochanteric and fractures below the lesser trochanter are described as subtrochanteric (Figure 5-41 ▶).
>
> Hip fractures account for nearly 30% of orthopaedic hospital admissions. Up to 80% of hip fractures occur in women. Results often are disabling because many patients are elderly and have underlying cardiac disease, osteoporosis, and senility. Mortality from all causes is 20% in the first 6 months following a hip fracture. Treatment depends on the portion of the proximal femur that is injured.
>
> Dislocations of the hip joint commonly occur from a fall or during a motor vehicle collision in which the knee impacts the dashboard. The force of the impact is transmitted posteriorly to the hip, resulting in posterior dislocation. Anterior hip dislocations are less common.

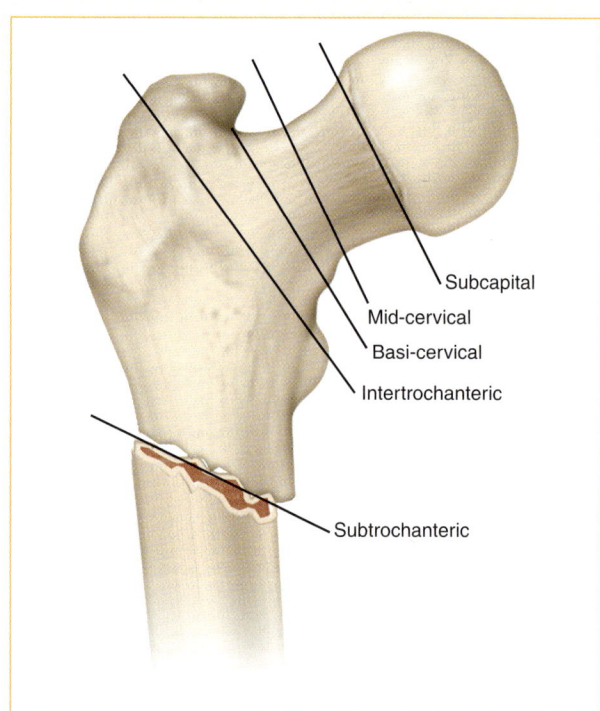

Figure 5-41 Fractures of the hip.

thicker of the two bones and is situated on the anterior surface of the leg. The anterior portion of the tibia, covered only by skin, is commonly called the shin. The flat medial and lateral condyles of the proximal tibia articulate with the condyles of the femur at the knee. The intercondylar eminence, which is a site of ligament attachment, is situated between the condyles. The medial malleolus, which forms the medial side of the ankle joint, lies at the distal end of the tibia.

The second of the two leg bones, the fibula, is posterior to the tibia and does not articulate directly with the femur, but rather with the tibia at the head. An enlargement of the distal end of the fibula forms the lateral wall of the ankle joint, the lateral malleolus.

The Leg

At the distal end of the femur, the lateral and medial condyles articulate with the proximal tibia at the knee (Figure 5-42 ▶). The medial and lateral epicondyles are important sites of muscle and ligament attachment. The patella, or kneecap, is the largest sesamoid bone in the body. It lies within the major anterior tendon of the thigh muscles and articulates with the trochlear groove of the femur.

The leg is made of the tibia and fibula, and extends from the knee to the ankle. The tibia is the longer and

The Knee

The knee joint is traditionally classified as a hinge joint and is unusual because it contains ligaments within the joint. The distal end of the femur articulates with the condyles of the proximal tibia. Thick crescent-shaped articular disks, menisci, cover the margins of the tibia to cushion the articular surface. The anterior and posterior cruciate ligaments extend between the intercondylar eminence of the tibia and the fossa of the femur. The anterior cruciate ligament prevents abnormal anterior movement (hyperextension) of the tibia. The

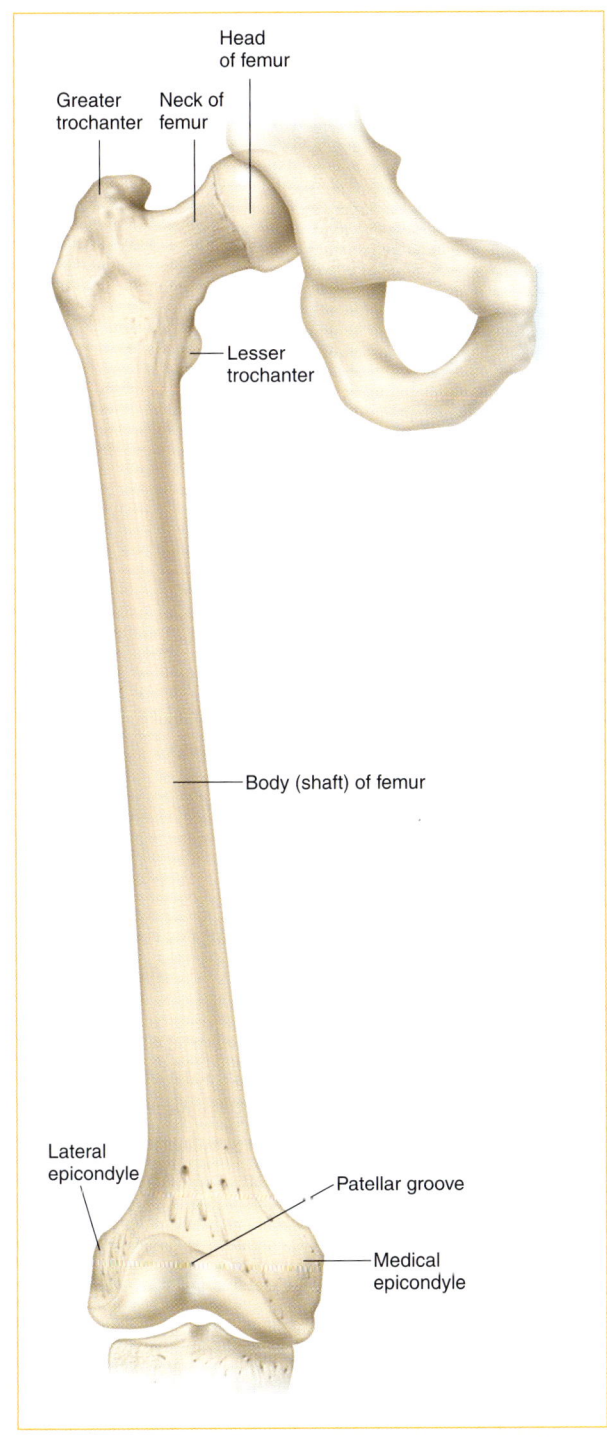

Figure 5-42 The femur.

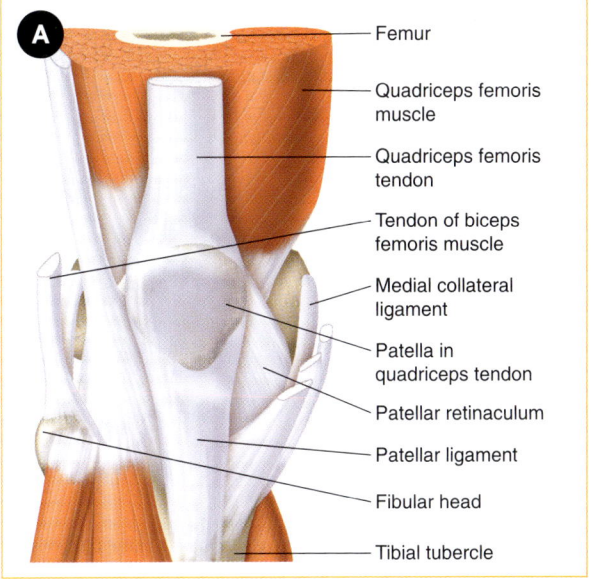

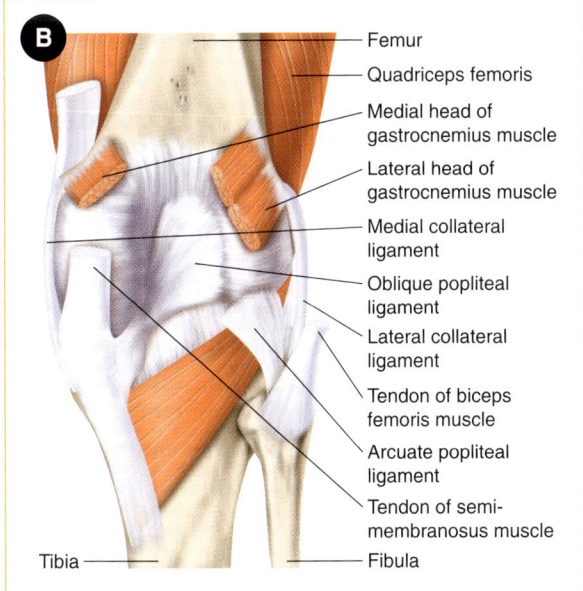

Figure 5-43 **A.** Anterior view of the knee. **B.** Posterior view of the knee.

The Ankle

The talus articulates with the tibia and fibula to form the ankle Figure 5-44 ▶ . The calcaneus, or heel bone, lies inferior and lateral to the talus, providing additional support. A fibrous capsule surrounds the ankle joint; the medial and lateral portions are thickened to form ligaments. Movements include dorsiflexion and plantar flexion, as well as limited inversion and eversion.

The metatarsals and phalanges of the foot are arranged much like the bones of the hand Figure 5-45 ▶ . The

posterior cruciate ligament prevents abnormal posterior displacement of the tibia. Several tendons, as well as collateral ligaments, lend further strength to the knee joint. The knee is surrounded by several fluid-filled bursae, the largest of which is the suprapatellar bursa Figure 5-43 ▶ .

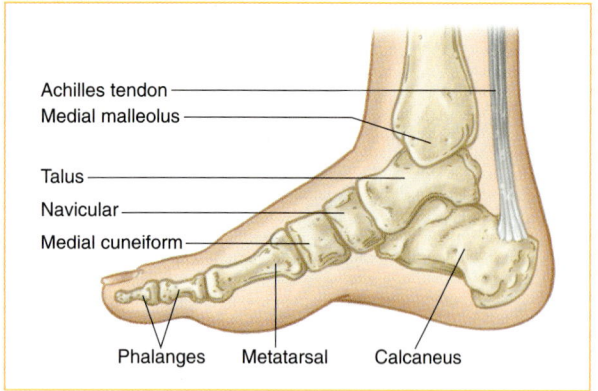

Figure 5-44 The medial side of the foot and ankle.

toes have three phalanges each, except the big toe, which has two phalanges. The ball of the foot is the junction between the metatarsals and the phalanges. Natural dorsal convexity and ventral concavity form the arches.

Cartilage, Tendons, and Ligaments

Cartilage, tendons, and ligaments are important connective tissues that work with bones to provide the support framework of the skeleton. Shiny connective tissue called cartilage is lubricated by a transparent viscous joint fluid (synovial fluid) that is secreted by the synovial membrane in an articulation to provide a slippery surface over which the bones may move. In addition to lubricating the joint, synovial fluid contains white blood cells to fight infections and provides nourishment to the cartilage covering the bone. Synovial fluid is found in the joint cavity, the space between the joint capsule (a connective tissue capsule that surrounds the bones) and the bones. Although there are several different types of cartilage, hyaline cartilage is the type most commonly associated with bone. A double-layered connective tissue membrane known as the perichondrium surrounds the cartilage.

Tendons are specialized tough cords or bands of dense white connective tissue that are continuous with the periosteum of the bone, the double-layer membrane that covers all bones except the articular surfaces. Tendons connect muscles to bones. Ligaments are tough white bands of tissue that connect bones to each other. Tendons and ligaments are composed of densely packed fibers of collagen, a twisted rope-like protein. The collagen fibrils in ligaments often are less compact than those in tendons. Ligaments usually are more flattened than tendons, forming sheets or bands of tissue. A sprain occurs when the bone ends partially or temporarily dis-

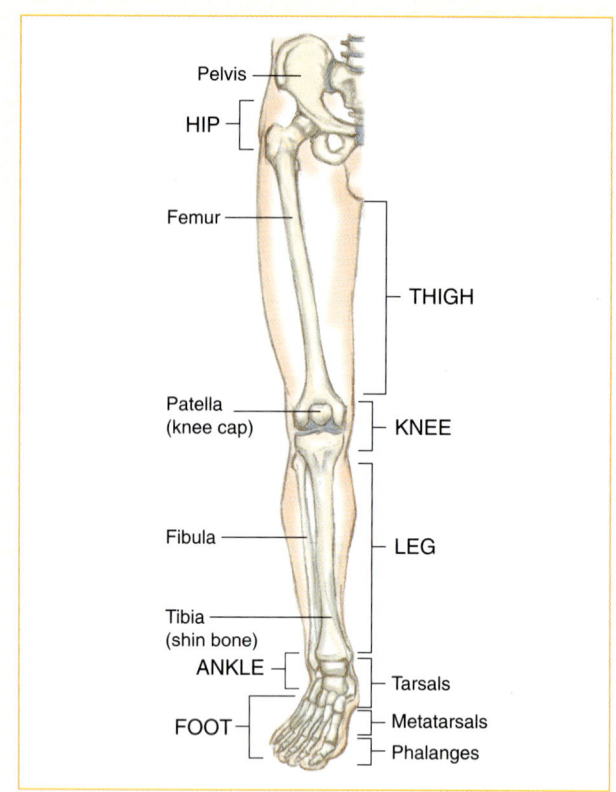

Figure 5-45 Dorsal view of the foot.

locate and the supporting ligaments are partially stretched or torn. Following a sprain, the joint surfaces generally fall back into alignment.

When a muscle contracts, tendon pulls on bone, resulting in motion at the joint, the point where two or more bones come together, allowing movement to occur. A strain, or muscle pull, occurs when a muscle is stretched or torn, resulting in pain, swelling, and bruising of surrounding soft tissues. No ligament or joint damage occurs with a strain. Sprains and strains are graded based on their severity and physical findings during examination Table 5-2 .

Bones: Their Growth and Organization

Bone is a specialized form of connective tissue. Bones protect internal organs and, with muscles, enable movement. Bone also serves as a storage site for minerals, particularly calcium, and has a role in the formation of blood cells and platelets. Bones consist of collagen and the mineral hydroxyapatite, a compound that contains calcium and phosphate. The collagen fibers in bone act much like reinforcing rods in a concrete structure, lending flexible strength to the bone. The mineral compo-

TABLE 5-2 Strains and Sprains

Grade	Degree of Damage	Clinical Findings and Implications
Strains		
Grade I	Minimal damage or disruption	■ Tender without substantial swelling ■ Minimal or no bruising or palpable defect ■ Active contraction and passive stretch are painful ■ Prognosis is good with minimal impairment
Grade II	Moderate damage	■ Tender with swelling ■ Mild to moderate bruising ■ Passive movement and attempted active movement are painful ■ Joint ROM limited due to pain ■ Prognosis usually is good with minimal impairment but requires a longer healing/rehabilitation period
Grade III	Complete disruption of muscle, tendon, or both	■ Substantial tenderness with swelling ■ Palpable defect may be present ■ Complete loss of muscle function ■ No increase in pain with passive stretch (nerve fibers are completely torn) ■ Prognosis is variable (injury may require surgery) ■ Requires a prolonged healing/rehabilitation period
Sprains		
Grade I	Minimal damage or disruption	■ Tender without substantial swelling ■ Minimal or no bruising ■ Active and passive range of motion are painful ■ Prognosis is good with no expectation of instability or functional loss
Grade II	Moderate damage	■ Moderate swelling and bruising ■ Very tender with more diffuse tenderness than grade I ■ Range of motion is restricted by pain ■ Joint may be unstable, and functional loss may result
Grade III	Complete disruption of the ligament	■ Severe swelling and bruising ■ Structural instability with abnormal motion (due to a complete tear of the ligament) ■ Pain on passive range of motion may be less than lower grades ■ Significant functional loss that may require surgery to restore

nents of the bone supply strength for bearing weight, much like concrete does in a structure. Bone without the necessary amount of mineral is very flexible; bone without enough collagen is extremely brittle.

Bones are a living substance with cells requiring a blood supply. During fetal development the skeleton is formed from hyaline cartilage, which is then converted to bone. During life, bones are constantly remodeled to meet the stresses that are placed on them. The level of a person's activity directly affects how the bones are remodeled. Increased activity levels such as walking or running causes compact bone to thicken to meet the increased stresses on the bones. Decreased activity or sedentary periods lead to decreased bone thickness.

Growth hormone (GH) produced by the anterior pituitary works with thyroid hormones to control normal growth. GH increases the rate of growth of the skeleton by causing cartilage cells and bone cells to reproduce and lay down their intercellular matrix, as well as stimulating the deposition of mineral within this matrix. GH also stimulates muscles to grow.

Bones play a significant role in maintaining proper blood calcium levels. The two hormones, calcitonin and parathormone, regulate the bone remodeling and control of blood calcium levels. Calcium-rich foods, vitamin D, which helps the body to absorb calcium, and exercise all help to maintain good bone health and prevent osteoporosis in women and men.

In postmenopausal women especially, weight-bearing activities and efficient maintenance of estrogen and calcium levels are significant factors in slowing bone deterioration and osteoporosis.

Cells called osteoblasts produce bone tissue. Bony matrix (connective tissue) that surrounds an osteoblast creates an osteocyte. Osteoclasts are large, multinucleated cells that dissolve bone tissue. Osteoclasts play a major role in bone remodeling, the removal of old bone and the deposition of new bone.

Bone tissue is organized into thin sheets or layers called lamellae. Each osteocyte is contained within a portion of matrix known as a lacuna, a minute cavity in the bone or cartilage. Minute canals in the structure, known as canaliculi, connect concentric sheets of lamella Figure 5-46 ▼.

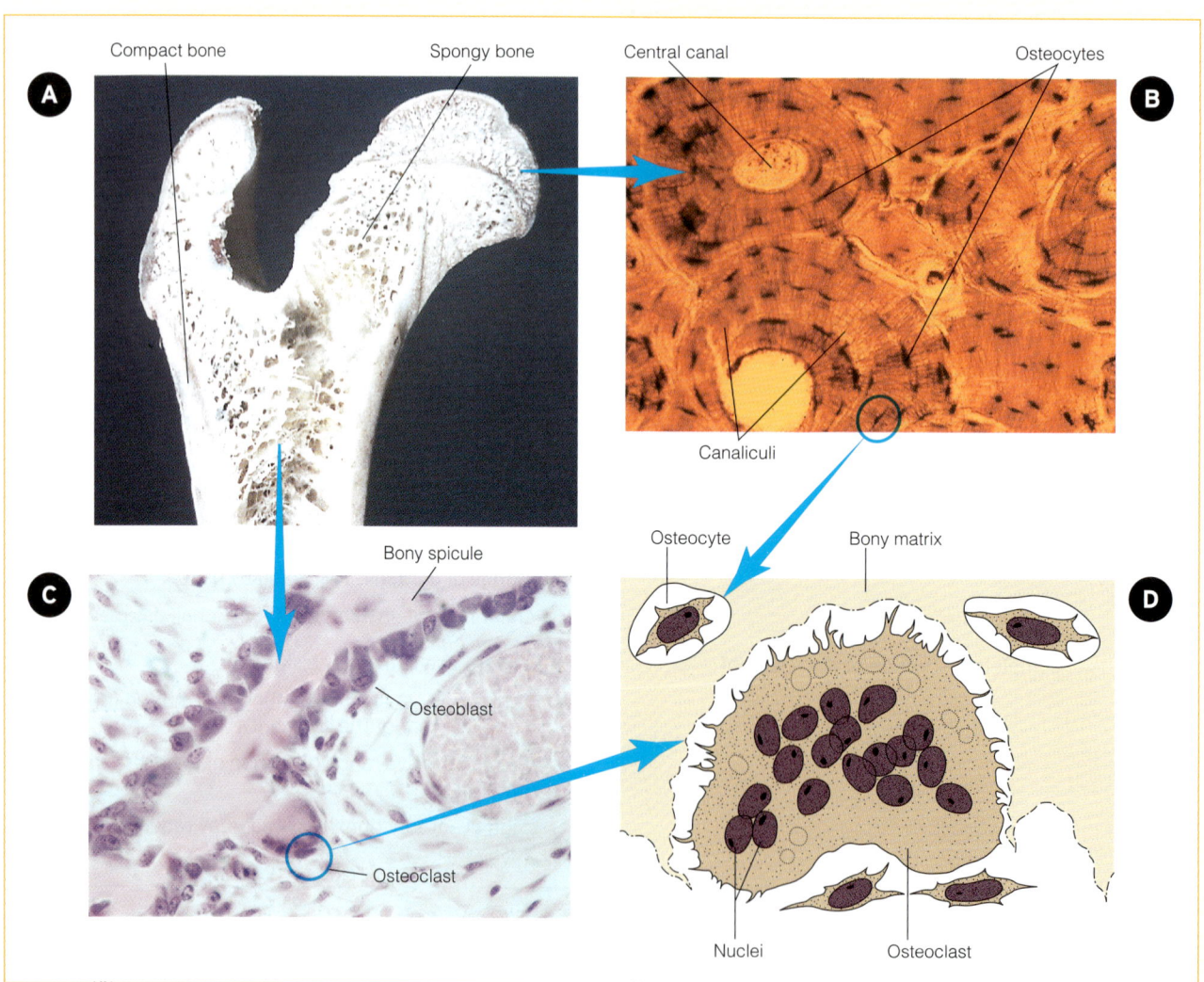

Figure 5-46 Bone. **A.** Compact and spongy bone of the humerus. **B.** Light micrograph of the lamella (concentric circles) showing the osteocytes and canaliculi. **C.** Photomicrograph of spongy bone showing osteoblasts and osteoclasts. **D.** An osteoclast digesting the surface of a bony spicule (sharp body or spike).

Bones are classified according to their shape . Long bones are longer than they are wide and include most bones of the upper and lower extremities, including the femur, tibia, fibula, ulna, radius, and humerus. Short bones are approximately as broad as they are long and often are cube-shaped or round, as exemplified by the bones of the wrist or of the ankle. Flat bones are relatively thin and flattened and include certain skull bones, ribs, the sternum (breastbone), and the scapulae (shoulder blades).

Long bones consist of a shaft, the diaphysis; the ends, or epiphyses; and the growth plate or epiphyseal plate (the physis), which is the major site of bone elongation . The epiphyseal plate is located just proximal to the epiphysis. The metaphysis is the region where the diaphysis and epiphyses converge. The periosteum, which consists of a double layer of connective tissue, lines the outer surface of the bone, and the inner surfaces are lined with endosteum.

The diaphysis of many bones includes the medullary cavity, an internal cavity that contains a substance known as bone marrow. In adults, most bone marrow in the long bones in the extremities contains adipose (fat) tissue and is, therefore, called yellow marrow. The bones of the axial skeleton and girdles contain red marrow, where most red blood cells are manufactured.

EMT-I Tips

Dysfunction or suppression of the bone marrow may develop in individuals who have adverse reactions to certain drugs, such as nonsteroidal anti-inflammatory drugs (NSAIDs), or who receive chemotherapy treatments for cancer. Use of chemotherapy and NSAIDs can result in anemia caused by a decrease in the number of red blood cells produced by the marrow, increased susceptibility to infection caused by a decrease in the number of infection-fighting white blood cells, and a tendency for internal or external bleeding caused by a decrease in the number of platelets (blood-clotting cells).

Geriatric Needs

Fractures are more common in older individuals because of a decrease in bone mineral density. The result is weaker bones.

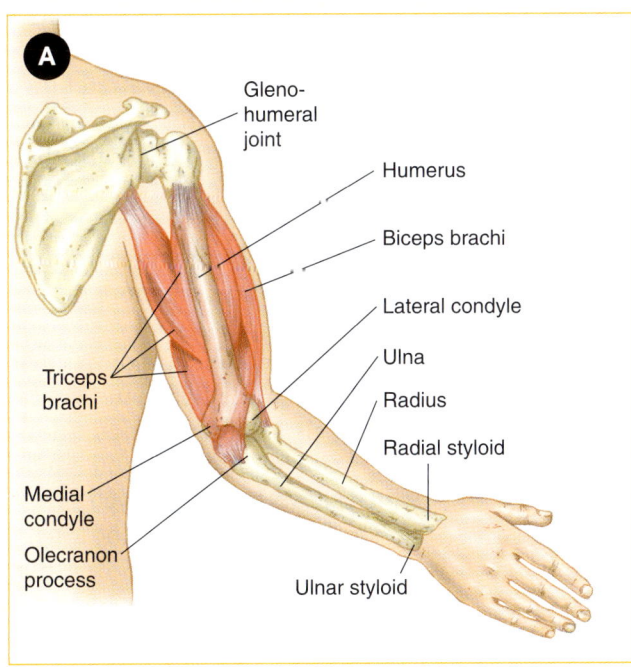

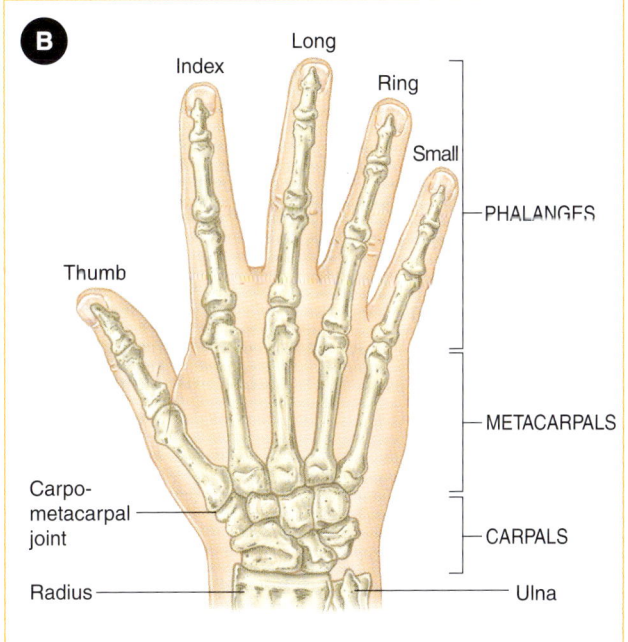

Figure 5-47 Bones are classified according to their shape. **A.** The scapula is a flat bone, and the humerus, ulna, and radius are long bones. **B.** The carpals, or wrist bones, are short bones.

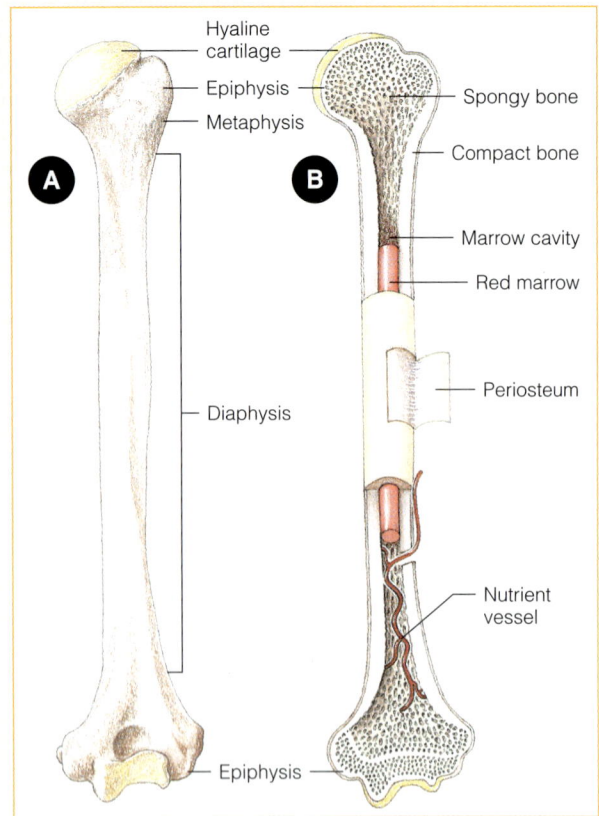

Figure 5-48 The components of the long bone. **A.** Drawing of the humerus. Notice the long shaft and dilated ends. **B.** Longitudinal section of the humerus showing compact bone, spongy bone, and marrow.

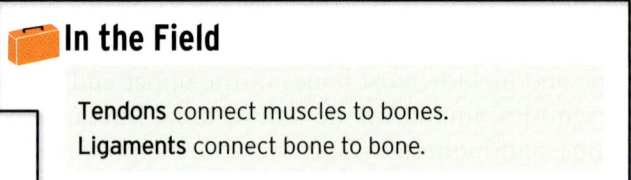

In the Field

Tendons connect muscles to bones.
Ligaments connect bone to bone.

Joints

Wherever two bones come in contact, a joint (articulation) is formed. A joint consists of the ends of the bones that make up the joint and the surrounding connecting and supporting tissue Figure 5-50 . Most joints in the body are named by combining the names of the two bones that form that joint. For example, the sternoclavicular joint is the formation between the sternum and the clavicle. Most joints allow motion—for example, the knee, hip, or elbow—whereas some bones fuse with one another at joints to form a solid, immobile, bony structure. For instance, the skull is composed of several bones that fuse as a child grows. An infant, whose skull bones are not yet fused, has fontanels (soft spots) between the bones. The fontanels close as the bones fuse together, usually by the time the infant reaches the age of two years. Some joints have slight, limited motion in which the bone ends are held together by fibrous tissue. Such a joint is called a symphysis.

A fibrous sac with a synovial lining, called the joint capsule, holds the bone ends of a joint together. At certain points around the circumference of the joint, the capsule is lax and thin so that motion can occur. In other areas, it is quite thick and resists stretching or bending. These bands of tough, thick tissue are called ligaments. A joint such as the sacroiliac joint that is virtually surrounded by tough, thick ligaments will have little motion, whereas a joint such as the shoulder, with few ligaments, will be free to move in almost any direction (and will, as a result, be more prone to dislocation).

The degree of freedom of motion of a joint is determined by the extent to which the ligaments hold the bone ends together and also by the configuration of the bone ends themselves. The shoulder joint is a ball-and-socket joint, which allows rotation as well as bending Figure 5-51 . The finger joints and the knee are hinge joints, with motion restricted to one plane Figure 5-52 . They can only flex (bend) and extend (straighten). Rotation is not possible because of the shape of the joint surfaces and the strong restraining ligaments on both sides of the joint. Thus, although the amount of motion varies from joint to joint, all joints have a definite limit beyond which motion cannot

The two main types of bone are compact bone and cancellous bone. Compact bone is mostly solid, with few spaces; cancellous bone consists of a lacy network of bony rods called trabeculae. The trabeculae are oriented along the lines of stress to increase the weight-bearing capacity of the long bones.

Blood vessels typically do not penetrate trabeculae. Thus, cancellous bone receives its nutrients via canaliculi. However, blood vessels do directly penetrate compact bone. The lamellae are oriented around these blood vessels in units called osteons or haversian systems. The blood vessels of the haversian canals are interconnected by a series of vessels called perforating canals Figure 5-49 .

Bones grow in two ways: appositional growth, the formation of new bone on the surface of a bone, or endochondral growth, the growth of cartilage in the epiphyseal plate and its eventual replacement by bone. As an individual grows, old bone is removed by osteoclasts and new bone is deposited by osteoblasts, resulting in changes in the bone's shape, a process known as bone remodeling.

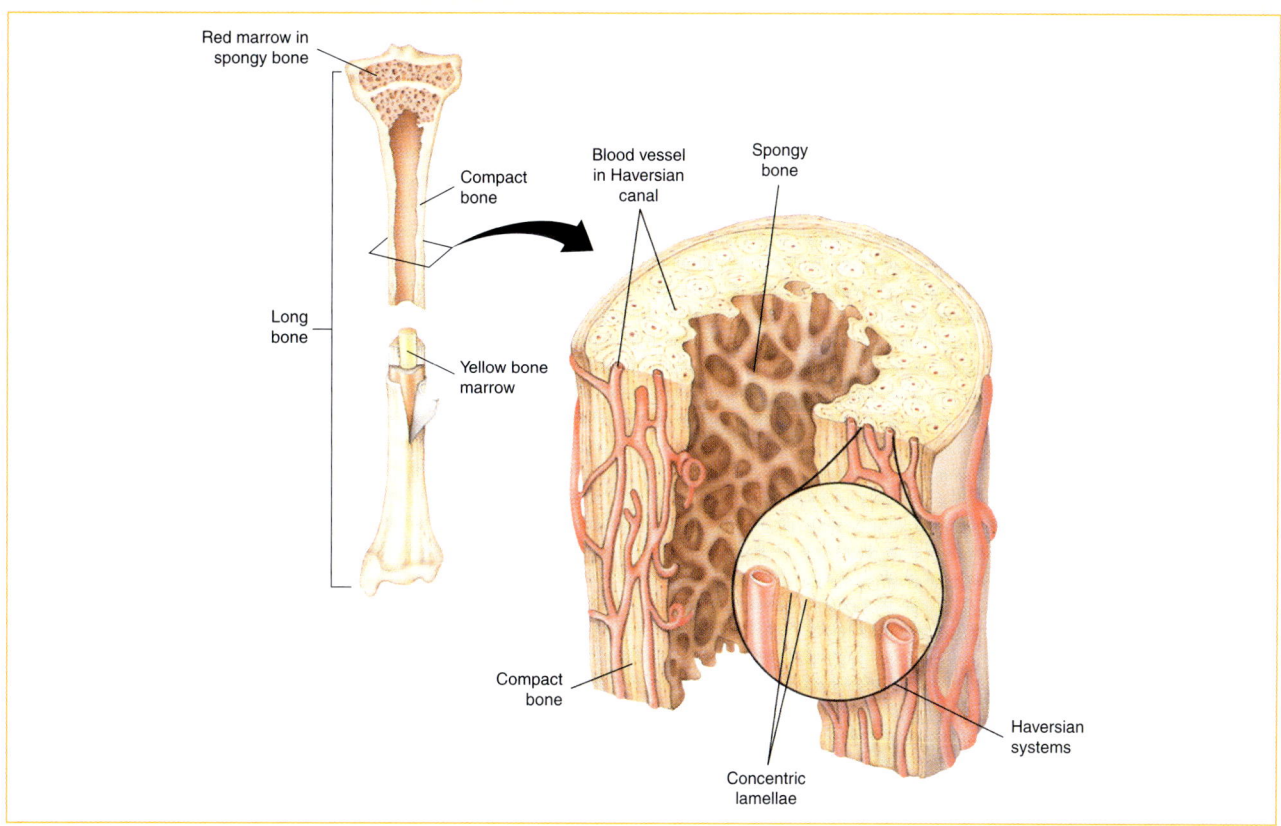

Figure 5-49 The shaft of the bone, shown at three levels of detail. The shaft is dense and compact, giving the bone strength. The ends of the bone and lining of the cavity within the long bone are spongy, with more open lattice areas. Blood cells are formed within red bone marrow that fills the lattice at the ends of the bone. Inset shows a magnified haversian system with its concentric lamellae. Yellow bone marrow fills the cavity in the shaft of the long bone.

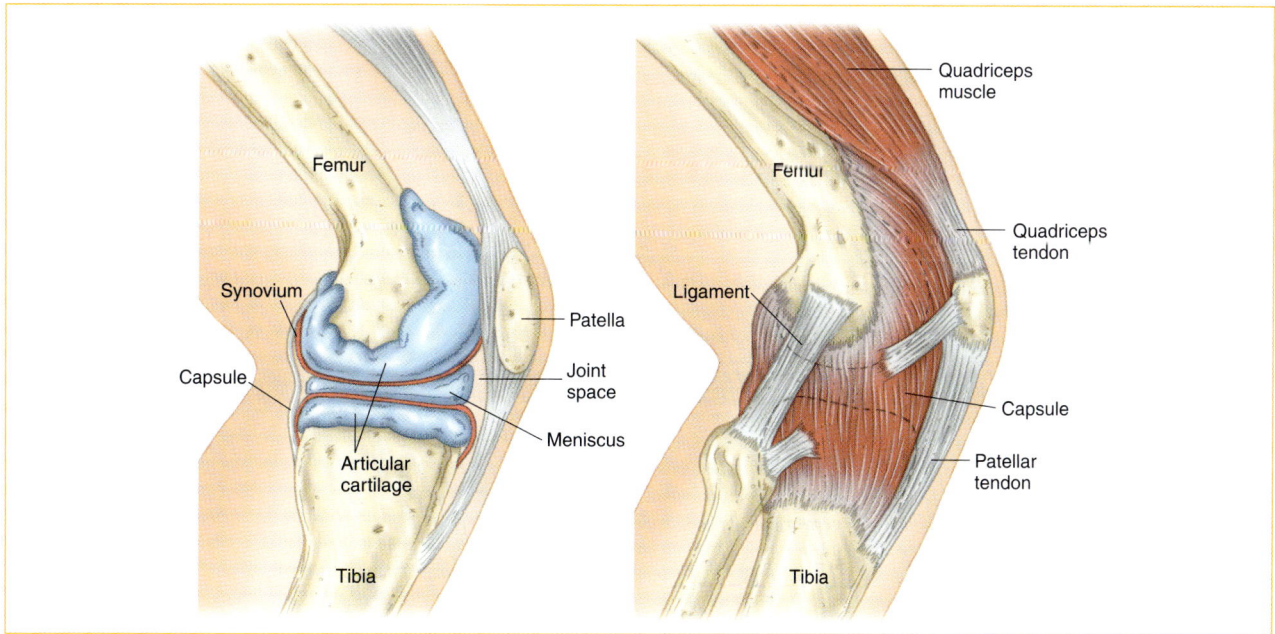

Figure 5-50 A joint consists of bone ends, the fibrous joint capsule, and ligaments. The directions and degree to which a joint can move are determined by how the ligaments hold the bone ends and by the configuration of the bones themselves.

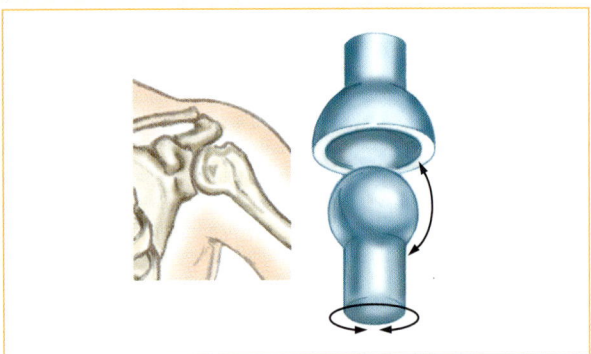

Figure 5-51 The shoulder is a ball-and-socket joint.

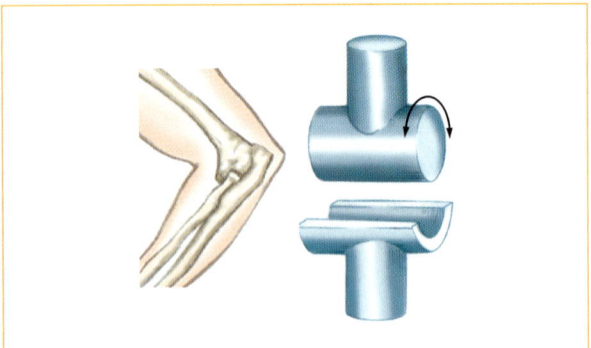

Figure 5-52 The elbow joints are hinge joints, which allow motion in only one plane.

occur. When a joint is forced beyond this limit, damage to some structure will occur. Either the bones that form the joint will break, or the supporting capsule and ligaments will be disrupted.

The Musculoskeletal System

The human body is a well-designed system whose form, upright posture, and movement are provided by the <u>musculoskeletal system</u>. As its combination form suggests, the term musculoskeletal refers to the bones and voluntary muscles of the body. The musculoskeletal system also protects the vital internal organs of the body. Muscles are a form of tissue that allows body movement. Although there are more than 600 muscles in the musculoskeletal system, they are generally divided into three types: skeletal, smooth, and cardiac (Figure 5-53 ▶).

Skeletal Muscle

<u>Skeletal muscle</u>, so named because it attaches to the bones of the skeleton, forms the major muscle mass of the body. It is also called <u>voluntary muscle</u>, because all skeletal muscle is under direct voluntary control of the brain and can be stimulated to contract or relax at will. Skeletal muscle is also called <u>striated muscle</u>, because

You are the Provider   Part 6

Your third victim is the elderly driver of the passenger vehicle. He was unrestrained and is complaining of severe pain in his right hip and leg. You suspect that his knee hit the dashboard during the collision. You note the following:

Initial Assessment	Recording Time: Zero Minutes
Appearance	In severe pain
Level of consciousness	Conscious and alert
Airway	Open and clear
Breathing	Increased respiratory rate, adequate depth
Circulation	Skin, warm and dry to touch; radial pulse present

9. What are the bones of the lower extremity?
10. What are the common causes of hip dislocations that the EMT-I should be aware of?

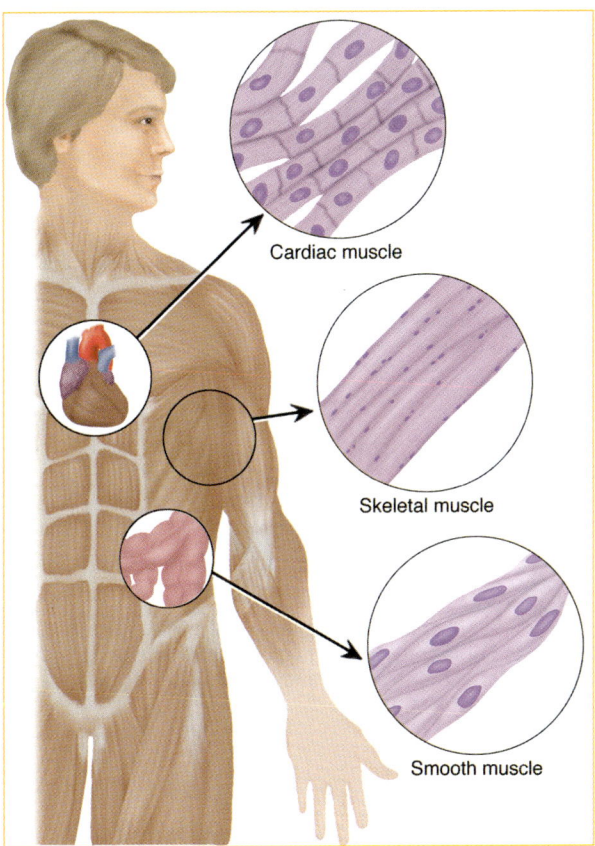

Figure 5-53 The three types of muscle are skeletal, smooth, and cardiac.

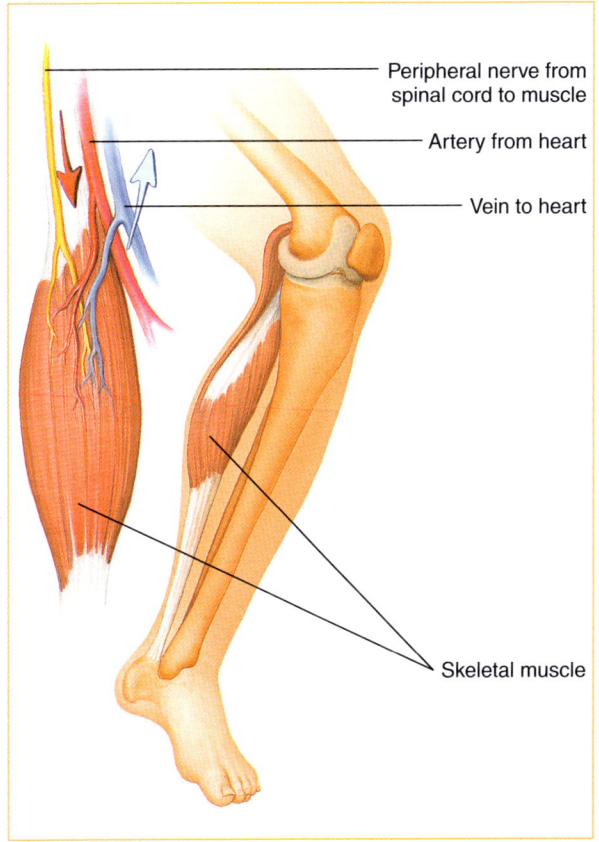

Figure 5-54 All skeletal muscles are supplied with arteries, veins, and nerves.

when viewed under the microscope, it has characteristic stripes (striations). All body movement results from skeletal muscle contraction or relaxation. Usually, a specific motion is the result of several muscles contracting and relaxing simultaneously.

All skeletal muscles are supplied with arteries, veins, and nerves Figure 5-54 . Arterial blood brings oxygen and nutrients to the muscle, and the veins carry away the waste products of muscular contraction (carbon dioxide and water). Muscles cannot function without this ongoing supply of oxygen and nutrients and removal of waste products. Muscle cramps result when insufficient oxygen or food is carried to the muscle or when acidic waste products accumulate and are not carried away.

Skeletal muscle is under the direct control of the nervous system and responds to a command from the brain to move a specific body part. Specific nerves pass directly from the brain to the spinal cord. There, they connect with other nerves that exit from the spinal cord and pass to each skeletal muscle. Electrical impulses are carried from the cells in the brain and spinal cord along the peripheral nerves to each muscle, signaling it to contract. When this normal nerve supply is lost through injury to the brain, spinal cord, or peripheral nerves, the voluntary control of the muscle is lost, and the muscle becomes paralyzed.

Most skeletal muscles attach directly to bone by tough, ropelike cords of fibrous tissue called tendons, which continue the fascia that covers all skeletal muscles. The fascia is much like the skin of a sausage in that it encases the muscle tissue. At either end of the muscle, the fascia extends beyond the muscle to attach to a bone. This musculotendinous unit crosses a joint and is responsible for the motion of that joint. The proximal point of attachment of the musculotendinous unit is its origin, and the distal bony attachment is called the insertion of the muscle. When a muscle contracts, a line of force is created between the origin and the insertion, which pulls the points of origin and insertion closer together Figure 5-55 . This motion occurs at the joint between the two bones.

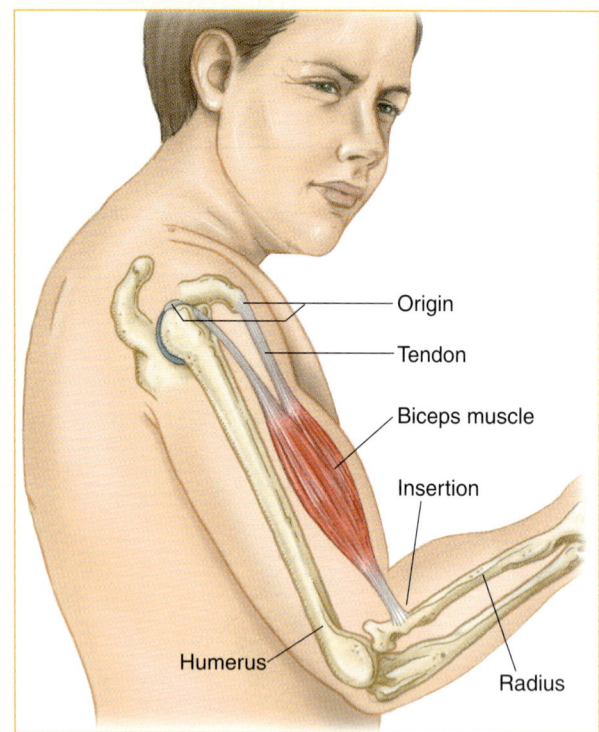

Figure 5-55 The biceps muscle causes the elbow to bend when it contracts. Note the points of tendon origin and insertion. As the muscle contracts and shortens, these points are pulled closer together, with motion occurring at the elbow joint.

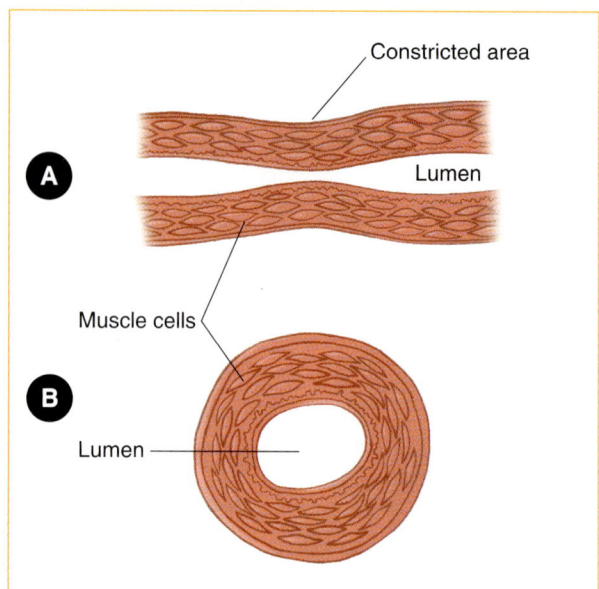

Figure 5-56 A. Smooth muscle lines the walls of the tubular structures of the body. **B.** Contraction of the muscles narrows the diameter of the structure, and relaxation allows the diameter to increase in size.

Smooth Muscle

Smooth muscle carries out much of the automatic work of the body; therefore, it is also called involuntary muscle. Smooth muscle is found in the walls of most tubular structures of the body, such as the gastrointestinal tract, the urinary system, the blood vessels, and the bronchi of the lungs. Contraction and relaxation of smooth muscle propel or control the flow of the contents of these structures along their course. For example, the rhythmic contraction and relaxation of the smooth muscles of the wall of the intestine propel ingested food through it, and smooth muscle in the walls of a blood vessel can alter the diameter of the vessel to control the amount of blood flowing through it Figure 5-56.

Smooth muscle responds only to primitive stimuli such as stretching, heat, or the need to relieve waste. An individual cannot exert any voluntary control over this type of muscle.

Cardiac Muscle

The heart is a large muscle composed of a pair of pumps of unequal force: one of lower pressure and one of higher pressure. The heart must function continuously from birth to death. It is a specially adapted involuntary muscle with a very rich blood supply and its own electrical system, which makes it different from both skeletal and smooth muscle. Another difference is that cardiac muscle has the property of "automaticity," which means that the heart muscle can generate and conduct electricity without influence from the brain. This property is unique to heart muscle. Cardiac muscle can tolerate an interruption of its blood supply for only a few seconds. It requires a continuous supply of oxygen and glucose for normal function. Because of its special structure and function, cardiac muscle is placed in a separate category.

The Nervous System

The nervous system is a complex array of structures that help control both voluntary and involuntary body functions. The central nervous system, the peripheral nervous system, and the autonomic nervous system comprise the major divisions of the nervous system. Together, these divisions integrate information throughout the entire body, allowing normal function.

The nervous system is composed of specialized tissue that conducts electrical impulses between the brain and the rest of the body. Neural tissue contains two basic types of cells: nerve cells, which are known as neurons and contain projections called axons and dendrites that make connections between adjacent cells (see Figure 5-12), and neuroglia, which are supporting cells that have five basic functions. Neuroglia provide a supporting skeleton for neural tissue, isolate and protect the cell membranes of neurons, regulate the composition of interstitial fluid, defend neural tissue from pathogens, and aid in the repair of injury.

Between the nerve cells lies a gap called the **synapse**, which consists of a terminal bouton or other type of axon terminal, the synaptic cleft, and the membrane of the postsynaptic cell. The **presynaptic terminal** is at one end of a nerve. The **synaptic cleft** is the space between neurons. Opposite of the presynaptic terminal, across the synaptic cleft, is the **postsynaptic terminal**. Electrical impulses travel down the nerve and trigger the release of chemicals known as **neurotransmitters** from the presynaptic terminal. These neurotransmitters cross the synaptic cleft to stimulate an electrical reaction in adjacent neurons. Neurotransmitters are contained within **synaptic vesicles** and are released into the synaptic cleft at the presynaptic terminal. This electrical reaction passes through the neuron to the next synapse, and the process is repeated **Figure 5-57 ▼**.

Groups of nerve cells are bundled together to form **nerve fibers**. Groups of nerve fibers are bundled together to form a **nerve**, which is tissue that connects the nervous system with body parts or organs. The nervous system is divided into the central nervous system (CNS), the peripheral nervous system (PNS), and the autonomic nervous system (ANS). The CNS is composed of the brain and spinal cord. The CNS includes the 12 pairs of cranial nerves that branch directly from the brain. The 31 pairs of spinal nerves that exit the spinal cord via the vertebral column are part of the PNS. The ANS is responsible for the "fight-or-flight" response, when the body is in a state of conflict or threat. It also is responsible for the "feed-or-breed" response, which is when the body is in a relaxed state. Autonomic functions are not under conscious control and include such activities as maintaining heart rate and blood pressure, intestinal motility, and pupillary response.

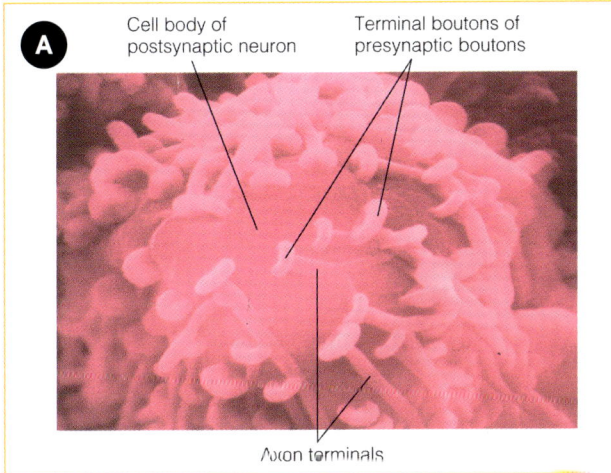

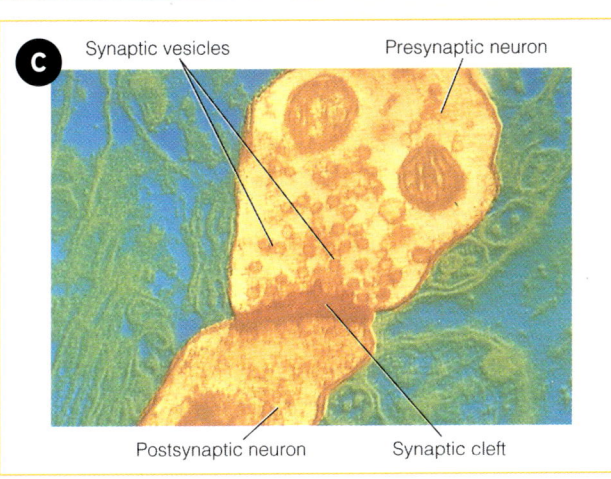

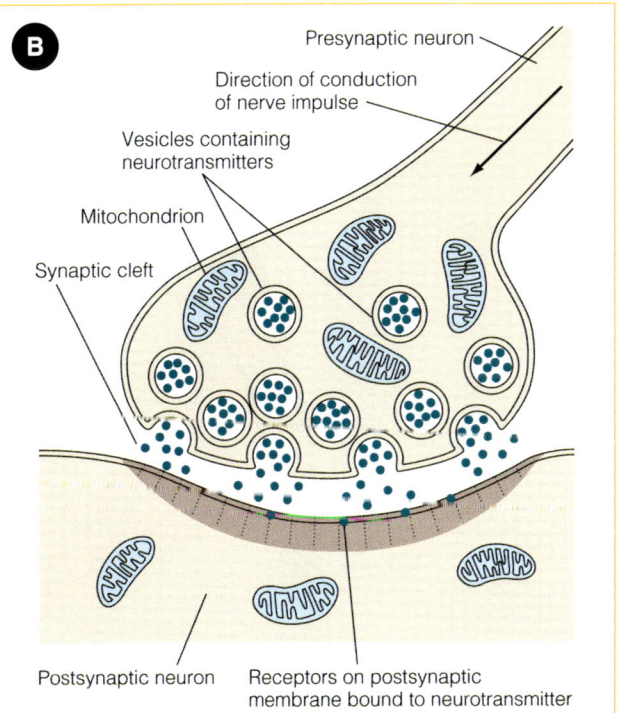

Figure 5-57 The function of neurotransmitters in the synaptic cleft. **A.** A scanning electron micrograph showing the terminal boutons of an axon ending on the cell body of another neuron. **B.** The arrival of the impulse stimulates the release of neurotransmitters held in synaptic vesicles in the axon terminals. Neurotransmitter diffuses across the synaptic cleft and binds to the postsynaptic membrane, where it elicits another action potential that travels down the dendrite to the cell body. **C.** A transmission electron micrograph showing the details of the synapse.

The Central Nervous System

The central nervous system (CNS) consists of the brain and the spinal cord, both of which are encased in and protected by bone. The brain is located within the cranial cavity and contains billions of neurons that serve a variety of vital functions. The major regions of the adult's brain are the cerebrum, diencephalon (thalamus and hypothalamus), mesencephalon (midbrain), pons, cerebellum, and medulla oblongata. The medulla oblongata often is just called the medulla. Collectively, the midbrain, pons, and medulla are referred to as the brainstem Figure 5-58. The largest portion of the brain is the cerebral cortex or cerebrum Figure 5-59.

The cerebrum controls higher thought processes and is divided into right and left hemispheres, or halves, by a longitudinal fissure. Numerous folds, called gyri, greatly increase the surface area of the cortex. Between the gyri are grooves called sulci.

Within each hemisphere are subdivisions known as lobes. Each lobe is named for the bone of the skull that overlies it. The frontal lobe is important in voluntary motor action, as well as personality traits. The parietal lobe is the site for reception and evaluation of some sensory information, excluding smell, hearing, and vision, and is separated from the frontal lobe by the central sulcus. Posteriorly, the occipital lobe is responsible for the processing of visual information. The temporal lobe plays an important role in hearing and memory and is separated from the rest of the cerebrum by a lateral fissure. The functions of various areas of the cerebral cortex differ by location.

> **EMT-I Tips**
>
> A lesion of the substantia nigra, a layer of gray matter in the midbrain that helps produce dopamine, is believed to be responsible for Parkinson's disease, a disorder resulting in tremor and decreased coordination.

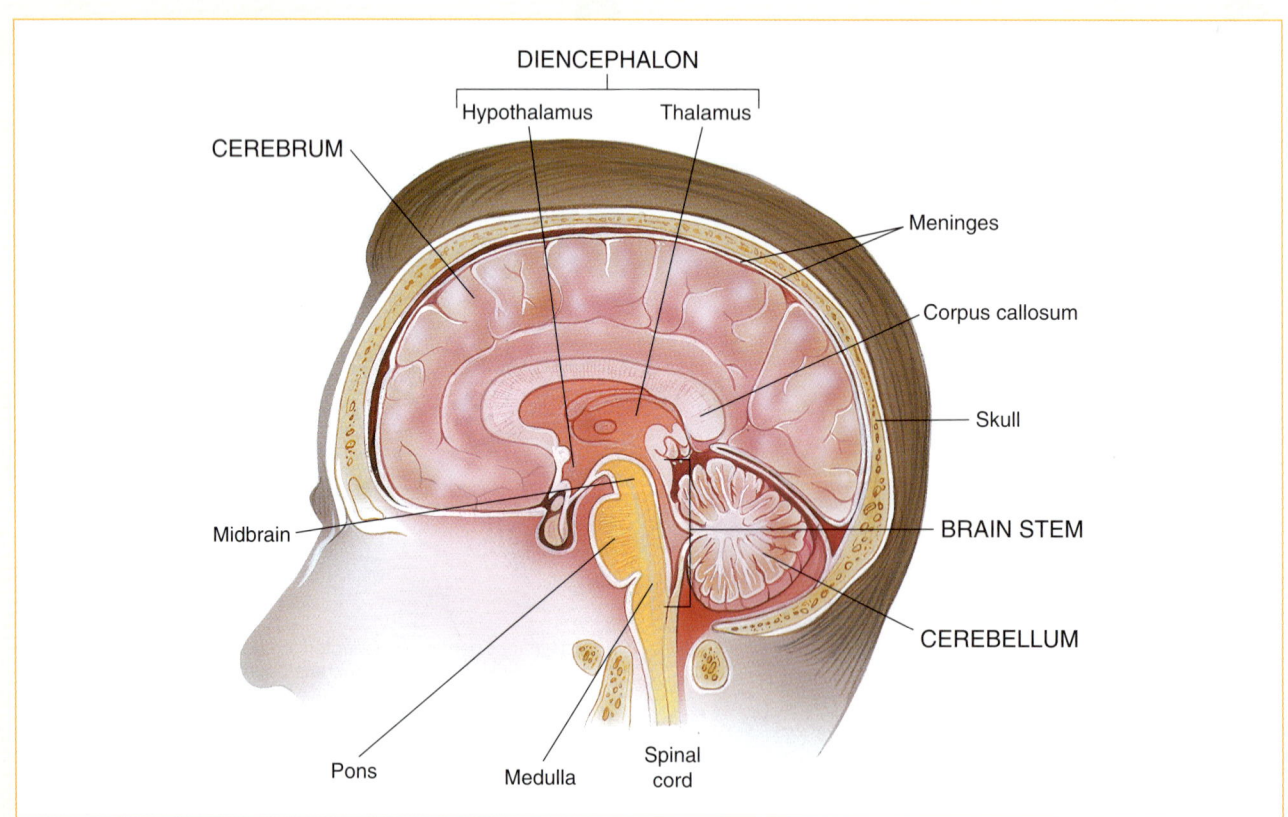

Figure 5-58 The major regions of the central nervous system.

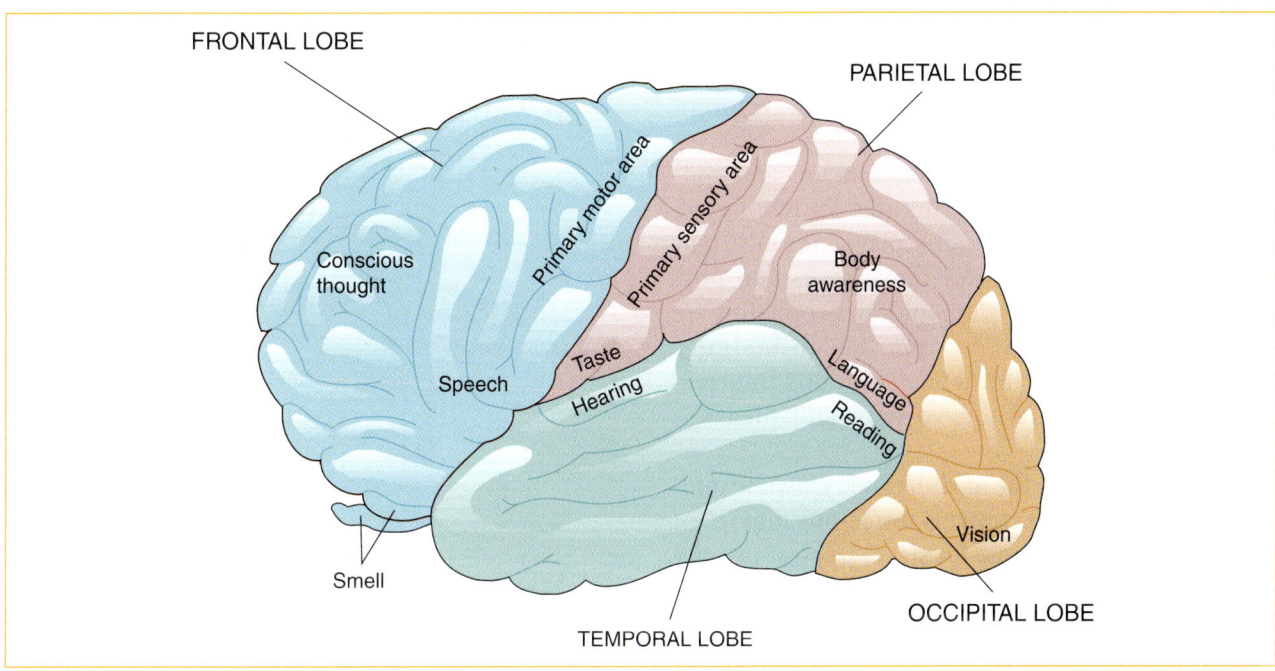

Figure 5-59 The cerebral cortex.

> **EMT-I Tips**
>
> In the brainstem, most nerves cross from one side to the other. Motor and sensory nerves on the left side of the brain, for example, serve the right side of the body. This is why an individual who has had a stroke or trauma in one hemisphere has nerve deficits on the opposite side of the body. Because the cranial nerves are above this crossover point, their function will be affected on the same side of the face as the injury or stroke.

The Diencephalon

The diencephalon is located between the brain stem and the cerebrum and includes the thalamus, subthalamus, hypothalamus, and epithalamus Figure 5-60 ▶. The thalamus processes most sensory input and influences mood and general body movements, especially those associated with fear or rage. The subthalamus is involved in controlling motor functions. The functions of the epithalamus, especially the pineal body, are unclear. The most inferior portion of the diencephalon is the hypothalamus. This organ is vital in the control of many body functions, including heart rate, digestion, sexual development, temperature regulation, emotion, hunger, thirst, and regulation of the sleep cycle.

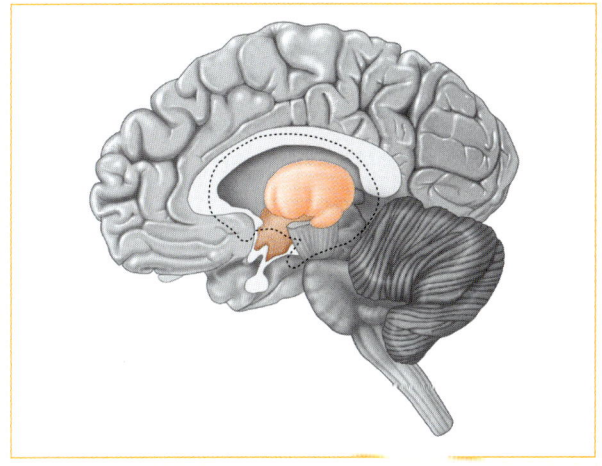

Figure 5-60 The diencephalon.

The Brainstem

The brainstem connects the spinal cord to the rest of the brain. The brainstem consists of the medulla, pons, and midbrain. It is vital for many very basic body functions. Damage to portions of the brainstem can easily result in death. All but two of the 12 cranial nerves exit from the brainstem. The midbrain lies immediately below the diencephalon and is the smallest region of the brainstem.

Deep within the cerebrum, diencephalon, and midbrain is a set of important structures known as the basal ganglia. The basal ganglia plays an important role in coordination of motor movements and posture. Portions of the cerebrum and diencephalon are referred to as the limbic system, which includes several structures that influence emotions, motivation, mood, and sensations of pain and pleasure Figure 5-61.

The pons lies above the medulla and below the midbrain Figure 5-62. It contains numerous important nerve fibers, including those for sleep, respiration, and the medullary respiratory center.

The inferior portion of the midbrain, the medulla, is continuous inferiorly with the spinal cord (see Figure

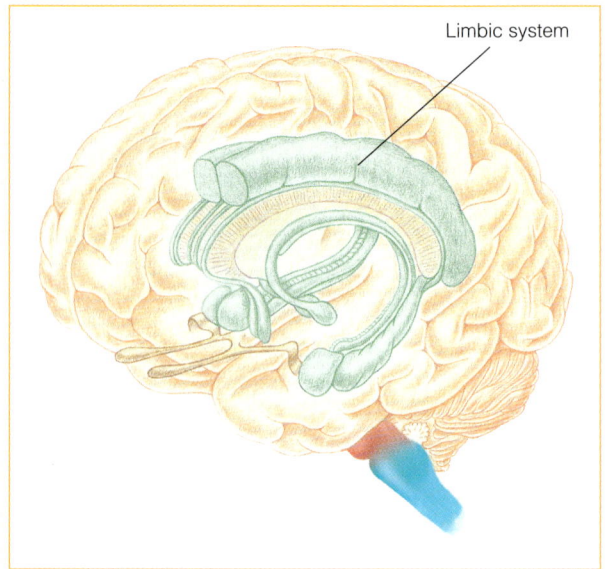

Figure 5-61 The limbic system is the seat of emotions, instincts, and other functions.

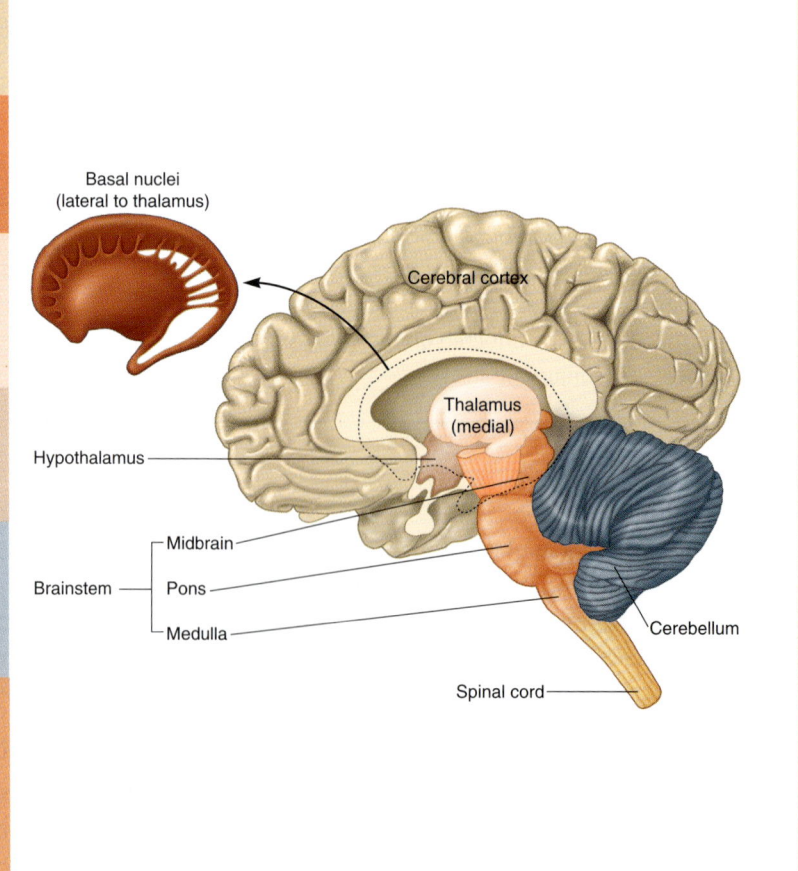

Cerebral cortex
- Receives sensory information from skin, muscles, glands, and organs
- Sends messages to move skeletal muscles
- Integrates incoming and outgoing nerve impulses
- Performs associative activities such as thinking, learning, and remembering

Basal nuclei
- Plays a role in the coordination of slow, sustained movements
- Suppresses useless patterns of movement

Thalamus
- Relays most sensory information from the spinal cord and certain parts of the brain to the cerebral cortex
- Interprets certain sensory messages such as those of pain, temperature, and pressure

Hypothalamus
- Controls various homeostatic functions such as body temperature, respiration, and heartbeat
- Directs hormone secretions of the pituitary

Cerebellum
- Coordinates subconscious movements of skeletal muscles
- Contributes to muscle tone, posture, balance, and equilibrium

Brainstem
- Origin of many cranial nerves
- Reflex center for movements of eyeballs, head, and trunk
- Regulates heartbeat and breathing
- Plays a role in consciousness
- Transmits impulses between brain and spinal cord

Figure 5-62 The pons.

5-58). The medulla is a conduction pathway for both ascending and descending nerve tracts. It also coordinates breathing, heart rate, blood vessel diameter, swallowing, coughing, sneezing, and vomiting. The pons and medullary respiratory center are responsible for all respiratory movements.

Several structures associated with the ascending reticular activating system are located throughout the brainstem. The ascending reticular activating systems is responsible for maintaining consciousness. Therefore, a sharp blow to the back of the neck, as with a karate chop, may result in unconsciousness.

The Cerebellum

The cerebellum communicates with the other regions of the CNS through the cerebellar peduncles, a set of three bands of nerve fibers. The cerebellum is essential in coordinating muscle movements of the body. Normal cerebellar function is necessary for proper balance and movement.

The Meninges

The entire CNS is enclosed by a set of three tough membranes known as the meninges (Figure 5-63 ▼). The outer membrane is the dura mater and is the toughest membrane. The second layer is called the arachnoid because the blood vessels it contains appear like a spider web. The innermost layer, resting directly on the brain or spinal cord, is the pia mater. When a hematoma develops, it can be classified according to its location in respect to the meninges (an epidural or a subdural hematoma). The meninges float in cerebrospinal fluid (CSF), which is manufactured in the ventricles of the brain and flows in the subarachnoid space. The subarachnoid space is located between the pia mater and the arachnoid mater.

CSF is manufactured by specialized cells within the choroid plexus in the ventricles, specialized hollow areas in the brain. These areas normally are interconnected, and CSF flows freely between them. CSF is similar in composition to plasma. The meninges and CSF form a fluid-filled sac that cushions and protects the brain and spinal cord.

> **A to Z** **Terminology Tips**
>
> Remember that the *meninges* are the protective covering of the brain and spinal cord. The suffix *-itis* means inflammation. Therefore, *meningitis* is an inflammation of the covering of the brain and spinal cord.

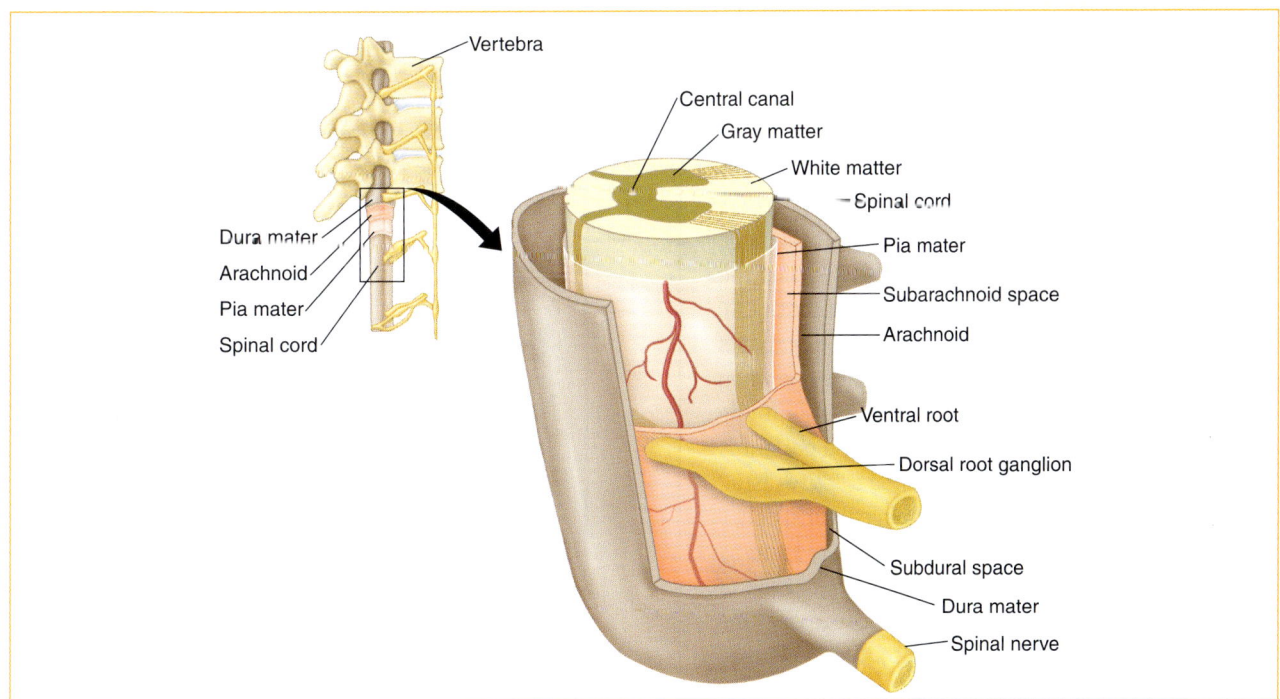

Figure 5-63 Section through the spinal cord. The meninges enclose the brain and the spinal cord.

The Spinal Cord

At the base of the brain, the spinal cord represents the continuation of the central nervous system. The spinal cord is composed of bundles of nerve fibers and leaves the skull through a large opening at the base called the foramen magnum (Figure 5-64 ▶).

The spinal cord extends to the level of the second lumbar vertebra. At this point, it gives rise to numerous individual nerve roots, called the cauda equina. Throughout its length, the spinal cord is encased in the bony vertebral canal formed by the individual vertebrae. Nerves branch off at regular intervals between vertebrae and are numbered according to the level at which they exit the spinal canal. Within the spinal cord are numerous tracts, or pathways, that contain nerve fibers 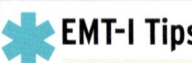.

Ascending fibers (afferent tracts) carry sensory information in the form of action potentials, from the periphery back to the brain. Descending fibers (efferent tracts) carry motor impulses, also in the form of action potentials, from the brain to the fibers of the peripheral nervous system.

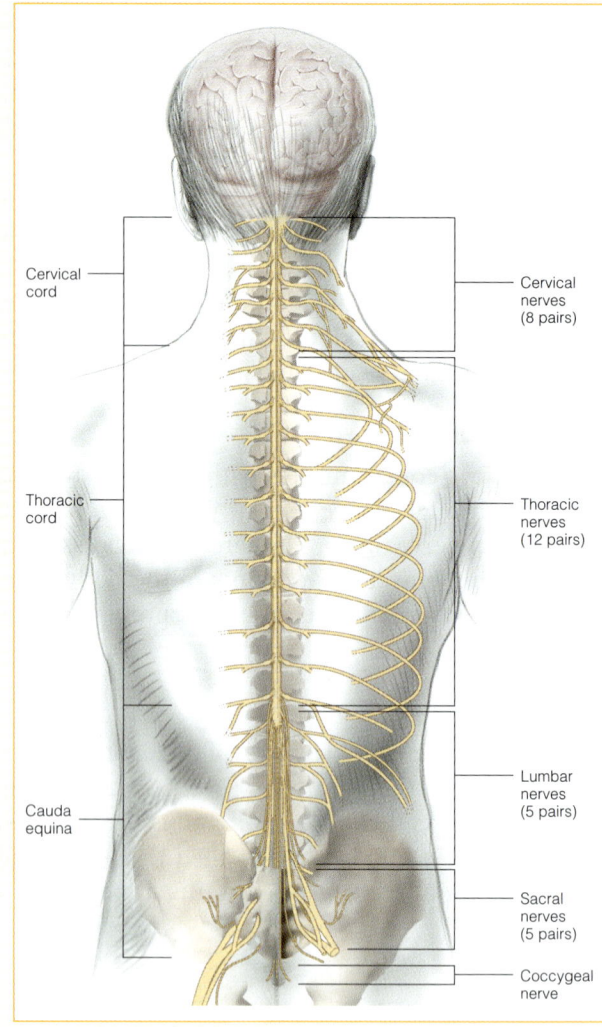

Figure 5-64 The spinal cord.

EMT-I Tips

Bleeding can occur between the meninges and the brain, usually as a result of trauma. The most common type of bleeding occurs with a subarachnoid hemorrhage, in which the blood lies between the arachnoid and the pia mater.

In the Field

In patients with a fracture at the base of the skull, CSF can leak into the eustachian tubes, past the eardrums, and out through the ears. Because CSF does not mix well with blood, it sometimes appears as a halo of clear fluid around drops of blood when it leaks onto a gauze pad. CSF that leaks into the back of a patient's throat because the patient is seated, often is described as having a "salty taste." Ironically, CSF is of the same chemical consistency as seawater, thus accounting for its salty taste.

Perform a halo test to determine leakage of CSF. This is done by placing a 4x4 gauze over the ear. Blood will collect in the center of the piece of gauze. If CSF is present, it will appear as a clear halo of liquid around the blood.

EMT-I Tips

Spinal reflex arcs are automatic reactions to stimuli that occur without conscious thought (Figure 5-66 ▶). For example, the tendon stretch reflex occurs when the patella is tapped gently with a reflex hammer. The lower leg first moves sharply forward, then backward (extends and flexes). The flexor reflex is a withdrawal reflex, which affects the muscles of a limb, as when someone touches a very hot object or other unpleasant stimulus, the hand rapidly withdraws without any conscious action. These reactions are mediated locally within the spinal cord, although impulses from higher centers in the CNS normally regulate reflex activity.

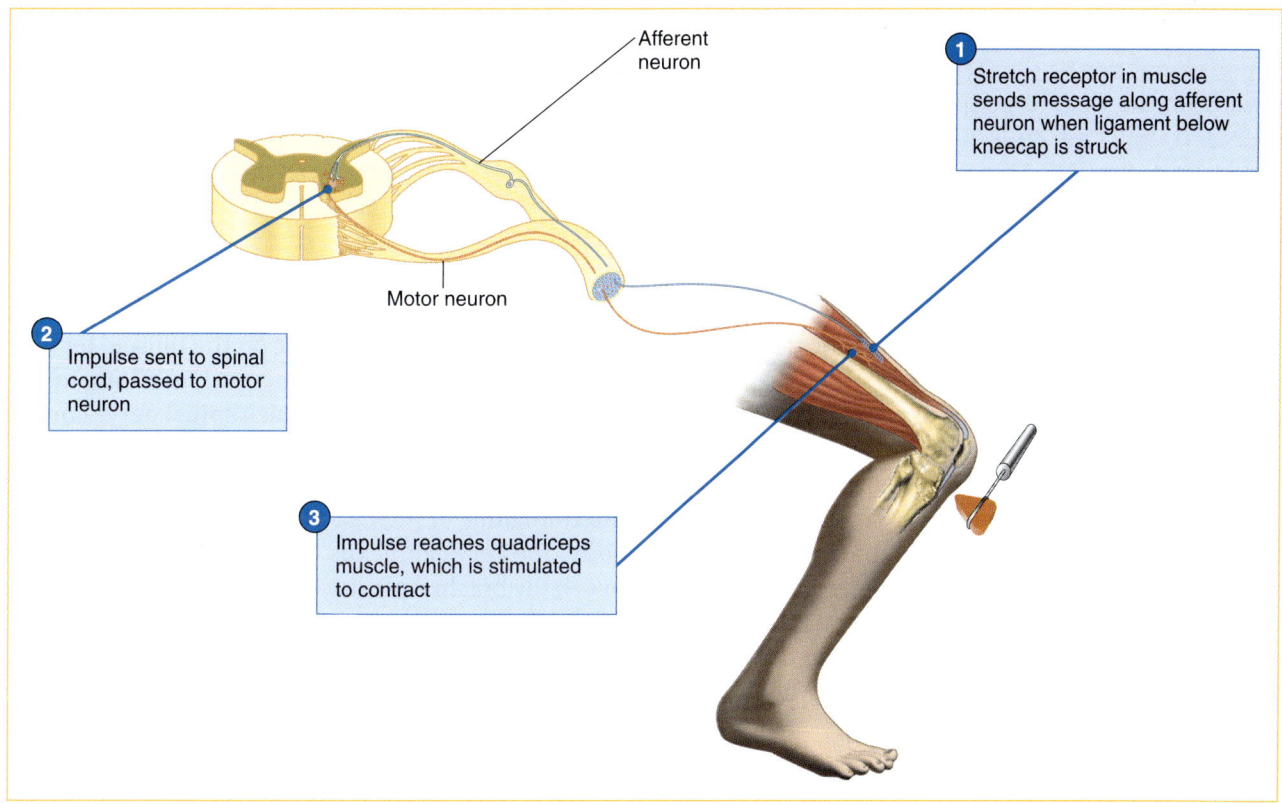

Figure 5-65 The spinal cord nerve tracts.

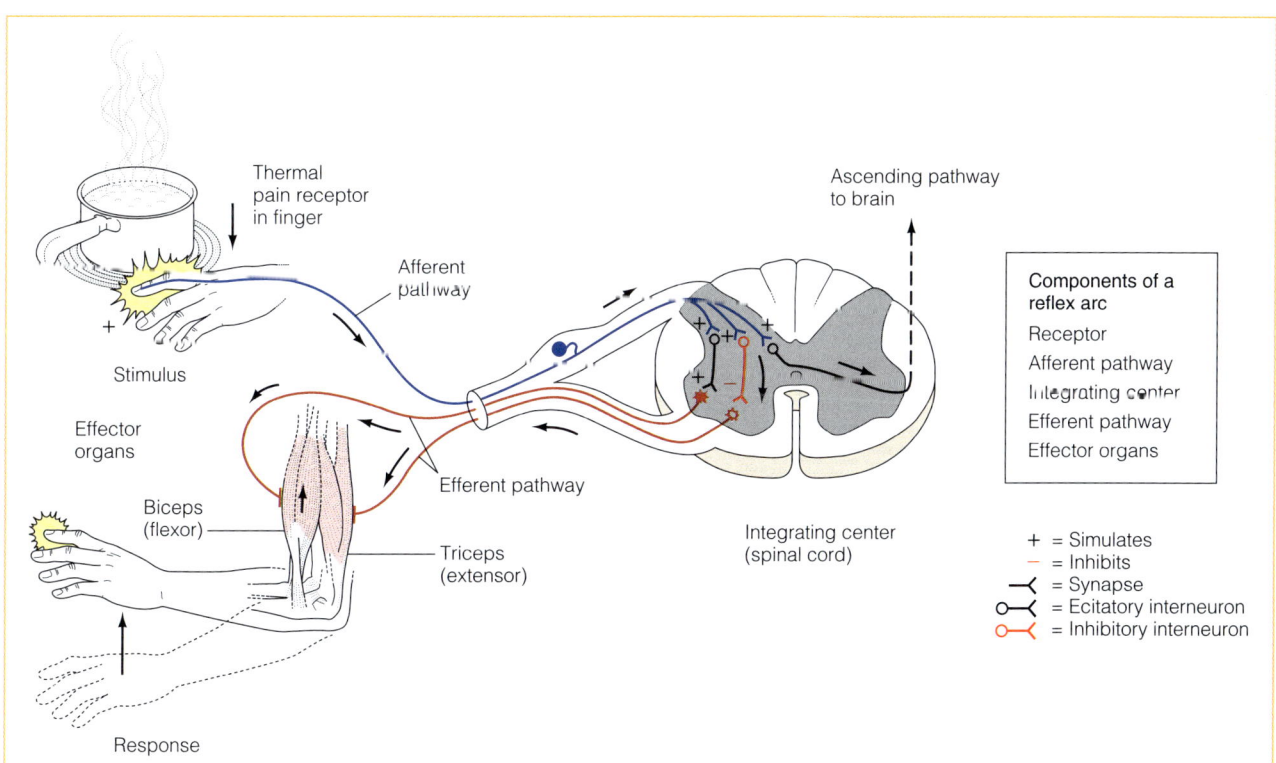

Figure 5-66 Components of a reflex arc.

The Peripheral Nervous System

The peripheral nervous system consists of nerves that extend from the CNS to peripheral structures outside the CNS. Ganglia are collections of nerve cell bodies located outside the CNS. Spinal nerves arise from numerous small nerves called rootlets along the dorsal and ventral surfaces of the spinal cord. Roughly six to eight rootlets combine to form a ventral root; a dorsal root is formed in the same manner by other rootlets. The roots join together to form the spinal nerve. The dorsal root contains the dorsal root ganglion (Figure 5-67 ▼).

With the exception of the first pair of spinal nerves and those in the sacrum, the remaining spinal nerves exit the vertebral column through openings between successive vertebrae, called the intervertebral foramen. There are eight pairs of spinal nerves in the cervical region, twelve in the thoracic region, five in the lumbar region, five in the sacral region, and one in the coccygeal region. Each of these pairs is numbered based on the vertebral level at which it exits the spinal canal (C1, T12).

The peripheral nervous system is made up of two types of nerves: sensory and motor nerves. Sensory nerves, or afferent nerves, carry impulses from the body to the brain and provide input to the brain about sensations that are felt, such as touch, pain, pressure, and temperature. A dermatome is the area of skin supplied by a given pair of spinal sensory nerves. Except for C1, each spinal nerve has a specific sensory distribution on the surface of the body.

Motor nerves, or efferent nerves, carry commands from the brain to the receptor on the muscle for nerve impulses (neuromuscular junction), resulting in muscle contraction and motion. Each spinal nerve contains both afferent and efferent components.

Several nerves come together to form an organized intermingling, or plexus. There are four plexuses in the body: the cervical plexus consists of spinal nerves C1 to C4; the brachial plexus, C5 to T1; the lumbar plexus, L1 to L4; the sacral plexus, L4 to S4. The plexuses give rise to the peripheral nerves, which branch and eventually supply motor function and sensation to many areas of the body.

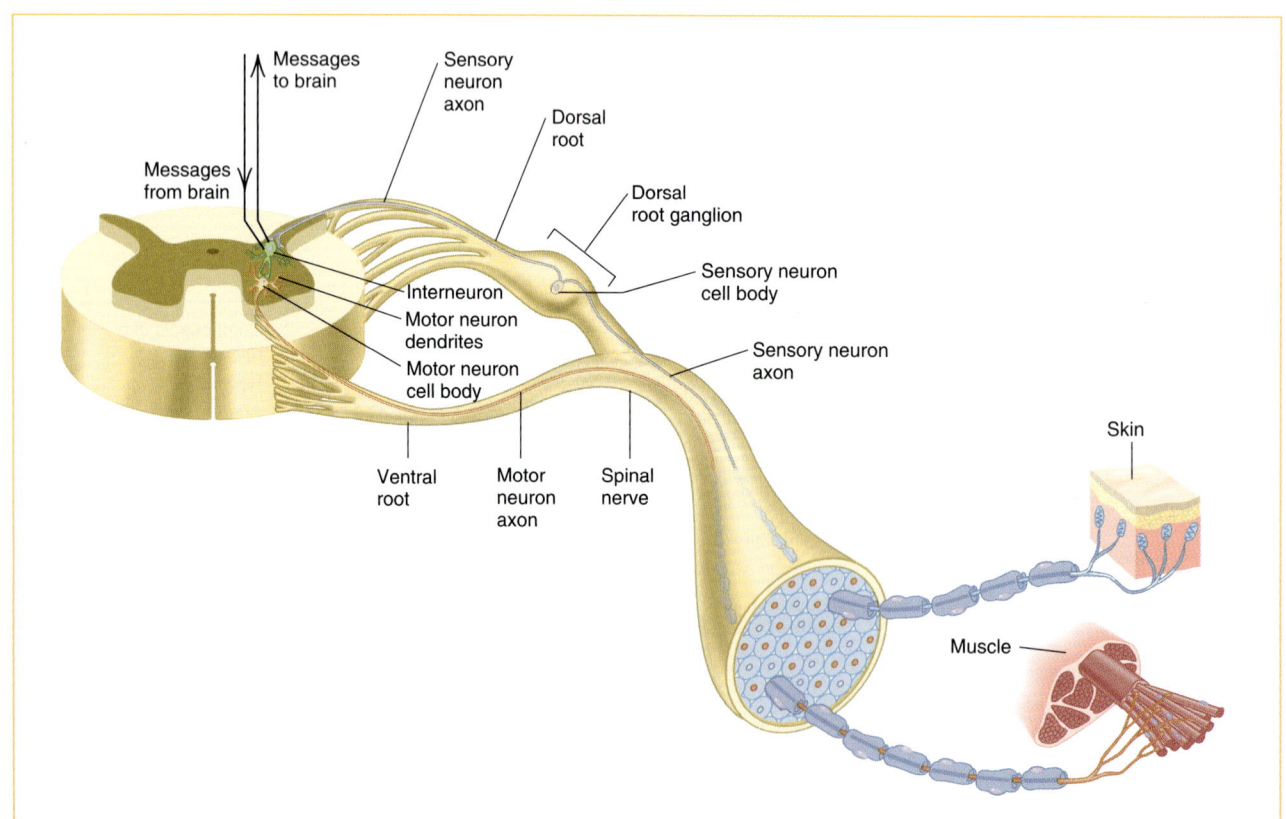

Figure 5-67 The dorsal root ganglion.

> **EMT-I Safety**
>
> CSF is a clear body fluid that can carry the same infectious diseases as blood. The risk of exposure to infectious agents from CSF can be even greater than from blood, because its presence is not as obvious as blood at first sight. To avoid exposure to infectious agents, the EMS provider should always wear gloves when making patient contact.

The Cervical Plexus

The cervical plexus provides innervation to the neck and posterior portion of the head. The most important nerve of the cervical plexus is the phrenic nerve as shown in Figure 5-68. It enters the thorax and innervates the diaphragm. Contraction of the diaphragm occurs during breathing.

The Brachial Plexus

The brachial plexus is divided into rami, trunks, divisions, cords, and branches. Together, the nerves in these divisions innervate the shoulder and upper extremity. The major nerves emanating from the brachial plexus are the axillary, radial, musculocutaneous, ulnar, and median nerves.

The axillary nerve supplies the deltoid and teres minor muscles, enabling arm abduction and lateral rotation. The radial nerve supplies the muscles that extend the elbow (brachioradialis and triceps brachii), supinate the forearm (supinator), and extend the wrist (extensor carpi muscles), fingers (extensor digitorum), and thumb muscles.

The musculocutaneous nerve innervates muscles that flex the shoulder and elbow (coracobrachialis, biceps brachii, and brachialis). The median nerve supplies the pronator muscles of the forearm, as well as those that flex the wrist (flexor carpi muscles and palmaris longus), the fingers (flexor digitorum muscles), and the thumb (flexor pollicis longus). The ulnar nerve innervates muscles that flex the wrist (flexor carpi ulnaris) and fingers (flexor digitorum muscles) and abduct and adduct the fingers and thumb (interossei, adductor pollicis, and the abductor pollicis).

In terms of sensory distribution, the axillary nerve innervates a small patch of skin on the lateral border of the proximal arm. The radial nerve provides sensation to the posterior arm and forearm as well as to the lateral two thirds of the dorsum of the hand. The musculocutaneous nerve provides sensation to the lateral surface of the forearm, and the ulnar nerve provides sensation to the medial one third of the hand, the little finger, and the medial one half of the ring finger. The median nerve provides sensation to the lateral two thirds of the palm of the hand, including the lateral half of the ring finger Figure 5-69.

The Lumbosacral Plexus

Four major nerves exit the lumbosacral plexus and supply the lower extremity: the obturator, femoral, tibial, and common peroneal nerves. Other nerves supply the lower back, hip, and lower abdomen.

The obturator nerve innervates muscles that adduct the thigh (adductor muscles and the gracilis) and rotate it laterally (obturator externus). The femoral nerve innervates the muscles that flex the hip (psoas major and

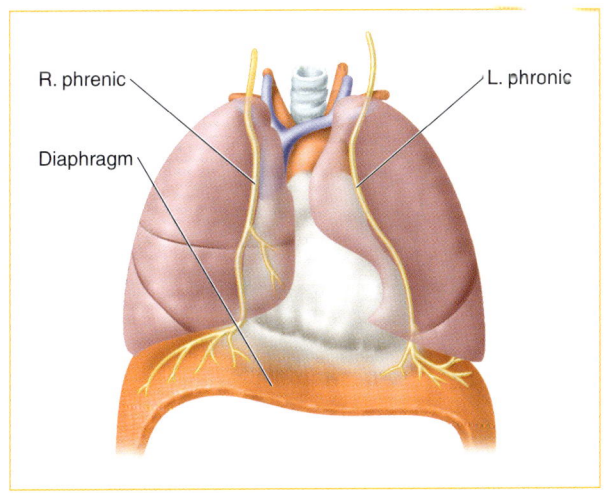

Figure 5-68   The phrenic nerve.

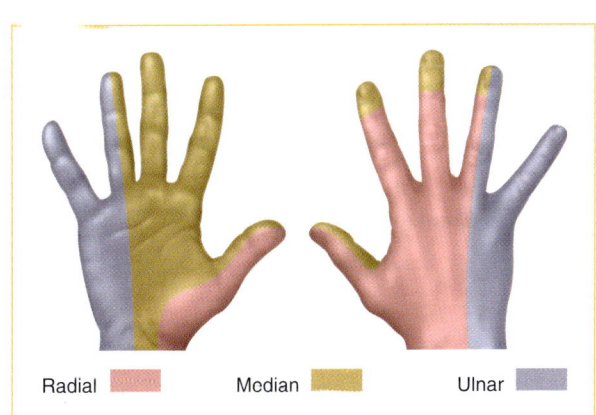

Figure 5-69   The nerves of the hand.

sartorius) and extend the knee (rectus femoris and the vastus muscles). The tibial nerve innervates muscles that extend the hip and flex the knee (biceps femoris, semitendinosus, semimembranosus, and popliteus), plantar flex the ankle (gastrocnemius, soleus, plantaris, and tibialis posterior), and flex the toes (flexor muscles).

The common peroneal branch of the sciatic nerve innervates the short head of the biceps femoris muscle, causing extension of the hip and flexion of the knee. Along with the tibial nerve, the common peroneal nerve travels within a connective tissue sheath for the length of the thigh. Combined, these two nerves often are called the sciatic nerve. The sciatic nerve is the largest peripheral nerve in the body Figure 5-70 .

After wrapping around the neck of the fibula below the knee joint, the common peroneal nerve branches into the deep peroneal nerve and the superficial peroneal nerve. The deep branch innervates muscles that dorsiflex the ankle (tibialis anterior) and extend the toes (extensor muscles). The superficial branch stimulates the muscles of plantar foot eversion (peroneus muscles).

The obturator nerve provides sensation to the upper medial side of the thigh. Sensory branches of the femoral nerve supply the thigh, medial leg, and medial aspect of the ankle. The tibial nerve provides sensation to the sole of the foot as well as to the posterior leg. The common peroneal nerve and its branches provide sensation

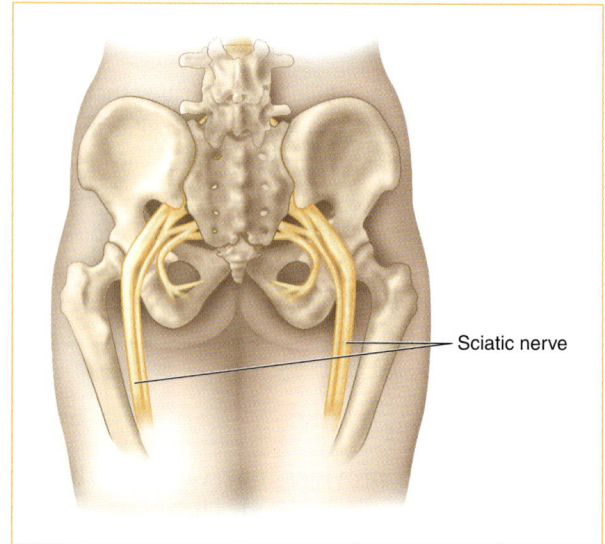

Figure 5-70 The sciatic nerve.

over the lateral surface of the knee, the skin over the great and second toes, the dorsum of the foot, and the distal anterior one third of the leg.

The Cranial Nerves

Twelve pairs of cranial nerves arise from the base of the brain. All but two pairs, the olfactory nerves and the optic nerves, exit from the brainstem Figure 5-71 .

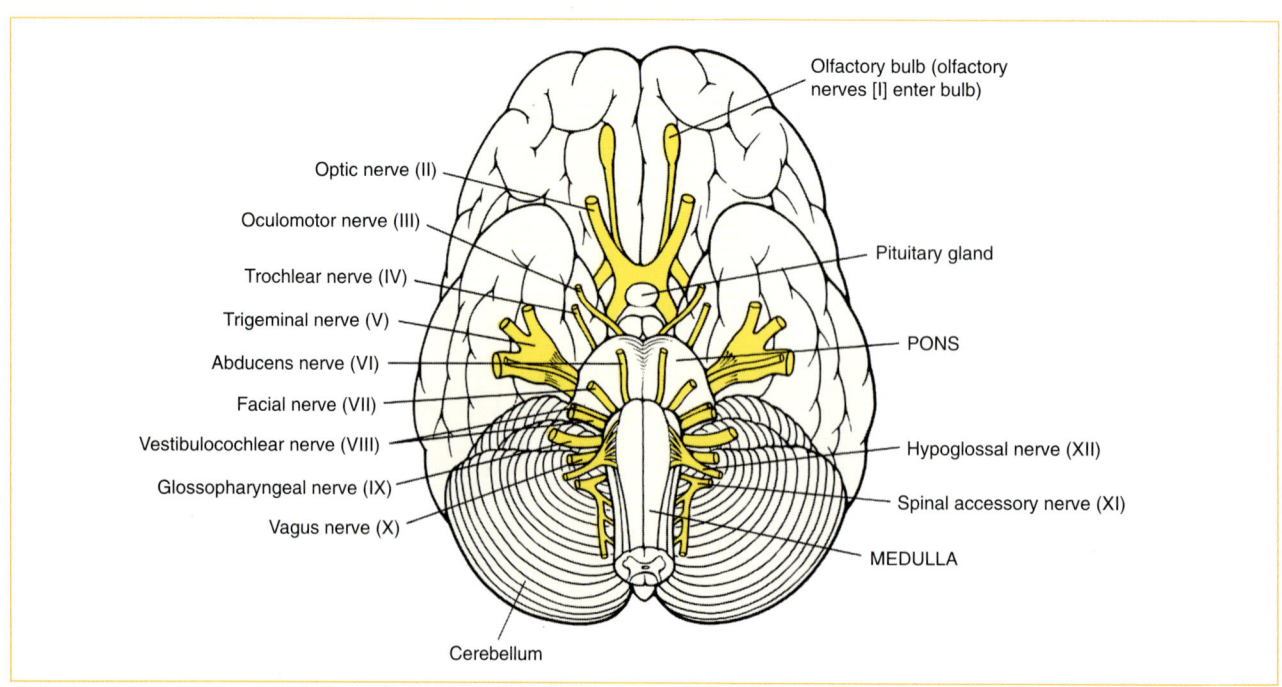

Figure 5-71 The cranial nerves.

Some of the cranial nerves carry only sensory fibers (I, II, and VIII), and others carry only motor fibers (III, IV, VI, XI, and XII). Many are mixed nerves, carrying a combination of sensory fibers and motor fibers (V, VII, IX, and X). Some cranial nerves also carry nerves of the parasympathetic nervous system in combination with motor, sensory, or both types of nerves (III, VII, IX, and X). Each nerve passes from the brain through a foramen in the skull to reach its endpoint.

Functions of the Cranial Nerves The olfactory nerve (I) provides the sense of smell. The nerve arises at the base of the brain as the olfactory tract. The tract forms the olfactory bulb, which lies on the cribriform plate of the ethmoid bone. Nerve fibers penetrate the cribriform plate providing sensations of smell to the nose.

The optic nerve (II) provides the sense of vision. The optic tracts arise at the base of the brain, forming the optic chiasma, anterior to the pituitary gland. The optic nerves extend from the optic chiasma to each eyeball, passing through the optic foramina (Figure 5-72▼).

The oculomotor nerve (III) innervates the muscles that cause motion of the eyeballs and upper lid. The oculomotor nerve also carries parasympathetic nerve fibers that cause constriction of the pupil (sphincter muscle), and accommodation of the lens (ciliary muscle).

The trochlear nerve (IV) innervates the superior oblique muscle of the eyeball, which allows a downward gaze. The trigeminal nerve (V) supplies sensation to the scalp, forehead, face, and lower jaw via three branches: the ophthalmic, maxillary, and mandibular divisions. The trigeminal nerve also provides motor innervation to the muscles of mastication (chewing), the throat, and the inner ear.

The abducens nerve (VI) supplies the lateral rectus muscle of the eyeball (lateral movement). The facial nerve (VII) supplies motor activity to all muscles of facial expression, the sense of taste to the anterior two thirds of the tongue, and cutaneous sensation to the external ear, tongue, and palate. The facial nerve also carries parasympathetic stimulation to the salivary glands, lacrimal gland, and the glands of the nasal cavity and palate.

The vestibulocochlear nerve (VIII) passes through the internal auditory meatus and provides the senses of hearing and balance. The glossopharyngeal nerve (IX) supplies motor fibers to the pharyngeal muscles. It provides taste sensation to the posterior portion of the tongue and carries parasympathetic fibers to the salivary glands (parotid glands) located on each side of the face.

The vagus nerve (X) provides motor functions to the soft palate, pharynx, and larynx (voice). The vagus nerve carries sensory fibers from the inferior pharynx, larynx, thoracic, and abdominal organs, taste bud fibers from the posterior tongue, and parasympathetic fibers to thoracic and abdominal organs.

The spinal accessory nerve (XI) provides motor innervation to the muscles of the soft palate and the pharynx and to the sternocleidomastoid and trapezius muscles. The spinal accessory nerve controls swallowing, speech, and head and shoulder movements. The hypoglossal nerve (XII) provides motor function to the muscles of the tongue and throat and contains fibers from C1 to C3 of the upper spinal cord.

The Autonomic Nervous System

Efferent neurons are separated into somatomotor and autonomic divisions. The somatomotor division comprises the nerves of the peripheral nervous system. The autonomic division, the autonomic nervous system (ANS) operates without conscious control and regulates the function of the internal organs, glands, and smooth muscle. The two divisions of the autonomic nervous system are the parasympathetic division and the sympathetic division.

The sympathetic pathway is responsible for the body's response to shock and stress. This response is associated with the release of adrenaline from the adrenal glands. Sympathetic responses include shunting of blood from the extremities to the vital core organs, increasing the heart rate and respirations, increasing blood pressure, dilation of the pupils, and reduction of digestive system activity.

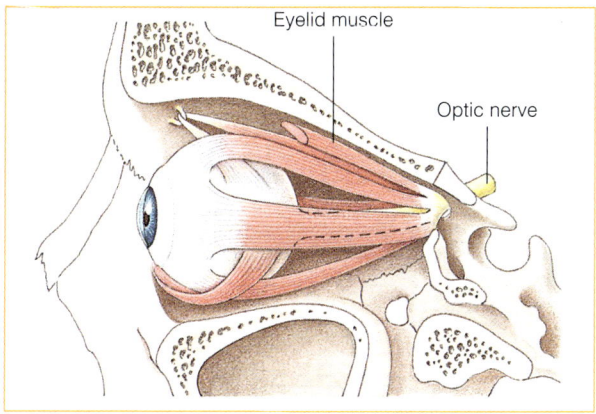

Figure 5-72 The optic nerve.

The parasympathetic nervous system relaxes the body. The parasympathetic responses include slowing the heart and respiratory rates, lowering the blood pressure, constricting the pupils, and increasing digestive system activity.

Preganglionic and Postganglionic Neurons

Although somatomotor nerves (sensory and motor nerves of the peripheral nervous system) extend directly from the CNS to skeletal muscle, nerves of the ANS contain two neurons in a series located between the CNS and the organs that are innervated. The first nerve, or preganglionic neuron, is separated from the second, the postganglionic neuron, by a ganglionic synapse. The preganglionic cell bodies are located within the central gray matter of the brainstem (the parasympathetic nervous system) and the spinal cord (the parasympathetic and sympathetic nervous systems). The cell bodies of the postganglionic neurons are located in autonomic ganglia and send their axons through nerves to various organs, where they synapse with the neuroeffector cells (target tissues).

Neurotransmitters and Receptors

The sympathetic and parasympathetic divisions secrete one of two neurotransmitters. A neuron that secretes acetylcholine is a cholinergic fiber. A neuron that secretes norepinephrine is an adrenergic fiber.

Both sympathetic and parasympathetic nerves release acetylcholine molecules from preganglionic fibers into the synaptic cleft. These molecules diffuse across to nicotinic receptors in the postganglionic neuron. These receptors are so named because they can be stimulated in the laboratory by the alkaloid nicotine. The impulse travels down the postganglionic neuron to reach the synapse at the target tissue with the neuroeffector cell. Acetylcholine is normally then rapidly destroyed by an enzyme, acetylcholinesterase.

At the target tissue, parasympathetic nerves release acetylcholine, which stimulates muscarinic receptors. Muscarinic receptors can be stimulated in the laboratory by the compound extracted from muscarine mushrooms. Sympathetic fibers release either norepinephrine, stimulating adrenergic receptors, or acetylcholine, stimulating muscarinic receptors.

All preganglionic neurons of the sympathetic and parasympathetic divisions and all postganglionic neurons of the parasympathetic division are cholinergic. Most postganglionic neurons of the sympathetic division are adrenergic, but a few, such as the postganglionic neurons that innervate sweat glands and a few blood vessels, are cholinergic.

Adrenergic receptors are classified into two structural and functional categories: alpha receptors and beta receptors. Norepinephrine binds to both but has somewhat greater affinity for alpha receptors. The substance epinephrine (adrenaline) is secreted by the adrenal gland and has nearly equal affinity for both receptor types. Alpha and beta receptors are also subdivided into $alpha_1$, $alpha_2$, $beta_1$, and $beta_2$ receptors.

Stimulation of various alpha and beta receptors can have either excitatory or inhibitory effects, depending on the location and type of the receptor. The primary type of stimulation in the heart involves $beta_1$ fibers. Such stimulation results in enhancement of myocardial contraction and increased heart rate. $Beta_2$ stimulation primarily affects the lungs, causing bronchodilation. Most alpha effects occur in the peripheral blood vessels, causing vasoconstrictions ($alpha_1$), and in the brain, having variable effects ($alpha_2$).

You are the Provider — Part 7

You assess of the third patient's vital signs, which reveals the following:

Vital Signs	Recording Time: 2 Minutes After Patient Contact
Respirations	20 breaths/min, unlabored
Pulse	88 beats/min, regular
Blood pressure	140/90 mm Hg
Sao_2	97% on supplemental oxygen

11. What is the function of the medulla in the brain?

The Endocrine System

The endocrine system is made up of various glands located throughout the body. Glands are cells or organs that selectively remove, concentrate, or alter materials in the blood and then secrete them back into the body. Glands secrete proteins called hormones that regulate many body functions, including growth, reproduction, temperature, metabolism, and blood pressure. Hormones move through the bloodstream to their target tissues. Endocrine cells and neurosecretory cells manufacture and secrete hormones that are released into the bloodstream. Endocrine glands secrete hormones directly into the blood, and exocrine glands, such as the sweat glands, secrete products through ducts, usually onto epithelial surfaces (Figure 5-73 ▶).

Prostaglandins are a group of hormone-like fatty acids that are produced in body tissues such as the uterus, brain, and kidneys. Semen also contains prostaglandins. Prostaglandins act on target organs to produce wide-ranging effects such as uterine contraction, regulation of blood pressure, smooth muscle contraction, pain, and inflammation. Aspirin and nonsteroidal anti-inflammatory drugs are believed to act by interfering with the synthesis of certain prostaglandins.

Hormones, regardless of their source, act by binding to receptors. Steroids and thyroid hormones bind to receptors located within cells. All other hormones, as a rule, bind to receptors located on the surface of cells. Hormones stimulate the production of intracellular proteins and other substances that carry out the next task in whatever body process the particular hormone is involved (Figure 5-74 ▼).

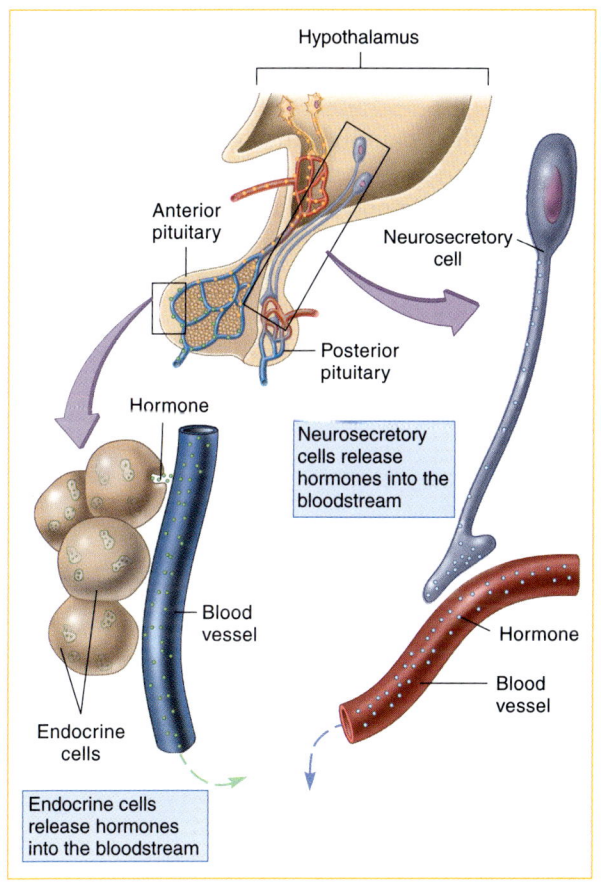

Figure 5-73 Hormones are released from neurosecretory cells or endocrine cells. Endocrine glands release their secretions into the bloodstream.

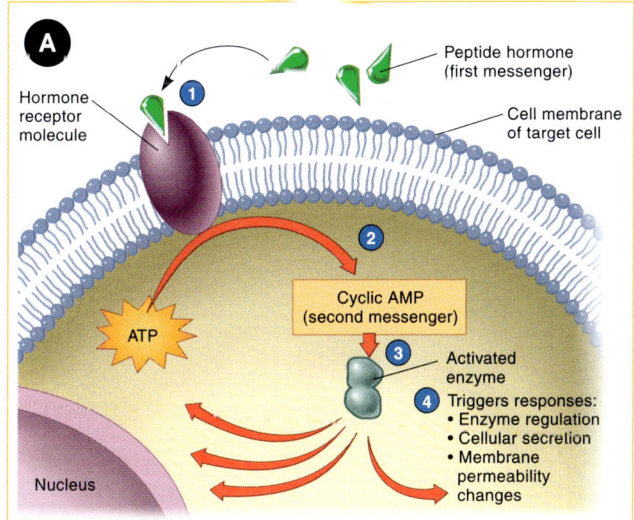 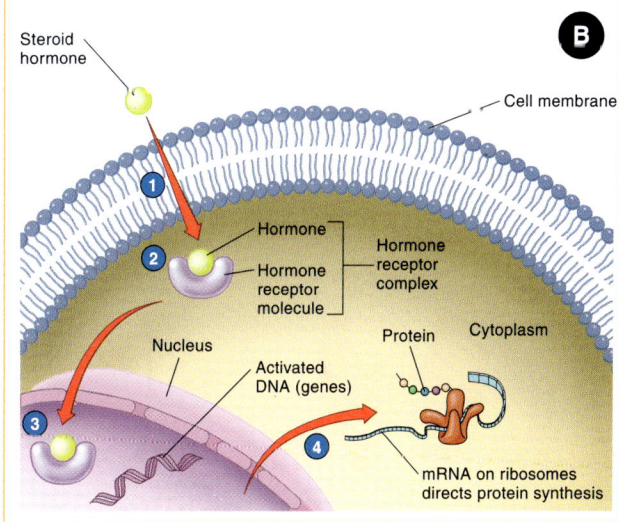

Figure 5-74 The mechanism of action of hormones. **A.** Peptide hormones. **B.** Steroid hormones.

In the absence of disease, hormones interact with each other to maintain homeostasis, or balance, in the body. Typically, this interaction involves positive feedback and negative feedback, or feedback inhibition. Negative feedback implies that when a hormone has exerted its desired effect, the result inhibits further production of the hormone until it is needed again (ie, the cessation of insulin production because of a low blood glucose concentration). Most feedback mechanisms in the human body are negative.

A few hormones, such as progressive labor and blood clotting hormones, work with positive feedback, in which the desired effect increases production of the hormone.

The Pituitary Gland and Hypothalamus

The pituitary gland, or hypophysis, is known as the master gland. The pituitary gland is located at the base of the brain in the cranial cavity, and it secretes hormones that regulate the function of many other glands in the body. The hypothalamus, the basal portion of the diencephalon, regulates the function of the pituitary gland. Compounds called releasing factors or inhibiting factors travel from the hypothalamus to the pituitary gland in a specialized set of blood vessels, the hypothalamohypophyseal portal system. The interactions of the hypothalamus and the pituitary gland often are referred to as the hypothalamic-pituitary axis.

The pituitary gland is located below the hypothalamus and is connected to it by a stalk, or infundibulum. The pituitary gland consists of two portions, the anterior pituitary lobe (adenohypophysis) and the posterior pituitary lobe (neurohypophysis) Figure 5-75 ▼.

The Posterior Pituitary Lobe

The posterior portion of the pituitary gland is directly connected to and continuous with the brain. Because this area of the pituitary gland is an extension of the central

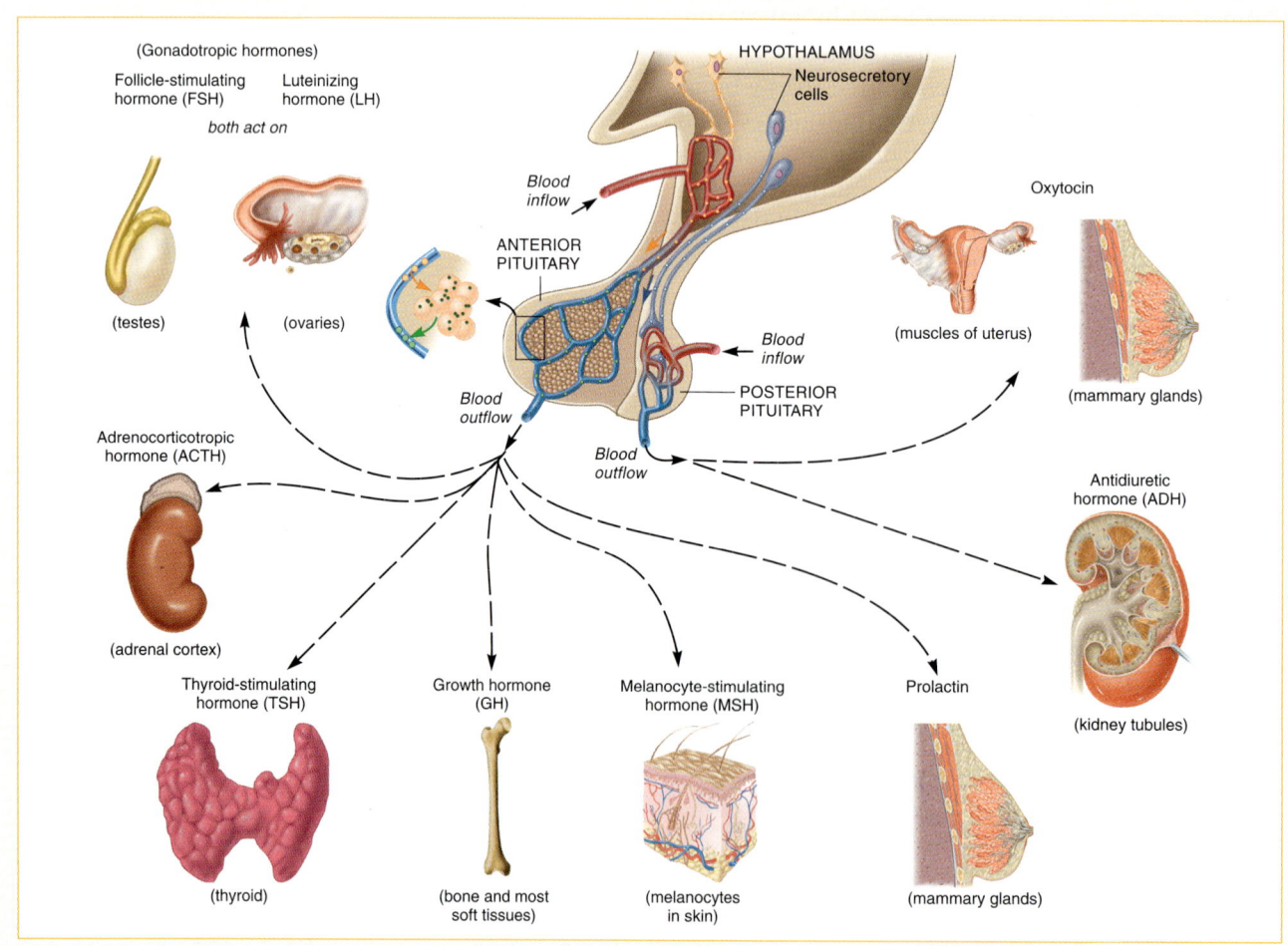

Figure 5-75 The pituitary gland secretes hormones from its two portions, the anterior pituitary lobe and the posterior pituitary lobe.

nervous system, hormones produced by this region are called neurohormones. The two major hormones stored and secreted by the neurohypophysis are antidiuretic hormone and oxytocin. Each of these hormones is secreted by different cells of the hypothalamus; however, both hormones are stored in and released by the posterior pituitary lobe.

Antidiuretic hormone (ADH) is also called vasopressin. In high concentrations, ADH constricts blood vessels and raises the blood pressure. Its primary target tissue is the kidney, where it promotes retention of water and reduction in urine volume. The secretion of ADH changes in response to signals given to the brain by specialized neurons, called osmoreceptors, as well as by blood pressure receptors in the blood vessels.

Oxytocin causes the smooth muscles of the pregnant uterus to contract and milk to be released from the breasts of lactating women. Preparations of oxytocin sometimes are used to induce or augment labor or to contract uterine musculature after childbirth to reduce or prevent bleeding.

The Anterior Pituitary Lobe

Because the anterior pituitary lobe of the pituitary gland is not considered part of the central nervous system, the hormones it produces are not neurohormones. However, hormones from the hypothalamus that inhibit or augment their release influence their secretion.

Growth Hormone

Growth hormone (GH), or somatotropin, stimulates growth in most tissues, especially of long bones in the extremities. GH also increases protein synthesis and the use of fats for energy. GH stimulates the production of proteins called somatomedins by the liver, skeletal muscle, and other tissues. Somatomedins circulate in the blood and affect target tissues. Both somatomedins and GH appear to be necessary for achieving the fullest effects.

Growth hormone-releasing hormone, produced by the hypothalamus, stimulates secretion of GH. Growth hormone release-inhibiting hormone, or somatostatin, inhibits its release. Body stresses such as shock or low blood glucose levels increase the secretion of GH, whereas high blood glucose levels decrease it.

Thyroid-Stimulating Hormone

Thyroid-stimulating hormone (TSH), or thyrotropin, controls the release of thyroid hormone from the thyroid gland into the bloodstream. TSH is influenced by thyrotropin-releasing factor from the hypothalamus.

Adrenocorticotropic Hormone

Adrenocorticotropic hormone (ACTH) is one of several molecules derived from a common precursor, proopiomelanocortin. ACTH is essential for development of the cortex of the adrenal gland and its secretion of corticosteroids. ACTH secretion is stimulated by stress, trauma, major surgery, fever, and other conditions. Beta-endorphins are proteins that have the same effects as opiate drugs such as morphine and also are derived from proopiomelanocortin.

Reproduction-Regulating Hormones

Luteinizing hormone (LH) and follicle-stimulating hormone (FSH) regulate the production of both eggs and sperm, as well as production of reproductive hormones (estrogen and progesterone in women, and testosterone in men). Gonadotropin-releasing hormone produced by the hypothalamus influences the release of both LH and FSH. Prolactin plays an important role in milk production in women; however, no role has been described in men. Prolactin-releasing hormones and prolactin-inhibiting hormones are released by the hypothalamus and influence the release or inhibition of prolactin.

The Thyroid Gland

The large gland at the base of the neck is called the thyroid gland. It consists of two lobes that are connected by a narrow band of tissue, the isthmus. The isthmus extends anteriorly across the trachea. The thyroid gland manufactures and secretes hormones that have a role in growth, development, and metabolism.

Microscopically, the thyroid gland contains numerous small cavity glands called follicles that are filled with thyroglobulin, a protein to which thyroid hormones are bound. Between the follicles are parafollicular cells that produce the hormone calcitonin, which is important in regulating calcium levels in the body. Calcitonin decreases the breakdown of bone by osteoclasts, resulting in a decrease in blood calcium and phosphate levels (Figure 5-76 ▶).

The two major hormones that the thyroid gland produces are triiodothyronine (T_3) and tetraiodothyronine (T_4). These hormones are produced in response to stimulation from the anterior pituitary lobe by TSH. In the blood, both T_3 and T_4 bind to a protein synthesized in the liver, thyroxine-binding globulin. T_3 interacts mostly with target tissues. Approximately 40% of T_4 is converted to T_3 in the body tissues. Both hormones are essential for normal growth and development in children. They also play an important role in the regulation of body metabolism.

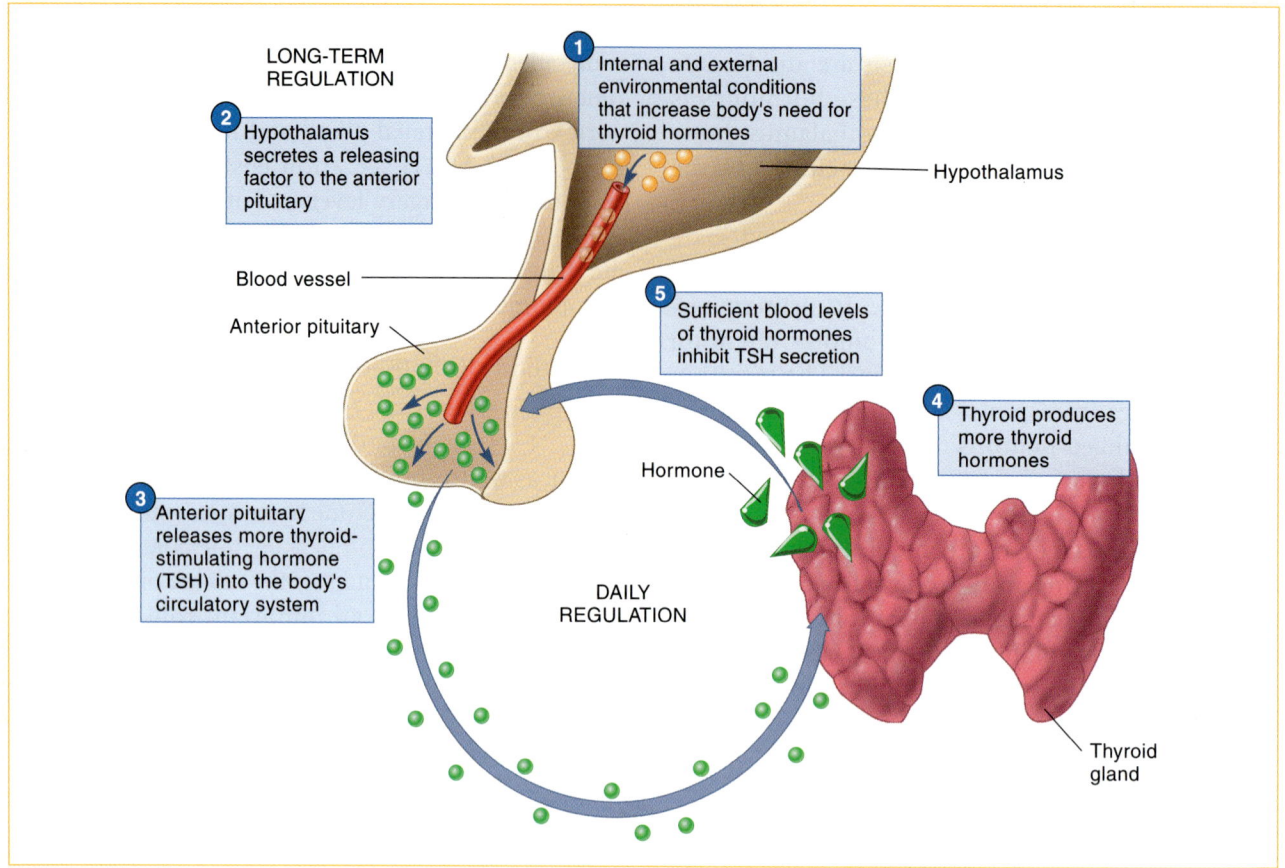

Figure 5-76 The thyroid gland. Production of thyroid hormone is controlled by the anterior pituitary with input from the hypothalamus and circulating plasma.

The Parathyroid Glands

The parathyroid glands, usually four in number, are embedded in the posterior portion of each lobe of the thyroid. They produce and secrete parathyroid hormone, which maintains normal levels of calcium in the blood and normal neuromuscular function (see Figure 5-76). Parathyroid hormone effects are opposite to those of calcitonin.

The Pancreas

The pancreas is an organ of both the endocrine and digestive systems. The pancreas lies between the greater curvature of the stomach and the duodenum in the retroperitoneum, or space behind the peritoneum (Figure 5-77 ▶). The head of the pancreas rests near the duodenum; the body and tail of the pancreas project toward the spleen.

The pancreas produces digestive enzymes, and also produces the hormones insulin and glucagon, which play important roles in controlling metabolism and blood glucose level. Insulin and glucagon are produced in specialized groups of cells known as the islets of Langerhans (see Figure 5-77 B and C). Within each islet are alpha cells that secrete glucagon and beta cells that secrete insulin. The function of the remaining cells, delta cells, is currently unknown.

Insulin and glucagon perform opposite functions. Insulin causes foodstuffs (sugar, fatty acids, and amino acids) to be taken up and metabolized by cells. Insulin also stimulates the storage of unmetabolized food and the conversion of glucose into a long polymer called glycogen. Fatty acids are converted into triglycerides and stored as fat. Amino acids are metabolized into proteins or glucose to be used for energy.

Glucagon stimulates the breakdown of glycogen to glucose by a process known as glycogenolysis. In addition, glucagon stimulates both the liver and the kidneys to produce glucose from noncarbohydrate molecules by a process known as gluconeogenesis. In addition,

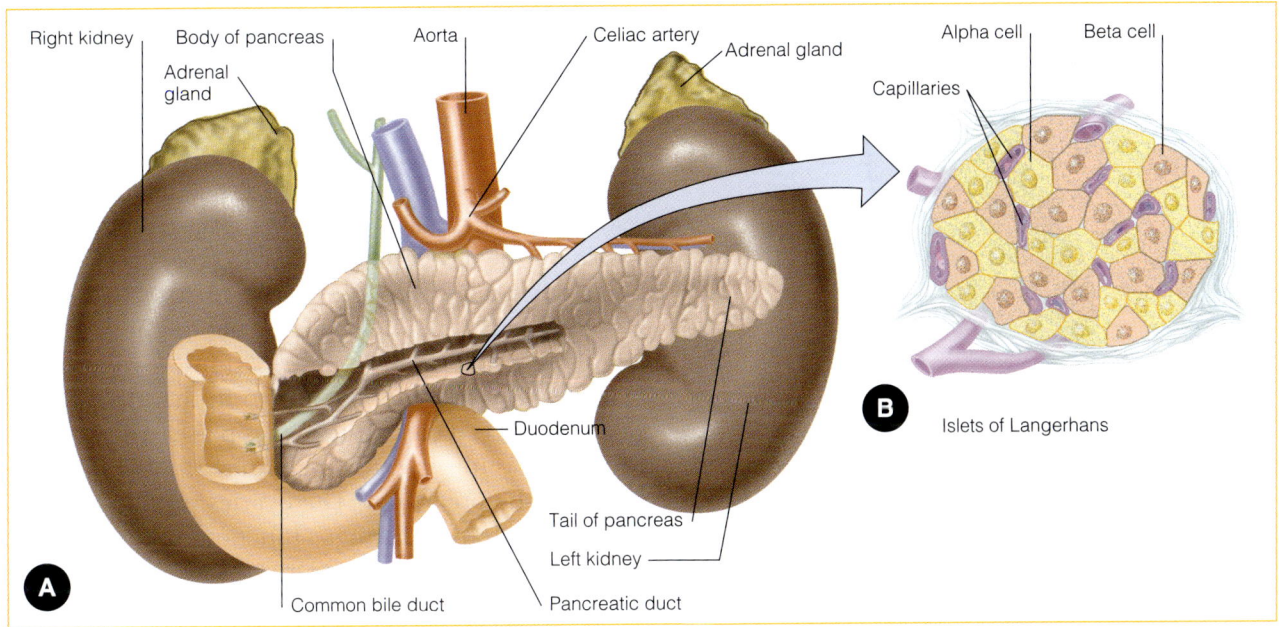

Figure 5-77 The pancreas. **A.** The pancreas produces two hormones, insulin and glucagon, as well as digestive enzymes. **B.** Hormones are produced by specialized cells within the islets of Langerhans. **C.** The islets of Langerhans are located among the acini, very small groups of digestive-enzyme-producing cells of the pancreas.

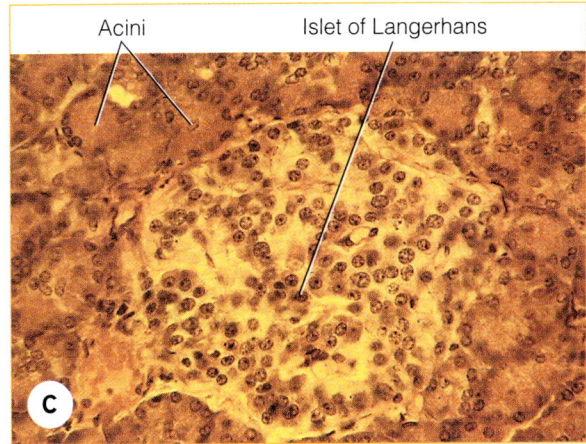

glucagon activates an enzyme, hormone sensitive lipase, which breaks triglycerides down into free fatty acids and glycerol. Depending on the metabolic needs of the body, the free fatty acids and glycerol may be metabolized directly or converted to ketones. In small amounts, ketone production is normal. In disease states, such as diabetic ketoacidosis, increased plasma glucagon concentrations and unopposed glucagon activity lead to excessive production, resulting in possible harm to the patient.

The Adrenal Glands

The adrenal glands, sometimes called the supra-renal glands, are located on top of each kidney. The adrenal gland manufactures and secretes certain sex hormones, as well as other hormones that are vital in maintaining the body's water and salt balance. The adrenal glands produce adrenaline (also called epinephrine), which mediates the "fight-or-flight" response of the sympathetic nervous system when the body is under stress.

The inner portion, or medulla, of the adrenal glands produces epinephrine and norepinephrine. These hormones are vital in the function of the sympathetic nervous system. The remainder of adrenal tissue, known as the adrenal cortex, is divided into three areas, or zones: the zona glomerulosa, zona fasciculata, and zona reticularis (Figure 5-78 ▶).

The zona glomerulosa produces mineralocorticoids. These hormones are important in regulating the water and salt balance of the body. The most important mineralocorticoid is aldosterone. This compound

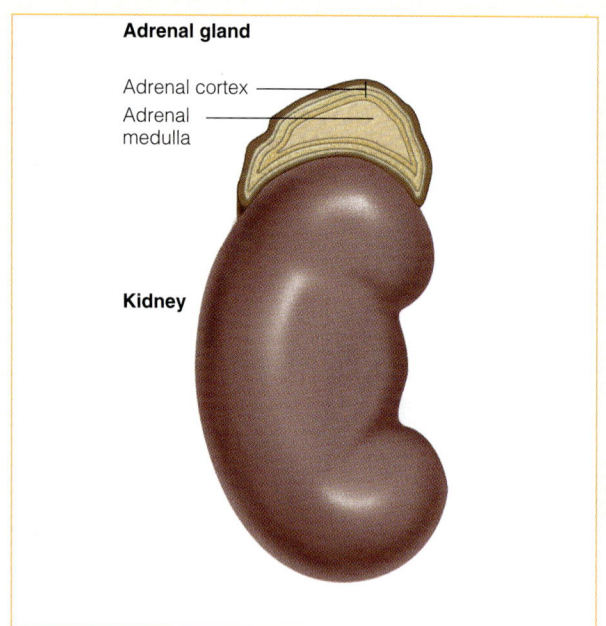

Figure 5-78 The adrenal glands sit on top of the kidney and consist of the adrenal medulla and adrenal cortex.

The Reproductive Glands and Hormones

The gonads are the reproductive glands and consist of the ovaries in women and the testes in men. Testosterone is the major androgen manufactured by the testes. Testosterone also is produced in small amounts in the adrenal glands and in the ovaries. Testosterone is responsible for the development of male secondary sex characteristics, such as a deep voice and facial hair.

The three major female hormones are estrogen, progesterone, and human chorionic gonadotropin (hCG). The developing embryo in the uterus manufactures hCG if conception takes place to keep the lining of the uterus (endometrium) thick and able to sustain the pregnancy. The ovaries produce estrogen and progesterone. Estrogen functions in the menstrual cycle and in the development of secondary sex characteristics, such as breast development in adolescence. Progesterone, which is produced by the corpus luteum of the ovary, prepares the uterus for implantation of a fertilized egg. In men, small amounts of estrogen and progesterone also are produced in the testes and adrenal glands.

increases the absorption of sodium by the kidneys. In addition, aldosterone increases the rate at which water is reabsorbed. The result is an increase in both the blood volume and the concentration of sodium within the plasma. Secretion of aldosterone also increases the excretion of potassium by the kidneys.

The zona fasciculata secretes glucocorticoids, which are also known as corticosteroids. The most important of these compounds is cortisol. Cortisol has a myriad of roles in the body, including regulation of blood glucose, metabolism of fat tissue, and inhibition of inflammation. Secretion of corticosteroids is regulated by the hypothalamic-pituitary-adrenal axis, a complex set of interactions involving chemical signals delivered through the bloodstream from the brain to the adrenal glands.

The zona reticularis secretes a few relatively weak male sex hormones, or androgens. Androgens are produced in both women and men, but in different quantities. The most common androgen is androstenedione. Adrenal androgens stimulate growth of pubic and axillary hair, as well as sexual drive in women. In men, their effects are insignificant compared to the sex hormones produced by the gonads.

Blood and Its Components

Plasma and Formed Elements (Cells)

Blood is the substance that is pumped by the heart through the arteries, veins, and capillaries (Figure 5-79 ▶). Blood consists of plasma and formed elements or cells that are suspended in the plasma. These cells include red blood cells, white blood cells, and platelets. The purpose of blood is to carry oxygen and nutrients to the tissues and carry cell waste products away from the tissues. In addition, the formed elements are the mainstay of numerous other body functions such as fighting infection and controlling bleeding. Human adult male bodies contain approximately 70 mL/kg, or about 5 L, of blood, whereas female bodies contain approximately 65 mL/kg.

Plasma is a watery, straw-colored fluid that accounts for more than half of the total blood volume. Plasma is made up of 92% water and 8% dissolved substances such as chemicals, minerals, and nutrients. Water enters the plasma from the digestive tract, from fluids between cells, and as a by-product of metabolism.

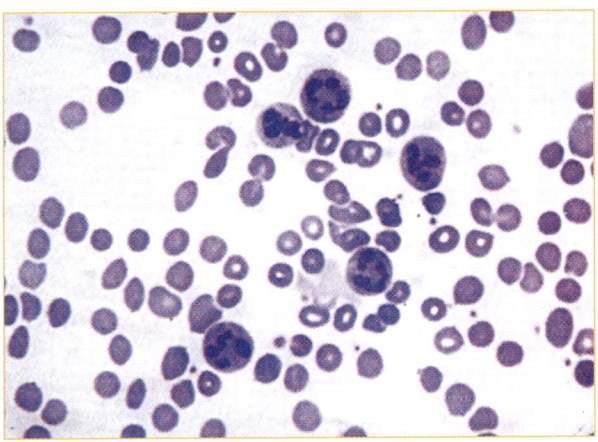

Figure 5-79 Components of blood include plasma and formed elements or cells, including red blood cells, white blood cells, and platelets.

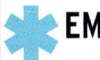 **EMT-I Tips**

Any decrease in the number of red blood cells in the body is called <u>anemia</u>. Anemia may be caused by inadequate nutrition (such as iron deficiency), inadequate production of erythrocytes by bone marrow, increased destruction of red blood cells by the body (hemolysis), or bleeding.

Red Blood Cells

Red blood cells carry oxygen to the tissues. They are disk-shaped, and are also known as <u>erythrocytes</u>. These are the most numerous of the formed elements. An average human has between 4.2 and 5.8 million erythrocytes per cubic millimeter of blood. Erythrocytes are unable to move on their own; the flowing plasma passively propels them. Red blood cells contain a protein known as <u>hemoglobin</u>, which gives them their reddish color. Hemoglobin carries oxygen from the lungs and to the tissues by binding to it.

<u>Erythropoiesis</u> is the ongoing process by which red blood cells are made. Approximately 25 trillion erythrocytes are contained in the normal adult circulation; of these, 2.5 million erythrocytes are destroyed every second.

Red blood cells have a finite lifespan of 120 days. Those cells that are destined for destruction decompose in the spleen and other tissues that are rich in cells known as <u>macrophages</u>. Macrophages protect the body against infection. The body "recycles" some components of hemoglobin, such as the protein, globin, and iron. The part of hemoglobin that is not recycled is converted to <u>bilirubin</u>, which is a waste product that undergoes further metabolism in the liver. Normally, a chemical derivative of bilirubin, urobilinogen, is excreted in the stool and in the urine.

Erythrocytes contain <u>antigens</u> on their surface, which are proteins recognized by the immune system. Within the plasma are <u>antibodies</u>, which are proteins that react with antigens. Individuals are classified as having one of four blood types based on the presence or absence of these specific antigens. This process of classification is referred to as blood typing, or determining the ABO blood group.

Type A blood contains erythrocytes with type A surface antigens and plasma containing type B antibodies; type B blood contains type B surface antigens and plasma containing type A antibodies. Type AB blood contains both types of antigens but the plasma contains no ABO antibodies. Type O contains neither A nor B antigens but contains both A and B plasma antibodies. A person's blood type determines which type of blood he or she may receive in a blood transfusion.

Rh blood groups involve a complex of antigens first discovered in rhesus monkeys. The presence of any of the 18 separate Rh antigens makes an individual's blood Rh positive. If an individual with Rh-negative blood were to be exposed to Rh-positive blood, antibodies to the antigens could be produced.

White Blood Cells

White blood cells are also known as <u>leukocytes</u>. There are several different types of white blood cells and each has a different function. The primary function of all white blood cells is to fight infection. Antibodies to fight infection may be produced, or leukocytes may directly attack and kill bacterial invaders. Leukocytes are larger than erythrocytes. Most leukocytes are motile and leave the blood vessels by a process known as <u>diapedesis</u> to move toward the tissue where they are needed most.

Leukocytes are named according to their appearance in a stained preparation of blood. In general, <u>granulocytes</u> have large cytoplasmic granules that are easily seen with a simple light microscope; <u>agranulocytes</u> are leukocytes that lack these granules. There are three types of granulocytes (neutrophils, eosinophils, and basophils) and two types of agranulocytes (monocytes and lymphocytes).

Neutrophils are normally the most common type of granulocyte in the blood. Their nuclei are commonly multilobed, resembling a string of baseballs held together by a thin strand of thread. For this reason, these cells often are called polymorphonuclear cells or "polys." Neutrophils destroy bacteria, antigen-antibody complexes, and foreign matter (Figure 5-80 ▼). Eosinophils are granulocytes that contain granules that stain bright red with the acidic stain, eosin. Eosinophils function in the body's allergic response and are, thus, increased in individuals with allergies. Certain parasitic infections, such as trichinosis, also result in an increase in the number of eosinophils present. Basophils are the least common of all granulocytes and play a role in both allergic and inflammatory reactions. Basophils contain large amounts of histamine, a substance that increases tissue inflammation, and heparin, a substance that inhibits blood clotting.

Lymphocytes are the smallest of the agranulocytes. Lymphocytes originate in the bone marrow but migrate through the blood to the lymphatic tissues. Most lymphocytes are located in the lymph nodes, spleen, tonsils, lymph nodules, and thymus.

Monocytes and macrophages are one of the first lines of defense in the inflammatory process. Monocytes migrate out of the blood and into the tissues in response to an infection. They engulf microbes and digest them in a process called phagocytosis. Unlike their counterparts, the neutrophils, which are short-lived, once in the tissues monocytes mature into long-lived macrophages.

Platelets and Blood Clotting

Platelets are small cells in the blood that are necessary for the series of chemical reactions that occur to form a clot. The blood clotting or coagulation process is a complex set of events involving platelets, clotting proteins in the plasma (clotting factors), other proteins, and calcium. The process begins with platelets clumping together. Then clotting proteins produced by the liver solidify the remainder of the clot, which eventually includes red and white blood cells.

Following injury to a blood vessel wall, a predictable series of events takes place, resulting in hemostasis (cessation of bleeding) and formation of the final blood clot. Chemicals released from the vessel wall cause local vasoconstriction, as well as activation of the platelets. The combination of vessel contraction and loose platelet aggregation forms a temporary "plug." Other factors released by the tissues, known as tissue thromboplastin, activate a cascade of clotting proteins. Eventually, thrombin is formed. This causes the conversion of fibrinogen to fibrin, which binds to the platelet plug, forming the final mature clot (Figure 5-81 ▼).

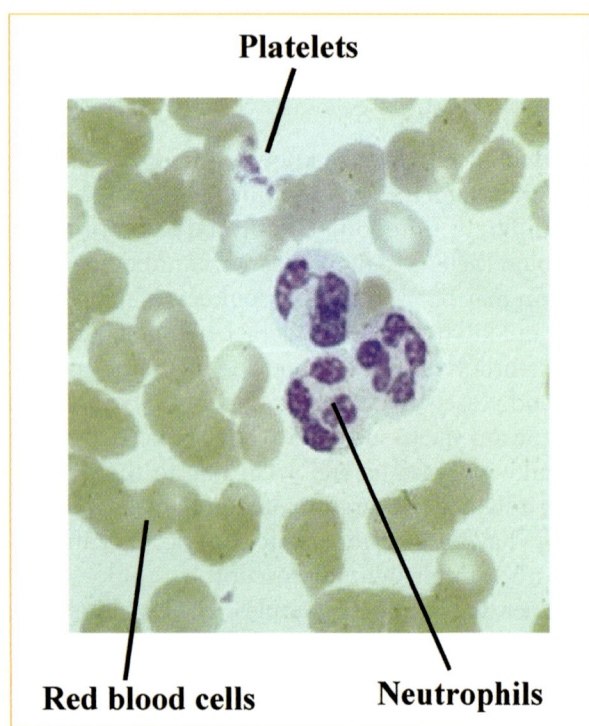

Figure 5-80 The blood cells.

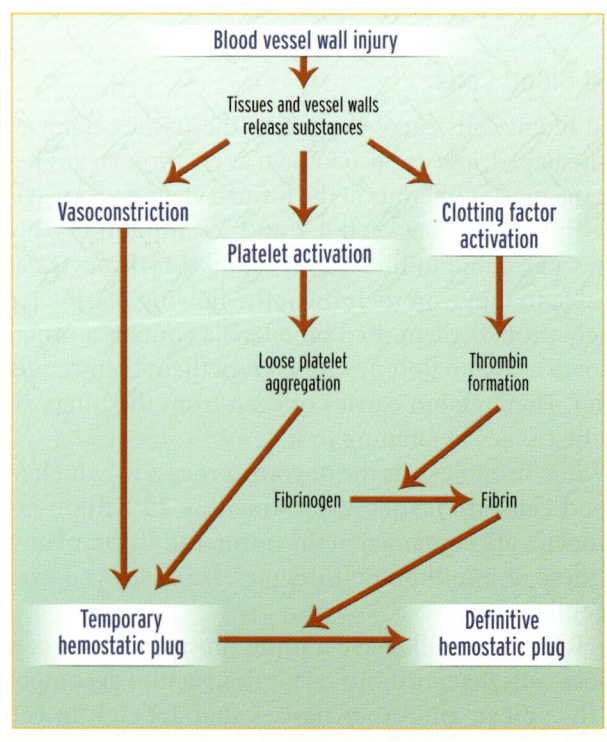

Figure 5-81 Algorithm showing the reactions in hemostasis.

The body also has two systems to counterbalance the clotting system. One, the fibrinolytic system, lyses or disrupts clots that already have formed. The main steps in the fibrinolytic system are the activation of tissue plasminogen activator (t-PA), which then converts plasminogen to plasmin.

The other counterbalance to the clotting system consists of three naturally occurring blood thinners (anticoagulants), protein S, protein C, and antithrombin III, that are activated if a blood clot begins to form in an abnormal location, such as the coronary artery.

Together, the fibrinolytic system and the body's own anticoagulants attempt to provide a balance between clotting and bleeding; however, neither system is absolutely effective (for example, in patients with thrombotic conditions, such as myocardial infarction or stroke, as well as in patients with spontaneous bleeding, such as subarachnoid hemorrhage).

The Heart

Location and Major Structures of the Heart

The heart is a muscular organ that pumps blood throughout the body. The heart is located behind the sternum and is about the size of the closed fist of the person it belongs to, roughly 5″ long, 3″ wide, and 2″ thick. It weighs 10 to 12 oz in male adults and 8 to 10 oz in female adults (Figure 5-82 ▶). Approximately two thirds of the heart lies in the left part of the mediastinum, the area between the lungs that also contains the great vessels.

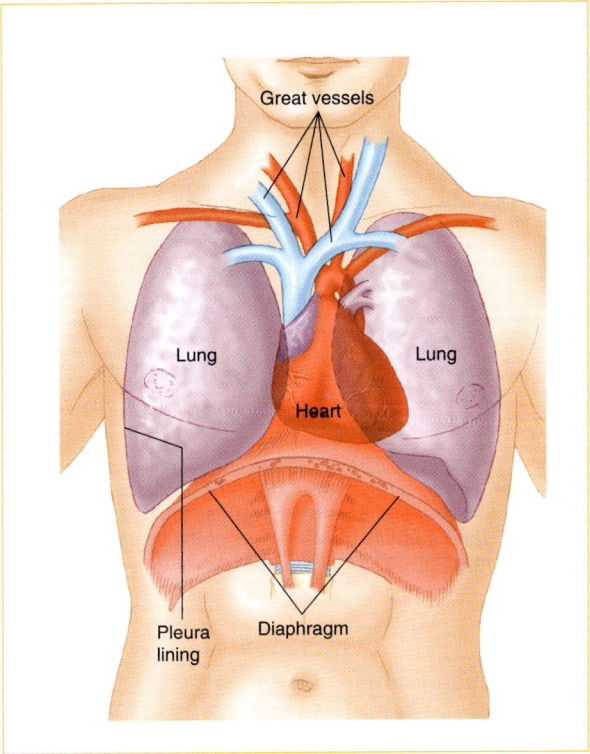

Figure 5-82 The anterior aspect of the thorax shows the relative position of the heart beneath the surface.

Heart muscle is called myocardium. The term "myo" means muscle and "cardium" means heart. The pericardium, also called the pericardial sac, is a thick, fibrous membrane that surrounds the heart (Figure 5-83 ▶). The pericardium anchors the heart within the mediastinum and prevents overdistention of the heart. The inner membrane of the pericardium is the serous pericardium.

You are the Provider   Part 8

The fourth patient is an elderly woman who was a passenger in the second vehicle. She also was unrestrained. She has a large right temporal laceration. You note the following:

Initial Assessment	Recording Time: Zero Minutes
Appearance	Bleeding from a large head laceration
Level of consciousness	Confused
Airway	Open and clear
Breathing	Increased respiratory rate with adequate depth
Circulation	Skin, pink and warm and dry to touch; radial pulse present

12. How does the body respond when a patient loses blood?

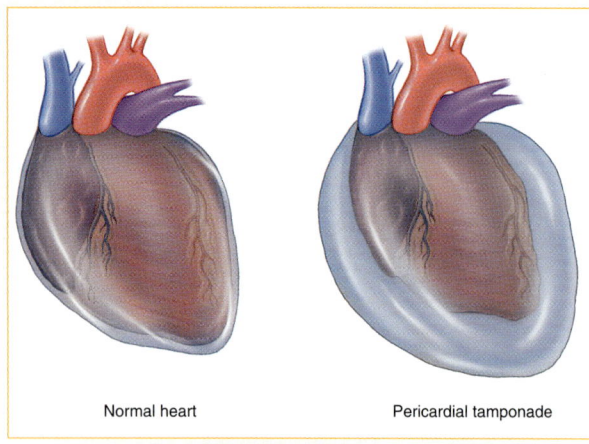

Figure 5-83 The pericardial sac surrounds the heart. When the pericardial sac fills with too much fluid (pericardial effusion), a life-threatening state of cardiac tamponade can develop. In this situation, the chambers of the heart are unable to expand and contract properly. Death can rapidly result.

This inner membrane contains two layers: the visceral layer and the parietal layer. The visceral layer of the pericardium lies closely against the heart and is also called the epicardium. The second layer of the pericardium, the parietal layer, is separated from the visceral layer by a small amount of pericardial fluid that reduces friction within the pericardial sac.

> **EMT-I Tips**
>
> Complete blockage of an artery that supplies oxygen to the heart results in death to a portion of the myocardium, or a myocardial infarction.

The normal human heart consists of four chambers: two atria and two ventricles. The upper chambers are the atria, and the lower chambers are the ventricles. Each side of the heart contains one atrium and one ventricle. A membrane, the interatrial septum, separates the two atria; a thicker wall, the interventricular septum, separates the right and left ventricles. Each atrium receives blood that is returned to the heart from other parts of the body; each ventricle pumps blood out of the heart. The upper and lower portions of the heart are separated by the atrioventricular valves, which prevent blood from flowing backward. There are also valves located between the ventricles and the arteries into which they pump blood. These are called the semilunar valves 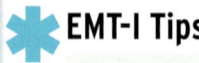 Figure 5-84 ▶ .

Blood enters the right atrium via the superior and inferior venae cavae and the coronary sinus, which consists of veins that collect blood that is returning from the walls of the heart. Blood from four pulmonary veins enters the left atrium. Between the right and left atria is a depression, the fossa ovalis, which represents the former location of the foramen ovale, an opening between the two atria that is present in the fetus.

Valves of the Heart

Blood passing from the atria to the ventricles flows through one of two atrioventricular valves. The tricuspid valve separates the right atrium from the right ventricle, and the mitral valve, a bicuspid valve, separates the left atrium from the left ventricle. The valves consist of flaps called cusps. Papillary muscles attach to the ventricles and send small muscular strands called chordae tendineae cordis to the cusps. When the papillary muscle contracts, these strands tighten, preventing regurgitation of blood through the valves from the ventricles to the atria.

Two semilunar valves, the aortic valve and the pulmonic valve, divide the heart from the aorta and the pulmonary artery. The pulmonic valve regulates blood flow from the right ventricle to the pulmonary artery. The aortic valve regulates blood flow from the left ventricle to the aorta. The semilunar valves are not attached to papillary muscles. When these valves close, they prevent backflow from the aorta and pulmonary artery into the left and right ventricles, respectively.

Blood Flow Within the Heart

Two large veins, the superior vena cava and the inferior vena cava, return deoxygenated blood from the body to the right atrium. Blood from the upper part of the body returns to the heart through the superior vena cava, and blood from the lower part of the body returns through the inferior vena cava. The inferior vena cava is the larger of the two veins. From the right atrium, blood passes through the tricuspid valve into the right ventricle. Blood is then pumped by the right ventricle through the pulmonic valve into the pulmonary artery and to the lungs. In the lungs, various processes take place that return oxygen to the blood, and at the same time, remove carbon dioxide and other waste products.

Freshly oxygenated blood is returned to the left atrium through the pulmonary veins. Blood then flows through the mitral valve into the left ventricle, which pumps the oxygenated blood through the aortic valve,

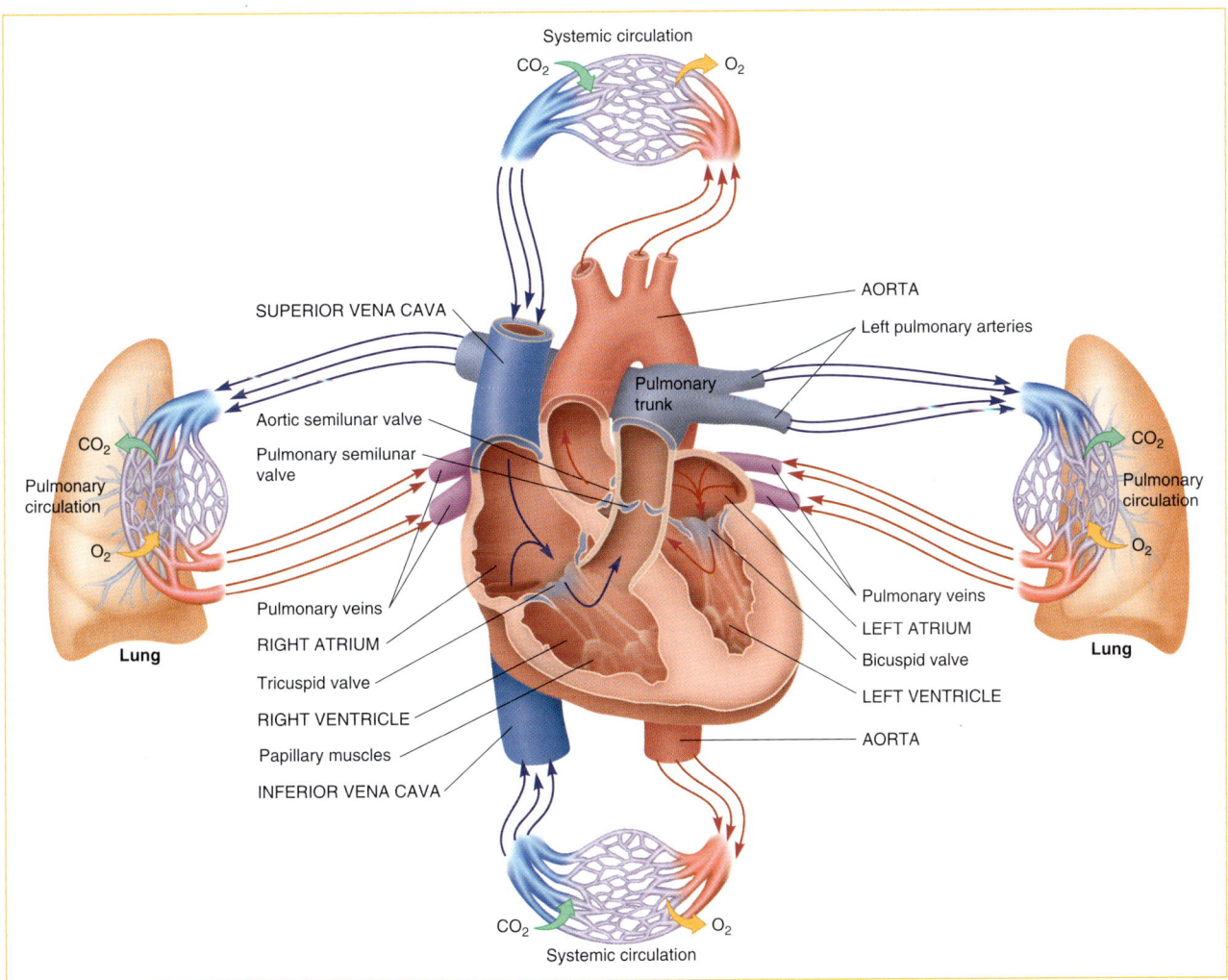

Figure 5-84 Blood flow through the heart.

into the aorta, the body's largest artery, and then to the entire body. The left ventricle is the strongest and largest of the four cardiac chambers because it is responsible for pumping blood through blood vessels throughout the body.

Heart sounds are created by the contraction and relaxation of the heart and flow of blood. These sounds can be heard during auscultation with a stethoscope. Normal heart sounds are often described as sounding like "lub-DUB, lub-DUB, lub-DUB...." The "lub" is called the first heart sound or S1, and the "DUB" is called the second heart sound or S2 (Figure 5-85). S2 ("DUB") is often louder than S1 ("lub"). The sudden closure of the mitral and tricuspid valves at the start of ventricular contraction causes S1. The closure of both the aortic and pulmonic valves at the end of a ventricular contraction causes S2.

Two other heart sounds, S3 and S4, usually are not heard in individuals with normal heart sounds (Figure 5-86). The S3 or third heart sound is a soft, low-pitched heart sound that occurs about one third of the way through diastole (the period during which the ventricles are relaxed). When an S3 sound is present, the heart beat cycle is described as sounding like "lub-DUB-da." This sound may correlate to a period of rapid ventricular filling. Although the S3 sound sometimes is present in healthy young individuals, it most commonly is associated with abnormally increased filling pressures in the atria secondary to moderate to severe heart failure.

The S4 heart sound is a medium pitched sound that occurs immediately before the normal S1 sound. When an S4 sound is present, the heart contraction cycle sounds like "bla-lub-DUB." The S4 sound represents either

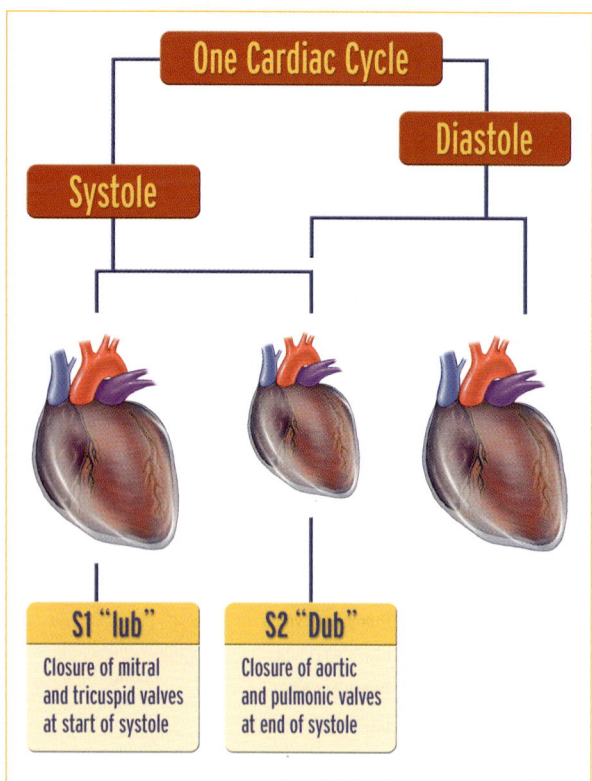

Figure 5-85 The normal S1 and S2 heart sounds.

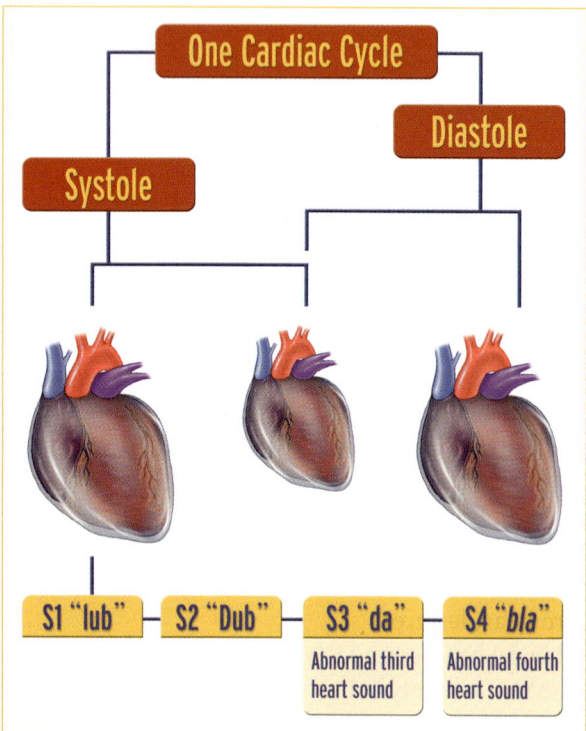

Figure 5-86 The abnormal S3 and S4 heart sounds.

decreased stretching (compliance) of the left ventricle or increased pressure in the atria. An S4 heart sound almost always is abnormal.

Four other sounds, all abnormal, may be heard when auscultating the heart and great vessels. Some of these sounds are very easy to hear; others may require years of experience to identify. These additional abnormal sounds include murmurs, bruits, clicks, and snaps. A murmur is an abnormal "whooshing-like" sound heard over the heart that indicates turbulent blood flow within the heart. Although many murmurs are "functional" (benign) and often go away, several are characteristic of heart disease. A bruit is an abnormal "whooshing-like" sound heard over a main blood vessel that indicates turbulent blood flow within the blood vessel. A bruit often indicates localized atherosclerotic disease (plaque formation in the arteries). Both clicks and snaps indicate abnormal cardiac valve function. They occur at different times in the cardiac cycle, depending on which valve is diseased. Although these sounds are significant, most of these sounds are fleeting and difficult to hear.

Electrical Properties of the Heart and Conduction System

The mechanical pumping action of the heart can only occur in response to an electrical stimulus. This impulse causes the heart to beat via a set of complex chemical changes within the myocardial cells. The brain partially controls the heart's rate and strength of contraction via the autonomic nervous system. The myocardium is the only muscle that has the property of automaticity, or the ability to generate its own electrical impulses. Therefore, the contractions are initiated within the heart itself, in a group of complex electrical tissues that are part of a conduction system. The cardiac conduction system consists of six parts: the sinoatrial (SA) node, the atrioventricular (AV) node, the bundle of His, the right and left bundle branches, and the Purkinje fibers Figure 5-87 ▶ .

The sinoatrial (SA) node is located high in the right atrium and is the normal site of origin of the electrical impulse. It is the heart's natural pacemaker. Impulses originating in the SA node travel through the right and left atria, resulting in atrial contraction. The impulse then travels to the atrioventricular (AV) node, located in the right atrium adjacent to the septum, where it transiently slows. Electrical stimulation of the heart muscle then continues toward the bundle of His, which is a continuation of the AV node. From here, it proceeds rapidly to the right and left bundle branches, stimulat-

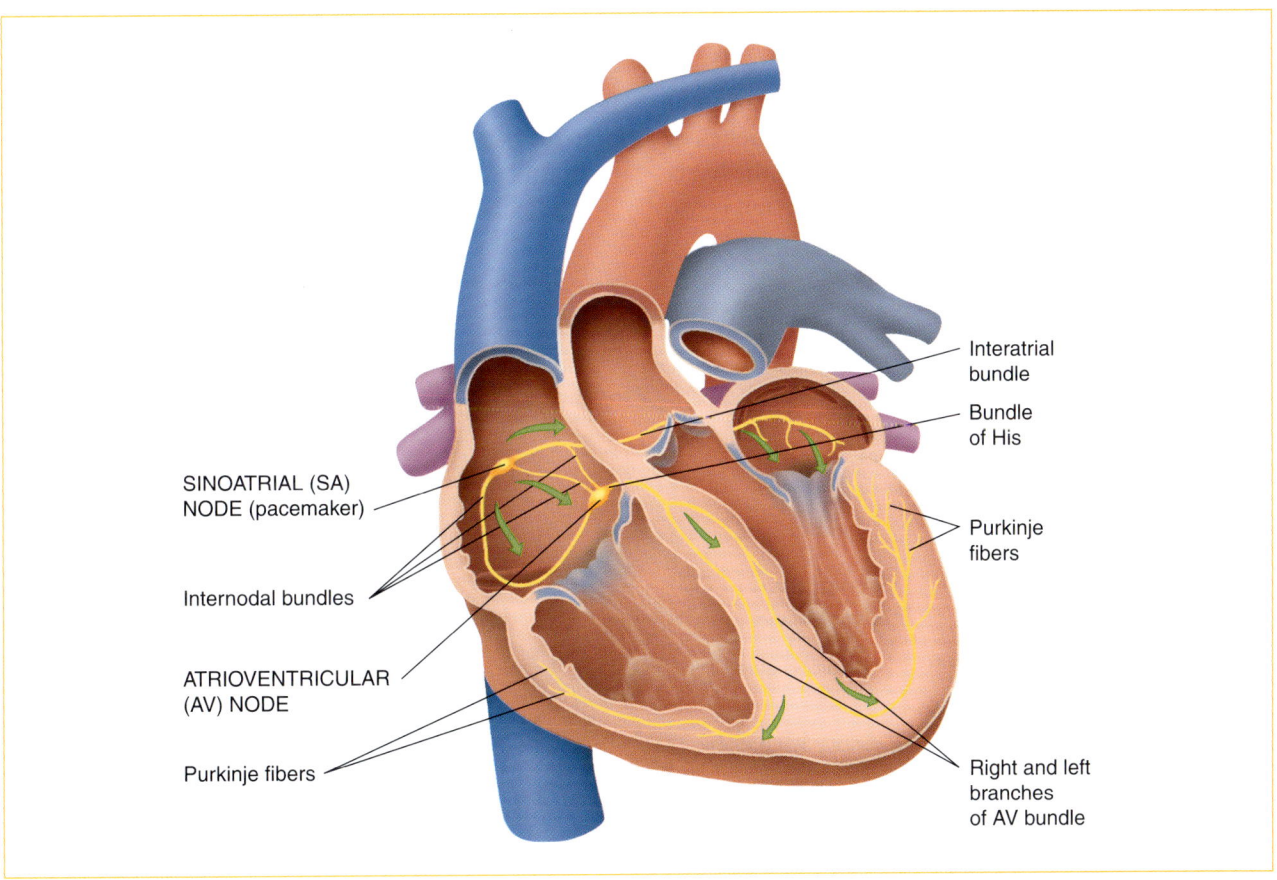

Figure 5-87 The cardiac conduction system. Specialized groups of cardiac muscle cells initiate an electrical impulse throughout the heart. The normal conduction pathway travels through the six parts of the cardiac conduction system. The impulse begins in the SA node and spreads through internodal bundles to the AV node. The AV node slows the impulse and initiates a signal that is conducted through the ventricles by way of the bundle of His, right and left bundle branches, and the Purkinje fibers.

ing the intraventricular septum. The impulse then spreads out, via the Purkinje fibers, to the left, then the right ventricular myocardium, resulting in ventricular contraction or systole.

Special Electrical Properties of Cardiac Cells

The ability of cells to respond to electrical impulses is referred to as the property of excitability. The ability of the cells to conduct electrical impulses is referred to as the property of conductivity. Cardiac cells possess an ability to generate an impulse to contract even when there is no external nerve stimulus, a process called intrinsic automaticity.

Regulation of Heart Function

The heart's chronotropic state (control of the rate of contraction), dromotropic state (control of the rate of electrical conduction), and inotropic state (control of the strength of contraction) are provided by the brain via the autonomic nervous system, the hormones of the endocrine system, and the heart tissue Table 5-3. Receptors in the blood vessels, kidneys, brain, and heart constantly monitor body functions to help maintain homeostasis. Baroreceptors and chemoreceptors are also involved in regulation of heart function. Baroreceptors respond to changes in pressure, usually within the heart or the main arteries. Chemoreceptors sense changes in the chemical composition of the blood. If either of these types of receptors sense abnormalities, they transmit nerve signals to the appropriate organs. As a result,

TABLE 5-3 Regulation of Heart Function
Chronotropic state = the heart's rate of contraction
Dromotropic state = the heart's rate of conduction
Inotropic state = the heart's strength of contraction

hormones or neurotransmitters are released to correct the situation. The transmission of nerve signals stops when conditions return to normal.

Stimulation of receptors often causes activation of either the parasympathetic or sympathetic branches of the autonomic nervous system, affecting both the heart rate and the strength of heart muscle contraction (contractility). Parasympathetic stimulation slows the heart rate, primarily by affecting the AV node. Sympathetic stimulation has two potential effects, alpha effects or beta effects, depending on which nerve receptor is stimulated (Figure 5-88 ▼). Alpha effects occur when alpha receptors are stimulated, resulting in vasoconstriction. Beta effects occur when beta receptors are stimulated,

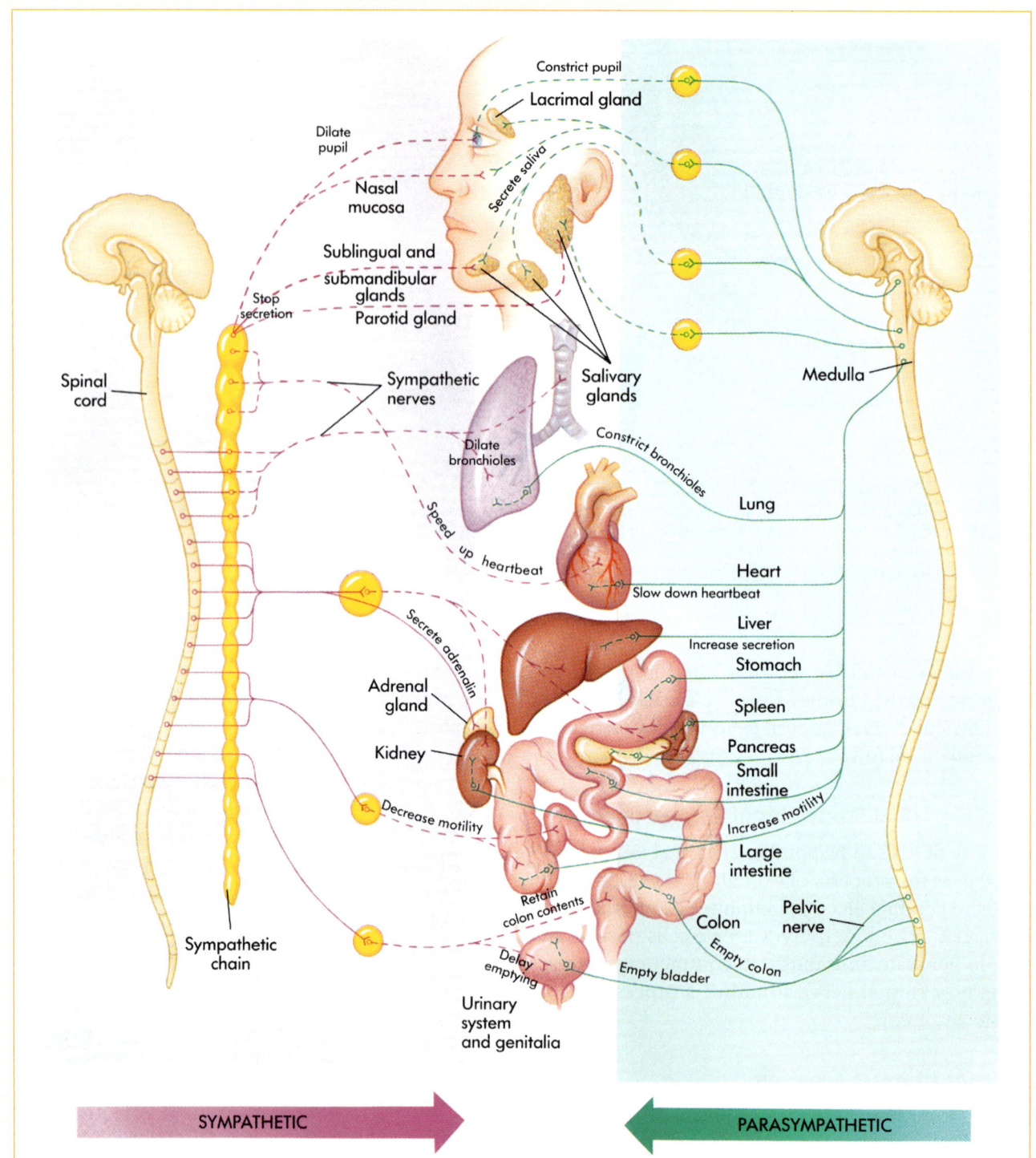

Figure 5-88 The autonomic receptors. Stimulation of the alpha receptors causes vasoconstriction of the organs they affect. Stimulation of beta receptors is split into beta$_1$, which causes increased heart rate and contractility, and beta$_2$, which causes bronchodilation.

resulting in increased inotropic, dromotropic, and chronotropic states.

Epinephrine and norepinephrine, also referred to as catecholamines, are naturally occurring (endogenous) hormones that also may be given as cardiac drugs. Epinephrine has a greater stimulatory effect on beta receptors, and norepinephrine has predominant stimulatory actions on alpha receptors.

The Cardiac Cycle

The process that creates the pumping of the heart is known as the cardiac cycle. This cycle begins with myocardial contraction and concludes at the beginning of the next contraction. The heart's contraction results in pressure changes within the cardiac chambers, resulting in the movement of blood from areas of high pressure to areas of low pressure.

Systole is a term that refers to the contraction of the ventricular mass and the pumping of blood into the systemic circulation. During systole, a pressure is created within the arteries that can be recorded and is known as the systolic blood pressure. A normal systolic blood pressure in an adult is between 110 and 140 mm Hg. A pressure also exists in the vessels during diastole, the relaxation phase of the heart cycle, and is called the diastolic blood pressure. A normal diastolic blood pressure in an adult is between 70 and 90 mm Hg.

Blood pressure is noted as a fraction, and the systolic reading is placed above the diastolic reading (for example, a systolic reading of 140 and a diastolic reading of 70 would be noted as 140/70 mm Hg). The unit of measure mm Hg refers to millimeters of mercury and describes the height, in millimeters, to which the blood pressure elevates a column of liquid mercury in a glass tube. Although many blood pressure measurement devices now use dials, blood pressure is still described in millimeters of mercury.

The pressure in the aorta against which the left ventricle must pump blood is called the afterload. The greater the afterload, the harder it is for the ventricle to eject blood into the aorta, reducing the stroke volume, or the amount of blood ejected per contraction. To a large degree, afterload is governed by arterial blood pressure. Afterload is greater with vasoconstriction and less with vasodilation.

Cardiac output is the amount of blood pumped through the circulatory system in 1 minute. Cardiac output is expressed in liters per minute (L/min). The cardiac output equals the heart rate multiplied by the stroke volume:

Cardiac Output = Stroke Volume × Heart Rate

Factors that influence the heart rate, the stroke volume, or both will affect cardiac output and, thus, oxygen delivery (perfusion) to tissue.

To a point, increased venous return to the heart stretches the ventricles, resulting in increased cardiac contractility. This relationship was first described by the British physiologist Dr Ernest Henry Starling and has become known as Starling's law of the heart.

In a mechanical piston pump, the stroke volume is a fixed quantity related to the distance traveled by the piston. The heart, by contrast, has several ways of increasing stroke volume. To begin with, one of the characteristics of cardiac muscle is that when it is stretched, it contracts with greater force. That property is called the Frank-Starling mechanism, or Starling's law, after the man who first described it. If for any reason an increased volume of blood is returned from the systemic veins to the right heart, or from the pulmonary veins to the left heart, the muscle surrounding the cardiac chambers will have to stretch to accommodate the larger volume; the more the cardiac muscle stretches, the greater will be the force of its contraction, the more completely it will empty, and therefore the greater will be the stroke volume. The amount of blood returning to the right atrium may vary somewhat from minute to minute, but the normal heart continues to pump out the same percentage of blood returned. This is called the ejection fraction.

If we recall our equation:

Cardiac Output = Stroke Volume × Heart Rate

it is clear that any increase in stroke volume, with the heart rate held constant, will cause an increase in the

EMT-I Tips

Starling's Law of the Heart states that primarily the length of the fibers constituting its muscular wall determines the force of the heartbeat. In other words, an increase in diastolic filling increases the force of the contraction.

Terminology Tips

To determine the meaning of the word *pericarditis*, break it down into individual components: *Peri* = around, *card* = heart, *itis* = inflammation. Pericarditis is an inflammation of the *pericardium* (the lining around the heart) that causes severe chest pain.

overall cardiac output. The pressure under which a ventricle fills is called the preload and is influenced by the volume of blood returned by the veins to the heart. In situations of increased oxygen demand, the body returns more blood to the heart (preload increases), and cardiac output therefore increases through the Frank-Starling mechanism. In the diseased heart, the same mechanism is used to achieve a normal resting cardiac output (that is why some diseased hearts become enlarged).

The Vascular System

The General Scheme of Blood Circulation

Blood is transported through the body in the arteries, which carry blood away from the heart, and veins, which carry blood back to the heart. Arteries become smaller as they get farther from the heart. Eventually, they branch into many small arterioles that divide even further into capillaries, which are microscopic, thin-walled blood vessels. Oxygen and nutrients pass out of the capillaries into the cells, and carbon dioxide and waste products pass from the cells into the capillaries in a process called diffusion Figure 5-89 .

Once oxygenated blood has been delivered in the capillaries, deoxygenated blood is returned to the heart, starting from the capillaries. The capillaries eventually enlarge to form venules, which merge together and form veins. Eventually the veins empty into the heart, where blood is reoxygenated and the process begins again Figure 5-90 .

The walls of the blood vessels are composed of three layers of tissue Figure 5-91 . The smooth, thin, inner lining is called the tunica intima, or endothelium. The middle layer, the tunica media, is composed of elastic tissue and smooth muscle cells that allow the vessels to expand or contract in response to changes in blood pressure and tissue demand. It is the thickest of the three tissue layers. The outer layer of tissue is called the tunica adventitia and consists of elastic and fibrous connective tissue.

Circulation to the Heart

The heart, like any other muscle, requires oxygen and nutrients. These are supplied via the coronary arteries, which arise from the aorta shortly after it leaves the left ventricle. The coronary circulation emanates from the left and right coronary arteries Figure 5-92 .

The right coronary artery divides into nine important branches: the conus branch, sinus node branch, right ventricular branch, atrial branch, acute marginal branch, atrioventricular node branch, posterior descending branch, left ventricular branch, and left atrial branch.

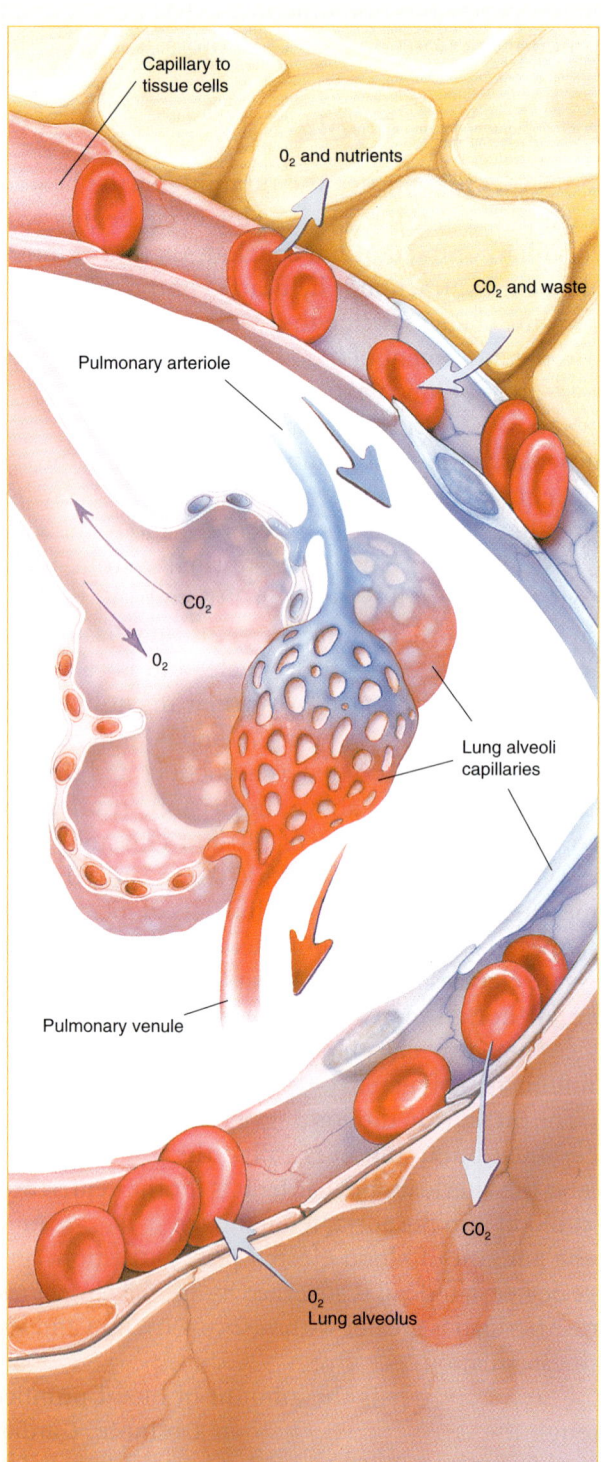

Figure 5-89 Diffusion. Oxygen and nutrients pass easily from the capillaries into the cells, and waste and carbon dioxide pass from the cells into the capillaries.

Not all branches are always present in all people. These branches supply blood to the walls of the right atrium and ventricle, a portion of the inferior part of the left ventricle, and portions of the conduction system (the sinus and AV nodes). When vessels to the conduction system fail to arise from the right coronary artery, they originate from the left side instead.

The left main coronary artery is the largest and shortest of the myocardial blood vessels. It rapidly divides into two branches, the left anterior descending (LAD) and the circumflex coronary arteries. These arteries subdivide further, supplying blood to most of the left ventricle, the intraventricular septum, and, at times, the AV node.

The Pulmonary Circulation

Within the body, the pulmonary circulation carries blood from the right side of the heart to the lungs and back to the left side of the heart, and the systemic circulation is responsible for blood flow throughout the body. Deoxygenated blood from the right ventricle is pumped through the pulmonic valve into the pulmonary artery. This artery rapidly divides into the right and left pulmonary arteries. These arteries transport the blood to the right and left lungs. Inside the lungs, the arteries branch, becoming smaller and smaller. At the level of the capillary, waste products are exchanged and the blood is reoxygenated. The reoxygenated blood travels through venules into the pulmonary veins. The four pulmonary veins empty into the left atrium, two from each lung (see Figure 5-84).

Systemic Arterial Circulation

Oxygenated blood leaves the heart through the aortic valve and passes into the aorta. From the aorta, blood is distributed to all parts of the body. All arteries of the body are derived from the aorta. The aorta is divided into three portions: the ascending aorta, the aortic arch, and the descending aorta.

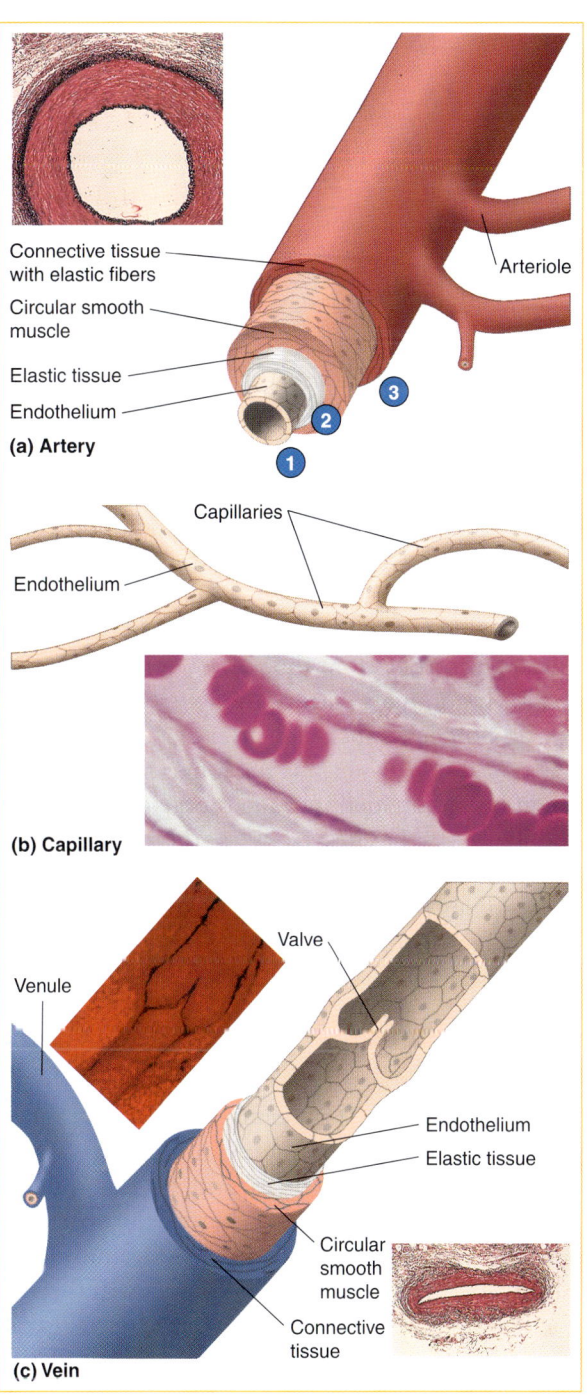

Figure 5-91 The walls of the blood vessels are composed of three layers of tissue: the endothelium, elastic tissue, and the connective tissue. **A.** Artery. **B.** Capillary. **C.** Vein.

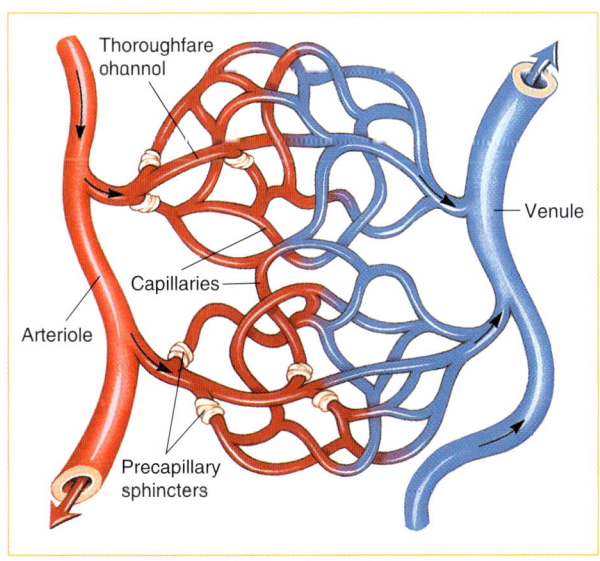

Figure 5-90 The scheme of circulation.

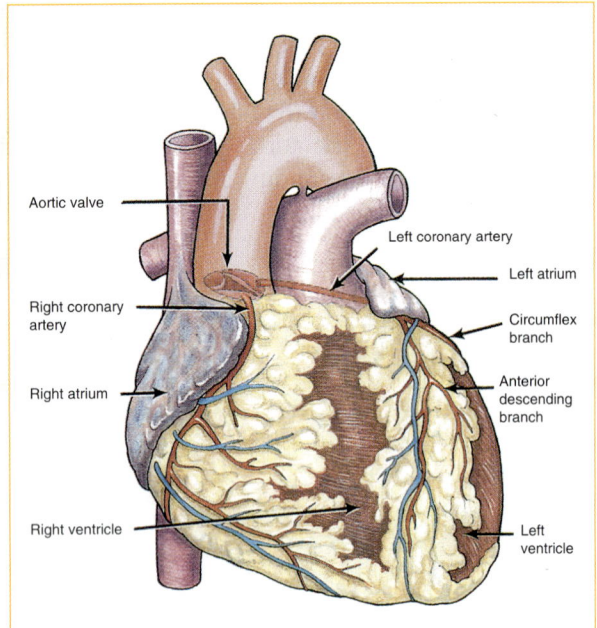

Figure 5-92 The coronary arteries supply oxygen and nutrients to the heart.

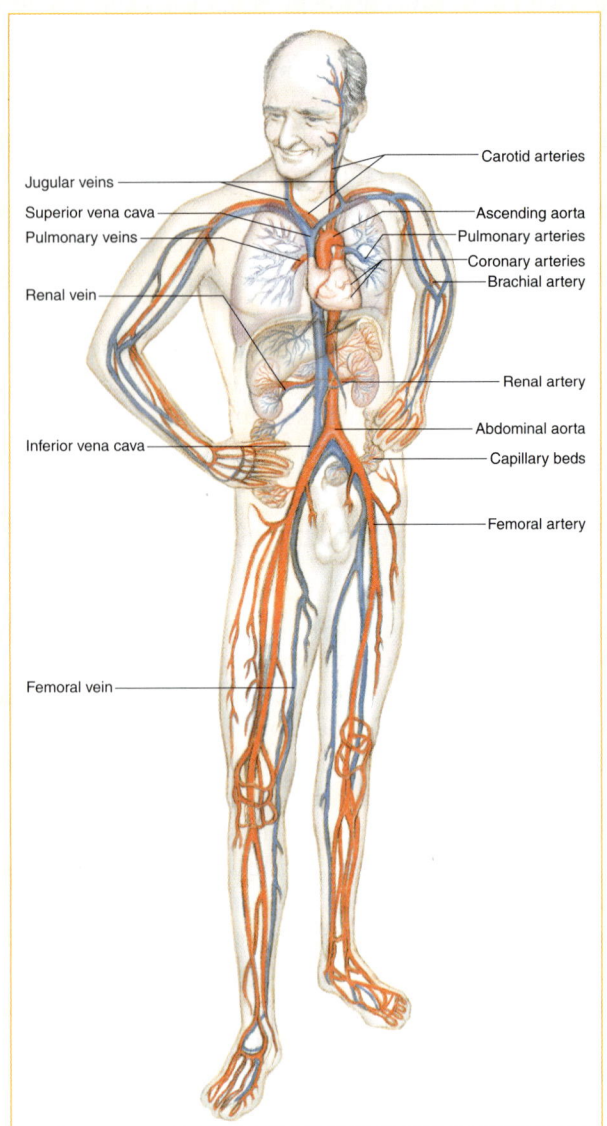

Figure 5-93 The cardiovascular system. The systemic arterial circulation is noted in red, and the systemic venous system is noted in blue.

The <u>ascending aorta</u> arises from the left ventricle and consists of only two branches, the right and left main coronary arteries (Figure 5-93 ▶). The aorta then arches posteriorly and to the left, forming the aortic arch. Three major arteries arise from the <u>aortic arch</u>: the brachiocephalic (innominate) artery, the left common carotid artery, and the left subclavian artery.

The <u>descending aorta</u> is the longest portion of the aorta and is subdivided into the thoracic aorta and the abdominal aorta. The descending aorta extends through the thorax and abdomen into the pelvis. In the pelvis, the descending aorta divides into the two common iliac arteries, which further divide into the internal and external iliac arteries.

The Head and Neck

The brachiocephalic artery is the first vessel to branch from the aortic arch. It is relatively short and rapidly divides into the right common carotid artery and the right subclavian artery. The carotid arteries transport blood to the head and neck, whereas the subclavian arteries transport blood to the upper extremities.

Each common carotid artery branches at the angle of the mandible into the internal and external carotid arteries. This point of division is called the <u>carotid bifurcation</u>. Here, a slight dilatation, the carotid sinus, contains structures that are important in regulating blood pressure. Branches of the external carotid artery supply blood to the face, nose, and mouth. The internal carotid arteries, together with the vertebral arteries (branches of the subclavian arteries), supply blood to the brain (Figure 5-94 ▶).

Circulation to the brain is provided through the vertebral arteries and the internal carotid arteries. The left and right vertebral arteries enter the cranial vault through the foramen magnum. They then unite to form the <u>basilar artery</u>. After branching to the pons (the mass of nerve fibers at the end of the medulla oblongata) and the cerebellum (the part of the brain that is dorsal to the pons and is responsible for coordination and balance), the basilar artery bifurcates into the posterior cerebral arteries. These arteries supply the posterior portion of the brain.

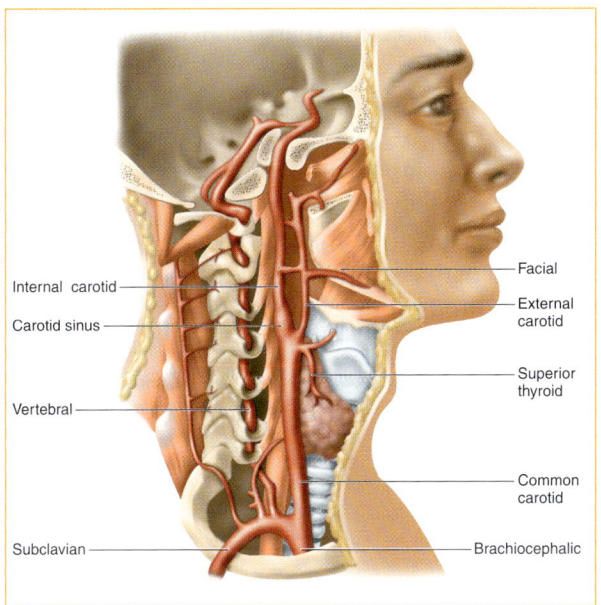

Figure 5-94 The arteries of the head and neck.

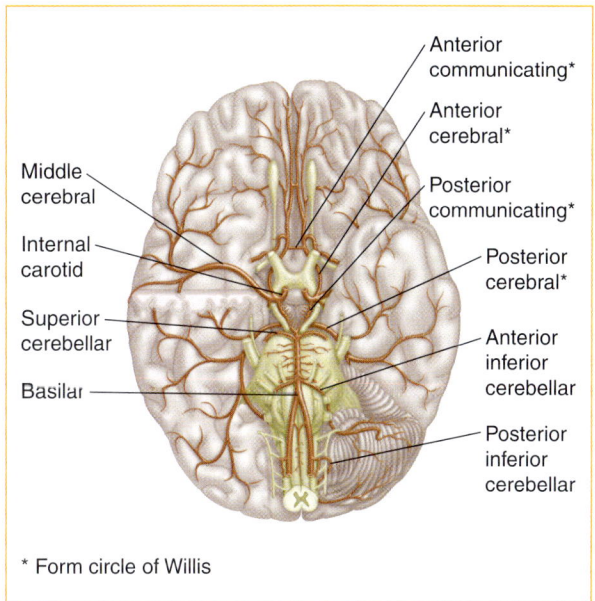

* Form circle of Willis

Figure 5-95 The circulation to the brain.

The carotid arteries enter the cranial vault through the <u>carotid canals</u> and soon give rise to the middle <u>cerebral arteries</u>, which supply blood to large portions of the brain cortex. The middle cerebral arteries give rise to several important branches. The posterior communicating arteries connect with the posterior cerebral arteries. The anterior cerebral arteries interconnect via the anterior communicating artery. This interconnection of arteries forms a collateral network to deliver circulation to the brain, known as the <u>circle of Willis</u> (Figure 5-95 ▶). This helps ensure that circulation to any portion of the brain is not interrupted if a single major artery leading to the brain becomes occluded.

The Upper Extremity

The <u>subclavian artery</u> supplies blood to the brain, neck, anterior chest wall, and shoulder. Shortly after its point of origin, the subclavian artery gives rise to the vertebral arteries. The subclavian system then continues from the thorax into the upper extremity. At the shoulder joint, it becomes the axillary artery, then the <u>brachial artery</u> below the head of the humerus. The transitions from subclavian to axillary to brachial are continuous and not due to branching. The brachial artery divides into the ulnar and radial arteries. These arteries form the two <u>palmar arches</u> of vessels within the hand: the superficial palmar arch and the deep palmar arch. Digital arteries extend from the superficial palmar arch to each digit (Figure 5-96 ▶).

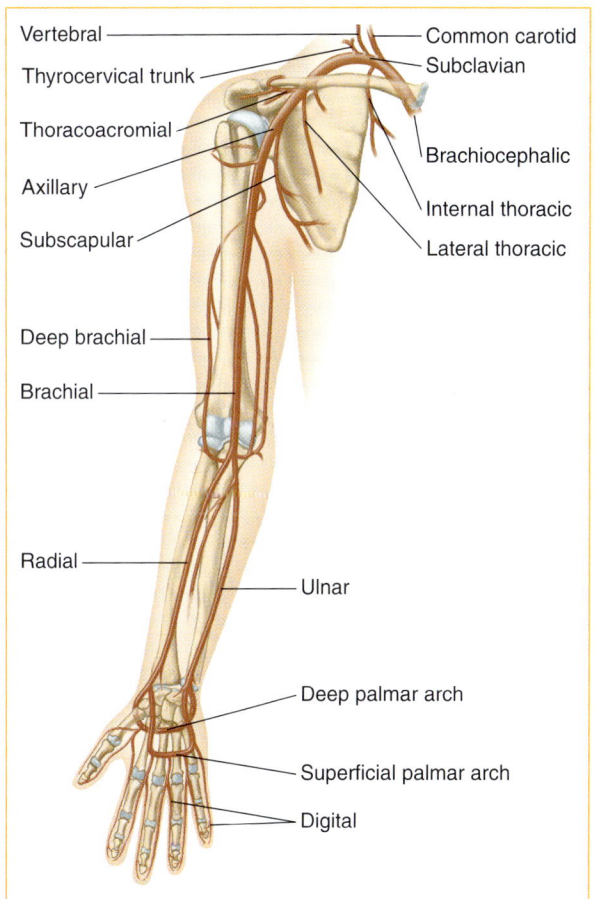

Figure 5-96 The arteries of the upper extremity.

The Thoracic Aorta

Two types of branches of arteries make up the thoracic aorta: the visceral arteries and the parietal arteries. Visceral arteries supply blood to the thoracic organs, and parietal arteries supply blood to the thoracic wall.

Intercostal arteries run along the ribs and provide circulation to the chest wall. Intercostal arteries branch into anterior and posterior intercostal arteries. The anterior intercostal arteries originate as branches of the subclavian system. The posterior intercostal arteries arise directly from the aorta. Visceral branches of the thoracic aorta supply the bronchial arteries in the lungs and the esophageal arteries (Figure 5-97).

The Abdominal Aorta

Like their thoracic counterpart, branches of the abdominal aorta are divided into visceral and parietal portions. The visceral arteries are subdivided into paired and nonpaired arteries. The three major unpaired branches of the abdominal aorta's visceral arteries include the celiac trunk, the superior mesenteric, and the inferior mesenteric arteries (Figure 5-98). The celiac trunk supplies blood to the esophagus, stomach, duodenum, spleen, liver, and pancreas (Figure 5-99). The superior mesenteric artery and its branches supply blood to the pancreas, small intestine, and colon. The inferior mesenteric artery and its

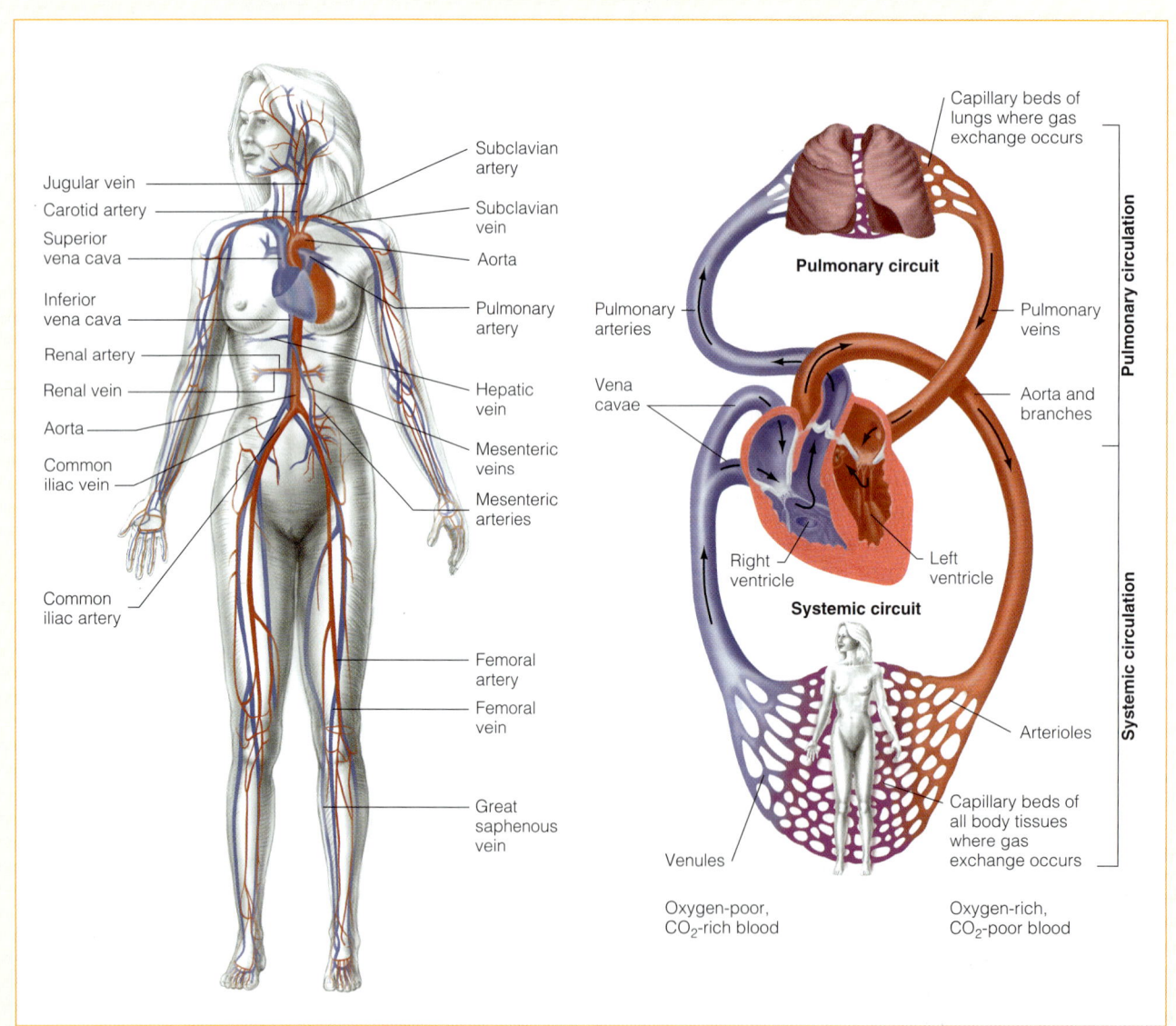

Figure 5-97 Systemic circulation rising from the aorta.

branches supply blood to the descending colon and rectum. Paired branches of the visceral abdominal aorta supply blood to the kidneys, adrenal gland, and gonads. The parietal branches supply blood to the diaphragm and abdominal wall.

The Pelvis and Lower Extremity

At the level of the fifth lumbar vertebra, the aorta divides into the two common iliac arteries. These arteries further divide into the internal iliac arteries, which supply blood to the pelvis, and the external iliac arteries, which enter the lower extremity (Figure 5-100 ▶). The internal iliac artery sends out visceral branches to the rectum, vagina, uterus, and ovary. Parietal branches supply blood to the sacrum, gluteal muscles of the buttocks region, the pubic region, rectum, external genitalia, and proximal thigh.

Like the upper extremity, the vessels of the lower extremity form a continuum. The external iliac arteries become the femoral arteries. Each femoral artery supplies blood to the thigh, external genitalia, anterior abdominal wall, and knee. The femoral artery becomes the popliteal artery in the lower thigh. Each popliteal artery then trifurcates, branching into anterior and posterior tibial and peroneal arteries. At the foot, the anterior tibial artery becomes the dorsalis pedis artery. Plantar arteries arise from the posterior tibial artery and subdivide into digital branches that supply blood to the toes (Figure 5-101 ▶).

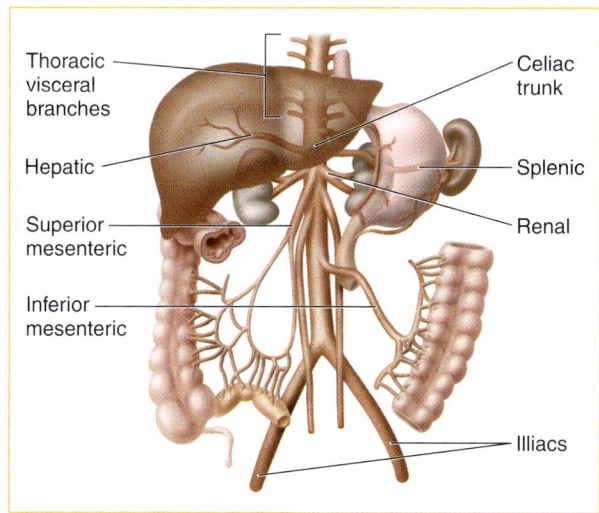

Figure 5-98 The branches of the abdominal aorta.

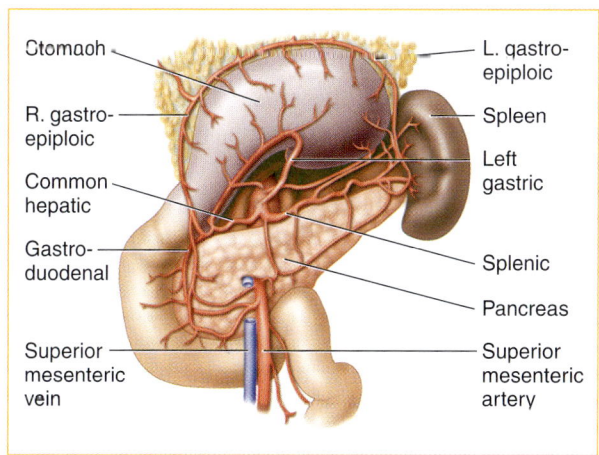

Figure 5-99 The celiac trunk and superior mesenteric vessels.

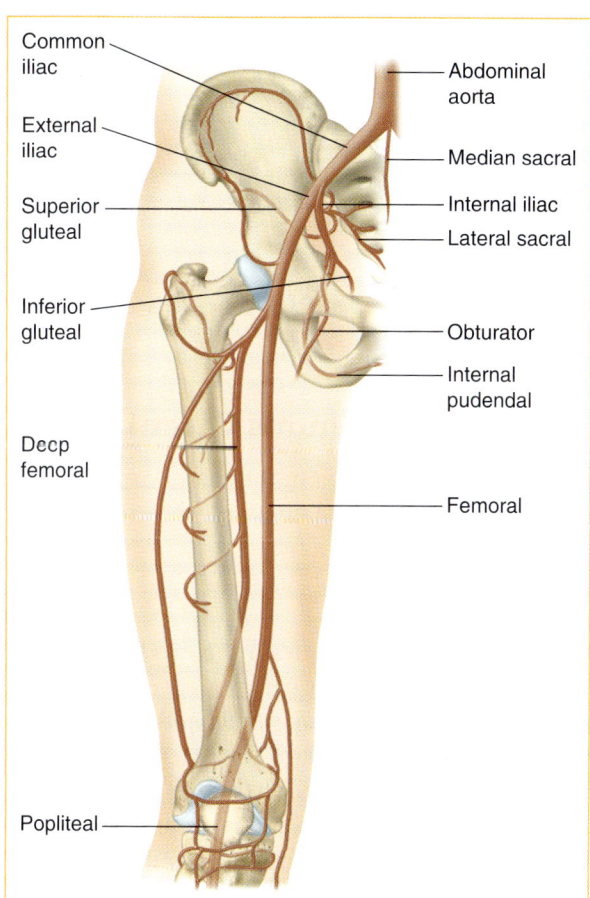

Figure 5-100 The arteries of the pelvis and thigh.

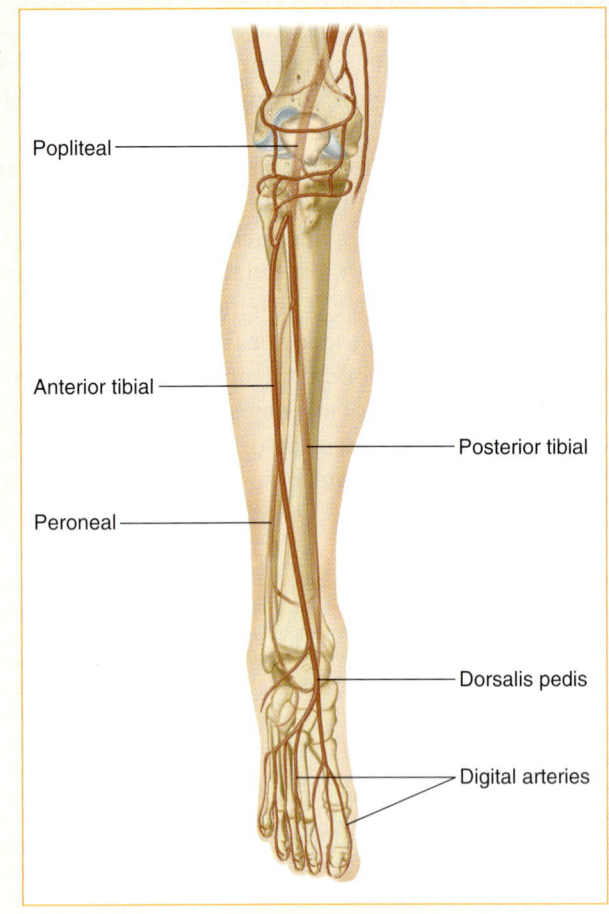

Figure 5-101 The arteries of the lower extremity.

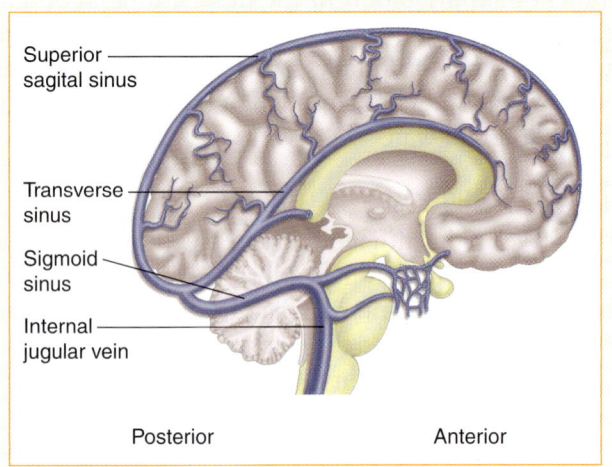

Figure 5-102 Venous drainage of the brain.

The Systemic Venous Circulation

As a rule, veins accompany the major arteries. Many veins have the same names as the arteries they accompany.

The Head and Neck

The two major veins that drain the head and neck are called the external and internal jugular veins. The external jugular vein is more superficial and often is visible immediately beneath the skin. The external jugular vein primarily drains the posterior head and neck. The internal jugular vein drains the cranial vault as well as the anterior portion of the head, face, and neck. Spaces between membranes surrounding the brain form venous sinuses. These sinuses are the primary means of venous drainage from the brain and feed into the internal jugular vein (Figure 5-102 ▶).

The external and internal jugular veins join the subclavian veins (the proximal part of the main vein of the arm) (Figure 5-103 ▶) to form the brachiocephalic veins, which drain into the superior vena cava.

The Upper Extremity

The veins of the upper extremity vary somewhat from individual to individual (Figure 5-104 ▶). The names of the veins of the hands, wrists, and forearm follow the arteries of the same name. In the upper forearm, these veins combine to form the basilic vein and the cephalic vein, the major veins of the arm. The basilic and cephalic veins combine to form the axillary vein, which drains into the subclavian vein.

The Thorax

In the thorax, venous drainage begins at the anterior and posterior intercostal veins. The intercostal veins empty into the azygos vein on the right side of the thorax and the hemiazygos vein on the left. These veins, along with the right and left brachiocephalic veins, provide the major source of flow into the superior vena cava.

The Abdomen and Pelvis

Ultimately, all venous drainage from the lower part of the body passes through the inferior vena cava. The inferior vena cava returns deoxygenated blood from the lower parts of the body to the right atrium for oxygenation. Within the abdominal and pelvic cavities, veins of the same name accompany the major arteries,

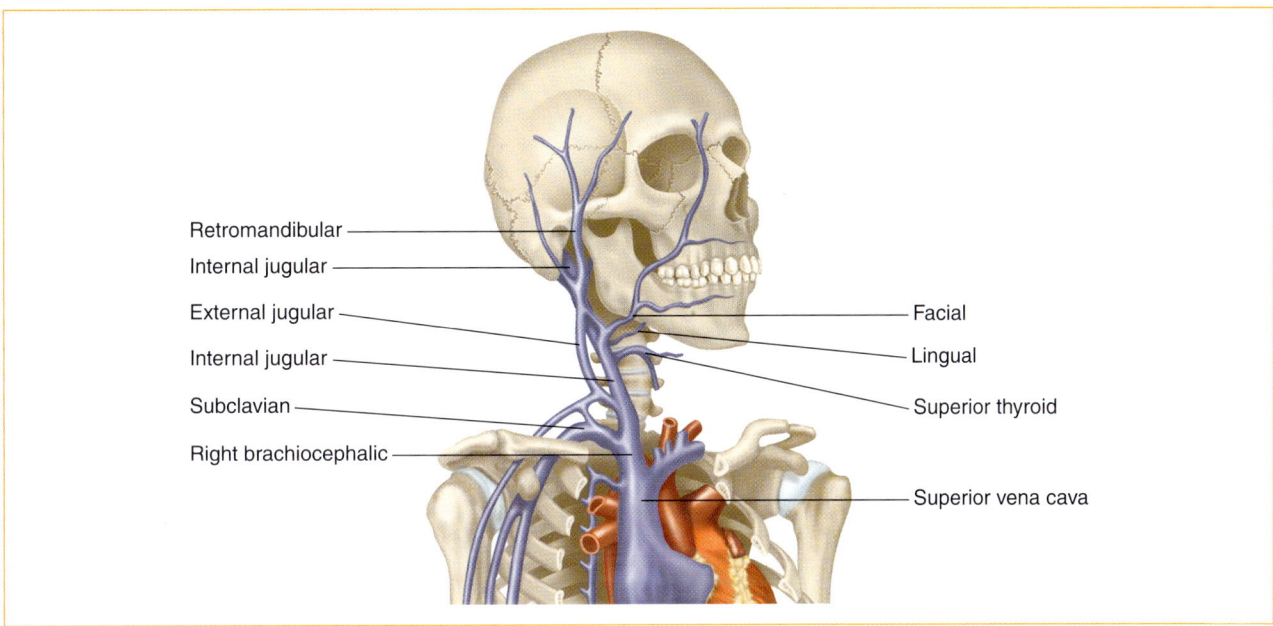

Figure 5-103 The veins of the head and neck.

providing venous drainage from structures including the kidney, adrenal glands, gonads, and diaphragm. The internal iliac veins drain the pelvis, and the external iliac veins drain the lower limbs. The internal and external iliac veins combine together in the pelvis, forming the common iliac veins, which combine to form the inferior vena cava.

The hepatic portal system is a specialized part of the venous system that drains blood from the liver, stomach, intestines, and spleen (Figure 5-105 ▶). Blood from the system flows first through the liver, where blood collects in sinusoids. In the sinusoids, the liver extracts nutrients, filters the blood, and metabolizes various drugs. The blood then empties into the hepatic veins, which join the inferior vena cava.

The Lower Extremity

The longest vein in the body is the great saphenous vein. It drains the foot, leg, and thigh. The saphenous vein originates over the dorsal and medial side of the foot, ascends along the medial side of the leg and thigh, and empties into the femoral vein, which then drains into the external iliac vein. Laterally, the small saphenous vein helps drain the leg and lateral side of the foot. The veins of the feet also drain into the anterior and posterior tibial veins, which accompany their respective arteries, uniting at the knee to form the popliteal vein. The popliteal vein ascends through the thigh, becoming the femoral vein (Figure 5-106 ▶).

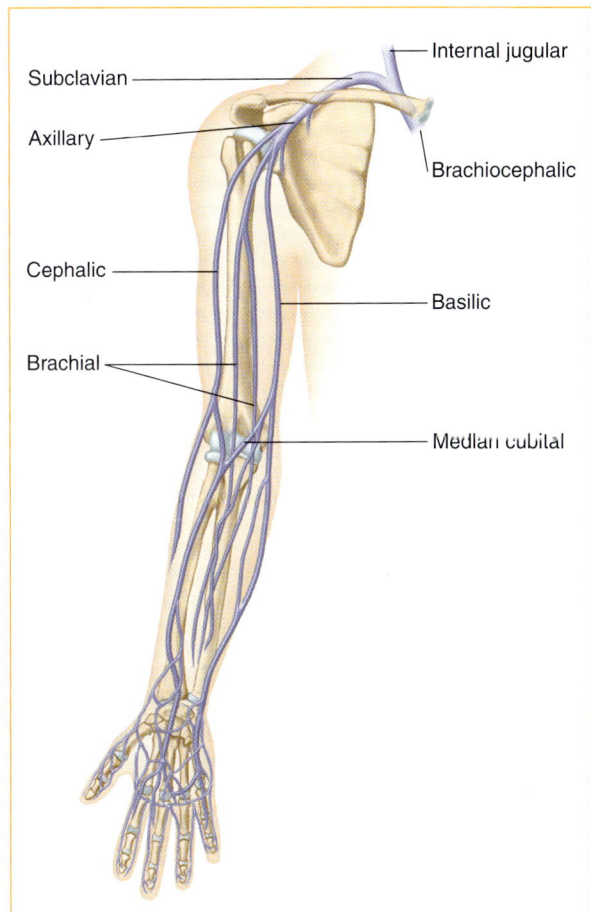

Figure 5-104 The veins of the upper extremity.

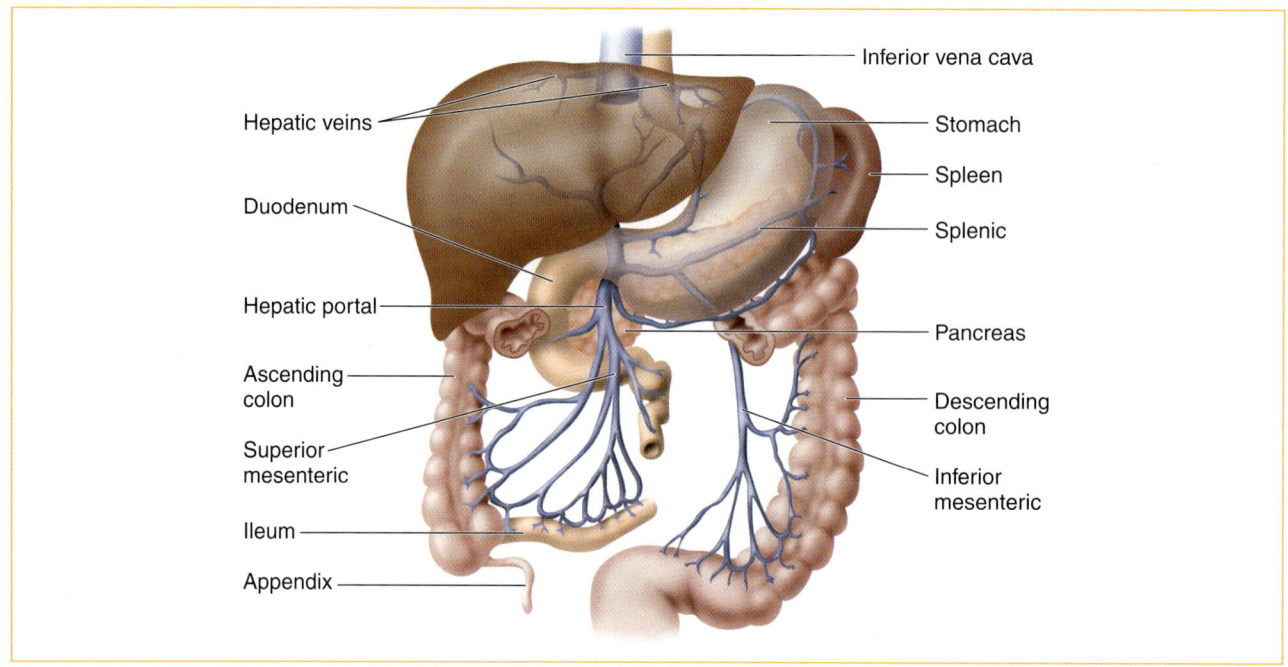

Figure 5-105 The hepatic portal system.

Physiology of the Circulatory System

The pulse, which is palpated most easily at the neck, wrist, or groin, is created by the forceful pumping of blood out the left ventricle and into the major arteries. It is present throughout the entire arterial system. It can be felt most easily where the larger arteries are near the skin. The central pulses are the carotid artery pulse, which can be felt at the upper portion of the neck, and the femoral artery pulse, which is felt in the groin. The peripheral pulses are the radial artery pulse, which is felt at the wrist at the base of the thumb; the brachial artery pulse, which is felt on the medial aspect of the arm, midway between the elbow and shoulder; the posterior tibial artery pulse, which is felt posterior to the medial

You are the Provider — Part 9

Your treatment of the fourth patient included 100% oxygen and an IV of normal saline. Your assessment of this patient's vital signs reveals the following:

Vital Signs	Recording Time: 2 Minutes After Patient Contact
Respirations	24 breaths/min, adequate depth
Pulse	110 beats/min, regular
Blood pressure	102/70 mm Hg
Sao$_2$	96% on 15 L/min of O$_2$ via nonrebreathing mask

13. Body fluid is divided into two main compartments. What are they and where are they found?

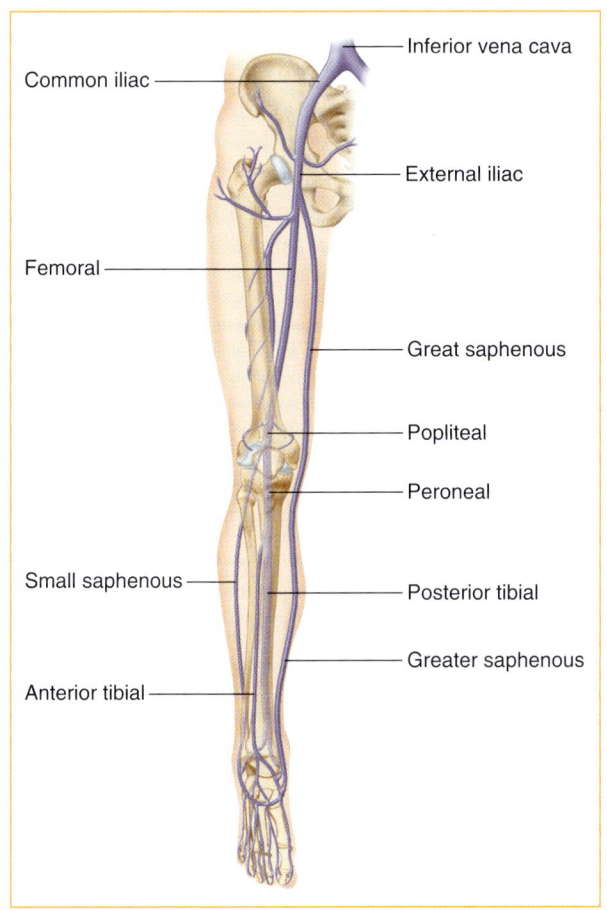

Figure 5-106 The veins of the lower extremity.

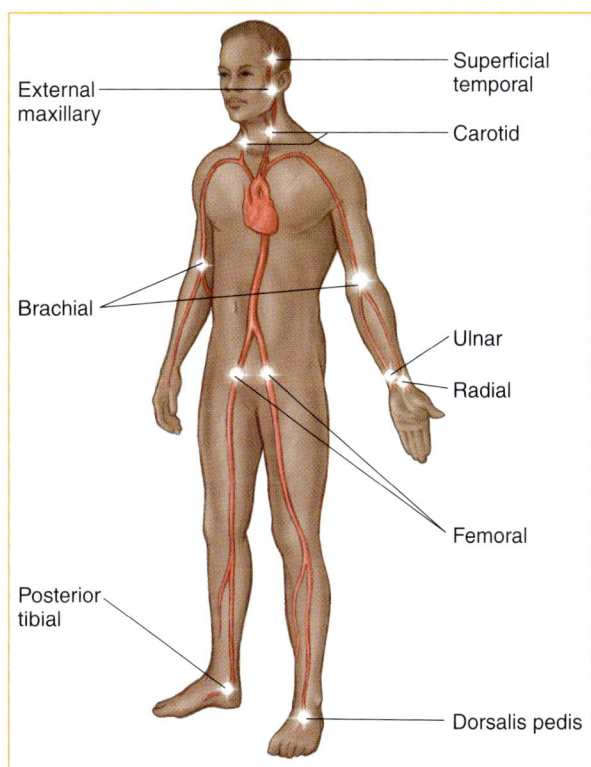

Figure 5-107 The central and peripheral pulses can be felt where the large arteries are near the skin.

malleolus; and the dorsalis pedis artery pulse, which is felt on the top of the foot (Figure 5-107).

Blood pressure is the pressure that the blood exerts against the walls of the arteries as it passes through them. When the left ventricle contracts, it pumps blood from the ventricle into the aorta. This muscular contraction phase is called systole. When the muscle of the ventricle relaxes, the ventricle fills with blood. This phase is called diastole. The pulsed forceful ejection of blood from the left ventricle of the heart into the aorta is transmitted through the arteries as a pulsatile pressure wave. This pressure wave keeps the blood moving through the body. The high and low points of the wave can be measured with a sphygmomanometer (blood pressure cuff) and are expressed numerically in millimeters of mercury (mm Hg). The high point is called the systolic blood pressure (measured as the heart muscle is contracting). The low point is called the diastolic blood pressure (measured when the heart muscle is in its relaxation phase).

The average adult has approximately 5 L of blood in the vascular system. Children have less, 2 to 3 L, depending on their age and size. Infants have only about 300 mL. The loss of an amount of blood that may be negligible for an adult could be fatal for an infant.

Normal Circulation in Adults

In all healthy people, the circulatory system is automatically adjusted and readjusted constantly so that 100% of the capacity of the arteries, veins, and capillaries holds 100% of the blood at that moment. Never are all the vessels fully dilated or constricted. The size of arteries and veins is controlled by the nervous system, according to the amount of blood that is available and many other factors to keep blood pressure normal at all times. Under the condition of normal pressure, with a system that can hold just 100% of the blood available, all parts of the system will have adequate blood supply all of the time.

Perfusion is the circulation of blood within an organ or tissue in adequate amounts to meet the cells' current needs. Blood enters an organ or tissue through the arteries and leaves it through the veins Figure 5-108 ▼. Loss of normal blood pressure is an indication that the blood is no longer circulating efficiently to every organ in the body. There are many reasons for loss of blood pressure. The result in each case is the same: Organs, tissues, and cells are no longer adequately perfused or supplied with oxygen and food, and wastes can accumulate. Under these conditions, cells, tissues, and whole organs may die. The state of inadequate circulation, when it involves the entire body, is called shock or hypoperfusion.

Inadequate Circulation in Adults

When a patient loses a small amount of blood, the arteries, veins, and heart automatically adjust to the smaller new volume. The adjustment occurs in an effort to maintain adequate pressure throughout the circulatory system and thereby maintain circulation for every organ.

The adjustment occurs very rapidly after the loss, usually within minutes. Specifically, the vessels constrict to provide a smaller bed for the reduced volume of blood to fill. And the heart pumps more rapidly to circulate the remaining blood more efficiently. As the blood pressure falls, the pulse increases to attempt to keep the cardiac output constant at 5 to 6 L per minute. If the loss of blood is too great, the adjustment fails, and the patient goes into shock.

> **EMT-I Tips**
>
> If a patient is bleeding or severely dehydrated, baroreceptors sense the abnormally low volume. Although several different body responses occur at once, a major response is the release of epinephrine and norepinephrine for the adrenal glands, causing sympathetic (adrenergic) stimulation, resulting in an increased heart rate, as well as increased myocardial contractility.

The Lymphatic System

The lymphatic system transports lymph by passive circulation. Lymph is a thin plasma-like fluid formed from interstitial or extracellular fluid that bathes the tissues of the body. Lymphatic capillaries pick up the lymph and drain it into larger vessels. Lymph circulates through the body in thin-walled lymph vessels that travel close to the major arteries and veins. Like veins, lymphatic vessels contain valves that limit backflow. Foreign material such as debris or bacteria is filtered from the lymph in the lymph nodes, round or bean-shaped structures that are interspersed along the course of the lymph vessels, and returns to the main circulatory system via the thoracic duct, one of two great lymph vessels, which empties into the junction of the left subclavian vein and the left internal jugular vein Figure 5-109 ▶. The lymphatic system helps absorb fat from the digestive tract, maintain fluid balance in the body, and fight infection.

Lymphatic Vessels

Lymphatic vessels only carry fluid away from the tissues. In the lymphatic capillaries, the epithelial cells contain one-way valves that allow fluid to enter the vessel but prevent it from flowing back into the tissues.

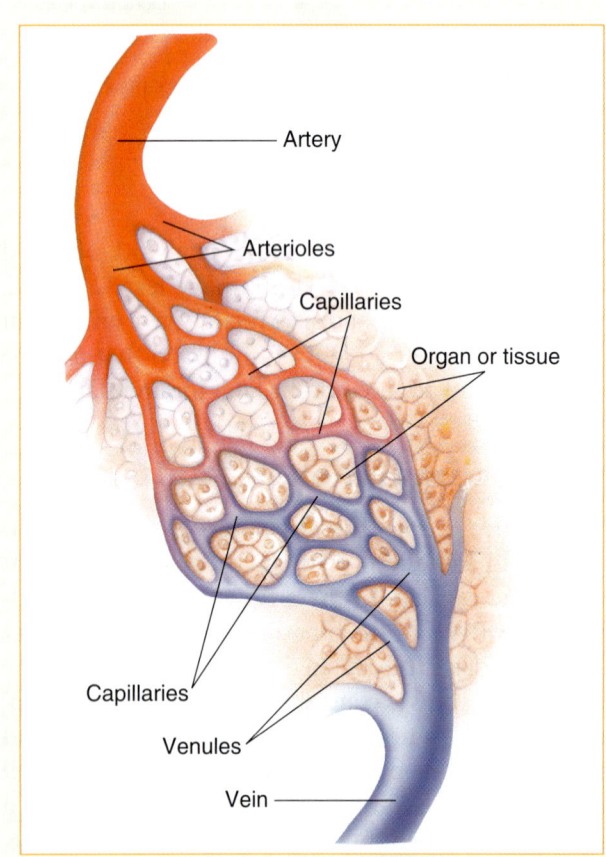

Figure 5-108 Blood enters an organ or tissue through the arteries and leaves through the veins. This process, called perfusion, provides adequate blood flow to the tissue to meet the cells' needs.

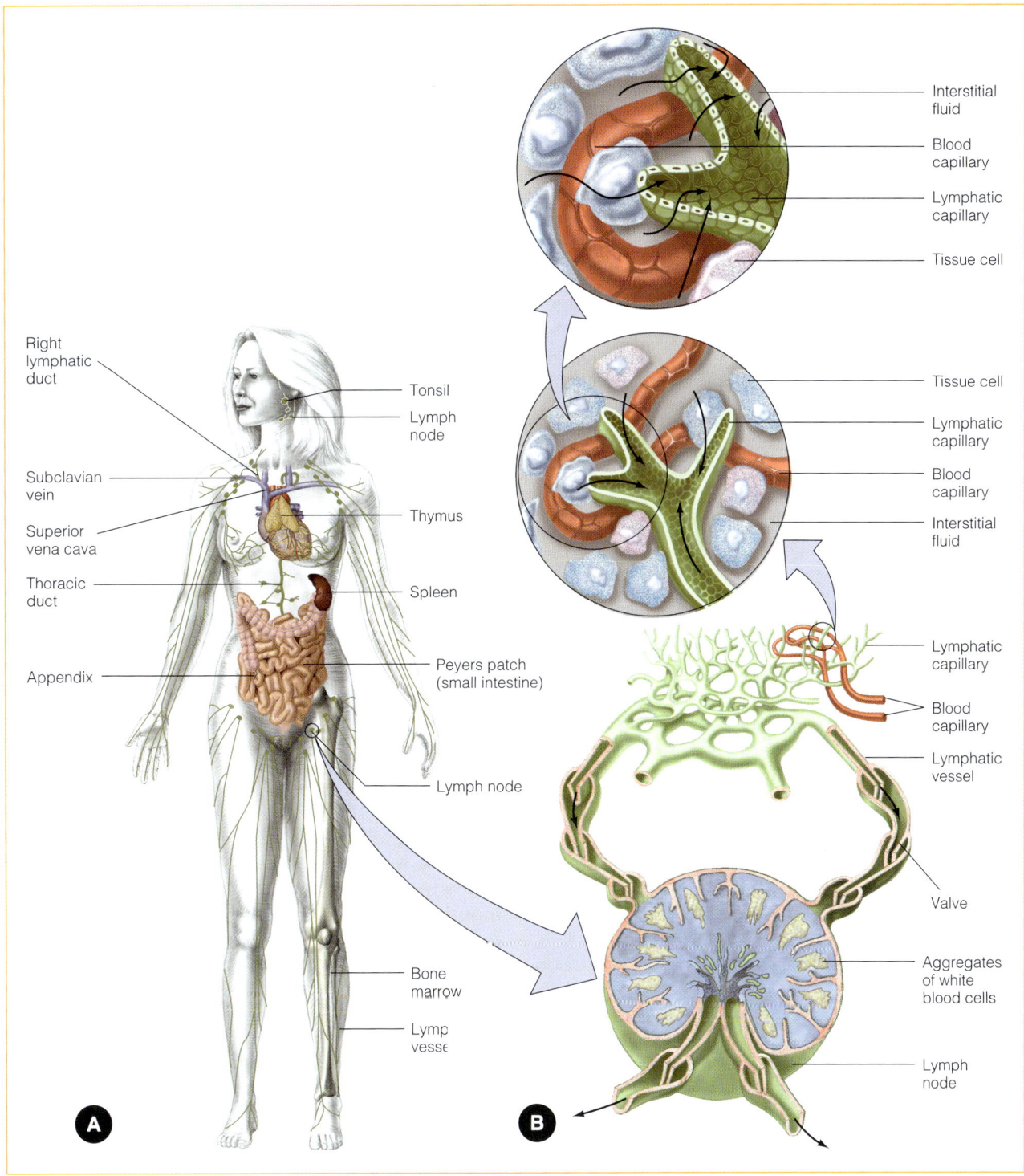

Figure 5-109 The lymphatic system. **A.** The lymphatic system consists of vessels that transport lymph back to the circulatory system. **B.** Lymph nodes interspersed along the vessels filter the lymph.

Lymphatic capillaries are present in all tissues except the central nervous system, bone marrow, cartilage, epidermis, and cornea. Generally, fluid flows from the blood capillaries to the tissues, then out of the tissue spaces into lymph capillaries. In the major blood capillary beds of the body, the internal hydrostatic "water" pressure allows a normal and continuous leak of a total of 3 to 4 mL/min of fluid into the interstitial spaces. To prevent the tissues from becoming edematous, the lymphatic vessel must absorb this excess fluid and return it to the central venous circulation (Figure 5-110).

Much like veins, lymph capillaries join to form larger lymph vessels. Lymph vessels tend to follow with the course of an associated artery and vein. Valves prevent backflow through these vessels when the lymph vessels are compressed. Muscle movements, as well as changes in the intrathoracic pressure during breathing, cause compression of the lymph vessels. Eventually, the lymphatic vessels empty into either the right or left subclavian vein. Vessels from the right upper extremity and right side of the head and neck enter via the lymphatic duct, the second of the great lymph vessels in the body, which empties into the junction of the right subclavian vein and the right internal jugular vein. Vessels from the remaining parts of the body enter the thoracic duct. Lymph vessels pass through at least one lymph node before entering the bloodstream, where lymphocytes normally filter the lymph. Lymphocytes are a type of white blood cell that helps fight infection and provide immunity to certain types of infection.

Lymph Organs

Diffuse lymphatic tissue is tissue with no clear boundary that blends with surrounding tissues and contains lymphocytes and other cells. Denser arrangements of lymphoid tissue are called lymph nodules and are found in the loose connective tissue of the digestive, respiratory, and urinary systems. They also are found in lymph nodes and the spleen. A protective membrane called the capsule surrounds each lymph node. Major collections of lymph nodes are located in the axilla (axillary nodes), neck (cervical nodes), and groin (inguinal nodes).

Three sets of lymphatic organs comprise the tonsils: the palatine tonsils, the pharyngeal tonsils (adenoids), and the lingual tonsils. The tonsils are located in the back of the throat and nasopharynx and protect the body from bacteria introduced through the nose and mouth. In most adults, the tonsils have decreased in size since childhood; in some, they have actually disappeared.

The palatine tonsils are located in the back of the throat, on each side of the posterior opening of the oral cavity. The pharyngeal tonsils (or adenoids) are located near the internal opening of the nasal cavity. The lingual tonsils are located on the posterior margin of the tongue (Figure 5-111).

The spleen is located in the left upper quadrant of the abdomen and consists of two types of lymph tissue: red pulp and white pulp. The red pulp is associated with the venous drainage of the spleen; the white pulp is associated with arterial drainage. Virtually all of the blood in the body transverses the splenic tissue, where it is filtered and worn out blood cells, foreign substances, and bacteria are removed.

The thymus is a triangular-shaped gland located below the sternum in the superior mediastinum. It is

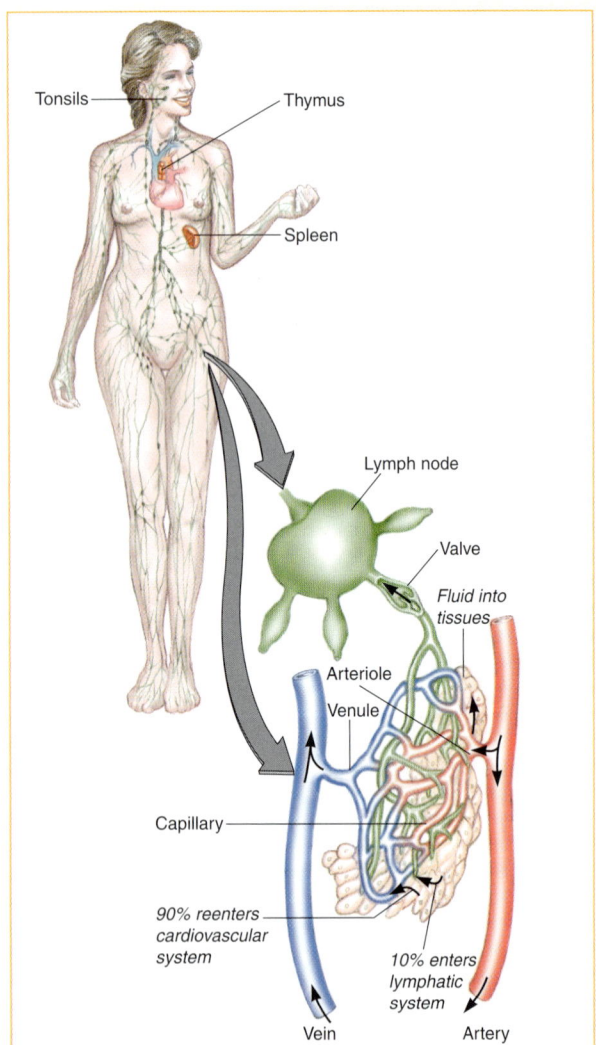

Figure 5-110 The lymphatic vessel. The enlarged diagram of a lymph node and vessels shows the path of the excess fluid that leaves the capillary, enters the adjacent tissue spaces, and is absorbed by lymphatic capillaries.

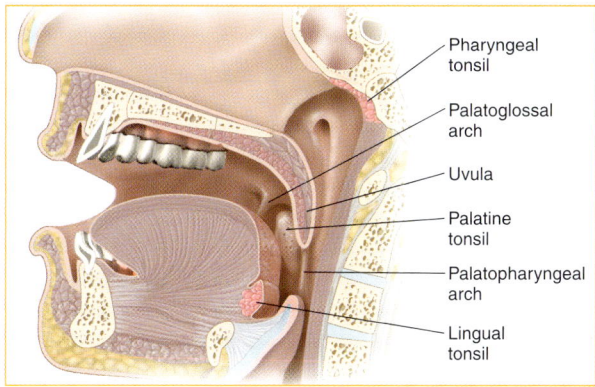

Figure 5-111 The tonsils.

The Respiratory System

The respiratory system is associated with breathing, gas exchange, and the entrance of air into the body. The organs and structures in the respiratory system are divided into the upper and lower airways. The upper airway includes the mouth, nasal cavity, and oral cavity, and the lower airway includes the larynx, trachea, bronchi, bronchioles, and alveoli.

The Upper Airway

A human can breathe air into the body through either the nose, also called the nasal cavity or nasopharynx, or through the mouth, also called the oral cavity or oropharynx. The nasopharynx and oropharynx connect posteriorly to form a cavity called the pharynx Figure 5-112 ▼.

The nasopharynx extends from the internal nares to the uvula (a small fleshy mass that hangs from the soft palate). The oropharynx extends from the uvula to the

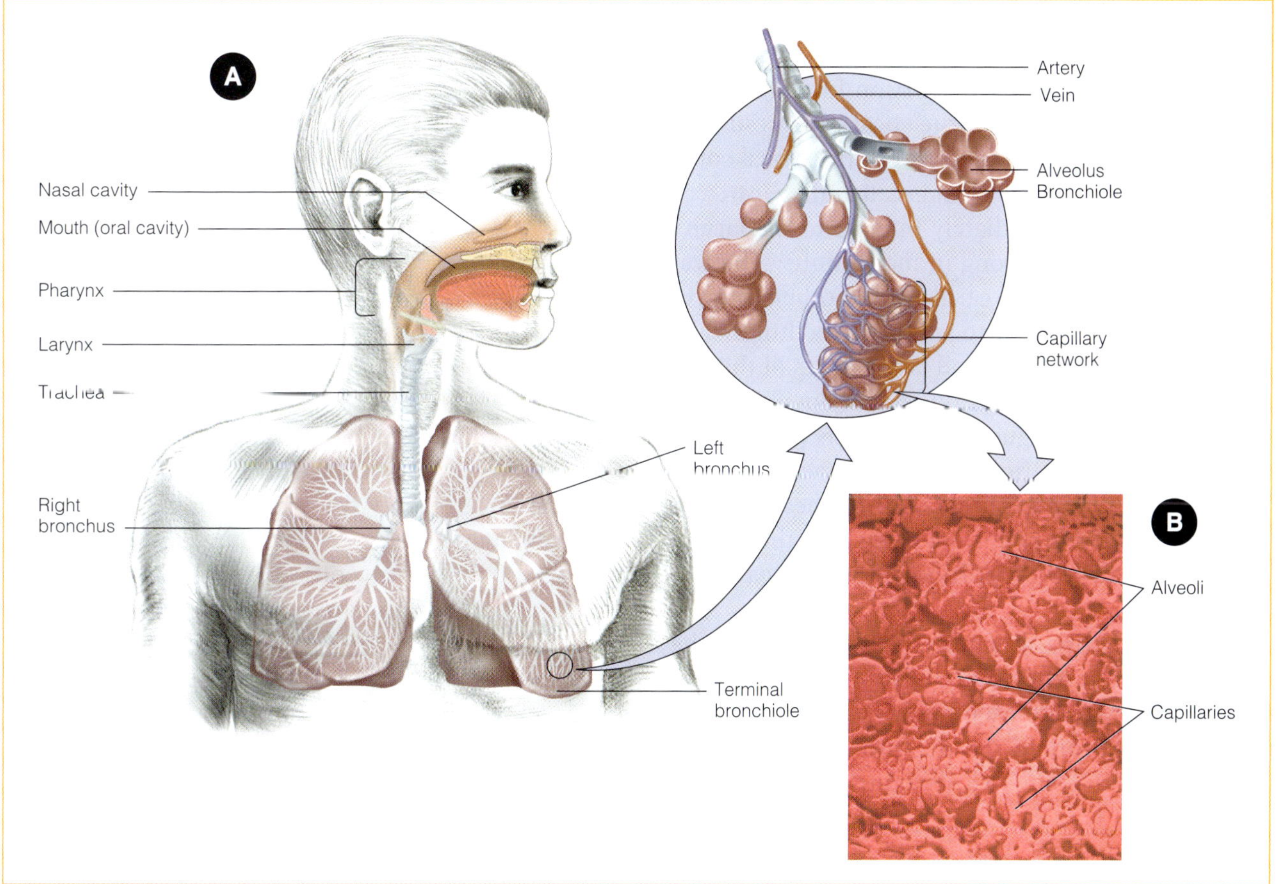

quite large in the infant and decreases in size with age. Often, there is no discernible thymic tissue in older adults. The thymus produces lymphocytes, which move to other lymph tissues to help fight infection. The thymus plays a major role in immunity, especially in early life.

Figure 5-112 The respiratory system. **A.** The upper and lower airway divisions of the respiratory system. The insert shows a higher magnification of the alveoli, where oxygen and carbon dioxide exchange occurs. **B.** A scanning electron micrograph of the alveoli, showing the rich capillary network surrounding them.

epiglottis, the thin plate of cartilage that closes over the glottic opening during swallowing. Inferiorly, the pharynx leads to the separate openings of the respiratory system (larynx) and the digestive system (esophagus).

The external openings of the nasopharynx are the external nares or nostrils. The interior nares comprise the posterior opening from the nasopharynx into the pharynx. The nasal septum separates the nasopharynx into two parts. The floor of the nasal cavity is the hard palate. The lateral walls of the nasopharynx contain three bony ridges, the conchae. Together, the conchae form a set of bony convolutions, called the turbinates, which help to maintain laminar (smooth) airflow. Below each turbinate is a passageway called a meatus. Each meatus contains the drainage opening from the sinus and the nasolacrimal ducts (the ducts that drain tears from the lacrimal sac).

The Lower Airway

The beginning of the lower airway, the larynx, consists of several sections of cartilage held together by ligaments (Figure 5-113). The larynx includes two pairs of ligaments that form the vocal cords. The superior portion of the vocal cords forms the vestibular folds, or false vocal cords; the inferior portion forms the true vocal cords. Vibration of the true vocal cords results in production of sounds and speech. The true vocal cords plus the opening between them is called the glottis.

The trachea is immediately inferior to the larynx and is approximately 4" long in most adults. The trachea is a tube made up of cartilage and other connective tissue and conveys air to and from the lungs. The cartilage forms the anterior and lateral sides of the trachea, providing both protection and an open passageway for air. The esophagus is immediately posterior to the cartilage-free posterior wall of the trachea. At the level of the fifth thoracic vertebra, the trachea branches into the right and left mainstem bronchi at the carina, a projection of the lowest portion of the tracheal cartilage (Figure 5-114).

Beyond the carina, air enters the lungs through the mainstem bronchi. The point of entry for the bronchi, vessels, and nerves into each lung is called the hilum. The mainstem bronchi divide into the secondary bronchi, each one going to a separate lobe of the lung (see Figure 5-114).

Secondary bronchi branch into tertiary bronchi, which continue to branch several times. After several generations of successive branching, bronchioles, very small subdivisions of the bronchi, are formed. Respiratory bronchioles develop from the final branching

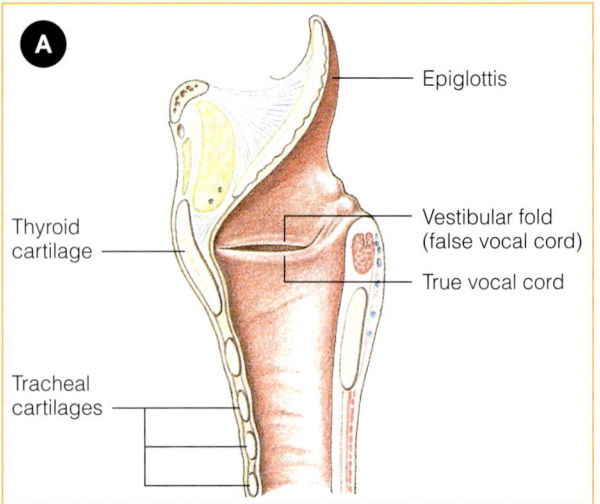
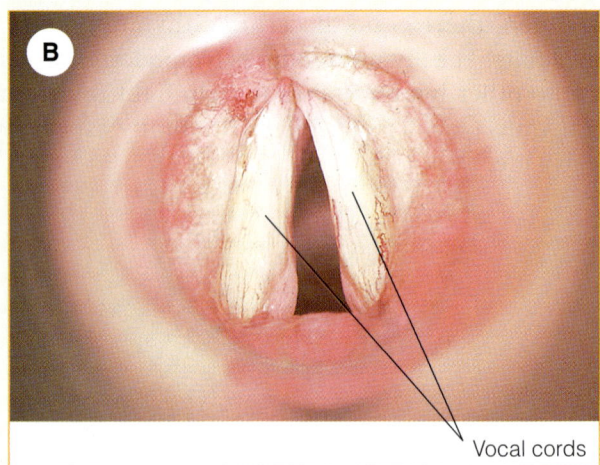

Figure 5-113 The larynx. **A.** Longitudinal section of the larynx showing the location of the vocal cords. Note the presence of the false vocal cord. **B.** View into the larynx showing the true vocal cords from above.

of the bronchiole. Each respiratory bronchiole divides to form alveolar ducts. Each alveolar duct ends in clusters known as alveoli, tiny sacs of lung tissue in which gas exchange takes place. The lung contains approximately 300 million alveoli; each alveolus is about 0.33 mm in diameter. Capillaries cover the alveoli. The alveolocapillary membrane lies between the alveolus and the capillary and is very thin, consisting of only one cell layer. Respiratory exchange between the lung and blood vessels occurs in the alveoli at the alveolocapillary membrane.

The lungs are the primary organs of breathing. The right lung contains three lobes (the upper, middle, and lower lobes); the left lung contains only two (the upper and lower lobes). In the left lung, a portion known as the lingula forms the equivalent of the middle lobe in the right lung. The lungs are surrounded by a mem-

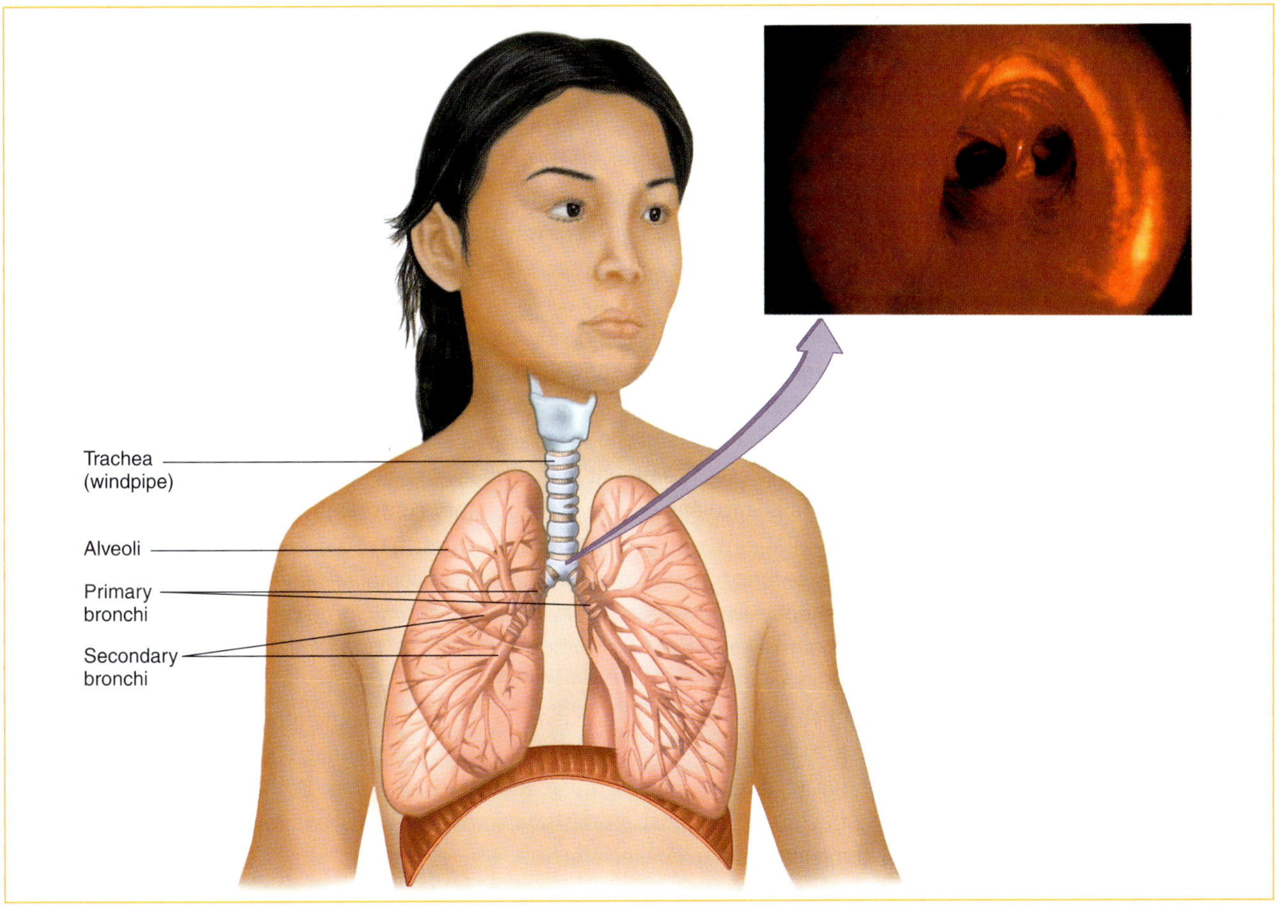

Figure 5-114 The mainstem bronchi. The upper insert shows the bifurcation of the trachea at the carina into the right and left mainstem bronchi.

brane of connective tissue known as pleura. Another pleural membrane lines the inner borders of the rib cage, or pleural cavity.

The pleural membrane that covers the lungs is referred to as the visceral pleura, and the pleural membrane that lines the pleural cavity is the parietal pleura. A potential space known as the pleural space exists between the visceral and parietal pleura. Normally, the two membranes are close together and a space does not exist. Both layers of pleura work together to help maintain normal expansion and contraction of the lung. Under certain disease conditions or following trauma, fluid and/or air may accumulate in the pleural space, resulting in hemothorax (a collection of blood in the pleural space) or hemopneumothorax (a collection of blood and air in the pleural space), potentially causing respiratory problems Figure 5-115 ▶.

The lungs receive blood in two ways. Deoxygenated blood flows from the right ventricle via the pulmonary arteries. This blood flows through pulmonary capillaries, is reoxygenated at the alveoli, and then returns to the heart via the pulmonary veins.

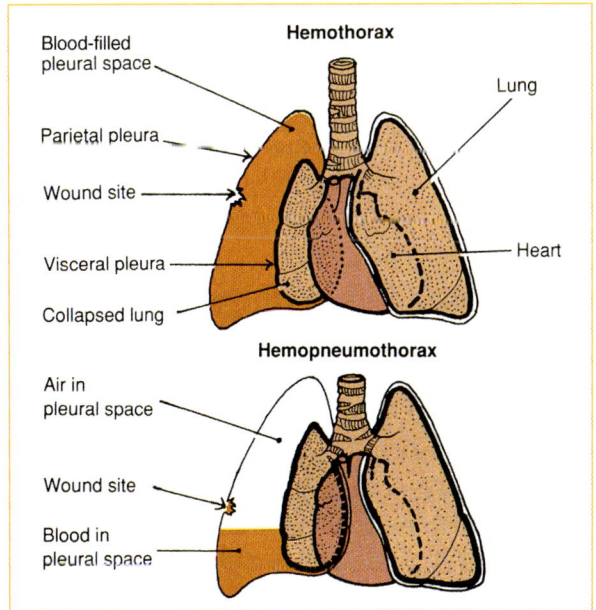

Figure 5-115 The pleural membranes. Normally, there is no space between the pleural membranes. When air, blood, or both enter the potential space, a potentially life-threatening condition can develop.

EMT-I Tips

Acute asthma is a recurring condition of reversible acute airflow obstruction in the lower airway. About 8.9 million people in the United States have asthma, and thousands with asthma die each year. It is the most common chronic disease of childhood. Four distinct events occur in an asthma attack. Smooth muscle spasm occurs when the muscle layers around the airways constrict (<u>bronchospasm</u>), resulting in narrowing of the airway diameter. Increased secretion of mucus causes mucus plugging, further decreasing the airway diameter, and finally, inflammatory cell proliferation occurs. White blood cells accumulate in the airway and secrete substances that worsen the muscle spasm and increase mucus production.

The most common cause of an asthma attack is an upper respiratory infection, such as bronchitis or a cold. Other causes include changes in environmental conditions; emotions, especially stress; allergic reactions to pollens, foods (chocolate, shellfish, milk, nuts) or drugs (penicillin, local anesthetics); and occupational exposures.

The severity of asthma attacks varies among patients. In very severe cases (status asthmaticus), the patient may die as a result of respiratory failure. In other cases, treatment may produce rapid improvement and resolution of the asthmatic crisis. The patient's level of compliance and degree of ambulatory control may be a strong mitigating factor in the development of complications. Patients with potentially fatal asthma have a greater likelihood of a shorter duration of premonitory symptoms, worse lung function, and medication noncompliance.

Understanding the underlying pathophysiology has radically impacted chronic drug therapy of asthma. Inhaled corticosteroids are now considered a mainstay of preventive therapy primarily for their anti-inflammatory effect. Oral and IV steroids have been used for the same purpose in acute attacks for many years. In addition, drugs are constantly being developed that block other inflammatory compounds involved in an acute attack. One newly available drug, zileuton, inhibits 5-lipoxygenase, an enzyme that catalyzes formation of leukotrienes, known inflammatory mediators in asthma. Another drug, zafirlukast, directly inhibits the actions of leukotrienes. Both drugs are approved by the FDA in the chronic treatment of asthma. The most promising combination of drugs for chronic therapy is an inhaled long-acting beta$_2$ agonist combined with an inhaled steroid.

In addition, <u>bronchial arteries</u> branch off of the thoracic aorta and supply the lung tissues themselves with blood. Deoxygenated blood returns to the heart via the <u>bronchial veins</u> and the azygos system. Peripherally in the lungs, venous blood from the bronchi enters the pulmonary veins, returning with oxygenated blood from the alveoli.

Respiratory Physiology

The primary function of the respiratory system is to exchange gases at the alveolocapillary membrane. Oxygen is essential for the body to function. The amount of oxygen in inspired air is approximately 21%. The primary waste product of metabolism is carbon dioxide, which is carried in the blood to the lungs. <u>Ventilation</u> is the process of moving air in and out of the lungs.

<u>Pulmonary function tests</u> assess volumes of air that move into and out of the lungs. Usually, measurement involves the use of a <u>spirometer</u>, a device that records the amount and rate of air that is breathed in and out over a specific period of time. Some commonly measured parameters include <u>tidal volume</u> (the volume of air inspired during normal inspiration), <u>residual volume</u> (the volume of air remaining in the respiratory passages and lungs after a forceful expiration), <u>vital capacity</u> (the amount of air moved in and out of the lungs with maximum inspiration and expiration), and <u>forced expiratory vital capacity (FEVI)</u> (the volume of air exhaled from the lung following a forceful exhalation).

At the alveolocapillary exchange surface, the alveolus and the red blood cells are located very close together. Diffusion is the process by which a gas dissolves in a liquid. Through the process of diffusion, the gases move from a higher concentration to a lower concentration. Therefore, oxygen moves across the membrane into the capillaries where it attaches to the hemoglobin. Likewise, carbon dioxide moves into the alveoli where the concentration is lower. Oxygenated blood enters the left side of the heart and is pumped to the tissues. Oxygen is "offloaded" from the red blood cells to the tissues as carbon dioxide and waste products from the tissues are "loaded" into the bloodstream. Venous blood returns to the right side of the heart and the pulmonary capillary bed (via the pulmonary arteries). The carbon dioxide diffuses into the alveoli and is released into the atmosphere as the individual exhales (Figure 5-116 ▼).

Because there are so many alveoli, a fairly large surface area exists for respiratory exchange to occur in the context of the relatively limited size of the thoracic cavity. The total surface area created around the alveoli is more than 85 m² 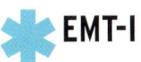. This is significantly more than would exist if each lung consisted of only a single sphere, like a large balloon. In that case, the surface area would be only 0.01 m² (1 m = 39.37″).

Respiration is controlled by the brain. The <u>respiratory center</u> is located in the medulla oblongata. A complicated interaction of signals provides feedback to the respiratory center, allowing it to continuously control respiration. The main respiratory stimulus is accumulation of carbon dioxide in the blood. Typically, this is measured as the Pa_{CO_2} on the arterial blood gases. Increases in the Pa_{CO_2} result in decreased pH levels in the respiratory center, which triggers an increase in ventilation. Decreases in the Pa_{CO_2} result in increased pH levels in the respiratory center and a decrease in ventilation. Low blood oxygen levels also stimulate breathing, but normally have much less of an effect than does the Pa_{CO_2}.

> **EMT-I Tips**
>
> Individuals with reversible restrictive lower airway disease, such as <u>asthma</u>, or progressive, irreversible airway disease resulting from <u>emphysema</u> (destruction of alveolar walls), <u>black lung disease</u> (consistent inhalation of coal dust), <u>asbestosis</u> (inhalation of asbestos particles), or <u>chronic bronchitis</u> (excess mucus production that blocks the airway) demonstrate typical abnormalities on pulmonary function testing. Residual volume often is increased, and the forced expiratory volume in the first second is decreased. Abnormalities of these parameters indicate chronic obstructive lung disease. Often, the technician measures lung function before and following administration of a <u>bronchodilator</u>, medication that is designed to decrease airway resistance and thereby improve lung function. Individuals with black lung disease, asbestosis, or other forms of lung scarring may demonstrate a significant decrease in the vital capacity, indicating <u>restrictive lung disease</u>.

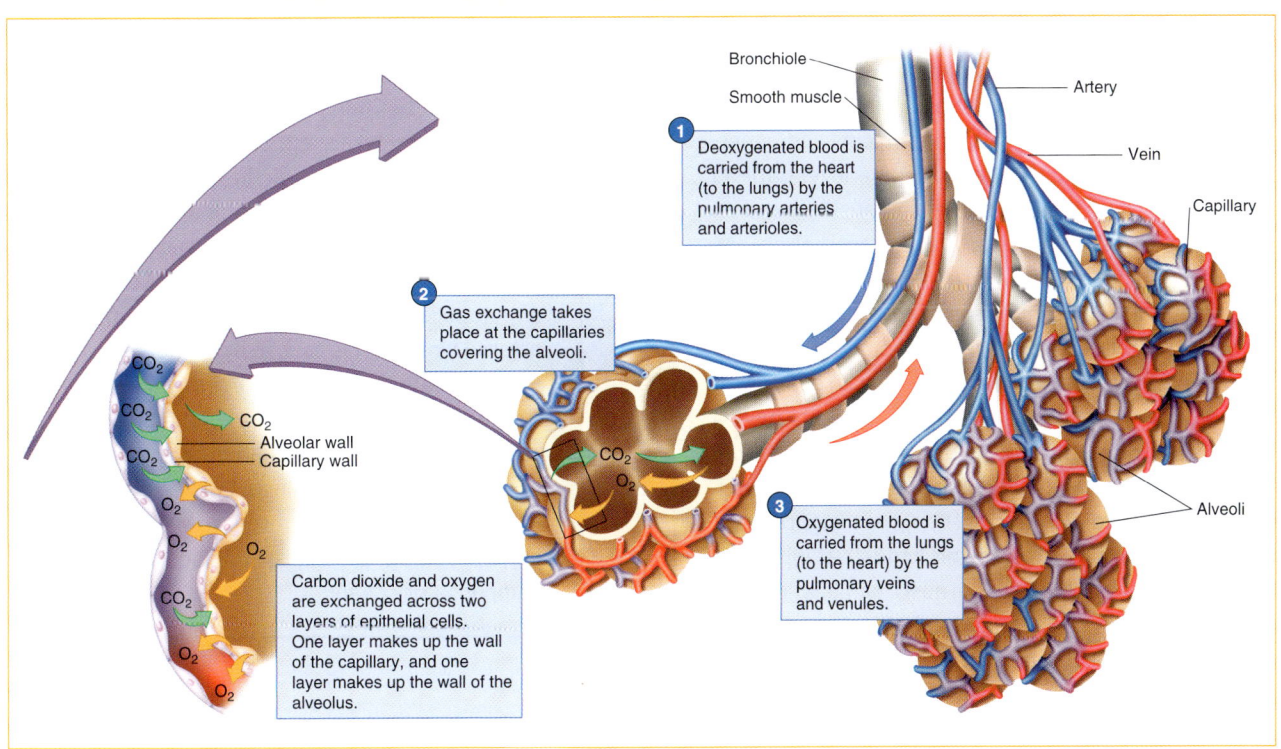

Figure 5-116 Exchange of gases in the lungs.

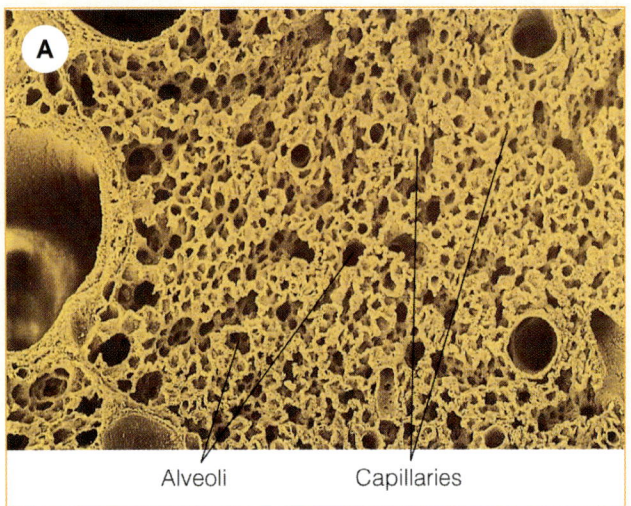 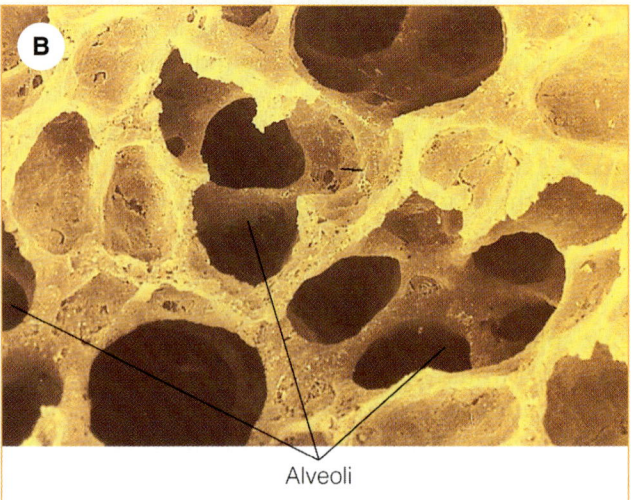

Figure 5-117 **A.** A scanning electron micrograph of the lung showing many alveoli. The smallest openings are capillaries surrounding the alveoli. **B.** A higher magnification scanning electron micrograph of lung tissue showing alveoli.

EMT-I Tips

<u>Chronic obstructive pulmonary disease (COPD)</u> is a progressive, irreversible disease of the airway marked by decreased inspiratory and expiratory capacity of the lungs. COPD may result from chronic bronchitis (excess mucus production) or emphysema (lung tissue damage with loss of elastic recoil of the lungs). Patients with COPD usually have a combination of both problems and generally function at a certain baseline level until an event occurs that causes decompensation and an acute COPD episode (or acute exacerbation). As with asthma, inflammation recently has been shown to play a significant role in COPD.

Chronic bronchitis results from overgrowth of the airway mucous glands and excess secretion of mucus, which blocks the airway. Patients have a chronic productive cough. Emphysema results from destruction of the alveolar walls, which creates resistance to expiratory airflow. The major cause of COPD is cigarette smoking. Industrial inhalants (such as asbestos and coal dust), air pollution, and tuberculosis can also lead to COPD. The patient in an acute COPD episode will complain of shortness of breath with gradually increasing symptoms over a period of days.

EMT-I Tips

Arterial blood gas tests measure the <u>partial pressure of oxygen (Pa_{O_2})</u> and the <u>partial pressure of carbon dioxide (Pa_{CO_2})</u> in the blood, as well as the <u>pH</u>, (the degree of acidity or alkalinity). Deviations from normal values occur in many different disease states. Essentially, Pa_{CO_2} acts as "respiratory acid." Changes in the Pa_{CO_2} value rapidly change the pH levels, either making it more basic (increased) or more acidic (decreased). Changes in the Pa_{CO_2} can be the result of diseases such as asthma, COPD exacerbation, or drug overdose or secondary to a change in the blood pH because of a metabolic problem. A decrease in the pH of the arterial blood that is caused by an elevation in the Pa_{CO_2} is called a primary respiratory acidosis, whereas an increase in the pH of the blood that is caused by excessive exhalation of CO_2 is called a primary respiratory alkalosis. Conversely, changes in the Pa_{CO_2} that occur in response to primary metabolic problems (alkalosis or acidosis) are called compensatory changes.

During inhalation, the diaphragm contracts and negative pressure is created in the chest cavity. The negative pressure results in air being "sucked" in, and the air fills the lungs. Air is expired when the lung tissue, characterized by elasticity, collapses. Exhalation is a passive process that does not normally require effort.

EMT-I Safety

A cough is the perfect mechanism for aerosolizing infectious materials. Whenever possible, minimize the risk of exposure by placing an oxygen mask on a patient with a cough.

We also have a "backup system" to control respiration called the <u>hypoxic drive</u>. When oxygen levels fall, this system will also stimulate breathing. There are areas in the brain, the walls of the aorta, and the carotid arteries that act as oxygen sensors. Minimal levels of oxygen in the arterial blood easily satisfy these sensors. Therefore, our backup system, the hypoxic drive, is much less sensitive and less powerful than the carbon dioxide sensors in the brain stem.

Pediatric Needs

The anatomy of the respiratory system in children is proportionally smaller and less rigid than that in an adult (Figure 5-118 ▶). A child's nose and mouth are much smaller than those of an adult. The larynx, cricoid cartilage, and trachea are smaller, softer, and more flexible as well. This makes the mechanics of breathing much more delicate. A child's pharynx is also smaller and less deeply curved. The tongue takes up proportionally more space in a child's mouth than in an adult's mouth.

These anatomic differences are important for your assessment. For example, the smaller larynx of a child becomes obstructed more easily. The chest wall in children is softer. Therefore, children depend more heavily on the diaphragm for breathing. You will notice that the abdomen moves in and out considerably with each breath, especially in an infant. Young infants do not know how to breathe through the mouth. Therefore, as you assess an infant or a child, you must carefully consider these differences.

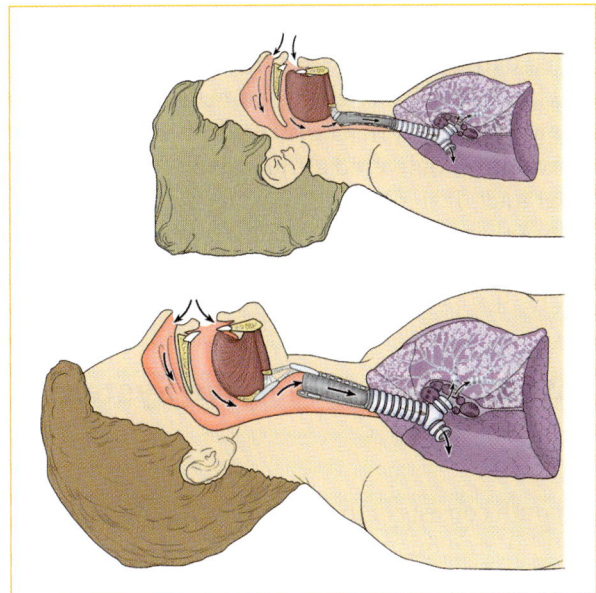

Figure 5-118 The respiratory system of a child is proportionally smaller and less rigid than that of an adult.

The Digestive System

The digestive system is composed of the gastrointestinal tract (stomach and intestines), mouth, salivary glands, pharynx, esophagus, liver, gallbladder, pancreas, rectum, and anus. The function of this system is <u>digestion</u>: the processing of food that nourishes the individual cells of the body.

How Digestion Works

Digestion of food, from the time it is taken into the mouth until essential compounds are extracted and delivered by the circulatory system to nourish all of the cells in the body, is a complicated chemical process. In succession, different secretions, primarily enzymes, are added to the food by the salivary glands, the stomach, the liver, the pancreas, and the small intestine to convert the food into basic sugars, fatty acids, and amino acids. These basic products of digestion are carried across the wall of the intestine and transported through the portal vein to the liver. In the liver, the products are processed further and then stored or transported to the heart through veins draining the liver. The heart then pumps the blood with these nutrients throughout the arteries and then to the capillaries, where the nutrients pass through the capillary walls to nourish the body's individual cells.

In normal routine activity, without any food or fluid ingestion at all, between 8 to 10 L of fluid is secreted daily into the gastrointestinal tract. This fluid comes from the salivary glands, stomach, liver, pancreas, and small intestine. In a normal adult, about 7% of the body weight is delivered as fluid daily to the gastrointestinal tract. If significant vomiting or diarrhea occurs for more than 2 or 3 days, the patient will lose a very substantial portion of body composition and become severely ill.

Anatomy of the Digestive System

Mouth

The mouth consists of the lips, cheeks, gums, teeth, and tongue. A mucous membrane lines the mouth. The hard and soft palates form the roof of the mouth. The hard palate is a bony plate lying anteriorly; the soft palate is a fold of mucous membrane and muscle that extends posteriorly from the hard palate into the throat. The soft palate is designed to hold food that is being chewed within the mouth and to help initiate swallowing.

Salivary Glands

There are two salivary glands located under the tongue, one on each side of the lower jaw, and one inside each cheek. They produce nearly 1.5 L of saliva daily. Saliva is approximately 98% water. The remaining 2% is composed of mucus, salts, and organic compounds. Saliva serves as a binder for the chewed food that is being swallowed and as a lubricant within the mouth.

Oropharynx

The oropharynx is a tubular structure about 5" long that extends vertically from the back of the mouth to the esophagus and trachea. An automatic movement of the pharynx during swallowing lifts the larynx to permit the epiglottis to close over it so that liquids and solids are moved into the esophagus and away from the trachea.

Esophagus

The esophagus is a collapsible tube about 10" long that extends from the end of the pharynx to the stomach and lies just anterior to the spinal column in the chest. Contractions of the muscle in the wall of the esophagus propel food through it to the stomach. Liquids will pass with very little assistance.

Stomach

The stomach is located in the left upper quadrant of the abdominal cavity, largely protected by the lower left ribs. Muscular contractions in the wall of the stomach and gastric juice, which contains much mucus, convert ingested food to a thoroughly mixed semi-solid mass. The stomach produces approximately 1.5 L of gastric juice daily for this process. The principal function of the stomach is to receive food in large quantities intermittently, store it, and provide for its movement into the small bowel in regular, small amounts. In 1 to 3 hours, the semisolid food mass derived from one meal is propelled by muscular contraction into the duodenum, the first part of the small intestine.

Pancreas

The pancreas, a flat, solid organ, lies below and behind the liver and stomach and behind the peritoneum. It is firmly fixed in position, deep within the abdomen, and is not easily damaged. It contains two kinds of glands. One set of glands secretes nearly 2 L of pancreatic juice daily. This juice contains many enzymes that aid in the digestion of fat, starch, and protein. Pancreatic juice flows directly into the duodenum through the pancreatic ducts. The other gland is the islets of Langerhans, which produces insulin. Insulin regulates the amount of glucose in the blood.

Liver

The liver is a large, solid organ that takes up most of the area immediately beneath the diaphragm in the right upper quadrant. It is the largest solid organ in the abdomen and has several functions. Poisonous substances produced by digestion are brought to the liver and rendered harmless. Factors that are necessary for blood clotting and for the production of normal plasma are formed here. Between 0.5 and 1 L of bile is made by the liver daily to assist in the normal digestion of fat. The liver is the principal organ for the storage of sugar or starch for immediate use by the body for energy. It also produces many of the factors that aid in the proper regulation of immune responses. Anatomically, the liver is a large mass of blood vessels and cells, packed tightly together. It is fragile and, because of its size, relatively easily injured. Blood flow in the liver is high, because all of the blood that is pumped to the gastrointestinal tract passes into the liver, through the portal vein, before it returns to the heart. In addition, the liver has a generous arterial blood supply of its own. Ordinarily, approximately 25% of the cardiac output of blood (1.5 L) passes through the liver each minute.

Bile Ducts

The liver is connected to the intestine by the bile ducts. The gallbladder is an outpouching from the bile ducts that serves as a reservoir and concentrating organ for bile produced in the liver. Together, the bile ducts and gallbladder form the biliary system. The gallbladder discharges stored and concentrated bile into the duodenum through the common bile duct. The presence of food in the duodenum triggers a contraction of the gallbladder to empty it. The gallbladder usually contains about 60 to 90 mL of bile.

Small Intestine

The small intestine is the major hollow organ of the abdomen. The cells lining the small intestine produce enzymes and mucus to aid in digestion. Enzymes from the pancreas and the small intestine carry out the final processes of digestion. More than 90% of the products of digestion (amino acids, fatty acids, and simple sugars), together with water, ingested vitamins, and minerals are absorbed across the wall of the lower end of the small intestine into veins to be transported to the liver. The small intestine is composed of the duodenum, the jejunum, and the ileum. The duodenum, which is about 12″ long, is the part of the small intestine that receives food from the stomach. Here, food is mixed with secretions from the pancreas and liver for further digestion. Bile, produced by the liver and stored in the gallbladder, is emptied as needed into the duodenum. It is greenish black, but through changes during digestion, it gives feces its typical brown color. Its major function is in the digestion of fat. The jejunum and ileum together measure more than 20′ on average to make up the rest of the small intestine.

Large Intestine

The large intestine, another major hollow organ, consists of the cecum, the colon, and the rectum. About 5′ long, it encircles the outer border of the abdomen around the small bowel. The major function of the colon, the portion of the large intestine that extends from the cecum to the rectum, is to absorb the final 5% to 10% of digested food and water from the intestine to form solid stool, which is stored in the rectum and passed out of the body through the anus.

Appendix

The appendix is a tube 3″ to 4″ long that opens into the cecum (the first part of the large intestine) in the right lower quadrant of the abdomen. It may easily become obstructed and, as a result, inflamed and infected. Appendicitis, which is the term for this inflammation, is one of the major causes of severe abdominal distress. The appendix has no known function.

Rectum

The lowermost end of the colon is the rectum. It is a large, hollow organ that is adapted to store quantities of feces until it is expelled. At its terminal end is the anus, a 2″ canal lined with skin. The rectum and anus are supplied with a complex series of circular muscles called sphincters that control, both voluntarily and automatically, the escape of liquids, gases, and solids from the digestive tract.

The Urinary System

The urinary system controls the discharge of certain waste materials filtered from the blood by the kidneys. In the urinary system, the kidneys are solid organs; the ureters, bladder, and urethra are hollow organs ▶ Figure 5-119 ▶). Ordinarily, we consider the urinary and genital systems together, because they share many organs.

The body has two kidneys that lie on the posterior muscular wall of the abdomen behind the peritoneum in the retroperitoneal space. These organs rid the blood of toxic waste products and control its balance of water and salt. Blood flow in the kidneys is high. Nearly 20% of the output of blood from the heart passes through the kidneys each minute. Large vessels attach the kidneys directly to the aorta and the inferior vena cava. Waste products and water are constantly filtered from the blood to form urine. The kidneys continuously concentrate this filtered urine by reabsorbing the water as it passes through a system of specialized tubes within them. The tubes finally unite to form the renal pelvis, a cone-shaped collecting area that connects the ureter and the kidney. Normally, each kidney drains its urine into one ureter through which the urine passes to the bladder.

A ureter passes from the renal pelvis of each kidney along the surface of the posterior abdominal wall behind the peritoneum to drain into the urinary bladder. The ureters are small (0.2″ in diameter), hollow, muscular tubes. Peristalsis, a wave-like contraction of smooth muscle, occurs in these tubes to move the urine to the bladder.

The urinary bladder is located immediately behind the pubic symphysis in the pelvic cavity and is composed of smooth muscle with a specialized lining membrane. The two ureters enter posteriorly at its base on

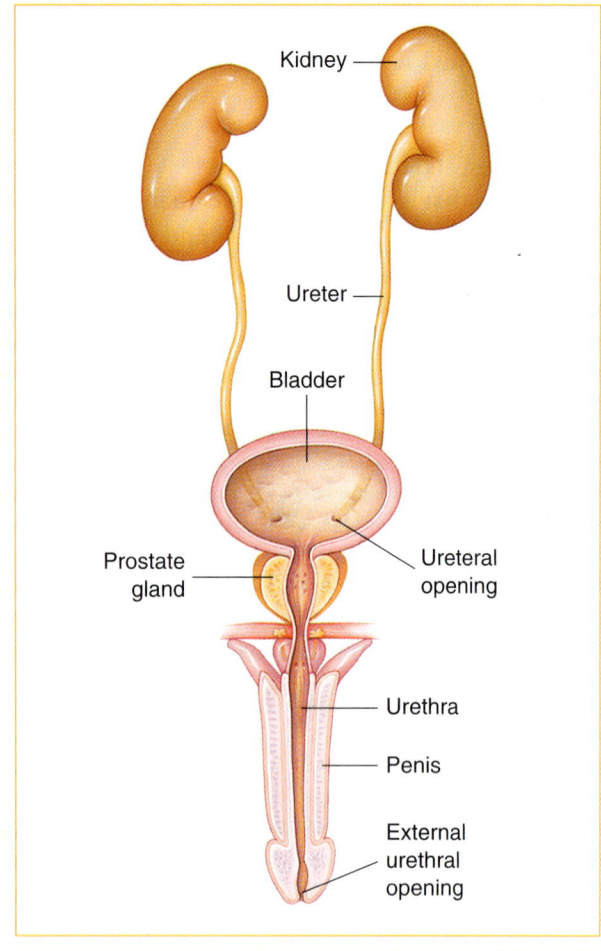

Figure 5-119 The urinary system lies in the retroperitoneal space behind the organs of the digestive system. The urinary system in males and females includes the kidneys, ureters, bladder, and urethra. This diagram shows the male urinary system.

either side. The bladder empties to the outside of the body through the urethra. In the male, the urethra passes from the anterior base of the bladder through the penis. In the female, the urethra opens at the front of the vagina. The normal adult forms 1.5 to 2 L of urine every day. This waste is extracted and concentrated from the 1,500 L of blood that circulate through the kidneys daily.

The Genital System

The genital system controls the reproductive processes by which life is created. The male genitalia, except for the prostate gland and the seminal vesicles, lie outside the pelvic cavity. The female genitalia are contained entirely within the pelvis. The male and female reproductive organs have certain similarities and, of course, basic differences. They allow the production of sperm and egg cells and appropriate hormones and the act of sexual intercourse and reproduction.

The Male Reproductive System and Organs

The male reproductive system consists of the testicles, vasa deferentia, seminal vesicles, prostate gland, urethra, and penis (Figure 5-120 ▶). Each testicle contains specialized cells and ducts; some of these produce male hormones, and others develop sperm. The hormones are absorbed directly into the bloodstream from the testicles. The vasa deferentia (or vas deferens) are ducts that travel from the testicles up beneath the skin of the abdominal wall for a short distance. They then pass through an opening into the abdominal cavity and into the prostate gland to connect with the urethra. The vasa deferentia carry the sperm from the testicles to the urethra. The seminal vesicles are small storage sacs for sperm and seminal fluid. The vesicles also empty into the urethra, at the prostate.

Semen, also called seminal fluid, contains sperm cells that are carried up each vas from each testicle to be mixed with fluid from the seminal vesicles and prostate gland. The prostate gland surrounds the urethra where it emerges from the urinary bladder. Fluids from the prostate gland and from the seminal vesicles mix during sexual intercourse. During intercourse, special mechanisms in the nervous system prevent the passage of urine into the urethra. Only seminal fluid, prostatic fluid, and sperm pass from the penis into the vagina during ejaculation.

The penis contains a special type of tissue called erectile tissue. This specialized tissue is largely vascular and, when filled with blood, causes the penis to distend into a state of erection. As the vessels fill under pressure from the circulatory system, the penis becomes a large, rigid organ that can enter the vagina. Certain spinal injuries and some diseases can cause a painful continuous erection called priapism.

The Female Reproductive System and Organs

The female reproductive organs include the ovaries, fallopian tubes, uterus, cervix, and vagina (Figure 5-121 ▶). The ovaries, like the testicles, produce sex hormones and

Chapter 5 The Human Body 211

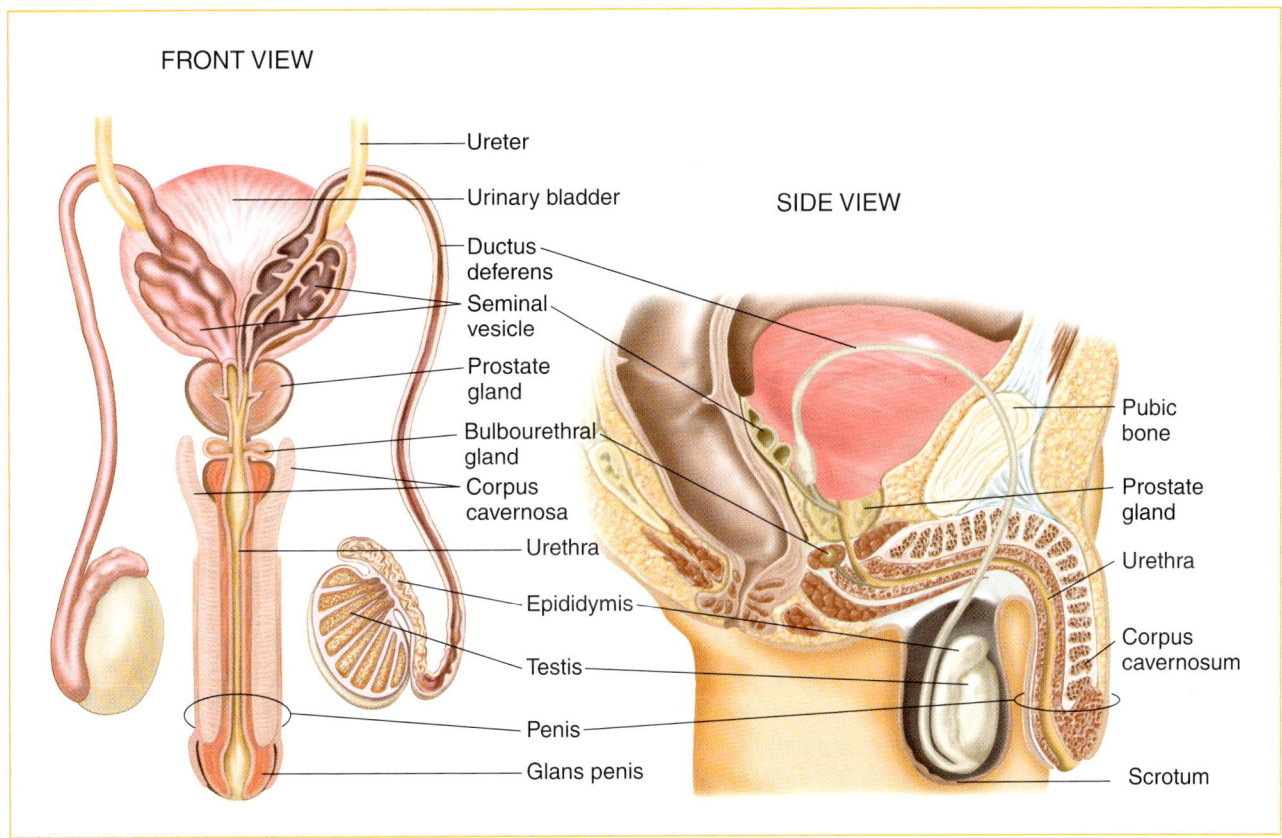

Figure 5-120 The male reproductive system consists of the testicles, vasa deferentia, seminal vesicles, prostate gland, urethra, and penis.

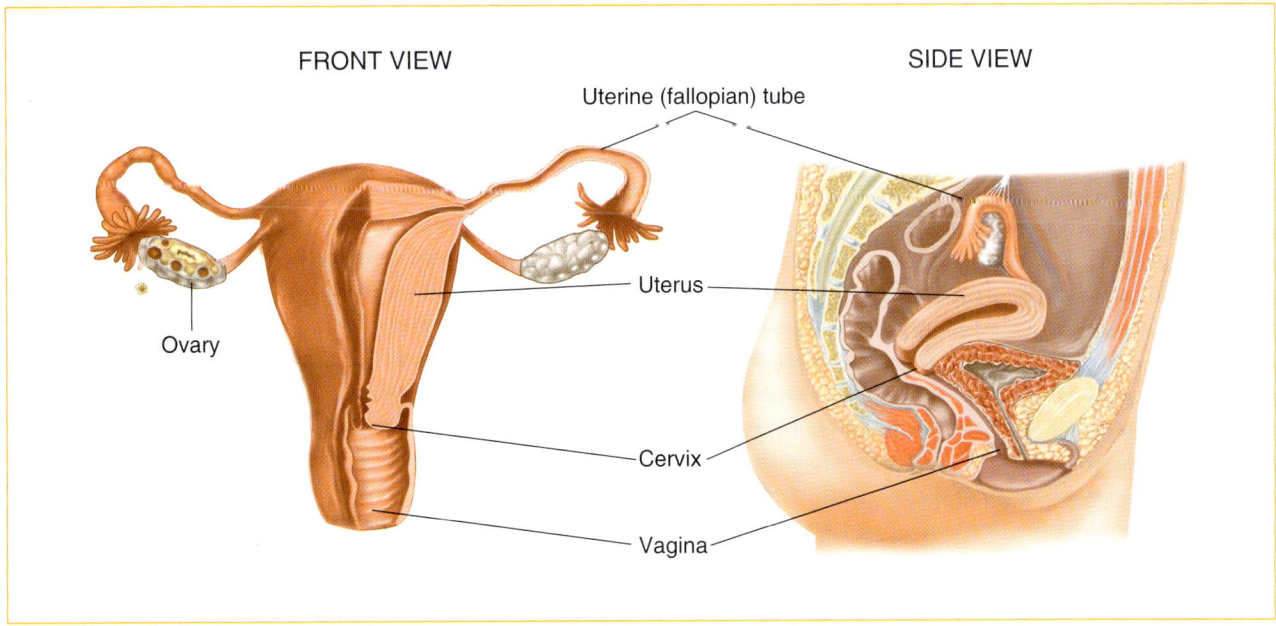

Figure 5-121 The female reproductive system consists of the ovaries, fallopian tubes, uterus, cervix, and vagina.

specialized cells for reproduction. The female sex hormones are absorbed directly into the bloodstream. A specialized ovum, or egg cell, is produced regularly during the adult female's reproductive years. The ovaries release a mature egg approximately every 28 days. This egg travels through the fallopian tubes to the uterus.

The fallopian tubes connect with the uterus and carry the ovum into the cavity of this organ. The uterus is pear-shaped and hollow, with muscular walls. The narrow opening from the uterus to the vagina is the cervix. The vagina (birth canal) is a muscular distensible tube that connects the uterus with the vulva (the external female genitalia). The vagina receives the penis during sexual intercourse, when semen is deposited in it. The sperm in the semen may pass into the uterus and fertilize an egg, causing pregnancy. Should the pregnancy come to completion at the end of nine months, the baby will pass through the vagina and be born. The vagina also channels the menstrual flow from the uterus out of the body.

Fluids and Electrolytes

Body Fluid Balance

The total body water content of the average adult ranges from 50% to 70% of total body weight, depending on age and sex. A newborn's total body water content may be as high as 75% to 80% of total body weight.

Body fluid is divided into two main compartments: intracellular fluid and extracellular fluid. Intracellular fluid (ICF) exists within individual cells and equals approximately 40% to 45% of total body weight. The intracellular fluid makes up approximately 75% of all body fluid. Extracellular fluid (ECF) exists outside of the cell membranes. It equals approximately 15% to 20% of the total body weight, or 25% of all body fluid. Extracellular fluid is further divided into intravascular fluid and interstitial fluid. Intravascular fluid (plasma), the fluid portion of blood, is found within the blood vessels and accounts for approximately 4.5% of total body weight. Interstitial fluid is located outside of the blood vessels, in the spaces between the body's cells. It accounts for approximately 10.5% of total body weight. There is a delicate balance among the various fluid compartments of the body that is essential to maintain homeostasis.

If fluid is lost from anywhere in the body, there can be serious ramifications because this disturbs the balance among various fluid compartments (homeostasis). The result can be shock. Under normal conditions, the total volume of water in the body and its distribution in the body compartments remain relatively constant, even though there are fluctuations in the amount of water that enters and is excreted from the body each day. Fluid balance is the process of maintaining homeostasis through equal intake (water taken into the body) and output (water excreted from the body) of fluids.

There are mechanisms in the body that maintain the balance between what is taken in and what is excreted. For example, when the fluid volume drops, the pituitary gland secretes antidiuretic hormone (ADH) Figure 5-122 . ADH causes the kidney tubules to reabsorb more water into the blood and excrete less urine, allowing fluid volume in the body to build up. Thirst also regulates fluid intake. The sensation of thirst occurs when body fluids become decreased, stimulating an individual to take in more fluids. Conversely, when too many fluids enter the body, thirst decreases, the kidneys are activated, and more urine is excreted, eliminating the excess fluid.

It is important to maintain the proper balance of fluids and electrolytes within the body, because this is necessary for life. An individual's body can become depleted of fluids and electrolytes for several reasons, including severe burns or dehydration. The body can maintain fluid balance by shifting water from one compartment to another. Water moves in response to osmotic forces as well as hormonal stimuli such as ADH. For a patient whose fluids or electrolytes are depleted, rapid restoration of fluid balance may mean the difference between life and death Table 5-4 .

> **EMT-I Tips**
>
> The kidneys also are important in the regulation of the body's fluid balance and blood pressure. They perform these vital functions in conjunction with complex hormone-driven mechanisms. Fluid balance is controlled by the effects of ADH on the kidney. The blood pressure effects are influenced by the renin-angiotensin system, of which the kidneys are an important part.

TABLE 5-4	Major Mechanisms for Fluid Homeostasis
■ Antidiuretic hormone (ADH)	
■ Thirst	
■ Kidneys	
■ Water shifts	

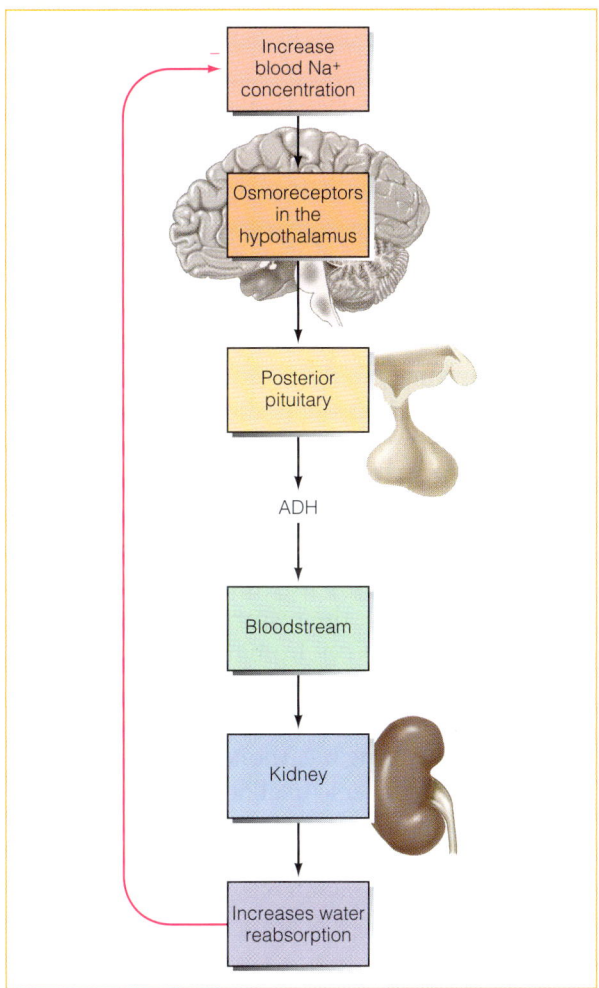

Figure 5-122 The role of ADH in regulating fluid levels.

Terminology Tips

Intra = within
Extra = outside of
Inter = between

Intracellular and *intravascular* fluids are *within* the cells and vessels respectively. *Extravascular* and *extracellular* fluids are *outside* of the vessels and cells, and *interstitial* fluid is *between* the cells.

EMT-I Tips

Sodium (Na^+) and potassium (K^+) are two of the most important electrolytes (dissolved chemicals) in the blood. Most of the body's supply of potassium is contained in the intracellular fluid (ICF). On the other hand, most of the body's supply of sodium resides in the extracellular fluid (ECF). Both fluids and electrolytes may move between the ICF and ECF, depending on many factors. Abnormal concentrations of either sodium or potassium in the ECF may result in life-threatening conditions. Measured levels of sodium or potassium may be normal, high, or low. The most common causes of electrolyte abnormalities are abnormalities in the body's fluid balance such as caused by dehydration, overhydration, or drugs. Failure to recognize and promptly treat any of these abnormalities may result in harm to the patient.

Acid-Base Balance

An acid is a substance that increases the concentration of hydrogen ions in a water solution. A base is a substance that decreases the concentration of hydrogen ions.

Whether the blood or body fluid is acidic, basic, or neutral depends on the concentration of dissolved hydrogen (H^+). Hydrogen is an acid. This means that the higher the concentration, the more acidic the blood will be; conversely, the lower the H^+ concentration, the more basic (less acidic) the blood will be. Normal homeostatic functions keep the concentration of H^+ within a fairly narrow range.

The most common expression of acidity is pH, which is a value calculated from H^+ concentration:

pH = concentration of hydrogen ions

Therefore, the lower the hydrogen ion concentration, the greater the pH (more basic) will be, and the higher the hydrogen ion concentration, the lower the pH (more acidic) will be. pH ranges from 0 (most acidic) to 14 (most basic), with 7.0 being neutral. (The pH of pure water, which is considered neutral, is 7.0.) The pH of the human body is normally slightly basic, or alkaline, ranging approximately 7.35 to 7.45. When pH is higher than this, the blood is too basic, or alkalotic. When pH is lower, the blood is too acidic, or acidotic **Figure 5-123**.

Buffer Systems

A buffer is a substance that can absorb or donate H^+. Buffers absorb hydrogen ions when they are in excess and donate hydrogen ions when they are depleted.

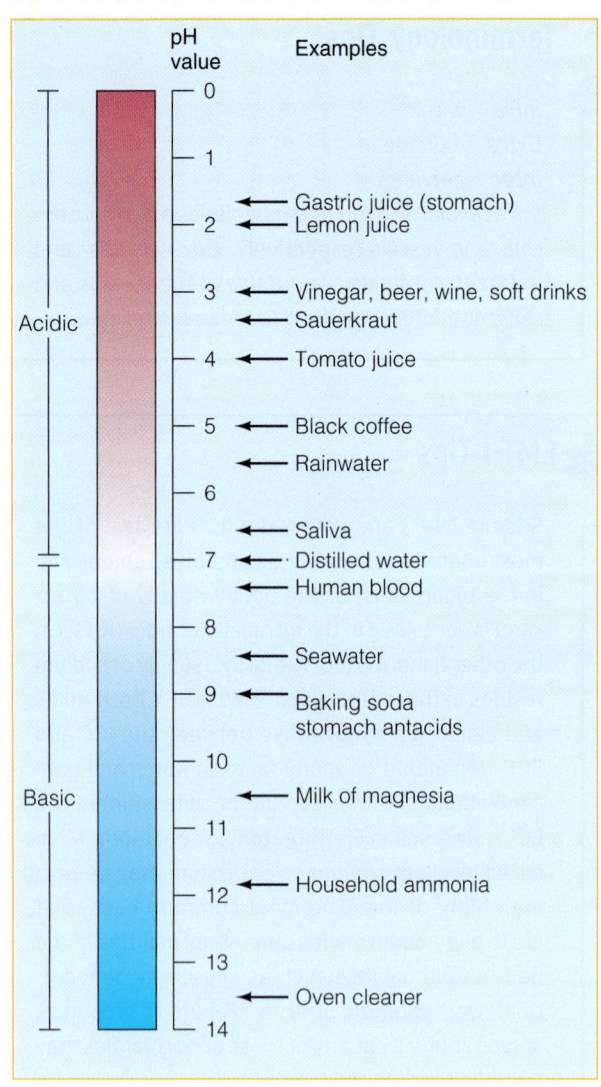

Figure 5-123 The pH scale.

Therefore, <u>buffer systems</u> act as fast defenses for acid-base changes, providing almost immediate protection against changes in the hydrogen ion concentration of the extracellular fluid. The generic reaction is expressed as follows:

$$H^+ + Buffer \leftrightarrow H\text{-}Buffer$$

Free H^+ (acid) binds with the buffer to form a weak acid (H-Buffer). This reaction can shift to the right or left depending on the hydrogen ion concentration. When the H^+ concentration increases and buffer is available, the reaction is forced to the right and more H-Buffer is formed. When the H^+ concentration decreases, the reaction shifts toward the left, and H^+ disassociates from the buffer, leaving H^+ and buffer.

The respiratory system and the renal system work in conjunction with the bicarbonate buffer to maintain homeostasis. The fastest way the body can get rid of excess acid is through the respiratory system. Excess acid can be expelled as CO_2 from the lungs. Conversely, slowing respirations will increase CO_2 in alkalotic states. The renal system regulates pH by filtering out more hydrogen and retaining bicarbonate in acidotic states, and doing just the reverse in alkalotic states. This will be discussed in more detail in upcoming chapters.

You are the Provider   Summary

1. How does each body system respond when another body system is damaged from illness or injury?

Maintenance of the internal environment of the cell is regulated by elaborate systems of checks and balances. As systems in the body become imbalanced and begin to shift, feedback systems create an appropriate response to return the internal environment to normal. This normally balanced condition is referred to as homeostasis, or the resistance to change.

2. What is anatomy, physiology, and pathophysiology?

Anatomy refers to the study of the structure of an organism and its parts. Gross anatomy includes body parts that are generally visible to the naked eye—the bones, the muscles, and the organs. Microscopic anatomy involves components of the body that are small, often visible only through a microscope. Physiology examines the body functions of the living organism. Pathophysiology is the study of the body functions of a living organism in an abnormal state, such as a disease.

3. How can knowledge of medical terminology help the EMT-I care for this patient?

EMT-Is must be familiar with the language of topographic anatomy. By using the proper medical terms, you will be able to communicate correct information with the least possible confusion to other members of the health care team.

4. How can knowledge of anatomy and physiology help the EMT-I care for patients?

Familiarity with the structures and function of the body's systems will allow you to better assess a patient as well as predict potential complications resulting from occult injuries (those not visible to the eye).

5. What is the function of the skeletal system?

The skeleton gives us our recognizable human form and protects our vital internal organs.

6. What is the musculoskeletal system designed to do?

The skeleton is designed to allow motion of the body. It involves coordinated function of the muscles and the skeleton.

7. What is the most common method used to describe the abdomen?

The simplest and most common method of describing the portions of the abdomen is by quadrants, the four equal areas formed by two imaginary lines that intersect at right angles at the umbilicus. On the anterior abdominal wall, the quadrants thus formed are the right upper, right lower, left upper, and left lower. The terms "right quadrant" and "left quadrant" refer to the patient's right and left as you face them, not to your right and left sides.

8. Why is it important for the EMT-I to use these designations?

Pain or injury in a given quadrant usually arises from or involves the organs that lie in that quadrant. This simple means of designation will allow you to identify injured or diseased organs that require emergency attention.

9. What are the bones of the lower extremity?

The lower extremity includes the hip, thigh, knee, leg, ankle, foot, and toes.

10. What are the common causes of hip dislocations that the EMT-I should be aware of?

Dislocations of the hip joint commonly occur from a fall or during a motor vehicle collision in which the knee impacts the dashboard. The force of the impact is transmitted posteriorly to the hip, most commonly resulting in posterior dislocation.

11. What is the function of the medulla in the brain?

The medulla serves as a conduction pathway for both ascending and descending nerve tracts. It also coordinates heart rate, blood vessel diameter, breathing, swallowing, vomiting, coughing, and sneezing. The pons and medullary respiratory center are responsible for all respiratory movements.

12. How does the body respond when a patient loses blood?

When a patient loses a small amount of blood, the arteries, veins, and heart automatically adjust to the smaller new volume. The adjustment occurs in an effort to maintain adequate pressure throughout the circulatory system and thereby maintain circulation for every organ. The adjustment occurs very rapidly after the loss, usually within minutes. Specifically, the vessels constrict to provide a smaller bed for the reduced volume of blood to fill. And the heart pumps more rapidly to circulate the remaining blood more efficiently.

13. Body fluid is divided into two main compartments. What are they and where are they found?

Body fluid is divided into two main compartments: intracellular fluid and extracellular fluid. Intracellular fluid (ICF) is found within individual cells and equals approximately 40% to 45% of total body weight. The intracellular fluid makes up approximately 75% of all body fluid. Extracellular fluid (ECF) is the fluid found outside of the cell membranes. It equals approximately 15% to 20% of the total body weight, or 25% of all body fluid. Extracellular fluid is further divided into intravascular fluid and interstitial fluid. Intravascular fluid (plasma), the fluid portion of blood, is noncellular and is found within the blood vessels. It equals approximately 4.5% of total body weight. Interstitial fluid is the fluid located outside of the blood vessels, in the spaces between the body's cells. It comprises approximately 10.5% of total body weight. There is a delicate balance among the various fluid compartments of the body that is essential in maintenance of homeostasis.

Prep Kit

Ready for Review

- To do your work as an EMT-I, you must have a working knowledge of human anatomy so that you can communicate with hospital personnel and other health care providers.
- You must be able to identify superficial landmarks of the body and know what lies underneath the skin so that you can perform an accurate assessment. Hospital personnel will use these terms to ask you questions about a patient; therefore, it is critical for the well-being of your patient that you learn them and can use them correctly.
- You must also have an understanding of physiology. Each body system works together to maintain homeostasis of the entire organism. Disruption in any system can lead to illness or even death. Knowledge of body systems and how they work will allow you to better assess and treat your patient.

Vital Vocabulary

abdomen The body cavity that contains the major organs of digestion and excretion.

abducens nerve The cranial nerve (VI) that supplies the lateral rectus muscle of the eyeball (lateral movement).

abduction Motion of a limb away from the midline.

acetabulum The depression on the lateral pelvis where its three component bones join, in which the femoral head fits snugly.

acetylcholine A neurotransmitter secreted by the autonomic nervous system.

acetylcholinesterase An enzyme that rapidly destroys acetylcholine once it has reached the target tissue.

acid A substance that increases the concentration of hydrogen ions in a water solution.

acidotic Blood that is too acidic.

acromioclavicular (AC) joint The point at which the clavicle attaches to the acromion process.

acromioclavicular (AC) separation One or more torn ligaments in the AC joint, resulting in a separated shoulder.

acromion process The tip of the shoulder and the site of attachment for both the clavicle and various shoulder muscles.

action potential A change in electrical potential that occurs when a cell or tissue has been activated by a stimulus.

Adam's apple The firm prominence in the upper part of the larynx formed by the thyroid cartilage. It is more prominent in men than in women.

adduction Motion of a limb toward the midline.

adenosine triphosphate (ATP) The major source of energy for all chemical reactions of the body.

adipose tissue A type of connective tissue that contains large amounts of fat.

adrenal cortex The outer layer of the adrenal gland; it produces hormones that are important in regulating the water and salt balance of the body.

adrenal glands Glands located on top of each kidney that produce and secrete certain sex hormones, as well as other hormones that are vital to maintaining the body's water and salt balance; also called suprarenal glands.

adrenaline Hormone produced by the adrenal glands that mediates the "fight-or-flight" response of the sympathetic nervous system; also called epinephrine.

adrenergic Description of a neuron that secretes the neurotransmitter norepinephrine.

adrenergic receptor A receptor stimulated by the neurotransmitter norepinephrine.

adrenocorticotropic hormone (ACTH) One of several molecules derived from a common precursor, proopiomelanocortin, that is essential for development of the cortex of the adrenal gland and its secretion of corticosteroids.

aerobic metabolism A biochemical process that occurs in the presence of oxygen and results in the production of energy in the form of ATP; also called cellular respiration.

Technology

- Interactivities
- Vocabulary Explorer
- Anatomy Review
- Web Links
- Online Review Manual

afferent nerves Nerves that carry impulses from the body to the brain and provide input to the brain about sensations; also called sensory nerves.

afterload The pressure in the aorta against which the left ventricle must pump blood.

agranulocytes Leukocytes that lack granules.

aldosterone A steroid hormone produced by the adrenal glands that increases the rate of sodium and water resorption from the distal tubules back into the blood.

alkalotic Blood that is too basic.

alpha cells Cells located in the islets of Langerhans that secrete glucagon.

alpha effects Stimulation of alpha receptors that results in vasoconstriction.

alpha receptors One of two adrenergic receptors classified into two structural and functional categories; are further subdivided into $alpha_1$ and $alpha_2$ receptors.

alveolar ducts Ducts formed from division of the respiratory bronchioles in the lower airway; each ducts ends in clusters known as alveoli.

alveoli The air sacs of the lungs in which the exchange of oxygen and carbon dioxide takes place.

alveolocapillary membrane The very thin membrane, consisting of only one cell layer, that lies between the alveolus and capillary, through which respiratory exchange between the alveolus and the blood vessels occurs.

anabolism The productive component of metabolism associated with the build-up of energy stores and body tissues.

anaerobic metabolism An alternate form of metabolism that occurs when oxygen levels are low and less energy is produced than during aerobic respiration; lactic acid is produced as a waste product during this process.

anatomic position The position of reference in which the patient stands facing you, arms at the side, with the palms of the hands forward.

anatomy The study of the structure of an organism and its parts.

androgens Male sex hormones.

androstenedione A steroid sex hormone secreted by the adrenal cortex, testes, and ovaries.

anemia A decrease in the number of red blood cells, for any reason.

angle of Louis A ridge on the sternum that lies at the level where the second rib is attached to the sternum; provides a constant and reliable bony landmark on the anterior chest wall.

anterior The front surface of the body; the side facing you in the standard anatomic position.

anterior pituitary lobe (adenohypophysis) One of the two portions of the pituitary gland; it produces hormones that are not neurohormones; also called the adenohypophysis.

anterior superior iliac spines The bony prominences of the pelvis (ilium) at the front on each side of the lower abdomen just below the plane of the umbilicus.

antibodies Proteins within plasma that react with antigens.

antidiuretic hormone (ADH) A hormone released by the pituitary gland that causes the kidney to reabsorb more water into the blood and excrete less urine.

antigens Substances on the surface of erythrocytes that are recognized by the immune system.

aorta The principal artery leaving the left side of the heart and carrying freshly oxygenated blood to the body.

aortic arch One of the three described portions of the aorta; the section of the aorta between the ascending and descending portions that gives rise to the right brachiocephalic (innominate), left common carotid, and left subclavian arteries.

aortic valve The semilunar valve that regulates blood flow from the left ventricle to the aorta.

apex (plural: apices) The tip or the topmost portion of a structure.

appendicular skeleton The upper and lower extremities and the girdles that attach them to the axial skeleton.

appendix A small tubular structure that is attached to the lower border of the cecum in the lower right quadrant of the abdomen.

appositional growth The formation of new bone on the surface of a bone; one of the ways a bone grows.

Prep Kit continued...

arachnoid The middle membrane of the three meninges that enclose the brain and spinal cord.

arteries The blood vessels that carry blood away from the heart.

arteriole The smallest branch of an artery leading to the vast network of capillaries.

asbestosis A disease of the lungs caused by inhalation of asbestos particles.

ascending aorta The first of three portions of the aorta; originates from the left ventricle and gives rise to two branches, the right and left main coronary arteries.

ascending fibers (afferent tracts) Fibers that carry sensory information from the periphery to the brain; also called afferent tracts.

ascending reticular activating system Several structures located throughout the brainstem that are responsible for maintenance of consciousness.

asthma A reversible restrictive lower airway disease.

atlanto-occipital joint The location where the atlas articulates with the occipital condyles.

atlas The first cervical vertebra (C1), which provides support for the head.

atrioventricular (AV) node The site located in the right atrium adjacent to the septum that is responsible for transiently slowing electrical conduction.

atrioventricular valves The two valves through which blood flows from the atria to the ventricles.

atrium Upper chamber of the heart.

auditory ossicles The bones that function in hearing and are located deep within cavities of the temporal bone.

automaticity The ability of cardiac cells to generate an impulse to contract even when there is no external nervous stimulus.

autonomic nervous system (ANS) The part of the nervous system that regulates functions, such as digestion and sweating, that are not controlled voluntarily.

axial skeleton The portion of the skeleton that includes the torso.

axillary nerve One of the major nerves emanating from the brachial plexus; it supplies the deltoid and teres minor muscles, enabling arm abduction and lateral rotation.

axillary nodes A large collection of lymph nodes located in the axilla (armpit).

axillary vein The vein that is formed from the combination of the basilic and cephalic veins; it drains into the subclavian vein.

axis The second cervical vertebra; the point that allows the head to turn.

axon A projection from a neuron that makes connections with adjacent cells.

ball-and-socket joint A joint that allows internal and external rotation as well as bending.

baroreceptors Receptors in the blood vessels, kidneys, brain, and heart that respond to changes in pressure in the heart or main arteries to help maintain homeostasis.

basal ganglia Structures located deep within the cerebrum, diencephalon, and midbrain that play an important role in coordination of motor movements and posture.

base A substance that decreases the concentration of hydrogen ions.

basilar artery The artery that is formed when the left and right vertebral arteries unite after entering the brain through the foramen magnum.

basilic vein One of the two major veins of the arm; it combines with the cephalic vein to form the axillary vein.

basophil A white blood cell that may play a role following infection of various areas in the body.

beta cells Cells located in the islets of Langerhans that secrete insulin.

beta effects Stimulation of beta receptors that results in inotropic, dromotropic, and chronotropic states.

beta-endorphins Proteins that have the same effects as opiate drugs such as morphine.

beta receptors One of two adrenergic receptors classified into two structural and functional categories; further subdivided into beta$_1$ and beta$_2$ receptors.

bilateral A body part that appears on both sides of the midline.

bile ducts Ducts that convey bile between the liver and the intestine.

bilirubin A waste product of red blood cell destruction that undergoes further metabolism in the liver.

black lung disease A disease of the lung caused by consistent inhalation of coal dust.

blood The fluid tissue that is pumped by the heart through the arteries, veins, and capillaries and consists of plasma and formed elements or cells, such as red blood cells, white blood cells, and platelets.

blood pressure (BP) The pressure that the blood exerts against the walls of the arteries as it passes through them.

blowout fracture A fracture of the floor of the orbit usually caused by a blow to the eye.

bone marrow The substance located within the medullary cavity of a bone that consists of adipose tissue (yellow marrow) or red-blood-producing cells in bones in the axial skeleton and girdles (red marrow).

brachial artery The major vessel in the upper extremity that supplies blood to the arm.

brachial plexus The plexus of spinal nerves that consists of nerves C5 to T1 and innervates the shoulder and upper extremity.

brain The controlling organ of the body and center of consciousness; functions include perception, control of reactions to the environment, emotional responses, and judgment.

brainstem The area of the brain between the spinal cord and cerebrum, surrounded by the cerebellum; controls functions that are necessary for life, such as respirations.

bronchial arteries Arteries that branch off of the thoracic aorta and supply the lung tissues with blood.

bronchial veins Veins that return deoxygenated blood to the heart from the lungs.

bronchioles Fine subdivisions of the bronchi that give rise to the alveolar ducts.

bronchodilator Medication that is designed to improve lung function.

bronchospasm Constriction of the airway passages of the lungs that accompanies muscle spasms.

bruit An abnormal "whooshing-like" sound indicating turbulent blood flow within a blood vessel.

bruxism Grinding together of the upper and lower teeth.

buffer Any substance that can reversibly bind H^+.

buffer systems Fast-acting defenses for acid-base changes, providing almost immediate protection against changes in the hydrogen ion concentration of extracellular fluid.

bundle of His Part of the conduction system of the heart; a continuation of the atrioventricular node.

bursa A small fluid-filled sac located between a tendon and a bone that cushions and protects the joint.

calcitonin A hormone produced by the parafollicular cells of the thyroid gland that is important in the regulation of calcium levels in the body.

canaliculi A minute canal in a compact bone.

cancellous bone A lacy network of bony rods called trabeculae.

capillary The fine end-divisions of the arterial system that allow contact between cells of the body tissues and the plasma and red blood cells.

cardiac cycle The repetitive pumping process that begins with the onset of cardiac muscle contraction and ends just prior to the beginning of the next contraction.

cardiac muscle Muscle that is found only in the heart, providing the contractions needed to propel the blood through the circulatory system.

cardiac output The amount of blood pumped through the circulatory system in 1 minute.

carotid artery The major artery that supplies blood to the head and brain.

carotid bifurcation The point of division at which the common carotid artery branches at the angle of the mandible into the internal and external carotid arteries.

carotid canals An opening in the cranial vault through which the carotid arteries enter.

carpometacarpal joint The joint between the wrist and the metacarpal bones; the thumb joint.

cartilage Plates of shiny connective tissue that are lubricated by synovial fluid to provide a slippery surface over which bones may move freely.

catabolism The destructive component of metabolism associated with the breakdown of larger molecules into smaller molecules.

Prep Kit continued...

cauda equina Numerous individual nerve roots that extend from the spinal cord at the level of the second lumbar vertebra.

caudad Toward the feet.

cecum The first part of the large intestine, into which the ileum opens.

cell membrane The cell wall; the cell membrane is selectively permeable.

cells The basic building blocks of life; made up of protoplasm or cytoplasm, specialized for particular functions.

cellular respiration A biochemical process resulting in the production of energy in the form of ATP.

central nervous system (CNS) The brain and spinal cord.

cephalad Situated toward the head.

cephalic vein One of the two major veins of the arm that combine to form the axillary vein.

cerebellar peduncles One of three bands of nerve fibers through which the cerebellum communicates with other regions of the CNS.

cerebellum One of the three major subdivisions of the brain, sometimes called the "little brain"; coordinates the various activities of the brain, particularly body movements.

cerebral arteries The arteries that supply blood to large portions of the cerebral cortex of the brain.

cerebrospinal fluid (CSF) Fluid produced in the ventricles of the brain that flows in the subarachnoid space and bathes the meninges.

cerebrum The largest part of the three subdivisions of the brain, sometimes called the "gray matter"; made up of several lobes that control movement, hearing, balance, speech, visual perception, emotions, and personality.

cervical nodes A large collection of lymph nodes located in the neck.

cervical spine The portion of the spinal column consisting of the first seven vertebrae that lie in the neck.

chemoreceptors Receptors in the blood vessels, kidneys, brain, and heart that respond to changes in chemical composition of the blood to help maintain homeostasis.

cholinergic Description of a neuron that secretes the neurotransmitter acetylcholine.

chordae tendineae cordis Small muscular strands that attach the ventricles and the valves, preventing regurgitation of blood through the valves from the ventricles to the atria.

choroid plexus Specialized cells within hollow areas in the ventricles of the brain that produce CSF.

chronic bronchitis Chronic inflammatory condition affecting the bronchi that is associated with excess mucus production that results from overgrowth of the mucous glands in the airways.

chronic obstructive pulmonary disease (COPD) A progressive and irreversible disease of the airway marked by decreased inspiratory and expiratory capacity of the lungs.

chronotropic state Related to the control of the heart's rate of contraction.

circle of Willis An interconnection of the anterior cerebral arteries and the anterior communicating artery, which forms an important source of collateral circulation to the brain.

circulatory system The complex arrangement of connected tubes, including the arteries, arterioles, capillaries, venules, and veins, that moves blood, oxygen, nutrients, carbon dioxide, and cellular waste throughout the body.

circumflex coronary artery One of the two branches of the left main coronary artery.

clavicle The collarbone; it is lateral to the sternum and medial to the scapula.

coccyx The last three or four vertebrae of the spine; the tailbone.

common peroneal nerve A major nerve of the leg, providing sensation to the lateral leg and dorsum of the foot and motor activity to hip extensors, knee flexors, ankle dorsiflexors, and toe extensors.

compact bone Bone that is mostly solid, with few spaces.

concentration gradient The difference in concentrations of a substance on either side of a selectively permeable membrane.

conchae Three bony ridges contained within the lateral walls of the nasopharynx.

conduction system A group of complex electrical tissues within the heart that initiate and transmit stimuli that result in contractions of myocardial tissue.

conductivity The ability of cardiac cells to conduct electrical impulses.

contractility The strength of heart muscle contraction.

contralateral On the opposite side.

coronal suture The point where the parietal bones join together with the frontal bone.

coronary arteries Arteries that arise from the aorta shortly after it leaves the left ventricle and supply the heart with oxygen and nutrients.

coronary sinus Veins that collect blood that is returning from the walls of the heart.

corticosteroids Any of several steroids secreted by the adrenal gland.

cortisol The most important corticosteroid secreted by the zona fasciculata.

costal arch A bridge of cartilage that connects the ends of the sixth through tenth ribs with the lower portion of the sternum.

costochondritis Inflammation of the costocartilages, which attach the ribs to the sternum.

costovertebral angle An angle that is formed by the junction of the spine and the tenth rib.

cranial Related to or toward the skull.

cranial nerves The 12 pairs of nerves that arise from the base of the brain.

cranial vault The bones that encase and protect the brain, including the parietal, temporal, frontal, occipital, sphenoid, and ethmoid bones.

cranium The area of the head above the ears and eyes; the skull. The cranium contains the brain.

crenation Shrinkage of a cell that results when too much water leaves the cell through osmosis.

crepitus A grinding sound or sensation.

cribriform plate A horizontal bone perforated with numerous foramina for the passage of the olfactory nerve filaments from the nasal cavity.

cricoid cartilage A firm ridge of cartilage that forms the lower part of the larynx.

cricothyroid membrane A thin sheet of fascia that connects the thyroid and cricoid cartilages that make up the larynx.

crista galli A prominent bony ridge in the center of the anterior fossa to which the meninges are attached.

cusps The flaps that comprise the heart valves.

deep Further inside the body and away from the skin.

deep peroneal nerve A component and branch of the common peroneal nerve that innervates the muscles that dorsiflex the foot and extend the toes.

dendrite A projection from a neuron that makes connections with an adjacent cell.

dermatome An area of skin supplied by a given spinal nerve.

dermis The inner layer of the skin, containing hair follicles, sweat glands, nerve endings, and blood vessels.

descending aorta One of the three portions of the aorta, it is the longest portion and extends through the thorax and abdomen into the pelvis.

descending fibers (efferent tracts) Fibers that carry motor impulses from the brain to the fibers of the peripheral nervous system; also called efferent tracts.

diapedesis A process whereby leukocytes leave blood vessels to move toward tissue where they are needed most.

diaphragm A muscular dome that forms the undersurface of the thorax, separating the chest from the abdominal cavity. Contraction of the diaphragm (and the chest wall muscles) brings air into the lungs. Relaxation allows air to be expelled from the lungs.

diaphysis The shaft of a long bone.

diastole The relaxation, or period of relaxation, of the heart, especially of the ventricles.

diencephalon The part of the brain between the brainstem and the cerebrum that includes the thalamus, the subthalamus, hypothalamus, and epithalamus.

diffuse lymphatic tissue Tissue with no clear boundary that blends with surrounding tissues and contains lymphocytes and other cells.

diffusion Movement of particles or solutes.

digestion The processing of food that nourishes the individual cells of the body.

distal Structures that are farther from the trunk or nearer to the free end of the extremity.

dorsal The posterior surface of the body, including the back of the hand.

dorsal root One of two roots of a spinal nerve that passes posteriorly into the spinal cord and contains the dorsal root ganglion.

Prep Kit continued...

dorsal root ganglion A ganglion on the dorsal root of each spinal nerve.

dorsalis pedis artery The artery on the anterior surface of the foot between the first and second metatarsals.

dromotropic state Related to the control of the heart's conduction rate.

dura mater The outermost of the three meninges that enclose the brain and spinal cord; it is the toughest membrane.

efferent nerves Nerves that carry commands from the brain to peripheral muscles also called motor nerves.

ejection fraction The portion of the blood ejected from the ventricle during systole.

electrolytes Salt or acid substances that become ionic conductors when dissolved in a solvent (ie, water); chemicals dissolved in the blood.

emphysema Destruction of the walls of the alveoli, which creates resistance to expiratory airflow.

endochondral growth The growth of cartilage in the epiphyseal plate and its eventual replacement by bone; one of the ways a bone grows.

endocrine glands Glands that empty secretions (hormones) directly into the blood.

endocrine system The complex message and control system that integrates many body functions, including the release of hormones.

endocytosis The uptake of material through the cell membrane by a membrane-bound droplet or vesicle formed within the cell's protoplasm.

endosteum The lining of the inner surfaces of a long bone.

eosinophils A leukocyte that may play a role following infection in various areas in the body.

epicardium The layer of the serous pericardium that lies closely against the heart. Also called the visceral pericardium.

epidermis The outer layer of skin, which is made up of cells that are sealed together to form a watertight protective covering for the body.

epiglottis A thin, leaf-shaped valve that allows air to pass into the trachea but prevents food or liquid from entering.

epinephrine A naturally occurring hormone with a greater stimulatory effect on beta receptors that also may be given as a cardiac drug.

epiphyses The ends of a long bone.

epithalamus Part of the diencephalon with uncertain functions.

erythrocytes Disk-shaped cells that carry oxygen to the tissues; also known as red blood cells.

erythropoiesis The process by which red blood cells are made.

esophagus A collapsible tube that extends from the pharynx to the stomach; contractions of the muscle in the wall of the esophagus propel food and liquids through it to the stomach.

estrogen Produced by the ovaries, it is one of three major female hormones.

excitability A property of cardiac cells that provides the cells with the ability to respond to electrical impulses.

exocrine glands Glands that empty their products through ducts, usually onto epithelial surfaces.

exocytosis The release of secretions from cells that have been accumulated in vesicles.

extend To straighten.

extension Return of a joint from a flexed position to an anatomic position.

external auditory meatus An opening in the temporal bone that contains the ear canal.

external nares The external openings to the nasal cavity; also called the nostrils.

external rotation Rotating an extremity at its joint away from the midline.

extracellular fluid (ECF) Fluid outside of the cell, in which most of the body's supply of sodium is contained.

facial nerve The cranial nerve (VII) that supplies motor activity to all muscles of facial expression, the sense of taste to the anterior two thirds of the tongue, and cutaneous sensation to the external ear, tongue, and palate.

facilitated diffusion Process whereby a carrier molecule moves substances in or out of cells from areas of higher to lower concentration.

fallopian tube Long, slender tube that extends from the uterus to the region of the ovary on the same side, and through which the ovum passes from ovary to uterus.

fascia A sheet or band of tough fibrous connective tissue that covers, supports, and separates muscles.

feedback inhibition The concept that once the desired effect of a hormone has been achieved, further production of the hormone is inhibited until it is needed again; also referred to as negative feedback.

femoral artery The principal artery of the thigh, a continuation of the external iliac artery. It supplies blood to the lower abdominal wall, external genitalia, and legs. It can be palpated in the groin area.

femoral head The proximal end of the femur, articulating with the acetabulum to form the hip joint.

femoral nerve The branch of the lumbosacral plexus that innervates the muscles that flex the hip and extend the knee.

femoral vein A continuation of the saphenous vein that drains into the external iliac vein.

femur The thighbone; the longest and one of the strongest bones in the body.

fibrin A white insoluble protein formed in the clotting process.

fibula The long bone on the posterior surface of the lower leg.

flat bones Type of bone that is relatively thin and flattened.

flex To bend.

flexion In the anatomic position, moving a distal point of an extremity closer to the trunk.

flexor reflex A withdrawal reflex in the flexor muscles of the limbs that contract in response to an unpleasant stimulus.

floating ribs The eleventh and twelfth ribs, which do not attach to the sternum through the costal arch.

fluid balance The process of maintaining homeostasis through equal intake and output of fluids.

follicles Small cavity glands within the thyroid gland that contain thyroglobulin.

follicle-stimulating hormone (FSH) Hormone that regulates the production of both eggs and sperm, as well as production of reproductive hormones.

fontanelles The soft spots in the skull of a newborn and infant where the sutures of the skull have not yet grown together.

foramen magnum A large opening at the base of the skull through which the brain connects to the spinal cord.

foramen ovale An opening between the two atria that is present in the fetus but closes shortly after birth.

foramina Small openings, perforations, or orifices in the bones of the cranial vault.

forced expiratory vital capacity (FEVI) The volume of air exhaled from the lung following a forceful exhalation.

fossa ovalis A depression between the right and left atria that indicates where the foramen ovale had been located in the fetus.

Fowler's position The position in which the patient is sitting up with the knees bent.

frontal lobe The portion of the brain that is important in voluntary motor actions and personality traits.

frontal plane The plane parallel to the anterior surface of the body.

gallbladder A sac on the undersurface of the liver that collects bile from the liver and discharges it into the duodenum through the common bile duct.

ganglia Collections of nerve cell bodies located outside the CNS.

ganglionic synapse A separation between two nerves (preganglionic and postganglionic neurons), in a series between the CNS and the organs innervated.

genital system The male and female reproductive systems.

gland A cell, group of cells, or an organ that selectively removes, concentrates, or alters materials in the blood and secretes them back into the body.

glenoid fossa The part of the scapula that forms the socket in the ball-and-socket joint of the shoulder.

glossopharyngeal nerve The cranial nerve (IX) that supplies motor fibers to the pharyngeal muscle, providing taste sensation to the posterior portion of the tongue, and carrying parasympathetic fibers to the parotid gland.

glottis The opening into the lower airway between the true vocal cords.

glucagon Hormone produced by the pancreas that is vital to the control of the body's metabolism and blood glucose level.

Prep Kit continued...

glucocorticoids Hormones secreted by the zona fasciculata that play an important role in metabolism and inhibit inflammation.

gluconeogenesis A process that stimulates both the liver and the kidneys to produce glucose from non-carbohydrate molecules.

glycogen A long polymer from which glucose is converted in the liver (animal starch).

glycogenolysis The breakdown of glycogen to glucose.

gonadotropin-releasing hormone A hormone released by the hypothalamus that influences the release of LH and FSH.

gonads The reproductive glands.

granulocytes A type of leukocyte that has large cytoplasmic granules that are easily seen with a simple light microscope.

greater trochanter A bony prominence on the proximal lateral side of the thigh, just below the hip joint.

growth hormone (GH) Hormone that stimulates growth in most tissues, especially of long bones in the extremities; also called somatotropin.

growth hormone release-inhibiting hormone Hormone released by the hypothalamus that inhibits the secretion of growth hormone; also called somatostatin.

growth hormone-releasing hormone A hormone released by the hypothalamus that stimulates the secretion of growth hormone.

gyri The numerous folds in the cerebrum, which greatly increase the surface area of the cortex.

hair follicles The small organs in the skin that produce hair.

hard palate The bony anterior part of the palate, which forms the roof of the mouth.

haversian systems A unit of compact bone consisting of a tube (haversian canal) with the laminae of bone that surrounds it.

heart A hollow muscular organ that receives blood from the veins and propels it into the arteries.

hemoglobin An iron-containing pigment found in red blood cells, carries 97% of oxygen.

hemostasis Control of bleeding by formation of a blood clot.

heparin A substance found in large amounts in basophils that inhibits blood clotting.

hepatic portal system A specialized part of the venous system that drains blood from the stomach, intestines, and spleen.

hepatic veins The veins to which blood empties after liver cells in the sinusoids of the liver extract nutrients, filter the blood, and metabolize various drugs.

hilium The point of entry for the bronchi, vessels, and nerves into each lung.

hinge joints Joints that can bend and straighten but cannot rotate; they restrict motion to one plane.

histamine A substance found in large amounts in basophils that increases tissue inflammation.

homeostasis The maintenance of a relatively stable internal physiologic environment.

hormone sensitive lipase An enzyme that is activated by glucagons; it breaks triglycerides down into free fatty acids and glycerol.

hormones Proteins secreted by glands to regulate body functions.

human chorionic gonadotropin (hCG) One of three major female hormones; it is produced by a developing embryo after conception.

humerus The supporting bone of the arm.

hydroxyapatite A mineral compound containing calcium and phosphate that, along with collagen, comprises the structural element of bone.

hyoid bone A bone at the base of the tongue that supports the tongue and its muscles.

hyperextension Extension of a body part to a maximum level or past the position of normal extension.

hyperflexion Flexion of a body part to a maximum level or past the position of normal flexion.

hyperosmolar hyperglycemic nonketotic coma (HHNC) A diabetic emergency that occurs from a relative insulin deficiency, resulting in marked hyperglycemia but the absence of ketones and acidosis.

hypoglossal nerve The cranial nerve (XII) that provides motor function to the muscles of the tongue and throat.

hypophysis The gland that secretes hormones that regulate the function of many other glands in the body; also called the pituitary gland.

hypothalamic-pituitary-adrenal axis A complex set of interactions that regulates the secretion of corticosteroids.

hypothalamic-pituitary axis The interactions of the hypothalamus and the pituitary gland.

hypothalamohypophyseal portal system A specialized set of blood vessels that carry releasing factors from the hypothalamus to the anterior pituitary lobe.

hypothalamus The basal part of the diencephalons; it regulates the function of the pituitary gland.

hypoxic drive A "backup system" to control respiration; senses drops in the oxygen level in the blood.

iliac crest The rim, or wing, of the pelvic bone.

ilium One of three bones that fuse to form the pelvic ring.

inferior The part of the body, or any body part, nearer to the feet.

inferior vena cava One of the two largest veins in the body; carries blood from the lower extremities and the pelvic and the abdominal organs into the heart.

inguinal ligament The tough, fibrous ligament that stretches between the lateral edge of the pubic symphysis and the anterosuperior iliac spine.

inguinal nodes A large collection of lymph nodes located in the groin.

inhibiting factors Compounds that travel from the hypothalamus to the pituitary gland in a specialized set of blood vessels; also called releasing factors.

inotropic state Related to the strength of the heart's contraction.

insulin Hormone produced by the pancreas that is vital in the control of the body's metabolism and blood glucose level.

integumentary system The body's external surface, including the skin, nails, hair, and sweat and oil glands.

interatrial septum A membrane that separates the right and left atria.

interior nares The posterior opening from the nasopharynx into the pharynx.

internal auditory meatus A short canal through which auditory and facial nerves pass.

internal rotation Rotating an extremity medially toward the midline.

interstitial fluid The fluid located outside of the blood vessels in the spaces between the body's cells.

interventricular septum A thick wall that separates the right and left ventricles.

intervertebral foramen The opening between each vertebra through which the spinal (peripheral) nerves pass from the spinal cord.

intracellular fluid (ICF) Fluid within cells in which most of the body's supply of potassium is contained.

intravascular fluid (plasma) The noncellular portion of blood found within the blood vessels; also called plasma.

involuntary Not normally under conscious control.

involuntary muscle Muscle that continues to contract, rhythmically, regardless of the conscious will of the individual.

ipsilateral On the same side.

islets of Langerhans A specialized group of cells in the pancreas where insulin and glucagon are produced.

isthmus A narrow bank of tissue that connects the two lobes of the thyroid gland.

joint (articulation) The place where two bones come into contact.

joint capsule The fibrous sac with synovial lining that encloses a joint.

jugular veins The two main veins that drain the head and neck.

kidneys Two retroperitoneal organs that excrete the end products of metabolism as urine and regulate the body's salt and water content.

Krebs cycle A sequence of reactions in an organism in which oxidation of acids provides energy for storage in phosphate bonds (as in ATP); also called the tricarboxylic acid cycle.

lacuna One of the minute cavities in bone or cartilage occupied by osteocytes.

lambdoid suture The point where the occipital bones attach to the parietal bones.

lamellae Thin sheets or layers into which bone tissue is organized.

large intestine The portion of the digestive tube that encircles the abdomen around the small bowel, consisting of the cecum, the colon, and the rectum.

Prep Kit continued...

larynx The opening of the lower airway, which consists of several cartilaginous structures held together by ligaments.

lateral Parts of the body that lie farther from the midline; also called outer structures.

lateral malleolus An enlargement of the distal end of the fibula, which forms the lateral wall of the ankle joint.

lateral recumbent position Lying on the side.

left anterior descending One of the two branches of the left main coronary artery that is the largest and shortest of the myocardial blood vessels. The LAD and the circumflex coronary arteries supply blood to the left ventricle and other areas.

leukocytes White blood cells that are responsible for fighting infection.

ligament A band of the fibrous tissue that connects bones to bones; it supports and strengthens a joint.

limbic system Structures within the cerebrum and diencephalon that influence emotions, motivation, mood, and sensations of pain and pleasure.

lingual tonsils One of three sets of lymphatic organs that comprise the tonsils; they are located on the posterior margin of the tongue and help protect the body from bacteria introduced into the mouth and nose.

lingula A small portion of the left lung that is the equivalent of the middle lobe in the right lung.

liver A large solid organ that lies in the right upper quadrant immediately below the diaphragm; it produces bile, stores sugar for immediate use by the body, and produces many substances that help regulate immune responses.

lobes Subdivisions within each hemisphere of the cerebrum; each lobe is named for the bone of the skull that overlies it.

long bones Type of bone that is longer than it is wide.

longitudinal fissure The crevasse that separates the right and left hemispheres of the cerebrum.

lumbar spine The lower part of the back, formed by the lowest five nonfused vertebrae; also called the dorsal spine.

lumbar vertebrae Vertebrae of the lumbar spine.

lumbosacral plexus A combination of the lumbar plexus and the sacral plexus and the coccygeal root.

lungs The two primary organs of breathing.

luteinizing hormone (LH) A hormone released from the pituitary gland at roughly monthly intervals that helps to stimulate one oocyte to undergo meiosis.

lymph A thin, plasma-like liquid formed from interstitial or extracellular fluid that bathes the tissues of the body.

lymph nodes Round or bean-shaped structures interspersed along the course of the lymph vessels, which filter the lymph and serve as a source of lymphocytes.

lymph nodules Tissue that is denser than diffuse lymphatic tissue, found in the loose connective tissue of the digestive, respiratory, and urinary systems.

lymph vessels Thin-walled vessels through which lymph circulates through the body; they travel close to the major veins.

lymphatic capillaries Vessels of the lymphatic system that carry fluid away from the tissues.

lymphatic duct One of two great lymph vessels; it empties into the subclavian vein.

lymphatic system A passive circulatory system that transports a plasma-like liquid called lymph, a thin fluid that bathes the tissues of the body.

lymphocytes The smallest of the agranulocytes, they originate in the bone marrow but migrate through the blood to the lymphatic tissues.

lysis The process of disintegration or breakdown of cells that occurs when excess water enters the cell through osmosis.

macrophages Cells that are responsible for protecting the body against infection.

mainstem bronchi The part of the lower airway below the larynx through which air enters the lungs.

mandible The bone of the lower jaw.

manubrium The upper quarter of the sternum.

mastoid process A prominent bony mass at the base of the skull behind the ear.

maxillae The upper jawbones that assist in the formation of the orbit, the nasal cavity, and the palate, and lodge the upper teeth.

meatus A passage located below each turbinate.

medial Parts of the body that lie closer to the midline; also called inner structures.

medial malleolus The distal end of the tibia, which forms the medial side of the ankle joint.

median nerve The nerve in the brachial plexus that innervates the pronator muscles of the forearm, as well as those that flex the wrist, fingers, and thumb.

median plane An imaginary longitudinal line that divides the human body into left and right parts; also called the midsagittal plane or the midline.

mediastinum The space between the lungs, in the center of the chest, that contains the heart, trachea, mainstem bronchi, part of the esophagus, and large blood vessels.

medulla (endocrine system) the inner portion of the adrenal glands, which produce epinephrine and norepinephrine.

medulla (nervous system) The inferior portion of the midbrain, which serves as a conduction pathway for both ascending and descending nerve tracts.

medullary cavity The internal cavity of the diaphysis of a long bone that contains bone marrow.

meninges A set of three tough membranes, the dura mater, arachnoid, and pia mater, that enclose the entire brain and spinal cord.

metabolism The sum of all the physical and chemical processes of living organisms; the process by which energy is made available for the uses of the organism.

metacarpal bones The bones that form the hand.

metaphysis The area of a long bone where the diaphysis and epiphysis converge; the epiphyseal plate is located here.

midaxillary line An imaginary vertical line drawn through the middle of the axilla (armpit), parallel to the midline.

midclavicular line An imaginary vertical line drawn through the middle portion of the clavicle and parallel to the midline.

midline An imaginary vertical line drawn from the middle of the forehead through the nose and the umbilicus (navel) to the floor.

mineralocorticoids Hormones produced in the zona glomerulosa that are important in the regulation of water and salt balance in the body.

mitochondria Small rod-like organelle that functions as the metabolic center of the cell and produce ATP.

mitral valve The valve in the heart that separates the left atrium from the left ventricle.

monocytes Migrate out of the blood and into the tissues in response to an infection.

motor nerves Nerves that carry information from the central nervous system to the muscles of the body.

mucous membranes The lining of body cavities and passages that communicate directly or indirectly with the environment outside the body.

mucus The opaque, sticky secretion of the mucous membranes that lubricates the body openings.

murmur An abnormal heart sound, heard as a "whooshing-like" sound indicating turbulent blood flow within the heart.

muscarinic receptors Receptors at the target tissue that are stimulated by acetylcholine and can also be stimulated in the laboratory by the compound extracted from muscarine mushrooms.

musculocutaneous nerve A nerve in the upper extremity that innervates muscles that flex the arm and forearm.

musculoskeletal system The bones and voluntary muscles of the body.

myocardial infarction Blockage of the arteries that supply oxygen to the heart, resulting in death to a portion of the myocardium.

myocardium The heart muscle.

nasal cavity The chamber inside the nose that lies between the floor of the cranium and the roof of the mouth.

nasal septum The separation between the right and left nostrils.

nasolacrimal ducts The ducts that drain tears from the lacrimal sac to the meatus.

nasopharynx The part of the pharynx that lies above the level of the roof of the mouth, or soft palate.

negative feedback The concept that once the desired effect of a hormone has been achieved, further production of the hormone is inhibited until it is needed again; also called feedback inhibition.

nerve Nervous tissue that connects the nervous system with body parts or organs.

nerve fibers Groups of nerves cells bundled together.

nervous system The system that controls virtually all activities of the body, both voluntary and involuntary.

Prep Kit continued...

neuroeffector cells The target tissues of the autonomic nervous system.

neuroglia Collectively, the name for the connective and supporting tissues of the nervous tissue.

neurohormones Hormones secreted by the posterior pituitary lobe.

neuromuscular junction The junction between a motor neuron and a muscle fiber; one type of a synapse.

neurons The main functional units of the nervous system.

neurotransmitters Chemical substances that transmit nerve impulses across a synapse.

neutrophils One of the three types of granulocytes; they have multi-lobed nuclei that resemble a string of baseballs held together by a thin strand of thread; they destroy bacteria, antigen-antibody complexes, and foreign matter.

nicotinic receptors Receptors in the postganglionic neuron that can be stimulated in the laboratory by the alkaloid nicotine.

nonstriated Smooth muscle tissue.

norepinephrine A naturally occurring hormone with a greater stimulatory effect on alpha receptors that also may be given as a cardiac drug.

obturator nerve A nerve emanating from the lumbosacral plexus that innervates muscles that adduct the thigh and rotate it medially.

occipital condyles Articular surface on the occipital bone where the skull articulates with the atlas on the vertebral column.

occipital lobe The portion of the brain that is responsible for the processing of visual information.

oculomotor nerve The cranial nerve (III) that innervates the muscles that cause motion of the eyeballs and upper lid.

olfactory bulb The cranial nerve for smell.

olfactory nerve The cranial nerve (I) that transmits information about the sense of smell.

olfactory tract The part of the olfactory nerve that arises at the base of the brain.

optic chiasma A continuation of the optic nerve, which forms an "X" under the hypothalamus.

optic foramina The openings through which the optic nerves pass to reach each eyeball.

optic nerve The cranial nerve (II) that transmits visual information to the brain.

optic tracts The parts of the optic nerve that arise at the base of the brain, forming the optic chiasma.

orbit The eye socket, made up of the maxilla and zygoma.

organ Different types of tissues working together to perform a particular function.

organism Any living thing considered as a whole, made up of various organ systems.

organ system A group of organs that have a common purpose, such as the skeleton, muscles, and the circulatory and respiratory systems, among others.

oropharynx A tubular structure that extends vertically from the back of the mouth to the esophagus and trachea.

osmoreceptors Specialized neurons in the brain that regulate the secretion of ADH.

osmosis The movement of a solvent, such as water, from an area of low solute concentration to one of high concentration through a selectively permeable membrane to equalize concentrations of a solute on both sides of the membrane.

osmotic pressure The tendency of water to move by osmosis across a membrane.

ossicles The three small bones in the middle ear: the malleus, incus, and stapes.

osteoblasts Bone-forming cells.

osteoclasts Large, multinucleated cells that dissolve bone tissue and play a major role in bone remodeling.

osteocyte An osteoblast that becomes surrounded by bony matrix.

osteons Unit within a compact bone in which blood vessels are located; also called the haversian system.

ovary A female gland that produces sex hormones and ova (eggs).

oxytocin A hormone that causes the smooth muscles of the pregnant uterus to contract and milk to be released from the breasts of lactating women.

palatine bone An irregularly shaped bone found in the posterior part of the nasal cavity.

palatine tonsils One of three sets of lymphatic organs that comprise the tonsils; they are located in the back of the throat, on each side of the posterior opening of the oral cavity, and help protect the body from bacteria introduced into the mouth and nose.

palmar The front region of the hand.

palmar arches The two arches formed from the radial and ulnar vessels within the hand, creating the superficial and deep palmar arches.

pancreas A flat, solid organ that lies below the liver and the stomach; it is a major source of digestive enzymes and produces the hormone insulin.

papillary muscles Specialized muscles that attach the ventricles to the cusps of the valves by muscular strands called chordae tendineae cordis.

parafollicular cells Cells located between the follicles in the thyroid gland that produce the hormone calcitonin.

paranasal sinuses The sinuses, or hollowed sections of bone in the front of the head, which are lined with mucous membrane and drain into the nasal cavity.

parasympathetic nervous system The part of the autonomic nervous system that relaxes the body.

parathyroid glands Four glands that are embedded in the posterior portion of each lobe of the thyroid; they produce and secrete parathyroid hormone.

parathyroid hormone Hormone produced and secreted by the parathyroid glands; it maintains normal levels of calcium in the blood and normal neuromuscular function.

parietal layer One of two layers of the serous pericardium; it is separated from the visceral pericardium by a small amount of pericardial fluid.

parietal lobe The portion of the brain that is the site for reception and evaluation of most sensory information, except smell, hearing, and vision.

parietal pleura The pleural membrane that lines the pleural cavity.

partial pressure of carbon dioxide (Paco$_2$) A measurement of the amount of carbon dioxide in the blood.

partial pressure of oxygen (Pao$_2$) A measurement of the amount of oxygen in the blood.

patella The kneecap; a specialized bone that lies within the tendon of the quadriceps muscle.

pathophysiology The study of body functions of a living organism in an abnormal state.

pelvis The attachment of the lower extremities to the body, consisting of the sacrum and two pelvic bones.

perfusion The circulation of blood within an organ or tissue in adequate amounts to meet the cells' current needs.

pericardial fluid A serous fluid that fills the space between the visceral pericardium and the parietal pericardium and helps to reduce friction.

pericardial sac The potential space between the layers of the pericardium.

pericardium The serous membranes that surround the heart.

periosteum The membrane, made up of a double layer of connective tissue, that covers all bones, except the articular surfaces.

peripheral nerves The nerves that extend from the brain and spinal cord to various parts of the body by exiting between the vertebrae of the spine.

peripheral nervous system The part of the nervous system that consists of 31 pairs of spinal nerves and 12 pairs of cranial nerves; these peripheral nerves may be sensory nerves, motor nerves, or connecting nerves.

peristalsis The wave-like contraction of smooth muscle by which the ureters or other tubular organs propel their contents.

pH The measure of acidity or alkalinity of a solution.

phagocytosis Endocytosis involving solid particles.

phalanges The small bones of the digits of the fingers and toes.

pharyngeal tonsils One of three sets of lymphatic organs that comprise the tonsils; they are located near the internal opening of the nasal cavity and help protect the body from bacteria introduced into the mouth and nose. Also called adenoids.

pharynx The cavity formed by the posterior connection of the oropharynx and nasopharynx.

physiology The study of the body functions of the living organism.

Prep Kit continued...

physis The major site of bone elongation, located just proximal to the bone ends; also called the growth plate.

pia mater The innermost of the three meninges that enclose the brain and spinal cord; it rests directly on the brain and spinal cord.

pineal body Part of the epithalamus in the diencephalon.

pinocytosis Endocytosis involving liquid.

pituitary gland An endocrine gland, located in the sella turcica of the brain, responsible for directly or indirectly affecting all body functions.

planes Imaginary surfaces used as references to identify parts of the body.

plantar The bottom of the foot.

plasma A sticky, yellow fluid that carries the blood cells and nutrients and transports cellular waste material to the organs of excretion.

plasmin An enzyme that dissolves the fibrin in blood clots.

platelets Tiny, disk-shaped elements that are much smaller than the cells; they are essential in the initial formation of a blood clot, the mechanism that stops bleeding.

pleura The serous membrane covering the lungs and lining the thoracic cavity, completely enclosing a potential space known as the pleural space.

pleural cavity The potential space between the visceral and parietal pleura.

pleural space The potential space between the parietal pleura and the visceral pleura. It is described as "potential" because under normal conditions, the lungs fill this space.

plexus An organized intermingling formed by several nerves.

pons The mass of nerve fibers at the end of the medulla oblongata.

popliteal artery A continuation of the femoral artery at the knee.

popliteal vein The vein that forms when the anterior and posterior tibial veins unite at the knee.

positive feedback The concept that once the desired effect of a hormone has been achieved, production of the hormone is continued.

posterior The back surface of the body; the side away from you in the standard anatomic position.

posterior pituitary lobe (neurohypophysis) One of the two portions of the pituitary gland; it is an extension of the central nervous system and produces hormones called neurohormones; also called the neurophypophysis.

posterior tibial artery The artery just posterior to the medial malleolus; supplies blood to the foot.

postganglionic neuron The second of two nerves, separated by a ganglionic synapse, in a series between the CNS and the organs that are innervated.

postsynaptic terminal The proximal portion of the muscle fiber in the neuromuscular junction.

preganglionic neuron The first of two nerves, separated by a ganglionic synapse, in a series between the CNS and the organs that are innervated.

preload The volume of blood returned to the heart.

presynaptic terminal The distal end of the nerve fiber in the neuromuscular junction.

priapism A continuous and painful erection of the penis caused by certain spinal injuries and some diseases.

progesterone A hormone released from the ovaries that stimulates the uterine lining during the menstrual cycle.

prolactin Hormone that plays an important role in milk production in women.

prolactin-inhibiting hormones Hormones released by the hypothalamus that influence inhibition of prolactin.

prolactin-releasing hormones Hormones released by the hypothalamus that influence the release of prolactin.

pronation When the palm faces downward.

prone position The position in which the body is lying face down.

prostaglandins A group of hormone-like fatty acids that are produced in many body tissues, including the uterus, brain, and kidneys.

prostate gland A small gland that surrounds the male urethra where it emerges from the urinary bladder; it secretes a fluid that is part of the ejaculatory fluid.

proximal Structures that are closer to the trunk.

pubic symphysis A hard bony prominence that is found in the midline in the lowermost portion of the abdomen.

pulmonary artery The major artery leading from the right ventricle of the heart to the lungs; it carries oxygen-poor blood.

pulmonary circulation The circulatory system in the body that carries blood from the right side of the heart to the lungs, and back to the left side of the heart.

pulmonary function tests Tests that assess volumes of air that move into and out of the lungs.

pulmonary veins The four veins that return oxygenated blood from the lungs to the left atrium of the heart.

pulmonic valve The semilunar valve that regulates blood flow between the right ventricle and the pulmonary artery.

pulse The wave of pressure created as the heart contracts and forces blood out the left ventricle and into the major arteries.

radial artery The major artery in the forearm; it is palpable at the wrist on the thumb side.

radial nerve One of the major nerves in the upper extremity; it supplies muscles that extend the elbow, supinate the forearm, and extend the wrist, fingers, and thumb.

radius The bone on the thumb side of the forearm.

rami The posterior vertical parts of the lower jaw that join the mandible.

range of motion (ROM) The arc of movement of an extremity at a joint in a particular direction.

rectum The lowermost end of the colon.

red blood cells Cells that carry oxygen to the body's tissues; also called erythrocytes.

releasing factors Compounds that travel from the hypothalamus to the pituitary gland in a specialized set of blood vessels; also called inhibiting factors.

renal pelvis A cone-shaped collecting area that connects the ureter and the kidney.

renin-angiotensin system System located in the kidney that helps to regulate fluid balance and blood pressure.

residual volume The volume of air remaining in the respiratory passages and lungs after a forceful expiration.

respiratory bronchioles Structures formed by the final branching of the bronchioles.

respiratory center The part of the brain located in the medulla oblongata that controls the respiratory stimulus.

respiratory system All the structures of the body that contribute to the process of breathing, consisting of the upper and lower airways and their component parts.

restrictive lung disease Diseases such as black lung disease, asbestosis, that result in stiffening of the lungs and significantly decreased vital capacity.

retroperitoneal Behind the abdominal cavity.

retroperitoneum The space behind the peritoneum.

rootlets Small nerves.

sacrum One of three bones (sacrum and two pelvic bones) that make up the pelvic ring; consists of five fused sacral vertebrae.

saddle joint Two saddle-shaped articulating surfaces oriented at right angles to each other so that complementary surfaces articulate with each other, such as is the case with the thumb.

sagittal plane A vertical plane that is parallel to the midline and divides the body into unequal left and right parts.

sagittal suture The point of the skull where the parietal bones join together.

salivary glands The glands that produce saliva to keep the mouth and pharynx moist.

saphenous vein The longest vein in the body, it drains the leg, thigh, and dorsum of the foot.

scalp The thick skin covering the cranium, which usually bears hair.

scapula The shoulder blade.

sciatic nerve The longest peripheral nerve in the body, formed by the combination of the common peroneal nerve and the tibial nerve.

sebaceous glands Glands that produce an oily substance called sebum, which discharges along the shafts of the hairs.

secondary bronchi Airway passages in the lungs that are formed from the division of the right and left mainstem bronchi.

Prep Kit continued...

selective permeability Allowing some but not all substances to pass through a membrane to maintain homeostasis.

sella turcica A depression in the middle of the sphenoid bone where the pituitary gland is located.

semen Seminal fluid ejaculated from the penis and containing sperm.

semi-Fowler's position The position in which the patient is sitting up at a 45° angle with the knees bent.

semilunar valves The two valves, the aortic and pulmonic valves, that divide the heart from the aorta and pulmonary arteries.

seminal vesicles Storage sacs for sperm and seminal fluid, which empty into the urethra at the prostate.

sensory nerves The nerves that carry sensations of touch, taste, heat, cold, pain, or other modalities from the body to the central nervous system.

serous pericardium The inner membrane of the pericardium, which contains two layers called the visceral pericardium and the parietal pericardium.

serum osmolality The number of osmotically active particles in serum.

shock position The position that has the head and torso (trunk) supine and the lower extremities elevated 8" to 12". This helps to increase blood flow to the brain; also referred to as the modified Trendelenburg's position.

short bones Type of bone that is as broad as it is long.

shoulder girdle The proximal portion of the upper extremity, made up of the clavicle, the scapula, and the humerus.

shoulder joint A ball-and-socket joint consisting of the head of the humerus and the glenoid fossa.

sinoatrial (SA) node The normal site of the origin of electrical impulses; located high in the right atrium, it is the heart's natural pacemaker.

sinusitis An inflammation of the paranasal sinuses.

sinusoids The part of the hepatic portal system in which blood collects within the liver and the liver cells extract nutrients from the blood, filter the blood, and metabolize various drugs.

skeletal muscle Muscle that is attached to bones and usually crosses at least one joint; striated, or voluntary, muscle.

skeleton The framework that gives us our recognizable form; also designed to allow motion of the body and protection of vital organs.

skull The structure at the top of the axial skeleton that houses the brain and consists of the 28 bones that comprise the auditory ossicles, the cranium, and the face.

small intestine The portion of the digestive tube between the stomach and the cecum, consisting of the duodenum, jejunum, and ileum.

smooth muscle Nonstriated, involuntary muscle; it constitutes the bulk of the gastrointestinal tract and is present in nearly every organ to regulate automatic activity.

solutes Particles, such as salts, that are dissolved in a solvent.

somatomedins Proteins produced in the liver, skeletal muscle, and other tissues that are stimulated by growth hormone.

somatostatin A hormone released by the hypothalamus that inhibits the secretion of growth hormone; also called growth hormone release-inhibiting hormone.

somatotropin Hormone that stimulates growth in many tissues, especially of long bones in the extremities; also called growth hormone (GH).

spinal accessory nerve The cranial nerve (XI) that provides motor innervation to the muscles of the soft palate and the pharynx and to the sternocleidomastoid and trapezius muscles.

spinal cord An extension of the brain, composed of virtually all the nerves carrying messages between the brain and the rest of the body; it lies inside of, and is protected by, the spinal canal.

spinal nerves Nerves in the peripheral nervous system that arise from numerous rootlets along the dorsal and ventral surfaces of the spinal cord.

spinal reflex arcs Automatic reactions to stimuli that occur without conscious thought.

spirometer A device used in pulmonary function testing that measures air entering and leaving the lungs over a specific period of time.

spleen An organ of the lymphatic system that is located in the left upper quadrant of the abdomen and consists of two types of lymph tissue that are associated with drainage of the spleen.

Starling's Law of the Heart The force of the heartbeat is determined primarily by the length of the fibers constituting its muscular wall. An increase in diastolic filling equals an increase in the force of the heartbeat.

sternocleidomastoid muscles The muscles on either side of the neck that allow movement of the head.

sternum The breastbone.

striated Striped.

striated muscle Muscle that has characteristic stripes, or striations, under the microscope; voluntary, or skeletal, muscle.

stroke volume The amount of blood that the left ventricle ejects into the aorta per contraction.

styloid process Several long, slender, and pointed bones that project downward and forward from the temporal bone; also, the small bony protrusion to which the ligaments of the wrist are attached.

subarachnoid hemorrhage A hemorrhage between the arachnoid membrane and the pia mater.

subarachnoid space The space located between the pia mater and the arachnoid mater.

subclavian artery The proximal part of the main artery of the arm, which supplies the brain, neck, anterior chest wall, and shoulder.

subclavian veins The proximal part of the main vein of the arm, which unites with the internal jugular vein.

subcutaneous tissue Tissue, largely fat, that lies directly under the dermis and serves as an insulator of the body.

substantia nigra A layer of gray matter located in the midbrain.

subthalamus The part of the diencephalon that is involved in controlling motor functions.

sulci Grooves located between the gyri in the cerebrum.

superficial Closer to or on the skin.

superficial peroneal nerve The nerve in the leg that innervates the muscles of foot eversion.

superior The part of the body, or any body part, nearer to the head.

superior oblique muscle The muscle that controls the downward gaze of the eyeball.

superior vena cava One of the two largest veins in the body; carries blood from the upper extremities, head, neck, and chest into the heart.

supination When the palm faces upward.

supine position The position in which the body is lying face up.

sutures Attachment points in the skull where the cranial bones join together.

sweat glands The glands that secrete sweat.

sympathetic pathway The part of the autonomic nervous system that is responsible for the body's response to shock and stress.

synapse A gap between nerve cells across which nervous stimuli are transmitted.

synaptic cleft The space between nerves and muscles in the neuromuscular junction across which a nerve impulse is transmitted by a neurotransmitter.

synaptic vesicles Vesicles that contain neurotransmitters.

synovial fluid The transparent viscous lubricating fluid secreted by the synovial membrane in an articulation.

systemic circulation The circulatory system in the body that is responsible for blood flow in all areas of the body, except for areas covered by the pulmonary circulation (blood flow from the right side of the heart to the lungs, and back to the left side of the heart).

systole The contraction, or period of contraction, of the heart, especially that of the ventricles.

target tissues Selected tissues to which hormones are directed to act on.

temporal lobe The portion of the brain that plays an important role in hearing and memory.

temporomandibular joint (TMJ) The joint where the mandible meets with the temporal bone of the cranium just in front of each ear.

tendons Specialized tough cords or bands of dense white connective tissue that attaches muscles to bones.

tertiary bronchi Airway passages in the lungs that are formed from branching of the secondary bronchi.

Prep Kit continued...

testes The male reproductive organs that produce sperm and secrete male hormones; also called testicles.

testicle A male genital gland that contains specialized cells that produce hormones and sperm.

tetraiodothyronine One of the two major hormones produced by the thyroid gland; it is essential for normal growth and development in children, as well as regulation of body metabolism.

thalamus The part of the diencephalon that processes most sensory input and influences mood and general body movements, especially those associated with fear or rage.

thoracic cage The chest or rib cage.

thoracic duct One of two great lymph vessels; it empties into the superior vena cava.

thoracic spine The 12 vertebrae that lie between the cervical vertebrae and the lumbar vertebrae. One pair of ribs is attached to each of the thoracic vertebrae.

thorax The chest cavity that contains the heart, lungs, esophagus, and great vessels (the aorta and the two venae cavae).

thrombin An enzyme that causes the conversion of fibrinogen to fibrin, which binds to the platelet plug, forming the final mature clot.

thymus A triangular-shaped gland located below the sternum in the superior mediastinum; it produces lymphocytes.

thyroglobulin A protein to which thyroid hormones are bound.

thyroid cartilage A firm prominence of cartilage that forms the upper part of the larynx; the Adam's apple.

thyroid gland A large endocrine gland that is located at the base of the neck and produces and excretes hormones that influence growth, development, and metabolism.

thyroid-stimulating hormone (TSH) Hormone that controls the release of thyroid hormone from the thyroid gland; also called thyrotropin.

thyrotropin Hormone that controls the release of thyroid hormone from the thyroid gland; also called thyroid-stimulating hormone.

thyroxine-binding globulin A protein synthesized in the liver that binds to hormones T_3 and T_4.

tibia The shinbone, the larger of the two bones of the lower leg.

tibial nerve The nerve in the leg that innervates the muscles that extend the hip and flex the knee, plantar flex the foot, and flex the toes.

tibial veins A continuation of the veins of the feet that unite at the knee to form the popliteal vein, which then drains into the femoral vein.

tidal volume The volume of air inspired during normal inspiration.

tinnitus A ringing in the ears.

tissue Groups of similar cells working together for a common function.

tissue plasminogen activator (t-PA) A major component in the fibrinolytic system, in which clots that have already formed are lysed or disrupted, converting plasminogen to plasmin.

tonsils Three sets of lymphatic organs—the palatine tonsils, pharyngeal tonsils, and lingual tonsils—that are located in the back of the throat and nasopharynx and protect the body from bacteria introduced into the mouth and nose.

topographic anatomy The superficial landmarks of the body that serve as guides to the structures that lie beneath them.

torso The trunk without the head and limbs.

trabeculae Bony rods that make up cancellous bone and are oriented to increase weight-bearing capacity of long bones.

trachea The windpipe; the main trunk for air passing to and from the lungs.

tracts Pathways within the spinal cord that contain nerves.

transverse plane A cross-horizontal sectioning that divides the body into the upper and lower parts.

Trendelenburg's position The position in which the body is supine with the head lower than the feet.

tricuspid valve The heart valve that separates the right atrium from the right ventricle.

trigeminal nerve The cranial nerve (V) that supplies sensation to the scalp, forehead, face, and lower jaw and innervates the muscles of mastication, throat, and inner ear.

triiodothyronine One of the two major hormones produced by the thyroid gland, it is essential for normal growth and development in children, as well as regulation of body metabolism.

trismus Spasm of the muscles of chewing.

trochlear nerve The cranial nerve (IV) that innervates the superior oblique muscle of the eyeball, which allows a downward gaze.

true vocal cords The inferior portion of the vocal cords that vibrate to produce sound.

tunica adventitia The outer layer of tissue of a blood vessel wall, composed of elastic and fibrous connective tissue.

tunica intima The smooth, thin, inner lining of a blood vessel.

tunica media The middle and thickest layer of tissue of a blood vessel wall, composed of elastic tissue and smooth muscle cells that allow the vessel to expand or contract in response to changes in blood pressure and tissue demand.

turbinates A set of bony convolutions formed by the conchae in the nasopharynx that help to maintain smooth airflow.

ulna The inner bone of the forearm, on the side opposite the thumb.

ulnar nerve The nerve in the arm that innervates muscles that flex the wrist and fingers and abduct and adduct the fingers and thumb.

ureter A small, hollow tube that carries urine from the kidneys to the bladder.

urethra The canal that conveys urine from the bladder to outside the body.

urinary bladder A sac behind the pubic symphysis made of smooth muscle that collects and stores urine.

urinary system The organs that control the discharge of certain waste materials filtered from the blood and excreted as urine.

uvula A small fleshy mass that hangs from the soft palate.

vagina A muscular distensible tube that connects the uterus with the vulva (the external female genitalia); also called the birth canal.

vagus nerve The cranial nerve (X) that provides motor functions to the soft palate, pharynx, and larynx and carries taste bud fibers from the posterior tongue, sensory fibers from the inferior pharynx, larynx, thoracic, and abdominal organs, and parasympathetic fibers to thoracic and abdominal organs.

vasa deferentia (vas deferens) The spermatic duct of the testicles; also called vas deferens.

vasopressin A hormone secreted by the posterior pituitary lobe of the pituitary gland, it constricts blood vessels and raises the blood pressure; also called antidiuretic hormone (ADH).

veins The blood vessels that transport blood back to the heart.

venous sinuses Spaces between the membranes surrounding the brain that are the primary means of venous drainage from the brain.

ventilation The process of moving air into and out of the lungs.

ventral The anterior surface of the body.

ventral root One of two roots of a spinal nerve that is formed from six to eight rootlets.

ventricle Lower chamber of the heart; also used to refer to specialized hollow areas in the brain.

vertebrae The 33 bones that make up the spinal column.

vertebral canal The bony canal formed by vertebrae that houses and protects the spinal cord.

vertebral column The spine or primary support structure of the body, which houses the spinal cord and the peripheral nerves.

vestibular folds The superior portion of the vocal cords. Also called the false vocal cords.

vestibulocochlear nerve The cranial nerve (VIII) that passes through the internal auditory meatus and transmits information important to the senses of hearing and balance.

visceral layer The layer of the serous pericardium that lies closely against the heart; also called the epicardium.

visceral pleura The pleural membrane that covers the lungs.

Prep Kit continued...

vital capacity The amount of air moved in and out of the lungs with maximum inspiration and exhalation.

voluntary Consciously controlled, as in skeletal muscle tissue.

voluntary muscle Muscle that is under direct voluntary control of the brain and can be contracted or relaxed at will; skeletal, or striated, muscle.

white blood cells Blood cells that play a role in the body's immune defense mechanisms against infection; also called leukocytes.

xiphoid process The narrow, cartilaginous lower tip of the sternum.

zona fasciculata One of three divisions of the adrenal cortex; it produces corticosteroids.

zona glomerulosa One of three divisions of the adrenal cortex; it produces mineralocorticoids.

zona reticularis One of three divisions of the adrenal cortex; it secretes a few relatively weak male sex hormones, or androgens.

zygomatic arch The bone that extends along the front of the skull below the orbit.

Assessment in Action

You and your partner are dispatched for a medical emergency. Upon arrival you see an older woman sitting in a chair. She tells you that she has not been feeling well for a few days. Your partner begins to obtain her vital signs.

You ask her to indicate where she is feeling pain. She points to her upper left abdomen, where she has point tenderness. She also tells you that she has pain in her lower back that radiates to either side. As you continue your assessment, you begin to think about what may be wrong. What organs may be involved?

1. The study of the body functions of a living organism to an abnormal state such as a disease is called:
   A. anatomy.
   B. physiology.
   C. pathophysiology.
   D. biology.

2. The human body is made up of trillions of building blocks. These building blocks are the basis for life and are called:
   A. tissues.
   B. organs.
   C. organ systems.
   D. cells.

3. The directional term used when referring to the back of the body is called:
   A. ventral.
   B. dorsal.
   C. superior.
   D. medial.

4. The separation of the extracellular and intracellular area by a selectively permeable membrane helps to maintain:
   A. homeostasis.
   B. equilibrium.
   C. selective permeability.
   D. diffusion.

5. Chemical reactions that take place within the body that provide energy are called:
   A. homeostasis.
   B. metabolism.
   C. xiphoid process.
   D. diffusion.

6. The organs of the left upper quadrant include the:
   A. liver, gallbladder, and parts of the small and large intestine.
   B. stomach, spleen, appendix, and parts of the small and large intestine.
   C. pancreas, spleen, liver, and parts of the small and large intestine.
   D. stomach, spleen, and parts of the small and large intestine.

7. The lower midportion of the pelvic ring where the left and right sides fuse together is called the:
   A. sacrum.
   B. pubic symphysis.
   C. ileum.
   D. ischium.

8. The part of the brain responsible for heart rate, vessel dilation and constriction, swallowing, vomiting, coughing, and sneezing is the:
   A. cerebrum.
   B. medulla.
   C. cerebellum.
   D. pons.

9. The large gland at the base of the neck that consists of two lobes is called the:
   A. isthmus.
   B. pancreas.
   C. pituitary.
   D. thyroid.

Assessment in Action

10. A thin plasma-like fluid formed from the interstitial or extracellular fluid that bathes the tissues of the body is known as:

    A. hemoglobin.
    B. lymph.
    C. synovial fluid.
    D. blood.

11. The system that includes the organs and structure associated with breathing, gas exchange, and entrance of air into the body is called the:

    A. digestive system.
    B. integumentary system.
    C. respiratory system.
    D. equilibrium system.

12. The organ that detoxifies poisonous substances produced by digestion is called the:

    A. pancreas.
    B. spleen.
    C. stomach.
    D. liver.

Points to Ponder

Your agency requires that you attend continuing education sessions each month. Included in each session is a section on anatomy and physiology, which you think is a waste of time. On your last shift, you brought in a patient complaining of severe abdominal pain. Later on that day you saw the emergency department physician and you asked him about your patient's condition. The doctor told you that she had an obstruction in the ileum. On your way back to your station you tell your partner that the patient you had earlier had some problem with her pelvis. Did you understand what the doctor explained to you? Was he referring to the pelvis or to the small intestine?

Issues: Understanding Anatomy and Physiology Terms, Communicating With Health Care Providers

Pharmacology and Intravenous Therapy

Section 2

6	**Pharmacology**	**242**
7	**Intravenous Access**	**284**
8	**Medication Administration**	**326**

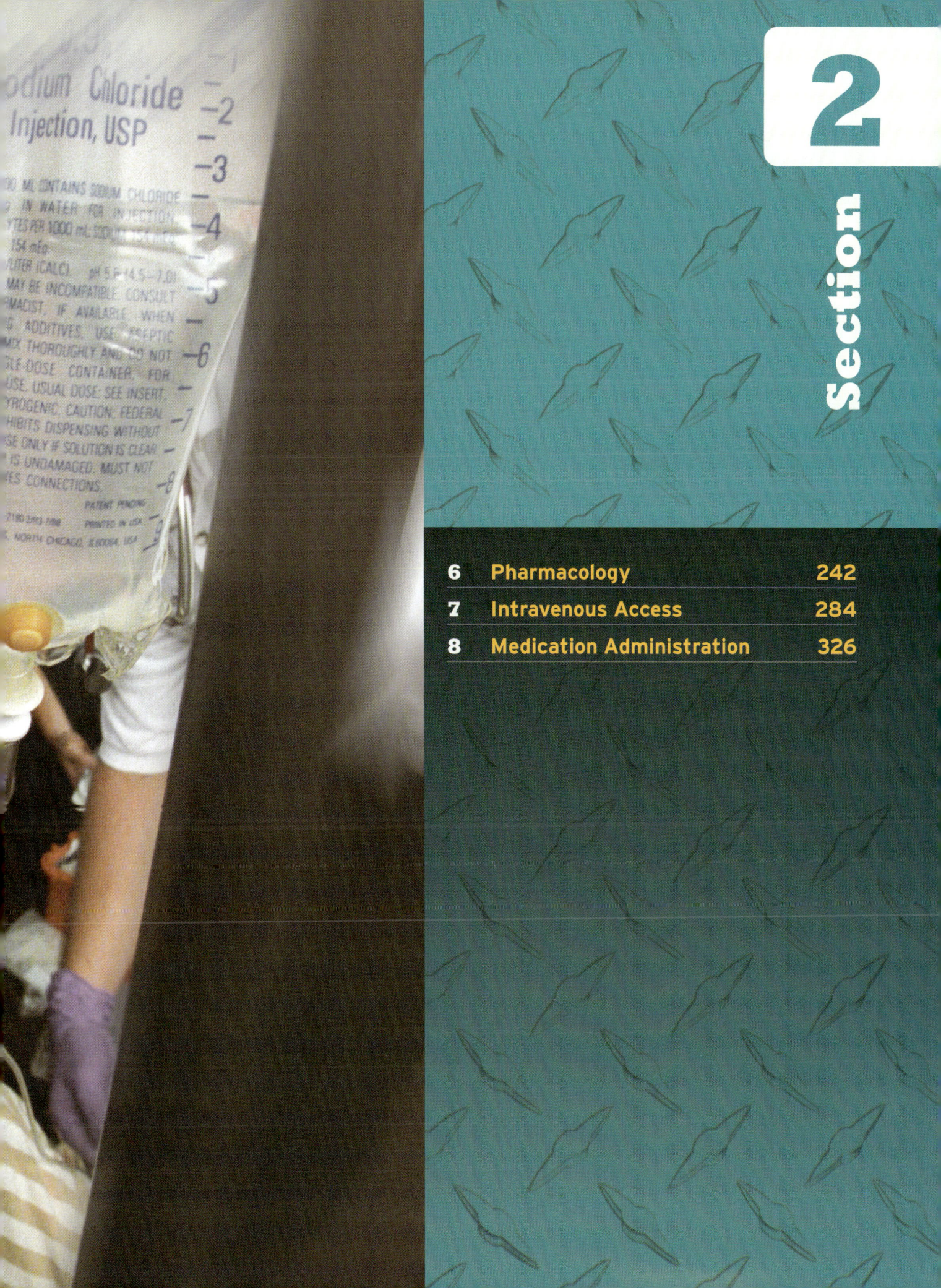

Pharmacology

1999 Objectives

Cognitive

1-3.1 Review the specific anatomy and physiology pertinent to pharmacology. (p 256)
1-3.2 Discuss the standardization of drugs. (p 246)
1-3.3 Differentiate among the chemical, generic (nonproprietary), and trade (proprietary) names of a drug. (p 245)
1-3.4 List the four main sources of drug products. (p 245)
1-3.5 Describe how drugs are classified. (p 246)
1-3.6 List the authoritative sources for drug information. (p 245)
1-3.7 Discuss special consideration in drug treatment with regard to pregnant, pediatric, and geriatric patients. (p 251, 254)
1-3.8 Discuss the EMT-Intermediate's responsibilities and scope of management pertinent to the administration of medications. (p 247)
1-3.9 List and describe general properties of drugs. (p 250)
1-3.10 List and describe liquid, solid, and gas drug forms. (p 250)
1-3.11 List and differentiate routes of drug administration. (p 254)
1-3.12 Differentiate between enteral and parenteral routes of drug administration. (p 255)
1-3.13 Describe mechanisms of drug action. (p 255)
1-3.14 List and differentiate the phases of drug activity, including the pharmaceutical, pharmacokinetic, and pharmacodynamic phases. (p 256)
1-3.15 Describe pharmacokinetics, pharmacodynamics, theories of drug action, drug-response relationship, factors altering drug responses, predictable drug responses, iatrogenic drug responses, and unpredictable adverse drug responses. (p 257, 259)
1-3.16 Discuss considerations for storing drugs. (p 262)
1-3.17 List the components of a drug profile. (p 244)
1-3.18 List and describe drugs which the EMT-Intermediate may administer in a pharmacological management plan according to local protocol. (p 262)
1-3.19 Discuss procedures and measures to ensure security of controlled substances the EMT-Intermediate may administer. (p 262)

Affective

1-3.20 Defend medication administration by an EMT-Intermediate to effect positive therapeutic affect. (p 244)

Psychomotor

None

1985 Objectives

There are no 1985 objectives for this chapter.

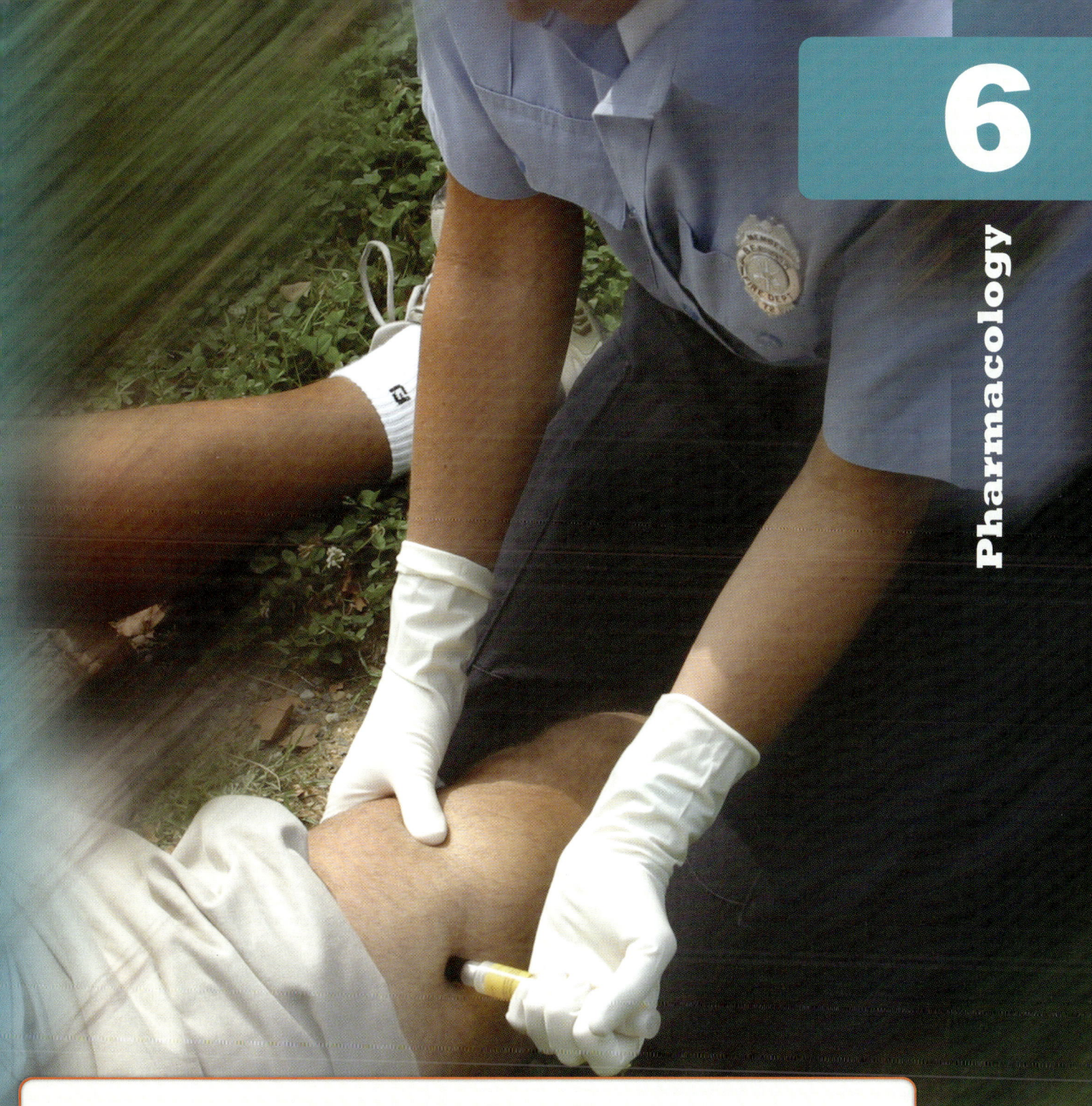

6

Pharmacology

You are the Provider

You and your partner are dispatched to 2201 4th Avenue for a 50-year-old man complaining of chest pain. You arrive to find the man sitting in a chair, clutching his chest. He is conscious and alert and his skin is pale and sweaty.

1. Given that this patient has cardiac-related chest pain, what drugs are potentially indicated for administration?
2. What mnemonic can assist you in remembering these medications?

Pharmacology

Administering medications is a serious business. Used appropriately, a medication may alleviate pain, ease suffering, and improve a patient's well-being. However, used inappropriately, medication may cause harm and even death. As an EMT-I, you will be responsible for administering certain medications to patients and helping them to self-administer others. You will ask patients about their medication allergies, and you will report this information to hospital personnel. To act without understanding how medications work will place patients and you in danger.

This chapter describes the various forms of medications, the different ways in which they can be administered, and their mechanisms of action. It then takes a close look at each of the medications you may be called on to administer or help patients to self-administer. Table 6-1 lists components of a drug profile and serves as an introduction to the type of information covered in this chapter.

How Medications Work

Pharmacology is the study of the properties (characteristics) and effects of drugs and medications on the body. Drugs are chemical agents used in the diagnosis, treatment, and prevention of disease. Although the terms drugs and medications are often used interchangeably, "drugs" may make some people think of narcotics or illegal substances. For this reason, you should try to use the word "medications," especially when interviewing patients and families. In general terms, a medication is a chemical substance that is used to treat or prevent disease or relieve pain.

The dose is the amount of the medication that is given. The dose depends on the patient's size and age; adults and children will get different amounts of the same medication. It also depends on the desired action of the medication. The action is the therapeutic effect that a medication is expected to have on the body. For example, nitroglycerin relaxes the walls of the blood vessels and may dilate the arteries. This increases the blood flow and, thus, the supply of oxygen to the heart muscle. In this way, nitroglycerin relieves the squeezing or crushing pain that occurs with angina. Nitroglycerin is, therefore, indicated for chest pain associated with angina. Indications are the therapeutic uses for a particular medication.

There are times when you should not give a patient medication, even if it usually is indicated for that person's condition. Such situations are called contraindi-

---

TABLE 6-1 Components of a Drug Profile

A drug profile gives all of the specifics about the drug. This is the information included on the package insert and listed in various pharmaceutical publications. As an EMT-I, you should familiarize yourself with the drug profiles of the medications you may be expected to administer. A typical drug profile includes the following:

- **Drug names**—This includes the generic name, trade name, and chemical name.
- **Classification**—What type of drug is this? What is it used for?
- **Mechanisms of action**—How does it work? What is its intended purpose?
- **Indications**—What are the reasons for taking this drug?
- **Contraindications**—When should the drug not be given? Does it affect certain medical conditions or react with other medications adversely?
- **Pharmacokinetics**—How is it absorbed, metabolized, and so forth? What is its half-life?
- **Side and adverse effects**—Are there any side effects? What are the adverse effects?
- **Routes of administration**—How is it given?
- **How supplied**—What is the total quantity of the medication? What form?
- **Dosages**—This generally includes proper dosages for adult, pediatric, and special considerations, such as when to modify the dosage based on the patient's history.

There are also considerations for certain groups such as pediatric, geriatric, and pregnant patients and other special patient groups. The drug profile may also include any other information that is vital to the user.

Technology

- Interactivities
- Vocabulary Explorer
- Anatomy Review
- Web Links
- Online Review Manual

www.EMSzone.com/EMTI

cations. A medication is contraindicated when it would harm the patient or have no positive effect on the patient's condition. For example, giving activated charcoal is indicated when a patient has swallowed a poison. Generally, activated charcoal, mixed with water, is used to prevent the body from absorbing a poison. However, activated charcoal would be contraindicated if the patient were unresponsive and could not swallow.

> **A to Z Terminology Tips**
>
> An *indication* is a reason for giving a drug. A *contraindication* is a reason not to give a drug. The number 1 contraindication for any medication is hypersensitivity (allergy) to that drug.

Side effects are any actions of a medication other than the desired ones. Side effects may occur even when a medication is administered properly and under the appropriate circumstances. For example, giving epinephrine to a patient who is having an allergic reaction should dilate the bronchioles and decrease wheezing. However, two side effects of epinephrine are cardiac stimulation and constriction of the arteries, which may elevate the patient's heart rate and blood pressure. These side effects are predictable; others are not. An idiosyncratic reaction is one that is a peculiar or individual reaction to a drug.

Medication Names

Medications have been identified or derived from four major sources: plants (alkaloids, glycosides, gums, oils), animals and humans, minerals and mineral products, and chemical and synthetic substances made in the laboratory. Morphine and atropine are derived from plants, insulin from animals and humans, and iron from minerals. Lidocaine is a synthetic produced from chemicals in a laboratory.

Medications have different types of names. A trade name is the brand name that a manufacturer gives to a medication, such as Tylenol and Lasix. As a proper noun, a trade name begins with a capital letter. Trade names are used in every aspect of our daily lives, not just in medications. Well-known examples include Jell-O gelatin, Band-Aid adhesive bandages, and Hershey chocolate candy. A medication may have many different trade names, depending on how many companies manufacture it. Advil, Nuprin, and Motrin all are trade names for the same generic medication, ibuprofen.

The generic name of a medication (such as ibuprofen) is usually its original chemical name, which is not capitalized, and is usually suggested by the first manufacturer and approved by the US Food and Drug Administration, or FDA. Sometimes a medication is called by its generic name more often than by any of its trade names. For example, you may hear the term "nitroglycerin" used more often than the trade names Isordil and Nitrostat. All medications that are licensed for use in the United States are listed by their generic names in the *United States Pharmacopeia* (or *USP*).

The chemical name of a medication is a precise description of the drug's chemical composition and molecular structure. The official name is the name assigned by the USP. In most cases, the official name is generally the generic name followed by "USP."

Examples of the four names for a drug are as follows:

- Chemical name: 9-chloro-11β,17,21-trihydroxy-16β-methylpregna-1,4-diene-3,20-dione 17,21-dipropionate
- Generic name: beclomethasone dipropionate
- Trade name: Vanceril
- Official name: beclomethasone dipropionate, USP

Medications may be prescription medications or over-the-counter (OTC) medications. Only pharmacists, according to a physician's order, can legally distribute prescription medications to patients. However, OTC medications may be purchased directly from a wholesale or retail source, such as a discount store or supermarket, without a prescription. In recent years, the number of prescription medications that have become available OTC has increased dramatically. Therefore, many of the problems that are attributable to prescription medications may become more common. You may also come into contact with patients who have taken "street" drugs such as heroin or cocaine. Although street drugs lack the pharmaceutical purity of OTC or prescribed medications, they are still pharmacologically active and will cause an effect.

There are numerous references to learn more about a particular drug. Publications include the *American Medical Association (AMA) Drug Evaluation* and the *Physician's Desk Reference* (also called the *PDR*). Information regarding drugs can also be obtained through the use of a hospital formulary—a local publication that delineates which drugs are used in a particular facility. Medications come packaged with drug inserts that give information specific to preparation, dosage, effects, possible side effects, and other information. There are also numerous other texts and sources including the Internet. EMT-Is should be familiar with these resources and other field references, particularly regarding medications commonly encountered in the prehospital setting.

> **EMT-I Safety**
>
> Assume that any needle withdrawn from a patient's skin after giving an injection is contaminated with potentially infectious fluids. Handle contaminated "sharps" accordingly, and dispose of them immediately according to your service's procedures for preventing infectious exposures.

Methods of Drug Classification

Drugs or medications can be classified into three categories:

- **By body system:** Classification by body system is simply categorizing by the system affected by that drug. Nitroglycerin is a vasodilator that is used predominantly for cardiac ischemia; therefore, it is classified as a cardiac drug. Understanding which systems are affected by which drugs will help you make the appropriate decisions for patient care.
- **Class of agent:** The class of a medication tells how it affects the system. For example, an antipyretic is given to reduce fever, and an antiemetic is used to control vomiting.
- **Mechanism of action:** The mechanism of action leads to the desired effect. It is the function of a drug or the particular action of a drug on an organism. Again using the example of nitroglycerin, it is a potent vasodilator given for cardiac ischemia because is opens the vessels to allow oxygenated blood to pass through.

Standardization of Drugs

The manufacture and distribution of medications in the United States and most other countries is subject to strict rules and regulations that help to ensure that drugs issued by various manufacturers are of uniform strength and purity. To determine whether a drug meets the standards, it must go through regimented testing. Two of these testing methods are known as assay and bioassay.

- **Assay**—the analysis of a substance to determine its constituents and the relative proportion of each.
- **Bioassay**—the determination of the strength of a drug by comparing its effect on a live animal or an isolated organ preparation with that of a standard preparation.

In the United States, drug standards are published in the *USP*. There are also numerous laws to protect people from unsafe substances and unscrupulous manufacturers and distributors.

You are the Provider   Part 2

You perform an initial assessment of the patient as your partner applies 100% oxygen via nonrebreathing mask. A cardiac monitor is applied and reveals a normal sinus rhythm.

Initial Assessment	Recording Time: 1 Minute After Patient Contact
Appearance	Conscious, pale, and diaphoretic
Level of consciousness	Alert to person, place, and time
Airway	Open and clear
Breathing	Increased rate, adequate depth and unlabored
Circulation	Pulse, normal rate and regular; skin, cool and clammy

3. Other than oxygen, what is the first drug given for patients with suspected cardiac chest pain?
4. What should you consider before administering this drug, and how should the drug be administered?

The Scope of Practice

As an EMT-I you are legally, morally, and ethically responsible for each drug you administer. You must have a good foundation of knowledge of OTC and prescription medications that may interact with drugs you may give, and you must have enough knowledge to obtain a medical history for patients who are unable to communicate.

Drug administration must be safe and therapeutically effective. You should always keep a field guide or other medication reference handy to look up medications you are not familiar with. Follow the standardized national guidelines listed in 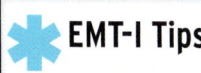 when providing drug therapy.

Nervous System Divisions

As discussed in Chapter 5, the nervous system is the body's principal control system. It comprises the central nervous system (CNS), made up of the brain and spinal cord, and the peripheral nervous system that includes all of the nervous tissue outside the CNS. The peripheral nervous system is further broken down into the somatic nervous system that controls all voluntary, or motor, functions and the <u>autonomic nervous system (ANS)</u> that controls all of the automatic, or involuntary, functions.

The ANS operates without conscious control and regulates the functions of the internal organs, glands, and smooth muscle. The two functional divisions of the ANS are the sympathetic nervous system and the parasympathetic nervous system. The <u>sympathetic</u>

TABLE 6-2 Guidelines for Providing Drug Therapy

- Understand pharmacology.
- Use correct precautions and techniques.
- Observe and document the effects of drugs, good or bad.
- Obtain a drug history from patients, including prescribed medications (name, strength, and daily dosage), OTC medications, vitamins, herbal preparations, and drug reactions.
- Perform an evaluation to identify drug indications and contraindications.
- Establish and maintain professional relationships.
- Keep your knowledge base current for changes and trends in pharmacology.
- Seek drug reference literature.
- Consult with medical direction.

EMT-I Tips

Drug Therapy in Pregnant Patients

Before administering any medications to a female of childbearing age, the patient should be asked about the possibility of being pregnant. In an emergency situation, the health of the mother is primary. However, before using any drug during pregnancy, the expected benefits should be considered against the possible risk to the fetus. Drugs, whether prescription or OTC, have the potential to harm the fetus by crossing the placental barrier, as well as through lactation. A <u>teratogenic</u> drug is one that poses a risk to the normal development or health of the unborn fetus.

Changes in the mother's body also affect the way drugs are processed and may increase the chance of harm to the baby. Metabolism of drugs in the liver is decreased during pregnancy, along with an increased rate of excretion owing to increased cardiac output.

The FDA has established the following scale with the categories A, B, C, D, and X to indicate drugs that have documented problems in animals and/or humans during pregnancy:

- *Category A*: No documented risk to the human fetus at any point throughout the pregnancy.
- *Category B*: Studies in animals have not demonstrated a risk to the fetus; however, adequate studies have not been performed in humans. Drugs in this category also include those in which human studies have not demonstrated adverse effects in the first or third trimesters; however, studies in animals have demonstrated adverse effects during these same time periods.
- *Category C*: Studies in animals have demonstrated adverse effects; however, studies have not been conducted in humans. Drugs in this category also include those in which adequate studies have not been conducted in animals or humans.
- *Category D*: Risk to the human fetus has been demonstrated; however, administration of the drug may outweigh the risk of potential adverse effects in certain circumstances.
- *Category X*: Risk of adverse effects has clearly been demonstrated in humans; therefore, these drugs should not be administered to pregnant or potentially pregnant women.

There are still many drugs used with unknown effects during pregnancy. For this reason, it is better to delay pharmacologic treatments for pregnant patients until they reach the hospital, except in life-threatening situations.

pathway (or nervous system) is responsible for the body's response to shock and stress and is known as the "fight or flight" division. This response is associated with the release of adrenaline from the adrenal glands. Sympathetic responses include shunting of blood from the extremities to the vital core organs, increasing the heart rate and respirations, increasing blood pressure, dilation of the pupils, and reduction of digestive system activity.

The parasympathetic nervous system relaxes the body. It controls automatic functions during nonstressful times and is referred to as the "rest and relax" division. The parasympathetic responses include slowing the heart and respiratory rates, lowering the blood pressure, constricting the pupils, and increasing digestive system activity.

The sympathetic and parasympathetic divisions work in constant opposition to each other to maintain basic harmony in the body, with each division taking more precedence in the proper circumstances. Figure 6-1 ▼ summarizes the organization of the nervous system.

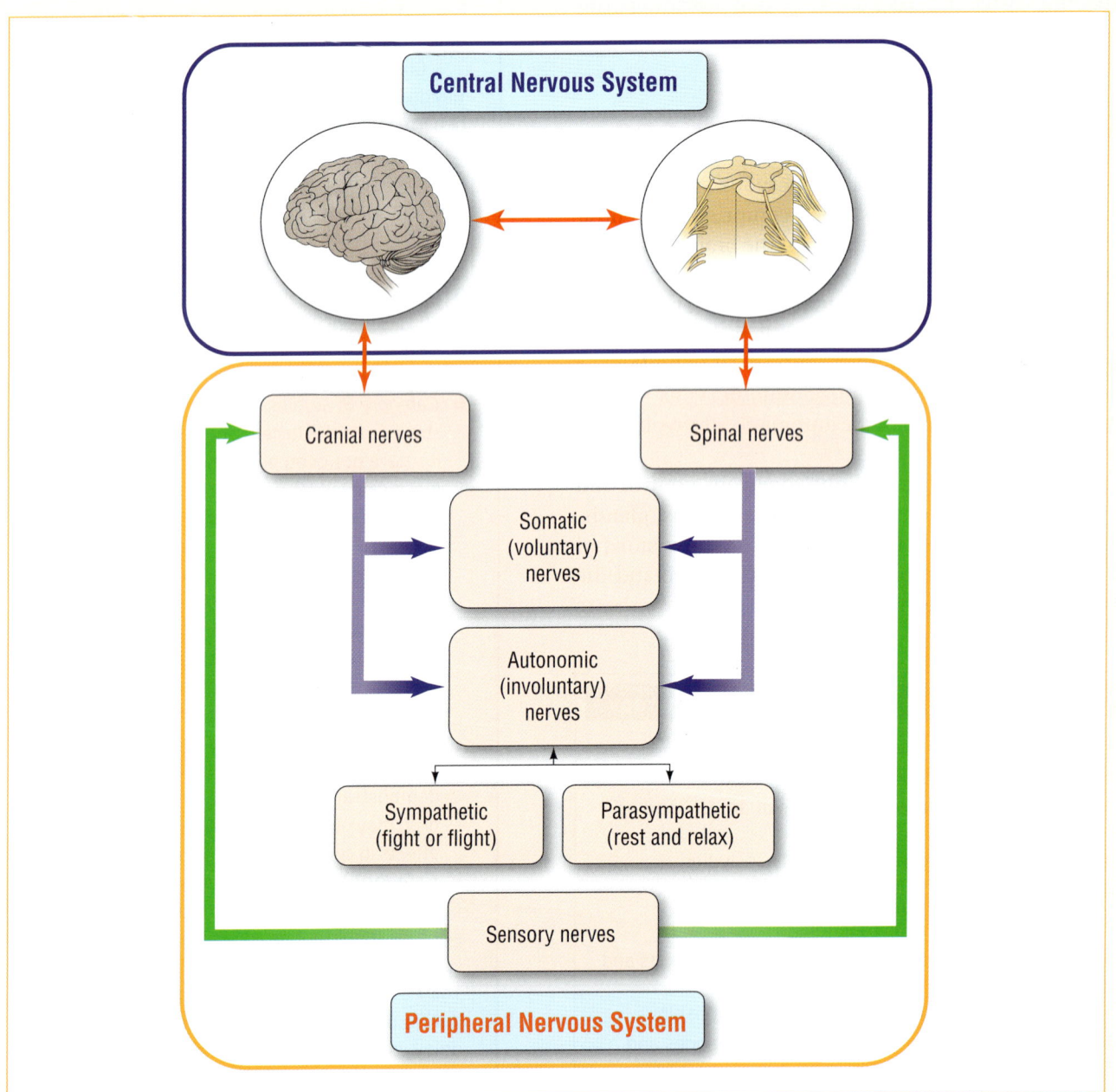

Figure 6-1 Organization of the nervous system.

The key to understanding the workings of the ANS lies in understanding the terminology. The sympathetic division is also known as the *adrenergic* division because a neuron that secretes norepinephrine is an adrenergic fiber. All of the stimulation of the sympathetic nervous system works to ready the body for a stressful situation. The nerves of the sympathetic ganglia accomplish this stimulation, or innervation. In addition, special preganglionic sympathetic nerve fibers innervate the adrenal medulla that, in turn, releases the hormones epinephrine (adrenaline) and norepinephrine (noradrenaline). When stimulated, the sympathetic ganglia, composed of the sympathetic chain ganglia and collateral ganglia, have the following effects:

- Stimulation of secretion by sweat glands
- Constriction of blood vessels in the periphery
- Increased blood flow to skeletal muscles
- Increased heart rate, contractility, automaticity, and conductivity
- Bronchodilation
- Increased energy production
- Reduction of blood flow to abdominal organs
- Decreased digestive activity
- Relaxation of the urinary bladder
- Release of glucose stores (glycogen) from the liver

Hormones released by stimulation of the adrenal medulla are carried throughout the body where they cause their intended effects by acting directly on hormone receptors. This stimulates tissues that are not innervated by sympathetic nerves and also prolongs the effects of direct sympathetic stimulation. Adrenergic receptors are located throughout the body and, once stimulated by the appropriate hormone, they cause a response in the target organ. Adrenergic receptors are generally divided into four types 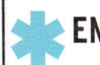.

Drugs can be given that produce the same effects on a body system as the hormones of the sympathetic nervous system that are released naturally in the body. These drugs are known as **sympathomimetics** because they *mimic* the effects of the sympathetic nervous system. Medications that have the opposite effect, or inhibit the sympathetic nervous system, are known as **sympatholytics** (also known as antiadrenergics), which antagonize, or fight against, the effects of the sympathetic nervous system. Some medications stimulate alpha and beta receptors, while others are selective to specific receptors. For example, beta-2 selective drugs cause bronchodilation with little effect on the heart, which only has beta-1 receptor sites.

> **EMT-I Tips**
>
> Think of the hormones of the sympathetic nervous system as a key that starts a car. When the key is placed in the ignition (or the hormone is placed in the receptor site) and the key is turned, a certain sequence of events occurs to start the car. If you have a duplicate key made and use it to start the car, the same sequence of events takes place. This is exactly what happens when a sympathomimetic drug (the duplicate key) is introduced into the body. The same sequence of events takes place when the duplicate is joined with the receptor site.

 Terminology Tips

> *Sympathomimetic:* Think of what a *mime* does— mimics. A sympathomimetic *mimics* the effects of the sympathetic nervous system.

To give the best patient care, it is imperative for the EMT-I to recognize certain medications and how they affect the body. Numerous drugs affect the ANS directly or indirectly. Many patients are taking medications that belong to the **beta-blocker** class. They are used to control blood pressure in some patients and heart rhythm disturbances in others. Beta-blockers work by filling a portion of the beta receptor sites to prevent binding by beta stimulators that occur naturally in the body (endogenous) and can be introduced as a medication.

TABLE 6-3	Alpha and Beta Responses
Alpha 1 (α_1)	■ Peripheral vasoconstriction
Alpha 2 (α_2)	■ Peripheral vasodilation ■ Little or no bronchoconstriction
Beta 1 (β_1)	■ Increased heart rate ■ Increased automaticity ■ Increased contractility ■ Increased conductivity
Beta 2 (β_2)	■ Bronchodilation

> **EMT-I Tips**
>
> Imagine beta-blockers as the plastic plugs that are placed in electric sockets to prevent children from sticking things into the sockets. The plugs do not do anything; they only plug up the holes. Beta-blockers work the same way. They have no effect on the body; they only plug up the receptor sites, preventing beta agonists from binding.

> **EMT-I Tips**
>
> Atropine is a potent *parasympatholytic* that is used to increase heart rate in symptomatic bradycardia. Because increasing the heart rate is an effect of the sympathetic nervous system, it would stand to reason that atropine should be classified as a sympathomimetic. However, atropine has no effect on the heart itself. Its mechanism of action is to block the vagus nerve and prevent innervation by acetylcholine. Think of it as a roadblock. It does not directly affect the target organ, in this case the heart, but simply blocks the road and prevents anything from passing through. Because its action is directed at decreasing the effects of the parasympathetic nervous system (which slows the heart rate), it is an antagonist to the parasympathetic division, or a parasympatholytic.

The parasympathetic nervous system arises from the brain stem and the sacral segments of the spinal cord, with the majority of innervation coming from the vagus nerve (the 10th cranial nerve). Acetylcholine is the neurotransmitter for the parasympathetic division. Stimulation of the parasympathetic division results in effects opposite from those of the sympathetic division. Pupils constrict, digestive activity increases, bronchioles constrict, and the heart rate and cardiac contractile force decrease.

Like the sympathetic division, antagonists to the parasympathetic nervous system are known as **parasympatholytics**, and agonists are known as **parasympathomimetics**. One of the most commonly used parasympatholytics (also known as an anticholinergic) is the drug atropine that is used for symptomatic bradycardia and exposure to organophosphates and certain chemical nerve agents. Atropine works by binding with acetylcholine receptors and preventing the acetylcholine from exerting its effect.

> **Terminology Tips**
>
> *Agonists* aid or increase effects. *Antagonists* antagonize or fight against.

one example of the action of epinephrine on the heart. The interaction of drugs with receptors has varying effects.

Once administered, drugs go through four stages: absorption, distribution, metabolism, and excretion. These are covered in the section on pharmacokinetics.

Drug Forms

The form that a medication comes in usually dictates its route of administration. For example, a tablet or a spray cannot be administered through a needle. The manufacturer chooses the form to ensure the proper route for the medication, the timing of its release into the bloodstream, and its effects on the target organs or body systems. As an EMT-I, you should be familiar with the following seven medication forms.

Drug Properties

Drugs are generally classified by the effects they have on the body. Drugs modify existing functions of tissues and organs. They do not give new functions to tissues or organs. Also, drugs in general cause multiple actions rather than a single effect. A drug action, as previously discussed, is the result of a physiochemical interaction between the drug and a functionally important molecule in the body, such as a receptor. An increase in rate is

Solid Drugs

Most medications that are given by mouth to adult patients are in tablet or capsule form (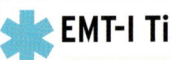). Capsules are gelatin shells filled with powdered or liquid medication. If the capsule contains liquid, the shell is sealed and usually soft. If the capsule contains powder, the shell can usually be pulled apart. Tablets often contain other materials that are mixed with the medication and compressed under high pressure.

Pediatric Needs

When treating pediatric patients, it is imperative to remember that they are not just little adults. Medication dosage is usually based on a child's weight or body surface area as opposed to age because size varies greatly from child to child. If possible, determine the exact weight of the child by asking the parent or guardian. With infants and toddlers, a length-based resuscitation tape, works well for estimating and also gives accurate dosage information for most emergency drugs, as well as sizes for endotracheal tubes and IV catheters.

When dealing with neonates, it is important to remember that they have immature body systems and are unable to metabolize drugs as quickly as an older child or adult can. Medications tend to remain in the system for longer periods, resulting in lengthened times of drug effect. Dosages may need to be altered to prevent inadvertent overdose.

Terminology Tips

Effects of Drug-Receptor Interaction
- **Agonists**—Drugs that interact with a receptor to stimulate a response
- **Antagonists**—Drugs that attach to a receptor to block a response
- **Partial agonists**—Drugs interact with a receptor to stimulate a response but inhibit other responses

Some tablets are designed to dissolve very quickly in small amounts of liquid so that they can be given sublingually and absorbed rapidly. An example is the sublingual nitroglycerin tablet used for chest pain by patients with cardiac conditions. These medications are especially useful in emergency situations. Tablets may also be ground into a powder, allowing them to be absorbed more quickly. Generally, a medication that must be swallowed is less useful in an emergency because the digestive tract provides a slower route of delivery. For example, an oral pain medication is less useful than an IV pain medication when pain relief is needed within minutes.

Suppositories are another form of solid drugs. They are made up of medication mixed in a firm base that will dissolve gradually at body temperature. They are usually inserted vaginally or rectally. These medications are more rapidly absorbed than those that must travel through the upper portion of the digestive tract.

Liquid Drugs

A **solution** is a liquid mixture of one or more substances that cannot be separated by filtering or allowing the mixture to stand. Solutions can be given by almost any route. When given by mouth, solutions may be absorbed from the stomach fairly quickly because the medication is already dissolved. Solutions that irritate the stomach may be given rectally, applied topically to the skin, sprayed sublingually, or inhaled. For example, you may need to assist in the sublingual (SL) delivery of a nitroglycerin spray (Figure 6-3). Many solutions can be given as an IV, intramuscular (IM), or subcutaneous (SC) injection. If a patient has a severe allergic reaction,

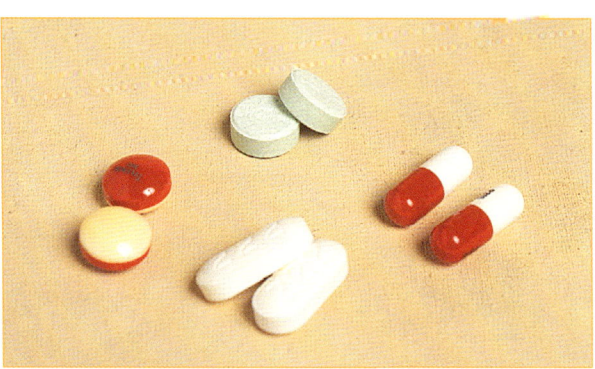

Figure 6-2 Tablets and capsules are typically taken by mouth and enter the bloodstream through the digestive system.

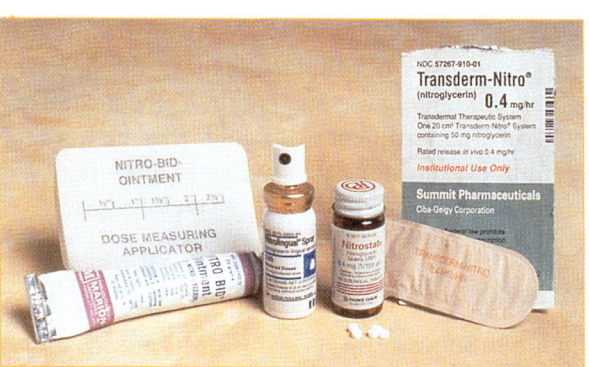

Figure 6-3 Nitroglycerin, which is prescribed for chest pain, is often given sublingually as a spray or as a tablet.

you may help to administer a solution of epinephrine intramuscularly, using an auto-injector.

Many substances do not dissolve well in liquids. Some of these can be ground into fine particles and evenly distributed throughout a liquid by shaking or stirring. This type of mixture is called a suspension. An example is activated charcoal, which you may give to patients who have taken overdoses of certain medications or ingested certain poisons.

> **EMT-I Tips**
>
> Suspensions separate if they stand or are filtered. It is very important that you shake a suspension well before administering it to ensure that the patient receives the right amount of medication.

Suspensions usually are administered by mouth but sometimes are given rectally. Occasionally, suspensions are applied directly to the skin to treat skin problems. You may have used calamine lotion in this way. Injectable suspensions are given via IM or SC injection only. Certain hormone shots or vaccinations are given this way because of the suspended particles. They cannot be given via IV injection because the suspended particles do not remain dissolved.

There are several other types of liquid drugs that you may encounter from time to time that include alcohol in their preparation. Tinctures are liquid preparations that are alcohol-based. The name of the material contained in the tincture other than alcohol is added to the name of the tincture, such as tincture of iodine. Spirits are also alcohol solutions that are volatile. Elixirs constitute one of the most common types of medicinal preparations taken orally in liquid form and are made up of a sweetened, aromatic, hydroalcoholic liquid.

Syrups are mixtures with a high sugar content that are designed to disguise the taste of the medication. These are most commonly used for children's medications. An emulsion is a mixture of two liquids that are not mutually soluble. Emulsions are generally a mixture of water and oil that must be thoroughly shaken to mix.

Metered-Dose Inhalers

If liquids or solids are broken into small enough droplets or particles, they can be inhaled. A metered-dose inhaler (MDI) is a miniature spray canister used to direct such substances through the mouth and into the lungs 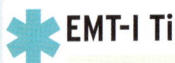. An MDI delivers the same amount of medication each time it is used. Because an inhaled medication usually is a suspension, the MDI must be shaken vigorously before the medication is administered. Patients with respiratory illnesses such as asthma and emphysema often use MDIs.

Topical Medications

Lotions, creams, and ointments all are topical medications, that is, they are applied to the surface of the skin and affect only that area. Lotions contain the most water, and ointments contain the least. You have probably noticed that OTC lotions are oilier than prescribed lotions. This is a result of a smaller amount of water used in the preparation, resulting in a slower rate of absorption of the medication. For example, hand lotions usually are absorbed faster than facial creams. Calamine lotion, on the other hand, is an example of a medical lotion. Creams, in turn, are absorbed faster than ointments such as Neosporin first-aid ointment. Hydrocortisone cream, used to diminish skin itching, is an example of a medical cream that can also be given in ointment form.

Transcutaneous Medications

Transdermal medications or transcutaneous medications are designed to be absorbed through the skin, or transcutaneously. Medications such as nitroglycerin paste usually have properties or delivery systems that help to dilate the blood vessels in the skin, thus speeding absorption into the bloodstream. In contrast to most topical medicines, which work directly on the application site, transdermal medications are usually intended for systemic effects. A note of caution: If you touch

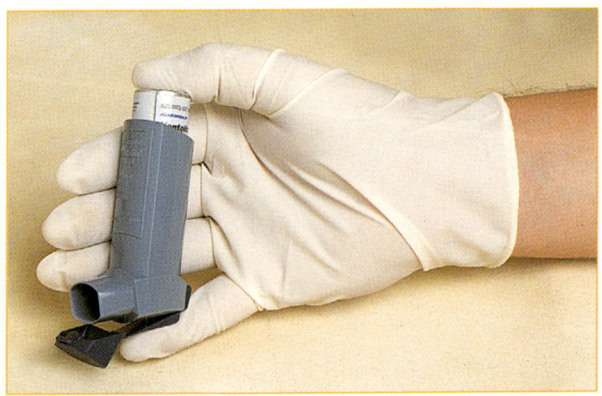

Figure 6-4 Some medications are inhaled into the lungs with an MDI so that they can be absorbed into the bloodstream more quickly.

such a medication with your bare skin while administering it, you will absorb it just as readily as the patient will.

Newer delivery systems for transcutaneous medications include the adhesive patch. Patches attach to the skin and allow even absorption of a medication for a specific time (Figure 6-5 ▶). Both prescription and OTC medications come in this form. Two common examples are nitroglycerin and nicotine.

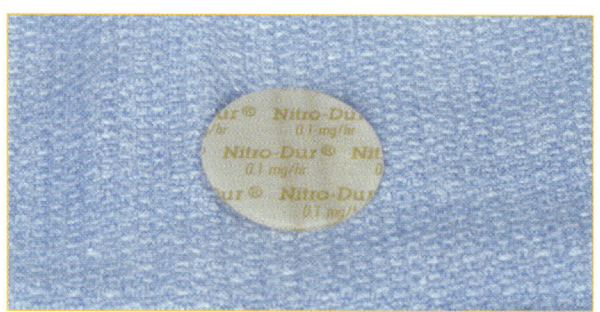

Figure 6-5 Some medications are transcutaneous, or administered through the skin, such as the nitroglycerin patch shown.

 EMT-I Safety

When removing a medication patch from a patient's skin, be sure not to touch the medication even with your gloves on. Grasp the edge with your fingers and gently pull it away from the skin. Use 4 × 4s to wipe the excess medication off the patient.

Gels

A <u>gel</u> is a semiliquid substance that is administered orally through capsules or plastic tubes. Gels usually have the consistency of pastes or creams but are transparent (clear). "Gelatinous" means thick and sticky, like gelatin. Depending on your local protocol, as an EMT-I, you may give <u>oral glucose</u> in gel form to a patient with a low blood sugar level (Figure 6-6 ▶).

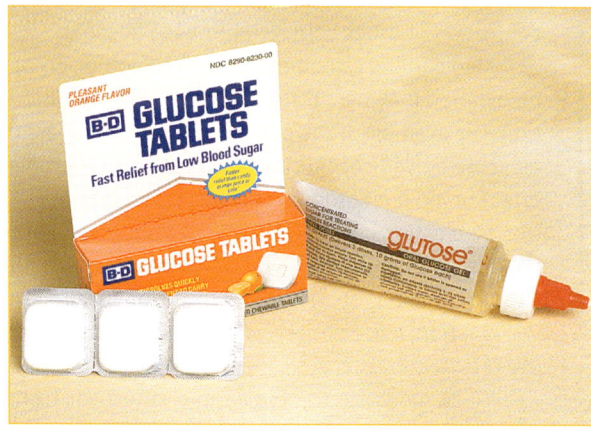

Figure 6-6 Oral glucose, used in diabetic emergencies, is available in gel and tablet form.

You are the Provider — Part 3

The patient describes his pain as a 7 on a scale of 0 to 10. As you are performing a focused history and physical exam, your partner obtains the following vital signs:

Vital Signs	Recording Time: 5 Minutes After Patient Contact
Respirations	24 breaths/min, adequate depth and unlabored
Pulse	86 beats/min, strong and regular
Blood pressure	130/72 mm Hg
Sao$_2$	98% (on supplemental oxygen)

5. What initial drug should you administer to this patient to relieve his chest pain?
6. What must you determine prior to its administration? Why is this important?

Geriatric Needs

Geriatric patients often take many medications. They might also save medications left over from previous medical conditions to use if they need them in the future. Make every effort to identify which medications are current and what conditions they are being used to treat. Ask family members to help distinguish current from outdated medications, or look at the expiration dates on the medication labels. Take a list of the current medications or the drugs themselves with you to the emergency department.

Elderly patients can become confused about their medication regimen. Uncertainty about whether they missed a dose may cause them to repeat the medication, possibly leading to an overdose. If you think an overdose has occurred, contact medical control.

Along with the potential for overdosing, the physiologic effects of aging can lead to altered pharmacodynamics and pharmacokinetics. As the body ages and organs (such as the liver and kidneys) function less effectively, medications are not processed and filtered out of the system as quickly as in a younger person. Each time a dose of a particular drug is taken, it results in overaccumulation of that drug in the body. Decreased gastric motility can result in greater absorption time, and a decrease in total body water along with an increase in fat can lead to a greater concentration of drugs with weight-based dosages.

Medications can interact with each other, creating potentially harmful conditions for the patient. Even though a medication may be indicated for a certain condition, it might be contraindicated in the presence of another medication. For example, if the patient is taking the heart medication propranolol (Inderal), which is a beta-blocker, and has an acute episode of shortness of breath, any asthma remedy might be rendered ineffective. Bronchodilation is a beta effect of most emergency asthma medications.

Medications such as sildenafil (Viagra), tadalafil (Cialis), and vardenafil (Levitra)—medications used to treat erectile dysfunction—can have potentially fatal interactions with common heart medications, specifically nitroglycerin. If used in combination with any of these medications, nitroglycerin can cause life-threatening hypotension due to severe vasodilation. Ask a patient who has been prescribed nitroglycerin if he or she has used Viagra, Cialis, or Levitra within the previous 24 hours. Report this to medical control.

While medications help people to recover from acute conditions and adjust to chronic diseases, they can pose serious problems for geriatric patients. You should distinguish current from previous medications, suspect accidental or intentional overdoses, and be prepared for potentially lethal medication interactions. Document all findings, and inform medical control.

Gases

Gaseous medications are neither solid nor liquid and most often are delivered in an operating room. The medication that is most commonly used in gas form in the prehospital setting is <u>oxygen</u>. You might not think of oxygen as a medication because it is all around us and we all use it. However, in its concentrated form, it is a potent medication that has systemic effects. You will usually administer oxygen through a nonrebreathing mask or bag-valve-mask device when ventilating a patient.

Overview of the Routes of Drug Administration

The route of drug administration affects the rate at which the onset of action occurs and may affect the therapeutic response that results. The choice of the route of administration is crucial in determining the suitability of a drug. Drugs are given for their local or systemic effects. Absorption is the process by which medications travel through body tissues until they reach the bloodstream. Categories of the routes of drug administration are the inhalation route, enteral route, and parenteral route.

Drugs administered by the <u>inhalation</u> route are aerosolized and drawn into the lungs as the patient breathes. These include nebulized medications and MDIs. Some medications are inhaled into the lungs so that they can be absorbed into the blood more quickly. Others are inhaled because they actually work in the lungs. Generally, inhalation helps to minimize the effects of the medication in other body tissues. Such medications come in the form of aerosols, fine powders, and sprays.

Several drugs may be given via an ET tube. When giving a drug through an ET tube, the dosage must be increased. The rule of thumb is 2 to $2^1/_2$ times the dose that would be given by the IV route. You also need to use a flush of normal saline to make sure the medication reaches the lungs and does not adhere to the sides of the tube.

Enteral drugs are those that are administered along any portion of the gastrointestinal tract, including the sublingual, buccal, oral, rectal, and nasogastric routes. Enteral routes are summarized in Table 6-4.

Parenteral drugs are those that are administered through any route other than the gastrointestinal tract. Parenteral routes include IV, intramuscular (IM), intraosseous (IO), subcutaneous (SC), transdermal or transcutaneous, intrathecal, inhalation, intralingual, intradermal, and umbilical injection. Parenteral routes are summarized in Table 6-5.

In the Field

The mnemonic LEAN will help you remember the drugs that may be administered via the ET route.
- L—Lidocaine
- E—Epinephrine
- A—Atropine
- N—Naloxone (Narcan)

Mechanism of Action

To produce optimal desired or therapeutic effects, a drug must reach appropriate concentrations at its site of action. Molecules of the chemical compound must proceed from the point of entry into the body to the tissues with which they react. The magnitude of the response depends on the dose and the time that it takes the drug to travel in the body.

Drugs may produce their effects locally, systemically, or both. Local effects are those that result from the direct application of a drug to a tissue. An example of a local effect would be when cortisone cream is applied

Terminology Tips

To differentiate between *pharmacokinetic* and *pharmacodynamic*, break the words down.
pharmaco—Drug, medicine
kinetic—Kinetic energy is the energy of motion
dynamic—Ever changing
Pharmacokinetic is the "movement" of the medication through the body: how it enters, where it goes, how it leaves.
Pharmacodynamic is how the medication "changes" the body: its mechanism of action.

TABLE 6-4	Enteral Routes of Drug Administration
Route	Description
Sublingual (SL)	"Sublingual" means "under the tongue." Medications that take the SL route, such as nitroglycerin tablets, are absorbed by the venous plexus under the tongue and enter the bloodstream through the oral mucous membranes within minutes. This route not only is faster, but it also protects medications from chemicals in the digestive system, such as acids that can weaken or inactivate them.
Buccal	The buccal route is similar to the sublingual route. The medication is placed between the cheek and gums, where it is absorbed into the bloodstream. This is a common route for glucose gel.
Oral	Many medications are taken by mouth, per os (PO), and enter the bloodstream through the digestive system. This process can take as long as 1 hour.
Per rectum (PR)	"Per rectum" means "by rectum." This route of delivery is frequently used with children because of easier administration and more reliable absorption. (Children often regurgitate some or all of a medication.) For similar reasons, many medications that are used for nausea and vomiting come in a rectal suppository form. Some medications to control seizures are administered PR when intravenous access is not available.
Nasogastric	The medication must be in liquid form and is injected through the nasogastric tube into the stomach.

to the skin to relieve itching. Systemic effects occur after the drug is absorbed by any route and distributed by the bloodstream. Systemic effects almost always involve more than one organ, although the response of one or another organ may predominate.

The concentration of the drug at its site of action is influenced by various processes, which are divided into three phases of drug activity:

- Pharmaceutical
  - Disintegration of dosage form
  - Dissolution of drug
- Pharmacokinetic
  - Absorption
  - Distribution
  - Metabolism
  - Excretion
- Pharmacodynamic
  - Drug-receptor interaction

TABLE 6-5 Parenteral Routes of Drug Administration

Route	Description
Intravenous (IV) injection	"Intravenous" means "into the vein." Medications that need to enter the bloodstream immediately may be injected directly into a vein. This is the fastest way to deliver a medication, but the IV route cannot be used for all medications. For example, aspirin, oxygen, and charcoal cannot be given by the IV route.
Intramuscular (IM) injection	"Intramuscular" means "into the muscle." Usually medications that are administered via IM injection are absorbed quickly because muscles are highly vascular. Some types of medications, though, are designed for a slower, sustained release from the muscle. Many such medications have the prefix "depo" in their names, meaning that they form a deposit in the muscle after being injected. However, not all medications can be administered intramuscularly. Intramuscular injections can cause damage to muscle tissue and result in uneven, unreliable absorption. This is especially true in people who are experiencing decreased peripheral perfusion (as in shock).
Intraosseous (IO)	"Intraosseous" means "into the bone." Medications that are delivered via this route reach the bloodstream through the bone marrow. To get medication into the marrow requires drilling a needle through the bone cortex. Because this is painful, the IO route of delivery is used most often in patients who are unresponsive as a result of cardiac arrest or extreme shock. Most commonly, the IO route is reserved for children who have less available (or difficult to access) IV sites.
Subcutaneous (SC) injection	"Subcutaneous" means "beneath the skin." An SC injection is given into the tissue between the skin and the muscle. Because there is less blood here than in the muscles, medications that are delivered via this route are generally absorbed more slowly, and their effects last longer. A SC injection is a useful way to deliver medications that cannot be taken by mouth, as long as they do not irritate or damage the tissue. Commonly, a daily insulin shot is given this way to a patient with diabetes. Also, epinephrine can be given by this route. Like the IM route, SC-administered medications would not be appropriate for patients with decreased peripheral perfusion.
Transdermal or transcutaneous	"Transcutaneous" means "through the skin." Some medications can be absorbed transcutaneously, such as the nicotine in "nicotine patches" used by individuals who are trying to quit smoking. On occasion, a medication that comes in another form is administered transcutaneously to achieve a slower, longer-lasting effect. An example is an adhesive patch containing nitroglycerin.
Intrathecal	"Intrathecal" means "within the spinal canal." The drug is injected through the sheath of the spinal canal, into the subarachnoid space.
Inhalation	The inhalation route introduces drugs into the respiratory system by way of nasal inhalation through the mucosa of the nose or injection through an endotracheal tube.
Intralingual	"Intralingual" means "within the tongue." The drug is injected into the tongue.
Intradermal	"Intradermal" means "within the skin." This is injection of a drug within the dermis. Tuberculosis (TB) tests are injected intradermally.
Umbilical	The drug is injected through the umbilical vein in a newborn.

Pharmacokinetics: Movement of Drugs Through the Body

Pharmacokinetics is defined as the study of the metabolism and action of drugs with particular emphasis on the time required for absorption, duration of action, distribution in the body, and method of excretion. As drugs move through the system, they undergo various changes before they are excreted. The processing of the drugs involves active and passive transport across the cell membranes.

Drug Absorption

The passage of a substance through some surface of the body into body fluids and tissues is known as absorption. Absorption usually takes place in the mouth, through the lining of the stomach, through the skin, in the subcutaneous tissue, in the blood vessels of the muscles, through the large or small intestine, or through the rectum. Numerous variables affect drug absorption, including the nature of the absorbing surface, blood flow to the site of administration, solubility of the drug, pH, drug concentration, dosage form, route of administration, bioavailability, diffusion, osmosis, and filtration. Table 6-6 describes these primary factors.

TABLE 6-6 Primary Factors of Drug Absorption

Factor	Discussion
Nature of the absorbing surface	Some surfaces are highly permeable. It is much easier for a drug to travel through a single layer of cells than through multiple layers. The greater the surface area exposed to the substance, the greater the absorption.
Blood flow to the site of administration	Blood flow to a particular area regulates how fast the medication is absorbed into the central circulation. This is why administering medications IM to a patient having a seizure produces a minimal effect. Because of the seizure activity, blood flow to the extremities is diminished. Medications introduced intramuscularly tend to stay in the tissues until the seizure activity stops. When blood flow resumes, the patient may experience the effects of an overdose if multiple doses were given.
Solubility of the drug	The more soluble the drug, the faster it enters the circulatory system.
pH	The pH of the body and that of the drug can affect the rate of absorption. Some medications are coated to keep them from being absorbed before they reach the small intestine because the acid environment of the stomach can destroy the drug.
Drug concentration	The more of a drug available for absorption, the more that will be absorbed and the more that will remain in the system. Often a loading dose (bolus) of a medication is given, followed by a continuous infusion to maintain a constant therapeutic level.
Dosage form	Form has a lot to do with the speed of absorption. A liquid will be absorbed much more quickly than a pill, which must be dissolved before it is absorbed.
Routes of drug administration	IV administration is the most rapid route for delivering drugs in the prehospital environment. The medication bypasses the absorption process because it is introduced directly into the vascular system. Intramuscular and subcutaneous routes are much slower because they depend on blood flow to the area in which the medication is administered.
Bioavailability	Bioavailability is the rate and extent to which an active drug enters the general circulation, permitting access to the site of action. It is determined by measurement of the concentration of the drug in body fluids or by the magnitude of the pharmacologic response.
Diffusion	Diffusion is the movement of solutes (molecules) from an area of higher concentration to an area of lower concentration.
Osmosis	Osmosis is the movement of a solvent (fluid) from an area of lower solute concentration to an area of higher solute concentration.
Filtration	Filtration is the removal of particles from a solution by allowing the liquid portion to pass through a membrane or other partial barrier. The semipermeability of the membrane allows fluid to pass through, but the openings are too small for solid particles.

Drug Distribution

Drugs pass freely and quickly out of the vascular space and into the interstitial fluid. Therefore, blood flow to the area determines the amount of a drug reaching a particular part of the body. Most drugs tend to pass fairly easily from the intravascular compartment, through the interstitial spaces, and on to their target tissue. These drugs tend to have a rapid onset and a short duration of action. Other drugs become bound to serum proteins in the blood and are not immediately available to act on receptor sites. With the drug bound to the protein, it cannot produce an effect in a receptor site, nor can it diffuse through the tissues.

Some areas of the body, such as the brain and placenta, are less accessible to certain drugs than others. Drugs that are protein-bound or in an ionized form are weak penetrators of the blood-brain barrier. The blood-brain barrier and the placental barrier are both less permeable to provide protection to the brain and fetus respectively.

Biotransformation

Many drugs are inactive when administered and only become active once they have been absorbed and converted into an active form in the blood or by the target tissue. The chemical alteration that a substance undergoes in the body is known as biotransformation. The primary organ for biotransformation is the liver. If the liver is diseased, inactivation (detoxification) of drugs may be impaired. This will also increase elimination time of the drug from the body, possibly resulting in toxic blood levels. The liver performs synthetic reactions that yield inactive products (metabolites) that can be secreted by the kidneys and nonsynthetic reactions, which may result in products that are more active, charged in activity, or less active. The drugs that are biotransformed to an inactive metabolite very quickly have limited effects on the body and must be administered frequently to continue the effect. Epinephrine during cardiac arrest is an example of a drug that is rendered inactive very quickly and must be administered every 3 to 5 minutes as needed.

Drug Elimination

Excretion is the elimination of waste products from the body. Drugs are eliminated in their original forms or as metabolites. Organs of excretion include the kidneys via the urine, the intestines through the feces, the lungs via respiration, sweat through the salivary glands, and the mammary glands through breast milk. The rate of elimination varies with the amount of drug in the body and the underlying condition of the excretion organs. During shock, when the kidneys are poorly perfused, drugs will remain in the body for longer periods. This also holds true for geriatric patients whose kidneys may not function as well owing to the normal deterioration associated with aging and for patients with chronic renal impairment. This may lead to an accumulation of the drug if subsequent doses are given, resulting in toxic effects.

You are the Provider — Part 4

Your partner initiates an IV of normal saline. So far, you have administered 325 mg of aspirin and 2 doses of 0.4 mg of nitroglycerin sublingually. The patient, however, still describes his pain as a 5.

Reassessment	Recording Time: 9 Minutes After Patient Contact
Level of consciousness	Conscious and alert to person, place, and time
Respirations	24 breaths/min, adequate depth and unlabored
Pulse	88 beats/min, strong and regular
Blood pressure	122/64 mm Hg
Sao_2	99% (on supplemental oxygen)

7. How many doses of nitroglycerin can you give and in what time frame?
8. What are some important considerations to note about the effectiveness of nitroglycerin when administered by the patient prior to your arrival? What other forms of nitroglycerin are commonly used?

Pharmacodynamics: Drug Actions

The study of drugs and their actions on living organisms is known as pharmacodynamics. Once a drug has arrived at its target tissue, it must induce the desired response. This is accomplished by binding with receptor sites. Drug receptors are generally proteins present on the surface of the cell membrane. Receptor sites are like locks that take an appropriate key, the drug, to open or initiate a response. Ideally, this will produce the desired therapeutic effect of the drug. Drugs that bind to a receptor and create a response are known as agonists. Some drugs will bind with a receptor site without creating a response. Instead, they block other drugs from binding. Drugs such as these are known as antagonists.

There are various types of receptors, and among those are the alpha, beta, and dopaminergic. The efficacy of the drug is directly related to the amount that is required by the receptor to produce the desired response. If the drug administered has a great affinity for the receptors, the concentration necessary to produce a response may be smaller. Receptors are also responsible for selective drug action. The molecular structure of the drug determines its ability to bind, so a change in the structure of a drug may affect its affinity for specific receptor sites.

Drug-response Relationship

For a medication to be effective, it must reach the target tissue in a certain concentration. The minimal concentration required to produce the desired response is referred to as the therapeutic threshold or the minimum effective concentration. A concentration lower than the therapeutic threshold will not induce a clinical response. A concentration higher than the therapeutic threshold can be detrimental and possibly fatal. The goal of drug therapy is to give the minimum concentration of a drug that will produce the desired effects. The difference between the minimum effective concentration and a toxic level is referred to as the therapeutic index. Drugs with a very narrow range between the effective dose and a toxic dose are said to have a low therapeutic index. Likewise, those with a large difference between the effective dose and a toxic level are said to have a high therapeutic index.

The plasma level profile of a drug also affects the drug-response relationship. The plasma level profile refers to the particular drug's rate of absorption, distribution, biotransformation, and excretion. The biologic half-life is the final factor. This is the time it takes for the body to metabolize half of the administered dose. Adenosine, for example, has a very short half-life (approximately 15 seconds) and can be repeated in 1 to 2 minutes from the time the initial dose is given. This is an important consideration in determining the proper dose of drug and frequency of administration.

There are many factors that influence drug responses. The most common factors are age, body mass, sex, environmental conditions and time of administration, genetic factors, and psychologic factors. Table 6-7 ▶ describes these factors.

Predictable Responses

Along with adverse and unusual reactions to medications, there are also predictable responses. A drug is given for its desired action, but there are certain adverse responses, known as side effects, that may be unavoidable. An example of this would be a patient experiencing a severe headache after administration of nitroglycerin. Because of nitroglycerin's vasodilatory effect, vessels in the head are also dilated, which usually causes the patient to experience a headache. Side effects are usually predictable and may be harmless or potentially harmful.

Iatrogenic Responses

An iatrogenic response is an adverse condition induced in a patient by the treatment given. An example of this would be the patient who develops a urinary tract infection after insertion of an indwelling (for example, Foley) catheter. When administration of drugs leads to symptoms that mimic naturally occurring disease states, it is known as an iatrogenic drug response.

Unpredictable Adverse Responses

Even though the doses of medications are carefully tested and designed for specific conditions, some patients have adverse effects regardless of how well they comply with the drug regimen. These are described as adverse responses and include drug allergy, anaphylactic reaction, delayed reaction, hypersensitivity, idiosyncrasy, tolerance, cross-tolerance, cumulative effect, drug dependence, drug interaction, drug antagonism, summation (addition or additive effect), synergism, and potentiation. Descriptions of these adverse responses are given in Table 6-8 ▶.

TABLE 6-7	Factors Altering Drug Responses
Factor	**Description**
Age	As the body ages, metabolism slows and the organs of excretion do not always function as well as those in younger patients. This can cause a toxic level of drugs in the system if not taken into account when administering multiple doses. Likewise, infants and small children have immature organs and systems and cannot metabolize the same amount of drug as an adult.
Body mass	Many medications are given based on the patient's weight. This is especially true of children. To have a therapeutic dose, concentrations within the tissues must meet the desired level.
Sex	Owing to different body compositions of fat, water, and hormones, certain medications affect males and females differently and must be adjusted accordingly.
Environmental conditions and time of administration	Factors such as time of day, temperature, altitude, and even noise may alter the body's response to a drug.
Genetic factors	Patients who may already have some compromise in function due to an existing condition may not be adversely affected by certain medications owing to changes in absorption, distribution, metabolism, and excretion.
Psychologic factors	Mental stresses can have negative effects on the entire system, resulting in an inability to properly metabolize medications.

Factors Influencing Drug Interactions

There are many variables that influence drug interactions. Some of these include intestinal absorption, competition for plasma protein binding, drug metabolism or biotransformation, action at the receptor site, renal excretion, and an alteration of electrolyte balance. Other variables include drug-to-drug interactions, drug-induced malabsorption of drugs, food-induced malabsorption of drugs, alteration of enzymes, alcohol consumption, cigarette smoking, food-initiated alteration of drug excretion, and drug incompatibilities that may occur when drugs are mixed before administration.

When administering medications, it is important to know not only how they affect the patient, but also how they may affect other medications that were previously

You are the Provider   Part 5

The patient is loaded into the ambulance and transport is begun to a local hospital. The patient has received the maximum dose of nitroglycerin; however, he still describes his pain as a 4. After reassessing the patient, you prepare to administer morphine sulfate.

Reassessment	Recording Time: 14 Minutes After Patient Contact
Level of consciousness	Conscious and alert to person, place, and time
Respirations	22 breaths/min, adequate depth and unlabored
Pulse	90 beats/min, strong and regular
Blood pressure	118/60 mm Hg
SaO_2	98% on supplemental oxygen

9. What is the dose and route for morphine? What are its potential side effects?
10. Why is morphine so effective in the treatment of cardiac-related chest pain?

TABLE 6-8 Unpredictable Adverse Responses

Adverse Response	Description
Drug allergy	An allergy develops when a person has previously been exposed to a particular antigen and develops antibodies against that substance (sensitization). After a person has become sensitized, subsequent exposure to that same substance results in hypersensitivity. Reactions may range from mild rashes to anaphylactic shock. The reaction may also be immediate or delayed. As a general rule, the more rapid the reaction, the more severe it tends to be. Before administering any medication, question the patient carefully about any known drug allergies.
Anaphylactic reaction	Anaphylaxis is an acute systemic reaction that is usually life threatening. Anaphylaxis occurs after an individual has been sensitized to a particular substance and then comes in contact with it again.
Delayed reaction (also known as "serum sickness")	This type of reaction is a hypersensitivity similar to an allergy. It is a reaction occurring a considerable time after a stimulus, especially a reaction such as a skin inflammation occurring hours or days after exposure to the allergen. Unlike other allergic reactions to drugs that occur very soon after administration, serum sickness can develop 7 to 14 days after the first exposure to a medication.
Hypersensitivity	An allergy to a drug occurring after previous exposure to the drug.
Idiosyncrasy	An abnormal sensitivity or reaction to a drug or other substance that is peculiar to an individual.
Tolerance	The capacity for enduring a large amount of a substance without experiencing adverse effects and showing a decreased sensitivity to subsequent doses of the same substance. It is a progressive decrease in susceptibility to the effects of a drug after repeated doses.
Cross-tolerance	Tolerance to a particular drug that "bleeds over" to other drugs in the same class. A person who develops a tolerance to a particular drug will also show a tolerance for other drugs in that class.
Cumulative effect	Action of increased intensity after administration of several doses of a drug.
Drug dependence	A psychologic and sometimes physical state resulting from continued use of a substance. Characteristic behavioral and other responses include a compulsion to take the drug on a continuous or periodic basis to experience its effects or to avoid the discomfort of its absence.
Drug interaction	The combined effect of drugs taken concurrently. The result may be antagonism or synergism and, consequently, may be lethal is some cases.
Drug antagonism	A decrease in the action of a drug by the administration of another drug. A beta-blocker is an example of an antagonist. It binds with beta receptors, preventing a beta agonistic drug from producing the intended results. Therefore, when administering a beta agonist such as epinephrine, a beta-blocker (antagonist) such as propranolol (Inderal) would antagonize, or block, its effects.
Summation (addition or additive effect)	Increased effect that may occur when two drugs that have the same or similar actions are given together.
Synergism	Combined effect of two drugs that is greater than the sum of their individual effects.
Potentiation	Enhancement of the action of one drug by the action of another drug.

administered. An interaction between drugs occurs whenever the actions of one drug on the body are in some way modified by another chemical substance. This chemical substance may be another prescription medication or something like nicotine from cigarette smoking, something in the diet, or anything the person is exposed to. An example of this would be the use of bronchodilators that may be exacerbated by ingesting caffeine. The caffeine stimulates the central nervous system and may produce adverse effects.

It is important to be aware of the potential interactions of drugs that are prescribed and those that the patient may be self-administering. Many patients, especially elderly patients, may take several medications each day (polypharmacy). The chance of developing an undesired drug interaction increases rapidly with the number of drugs used. This also holds true when patients take medications that may interact with other substances such as particular foods and alcohol. Warning labels on prescription bottles serve to warn against the substances that may cause interactions. Unfortunately, however, many people do not read the warning labels.

Drug Storage and Security of Controlled Substances

All drug containers or "boxes" should be carefully guarded against possible theft. This requires that the boxes not only be locked, but also secured within the ambulance. Certain precepts should guide the manner in which drugs are secured, stored, distributed, and accounted for. Your local protocols will dictate the manner in which the drugs are maintained.

If controlled substances, such as narcotics, are administered, the records must be kept separate from other paperwork. The Drug Enforcement Administration (DEA) strictly regulates these substances. If drugs are lost or stolen, the supervisor and law enforcement personnel must be notified immediately. Controlled substances are classified by the DEA as follows:

- *Schedule I:* No accepted medical use; high abuse and dependence potential (ie, heroin, marijuana, LSD)
- *Schedule II:* Accepted medical uses; high abuse and dependence potential (ie, morphine, demerol)
- *Schedule III:* Accepted medical uses; moderately high abuse and dependence potential (ie, Tylenol with Codeine, paregoric)
- *Schedule IV:* Accepted medical uses; moderate abuse and dependence potential (ie, valium, phenobarbital)
- *Schedule V:* Accepted medical uses; low abuse and dependence potential (ie, Robitussin A-C [less than 100 mg codeine per 100 mL])

All medications should be stored in an environment with a constant temperature if possible. Temperature, light, moisture, shelf life, and exposure to air all affect the potency of medications. If controlled medications are not used before their expiration dates, they must be destroyed. The destruction must be witnessed by two employees and documented on the proper forms.

EMT-I Tips

Know These Medications

An EMT-I certified at the 1985 level is allowed to administer or help patients self-administer the following seven medications.

You may be called on to administer:
- Oxygen
- Activated charcoal
- Oral glucose
- $D_{50}W$ (50% dextrose)

You may help patients self-administer:
- Epinephrine
- MDI medications
- Nitroglycerin

However, you may administer or help to administer these medications only under the following conditions:
- A licensed physician gives you a direct order to administer a medication and/or the local medical protocols under which you are working permit you to administer that medication. Some local protocols exclude one or more of the seven medications in the preceding list.
- The local medical protocols under which you are working include standing orders for the use of a medication in defined situations. It is imperative that you do not give or help patients take any other medications under any circumstances.

Activated Charcoal

Many poisoning emergencies involve an overdose of medications taken by mouth. Fortunately, many medications are adsorbed by activated charcoal, which delays digestion and keeps the medications from being absorbed by the body. Adsorption means to bind to or stick to a surface. Activated charcoal is ground into a very fine powder to provide the greatest possible surface area for binding. You will probably carry a container with a premixed suspension of activated charcoal powder and water in the EMS unit, if allowed by local protocol.

The bond between medication and charcoal is not permanent. Because the medication may break free and be absorbed into the bloodstream if activated charcoal remains in the digestive system throughout a normal day, charcoal is frequently suspended with another medication called sorbitol (a complex sugar). This suspension has a laxative effect that causes the entire mixture, including the medication, to move quickly through the digestive system.

Activated charcoal is given by mouth. Although sorbitol sweetens the suspension, the black charcoal makes it look unappealing. For this reason, you should use a covered container and ask the patient to drink the fluid through a straw.

> **Documentation Tips**
>
> When documenting administration of a medication, the proper form includes the name of the medication, dose and route, and vital signs before and after administration. For example:
> 10:30 AM VS: P, 88; R, 18; BP, 128/68;
>   nitroglycerin, 0.4 mg SL
> 10:35 AM VS: P, 80; R, 18; BP, 124/60

General Steps in Administering Medication

As an EMT-I, you must be familiar with the general steps of administering any medication to a patient:

1. **Obtain an order from medical control.** This order may be given to you directly, through online medical control via telephone or radio. Or it may be indirect, through protocols that contain standing orders for the administration of certain medications. For example, your system may use a protocol that describes how the medical director wants you to deal with a patient who is having respiratory difficulties. Part of this protocol may direct you to use a nonrebreathing mask to deliver oxygen to such a patient at 15 L/min. You may do this without calling online medical control if the patient meets the criteria of the protocol.
2. **Repeat the order**, word for word, back to the physician. This will ensure that you understand the order and that the physician did not inadvertently give you an incorrect dosage order.
3. **Inquire about any medication allergies** the patient may have.
4. **Verify the proper medication and prescription.** You have received and confirmed the medication order and determined that the patient is still a candidate for the medication. You must now make sure that the medication you are about to give is the correct medication. Carefully read the label. If it is the patient's own prescription, the bottle may show the trade name or the generic name. If you have any questions at all, contact online medical control. Make sure that the medication is, indeed, the patient's own and does not belong to a friend or relative. You should never give a medication to a patient that has been prescribed for someone else.
5. **Verify the form, dose, and route of the medication.** You have confirmed your order and verified that the medication is the one you want to give. Now you must make sure that the form of the medication, the dose, and the route are all consistent with the order you received. For example, suppose that you are told to give the patient a sublingual nitroglycerin tablet. The patient's nitroglycerin bottle is empty, but he has another bottle of nitroglycerin capsules. These are to be swallowed four times a day. The medication is the same, but the form, dose, and route of delivery are different from the order given. You may not substitute the capsules for the tablets without specific orders from medical control.
6. **Check the expiration date and condition of the medication.** The last step before administering a medication is to make sure the expiration date has not passed. Prescription and OTC medications alike should have an expiration date on their labels. Check the date. If no date can be found, you should examine the medication with suspicion. In addition, if you find discoloration, cloudiness, or particles in a liquid medication, you should not administer it. If a patient with asthma gives you an MDI and the expiration date on it is smudged, you should not administer it.
7. **Reassess the vital signs**, especially heart rate and blood pressure, at least every 5 minutes or as the patient's condition warrants.
8. **Document.** Remember the EMS rule: The work is not done until the paperwork is done. Once the medication has been given, you must document your actions and the patient's response. This includes the time you gave the medication and the name, dose, and route of administration. Did

the patient's condition improve, get worse, or not change at all? Were there any side effects? A second EMS rule says, "If you did not write it down, it did not happen." If your performance should ever be questioned, documentation is your best defense.

This chapter concludes with a listing of information on drugs that may be administered by EMT-Is certified at the 1999 level (Table 6-9 ▼). Use may vary depending on local protocol; check your local protocol regarding which drugs an EMT-I may administer in your area.

EMT-I Tips

General Steps in Administering Medication
1. Obtain an order from medical control.
2. Repeat the order, word for word.
3. Determine whether the patient has any drug allergies.
4. Verify the proper medication and prescription.
5. Verify the form, dose, and route of the medication.
6. Check the expiration date and condition of the medication.
7. Reassess the vital signs, especially heart rate and blood pressure, at least every 5 minutes or as the patient's condition changes.
8. Document accordingly.

TABLE 6-9 Drugs Used in Pharmacologic Management Plans*

Drug Name (Generic)	Characteristics	Descriptions and Trade Names
Acetylsalicylic acid (ASA)	Brand name(s)	Bayer Aspirin, St Joseph Aspirin, Empirin, Ascriptin, Acuprin 81, Anacin, Bufferin
	Classification	Antithrombic, antipyretic
	Mechanism of action	Blocks formation of thromboxane A_2, which decreases platelet aggre-gation and vasoconstriction; reduces risk of death or nonfatal myocardial infarction in patients with previous or unstable angina; reduces fever.
	Onset of action	15-30 min
	Indications	Unstable angina or suspected acute myocardial infarction (acute coronary syndromes); should be given as soon as possible
	Contraindications	Hypersensitivity to salicylates or nonsteroidal anti-inflammatory agents, hemophilia, bleeding ulcers; caution in asthmatics and patients with severe hepatic disease
	Side effects	Gastrointestinal upset, heartburn, rash, prolonged bleeding
	Significant interactions	Enhanced effects of warfarin and other anticoagulants; can increase blood level of phenytoin and sulfonylureas
	Route and method of administration	Chewable tablet(s) given by mouth
	How supplied	Various strengths of tablets ranging from 81-325 mg
	Dose	162-325 mg
	Special considerations	Patients with stomach ulcers, currently taking anticoagulants, currently taking other aspirin-based medications; strong vinegar smell indicates tablets have started to degrade, and they should be replaced

*Note: There may be other medications carried by your service not listed in this table. You should be familiar with those drugs and follow local protocols for administration.

TABLE 6-9 Drugs Used in Pharmacologic Management Plans—cont'd

Drug Name (Generic)	Characteristics	Descriptions and Trade Names
Adenosine	Brand name(s)	Adenocard
	Classification	Antiarrhythmic
	Mechanism of action	Slows conduction through the AV node; Inhibits reentry through the AV node
	Onset of action	10-15 seconds
	Indications	Conversion of paroxysmal supraventricular tachycardia and supraventricular tachycardia to regular sinus rhythm
	Contraindications	Second- or third-degree heart block, sick sinus syndrome
	Side effects	Brief periods of asystole or bradycardia, ventricular ectopy, dyspnea, flushing, chest pain or pressure, dizziness, headache, palpitations, metallic taste, apprehension
	Significant interactions	Carbamazepine and dipyridamole may potentiate and prolong adenosine's effect, requiring smaller doses. Theophylline and related drugs can reduce the effectiveness of adenosine, requiring larger doses. Use with caution if patient is taking digoxin.
	Route and method of administration	IV or IO; rapidly
	How supplied	3 mg/mL in 2-mL vials (total = 6 mg)
	Dose	*Adult*: 6 mg rapid IV push over 1 to 3 seconds, immediately flushed with 20 mL of saline. If no response in 1 to 2 min, repeat at 12 mg up to 2 times; total adult dose = 30 mg. *Pediatric*: 0.1 mg/kg rapid IV push (up to 6 mg); may repeat in 1 to 2 min at 0.2 mg/kg; maximum single dose of 12 mg
	Special considerations	Monitor patient in the record mode to capture change in rhythm. Elevate the arm before administration. If drug is refrigerated or in a cold environment, crystals can form. Warming should cause crystals to dissolve.
Amiodarone hydrochloride	Brand name(s)	Cordarone
	Classification	Antiarrhythmic
	Mechanism of action	Acts on the supraventricular and ventricular myocardium, increases the duration of the myocardial cells' action potential and refractory period, decreases sinus node discharge, increases PR and QT intervals
	Onset of action	Immediate
	Indications	Supraventricular dysrhythmias (supraventricular tachycardia, atrial fibrillation, atrial flutter) and ventricular dysrhythmias (ventricular fibrillation [V-fib], ventricular tachycardia [V-tach] with and without a pulse)
	Contraindications	Sinoatrial dysfunction, bradycardia, second- and third-degree heart block
	Side effects	Hypotension, weakness, nausea, tremors, premature ventricular complexes (PVCs)

TABLE 6-9 Drugs Used in Pharmacologic Management Plans—cont'd

Drug Name (Generic)	Characteristics	Descriptions and Trade Names
Amiodarone hydrochloride (continued)	Significant interactions	May increase the effects of anticoagulants (ie, Coumadin), can potentiate the effects of beta-blockers (ie, Inderal), causing significant bradycardia and hypotension
	Route and method of administration	IV or IO; rapidly
	How supplied	3 mL ampules and prefilled syringes containing 50 mg/mL; 900 mg vials
	Dose	**Cardiac arrest (V-fib or pulseless V-tach)** *Adult*: 300 mg rapid IV push (initial dose); may repeat in 3 to 5 min at 150 mg rapid IV push *Pediatric*: 5 mg/kg; maximum dose of 15 mg/kg **Supraventricular and Ventricular Tachycardia (Stable)** *Adult* <u>Rapid infusion</u>: 150 mg IV over 10 min (15 mg/min); may repeat every 10 min as needed <u>Slow infusion</u>: 360 mg over 6 h (1.0 mg/min) <u>Maintenance infusion</u>: 540 mg over 18 h (0.5 mg/min); maximum cumulative dose of 2.2 g/24 h *Pediatric* 5 mg/kg IV bolus Can repeat up to total dose of 15 mg/kg IV per 24 hours. Max single dose: 300 mg. Pediatric dose for perfusing SVT and V-tach is 5 mg/kg IV/IO bolus over 20 to 60 minutes (max single dose: 300 mg). Can repeat to total dose of 15 mg/kg IV per 24 hours.
	Special considerations	Must dilute amiodarone in 20 to 30 mL of D_5W prior to administration (both in patients with a pulse and patients in cardiac arrest); use with caution in patients with congestive heart failure, draw up slowly
Atropine sulfate	Brand name(s)	Atropine
	Classification	Anticholinergic (parasympathetic blocker)
	Mechanism of action	Direct vagolytic action increases sinus node automaticity and faster conduction through the AV node
	Onset of action	1–5 min
	Indications	Symptomatic bradycardia (may not be effective in second-degree type II or third-degree AV block), asystole, bradycardic (<60 beats/min) pulseless electrical activity (PEA), organophosphate poisoning
	Contraindications	Angle-closure glaucoma, tachycardia. In acute myocardial infarction, increases oxygen demand and can worsen ischemia
	Side effects	Headache, hot flushed skin, disorientation, tachycardia, dry mouth, blurred vision, urinary retention, pupillary dilation
	Significant interactions	Additive with other drugs having anticholinergic properties
	Route and method of administration	IV, IO, ET; rapidly
	How supplied	Various sizes of vials and prefilled syringes; strengths ranging from 0.05 to 1.0 mg/mL

TABLE 6-9 Drugs Used in Pharmacologic Management Plans—cont'd

Drug Name (Generic)	Characteristics	Descriptions and Trade Names
Atropine sulfate (continued)	Dose	**Symptomatic bradycardia** *Adult*: 0.5 mg rapid IV push; repeat every 3-5 min as needed; maximum dose, 3 mg *Pediatric*: 0.02 mg/kg IV, IO, or ET; minimum single dose, 0.1 mg; maximum total dose, 1 mg for a child and 2 mg for an adolescent **Asystole or bradycardic PEA** *Adult*: 1.0 mg IV or ET; repeat every 3-5 min; maximum dose, 3 mg *Pediatric*: Safety and efficacy not established **Organophosphate poisoning** *Adult*: 2-4 mg IV or IM every 5-15 min; repeat as needed until secretions clear *Pediatric*: 0.05 mg/kg per dose IV (usual dose, 1-5 mg); repeat every 20 min as needed until secretions clear
	Special considerations	Use care in hot environments. Owing to increased heart rate, can increase oxygen demand. Use cautiously in myocardial ischemia or infarction. VF or VT occurs rarely following IV use. If necessary, can be administered directly into the tracheobronchial tree via an ET tube at 2-2.5 times the standard IV dose. May cause paradoxical bradycardia if pushed too slowly or when given in doses of less than 0.5 mg.
50% dextrose solution	Brand name(s)	$D_{50}W$, D_{50}
	Classification	Carbohydrate (hypertonic solution)
	Mechanism of action	Supplies carbohydrate; increases circulating blood glucose levels
	Onset of action	1 min; may be longer with severe hypoglycemia
	Indications	Hypoglycemia, altered level of consciousness, coma of unknown cause, seizures of unknown cause
	Contraindications	Anuria, intraspinal or intracranial hemorrhage, increased intracranial pressure, stroke without hypoglycemia; delirium tremens
	Side effects	Burning or pain during infusion, thrombophlebitis, nausea, vomiting
	Significant interactions	Do not administer in the same line with blood.
	Route and method of administration	IV; slowly
	How supplied	25 g/50 mL prefilled syringe (500 mg/mL)
	Dose	*Adult*: 25-50 mL (12.5-25 g) of 50% solution *Pediatric*: 0.5-1.0 g/kg IV or IO
	Special considerations	Patient may need additional carbohydrates after awakening. D_{25} solution normally used for pediatric patients; D_{10} solution for neonates. May precipitate Wernicke encephalopathy in thiamine-deficient patients (ie, alcoholics). Therefore, 100 mg of thiamine IV should be given before dextrose.

TABLE 6-9 Drugs Used in Pharmacologic Management Plans—cont'd

Drug Name (Generic)	Characteristics	Descriptions and Trade Names
Diazepam	Brand name(s)	Valium
	Classification	Benzodiazepine
	Mechanism of action	Exact sedative mechanism unknown, suppresses seizure activity across the cerebral motor cortex
	Onset of action	IV: 1-5 min; IM: 15-30 min
	Indications	To provide sedation or to treat seizures
	Contraindications	Acute angle-closure glaucoma, hypersensitivity to benzodiazepines, shock, respiratory depression
	Side effects	Sedation, ataxia, hypotension, possible respiratory depression, confusion, nausea
	Significant interactions	Potentates other sedative drugs, including alcohol. Cimetidine and disulfiram can increase diazepam effects. May worsen symptoms of Parkinson patient taking levodopa. Potentially increases digoxin blood levels.
	Route and method of administration	IV or IM; slowly
	How supplied	Various sizes of vials, 5 mg/mL
	Dose	*Adult*: 2-10 mg over 5-10 min; maximum dose, 30 mg *Pediatric*: Up to 5 years: 0.2-0.5 mg every 2-5 min; maximum dose, 5.0 mg Older than 5 years: 1 mg every 2-5 min; maximum dose, 10 mg
	Special considerations	Controlled substance; should be administered through large vein or into line with adequate flow of fluids to minimize trauma to vein. Incompatible with most IV solutions (give into an IV of normal saline)
Epinephrine hydrochloride (1:1,000)	Brand name(s)	Adrenalin
	Classification	Sympathomimetic
	Mechanism of action	Alpha and beta agonist; increases systemic vascular resistance, arterial pressure, cardiac contractility; relieves bronchospasm
	Onset of action	SC: 5-10 min
	Indications	Mild to moderate asthma and allergic reactions
	Contraindications	Caution with hypertension, hyperthyroidism, angle-closure glaucoma
	Side effects	Headache, restlessness, palpitations, tachycardia, anginal pain, dysrhythmias
	Significant interactions	Potentiates other sympathomimetics, tricyclic antidepressants, monoamine oxidase inhibitors; beta-blockers decrease effects
	Route and method of administration	SC; slowly
	How supplied	1-mL ampules (1.0 mg/mL); 30-mL vials (1 mg/mL)

TABLE 6-9 Drugs Used in Pharmacologic Management Plans—cont'd

Drug Name (Generic)	Characteristics	Descriptions and Trade Names
Epinephrine hydrochloride (1:1,000) (continued)	Dose	**Mild to moderate asthma and allergic reactions** *Adult*: 0.3-0.5 mL (0.3-0.5 mg) *Pediatric*: 0.01 mL/kg (0.01 mg/kg); maximum dose, 0.3 mL (0.3 mg)
	Special considerations	Store in a dark place. Use only clear solution. Use with caution in elderly patients. Watch for extravasation. If necessary, may be administered directly into the tracheobronchial tree via an ET tube.
Epinephrine hydrochloride (1:10,000)	Brand name(s)	Adrenalin
	Classification	Sympathomimetic
	Mechanism of action	Alpha and beta agonist; increases systemic vascular resistance, arterial pressure, cardiac contractility; relieves bronchospasm
	Onset of action	Seconds
	Indications	Cardiac arrest, anaphylactic shock
	Contraindications	Caution with hypertension, hyperthyroidism, angle-closure glaucoma
	Side effects	Headache, restlessness, palpitations, tachycardia, anginal pain, dysrhythmias
	Significant interactions	Potentiates other sympathomimetics, tricyclic antidepressants, monoamine oxidase inhibitors; beta-blockers decrease effects
	Route and method of administration	IV, IO, ET; rapidly
	How supplied	0.1 mg/mL prefilled syringe
	Dose	**Cardiac arrest** *Adult*: 1 mg (10 mL) IV or ET every 3-5 min; administer 2-2.5 mg, diluted in 10 mL of normal saline if given ET *Pediatric*: Initial dose: 0.01 mg/kg (0.1 mL/kg) IV or IO; 0.1 mg/kg (0.1 mL/kg) of a 1:1,000 solution if given ET; repeat every 3-5 min **Symptomatic bradycardia** *Adult*: 2-10 µg/min as an IV infusion *Pediatric*: 0.01 mg/kg (0.1 mL/kg); may repeat as needed. **Anaphylactic shock or severe bronchospasm** *Adult*: 1-2 mL (0.1-0.2 mg) slow IV push *Pediatric*: 0.05-0.15 µg/kg per minute as an IV infusion
	Special considerations	Store in a dark place. Use only clear solution. Use with caution in elderly patients. Watch for extravasation. If necessary, may be administered directly into the tracheobronchial tree via an ET tube.
Furosemide	Brand name(s)	Lasix
	Classification	Loop diuretic

TABLE 6-9 Drugs Used in Pharmacologic Management Plans—cont'd

Drug Name (Generic)	Characteristics	Descriptions and Trade Names
Furosemide (continued)	Mechanism of action	Inhibits reabsorption of sodium and chloride in proximal tubules and loop of Henle; can also reduce cardiac preload and decrease afterload by increasing venous capacitance
	Onset of action	Diuretic effects: within 15-20 min; vascular effects: within 5 min
	Indications	Acute pulmonary edema and congestive heart failure
	Contraindications	Anuria, hepatic coma, severe electrolyte depletion, hypovolemia; caution if allergic to sulfonamides
	Side effects	Headache, tinnitus, dizziness, hypotension, dehydration, electrolyte imbalance, increased blood glucose level
	Significant interactions	Potential additive adverse effects if administered with aminoglycoside antibiotics (such as gentamicin, tobramycin); increases effects of other diuretics and antihypertensives; decreases serum potassium level; increases serum lithium level
	Route and method of administration	IV; slowly
	How supplied	Various sizes of vials, 10 mg/mL
	Dose	*Adult*: 20-40 mg (0.5-1.0 mg/kg) over 1-2 min; do not exceed 20 mg/min; if no response, give 2 mg/kg over 1-2 min *Pediatric*: 1 mg/kg per dose; maximum dose, 6 mg/kg
	Special considerations	In certain situations, doses can exceed 1 mg/mL; may cause fetal abnormalities; should be protected from light; may need to increase dose in patients who are taking furosemide; give slowly to avoid ototoxicity
Lidocaine HCl 2%	Brand name(s)	Xylocaine
	Classification	Antiarrhythmic
	Mechanism of action	Sodium channel blocker; decreases automaticity, increases ventricular fibrillation (VF) threshold and electrical stimulation threshold of ventricle during diastole
	Onset of action	1-5 min
	Indications	VF or pulseless ventricular tachycardia (VT)
	Contraindications	Hypersensitivity to amide local anesthetics, bradycardia (<60 beats/min), Stokes-Adams syndrome, Wolff-Parkinson-White syndrome, AV or intraventricular block in patient without artificial pacemaker; use with caution in congestive heart failure, renal and hepatic disease, elderly patients, and patients with digoxin toxicity accompanied by AV block.
	Side effects	Tachycardia, nystagmus, labile blood pressure, possible malignant hyperthermic crisis, dizziness, seizures, respiratory depression, slurred speech, cardiovascular collapse
	Significant interactions	Beta-blockers (for example, propranolol [Inderal], metoprolol [Lopressor]) and cimetidine decrease lidocaine clearance; in higher doses, potentiates effects of succinylcholine (a neuromuscular blocker [paralytic])

TABLE 6-9 Drugs Used in Pharmacologic Management Plans—cont'd

Drug Name (Generic)	Characteristics	Descriptions and Trade Names
Lidocaine HCl 2% (continued)	Route and method of administration	IV or ET; rapidly
	How supplied	Prefilled syringes: 100 mg/5 mL (20 mg/mL); 1- and 2-g additive syringes; ampules: 100 mg/5 mL (20 mg/mL); 1- and 2-g vials in 30-mL solution
	Dose	**Cardiac arrest (VF or pulseless VT)** *Adult*: 1.0-1.5 mg/kg IV repeated every 5-10 min in a dose of 0.5-0.75 mg/kg; give 2-2.5 times the IV dose if administered ET; maximum dose, 3.0 mg/kg (IV or ET) *Pediatric*: 1.0 mg/kg rapid IV/IO push (maximum dose, 100 mg) **IV infusion following resuscitation** *Adult*: 1-4 mg/min (30-50 µg/kg per minute); can dilute in D_5W or normal saline *Pediatric*: 20-50 µg/kg per minute; administer bolus dose of 1.0 mg/kg when infusion initiated if bolus dose not given within the previous 15 min
	Special considerations	Reduce infusion dose by 50% in patients older than 70 years and in patients with renal or hepatic dysfunction.
Morphine sulfate (MSO_4)	Brand name(s)	Morphine, Duramorph, Astromorph
	Classification	Narcotic (opioid) analgesic
	Mechanism of action	Opiate receptor agonist; reduces pain of myocardial ischemia, anxiety, and extension of ischemia by reducing myocardial oxygen demand; alleviates pulmonary edema by promoting venous pooling and decreasing cardiac preload and afterload
	Onset of action	1-2 min
	Indications	Pain management, especially from burns or myocardial infarction; sedation; pulmonary edema
	Contraindications	Hypersensitivity to opiates, acute bronchial asthma, upper airway obstructive disease, central nervous system (CNS) depression, head injury with increased intracranial pressure, undiagnosed abdominal pain
	Side effects	Dizziness, hypotension, bradycardia, respiratory depression, sedation, nausea, vomiting, sweating, euphoria, bronchospasm, arrhythmias, miosis, decreased cough reflex
	Significant interactions	Potentiates other CNS depressants, including alcohol
	Route and method of administration	IV; slowly
	How supplied	Ampules or prefilled syringes; 10 mg/mL
	Dose	*Adult*: 2-4 mg over 1-5 min every 5-30 min; titrated to effect *Pediatric*: 0.1-0.2 mg/kg; maximum dose, 15 mg
	Special considerations	Schedule II controlled substance; may obscure diagnosis of head or abdominal injuries. Naloxone should be readily available to reverse CNS depression if it occurs.

TABLE 6-9　Drugs Used in Pharmacologic Management Plans—cont'd

Drug Name (Generic)	Characteristics	Descriptions and Trade Names
Naloxone hydrochloride	Brand name(s)	Narcan
	Classification	Narcotic (opioid) antagonist
	Mechanism of action	Binds to opiate receptor sites
	Onset of action	Within 2 minutes
	Indications	Reversal of narcotic-induced central nervous system depression (for example, hypoventilation, bradycardia, hypotension), coma of unknown etiology
	Contraindications	Hypersensitivity; cautious use in narcotic-addicted patients (acute withdrawal seizures may occur)
	Side effects	Reversal of narcotic depression could lead to nausea, vomiting, sweating, tachycardia, increased blood pressure, premature ventricular contractions
	Significant interactions	If preparing a continuous infusion, do not mix other drugs in the same IV bag.
	Route and method of administration	IV, IM, SC, ET; slowly
	How supplied	Ampules or vials: 0.02, 0.4, and 1 mg/mL
	Dose	*Adult*: 0.4-2.0 mg over 2-3 min, up to 10 mg total *Pediatric*: 5 years or younger or less than 20 kg: 0.1 mg/kg; repeat as needed to achieve desired effect Older than 5 years or more than 20 kg: 2.0 mg
	Special considerations	In an addicted patient, the dose is normally titrated to improve respiration only, not to fully arouse the patient. If necessary, may be given IM or SC.
Nitroglycerin (NTG)	Brand name(s)	Nitroglycerin, Nitrostat, Nitro-bid, Isordil
	Classification	Vasodilator
	Mechanism of action	Decreases pain of ischemia, venous blood return to heart, preload and cardiac oxygen consumption; increases venous capacitance; dilates coronary arteries
	Onset of action	2-5 min
	Indications	Angina pectoris, suspected acute myocardial infarction
	Contraindications	Hypersensitivity, severe anemia, closed-angle glaucoma, head trauma, systolic blood pressure <90 mm hg, recent (within 24 h) use of sildenafil (Viagra), tadalafil (Cialis), or vardenafil (Levitra)
	Side effects	Headache, flushing, nausea, vomiting, involuntary passing of urine or feces, palpitations, hypotension
	Significant interactions	May potentiate antihypertensive medications
	Route and method of administration	SL; rapid absorption
	How supplied	Tablets for SL use: 0.3, 0.4, and 0.6 mg; metered spray: 0.4 mg per spray

TABLE 6-9 Drugs Used in Pharmacologic Management Plans—cont'd

Drug Name (Generic)	Characteristics	Descriptions and Trade Names
Nitroglycerin (NTG) (continued)	Dose	*Adult*: Tablet: 0.3-0.4 mg SL; may repeat twice; metered spray: 0.4 mg per spray SL; may repeat twice *Pediatric*: Not recommended
	Special considerations	Tablets may cause a burning or sweet sensation under the tongue. Store tablets in a cool, dark, dry environment. Tolerance to nitrates can develop.
Vasopressin	Brand name(s)	Pitressin synthetic
	Classification	Hormone (antidiuretic hormone [ADH])
	Mechanism of action	Nonadrenergic vasoconstrictor (in high doses)
	Onset of action	5 min
	Indications	Alternative drug to the first or second dose of epinephrine in cardiac arrest from ventricular fibrillation, pulseless ventricular tachycardia, PEA, or asystole
	Contraindications	None, when given for cardiac arrest
	Side effects	Uncommon with low doses
	Significant interactions	Carbamazepine, chlorpropamide, or clofibrate may increase the antidiuretic effects of vasopressin.
	Route and method of administration	IV; rapid
	How supplied	2-mL vials and ampules containing 20 units/mL
	Dose	*Adult*: 40 units via IV push (one-time dose only) *Pediatric*: Not indicated
	Special considerations	Must wait 10 to 20 min after administering vasopressin before initiating/continuing epinephrine therapy
Medications Used to Treat Respiratory Diseases and Bronchospasm		
Albuterol sulfate	Brand name(s)	Proventil, Ventolin
	Classification	Sympathomimetic, bronchodilator
	Mechanism of action	Selective beta-2 adrenergic stimulation
	Onset of action	5-15 min after inhalation
	Indications	Bronchospasm associated with asthma, emphysema, or allergic reaction
	Contraindications	Caution with history of seizures, diabetes, hyperthyroidism
	Side effects	Tremors, increased heart rate and blood pressure, dizziness, dysrhythmias, nausea
	Significant interactions	Beta-blockers can antagonize effects; caution with other sympathomimetics because effects may be additive
	Route and method of administration	Nebulizer or MDI; inhaled into the lungs

TABLE 6-9 Drugs Used in Pharmacologic Management Plans—cont'd

Drug Name (Generic)	Characteristics	Descriptions and Trade Names
Albuterol sulfate (continued)	How supplied	MDI: 90 μg per metered spray; 17-g canister with 200 inhalations Solution for nebulization: 0.5% (5 mg/mL); 0.083% (2.5 mg) in 3 mL unit-dose per nebulizer
	Dose	*Adult*: MDI: Up to 3 inhalations (90 μg each); repeated at 15 min intervals Nebulizer: 2.5 mg (0.5 mL of a 0.5% solution diluted in 3 mL of normal saline); repeat every 15 min as needed *Pediatric*: Younger than 12 years: 0.03 mL/kg (0.5% solution); up to 1 mL over 5-10 min Older than 12 years: adult dose
	Special considerations	Do not allow solution to freeze. Avoid storage in excessive heat.
Ipratropium bromide	Brand name(s)	Atrovent
	Classification	Anticholinergic
	Mechanism of action	Inhibits interaction of acetylcholine at muscarinic receptor sites on bronchial smooth muscle, resulting in bronchodilation and drying of secretions
	Onset of action	10-15 min
	Indications	Bronchospasm associated with asthma, chronic bronchitis, and emphysema
	Contraindications	Hypersensitivity to ipratropium, atropine, peanuts, soybean proteins
	Side effects	Dry mouth, bitter taste, cough, nausea, blurred vision, tachycardia, headache
	Significant interactions	Minimally absorbed; no significant drug interactions reported
	Route and method of administration	Inhalation; MDI or nebulizer
	How supplied	MDI: 18 μg/actuation Solution for nebulization: 0.02% solution
	Dose	*Adult*: MDI: 2 inhalations (36 μg); repeat as needed Nebulizer: 0.5 mg in 3.0 mL normal saline; repeat as needed *Pediatric*: Older than 12 years: 0.125-0.250 mg in 3.0 mL of normal saline or 1-2 inhalations from MDI Younger than 12 years: not recommended
	Special considerations	Not commonly used as the sole agent in acute situations; may be combined with albuterol
Isoetharine	Brand name(s)	Isoetharine Inhalation Solution (formerly marketed as Bronkosol and Bronkometer in the United States; currently, only the solution available in the United States)
	Classification	Bronchodilator
	Mechanism of action	Beta-2 adrenergic stimulation
	Onset of action	Immediate

TABLE 6-9 Drugs Used in Pharmacologic Management Plans—cont'd

Drug Name (Generic)	Characteristics	Descriptions and Trade Names
Isoetharine (continued)	Indications	Bronchospasm associated with obstructive airway diseases, including asthma, chronic bronchitis, and emphysema
	Contraindications	Known hypersensitivity, use caution with history of seizures, diabetes, hyperthyroidism
	Side effects	Tremors, increased heart rate and blood pressure, palpitations, dizziness, dysrhythmias, nausea, headache
	Significant interactions	Beta-blockers can antagonize effects; use with caution with other sympathomimetics because effects may be additive
	Route and method of administration	Inhalation; MDI or nebulizer
	How supplied	Various concentrations ranging from 0.1% to 1% solutions
	Dose	*Adult*: MDI: 1-2 inhalations Nebulizer: dilute 0.5 mL of 1% solution 1:3 with saline; give dose over 15-20 min; solutions other than 1% may be used undiluted *Pediatric*: Older than 12 years: same as adult dose Younger than 12 years: not recommended
	Special considerations	None
Metaproterenol sulfate	Brand name(s)	Alupent, Metaprel
	Classification	Bronchodilator
	Mechanism of action	Beta-2 adrenergic stimulation, relaxation of bronchial smooth muscle
	Onset of action	1-2 min following inhalation
	Indications	Bronchospasm associated with obstructive airway diseases, including asthma, chronic bronchitis, and emphysema
	Contraindications	Hypersensitivity; use caution with history of seizures, diabetes, hyperthyroidism, or dysrhythmias
	Side effects	Tremors, restlessness, apprehension, cough, increased heart rate and blood pressure, palpitations, dizziness, dysrhythmias, nausea
	Significant interactions	Beta-blockers can antagonize effects; use with caution with other sympathomimetics because effects may be additive
	Route and method of administration	Inhalation; MDI or nebulizer
	How supplied	MDI: 0.65 mg per spray (15-mL inhaler); solution for nebulization: 0.4%, 0.6%, and 5.0%
	Dose	*Adult*: MDI: 2-3 inhalations (2 minutes apart) Nebulizer: 2.5 mL of 0.4% or 0.6% solution (or dilute 5.0% solution), repeated in 4 to 6 h if needed *Pediatric*: MDI: Older than 12 years: same as adult dose Younger than 12 years: not recommended Nebulizer: Older than 6 years: same as adult dose Younger than 6 years: not recommended
	Special considerations	Shake well before use, do not use if solution is brown or contains precipitate

TABLE 6-9 Drugs Used in Pharmacologic Management Plans—cont'd

Drug Name (Generic)	Characteristics	Descriptions and Trade Names
Methylprednisolone sodium succinate	Brand name(s)	Solu-Medrol
	Classification	Steroid; synthetic glucocorticoid
	Mechanism of action	Glucocorticoid effects; anti-inflammatory
	Onset of action	1-2 h or longer
	Indications	Bronchodilator for refractory asthma, anaphylaxis; acute spinal cord injury
	Contraindications	Hypersensitivity, active ocular herpes simplex infection, systemic fungal infection; use with caution in hypothyroidism, seizure disorders, cirrhosis, thromboembolic disorders
	Side effects	Short-term administration of even high doses is not likely to produce harmful effects. Patient may exhibit myopathy, headache, vertigo, sodium and fluid retention with potassium loss, rise in blood glucose level.
	Significant interactions	Severe weakness in patients with myasthenia gravis who are taking anticholinesterase agents such as neostigmine or pyridostigmine. Increased potassium loss in patients taking furosemide or other potassium-depleting drugs.
	Route and method of administration	IV; slowly
	How supplied	"Mix-a-vials" with 40, 125, 500, and 1,000 mg (requires reconstitution before use) and 20 mg/mL vials
	Dose	*Adult*: Bronchospasm: 40-125 mg IV push; higher doses given by slow IV push or IV infusion Spinal cord injury: 30 mg/kg followed by infusion of 5.4 mg/kg/h *Pediatric*: 1-2 mg/kg IV push
	Special considerations	None
Salmeterol	Brand name(s)	Serevent
	Classification	Bronchodilator
	Mechanism of action	Beta-2 adrenergic stimulation
	Onset of action	10-20 min
	Indications	Asthma
	Contraindications	Caution with history of seizures, diabetes, hyperthyroidism
	Side effects	Dental pain, headache, tremors, increased heart rate and blood pressure, dizziness, dysrhythmias, nausea
	Significant interactions	Beta-blockers can antagonize effects; use with caution with other sympathomimetics because effects may be additive
	Route of administration	Inhalation
	How supplied	Metered-spray aerosol
	Dose	Two inhalations; repeat in 12 h if needed
	Special considerations	Not normally used for acute attacks

TABLE 6-9 Drugs Used in Pharmacologic Management Plans—cont'd

Drug Name (Generic)	Characteristics	Descriptions and Trade Names
Terbutaline	Brand name(s)	Brethine, Brethaire
	Classification	Bronchodilator
	Mechanism of action	Beta-2 adrenergic stimulation resulting in relaxation of bronchiole smooth muscle
	Onset of action	5-15 min
	Indications	Bronchospasm associated with obstructive airway diseases, such as asthma, chronic bronchitis, and emphysema
	Contraindications	Known hypersensitivity; use with caution with history of seizures, diabetes, hyperthyroidism
	Side effects	Tremors, premature ventricular contractions, palpitations, flushing, sweating, increased heart rate and blood pressure, dizziness, nausea, headache
	Significant interactions	Beta-blockers can antagonize effects; use with caution with other sympathomimetics because effects may be additive
	Route and method of administration	SC or MDI
	How supplied	MDI: 0.2 mg per inhalation; ampule: 1 mg/mL
	Dose	*Adult*: MDI: 1-2 inhalations every 4-6 h (1 min between inhalations) SC: 0.25 mg repeated in 15-30 min if needed. *Pediatric*: Older than 12 years: same as adult dose Younger than 12 years: not recommended
	Special considerations	Do not administer IV
Triamcinolone	Brand name(s)	Azmacort
	Classification	Steroid; synthetic glucocorticoid
	Mechanism of action	Glucocorticoid effects; anti-inflammatory
	Onset of action	Hours or longer
	Indications	Asthma
	Contraindications	Hypersensitivity, systemic fungal infection
	Side effects	Dysphonia, cough, wheezing, dry mouth
	Significant interactions	Because absorption is minimal, no significant interactions are anticipated.
	Route of administration	Inhalation
	How supplied	Inhaler delivering metered doses
	Dose	*Adult*: 2-4 sprays repeated in 4 or more h if needed *Pediatric*: 6-12 years old, 1-2 sprays; not normally used with children younger than 6 years
	Special considerations	Not recommended as primary agent in acute asthma attacks

You are the Provider — Summary

1. Given that this patient has cardiac-related chest pain, what drugs are potentially indicated for administration?

Oxygen, aspirin, nitroglycerin, and morphine are drugs that you will potentially administer to a patient with suspected cardiac chest pain. (Morphine sulfate is not part of every EMT-I scope of practice; therefore, always adhere to local protocols.)

2. What mnemonic can assist you in remembering these medications?

Although not given in this order, the mnemonic MONA is helpful is remembering the appropriate medications to administer to patients with suspected cardiac chest pain. The appropriate order of these medications is oxygen, aspirin, nitroglycerin, and morphine.

3. Other than oxygen, what is the first drug given for patients with suspected cardiac chest pain?

Aspirin is usually the first drug given to cardiac patients after oxygen. The recommended dose of aspirin is 162 to 325 mg. In this dosing range, aspirin effectively blocks the formation of thromboxane A_2, thus inhibiting platelet aggregation and coronary vasoconstriction.

4. What should you consider before administering this drug, and how should the drug be administered?

Prior to administering aspirin, you must confirm that the patient is not allergic to it and does not have a history of bleeding disorders or ulcers. Caution should be used when administering aspirin to asthmatics. To achieve the fastest therapeutic blood level, you should instruct the patient to chew the aspirin prior to swallowing it.

5. What initial drug should you administer to this patient to relieve his chest pain?

Nitroglycerin is usually the initial drug administered to patients with suspected cardiac chest pain.

6. What must you determine prior to its administration? Why is this important?

There are several important questions to ask the patient prior to administering nitroglycerin. First, you must determine if the patient has prescribed nitroglycerin. If so, determine how many doses he or she self-administered prior to your arrival. Second, you must ensure that the patient's systolic BP is at least 90 mm Hg; nitroglycerin is a vasodilator and may cause hypotension in some people. Last, you must determine if the patient has taken Viagra, Cialis, or Levitra within the past 24 hours. These drugs, used to treat erectile dysfunction, can cause life-threatening hypotension if administered concomitantly with nitroglycerin. *If the patient has taken any of these medications within the past 24 hours, nitroglycerin is contraindicated.*

7. How many doses of nitroglycerin can you give and in what time frame?

Nitroglycerin can be given up to 3 times (0.4 mg per dose), waiting 3 to 5 minutes in between doses. You must also take into consideration how many doses, if any, the patient self-administered prior to your arrival.

You are the Provider continued

Summary

8. What are some important considerations to note about the effectiveness of nitroglycerin when administered by the patient prior to your arrival? What other forms of nitroglycerin are commonly used?

Nitroglycerin is photosensitive as well as sensitive to air. If a patient has taken nitroglycerin prior to your arrival, examine the bottle from which it was administered. If the patient has removed the tablets from the original bottle and/or replaced the rayon ball with a cotton ball, the effectiveness of the drug may be reduced. If the patient tells you that he or she has not experienced any relief from the pain after taking nitroglycerin, inspect the bottle or canister to confirm that the drug is not out of date. Additionally, if the patient does not complain of a headache or a bitter taste under the tongue (common side effects), the drug may no longer be effective. Nitroglycerin is also administered via metered-dose spray (more common now than the bottle), transdermal paste, or a transdermal patch.

9. What is the dose and route for morphine? What are its potential side effects?

The recommended dose of morphine is 2 to 4 mg via slow IV push. Although relatively uncommon in this low dosing range, morphine can cause respiratory depression, bradycardia, and hypotension (signs of CNS depression) in some patients. Therefore, be prepared to administer naloxone (Narcan) if these signs are observed.

10. Why is morphine so effective in the treatment of cardiac-related chest pain?

Morphine reduces cardiac preload and afterload, thus promoting systemic venous pooling of blood, decreased myocardial workload, and decreased myocardial oxygen demand and consumption. As a narcotic analgesic, morphine is effective in relieving pain—an important aspect in the treatment of a patient with suspected cardiac compromise.

Prep Kit

Ready for Review

- Drugs are chemical agents used in the diagnosis, treatment, and prevention of disease. As an EMT-I you must be familiar with the various names of drugs, the sources of drugs, their classification, and sources where information on drugs may be obtained.
- Drugs are standardized for the protection of the consumer.
- There are special considerations for certain groups of patients when administering medications: geriatric, pediatric, and pregnant patients.
- As an EMT-I, you are held responsible for safe and therapeutically effective drug administration. This includes legal, moral, and ethical considerations.
- To understand the effects drugs have on the body, you must first have an understanding of the nervous system. Next, you must understand the general properties of drugs and the various forms in which they are dispensed.
- You should also know the various routes of medication administration and which routes are used for the drugs you may administer in the prehospital setting.
- The mechanism of drug action is the desired effect of a medication. An understanding of pharmacodynamics and pharmacokinetics helps to make the decision of which drug will work best for which patient. Before administering a medication, you must also know what to expect from a particular medication and what to do to offset an adverse reaction.
- Overall, it is important to learn as much as you can about the drugs you may be allowed to administer in your area. Carry a pharmacologic reference to look up drugs that may be unfamiliar.
- You should also be aware of proper drug storage and security. Follow local protocols for drug administration, and review pharmacology often.

Vital Vocabulary

absorption The process by which medications travel through body tissues until they reach the bloodstream.

action The expected therapeutic effect of a medication on the body.

activated charcoal An oral medication that binds and adsorbs ingested toxins in the gastrointestinal tract, for treatment of some poisonings and medication overdoses. Charcoal is ground into a very fine powder that provides the greatest possible surface area for binding medications that have been taken by mouth; it is carried on the EMS unit.

adrenal glands Endocrine glands located on top of the kidneys that release adrenaline when stimulated by the sympathetic nervous system.

adsorption To bind or stick to a surface.

agonists Drugs that bind to a receptor and cause a response.

antagonists In the pharmacologic sense, drugs that counteract the action of something else, such as a muscle or drug.

autonomic nervous system (ANS) The part of the nervous system that regulates functions, such as digestion and sweating, that are not controlled voluntarily.

beta-blocker A common class of cardiac drugs that blocks beta effects, causing a decrease in the workload of the heart by reducing the speed of contraction, as well as reducing blood pressure.

bioavailability The rate and extent to which an active drug enters the general circulation, permitting access to the site of action.

biotransformation The chemical alteration that a substance undergoes in the body.

buccal A medication route in which the medication is placed between the cheek and gums, where it is absorbed into the bloodstream.

chemical name Precise description of a drug's chemical composition and molecular structure.

contraindications Situations in which a medication should not be given because it would not help or may actually harm a patient.

Technology

- Interactivities
- Vocabulary Explorer
- Anatomy Review
- Web Links
- Online Review Manual

www.EMSzone.com/EMTI

cross-tolerance A tolerance to a particular drug that crosses over to other drugs in the same class.

cumulative effect Action of increased intensity after administration of several doses of a drug.

diffusion The movement of solutes (molecules) from an area of higher concentration to an area of lower concentration.

dose The amount of medication given on the basis of the patient's size and age.

drug antagonism A decrease in the action of a drug by the administration of another drug.

drugs Chemical agents used in the diagnosis, treatment, and prevention of disease.

efficacy The ability to produce a desired effect.

enteral Drugs that are administered along any portion of the gastrointestinal tract, including the sublingual, buccal, oral, rectal, and nasogastric routes.

epinephrine Medication that increases heart rate and blood pressure but also eases breathing problems by decreasing muscle tone of the bronchiole tree; the EMT-I may be allowed to help the patient self-administer the medication.

excretion The elimination of waste products from the body.

filtration The removing of particles from a solution by allowing the liquid portion to pass through a membrane or other partial barrier.

gel A semiliquid substance that is administered orally through capsules or plastic tubes.

generic name The original chemical name of a medication (in contrast with one of its trade names); not capitalized.

half-life The time required by the body, tissue, or organ to metabolize or inactivate half the amount of a substance taken in. This is an important consideration in determining the proper dose of drug and frequency of administration.

iatrogenic response An adverse condition induced in a patient by the treatment given.

idiosyncrasy An abnormal sensitivity or reaction to a drug or other substance that is peculiar to an individual.

idiosyncratic reaction A peculiar or individual response to a drug or medication through unusual susceptibility.

indications Therapeutic uses for a specific medication.

inhalation Breathing into the lungs; a medication delivery route.

intradermal Into the skin; a medication delivery route.

intralingual Into the tongue; a medication delivery route.

intramuscular (IM) injection Injection into a muscle; a medication delivery route.

intraosseous (IO) Into the bone; a medication delivery route.

intrathecal Into the spine; a medication delivery route.

intravenous (IV) injection Injection directly into a vein; a medication delivery route.

metered-dose inhaler (MDI) A miniature spray canister through which droplets or particles of medication may be inhaled.

nasal Into the nasal mucosa; a medication delivery route.

nasogastric A medication delivery route in which liquid medication is injected through a nasogastric tube into the stomach.

nitroglycerin Medication that increases cardiac perfusion by causing arteries to dilate; the EMT-I may be allowed to help the patient self-administer the medication.

official name Drug name assigned by the United States Pharmacopeia (USP), generally the generic name followed by USP.

oral By mouth; a medication delivery route.

oral glucose A simple sugar that is readily absorbed by the bloodstream; it is carried on the EMS unit.

osmosis The movement of a solvent (fluid) from an area of lower solute concentration to an area of higher solute concentration.

over-the-counter (OTC) medications Medications that may be purchased directly by a patient without a prescription.

oxygen A gas that all cells need to metabolize; the heart and brain, especially, cannot function without oxygen.

parasympathetic nervous system The part of the autonomic nervous system that relaxes the body.

parasympatholytics Drugs that block the actions of the parasympathetic nervous system; also known as anticholinergics.

parasympathomimetics Drugs that produce the same effects as those of the parasympathetic nervous system; also known as cholinergics.

Prep Kit continued...

parenteral Drug administration through any route other than through the gastrointestinal tract. Parenteral routes include intravenous, intramuscular, intraosseous, subcutaneous, transdermal, intrathecal, inhalation, intralingual, intradermal, and umbilical.

partial agonists Drugs that interact with a receptor to stimulate a response but inhibit other responses.

per os (PO) Through the mouth; a medication delivery route; same as oral.

per rectum (PR) Through the rectum; a medication delivery route.

pH The measure of acidity and alkalinity of a solution.

pharmacodynamics The study of drugs and their actions on living organisms.

pharmacokinetics The study of the metabolism and action of drugs with a particular emphasis on the time required for absorption, duration of action, distribution in the body, and method of excretion.

pharmacology The study of the properties and effects of medications.

polypharmacy The use of many drugs by the same patient.

potentiation Enhancement of the action of a drug by the administration of another drug.

prescription medications Medications that are distributed to patients only by pharmacists according to a physician's order.

side effects Any effects of a medication other than the desired ones.

solution A liquid mixture that cannot be separated by filtering or allowing the mixture to stand.

subcutaneous (SC) injection Injection into the tissue between the skin and muscle; a medication delivery route.

sublingual (SL) Under the tongue; a medication delivery route.

summation Increased effect that may occur when two drugs that have the same or similar action are given together.

suspension A mixture of ground particles that are distributed evenly throughout a liquid but do not dissolve.

sympathetic pathway (or nervous system) Part of the autonomic nervous system that is responsible for the body's response to shock and stress.

sympatholytics Drugs that block the actions of the sympathetic nervous system.

sympathomimetics Drugs that produce the same effects as the hormones of the sympathetic nervous system.

synergism Combined effect of two drugs that is greater than the sum of their individual effects.

teratogenic Poses a risk to the normal development or health of the unborn fetus.

therapeutic effect Beneficial action of a drug to correct a body dysfunction.

therapeutic index The difference between the minimum effective concentration and the toxic level of a drug.

therapeutic threshold The minimal concentration of a drug necessary to cause the desired response.

tolerance The capacity for enduring a large amount of a substance without an adverse effect and showing decreased sensitivity to subsequent doses of the same substance.

topical medications Lotions, creams, and ointments that are applied to the surface of the skin and affect only that area; a medication delivery route.

trade name The brand name that a manufacturer gives a medication; capitalized.

transcutaneous Through the skin; a medication delivery route.

transdermal medications Medications that are designed to be absorbed through the skin (transcutaneously).

umbilical Into the umbilical vein; a medication delivery route.

Points to Ponder

Mr. Reese is a diabetic. He is a carpenter by trade, and although he takes his insulin regularly, he "works" it off too quickly. This results in frequent calls to 9-1-1 when his blood glucose level falls too low.

Today, you arrive to find him conscious but confused. He is cool to the touch, yet sweaty and drooling. Your glucometer shows a blood glucose level of 36. You consider giving Mr. Reese oral glucose but recognize that his level of consciousness has fallen to a point that the medication might cause airway compromise. Your partner administers oxygen, and then applies the electrocardiographic monitor while you gain IV access. You administer 25 g of $D_{50}W$ per protocol. Within seconds, Mr. Reese is back to normal. He is alert and oriented to person, place, and time. You encourage him to go with you to the emergency department, and he finally agrees.

Issues: Increased Danger in Administering PO Medications in Patients With a Decreased Level of Consciousness, Understanding How to Use Different Medication Routes

Assessment in Action

You are called to the home of Mrs. Reynolds who complains of chest pain. She tells you the pain started while she was mopping her kitchen floor about 30 minutes ago. She describes the pain as a tightening in her chest, places it as an "8" on a 0 to 10 pain scale, and tells you that it seems to run down her left arm. She had a coronary artery bypass 2 years ago and frequently suffers angina.

In your ambulance, your partner assesses her vital signs and finds: BP, 164/108; HR, 92; and RR, 20. She is pale, cool, and diaphoretic. You administer oxygen at 15 L/min via nonrebreathing mask and initiate IV access. Her electrocardiogram reveals a sinus rhythm with occasional premature ventricular contractions. Per your protocol, you administer aspirin and nitroglycerin. After 3 doses of nitroglycerin, Mrs. Reynolds says the pain is still a "5." Her vital signs are now as follows: BP, 152/90 mm Hg; HR, 88 beats/min; and RR, 20 breaths/min. Medical control authorizes administration of morphine for the pain. As you prepare the morphine, your partner removes the naloxone from the shelf and places it within your reach. You administer the morphine as ordered. Mrs. Reynolds tells you her pain is gone. There is no need to administer the naloxone. She is transferred to the emergency department without any further changes in her condition.

1. Mrs. Reynolds received several medications. Which administration route did you not use in giving these medications?
   A. PO
   B. IV
   C. SL
   D. SC

2. Therapeutic uses for a particular medication are known as:
   A. indications.
   B. interactions.
   C. contraindications.
   D. actions.

3. You gave Mrs. Reynolds "Bayer" aspirin. This is a:
   A. generic name.
   B. chemical name.
   C. trade name.
   D. official name.

4. Your partner placed naloxone within your reach as you gave morphine. The reason for this is that naloxone is a narcotic:
   A. agonist.
   B. antagonist.
   C. contragonist.
   D. beta-blocker.

5. Mrs. Reynolds' vital signs must be monitored carefully because both nitroglycerin and morphine can lower the blood pressure. This is a _____ of the two drugs.
   A. side effect
   B. indication
   C. contraindication
   D. consideration

6. What is the most rapid route for delivering drugs in the prehospital environment?
   A. PO
   B. SC
   C. IV
   D. IM

Intravenous Access

1999 Objectives

Cognitive

1-4.7 Calculate intravenous infusion rates for adults, infants, and children. (p 312)
1-4.10 Discuss medical asepsis and the differences between clean and sterile techniques. (p 296)
1-4.11 Describe use of antiseptics and disinfectants. (p 296)
1-4.13 Describe the indications, equipment needed, techniques utilized, precautions, and general principles of peripheral venous cannulation. (p 298)
1-4.14 Describe the indications, equipment needed, techniques utilized, precautions, and general principles of intraosseous needle placement and infusion. (p 309)
1-4.22 Describe the purpose, equipment needed, techniques utilized, complications, and general principles for obtaining a blood sample. (p 304)
1-4.23 Describe disposal of contaminated items and sharps. (p 304)

Affective

1-4.27 Comply with universal precautions and body substance isolation (BSI). (p 296)
1-4.29 Serve as a model for medical asepsis. (p 304)
1-4.31 Serve as a model for disposing of contaminated items and sharps. (p 308)

Psychomotor

1-4.33 Demonstrate cannulation of peripheral veins. (p 305)
1-4.34 Demonstrate intraosseous needle placement and infusion. (p 309)
1-4.40 Demonstrate preparation and techniques for obtaining a blood sample. (p 304)
1-4.41 Perfect disposal of contaminated items and sharps. (p 308)

1985 Objectives

1.6.46 Describe which laboratory samples are drawn in the field when the IV is started and their usefulness. (p 304)
1.8.10 Discuss body fluids based on total body water, intracellular fluid, and extracellular fluid. (p 289)
1.8.11 Identify the significant anions and cations in the body. (p 287)
1.8.12 Describe the role of protein. (p 295)
1.8.13 Discuss osmosis. Define semi-permeable membranes, and discuss their function. (p 288)
1.8.14 Define isotonic fluids, hypotonic fluids, and hypertonic fluids. (p 289)
1.8.15 Define and discuss diffusion. (p 288)
1.8.16 Define active transport. (p 288)
1.8.17 Describe the mechanisms of concentration of electrolytes. (p 287)
1.8.32 Discuss fluid replacement, the types of fluid that are available, the benefits and detrimental effects of each. (p 293)
1.8.33 Discuss how fluid replacement is monitored and controlled. (p 297)
1.8.34 Discuss the routes of fluid replacement and the advantages and disadvantages of each. (p 300)
1.8.37 Demonstrate the proper technique to insert an intravenous catheter. (p 303)

7

Intravenous Access

You are the Provider

You and your partner are dispatched to a motor vehicle crash at the intersection of Highway 12 and Anvil Road. A few moments after you respond, the dispatcher informs you that a state trooper is on the scene. He confirms that one vehicle and one patient are involved. He further states that the vehicle has struck a tree and the man inside is awake and complaining of severe pain in both legs. Engine 11 was also dispatched simultaneously for a potential fire, spill, and/or vehicle extrication.

1. On the basis of the MOI and the chief complaint, what injuries do you suspect?
2. What should you do while you are en route to the scene?

Intravenous Access

Intravenous (IV) therapy is one of the most invasive procedures an EMT-I learns. During your career in EMS, few procedures will require more training or practice. Proficiency in IV therapy and technique is required for most procedures administered in advanced life support.

A medical problem of any type alters an individual's established balance among the systems of the body. This balance, called homeostasis, produces optimal physical performance. It is the job of health care providers to fully assess a patient's condition and to find and treat life-threatening injuries and illnesses that alter homeostasis. EMT-Is are often first on the scene and provide the first line of defense for individuals who need to have their homeostatic balance restored.

Basic Cell Physiology

A human cell can exist only in a special balanced environment. Understanding how this environment is created and maintained will give you the foundation you need to perform IV therapy.

Because the cell is completely enclosed by a cell membrane, compounds must move through the membrane to enter the cell. Small compounds such as water (H_2O), carbon dioxide (CO_2), hydrogen ions (H^+), and oxygen (O_2) can easily pass through the membrane. Larger charged compounds need assistance to cross the cell membrane and enter the cell.

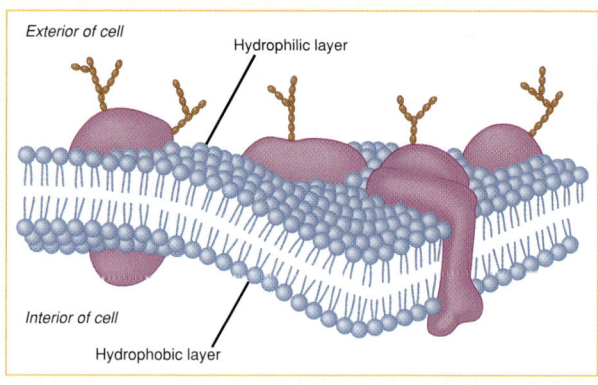

Figure 7-1 The phospholipid bilayer.

The cell membrane is a selective barrier. It chooses which compounds to allow across, depending on the needs of the cell. This selective permeability of the cell membrane is due to its composition Figure 7-1 ▲. The cell membrane is a phospholipid bilayer, that is, it has two parts:

- A hydrophilic outer layer made up of phosphate groups
- A hydrophobic inner layer made up of lipids or fatty acids

This bilayer is a very important barrier to fluid movement and the acid-base balance. Everything discussed in this text will in some way be related to the cell membrane barrier and movement across it.

Electrolytes

Atoms carry charges—some positive, some negative. Two or more atoms that bond together form a molecule. When atoms bond together, they share and disperse their charges throughout the molecule. Molecules containing carbon atoms—for example, table sugar ($C_6H_{12}O_6$)—are called organic molecules. Molecules created without carbon—for example, table salt (NaCl)—are called inorganic molecules. Inorganic molecules give rise to electrolytes when they disassociate in water into their charged components. For example, table salt disassociates into sodium (Na^+) and chloride (Cl^-).

Charged atoms and charged compounds are called electrolytes because of their ability to conduct electricity. Electrolytes, also called ions, are reactive and dangerous if left to circulate in the body, but the body uses the energy stored in these charged particles. Electrolytes help to regulate everything from water levels to cardiac

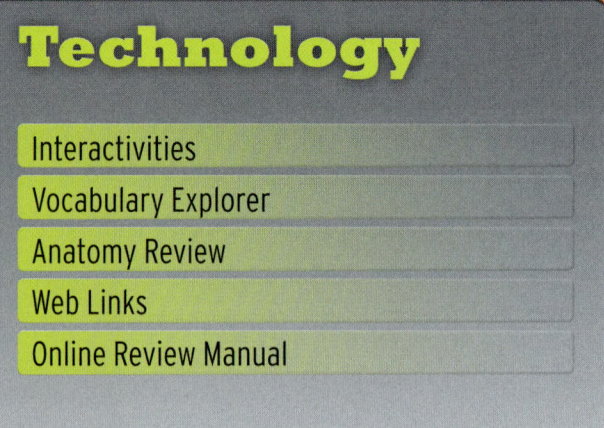

function and muscle contractions. Water in the body helps to stabilize the electrolyte charges so that the electrolytes can be used to perform the metabolic functions that are necessary to life.

Each electrolyte has a unique property or value to the body and is used in a different way. If the electrolyte has an overall positive charge, it is called a cation; an electrolyte with an overall negative charge is called an anion. The major cations of the body include sodium, potassium, and calcium; bicarbonate, chloride, and phosphorus are the major anions.

Sodium

Sodium (Na^+) is the principal extracellular cation needed to regulate the distribution of water throughout the body in the intravascular and interstitial fluid compartments, making it a major factor in adequate cellular perfusion. This gives rise to the saying, "Where sodium goes, water follows." Sodium is also a major component of the circulating buffer, sodium bicarbonate ($NaHCO_3$).

Potassium

About 98% of all the body's potassium (K^+) is found inside the cells of the body, making it the principal intracellular cation. Potassium plays a major role in neuromuscular function as well as in the conversion of glucose into glycogen. Cellular potassium levels are regulated by insulin. The sodium/potassium (Na^+/K^+) pump is helped by the presence of insulin and epinephrine. Low potassium levels—hypokalemia—in the serum (blood plasma) can lead to decreased skeletal muscle function, gastrointestinal (GI) disturbances, and alterations in cardiac function. High potassium levels in the serum—hyperkalemia—can lead to hyperstimulation of neural cell transmission, resulting in cardiac arrest.

Calcium

Calcium (Ca^{++}) is the principal cation needed for bone growth. It plays an important part in the functioning of heart muscle, nerves, and cell membranes and is necessary for proper blood clotting.

Low serum calcium levels—hypocalcemia—can lead to overstimulation of nerve cells, resulting in the following signs and symptoms:
- Skeletal muscle cramps
- Abdominal cramps
- Carpopedal spasms
- Hypotension
- Vasoconstriction

High serum calcium levels—hypercalcemia—can lead to decreased stimulation of nerve cells, resulting in the following signs and symptoms:
- Skeletal muscle weakness
- Lethargy
- Ataxia
- Vasodilation
- Hot, flushed skin

Bicarbonate

Bicarbonate (HCO_3^-) levels are the determining factor between acidosis and alkalosis in the body. Sodium bicarbonate is the primary buffer used in all circulating body fluids.

Chloride

Chloride (Cl^-) primarily regulates the pH of the stomach. It also regulates extracellular fluid levels.

Phosphorus

Phosphorus (P) is an important component in the formation of adenosine triphosphate (ATP), the powerful energy supplier of the body.

Fluid and Electrolyte Movement

Water and electrolytes move among the body's fluid compartments according to some basic chemical and biologic tenets. One of these governing principles is that unequal concentrations on different sides of a cell membrane will move to balance themselves equally on both sides of the membrane. Balance across a cell membrane has two components:
- Balance of compounds (water, electrolytes, etc) on either side of the cell membrane
- Balance of charges (the + or − charges carried on the atoms) on either side of the cell membrane

When concentrations of charges or compounds are greater on one side of the cell membrane than on the other, a gradient is created. The natural tendency for materials is to flow from an area of higher concentration to one of lower concentration. This movement establishes a concentration gradient. Gradients are categorized according to the type of material that flows down them; chemical compounds flow down chemical gradients; electrical currents flow down electrical gradients. The process of flowing down a gradient depends on whether the cell membrane will allow the material to pass through it. Certain compounds can travel freely across the cell membrane, a kinetically favorable situation that requires little energy, while others require active transport across the membrane, either because of the size of the compound or because of an incompatible charge.

Diffusion

Compounds or charges concentrated on one side of a cell membrane will move across it to an area of lower concentration to balance themselves across the membrane, a process called diffusion. To visualize this, imagine that too many people show up for a theater performance. The management decides to open another seating area to accommodate the crowd. Patrons (charges or compounds) are concentrated in the small seating area (the cell) outside the door (the cell membrane) leading to the new seating area. When the theater manager opens the door, patrons can move through (selective cell membrane permeability) from the congested seating area (down a concentration gradient). The patrons spread themselves out evenly (diffuse) throughout the total area, some choosing to stay behind in the original seating area as others move into the new area, so that they all have an equal amount of room.

Filtration

Filtration is another type of diffusion, commonly used by the kidneys to clean blood. Water carries dissolved compounds across the cell membranes of the tubules of the kidney. The tubule membrane traps these dissolved compounds but lets the water pass through in much the same way that a coffee filter traps the grounds as water passes through it. This cleans the blood of wastes and removes the trapped compounds from circulation so they can be flushed out of the body. The antidiuretic hormone (ADH) prevents the loss of water from the kidneys by causing its reabsorption into the tubules. ADH plays an important role in diabetes insipidus.

Active Transport

Often, the cell must maintain an imbalance of compounds across its membrane to achieve some metabolic purpose. An example of such an imbalance is the sodium/potassium pump. The cell uses sodium outside the cell and potassium inside the cell for an important cellular function called depolarization. To maintain this imbalance, the cell must use energy in the form of ATP and actively transport compounds across its membrane. Even though active transport demands a high-energy expenditure, the benefits outweigh the initial utilization of ATP. Pumping sodium out of the cell and potassium into the cell has the added benefit of moving glucose into the cell at the same time.

Osmosis

Osmosis is the diffusion of water across a cell membrane. When molecules of solute are added to a solution, an equal number of molecules of solvent are displaced from the solution. For example, if 10 sodium ions are added to the fluid surrounding the cell, 10 molecules of water are displaced from that fluid. Therefore, the fluid surrounding the cell contains 10 fewer water molecules relative to the fluid within the cell. Water will diffuse down its concentration gradient to balance itself across the cell membrane. In this example, 5 water molecules will diffuse out of the cell into the surrounding fluid. Increasing the concentration of sodium in the surrounding (extracellular) fluid decreases the concentration of water in that fluid. Water diffuses out of the cell to create a balance of water molecules and to dilute the increased concentrations of sodium. Remember, where sodium goes, water follows.

The diffusion of water adds additional molecules to the extracellular compartment to create a balanced solution. This increased, yet balanced, volume puts pressure against the cell wall, called osmotic pressure. Osmotic pressure drives several important metabolic functions in the body, including cellular perfusion.

The effects of osmotic pressure on a cell are referred to as the tonicity of the solution Figure 7-2 ▼. Tonicity is related to the concentration of sodium in a solution and the movement of water in relation to the sodium levels inside and outside the cell:

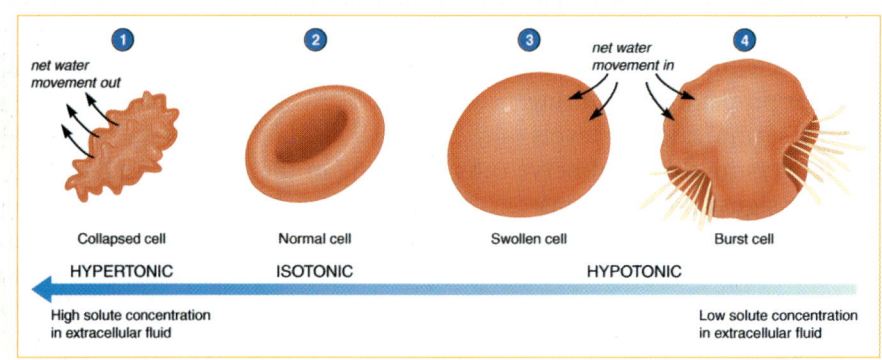

Figure 7-2 Tonicity.

- An <u>isotonic solution</u> has the same concentration of sodium as does the cell. In this case, water doesn't shift, and no change in cell shape occurs.
- A <u>hypertonic solution</u> has a greater concentration of sodium than does the cell. Water is drawn out of the cell, and the cell collapses from the increased extracellular osmotic pressure.
- A <u>hypotonic solution</u> has a lower concentration of sodium than does the cell. Water flows into the cell, causing it to swell and possibly burst from the increased intracellular osmotic pressure.

IV fluids introduced into the circulatory system can affect the tonicity of the extracellular fluid, resulting in dire consequences unless care is used.

> **EMT-I Tips**
>
> In osmosis, water diffuses across the cell membrane to reach a balance of equal concentration of water on either side of the cell membrane.

Fluid Compartments

The body stores water in various locations called fluid compartments. The fluid compartments are defined by their relationship to cells—the water is either inside the cell (intracellular) or outside the cell (extracellular). Although water levels in these compartments constantly shift, homeostatic control mechanisms ensure that balance is restored whenever water is lost.

The body's circulatory (vascular) system functions as a fluid highway, but it also contains cells. Thus, it can be thought of as another fluid compartment. Blood cells contain intracellular water and are surrounded by extracellular water. To differentiate between these two cellular areas, the extracellular compartment is broken down into:

- *Intravascular:* The water portion of the circulatory system surrounding the blood cells (for example in the heart, arteries, or veins)
- *Interstitial:* Water outside the vascular system and between surrounding cells (for example, between the membranes of two cells in muscle tissue)

In summary, there are three fluid compartments in the human body: intravascular (extracellular), interstitial (extracellular), and intracellular 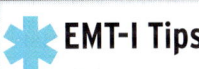. The fluids within these compartments account for 60% of total body weight.

Intracellular fluid (ICF) accounts for 40% of total body weight, or 75% of all fluid weight. ICF is within all the cells of the body. Large proteins within the cell can draw fluid into the cell because their overall negative charge attracts positively charged atoms like potassium, sodium, and the positive end of the water molecule (H_2O). The cell membrane prevents too many positively charged compounds, including water, from entering the cell and causing it to rupture. The sodium ions drawn into the cell are quickly removed via the sodium/potassium pump to prevent cellular <u>lysis</u>.

Extracellular fluid (ECF) occupies any area that is not inside the cells and equals 20% of the total body weight, or 25% of all fluid weight. ECF compartments act as conduits for transferring gases and nutrients between the vascular and ICF compartments. ECF is found in the interstitial and intravascular compartments. ECF levels in the intravascular and interstitial compartments are regulated by the presence of sodium. Interstitial fluid accounts for 16% of total body weight and occupies the microscopic spaces between the cells. Interstitial fluid consists of a gel-type protein that helps disperse the water evenly throughout the interstitial compartment. This protein gel helps move water freely between the cells and vasculature. Intravascular fluid is also called plasma and accounts for 4% of total body weight. Perfusion occurs in the capillaries as a result of high hydrostatic pressures and osmosis in the <u>capillary beds</u>. The high arterial capillary pressures (hydrostatic pressures) placed on the capillary beds push fluids from the vascular compartment into the interstitial compartment.

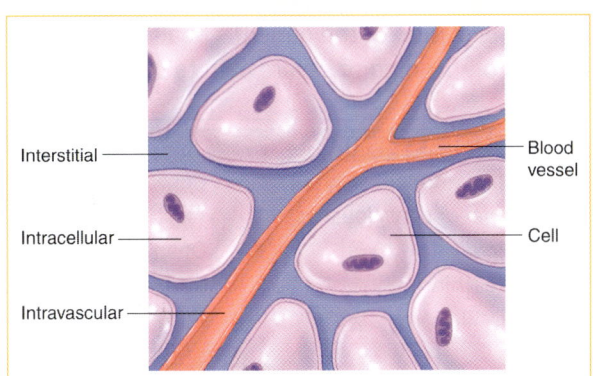

Figure 7-3 The three fluid compartments in the body.

TABLE 7-1	Daily Fluid Balances			
Fluid Gains	Daily Intake, mL		Fluid Losses	Daily Output, mL
Actual fluid intake	500-1,700		Water vapor	850-1,200
Fluid from solid food	800-1,000		Urine	600-1,600
Metabolism	200-300		Feces	50-200
Totals	1,500-3,000		Totals	1,500-3,000

Dissolved oxygen and nutrients are carried along with the fluids. The resulting shift of fluids from the vascular system creates a high concentration of blood proteins in the venous side of the capillary, which pulls fluid back into the capillary circulation via osmosis.

Fluid Balance

Several factors influence the balance between ICF and ECF. The balance among intracellular, intravascular, and interstitial compartments is dynamic. Changes always occur, and the body adjusts to these changes by retaining or eliminating water. Fluid levels in the body are balanced when intakes equal outputs. Daily intakes of water include fluid from liquid, food, and cellular metabolism; daily outputs occur from respiration and excretion of urine and feces. Table 7-1 demonstrates how fluid levels are controlled in the body. Amounts shown are estimates for fluid intake versus fluid output.

The interstitial compartment is unique because it acts as the buffer between the other compartments. As fluid levels fluctuate between the intravascular and intracellular compartments, the interstitial compartment first responds by shifting fluid reserves between the two compartments Figure 7-4. One clinical manifestation of a fluid imbalance is edema, which is defined as increased interstitial fluid levels.

Causes of edema include:

- Increased arterial capillary pressures that push fluid out into the tissues (heart failure and/or unmonitored IV lines are possible causes)

You are the Provider   Part 2

At the scene, a police officer directs you to an area off of the road where you note skid marks that leave the pavement. The vehicle, a 4-door sedan, has struck a large tree. Your partner provides inline stabilization of the patient's head as you perform an initial assessment. The patient, a 40-year-old man, is complaining of severe pain to both of his legs.

Initial Assessment	Recording Time: Zero Minutes
Appearance	Conscious, in severe pain
Level of consciousness	Alert to person and place, but not to time or event
Airway	Open and clear
Breathing	Respirations, increased; adequate depth
Circulation	Radial pulses, increased and weak; skin, cool and clammy; no gross bleeding

3. What is your impression of the initial assessment findings?
4. What does the presence of skid marks tell you about the patient?

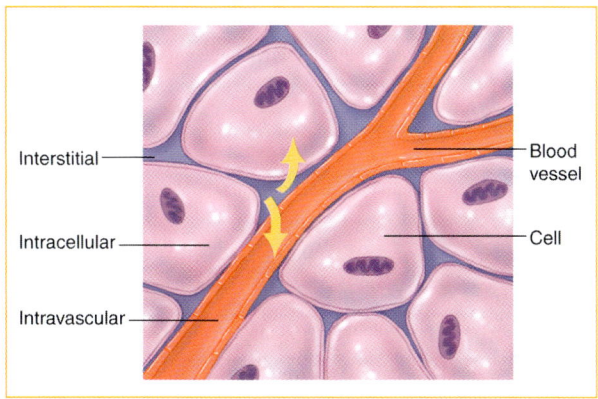

Figure 7-4 The interstitial compartment shifts fluid reserves.

- Decreased production of circulating blood proteins created in the liver, as seen with advanced liver diseases and severe burns
- Increased capillary permeability associated with capillary-dilating compounds, such as histamines released during allergic reactions

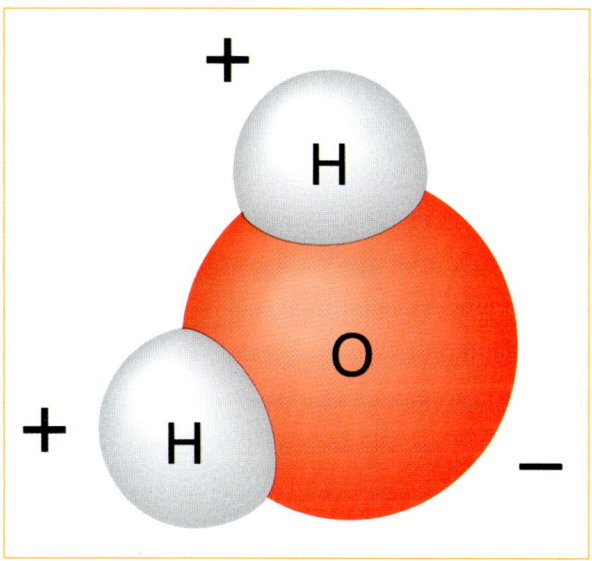

Figure 7-5 Water is a polar molecule with two positive poles and one negative pole.

Principles of Fluid Balance

The role of water in the body is diverse; it plays a part both in cellular metabolism and in the maintenance of homeostasis. Without the presence of water in the body, people would quickly succumb to illness and disease, cellular function would cease, and body systems would shut down.

The role water plays in helping to maintain homeostasis is related to the size of the water molecule itself. Composed of only three atoms (two hydrogens and one oxygen) water has some unique properties (Figure 7-5 ▶). Water is a polar molecule; that is, it has two positive poles (hydrogen) and a negative pole (oxygen). This property means that water can surround charged particles and stabilize their charges, allowing the particles to remain in solution. Water can also move across cell membranes easily, because it is a relatively small molecule.

Internal Environment of the Cell

The environment of the cells is one of water; some form of water surrounds all cells. Cells survive as long as this environment remains stable and is compatible for the life of the cell; any alteration in the supply of water, nutrients, oxygen, or food can lead to cellular death. Water exists both inside and outside the cell.

Homeostasis

Maintenance of the internal environment of the cell is regulated by elaborate systems of checks and balances. As systems in the body become imbalanced and begin to shift, feedback systems create an appropriate response to return the internal environment to normal. This normally balanced condition is referred to as homeostasis, or the resistance to change. These checks and balances can be seen in the way that the body regulates blood glucose: too little circulating blood glucose and the feedback system responds to create glucose; too much circulating blood glucose and the feedback system responds to store the excess glucose. When disturbances in homeostasis occur as a result of water shifting within the body, certain conditions develop related to the type of shifting that occurs.

Dehydration

Dehydration is defined as depletion of the body's total systemic fluid volume (Figure 7-6 ▶). Dehydration is usually a chronic condition of the elderly or the very young and may take days to manifest. As fluid is lost from the vascular compartment, the body reacts by shifting interstitial fluid into the vascular area. This then forces a shift of fluid from the intracellular to the

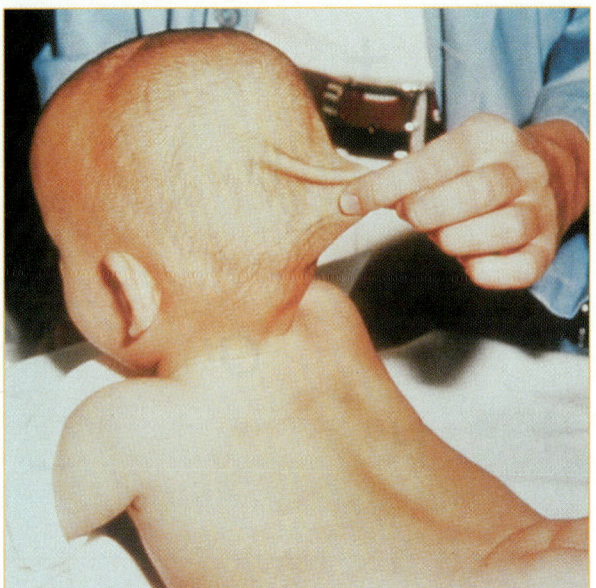

Figure 7-6 Dehydration.

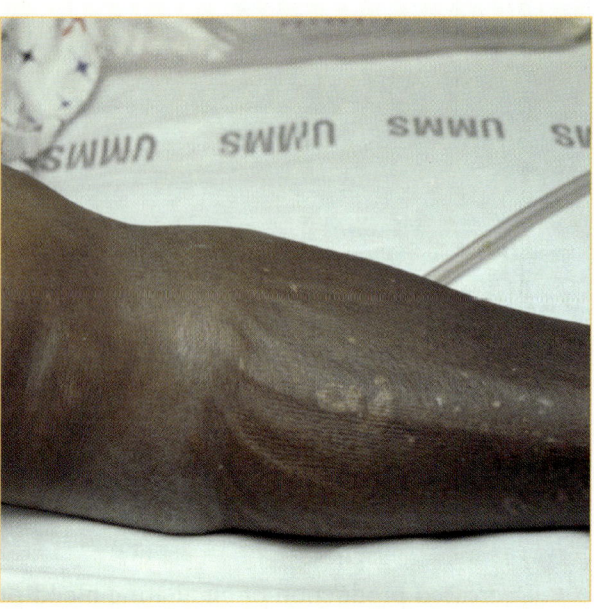

Figure 7-7 In an overhydrated patient, fluid backup occurs.

extracellular compartments. A total systemic fluid deficit occurs.

Signs and symptoms of dehydration include:
- Decreased level of consciousness (LOC)
- Postural hypotension
- Tachypnea
- Dry mucous membranes
- Tachycardia
- Poor skin turgor
- Flushed, dry skin

Causes of dehydration include:
- Diarrhea
- Vomiting
- GI drainage
- Hemorrhage
- Insufficient fluid/food intake

Overhydration

When the body's total systemic fluid volume increases, overhydration occurs. Fluid fills the vascular compartment, filters into the interstitial compartment, and finally is forced from the engorged interstitial compartment into the intracellular compartment. Fluid backup occurs, and the patient can succumb from these increased fluid levels Figure 7-7 ▶.

Signs and symptoms of overhydration include:
- Shortness of breath
- Puffy eyelids
- Edema
- Polyuria
- Moist crackles (rales)
- Acute weight gain

Causes of overhydration include:
- Unmonitored IVs
- Kidney failure
- Prolonged hypoventilation

Body Fluid Composition

The fluids found in the body are composed of dissolved elements and water, a combination known as a solution. A solution is a mixture of two things:
- *Solvent*: The fluid that does the dissolving, or the solution that contains the dissolved components (in the body, the solvent is water)
- *Solute*: The dissolved particles contained in the solvent

A good example of making a solution is the process of brewing a cup of coffee. Passing hot water (solvent) over the coffee grounds leaches out the oils (the solute) to create the solution known as coffee. Remember, as the solute concentration increases, the solvent concentration decreases. Is a strong cup of coffee created by using less water (solvent) or by adding more coffee (solute)? Either one could be true, as they both end up creating stronger coffee.

IV Fluid Composition

IV solutions are tools designed to facilitate patient treatment. The use of IV fluids can significantly alter the patient's condition. It is critical that each bag of IV solution is sterile and safe; therefore, each bag of IV solution is individually sterilized Figure 7-8. Compounds and ions dissolved in the solution are identical to the ones found in the body. Each solution is a concentration of solute and solvent.

Because sodium is the primary extracellular cation and regulates water levels in the body, it is used as the benchmark to calculate a solution's tonicity. The concentration of sodium in the cells of the body is approximately 0.9%. Altering the concentration of sodium in the IV solution can move the water into or out of any fluid compartment in the body. Remember, where sodium goes, water follows.

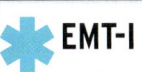

EMT-I Tips

Remember, *cations* have a positive charge and *anions* have a negative charge.

Types of IV Solutions

There are five basic types of IV solutions, each with a different tonicity and dissolved components. The five basic types are isotonic, hypotonic, hypertonic, crystalloid, and colloid. IV fluids use combinations of these five types of solutions to create the desired effects inside the body.

Isotonic Solutions

Isotonic solutions such as normal saline (0.9% sodium chloride), possess close to the same osmolarity as serum and other body fluids. Because there is no alteration of serum osmolarity, the fluid stays inside the intravascular compartment. Isotonic solutions expand the contents of the intravascular compartment without shifting fluid to or from other compartments. Awareness of this fact is useful when dealing with hypotensive or hypovolemic patients. Because this fluid remains in the vascular compartment, you must be careful to avoid fluid overloading. Patients with *hypertension* and *congestive heart failure* are at greatest risk of fluid overload. The extra fluid increases the workload of the heart, creating fluid backup in the lungs. Lactated Ringer's (LR) solution is generally used in the field for patients who have lost large amounts of blood. It contains the buffering compound lactate, which is metabolized in the liver to form bicarbonate—the key buffer that combats the intracellular acidosis associated with severe blood loss. LR solution should not be given to patients with liver problems because they cannot metabolize the lactate.

D_5W, 5% dextrose in water, is a special type of isotonic solution. As long as it remains in the bag, it is considered an isotonic solution. Once it is administered, the dextrose is quickly metabolized, and the solution becomes hypotonic.

Hypotonic Solutions

A hypotonic fluid has an osmolarity less than that of serum, which means the fluid has less sodium ion concentration than serum. When this fluid is placed in the vascular compartment, it begins diluting the serum. Soon the serum osmolarity is less than the interstitial

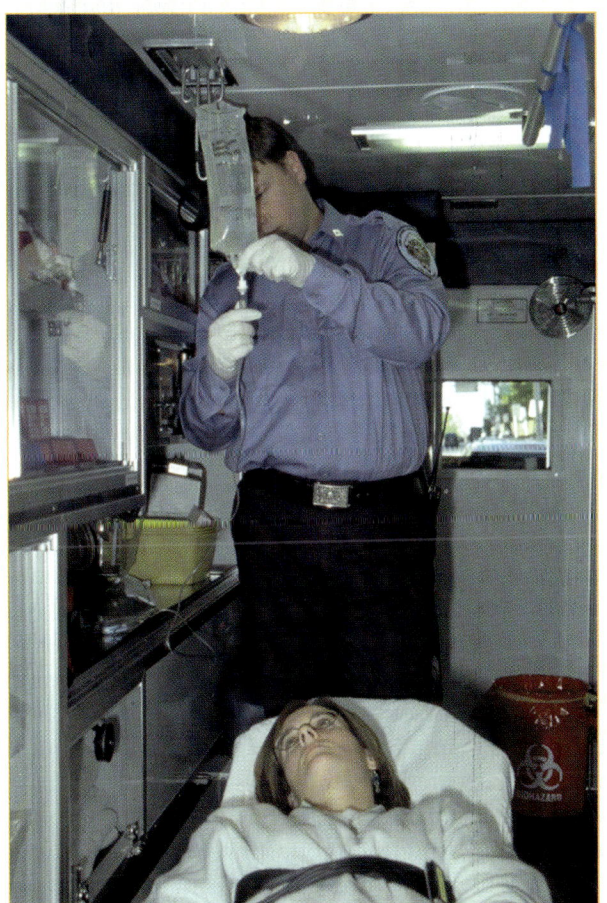

Figure 7-8 It is imperative that each bag of IV solution be sterile and safe.

fluid; water is pulled from the vascular compartment into the interstitial fluid compartment and eventually the same process is repeated, pulling water from the interstitial compartment into the cells.

Hypotonic solutions hydrate the cells while depleting the vascular compartment. These solutions may be needed for a patient on dialysis when diuretic therapy dehydrates the cells. They may also be used for hyperglycemic conditions such as diabetic ketoacidosis, in which high serum glucose levels draw fluid out of the cells and into the vascular and interstitial compartments. Hypotonic solutions can be dangerous to use because they can cause a sudden fluid shift from the intravascular space to the cells, causing cardiovascular collapse and increased intracranial pressure (ICP) from shifting fluid into the brain cells. For example, giving D_5W for an extended period can cause increased ICP. This makes hypotonic solutions dangerous to use with patients experiencing a stroke or any head trauma. Using hypotonic solutions on patients with burns, trauma, malnutrition, or liver disease is also hazardous, because these patients are at risk for developing third spacing, an abnormal fluid shift into the serous linings of the body.

EMT-I Tips

Examples of the various types of IV solutions include:
Isotonic: 0.9% sodium chloride (normal saline), lactated Ringer's
Hypotonic: 5% dextrose in water D_5W
Hypertonic: 9.0% saline, D_5W (when introduced into the body), blood products, and albumin

Hypertonic Solutions

A hypertonic solution has an osmolarity higher than serum, which means the solution has more ionic concentration than serum and pulls fluid and electrolytes from the intracellular and interstitial compartments into the intravascular compartment. Hypertonic solutions shift body fluids into the vascular spaces and help stabilize blood pressure, increase urine output, and reduce edema. These fluids are rarely, if ever, used in the prehospital setting. Often, the term hypertonic refers to solutions that contain high concentrations of proteins. They have the same effect on fluid as sodium. Careful monitoring is needed to guard against fluid overloading when using hypertonic fluids, especially with patients who suffer from impaired heart or kidney function. Also, hypertonic solutions should not be given to patients with diabetic ketoacidosis or others at risk of cellular dehydration. Hypertonic solutions have been studied in the treatment of patients experiencing hemorrhaging to help restore blood pressure while minimizing fluid overloading. Fluid movement across a cell membrane resulting from hypertonic, isotonic, and hypotonic solutions is shown in 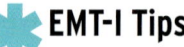 Figure 7-9.

Terminology Tips

When deciding on a type of IV fluid, use the prefixes to help make the decision:
- *iso* means equal
- *hypo* means low
- *hyper* means high

We are comparing the osmolarity of the fluid to the patient's blood. An *isotonic* solution will remain in the vascular space, a *hypotonic* solution will quickly leave the vascular space, and a *hypertonic* solution will draw fluid into the vascular space.

Crystalloid Solutions

Crystalloid solutions are dissolved crystals (for example, salts or sugars) in water. They contain compounds that quickly disassociate in solution. The ability of these fluids to cross membranes and alter the various fluid levels makes them the best choice for the prehospital care of injured patients who need fluid replacement for body fluid loss. When using an isotonic crystalloid for fluid replacement to support blood pressure from blood loss, remember the 3 to 1 replacement rule: *3 mL of isotonic crystalloid solution is needed to replace 1 mL of patient blood.* This amount is needed because approximately two thirds of the infused isotonic crystalloid solution will leave the vascular spaces in about 1 hour.

When replacing lost volume, it is imperative to remember that crystalloid solutions do not have the capability of carrying oxygen. Boluses of 20 mL/kg should be given to maintain perfusion (radial pulses), but not to raise blood pressure. Increasing blood pressure with IV solutions not only dilutes remaining blood volume, thereby decreasing the proportion of hemoglobin, but also may increase internal bleeding by interfering with hemostasis—the body's internal blood-clotting mechanism.

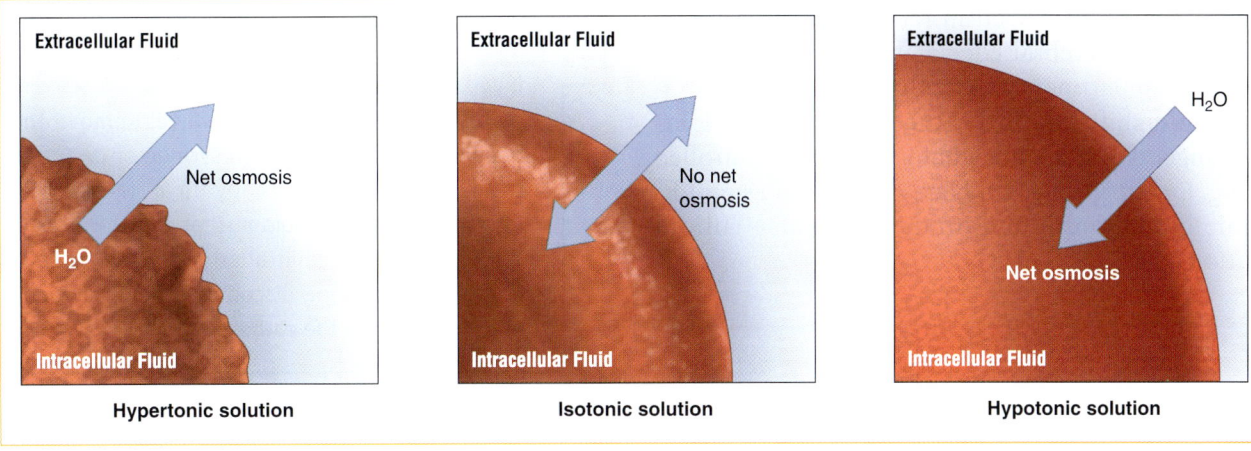

Figure 7-9 Fluid movement with hypertonic, isotonic, and hypotonic solutions.

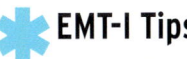 **EMT-I Tips**

Standard IV solutions replace volume, but do not have the capacity to carry oxygen. Replace lost volume to maintain perfusion, but recognize the need for rapid transport.

Colloid Solutions

Colloid solutions contain molecules (usually proteins) that are too large to pass out of the capillary membranes and therefore remain in the vascular compartment. The very large protein molecules give colloid solutions a very high osmolarity. As a result, they draw fluid from the interstitial and intracellular

You are the Provider   Part 3

You apply 100% oxygen via nonrebreathing mask and rapidly extricate the patient from his car. Next, you perform a rapid trauma assessment, during which you note deformity to both of the patient's femurs. The patient is fully immobilized and placed into the ambulance. As your partner obtains vital signs, you prepare to initiate an IV.

Vital Signs	Recording Time: 7 Minutes After Patient Contact
Respirations	28 breaths/min, adequate depth
Pulse	120 beats/min, weak and regular
Blood pressure	90/60 mm Hg
SaO_2	97% (on supplemental oxygen)

5. What size IV catheter should you use?
6. What type of IV tubing is appropriate for this patient?

compartments into the vascular compartments. Colloid solutions work very well in reducing edema (as in pulmonary or cerebral edema) while expanding the vascular compartment. These fluids could cause dramatic fluid shifts and place the patient in considerable danger if they are not administered in a controlled setting. Examples of colloids are albumin and steroids. Whole blood and blood products are also colloid solutions.

IV Techniques and Administration

The most important point to remember about IV techniques and fluid administration is to keep the IV equipment sterile. Forethought will help prevent mental and procedural errors while starting the IV.

One way to ensure proper technique is to develop a routine to follow as you assemble the appropriate equipment. A routine will help you keep track of your equipment and the steps necessary to complete a successful IV.

Assembling Your Equipment

To avoid delays or the possibility of IV site contamination, gather and prepare all your equipment before you attempt to start an IV. Sometimes the condition and presentation of the patient make full preparation difficult.

> **In the Field**
>
> If you have trouble getting a catheter to feed completely, it may be against a valve. Remove the needle and attach the flush syringe or IV line to the hub of the catheter. Gently "float" the catheter into the vein as the fluid pushes the valve open. Watch carefully for infiltration around the site and if swelling is present, discontinue the IV immediately and remove the catheter.

This is where working as a team becomes critical. It is often the members of your own crew who, by anticipating your needs, help make the IV equipment assembly possible. Table 7-2 shows a logical sequence of steps in assembling your equipment; each will be described in this chapter.

> **In the Field**
>
> **Helpful IV Hints**
> - Allow the hand or arm to hang off the stretcher.
> - Pat or rub the area.
> - Apply chemical hot packs.
> - If you meet resistance from a valve, elevate the extremity.
> - After 2 misses, let your partner try.
> - Try sticking without the tourniquet if the vein keeps infiltrating.
> - Never pull the catheter back over or through the needle.
> - The more IVs you perform, the more proficient you become.

TABLE 7-2	Steps in Assembling IV Equipment

1. Always wear gloves! BSI precautions cannot be emphasized strongly enough.
2. Choose a solution. Check the solution for clarity and the expiration date and to ensure it is the correct one.
3. Choose an administration set appropriate for the needs of the patient.
4. Choose an appropriate IV site.
5. Choose an appropriately sized catheter.
6. Recheck your work before you go any further.
7. Tear tape for securing the IV site.
8. Have blood tubes close by.
9. Set up the Luer adapter and the Vacutainer barrel, or have a syringe close by for drawing blood, if indicated.
10. Have a couple of catheters ready for insertion.
11. Open an alcohol wipe.
12. Have 4" x 4" pieces of gauze ready for catching blood.
13. Then, and only then, apply a constricting band. (It is the last thing done before inserting the IV.)
14. Insert the catheter and draw blood, if indicated.
15. Hook up the IV tubing and adjust the flow.
16. Secure the site and the blood tubes.
17. Administer medication if necessary.
18. Adequately dispose of sharps.
19. Document every procedure.

Choosing an IV Solution

Prehospital patient care and IV therapy center on identifying the type of situation and the needs of the patient. Ask yourself:

- Is the patient critical?
- Is the patient stable?
- Does the patient need fluid replacement?

In the prehospital setting, the choice of IV solution is limited to the isotonic crystalloids normal saline and lactated Ringer's solution. D_5W (5% dextrose in water) is often reserved for administering medication because the presence of dextrose has the potential to alter fluid and electrolyte levels in the body.

Each IV solution bag is wrapped in a protective sterile plastic bag and is guaranteed to remain sterile until the posted expiration date. Once the protective wrap is torn and removed, the IV solution has a shelf-life of 24 hours. The bottom of each IV bag has two ports: an injection port for medication and an access port for connecting the administration set. A removable pigtail that represents a point-of-no-return line protects the sterile access port. Once this pigtail is removed, the bag must be used immediately or discarded.

IV solution bags come in different fluid volumes Figure 7-10 ▼. Volumes commonly used in hospitals are 1,000 mL, 500 mL, 250 mL, and 100 mL; the more common prehospital volumes are 1,000 mL and 500 mL. The smaller volumes (250 mL and 100 mL) more commonly contain D_5W and are used for mixing

In the Field

Whether the patient is a trauma patient or medical patient has nothing to do with the amount of fluid that needs to be administered. Instead, consider how much fluid the patient has lost. Any patient who has lost a significant amount of fluid needs rapid replacement with large-bore IV catheters. This applies to a medical patient with gastrointestinal bleeding as well as a trauma patient with an unstable pelvis and bilateral femur fractures.

and administering medication via IV "piggyback" administration.

Choosing an Administration Set

An administration set moves fluid from the IV bag into the patient's vascular system. As with IV solution bags, IV administration sets are sterile as long as they remain in their protective packaging. Once they are removed from the packaging, their sterility cannot be guaranteed. Each IV administration set has a piercing spike protected by a plastic cover. Again, once the piercing spike is exposed and the seal surrounding the cap is broken, the set must be used immediately or discarded.

There are different sizes of administration sets for different situations and patients. Most drip sets have a number visible on the package Figure 7-11 ▼, which

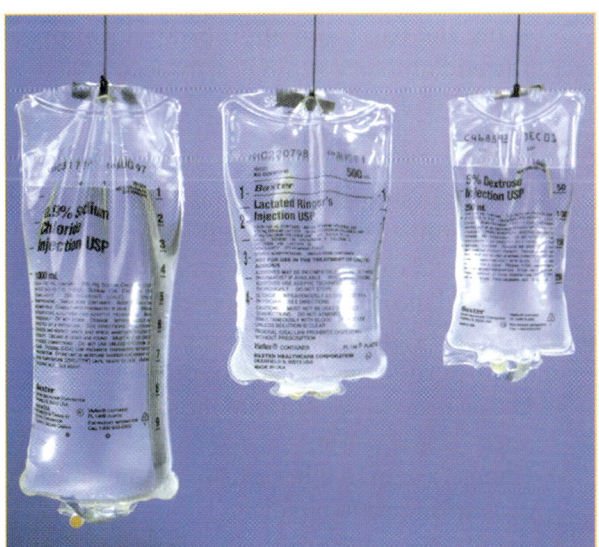

Figure 7-10 IV solution bags come in different fluid volumes.

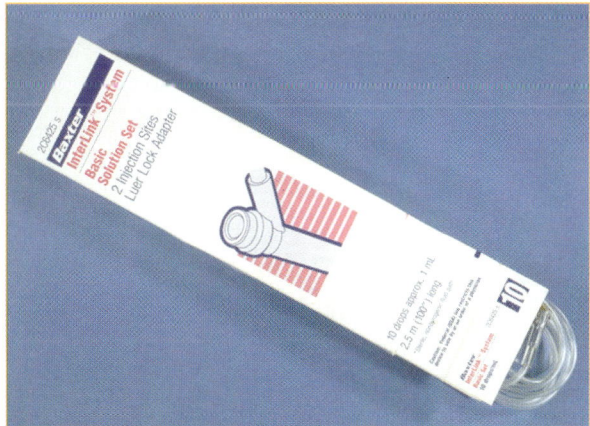

Figure 7-11 The number visible on the drip set refers to the number of drops it takes for a milliliter of fluid to pass through the orifice and into the drip chamber.

indicates the number of drops it takes for a milliliter of fluid to pass through the orifice and into the drip chamber. Drip sets come in two primary sizes: microdrip and macrodrip. Microdrip sets allow 60 gtt (drops)/mL through the small, needlelike orifice inside the drip chamber. Microdrips are ideal for medication administration or pediatric fluid delivery because it is easy to control their fluid flow. Macrodrip sets allow 10 to 15 gtt/mL through a large opening between the piercing spike and the drip chamber. Macrodrip sets are best used for rapid fluid replacement.

> **A to Z Terminology Tips**
>
> To differentiate between macrodrip and microdrip sets, remember that the prefixes refer to the size of the drops, not the size of the tubing.
>
> **Macro** means *large*. A 10 gtt set, which is a macrodrip set, has 10 drops that equal 1 mL of fluid.
> **Micro** means *small*. A 60 gtt set, which is a microdrip set, has 60 drops that equal 1 mL of fluid.

A blood set is a special type of macrodrip set designed to facilitate rapid fluid replacement by manual infusion of either multiple IV bags or IV/blood replacement combinations. Most blood sets have dual piercing spikes that allow two bags of fluid to be hung at once on the same patient (Figure 7-12 ▼). The central drip chamber has a special filter designed to filter the blood during transfusions.

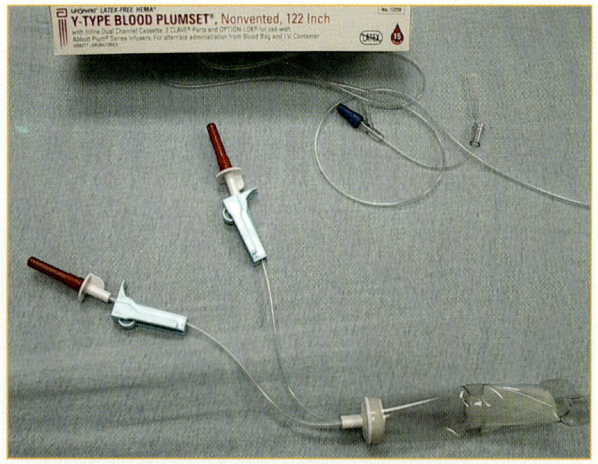

Figure 7-12 Most blood sets have dual piercing spikes that allow two bags of fluid to be hung at once on the same patient.

Preparing an Administration Set

After choosing the IV administration set and the IV solution bag, verify the expiration date of the solution and check for solution clarity. Prepare to spike the bag with the administration set. The steps for this procedure are indicated in (Skill Drill 7-1 ▶) as follows:

1. **Remove the rubber pigtail found on the end of the IV bag** by pulling on it. The bag is still sealed and will not leak until the IV punctures this port.
   Remove the protective cover from the piercing spike. (Remember, this spike is sterile!) (**Step 1**).
2. **Slide the spike into the IV bag port** until you see fluid enter the drip chamber (**Step 2**).
3. **Allow the solution to run freely through the drip chamber** and into the tubing to prime the line and flush the air out of the tubing (**Step 3**).
4. **Twist the protective cover on the opposite end of the IV tubing to allow air to escape.** Do not remove this cover yet, because the cover keeps the tubing end sterile until it is needed. Let the fluid flow until air bubbles are removed from the line before turning the roller clamp wheel to stop the flow (**Step 4**).
5. **Next, go back and check the drip chamber; it should be only half filled.** The fluid level must be visible to calculate drip rates. If the fluid level is too low, squeeze the chamber until it fills; if the chamber is too full, invert the bag and the chamber and squeeze the chamber to empty the fluid back into the bag (**Step 5**).
   Hang the bag in an appropriate location with the end of the IV tubing easily accessible.

Choosing an IV Site

It is important to select the most appropriate vein for IV catheter insertion. Avoid areas of the vein that contain valves because a catheter will not pass through these areas easily and the needle may cause damage. Valves can be recognized as small bumps located in the vein. Use the following criteria to select a vein:

- Locate the vein section with the straightest appearance (Figure 7-13 ▶).
- Choose a vein that has a firm, round appearance or is springy when palpated.
- Avoid areas where the vein crosses over joints.
- Avoid edematous extremities, or any extremity with a dialysis fistula or history of a mastectomy.

Chapter 7 Intravenous Access

Skill Drill 7-1: Spiking the Bag

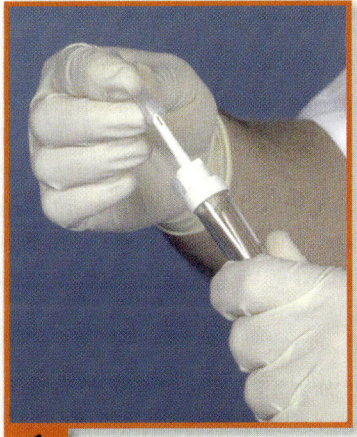

1 Pull on the rubber pigtail on the end of the IV bag to remove it.
Remove the protective cover from the piercing spike.

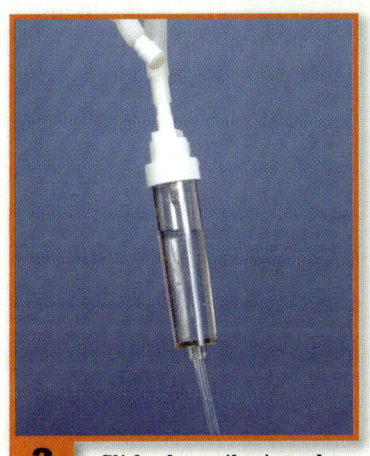

2 Slide the spike into the IV bag port until you see fluid enter the drip chamber.

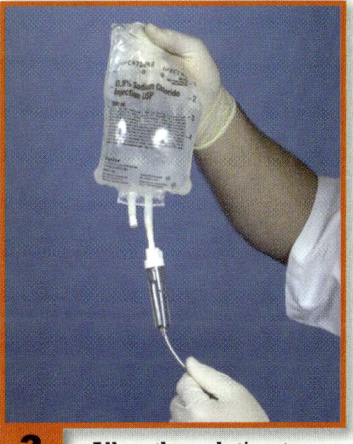

3 Allow the solution to run freely through the drip chamber and into the tubing to prime the line and flush the air out of the tubing.

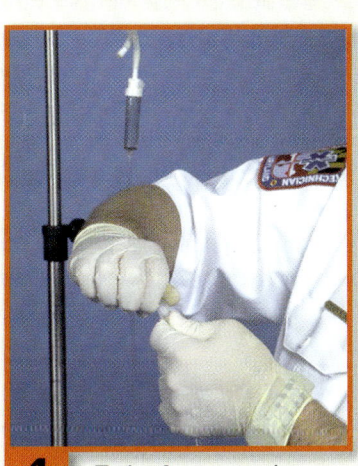

4 Twist the protective cover on the opposite end of the IV tubing to allow air to escape. Do not remove this cover yet. Let the fluid flow until air bubbles are removed from the line before turning the roller clamp wheel to stop the flow.

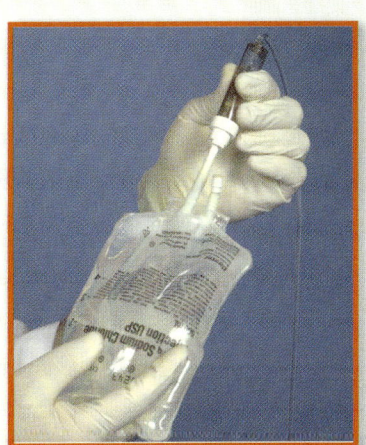

5 Check the drip chamber; it should be only half filled. If the fluid level is too low, squeeze the chamber until it fills; if the chamber is too full, invert the bag and the chamber and squeeze the chamber to empty the fluid back into the bag.
Hang the bag in an appropriate location.

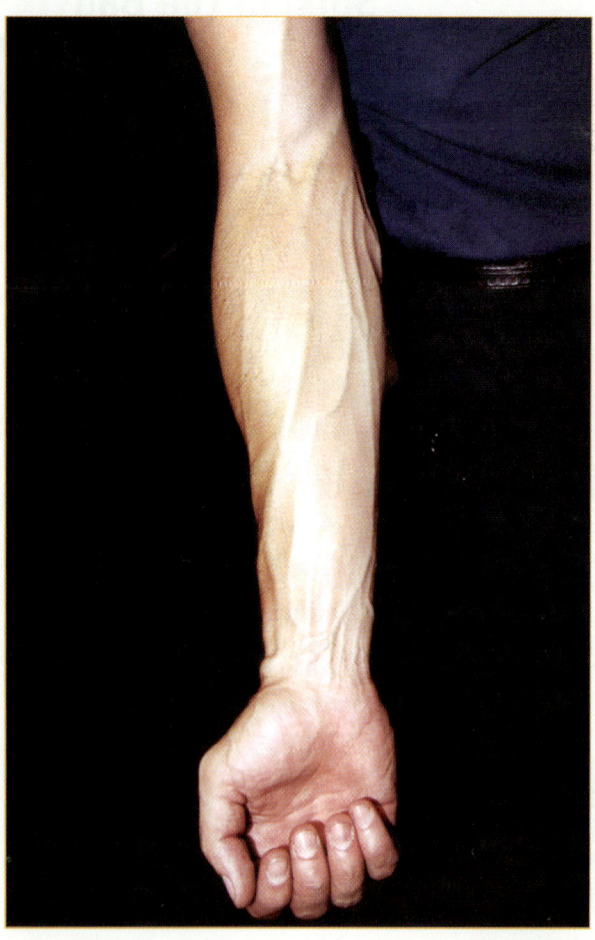

Figure 7-13 Look for veins that are relatively straight and spring back when palpated.

If the IV treatment is for a life-threatening illness or injury, choice is often limited to the areas that remain open during hypoperfusion. Otherwise, limit IV access to the more distal areas of the extremities. An important concept to remember is *Choose distally, work medially*. First, select areas that are as distal as possible. If the distal site ruptures, or infiltrates, you can move up the extremity to the next appropriate site. Because the failed cannulation creates a possibility of leakage into the surrounding tissues, any fluid introduced immediately below an open wound has the potential to enter the tissue and possibly cause damage.

Large protruding arm veins can be deceiving in terms of their ease of cannulation. Often these bulging veins can roll and infiltrate, which means they will move from side to side during cannulation, causing you to miss the vein. A remedy is to apply manual traction to the vein to lock it into position. Traction techniques differ depending on the location chosen for cannulation. Hold hand veins in place by pulling the skin over the vein taut with the thumb of your free hand as you flex the patient's hand (Figure 7-14 ▶). Stabilize wrist veins by flexing the wrist and pulling the skin taut over the vein. Applying lateral traction to the vein with your free hand can stabilize veins in the forearm and antecubital areas.

The patient's opinion should also be considered when selecting an IV site, because he or she may know an IV location that has worked in the past. Avoid attempts to insert an IV in an extremity if it shows signs of trauma, injury, or infection; if it has an arteriovenous shunt for

You are the Provider — Part 4

You begin transport to a local trauma center and successfully establish two large-bore IVs of normal saline and administer the appropriate volume of fluid. You reassess the patient and note the following:

Reassessment	Recording Time: 12 Minutes After Patient Contact
Level of consciousness	Conscious and alert to person and place, but not to time and event
Respirations	26 breaths/min, adequate depth
Pulse	114 beats/min, regular and stronger
Blood pressure	100/60 mm Hg
Sao_2	98% (on supplemental oxygen)

7. Is it acceptable to delay transport of a critically injured patient in order to start an IV?

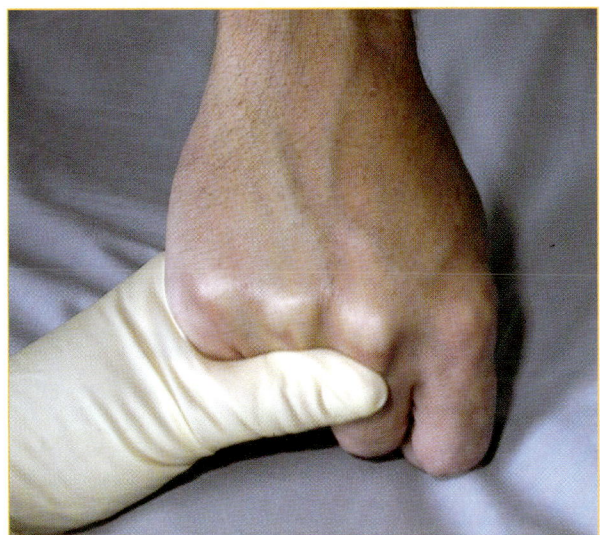

Figure 7-14 Hold hand veins in place by pulling the skin over the vein taut with the thumb of your free hand as you flex the patient's hand.

renal dialysis; or if it is on the same side as a mastectomy. Also pay careful attention to areas of the vein that have track marks, because this is usually a sign of sclerosis caused by frequent cannulation or puncture of the vein.

Some protocols allow cannulation of leg veins for IV starts. Caution must be used when cannulating these areas, because they can place the patient at greater risk of venous thrombosis and pulmonary embolus.

Choosing a Catheter

A catheter is a hollow, laser-sharpened needle inside a hollow plastic tube inserted into a vein to keep the vein open Figure 7-15 ▶ . The most common types of catheters found in the prehospital setting are butterfly catheters and over-the-needle catheters Figure 7-16 ▶ . Catheter selection should reflect the need for the IV, the age of the patient, and the location for the IV.

Catheters are sized by their diameter and referred to by the gauge of the catheter. The larger the diameter of the catheter, the smaller the gauge. Thus, a 14-gauge catheter has a greater diameter than a 22-gauge catheter. The larger the diameter, the more fluid can be delivered through the catheter.

Select the largest-diameter catheter that will fit the vein you have chosen or that will be the most appropriate and comfortable for the patient. A good rule of thumb to follow is: *The more distal the IV site, the smaller*

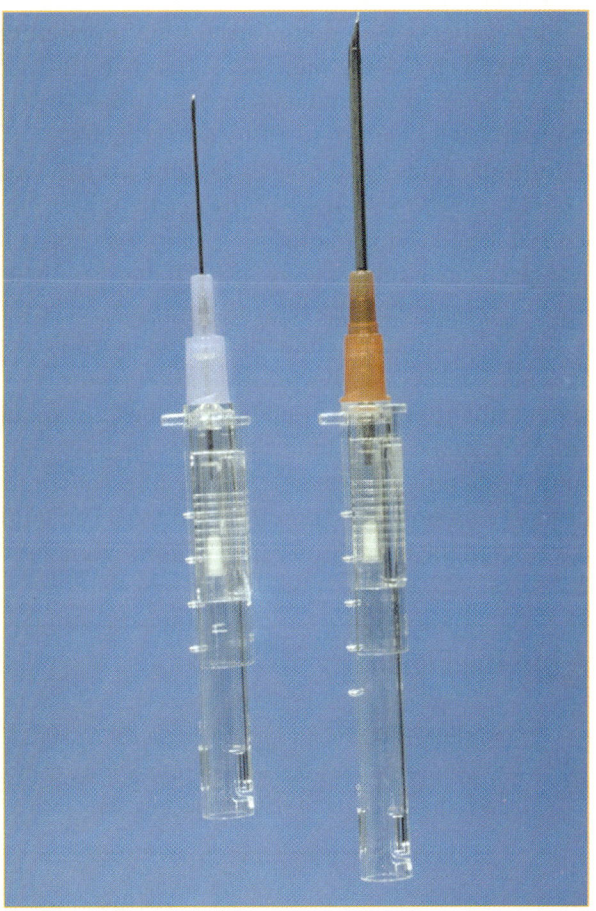

Figure 7-15 A catheter is a hollow tube that is inserted into a vein in order to keep the vein open, allowing a passageway into the vein.

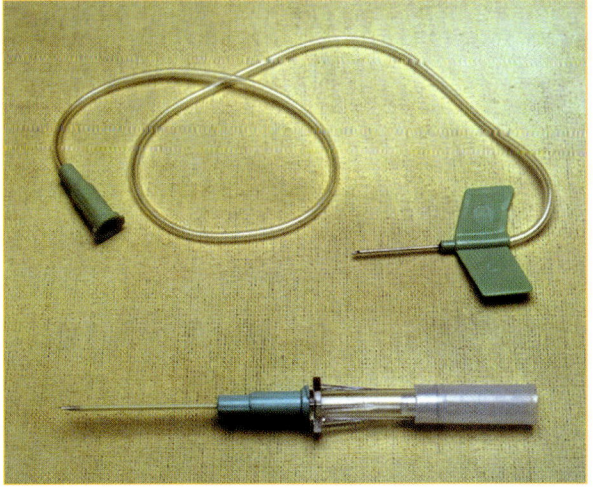

Figure 7-16 The most common types of catheters found in the prehospital setting are butterfly catheters and over-the-needle catheters.

the catheter. An 18-gauge catheter is usually a good size for adult patients who do not need fluid replacement. Metacarpal veins of the hand accommodate 18- to 20-gauge catheters; antecubital veins of the upper arm can accommodate larger 16- to 14-gauge catheters.

Butterfly catheters derive their name from the plastic tabs attached to the sides of the needle. These allow for a stable anchoring platform. 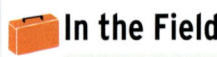 lists the advantages and disadvantages of using butterfly catheters.

Over-the-needle catheters (<u>angiocaths</u>) can be used for all adults and most children for long-term IV therapy Figure 7-17 ▶ . The plastic catheter allows for greater patient movement and often does not require immobilizing the entire limb. Over-the-needle catheters come in different gauges as well as in different lengths. The most common lengths are 2¼" and 1¼". The shorter the catheter, the more fluid can flow through it.

> **In the Field**
>
> Always start low and work your way up. For patients who need rapid fluid replacement, or are in cardiac arrest, the antecubital vein should be used.

In recent years, an attempt has been made to create over-the-needle catheters that minimize the risk of a contaminated stick. A <u>contaminated stick</u> occurs when the EMT-I punctures his or her skin with the same catheter that was used to cannulate the vein of a patient. Newer over-the-needle catheters use several different methods to protect the EMT-I from the possibility of a contaminated stick. One of the more common methods is automatic needle retraction after insertion, usually accomplished with a locking slide mechanism or a spring-loaded slide mechanism. As with the butterfly catheter, there are advantages and disadvantages with the over-the-needle catheters Table 7-4 ▼ .

Occasionally, cannulation of an artery occurs. Cannulation of an artery is easily recognized because bright red blood is quickly seen in the IV tubing and the IV bag

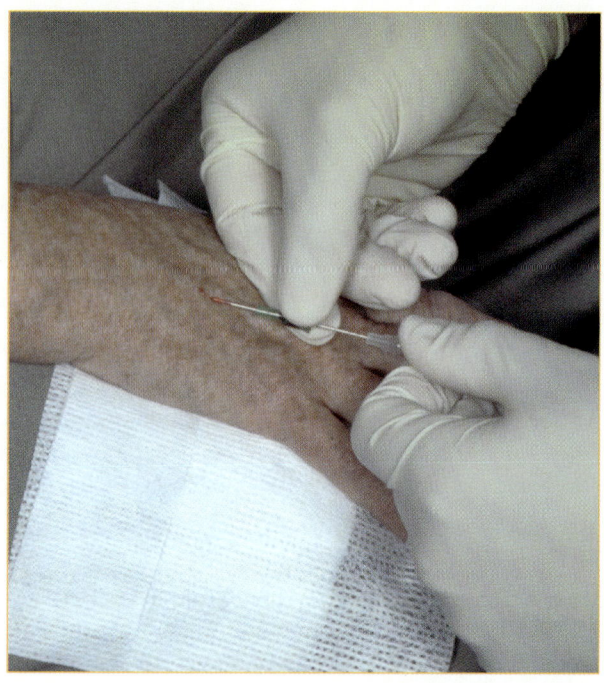

Figure 7-17 The over-the-needle sheath slides off the needle during cannulation and remains inside the vein to keep the vein open.

TABLE 7-3	Advantages and Disadvantages of Butterfly Catheters
Advantages	**Disadvantages**
Easiest venipuncture device to insert	May easily cause infiltration
Useful for scalp veins in infants and small, difficult veins in geriatric patients who only require blood drawings	Possible blood cell damage when drawing blood through the butterfly catheter
Small, short needles	Small-gauge needles limit fluid flow

TABLE 7-4	Advantages and Disadvantages of Over-the-Needle Catheters
Advantages	**Disadvantages**
Less likely to puncture a vein than the butterfly catheter	Risk of resticking the rescuer with contaminated needle
More comfortable once in position	More difficult to insert than other devices
Radiopaque for easy identification during x-ray	Possibility of catheter shear

because of the high pressure that exists in the arteries Figure 7-18 ▼. If cannulation of an artery occurs, you must stop the IV, remove the catheter, and apply direct pressure to the site until any bleeding is controlled.

Inserting the IV Catheter

Each EMT-I has a unique technique to insert an IV, and it is important for you to observe many different techniques to determine what works best for you. The following considerations, however, are common with any technique:

- Keep the beveled side of the catheter up when inserting the needle in a vein Figure 7-19 ▶.
- Maintain adequate traction on the vein during cannulation.

Apply a constricting band above the site you have chosen for the insertion to allow blood to fill the veins. A constricting band is used to help create additional vascular pressure to engorge the veins with blood below the constricting band. Constricting bands should be snug enough to significantly diminish venous flow but should not hamper arterial flow. The constricting band should be left in place only long enough to complete the IV insertion, blood draws, and line attachment. *Do not leave the constricting band applied while you assemble IV equipment.*

Constricting bands can be difficult to manage, especially if you are wearing gloves. You should develop a technique that will allow you to release the constricting band with a small tug on one end. Constricting bands can be made of any available material, such as:

- Penrose drains
- Blood pressure cuffs Figure 7-20 ▼
- Gloves
- Surgical hose

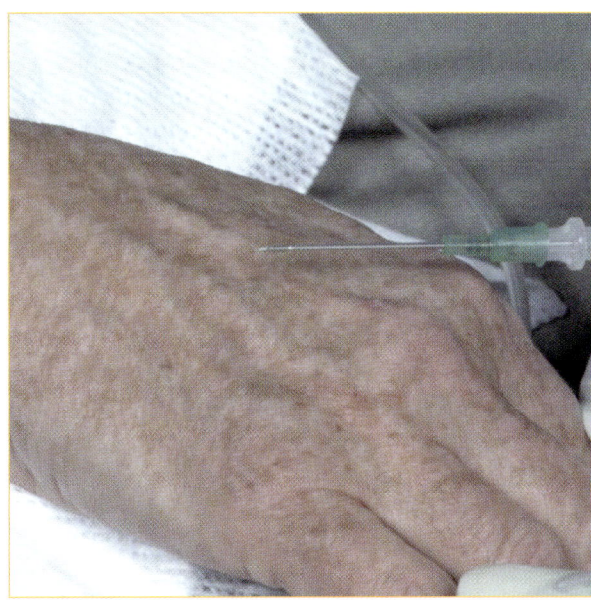

Figure 7-19 Keep the beveled side of the catheter up when inserting the needle in a vein.

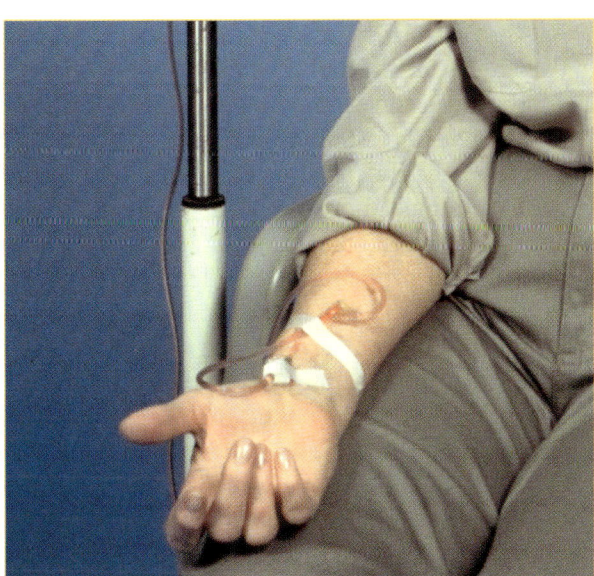

Figure 7-18 A cannulated artery can be recognized by the bright red blood quickly seen through the IV tubing due to the pressure that exists in the arteries.

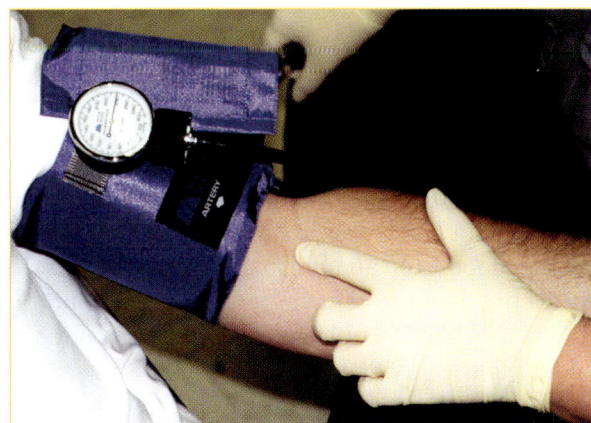

Figure 7-20 A blood pressure cuff may be used in the absence of a constricting band.

> **✱ EMT-I Tips**
>
> Use an aseptic technique when cleansing the site (Figure 7-21▶). With an alcohol prep or iodine swab, start from the center of the area you intend to stick and wipe in a circular motion from the inside out. Take a second swab and wipe straight down the center.

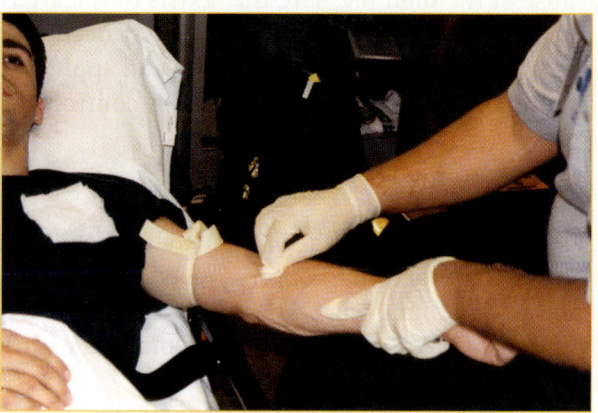

Figure 7-21 Always use an aseptic technique when cleansing the site for IV cannulation. Use the first alcohol pad to clean in a circular motion from the inside out, then use the second to wipe straight down the center.

Once you have selected an insertion site, prep it with an alcohol or iodine swab. Apply gentle downward or lateral traction on the vein with your free hand while holding the catheter, bevel side up, in your dominant hand. Take care as you apply traction to avoid collapsing the vein. Begin by establishing an insertion angle of about 45°. Advance the catheter through the skin until the vein is pierced (there may or may not be a flash of blood in the catheter 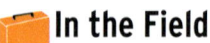flash chamber); then immediately drop the angle down to about 15° and advance the catheter a few more centimeters to ensure the catheter sheath is in the vein. Slide the sheath off the needle and into the vein; do not advance the needle too far because it can lacerate the vein. After the catheter is fully advanced, apply pressure to the vein just proximal to the end of the indwelling catheter, remove the needle, and dispose of it in a sharps container.

> **🧰 In the Field**
>
> Iodine helps to make veins more visible in dark-skinned individuals.

Drawing Blood

Drawing blood, while preferable, is not always possible. Often a patient is so compromised that it is impossible to obtain blood draws. If you are having difficulty drawing blood, stop and finish the IV. Do not allow the constricting band to remain tied too long around the patient's arm because this will allow waste products to build up in the blood and will skew lab results. Attach the Vacutainer to the hub of the catheter sheath and release the hand holding pressure because you now have a sealed system. Grasp the Vacutainer in one hand to stabilize it while you insert the tubes for the blood draws. If you do not have a Vacutainer setup, you can draw blood from the IV site through a 15- to 20-mL syringe. It is important to remember that for the tubes to be viable for testing, they need to be at least three quarters full. Follow local protocols for the types of blood tubes to draw. The tube tops usually come in red, blue, green, and lavender. You can use the following mnemonic to help remember the order for filling the tubes:

- *Red*—red top
- *Blood*—blue top
- *Gives*—green top
- *Life*—lavender top

Fill the red-topped tube first because it contains no additives and is intended to clot if blood typing is needed. The blue-topped tube should be filled next. It contains the preservative EDTA (ethylenediaminetetraacetic acid) and is used to help determine a patient's prothrombin time (PT) and partial prothrombin time (PPT). These values are used to calculate the patient's blood clotting time. The green-topped tube is filled with heparin to prevent clotting and is used to evaluate the patient's electrolyte and glucose levels. Lavender-topped tubes are filled with sodium citrate and are often used for a CBC (complete blood count) panel, including hematocrit and hemoglobin levels.

Once the blood tubes are filled, gently turn them back and forth several times to mix the anticoagulant and blood evenly. *Note:* The exception is the red-topped tube, which is intended to separate the serum from the other blood components. There is no need to invert this tube because there is no additive to mix and the blood clots fairly quickly. Avoid shaking this tube after the blood has clotted, as this may destroy the sample.

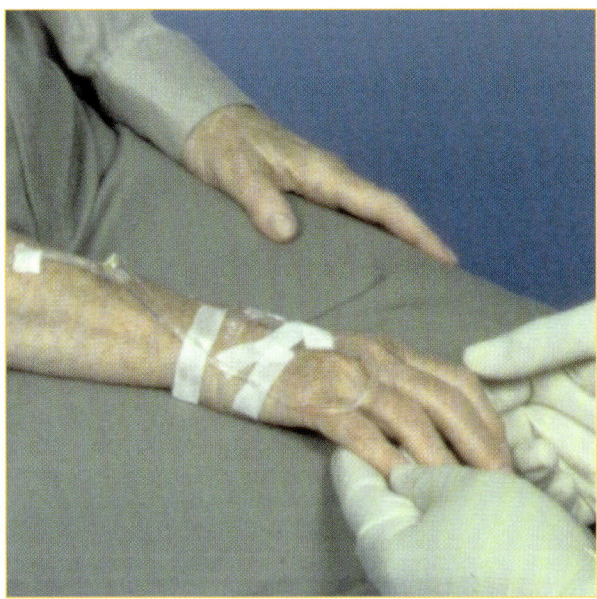

Figure 7-22 Tape the area so that the catheter and tubing are securely anchored.

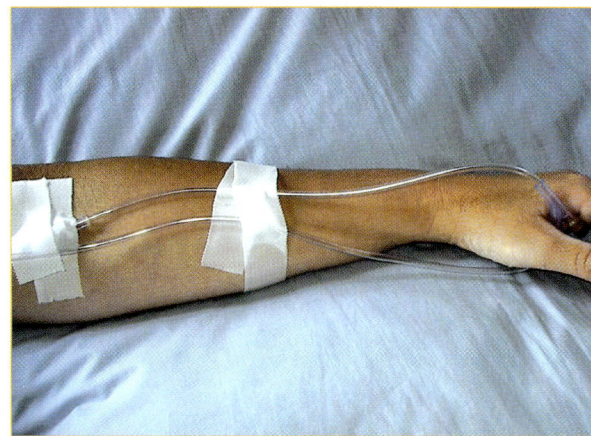

Figure 7-23 Loosely wrap the IV line around the patient's thumb and secure it to the forearm.

Label all the tubes with patient's name, the date, the time, and your name as soon as possible to avoid mixing tubes with those of another patient.

Securing the Line

Once the catheter is in position and the contents of the IV bag are flowing properly, the site must be secured. Tape the area so that the catheter and tubing are securely anchored in case of a sudden pull on the line (Figure 7-22 ▲). You should tear the tape before you start the IV, because you will need one hand to stabilize the site while you tape the IV. Double back the tubing to create a loop that will act as a shock absorber if the line gets pulled accidentally. If you are required to apply an opsite over the catheter site, use the tape to secure the site. Avoid any circumferential taping around any extremity, because circumferential taping can act like a constricting band and may impair circulation.

> 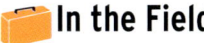 **In the Field**
>
> To further stabilize the IV line, loosely wrap it around the patient's thumb and secure it to the forearm. This will prevent disruption of the IV if the line is pulled (Figure 7-23 ▶).

The steps in performing IV therapy are as follows (Skill Drill 7-2 ▶):

1. Choose the appropriate fluid and examine for clarity and expiration date (**Step 1**). Make sure there are no particles floating in the fluid and that the fluid is appropriate for the patient's condition.
2. Choose the appropriate drip set and attach it to the fluid (**Step 2**). A macrodrip set (example: 10 gtt/mL) should be used for a patient who needs volume replacement and a microdrip set (example: 60 gtt/mL) should be used for a patient who predominantly needs a medication route.
3. Fill the drip chamber by squeezing it together (**Step 3**).
4. Flush or "bleed" the tubing to remove any air bubbles by opening the roller clamp (**Step 4**). Make sure no errant bubbles are floating in the tubing.
5. Tear tape prior to venipuncture or have a commercial device available (**Step 5**).
6. Apply gloves prior to contact with the patient. Palpate a suitable vein (**Step 6**). Veins should be "springy" when palpated. Stay away from areas that are hard when palpated.
7. Apply the constricting band above the intended IV site (**Step 7**). It should be placed approximately 6″ to 10″ above the intended site.
8. Clean the area using an aseptic technique. Use an alcohol pad to cleanse in a circular motion from the inside out. Use a second alcohol pad to wipe straight down the center (**Step 8**).

9. Choose the appropriate sized catheter, twist the catheter to break the seal; however, do not advance the catheter upward as this may cause the needle to shear the catheter. Examine the catheter for any imperfections (**Step 9**). Occasionally you will find "burrs" on the edge of the catheter. Discard any catheter that has an imperfection.
10. Insert the catheter at approximately 45° with the bevel up while applying distal traction with the other hand (**Step 10**). This traction will stabilize the vein and help to keep it from "rolling" as you stick.
11. Observe for "flashback" as blood enters the catheter (**Step 11**). The clear chamber at the top of the catheter should fill with blood when the catheter enters the vein. If you note only a drop or two, you should gently advance the catheter farther into the vein.
12. Occlude the catheter to prevent blood leaking while removing the stylet (**Step 12**). Place the thumb of the hand not holding the catheter over the end of the catheter that is currently situated inside the vein to prevent blood running out when you remove the needle. With practice you will be able to feel the catheter.
13. Immediately dispose of all sharps in the proper container (**Step 13**).
14. Attach the prepared IV line (**Step 14**).
15. Remove the constricting band (**Step 15**).
16. Open the IV line to ensure fluid is flowing and the IV is patent. Observe for any swelling or infiltration around the IV site (**Step 16**). If the fluid does not flow, check to see if the constriction band has been released. If infiltration is noted, immediately stop the infusion and remove the catheter while holding pressure over the site to prevent bleeding.
17. Secure the catheter with tape or a commercial device (**Step 17**).
18. Secure IV tubing and adjust the flow rate while monitoring the patient (**Step 18**).

Discontinuing the IV Line

To discontinue the IV line, shut off the flow from the IV with the roller clamp. Gently peel the tape back *toward* the IV site. As you get closer to the site and the catheter, stabilize the catheter while you loosen all the remaining tape holding the catheter in place. Do not remove the IV tubing from the hub of the catheter.

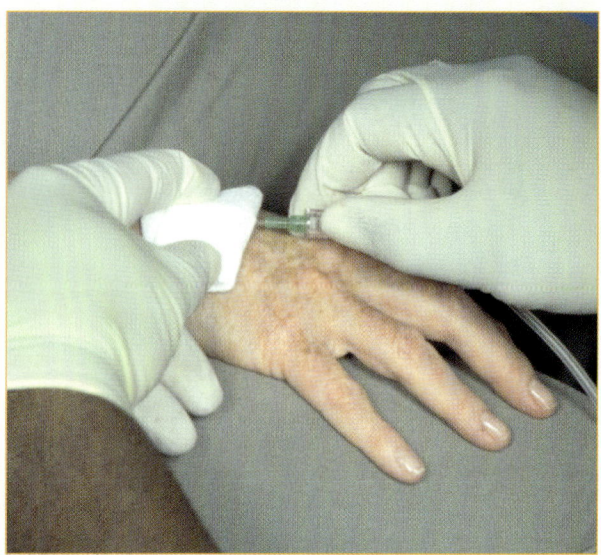

Figure 7-24 When removing a catheter and IV line, pull gently and apply pressure to control bleeding.

Fold a 4″ × 4″ piece of gauze and place it over the site, holding it down while you pull back on the hub of the catheter. Gently pull the catheter and the IV line from the patient's vein while applying pressure to control bleeding (**Figure 7-24**).

Alternative IV Sites and Techniques

Some additional IV sites and techniques available to prehospital providers require training beyond the scope of this chapter. However, because you may need to assist in these types of IV administration, you can benefit from understanding how they work.

Saline Locks

Saline locks (buff caps, Hep-locks, INTs) are a way to maintain an active IV site without having to run fluids through the vein. These access devices are used primarily for patients who do not need additional fluids but may need rapid medication delivery. Saline locks are access ports commonly used with patients who have disorders such as congestive heart failure (CHF) or pulmonary edema. A saline lock is attached to the end of an IV catheter and filled with approximately 2 mL of normal saline to keep blood from clotting at the end of the catheter (**Figure 7-25**). Because this is a sealed-access site, the saline remains in the port without entering the vein, thus preventing clotting. These are also known as intermittent, or INT sites because they

IV Therapy

Skill Drill 7-2

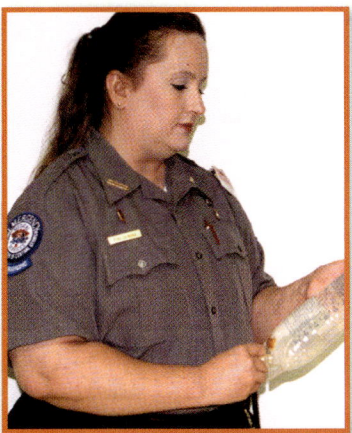
1. Choose the appropriate fluid and examine for clarity and check the expiration date.

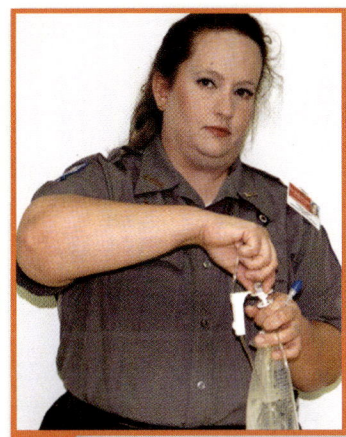
2. Choose the appropriate drip set and attach it to the fluid.

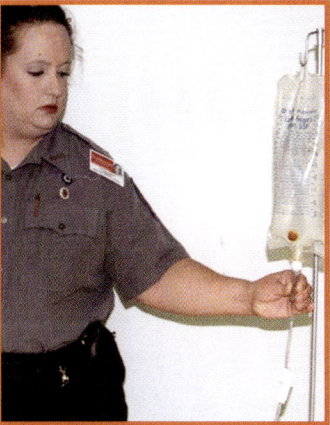
3. Fill the drip chamber by squeezing it together.

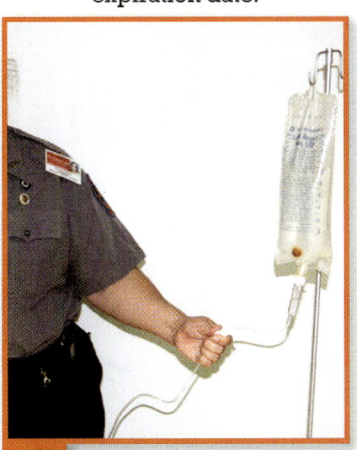
4. Flush or "bleed" the tubing to remove any air bubbles by opening the roller clamp.

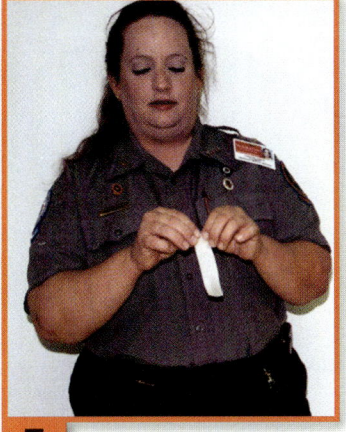
5. Tear tape prior to venipuncture or have a commercial device available.

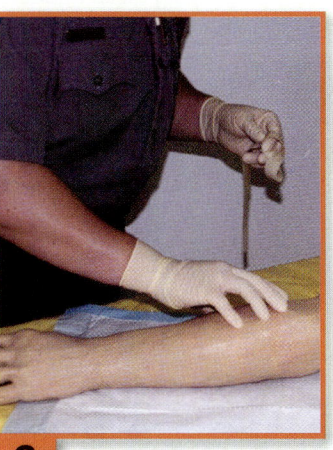
6. Apply gloves prior to contact with patient. Palpate a suitable vein.

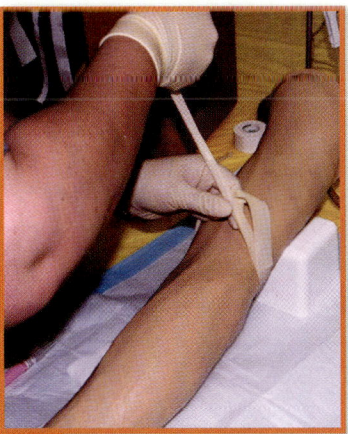
7. Apply the constricting band above the intended IV site.

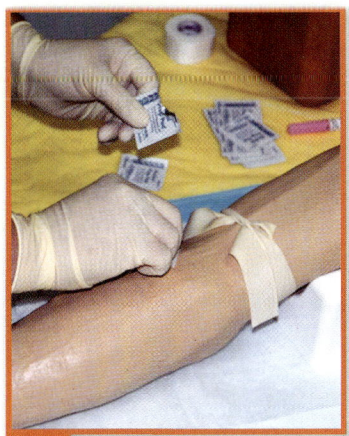
8. Clean the area using an aseptic technique. Use an alcohol pad to cleanse in a circular motion from the inside out. Use a second alcohol pad to wipe straight down the center.

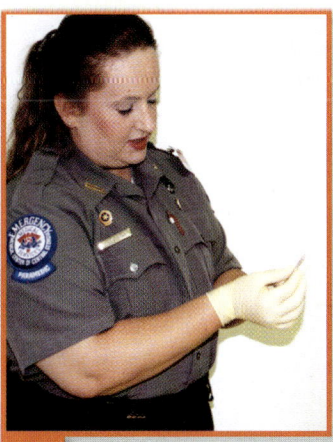
9. Choose the appropriate sized catheter and examine it for any imperfections.

IV Therapy (continued)

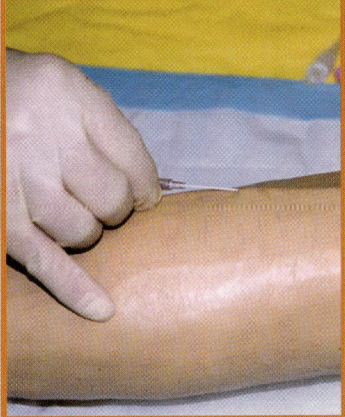
10 Insert the catheter at approximately 45° with the bevel up while applying distal traction with the other hand.

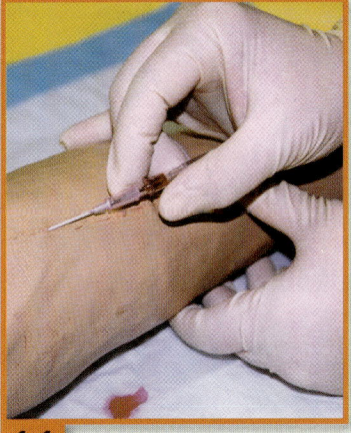
11 Observe for "flashback" as blood enters the catheter.

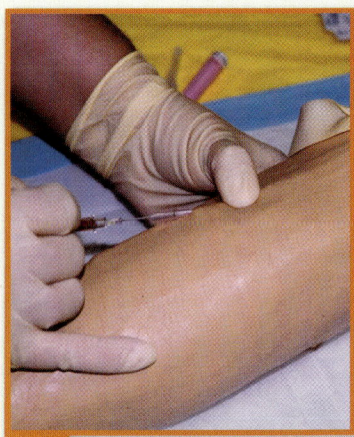
12 Occlude the catheter to prevent blood leaking while removing the stylet.

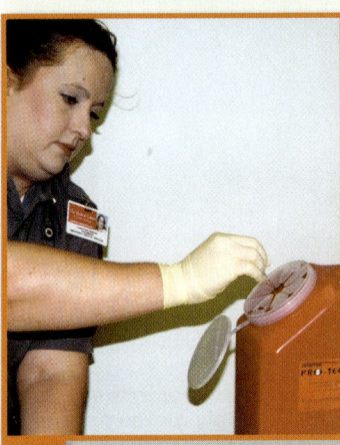
13 Immediately dispose of all sharps in the proper container.

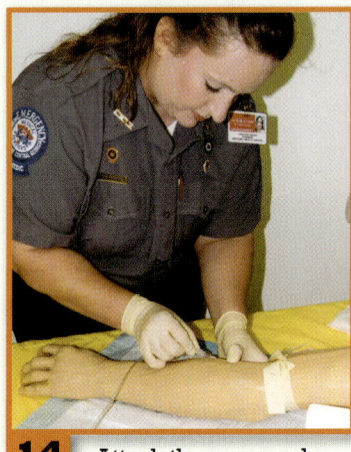
14 Attach the prepared IV line.

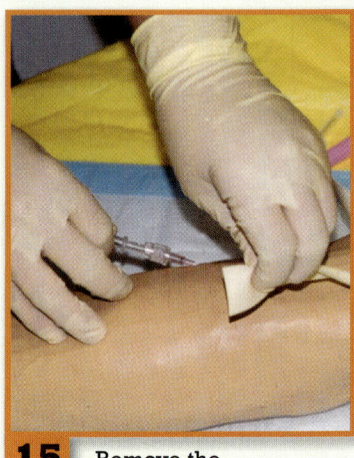
15 Remove the constricting band.

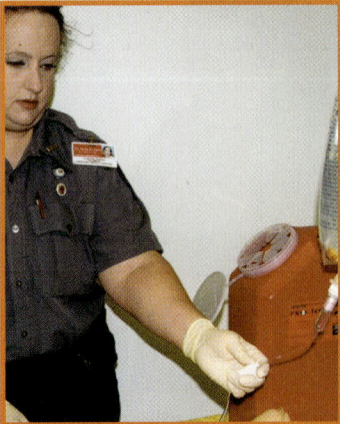
16 Open the IV line to ensure fluid is flowing and the IV is patent. Observe for any swelling or infiltration around the IV site.

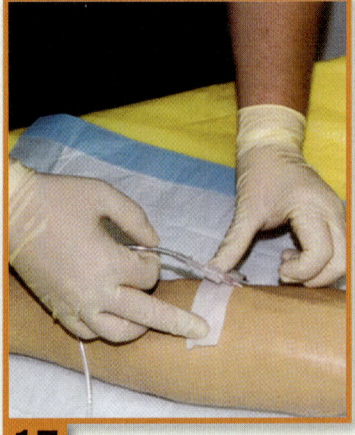
17 Secure the catheter with tape or a commercial device.

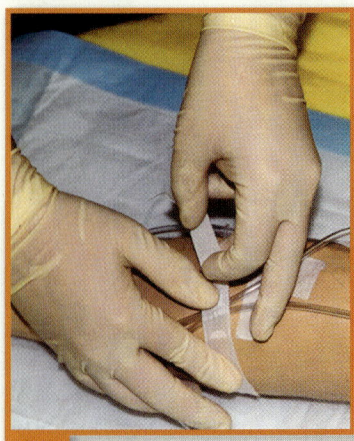
18 Secure IV tubing and adjust the flow rate while monitoring the patient.

is attached to this catheter. Anything that flows through a normal IV can be infused through an IO line. Once established, these lines work as well as peripheral IV lines. Intraosseous lines require full and careful immobilization because they rest at a 90° angle to the bone and are easily dislodged. Stabilization is critical for these lines to maintain adequate flow. Stabilize the IO needle in the same manner that you would any impaled object, with the following steps (Skill Drill 7-3 ▶):

1. Check selected IV fluid for proper fluid, clarity, and expiration date. Look for any discoloration or particles floating in the fluid. If found, discard and choose another bag of fluid.
2. Select the appropriate equipment, including an IO needle, syringe, saline, and extension set (**Step 1**). A three-way stopcock may also be used to facilitate easier fluid administration.
3. Select the proper administration set. Connect the administration set to the bag. Prepare the administration set. Fill the drip chamber and flush the tubing. Make sure all air bubbles are removed from the tubing.
4. Prepare the syringe and extension tubing (**Step 2**).
5. Cut or tear the tape. This can be done at any time before IO puncture.
6. Take body substance isolation precautions. This must be done prior to IO puncture.
7. Identify the proper anatomical site for IO puncture (**Step 3**). In order to miss the epiphyseal plate you should measure two fingerwidths below the knee on the medial side of the leg.
8. Cleanse the site appropriately. Follow an aseptic technique by cleansing in a circular manner from the inside out.
9. Perform the IO puncture, involving the following steps:
   Stabilize the tibia. Place a folded towel underneath the knee and hold in such a manner as to keep your fingers away from the site of puncture.
10. Insert the needle at a 90° angle to the leg. Advance the needle with a twisting motion until a "pop" is felt (**Step 4**). Unscrew the cap and remove the stylet from the needle (**Step 5**).
11. Attach the syringe and extension set to the IO needle. Pull back on the syringe to aspirate blood and particles of bone marrow to ensure placement.

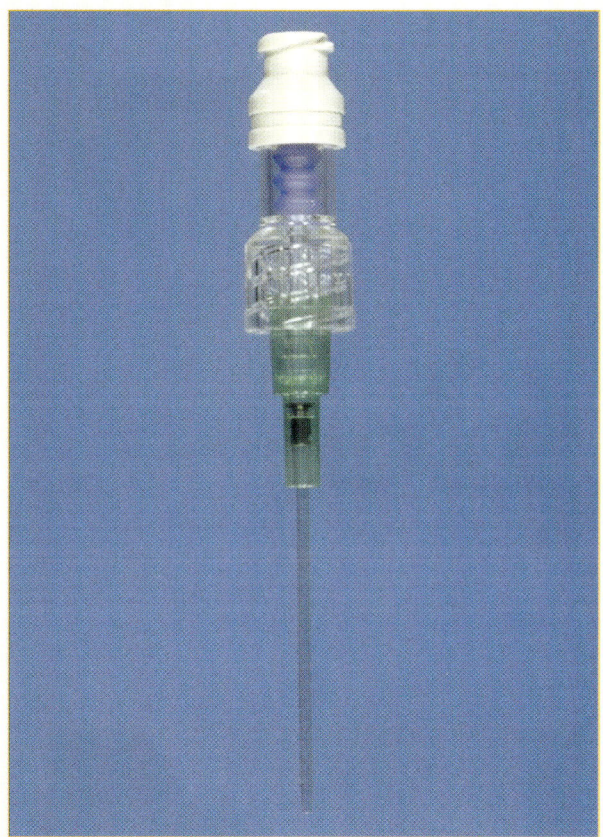

Figure 7-25 A saline lock is attached to the end of an IV catheter and filled with approximately 2 mL of normal saline in order to keep blood from clotting at the end of the catheter.

eliminate the need to completely reestablish an IV each time the patient needs medication or fluid.

Intraosseous Lines

Intraosseous lines (IOs) are used for emergency venous access in pediatric patients as defined by protocol when immediate IV access is difficult or impossible. The rule of thumb is an inability to gain IV access in three tries or 90 seconds in a critical pediatric patient. Often these children are experiencing a life-threatening situation such as cardiac arrest, status epilepticus, or progressive shock. IOs are contraindicated in tibias that are fractured. IOs are established in the proximal tibia with a rigid boring catheter, commonly known as a Jamshedi needle. This double needle, consisting of a solid boring needle inside a sharpened hollow needle, is pushed into the bone with a screwing, twisting action. Once the needle pops through the bone, the solid needle is removed, leaving the hollow steel needle in place. The IV tubing

Pediatric Intraosseous Infusion

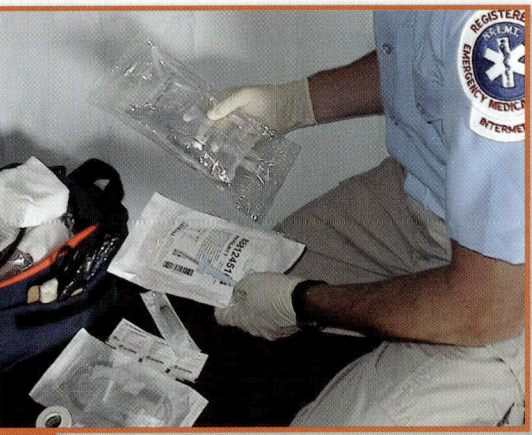

1 Check selected IV fluid for proper fluid, clarity, and expiration date.

Select the appropriate equipment, including an IO needle, syringe, saline, and extension.

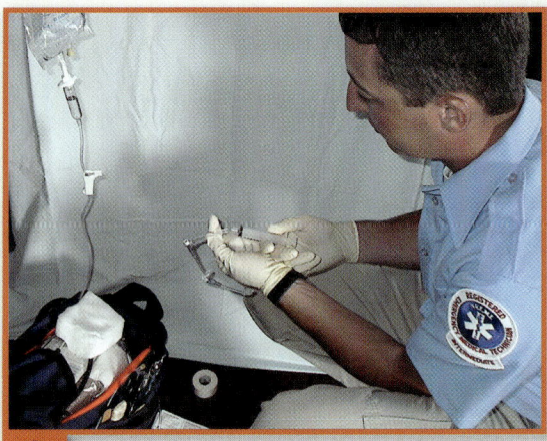

2 Select the proper administration set. Connect the administration set to the bag. Prepare the administration set, syringe, and extension tubing.

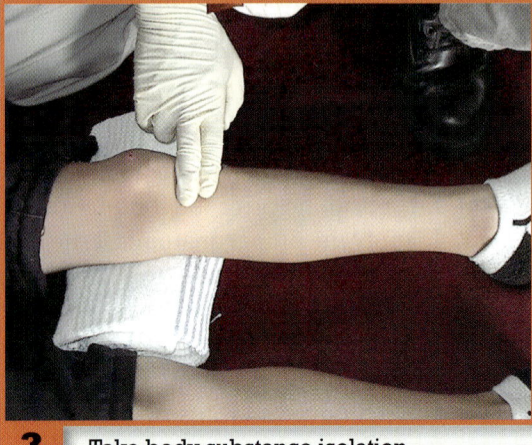

3 Take body substance isolation precautions.

Identify the proper anatomical site for IO puncture.

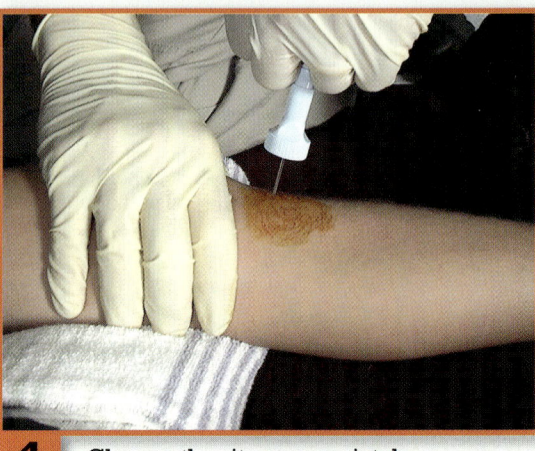

4 Cleanse the site appropriately.

Stabilize the tibia and insert the needle at a 90° angle, advancing it with a twisting motion until a "pop" is felt.

12. Slowly inject saline to ensure proper placement of the needle. Watch for infiltration and stop the infusion immediately if noted. It is possible to fracture the bone during insertion of the IO. If this happens you should remove the IO and switch to the other leg.

13. Connect the administration set and adjust the flow rate as appropriate (**Step 6**). Fluid does not flow well through an IO, and boluses are given by administering the fluid using the syringe.

14. Secure the needle with tape and support it with a bulky dressing. Stabilize in place in the same

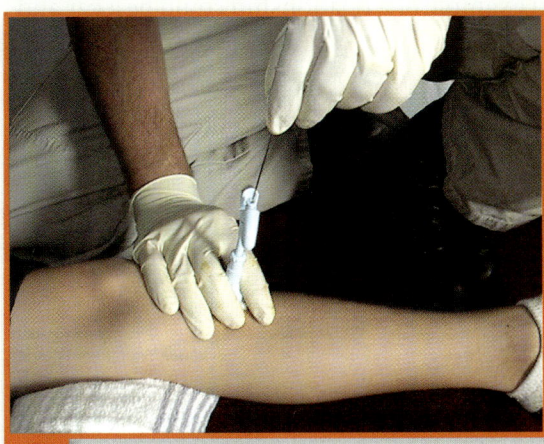

5 Unscrew the cap and remove the stylet from the needle.

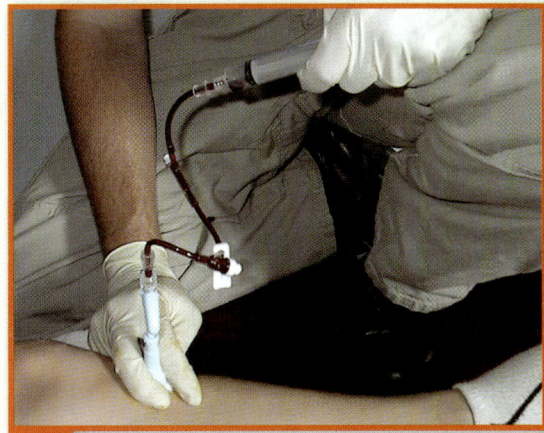

6 Attach the syringe and extension set to the IO needle.

Pull back on the syringe to aspirate blood and particles of bone marrow to ensure placement.

Slowly inject saline to ensure proper placement of the needle.

Watch for infiltration and stop the infusion immediately if noted.

Connect the administration set and adjust the flow rate as appropriate.

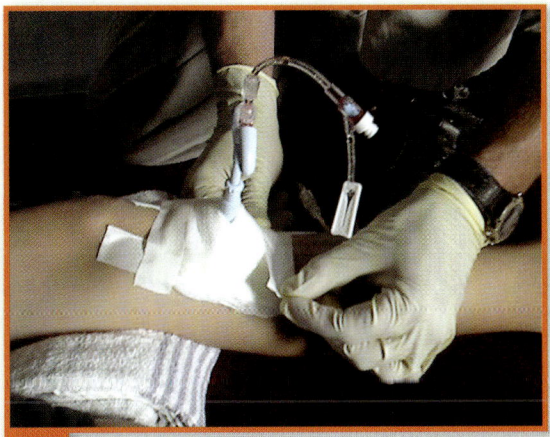

7 Secure the needle with tape and support it with a bulky dressing.

manner that an impaled object is stabilized. Use bulky dressings around the catheter and tape securely in place. Be careful not to tape around the entire circumference of the leg, which could impair circulation, resulting in a compartment syndrome (**Step 7**).

15. Dispose of the needle in the proper container.

External Jugular IVs

<u>External jugular IVs</u> provide venous access through the external jugular veins of the neck. These are the same veins used to assess jugular vein distention (JVD). The vein is tamponaded by placing a finger or the edge of a tongue depressor on the vein just above the clavicle, causing the vein to fill. If the vein is difficult to find,

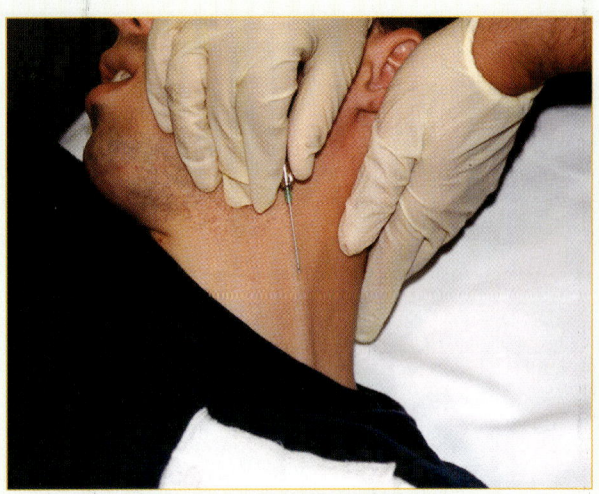

Figure 7-26 The external jugular IV requires a very specific insertion site midway between the angle of the jaw and the midclavicular line with the catheter pointed toward the shoulder on the same side as the puncture.

place the patient in the Trendelenburg position to facilitate venous return. The catheter is inserted into the vein in the same manner as a normal IV, except the insertion point is very specific. The catheter is inserted midway between the angle of the jaw and the midclavicular line, with the catheter pointed toward the shoulder on the same side as the puncture site 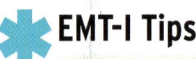. These punctures are difficult because a very tough fibrous sheath that makes access difficult surrounds these veins.

These techniques require more advanced education and training than this chapter will provide. Understanding their application and use is important because you may need to assist with these procedures.

> **EMT-I Tips**
>
> **ALWAYS** feel very carefully for a pulse prior to cannulating an external jugular vein. It is imperative not to pierce the carotid artery.

Dimensional Analysis

One of the easiest ways to figure out drip rates, dose calculations, weight-based calculations, and drug concentration equations is to use dimensional analysis. Dimensional analysis uses the same simple conversions as equations, and you will not need to memorize the equation! Dimensional analysis allows you to compare seemingly unrelated items by setting up a relationship (that is, a comparison between two items).

An example of a relationship could be a car and the wheels on a car. Every car rides on four wheels, so there are four wheels for every car.

$$\frac{1 \text{ car}}{4 \text{ wheels}} = \frac{4 \text{ wheels}}{1 \text{ car}}$$

Another way to look at these comparisons is as a ratio, which is by nature a relationship. Dimensional analysis uses ratios as conversion factors.

Drip Rates

Use dimensional analysis to solve IV drip rates.
For this work you need to know:
- Which administration set to use
- Length of time for the infusion
- Amount to flow

You may need the conversion factor of 1 hour = 60 minutes.

Example:
- Order given is for 250 mL normal saline (NS) over 90 minutes.
- Administration set = macrodrip (10 gtt/mL).

Determine how many drops per minute should be given.

Set up the equation:

$$\frac{? \text{ gtt}}{\text{min}} = \frac{10 \text{ gtt}}{1 \text{ mL}} \times \frac{250 \text{ mL}}{90 \text{ min}}$$

Cancel out what you can and reduce the fractions:

$$\frac{? \text{ gtt}}{\text{min}} = \frac{\cancel{10} \text{ gtt}}{1 \cancel{\text{ mL}}} \times \frac{250 \cancel{\text{ mL}}}{\cancel{90} \text{ min}}$$

$$= \frac{1 \text{ gtt}}{1} \times \frac{250}{9 \text{ min}}$$

Multiply and divide:

$$= \frac{250 \text{ gtt}}{9 \text{ min}} = \frac{27.77 \text{ gtt}}{\text{min}} = 28 \text{ gtt}$$

> 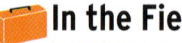 **In the Field**
>
> The volume in mL is the "doctor's order." The drip set is always drops per mL, and the time is always in minutes. Multiply the doctor's order (in mL) times the drip set (in drops per mL) and divide by the time (in minutes). This yields the number of drops per minute.

You will need to set the drip rate at 28 gtt/min normal saline to achieve the desired order.

Drops per Minute

Another useful formula to remember is a simple drip rate calculation that gives you the number of drops per minute:

$$\frac{(\text{volume in mL}) \times (\text{drip set})}{(\text{time in minutes})} = \frac{\text{gtt}}{\text{min}}$$

> **A to Z Terminology Tips**
>
> **KVO** means keep vein open; **TKO** means to keep open. Both are abbreviations for rates equal to about 8 to 15 drops per minute that are used to allow just enough fluid through the IV to keep blood from clotting at the end of the catheter.

Possible Complications of IV Therapy

Peripheral IV insertion carries associated risks. The problems associated with IVs can be categorized as either local or systemic reactions. Local reactions include problems such as infiltration and phlebitis. Systemic complications include allergic reactions and circulatory overload.

> **Documentation Tips**
>
> To document an IV, you need to include four things:
> - The gauge of the needle
> - The site
> - The type of fluid you are administering
> - The rate the fluid is running
>
> For an IV initiated in the left antecubital fossa with an 18-gauge needle and normal saline at a rate of 120 mL per hour, the documentation would look like this:
>
> 18g IV L ac c̄ NS @ 120 mL/h
>
> If you establish an intermittent site without running fluid it would be documented as follows:
>
> 18g INT Ⓛ ac

Local IV Site Reactions

Most local reactions require that you discontinue the IV, reestablish the IV in the opposite extremity, and document the event. Some examples of local reactions include:

- Infiltration
- Phlebitis
- Occlusion
- Vein irritation
- Hematoma
- Nerve, tendon, or ligament damage

You are the Provider — Part 5

You reassess the patient shortly before arriving at the trauma center. Upon arrival, you are met by the attending physician. After further assessment and management in the emergency department, the patient is taken to surgery to repair his fractured femurs.

Reassessment	Recording Time: 18 Minutes After Patient Contact
Level of consciousness	Conscious and alert to person, place, and time
Respirations	22 breaths/min, adequate depth
Pulse	108 beats/min, strong and regular
Blood pressure	104/62 mm Hg
Sao₂	98% (on supplemental oxygen)

8. What role do isotonic crystalloid solutions play in the management of a patient in shock?

Infiltration

Infiltration is the escape of fluid into the surrounding tissue. This escape of fluid causes a localized area of edema. Some of the more common reasons for infiltration include the following:

- The IV has passed completely through the vein and out the other side.
- The patient is moving excessively.
- The tape used to secure the area has become loose or dislodged.
- The catheter was started at an angle that is too shallow and has only entered the fascia surrounding the vein (this is more common with IVs in larger veins, such as those in the upper arm and neck).

Some of the associated signs and symptoms of infiltration include the following:

- Edema at the catheter site
- Continued IV flow after occlusion of the vein above the insertion point
- Patient complaints of tightness and pain around the IV site

To correct the infiltration, discontinue the IV and reestablish it in the opposite extremity or at a more proximal location on the same extremity. Apply direct pressure over the swollen area to reduce further swelling or bleeding into the tissue. Avoid wrapping tape around the extremity for direct pressure because this could create a constricting band.

Phlebitis

Phlebitis is inflammation of the vein. Phlebitis is not usually seen with the emergency prehospital patient, although you may encounter it in patients who abuse drugs when you attempt to establish an IV. Hospital outpatient treatment or home health care often allows the patient to receive IV therapy at home, which can also lead to phlebitis. Often phlebitis is associated with fever, tenderness, and red streaking up the associated vein. Hardening of the vein can occur if perforation of the vein is from repeated puncture, as seen with drug abuse. Some of the more common causes for phlebitis include localized irritation and infection from nonsterile equipment, prolonged IV therapy, or irritating IV solutions. If the phlebitis is associated with the IV you have started, discontinue the IV and reestablish it in another location, using new equipment.

Occlusion

Occlusion is the physical blockage of a vein or catheter. If the flow rate is not sufficient to keep fluid moving out of the catheter tip and if blood enters the catheter, a clot may form and occlude the flow. The first sign of a possible occlusion is a decreasing drip rate or the presence of blood in the IV tubing. A positional IV site can cause occlusion, which means that fluid flows at different rates depending on the position of the catheter within the vein. Close proximity to a valve is often the reason for positional IVs. Other causes can be related to patient movement that allows the line to become physically blocked from either resting on the line or crossing arms. Occlusion may also develop if the IV bag nears empty and the blood pressure overcomes the flow and backs up in the line.

Use the steps shown in **Skill Drill 7-4** to determine whether the IV should be reestablished:

1. Select and assemble a sterile 10-mL syringe and large-gauge needle (**Step 1**).
2. Select an injection port close to the IV site and wipe it with an alcohol wipe.
3. Depress the plunger of the syringe and insert the syringe into the port (**Step 2**).
4. Pinch the line between the IV site and the port and pull back on the plunger to draw clean IV fluid from the bag (**Step 3**).
5. Once the syringe is full, leave it in place and switch your hand from the tubing between the port and the IV site to between the port and the IV bag, then pinch the line.
6. Now you have a full syringe of clean IV fluid and a way to add pressure to the line. Gently apply pressure to the plunger to disrupt the occlusion and reestablish flow.
7. If flow is reestablished, ensure that the line is free and the rate is sufficient.
8. If the occlusion does not dislodge, discontinue the IV and reestablish it in the opposite extremity or at a proximal location on the same extremity (**Step 4**).

Vein Irritation

Occasionally, a patient will experience vein irritation in reaction to the fluid used for an IV. Patients who have this problem often complain immediately that the solution is bothering them. It may tingle, sting, or itch. Note these complaints and observe the patient closely

Determining if an IV is Viable

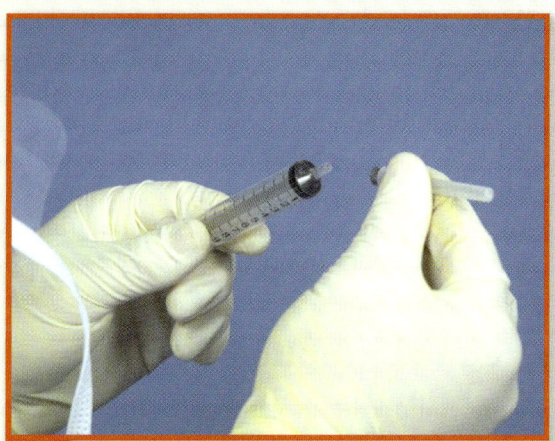

1 Select and assemble a sterile 10-mL syringe and large-gauge needle.

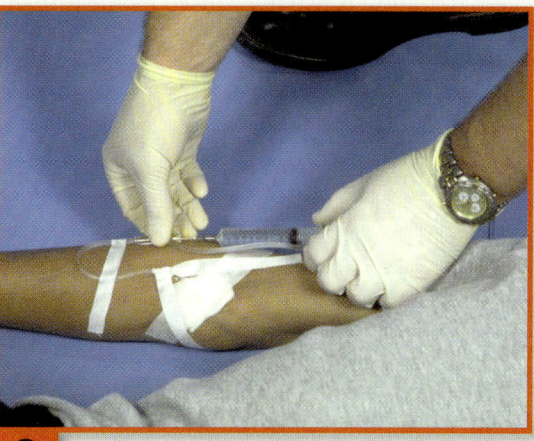

2 Select an injection port close to the IV site and wipe it with an alcohol wipe.

Depress the plunger of the syringe and insert the syringe into the port.

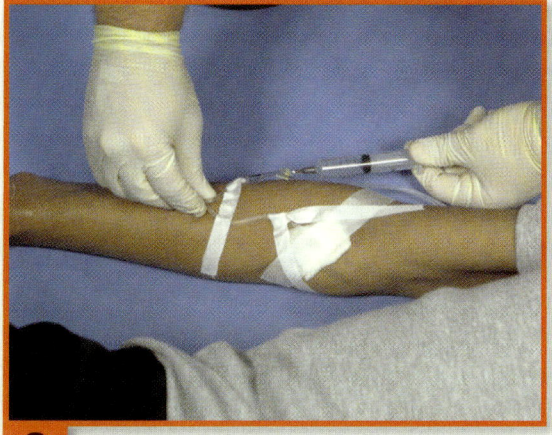

3 Pinch the line between the IV site and the port and pull back on the plunger to draw clean IV fluid from the bag.

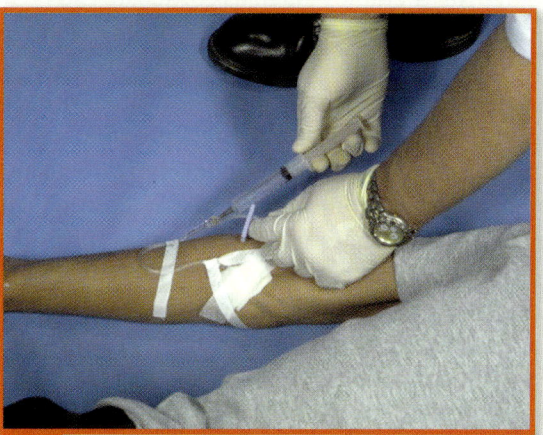

4 Once the syringe is full, leave it in place and switch your hand from the tubing between the port and the IV site to between the port and the IV bag, then pinch the line. Gently apply pressure to the plunger to disrupt the occlusion and reestablish flow. Ensure that the line is free and the rate is sufficient.

If the occlusion does not dislodge, discontinue the IV and reestablish it in the opposite extremity or at a proximal location on the same extremity.

Skill Drill 7-4

in case he or she develops a more serious allergic reaction to the fluid.

The vein irritation is usually caused by the infusion being too rapid. If redness develops at the IV site with rapidly developing phlebitis, discontinue the IV and save the equipment for later analysis. Reestablish the IV in the other extremity with all new equipment in case there were unseen contaminants in the old equipment. Be sure to document the event and the patient's response.

Hematoma

A hematoma is an accumulation of blood in the tissues surrounding an IV site. Hematomas result from vein perforation or improper catheter removal that allows blood to accumulate in the surrounding tissues. Blood can be seen rapidly pooling around the IV site, leading to tenderness and pain (Figure 7-27). Patients with a history of vascular diseases (diabetes) or patients receiving certain drug therapies (such as corticosteroids) can have a predisposition to vein rupture or have tendencies to develop hematomas rapidly on IV insertion.

If a hematoma develops while you are attempting to insert a catheter, stop and apply direct pressure to help minimize bleeding. If a hematoma develops after a successful catheter insertion, evaluate the IV flow and the hematoma. If the hematoma appears to be controlled and the flow is not affected, monitor the IV site and leave the line in place. If the hematoma develops as a result of discontinuing the IV, apply direct pressure with a 4″ × 4″ gauze pad to the site.

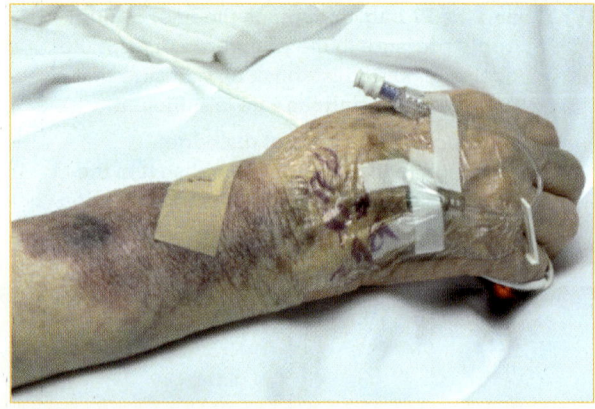

Figure 7-27 Hematomas can be caused by the improper removal of a catheter, resulting in the pooling of blood around the IV site, leading to tenderness and pain.

Nerve, Tendon, or Ligament Damage

Improper identification of anatomic structures around the IV site can lead to perforation of tendons, ligaments, or nerves. An IV site choice around joints increases the risk for perforation of these structures. Patients will experience sudden and severe shooting pain when a nerve, tendon, or ligament is perforated. Numbness in the extremity after the incident can be common. Immediately remove the catheter and select another IV site. Be sure to document the event.

Systemic Complications

Systemic complications can evolve from reactions or complications associated with IV insertion. Systemic complications usually involve other body systems and can be life-threatening. If the IV line is established and patent, do not remove it, because it may be needed for treatment of the patient. Common systemic complications are:

- Allergic reactions
- Circulatory overload
- Air embolus
- Vasovagal reactions
- Catheter shear

Allergic Reactions

Often, allergic reactions are minor, but <u>anaphylaxis</u> is possible and must be treated aggressively. Allergic reactions can be related to an individual's unexpected sensitivity to an IV fluid or medication. Such sensitivity could be an unknown condition to the patient; thus, vigilance must be maintained with any IV for a possible reaction.

Patient presentation depends on the extent of the reaction. Common signs and symptoms of an allergic reaction include:

- Itching
- Shortness of breath
- Edema of face and hands
- Urticaria
- Bronchospasm
- Anaphylaxis
- Wheezing

If an allergic reaction occurs, discontinue the IV and remove the solution. Leave the catheter in place as an emergency medication route. Notify medical control immediately and maintain an open airway. Monitor the patient's ABCs and vital signs. Document the event and keep the solution or medication for evaluation by the hospital. Further treatment for anaphylaxis is covered in Chapter 22.

Air Embolus

Healthy adults can tolerate as much as 200 mL of air introduced into the circulatory system, but patients who are already ill or injured can be affected if any air is introduced into the IV line. Properly flushing an IV line will help eliminate any potential of introducing air into a patient. IV bags are designed to collapse as they empty to help prevent this problem, but collapse does not always occur. Be sure to replace empty IV bags with full ones.

If your patient begins developing respiratory distress with unequal breath sounds, consider the possibility of an air embolus. Other associated signs and symptoms include:

- Cyanosis (even in the presence of high-flow oxygen)
- Signs and symptoms of shock
- Loss of consciousness
- Respiratory arrest

Treat a patient with a suspected air embolus by placing the patient on his or her left side with the head down to trap any air inside the right atrium or right ventricle and rapidly transport to the closest most appropriate facility. Be prepared to assist ventilations if the patient experiences increasing shortness of breath or inadequate tidal volume. Document the event.

Catheter Shear

Catheter shear occurs when part of the catheter is pinched against the needle, and the needle slices through the catheter, creating a free-floating segment. This allows the catheter segment to travel through the circulatory system and possibly end up in the pulmonary circulation, causing a pulmonary embolus.

Treatment involves surgical removal of the sheared tip. Catheter hubs are radiopaque (that is, they will appear white in an x-ray) to aid in diagnosing this type of problem. Never rethread a catheter. Dispose of the used one and use a new one.

Patients who have experienced catheter shear with pulmonary artery occlusion present with sudden dyspnea, shortness of breath, and possibly diminished breath sounds. They will mimic the presentations of the air embolus patient and can be treated the same way. Such patients will need continued IV access, and you must try to obtain an IV site in the other extremity.

> **In the Field**
>
> When starting an IV on a patient who is frightened of needles, make sure he or she is in a supine position prior to sticking. Advise the patient of each step—even when you are only cleansing the site.

Circulatory Overload

An unmonitored IV bag can lead to circulatory overload. Healthy adults can handle as much as 2 to 3 extra liters of fluid without compromise. Problems occur when the patient has cardiac, pulmonary, or renal dysfunction. These types of dysfunction do not tolerate any additional demands from increased circulatory volume. The most common cause of circulatory overload in the prehospital setting is failure to readjust the drip rate after flushing an IV line immediately after insertion. Always monitor IV bags to ensure the proper drip rate.

Patient presentation includes dyspnea, JVD, and increased blood pressure. Crackles are often heard when evaluating breath sounds. Acute peripheral edema can also be an indication of circulatory overload.

To treat a patient with circulatory overload, slow the IV rate to keep the vein open and raise the patient's head to ease respiratory distress. Administer high-flow oxygen and monitor vital signs and breathing adequacy. Contact medical control immediately and inform them of the developing problem, because there are drugs that can be given to reduce the circulatory volume. Document the event.

Vasovagal Reactions

Some patients have anxiety concerning needles or to the sight of blood. Such anxiety may cause vasculature dilation, leading to a drop in blood pressure and patient collapse. Patients can present with anxiety, diaphoresis, nausea, and syncopal episodes.

Treatment for patients with vasovagal reactions (also known as 'vagaling down') centers on treating them for shock:

1. Place patient in shock position.
2. Apply high-flow oxygen.
3. Monitor vital signs.
4. Establish an IV in case fluid resuscitation is needed.

Troubleshooting

Several factors can influence the flow rate of an IV. For example, if the IV bag is not hung high enough, the flow rate will not be sufficient. It is always helpful to perform the following checks after completing IV administration. Also, if there is a flow problem, rechecking these items will help determine the problem.

- Check your IV fluid.
  Thick, viscous fluids such as blood products and colloid solutions infuse slowly and may be diluted to help speed delivery. Cold fluids run slower than warm fluids. If you can, warm IV fluids before administering them in cold weather.
- Check your administration set.
  Macrodrips are used for rapid fluid delivery, whereas microdrips are designed to deliver a more controlled flow.
- Check the height of your IV bag.
  The IV bag must be hung high enough to overcome the patient's own blood pressure. Hang the bag as high as possible.
- Check the type of catheter used.
  The wider the catheter (the smaller the gauge), the more fluid can be delivered; 14 gauge is the widest, 27 gauge the narrowest.
- Check your constricting band.
  One of the most overlooked factors is leaving the constricting band on the patient's arm after completing the IV.

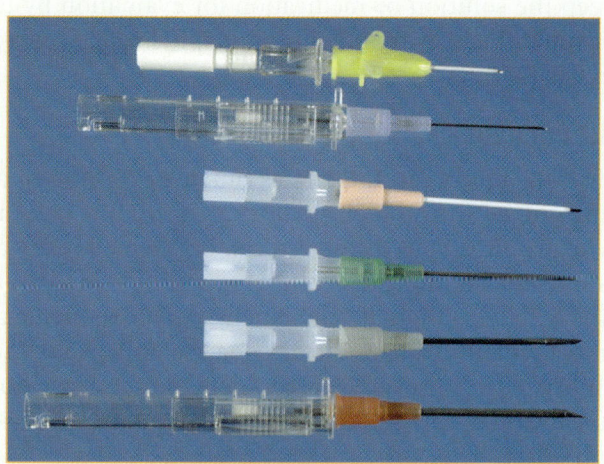

Figure 7-28 Note the difference in sizes of catheters.

Pediatric Considerations

The same IV solutions and equipment can be used on pediatric patients as on adults, with a few exceptions.

Catheters

If you are using over-the-needle catheters to start a pediatric IV, the 20-, 22-, 24-, or 26-gauge catheters are best for insertions **Figure 7-28**. Butterfly catheters are ideal for pediatric patients and can be placed in the same locations as over-the-needle catheters as well as in visible scalp veins. Scalp veins are best used in young infants.

Volutrol IV Sets

Fluid control for pediatric patients is important. A special type of microdrip set called a Volutrol IV allows you to fill the large drip chamber with a specific amount of fluid and administer only this amount to avoid fluid overload. The 100-mL calibrated drip chamber can be shut off from the IV bag.

IV Locations

When starting the IV, explain what you are doing to both the child and the parent. A parent can become as stressed as a child, so take time to thoroughly explain the procedure.

The younger the pediatric patient, the fewer choices you have for IV sites. Hand veins are painful and difficult to manage in younger pediatric patients but remain the location of choice for starting peripheral IVs. Protecting the IV site after it has been established is critical and is sometimes best accomplished by immobilizing the site before cannulation with an arm board. One of the better techniques for starting pediatric IVs is to use a penlight to illuminate the veins on the back of the hand. Shine the light through the palm side of the hand to illuminate the veins on the backside of the hand. Once a suitable site is located, slightly graze the surface of the hand with your fingernail so you can find the location after you turn off the penlight. Proceed with the IV, using the mark you created as a guide. Sometimes the best choice is an AC (antecubital vein) line with full arm immobilization to avoid dislodging the IV.

Scalp vein cannulation is often aesthetically unpleasant for both the child and the parents and can produce apprehension in both simply because of the location. In addition, scalp veins can be difficult to cannulate and do not allow for rapid fluid resuscitation. When securing a scalp vein, tape a paper cup over the site to avoid applying any direct pressure to the butterfly catheter.

Pressure may cause the needle to puncture the other side of the vein and let fluids escape into the tissues (extravasation).

Geriatric Considerations

Smaller catheters may be preferable with the elderly patient unless rapid fluid replacement is needed. Some medications commonly used by the elderly patient have the tendency to create fragile skin and veins. Often, simply puncturing the vein will cause a massive hematoma. The use of tape can lead to skin damage, so be careful when establishing IVs on the elderly.

Catheters

Try using the smaller catheters (such as 20-, 22-, or 24-gauge), because they may be more comfortable for the patient and can reduce the risk of extravasation. If fluid resuscitation is necessary, choose an appropriately sized catheter.

IV Sets

Be careful when using macrodrips, because they can allow rapid infusion of fluids, which may lead to edema if they are not monitored closely. With both geriatric and pediatric patients, fluid overloading is potentially serious. If necessary, use the Volutrol IV set to prevent fluid overload **Figure 7-29**.

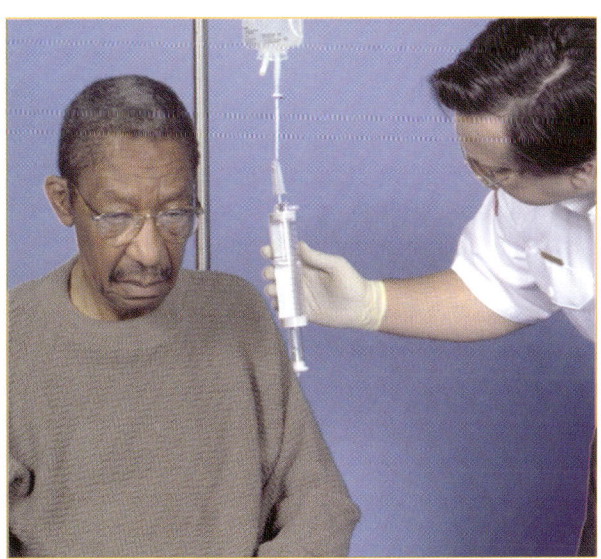

Figure 7-29 If necessary, use the Volutrol IV set to prevent fluid overload.

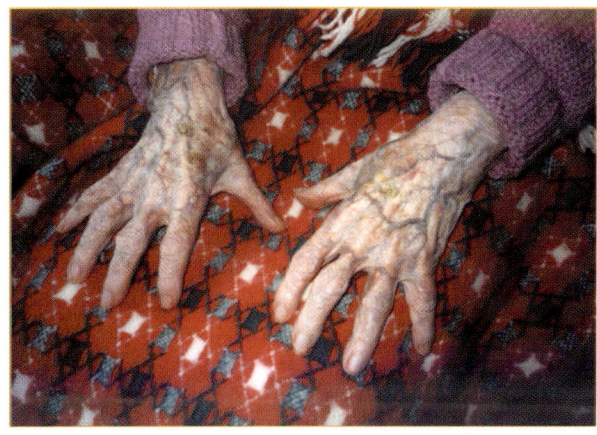

Figure 7-30 When you are looking for an IV site, avoid small spidery veins and varicose veins.

Locations

In choosing an IV site, you should consider the possibility of poor vein elasticity. One of the consequences of aging is the loss of elasticity in the body tissues. Veins become sclerosed, making them brittle. Certain medications, like prednisone, can also affect the structure of the vein, making the veins of geriatric patients even more fragile and easily ruptured. Avoid small spidery veins that weave back and forth **Figure 7-30** because they may rupture easily. Be careful of varicose veins; although they often appear to be ideal choices for IV starts, they are almost completely closed off and allow very little circulation.

> **EMT-I Tips**
>
> Because geriatric patients have more delicate skin, use extra care when establishing IVs and when applying tape to stabilize IVs.

You are the Provider: Summary

1. On the basis of the MOI and patient's complaint, what injuries do you suspect?

Given the MOI and the patient's complaint of leg pain, you should suspect lower extremity and pelvic injuries, probably as a result of striking the dashboard with his knees. You will be able to obtain additional information regarding potential injuries when you see the vehicle.

2. What should you do while you are en route to the scene?

You and your partner should discuss who will do what upon arriving at the scene. If time permits, you should consider alerting the local trauma center to prepare them for a potentially critical patient.

3. What is your impression of the initial assessment findings?

The patient's vital functions—pulse, respirations, and level of consciousness—are abnormal and suggest the presence of shock. Therefore, you should be alert to the possibility of internal bleeding.

4. What do the presence of skid marks tell you about the patient?

The skid marks indicate that the patient was conscious and alert enough to brake or maneuver the car prior to impacting the tree. This is an important finding since underlying medical conditions that alter a patient's level of consciousness (ie, stroke, hypoglycemia, seizures) often result in the crash. Always consider the possibility of an underlying medical cause when evaluating a trauma patient.

5. What size IV catheter should you use?

For critically injured patients, you should use a large-bore (14- or 16-gauge) IV catheter. Large-bore IV catheters will allow you to deliver large amounts of volume over a short period of time, if needed to maintain adequate perfusion.

6. What type of IV tubing is appropriate for this patient?

A macrodrip administration set (10 gtts/mL) should be used in conjunction with large-bore IV catheters for critically injured patients. Macrodrip tubing, like large-bore IV catheters, will also allow you to administer large volumes of fluid over a short period of time.

7. Is it acceptable to delay transport of a critically injured patient in order to start an IV?

Time-consuming procedures, such as IV therapy, should be performed en route to the hospital when managing a critically injured patient. The only exception to this is if the patient will require prolonged extrication and you can access an upper extremity for IV insertion. Remember that definitive care cannot be provided in the prehospital setting for a critically injured patient; the quicker you get the patient to a trauma center, the better.

8. What role do isotonic crystalloid solutions play in the management of a patient in shock?

Crystalloid IV solutions (ie, normal saline, lactated Ringer's) increase circulating volume and maintain adequate perfusion to the tissues and cells of the body. However, unlike whole blood or packed red blood cells, crystalloids do not have the ability to carry oxygen. It is important to remember that crystalloids should be administered to maintain adequate perfusion (ie, radial pulses); they are not used to rapidly increase the patient's blood pressure. Doing so may interfere with the body's hemostatic effect and exacerbate internal bleeding.

Prep Kit

Ready for Review

- The cellular environment contains ions, or electrolytes, that are used by the cell for different purposes, depending on its needs. These ions include sodium, potassium, calcium, bicarbonate, chloride, and phosphorus. Their electrical charges must remain in balance on either side of the cell membrane.
- There must be a balance of compounds on either side of the cell membrane. If an imbalance occurs, the cell can move chemicals or charges across its membrane by various methods, including diffusion, filtration, active transport, and osmosis.
- Understanding the workings of extracellular and intracellular chemicals and charges will provide you with a better foundation for understanding why different types of IV fluids are administered for different conditions.
- Becoming familiar with the various types of IV solutions will give you an understanding of their use in relation to patient conditions.
- Successful IV technique takes practice. Several factors, from the patient's condition to the available IV equipment, influence every IV start. Mastery of IV skills comes when you understand and can overcome all the variables. Take your time when practicing IV starts and gain a solid understanding of what you are doing. This understanding will be useful when you need to perform a quick and flawless IV start in less than optimum conditions.
- Administering IVs to pediatric and geriatric patients requires special care. Both populations are at a higher risk for certain medical conditions that can affect both the patient's need for IV therapy and the effectiveness of the therapy. By understanding the risks and concerns of these populations, you will be better equipped to properly administer IV therapy. Finally, in any medical situation involving pediatric or geriatric patients, remember to be sensitive to the patient's personal issues.

Vital Vocabulary

access port A sealed hub on an administration set designed for sterile access to the IV fluid.

acidosis A pathologic condition resulting from the accumulation of acids in the body.

administration set Tubing that connects to the IV bag access port and the catheter in order to deliver the IV fluid.

alkalosis A pathologic condition resulting from the accumulation of bases in the body.

anaphylaxis An extreme, life-threatening systemic allergic reaction that may include shock and respiratory failure.

angiocath An over-the-needle catheter.

anion An ion that contains an overall negative charge.

antecubital The anterior aspect of the elbow.

anticoagulant A substance that prevents blood from clotting.

antidiuretic hormone (ADH) A hormone produced by the pituitary gland that signals the kidneys to prevent excretion of water.

ataxia A staggered walk or gait caused by injury to the brain or spinal cord.

buffer A substance or group of substances that controls the hydrogen levels in a solution.

butterfly catheter A rigid, hollow, venous cannulation device identified by its plastic "wings" that act as anchoring points for securing the catheter.

cannulation The insertion of a hollow tube into a vein to allow for fluid flow.

Technology

Interactivities
Vocabulary Explorer
Anatomy Review
Web Links
Online Review Manual

Prep Kit continued...

capillary beds The terminal ends of the vascular system where fluids, food, and wastes are exchanged between the vascular system and the cells of the body.

carpopedal spasms Hand/foot spasms; usually the result of hyperventilation or hypocalcemia.

catheter A flexible, hollow structure that delivers fluid.

cation An ion that contains an overall positive charge.

cellular perfusion The ability of a cell to take in oxygen and remove carbon dioxide.

concentration gradient The natural tendency for substances to flow from an area of higher concentration to an area of lower concentration, either within the cell or outside the cell.

contaminated stick The puncturing of an emergency care provider's skin with a catheter that was used on a patient.

crystalloid solution A type of intravenous solution that contains compounds that quickly disassociate in solution and can cross membranes; considered the best choice for prehospital care of injured patients who need fluids to replace lost body fluid.

D_5W An intravenous solution made up of 5% dextrose in water.

depolarization The rapid movement of electrolytes across a cell membrane that changes the cell's overall charge. This rapid shifting of electrolytes and cellular charges is the main catalyst for muscle contractions and neural transmissions.

diabetes insipidus A form of diabetes characterized by polyuria and polydipsia (excessive thirst) that often results from decreased or absent ADH production.

diffusion A process in which molecules move from an area of higher concentration to an area of lower concentration.

drip chamber The area of the administration set where fluid accumulates so that the tubing remains filled with fluid.

drip rate Number of drops per minute.

drip set Another name for an administration set.

electrolyte A charged atom or compound that results from the loss or gain of an electron. These are ions that the body uses to perform certain critical metabolic processes.

epinephrine A hormone (adrenaline) produced by the body and a drug produced by pharmaceutical companies to increase pulse and blood pressure; the drug of choice for an anaphylactic reaction.

external jugular IV IV access established in the jugular veins of the neck.

fascia The fiber-like connective tissue that covers arteries, veins, tendons, and ligaments.

flash chamber The area of a catheter that fills with blood to help indicate when a vein is cannulated.

gtt A measurement that indicates drops.

homeostasis The balance of all systems of the body; also known as homeostatic balance.

hydrophilic Water-loving.

hydrophobic Water-fearing.

hypercalcemia High serum calcium levels.

hyperkalemia High serum levels of potassium.

hypertonic solution A solution that has a greater concentration of sodium than does the cell; the increased extracellular osmotic pressure can draw water out of the cell and cause it to collapse.

hypocalcemia Low serum calcium levels.

hypokalemia Low levels of potassium.

hypotonic solution A solution that has a lower concentration of sodium than does the cell; the increased intracellular osmotic pressure lets water flow into the cell, causing it to swell and possibly burst.

infiltration The escape of fluid into the surrounding tissue.

interstitial Water between the vascular system and the surrounding cells (for example, between the membranes of two cells located outside the vascular compartment in the body).

intraosseous (IO) Within a bone.

intravascular The water portion of the circulatory system surrounding the blood cells (for example, in the heart, arteries, or veins).

ion A charged atom or compound that results from the loss or gain of an electron.

ionic concentration The amount of charged particles found in a particular area.

isotonic solution A solution that has the same concentration of sodium as does the cell. In this case, water does not shift, and no change in cell shape occurs.

Jamshedi needle A type of intraosseous double needle consisting of a solid boring needle inside a sharpened hollow needle.

lactated Ringer's (LR) solution A sterile crystalloid isotonic intravenous solution of specified amounts of calcium chloride, potassium chloride, sodium chloride, and sodium lactate in water.

local reaction Mild to moderate allergic reaction occurring in a localized area.

lysis The rupturing of a cell caused by either the presence of certain enzymes or the uncontrolled influx of material into the cell.

macrodrip set An administration set named for the large orifice between the piercing spike and the drip chamber; allows for rapid fluid flow into the vascular system.

metabolic The breakdown of ingested foodstuffs into smaller and smaller molecules and atoms that are used as energy sources for cellular function.

microdrip set An administration set named for the small orifice between the piercing spike and the drip chamber; allows for carefully controlled fluid flow and is ideally suited for medication administration.

normal saline 0.9% sodium chloride; an isotonic crystalloid.

occlusion Blockage, usually of a tubular structure such as a blood vessel.

opsite A type of sterile covering for IV sites.

osmolarity The ability to influence the movement of water across a semipermeable membrane.

osmosis The movement of water across a cell membrane from an area of lower to higher solute molecules.

osmotic pressure Pressure created against the cell wall by the presence of water.

over-the-needle catheter The prehospital standard for IV cannulation. It consists of a hollow tube over a laser-sharpened steel needle; also referred to as an angiocath.

penrose drain A type of surgical drain often used as a constricting band.

pH A measure of the acidity of a solution. (Potential of hydrogen)

phospholipid bilayer The cell membrane's double layer, consisting of a hydrophilic outer layer composed of phosphate groups, and a hydrophobic inner layer made up of lipids, or fatty acids. It is this structure and composition that allows the cell membrane to have selective permeability.

piercing spike The hard, sharpened plastic spike on the end of the administration set designed to pierce the sterile membrane of the IV bag.

"piggyback" administration The addition of a second IV administration set to a primary line via an access port.

polyuria The passage of an unusually large volume of urine in a given period. In diabetes, polyuria can result from excreting excess glucose in the urine.

postural hypotension Symptomatic drop in blood pressure related to the patient's body position, detected by measuring pulse and blood pressure while the patient is lying supine, sitting up, and standing. An increase in pulse rate and a decrease in blood pressure in any one of these positions is considered a positive sign for this condition.

pulmonary embolus A blood clot trapped within the pulmonary circulation.

saline lock A special type of IV, also called a buff cap or heparin cap.

sclerosis The hardening of a vein from scar tissue after repeated cannulation.

selective permeability The ability of the cell membrane to selectively allow compounds into the cell based on the cell's current needs.

serous linings Single-cell thick membranes found covering organs.

sodium/potassium (Na^+/K^+) pump The mechanism by which the cell brings in two potassium (K^+) ions and releases three sodium (Na^+) ions.

syncopal episode Fainting; brief loss of consciousness caused by transiently inadequate blood flow to the brain.

systemic complications Moderate to severe allergic reaction affecting the systems of the body.

Prep Kit continued...

tachycardia Rapid heart rhythm, more than 100 beats/min.

tachypnea Rapid respirations.

third spacing The shifting of fluid into the tissues, creating edema.

tonicity The osmotic pressure of a solution, based on the relationship between sodium and water inside and outside the cell, that takes advantage of their chemical and osmotic properties to move water to areas of higher sodium concentration.

track marks The visible scars from repeated cannulation of a vein associated with illicit drug use.

tubule A section of the kidney where the filtration of wastes, electrolytes, and water is controlled.

vacutainer A device that connects to a catheter to assist with blood collection.

varicose veins Veins on the leg which are large, twisted, and ropelike, and can cause pain, swelling, or itching.

vasovagal reaction A reaction consisting of precordial distress, anxiety, nausea, and sometimes syncope.

venous thrombosis The development of a stationary blood clot in the venous circulation.

Points to Ponder

You are called to respond to a pediatric emergency. As you arrive on scene you find a young woman holding the infant in her arms. She tells you that her daughter has had vomiting and diarrhea for the last two days and that she is now so sick that she can barely move. You assess the infant and find that she has a decreased LOC and that she is tachycardic and tachypneic. Her eyes are dry and sunken and her mucous membranes are dry. You recognize that the patient is dehydrated. You move her to the ambulance and place her on oxygen. You attempt a peripheral IV but are unable to obtain one so you move to an IO line. You administer a bolus of 20 mL/kg per protocol and place her on the ECG monitor. Transport is uneventful.

Issues: Recognizing the Need for Venous Access in the Critical Pediatric Patient, Recognizing the Need to Move to IO Placement if IV Placement Is Not Possible

Assessment in Action

Mr. Gibbs has a history of cancer that has metastasized to the liver. He has recently noticed that he has more swelling to his legs and his abdomen. Over the last few nights he has had to sleep on an additional pillow to breathe easier. When you are called to his home, you find him to be very short of breath and anxious. He is sweaty and pale with cyanosis to his lips. You note significant edema to his lower extremities and to his abdomen.

You determine that Mr. Gibbs must go to the hospital for definitive care due to his condition. You move him to your ambulance and place him on oxygen. En route to the hospital, you establish IV access and monitor his electrocardiogram.

1. _____ primarily regulates the pH of the stomach and regulates extracellular fluid levels.
   A. Bicarbonate
   B. Calcium
   C. Chloride
   D. Phosphorus

2. Edema is caused by:
   A. increased arterial capillary pressures that push fluid out into the tissues.
   B. decreased production of circulating blood proteins created in the liver.
   C. increased capillary permeability associated with capillary-dilating compounds.
   D. All of the above

3. Colloid solutions:
   A. contain molecules that are too large to pass out of the capillary membrane and therefore remain in the vascular compartment.
   B. work very well in reducing edema while expanding the vascular compartment.
   C. can cause dramatic fluid shifts and place the patient in considerable danger if not administered in a controlled setting.
   D. All of the above

4. Patients like Mr. Gibbs can prove to be difficult IV sticks. A helpful tip would be to:
   A. apply a cold pack to the area.
   B. pat or rub the area.
   C. never stick what you can't see.
   D. tighten the tourniquet and try again.

5. When you are comparing macrodrip and microdrip sets, you should consider that:
   A. the number on the package refers to the number of drops per minute.
   B. the number on the package refers to the number of drops for 1 mL of fluid to pass through the orifice and into the drip chamber.
   C. macrodrips are better for medication administration because it is easy to control their fluid flow.
   D. microdrips are better for fluid replacement because they deliver 60 drops per minute instead of 10.

6. When you are choosing an IV site, you should:
   A. try to find a vein that crosses over a joint.
   B. choose a flat vein because it will not "roll" as much.
   C. avoid any extremity with edema or a dialysis fistula.
   D. start medially and work distally.

www.EMSzone.com/EMTI

Medication Administration

1999 Objectives

Cognitive

1-4.1 Review the specific anatomy and physiology pertinent to medication administration. (p 343)
1-4.2 Review mathematical principles. (p 328)
1-4.3 Review mathematical equivalents. (p 329)
1-4.4 Differentiate temperature readings between the centigrade and Fahrenheit scales. (p 331)
1-4.5 Discuss formulas as a basis for performing drug calculations. (p 329)
1-4.6 Calculate oral and parenteral drug dosages for all emergency medications administered to adults, infants, and children. (p 331)
1-4.8 Discuss legal aspects affecting medication administration. (p 334)
1-4.9 Discuss the "six rights" of drug administration and correlate these with the principles of medication administration. (p 335)
1-4.12 Describe the use of universal precautions and body substance isolation (BSI) procedures when administering a medication. (p 338)
1-4.15 Describe the indications, equipment needed, techniques utilized, precautions, and general principles of administering medications by the inhalation route. (p 336)
1-4.16 Differentiate among the different dosage forms of oral medications. (p 337)
1-4.17 Describe the equipment needed and general principles of administering oral medications. (p 338)
1-4.18 Describe the indications, equipment needed, techniques utilized, precautions, and general principles of rectal medication administration. (p 338)
1-4.19 Differentiate among the different parenteral routes of medication administration. (p 340)
1-4.20 Describe the equipment needed, techniques utilized, complications, and general principles for the preparation and administration of parenteral medications. (p 340)
1-4.21 Differentiate among the different percutaneous routes of medication administration. (p 340)
1-4.24 Synthesize a pharmacologic management plan including medication administration. (p 335)
1-4.25 Integrate pathophysiological principles of medication administration with patient management. (p 336, 338, 349, 351)

Affective

1-4.26 Comply with EMT-Intermediate standards of medication administration. (p 328, 335)
1-4.28 Defend a pharmacologic management plan for medication administration. (p 335)
1-4.30 Serve as a model for advocacy while performing medication administration. (p 335)

Psychomotor

1-4.32 Use universal precautions and body substance isolation (BSI) procedures during medication administration. (p 338)
1-4.35 Demonstrate clean technique during medication administration. (p 335)
1-4.36 Demonstrate administration of medications by the inhalation route. (p 336)
1-4.37 Demonstrate administration of oral medications. (p 338)
1-4.38 Demonstrate rectal administration of medications. (p 338)
1-4.39 Demonstrate preparation and administration of parenteral medications. (p 341)
2-1.74 Perform medication administration with an in-line small-volume nebulizer. (p 336)

1985 Objectives

There are no 1985 objectives for this chapter.

8

Medication Administration

You are the Provider

You and your partner are dispatched to a bus stop in front of 3505 NW Berry Street for a 45-year-old man, unknown medical problem. You arrive to find a man seated on a bench who is confused, sweaty, and slurring his words. You see no signs of trauma, and a bystander tells you he called 9-1-1 because "the guy was acting funny."

As an EMT-I, you will often assess patients with altered mental status; some patients will require medication therapy to treat their condition. This chapter will introduce the principles of math as they relate to pharmacology, teach you how to calculate medication doses, and demonstrate the various techniques used to administer medications. In addition, it will help you answer the following questions:

1. What are the "six rights" of medication administration?
2. Why is it important to conduct a thorough patient assessment before giving medications?

Medication Administration

Before administering *any* medication to a patient, you must have a thorough understanding of how the medication will affect the human body—both negatively and positively. This includes familiarity with the medication's mechanism of action, indications, contraindications, route(s) of administration, dose, and antidotes for adverse reactions; this information was discussed in Chapter 6.

The first rule of medicine—*primum non nocere*—is a Latin term that means "*The first thing (is) to do no harm.*" For example, administering the drug atropine to a patient with *asymptomatic* bradycardia could result in undesirable tachycardia and potential hemodynamic compromise. As a result, you have caused harm to the patient, who otherwise did not need the drug. It is, therefore, paramount to ensure that a particular drug is clearly indicated to treat the patient's condition. A careful assessment of the patient will help ensure that you do this (Figure 8-1).

In addition to knowledge of the medications you may administer as an EMT-I, you must also have an understanding of basic math for pharmacology to calculate the appropriate medication dose. This chapter begins with a review of basic mathematical principles as they apply to pharmacology and concludes with the various methods of medication administration.

Drug doses and flow rate calculations are common areas of confusion for many prehospital personnel, yet they are skills you will need to perform frequently, in the field and during your initial training, while practicing at skill stations. As an EMT-I, you must learn to quickly

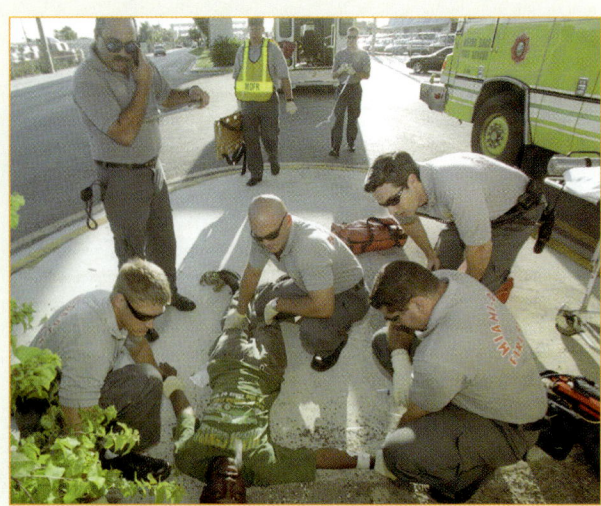

Figure 8-1 Carefully assess the patient before administering a drug.

and accurately calculate doses to maximize the chance for a positive patient outcome. Disastrous results, including death, may be the outcome if you administer an inappropriate drug or dose, give it by the wrong route, or give the medication too rapidly or too slowly.

Mathematical Principles Used in Pharmacology

The Metric System

The metric system is a decimal system based on multiples of ten. It is used to measure length, volume, and weight, which are represented as follows:

- Meter (m): The basic unit of length
- Liter (L): The basic unit of volume
- Gram (g): The basic unit of weight

In the metric system, prefixes demonstrate the fraction of the base being used. Commonly used prefixes, from smallest to largest, include the following:

- micro- = 0.000001
- milli- = 0.001
- centi- = 0.01
- kilo- = 1,000.0

(Table 8-1) illustrates the symbols of weight and volume used in the metric system. It is important to be able to recognize these symbols, because drugs will be supplied in a variety of weights and volumes, and you will be required to convert these weights to volume to administer the appropriate dose of a medication to your patient.

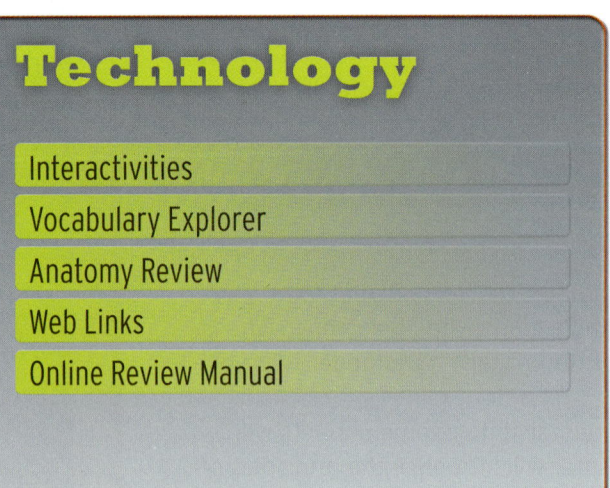

Technology

- Interactivities
- Vocabulary Explorer
- Anatomy Review
- Web Links
- Online Review Manual

www.EMSzone.com/EMTI

TABLE 8-1	Symbols Used in the Metric System

Symbols of weight (smallest to largest)
- microgram = μg (or mcg)
- milligram = mg
- gram = g (or gm)
- kilogram = kg

Symbols of volume (smallest to largest)
- milliliter = mL
- deciliter = dL
- liter = L

TABLE 8-2	Metric Units and Their Equivalents

Units of weight (smallest to largest)
- 1 μg = 0.001 mg
- 1 mg = 1,000 μg
- 1 g = 1,000 mg
- 1 kg = 1,000 g

Units of volume (smallest to largest)
- 1 mL = 1 cc*
- 100 mL = 1 dL
- 1,000 mL = 1 L

* Cubic centimeter (cc) is a unit also used to represent milliliters (mL); therefore, 1 cc is the same as 1 mL (1 cc = 1 mL).

Table 8-2 illustrates the metric units of weight and volume and their equivalents. Again, you must be able to understand these metric unit equivalents for proper drug conversion and subsequent administration.

> **EMT-I Tips**
>
> In the administration of drugs, a working knowledge of the metric system is imperative.

Weight and Volume Conversion

To administer the appropriate dose of a medication to a patient, you must be able to convert larger units of weight to smaller ones (for example, g to mg) and larger units of volume to smaller ones (for example, L to mL). Conversely, you must also be able to convert smaller units of weight to larger ones (for example, mg to g) and smaller units of volume to larger ones (for example, mL to L).

Drugs are packaged in different units of weight and volume; however, the weight (for example, μg, mg, g) and volume (for example, mL) of the drug to be administered is usually only a fraction of the total amount of its packaged form. For example, a physician may order 50 mg of a drug for a patient, but the drug is packaged in grams. Therefore, you must be able to convert grams to milligrams and then determine how much volume is required to achieve the desired dose.

Weight Conversion

Converting weight is simply a matter of multiplying or dividing by 1,000 *or* moving the decimal point 3 places to the right or left. To convert a larger unit of weight to a smaller one, multiply the larger unit of weight by 1,000

You are the Provider — Part 2

You perform an initial assessment of the patient, which reveals the following:

Initial Assessment	Recording Time: Zero Minutes
Level of consciousness	Conscious but disoriented; slurred speech
Airway	Open and clear
Breathing	Respirations, increased and shallow
Circulation	Radial pulses, weak and rapid; skin, cool and clammy; no gross bleeding

3. How should you manage this patient initially?
4. Other than oxygen, are any other medications indicated at this particular time?

or simply move the decimal point 3 places to the right, as demonstrated in the following examples:

> Example 1:
> Converting 2 g to mg (2g = X mg)
> 2 g × 1,000 = 2,000 mg   or   2.000 = 2,000 mg
>
> Example 2:
> Converting 5 mg to μg (5 mg = X μg)
> 5 mg × 1,000 = 5,000 μg   or   5.000 = 5,000 μg

Conversely, to convert a smaller unit of weight to a larger one, divide the smaller unit of weight by 1,000 *or* simply move the decimal point 3 places to the left, as demonstrated in the following examples:

> Example 1:
> Converting 200 μg to mg (200 μg = X mg)
> 200 μg ÷ 1,000 = 0.2 mg   or   200. = 0.2 mg
>
> Example 2:
> Converting 250 mg to g (250 mg = X g)
> 250 mg ÷ 1,000 = 0.25 g   or   250. = 0.25 g

Volume Conversion

In the prehospital setting, you will usually be dealing with only two measurements of volume: milliliters and liters. The formula is the same as with converting units of weight—simply dividing or multiplying by 1,000 *or* moving the decimal point 3 places to the left or right.

When converting a smaller unit of volume to a larger one (for example, mL to L), divide the smaller unit of volume by 1,000 *or* simply move the decimal point 3 places to the left, as demonstrated in the following examples:

> Example 1:
> Converting 100 mL to L (100 mL = X L)
> 100 mL ÷ 1,000 = 0.1 L   or   100. = 0.1 L
>
> Example 2:
> Converting 250 mL to L (250 mL = X L)
> 250 mL ÷ 1,000 = 0.25 L   or   250. = 0.25 L

Conversely, when converting a larger unit of volume to a smaller one (for example, L to mL), multiply the larger unit of volume by 1,000 *or* simply move the decimal point 3 places to the right, as demonstrated in the following examples:

> Example 1:
> Converting 1.5 L to mL (1.5 L = X mL)
> 1.5 L × 1,000 = 1,500 mL   or   1.500 = 1,500 mL
>
> Example 2:
> Converting 25 L to mL (25 L = X mL)
> 25 L × 1,000 = 25,000 mL   or   25.000 = 25,000 mL

> **EMT-I Tips**
>
> When converting units of weight or volume, remember these basic rules:
>
> *Weight conversion*
> *Smaller to larger (for example, μg to mg, mg to g):* Divide the smaller unit by 1,000 *or* move the decimal point 3 places to the left.
> *Larger to smaller (for example, mg to μg, g to mg):* Multiply the larger unit by 1,000 *or* move the decimal point 3 places to the right.
>
> *Volume conversion*
> *Smaller to larger (for example, mL to L):* Divide the smaller unit by 1,000 *or* move the decimal point 3 places to the left.
> *Larger to smaller (for example, L to mL):* Multiply the larger unit by 1,000 *or* move the decimal point 3 places to the right.

Converting Pounds to Kilograms

It would be a luxury if your patients were able to tell you how much they weighed in kilograms (kg); however, the chances of this happening are slim to none. For patients who do not know their weight in pounds or who are unconscious and unable to provide you with this information, you must do the following:

1. Estimate the patient's weight in pounds (lb)
2. Convert pounds to kilograms (kg)

Although many of the drugs given in emergency medicine are administered in a standard dose (for example, 1 mg of epinephrine), others are administered based on the patient's weight in kilograms (for example, 1–1.5 mg/kg of lidocaine). In addition, most drugs administered to pediatric patients are based on their weight in kilograms.

There are two formulas that can be used to convert pounds to kilograms; use the one that is easiest for you to remember.

Formula 1: Divide the patient's weight in pounds by 2.2 (1 kg = 2.2 lb)

For example, when converting a 170-lb man's weight to kilograms, the formula would be as follows:

$$170 \text{ lb} \div 2.2 = 77.27 \text{ kg}$$

Because the value following the decimal point in the preceding example is less than 0.5, you may round the patient's weight in kg to 77.0. If the value after the decimal point had been greater than 0.5, you would round the weight in kg to 78.0. Although this may seem negligible, it is important to administer the *most* appropriate amount of the drug to the patient; it's good practice.

Formula 2: Divide the patient's weight in pounds by 2 and subtract 10%

For example, when converting a 120-lb woman's weight to kg, the formula would be as follows:

Step 1: 120 lb ÷ 2 = 60 lb
Step 2: 60 lb × 10% = 6
Step 3: 60 − 6 = 54 kg

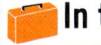

In the Field

Carry a calculator or EMS field guide to assist you in converting pounds to kilograms.

The Apothecary System

The apothecary system was formerly used by physicians and pharmacists but has now been replaced by the metric system.

It is based on 480 grains (gr) to 1 oz and 16 oz to 1 lb. The grain (gr) is the basic unit of weight and is approximately the weight of a drop of water. The minim is the unit of volume and is approximately the volume of a drop of water. Additional units of volume are the pint (pt), quart (qt), and gallon (gal), which are the units most familiar to people in the United States. Fractions are used in the apothecary system.

Fahrenheit and Celsius Scales

The Fahrenheit and Celsius (or centigrade) scales are commonly used to measure temperature. On the Celsius scale, water freezes at 0° and boils at 100°. On the Fahrenheit scale, water freezes at 32° and boils at 212°.

Although there are several methods to convert Fahrenheit temperature readings to Celsius and Celsius to Fahrenheit, the following represents a common conversion method:

Converting Fahrenheit to Celsius
°C = (°F − 32) × 5 ÷ 9

For example, to convert 212°F (the boiling point of water on the Fahrenheit scale) to Celsius, subtract 32 from 212 (180), multiply 180 by 5 (900), and divide 900 by 9. Following this equation, 212°F equals 100°C (the boiling point of water on the Celsius scale).

Converting Celsius to Fahrenheit
°F = (°C × 9) ÷ 5 + 32

For example, to convert 37°C to Fahrenheit, multiply 37 by 9 (333), divide 333 by 5 (66.6), and add 32. In this equation, 37°C equals 98.6°F (normal body temperature).

Calculating Medication Doses

There are multiple formulas for calculating medication doses. It is beyond the scope of this chapter to demonstrate *every* one of these calculation formulas. Therefore, the discussion in this chapter will be limited to formulas that most students find easy to understand. For other calculation formulas, the EMT-I is encouraged to consult with his or her instructor. The method of drug dose calculation demonstrated in this chapter will be based on the following three factors:

1. Desired dose
2. Concentration of the drug available (dose on hand)
3. Volume to be administered

Desired Dose

The desired dose (that is, the drug order) is the amount of a drug that the physician orders you to give to a patient. It may be expressed as a standard dose (for

EMT-I Tips

Although many drug doses are based on standard protocols, such as those outlined in the Advanced Cardiac Life Support (ACLS) algorithms, you must always follow your local protocols and contact medical control as needed.

example, 10 mg of diazepam [Valium]; 25 g of dextrose), or it may be expressed as a specific number of grams or milligrams per kilogram of body weight (for example, 1–1.5 mg/kg of lidocaine [Xylocaine]).

Drug Concentrations

After receiving a drug order (that is, the desired dose), you must determine how much of the drug that you have available. In other words, you must know its <u>concentration</u>—the total weight (μg, mg, or g) of the drug contained in a specific volume (mL or L). The following are examples of common prepackaged drug concentrations:

- Lidocaine, 100 mg/10 mL
- Epinephrine, 1 mg/10 mL
- Furosemide (Lasix), 40 mg/4 mL
- Adenosine, 6 mg/2 mL
- 50% Dextrose, 25 g/50 mL

In the preceding examples, you will notice that the drugs are contained in different volumes of solution. *However, to administer a drug, you must know the weight of the drug that is present in each milliliter.* This will tell you the concentration of the drug that you have on hand. The formula for calculating this is as follows:

Total Weight of the Drug ÷ Total Volume in Milliliters = Weight per Milliliter

By using the preceding formula and the examples of common prepackaged drugs, you will calculate how much of the drug is contained in each milliliter (dose on hand).

<u>Lidocaine, 100 mg/10 mL:</u>
100 mg (total weight) ÷ 10 mL (total volume) = 10 mg/mL

<u>Epinephrine, 1 mg/10 mL:</u>
1 mg (total weight) ÷ 10 mL (total volume) = 0.1 mg/mL

<u>Furosemide, 40 mg/4 mL:</u>
40 mg (total weight) ÷ 4 mL (total volume) = 10 mg/mL

<u>Adenosine, 6 mg/2 mL:</u>
6 mg (total weight) ÷ 2 mL (total volume) = 3 mg/mL

<u>Dextrose, 25 g/50 mL:</u>
25 g (total weight) ÷ 50 mL (total volume) = 0.5 gm/mL

Volume to be Administered

After determining the concentration of the drug present in each milliliter (dose on hand), you must calculate how much volume is needed to give the amount of the drug ordered (desired dose). Use the following formula to calculate the volume to be administered:

Desired Dose (μg, mg, g) ÷ Dose on Hand (mg/mL) = Volume to be Administered (mL)

On the basis of the preceding formula, you will be able to determine how much volume to give to achieve the required dose. Here are some examples.

Example 1: Medical control orders you to administer 5 mg of diazepam to your patient for sedation. You have a vial of diazepam, which contains 20 mg in 5 mL. How many mL of diazepam must you give to achieve the ordered dose of 5 mg?
Step 1: Determine the concentration/dose on hand (in mg/mL)
- 20 mg ÷ 5 mL = 4 mg/mL (dose on hand)

Step 2: Determine how much volume to administer
- 5 mg (desired dose) ÷ 4 mg/mL (dose on hand) = 1.25 mL

Example 2: A patient requires 0.5 mg of atropine for the treatment of unstable bradycardia. You have a prefilled syringe, which contains 1 mg of atropine in 10 mL. How many milliliters of atropine will you give?
Step 1: Determine the concentration/dose on hand (in mg/mL)
- 1 mg ÷ 10 mL = 0.1 mg/mL (dose on hand)

Step 2: Determine how much volume to administer
- 0.5 mg (desired dose) ÷ 0.1 mg/mL (dose on hand) = 5 mL

Example 3: You are ordered to administer 12.5 g of dextrose to a hypoglycemic patient. You have a prefilled syringe of 50% dextrose containing 25 g in 50 mL. How many milliliters of dextrose will you give?

EMT-I Tips

Drugs represented as a percentage, such as 50% dextrose, indicate the number of grams per 100 mL (1 dL) of volume. Therefore, 50% dextrose contains 50 g of glucose per 100 mL of volume. Other examples include 2% lidocaine, which contains 2 g of lidocaine in 1 dL, and 0.9% (0.9 g or 900 mg) sodium chloride contains 900 mg/dL.

Step 1: Determine the concentration/dose on hand (in g/mL)
- 25 g ÷ 50 mL = 0.5 g/mL (dose on hand)

Step 2: Determine how much volume to administer
- 12.5 g (desired dose) ÷ 0.5 g/mL (dose on hand) = 25 mL

Weight-Based Drug Doses

As previously discussed, some medication doses are based on the patient's weight in kilograms. Determining the appropriate dose for the patient requires simply converting the patient's weight in pounds to kilograms and then proceeding with the formula that we just discussed. Remember, 1 kg equals 2.2 lb.

The following are some examples of how to calculate the appropriate drug dose based on the patient's weight:

Example 1: You are ordered to give 1 mg/kg of lidocaine to your 170-lb patient who has ventricular fibrillation. You have a prefilled syringe of lidocaine containing 100 mg in 10 mL. How many milligrams will you give to this patient (that is, what is the drug order)? How much volume will you give to achieve the required dose?

Step 1: Convert the patient's weight in pounds to kilograms
- Formula 1: 170 lb ÷ 2.2 = 77.27 kg (round to 77 kg)
- Formula 2: 170 lb ÷ 2 − 10% = 76.5 (round to 77 kg)

Step 2: Determine the desired dose
- 1 mg × 77 kg = 77 mg (desired dose)

Step 3: Determine the concentration/dose on hand (in mg/mL)
- 100 mg ÷ 10 mL = 10 mg/mL (dose on hand)

Step 4: Determine how much volume to administer
- 77 mg (desired dose) ÷ 10 mg/mL (dose on hand) = 7.7 mL (round to 8 mL)

Example 2: A 4-year-old boy in asystole requires 0.01 mg/kg of epinephrine. You have a prefilled syringe of epinephrine containing 1 mg in 10 mL. The child's mother tells you that he weighs 35 lb. How many milligrams will you give to this patient (that is, what is the desired dose)? How much volume will you give to achieve the required dose?

Step 1: Convert the patient's weight in pounds to kilograms
- Formula 1: 35 lb ÷ 2.2 = 15.9 kg (round to 16 kg)
- Formula 2: 35 lb ÷ 2 − 10% = 15.75 kg (round to 16 kg)

Step 2: Determine the desired dose
- 0.01 mg × 16 kg = 0.16 mg (desired dose)

Step 3: Determine the concentration/dose on hand (in mg/mL)
- 1 mg ÷ 10 mL = 0.1 mg/mL (dose on hand)

Step 4: Determine how much volume to administer
- 16 mg (desired dose) ÷ 0.1 mg/mL (dose on hand) = 1.6 mL (round to 2 mL)

Calculating the Dose and Rate for a Medication Infusion

Following the administration of certain drugs, you may need to begin a continuous infusion to maintain a therapeutic blood level of the drug to prevent a recurrence of the condition. Medication infusions are usually ordered to be administered in a specified period of time, usually per minute.

To calculate a continuous medication infusion, you must know the following information in advance:
1. The desired dose (μg/min or mg/min)
2. The rate for the intravenous (IV) administration set (drops [gtt]/mL)

You will use the same formula to calculate a drug dose as previously discussed; however, you will then calculate the desired dose to be administered continuously, usually a certain number of micrograms (μg) or milligrams (mg) per minute.

For example, you have just administered 75 mg of lidocaine to your patient in cardiac arrest, after which time his heart rhythm converts to a perfusing rhythm. Medical control then orders you to begin a continuous lidocaine infusion at 2 mg/min.

By using the formulas previously discussed, we must determine how many drops (gtt) per minute to set the IV drip rate to deliver the 2 mg/min desired dose.

To do this, add a certain amount of lidocaine into a bag of IV fluid. For demonstrative purposes, we will add 2 g (2,000 mg) of lidocaine to a 500-mL bag of normal saline, a common combination. The formula to calculate the continuous infusion rate would be as follows:

Step 1: Determine the concentration/dose on hand
- 2,000 mg (2 g) of lidocaine ÷ 500 mL normal saline = 4 mg/mL (dose on hand)

Step 2: Determine the amount of volume to infuse per minute (mL/min)

To do this, you must recall the number of milligrams the physician ordered you to infuse per minute. In this case, it is 2 mg/min. Therefore, to determine the number of mL/min, the calculation continues as follows:

- 2 mg (desired dose) ÷ 4 mg/mL (dose on hand) = 0.5 mL/min

Step 3: Determine how many drops per minute (gtt/min) at which to set the IV flow rate

To do this, you must know the number of drops per milliliter (gtt/mL) that your IV administration set delivers—a microdrip (60 gtt/mL) or a macrodrip (10 gtt/mL). Microdrip infusion sets are typically used when administering a continuous medication infusion. For a microdrip set, the number of drops per minute for the IV flow rate would be calculated as follows:

- 0.5 mL/min × 60 gtt/mL ÷ total time in minutes (1) = 30 gtt/min

Pediatric Doses

There are numerous methods for determining the appropriate dose of medication for a pediatric patient. Many rescuers use length-based resuscitation tapes; others may carry a field guide with tables or charts for reference. Most drugs used in pediatric emergency medicine are based on the child's weight in kilograms. The calculations for pediatric drug dosing and medication infusions are the same as they are for adults, but the doses and volumes will be obviously smaller.

EMT-I Tips

When administering a continuous medication infusion, remember these rules:

1. When adding a certain number of grams of a drug to a bag of IV fluid, *you must convert the drug into milligrams*. For example, if you place 2 g of lidocaine into the IV fluid, you must use 2,000 mg (2 g) to determine the concentration/dose on hand.
2. Always divide the amount of the drug by the *total number of minutes* over which the medication will be infused. For example, do not divide by 1 hour, divide by 60 minutes.

Medical Direction

Medication administration is governed by the EMT-I's local protocols and/or online medical direction. The medical director for your service may allow the administration of certain medications as long as the patient meets certain criteria. For example, for a patient with a cardiac history experiencing chest pain and a systolic blood pressure of at least 90 mm Hg, the EMT-I may be allowed by written protocols or online medical control

You are the Provider — Part 3

As your partner obtains vital signs, you perform a blood glucose test. You find that his blood glucose level is 40 mg/dL. According to your standing orders, you initiate an IV of normal saline and prepare to give 50% dextrose (D_{50}).

Vital Signs	Recording Time: 5 Minutes After Patient Contact
Blood pressure	100/68 mm Hg
Pulse	120 beats/min, weak and regular
Respirations	36 breaths/min and shallow (baseline); your partner is assisting ventilations with a bag-valve-mask device and 100% oxygen
Sao_2	98% (with assisted ventilations and 100% oxygen)

5. Because D_{50} is a hypertonic solution, what contraindications exist for administration of this medication?
6. What must be confirmed before administering this drug? Why is this important?

EMT-I Tips

It is important to administer the *most* appropriate dose of a drug to a child. Many parents or caregivers know how much their children weigh in pounds, which you can easily convert to kilograms (1 kg = 2.2 lb). If a parent or caregiver is available, simply ask the child's weight; do not attempt to estimate the child's weight if it is not necessary.

EMT-I Safety

Medical asepsis is the term applied to the practice of preventing contamination of the patient by using aseptic technique. This is a method of cleansing used to prevent contamination of a site when performing an invasive procedure such as starting an IV line or administering a medication. Medical asepsis may be accomplished through the use of sterilization of equipment used, antiseptics, or disinfectants.

to administer nitroglycerin up to three times as long as the blood pressure remains adequate. Local policies and procedures are designed to guide the EMT-I in specific situations. When questions or unusual situations arise, contact medical control for direction.

Principles of Medication Administration

Most EMS services carry "drug boxes" with a variety of cardiac drugs, pain medications, anticonvulsants, antiemetics, and other drugs specific to their service. The medical director generally makes the determination of what medications will be carried on the unit.

When requesting orders to give a particular medication, the EMT-I has the responsibility to make sure that the medication is indicated for the patient's condition. Once an order has been given by medical control, the EMT-I must repeat, word-for-word, the information to medical control for verification. If any medication order is unclear or seems inappropriate for the patient's condition, the EMT-I should voice the concerns to medical control, repeating pertinent patient information as necessary to ensure that he or she was heard correctly the first time. Before giving any drug, review the "six rights" of medication administration:

- Right patient
- Right drug
- Right dose
- Right route
- Right time
- Right documentation

You are the Provider — Part 4

You determine the IV line is patent and then administer the appropriate dose of D_{50}. You reassess the patient's condition for any changes. He resists assisted ventilation, so your partner applies a nonrebreathing mask at 15 L/min.

Reassessment	Recording Time: 8 Minutes After Patient Contact
Level of consciousness	Improved; patient is conscious and alert to person, place, and time
Blood pressure	130/70 mm Hg
Pulse	90 beats/min, strong and regular
Respirations	20 breaths/min, adequate depth
Sao_2	99% with oxygen at 15 L/min via nonrebreathing mask

7. You must know what routes of administration are appropriate for each and every drug you give. What is the reasoning behind this essential knowledge?
8. D_{50} is prepackaged as 25 g in 50 mL. How many milligrams are in each milliliter?

Medications Administered by the Inhalation Route

Many medications used in the treatment of respiratory emergencies are administered via the inhalation route. The most common inhaled medication is oxygen. Bronchodilator (beta-agonist) medications are often administered in the prehospital setting for patients experiencing respiratory distress caused by certain obstructive airway diseases, such as asthma, bronchitis, and emphysema. Check your drug reference guide or the package insert for indications, contraindications, and precautions before giving any medication.

A patient with a history of respiratory problems will usually have a metered-dose inhaler (also called MDI) to use on a regular basis or as needed (Figure 8-2). For more severe problems, liquid bronchodilators may be aerosolized in a nebulizer for inhalation. Small-volume nebulizers, also called updraft or handheld nebulizers, are the most commonly used method of administration of inhaled medications in the prehospital arena (Figure 8-3). Oxygen or a compressed air source is connected to the nebulizer to produce the aerosolized mist. The mist may be delivered through a mouthpiece held by the patient or by a mask for young children and those who are unable to hold the mouthpiece.

Drugs given through an endotracheal tube are also considered inhaled medications.

Follow the steps in (Skill Drill 8-1) to administer a medication via small-volume nebulizer:

1. Take BSI precautions.
2. Determine the need for an inhaled bronchodilator based on patient presentation.
3. Obtain a focused history and physical exam, including any drug allergies.
4. Follow standing orders, or contact medical control for permission.
5. Check the medication and its expiration date. Make sure you have the right medication and that it is not cloudy or discolored (**Step 1**).
6. If the medication is in a premixed package, add it to the bowl of the nebulizer. If not premixed, add the medication to the bowl and mix it with the specified amount of normal saline, usually 3 mL (**Step 2**).
7. Connect the T piece with the mouthpiece to the top of the bowl, or the mask to the bowl, and connect it to the oxygen tubing.
8. Set the flowmeter at 6 L/min to produce a steady mist (**Step 3**).
9. With the metered-dose inhaler (MDI) or handheld nebulizer in position, instruct the patient on the proper way to breathe. Have the patient breathe as deeply as possible and hold his or her breath for 3 to 5 seconds before exhaling. Continue to coach the patient as needed.
10. Monitor the patient's condition, and document the medication given, route, time of administration, and response of the patient (**Step 4**).
11. Cardiac monitoring is essential when administering a beta-agonist. If cardiac dysrhythmias are noted, stop the administration of the medication, administer high-flow oxygen, and contact medical control.

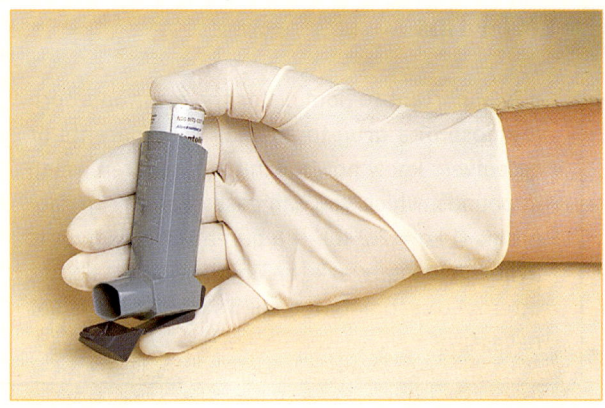

Figure 8-2 Some medications are inhaled into the lungs with a metered-dose inhaler so that they can be absorbed into the bloodstream more quickly.

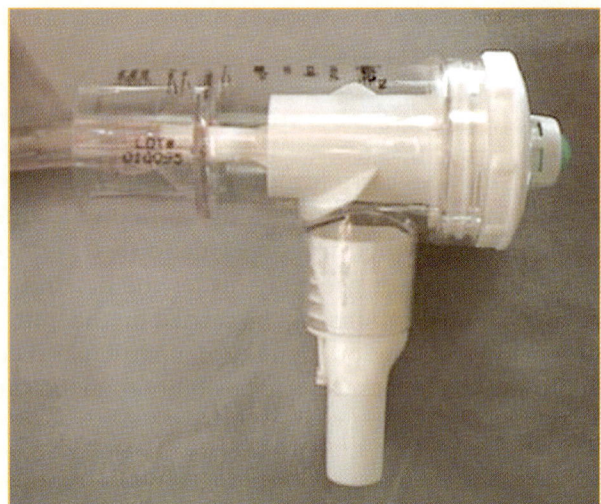

Figure 8-3 A small-volume nebulizer is used to deliver medications via aerosolized mist.

Skill Drill 8-1: Administering Medication Via Small-Volume Nebulizer

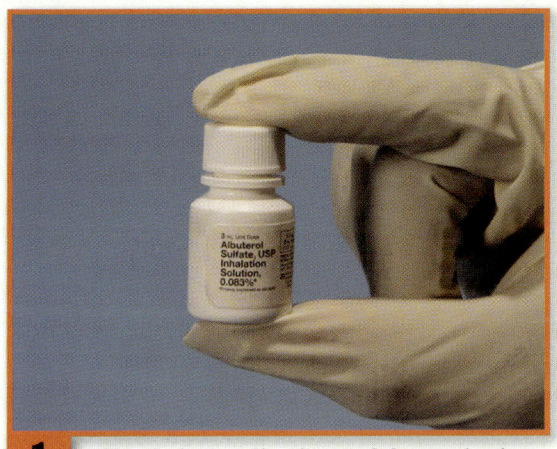
1. Check the medication and the expiration date.

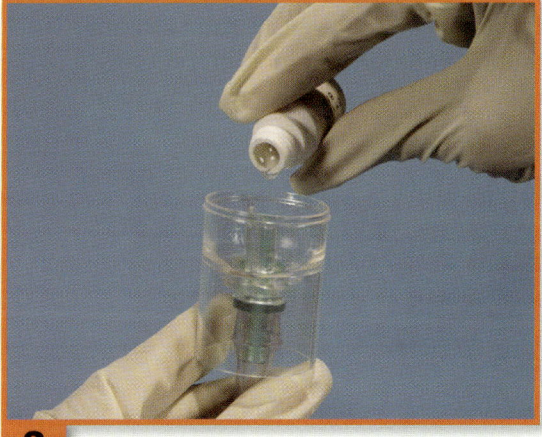
2. Add premixed medication to the bowl of the nebulizer.

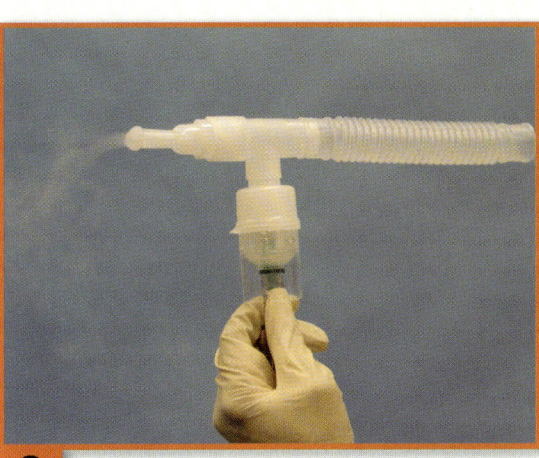
3. Connect the T piece with the mouthpiece to the top of the bowl, connect it to the oxygen tubing, and set the flowmeter at 6 L/min.

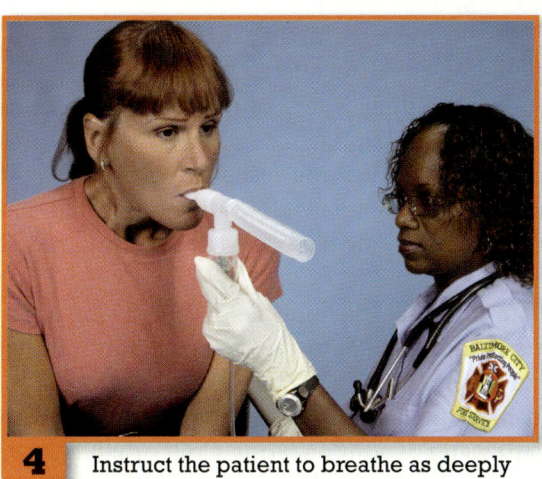
4. Instruct the patient to breathe as deeply as possible and hold his or her breath for 3 to 5 seconds before exhaling. Monitor the patient for effects.

Enteral Medication Administration

Enteral medications are those that are given through some portion of the digestive or intestinal tract. This includes orally, through a feeding tube, or rectally.

Oral Administration

Forms of solid and liquid oral medications include capsules, timed-release capsules, lozenges, pills, tablets, elixirs, emulsions, suspensions, and syrups Figure 8-4 ▶. These are discussed in Chapter 6.

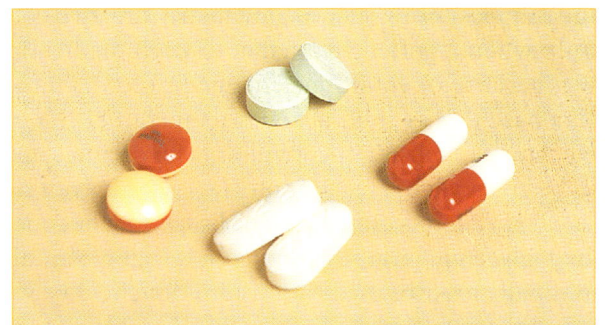

Figure 8-4 Tablets and capsules, oral medications typically taken by mouth, enter the bloodstream through the digestive system.

To give oral medications, you may use a small medicine cup, a medicine dropper, a teaspoon, an oral syringe, or a nipple. Gather the appropriate equipment for the form of medication you are administering. Check for indications, contraindications, precautions, and the six rights before administering any medication.

> **EMT-I Safety**
>
> BSI precautions should be used any time you are administering a medication.

Follow these steps when administering an oral medication Figure 8-5 :

1. Take BSI precautions.
2. Determine the need for the medication based on patient presentation.
3. Obtain a focused history and physical exam, including any drug allergies.
4. Follow standing orders, or contact medical control for permission.
5. Check the medication to be sure it is the right medication and not cloudy or discolored and that its expiration date has not passed. Check the six rights.
6. Determine the appropriate dose. If using a liquid medication, pour the desired amount into a calibrated cup.
7. Instruct the patient to swallow the medication with water, if administering a pill or tablet.
8. Monitor the patient's condition, and document the medication given, route, time of administration, and response of the patient.

Rectal Administration

Medications that may be given rectally come in various forms. Suppositories, such as antiemetics, are used commonly when a patient is unable to keep medication down because of vomiting. The medication is mixed into a base that is solid at room temperature. Liquid medications, such as anticonvulsants for seizures, may also be given via the rectal route. D_{50} is also given rectally when IV access cannot be established and the patient is hypoglycemic. The rectal mucosa is highly vascular and rapidly absorbs medications; it is an effective way to administer certain medications if IV or intraosseous (IO) access cannot be obtained Figure 8-6 . Check

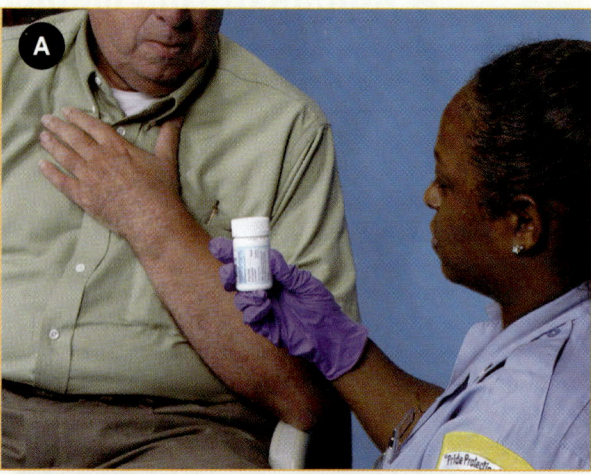
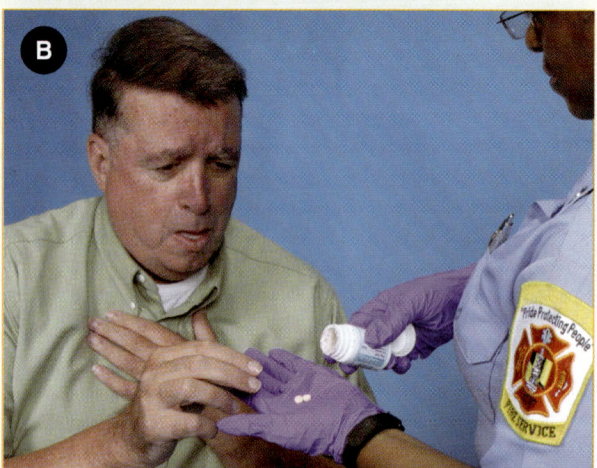

Figure 8-5 Administering an oral medication. **A.** Check the medication and its expiration date. **B.** Have the patient take the medication. Administer a cup of water if necessary.

for indications, contraindications, and precautions before giving any drug rectally.

Follow these steps to administer a drug rectally:

1. Take BSI precautions.
2. Determine the need for the medication based on patient presentation.
3. Obtain a focused history and physical exam, including any drug allergies.
4. Follow standing orders, or contact medical control for permission.
5. Determine the appropriate dose, and check that the medication is the right medication, there is no cloudiness or discoloration, and the expiration date has not passed.
6. When inserting a suppository, use a water-soluble gel for lubrication. Insert the supposi-

tory into the rectum approximately 1″ to 1½″ while instructing the patient to relax and not to bear down.

7. For medications that are in liquid form, some modifications are needed. You may use a nasopharyngeal airway or a small endotracheal tube as your delivery route.

   a. Lubricate the end of the nasal airway or endotracheal tube with a water-soluble gel, and gently insert it approximately 1″ to 1½″ into the rectum. Instruct the patient to relax and not to bear down Figure 8-7 ▼.

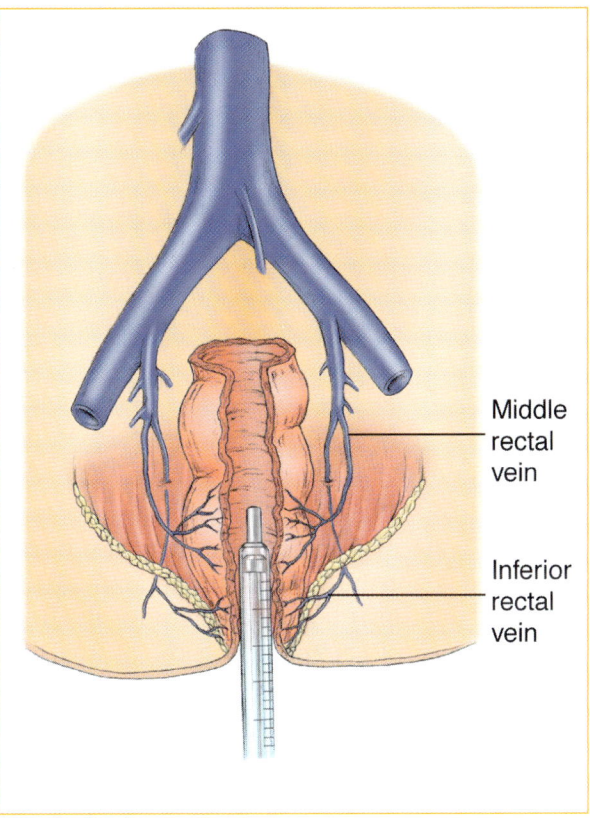

Figure 8-6 The rectal mucosa is highly vascular and rapidly absorbs medications.

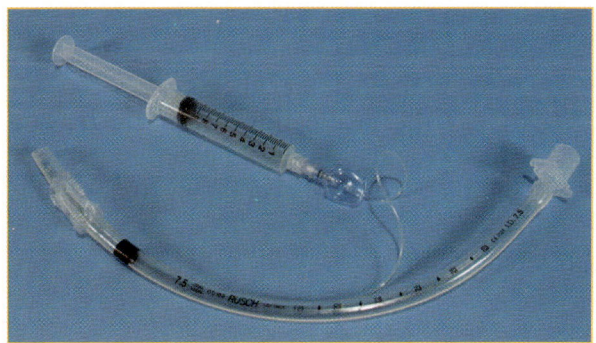

Figure 8-7 Syringe attached to an endotracheal tube.

You are the Provider   Part 5

Your patient's condition continues to improve. He is able to answer questions appropriately but is still unsure of the events leading up to his hypoglycemia. Your reassessment findings are as follows:

Reassessment	Recording Time: 12 Minutes After Patient Contact
Level of consciousness	Conscious and alert to person, place, and time
Blood pressure	128/74 mm Hg
Pulse	88 beats/min, strong and regular
Respirations	20 breaths/min, adequate depth
Sao_2	99% (with 100% oxygen via nonrebreathing mask)

9. Is further treatment required for this patient?
10. What does the "%" in 50% dextrose indicate?

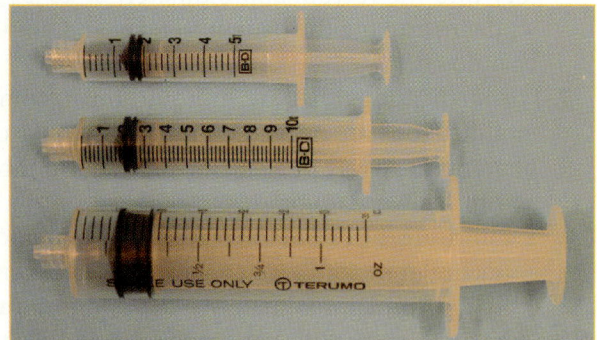

Figure 8-8 Syringes come in a variety of sizes. Some come with needles already attached, others without needles attached.

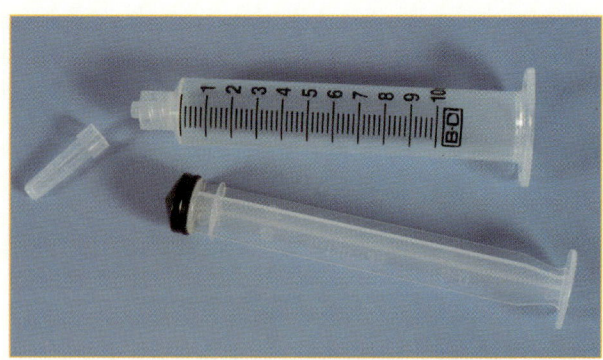

Figure 8-9 A syringe consists of a plunger, body or barrel, flange, and tip.

   b. With a needleless syringe, gently push the medication through the tube 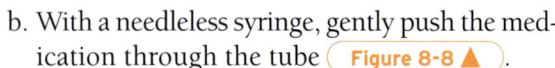.
   c. Once the medication has been delivered, remove and dispose of the tube.
8. Monitor the patient's condition, and document the medication given, route, time of administration, and response of the patient.

Parenteral Administration of Medications

Parenteral medications are those that are given through any route other than the gastrointestinal tract. Parenteral routes used by the EMT-I include subcutaneous, intramuscular, IV bolus, IO, sublingual, transcutaneous, and transdermal. Of the parenteral drug routes, IV administration is the most common route used in the prehospital setting and generally is the quickest route for getting medication into the central circulation.

> **EMT-I Tips**
>
> Any medication that is administered directly through the skin, such as the subcutaneous or intramuscular route, is referred to as "percutaneous" administration.

Equipment

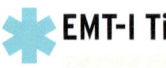

A variety of needles and syringes are used for administering parenteral medications. Most syringes come prepackaged in color-coded packs with a needle already attached. The needles and syringes may also be packaged separately. You must choose the appropriate size of syringe and appropriate needle length for the desired route. Syringes consist of a plunger, body or barrel, flange, and tip. All hypodermic syringes are marked with 10 calibrations per milliliter on one side of the barrel. Each small line represents 0.1 mL. The other side of the barrel is marked in minims (an apothecary measurement). The 3-mL syringe is the most common used for injections, but others are available as needed. Needle lengths vary from 3/8" to 1" for standard injections. The gauge of the needle refers to the diameter; the smaller the number, the larger the diameter.

Packaging of Parenteral Medications

Parenteral medications are most commonly packaged in ampules, vials, and prefilled syringes. Ampules are breakable sterile glass containers that are designed to carry a single dose of medication. Vials may contain single or multiple doses. Vials have a rubber-stopper top and are made of glass or plastic. Many drugs used in prehospital care are carried in vials. Prefilled syringes are designed for ease of use. It is much easier and quicker to use a prefilled syringe when you are treating a patient in cardiac arrest than it is to draw up each individual dose. There are also single-dose disposable cartridges that use a reusable syringe such as a Tubex or Aboject. Some medications may need to be reconstituted, such as methylprednisolone sodium succinate (Solu-Medrol) and glucagon. These come with two vials, one with a powdered form of the drug and one with sterile water. Drug reconstitution involves injecting the sterile water

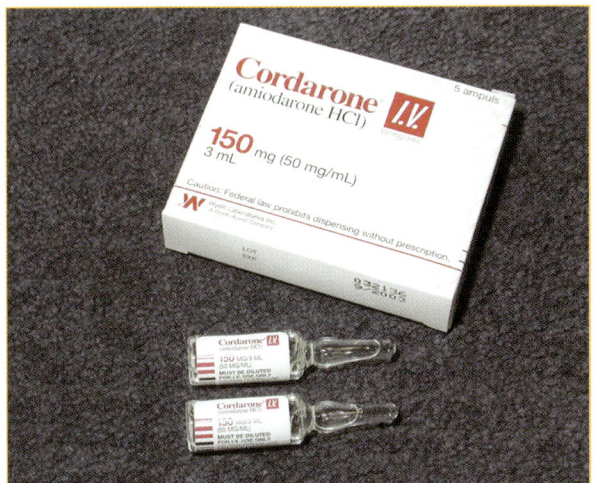

Figure 8-10 An ampule.

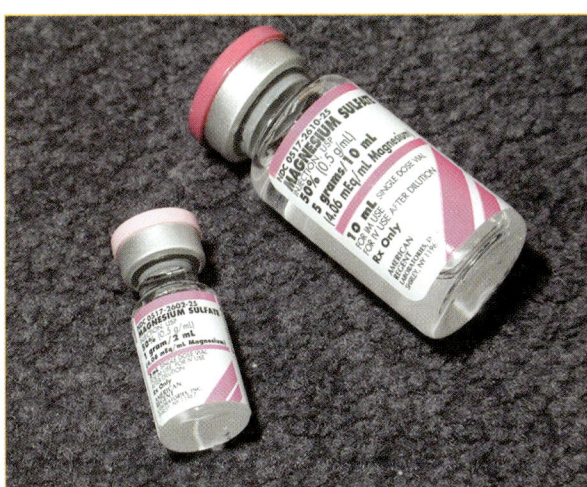

Figure 8-11 Vials (single-dose and multidose).

> ### EMT-I Safety
>
> Any time you are using a needle to draw up medication or to inject blood into blood tubes, always hold the syringe against your palm with the needle pointing up and draw the vial or blood tube down onto the needle using the thumb and forefinger of the palm the syringe is braced against to avoid sticking yourself. This especially applies if you are in a moving ambulance.

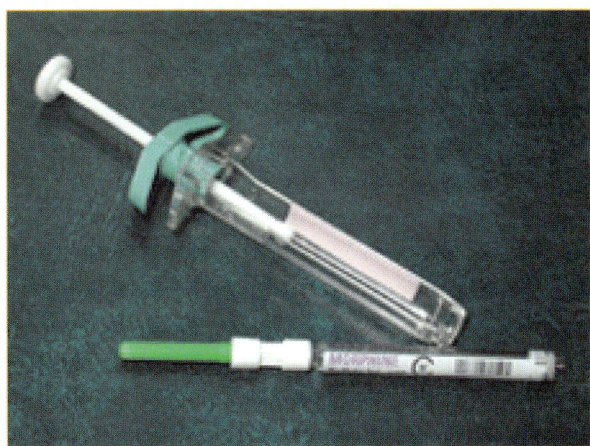

Figure 8-12 A Tubex syringe.

from one vial into the vial that contains the powder, making a solution for injection.

Ampules

When drawing a medication from an ampule, follow the steps in **Skill Drill 8-2**:

1. Check the medication to be sure that the expiration date has not passed, and that it is the correct drug and concentration.
2. Shake the medication down into the base of the ampule. If some of the drug appears to be stuck in the neck, gently thump or tap the stem (**Step 1**).
3. Using a 4″ × 4″ gauze pad or an alcohol prep, grip the neck of the ampule and snap it off. Drop the stem in the sharps container (**Step 2**).
4. Insert the needle into the ampule without touching the outer sides of the ampule. Draw the solution into the syringe, and dispose of the ampule in the sharps container (**Step 3**).
5. Hold the syringe with the needle pointing up, and gently tap the barrel to loosen air trapped inside and cause it to rise (**Step 4**). Press gently on the plunger to dispel any air bubbles (**Step 5**).
6. Recap the needle using the one-handed method and avoiding contamination.

Vials

When using a vial of medication, you must first determine how much of the drug you will need and how many doses are in the vial. For a single-dose vial,

Skill Drill 8-2

Drawing Medication From an Ampule

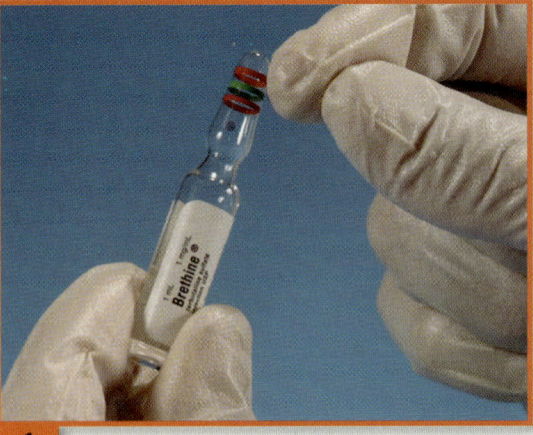

1. Gently thump or tap the stem of the ampule to shake medication down into the base.

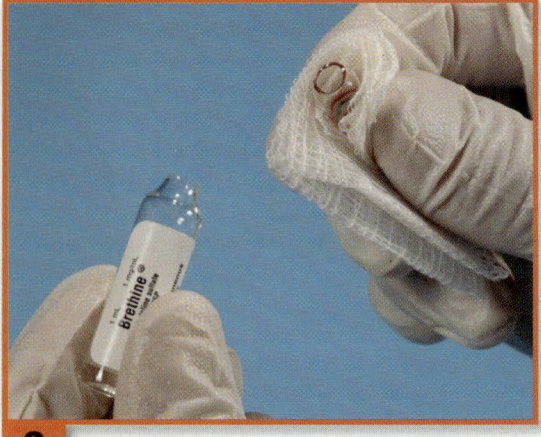

2. Grip the neck of the ampule using a 4″ × 4″ gauze pad and snap the neck off.

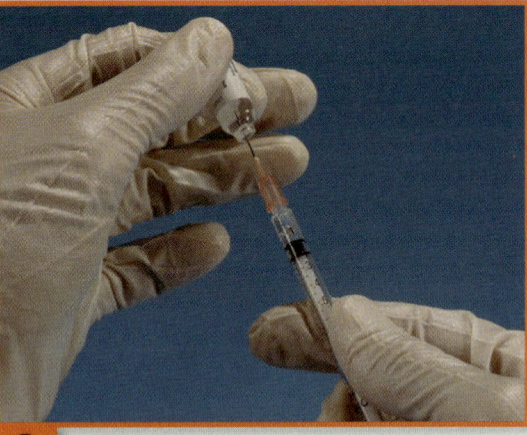

3. Without touching the outer sides of the ampule, insert the needle into the medication in the ampule, and draw the solution in the syringe.

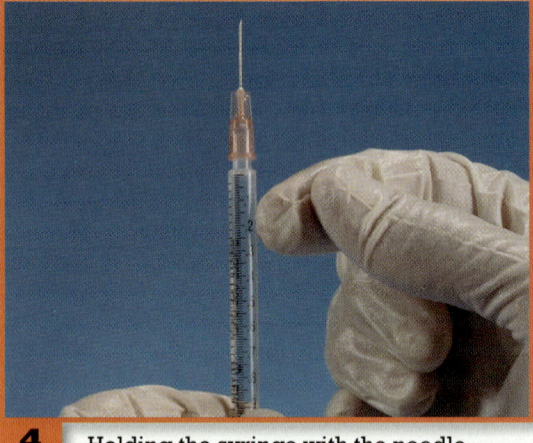

4. Holding the syringe with the needle pointing up, gently tap the barrel to loosen air trapped inside.

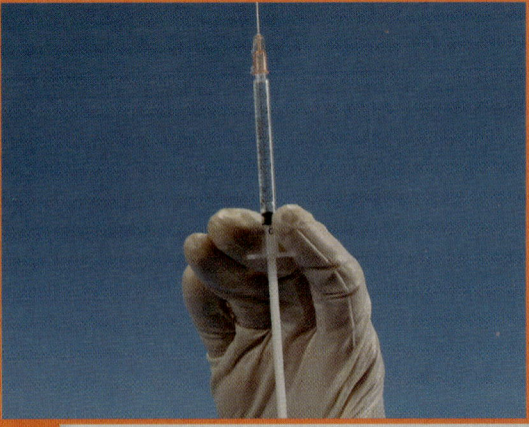

5. Gently press on the plunger to dispel any air bubbles, and recap the needle using the one-handed method.

you will draw up the entire amount in the vial. For multiple-dose vials, you should draw out only the amount needed. Remember that once you remove the cover from a vial, it is no longer sterile. If you need a second dose, the top of the vial should be cleaned with alcohol before withdrawing the medication.

When drawing medication from a vial, follow the steps in Skill Drill 8-3:

1. Check the medication to be sure that the expiration date has not passed, and that it is the correct drug and concentration (**Step 1**).
2. Remove the sterile cover, or clean the top with alcohol if it was previously opened.
3. Determine the amount of medication that you will need, and draw that amount of air into the syringe (**Step 2**). Allow a little extra room to expel some while removing air bubbles.
4. Invert the vial, and insert the needle through the rubber stopper into the medication. Expel the air in the syringe into the vial and then release the plunger, keeping the tip of the needle within the medication (**Step 3**).
5. Once you have the correct amount of medication in the syringe, withdraw the needle and expel any air in the syringe (**Step 4**).
6. Recap the needle using the one-handed method and avoiding contamination (**Step 5**).

Medications that need to be reconstituted come in two separate vials or in a single vial divided into two compartments by a rubber stopper. These may also be known as Mix-o-Vials Figure 8-13. With Mix-o-Vials, you simply squeeze the two vials together, which releases the center stopper and allows the contents to mix. Shake vigorously to mix the contents before drawing out the medication. To mix the contents of two separate vials, draw the fluid out of the first vial in the same manner described above. Insert the syringe into the top of the second vial, and expel all of the fluid into it. Shake vigorously to mix. Once the medication is reconstituted, regardless of the manner, draw up the medication as described for single- and multiple-dose vials.

Prefilled Syringe

Prefilled syringes come in tamper-proof boxes and are separated into the glass drug cartridge and a syringe Figure 8-14. Pop the tops off of the syringe and the drug cartridge, and screw them together. Remove the needle cover, and expel air in the manner previously described. Follow the steps for the route the medication is to be given.

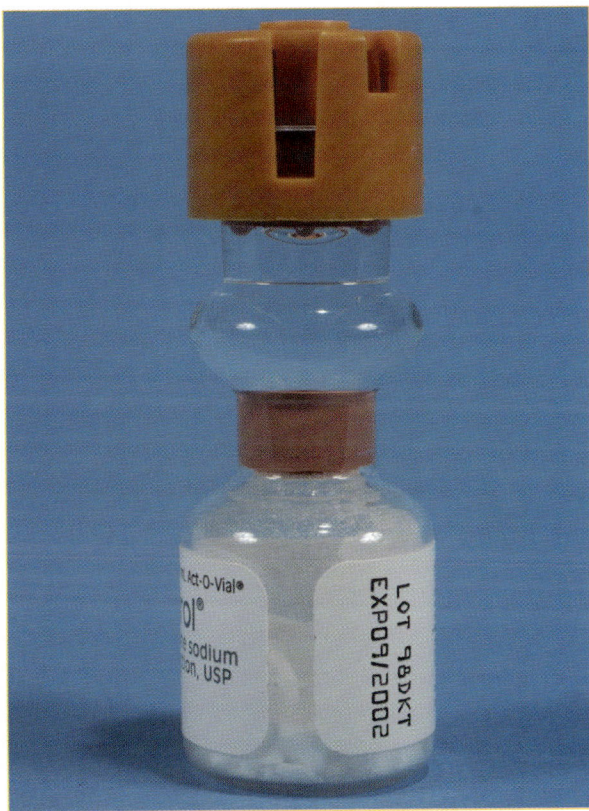

Figure 8-13 A Mix-o-Vial.

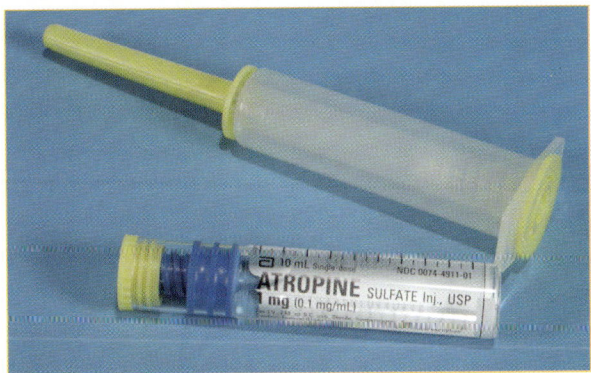

Figure 8-14 Prefilled syringes come in two parts, the glass drug cartridge and a syringe.

Administration of Medication by the Subcutaneous Route

<u>Subcutaneous</u> injections are given into the loose connective tissue between the dermis and the muscle layer Figure 8-15. Volumes of a drug administered subcutaneously are usually 1 mL or less. The injection is

Drawing Medication From a Vial

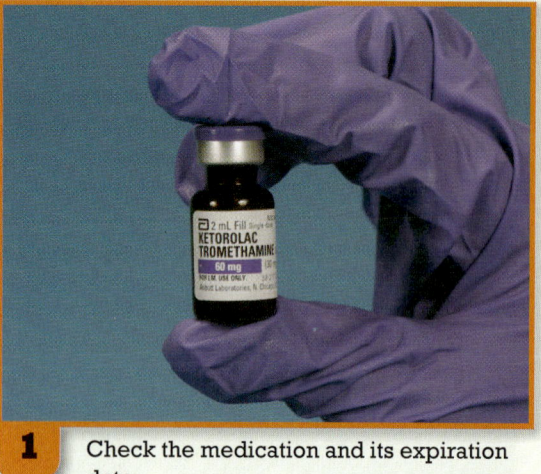

1 Check the medication and its expiration date.

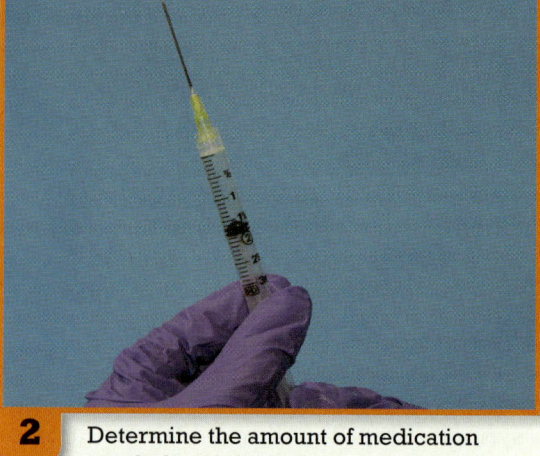

2 Determine the amount of medication needed, and draw that amount of air into the syringe.

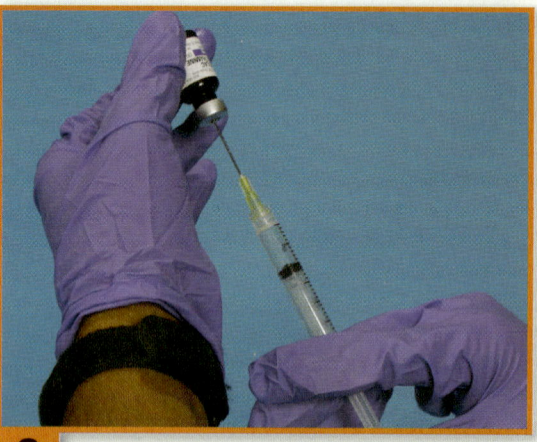

3 Invert the vial, and insert the needle through the rubber stopper. Expel the air in the syringe and release the plunger, keeping the tip of the needle within the medication.

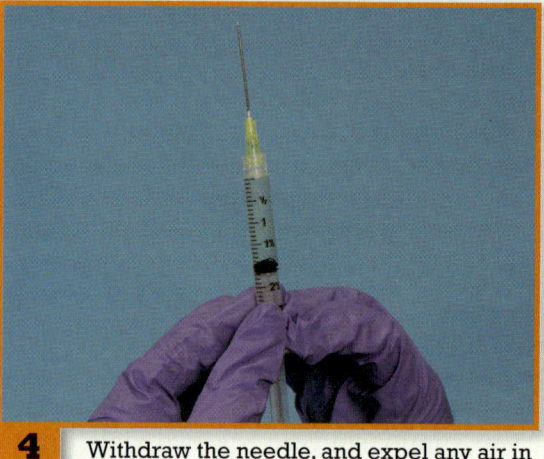

4 Withdraw the needle, and expel any air in the syringe.

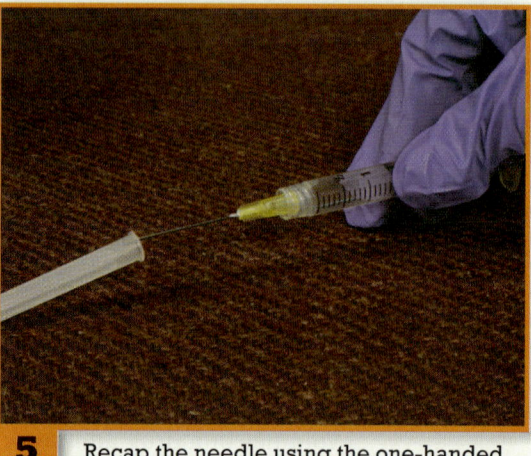

5 Recap the needle using the one-handed method.

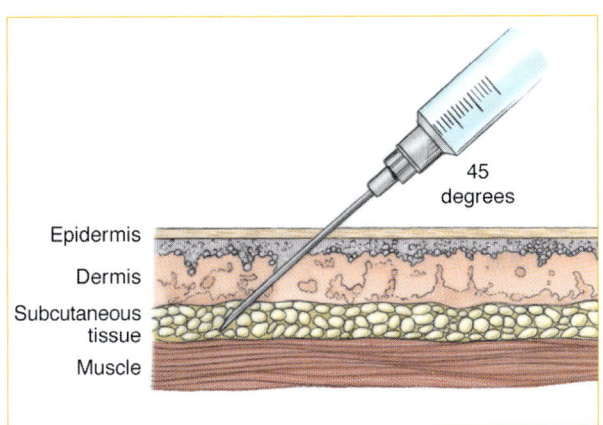

Figure 8-15 A subcutaneous injection is below the dermis and above the muscle.

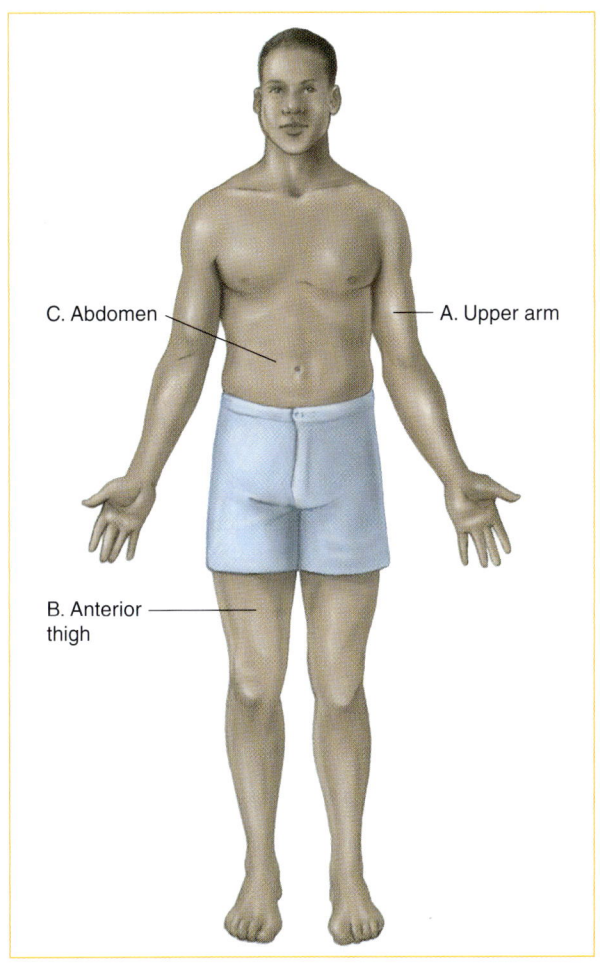

Figure 8-16 Common sites for subcutaneous injections. **A.** Upper arm. **B.** Anterior thigh. **C.** Abdomen.

performed using a 24- to 26-gauge ½″ to 1″ needle. Common sites include the upper arms, anterior thighs, and the abdomen (Figure 8-16 ▶). Patients who take insulin injections usually vary the sites owing to the multiple number of injections they require (usually daily).

Follow the steps in (Skill Drill 8-4 ▶) to administer a medication via the subcutaneous route:

1. Take BSI precautions.
2. Determine the need for the medication based on patient presentation.
3. Obtain a focused history and physical exam, including any drug allergies and vital signs.
4. Follow standing orders, or contact medical control for permission.

You are the Provider — Part 6

En route to the hospital, you continue to monitor the patient's condition. A reassessment of his blood glucose level reveals 110 mg/dL. You deliver the patient to the hospital in stable condition.

Reassessment	Recording Time: 20 Minutes After Patient Contact
Level of consciousness	Conscious and alert to person, place, and time
Blood pressure	128/70 mm Hg
Pulse	80 beats/min, strong and regular
Respirations	18 breaths/min, unlabored with adequate depth
Sao_2	99% (with 100% oxygen via nonrebreathing mask)

11. As with most medicines, doses for children vary from those for adults. If this scenario involved a child, the use of D_{25} would be required. How would you convert D_{50} to D_{25} if you did not have it in preloaded form?
12. According to knowledge about how carbohydrates are used in the body, what vitamin must be present for the body to benefit from the D_{50} you administer?

Administering Medication Via the Subcutaneous Route

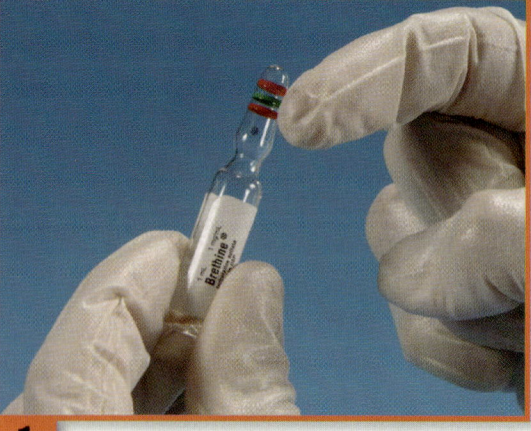

1. Check the medication to be sure that it is the correct one, that it is not discolored, and that the expiration date has not passed.

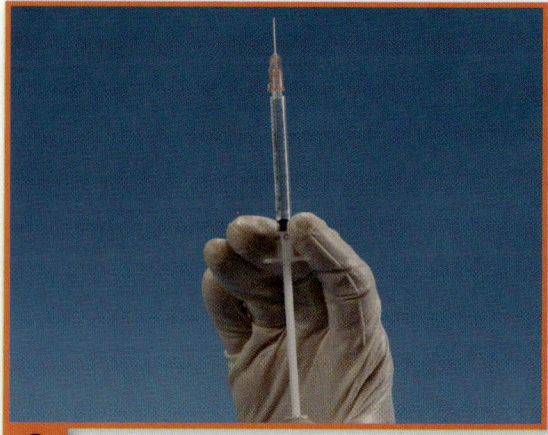

2. Assemble and check the equipment. Draw up the correct dose of medication.

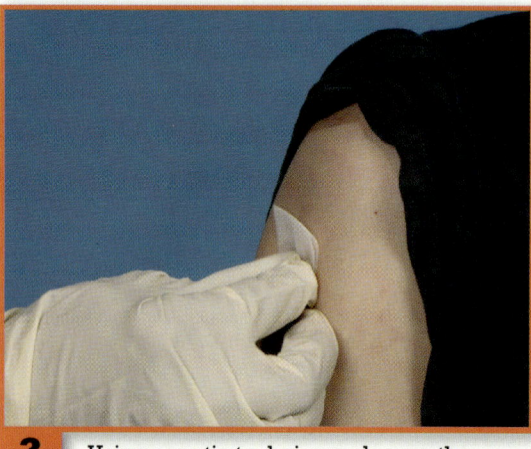

3. Using aseptic technique, cleanse the injection area.

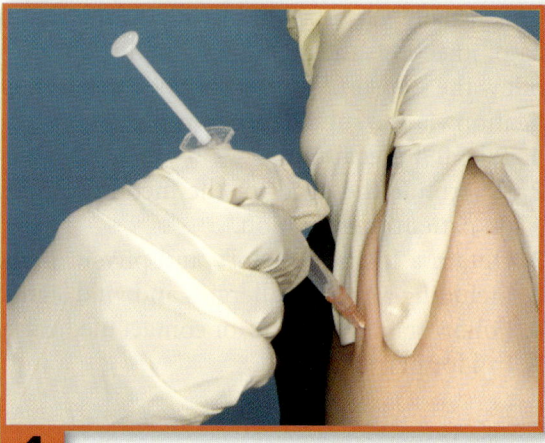

4. Pinch the skin surrounding the area, and insert the needle at a 45° angle. Pull back on the plunger to aspirate for blood. If there is no blood, inject the medication, remove the needle, and hold pressure over the area.

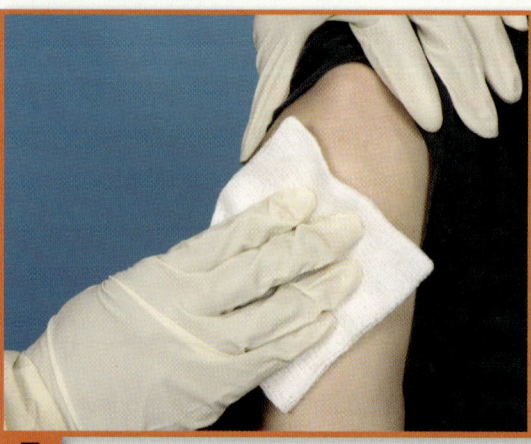

5. To disperse the medication, rub the area in a circular motion. Monitor the patient's condition.

5. Check the medication to be sure that it is not cloudy, that the expiration date has not passed, and that it is the correct drug and concentration, and determine the appropriate dose (**Step 1**).
6. Advise the patient of potential discomfort while explaining the procedure.
7. Assemble and check equipment needed: alcohol preps and a 3-mL syringe with a 24- to 26-gauge needle. Draw up the correct dose of medication (**Step 2**).
8. Cleanse the area for the administration (usually the upper arm or thigh) using aseptic technique (**Step 3**).
9. Pinch the skin surrounding the area, advise the patient of a stick, and insert the needle at a 45° angle.
10. Pull back on the plunger to aspirate for blood. The presence of blood in the syringe indicates you may have entered a vein. Remove the needle, and hold pressure over the site. Discard the syringe and needle in the sharps container. Prepare a new syringe and needle and select another site.
11. If there is no blood in the syringe, inject the medication and remove the needle. Immediately place it in the sharps container (**Step 4**).
12. To disperse the medication through the tissue, rub the area in a circular motion with your gloved hand.
13. Properly store any unused medication.
14. Monitor the patient's condition, and document the medication given, route, administration time, and response of the patient (**Step 5**).

Administration of Medication Via the Intramuscular Route

Intramuscular (IM) injections are made by penetrating a needle through the dermis and subcutaneous tissue into the muscle layer. This allows administration of a larger volume of medication (up to 5 mL) than the subcutaneous route. There is also the potential for damage to nerves because of the depth of the injection, so it is important to choose the appropriate site. Common anatomic sites for IM injections for adults and children include the following:

- Vastus lateralis muscle—the large muscle on the lateral side of the thigh
- Rectus femoris muscle—the large muscle on the anterior side of the thigh
- Gluteal area—the buttocks, specifically the upper lateral aspect of either side
- Deltoid muscle—the muscle of the upper arm that covers the prominence of the shoulder. The site for injection is approximately $1\frac{1}{2}''$ to $2''$ below the acromion process on the lateral side (**Figure 8-17**).

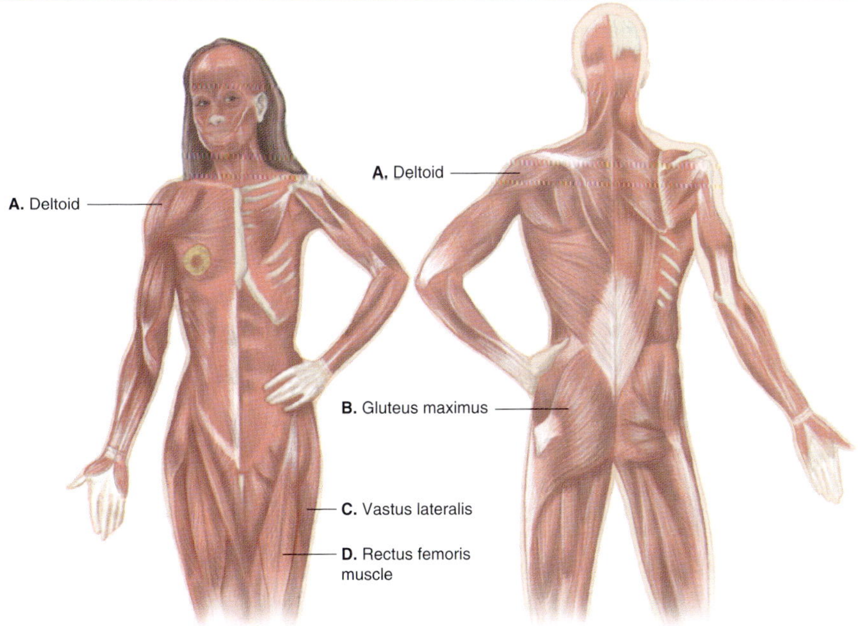

Figure 8-17 Common sites for intramuscular injections. **A.** Deltoid muscle. **B.** Gluteal area. **C.** Vastus lateralis muscle. **D.** Rectus femoris muscle.

Administering Medication Via the Intramuscular Route

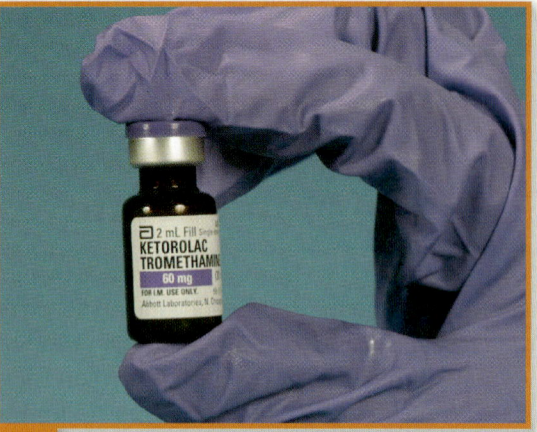

1 Check the medication to be sure it is the correct one, that it is not discolored, and that its expiration date has not passed.

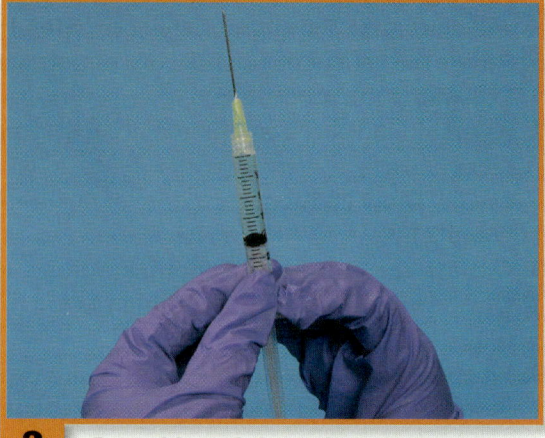

2 Assemble and check the equipment. Draw up the correct dose of medication.

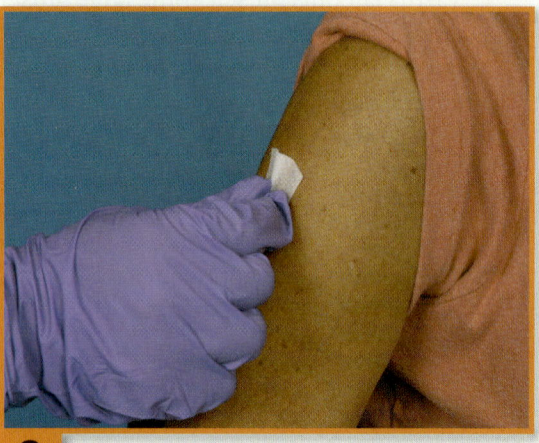

3 Using aseptic technique, cleanse the injection area.

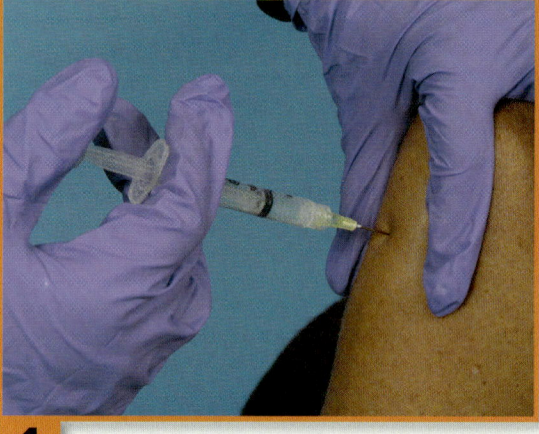

4 Stretch the skin over the area, and insert the needle at a 90° angle. Pull back on the plunger to aspirate for blood. If there is no blood, inject the medication and remove the needle.

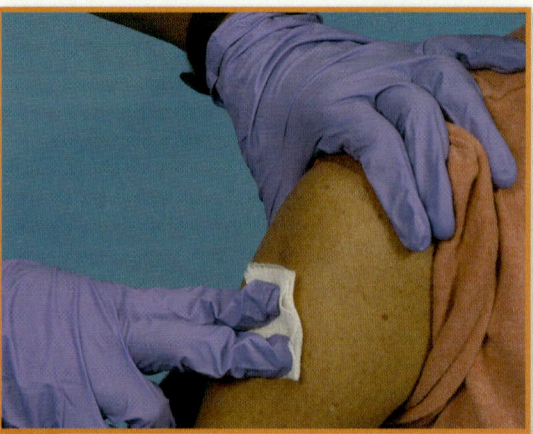

5 To disperse the medication, rub the area in a circular motion. Monitor the patient's condition.

Follow the steps in **Skill Drill 8-5** to administer an IM injection:

1. Take BSI precautions.
2. Determine the need for the medication based on patient presentation.
3. Obtain a focused history and physical exam, including any drug allergies and vital signs.
4. Follow standing orders, or contact medical control for permission.
5. Check the medication to be sure it is the correct one, that it is not discolored, and that the expiration date has not passed, and determine the appropriate dose (**Step 1**).
6. Advise the patient of potential discomfort while explaining the procedure.
7. Assemble and check equipment needed: alcohol preps and a 3- to 5-mL syringe with a 21-gauge, 1″ or 2″ needle. Draw up the correct dose of medication (**Step 2**).
8. Cleanse the area for the administration (usually the upper arm or the hip) using aseptic technique (**Step 3**).
9. Stretch the skin over the cleansed area, advise the patient of a stick, and insert the needle at a 90° angle.
10. Pull back on the plunger to aspirate for blood. The presence of blood in the syringe indicates you may have entered a blood vessel. Remove the needle, and hold pressure over the site. Discard the syringe and needle in the sharps container. Prepare a new syringe and needle, and select another site.
11. If there is no blood in the syringe, inject the medication and remove the needle. Immediately place it in the sharps container (**Step 4**).
12. To disperse the medication through the tissue, rub the area in a circular motion with your gloved hand (**Step 5**).
13. Store any unused medication properly.
14. Monitor the patient's condition, and document the medication given, route, administration time, and response of the patient.

EMT-I Tips

As an EMT-I, you must fully understand the properties of the medications you administer. This knowledge includes indications, contraindications, side and adverse effects, medication interactions, precautions, doses, routes, onset, half-life, and mechanism of action. Having complete knowledge of a drug helps ensure its safe use, including alternative methods of administration (should preferred methods be unavailable), and helps ensure that the patient receives full benefits of the medication.

Administration of Medication Via Intravenous Bolus

The intravenous (IV) route places the drug directly into the circulatory system. This is the fastest route of medication administration for EMT-Is to administer because it bypasses most barriers to drug absorption. This also means that there is no room for error. Drugs are administered by direct injection with a needle and syringe into an established peripheral IV line. Many services now use needleless systems to provide protection against needlesticks. When using a needleless system, the syringe simply screws into the injection port.

In terms of medication administration, a bolus is a single dose given by the IV route. A bolus (in one mass) can be a small or large quantity of a drug. Some medications require an initial bolus and then a continuous IV infusion to maintain a therapeutic level of the drug. This especially applies to cardiac medications (for example, lidocaine). Complications may arise from using the IV route. These include phlebitis (inflammation of a vein) or infection, extravasation of fluid or medication into the surrounding tissues, air in tubing that may lead to an air embolus, allergic reaction to a fluid or drug, pulmonary embolism, or a failure to infuse properly for any reason.

Follow the steps in **Skill Drill 8-6** when administering a medication via the IV bolus route:

1. Take BSI precautions.
2. Determine the need for the medication based on patient presentation.
3. Obtain a focused history and physical exam, including any drug allergies and vital signs.
4. Follow standing orders, or contact medical control for permission.
5. Check the medication to be sure that it is the correct one, that it is not cloudy or discolored, and that its expiration date has not passed, and determine the appropriate dose.

Administering Medication Via the Intravenous Bolus Route

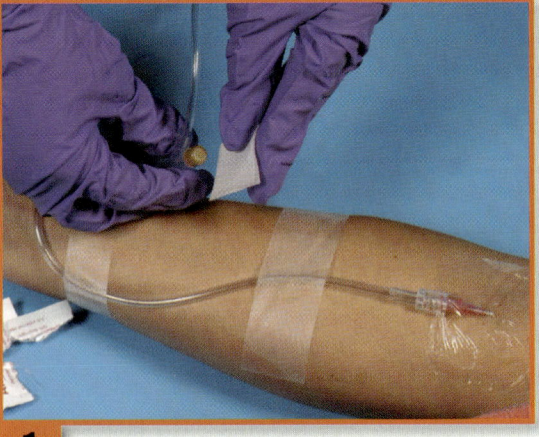

1 Assemble and check the equipment. Cleanse the injection port, or remove the protective cap if using the needleless system.

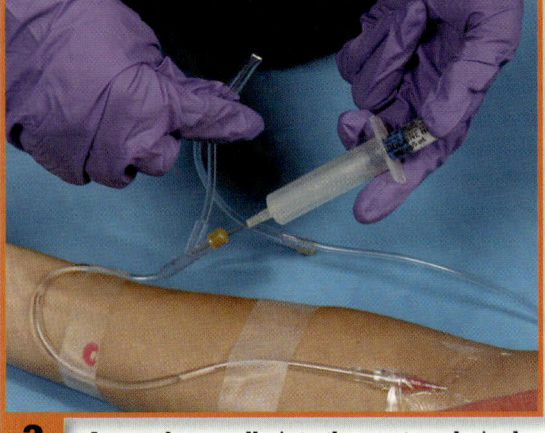

2 Insert the needle into the port, and pinch off the IV tubing proximal to the administration port. Administer the correct dose at the appropriate rate.

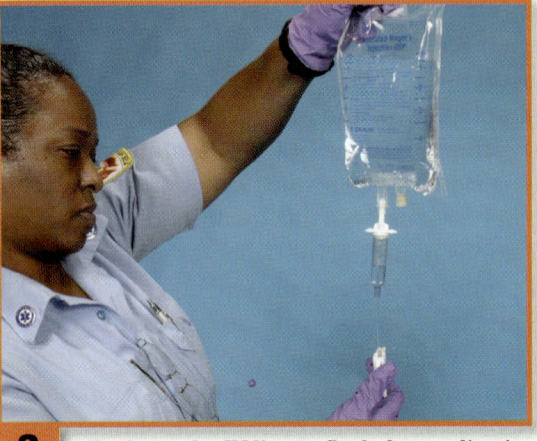

3 Unclamp the IV line to flush the medication into the vein, allowing it to run briefly wide open, or flush with a 20-mL bolus of normal saline.

Readjust the IV flow rate to the original setting, and monitor the patient's condition.

---

6. Explain the procedure to the patient and the need for the medication.
7. Assemble needed equipment, and draw up medication. Expel any air in the syringe. Draw up 20 mL of normal saline to use as a flush for the medication.
8. Cleanse the injection port with alcohol, or remove the protective cap if using the needleless system (**Step 1**).
9. Insert the needle into the port, and pinch off the IV tubing proximal to the administration port. Failure to shut off the line will result in the medication taking the pathway of least resistance and flowing into the bag instead of into the patient.
10. Administer the correct dose of the medication at the appropriate rate. Some medications must be administered very quickly, while others must

be pushed slowly to prevent adverse effects (**Step 2**).
11. Place the needle and syringe into the sharps container.
12. Unclamp the IV line to flush the medication into the vein. Allow it to run briefly wide open, or flush with a 20-mL bolus of normal saline.
13. Readjust the IV flow rate to the original setting (**Step 3**).
14. Properly store any unused medication.
15. Monitor the patient's condition, and document the medication given, route, time of administration, and response of the patient.

Follow these steps to administer a medication through a heparin or saline lock (Figure 8-18 ▶):
1. Take BSI precautions.
2. Determine the need for the medication based on patient presentation.
3. Obtain a focused history and physical exam, including any drug allergies and vital signs.
4. Follow standing orders, or contact medical control for permission.
5. Check the medication to be sure it is the correct one, that it is not cloudy or discolored, and that its expiration date has not passed, and determine the appropriate dose.
6. Explain the procedure to the patient and the need for the medication.
7. Assemble needed equipment, and draw up the medication. Draw up 20 mL of normal saline to use as a flush for the medication.
8. Cleanse the injection port with alcohol, or remove the protective cap if using the needleless system.
9. Insert the needle into the port while holding it carefully, or screw the syringe onto the port.
10. Pull back slightly on the syringe plunger, and observe for blood return. If blood appears, slowly inject the medication, watching for infiltration. If resistance is felt, or if the patient complains of any discomfort, discontinue administration immediately. A new site will need to be established.
11. Place the needle and syringe into the sharps container.
12. Clean the port, and insert the needle with the syringe containing the flush.
13. Flush the heparin lock, and place the needle in the sharps container.
14. Store any unused medication properly.
15. Monitor the patient's condition, and document the medication given, route, time of administration, and response of the patient.

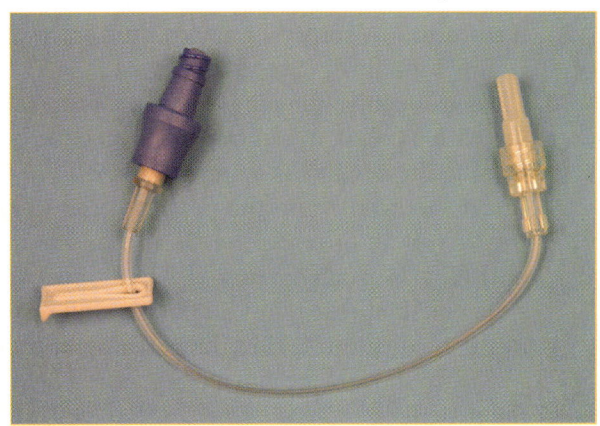

Figure 8-18 Heparin lock.

Administration of Medication Via the IO Route

Intraosseous (IO) routes are used for critically ill patients when IV access cannot be established within three attempts or 90 seconds. Any fluid or medication that may be given through an IV line can also be given by the IO route. Shock and status epilepticus are only two of the reasons for establishing IO access. Unlike an IV line, fluid does not flow well into the bone because of resistance; therefore, it is necessary to use a large syringe to infuse the fluid.

Complications of using the IO route are similar to those of the IV route. Along with the complications discussed in the previous section, there is also the potential for compartment syndrome if fluid leaks outside of the bone and into the osteofascial compartment, fracture of the tibia from improper technique, and pulmonary embolism due to the bone and fat particles.

Follow the steps in (Skill Drill 8-7 ▶) to administer a medication via the IO route:
1. Take BSI precautions.
2. Determine the need for the medication based on patient presentation.
3. Obtain a focused history and physical exam, including any drug allergies and vital signs.
4. Follow standing orders, or contact medical control for permission.
5. Check the medication to be certain that it is the correct one, that it is not cloudy or discolored, and that the expiration date has not passed, and determine the appropriate dose.
6. Explain the procedure to the patient and/or parent and the need for the medication.

7. Assemble needed equipment, and draw up the medication. Also draw enough fluid from the IV line for a flush (**Step 1**).
8. Cleanse the injection port of the extension tubing with alcohol, or remove the protective cap if using the needleless system (**Step 2**).
9. Insert the needle into the port, and clamp off the IV tubing proximal to the administration port. This is usually managed with a three-way stopcock. Failure to shut off the line will result in the medication taking the pathway of least resistance and flowing into the bag instead of into the patient.
10. Administer the correct dose of the medication at the proper push rate. Some medications must be administered very quickly, while others must be pushed slowly to prevent adverse effects (**Step 3**).
11. Place the needle and syringe into the sharps container.
12. Unclamp the IV line to flush the medication into the vein. Flush with at least a 20-mL bolus of normal saline (or the fluid being administered).
13. Readjust the IV flow rate to the original setting.
14. Store any unused medication properly.
15. Monitor the patient's condition, and document the medication given, route, time of administration, and response of the patient (**Step 4**).

Administering Medications Via the Sublingual Route

Sublingual medications get into the circulatory system much faster than those that travel through the enteral route. There is a vast network of vessels under the tongue (sublingual) and in the cheek (buccal). Medications given by the sublingual route come in tablet, liquid, and spray forms. Nitroglycerin is a drug that is commonly given via the sublingual route, and it comes in tablet and spray forms (Figure 8-19 ▲).

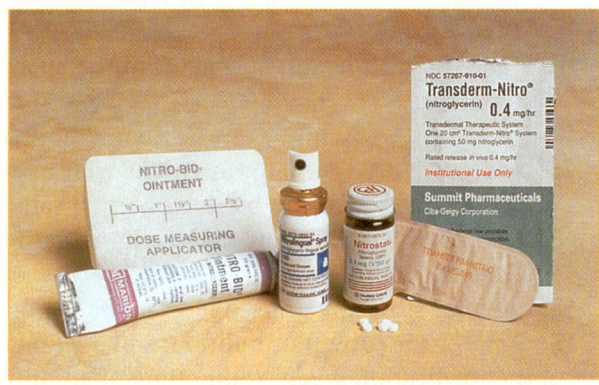

Figure 8-19 Nitroglycerin is often given sublingually as a spray or a tablet. It is also available as a transdermal ointment or patch.

To administer a sublingual medication, follow these steps (Skill Drill 8-8 ▶):

1. Take BSI precautions.
2. Determine the need for the medication based on patient presentation.
3. Obtain a focused history and physical exam, including any drug allergies and vital signs.
4. Follow standing orders, or contact medical control for permission.
5. Check the medication to make sure that it is the correct one and that its expiration date has not passed, and determine the appropriate dose.
6. Ask the patient to rinse his or her mouth with a little water if the mucous membranes are dry (**Step 1**).
7. Explain the procedure, and ask the patient to lift his or her tongue. Place the tablet or spray the dose under the tongue, or ask the patient to do so.
8. Advise the patient not to chew or swallow the tablet, but to let it dissolve slowly.
9. Monitor the patient's condition, and document the medication given, route, administration time, and response of the patient (**Step 2**).

Administering Medication Via the IO Route

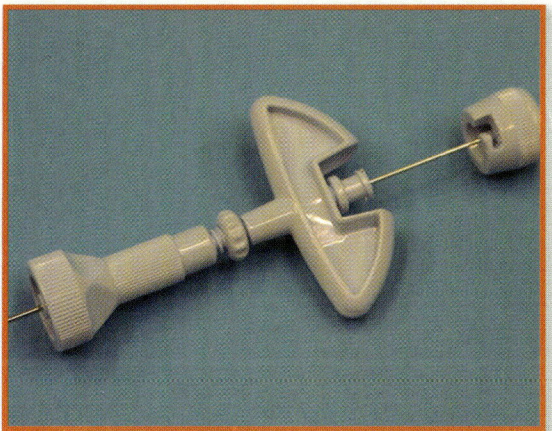

1 Check the medication to make sure it is the correct one, that it is not discolored, and that the expiration date has not passed.

Assemble the equipment, and draw up the medication. Draw enough fluid from the IV line for a flush.

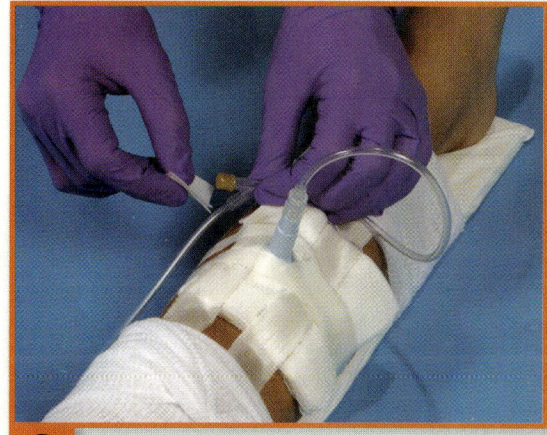

2 Cleanse the injection port, or remove the protective cap if using the needleless system.

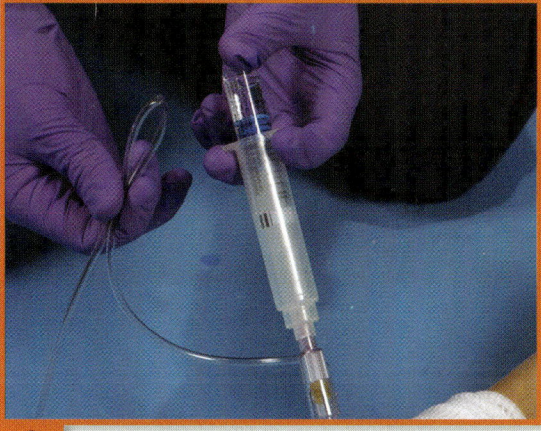

3 Insert the needle into the port, and pinch off the IV tubing proximal to the administration port. Administer the correct dose at the proper push rate.

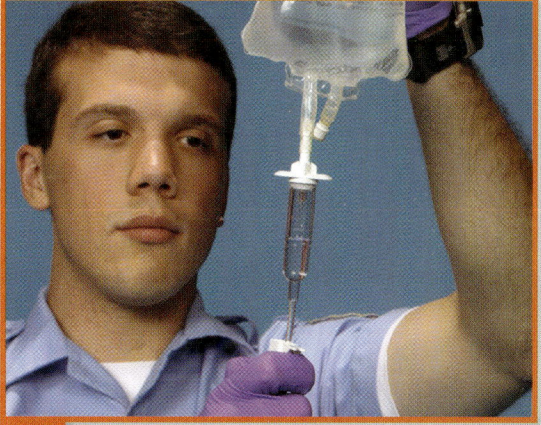

4 Unclamp the IV line to flush the medication into the vein, allowing it to run briefly wide open, or flush with a 20-mL bolus of normal saline (or the fluid being given).

Readjust the IV flow rate to the original setting, and monitor the patient's condition.

Administering Medication Via the Sublingual Route

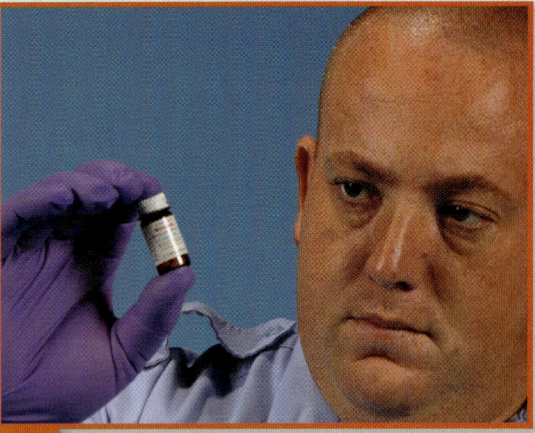

1. Check the medication for drug type and its expiration date, and determine the appropriate dose.

   Have the patient rinse his or her mouth with a little water if the mucous membranes are dry.

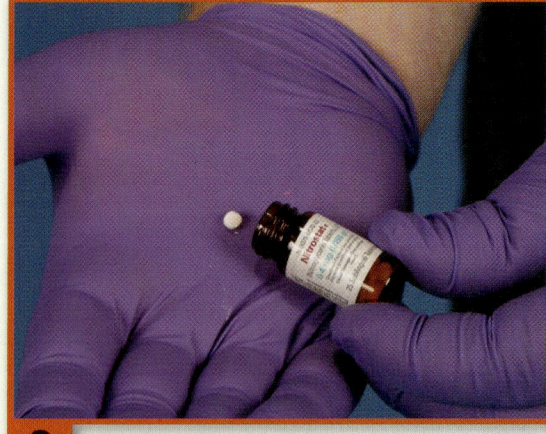

2. Explain the procedure and ask the patient to lift his or her tongue. Place the tablet or spray the dose underneath the tongue or have the patient do so.

   Advise the patient not to chew or swallow the tablet, but to let it dissolve slowly.

   Monitor the patient and document the medication given, the route, administration time, and the response of the patient.

You are the Provider — Summary

1. What are the "six rights" of medication administration?

- Right patient
- Right drug
- Right dose
- Right route
- Right time
- Right documentation

2. Why is it important to conduct a thorough patient assessment before giving medications?

Because medications, if given under inappropriate circumstances, can cause harm to the patient (including death), a careful and thorough assessment is crucial to determine whether the drug is indicated for the patient's condition. Many patients who present with various medical conditions do not require medication therapy other than oxygen.

3. How should you manage this patient initially?

Your initial assessment findings indicate that the patient has altered mental status and that his respirations are rapid and shallow (ie, reduced tidal volume). Therefore, initial management includes assisting his ventilations with a bag-valve-mask device and 100% oxygen.

4. Other than oxygen, are any other medications indicated at this particular time?

Because you have not performed a thorough assessment of the patient, you cannot determine which, if any, medications are required, other than oxygen. Further assessment of the patient will clearly be needed.

5. Because D_{50} is a hypertonic solution, what contraindications exist for administration of this medication?

Administering hypertonic solutions intravenously causes a shift in body fluids from the cell and into the vascular space. Knowing this, it makes sense that a hemorrhagic stroke, a potential cause of your patient's altered mental status, could be exacerbated after administering a hypertonic solution.

6. What must be confirmed before administering this drug? Why is this important?

You must confirm that the IV line is patent before administering 50% dextrose. Checking for ease of flow and lack of swelling around the IV site and/or obtaining blood when pulling back on a syringe in the IV line are techniques that must be used and documented. Failure to establish a patent IV with consequential extravasation of D_{50} into the surrounding tissues can cause tissue necrosis.

7. You must know what routes of administration are appropriate for each and every drug you give. What is the reasoning behind this essential knowledge?

Some drugs may not be given via certain routes because they will be ineffective and/or may cause harm, such as D_{50}. Knowing all of the routes of administration also gives you other options for administration should one method be unavailable.

Continued

You are the Provider continued

8. D_{50} is packaged as 25 g in 50 mL. How many milligrams are in each milliliter?

Recall that 50% dextrose means that there are 50 g (50,000 mg) in each 100 mL of fluid; with D_{50}, there is a total of 25 g (25,000 mg) in 50 mL. According to the formula to determine the concentration/dose on hand learned in this chapter, 500 mg/mL in D_{50} (25,000 mg [total weight] ÷ 50 mL [total volume] = 500 mg/mL).

9. Is further treatment required for this patient?

Because your patient's condition has clearly improved following the administration of 50% dextrose, further treatment is not required at this time. However, you must frequently reassess his condition, especially his mental status and blood glucose level, to determine whether further medication or other therapy is needed.

10. What does the "%" in 50% dextrose indicate?

The percentage (%) in 50% dextrose indicates the number of grams present in 100 mL (1 dL) of volume. However, because D_{50} is stored in only 50-mL volumes, there is 25 g present in the solution. If D_{50} were stored in 100-mL volumes, then there would be 50 g present.

11. As with most medicines, doses for children vary from those for adults. If this scenario involved a child, the use of D_{25} would be required. How would you convert D_{50} to D_{25} if you did not have it in preloaded form?

Unlike adult doses of D_{50} that are not dependent on body weight, child doses of IV dextrose are 0.5 to 1.0 g/kg of D_{25}. To convert D_{50} to D_{25} you would dilute equal parts of D_{50} and normal saline in a 1:1 solution (that is, 12.5 g [25 mL] in 25 mL of normal saline).

12. According to knowledge about how carbohydrates are used in the body, what vitamin must be present for the body to benefit from the D_{50} you administer?

The presence of thiamine (vitamin B_1) is necessary for the utilization of D_{50}. A provider who suspects that a hypoglycemic patient may be deficient in vitamin B_1 (seen in cases of alcoholism and malnourished states) should administer vitamin B_1 (typically 100 mg).

Summary

Prep Kit

Ready for Review

- Along with the dispensing of medications comes the responsibility to learn as much as possible about the medications. Carry a field guide or other reference to look up unfamiliar drugs and doses. The first rule of EMS is *Do no harm*.
- Good math skills, along with an understanding of the metric system, are imperative to providing the correct dose for the patient. Practice your math skills frequently to stay proficient. The "right" drug must be given at the "right" time to the "right" patient by the "right" route. Administering the wrong medication, using the wrong route, and giving the wrong dose can have disastrous effects.
- All equipment used in the administration of medication must be kept sterile to prevent contamination of the patient. Proper BSI procedures must be followed to protect the EMT-I as well. For further protection, Occupational Safety and Health Administration (or OSHA)-recommended needleless systems have made older needle systems increasingly obsolete in an effort to decrease the incidence of needlesticks.
- A good rule of thumb for administering medications is the adage that carpenters use: Measure twice, cut once. Applied to medication administration to prevent careless errors, it would read: Figure twice, then administer the medication.
- As an EMT-I, you should be familiar with the various routes of medication administration. This includes an understanding of the proper use of equipment and proper anatomic locations for administration.
- Enteral administration includes the administration of all drugs that may be given through any portion of the digestive tract. The parenteral route includes any method of drug administration that does not go through the digestive tract.
- The IO route is used when the EMT-I is unable to obtain IV access in a critically ill patient. Any medication or fluid that can be administered via the IV route can be given by the IO route. Owing to potential complications, it is imperative that the EMT-I practice IO skills, as well as the other routes of medication administration, on a regular basis.
- When in doubt, always follow local protocols or contact medical control for direction.

Vital Vocabulary

ampules Small glass containers that are sealed and the contents sterilized.

apothecary system A system of weights and measures.

aseptic technique A method of cleansing used to prevent contamination of a site when performing an invasive procedure, such as inserting an IV line.

bolus A term used to describe "in one mass"; in medication administration, a single dose given by the IV route; may be a small or large quantity of the drug.

buccal Relating to the cheek or mouth.

Celsius scale A scale for measuring temperature in which water freezes at 0° and boils at 100°.

concentration The total weight of a drug contained in a specific volume of liquid.

drug reconstitution Injecting sterile water (or saline) from one vial into another vial containing a powdered form of the drug.

enteral medications Medications that are given through a portion of the gastrointestinal tract.

Fahrenheit scale A scale for measuring temperature in which water freezes at 32° and boils at 212°.

gauge In the medication administration sense, the interior diameter of a catheter or needle.

inhalation Breathing into the lungs; a medication delivery route.

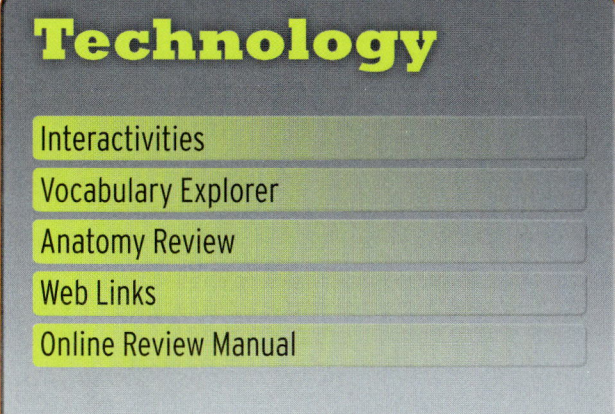

Technology
- Interactivities
- Vocabulary Explorer
- Anatomy Review
- Web Links
- Online Review Manual

Prep Kit continued...

intramuscular (IM) Into a muscle; a medication delivery route.

intraosseous (IO) Into the bone; a medication delivery route.

intravenous (IV) Into a vein; a medication delivery route.

medical asepsis A term applied to the practice of preventing contamination of the patient by using aseptic technique.

metric system A decimal system based on tens for the measurement of length, weight, and volume.

nebulizer A device for producing a fine spray or mist that is used to deliver inhaled medications.

parenteral medications Medications that are given through any route other than through the GI tract.

subcutaneous Into the tissue between the skin and muscle; a medication delivery route.

sublingual Under the tongue; a medication delivery route.

vials Small glass bottles for medications; may contain single or multiple doses.

Points to Ponder

Megan Norris is a 15-year-old girl with a history of asthma. She uses a metered-dose inhaler of albuterol as needed when she has an attack. She went to her grandmother's house for the weekend and forgot her inhaler. She experienced an asthma attack, and her grandmother called 9-1-1 for assistance.

You find Megan sitting in a tripod position at the dining room table. She has audible wheezing. You assess Megan and obtain a history from her grandmother while your partner obtains vital signs and gives her oxygen. You have a written protocol that allows you to administer albuterol by nebulizer. You check off your list of the "six rights" before administration.

You move Megan to the ambulance and begin the breathing treatment as you check her condition en route to the hospital. After completing the treatment, Megan is placed back on oxygen and transported to the hospital for further evaluation.

Issues: Understanding the Need to Verify the "Six Rights" of Medication Administration

Assessment in Action

Mr. Anderson is a 60-year-old man with a history of congestive heart failure. He began to experience chest pain after playing a game of catch with his grandson. You are called to his residence at 2:30 PM.

You find Mr. Anderson sitting on his front porch. He is in respiratory distress, is sweaty and pale, and is holding his chest. You obtain an appropriate history and move him to your ambulance. Your partner takes vital signs, and gives the patient oxygen. On the basis of your protocols, you administer nitroglycerin to the patient and call medical control for an order for furosemide (Lasix). Medical control approves your request and also advises you to give 5 mg of morphine IV. Mr. Anderson's level of distress decreases, and he is now pain free. He is transported to the emergency department without further incident.

1. Nitroglycerin is administered sublingually, which means:
   A. in the buccal cavity.
   B. under the tongue.
   C. swallowed.
   D. under the skin.

2. Before giving the nitroglycerin, you must ensure that you have met the "six rights" of medication administration. This includes all EXCEPT:
   A. right patient.
   B. right dose.
   C. right route.
   D. right doctor.

3. Lasix is a medication that comes in tablet and liquid form. Patients frequently take the tablet form in a maintenance dose at home. The benefits of giving the liquid form as an IV medication include all EXCEPT:
   A. it places the drug directly in the bloodstream.
   B. it bypasses most barriers of drug absorption.
   C. extravasation of fluid or medication.
   D. it is faster acting than oral administration.

4. The morphine on your ambulance is packaged as 10 mg/10 mL. Medical control ordered 5 mg. How many milliliters of the drug would you administer?
   A. 1.0
   B. 5.0
   C. 0.5
   D. 10.0

5. A single dose of a medication is known as a/an:
   A. bolus.
   B. infusion.
   C. ampule.
   D. multidose vial.

6. The term applied to the practice of preventing contamination of the patient is:
   A. decontamination.
   B. medical asepsis.
   C. medical direction.
   D. universal precautions.

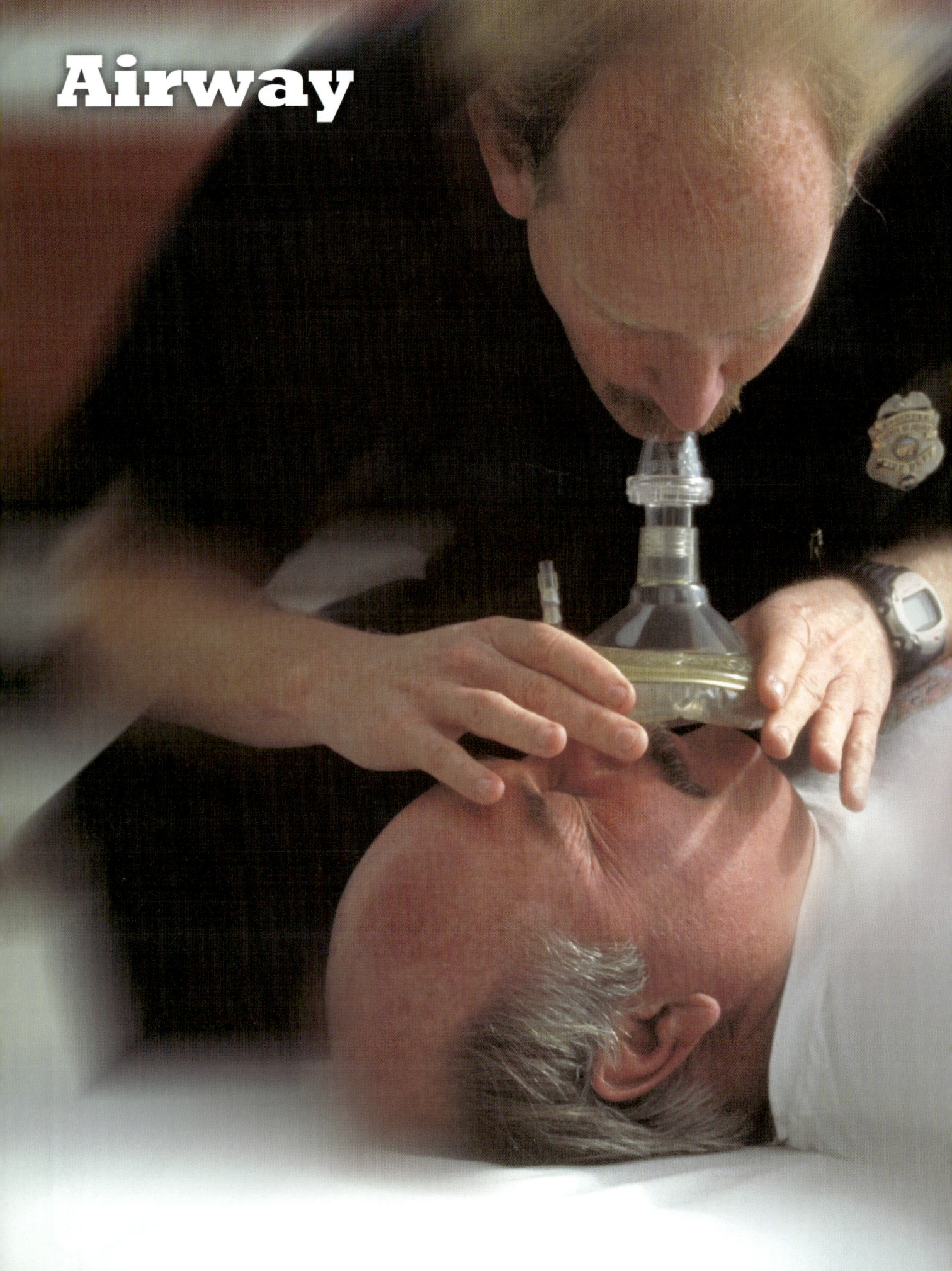
Airway

Section 3

| 9 | Airway Management and Ventilation | 362 |

Airway Management and Ventilation

1999 Objectives

Cognitive

2-1.1 Explain the primary objective of airway maintenance. (p 368)
2-1.2 Identify commonly neglected prehospital skills related to airway. (p 368)
2-1.3 Identify the anatomy and functions of the upper airway. (p 368)
2-1.4 Describe the anatomy and functions of the lower airway. (p 370)
2-1.5 Explain the differences between adult and pediatric airway anatomy. (p 371)
2-1.6 Define normal tidal volumes for the adult, child, and infant. (p 371)
2-1.7 Define atelectasis. (p 370)
2-1.8 Define FiO_2. (p 370)
2-1.9 Explain the relationship between pulmonary circulation and respiration. (p 372)
2-1.10 List factors which cause decreased oxygen concentrations in the blood. (p 373)
2-1.11 List the factors which increase and decrease carbon dioxide production in the body. (p 373)
2-1.12 Describe the measurement of oxygen in the blood. (p 374)
2-1.13 Describe the measurement of carbon dioxide in the blood. (p 374)
2-1.14 List the concentration of gases which compromise atmospheric air. (p 374)
2-1.15 List the factors which affect respiratory rate and depth. (p 374)
2-1.16 Describe the voluntary and involuntary regulation of respiration. (p 372)
2-1.17 Describe causes of upper airway obstruction. (p 388)
2-1.18 Define normal respiratory rates for adult, child, and infant. (p 376)
2-1.19 Describe causes of respiratory distress. (p 376)
2-1.20 Define and differentiate between hypoxia and hypoxemia. (p 376)
2-1.21 Define pulsus paradoxus. (p 377)
2-1.22 Describe the modified forms of respiration. (p 377)
2-1.23 Define gag reflex. (p 377)
2-1.24 Explain safety considerations of oxygen storage and delivery. (p 408)
2-1.25 Identify types of oxygen cylinders and pressure regulators (including a high-pressure regulator and a therapy regulator). (p 408)
2-1.26 List the steps for delivering oxygen from a cylinder and regulator. (p 410)
2-1.27 Describe the indications, contraindications, advantages, disadvantages, complications, liter flow range, and concentration of delivered oxygen for supplemental oxygen delivery devices. (p 412)
2-1.28 Describe the use, advantages, and disadvantages of an oxygen humidifier. (p 413)
2-1.29 Define, identify and describe a tracheostomy, stoma, and tracheostomy tube. (p 466)
2-1.30 Explain the risk of infection to EMS providers associated with ventilation. (p 414)
2-1.31 Describe the indications, contraindications, advantages, disadvantages, complications, and technique for ventilating a patient by:
  a. Mouth-to-mouth
  b. Mouth-to-nose
  c. Mouth-to-mask
  d. One person bag-valve-mask
  e. Two person bag-valve-mask
  f. Three person bag-valve-mask
  g. Flow-restricted, oxygen-powered ventilation device (p 411, 414, 415, 417, 418, 421)
2-1.32 Explain the advantage of the two-person method when ventilating with the bag-valve-mask. (p 417)
2-1.33 Describe indications, contraindications, advantages, disadvantages, complications, and technique for ventilating a patient with an automatic transport ventilator. (p 422)
2-1.34 Describe the Sellick (cricoid pressure) maneuver. (p 422)
2-1.35 Describe the use of cricoid pressure during intubation. (p 422)
2-1.36 Compare the ventilation techniques used for an adult patient to those used for pediatric patients. (p 419)
2-1.37 Define how to ventilate a patient with a stoma, including mouth-to-stoma and bag-valve-mask-to-stoma ventilation. (p 467)
2-1.38 Define complete airway obstruction. (p 391)
2-1.39 Define and explain the implications of a partial airway obstruction with good and poor air exchange. (p 391)
2-1.40 Describe complete airway obstruction maneuvers. (p 392)
2-1.41 Describe laryngoscopy for the removal of a foreign body airway obstruction. (p 396)

2-1.42 Identify types of suction catheters, including hard or rigid catheters and soft catheters. (p 398)
2-1.43 Explain the purpose for suctioning the upper airway. (p 397)
2-1.44 Identify types of suction equipment. (p 398)
2-1.45 Describe the indications for suctioning the upper airway. (p 398)
2-1.46 Identify techniques of suctioning the upper airway. (p 398)
2-1.47 Identify special considerations of suctioning the upper airway. (p 398)
2-1.48 Describe the technique of tracheobronchial suctioning in the intubated patient. (p 451)
2-1.49 Define gastric distention. (p 423)
2-1.50 Describe the indications, contraindications, advantages, disadvantages, complications, equipment, and technique for inserting a nasogastric tube and orogastric tube. (p 425, 430)
2-1.51 Describe manual airway maneuvers. (p 402)
2-1.52 Describe the use of an oral and nasal airway. (p 402, 405)
2-1.53 Describe the indications, contraindications, advantages, disadvantages, complications, and technique for inserting an oropharyngeal and nasopharyngeal airway. (p 402, 405)
2-1.54 Differentiate endotracheal intubation from other methods of advanced airway management. (p 438)
2-1.55 Describe the indications, contraindications, advantages, disadvantages, and complications of endotracheal intubation. (p 438)
2-1.56 Describe the visual landmarks for direct laryngoscopy. (p 443)
2-1.57 Describe the methods of assessment for confirming correct placement of an endotracheal tube. (p 445)
2-1.58 Describe methods for securing an endotracheal tube. (p 449)
2-1.59 Describe the indications, contraindications, advantages, disadvantages, complications, equipment, and technique for extubation. (p 451)
2-1.60 Describe methods of endotracheal intubation in the pediatric patient. (p 453)
2-1.61 Describe the indications, contraindications, advantages, disadvantages, complications, equipment, and technique for using a dual lumen airway. (p 431)
2-1.62 Define, identify, and describe a laryngectomy. (p 470)
2-1.63 Describe the special considerations in airway management and ventilation for patients with facial injuries. (p 430)
2-1.64 Describe the special considerations in airway management and ventilation for the pediatric patients. (p 453)

Affective

2-1.65 Defend oxygenation and ventilation. (p 406)
2-1.66 Defend the necessity of establishing and/or maintaining patency of a patient's airway. (p 368)
2-1.67 Comply with standard precautions to defend against infectious and communicable diseases. (p 414)

Psychomotor

2-1.68 Perform body substance isolation (BSI) procedures during basic airway management, advanced airway management, and ventilation. (p 414)
2-1.69 Perform pulse oximetry. (p 373)
2-1.70 Perform end-tidal CO_2 detection. (p 373)
2-1.71 Perform oxygen delivery from a cylinder and regulator with an oxygen delivery device. (p 410)
2-1.72 Deliver supplemental oxygen to a breathing patient using the following devices: nasal cannula, simple face mask, partial rebreathing mask, nonrebreathing mask, and venturi mask. (p 412)
2-1.73 Perform oxygen delivery with an oxygen humidifier. (p 413)
2-1.75 Demonstrate ventilating a patient by the following techniques:
   a. Mouth-to-mask ventilation
   b. One person bag-valve-mask
   c. Two person bag-valve-mask
   d. Three person bag-valve-mask
   e. Flow-restricted, oxygen-powered ventilation device
   f. Automatic transport ventilator
   g. Mouth-to-stoma
   h. Bag-valve-mask-to-stoma ventilation
   (p 415, 417, 418, 420, 422, 467, 471)
2-1.76 Perform the Sellick maneuver (cricoid pressure). (p 422)

Airway Management and Ventilation

2-1.77 Ventilate a pediatric patient using the one and two person techniques. (p 415)
2-1.78 Perform complete airway obstruction maneuvers, including:
   a. Heimlich maneuver
   b. Finger sweep
   c. Chest thrusts
   d. Removal with Magill forceps (p 392, 396, 397)
2-1.79 Perform retrieval of foreign bodies from the upper airway. (p 392)
2-1.80 Demonstrate suctioning the upper airway by selecting a suction device, catheter, and technique. (p 397)
2-1.81 Perform tracheobronchial suctioning in the intubated patient by selecting a suctioning device, catheter, and technique. (p 398)
2-1.82 Demonstrate insertion of a nasogastric tube. (p 425)
2-1.83 Demonstrate insertion of an orogastric tube. (p 427)
2-1.84 Perform gastric decompression by selecting a suction device, catheter, and technique. (p 423)
2-1.85 Perform manual airway maneuvers, including:
   a. Opening the mouth
   b. Head-tilt/chin-lift maneuver
   c. Jaw-thrust without head-tilt maneuver
   d. Modified jaw-thrust maneuver (p 385-388)
2-1.87 Demonstrate insertion of an oropharyngeal airway. (p 403)
2-1.88 Demonstrate insertion of a nasopharyngeal airway. (p 405)
2-1.89 Intubate the trachea by direct orotracheal intubation. (p 403)
2-1.90 Perform assessment to confirm correct placement of the endotracheal tube. (p 445)
2-1.91 Adequately secure an endotracheal tube. (p 449)
2-1.92 Perform extubation. (p 451)
2-1.93 Perform endotracheal intubation in the pediatric patient. (p 453)
2-1.94 Insert a dual lumen airway. (p 432)
2-1.95 Perform stoma suctioning. (p 472)
2-1.96 Perform replacement of a tracheostomy tube through a stoma. (p 472)

1985 Objectives

Cognitive

1.6.11 Describe the anatomy of the following: upper airway, tongue, hypopharynx, nasopharynx, oropharynx, larynx, vocal cords. (p 368)
1.6.12 Describe the function of the vocal cords. (p 369)
1.6.13 Describe the flow of air from outside the body into the trachea. (p 372)
1.6.14 Describe the reasons for and mechanisms of humidification and warming of the air as it passes through the naso- and oral pharynx. (p 372)
1.6.15 Describe the pathological conditions that can occur in the nose, pharynx, and larynx to obstruct or retard air flow and identify the complications of laryngeal fracture. (p 391)
1.6.16 Describe the methods of airway management. (p 384)
1.6.17 Describe the methods and management of an obstructed airway. (p 392)
1.6.18 Describe the mechanical methods of airway management including the benefits and limitations. Oral, nasal, and EOA. (p 402)
1.6.19 Describe how the cervical spine is protected throughout these maneuvers. (p 368)
1.6.20 Describe the anatomy of the following:
   a. Lungs
   b. Trachea
   c. Alveolus
   d. Diaphragm
   e. Thoracic wall
   f. Pleural space (p 368-370)
1.6.21 Describe how pulmonary ventilation (inhalation and exhalation) is accomplished. (p 372)
1.6.22 Describe the gaseous exchange across the alveoli-capillary membrane (O_2 and CO_2). (p 372)
1.6.23 Describe the pulmonary problems that can complicate exhalation and inhalation, the mechanisms by which they reduce ventilation, and management of each problem, including:
   a. Open pneumothorax
   b. Diaphragmatic injury
   c. Closed pneumothorax (simple and tension)
   d. Flail chest. (p 376)
1.6.24 Describe the problems of ventilation. (p 414)

1.6.25 Define mouth-to-mask ventilation, its benefits and limitations. (p 414)

1.6.26 Discuss the bag-valve-mask (BVM), its benefits and limitations. (p 415)

1.6.27 Discuss the techniques for evaluating the effectiveness of ventilation. (p 415)

1.6.32 Discuss ventilation with an EOA. (p 461)

*1.6.33 Discuss ventilation with an endotracheal tube. (p 438)

1.6.34 Describe the equipment and method of suctioning the airway, pharynx, and endotracheal tube. (p 398)

S1.6.60 Demonstrate effective mouth-to-mask ventilation. (p 415)

S1.6.61 Demonstrate effective bag-valve:
   a. Mask
   b. EOA
   *c. ET (p 414, 461)

S1.6.63 Demonstrate the manual methods of airway management. (p 385)

S1.6.64 Demonstrate the methods of management of an obstructed airway. (p 392)

S1.6.65 Demonstrate the mechanical methods of airway management:
   a. Nasal
   b. Oral
   c. EOA
   *d. ET (p 402, 405, 463)

S1.6.67 Demonstrate the use of various types of portable and fixed suction devices. (p 398)

1.7.1 Describe the anatomy of the following: upper airway, tongue, hypopharynx, nasopharynx, oropharynx, larynx, and vocal cords. (p 368)

1.7.2 Describe the relationship between:
   a. Cords and larynx
   b. Esophagus and larynx
   c. Epiglottis and larynx
   d. Tongue and larynx
   e. True cords and false cords
   f. Pharynx and larynx (p 368, 369)

1.7.3 Given a list of arterial oxygen concentrations, the student should be able to select the normal PO_2, for a young adult breathing air. (p 373)

1.7.4 Given a list of arterial carbon dioxide concentrations, the student should be able to select the normal PCO_2. (p 373)

1.7.5 Given an increase in arterial PCO_2, the student should be able to name this condition and describe its effect on respiratory activity and on blood pH in the normal individual. (p 380)

1.7.6 Given a decrease in arterial PO_2, the student should be able to name this condition and describe its effect on respiratory activity in the normal individual. (p 381)

1.7.7 Given an increase in CO_2 production, the student should be able to list at least two ways in which this increase may occur. (p 380)

1.7.8 Given an increase in CO_2 elimination, the student should be able to describe how this elimination can occur. (p 381)

1.7.9 Given a list of statements, the student should be able to identify the statement that best describes the purpose of suctioning a patient. (p 397)

1.7.10 Given a diagram of a piston-powered suction unit, the student should be able to label and describe the operation and cleaning of each component and attached part. (p 399)

1.7.11 Given that there are various types of suction units, the student should be able to list at least four different types of units determined by the method in which the suction effect is obtained. (p 399)

1.7.12 Given that there are various types of suction catheters, the student should be able to list at least three different types, determined by difference in use and material composition. (p 399)

1.7.13 Given a list of situations describing patients who require suctioning, the student should indicate which type of catheter should be used. (p 398)

1.7.14 Given a list of statements, the student should be able to identify the statement that best describes the purpose of using the esophageal obturator airway. (p 461)

1.7.15 Given a list of situations describing patients with airway maintenance problems or potential airway maintenance problems, the student should be able to identify situations in which the use of the esophageal obturator airway is indicated and contraindicated. (p 461)

1.7.16 Given a list of situations, the student should be able to identify those situations in which the esophageal airway may be removed. (p 463)

1.7.17 Given a list of advantages, the student should be able to identify the advantages of using the esophageal obturator airway over other methods of airway control. (p 461)

Airway Management and Ventilation

1.7.18 Given a list of airway adjuncts, advantages, and disadvantages, the student should be able to match the airway adjuncts with the advantages and disadvantages. (p 461)

S1.7.19 Given an adult manikin, oropharyngeal and nasopharyngeal airways, pocket mask, oxygen cylinder, and bag-valve-mask, the student should be able to demonstrate the procedure for administering intermittent positive pressure ventilation using:
  a. Pocket mask
  b. Bag-valve-mask and oropharyngeal airway
  c. Bag-valve-mask with oxygen
  d. Nasopharyngeal airway with bag-valve-mask (p 405, 414, 415)

S1.7.20 Given a bag-valve-mask, the student should be able to demonstrate the assembly, disassembly, and cleaning of the bag-valve-mask unit. (p 417)

S1.7.21 Given an adult manikin, an oropharyngeal airway, and a demand-valve unit, the student should be able to demonstrate the procedure for performing intermittent positive pressure ventilation. (p 416)

S1.7.22 Given a demand-valve unit, the student should be able to demonstrate the assembly, disassembly, and cleaning of the unit. (p 411)

1.7.23 Given a list of disadvantages, the student should be able to identify the disadvantages of using the esophageal obturator airway over other methods of airway control. (p 461)

1.7.24 Given a diagram of the esophageal obturator airway, the student should be able to label and describe the function of all component parts. (p 461)

1.7.25 Given a list of equipment and materials, the student should be able to identify those items that must be available before esophageal obturation is begun. (p 462)

1.7.26 Given that a patient requires an esophageal obturator airway, the student should be able to list the procedures for insertion of the esophageal airway, including all steps in the proper sequence. (p 462)

1.7.27 Given a list of errors, the student should be able to identify common errors involved in the use of the esophageal obturator airway. (p 462)

*1.7.28 Describe laryngoscope, suction, endotracheal tube, and bag-valve-mask. (p 415)

*1.7.29 Discuss indications and contraindications of endotracheal intubation. (p 438)

*1.7.30 Discuss alternatives to endotracheal intubation. (p 461)

*1.7.31 Discuss skill deterioration and methods of prevention. (p 384)

*1.7.32 Discuss need for rapid placement of the ET tube. (p 438)

*1.7.33 Discuss methods of assuring and maintaining correct placement of the ET tube. (p 445)

*1.7.34 Given that a patient needs suctioning and already has an endotracheal tube in place, the student should be able to describe the difference between endotracheal suctioning and oropharyngeal suctioning, including:
  a. Dangers
  b. Precautions (p 451)

*S1.7.35 Given an adult intubation manikin, an esophageal obturator airway, 30cc syringe, and a bag-valve unit, the student should be able to demonstrate the technique for the insertion of an esophageal airway. He should further be able to demonstrate endotracheal intubation with the esophageal obturator in place and subsequent correct removal of the obturator. (p 461)

*S1.7.36 Demonstrate placement of an ET within 45 seconds. (p 441)

*S1.7.37 Demonstrate ventilation with a bag-valve and endotracheal tube. (p 445)

*S1.7.38 Demonstrate method by assuring and maintaining correct placement of ET tube. (p 445)

*S1.7.39 Demonstrate reventilation for missed intubation. (p 449)

*S1.7.40 Demonstrate skills described above both on manikin and a live patient. (p 441, 445)

1.8.18 Define acid-base balance. (p 449)

1.8.19 Discuss acid-base balance based on hydrogen concentration, pH, and buffer systems. (p 378, 380)

1.8.20 Define and discuss the following:
  a. Respiratory acidosis
  b. Respiratory alkalosis
  c. Metabolic acidosis
  d. Metabolic alkalosis (p 380, 382)

*Indicates optional.
"S" indicates a skill objective.

9

Airway Management and Ventilation

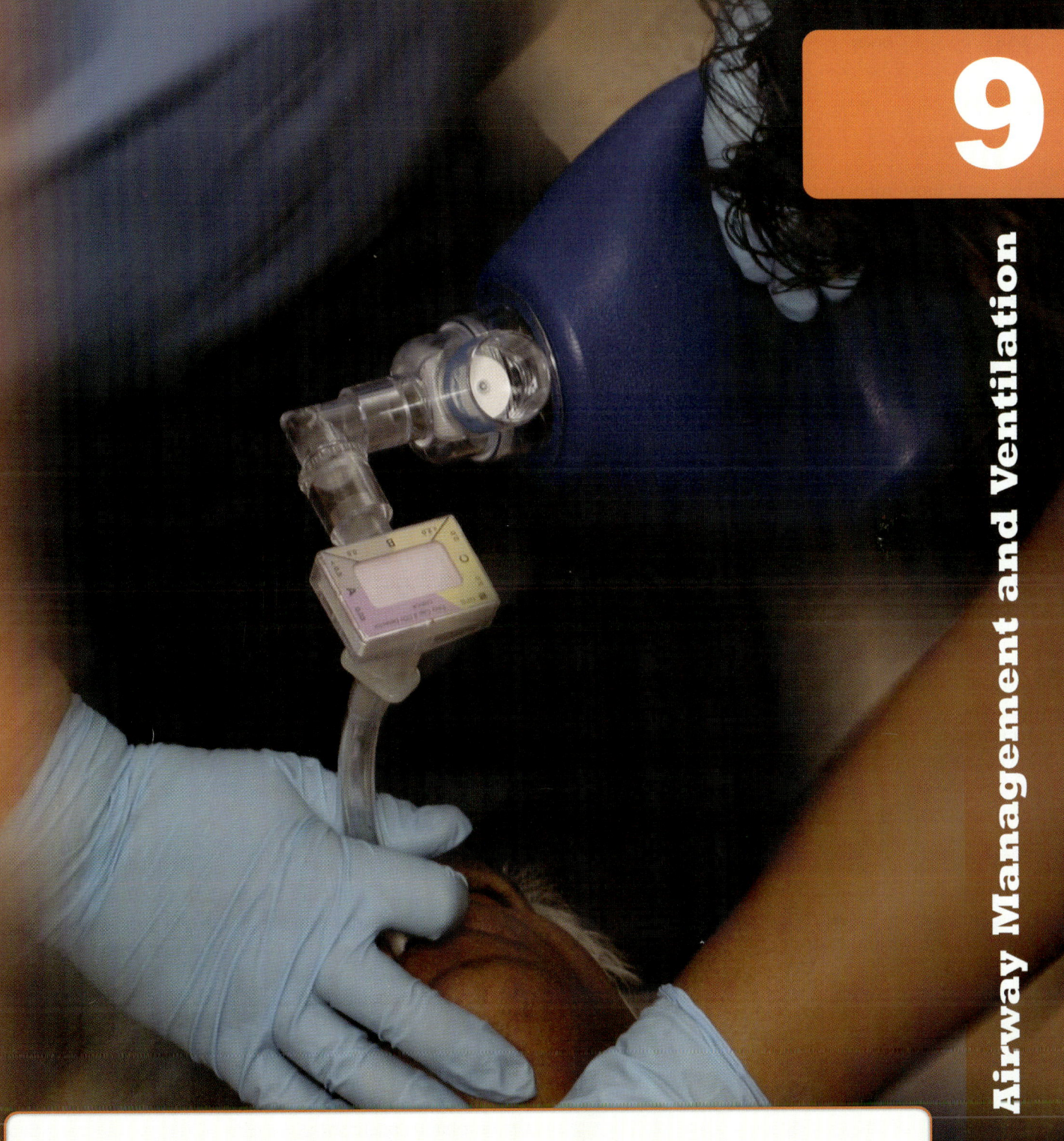

You are the Provider

You receive a call for an 82-year-old woman with difficulty breathing. You recognize the address because you have been there many times before. The patient is often admitted to the hospital and has a history of acute exacerbations of chronic obstructive pulmonary disease (COPD) with intensive care unit admissions.

　　Approximately one of every four calls to EMS are related to airway or respiratory problems. This chapter will help prepare you for these frequently encountered calls and will help you answer the following questions:

1. Why do airway and breathing assessment and care have such a prominent position in the realm of an EMT-I's scope of practice?
2. Why is it necessary that you be familiar with all the airway equipment on your ambulance?

Airway

The single most important steps in caring for any patient are to obtain and maintain a patent airway and to ensure that the patient is breathing adequately. Without a patent airway, effective patient care is not possible. All organs, body tissues, and cells require a constant supply of oxygen to survive. Within a few minutes of being deprived of oxygen, vital organs such as the heart and brain may not function normally.

Oxygen reaches body tissues and cells through two separate but related processes: breathing and circulation. As we inhale, oxygen moves from the atmosphere into our lungs and then passes from the alveoli in the lungs into the capillaries to oxygenate the blood. The blood, enriched with oxygen, travels through the body by the pumping action of the heart. At the same time, carbon dioxide, produced by cells in the tissues of the body, moves from the capillaries into the alveoli. The carbon dioxide then leaves our bodies as we exhale.

The primary objective of emergency care is to ensure optimal ventilation to facilitate the delivery of oxygen and elimination of carbon dioxide. Brain cell death occurs within 4 to 6 minutes after being deprived of oxygen. The major causes of preventable death in the prehospital setting can be intercepted by early detection, early intervention, and layperson education in basic life support (that is, CPR).

Airway maneuvers are often the most neglected of prehospital skills. Basic airway management skills tend to be taken for granted as more advanced skills are learned. Poor technique leads to ineffective ventilation and inadequate patient care. These include an inadequate mask-to-face seal, improper positioning of the patient for airway patency, equipment that is not readily available, and failure to reassess the patient frequently. As an EMT-I, you must be familiar with the respiratory system, understand how the system works, and be able to recognize which patients are breathing adequately and which ones are breathing inadequately. This will enable you to provide the most effective patient care.

This chapter will review the anatomy and physiology of the respiratory system. It will then describe how to assess patients quickly and carefully to determine their airway and ventilation status. The equipment, procedures, and guidelines that you will need to manage a patient's airway and breathing are described in detail. You will learn several ways to open a patient's airway and specific techniques for removing foreign objects or fluids that place the airway in jeopardy. Because artificial airway equipment can cause harm to the patient if used improperly, the chapter will thoroughly discuss airway adjuncts, oxygen therapy devices, definitive airway equipment, and artificial ventilation methods.

Anatomy of the Upper Airway

The airway is divided into both upper and lower airways. The major functions of the upper airway are to warm, filter, and humidify air brought into the body. Air enters the body through the mouth and nose. Warming protects the patient from becoming hypothermic. Humidification is accomplished as the air picks up moisture from the tissues of the airway.

The pharynx (throat) is the first portion of the upper airway and is composed of the nasopharynx and oropharynx. The hypopharynx is the lower portion of the pharynx that opens into the larynx anteriorly and the esophagus posteriorly.

Nasopharynx

The union of the facial bones forms the nasopharynx. The orientation of the nasal floor is toward the ear, not the eye. The nasopharynx is divided by the septum. The entire nasal cavity is lined with a ciliated mucosal membrane. The mucosal membranes trap dust and small particles and prevent them from entering the respiratory system. Cilia help move contaminants out of the body. During an illness, the body produces more mucus to trap potentially infectious agents.

Technology

- Interactivities
- Vocabulary Explorer
- Anatomy Review
- Web Links
- Online Review Manual

www.EMSzone.com/EMTI

From the lateral walls of the nose, three bony shelves called turbinates extend into the nasal passageway. They are parallel to the nasal floor. The turbinates serve to increase the surface area of the nasal mucosa, thereby improving filtration, warming, and humidification of inhaled air. The sinuses are cavities formed by the cranial bones. They seem to further trap bacteria and act as tributaries for fluid to and from the eustachian tubes and tear ducts and commonly become infected. Because the cranial bones form the sinus cavities, fractures of certain sinus bones may cause a leakage of cerebrospinal fluid (CSF) into the nasal passageways and auditory canal.

The tissues of the nasopharynx are extremely delicate and highly vascular. Improper or overly aggressive placement of airway devices may cause significant bleeding that cannot be controlled by direct pressure.

Oropharynx

The oropharynx, or oral cavity, begins with the mouth and teeth. There are 32 adult teeth, which are embedded in the gums in such a manner that significant force is required to dislodge them. However, trauma may result in fracture or avulsion, causing obstruction of the upper airway or aspiration into the lungs.

The tongue is a large muscle attached at the mandible and hyoid bone. The hyoid bone is a small bone located between the chin and the mandibular angle. The jaw, tongue, epiglottis, and thyroid cartilage attach at this point. The tongue is the most common cause of upper airway obstruction, especially in patients with altered mental status.

The palate forms the roof of the mouth and separates the oropharynx and nasopharynx. The anterior portion is the hard palate, and the posterior portion, beyond the teeth, is the soft palate. Aggressive insertion of oral airways may result in trauma to the hard or soft palate. The adenoids are located on the posterior nasopharyngeal wall. Adenoids are lymph tissue that filter bacteria and frequently become infected and swollen. Severe swelling of the tonsils and adenoids can also result in upper airway obstruction.

The superior border of the glottic opening is the epiglottis. The epiglottis is a leaf-shaped cartilaginous flap located at the base of the tongue and above the larynx that prevents food and liquid from entering the larynx during swallowing. When swallowing begins, laryngeal muscles contract to cause downward movement of the epiglottis and upward movement of the glottis. Combined with closure of the vocal cords, these actions protect the airway from aspiration during eating and drinking. The vallecula is the anatomic space, or "pocket," between the base of the tongue and the epiglottis and is an important landmark for endotracheal intubation.

Larynx

The glottic opening separates the upper and lower airways. The larynx is a complex structure formed by many independent cartilaginous structures that all work together. The shield-shaped thyroid cartilage is the major laryngeal structure. The posterior portion is made of smooth muscle. The thyroid cartilage is the first tracheal cartilage and is suspended from the hyoid bone by the thyroid ligament. It forms the anterior laryngeal prominence commonly known as the "Adam's apple." The glottic opening is directly posterior to the thyroid cartilage.

The glottic opening is the narrowest portion of the adult trachea. Airway patency in this area is heavily dependent on muscle tone. The lateral borders of the glottis are the vocal cords, which are white bands of tough, fibrous tissue. Voice is generated by air passing through the vibrating vocal cords. The arytenoid cartilage is a pyramid-like cartilaginous structure that forms the posterior attachment of the vocal cords. These cartilaginous structures are valuable landmarks for endotracheal intubation. The pyriform fossae are hollow "pockets" along the lateral borders of the larynx. Airway devices are occasionally inadvertently inserted into these pockets, resulting in "tenting" of the skin under the jaw.

The inferior aspect of the thyroid cartilage articulates with the cricoid cartilage. The cricoid cartilage is a signet-ring–shaped structure that is the only upper airway structure that forms a complete ring. It is the first tracheal ring and is completely cartilaginous. Compression of the cricoid cartilage, also known as the Sellick maneuver, occludes the esophagus, reducing gastric distention during ventilation and facilitating placement of an endotracheal tube. The anterior portion of the cricoid ring is the narrowest and is separated from the thyroid cartilage by the cricothyroid membrane—a thin, fibrous membrane located between the cricoid ring and the thyroid cartilage. It is the site for surgical and alternative airway placement.

Other associated structures of the lower airway include the thyroid gland, carotid arteries, and jugular veins. The thyroid gland is located below the cricoid cartilage and lies across the trachea and up both sides. Branches of the carotid arteries cross and lie closely alongside the trachea, as do the jugular veins. Because of its proximity to these structures, it is very important to locate the landmarks carefully when attempting airway access through the cricothyroid membrane.

Anatomy of the Lower Airway

The function of the lower airway is to exchange oxygen and carbon dioxide. It extends from the fourth cervical vertebra to the xiphoid process and, internally, from the glottic opening to the pulmonary capillary membrane.

The trachea begins immediately below the cricoid cartilage. It is 10 to 12 cm long and bifurcates at the carina into the right and left mainstem bronchi. The right branch has a lesser angle than the left, resulting in greater occurrences of foreign bodies entering the right mainstem bronchus. Endotracheal (ET) tubes that are advanced too far also commonly displace into the right mainstem bronchus. The bronchi are lined with mucous cells and beta-2 receptors that dilate the bronchioles.

All of the blood vessels and the mainstem bronchi enter each lung at the hilum. The right lung has three lobes, and the left lung has two lobes, each made of parenchymal tissue. The lungs are covered with a thin, slippery outer lining, known as the visceral pleura, which enables the delicate tissue to move along the inside of the chest without damage. In total, the lungs hold about 6 L of air. The parietal pleura lines the inside of the chest (thoracic) wall. There is a small amount of fluid located in the potential space between the two pleural layers, which decreases friction during the respiratory cycle.

After entering the lungs, the mainstem bronchi branch into narrowing secondary and tertiary bronchi that branch into bronchioles. The smaller bronchioles then branch into alveolar ducts that end at alveolar sacs. The alveoli are balloonlike clusters of single-layered air sacs that are the functional site for the exchange of oxygen and carbon dioxide. This gas exchange occurs by simple diffusion between the alveoli and the capillaries of the pulmonary circulatory system. Alveoli function to increase the surface area of the lungs. As the alveoli are expanded, during deep inhalation, they become even thinner, making diffusion easier.

The alveoli are lined with a proteinaceous substance known as surfactant, which decreases surface tension and helps keep the alveoli expanded. If the amount of surfactant is decreased or alveoli are not inflated, the alveoli collapse, which results in a condition known as atelectasis.

Lung and Respiratory Volumes

The average adult male has a total lung capacity of approximately 6 L, but not all of this air actually enters the alveoli. A minor diffusion of oxygen takes place in the alveolar ducts and terminal bronchioles. The percentage or fraction of oxygen in inspired air is known as the FIO_2. It increases with supplemental oxygen and is commonly documented as a decimal.

You are the Provider — Part 2

As you approach the patient, you notice that she has labored breathing with accessory muscle use. She is receiving oxygen via nasal cannula at 2 L/min. You perform an initial assessment, which reveals the following:

Initial Assessment	Recording Time: Zero Minutes
Appearance	Severe respiratory distress; pale and diaphoretic
Level of consciousness	Responsive verbally, appears fatigued, stares off into the distance
Airway	Open
Breathing	Respiratory rate, increased and labored
Circulation	Skin, appears pale, very clammy; radial pulse, rapid

3. What is your priority of care for this patient? Why?

Tidal volume, a measure of the depth of breathing, is the volume of air that is inhaled or exhaled during a single respiratory cycle. The normal tidal volume in an adult male is 5 to 7 mL/kg, or approximately 500 mL. The normal tidal volume for pediatric patients, infant or child, is 6 to 8 mL/kg. Breathing becomes deeper as tidal volume increases in response to the increased metabolic demand for oxygen and can increase as much as three or four times. At the end of inhalation, there is approximately 150 mL of air, or dead-space air, that remains in the air passageways and is unavailable for gas exchange. Dead space is the portion of the airway that does not contain air that can participate in respiration. This space is divided into two sections, the anatomic dead space and the physiologic dead space. The anatomic dead space consists of the trachea and larger bronchi. The air remaining in this area is simply the result of residual gas once the pressure inside the thoracic cavity equals that of atmospheric pressure. Air remaining in the physiologic dead space is the result of disease or obstruction. Conditions such as COPD and asthma contribute to air trapping.

Alveolar air is the amount of gas that reaches the alveoli with each breath. Alveolar air is equal to tidal volume minus dead-space volume and is approximately 350 mL. During artificial ventilation with a bag-valve-mask (BVM) or similar device, the volume of the mask increases the dead space. While this may seem to be a relatively small factor, a mask volume of only 50 mL can increase dead space by 25%.

Minute volume, or the amount of air moved in and out of the lungs per minute, is a computation of tidal volume minus dead-space volume multiplied by the respiratory rate. It is important to note that variations in tidal volume, respiratory rate, or both, will affect minute volume. For example, if a patient is breathing at a rate of 14 breaths/min, but the tidal volume is reduced (shallow breathing), minute volume will decrease. Likewise, if a patient is breathing at a rate of 14 breaths/min and the tidal volume is increased (deep breathing), minute volume will increase. Conversely, if a patient is breathing too rapidly with reduced tidal volume, inhaled air may only reach the dead space before it is exhaled, resulting in smaller volumes of air actually entering the lungs to participate in gas exchange (alveolar air). As a result, minute volume would decrease.

After an optimal inspiration, the amount of air that can be forced from the lungs in a single forced exhalation is known as the functional reserve capacity.

Even if you exhale forcefully, you cannot completely empty your lungs of air. The air that remains after maximal expiration is known as the residual volume, which is about 1,200 mL in the average adult male. The amount of air that you can exhale following a normal (relaxed) exhalation is referred to as the expiratory reserve volume; this amount is also about 1,200 mL. The inspiratory reserve volume, which is about 3,000 mL, is the amount of air you can inhale after a normal inhalation. This is the amount of gas that can be inspired in addition to the tidal volume.

> **Pediatric Needs**
>
> A proportionately smaller jaw in pediatric patients causes the tongue to encroach on the airway, resulting in easier blockage than in adults. The airway changes greatly during the early years of life. The epiglottis is floppy, contributing to airway problems. The tongue is larger in relation to the size of the mandible in younger children, and it is more rounded than in adults. These characteristics make the tongue a greater risk for obstruction. As children grow, the mandible grows and pulls the tongue forward, which flattens the tongue.
>
> The soft tissue in the posterior pharynx can also contribute to airway problems in infants and small children. The tonsils, adenoids, and soft palate, in combination with the tongue, produce a smaller opening for easy air movement. Upper respiratory infections can increase a child's work of breathing. Also, the trachea is softer, smaller, and narrower at all levels, making it more prone to collapse during increased work of breathing. The larynx lies more superior than in older children and adults and is funnel-shaped owing to the narrow, undeveloped cricoid cartilage. Before the age of 10 years, the narrowest point is at the cricoid ring. Further narrowing of the airway by tissue swelling or a foreign body results in a major increase in airway resistance. The cartilage that provides support matures as we grow; however, the trachea can be occluded from compression. Even during the head tilt–chin lift maneuver, the airway can be occluded if the head is extended too much or the maneuver is performed too aggressively.
>
> The ribs and cartilage are also softer and more pliable in children. Because of this, they cannot optimally contribute to lung expansion. Infants and children tend to depend more heavily on the diaphragm for breathing.

Ventilation

Ventilation is the movement of air into and out of the lungs. Adequate, continuous ventilation is essential for life and is, therefore, one of the highest priorities in treating any patient. If a patient is not breathing or is breathing inadequately, you must immediately intervene to ensure adequate ventilation.

Ventilation has two phases: inspiration and expiration. Inspiration is the process of air moving into the lungs. Expiration is the process of moving air out of the lungs. One ventilation cycle consists of one inspiration and one expiration.

Inspiration

The stimulus to breathe comes from the respiratory center located in the medulla. The involuntary control of breathing originates in the brain stem, specifically in the pons and medulla. The impulses for automatic breathing descend through the spinal cord and can be overridden (to a point) by voluntary control. The motor nerves of respiration are the phrenic nerves, which innervates the diaphragm, and the intercostal nerves, which innervate the external intercostal muscles (muscles between the ribs).

The diaphragm is the muscle of respiration and separates the thoracic cavity from the abdominal cavity. During inspiration, the diaphragm and intercostal muscles contract. When the diaphragm contracts, it flattens and descends, increasing the vertical dimension of the thoracic cage. When the intercostal muscles contract, they raise the ribs up and out. The combined actions of these structures enlarge the thorax in all directions, causing intrapulmonary pressure to fall slightly below atmospheric pressure. The air pressure outside the body, called the atmospheric pressure, is normally higher than the air pressure within the thorax. As the diaphragm and intercostal muscles contract and the thoracic cage expands, air pressure within the thorax decreases, creating a slight vacuum. This pulls air in through the trachea and fills the lungs, inflating the alveoli. When the air pressure outside the thorax equals the air pressure inside the thorax, air stops moving. Gases, such as oxygen, will move from an area of higher pressure to an area of lower pressure until the pressures are equal. At this point, the air stops moving, and we stop inhaling. Oxygen and carbon dioxide are then able to diffuse across the alveolar membrane.

Expiration

As the chest expands, mechanical receptors, known as stretch receptors, in the chest wall and bronchioles send a signal to the apneustic center via the vagus nerve to inhibit the inspiratory center, and expiration occurs. This feedback loop, a combination of mechanical and neural control, is known as the Hering-Breuer reflex and terminates inhalation to prevent overexpansion of the lungs. The diaphragm and intercostal muscles relax, which increases intrapulmonary pressure. The natural elasticity, or recoil, of the lungs passively removes the air.

Respiration

Respiration is defined as the exchange of gases between a living organism and its environment. The major gases of respiration are oxygen and carbon dioxide.

There are two types of respiration: external and internal. External (or pulmonary) respiration is the exchange of gases between the lungs and the blood cells in the pulmonary capillaries. Internal (or cellular) respiration is the exchange of gases between the blood cells and tissues.

The gas exchange during respiration occurs by a process of diffusion, in which a gas moves from an area of higher concentration to an area of lower concentration. Oxygen and carbon dioxide dissolve in water and pass through the alveolar membrane by diffusion.

> **In the Field**
>
> Remember that a pulse oximeter can detect only the saturation of hemoglobin. It cannot identify the gas that is saturating the hemoglobin. For example, a patient in an area rich with carbon monoxide may have a normal Sao_2. Carbon monoxide, which has a 200 times greater affinity for hemoglobin than oxygen, has similar characteristics to arterial blood. Therefore, the dual wavelengths of infrared light used by the pulse oximeter may not be able to distinguish between the two, producing a falsely high reading. It is essential to pay close attention to the scene survey and to treat the patient instead of the diagnostic equipment. The pulse oximeter is designed to detect gross abnormalities, not subtle changes.

Dissolved oxygen crosses the pulmonary capillary membrane and binds to the hemoglobin of the red blood cells. Without hemoglobin, there is no transport of oxygen. This is why replacing large amounts of lost blood with the standard intravenous fluids will be less effective in resuscitation. Isotonic crystalloid solutions that are carried by most emergency medical services lack the hemoglobin necessary for transport of oxygen. Approximately 97% of the total oxygen (O_2) is bound to hemoglobin; the remainder is dissolved in the plasma. A pulse oximeter reads the percentage of hemoglobin that is saturated, which is normally greater than 98% (SaO_2). The remaining oxygen that is dissolved in the plasma makes up the partial pressure of oxygen, also called the PaO_2 or PO_2.

Carbon dioxide (CO_2) is a by-product of cellular respiration. The majority of CO_2 is transported in the blood in the form of bicarbonate ions, with about 33% bound to the hemoglobin. As O_2 crosses from the alveoli into the blood, CO_2 diffuses from the blood into the alveoli. The CO_2 dissolved in the plasma makes up the partial pressure of CO_2, also called the $PaCO_2$ or PCO_2.

In addition to your physical examination of the patient, assessment of adequate respiration may be accomplished through the use of pulse oximetry, peak expiratory flow testing, end-tidal CO_2 monitoring, and other equipment. Again, it is imperative to use these devices as an assessment adjunct and to treat the patient as he or she presents.

Causes of Decreased Oxygen Concentrations in the Blood

There are numerous conditions that may contribute to a lower oxygen concentration in the bloodstream. A lower partial pressure of atmospheric oxygen, such as a smoke-filled environment, decreases the amount of oxygen available for use. Excessive bleeding causes decreased hemoglobin levels, thereby decreasing the oxygen-carrying capability of the blood and, in turn, decreasing the amount of oxygen available to the cells.

Any condition that reduces the surface area for gas exchange also decreases the available oxygen supply. Examples of these are flail chest, diaphragmatic injury, closed pneumothorax (simple or tension) (a partial or complete accumulation of air in the pleural space [the space between the visceral and parietal pleura of the lung]), open pneumothorax, hemothorax, and hemopneumothorax. With any of these conditions, increasing pressure decreases the ability of the lungs to expand, further decreasing the surface area of the alveoli for gas exchange. Treatment of each of these conditions is covered in Chapter 15, Thoracic Trauma.

Decreased mechanical effort also decreases the availability of oxygen for respiration. A person experiencing pain in the chest due to trauma or medical reasons tends to breathe as shallowly as possible to prevent movement of the chest wall and relieve pain. Traumatic asphyxia (caused by compression injuries to the chest) and hypoventilation from any cause also result in decreased oxygen levels in the blood.

Medical conditions that create a physical barrier to diffusion decrease available oxygen levels. Pneumonia, pulmonary edema, and COPD are conditions that decrease the surface area of the alveoli, through damage to the alveoli themselves or a buildup of fluid, which increases the distance between the alveoli and the capillaries. If the alveoli are not functional, carbon dioxide and oxygen will not be allowed to diffuse. Therefore, the blood will bypass the alveoli and will return to the left side of the heart in an unoxygenated state, a condition known as intrapulmonary shunting.

Carbon Dioxide in the Blood

Carbon dioxide levels in the blood fluctuate in relation to changes in breathing. Hypoventilation causes carbon dioxide to build up because the slow respiratory rate does not allow for removal of enough carbon dioxide. Conversely, hyperventilation rids the body of excessive amounts of carbon dioxide. Because carbon dioxide adds to our total acid-base balance and our stimulus to breathe, it is imperative to closely control carbon dioxide levels in the blood.

The Measurement of Gases

The percentage and the partial pressure of a given gas in a breathing mixture are important values. Understanding them requires an understanding of Dalton's law of partial pressure.

Dalton's law states that the total pressure of a gas is the sum of the partial pressure of the components of that gas, or the pressure exerted by a specific atmospheric gas. At sea level, the total pressure of air (100% of all atmospheric gases) is about 760 mm Hg, or 760 torr. The major components of air are nitrogen,

597.0 torr (78.62%); oxygen, 159.0 torr (20.84%); carbon dioxide, 0.3 torr (0.04%); and water vapor, 3.7 torr (0.50%). The partial pressure of each of these gases is proportional to the relative percentage of each.

The alveolar gas concentration is a measure of the partial pressure that each of the gases exerts in the alveoli. The major components of alveolar gas are nitrogen, 560.0 torr (74.9%); oxygen, 104.0 (13.7%); carbon dioxide, 40.0 torr (5.2%); and water vapor, 47.0 torr (6.2%).

> **In the Field**
>
> The blood does not use all the inhaled oxygen as it passes through the body. The air that we exhale contains approximately 16% oxygen and 3% to 5% carbon dioxide; the rest is nitrogen. Therefore, when you provide mouth-to-mouth (or mask) ventilation to a patient who is not breathing, the patient is receiving a 16% concentration of oxygen with each of your exhaled breaths.

Respiratory Rate

Neural Control

The respiratory rate is the number of times a person breathes in 1 minute. The neural control of breathing originates in the brain and brain stem. Primary control comes from the medulla and pons. The medulla is the primary involuntary respiratory center. It is connected to the respiratory muscles by the vagus nerve. The medullary respiratory centers control the rate, depth, and rhythm of breathing in a negative feedback interaction with centers in the pons.

The apneustic center of the pons is the secondary control center if the medulla fails to initiate respiration. The apneustic center influences the respiratory rate by increasing the number of inspirations per minute. This is balanced by the pneumotaxic center, which has an inhibitory influence on inspiration. The respiratory rate, therefore, results from the interaction between these two centers. In times of increased demand, the pneumotaxic center decreases its influence, thereby increasing the respiratory rate.

Chemical Stimuli

The goal of the respiratory system is to keep the blood's concentrations of oxygen and carbon dioxide and its acid-base balance within very narrow normal ranges. The body has a number of receptors that monitor variables and provide feedback to the respiratory centers to modify the respiratory rate and depth based on the body's needs. These chemoreceptors have important effects on respiratory rate and depth.

Chemoreceptors that constantly monitor the chemical composition of body fluids are located throughout the body to provide feedback on many metabolic processes. Three sets of chemoreceptors affect respira-

You are the Provider — Part 3

You apply a nonrebreathing mask set at 15 L/min and continue your assessment of the patient. Your partner obtains the following baseline vital signs:

Vital Signs	Recording Time: 2 Minutes After Patient Contact
Respirations	32 breaths/min, shallow
Pulse	120 beats/min, irregular
Skin	Pale and diaphoretic
Blood pressure	112/68 mm Hg
Sao_2	85% while receiving O_2 at 15 L/min via nonrebreathing mask

4. This patient is in obvious respiratory distress. What are some of the causes of respiratory distress that must be considered by the EMT-I?
5. What signs of respiratory distress should the EMT-I look for?

tory function. The first two, which monitor the carbon dioxide level in the blood and the pH of the CSF, have a much greater effect on ventilatory depth and rate than the third.

The chemoreceptors that measure the amount of CO_2 in arterial blood ($PaCO_2$) are located in the carotid bodies and the aortic arch. These receptors sense minute changes in the CO_2 level and send signals to the respiratory center via the glossopharyngeal nerve (9th cranial nerve) and the vagus nerve (10th cranial nerve).

Central chemoreceptors, which constantly monitor the pH of the CSF, are located adjacent to the respiratory centers in the medulla. The acidity of the CSF is an indirect measure of the $PaCO_2$ because the CO_2 in the blood readily diffuses across the blood-brain barrier and combines with water to form carbonic acid (H_2CO_3). The carbonic acid dissociates, and the pH drops as the hydrogen ion (H^+) concentration increases. An increase in the acidity of CSF triggers the central chemoreceptors to increase the rate and depth of respiration. These central chemoreceptors are very sensitive to small changes in pH and provide for "fine-tuning" of the body's acid-base balance.

While the primary control of ventilation is the pH of the CSF, the amount of O_2 dissolved in the plasma (PaO_2) has a secondary and protective role. The chemoreceptors located in the aortic arch and carotid bodies also respond to decreases in PaO_2 by sending messages to the respiratory control center to increase respiration. Under normal conditions, these chemoreceptors serve as a backup to the primary control of ventilation, which is based on the level of CO_2 in the blood and the pH of the CSF.

We also have a "backup system," called the hypoxic drive, to control respiration. This system stimulates breathing when the arterial O_2 level falls (hypoxemia). However, the nerves in the brain, the walls of the aorta, and the carotid arteries that act as oxygen sensors are easily satisfied with minimal levels of oxygen. Therefore, the hypoxic drive is much less sensitive and less powerful than the carbon dioxide sensors in the brain stem.

Normally, the stimulus to breathe is mediated by the acidity of the blood and CSF, which is directly related to the concentration of CO_2 in the blood. Patients with chronic lung diseases, such as bronchitis or emphysema, tend to maintain chronically elevated CO_2 levels. Eventually the sensitivity to the high $PaCO_2$ decreases, and the body uses another feedback loop to control breathing. These patients develop a hypoxic drive, which regulates the respiratory rate based on the O_2 content of the blood.

Control of Respiration by Other Factors

Numerous factors other than changes in pH influence respirations. Respirations increase or decrease based on the body's need at any given time. As body temperature rises, respirations increase in response to the increased metabolic activity. Certain medications cause the respiratory rate to increase or decrease,

You are the Provider — Part 4

You apply a cardiac monitor and establish an IV of normal saline set at a keep vein open (or KVO) rate. Shortly before transporting, you reassess the patient and note the following:

Reassessment	Recording Time: 5 Minutes After Patient Contact
Level of consciousness	Responsive to verbal stimuli only
Respirations	36 breaths/min, shallow
Pulse	130 beats/min, irregular
Skin	Pale and diaphoretic
Blood pressure	100/60 mm Hg
SaO_2	82% while breathing 100% O_2 via nonrebreathing mask

6. What is your rationale for administering 100% oxygen to a COPD patient?

depending on their physiologic action. Pain and strong emotions can also increase respirations. Hypoxia, which is a powerful stimulus to breathe, increases respirations in an effort to bring in more oxygen. Conversely, acidosis increases respirations as a compensatory response to increased carbon dioxide production in an effort to eliminate more carbon dioxide from the body. Respirations decrease as metabolism slows, such as during sleep.

TABLE 9-1	Normal Respiration Rate Ranges
Adults	12 to 20 breaths/min
Children	15 to 30 breaths/min
Infants	25 to 50 breaths/min

Note: These ranges are per the 2002 Airway Management supplement to the US DOT 1994 EMT-Basic National Standard Curriculum. Ranges presented in other courses or texts may vary.

Airway Evaluation

Essential Parameters

You can think of a normal breathing pattern as a bellows system. Breathing should appear easy, not labored. As with a bellows used to move air to start a fire, breathing should be a smooth flow of air moving into and out of the lungs. Generally speaking, if you can see or hear a patient breathe, there is a problem.

Normal respirations in the adult are characterized by a rate of between 12 and 20 breaths/min with adequate depth (tidal volume) and a regular pattern of inhalation and exhalation. Irregular respiratory patterns are clinically significant until proven otherwise. Breathing at rest should be effortless; changes may be subtle in rate or regularity. Patients often compensate for respiratory distress with preferential positioning, such as an upright sniffing position or semi-Fowler (semisitting) position. A patient experiencing breathing difficulty will avoid a supine position because this position increases respiratory distress.

Recognition of Airway Problems

An adult who is awake, alert, and able to talk to you in complete sentences has no immediate airway or breathing problems. However, you should always have supplemental oxygen and ventilation equipment close at hand to assist with breathing if this becomes necessary. An adult who is breathing normally will have respirations of 12 to 20 breaths/min Table 9-1 with a regular pattern of breathing and adequate depth (tidal volume). The adult patient who is breathing fewer than 12 times per minute or more than 20 times per minute should be evaluated for other signs of inadequate breathing, such as reduced tidal volume (shallow breathing), an irregular pattern of breathing, altered mentation, or abnormal airway sounds.

Respiratory distress may be the result of upper and/or lower airway obstruction, inadequate ventilation, impairment of the respiratory muscles, or impairment of the nervous system. Any difficulty in respiratory rate, regularity, or effort is defined as dyspnea. Dyspnea may be the result of or result in hypoxemia, which is a deficiency of oxygen in arterial blood. If left untreated, hypoxemia will progress to hypoxia, a lack of oxygen to the body's cells and tissues. Untreated hypoxia will lead to anoxia and death of the body's cells and tissues.

> **A to Z Terminology Tips**
>
> Remember that the prefix *hypo-* means *low*, and *a-* means *without*.
> - Hypoxia = low levels or a lack of oxygen to the cells and tissues
> - Anoxia = a total absence of oxygen
>
> The suffix *-emia* means *blood*.
> - Hypoxemia = low levels of oxygen in the arterial blood, which leads to a lack of oxygen to the tissues (hypoxia).

Recognition and treatment of dyspnea is crucial to patient survival. Careful assessment and management of the patient with dyspnea are essential. The brain can survive only a few minutes of anoxia. After 4 to 6 minutes without oxygen, brain cells and cells in the nervous system may be severely and permanently damaged and may even die. Dead brain cells can never be replaced. Management of the patient will be ineffective if the airway is not patent and the patient is not breathing adequately.

Evaluation of the patient includes the technique of look, listen, and feel. Visual techniques should be used at first sight of the patient. The following questions should be answered when assessing the patient for signs of respiratory distress:

- How is the patient positioned?
- Is he or she in a tripod position?
- Is the patient experiencing orthopnea (positional dyspnea)?
- Is there adequate rise and fall of the chest?
- Is the patient gasping?
- What is the color of the skin?
- Is there any flaring of the nares?
- Are the lips pursed?
- Do you note any retractions (skin pulling in around the ribs during inspiration):
  - Intercostal?
  - At the suprasternal notch?
  - At the supraclavicular fossa?
  - Subcostal?
- Is the patient using accessory muscles to breathe?

Next, auscultate breathing with and without a stethoscope. Is air movement noted at the mouth and nose? Can equal and bilateral breath sounds be heard over all lung fields?

Finally, feel for air movement at the mouth and nose. Observe the chest for symmetry, paradoxical motion, and retractions. If you are ventilating the patient with a BVM device, note any resistance or change in compliance with ventilation.

Evaluate for pulsus paradoxus, a condition in which the systolic blood pressure drops more than 10 mm Hg with inspiration. A change in pulse quality, or even the disappearance of a pulse, may also be detected. Pulsus paradoxus is generally seen in patients with decompensating COPD or severe pericardial tamponade. It may also indicate an increase in intrathoracic pressure.

A history of the present illness is a vital part of your assessment. Determine the evolution of this particular event:

- Was its onset sudden or gradual?
- Is there any known cause or "trigger" of the event?
- What is the duration?
- Is this a constant (chronic) or recurrent (episodic) problem?
- Are there any alleviating or exacerbating factors?
- Are there any other associated symptoms, such as a productive cough, chest pain, or fever?
- What interventions have been attempted before EMS arrival?
- Has the patient been evaluated or admitted to the hospital for this condition in the past?
- What medications does the patient take, and is he or she compliant with the prescribed regimens?

One of the most important questions to ask is whether the patient has ever been intubated for this problem. A condition bad enough to warrant intubation needs urgent attention to prevent a repeated occurrence.

Note any modified forms of respirations. Protective reflexes of the airway include coughing, sneezing, and gagging. A cough is a forceful, spastic exhalation that aids in clearing the bronchi and bronchioles. Sneezing clears the nasopharynx and is often caused by an irritant, such as dust. The gag reflex is a spastic pharyngeal and esophageal reflex due to a stimulus of the posterior pharynx to prevent foreign objects from entering the trachea.

Sighing and hiccuping are other modified forms of respiration. Sighing is an involuntary deep breath that increases opening of the alveoli, preventing atelectasis. The average person normally sighs about once per minute. Hiccuping is the intermittent spastic closure of the glottis and is caused by spasm of the diaphragm. Persistent hiccuping may be clinically significant.

Respiratory pattern changes indicate serious injury or illness. Table 9-2 shows various respiratory patterns and causes. Patients with inadequate breathing have inadequate minute volume and need to be treated with positive-pressure ventilation and 100% oxygen.

TABLE 9-2	Respiratory Pattern Changes
Cheyne-Stokes respirations	Gradually increasing rate and tidal volume followed by gradual decrease; associated with brain stem insult
Kussmaul respirations	Deep, gasping respirations; common in diabetic coma and ketoacidosis
Biot respirations	Irregular pattern, rate, and volume with intermittent periods of apnea (absence of breathing); results from increased intracranial pressure
Central neurogenic hyperventilation	Deep, rapid respirations similar to Kussmaul; also results from increased intracranial pressure
Agonal respirations	Slow, shallow, irregular respirations or occasional gasping breaths; results from brain anoxia. Agonal respirations may be seen when the heart has stopped but the brain continues to send signals to the muscles of respiration

Inadequate ventilation occurs when the body cannot compensate for increased oxygen demand or maintain an adequate oxygen–carbon dioxide balance. There are many causes, including infection, trauma, brain stem insult, a noxious or hypoxic atmosphere, and renal failure. There are also multiple symptoms, the most common of which are altered mental status and changes in respiratory rate, depth, and regularity. Regardless of the cause, a thorough assessment of the airway and prompt treatment are essential to patient survival.

Acid-Base Balance

Homeostasis requires a balance between the acids and bases in the body. An acid is any molecule that gives up a hydrogen ion and is often referred to as H^+. A base is any molecule that can accept a hydrogen ion and is often referred to as OH^-. Acids can be further classified as strong or weak, depending on how completely they dissociate in water. Strong acids like hydrochloric acid (an aqueous solution of hydrogen chloride, or HCl) dissociate almost completely, whereas weak acids like carbonic acid (H_2CO_3) only partially dissociate. It is the ability of weak acids to bond weakly to hydrogen ions that makes them ideal buffers because they can accept or donate hydrogen ions, depending on the needs of the body. Several mechanisms help regulate the acids and bases created during normal metabolism.

Defining the Acidity of a Solution

The acidity of a solution is defined by the amount of free hydrogen found in the solution. The measurement of hydrogen in solution is called pH. Measurement of pH is based on the ratio of the amount of acid (H^+) to the amount of base (OH^-). One H^+ removes one OH^- from solution, creating water (H_2O), so if there is exactly enough H^+ for every OH^-, the result is pure water (neither acidic nor basic) with a pH of 7. Thus, the definition of neutral pH is based on the equation:

$$[H^+] + [OH^-] \leftrightarrow [H_2O]$$

If there are more H^+ ions in solution than OH^-, the solution becomes acidic (pH below 7), and the pH drops. If there are fewer H^+ ions in solution than OH^-, the solution becomes basic (pH above 7), and the pH rises. Normal body functions work best within a very narrow range of pH: between 7.35 and 7.45. Cellular function deteriorates and death occurs when the pH drops below 6.9 or rises above 7.8.

It is important to note that concentrations of H^+ ions can be increased by adding more H^+ ions or by removing OH^-. To illustrate this concept, think of making coffee. To make strong coffee, you can add more coffee grounds or you can add less water. The reverse is also true to make the solution basic.

Ion Shifts

To function properly, acid-base balance, or a balance of charges, must exist on both sides of the cell. If excess H^+ ions exist in the extracellular fluid (fluid outside the cells), diffusion occurs, and H^+ ions move into the cell along the charge gradient between the extracellular and intracellular fluids. When hydrogen moves across the cell membrane into the cell, the cell starts taking on an overall positive charge. To return its overall charge to neutral, the cell begins to shift cations into the interstitial fluid. The H^+ ions moving into the cell force potassium to shift out into the extracellular fluid until no more potassium can safely be shifted out of the cell. This shift has significant consequences. A decreasing amount of intracellular potassium leads to problems with cellular depolarization. High serum (intravascular) potassium levels (hyperkalemia) mean the cell needs a greater stimulus to depolarize.

Calcium ions also shift out of the cell in response to the influx of hydrogen. Neural permeability is regulated by the presence of calcium ions. High serum calcium levels (hypercalcemia) decrease neural transmissions, whereas low serum calcium levels (hypocalcemia) lead to hypersensitive nerve cells and increased neural transmissions. In summary, an increase in extracellular H^+ ions results in acidosis; a decrease in extracellular H^+ ions results in alkalosis.

↑pH means ↓ H^+ ion concentration = alkalosis
↓pH means ↑ H^+ ion concentration = acidosis

Buffers

A buffer is a compound that can repeatedly neutralize excess acids or bases to prevent pH levels from exceeding acceptable levels. Several buffers and buffering sites exist in the body:

- Circulating proteins can bind with excess acids or bases, thus neutralizing their effects.
- Bone acts as a buffer by absorbing excess acids and bases and by releasing calcium into the circulation.

- The bicarbonate buffer system circulates in all fluid compartments of the body.

Any buffer system in the body may be best imagined as a bucket. Like a bucket, the buffer system can hold only a certain amount of acid before it reaches the point at which it is saturated and overflows. The body responds to shifts in pH levels by absorbing or releasing small amounts of acid into the blood. Problems begin when the amount of acid in circulation is too great and the buffer system becomes overwhelmed.

There are three main components to the buffer system found in the body:
- The circulating bicarbonate (HCO_3^-) buffer component
- The respiratory component
- The renal component

The following equation illustrates the balance among these three components:

$$CO_2 + H_2O \leftrightarrow H_2CO_3 \leftrightarrow HCO_3^- + H^+$$

Respiratory Component — Circulating Bicarbonate Buffer System — Renal Component

The Circulating Bicarbonate Buffer Component

This component is the "bucket" that holds and neutralizes excess acid. The circulating bicarbonate buffer system can be found in the intracellular and extracellular fluids and is the fastest acting segment of the buffer system.

$$H_2CO_3 \leftrightarrow H^+ + HCO_3^-$$

Carbonic acid (H_2CO_3) is a weak acid that can give up an extra H^+ ion to re-form as the bicarbonate ion (HCO_3^-). Through metabolic processes, the extra H^+ ion is then converted into compounds that are easily expelled from the body, eliminating the extra acid.

The Respiratory Component

$$H_2CO_3 \leftrightarrow CO_2 + H_2O$$

The fastest way the body can get rid of the excess H^+ ions is to create water (H_2O) and CO_2, which can be expelled as gases from the lungs. The preceding equation illustrates this process, which occurs in the lungs.

The main reason for breathing is to maintain the circulating level of carbon dioxide in the blood. Carbon dioxide combines with the circulating water of the blood to create H_2CO_3. Chemoreceptors in the brain sense the rising levels of carbonic acid and signal the respiratory center to increase ventilation and to reduce the available amount of circulating carbon dioxide. Tachypnea then reduces the level of carbon dioxide. Although the respiratory component reacts within minutes, it is much slower to respond than the circulating buffer system. Consider the buffer bucket example again; the respiratory component can be thought of as a large faucet that allows acid to spill out of the buffer bucket, returning the pH to normal levels.

$$\text{Excess } H^+ \rightarrow H_2CO_3 \rightarrow CO_2 \rightarrow \text{Tachypnea}$$

Anything that limits respirations can lead to acid retention and acidosis. Any time a patient is in respiratory distress or is unable to breathe, acidosis quickly develops.

$$\text{Bradypnea} \rightarrow \uparrow CO_2 \rightarrow \uparrow H_2CO_3 \rightarrow \text{Acidosis}$$

The preceding equation demonstrates how a patient experiencing respiratory difficulty drives the respiratory component back toward acid retention. The patient can also experience alkalosis if the respiratory rate is too high, as shown in the following equation:

$$\text{Tachypnea} \rightarrow \downarrow CO_2 \rightarrow \downarrow H_2CO_3 \rightarrow \text{Alkalosis}$$

The Renal Component

$$H_2CO_3 \leftrightarrow H^+ + HCO_3^-$$

Another smaller faucet connected to the buffer bucket is the renal component. The smaller faucet represents the slower nature by which the kidneys respond to increasing acid levels. The renal response could take from hours to days to restore the body's pH to normal. Kidneys account for every molecule, ion, and electrolyte found in the circulation; they maintain homeostasis by retaining certain products and filtering out others.

As with the respiratory system, the renal system can control increasing acid levels in the blood by excreting the acid. The kidneys excrete acid in an ionic form, unlike the respiratory system, which excretes acid as a gas.

$$\text{Excess } H^+ \rightarrow H_2CO_3 \rightarrow HCO_3^- + H^+ \text{ (urine)}$$

If the patient experiences decreased urine output, excess acid cannot be removed from the blood, and the patient can experience acidosis.

$$\text{Decreased Output} \rightarrow \uparrow H^+ \rightarrow \uparrow HCO_3^- \rightarrow \text{Acidosis}$$

If urine output becomes excessive, alkalosis can develop.

$$\text{Increased output} \rightarrow \downarrow H^+ \rightarrow \downarrow HCO_3^- \rightarrow \text{Alkalosis}$$

Compensatory Mechanisms

Acid-base disorders that are not immediately correctable by the body's buffering systems initiate compensatory mechanisms to help return levels to normal. Metabolic acidosis may create respiratory alkalosis as a compensatory response. Often, patient management involves treating more than one form of acid-base imbalance.

Clinical Presentations

There are two types of acid-base disorders: metabolic and respiratory.

- Fluctuations in pH due to available bicarbonate levels result in metabolic acidosis or alkalosis.
- Fluctuations in pH due to respiratory disorders result in respiratory acidosis or alkalosis.

Therefore there are four main clinical presentations:

- Respiratory acidosis
- Respiratory alkalosis
- Metabolic acidosis
- Metabolic alkalosis

Respiratory Acidosis

$$\downarrow \text{Breathing} \rightarrow \uparrow CO_2 \rightarrow \uparrow H_2CO_3 \rightarrow \downarrow pH$$

Respiratory acidosis is always related to hypoventilation of some type. Because the acidosis is a result of insufficient breathing, the compensatory mechanism is the slower reacting renal system. Some causes for respiratory acidosis are as follows:

- Airway obstruction
- Cardiac arrest
- Overdose of a central nervous system (CNS) depressant drug
- Drowning
- Respiratory arrest
- Pulmonary edema
- Closed head injury
- Chest trauma
- Carbon monoxide poisoning

Hypoventilation that develops from any of the conditions listed is considered a serious, life-threatening condition. The acidosis that results is quick, overwhelming, and usually fatal, making it impossible for the slower-reacting renal system to compensate in time for the pH shift. The increasing acidosis causes potassium ions to shift into the extracellular fluid, leading to a potentially fatal cardiac dysrhythmia. Calcium also shifts into extracellular spaces, resulting in hypercalcemia and decreased neural cell permeability and creating lethargy and a decreasing level of consciousness (LOC).

Signs and symptoms of respiratory acidosis include the following:

- Systemic or cerebral vasodilation or both
- Headaches
- Red, flushed skin
- Central nervous system (CNS) depression
- Bradypnea
- Nausea and vomiting
- Hypercalcemia

When assessing patients for respiratory acidosis, evaluate the following:

- LOC
- Skin color and temperature

You are the Provider — Part 5

You are transporting your patient to the emergency department and you note that her condition is not improving with 100% O_2 by nonrebreathing mask.

Reassessment	Recording Time: 7 Minutes After Patient Contact
Level of consciousness	Responsive to deep painful stimuli only
Respirations	40 breaths/min, shallow
Pulse	140 beats/min, irregular
Skin	Pale and diaphoretic, developing perioral cyanosis
Blood pressure	96/58 mm Hg
Sao_2	80% while receiving 100% O_2 via nonrebreathing mask

7. What intervention should the EMT-I consider next?

- Respiratory rate and effort
- Lung sounds
- Hydration status
- Cardiac rhythm

A Word About COPD

Chronic obstructive pulmonary disease creates respiratory acidosis over time. It is the slow onset that makes this form of respiratory acidosis survivable compared with other forms of respiratory acidosis. The gradual destruction of lung tissue inhibits the exchange of oxygen and carbon dioxide, creating acidosis. With COPD, the normal stimulus for this exchange is absent. Increasing carbon dioxide retention leads to increasing levels of carbonic acid, eventually making chemoreceptors unaware of the presence of metabolic acids. The hypoxic drive is then the only remaining stimulus for respiration. The hypoxic drive stimulates breathing based on the circulating oxygen level in the blood. The chronic nature of COPD allows the renal system enough time to moderate the acidosis, thus preventing the life-threatening cardiac dysrhythmias that may occur from acute acidosis.

Healthy individuals also respond to oxygen and carbon dioxide levels in the blood. When the oxygen level rises, the respiratory center suspends respiration until a rising carbon dioxide level stimulates the respiratory center to begin breathing again. With COPD, the rising carbon dioxide level no longer stimulates the respiratory center to regulate breathing. This presents a dilemma: COPD patients in respiratory distress need high-flow oxygen, even though it may suppress their respiratory drive and create respiratory arrest. Respiratory arrest, however, can be treated. It should be noted that respiratory arrest in COPD patients following the administration of high concentrations of oxygen is an uncommon occurrence. If a patient with COPD is in clinically unstable condition and has significant hypoxia, 100% oxygen should not be withheld.

Respiratory Alkalosis

$$\uparrow \text{Breathing} \to \downarrow CO_2 \to \downarrow H_2CO_3 \to \uparrow pH$$

Respiratory alkalosis is always the result of hyperventilation. The carbon dioxide level drops in the blood, forcing a reduction of circulating carbonic acid. The renal system then begins retaining H^+ ions to rebalance the depleted acid levels. As this is happening, H^+ ions begin to shift from the extracellular to the intracellular fluid compartment. Calcium shifts into the intracellular compartment to rebalance depleted hydrogen levels. Hypocalcemia leads to increased neural cell permeability. Muscle contractions create the classic signs of carpopedal spasms that accompany hyperventilation. Treatment for the classic hyperventilation syndrome focuses on restoring the normal respiratory rate to increase the carbon dioxide level. However, increasing the carbon dioxide level can aggravate other more serious medical conditions that cause hyperventilation. Therefore, you must carefully evaluate the patient to determine the underlying cause of the hyperventilation before you attempt to correct it.

Some effects of respiratory alkalosis include the following:
- Decreased cerebral perfusion
- Decreased LOC
- Lightheadedness
- Confusion
- Vertigo
- Blurred vision
- Hypocalcemia
- Nausea and vomiting

When assessing patients who are hyperventilating, evaluate the following:
- LOC
- Skin color and temperature
- Lung sounds
- Respiratory rate and effort
- Hydration status
- Cardiac rhythm

Some causes for hyperventilation and respiratory alkalosis can be the following:
- Drug overdoses, especially aspirin
- Fever
- Overzealous BVM ventilations

Metabolic Acidosis

$$\uparrow H_2CO_3 \to \uparrow H^+ + HCO_3^- \to \downarrow pH$$

Any acidosis that is not related to the respiratory system is considered metabolic in origin. Tachypnea is the compensatory mechanism for this condition as the respiratory system attempts to restore acid-base balance by eliminating carbon dioxide. Patient presentations for metabolic acidosis are similar to those for respiratory acidosis.

As with any acidosis, the extracellular hydrogen level increases, and the extracellular buffers attempt to neutralize the excess acid. Ion shifts occur, hydrogen leaks into the cell, and potassium shifts into the extracellular spaces, raising the serum potassium levels, which can lead to potentially life-threatening cardiac dysrhythmias. Along with the potassium ion shift, calcium also shifts into extracellular spaces. The resulting hypercalcemia leads to decreased neural cell permeability. Impulses sent to muscle and nerve cells are obstructed, and the patient becomes lethargic with a decreased LOC.

Major causes for metabolic acidosis include the following:

- Lactic acidosis created by anaerobic cellular respiration due to hypoperfusion of tissues and organs, as seen with shock and cardiac arrest.
- Ketoacidosis resulting when cells are forced to switch to metabolizing fatty acids for energy because they are unable to utilize glucose, either because of insulin insufficiency or desensitization of the cells to insulin. The by-products of fat metabolism are ketones, which are extremely acidotic.
- Aspirin (acetylsalicylic acid) overdose (10 to 30 g for adults). Acetylsalicylic acid directly stimulates the respiratory centers of the brain, creating tachypnea and leading to respiratory alkalosis. Compensatory mechanisms involve the renal system, resulting in metabolic acidosis.
- Alcohol ingestion. Ingestion of ethyl alcohol can lead to alcoholic ketoacidosis. Methanol (wood alcohol) and ethylene glycol can produce fatal forms of acidosis, often with amounts as small as 30 mL.
- Gastrointestinal losses. Diarrhea, for example, removes bases from the lower intestinal tract.

Signs and symptoms of metabolic acidosis include the following:

- Vasodilation
- CNS depression
- Headaches
- Hot, red, flushed skin
- Hypercalcemia
- Tachypnea
- Nausea and vomiting
- Dysrhythmias

When assessing patients with metabolic acidosis, evaluate the following:

- LOC
- Skin color and temperature
- Respiratory effort and rate
- Lung sounds
- Hydration status
- Cardiac rhythm

Metabolic Alkalosis

$\downarrow H^+ \rightarrow \downarrow H_2CO_3 \rightarrow \uparrow pH \rightarrow$ Bradypnea

Metabolic alkalosis results any time there is excessive loss of acid, either from excessive urination or from decreased acid levels in the stomach. Several factors related to upper GI losses can lead to metabolic alkalosis:

- Excessive vomiting
- Excessive water intake
- Nasogastric suctioning
- Excessive intake of base
- Eating disorders

Major causes for metabolic alkalosis are as follows:

- Upper GI losses of acid resulting from illness or anorexia. When the patient expels a great deal of acid from the stomach, a complex metabolic pathway can lead to metabolic alkalosis.
- Drinking large amounts of water during heavy exertion. The water not only dilutes the stomach acid, it also stimulates the digestive system to prepare for incoming food from the stomach. This stimulation causes a dump of very basic digestive enzymes into the lower GI tract, adding to the acid-base imbalance. As with respiratory alkalosis, there is a shift of calcium out of the cell—hypercalcemia—causing overstimulation of the nervous system and leading to muscle cramping. This cramping is analogous to carpopedal spasms, except it occurs in the abdominal area and is referred to as heat cramps.
- Excessive intake of basic substances such as antacids Figure 9-1 ▼ . This is important to remember when dealing with cardiac patients,

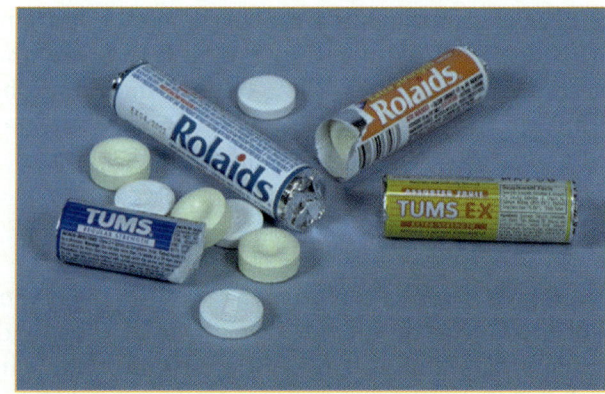

Figure 9-1 Excessive intake of basic substances such as antacids can result in metabolic alkalosis.

Placing a Patient in the Recovery Position

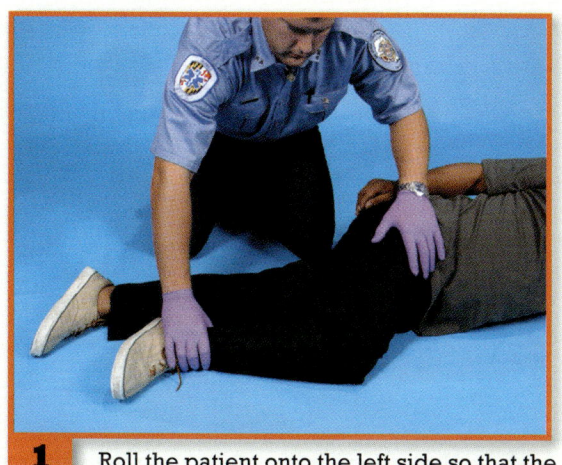

1 Roll the patient onto the left side so that the head, shoulders, and torso move at the same time without twisting.

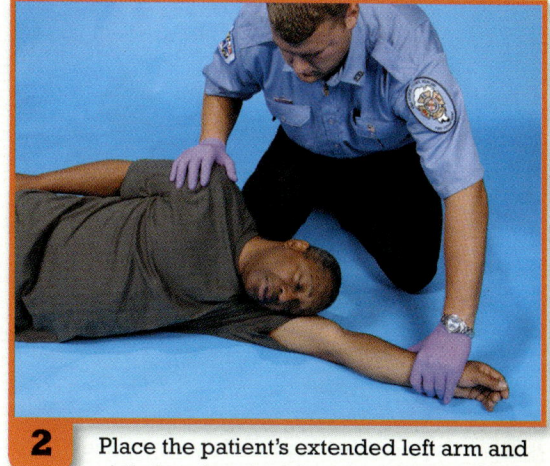

2 Place the patient's extended left arm and right hand under his or her cheek.

because one of their main complaints tends to be feelings of nausea or indigestion. Often, the patient has self-medicated for hours or days with over-the-counter antacids, which can result in metabolic alkalosis. Another cause of excessive base intake is the excessive administration of sodium bicarbonate ($NaHCO_3$) during resuscitation. Introducing excessive amounts of sodium bicarbonate intravenously can seriously alter pH levels.

The compensatory mechanism for metabolic alkalosis is the respiratory system. To correct the reduced hydrogen levels, bradypnea develops to retain carbon dioxide and drive up the levels of circulating acids.

Signs and symptoms of metabolic alkalosis include the following:

- Confusion
- Muscle tremors and cramps
- Bradypnea
- Hypotension

Maintaining the Airway

The recovery position is used to help maintain a clear airway in a patient who has not had traumatic injuries and is breathing on his or her own with a normal rate and adequate tidal volume (depth of breathing). Take the following steps to put the patient in the recovery position (Skill Drill 9-1):

1. **Roll the patient** onto the left side so that head, shoulders, and torso move at the same time without twisting (**Step 1**).
2. **Place the patient's extended left arm and right hand** under his or her cheek (**Step 2**).

Once patients have resumed spontaneous breathing after being resuscitated, the recovery position will prevent the aspiration of vomitus. However, this position is not appropriate for patients with suspected spinal trauma, nor is it adequate for patients who are unresponsive and require airway management. You must reposition such patients to provide access to the airway.

Skill Drill 9-2

Positioning an Unresponsive Patient

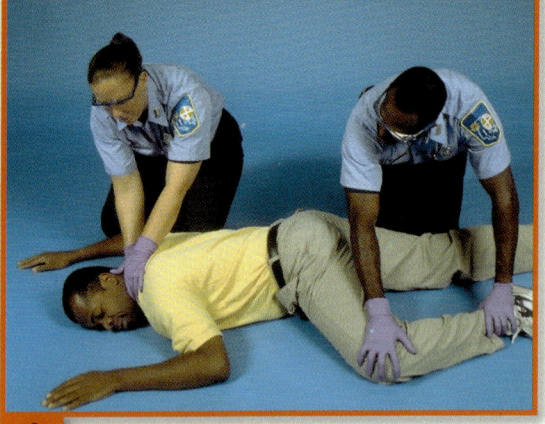

1 Support the head while your partner straightens the patient's legs.

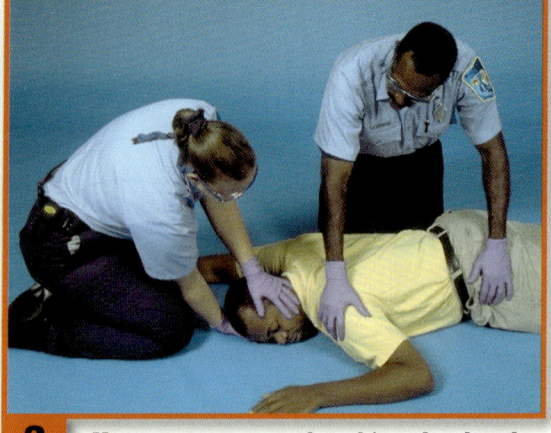

2 Have your partner place his or her hand on the patient's far shoulder and hip.

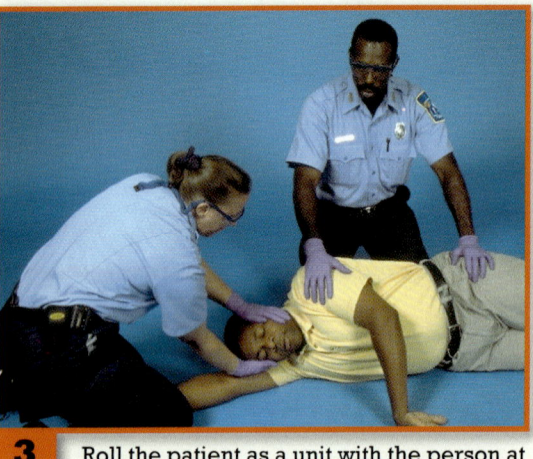

3 Roll the patient as a unit with the person at the head calling the count to begin the move.

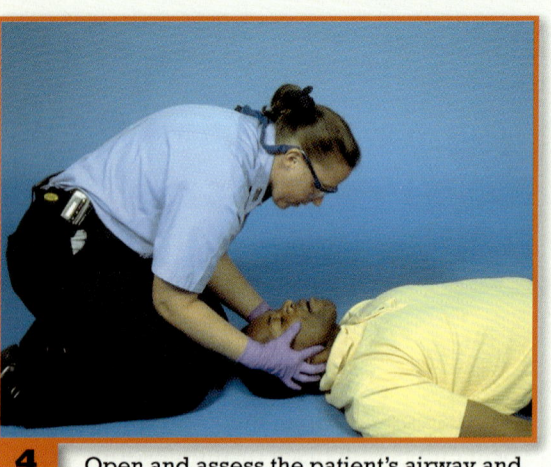

4 Open and assess the patient's airway and breathing status.

Airway Management

Emergency medical care begins with ensuring an open airway. The patient's airway and breathing status are the first steps in your initial assessment for a very good reason: Unless you can immediately open and maintain an airway, you will not be able to provide appropriate patient care. You must maintain your skills through constant practice.

When you respond to a call and find an unresponsive patient, you need to assess and determine immediately whether the patient has an open airway and breathing is adequate. To open the airway and to assess breathing, the patient needs to be in the supine position. If your patient is found in the prone (lying face down) position, he or she must be properly positioned to allow for assessment of airway and breathing and to begin CPR should it be necessary. The patient should be log rolled as a unit so the head, neck, and spine all move together without any twisting (Skill Drill 9-2 ▲):

1. **Kneel beside the patient.** Have your partner kneel far enough away so that the patient, when rolled toward you, does not come to rest in your lap. Rapidly straighten the patient's legs and move the nearer arm across the patient's chest to minimize movement. Place your hands behind the back of the patient's head and neck to provide in-line stabilization of the cervical spine (**Step 1**).

2. **Have your partner** place his or her hands on the patient's far shoulder and hip (**Step 2**).
3. **As you call the count** to control movement, have your partner turn the patient toward you by pulling on the far shoulder and hip. Control the head and neck so that they move as a unit with the rest of the torso. In this way, the head and neck stay in the same vertical plane as the back. This single motion will minimize aggravation of any spinal injury. Replace the patient's farther arm back at his or her side (**Step 3**).
4. **Once the patient is positioned**, maintain an open airway and check for breathing (**Step 4**).

In an unresponsive patient, the most common airway obstruction is the patient's tongue, which falls back into the throat when the muscles of the throat and tongue relax (**Figure 9-2**). Dentures (false teeth), blood, vomitus, mucus, food, and other foreign objects may also create a blockage. Therefore, you should always have a suction device available to help clear and maintain a patent airway.

Manual Maneuvers

Head Tilt–Chin Lift Maneuver

Opening the airway to relieve an obstruction can often be done quickly and easily by simply tilting the patient's head back and lifting the chin in what is known as the head tilt–chin lift maneuver. For patients who have not sustained trauma, this simple maneuver is sometimes all that is needed for the patient to resume breathing. **Table 9-3** lists indications, contraindications, advantages, disadvantages, and complications of the head tilt–chin lift maneuver.

To perform the head tilt–chin lift maneuver, follow these steps (**Skill Drill 9-3**):

1. With the patient in a supine position, **position yourself beside the patient's head** (**Step 1**).
2. Place one hand on the patient's forehead, and **apply firm backward pressure** with your palm to tilt the patient's head back (**Step 2**). This extension of the neck will move the tongue forward, away from the back of the throat and clear the airway if the tongue is blocking it.
3. **Place the tips of the fingers** of your other hand under the lower jaw near the bony part of the chin (**Step 3**). Do not compress the soft tissue under the chin because this may block the airway.
4. **Lift the chin upward**, bringing the entire lower jaw with it, helping to tilt the head back (**Step 4**). Do not use your thumb to lift the chin. Lift so that the teeth are nearly brought together, but avoid closing the mouth completely. Continue to hold the forehead to maintain the backward tilt of the head.

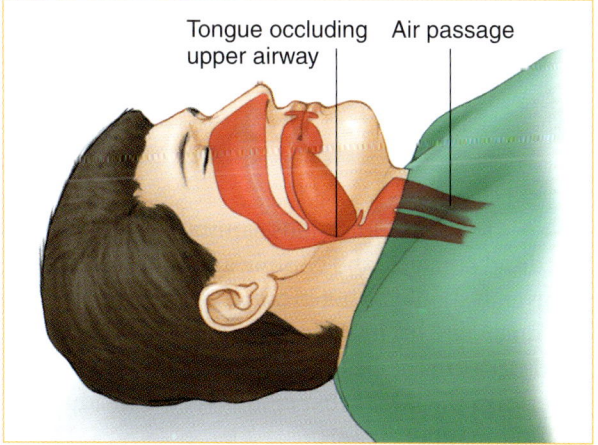

Figure 9-2 The most common airway obstruction is the patient's tongue, which falls back into the throat when the muscles of the throat and tongue relax.

TABLE 9-3	Head Tilt-Chin Lift Maneuver

Indications
- Soft-tissue upper airway obstruction
- Patient unable to protect his or her own airway for any reason
- Noisy respirations

Contraindication
- Possible cervical spine injury

Advantages
- No equipment required
- Simple
- Safe
- Noninvasive

Disadvantages
- No protection against aspiration
- Not equally effective for all patients

Complication
- Aspiration

Skill Drill 9-3

Head Tilt–Chin Lift Maneuver

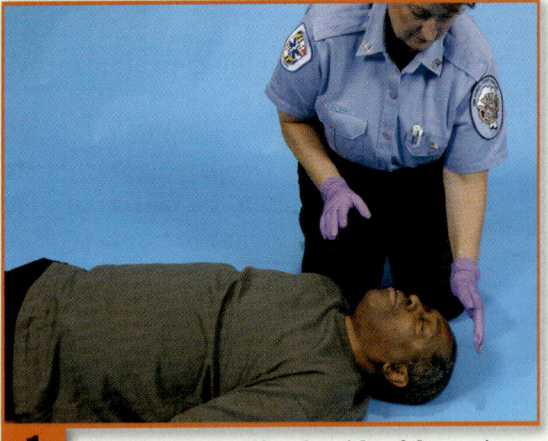

1 Position yourself at the side of the patient.

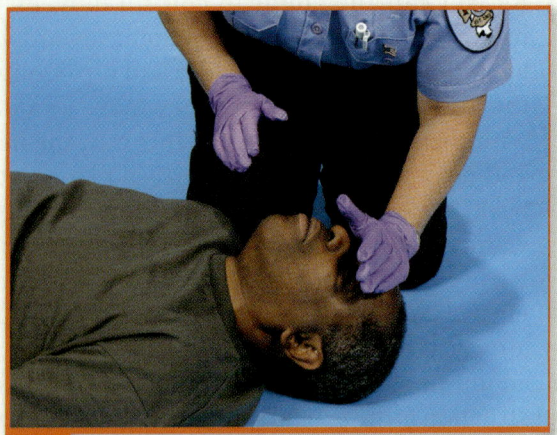

2 Place your hand closest to the patient's head on the forehead.

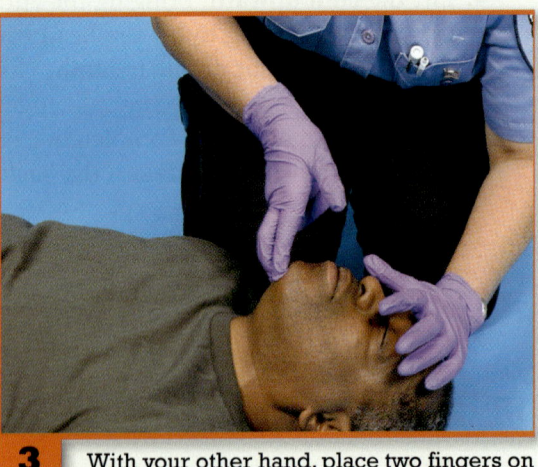

3 With your other hand, place two fingers on the underside of the patient's chin.

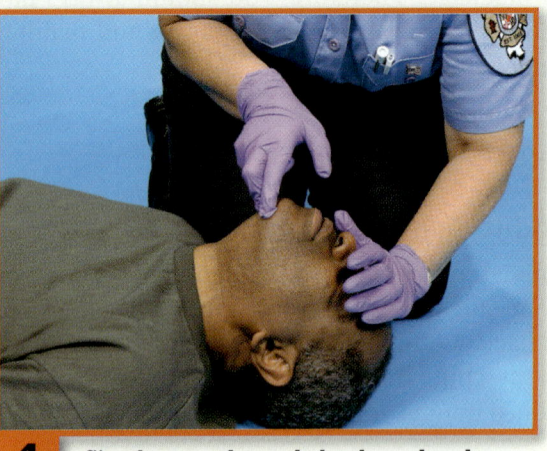

4 Simultaneously apply backward and downward pressure to the patient's forehead and lift the jaw straight up. Do not depress the submental triangle with your fingers, which causes the tongue to elevate, possibly pushing it against the roof of the mouth.

Jaw-Thrust Maneuver

The head tilt–chin lift will open the airway in most patients. If you suspect a cervical spine injury, use the jaw-thrust maneuver. The <u>jaw-thrust maneuver</u> is a technique to open the airway by placing the fingers behind the angle of the jaw and lifting the jaw upward. The jaw is displaced forward at the mandibular angle. You can easily seal a mask around the mouth while doing the jaw-thrust maneuver. This is the method of choice for patients with suspected cervical spine injury.

Table 9-4 ▶ lists indications, contraindications, advantages, disadvantages, and complications of the jaw-thrust maneuver. It should be noted that if the jaw-thrust maneuver is unsuccessful in opening the patient's airway, you should perform the head tilt-chin lift maneuver.

Perform the jaw-thrust maneuver on an adult in the following manner (Skill Drill 9-4 ▶):

1. **Kneel above the patient's head.** Place your fingers behind the angles of the lower jaw, and forcefully move the jaw upward. Use your thumbs to help position the lower jaw to

allow breathing through the mouth and nose (**Step 1**).
2. The completed maneuver should open the airway with the mouth slightly open and the jaw jutting forward (**Step 2**).

Once the airway has been opened, the patient may start to breathe on his or her own. Assess whether breathing has returned by using the look, listen, and feel technique.

With complete airway obstruction, there will be no movement of air. However, you may see the chest and abdomen rise and fall considerably with the patient's frantic attempts to breathe. This is why the presence of chest wall movement alone does not indicate breathing is present. Regular chest wall movement indicates that respiratory effort is present. Observing chest and abdominal movement is often difficult with a fully clothed patient. You may see little, if any, chest movement, even with normal breathing. This is particularly true in some patients with chronic lung disease. You must begin artificial ventilation immediately if you use the three-part approach—look, listen, and feel—and discover that there is no movement of air.

Jaw-Thrust Maneuver With Head Tilt

The jaw-thrust maneuver with head tilt is similar to the head tilt–chin lift maneuver, with a few exceptions. Kneel above the patient's head and place the meaty portion of the base of your thumbs on the zygomatic arches. Hook the tips of your index fingers under the angle of the mandible, in the indent below the ear. Lift the jaw upward, and tilt the patient's head back. Table 9-5 lists the indications, contraindications, advantages, disadvantages, and complications of the jaw-thrust maneuver with head tilt.

Perform the jaw-thrust maneuver with head tilt in the following manner (Skill Drill 9-5):
1. Position yourself at the top of the patient's head (**Step 1**).
2. **Place the meaty portion of the base of your thumbs on the zygomatic arches, and hook the tips of your index finders under the angle of the mandible**, in the middle indent below each ear (**Step 2**).
3. **Displace the jaw upward, and tilt the head back** (**Step 3**).

TABLE 9-4	Jaw-Thrust Maneuver

Indications
- Unresponsive patient
- Possible cervical spine injury
- Patient unable to protect his or her own airway
- Patient resistant to opening mouth

Contraindications
- Unable to open the patient's mouth
- Fractured jaw
- Awake patient
- Dislocated jaw

Advantages
- Noninvasive
- No special equipment required
- May use with cervical collar in place
- Second rescuer can ventilate the patient with positive pressure

Disadvantages
- Difficult to maintain for a long period
- No protection against aspiration

Complication
- Posterior mandibular bruising

TABLE 9-5	Jaw-Thrust Maneuver With Head Tilt

Indications
- Soft-tissue upper airway obstruction
- Unresponsive patient
- Patient unable to protect his or her own airway

Contraindications
- Unable to open the patient's mouth
- Fractured jaw
- Awake patient
- Dislocated jaw

Advantages
- May use as an alternative airway technique for any patient without a suspected spinal injury
- No special equipment required

Disadvantages
- Cannot be maintained if patient becomes responsive or combative
- Difficult to maintain for extended period
- No protection against aspiration

Complication
- Posterior mandibular bruising

Skill Drill 9-4: Jaw-Thrust Maneuver

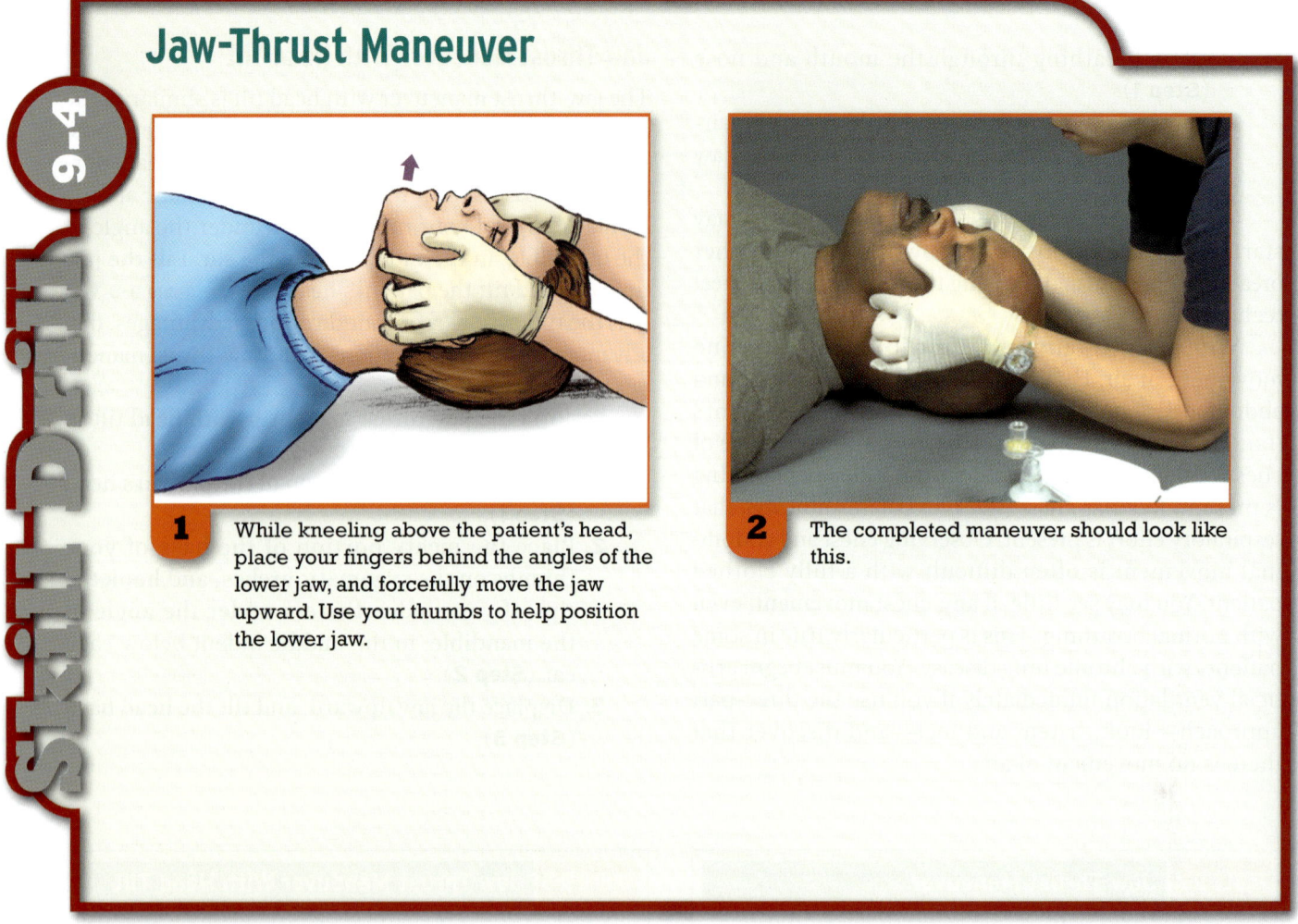

1. While kneeling above the patient's head, place your fingers behind the angles of the lower jaw, and forcefully move the jaw upward. Use your thumbs to help position the lower jaw.

2. The completed maneuver should look like this.

Tongue-Jaw Lift Maneuver

The tongue–jaw lift maneuver is used more frequently to open a patient's airway in order to facilitate oropharyngeal suctioning. It cannot be used to ventilate a patient because it will not allow for an adequate mask seal on the patient's face. To grip on the jaw, place your thumb in the patient's mouth and grasp the lower incisors or gums. The jaw is then lifted upward. Follow the steps in Skill Drill 9-6:

1. Position yourself at the side of the patient (**Step 1**).
2. Place the hand closest to the patient's head on the forehead (**Step 2**).
3. With your other hand, reach into the patient's mouth and hook your first knuckle under the incisors or gum line. While holding the patient's head and maintaining the hand on the forehead, lift the jaw straight up (**Step 3**).

Airway Obstructions

A foreign body that *completely* blocks the airway in a patient is a true emergency that will result in death if not treated immediately. In an adult, sudden foreign body airway obstruction usually occurs during a meal. In a child, it occurs while eating, playing with small toys, or crawling around the house. An otherwise healthy child who has sudden difficulty breathing has probably aspirated a foreign object.

By far, the most common airway obstruction in an unresponsive patient is the tongue, which relaxes and falls back into the throat, occluding the posterior pharynx. There are other causes of airway obstruction that do not involve foreign bodies in the airway. These include laryngeal edema (from infection or acute allergic reactions), laryngeal spasm, and trauma (tissue damage from injury). With airway obstruction from medical conditions such as infection and acute allergic reactions,

Skill Drill 9-5: Jaw-Thrust Maneuver With Head Tilt

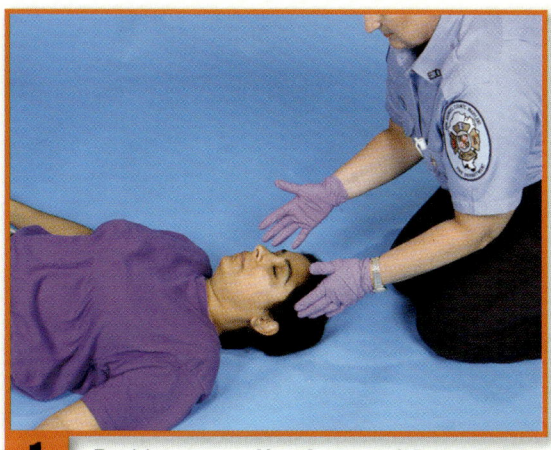

1 Position yourself at the top of the patient's head.

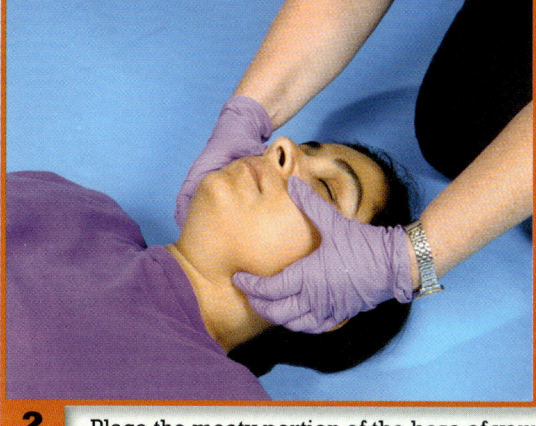

2 Place the meaty portion of the base of your thumbs on the zygomatic arches, and hook the tips of your index fingers under the angle of the mandible, in the middle indent below each ear.

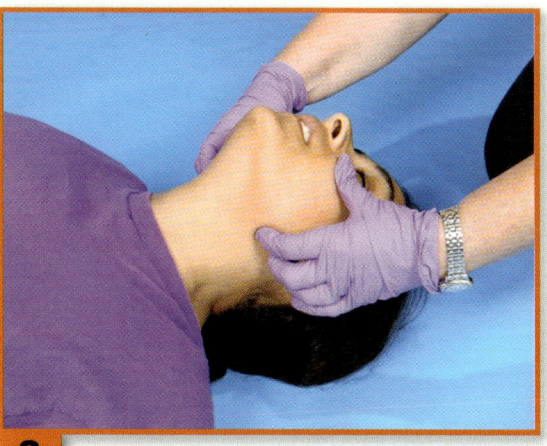

3 Displace the jaw upward, and tilt the head back.

---

repeated attempts to clear the airway as if there were a foreign body will be unsuccessful and potentially dangerous. These patients require specific emergency medical care and rapid transport to the hospital.

Possible Causes of Airway Obstruction

Obstruction of the airway is a true emergency. Without a patent airway, the patient will soon die. Learning the signs and symptoms of various causes of airway obstruction will allow you to promptly recognize and treat many conditions.

Tongue

The tongue is the most common cause of upper airway obstruction in a patient with altered mental status. With no muscle control, the tongue relaxes and falls back, covering the posterior pharynx and creating snoring respirations. This is the easiest of all airway obstructions to correct, requiring only a change in position. Opening the airway with the head tilt–chin lift

Skill Drill 9-6: Tongue-Jaw Lift Maneuver

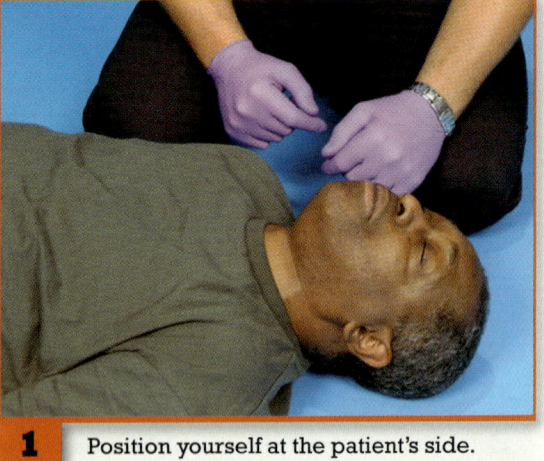

1 Position yourself at the patient's side.

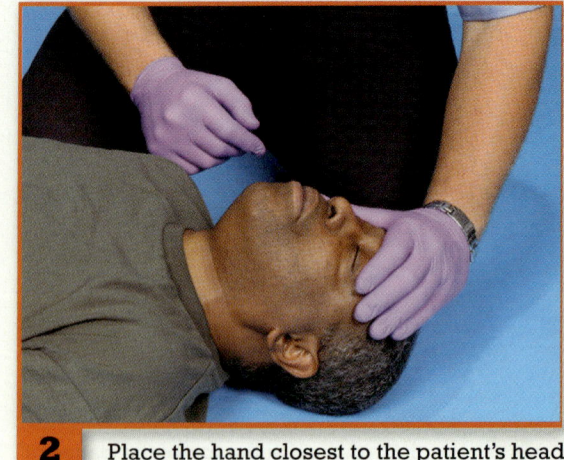

2 Place the hand closest to the patient's head on the forehead.

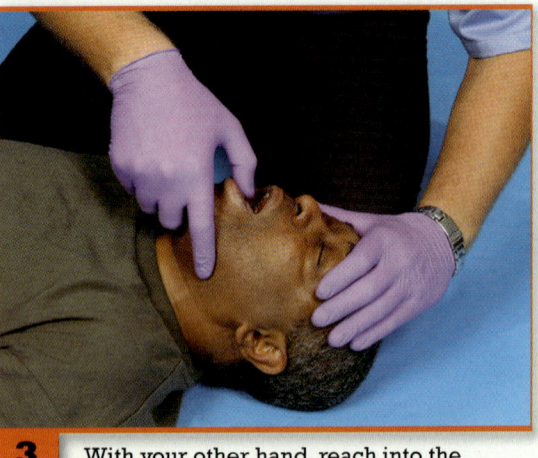

3 With your other hand, reach into the patient's mouth and hook your first knuckle under the incisors or gum line. While holding the patient's head and maintaining the hand on the forehead, lift the jaw straight up.

---

maneuver in a nontrauma patient or a jaw thrust in a trauma patient displaces the jaw anteriorly, pulling the tongue forward and away from the airway.

Foreign Body

A foreign body may cause a mild or severe airway obstruction, depending on the size of the object and the location of the obstruction. Signs may include choking, gagging, stridor, dyspnea, dysphonia (difficulty speaking), or aphonia (an inability to speak). As long as the patient is moving air effectively, no action should be taken. He or she should be encouraged to cough in an attempt to dislodge the obstruction. If the obstruction becomes severe (complete), the Heimlich maneuver (abdominal thrusts) should be performed. For the unresponsive patient, alternate chest compressions with attempts to ventilate. *Use the finger sweep only to remove a visible foreign body.*

Laryngeal Spasm and Edema

A laryngeal spasm results in the spasmodic closure of the vocal cords, completely occluding the airway. It is often caused by trauma from an over-aggressive technique during intubation and immediately upon extubation, especially when the patient is semiconscious.

Edema of the upper airway causes the glottic opening to become extremely narrow or totally obstructed. It is commonly caused by epiglottitis, anaphylaxis, or inhalation injury.

The obstruction may be relieved by aggressive ventilation or a forceful upward pull of the jaw in an attempt to reposition the airway. Muscle relaxant medications may also be effective for laryngeal spasms.

Fractured Larynx

Airway patency is dependent on good muscle tone to keep the trachea open. Fractured laryngeal tissue increases airway resistance by decreasing airway size secondary to decreasing muscle tone, laryngeal edema, and ventilatory effort.

Endotracheal intubation may be necessary to maintain the airway.

Aspiration

Aspiration of blood or other fluid significantly increases mortality. In addition to obstructing the airway, aspiration destroys delicate bronchiolar tissue, introduces pathogens into the lungs, and decreases the ability to ventilate. Suction should be readily available for any patient unable to maintain his or her own airway. Patients requiring emergency care should always be assumed to have a full stomach.

Recognition

Early recognition of airway obstruction is crucial for the EMT-I to be able to provide emergency medical care effectively. Obstruction from a foreign body can result in a mild airway obstruction or a severe airway obstruction.

Patients with a mild airway obstruction (partially obstructed airway) are still able to exchange air but will have varying degrees of respiratory distress. Great care must be taken to prevent a mild airway obstruction from becoming a severe airway obstruction.

With a mild airway obstruction, the patient can cough forcefully, although you may hear wheezing in between coughs. As long as the patient can breathe, cough forcefully, or talk, you should not interfere with the patient's efforts to expel the foreign object on his or her own. Continue to monitor the patient closely and encourage the patient to continue coughing. Abdominal thrusts are not indicated for patients with a mild airway obstruction. Furthermore, attempts to remove the object manually could force the object farther down into the airway and cause a severe obstruction. Continually reassess the patient's condition and be prepared to provide immediate treatment if the mild obstruction becomes a severe obstruction.

Patients with a severe airway obstruction (completely obstructed airway) cannot breathe, talk, or cough. One sure sign of a severe obstruction is the sudden inability to speak or cough immediately after eating. The person may clutch or grasp his or her throat (universal distress signal), begin to turn cyanotic, and make frantic attempts to breathe Figure 9-3. There is little or no air movement. Ask the conscious patient, "Are you choking?" If the patient nods "yes," provide immediate treatment. If the obstruction is not cleared quickly, the amount of oxygen in the patient's blood will decrease dramatically. If not treated, the patient will become unconscious and die.

Some patients with a severe airway obstruction will be unconscious during your initial assessment. You may not know that an airway obstruction is the cause of their condition. There are many other causes of unconsciousness and respiratory distress, including stroke, heart attack, trauma, seizures, and drug overdose. A complete and thorough patient assessment by you, therefore, is key in providing appropriate emergency medical care.

Any person found unconscious must be managed as if he or she has a compromised airway. You must first open the airway, assess breathing, and provide artificial

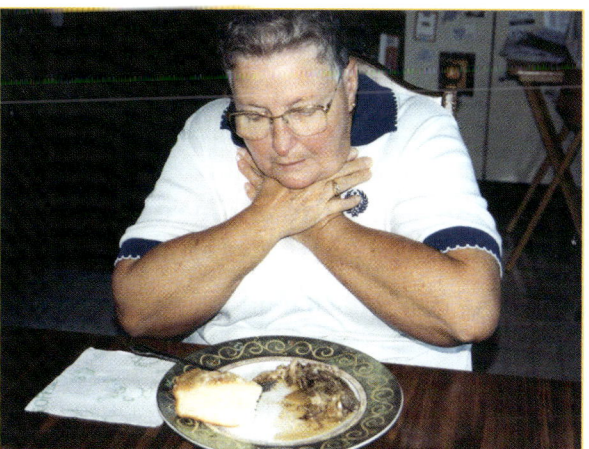

Figure 9-3 The universal sign of choking.

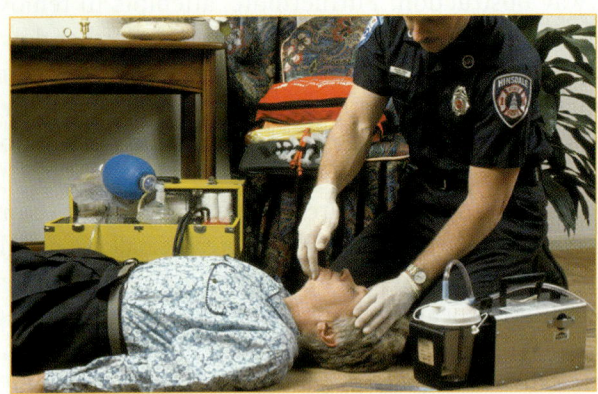

Figure 9-4 Securing and maintaining the airway and ensuring adequate breathing are among the most important steps in caring for an unconscious patient.

breathing if the patient is not breathing or is breathing inadequately (Figure 9-4). If, after opening the airway, you are unable to ventilate the patient after two attempts (the chest does not visibly rise), or you feel resistance when ventilating, consider the possibility of an airway obstruction. Resistance to ventilation can also be due to poor lung compliance. Lung compliance is the ability of the alveoli to expand when air is drawn in during inhalation; poor lung compliance is the inability of the alveoli to expand fully during inhalation.

EMT-I Tips

Possible Causes of Airway Obstruction
- Relaxation of the tongue in an unresponsive patient
- Foreign objects—food, small toys, dentures
- Blood clots, bone fragments, or damaged tissue after an injury
- Airway tissue swelling—infection, allergic reaction
- Aspirated vomitus (stomach contents)

Emergency Medical Care for Foreign Body Airway Obstruction

Perform the head tilt–chin lift maneuver to clear an obstruction that is caused by the tongue and throat muscles relaxing back into the airway in any person who is found unresponsive, has inadequate breathing or is not breathing, and is not suspected of having spinal trauma. If spinal trauma is suspected, you should open the airway with a jaw-thrust maneuver. Large pieces of vomited food, mucus, loose dentures, or blood clots in the mouth should be swept forward and out of the mouth with your gloved index finger. Once available, suctioning should be used to maintain a clear airway.

The steps for managing a severe airway obstruction in an unconscious adult or child are listed here and shown in Skill Drill 9-7:

1. Open the airway, and attempt ventilation (**Step 1**).
2. If unsuccessful, reopen the airway, and reattempt ventilation (**Step 2**).
3. Provide chest compressions (**Step 3**).
4. Open the patient's airway, look in the mouth, and attempt to visualize the foreign body. Perform a finger sweep *only* if the object is visible (**Step 4**).
5. Attempt to ventilate (**Step 5**). Repeat steps 3 through 5 until successful or help arrives.

The steps for managing a severe airway obstruction in an unconscious child are listed here and shown in Skill Drill 9-8:

1. Open the airway, and attempt ventilation (**Step 1**).
2. If unsuccessful, reopen the airway, and reattempt ventilation (**Step 2**).
3. Provide chest compressions (**Step 3**).
4. Open the patient's airway, look in the mouth and attempt to visualize the foreign body. Perform a finger sweep *only* if the object is visible (**Step 4**).
5. Attempt to ventilate (**Step 5**). Repeat steps 3 through 5 until successful or until help arrives.

The steps for managing a severe airway obstruction in an unconscious infant are listed here and shown in Skill Drill 9-9. Information on how to perform chest thrusts, which are a part of this skill, are discussed in Chapter 39, BLS Review.

1. Open the airway, and attempt ventilation (**Step 1**).
2. If unsuccessful, reopen the airway, and reattempt ventilation (**Step 2**).
3. Provide chest compressions (**Step 3**).
4. Open the patient's mouth airway, look in the mouth, and attempt to visualize the foreign body. Perform a finger sweep *only* if the object is visible (**Step 4**).
5. Attempt to ventilate (**Step 5**). Repeat steps 3 through 5 until successful or until help arrives.

Managing Severe Airway Obstruction in an Unconscious Adult or Child

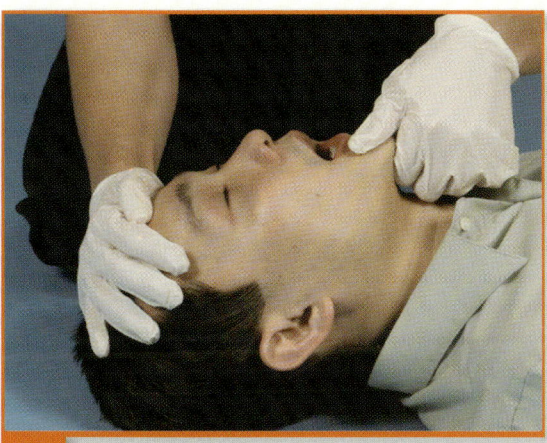

1 Open the airway, and attempt ventilation.

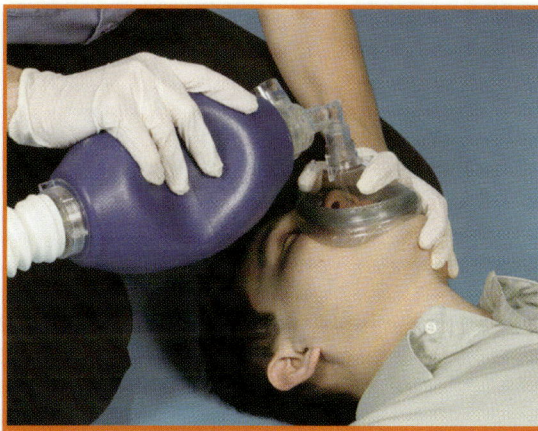

2 If unsuccessful, reopen the airway, and reattempt ventilation.

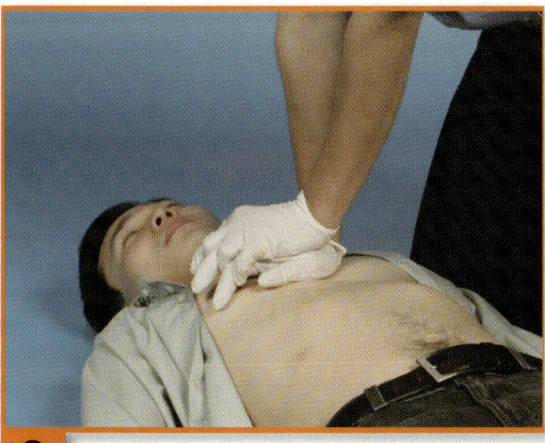

3 Provide chest compressions.

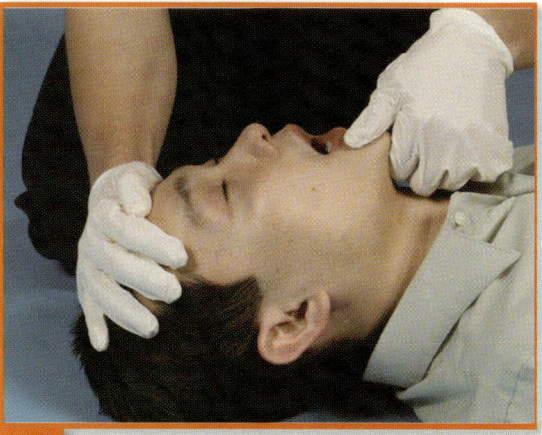

4 Open the patient's airway and perform a finger sweep if the object is visible.

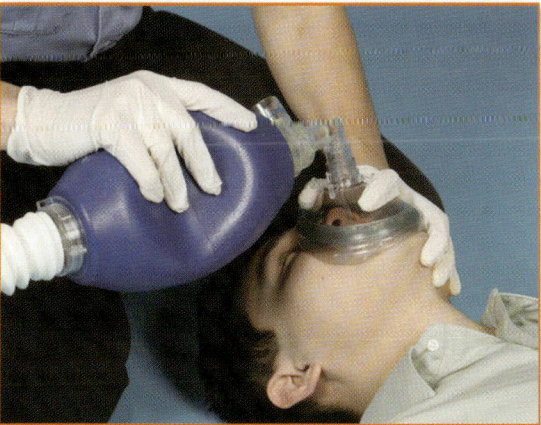

5 Attempt to ventilate.
Repeat steps 3 through 5 until successful or help arrives.

Skill Drill 8-6

Managing Severe Airway Obstruction in an Unconscious Child

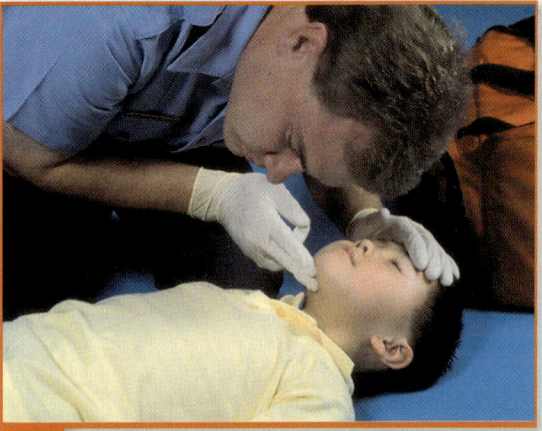

1 Open the airway, and attempt ventilation.

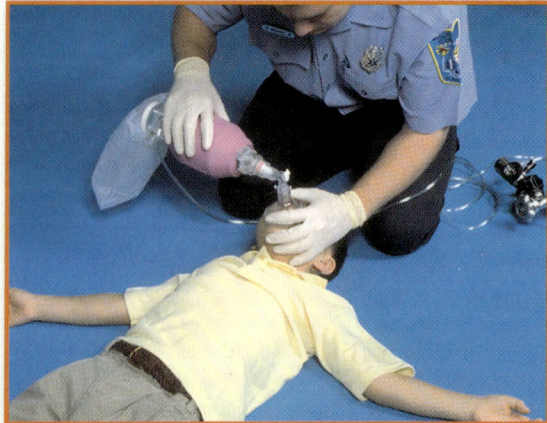

2 If unsuccessful, reopen the airway, and reattempt ventilation.

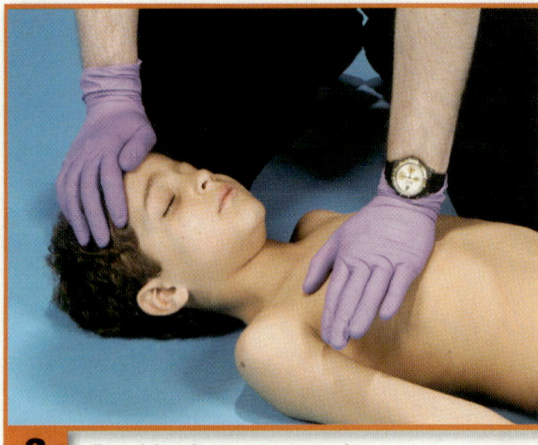

3 Provide chest compressions.

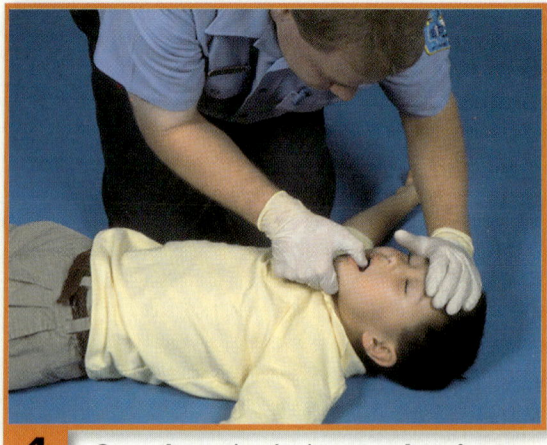

4 Open the patient's airway and perform a finger sweep if the object is visible.

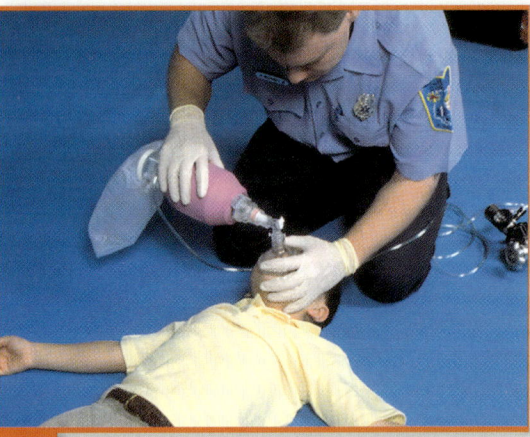

5 Attempt to ventilate.
Repeat steps 3 through 5 until successful or until help arrives.

Managing Severe Airway Obstruction in an Unconscious Infant

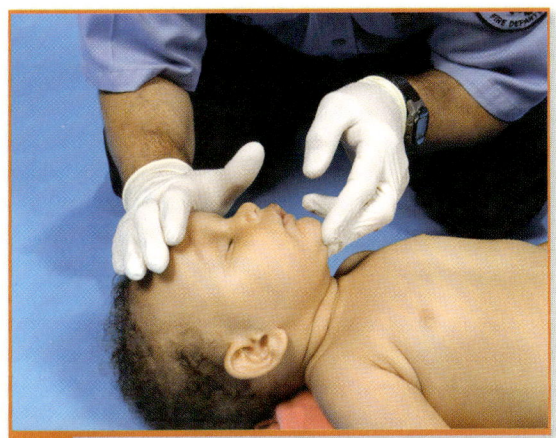
1. Open the airway, and attempt ventilation.

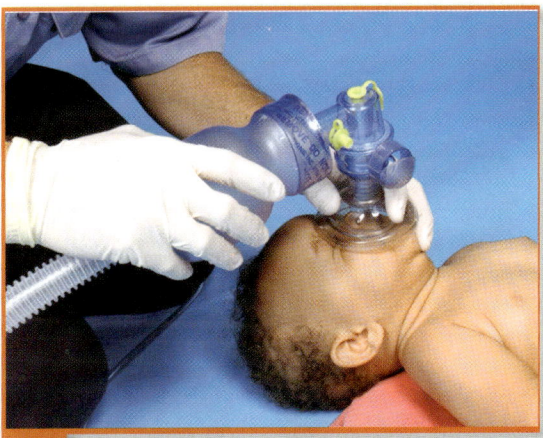
2. If unsuccessful, reopen the airway, and reattempt ventilation.

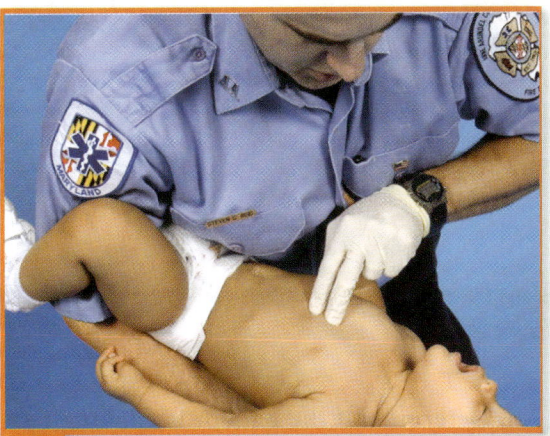
3. Provide chest compressions.

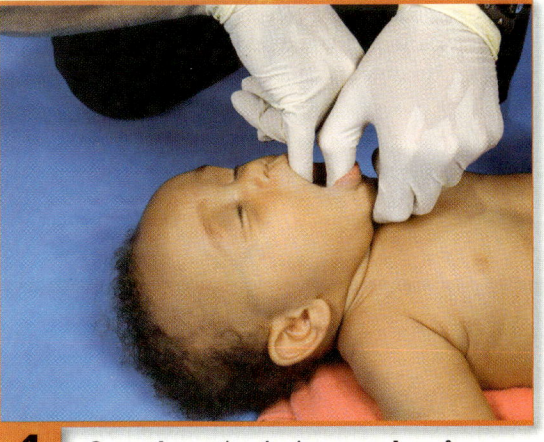
4. Open the patient's airway and perform a finger sweep if the object is visible.

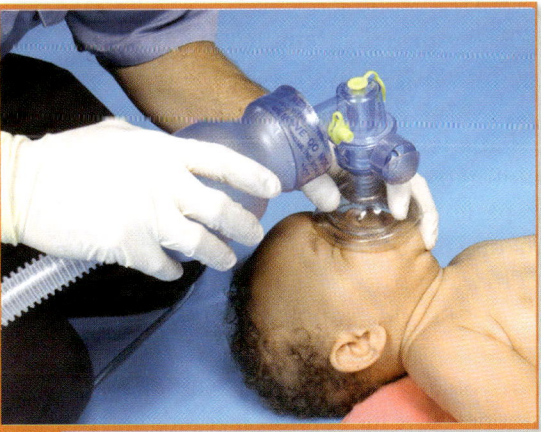
5. Attempt to ventilate.
Repeat steps 3 through 5 until successful or until help arrives.

Skill Drill 9-10

Managing Severe Airway Obstruction in a Conscious Adult or Child

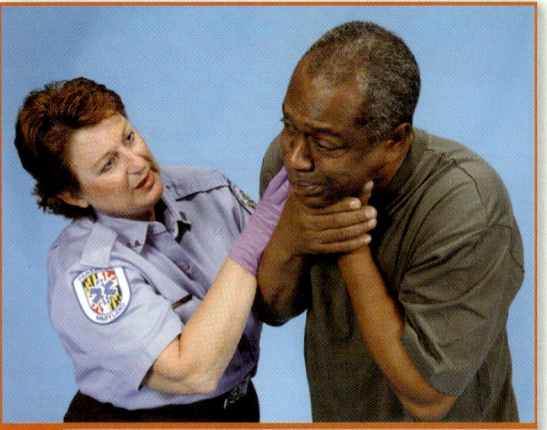

1 Determine if the patient is choking by asking, "Are you choking?" If the patient cannot talk and nods, "yes," immediate treatment is needed.

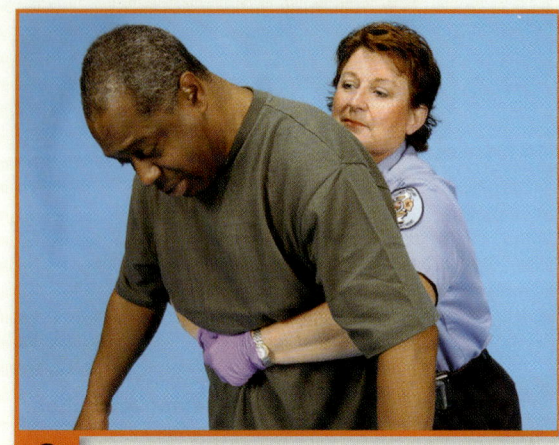

2 Perform the Heimlich maneuver until the object is expelled or the patient becomes unresponsive.

The Heimlich maneuver (abdominal thrusts) is the most effective method of dislodging and forcing an object out of the airway. Residual air, which is always present in the lungs, is compressed upward and used to expel the object. You should use the Heimlich maneuver in the conscious adult or child with a severe airway obstruction. Continue abdominal thrusts until the object is expelled or the patient becomes unconscious.

If you are unable to clear a severe airway obstruction with your initial attempts, begin rapid transport and continue your efforts at relief of the obstruction with abdominal thrusts en route to the hospital.

The steps for managing a severe airway obstruction in a conscious adult or child are listed here and shown in **Skill Drill 9-10**:

1. **Determine if the patient is choking** by asking, "Are you choking?" If the patient cannot talk and nods "yes," immediate treatment is needed (**Step 1**).
2. **Perform the Heimlich maneuver** until the object is expelled or the patient becomes unresponsive (**Step 2**).

Patients with a mild airway obstruction should be monitored closely for signs of a severe obstruction. If the patient is unable to clear the obstruction and remains conscious, support (or let the patient control) the airway position that is most effective and comfortable. Provide supplemental oxygen and transport to the hospital.

If you are unable to ventilate the patient and conventional basic life support methods fail, consider direct laryngoscopy for the removal of the foreign body in unresponsive patients. Insert the laryngoscope blade

Removal of an Upper Airway Obstruction With Magill Forceps

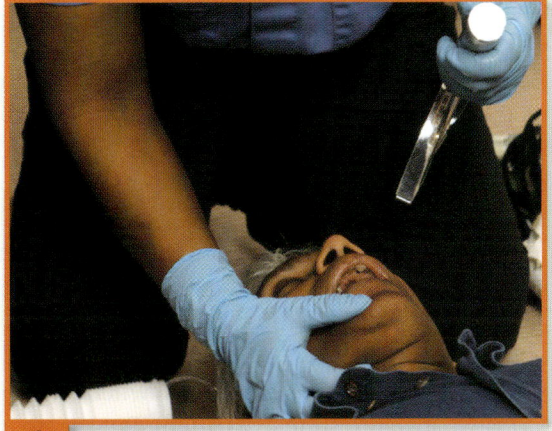

1 With the patient's head in the sniffing position, open the patient's mouth and insert the laryngoscope blade.

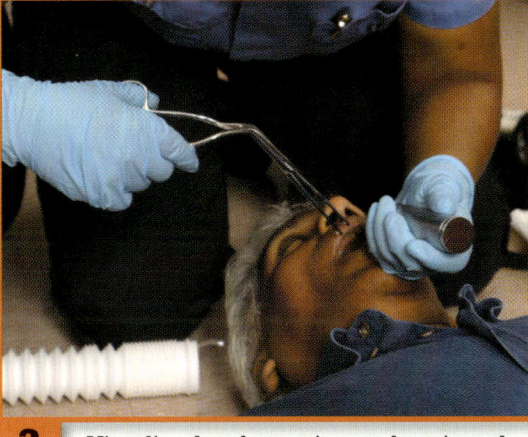

2 Visualize the obstruction, and retrieve the object with the Magill forceps.

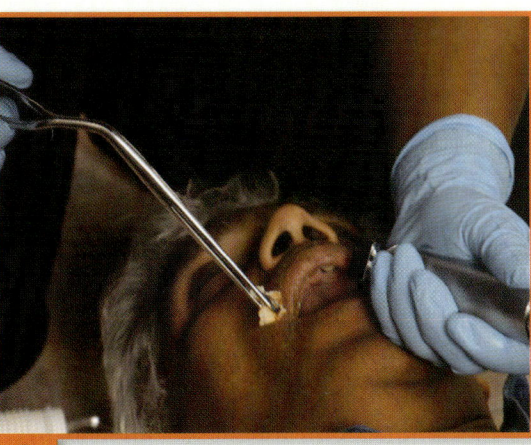

3 Remove the object with the Magill forceps.

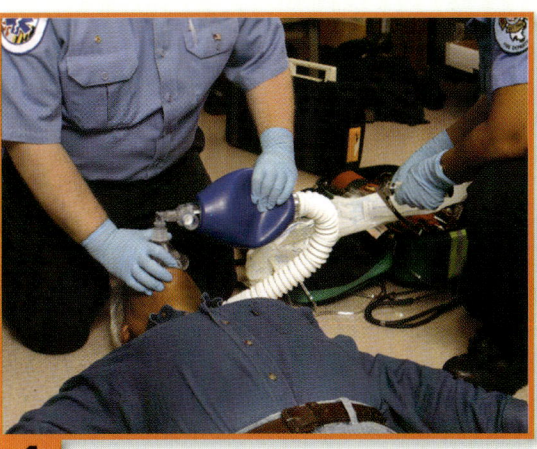

4 Reattempt to ventilate the patient.

into the patient's mouth. If the foreign body is visualized, carefully and deliberately remove the foreign body with Magill forceps. Also consider intubation to ventilate the patient. The steps for removal of an upper airway obstruction with Magill forceps are listed here and shown in **Skill Drill 9-11**:

1. With the patient's head in the sniffing position, **open the patient's mouth and insert the laryngoscope blade** (**Step 1**).
2. **Visualize the obstruction**, and retrieve the object with the Magill forceps (**Step 2**).
3. **Remove the object** with the Magill forceps (**Step 3**).
4. **Reattempt to ventilate** the patient (**Step 4**).

Suctioning

You must keep the airway clear so that you can ventilate the patient properly. If the airway is not clear, you will force material into the lungs and possibly cause a complete airway obstruction. Therefore, suctioning is your first priority. If you have any doubt about the situation, remember this rule: If you hear gurgling, the patient needs suctioning!

Suctioning Equipment

Portable, hand-operated, oxygen-powered, battery-operated, and fixed (mounted) suctioning equipment is essential for resuscitation (Figure 9-5 ▶). A portable suctioning unit must provide enough vacuum pressure and flow to allow you to suction the mouth and oropharynx effectively. Hand-operated suctioning units with disposable chambers are reliable, effective, and relatively inexpensive. A fixed suctioning unit should generate air flow of more than 40 L/min and a vacuum of more than 300 mm Hg when the tubing is clamped. There is also a type of suction unit called a piston-powered suction unit, used in the 1980s, but the vast majority have been replaced by the vacuum type. (Table 9-6 ▶) lists advantages and disadvantages of the most common types of suction devices.

A suctioning unit should be fitted with the following:
- Wide-bore, thick-walled, nonkinking tubing
- Plastic, rigid pharyngeal suction tips, called tonsil tips, or Yankauer tips
- Nonrigid plastic catheters, called French or whistle-tip catheters
- A nonbreakable, disposable collection bottle
- A supply of water for rinsing the tips

You should make sure that the suction yoke, the collection bottle, water for rinsing, and the suction tube are easily accessible at the patient's head.

A suction catheter is a hollow, cylindrical device that is used to remove fluids and secretions from the airway. Hard or rigid catheters include the Yankauer, or tonsil-tip, catheters. Tonsil tips are the best kind of catheter for suctioning the pharynx in adults and the preferred method for infants and children. These plastic tips have a large diameter and are rigid, so they do not collapse. Rigid catheters are capable of suctioning large volumes of fluid rapidly. Tips with a curved contour allow for easy, rapid placement in the pharynx (Figure 9-6 ▶).

When determining the length of a suction catheter for endotracheal suction, measure from the center of the lips to the earlobe to the xiphoid process (Figure 9-7 ▶).

You should use extreme caution when suctioning a responsive or semiresponsive patient. Put the tip in only as far as you can visualize. Be aware that suctioning may induce vomiting in these patients, resulting in possible aspiration.

Techniques of Suctioning

Follow these steps to operate the suction unit:
1. Check the unit for proper assembly of all its parts. Turn on the suctioning unit. Select and attach the appropriate catheter to the tubing. Use bulb suction or a soft catheter with the unit set at the low to medium setting when suctioning the nose.
2. Measure the catheter to ensure that you do not allow it to be inserted too deeply.
3. Open the patient's mouth using the cross-finger technique or the tongue-jaw lift maneuver. Insert

You are the Provider   Part 6

You are assisting the patient's ventilations with a BVM device and 100% oxygen and notice that her respirations have become "noisy" and are making a gurgling sound.

Reassessment	Recording Time: 8 Minutes After Patient Contact
Level of consciousness	Responsive to deep, painful stimuli only
Respirations	40 breaths/min and gurgling (baseline); assisted with a BVM device and 100% O_2
Pulse	144 beats/min, irregular
Skin	Remains pale and diaphoretic; facial cyanosis is worsening
Blood pressure	90/50 mm Hg
Sao_2	85% with assisted ventilations and 100% O_2

8. What must the EMT-I do next to maintain airway patency?

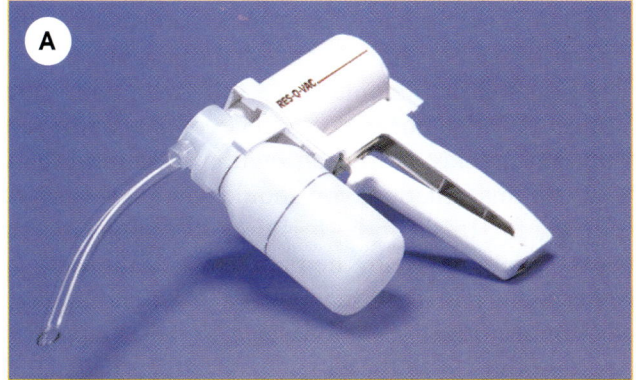
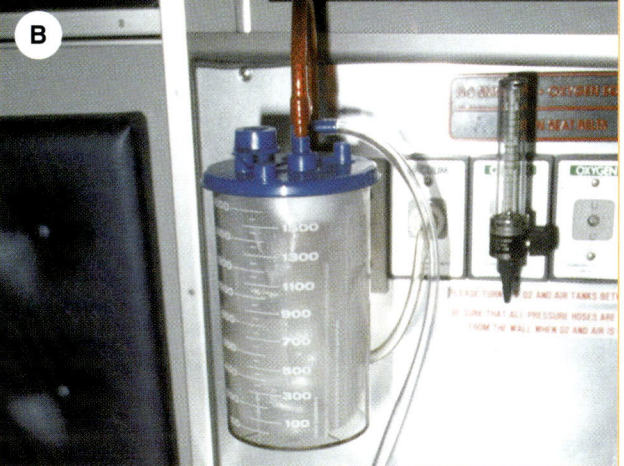
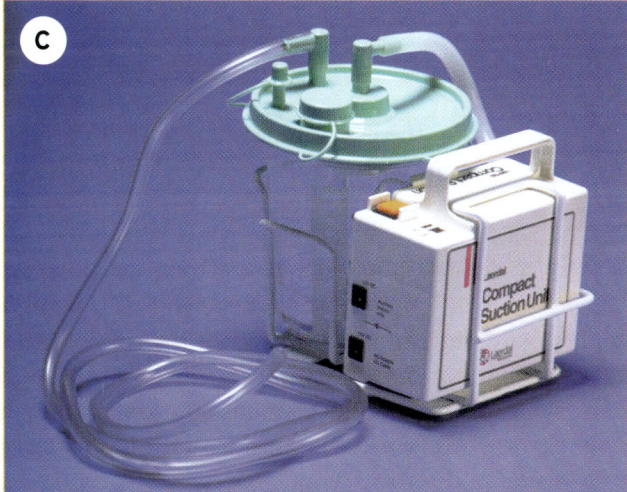

Figure 9-5 Suctioning equipment is essential for resuscitation. **A.** Hand-operated device. **B.** Fixed unit. **C.** Portable unit.

TABLE 9-6	Suction Devices	
Suction Device	**Advantages**	**Disadvantages**
Hand-powered	■ Lightweight ■ Portable ■ Mechanically simple ■ Inexpensive	■ Limited volume ■ Manually powered ■ Fluid contact components not disposable
Oxygen-powered portable	■ Lightweight ■ Small	■ Limited suctioning power ■ Uses a lot of oxygen for limited suctioning power
Battery-operated portable	■ Lightweight ■ Portable ■ Excellent suction power ■ May "field" troubleshoot most problems with the device	■ More complicated mechanics ■ May lose battery integrity over time ■ Some fluid contact components not disposable
Mounted vacuum-powered	■ Extremely strong vacuum ■ Adjustable vacuum power ■ Fluid contact components disposable	■ Not portable ■ Cannot "field service" or substitute power source

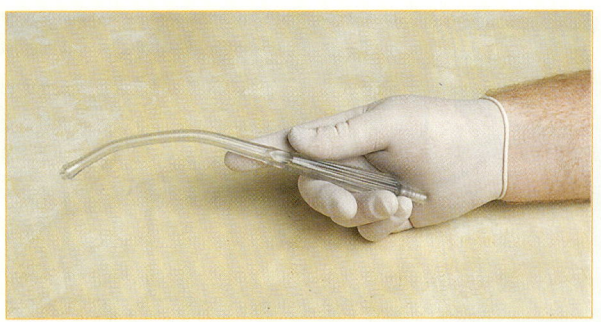

Figure 9-6 Tonsil-tip catheters are the best for suctioning the oropharynx because they have wide-diameter tips and are rigid.

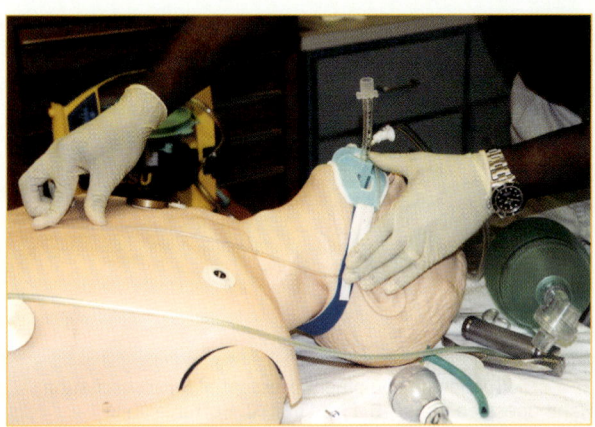

Figure 9-7 When determining the length of a suction catheter for endotracheal suction, measure from the center of the lips to the earlobe to the xiphoid process.

the suction tip along the roof of the mouth until you reach the pharynx. Do not use suction unless it is absolutely necessary. Insert the tip only to the base of the tongue.

4. After the tip is in place, apply suction as you withdraw the suction tip from the pharynx and mouth. Move the suction tip from side to side.

Never suction for more than 15 seconds at one time for adult patients, 10 seconds for children, and 5 seconds for infants. Suctioning removes oxygen from the airway along with obstructive material. Rinse the catheter and tubing with water to prevent clogging of the tube with dried vomitus or other secretions. Repeat suctioning only after the patient has been ventilated and reoxygenated.

At times, a patient may have secretions or vomitus that cannot be suctioned quickly and easily. There are also some suction units that are unable to effectively remove solid objects such as teeth, foreign bodies, and food. In these instances, you should remove the catheter from the patient's mouth, log roll the patient to the side, and then clear the mouth carefully with your gloved finger. A patient may also produce copious frothy secretions as quickly as you can suction them from the airway. In this situation, you should suction the patient's airway for 15 seconds (less time in infants and children), then ventilate the patient for 2 minutes. This alternating pattern of suctioning and ventilating should continue until all secretions have been cleared from the patient's airway or the patient has been intubated. Continuous ventilation is not appropriate if vomitus or other particles are present in the airway.

To properly suction a patient's airway **Skill Drill 9-12 ▶**):

1. **Turn on the assembled suction unit** (**Step 1**).
2. **Insert the catheter** to the correct depth by measuring the catheter from the corner of the patient's mouth to the tip of the earlobe (**Step 2**).
3. **Before applying suction**, open the patient's mouth by using the cross-finger technique or tongue-jaw lift, and insert the tip of the catheter to the depth measured without using force (**Step 3**).
4. **Apply suction** in a circular motion as you withdraw the catheter. Do not suction an adult for more than 15 seconds (**Step 4**).

Soft plastic, nonrigid catheters, sometimes called French or "whistle-tip" catheters, can be placed in the oropharynx or nasopharynx or down an ET tube. They come in various sizes that have a smaller inside diameter than hard-tip catheters. Soft catheters are used to suction the nose and liquid secretions in the back of the mouth and in situations in which you cannot use a rigid catheter, such as for a patient with a stoma **Figure 9-8 ▼**). For example, a rigid catheter could

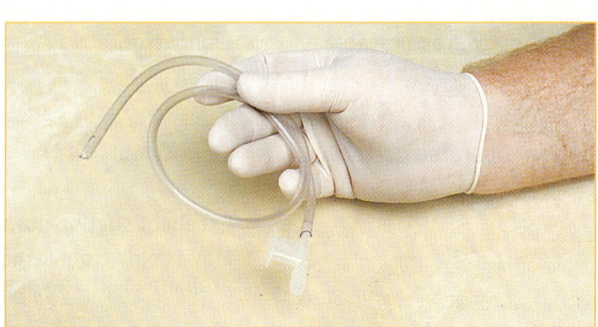

Figure 9-8 French, or whistle-tip, catheters are used in situations in which rigid catheters cannot be used, such as with a patient who has a stoma or if the patient's teeth are clenched.

Suctioning a Patient's Airway

Skill Drill 9-12

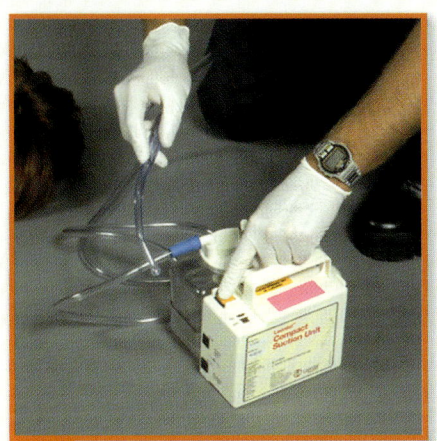

1. Make sure the suctioning unit is properly assembled, and turn on the suction unit.

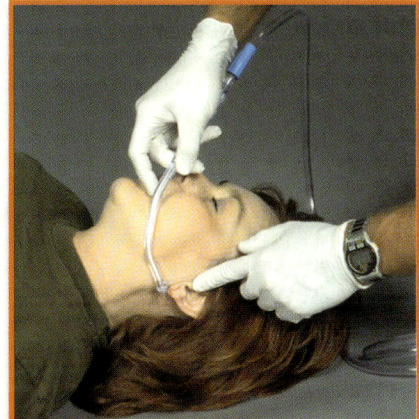

2. Measure the catheter from the corner of the mouth to the earlobe.

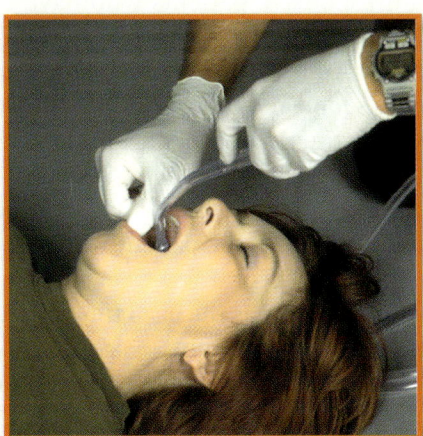

3. Open the patient's mouth, and insert the catheter to the depth measured without using force.

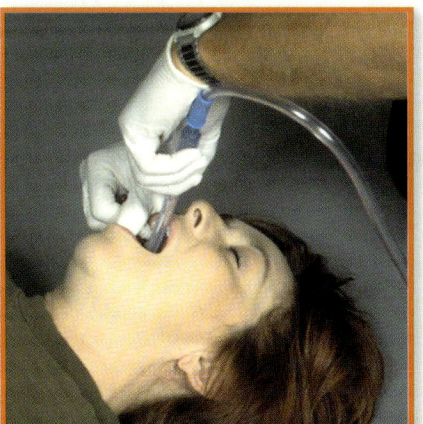

4. Apply suction in a circular motion as you withdraw the catheter. Do not suction an adult for more than 15 seconds.

break off a tooth, whereas a flexible catheter may be worked along the cheeks without injury. Suction tubing without the attached catheter facilitates suctioning of large debris in the oropharynx.

Suctioning of the upper airway to prevent aspiration is critical. Mortality increases significantly if aspiration occurs. Preoxygenate the patient if possible, and hyperoxygenate after suctioning. Soft-tip catheters must be prelubricated when suctioning the nasopharynx and through an ET tube. The catheter is inserted, and suction is applied during extraction to clear the airway. Reevaluate the patency of the airway, and continue to ventilate and oxygenate the patient.

Before you insert any catheter, make sure to measure for the proper size. Use the same technique as you would use when measuring for an oropharyngeal or nasopharyngeal airway. Never insert a catheter past the base of the tongue, as this may result in gagging and vomiting.

You should clean and decontaminate your suctioning equipment after each use according to the manufacturer's guidelines. You should also inspect this equipment regularly to make sure it is in proper working condition. Switch on the suction, clamp the tubing, and make sure that the unit generates a vacuum of more than 300 mm Hg. Check that a battery-charged unit has charged batteries.

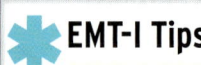

EMT-I Tips

Suctioning Time Limits
Adult 15 seconds
Child 10 seconds
Infant 5 seconds

Airway Adjuncts

Oral Airway

An <u>oropharyngeal (oral) airway</u> is a hard plastic airway designed to prevent the tongue from obstructing the glottis. It also makes it easier to suction the airway if necessary. Both functions are made possible by an opening down the center or along either side of the oropharyngeal airway (Figure 9-9 ▶). This type of airway is often used in conjunction with BVM ventilation.

EMT-I Safety

A mask and protective eyewear should be worn whenever airway management involves suctioning. Body fluids can become aerosolized, and exposure to the mucous membranes of the EMT-I's mouth, nose, and eyes can easily occur.

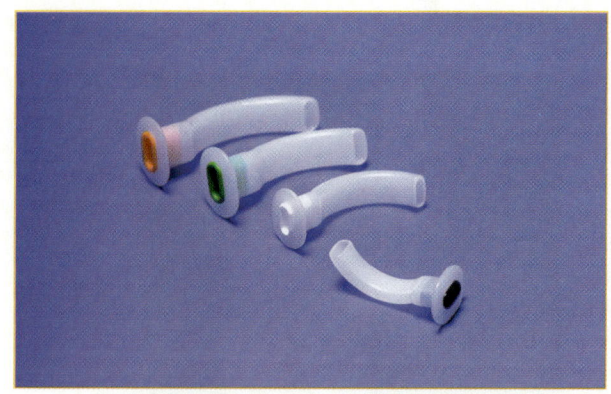

Figure 9-9 An oral airway is used for unconscious patients who have no gag reflex. It works to keep the tongue from blocking the airway and to facilitate suctioning the airway.

An oropharyngeal airway should be inserted promptly in unresponsive patients who have no gag reflex. These patients may or may not be breathing on their own. The <u>gag reflex</u> is a protective reflex mechanism that prevents food and other particles from entering the airway. Inserting an oral airway in a patient with a gag reflex may result in vomiting or a spasm of the vocal cords. An oral airway is a safe, effective way to help maintain the airway of the patient with a possible spinal injury. The use of an oral airway may make manual airway maneuvers such as the head tilt–chin lift and the jaw-thrust easier to maintain. (Table 9-7 ▶) lists indications, contraindications, advantages, disadvantages, and complications of using an oral airway.

You are the Provider — Part 7

You suction the patient's oropharynx to clear her airway of secretions. Following this intervention, you reassess her condition and note the following:

Reassessment	Recording Time: 9 Minutes After Patient Contact
Level of consciousness	Responsive to deep painful stimuli only
Respirations	30 breaths/min and shallow (baseline); assisted with a BVM device and 100% O_2
Pulse	124 beats/min, irregular
Skin	Remains pale and diaphoretic; cyanosis has improved
Blood pressure	98/64 mm Hg
Sao_2	88% with assisted ventilations and 100% O_2

9. What is the method you should use to determine the appropriate size of suction catheter?
10. What is the time limit for suctioning this patient?

Inserting an Oral Airway

Skill Drill 9-13

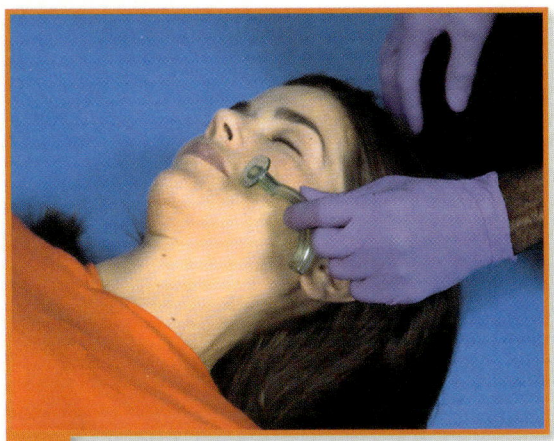

1 Determine the size of the airway by measuring the distance from the patient's earlobe to the corner of the mouth.

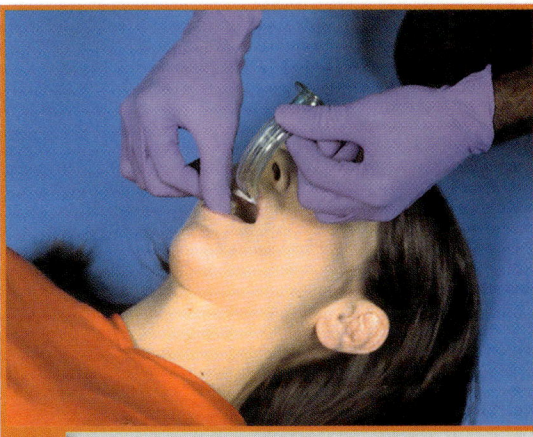

2 Open the patient's mouth with the cross-finger technique. Hold the airway upside down with your other hand. Insert the airway with the tip facing the roof of the mouth and slide it in until it touches the roof of the mouth.

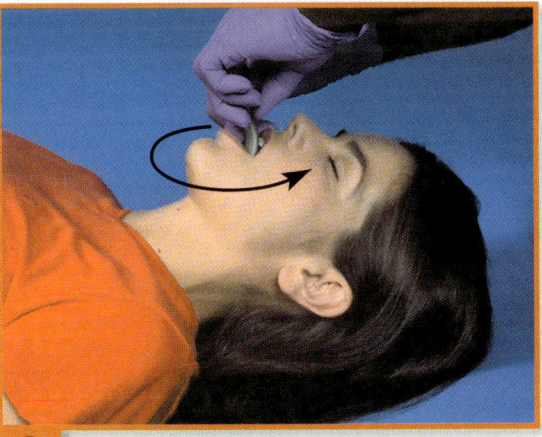

3 Rotate the airway 180°. Insert the airway until the flange rests on the patient's lips and teeth. In this position, the airway will hold the tongue forward.

You must be very clear on when and how this device is used. **Skill Drill 9-13** shows the steps for inserting an oral airway. If the oropharyngeal airway is not the proper size or is inserted incorrectly, it could actually push the tongue back into the pharynx, blocking the airway. The following steps should be used when inserting an oropharyngeal airway:

1. **To select the proper size**, measure the distance from the patient's earlobe to the corner of the mouth on the side of the face (**Step 1**).
2. **Open the patient's mouth** with the cross-finger technique. Hold the airway upside down with your other hand. Insert the airway with the tip facing the roof of the mouth (**Step 2**).
3. **Rotate the airway 180°**. When inserted properly, the airway will rest in the mouth with the curvature of the airway following the contour of the tongue. The flange should rest against the lips or teeth, with the other end opening into the pharynx (**Step 3**).

Take care to avoid injuring the hard palate as you insert the airway. Roughness can cause bleeding, which may aggravate airway problems or even cause vomiting.

Inserting an Oral Airway With a 90° Rotation

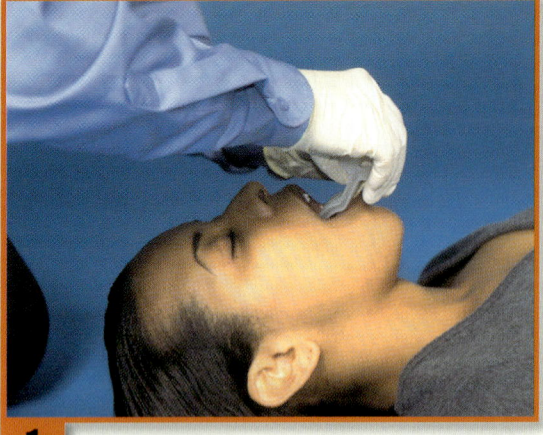

1. Depress the tongue with a tongue blade so the tongue remains forward.

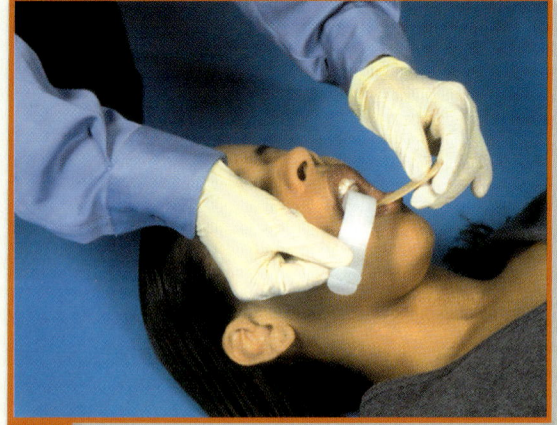

2. Insert the oral airway sideways from the corner of the mouth, until the flange reaches the teeth.

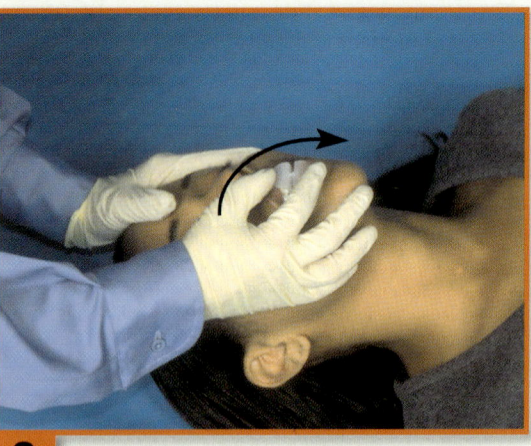

3. Rotate the oral airway 90°. Remove the tongue blade as you exert gentle backward pressure on the oral airway until it rests securely in place against the lips and teeth.

If you encounter difficulty while inserting the oral airway, an alternative method may be used by following these steps (Skill Drill 9-14):

1. **Use a tongue blade** to depress the tongue, ensuring that the tongue remains forward (**Step 1**).
2. **Insert the oral airway sideways** from the corner of the mouth, until the flange reaches the teeth (**Step 2**).
3. **Rotate the oral airway 90°**, removing the tongue blade as you exert gentle backward pressure on the oral airway until it rests securely in place against the lips and teeth (**Step 3**).

In some cases, a patient may become responsive and regain a gag reflex after you have inserted an oral airway. If this occurs, gently remove the airway by pulling it out, following the normal curvature of the mouth and throat. Be prepared for the patient to vomit. Have suction available, and log roll the patient onto his or her side to allow any fluids to drain out.

TABLE 9-7	Oral Airway

Indications
- Unresponsive patients
- Absent gag reflex

Contraindication
- Conscious patients

Advantages
- Noninvasive
- Easily placed
- Blockage of glottis by tongue prevented

Disadvantages
- Aspiration not prevented

Complications
- Vomiting possible after unexpected gag reflex
- Pharyngeal or dental trauma with poor technique

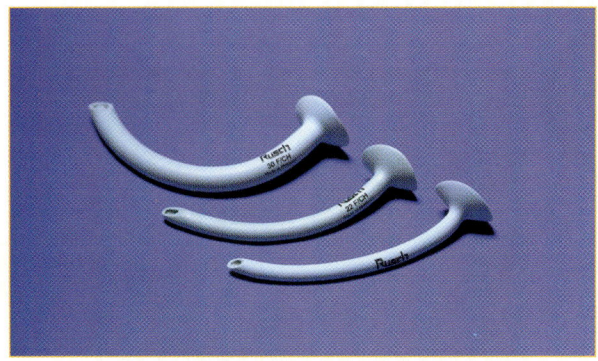

Figure 9-10 A nasal airway is better tolerated by patients who have an intact gag reflex.

 Pediatric Needs

In children, using a tongue blade to hold the tongue down while inserting the airway is the preferred method. Because the airways of children are less developed than in adults, rotating an oropharyngeal airway in the posterior pharynx may cause damage.

Nasal Airway

A nasopharyngeal (nasal) airway is soft rubber with a beveled tip and usually is used in a patient who has an intact gag reflex and is not able to maintain an airway (Figure 9-10). Patients with altered mental status or those who have just had a seizure may also benefit from this type of airway. If a patient has sustained severe trauma to the head or face, you should consult medical control before inserting a nasopharyngeal airway. Extreme care must be used with such trauma patients. If the airway is accidentally pushed through the hole caused by a skull fracture, it may penetrate through the cranium and into the brain.

This type of airway is usually better tolerated by patients who have an intact gag reflex. It is not as likely as the oropharyngeal airway to cause vomiting. The distal tip of the nasopharyngeal airway rests in the hypopharynx behind the tongue. You should coat the airway well with a water-soluble lubricant before it is inserted. Be aware that slight bleeding may occur even when the airway is inserted properly. However, you should never force the airway into place. Table 9-8 lists indications, contraindications, advantages, and disadvantages of using a nasal airway.

Follow these steps to ensure correct placement of the nasopharyngeal airway (Skill Drill 9-15):

1. **Before inserting the airway,** be sure you have selected the proper size. Measure the distance from the tip of the nostril to the earlobe. In almost all individuals, one nostril is larger than the other. The diameter should be roughly equal to the patient's little finger (**Step 1**).
2. **The airway should be placed** in the larger nostril, with the curvature of the device following the curve of the floor of the nose and the bevel facing the septum. Lubricate the tip with a water-soluble gel (**Step 2**).
3. **Place the bevel toward the septum** and insert gently along the nasal floor, parallel to the mouth. **DO NOT FORCE THE AIRWAY** (**Step 3**).
4. **When completely inserted,** the flange rests against the nostril. The other end of the airway opens into the posterior pharynx (**Step 4**).

The proper size may also be determined from the tip of the nostril to the angle of the jaw rather than the tip of the ear. If the nasopharyngeal airway is too long, it will obstruct the patient's airway. If the patient becomes intolerant of the nasal airway, you may have to remove it. Gently withdraw the airway from the nasal passage.

Skill Drill 9-15

Inserting a Nasal Airway

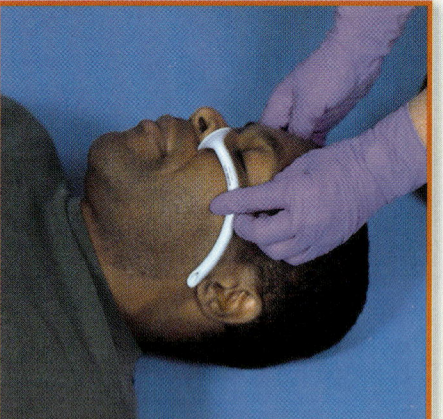

1 Determine the size of the airway by measuring the distance from the tip of the nose to the patient's earlobe. Coat the tip with a water-soluble lubricant.

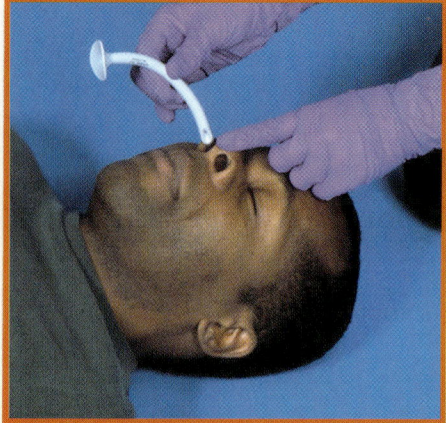

2 Insert the lubricated airway into the larger nostril with the curvature following the floor of the nose and the bevel facing the septum.

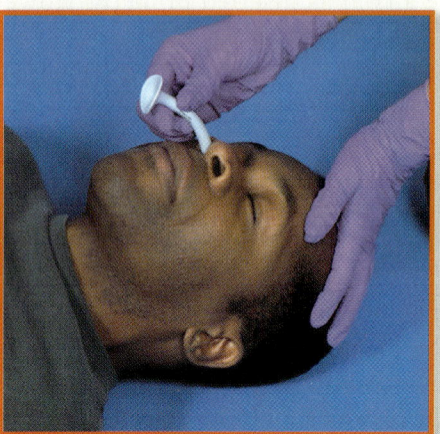

3 Gently advance the airway. If using the left nare, insert the nasopharyngeal airway until resistance is met. Then rotate the nasopharyngeal airway 180° into position. This rotation is not required if using the right nostril.

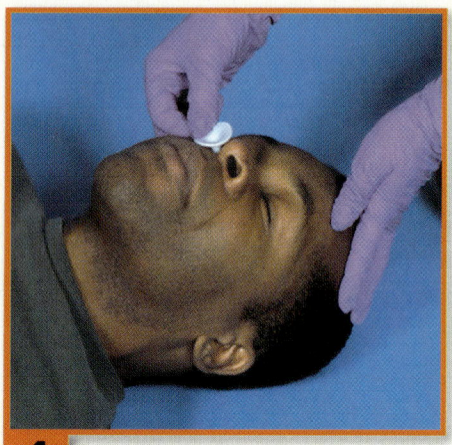

4 Continue until the flange rests against the skin. If you feel any resistance or obstruction, remove the airway and insert it into the other nostril.

Supplemental Oxygen

Supplemental oxygen should be administered to any patient with potential hypoxia, even if the patient's clinical appearance is otherwise normal. Consider the patients complaining of chest pain who have an oxygen saturation more than 95% while breathing room air. Lack of oxygen to the myocardium causes ischemic pain. By enriching atmospheric air with supplemental oxygen, you subsequently increase oxygen to the cells, thereby reducing pain and further damage to myocardial tissue. Increasing the available oxygen also enhances the body's compensatory mechanisms during shock and other distressed states. The oxygen-delivery method

TABLE 9-8	Nasal Airway

Indications
- Unresponsive patients
- Patients with altered mental status with an intact gag reflex

Contraindications
- Patient intolerance
- Caution in presence of facial fracture or skull fracture

Advantages
- Can suction through the airway
- Provides patent airway
- Can be tolerated by awake patients
- Can be safely placed "blindly"
- Does not require the mouth to be open

Disadvantages
- Severe bleeding a possible result of poor technique
  - Resulting epistaxis may be extremely difficult to control
- No protection from aspiration

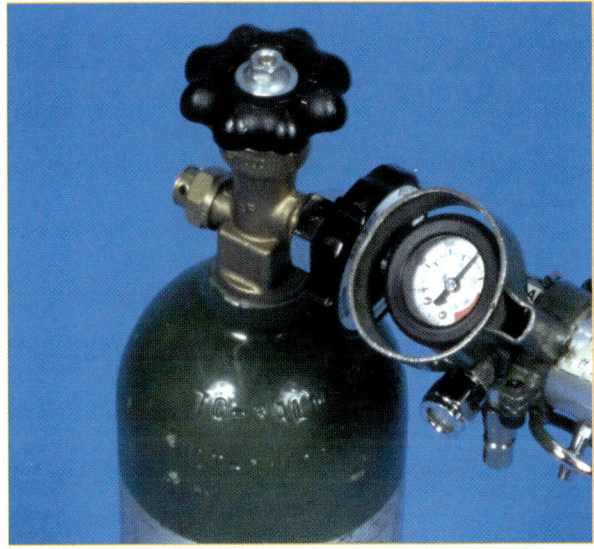

Figure 9-11 Oxygen tanks for medical use have a series of letters and numbers stamped into the metal on the collar of the cylinder.

must be reassessed frequently and adjusted accordingly based on the patient's clinical condition and breathing adequacy.

In addition to knowing when and how to give supplemental oxygen, you must understand how oxygen is stored and the various hazards associated with its use.

Oxygen Sources

The oxygen that you will give to patients is usually supplied as a compressed gas in green, seamless steel or aluminum cylinders. Some cylinders may be silver or chrome with a green area around the valve stem on top. Newer cylinders are often made of lightweight aluminum or spun steel; older cylinders are much heavier.

Check to make sure that the cylinder is labeled for medical oxygen. You should look for letters and numbers stamped into the metal on the collar of the cylinder **Figure 9-11**. Of particular importance are the month and year stamps, which indicate when the cylinder was last tested.

Oxygen cylinders are available in several sizes. The two sizes that you will most often use are the D (or super D) cylinder, which contains 400 L, and the M cylinder, which contains 3,450 L **Figure 9-12**. The D (or super D) cylinder can be carried from your unit to the patient. The M tank remains on board your unit as a main

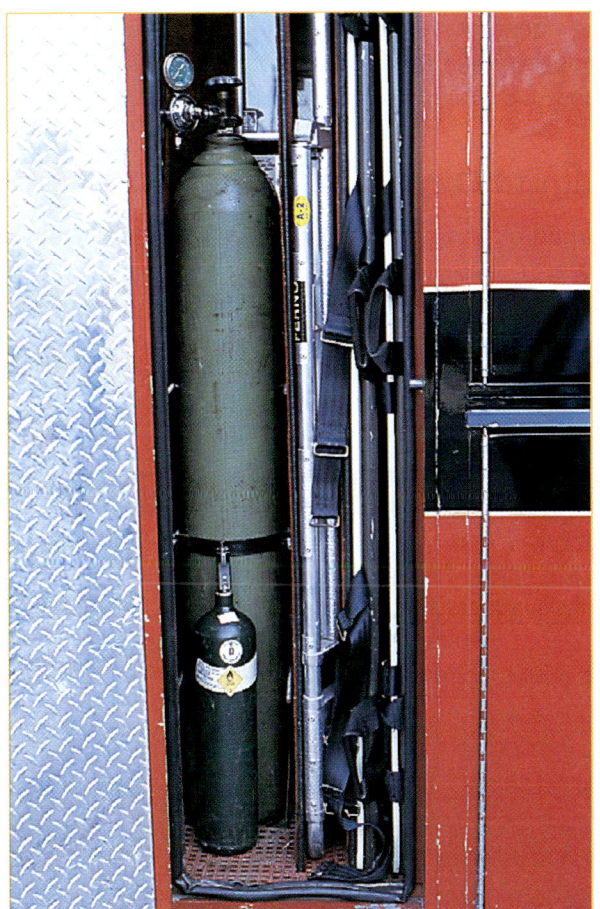

Figure 9-12 The cylinders most commonly found on an ambulance are the D (or super D) and M size cylinders.

supply tank. The E cylinder is another common size and holds 660 L.

Oxygen delivery is measured in liters per minute. The length of time you can use an oxygen cylinder depends on the pressure in the cylinder and the flow rate. A method of calculating cylinder duration, or tank life, is shown in Table 9-9.

Safety Considerations

Compressed gas cylinders must be handled very carefully because their contents are under pressure. Cylinders are fitted with pressure regulators to make sure that patients receive the right amount and type of gas. (See the subsequent section on the pin-indexing system for information on how regulators help ensure the right type of gas is given.) Make sure that the correct pressure regulator is firmly attached before you transport the cylinders. A puncture or hole in the tank can cause the cylinder to become a deadly missile. Do not handle a cylinder by the neck assembly alone. Cylinders should be secured with mounting brackets when they are stored on the ambulance. Oxygen cylinders that are in use during transport should be positioned and secured to prevent the tank from falling or from damage occurring to the valve-gauge assembly.

Liquid Oxygen

Liquid oxygen is oxygen that is cooled to its aqueous state. It converts to the gaseous state when warmed. There are advantages and disadvantages of liquid oxygen. A much larger volume of gaseous oxygen can be stored in the aqueous state. However, units for liquid oxygen generally require upright storage. There are also special requirements for large volume storage and cylinder transfer.

Pin-Indexing System

The compressed gas industry has established a pin-indexing system for portable cylinders to prevent an oxygen regulator from being connected to a carbon dioxide cylinder, and so on. When preparing to administer oxygen, always check to be sure that the pinholes on the cylinder exactly match the corresponding pins on the regulator.

The pin-indexing system features a series of pins on a yoke that must be matched with the holes on the valve stem of the gas cylinder. The arrangement of the pins and holes varies for different gases according to accepted national standards Figure 9-13. Other gases that are supplied in portable cylinders, such as acetylene, carbon dioxide, and nitrogen, use regulators and flowmeters that are very similar to those used with oxygen. Each cylinder of a specific gas has a given pattern and a given number of pins. These safety measures make it impos-

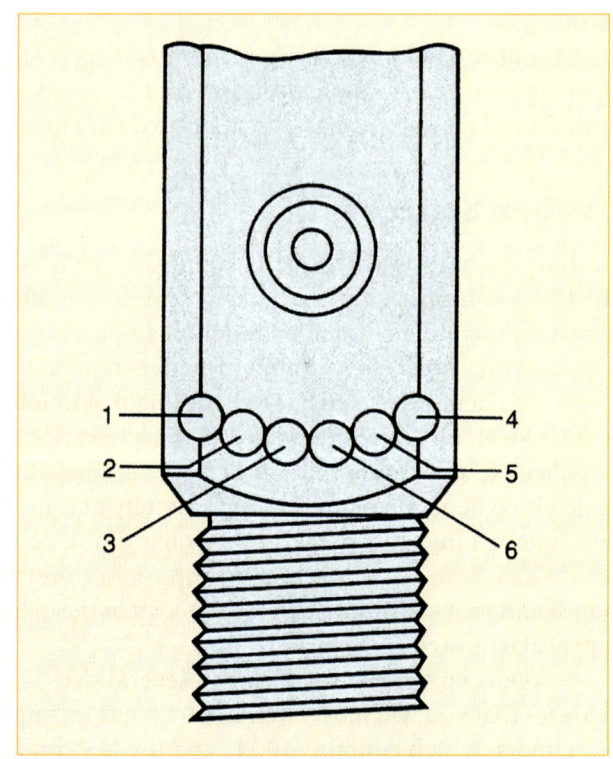

Figure 9-13 The locations of the pin-indexing safety system holes in a cylinder valve face. Each cylinder of a specific gas has a given pattern and a given number of pins.

TABLE 9-9	Oxygen Cylinders: Duration of Flow

Formula:

$$\frac{(\text{Tank pressure in psi} - 200 \text{ psi [the safe residual pressure]}) \times \text{cylinder constant}}{\text{Flow rate in L/min}} = \text{Duration of flow in minutes}$$

CYLINDER CONSTANT
D = 0.16   G = 2.41
E = 0.28   H = 3.14
M = 1.56   K = 3.14

Determine the life of an M cylinder that has a pressure of 2,000 psi and a flow rate of 10 L/min.

$$\frac{(2{,}000 - 200) \times 1.56}{10} = \frac{2{,}808}{10} = 281 \text{ min, or } 4 \text{ h } 41 \text{ min}$$

Note: psi indicates pounds per square inch.

sible for you to attach a cylinder of nitrous oxide to an oxygen regulator. The oxygen regulator will not fit.

The outlet valves on E size or smaller cylinders are designed to accept yoke-type pressure-reducing gauges, which conform to the pin-indexing system. The safety system for large cylinders is known as the American Standard System. In this system, cylinders larger than E sizes are equipped with threaded gas outlet valves. The inside and outside thread sizes of these outlets vary depending on the gas in the cylinder. The cylinder will not accept a regulator valve unless it is properly threaded to fit that regulator. The purpose of these safety devices is the same as in the pin-indexing system: to prevent the accidental attachment of a regulator to a wrong cylinder.

Regulators

High-pressure regulators are attached to the cylinder stem to deliver cylinder gas under high pressure. These regulators are used to transfer cylinder gas from tank to tank.

The pressure of gas in a full oxygen cylinder is approximately 2,000 psi. This is far too much pressure to be safe or useful for your purposes. Regulators reduce the pressure to a more useful range, usually 40 to 70 psi. Most pressure regulators that are in use today reduce the pressure in a single stage, although multistage regulators exist. A two-stage regulator will reduce the pressure first to 700 psi and then to 40 to 70 psi.

After the pressure is reduced to a workable level, the final attachment for delivering the gas to the patient is usually one of the following:

- A quick-connect female fitting that will accept a quick-connect male plug from a pressure hose or ventilator or resuscitator
- A flowmeter that will permit the regulated release of gas measured in liters per minute

Flowmeters

Flowmeters are usually permanently attached to pressure regulators on emergency medical equipment. The two types of flowmeters that are commonly used are pressure-compensated flowmeters and Bourdon-gauge flowmeters.

A pressure-compensated flowmeter incorporates a float ball within a tapered calibrated tube. The float rises or falls according to the gas flow within the tube. The flow of gas is controlled by a needle valve located downstream from the float ball. This type of flowmeter is affected by gravity and must always be maintained

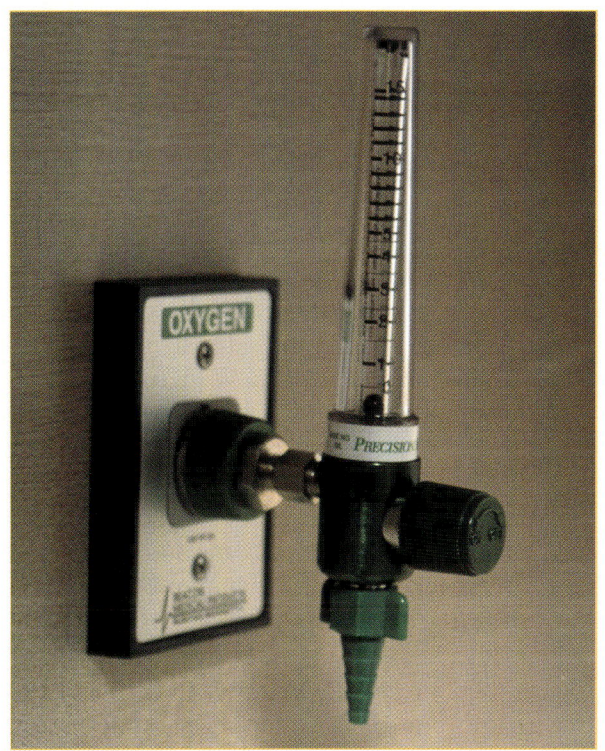

Figure 9-14 Pressure-compensated flowmeters contain a float ball that rises or falls according to the gas flow within the tube. It must be maintained in an upright position for an accurate reading.

in an upright position for an accurate flow reading Figure 9-14.

The Bourdon-gauge flowmeter is commonly used because it is not affected by gravity and can be used in any position. It is actually a pressure gauge that is calibrated to record flow rate Figure 9-15. The major disadvantage of this flowmeter is that it does not compensate for backpressure. Therefore, it will usually record

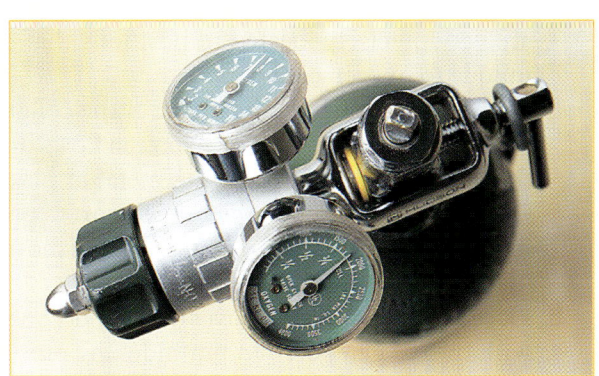

Figure 9-15 The Bourdon-gauge flowmeter is not affected by gravity and can be used in any position.

a higher flow rate when there is any obstruction to gas flow downstream.

Operating Procedures

Before placing an oxygen cylinder into service Skill Drill 9-16 ▶ :

1. **Inspect the cylinder** and its markings. If the cylinder was commercially filled, it will have a plastic seal around the valve stem covering the opening in the stem. Remove the seal, and inspect the opening to make sure that it is free of dirt and other debris. The valve stem should not be sealed or covered with adhesive tape or any petroleum-based substances. These can contaminate the oxygen and can contribute to spontaneous combustion when mixed with the pressurized oxygen.

    "Crack" the cylinder by quickly opening and then reclosing the valve to help make sure that dirt particles and other possible contaminants do not enter the oxygen flow. Never face the tank toward yourself or others when cracking the cylinder. Open the tank by attaching a tank key to the valve and rotating the valve counterclockwise. You should be able to clearly hear the rush of oxygen coming from the tank. Close the tank by rotating the valve clockwise (**Step 1**).

2. **Attach the regulator/flowmeter** to the valve stem after clearing the opening. On one side of the valve stem, you will find three holes. The larger one, on top, is a true opening through which the oxygen flows. The two smaller holes below it do not extend to the inside of the tank. They provide stability to the regulator. Following the design of a pin-indexing system, these two holes are very precisely located in positions that are unique to oxygen cylinders.

    Above the pins on the inside of the collar is the actual port through which oxygen flows from the cylinder to the regulator. A metal or plastic O-ring is placed around the oxygen port to optimize the airtight seal between the collar of the regulator and the valve stem (**Step 2**).

3. **Place the regulator collar** over the cylinder valve, with the oxygen port and pin-indexing pins on the side of the valve stem that has the three holes. Open the screw bolt just enough to allow the collar to fit freely over the valve stem. Move the regulator so that the oxygen port and the pins fit into the correct holes on the valve stem. The screw bolt on the opposite side should be aligned with the dimpled depression. As you hold the regulator securely against the valve stem, tighten the screw bolt until the regulator is firmly attached to the cylinder. At this point, you should not see any open spaces between the sides of the valve stem and the interior walls of the collar (**Step 3**).

4. **With the regulator firmly attached**, open the cylinder and read the pressure level on the regulator gauge. Most portable cylinders have a maximum pressure of approximately 2,000 psi. Most EMS services consider a cylinder with less than 500 to 1,000 psi to be too low to keep in service. Learn your department's policies in this regard and follow them.

    The flowmeter will have a second gauge or a selector dial that indicates the oxygen flow rate. Several popular types of devices are widely used. Attach the selected oxygen device to the flowmeter by connecting the universal oxygen connective tubing to the "Christmas tree" nipple on the flowmeter. Most oxygen-delivery devices come with this tubing permanently attached. Some oxygen masks do not. You must add this tubing to the oxygen-delivery device if it is not attached (**Step 4**).

Open the flowmeter to the desired flow rate. Flow rates will vary based on the oxygen-delivery device being used. Remember that you must be completely familiar with the equipment before attempting to use it on a patient. Once the oxygen is flowing at the desired rate, apply the oxygen device to the patient and make any necessary adjustments. Monitor the patient's reaction to the oxygen and to the oxygen device, and periodically recheck the regulator gauge to make sure there is sufficient oxygen in the cylinder. Disconnect the tubing from the flowmeter nipple and turn off the cylinder valve when oxygen therapy is complete or when the patient has been transferred to the hospital and has been switched to the hospital's oxygen system. In a few seconds, the sound of oxygen flowing from the nipple will cease. This indicates that all the pressurized oxygen has been removed from the flowmeter. Turn off the flowmeter. The gauge on the regulator should read zero with the tank valve closed. This confirms that there is no pressure left above the valve stem. As long as there is a pressure reading on the regulator gauge, it is not safe to remove the regulator from the valve stem.

Skill Drill 9-16: Placing an Oxygen Cylinder Into Service

1. Using an oxygen wrench, turn the valve counterclockwise to "crack" the cylinder.

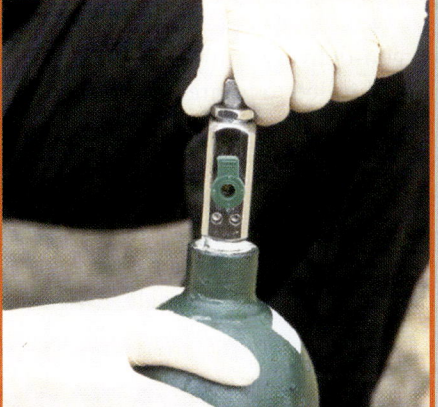

2. Attach the regulator/flowmeter to the valve stem using the two pin-indexing holes, and make sure that the washer is in place over the larger hole.

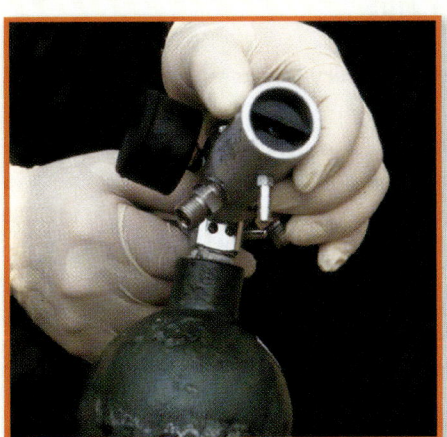

3. Align the regulator so that the pins fit snugly into the correct holes on the valve stem and hand tighten the regulator.

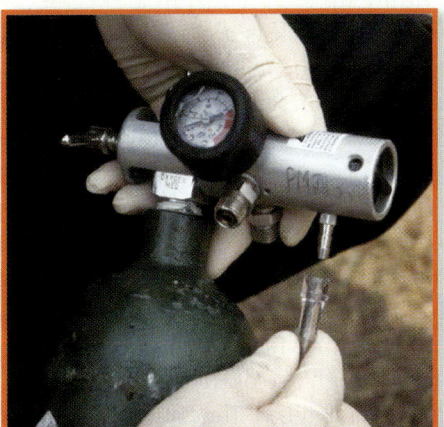

4. Attach the oxygen connective tubing to the flowmeter.

Hazards of Supplemental Oxygen

Oxygen does not burn or explode. However, it does support combustion. The more oxygen that is around, the faster the combustion process. A small spark, even a glowing cigarette, can become a flame in an oxygen-rich atmosphere. Therefore, you must keep any possible source of fire away from the area while oxygen is in use. Make sure the area is adequately ventilated, especially in industrial settings where hazardous materials may be present and where sparks are easily generated. Be extremely cautious in any enclosed environment in which oxygen is being administered because an oxygen-rich environment increases the chance of fire if a spark or flame is introduced. A bystander who is smoking or sparks generated from vehicle extrication are possible ignition sources. Never leave an oxygen cylinder standing unattended. The cylinder could be knocked over, injuring the patient or damaging the equipment.

Supplemental Oxygen-Delivery Devices

In general, the oxygen-delivery equipment that is used in the field should be limited to nonrebreathing masks, BVM devices, and nasal cannulas, depending on local protocol. However, you may encounter other devices during transports between medical facilities. Such devices include simple face masks, partial rebreathing masks, and Venturi masks. Small-volume nebulizers may also be used for oxygen delivery, in addition to delivering medications.

Nonrebreathing Mask

The nonrebreathing mask is the preferred device to use when giving oxygen in the prehospital setting. With a good mask-to-face seal and a flow rate of 15 L/min, it is capable of providing up to 90% inspired oxygen.

The nonrebreathing mask is a combination mask and reservoir bag system. The mask is similar to a simple face mask. Oxygen fills a reservoir bag that is attached to the mask by a one-way valve. The system is called a nonrebreathing mask because the exhaled gas escapes through flapper valve side ports covered by a one-way disk at the cheek areas of the mask (Figure 9-16). The valve also prevents the patient from rebreathing exhaled gases as the gas in the reservoir bag flows into the mask during inhalation. This provides the highest concentration of oxygen. Through use of the reservoir, a nonrebreathing mask delivers high volume and high oxygen enrichment. The patient inhales enriched oxygen from the reservoir bag rather than residual air.

In this system, you must be sure that the reservoir bag is full before the mask is placed on the patient. Adjust the flow rate so that the bag does not fully collapse when the patient inhales. This is about two thirds of the bag volume, or 15 L/min. Use a pediatric mask, which has a smaller reservoir bag, for infants and children because they inhale a smaller volume.

Indications for use of a nonrebreathing mask include any situation in which the patient needs delivery of the highest oxygen concentration and has sufficient tidal volume. Contraindications include apnea and poor respiratory effort. The nonrebreathing mask delivers oxygen passively and requires adequate tidal volume for the oxygen to be effectively drawn into the lungs. Because the device does not deliver oxygen by positive pressure, it would be ineffective for a patient with reduced tidal volume (shallow breathing).

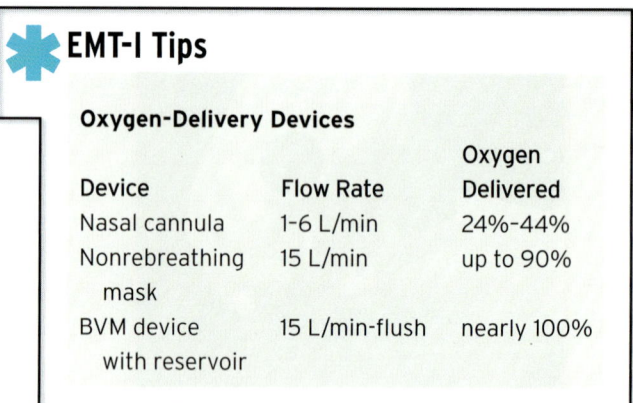

EMT-I Tips

Oxygen-Delivery Devices

Device	Flow Rate	Oxygen Delivered
Nasal cannula	1-6 L/min	24%-44%
Nonrebreathing mask	15 L/min	up to 90%
BVM device with reservoir	15 L/min-flush	nearly 100%

Nasal Cannula

A nasal cannula delivers oxygen through two small, tubelike prongs that fit into the patient's nostrils (Figure 9-17). This device can provide 24% to 44% inspired oxygen when the flowmeter is set at 1 to 6 L/min. For the comfort of your patient, flow rates above 6 L/min are not recommended with the nasal cannula.

A nasal cannula provides low to moderate oxygen enrichment and is used for long-term oxygen maintenance therapy. It is ineffective for patients with poor respiratory effort, severe hypoxia, apnea, or mouth breathing. The primary use of a nasal cannula in the prehospital setting is for a patient who will not tolerate a nonrebreathing mask. In addition, a nasal cannula would be appropriate for patients requiring long-term oxygen therapy for certain diseases (such as COPD) whose present complaint is unrelated to their respiratory disease.

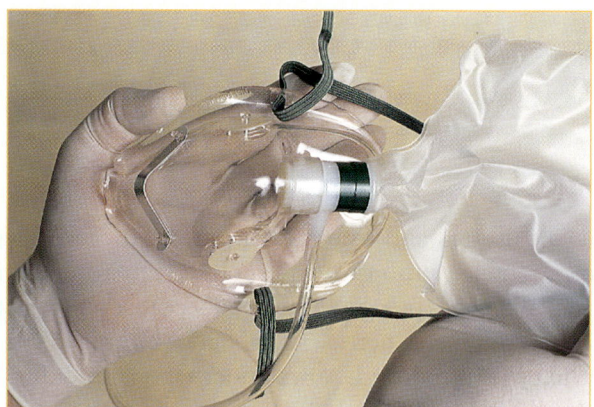

Figure 9-16 The nonrebreathing mask contains flapper valve ports at the cheek areas of the mask to prevent the patient from rebreathing exhaled air.

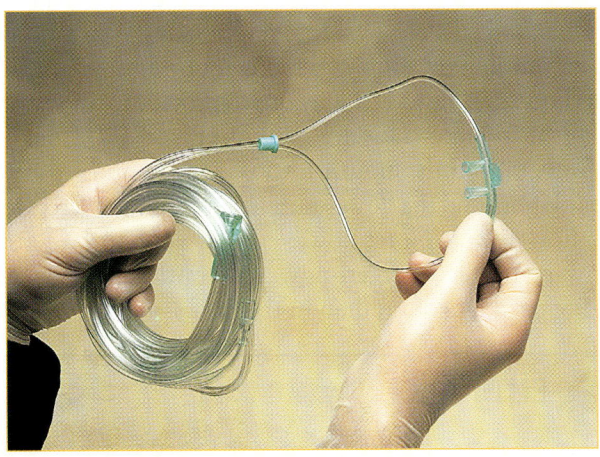

Figure 9-17 The nasal cannula delivers oxygen directly through the nostrils.

The advantage of a nasal cannula is that it is well tolerated. Even patients who are claustrophobic can tolerate the nasal cannula. Unfortunately, it does not deliver high volumes or high concentrations of oxygen.

The nasal cannula delivers dry oxygen directly into the nostrils. Therefore, when you anticipate a long transport time, you should use an oxygen humidifier to avoid drying and irritating the nasal mucosa.

Simple Face Mask

A simple face mask is a full airway enclosure with open side ports. Room air is drawn in through the side ports on inspiration, diluting the concentration of inspired oxygen. A simple mask is appropriate for a patient requiring a moderate to high oxygen concentration. It will deliver 40% to 60% at 10 L/min. A simple face mask delivers higher concentrations of oxygen than a nasal cannula. However, if there is a leak around the face, the oxygen concentration decreases. Increasing the flow rate beyond 10 L/min does not enhance oxygen concentrations because the oxygen is diluted with the air brought in through the open side ports.

Partial Rebreathing Mask

A partial rebreathing mask is a device with vent ports covered by one-way disks. The difference between a partial rebreathing mask and a nonrebreathing mask is the absence of the reservoir bag. Like the nonrebreathing mask, room air is not entrained with inspiration. However, residual expired air is mixed in the mask and rebreathed.

Contraindications are the same as for the nonrebreathing mask—any patient with inadequate tidal volume or apnea. Because inspired gas is not mixed with room air, higher concentrations of oxygen are attainable. Like the simple face mask, increasing delivery of volumes beyond 10 L/min does not enhance the oxygen concentration, and mask leak around the face decreases oxygen concentration.

Venturi Mask

A Venturi system is a mask with interchangeable adapters. The adapters have portholes that entrain room air as oxygen passes through them. The patient receives a highly specific concentration of oxygen. Air is entrained by the Venturi principle. The opening in the adapter is such that a preset amount of air is entrained when the flowmeter is set at a predetermined rate. This gives a more exact concentration than any other oxygen mask.

Small Volume Nebulizer

Nebulizers are used primarily to deliver aerosolized medication. Oxygen enters an aerosol chamber that contains 3 to 5 mL of fluid. The pressurized oxygen aerosolizes the fluid for inhalation.

Oxygen Humidifiers

Some EMS systems provide humidified oxygen to patients during transport 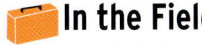, especially those receiving long-term oxygen therapy. A sterile water reservoir is needed for humidifying the oxygen. However, humidified oxygen is usually indicated only for long-term oxygen therapy, prolonged transport time, or conditions such as croup, epiglottitis, and bronchiolitis. Many EMS systems do not use humidified oxygen in the prehospital setting, especially if their transport times to the hospital are short. Always refer to medical control or local protocols for guidance involving patient treatment issues.

In the Field

A nebulizer with saline or sterile water placed in the medication chamber may be used in place of humidified oxygen. Simply attach an oxygen mask to the aerosol chamber and set the flowmeter at 6 L/min.

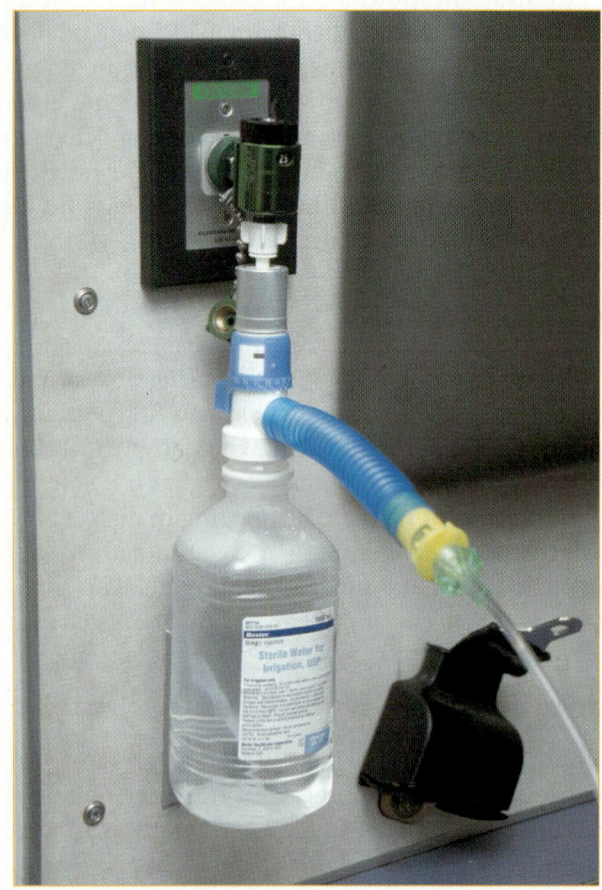

Figure 9-18 Giving humidified oxygen may be preferred with long transport times. However, this type of oxygen-delivery system is not used in all EMS systems.

Assisted and Artificial Ventilation

Obviously, a patient who is not breathing needs artificial ventilation and supplemental oxygen. But the same is true of patients who are breathing inadequately. Signs of inadequate breathing in the adult include a slow (less than 12 breaths/min) or fast (greater than 20 breaths/min) respiratory rate with reduced tidal volume (shallow breathing) or an irregular pattern of inhalation and exhalation. Keep in mind that fast, shallow breathing can be as dangerous as very slow breathing. Fast, shallow breathing moves air primarily in the larger airway passages (dead air space) and does not allow for adequate exchange of air and carbon dioxide in the alveoli. Patients with inadequate breathing require assisted ventilation with 100% oxygen.

Once you determine that a patient is not breathing or is breathing inadequately, you should follow body substance isolation (BSI) precautions and begin artificial ventilation immediately. There are several ways to provide artificial ventilation, some of which require equipment. The methods that an EMT-I may use to provide artificial ventilation include the one- or two-person BVM device; mouth-to-mouth, mouth-to-nose, and mouth-to-mask ventilation; and the flow-restricted, oxygen-powered ventilation device. Note, however, that ventilation with a flow-restricted, oxygen-powered ventilation device is being used less often than in the past.

> **EMT-I Tips**
>
> **Methods of Ventilation**
> (listed in order of preference)
> - Mouth-to-mask
> - Two-person BVM device
> - Flow-restricted, oxygen-powered ventilation device
> - One-person BVM device
>
> *Note: This order of preference has been stated because research has demonstrated that personnel who infrequently ventilate patients have great difficulty maintaining an adequate seal between the mask and the patient's face.*

Mouth-to-Mouth, Mouth-to-Nose, and Mouth-to-Mask Ventilation

As you learned in your CPR course, mouth-to-mouth ventilation is now routinely performed with a barrier device, such as a mask. A barrier device is a protective item that features a plastic barrier placed on a patient's face with a one-way valve to prevent the back flow of secretions, vomitus, and gases. Barrier devices provide adequate BSI. Mouth-to-mouth ventilation without a barrier device should be provided only in extreme circumstances, when no other means of ventilating the patient are available. Performing mouth-to-mask ventilation with a pocket mask with a one-way valve is a safer method of ventilation to prevent possible disease transmission.

Mouth-to-mouth is the most basic form of ventilation. Mouth-to-nose is simply ventilating through the nose rather than the mouth. Indications for this type of ventilation include apnea and when other ventilation devices are not available.

Although mouth-to-mouth or nose ventilation requires no special equipment and can deliver effective

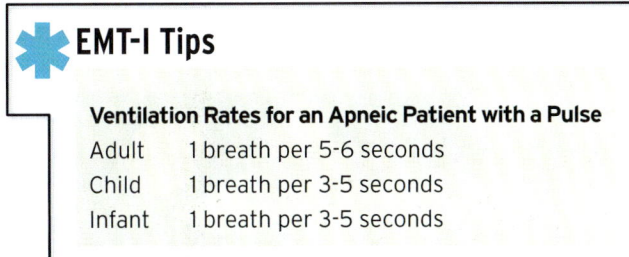

EMT-I Tips

Ventilation Rates for an Apneic Patient with a Pulse
Adult   1 breath per 5-6 seconds
Child   1 breath per 3-5 seconds
Infant 1 breath per 3-5 seconds

In the Field

Applying oxygen to the rescuer with a nasal cannula increases the oxygen concentration in expired air, thereby increasing oxygen to the patient during mouth-to-mouth or mouth-to-nose ventilation.

tidal volume, there are other methods of providing artificial ventilation that are safer for the rescuer. The disadvantages of the mouth-to-mouth or nose technique include psychological barriers from sanitary and communicable disease issues. There is the potential for exposure to blood and other body fluids through direct contact. There is also the risk of unknown communicable diseases at the time of the event.

Hyperinflation of the patient's lungs is a potential complication associated with mouth-to-mouth or mouth-to-nose ventilation, especially if the patient is small and the rescuer is overzealous. Gastric distention may also occur, increasing the risk of vomiting and aspiration. This also increases risk to the rescuer. Hyperventilation of the rescuer is another possible complication. Rapid, deep breathing decreases carbon dioxide levels and, in extreme cases, could cause the rescuer to lose consciousness.

Mouth-to-mask ventilation is preferred over the mouth-to-mouth or nose technique. Advantages of using a mask include placing a physical barrier between the rescuer's mouth and the patient's mouth. Most masks offer a one-way valve to prevent the rescuer's exposure to blood and body fluids. It is also easier to secure an effective seal with a mask because you are able to use both hands. This will enable you to provide adequate tidal volume to the patient.

It is prudent for the EMT-I to have access to a pocket face mask in case a BVM device is not readily available. Complications associated with using a pocket face mask are the same as for mouth-to-mouth ventilation, including hyperinflation of the patient's lungs and hyperventilation of the rescuer.

A mask with an oxygen inlet provides oxygen during mouth-to-mask ventilation to supplement the air from your own lungs. Remember that the gas you exhale contains 16% oxygen, which is adequate to sustain the patient's life. With the mouth-to-mask system, however, the patient gets the additional benefit of significant oxygen enrichment with inspired air.

The mask may be shaped like a triangle or a doughnut, with the apex (top) placed across the bridge of the nose. The base (bottom) of the mask is placed in the groove between the lower lip and the chin. In the center of the mask is a chimney with a 15-mm connector.

Follow these steps to use mouth-to-mask ventilation (Skill Drill 9-17 ▶):

1. **Kneel at the patient's head.** Open the airway by using the head tilt–chin lift maneuver or the jaw-thrust maneuver if indicated. Connect the one-way valve to the face mask. Place the mask on the patient's face. Make sure the top is over the bridge of the nose and the bottom is in the groove between the lower lip and the chin. Grasp the patient's lower jaw with the first three fingers on each hand. Place your thumbs on the dome of the mask. Make an airtight seal by applying firm pressure between the thumbs and the fingers. Maintain an upward and forward pull on the lower jaw with your fingers to keep the airway open (**Step 1**).
2. **Take a deep breath and exhale** through the open port of the one-way valve. Breathe into the mask for 1 second (**Step 2**).
3. **Remove your mouth**, and watch for the patient's chest to fall during passive exhalation (**Step 3**).

You know that you are providing adequate ventilation if you see the patient's chest rise and fall. Feel for resistance of the patient's lungs as they expand. You should also hear and feel air escape as the patient exhales. Make sure that you are providing the correct number of breaths per minute for the patient's age.

To increase the oxygen concentration, administer high-flow oxygen at 15 L/min through the oxygen inlet valve. This, when combined with your exhaled breath, will deliver approximately 55% oxygen to the patient.

One-Person BVM Device

Both mouth-to-mouth and mouth-to-mask ventilation can provide large volumes of inspired air—up to 4 L per breath, more than a patient needs. However, the concentration of oxygen delivered to the patient is only 16%. With mouth-to-mask ventilation connected to

Mouth-to-Mask Ventilation

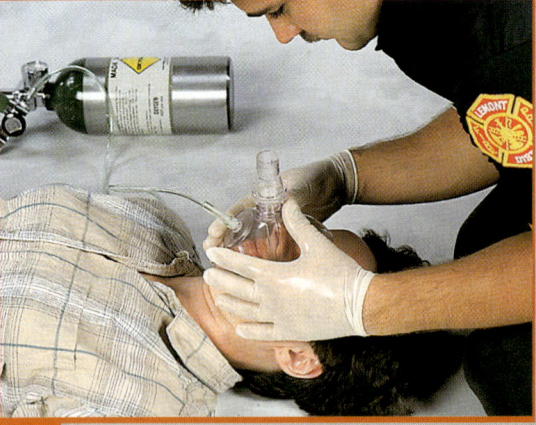

1 Once the patient's head is properly positioned, place the mask on the patient's face. Seal the mask to the face using both hands.

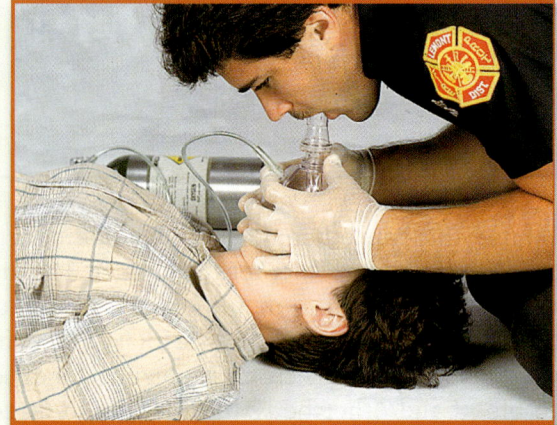

2 Exhale into the open port of the one-way valve for 1 second as you watch for chest rise.

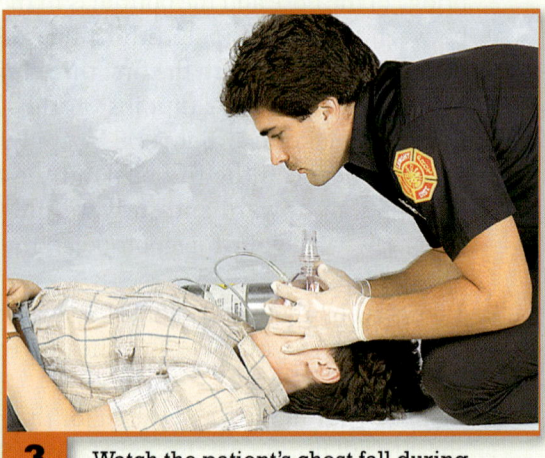

3 Watch the patient's chest fall during exhalation.

---

high-flow oxygen, the concentration of oxygen, at best, is only 55%. The BVM also protects the rescuer from blood and body fluids and allows the rescuer to ventilate for extended periods without fatigue.

With an oxygen flow rate of 15 L/min, a <u>bag-valve-mask (BVM) device</u> with an oxygen reservoir can deliver nearly 100% oxygen (Figure 9-19 ▶). Most BVM devices on the market include modifications or accessories (reservoirs) that permit the delivery of oxygen concentrations approaching 100%. However, the device can deliver only as much volume as you can squeeze out of the bag by hand. The BVM device provides less tidal volume than mouth-to-mask ventilation; however, it delivers a much higher oxygen concentration.

The BVM device is the most common method used to ventilate patients in the field. An experienced EMT-I will be able to supply adequate tidal volumes with a BVM device. Use of the device, however, is a difficult skill to master. Mask seal may be difficult to obtain and maintain with only one rescuer. The amount of tidal volume and concentration of oxygen delivered to the patient are dependent on mask seal integrity. Be sure to practice on ventilation manikins several times before using a BVM device on a patient.

A BVM device should be used when you need to deliver positive-pressure ventilation with high concentrations of oxygen to patients who are not breathing, are breathing inadequately, or are in cardiopulmonary

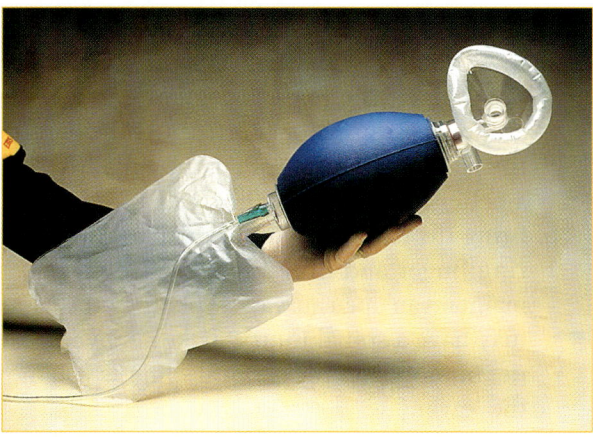

Figure 9-19 A BVM device with an oxygen reservoir can deliver nearly 100% oxygen if a good seal between the mouth and mask is achieved and if supplemental oxygen is used.

- An outlet valve that is a true valve for nonrebreathing
- An oxygen reservoir that permits delivery of a high oxygen concentration
- A one-way, no-jam inlet valve system that provides an oxygen inlet flow at a maximum of 30 L/min with standard 15/22-mm fittings for face mask and endotracheal (or other advanced airway adjunct) connection
- A transparent face mask
- Ability to perform under extreme environmental conditions, including extreme heat or cold

The total amount of gas in the reservoir bag of an adult BVM device is usually 1,200 to 1,600 mL. The pediatric bag contains 500 to 700 mL, and the infant bag holds 150 to 240 mL.

The volume of air (oxygen) to deliver to the patient is based on one key observation—visible chest rise. When using a BVM device, whether supplemental oxygen is attached to it or not, you should deliver each breath over a period of 1 second—just enough to produce visible chest rise—at the appropriate rate. Breaths that are delivered too forcefully or too fast can result in two negative effects: gastric distention (and the associated risks of vomiting and aspiration) and decreased blood return to the heart, secondary to increased intrathoracic pressure.

As noted earlier, a delivered tidal volume of 500 to 600 mL (6 to 7 mL/kg) per breath will produce visible chest rise in most adults. However, because it is not possible for the EMT-I to accurately measure tidal volumes in milliliters per kilogram for each patient ventilated in the field, the key is to watch for visible rise and fall of the chest—let these observations determine the appropriate amount of volume to deliver.

Inadequate tidal volume and decreased oxygen may be delivered owing to poor technique, an ineffective mask-to-face seal, or the presence of gastric distention. Training and practice are key to the proper use of a BVM.

arrest. The BVM device may be used with or without oxygen. However, it is most effective when used with supplemental oxygen and a reservoir. Depending on the patient's level of consciousness, you should use an oral or nasal airway adjunct in conjunction with the BVM device to maintain patency of the patient's airway. Generally, a BVM device should not be used on any patient who is intolerant of its use; however, if the patient is conscious or semiconscious and breathing inadequately (that is, reduced tidal volume), ventilatory assistance with a BVM device will be required to maintain adequate minute volume. In such cases, you must explain the procedure to the patient, advising that each time he or she takes a breath, you will squeeze the BVM to assist breathing efforts.

Two-Person BVM Ventilation Method

Two-person BVM ventilation is the most efficient method. This is especially useful for patients immobilized for cervical spine protection and patients on whom it is difficult to maintain an adequate mask-to-face seal. Two-person ventilation provides a superior mask seal and superior tidal volume and oxygen delivery.

Extra personnel are required for two-person ventilation, which may not be an option in all situations. Complications are a consideration as well. Hyperinfla-

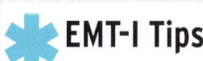

EMT-I Tips

Volume Capabilities of the BVM Device

Size	Amount, mL
Adult	1,200-1,600
Pediatric	500-700
Infant	150-240

Components

All adult BVM devices should have the following components and characteristics:
- A disposable self-refilling bag
- No pop-off valve, or if one is present, the capability of disabling the pop-off valve

tion of the patient's lungs and gastric distention may occur with overzealous ventilation. The first rescuer maintains an effective mask seal while the second rescuer squeezes the bag. Chest movement should be observed and lung compliance monitored with ventilation to avoid overinflation.

Three-Person BVM Ventilation

Three-person BVM ventilation works the same as two-person BVM ventilation. The major difference is that extra personnel are crowded around the airway. The first rescuer maintains the mask seal by the appropriate method, the second rescuer performs the Sellick maneuver, and the third rescuer squeezes the bag and monitors compliance.

Technique

Whenever possible, you and your partner should work together to provide ventilation with the BVM device. One EMT-I can maintain a good mask seal by securing the mask to the patient's face with two hands while the other EMT-I squeezes the bag.

Follow these steps to use the two-person BVM device technique:

1. Kneel above the patient's head. If possible, your partner should be at the side of the head to squeeze the bag while you hold a seal between the mask and the patient's face with two hands. (This assumes that you have enough personnel to do everything else that needs to be done at the same time, such as chest compressions, putting the stretcher in place, or helping to lift the patient onto the stretcher.)
2. Maintain the patient's neck in an extended position unless you suspect a cervical spine injury. In that case, you should immobilize the patient's head and neck and use the jaw-thrust maneuver. Have your partner hold the head, or, if you are alone, use your knees to immobilize the head.
3. Open the patient's mouth, and suction as needed. Insert an oropharyngeal or nasopharyngeal airway to maintain an open airway.
4. Select the proper mask size. It should seat from the bridge of the nose to the chin.
5. Place the mask on the patient's face. Make sure the top is over the bridge of the nose and the bottom is in the groove between the lower lip and the chin. If the mask has a large, round cuff around the ventilation port, center the port over the patient's mouth. Inflate the collar to obtain a better fit and seal to the face.
6. Bring the lower jaw up to the mask with your ring finger and little finger. This will help to maintain an open airway. If you think the patient may have a spinal injury, make sure your partner immobilizes the cervical spine as you move the lower jaw.
7. Hold the mask in position by placing the thumbs over the top part of the mask and the index and middle fingers over the bottom half. Make sure you do not grab the fleshy part of the neck because you may compress structures and create an airway obstruction.
8. Connect the bag to the mask if you have not already done so.
9. Hold the mask in place while your partner squeezes the bag with two hands over 1 second until the patient's chest visibly rises (Figure 9-20). Continue squeezing the bag once every 5 to 6 seconds for adults and once every 3 to 5 seconds for infants and children.
10. If you are alone, hold your index finger over the lower part of the mask, and secure the upper part of the mask with your thumb. This is known as the C-clamp technique and will maintain the seal (Figure 9-21). Use the head tilt–chin lift maneuver to make sure the neck is extended. Squeeze the bag with your other hand in a rhythmic manner once every 5 to 6 seconds for adults and once every 3 to 5 seconds for infants and children.
11. Observe for gastric distention, changes in compliance of the bag with ventilations, and improvement or deterioration of the patient's condition.

When using the BVM device to assist ventilation, you should squeeze the bag as the patient breathes in, ideally achieving a normal rate and depth of respiration.

As you are assisting ventilation with a BVM device, you should evaluate the effectiveness of your ventilation. Artificial ventilation is not adequate if the patient's chest does not rise and fall with each ventilation, the

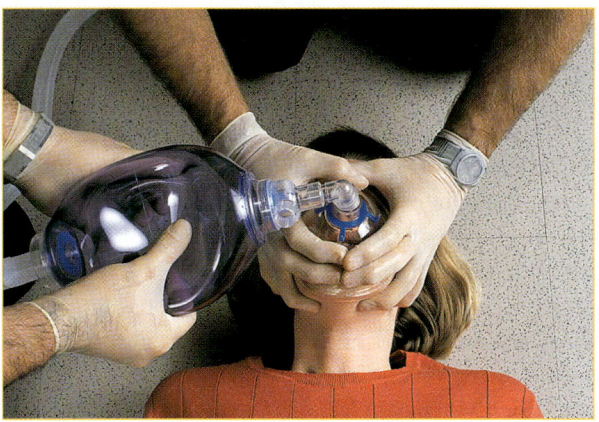

Figure 9-20 With two-person BVM device ventilation, you should hold the mask in place while your partner squeezes the bag with two hands until the patient's chest rises.

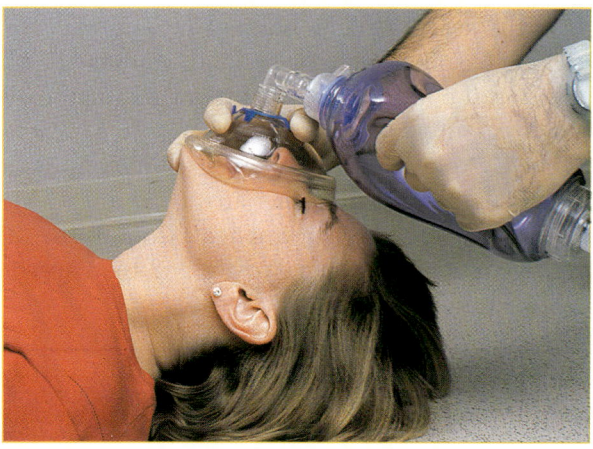

Figure 9-21 Maintain the seal of the mask to the face using the C-clamp technique if you must ventilate alone.

Pediatric Needs

Artificial Ventilation of the Pediatric Patient

The flat nasal bridge of the pediatric patient makes achieving an effective mask-to-face seal more difficult. Compressing the mask against the face to improve mask seal may result in obstruction. The best mask seal is achieved by the two-person ventilation method with jaw displacement.

A pediatric BVM device with a minimum tidal volume of 450 mL should be used for full-term neonates and infants. In children up to 8 years of age, consider the size of the child when determining bag size. An adult bag with a 1,500 mL-tidal volume may be used, but a pediatric BVM device is preferred. Children older than 8 years require the adult-sized BVM device for adequate ventilation. When deciding on size, assure a proper mask fit. The mask should reach from the bridge of the nose to the cleft of the chin. A length-based resuscitation tape may also be used to determine the proper size of the BVM device.

When ventilating a pediatric patient, ensure that there is a proper mask seal by using the EC-clamp technique. Place the mask over the mouth and nose. Take care to avoid compressing the eyes. With one hand, place the thumb on the mask at the apex (over the nose) and the index finger on the mask at the chin. This forms the "C." With gentle pressure, push down on the mask to establish an adequate seal. Maintain the airway by lifting the bony prominence of the chin with the remaining fingers, forming an "E." Avoid placing pressure on the soft area under the chin. You may use the one- or two- rescuer technique to ventilate the patient according to current standards.

Deliver each ventilation over 1 second—just enough to produce visible chest rise. **DO NOT OVERINFLATE**. Deliver one ventilation every 3 to 5 seconds and allow adequate time for exhalation.

While ventilating, look for adequate chest rise. Listen for lung sounds at the third intercostal space on the midaxillary line. Also assess for improvement in skin color and heart rate.

If needed, apply cricoid pressure to minimize gastric inflation and passive regurgitation. Locate the cricoid ring by palpating the trachea for a prominent horizontal band inferior to the thyroid cartilage and the cricothyroid membrane. Apply gentle downward pressure using one fingertip in infants and the thumb and index finger in children. Avoid excessive pressure because it may produce tracheal compression and obstruction in infants.

rate of ventilation is too slow or too fast for the patient's age, or the heart rate does not return to normal. If the patient's chest does not rise and fall, you may need to reposition the head, insert an airway adjunct, or use cricoid pressure.

The BVM device may also be used in conjunction with an ET tube or with other airway adjunct devices such as the esophageal tracheal Combitube, the Pharyngeotracheal Lumen Airway, and the Laryngeal Mask Airway.

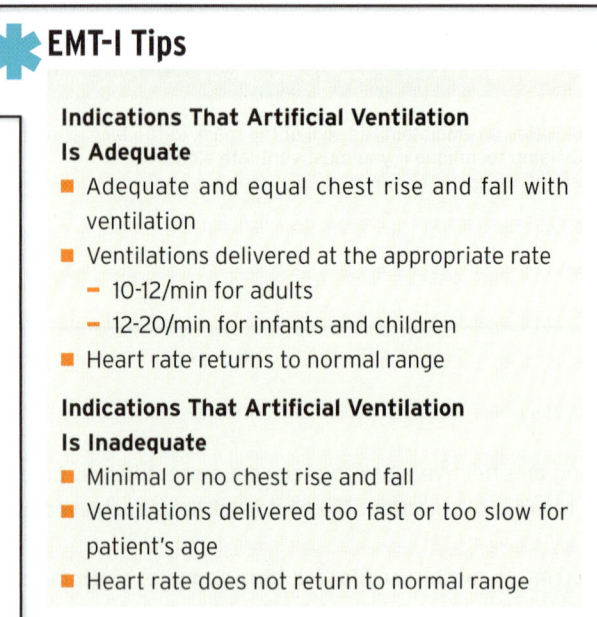

EMT-I Tips

Indications That Artificial Ventilation Is Adequate
- Adequate and equal chest rise and fall with ventilation
- Ventilations delivered at the appropriate rate
  - 10-12/min for adults
  - 12-20/min for infants and children
- Heart rate returns to normal range

Indications That Artificial Ventilation Is Inadequate
- Minimal or no chest rise and fall
- Ventilations delivered too fast or too slow for patient's age
- Heart rate does not return to normal range

Flow-Restricted, Oxygen-Powered Ventilation Devices

Another method of providing artificial ventilation is with the flow-restricted, oxygen-powered ventilation device (FROPVD), also referred to as manually triggered ventilation devices. They are mainly used to ventilate apneic or hypoventilating patients, although these devices can also be used to provide supplemental oxygen to breathing patients. The FROPVD has a "demand valve" that is triggered by the negative pressure generated by inhalation. This valve automatically delivers 100% oxygen as the patient begins to inhale and stops the flow of gas at the end of the inspiratory phase of the respiratory cycle. Because the FROPVD makes an airtight seal with the patient's face, the gas that the patient inspires is almost 100% oxygen.

Generally, patients find it most comfortable if they hold the mask to their face themselves. The FROPVD is an efficient way to conserve oxygen because it delivers only the volume needed by the patient during inspi-

ration, rather than wasting oxygen with a constant flow. These masks, however, are relatively expensive and typically not disposable. The entire unit should be properly disinfected following each use.

These devices are widely available and have been used in EMS for several years. However, recent findings suggest that they should not be used routinely because of the high incidence of gastric distention and possible damage to structures within the chest cavity. Flow-restricted, oxygen-powered devices *should not* be used for infants and children or for patients with suspected cervical spine or chest injury. *Cricoid pressure must be maintained whenever FROPVDs are used to ventilate a patient.* This will help to reduce the amount of gastric distention, the most common and significant complication associated with the use of the device.

The FROPVD delivers gas to the patient at a fixed flow rate of 40 L/min and has a pressure pop-off valve at approximately 30 cm of water. The valve opening pressure at the cardiac sphincter is approximately 30 cm of water. The FROPVD operates at or below 30 cm of water to prevent gastric distention. The device has been shown to reduce (but not eliminate) gastric distention significantly, compared with BVM ventilation. This limited pressure is also a disadvantage, however, for some patients who need greater pressure to overcome increased airway resistance. This can be a major problem in patients with disease processes that decrease lung compliance or in cases of increased airway resistance secondary to airway obstruction. Whenever you use the FROPVD, ensure that the patient is receiving enough volume by making sure that the chest is rising adequately.

Another disadvantage of the FROPVD is the inability to feel ventilatory compliance. Changes in compliance can be an important early indication of an impending problem. It is very important to closely monitor the patient being ventilated mechanically and to be vigilant about noticing changes in the patient's condition.

The plastic housing of the demand valve has a 22-mm adapter designed to fit onto standard ventilation masks. When the button on the top of the regulator is pressed, oxygen flows at a constant rate. Although the FROPVD solves the pressure and flow rate problems of BVM ventilation, one hand is still needed to press the button to ventilate, leaving only one hand to maintain the mask seal and the airway.

Table 9-10 ▶ lists the indications, contraindications, advantages, disadvantages, and complications of FROPVD ventilation for apneic patients. Table 9-11 ▶

TABLE 9-10	Using Flow-Restricted, Oxygen-Powered Ventilation for Apneic Patients

Indications
- Apneic patients
- Hypoventilating patients

Contraindications
- Small children or infants
- Patients with suspected cervical spine or thoracic injury

Advantages
- Delivers high-volume, high-concentration O_2
- O_2 volume delivery restricted to 30 cm of water, reducing gastric distention

Disadvantages
- Cannot monitor lung compliance
- Requires O_2 source

Complications
- Gastric distention
- Barotrauma
- Hypoventilation in patients with poor lung compliance, increased airway resistance, or airway obstruction

TABLE 9-11	Flow-Restricted, Oxygen-Powered Ventilation as Supplemental Oxygen to Breathing Patients

Indication
- Self-administration of 100% oxygen to conscious, breathing patients

Contraindications
- Inadequate tidal volume
- Small children
- Unresponsive patients or patients with an altered mental status

Advantages
- Can be self-administered
- Delivers high-volume, high-concentration O_2
- O_2 delivered in response to inspiratory effort (no O_2 wasting)

Disadvantage
- Requires the patient's cooperation

Complications
- None

lists the indications, contraindications, advantages, disadvantages, and complications of FROPVD ventilation to provide supplemental oxygen to breathing patients.

Components

Flow-restricted, oxygen-powered ventilation devices should have the following components (Figure 9-22 ▶):
- A peak flow rate of 100% oxygen of up to 40 L/min
- An inspiratory pressure safety release valve that opens at approximately 30 cm of water and vents any remaining volume to the atmosphere or stops the flow of oxygen
- An audible alarm that sounds whenever the relief valve pressure is exceeded
- The ability to operate satisfactorily under normal and varying environmental conditions
- A trigger (or lever) positioned so that both of your hands can remain on the mask to provide an airtight seal while supporting and tilting the patient's head and keeping the jaw elevated

Learning how to use these devices correctly requires proper training and considerable practice. As with BVM devices, you must make sure there is an airtight fit between the patient's face and the mask. The amount of pressure that is necessary to ventilate a patient adequately will vary according to the size of the patient, the patient's lung volume, and the condition of the lungs. A patient with COPD will need greater pressure to receive a given volume than would be necessary for a patient with normal lungs. Pressures that are too great can cause a pneumothorax. Always follow local medical protocols carefully when you use these devices.

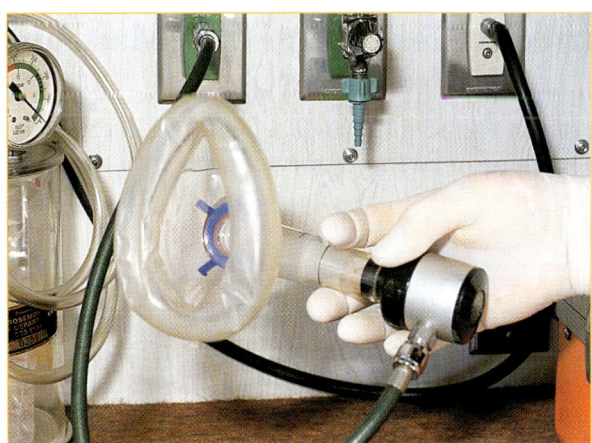

Figure 9-22 A flow-restricted oxygen-powered ventilation device can provide up to 100% oxygen.

Automatic Transport Ventilators

The main advantage of the FROPVD is the constant flow rate that subsequently controls the upper airway pressure. Unfortunately, one hand is still needed to press the button to ventilate the patient. Variations in the rate and duration of ventilation are also possible. The automatic transport ventilator (ATV) solves these problems (Table 9-12).

The ATV is essentially a FROPVD attached to a control box that allows the variables of ventilation to be set. Although the ATV lacks the sophisticated control of a hospital ventilator, it frees your hands to perform other tasks, such as maintaining a mask seal or ensuring continued patency of the airway. You can even perform other, non-airway-related tasks if the patient is intubated and being ventilated with the ATV.

Most models have adjustments for respiratory rate and tidal volume. In most cases, the respiratory rate is set at the midpoint or average for the patient's age. Tidal volume is usually estimated using the formula of 6 to 7 mL/kg because ATVs are oxygen-powered and provide oxygen-enriched breathing gas. The tidal volume can be adjusted based on the patient's chest rise and physiologic response. ATVs are considered volume-cycled–rate-controlled ventilators. This means that they deliver a preset volume at a preset ventilatory rate, although this does not guarantee that all of the volume is being delivered to the lungs.

Like the FROPVD, the ATV has a pressure relief valve, which can lead to hypoventilation in cases of poor lung compliance, increased airway resistance, or airway obstruction. (Table 9-13) lists the indications, contraindications, advantages, disadvantages, and complications of ATVs.

Cricoid Pressure/Sellick Maneuver

When using a BVM device or any other ventilation device in the nonintubated patient, be alert for gastric distention—inflation of the stomach with air. To prevent or alleviate gastric distention, use the Sellick maneuver. Applying cricoid pressure reduces gastric distention and can help prevent passive regurgitation with aspiration during BVM ventilation. To perform the Sellick maneuver, have an additional rescuer apply cricoid pressure on the patient by placing the thumb and index finger on either side of the cricoid cartilage (at the inferior border of the larynx). Apply firm, posterior pressure and maintain the pressure until the airway is secured with an ET tube. Occluding the esophagus will inhibit the flow of air into the stomach, thus reducing gastric distention, and reduce the chance of aspiration by helping block regurgitation of gastric contents up the esophagus. Cricoid pressure should be performed only on unresponsive patients.

If the patient's stomach, rather than the chest, seems to be rising and falling, you should reposition the head and use cricoid pressure. In a patient with a possible spinal injury, you should reposition the jaw rather than the head. If too much air is escaping from under the mask, reposition the mask for a better seal. If the patient's chest still does not rise and fall after you have made these corrections, check for an airway obstruction. If an obstruc-

TABLE 9-13 Automatic Transport Ventilator

Indication
- Extended periods of ventilation

Contraindications
- Poor lung compliance (such as with emphysema or significant pulmonary edema)
- Increased airway resistance (such as with asthma)
- Obstructed airway

Advantages
- Frees personnel to perform other tasks
- Lightweight
- Portable
- Durable
- Mechanically simple
- Adjustable tidal volume
- Adjustable rate
- Adapts to portable O_2 tank

Disadvantages
- Does not detect increasing airway resistance
- Difficult to secure
- Dependent on O_2 tank pressure

Complication
- Unrecognized hypoventilation

TABLE 9-12 Ventilating a Patient With an ATV

1. Attach the ATV to the wall-mounted oxygen source.
2. Set the tidal volume and ventilatory rate on the ATV as appropriate for the patient's condition.
3. Connect the ATV to the 15/22-mm fitting on the ET tube.
4. Auscultate the patient's breath sounds and observe for chest rise to ensure adequate ventilation.

TABLE 9-14	Use of the Sellick Maneuver

Indications
- Vomiting is imminent or occurring
- Patient cannot protect his or her own airway

Contraindication
- Use with caution in cervical spine injuries

Advantages
- Noninvasive
- Protects from aspiration as long as pressure is maintained

Disadvantages
- May have extreme emesis if pressure is removed
- Second rescuer required for BVM ventilation
- May further compromise injured cervical spine

Complications
- Laryngeal trauma with excessive force
- Esophageal rupture from unrelieved high gastric pressures
- Excessive pressure may obstruct the trachea in small children

tion is not present, you should attempt ventilation with another airway device. (Table 9-14) lists the indications, contraindications, advantages, disadvantages, and complications of using the Sellick maneuver.

Advanced airway techniques are beneficial when ventilation with basic means is not effective, the patient has a cervical spine injury, or the patient's condition warrants. Cricoid pressure can facilitate intubation by moving the larynx posteriorly and into direct view. Avoid the application of excessive pressure, which may result in laryngeal trauma and possible obstruction. Always follow local protocols and consult medical direction as needed.

Gastric Distention

Gastric distention occurs when artificial ventilation causes air to become trapped in the stomach. Although it most commonly affects children, it also affects adults. This is very common when ventilating nonintubated patients. As the stomach diameter increases, it pushes against the diaphragm, interfering with lung expansion. The abdomen becomes increasingly distended, and resistance to BVM ventilation is noted.

Gastric distention is most likely to occur when you ventilate the patient too forcefully or too often or when the airway is obstructed as a result of a foreign body or an improper head position. Slight gastric distention is not of concern; however, severe inflation of the stomach is dangerous because it may cause vomiting and increase the risk of aspiration during CPR. Gastric distention is a common complication associated with the use of FROPVDs—a key reason why this device is not highly recommended.

If the patient's stomach becomes distended as a result of rescue breathing, you should recheck and reposition the airway, apply cricoid pressure, and watch for rise and fall of the chest wall as you continue rescue breathing. The risk of gastric distention can be reduced by delivering each rescue breath over a period of 1 second—just enough to produce visible chest rise.

If gastric distention interferes with ventilation and lung expansion, further management may be required. The steps for manual gastric decompression are as follows (Skill Drill 9-18 ▶):

1. **Prepare for large volumes of emesis**; have suction ready (**Step 1**).
2. **Position the patient** on the left side (**Step 2**).
3. **Slowly apply pressure** to the epigastric region (**Step 3**).
4. **If vomiting occurs**, suction and/or wipe out the mouth with your gloved hand, and return the patient back to a supine position so that you can continue ventilation or CPR. Continue to suction as needed (**Step 4**).

Gastric Tubes

Invasive gastric decompression involves inserting a tube, called a gastric tube, into the stomach and then removing the contents with suction. In addition to decompressing the stomach, gastric tubes are also used for tube feeding in patients with decreased swallowing mechanisms, administering medications, and removing poisons from the stomach.

A gastric tube is a very effective tool for removing air and liquid from the stomach, which decreases the pressure on the diaphragm and virtually eliminates the risk of regurgitation and aspiration. The gastric tube can be inserted into the stomach through the mouth (if inserted through the mouth it is referred to as an orogastric [OG] tube) or through the nose (if inserted through the nose it is referred to as a nasogastric [NG] tube).

Skill Drill 9-18

Manual Gastric Decompression

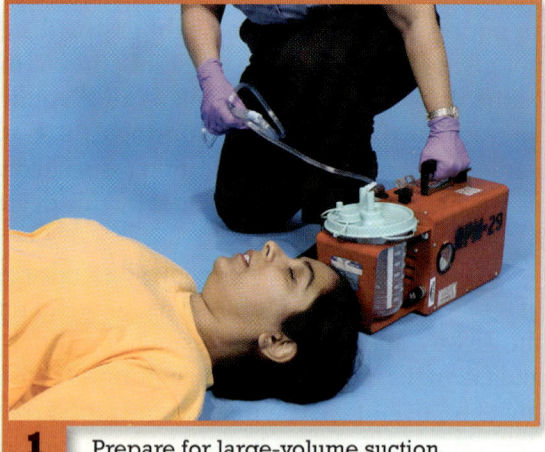
1. Prepare for large-volume suction.

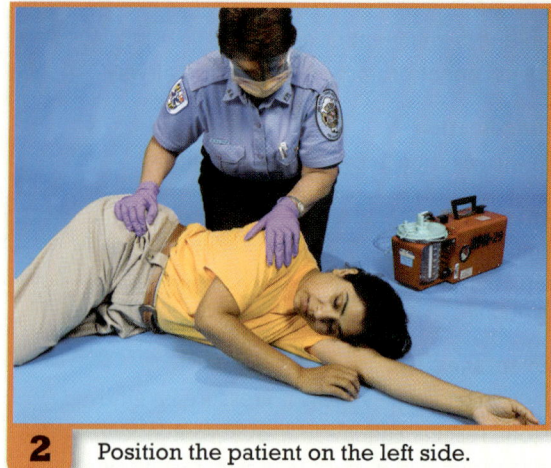
2. Position the patient on the left side.

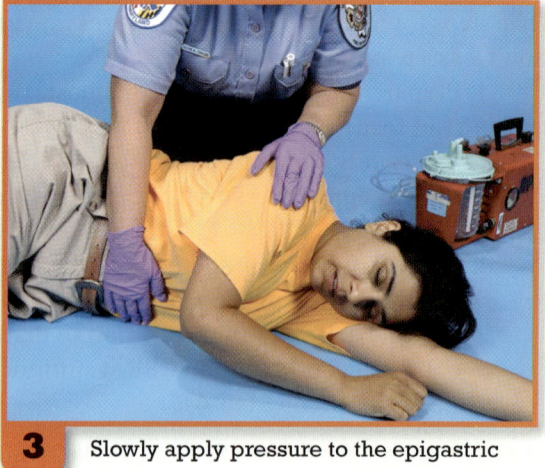
3. Slowly apply pressure to the epigastric region.

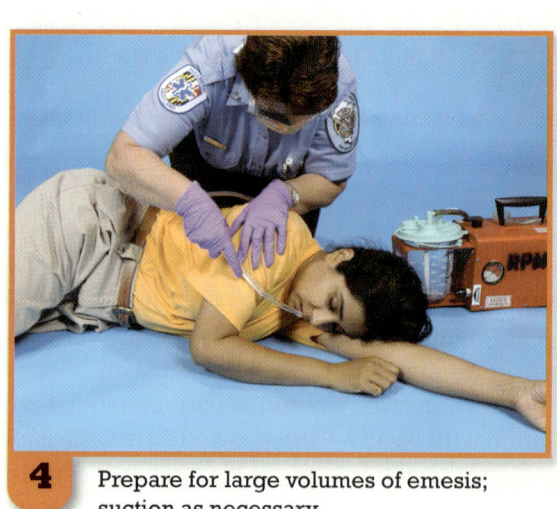
4. Prepare for large volumes of emesis; suction as necessary.

A gastric tube should be considered for any patient who will need ventilation for an extended period. Also, insert an NG or OG tube any time gastric distention is interfering with ventilations. This occurs commonly when children are receiving positive-pressure ventilation or have swallowed large volumes of air while breathing on their own.

Because both NG and OG tubes are inserted through the esophagus, they must be used with caution in any patient with known esophageal disease (such as tumors or varices). They should never be used in a patient whose esophagus is not patent. After insertion, you must be sure that the tube has been placed into the stomach. Occasionally the tube may remain in the esophagus or may have been inadvertently placed into the trachea.

NG Tube

An NG tube is a long tube inserted through the nose, into the nasopharynx, through the esophagus, and into the stomach Figure 9-23 ▶. For the purposes of airway management and ventilation, the tube is used to decompress the stomach, thereby decreasing pressure on the diaphragm and limiting the risk of regurgitation. Although an NG tube causes some discomfort, it is relatively well tolerated, even by patients who are awake. Patients can still talk with an NG tube in place, and, after a few hours, most patients get used to the feeling of having something in their noses and the back of their throats. For these reasons, the NG route of insertion is generally preferred for conscious patients.

The steps of nasogastric tube insertion are listed here and shown in (Skill Drill 9-19 ▶):

1. **Explain the procedure** to the patient, and oxygenate the patient, if necessary and possible. Suppress the gag reflex with a topical anesthetic spray (**Step 1**).
2. **Constrict the blood vessels in the nares** with a topical alpha agonist (**Step 2**).
3. **Measure the tube** for the correct depth of insertion (nose to ear to xiphoid process) (**Step 3**).
4. **Lubricate the tube** (**Step 4**).
5. **Advance the tube** gently along the nasal floor (**Step 5**).
6. **Encourage the patient to swallow or drink** to facilitate passage of the tube (**Step 6**).
7. **Advance the tube** into the stomach (**Step 7**).
8. **Confirm placement**: auscultate while injecting 30 to 50 mL of air and/or note gastric contents through the tube (**Step 8**).
9. **Apply suction** to the tube to aspirate the stomach contents, and secure the tube in place (**Step 9**).

During the insertion of an NG tube, most patients who are awake will gag and may even vomit. In a patient with a decreased level of consciousness, vomiting can seriously threaten the airway. Insertion of an NG tube in patients with severe facial injuries, particularly midface fractures and skull fractures, is contraindicated. Although it has happened rarely, NG tubes have been inadvertently inserted into the cranial vault of patients with severe facial and skull fractures. For patients with these conditions, use the OG route of insertion.

The NG tube in patients who are not intubated interferes with the mask's seal, which is a significant disadvantage. If you are unable to ventilate a patient because of serious gastric distention, however, you must make a difficult choice. You have to balance the benefit of gastric decompression against the risk of a poor mask seal and determine which has a higher priority.

(Table 9-15 ▼) lists the indications, contraindications, advantages, disadvantages, and complications of using a nasogastric tube.

TABLE 9-15	Nasogastric Tube

Indications
- Threat of aspiration
- A need to decrease the pressure of the stomach on the diaphragm

Contraindications
- Extreme caution in esophageal disease or esophageal trauma
- Facial trauma
- Esophageal obstruction

Advantages
- Tolerated by awake patients
- Does not interfere with intubation
- Mitigates recurrent gastric distention
- Patient can still talk

Disadvantages
- Uncomfortable for patient
- May cause patient to vomit during placement, even if gag reflex is suppressed
- Interferes with BVM seal

Complications
- Nasal, esophageal, or gastric trauma from poor technique
- Endotracheal placement
- Supragastric placement
- Tube obstruction

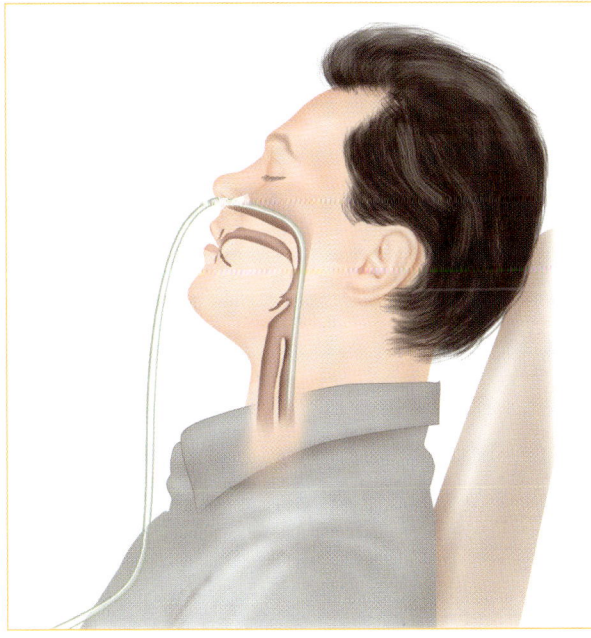

Figure 9-23 Nasogastric tube.

Nasogastric Tube Insertion in a Conscious Patient

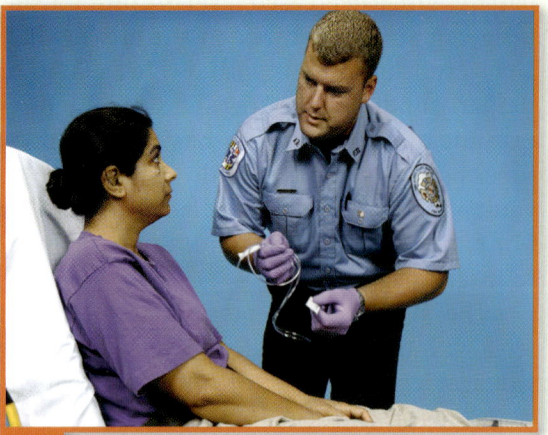
1 Explain the procedure to the patient, and oxygenate the patient if necessary. Suppress the gag reflex with a topical anesthetic spray.

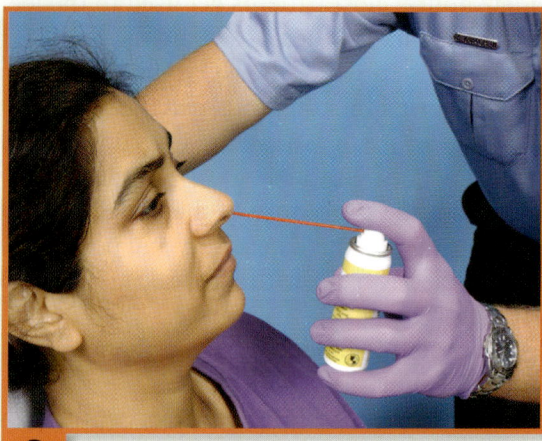
2 Constrict the blood vessels in the nares with a topical alpha agonist.

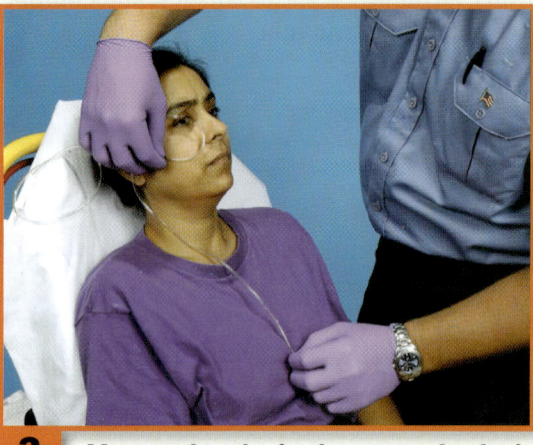
3 Measure the tube for the correct depth of insertion (nose to ear to xiphoid process).

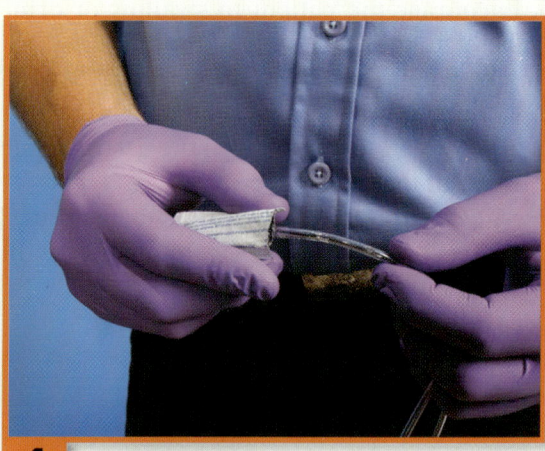
4 Lubricate the tube.

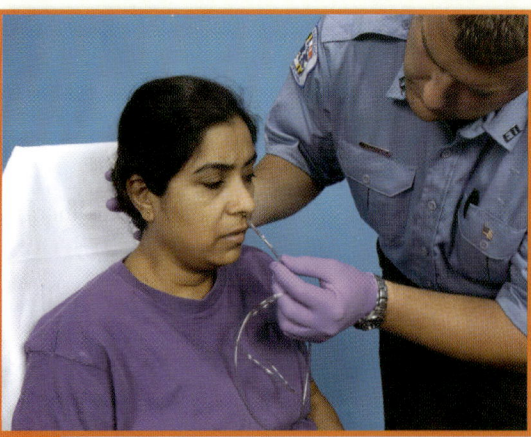
5 Advance the tube gently along the nasal floor.

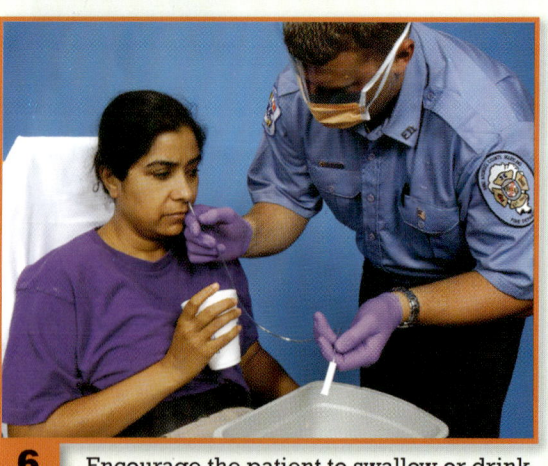
6 Encourage the patient to swallow or drink to facilitate passage of the tube.

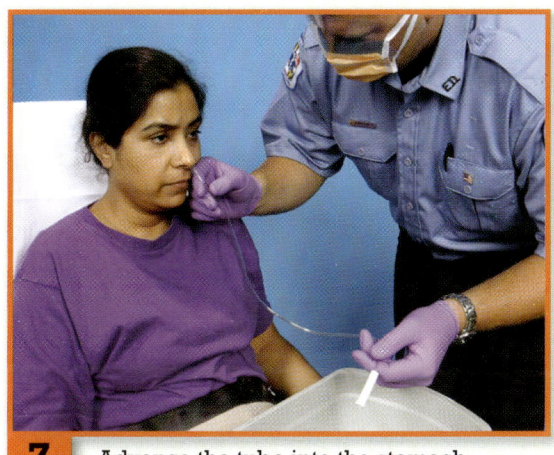

7 Advance the tube into the stomach.

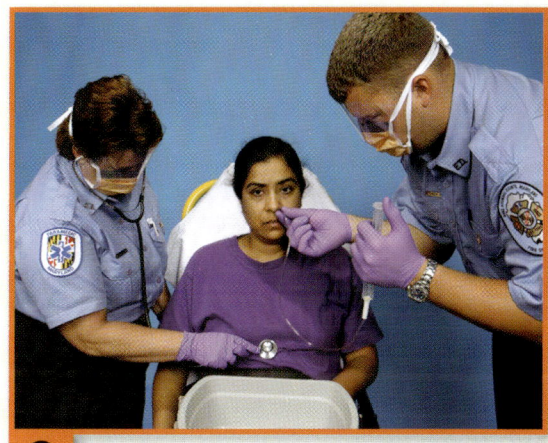

8 Confirm placement: auscultate while injecting 30 to 50 mL of air and/or note gastric contents through the tube.

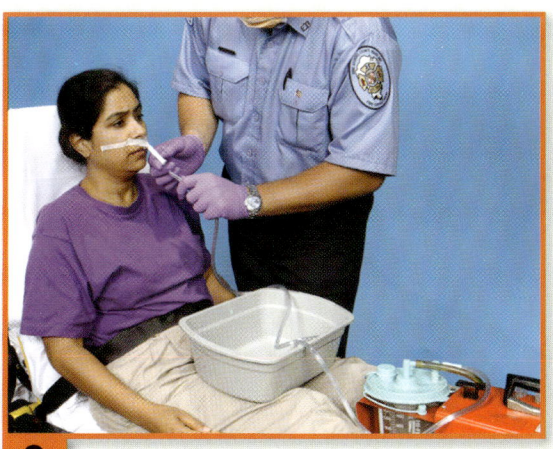

9 Apply suction to the tube to aspirate the stomach contents and secure the tube in place.

OG Tube

An OG tube is the same tube as an NG tube but is inserted through the mouth instead of the nose Figure 9-24 . It works the same way and has most of the same advantages and disadvantages. The major differences include the lower risk of nasal bleeding and increased safety in patients with severe facial trauma. The OG tube, however, is less comfortable for conscious patients, causes gagging much more often, and increases the possibility of vomiting. Considering these advantages and disadvantages, the OG route is generally preferred when a gastric tube is needed in an unconscious patient without a gag reflex. Because these patients obviously need aggressive airway management, the OG tube is almost always inserted after the patient's airway is protected with an ET tube.

The steps of OG tube insertion are listed here and shown in Skill Drill 9-20 :

1. **Position the patient's head** in a neutral or flexed position (**Step 1**).

Skill Drill 9-20: OG Tube Insertion

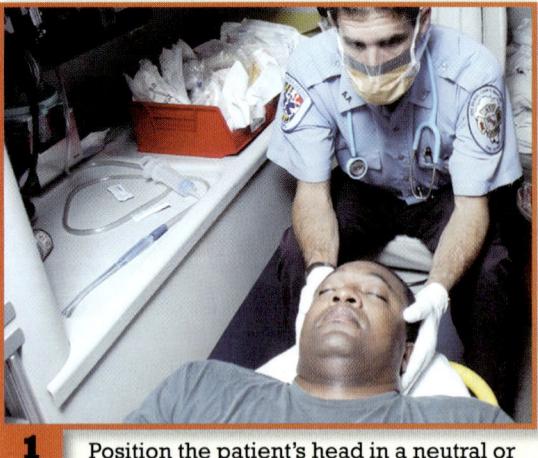
1. Position the patient's head in a neutral or flexed position.

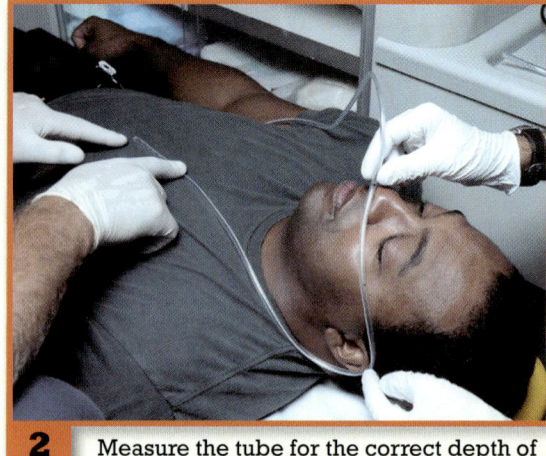
2. Measure the tube for the correct depth of insertion (nose to ear to xiphoid process).

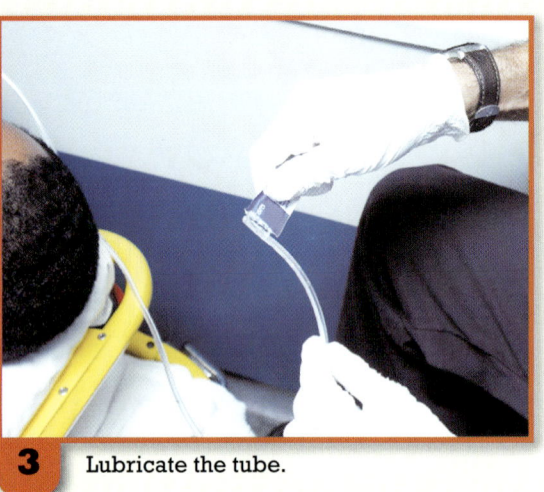
3. Lubricate the tube.

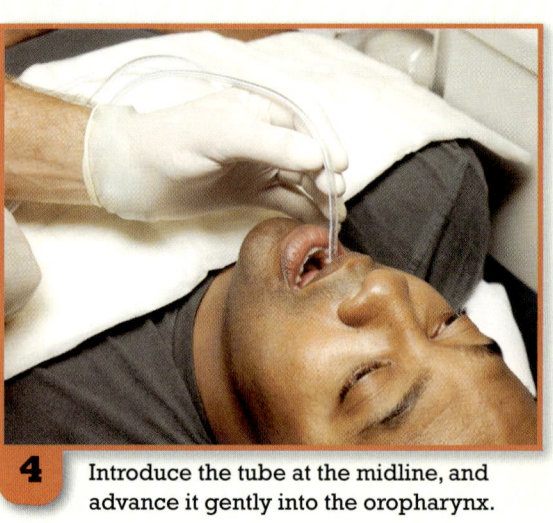
4. Introduce the tube at the midline, and advance it gently into the oropharynx.

2. **Measure the tube** for the correct depth of insertion (nose to ear to xiphoid process) (**Step 2**).
3. **Lubricate the tube** (**Step 3**).
4. **Introduce the tube** at the midline, and advance it gently into the oropharynx (**Step 4**).
5. **Advance the tube** into the stomach (**Step 5**).
6. **Confirm placement**: auscultate while injecting 30 to 50 mL of air and/or note gastric contents through the tube. There should be no reflux around the tube (**Step 6**).
7. **Apply suction** to the tube to aspirate the stomach contents, and secure the tube in place (**Step 7**).

Table 9-16 lists the indications, contraindications, advantages, disadvantages, and complications of using an OG tube.

Dental Appliances

Many dental appliances can cause an airway obstruction. If a dental appliance, such as a crown or bridge, dentures, or even a piece or section of braces, has become loose, you should manually remove it before providing ventilation. Simple manual removal may relieve the obstruction and allow the patient to breathe on his or her own.

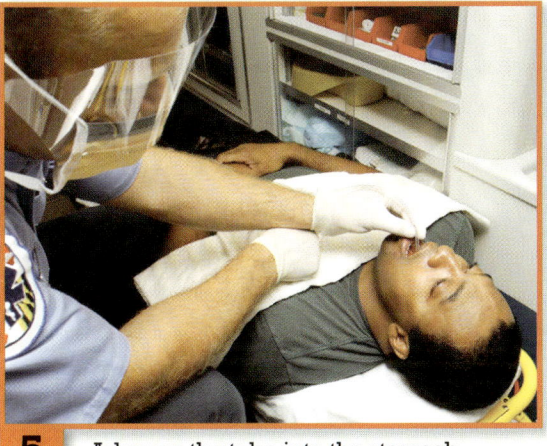
5 Advance the tube into the stomach.

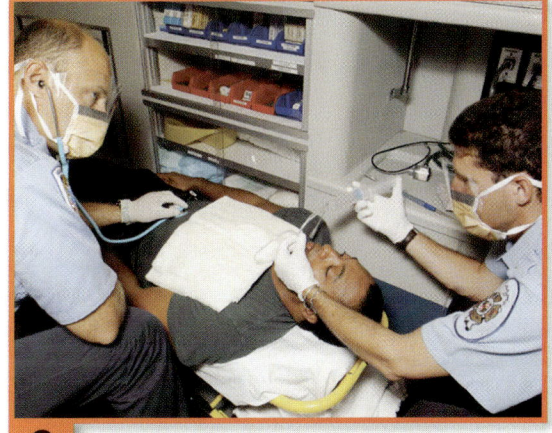
6 Confirm placement: auscultate while injecting 30 to 50 mL of air and/or note gastric contents through the tube. There should be no reflux around the tube.

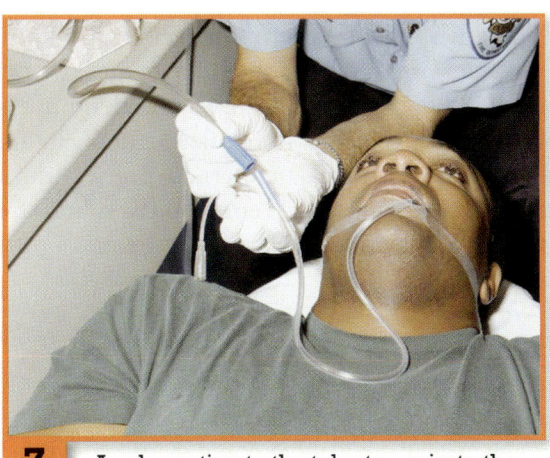
7 Apply suction to the tube to aspirate the stomach contents, and secure the tube in place.

Providing BVM device or mouth-to-mask ventilation is usually much easier when dentures can be left in place. Leaving the dentures in place provides more "structure" to the face and will generally assist you to provide a good face-to-mask seal. However, loose dentures make it much more difficult to perform artificial ventilation by any method and can easily obstruct the airway. Therefore, dentures and dental appliances that do not stay in place should be removed. Dentures and appliances may become loose or be completely out of place following an accident or as you are providing care. Periodically reassess the patient's airway to make sure the devices are firmly in place.

 In the Field

If a dental appliance fits well, leave it in place. If it is loose, remove it. A well-fitting appliance helps to maintain the shape of the mouth, which enhances your ability to maintain an effective mask-to-face seal and provide adequate ventilation.

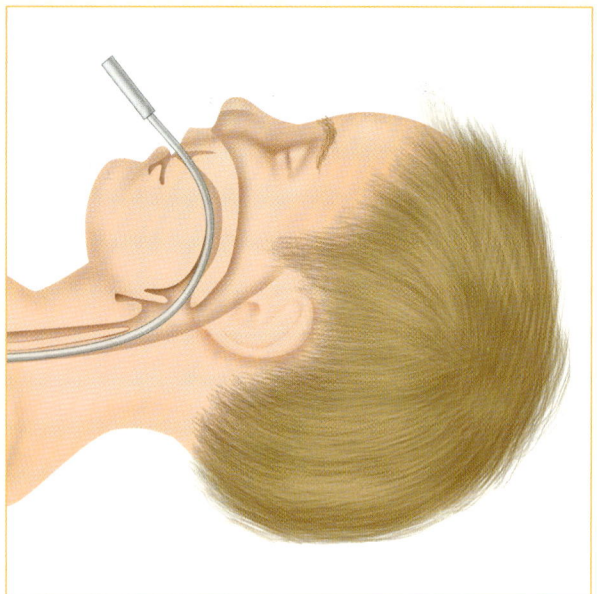

Figure 9-24 Orogastric tube.

TABLE 9-16	OG Tube

Indications
- Threat of aspiration
- A need to decrease the pressure of the stomach on the diaphragm
- Patient is unconscious

Contraindications
- Extreme caution with esophageal disease or esophageal trauma
- Esophageal obstruction

Advantages
- May use larger tubes
- Safer to insert in patients with facial fractures

Disadvantages
- Uncomfortable for conscious patients
- May cause retching and vomiting in patients with an intact gag reflex

Complication
- Patient may bite tube

Facial Bleeding

Airway problems can be especially challenging in patients with serious facial injuries Figure 9-25 ▶. Because the blood supply in the face is so rich, injuries to the face can result in severe tissue swelling and bleeding into the airway. Control bleeding with direct pressure and suction as necessary.

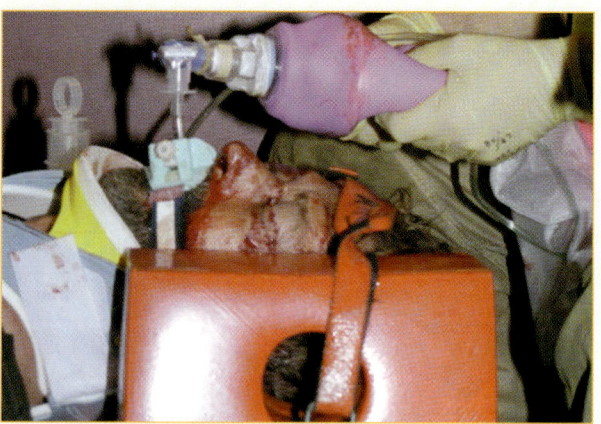

Figure 9-25 Airway problems can be especially challenging in patients with serious facial injuries.

Facial injuries also lend a high suspicion of cervical spine injury. When inserting any type of airway device, it is imperative to maintain in-line stabilization of the cervical spine. Use the trauma technique, the jaw-thrust or tongue–jaw lift, to open the airway for definitive airway placement. An inability to ventilate or orally intubate a patient requires a surgical or alternative airway device. Be alert for changes in ease of ventilation or sounds from the airway that may indicate laryngeal edema.

Multilumen Airways

Through the 1970s and 1980s, many people sought to develop an airway device that could be inserted blindly (obviating the need for laryngoscopy) and that would result in better airway management and ventilation. Two devices that have been developed are the Pharyngeotracheal Lumen Airway (PtL) and the Combitube Figure 9-26 ▶.

Both the PtL and the Combitube have a number of improvements over their predecessors. These devices have a long tube that is blindly inserted into the airway. In contrast with esophageal airways, the tube can be used for esophageal obturation (if it is inserted into the esophagus, as is usually the case) or as an ET tube (if it is inserted into the trachea). The other major improvement is the presence of an oropharyngeal balloon, which eliminates the need for a mask seal.

These two multilumen airways have two lumens, each with a 15/22-mm ventilation adapter. The proper port for ventilation depends on where the tube is located. Both multilumen airways have a proximal cuff, which is inflated in the oropharynx to eliminate the need for a face mask.

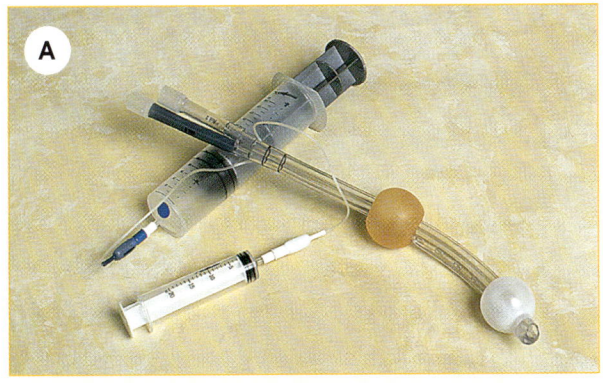

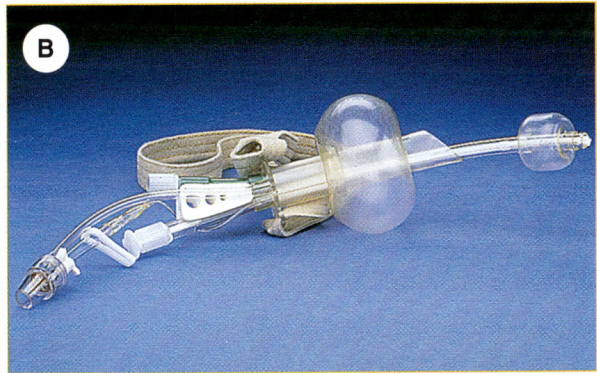

Figure 9-26 **A.** Combitube. **B.** Pharyngotracheal Lumen Airway (PtL).

Advantages and Disadvantages of Multilumen Airways

Multilumen airways have many of the advantages of esophageal airways and have been engineered to decrease some of the disadvantages. The major advantage is that insertion is technically easier than endotracheal intubation and requires less experience and technical skill. In effect, the airway cannot be improperly placed, because effective ventilation is possible if the tube goes into either the trachea or the esophagus. Because the procedure is performed with the patient in the neutral position, cervical spine movement is kept to a minimum. No mask seal is required to ventilate with either device.

Multilumen airways also provide some patency to the airway. If the tube is placed in the trachea, it functions exactly like an ET tube, and no upper airway positioning is required. If the tube is placed into the esophagus (as most commonly occurs), the pharyngeal balloon creates an airtight seal in the oropharynx, making the tongue position less of a factor in the maintenance of a patent airway. A jaw-thrust maneuver should easily alleviate any ventilatory difficulty that occurs if the epiglottis partially obstructs the airway.

Multilumen airways can be used only on deeply unresponsive patients with no gag reflex. If the patient regains consciousness, the device must be removed. You must pay strict attention to the assessment of ventilation because ventilation in the wrong port results in no pulmonary ventilation. Multilumen airways are usually considered temporary airways. Although in some cases they have been used for prolonged ventilation, these devices are generally replaced as soon as possible. Intubating the trachea via direct laryngoscopy with a multilumen airway in place can be challenging.

Indications for Multilumen Airways

Multilumen airways are indicated for the airway management of deeply unresponsive, apneic patients with no gag reflex, in whom endotracheal intubation is not possible, or has failed.

Contraindications for Multilumen Airways

Neither of the multilumen airways can be used in pediatric patients, and they should be used only for patients between 5 and 7 ft tall. (A smaller version of the Combitube, called the Combitube SA [small adult], can be used on adults more than 4 ft tall.) Because most of the time the tube is inserted into the esophagus, neither the PtL nor the Combitube should be used in patients who have a known pathologic condition of the esophagus or who have ingested a caustic substance.

Complications of Multilumen Airways

Multilumen airways address many of the design limitations of esophageal airways. Experience with the devices is still somewhat limited, however. It is reasonable to assume that laryngospasm, vomiting, and possible hypoventilation may occur. Trauma may also result from improper insertion technique.

Ventilation may be difficult if the pharyngeal balloon pushes the epiglottis over the glottic opening. A few cases of difficult ventilation have occurred with multilumen airways. In all cases, ventilation became easier when the device was withdrawn 2 to 4 cm.

Equipment for Multilumen Airways

The PtL consists of two tubes and two cuffs. The longer tube passes through the shorter, wider tube. The longer tube is 31 cm long and 8 mm in diameter and usually

Skill Drill 9-21

Insertion of the PtL

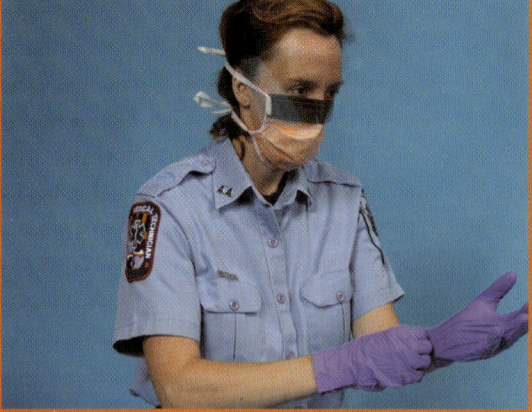

1 Take BSI precautions (gloves and face shield).

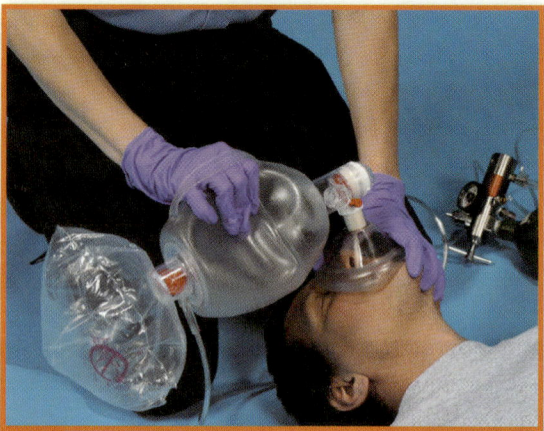

2 Preoxygenate the patient whenever possible with a BVM device and 100% oxygen.

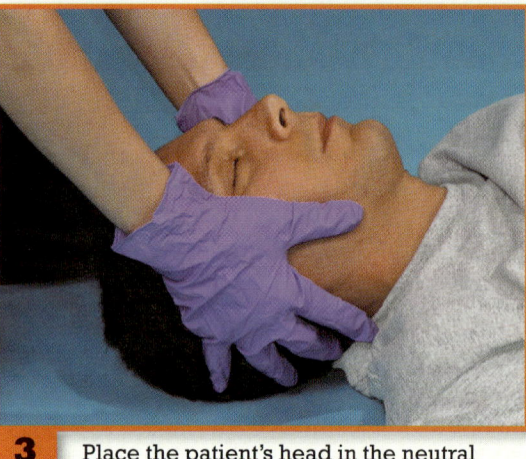

3 Place the patient's head in the neutral position.

4 Open the patient's mouth with a tongue–jaw lift maneuver, and insert the PtL in the midline of the patient's mouth.

---

is inserted into the esophagus. This tube is open at its distal tip and has a balloon at its distal end. A semirigid stylet maintains the curvature and rigidity of the long tube and occludes the tip. The shorter tube is 21 cm long and is designed to come to rest with its tip deep in the oropharynx. A large low-pressure cuff is inflated proximal to the tip of the shorter tube. Both cuffs are inflated simultaneously with an in-series valve system that can be inflated with a bag-valve device. The short tube is made of hard plastic to resist damage from biting, and a strap goes around the head to secure the device **Figure 9-27 ▶**. The steps for insertion of a PtL are listed here and shown in **Skill Drill 9-21 ▲**:

1. **Take BSI precautions** (gloves and face shield) (**Step 1**).
2. **Preoxygenate the patient** whenever possible with a BVM device and 100% oxygen (**Step 2**).
3. **Place the patient's head** in the neutral position (**Step 3**).
4. **Open the patient's mouth** with the tongue–jaw lift maneuver, and insert the PtL in the midline of the patient's mouth (**Step 4**).
5. **Inflate** the proximal and distal cuffs (**Step 5**).
6. **Ventilate the patient** through the pharyngeal (green) tube first. If the chest rises, continue to ventilate through the green tube (**Step 6**).
7. **If the chest does not rise**, remove the stylet from the clear tube and ventilate through the clear tube (**Step 7**).

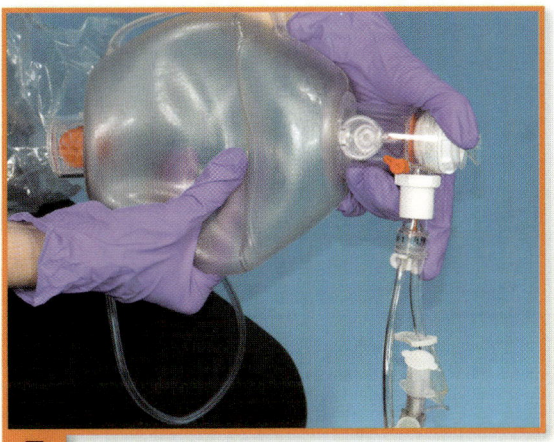

5 Inflate the proximal and distal cuffs.

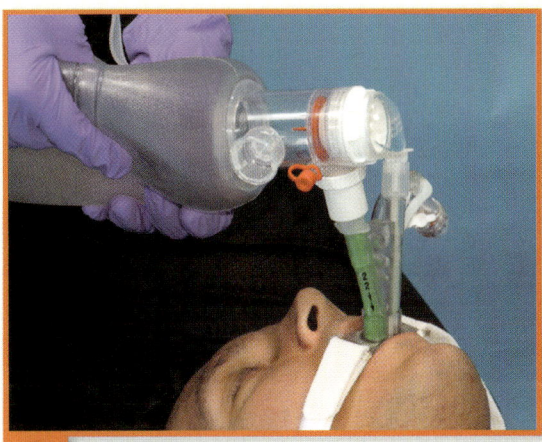

6 Ventilate the patient through the pharyngeal (green) tube first. If the chest rises, continue to ventilate through the green tube.

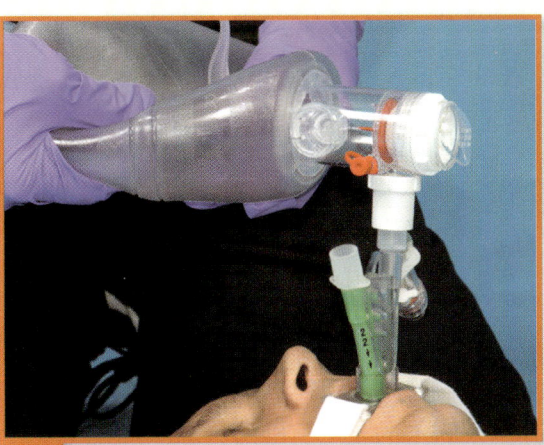

7 If the chest does not rise, remove the stylet from the clear tube and ventilate through the clear tube.

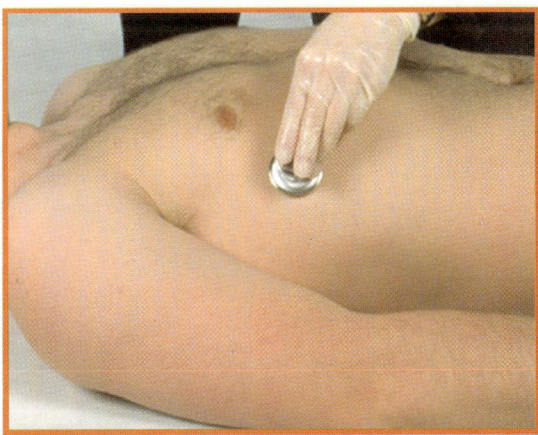

8 Confirm placement by listening for breath sounds over the lungs and for gastric sounds over the abdomen.

8. **Confirm placement by listening for breath sounds** over the lungs and for gastric sounds over the abdomen (**Step 8**).

The Combitube consists of a single tube with two lumens, two balloons, and two ventilation attachments. One of the lumens is open at its distal end, and the other is closed. The closed lumen has side holes distal to the pharyngeal balloon. The proximal balloon is designed to be inflated with 100 to 140 mL of air and provide a pharyngeal seal. The distal balloon is inflated with 15 mL of air and makes an airtight seal with the walls of the trachea (in case of tracheal placement) or leads to esophageal obturation (in case of esophageal placement) (Figure 9-28 ▶). The steps for insertion of

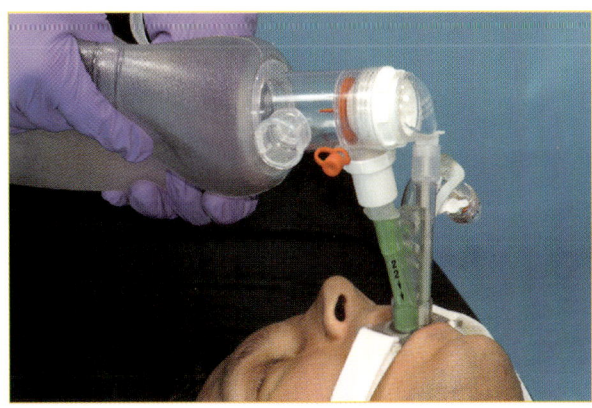

Figure 9-27 Ventilation with a PtL in place.

Insertion of the Combitube

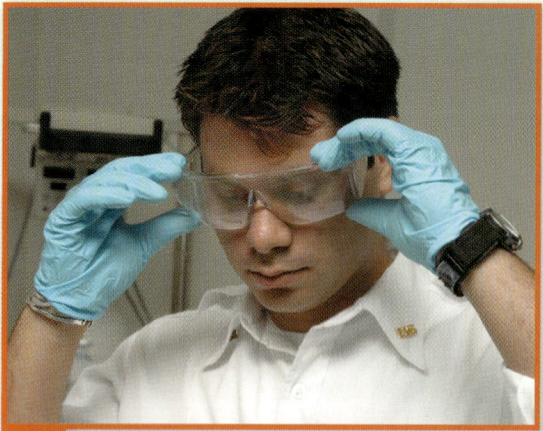

1 Take BSI precautions (gloves and face shield).

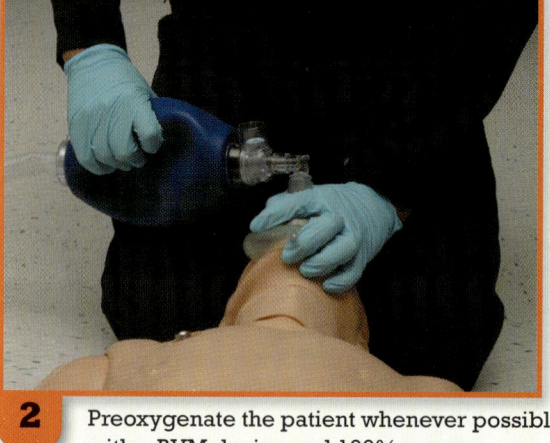

2 Preoxygenate the patient whenever possible with a BVM device and 100% oxygen.

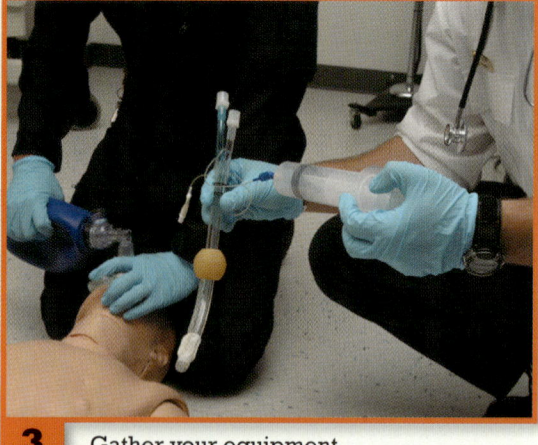

3 Gather your equipment.

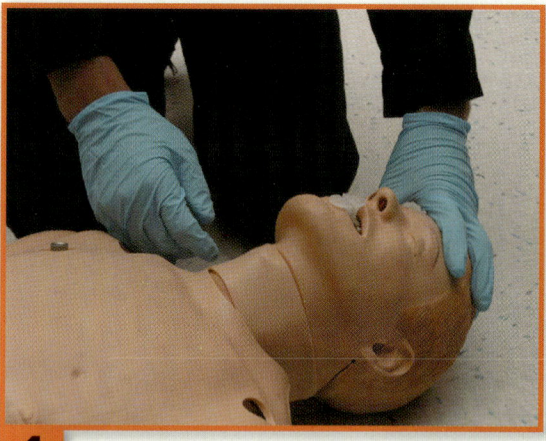

4 Place the patient's head in the neutral position.

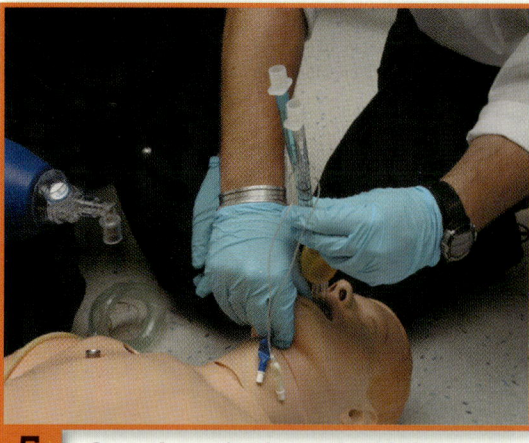

5 Open the patient's mouth with the tongue–jaw lift maneuver, and insert the Combitube in the midline of the patient's mouth. Insert the tube until the incisors or alveolar ridge lie between the two reference marks.

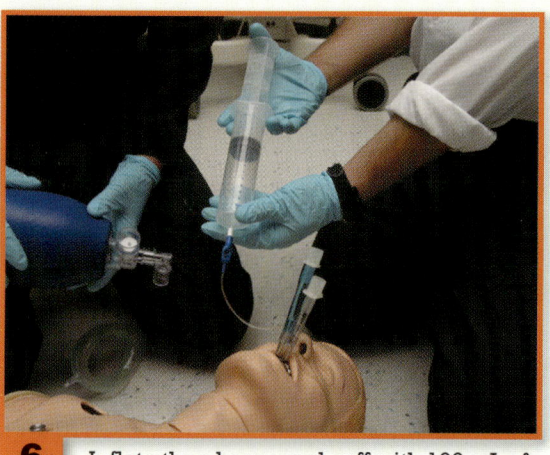

6 Inflate the pharyngeal cuff with 100 mL of air.

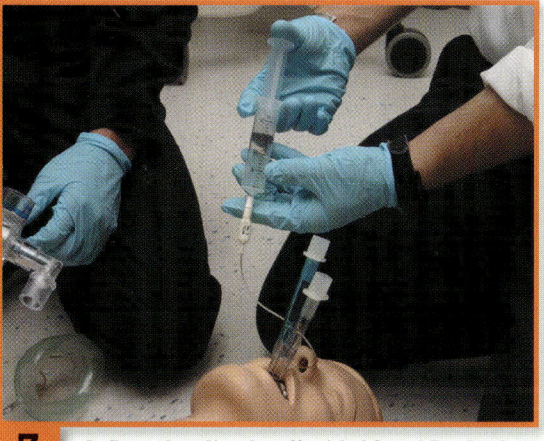

7 Inflate the distal cuff with 10 to 15 mL of air.

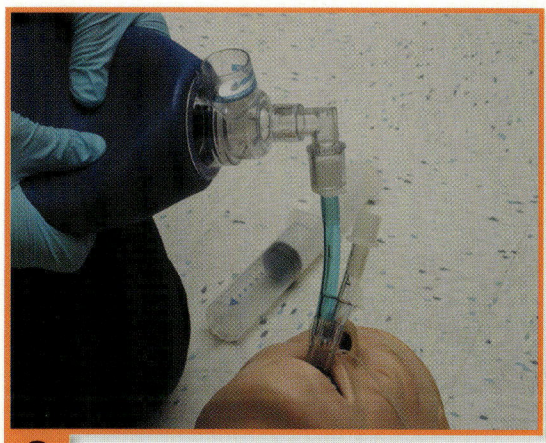

8 Ventilate the patient through the longest tube (pharyngeal) first. Chest rise indicates esophageal placement of distal tip (continue to ventilate).

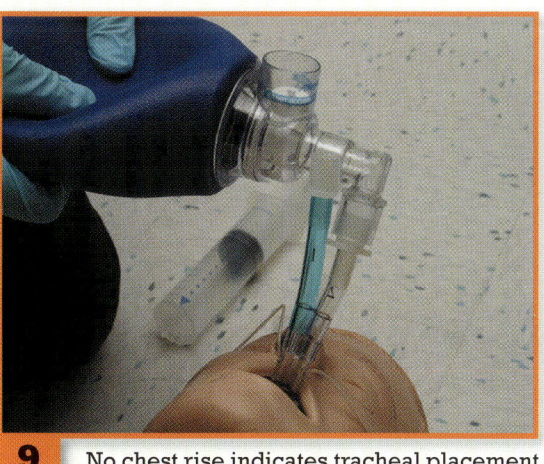

9 No chest rise indicates tracheal placement (switch ports and ventilate).

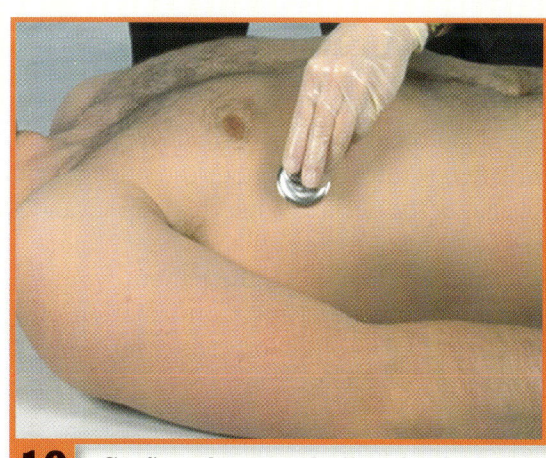

10 Confirm placement by listening for breath sounds over the lungs and for gastric sounds over the abdomen.

a Combitube are listed here and shown in Skill Drill 9-22 ▲):

1. **Take BSI precautions** (gloves and face shield) (**Step 1**).
2. **Preoxygenate the patient** whenever possible with a BVM device and 100% oxygen (**Step 2**).
3. **Gather your equipment** (**Step 3**).
4. **Place the patient's head** in the neutral position (**Step 4**).
5. **Open the patient's mouth** with the tongue–jaw lift maneuver, and insert the Combitube in the midline of the patient's mouth. Insert the tube until the incisors or alveolar ridge lie between the two reference marks (**Step 5**).
6. **Inflate the pharyngeal cuff** with 100 mL of air (**Step 6**).
7. **Inflate the distal cuff** with 10 to 15 mL of air (**Step 7**).
8. **Ventilate** the patient through the longest tube (pharyngeal) first. Chest rise indicates esophageal placement of distal tip (continue to ventilate) (**Step 8**).
9. No chest rise indicates tracheal placement (switch ports and ventilate) (**Step 9**).
10. **Confirm placement by listening for breath sounds** over the lungs and for gastric sounds over the abdomen (**Step 10**).

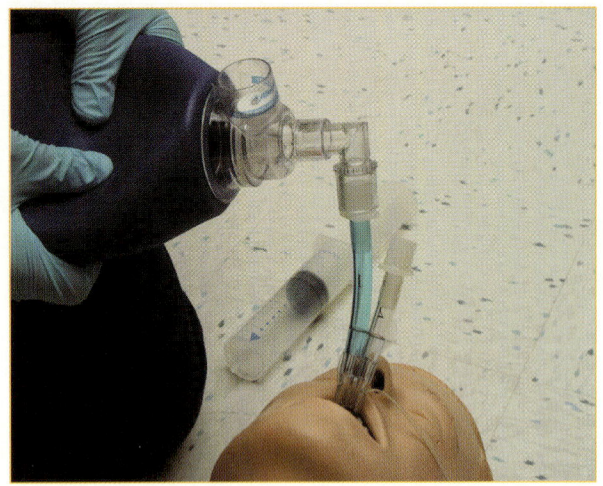

Figure 9-28 Ventilation with a Combitube in place.

Technique for Multilumen Airway Insertion

The advantage of multilumen airways is that you can use them to ventilate regardless of whether the tube goes into the esophagus or the trachea. While this is an advantage, it makes confirmation of ventilation very important. If you used the wrong port, the patient would receive no pulmonary ventilation. Confirmation of ventilation is a critical part of the procedure for using multilumen airways.

Procedures Before Insertion

Check and prepare all equipment. Check both cuffs, and ensure that they hold air. The patient should be pre-oxygenated before insertion. Ventilation should not be interrupted for longer than 30 seconds to accomplish airway placement. This is rarely a problem because the procedure is blind and relatively fast. For both PtL and Combitube insertion, the patient's head should be placed in the neutral position.

- **Forwardly displace the jaw.** With the patient's head in the neutral position, insert the thumb of your gloved nondominant hand into the patient's mouth and lift the jaw. This action lifts the hyoid bone and pulls the base of the tongue off the posterior pharyngeal wall.
- **Insert the device.** Following the curvature of the tube, insert the device blindly into the posterior pharynx. The Combitube is inserted until the incisors are between the two black lines printed on the tube. The PtL is inserted until the flange comes to rest on the teeth. Be gentle, and stop advancing the tube if you meet resistance.
- **Inflate the cuffs.** Both multilumen devices have two cuffs. In the PtL, the cuffs inflate together through an in-line valve system. Attach a bag-valve device to the inflation adapter, and inflate the cuffs until the pilot balloon is firm. Close the clamp to prevent air leakage. The Combitube has two independent inflation valves that must be inflated sequentially. The first inflation valve goes

You are the Provider — Part 8

Your patient suddenly develops respiratory arrest during transport to the emergency department. You continue to ventilate her with a BVM and 100% oxygen at a rate of 15 breaths/min. Your reassessment reveals the following:

Reassessment	Recording Time: 10 Minutes After Patient Contact
Level of consciousness	Unconscious and unresponsive
Respirations	Absent; ventilated with a BVM and 100% O_2 at a rate of 15 breaths/min
Pulse	110 beats/min, irregular
Skin	Remains pale and diaphoretic; still cyanotic in the face
Blood pressure	90/60 mm Hg
Sao_2	89% with assisted ventilation and 100% O_2

11. What is the next step to be considered in managing this patient's airway?

to the pharyngeal balloon and is inflated with 100 mL of air (this is printed on the pilot balloon). The second inflation valve inflates the distal balloon and is filled with 15 mL of air.

Procedures After Insertion

Following inflation of the balloons, begin to ventilate the patient. With the PtL, first ventilate the short tube (the one without the stylet); with the Combitube, ventilate the longer (blue) tube. Confirm the patient's chest rise and the presence of breath sounds. If there are no breath sounds and the chest does not rise and fall with ventilation, switch immediately to the other inflation port. Be sure to continuously monitor ventilation. Both multilumen airways are generally secure in the airway owing to the large pharyngeal balloons. Nevertheless, the head strap of the PtL should be attached because inadvertent removal of a multilumen airway would be extremely traumatic.

Table 9-17 ◀ summarizes the indications, contraindications, advantages, disadvantages, complications, and special considerations of PtL airway insertion.

Table 9-18 ▼ summarizes the indications, contraindications, advantages, disadvantages, complications, and special considerations of Combitube insertion.

TABLE 9-17 | PtL Airway Insertion

Indications
- Alternative airway control when conventional intubation procedures have been unsuccessful or equipment is unavailable

Contraindications
- Children (too small for the tube)
- Patient who is over 7' or under 5'
- Esophageal trauma or disease
- Caustic ingestion
- Known alcoholic (due to esophageal varices)

Advantages
- Can ventilate with tracheal or esophageal placement
- No face mask needed to seal
- No special equipment required
- Does not require the patient's head to be placed in the sniffing position

Disadvantages
- Cannot be used on patients who are awake
- Can be used only on adults
- Pharyngeal balloon mitigates but does not eliminate aspiration risk
- Can be inserted orally only
- Extremely difficult to perform endotracheal intubation with the device in place

Complications
- Pharyngeal or esophageal trauma can occur due to poor technique
- Unrecognized displacement of tracheal tube into the esophagus
- Displacement of the pharyngeal balloon

Special Considerations
- Good assessment skills essential to properly confirm placement
- Misidentification of placement possible
- Multiple confirmations of placement should be done

TABLE 9-18 | Combitube Insertion

Indications
- Alternative airway control when conventional intubation procedures have been unsuccessful or equipment is unavailable

Contraindications
- Children (too small for the tube)
- Patient who is over 7' or under 5'
- Esophageal trauma or disease
- Caustic ingestion
- Known alcoholic (due to esophageal varices)

Advantages
- Rapid insertion
- No face mask needed to seal
- No special equipment required
- Does not require the patient's head to be placed in the sniffing position

Disadvantages
- Impossible to suction the trachea when the tube is in the esophagus
- Cannot be used on patients who are awake
- Can be used only on adults
- Extremely difficult to perform endotracheal intubation with the device in place

Complications
- Pharyngeal or esophageal trauma can result from poor technique
- Unrecognized displacement of tracheal tube into the esophagus
- Displacement of the pharyngeal balloon

Special Considerations
- Good assessment skills essential to properly confirm placement
- Misidentification of placement possible
- Multiple confirmations of placement should be done

Advanced Airway Management

Endotracheal Intubation

For patients unable to maintain their own airway, endotracheal intubation provides not only airway management, but also a medication route for several prehospital drugs. The ET tube can also be used for deep tracheal suctioning when needed.

Endotracheal intubation involves placing a tube through the glottic opening and sealing the tube with a cuff inflated against the wall of the trachea. Endotracheal intubation provides an airtight seal between the patient's lungs and the ventilation device. A sealed cuff placed below the level of the vocal cords is the only form of definitive airway management. All other techniques of airway management are evaluated in comparison with the effectiveness of endotracheal intubation. A solid understanding of the basics of endotracheal intubation is needed when making urgent decisions about when and how to intubate a patient. Table 9-19 lists indications, contraindications, advantages, disadvantages, and complications of endotracheal intubation.

By definition, endotracheal intubation means simply placing a tube into the trachea Figure 9-29. In common usage, however, this term is used in a variety of contexts. For the purposes of this book, the phrase *endotracheal intubation* means the process of placing a tube into the trachea. It is a common error to consider the term endotracheal intubation as synonymous with direct laryngoscopy, the most common method of putting a tube in the trachea. Direct laryngoscopy is only one of many techniques used to place a tube into the trachea. The tube is passed into the trachea to provide externally controlled breathing through a BVM or other ventilation device.

Equipment

Endotracheal tubes Figure 9-30 range in size from 2.5 to 9.0 mm inside diameter, and the length ranges from 12 to 32 cm. Sizes ranging from 5.0 to 9.0 mm are cuffed to make an airtight seal with the tracheal wall. They have a proximal end 15/22-mm adapter that allows for ventilation with a standard device. There is also an inflation port with a pilot balloon at the proximal end. The distal cuff is inflated with a syringe attached to a one-way valve. The pilot balloon indicates whether the cuff is inflated or deflated once the distal end of the tube is inserted into the patient. Centimeter markings along the length of the tube provide a measurement of the depth of the tube. The distal end has a beveled tip to facilitate insertion.

TABLE 9-19 | Endotracheal Intubation

Indications
- Present or impending respiratory failure
- Apnea
- Inability of patient to protect own airway

Contraindications
- None in emergency situations

Advantages
- Provides a secure airway
- Protects against aspiration
- Provides a route for certain medications (as a last resort; absorption of medications is unpredictable at best)

Disadvantages
- Special equipment needed
- Bypasses physiologic function of upper airway
  - Warming
  - Filtering
  - Humidifying

Complications
- Bleeding
- Hypoxia
- Laryngeal swelling
- Laryngospasm
- Vocal cord damage
- Mucosal necrosis
- Barotrauma

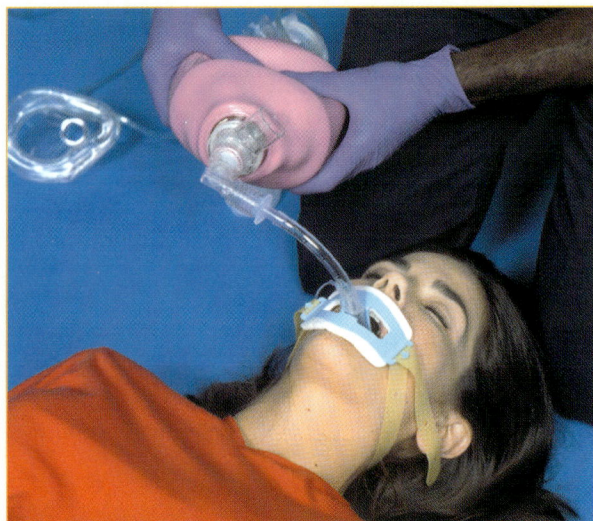

Figure 9-29 Endotracheal intubation.

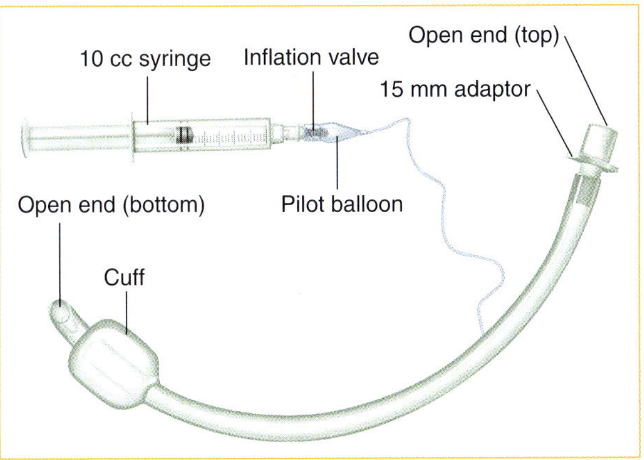

Figure 9-30 Endotracheal tube.

Tubes ranging from 2.5 to 5.0 mm are used in pediatric patients and are generally uncuffed. The narrowest portion of the pediatric airway is the cricoid ring. In children the cricoid ring is funnel-shaped and forms an anatomic seal with the ET tube, eliminating the need for a cuff. The proximal end still has a 15/22-mm adapter for use with standard ventilating devices. The distal end has a beveled tip with distal end depth markings. Because there is no balloon cuff, there is no pilot balloon.

Selecting the proper tube size is important. When the tube selected is too small for the patient, it increases the resistance to flow and, therefore, difficulty in ventilating. When the tube selected is too large, it can be difficult to insert and can cause trauma. The average-sized adult female uses a 7.0- to 8.0-mm tube. An average-sized adult male uses a 7.5- to 8.5-mm tube.

A number of anatomic clues can help determine the proper tube size for adults and children. First, the internal diameter of the nostril is a good approximation of the diameter of the glottic opening. The diameter of the little finger or the size of the thumbnail is also a good approximation of airway size.

There are many types of laryngoscope blades, each with its own advantages and disadvantages, depending on personal preferences. The two most common blades are the straight (Miller) and the curved (Macintosh) blades. Many other blade designs are manufactured for specialty purposes, with the Wisconsin blade having gained much popularity, especially for use in intubating children. Various blade designs have been shown to be effective, although the curved and straight blades are the most commonly used and readily available. In most emergency situations, it is unlikely that you will have immediate access to other blades.

Blade choice is mainly a matter of personal preference and is more related to experience than to functional differences. Nevertheless, the two blades are used differently. The straight blade is narrow and has a curved channel. Its tip is rounded and is designed to lift the epiglottis to provide the laryngoscopic view. The curved blade has a broad flange that is used to move the tongue out of the way. The tip of the curved blade is flat and broader and is designed to fit into the vallecula. Because of the hypoepiglottic ligament, upward pressure in the vallecula moves the epiglottis, providing the laryngoscopic view.

Blade sizes range from 0 to 4. Infants and children use sizes 0, 1, and 2, whereas 3 and 4 are considered adult sizes. In most adults of average size, a size 3 straight or curved blade provides the best visualization. For pediatric patients, blade sizes are often recommended based on patient age or height. Most providers choose the blade for adults based on experience and the size of the patient (3 for average-sized adults and 4 for larger persons).

Two other pieces of equipment have specific uses. The first is the stylet. It is common, especially in emergency situations, to be unable to obtain a full view of the glottic opening. The stylet enables you to guide the tip of the tube over the arytenoid cartilage, even if you cannot see the entire glottic opening. The second is the Magill forceps. Magill forceps have two uses in the emergency setting. First, they are used to remove obstructions from the airway under direct visualization. If you see a solid obstruction in the airway, hold the Magill forceps in your right hand and remove the obstruction. The Magill forceps can also be used to guide the tip of the ET tube through the glottic opening if you are unable to get the proper angle with simple manipulation of the tube.

> ### Pediatric Needs
>
> The formula to calculate the proper tube size for children is to add 16 to the child's age and divide that sum by 4 (for children older than 1 year). For pediatric patients, the patient's length (height) has been shown to be correlated with the airway size. A number of resuscitation tapes not only suggest tube and laryngoscope blade sizes, but also recommend emergency drug dosages. Because the pediatric tube is uncuffed, proper tube size is even more important. It is always useful to have tubes half a size larger and smaller immediately available.

Orotracheal Intubation by Direct Laryngoscopy

It is important to prepare and check the equipment before beginning the intubation attempt (Table 9-20). It is easy to become complacent with this step. With practice, you will find that most intubations are relatively easy and uncomplicated. In most cases, you do not use all of the extra equipment that you assemble for an intubation attempt. Unfortunately, this usual experience may lull you into a false sense of security. When you do encounter a difficult airway, you need to have the necessary extra equipment immediately available. Remember that you are preparing for difficulty, even though you hope that you have none. Even though you may use extra equipment only in a small percentage of cases, you will be glad to have it when you need it.

Body Substance Isolation

Intubation is a procedure that may expose you to body fluids, and, therefore, proper precautions should be taken. In addition to gloves, you should wear a mask and eye shield because your face will be relatively close to the patient's mouth and nose. The mask and eye shield will protect you if the patient vomits. Masks with eye protection included are inexpensive, easy to put on, and unobtrusive. They should be considered mandatory parts of your airway kit.

Preoxygenation

The importance of preoxygenation cannot be overstated. During an intubation attempt, the patient will undergo a period of forced apnea. The goal is to prevent hypoxia from occurring during this period in which the patient is not breathing or being ventilated. In general, patients in stable condition can undergo 2 to 3 minutes of apnea provided they are adequately preoxygenated. In the operating room, patients commonly go a few minutes between ventilations, although these patients are in hemodynamically and cardiovascularly stable condition. Their hemoglobin and hematocrit levels are known, and they are being closely monitored.

Unfortunately, this is not the case in the prehospital setting or even in the emergency department, where

TABLE 9-20 Preparing Equipment for Intubation

Equipment	What to Check, Prepare, and Assemble
Ventilation equipment	Have an assistant ventilate the patient while you are assembling, checking, and preparing your equipment. Check to make sure that the patient is being ventilated with 100% O_2 and that the pulse oximeter is reading 96% to 100%.
Endotracheal tube, stylet, 10-mL syringe (or appropriate size for the type of tube you are using), water-soluble lubricant	Select the proper size endotracheal tube (7.0 to 8.0 for adult female; 7.5 to 8.5 for adult male). Inject 10 mL of air into the cuff, and check that it holds air. Check to make sure that the 15/22-mm adapter is firmly inserted into the tube. Insert the stylet, and be sure that the tip is proximal to Murphy's eye. Bend it to be sure that the stylet does not protrude. Bend the tube/stylet into a hockey stick configuration. Increase the angle of the bend if you anticipate a difficult intubation.
Laryngoscope handle and blades	It is best to have an assortment of blades available because some patients are easier to intubate with one than another. Check the blade that you plan to use. Be sure that it is free from any nicks in the metal (which could easily cause a laceration). Check the bulb to be sure that the light is "bright, white, steady, and tight." The light should be bright enough that it is uncomfortable to look directly at it. It should be white, not yellow or dim. The light should not flicker, especially as the blade is moved on the handle. Most important, the bulb must be tightly screwed into the handle to prevent its loss in the airway.
Magill forceps	Have available to guide the tip of the tube into the trachea or to remove foreign body airway obstructions.
Tape or commercial tube-securing device	Have tape torn or the device ready before you start.
Suction	You will not need it in the majority of cases, but when you need it, you need it fast!
Towels	Needed to position the patient's head.

there is seldom the opportunity to do an extensive preintubation evaluation of the patient. Many patients requiring intubation are physiologically compromised. To prepare them for the apnea during intubation, they must be preoxygenated and the amount of time between breaths significantly limited.

Pulse oximetry has dramatically changed how patients are monitored before and during intubation. Pulse oximetry is performed by placing the probe of the pulse oximeter on the patient's finger. Ideally, the patient should have an oxygen saturation of 100% for 2 minutes before intubation, and it should never fall below 96% during an intubation attempt. Because we do not know the patient's baseline level before the crisis, we cannot rely entirely on the pulse oximeter reading, but nevertheless, it provides us with important trending information.

For patients who are breathing, it is first important to have them breathe 100% oxygen. Even if they have a 100% saturation level, more oxygen can be forced into the blood. Adequate preoxygenation delays desaturation and the resulting hypoxia. If a patient is apneic or hypoventilating, you should preoxygenate him or her for 2 to 3 minutes before intubation.

The consequences of brief periods of hypoxia can be disastrous. Do not rely too heavily on the pulse oximeter reading because it may be falsely high, even if the patient is profoundly hypoxic. Although some of the sequelae of hypoxia are dramatic and immediate, most are subtle and occur gradually. Clearly, some of the poor neurologic outcomes following aggressive airway management result from intubation-induced hypoxia. These incidents can be avoided by adequate preintubation hyperoxygenation.

Position the Patient

Proper positioning of the patient is one of the main keys to successful laryngoscopy. An understanding of the proper positioning for intubation by direct laryngoscopy depends on knowledge of basic airway anatomy. There are three axes of the airway: the mouth, pharynx, and larynx. Ordinarily these axes are at sharp angles, facilitating the entry of food into the esophagus and reducing the likelihood of food entering the airway. Although this is an obvious advantage for everyday life, the angles of these three axes make intubation difficult (Figure 9-31).

To facilitate visualization of the airway, you want to align the three axes to the extent possible. This is achieved by placing the patient in the "sniffing"

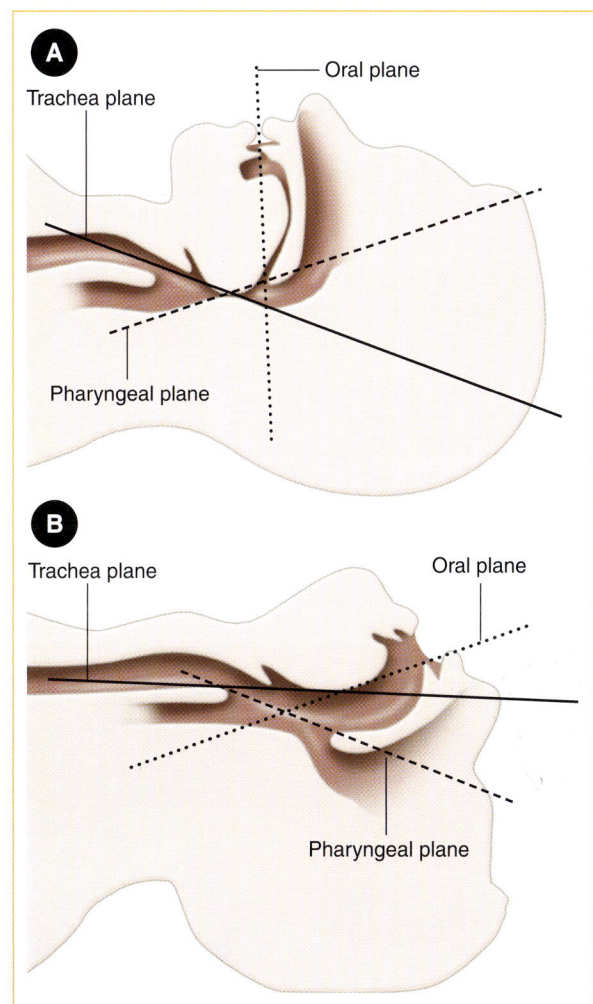

Figure 9-31 Three axes of the airway: oral, tracheal, and pharyngeal. **A.** Neutral position. **B.** Sniffing position.

EMT-I Safety

Intubation is a procedure that may expose you to body fluids, and, therefore, proper precautions should be taken. In addition to gloves, you should wear a mask and eye shield because your face will be relatively close to the patient's mouth and nose. The mask and eye shield help protect you if the patient vomits. Masks with eye protection included are inexpensive, easy to put on, and unobtrusive. They should be considered mandatory parts of your airway kit.

position. The sniffing position is so-named because this is the position of the head when intentionally sniffing. The position involves approximately a 20° extension of the atlanto-occipital joint and 30° flexion of the neck at C6 and C7.

In most supine patients, the sniffing position is achieved by extension of the head and elevation of the occiput 2.5 to 5 cm. The most practical guide to the amount of occipital elevation necessary in a given patient is to elevate the head until the ear is at the level of the sternum. Elevation of the head is best achieved with folded towels positioned under the head and/or neck Figure 9-32 . The advantage of using towels is that the thickness can easily be adjusted by changing the number of folds Figure 9-33 . In obese patients, however, padding under the head alone may not result in the sniffing position. You may need to pad also under the shoulders, neck, and head. When in doubt as to whether the patient is in a true sniffing position, looking at the person from the side usually provides the best view for evaluating the adequacy of the head tilt.

After the patient is in the sniffing position, have the assistant stop ventilating. The intubation attempt should take no more than 30 seconds. The attempt should be stopped at 30 seconds, if the oxygen saturation falls significantly, or if the patient's heart rate or rhythm changes dramatically.

If you abort an intubation attempt, simply reoxygenate the patient for 2 to 3 minutes with 100% oxygen and try again. Repeated attempts do not harm the patient, but prolonged attempts do.

Insert the Blade

The tongue is a sticky, amorphous structure that is a major hindrance to visualizing the airway. The proper use of the laryngoscope blade is critical to controlling the tongue; this is difficult to simulate in practice with manikins. Nevertheless, you need to develop excellent technique in manikins to help avoid difficulties in patients.

Position yourself at the top of the patient's head. If the patient is on a gurney, you can squat to put your head at the level of the patient's face. If the patient is on the floor or ground, you may need to kneel and lean forward or lie down on the floor to get into the proper position Figure 9-34 .

All laryngoscope handles and blades are held in the left hand. Some custom-made or specialty blades can be held in the right hand, but these are rare in tradi-

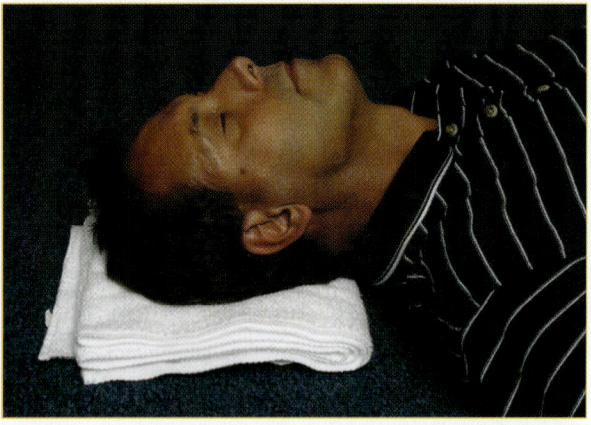

Figure 9-32 Head elevation is best achieved with folded towels positioned under the head and/or neck.

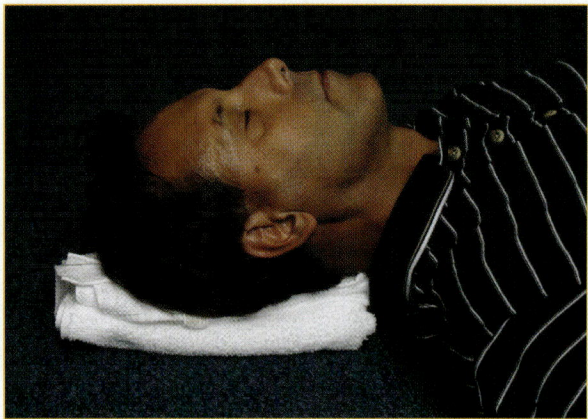

Figure 9-33 The advantage of using towels is that the thickness can easily be adjusted by changing the number of folds.

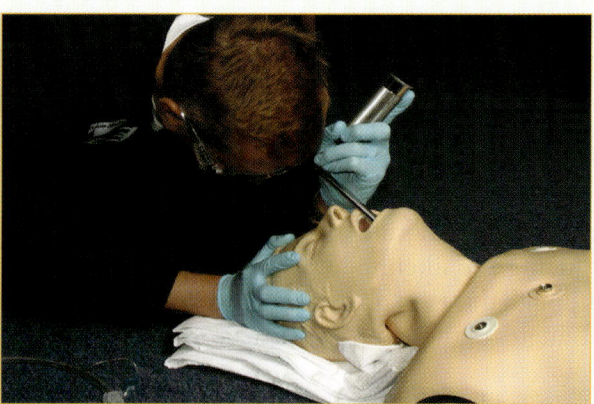

Figure 9-34 If the patient is on the floor or ground, you may need to kneel and lean forward or lie down on the floor to get into the proper position.

tional emergency settings. Hold the laryngoscope in your left hand and the prepared, lubricated tube like a pencil in your right hand.

Be sure the patient's mouth is open. Most patients' mouths naturally fall open when the head is placed in the sniffing position. If the patient's mouth is not open, the easiest technique is to place the side of your right-hand thumb just below the bottom lip and push the mouth open, or "scissor" your thumb and forefinger between the molars Figure 9-35 .

Regardless of the blade being used, it should be inserted into the right side of the patient's mouth. Use the flange of the blade to sweep the tongue to the left side of the mouth while the blade is moved into the midline. Moving the tongue from right to left is a critical step. If you simply insert the blade in the midline, the tongue will hang over both sides of the blade and you will see only the tongue Figure 9-36 .

If you are using a straight blade, insert the tip of the blade all the way to the posterior pharyngeal wall and then lift the jaw. If you are using a curved blade, insert the tip into the vallecula. With both, the goal is to lift the jaw. The most common beginning error is to pull the jaw back using the patient's teeth as a leverage point Figure 9-37 . This can break the teeth and does not provide a view of the glottis. Lifting the patient's jaw is accomplished by keeping your left wrist straight, elbow bent, and back straight Figure 9-38 . The correct motion is similar to holding a wine glass and offering a toast.

Visualize the Glottic Opening

Now is the stressful part. As you look down the blade, you should start to see some familiar airway landmarks. Identifying the epiglottis or the arytenoid cartilage is very important at this point. Identifying these

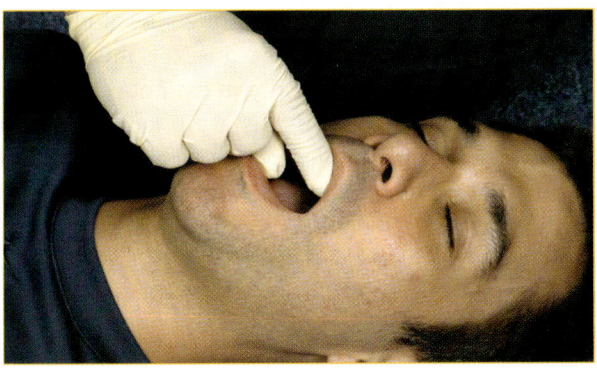

Figure 9-35 Place the side of your right-hand thumb just below the bottom lip and push the mouth open, or scissor your thumb and forefinger between the molars.

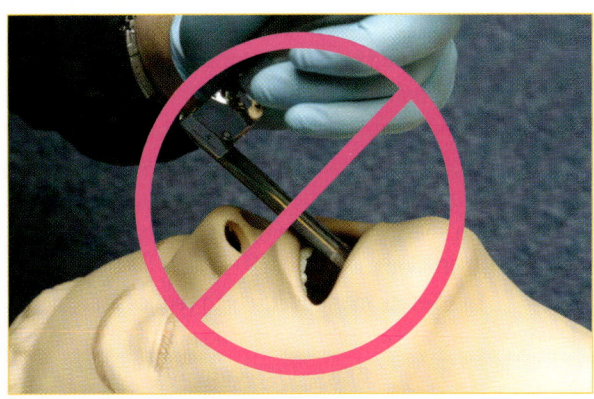

Figure 9-37 The most common beginning error is to pull the jaw back using the patient's teeth as a leverage point.

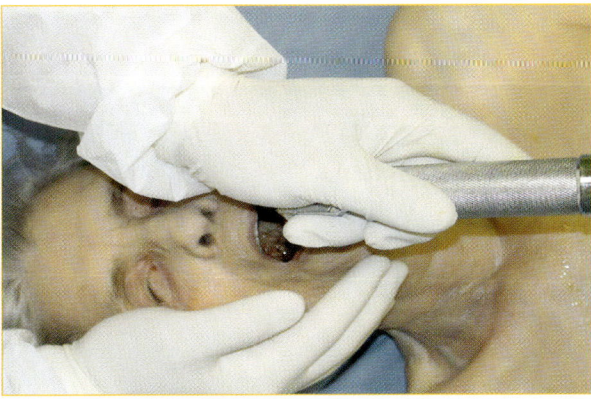

Figure 9-36 If you simply insert the blade in the midline, the tongue will hang over both sides of the blade and you will see only the tongue.

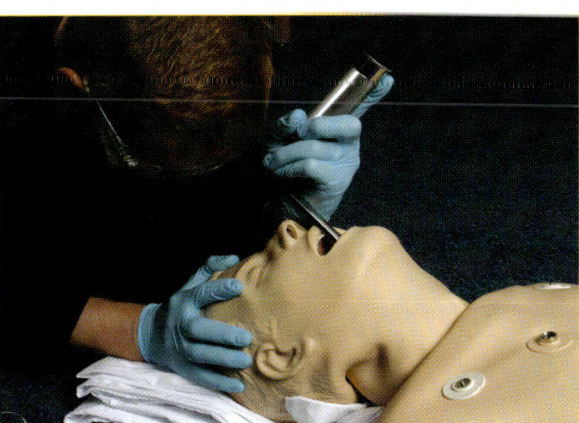

Figure 9-38 Lifting the patient's jaw is accomplished by keeping your left wrist straight, elbow bent, and back straight.

structures enables you to make small adjustments in the position of the blade to aid in visualization of the glottic opening. If you are not able to identify any familiar structures, it is generally fruitless to continue, and it may be better to start over. With the curved blade, it is best to walk the blade down the tongue because you know that the vallecula and the epiglottis lie at the base of the tongue. With the straight blade, insert the blade straight back until the tip touches the posterior pharyngeal wall. This is the proper depth of insertion.

As you continue to work the tip of the blade into the proper position (lifting the epiglottis or in the vallecula), the glottic opening should come into view as you lift. Do not be concerned if you do not have a full view of the glottic opening.

EMT-I Tips

Improving Your Laryngoscope View: The Sellick Maneuver and the BURP Maneuver
When the angle of the pharynx and the larynx is particularly acute, it is often difficult to see the entire glottic opening. You can do two things to increase the percentage of the glottic opening that you can see. You can use the Sellick maneuver or the BURP maneuver.

The Sellick maneuver, which reduces the incidence of gastric distention during positive-pressure ventilation, also moves the airway structures more posteriorly. If applied by an assistant during direct laryngoscopy, it reduces the acuity of the angle between the pharynx and larynx and can improve the laryngoscopic view Figure 9-39.

The BURP maneuver is an acronym for Backward, Upward, Rightward Pressure. If you are having difficulty seeing the glottic opening, take your right hand and locate the lower third of the thyroid cartilage. By applying backward, upward, and rightward pressure, you can often move the larynx into view Figure 9-40. Unfortunately, sometimes when you let go to pass the tube with your right hand, you will lose the view. If possible, once you have visualized the glottic opening, have an assistant hold the larynx in position as you pass the tube. The BURP maneuver can also be applied to the cricoid ring or the hyoid bone.

The gum bougie is an ingenious device that can make intubation possible in some difficult situations, especially when you have limited glottic visualization. The gum bougie is a flexible device that is roughly a centimeter in diameter. It is rigid enough to be able to be easily directed through the glottic opening, but flexible enough so that it does not cause damage to the tracheal walls. There is a slight angle at its distal tip.

The gum bougie is inserted through the glottic opening under direct visualization. Because it is much smaller than an ET tube, it is useful if you cannot obtain a full glottic view. The angle at its distal tip facilitates entry into the airway and enables you to "feel" the ridges of the tracheal wall. Once the gum bougie is placed deeply into the trachea, it becomes a guide for the ET tube. Simply slide the tube over the device and into the trachea. Remove the gum bougie, ventilate, and confirm placement.

Insert the Tube

Once you have visualized the glottic opening, the next step is to insert the tube. When you find the glottic opening, do not take your eye off it. Losing sight of the glottic opening is a major cause of failed intubation.

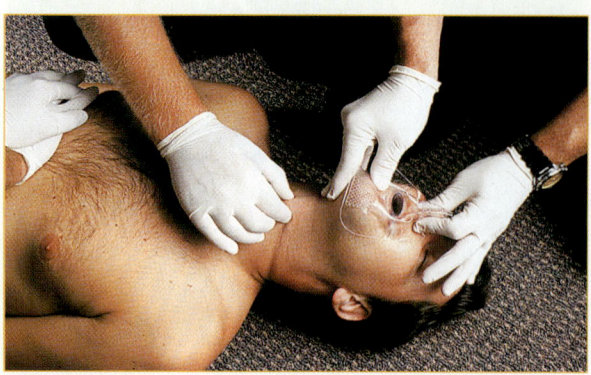

Figure 9-39 The Sellick maneuver.

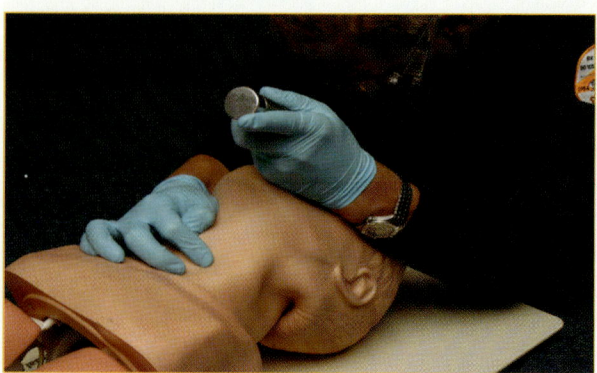

Figure 9-40 BURP maneuver.

Have the tube ready in your right hand so that you can advance it immediately on identification of the vocal cords.

A major mistake of beginners is to try to pass the tube down the barrel of the blade. The laryngoscope blade is not designed as a guide for the tube; it is a tool used only to visualize the glottic opening. Placing the tube down the blade obscures your view of the glottic opening (Figure 9-41 ▼). Pass the tube as far to the right as possible and at an angle that lets you watch the tip as you insert it through the vocal cords. Continue to insert the tube until the proximal end of the cuff is 1 to 2 cm past the cords. If you take your eye off the tip of the tube, even for a second, you significantly increase the likelihood of allowing the tube to slip into the esophagus.

Ventilate

After watching the tube pass between the patient's vocal cords, gently remove the blade, hold the tube with your right hand, and carefully remove the stylet. Fill the tube cuff with just enough air to stop the leaking sound around the tube and then detach the syringe from the inflation port. If the tube is properly sized, it will take 4 to 6 mL of air to achieve an airtight seal. Be careful to avoid cuff pressures in excess of 25 mm Hg because they can cause mucosal tissue necrosis. Have your assistant attach the ventilation device to the tube with an end-tidal carbon dioxide detector (note, if you are using an esophageal detection device, it is important to use it before the first breath is taken). As the first breaths are delivered, watch the patient's chest rise.

You should now listen to breath sounds as another way to confirm the tube location. You should listen to both lungs at both the apices and bases and to the stomach over the epigastrium. If the tube is properly positioned in the trachea, you will hear equal breath sounds bilaterally and a quiet epigastrium. Gurgling over the stomach suggests esophageal placement, and the tube should be immediately removed and the patient ventilated. Unilateral breath sounds generally indicate a mainstem intubation. Place your stethoscope over the quiet side of the chest and slowly withdraw the tube until you hear breath sounds return.

Ventilation should continue as indicated according to the patient's size and clinical condition. It is prudent to slightly hyperventilate the patient for 30 seconds to 1 minute immediately after intubation to eliminate any accumulated carbon dioxide.

A summary of the steps of orotracheal intubation by direct laryngoscopy is listed here, and the steps are shown in (Skill Drill 9-23 ▶):

1. **Use BSI precautions** (gloves and face shield) (**Step 1**).
2. **Preoxygenate the patient** whenever possible with a BVM device and 100% oxygen (**Step 2**).
3. **Check, prepare, and assemble your equipment** (**Step 3**).
4. **Place the patient's head** in the sniffing position (**Step 4**).
5. **Insert the blade** into the right side of the patient's mouth, and displace the tongue to the left (**Step 5**).
6. **Gently lift** the long axis of the laryngoscope handle until you can visualize the glottic opening and the vocal cords (**Step 6**).
7. **Insert the ET tube** through the right corner of the mouth, and place it between the vocal cords (**Step 7**).
8. **Remove the laryngoscope** from the patient's mouth (**Step 8**).
9. **Remove the stylet** from the ET tube (**Step 9**).
10. **Inflate the distal cuff** of the ET tube with 5 to 10 mL of air, and detach the syringe (**Step 10**).
11. **Attach the end-tidal carbon dioxide detector** to the ET tube (**Step 11**).
12. **Attach the bag-valve device**, ventilate, and auscultate over the apices and bases of both lungs and over the epigastrium (**Step 12**).
13. **Secure the ET tube** (**Step 13**).
14. **Place a bite block** in the patient's mouth (**Step 14**).

Confirm Placement

Watching the tube pass between the vocal cords is your first method of confirming tube placement. You must continue the process of gathering information to assess the location of the tube. Remember that a misplaced

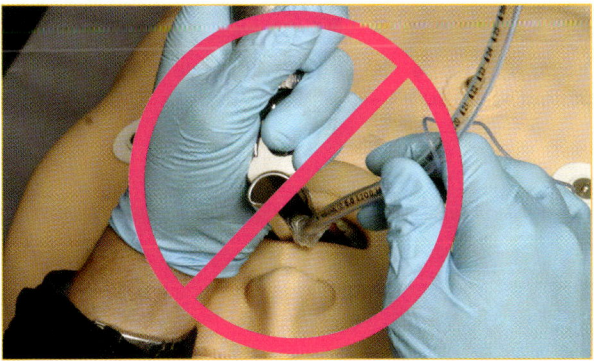

Figure 9-41 Placing the tube down the blade obscures your view of the glottic opening.

Intubation of the Trachea Using Direct Laryngoscopy

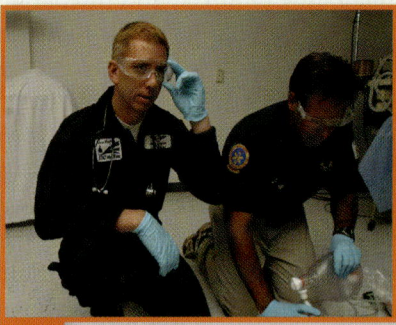

1 Use BSI precautions (gloves and face shield).

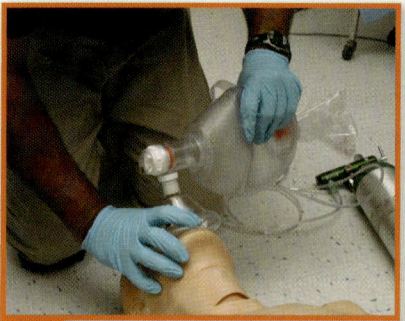

2 Preoxygenate the patient whenever possible with a BVM device and 100% oxygen.

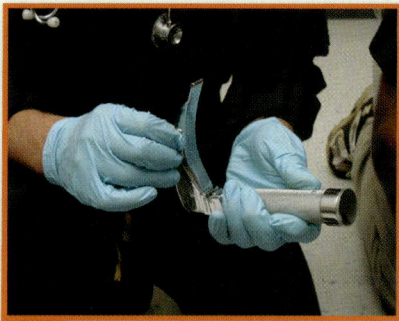

3 Check, prepare, and assemble your equipment.

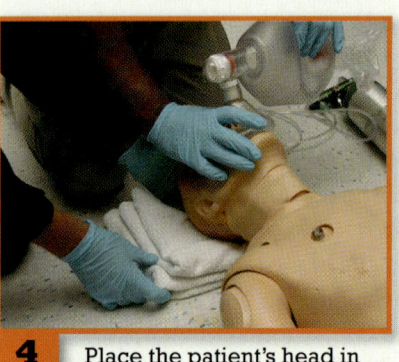

4 Place the patient's head in the sniffing position.

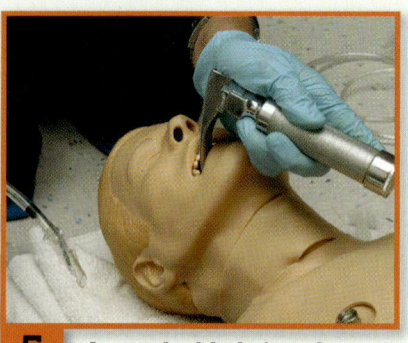

5 Insert the blade into the right side of the patient's mouth, and displace the tongue to the left.

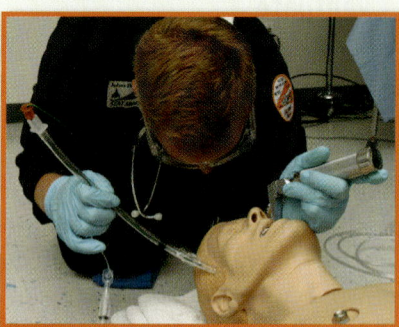

6 Gently lift the long axis of the laryngoscope handle until you can visualize the glottic opening and the vocal cords.

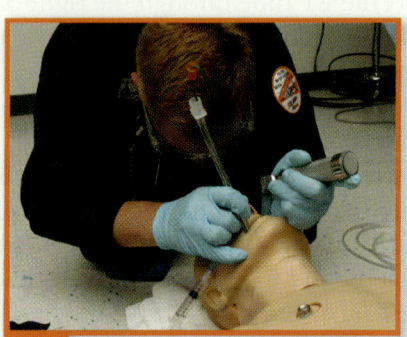

7 Insert the ET tube through the right corner of the mouth, and place it between the vocal cords.

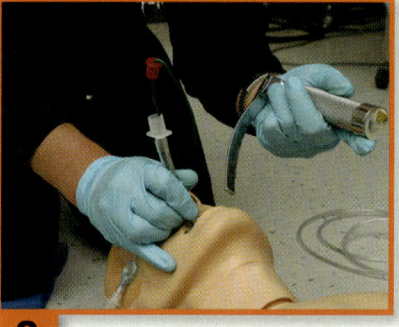

8 Remove the laryngoscope from the patient's mouth.

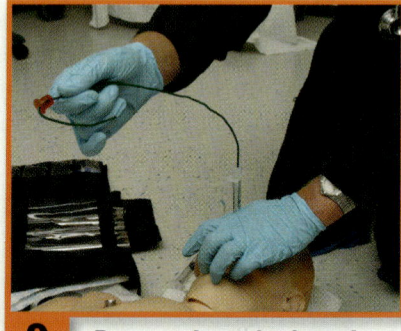

9 Remove the stylet from the ET tube.

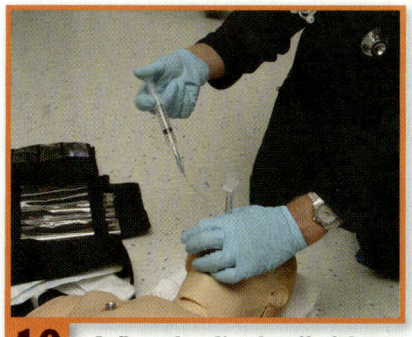

10 Inflate the distal cuff of the ET tube with 5 to 10 mL of air, and detach the syringe.

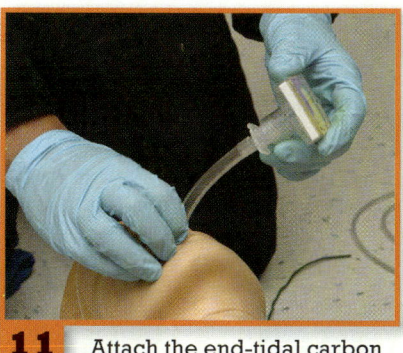

11 Attach the end-tidal carbon dioxide detector to the ET tube.

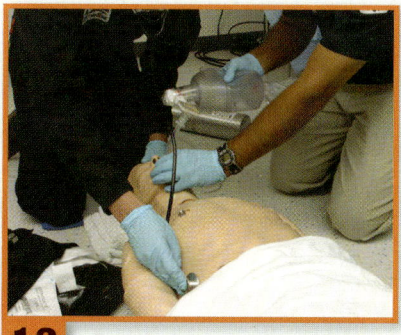

12 Attach the bag-valve device, ventilate, and auscultate over the apices and bases of both lungs and over the epigastrium.

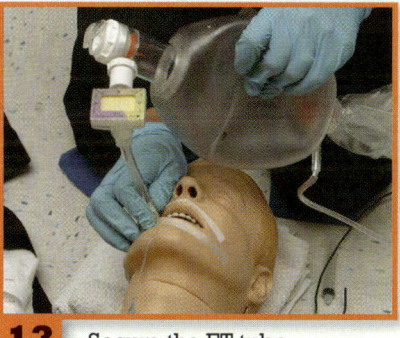

13 Secure the ET tube.

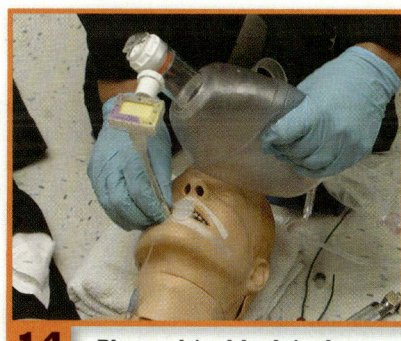

14 Place a bite block in the patient's mouth.

tube that goes undetected is a fatal error. You *must* incorporate multiple assessment findings into the determination of where the tube is located. If the tube must be repositioned or moved, be sure to remove the air from the cuff first.

After visualizing the tube passing through the glottis, note the depth of the markings on the tube. The average depth in adult males is 22 cm at the teeth, and the average depth in adult females is 21 cm at the teeth. Look for condensation in the tube. Condensation indicates correct placement in the trachea.

Auscultation over the lungs and epigastric area is the next step. Air entry into the stomach indicates esophageal placement, mandating immediate removal of the tube. Equal breath sounds should be heard over the apices of each lung and equal breath sounds and expansion over the bilateral bases. Unequal or absent breath sounds over the lung fields indicate esophageal placement, right mainstem placement, pneumothorax, or bronchial obstruction.

Palpation of the balloon cuff at the sternal notch by compressing the pilot balloon is another indication of correct placement. Pulse oximetry provides a measurement of oxygenation as long as other factors do not interfere with peripheral circulation. Carbon dioxide detectors (end tidal carbon dioxide) may also be used. They detect the presence of carbon dioxide in expired air **Figure 9-42**. These detectors may be colorimetric, digital, or digital/waveform. A capnographer attaches in between the ET tube and BVM device; it contains colorimetric paper, which should turn yellow during exhalation, indicating proper tube placement. A <u>capnometer</u> performs the same function; however, instead of using colorimetric paper, it attaches in the same way as a <u>capnographer</u>, but provides an LED readout of the patient's exhaled carbon dioxide, again indicating correct ET tube

Performing End-tidal Carbon Dioxide Detection

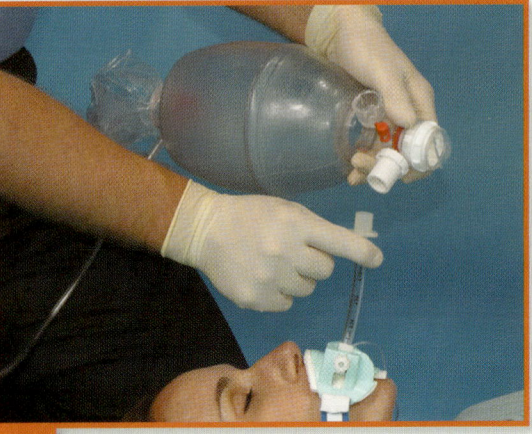

1. Detach the ventilation device from the ET tube.

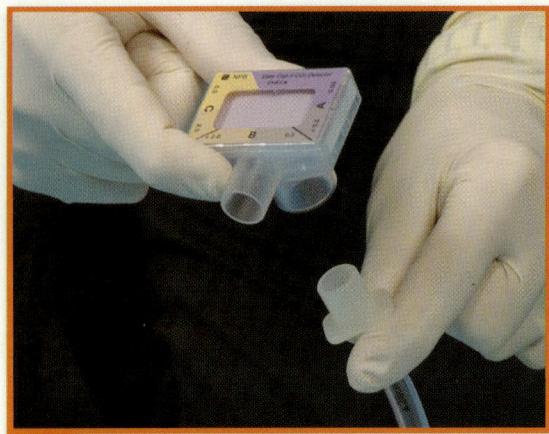

2. Attach an in-line capnographer or capnometer to the proximal adapter of the ET tube.

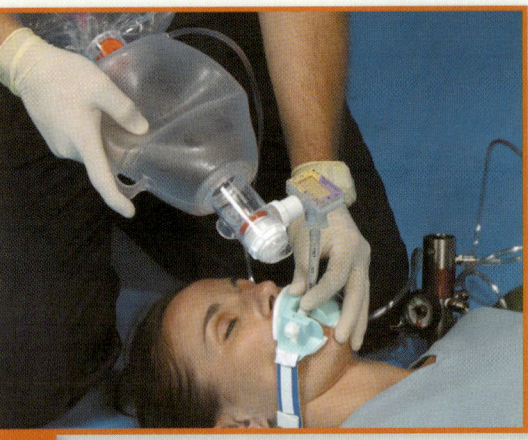

3. Reattach the ventilation device to the ET tube, and resume ventilations.

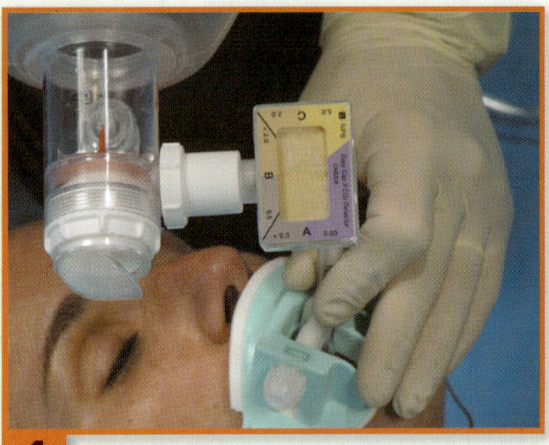

4. Monitor the capnographer or capnometer for appropriate reading (appropriate color change or digital reading).

placement. Because carbon dioxide is not present in the esophagus, use of carbon dioxide detectors is yet another method of determining correct tube placement. The steps are as follows (Skill Drill 9-24).

1. **Detach the ventilation device** from the ET tube (**Step 1**).
2. **Attach an in-line capnographer** or capnometer to the proximal adapter of the ET tube (**Step 2**).
3. **Reattach the ventilation device** to the ET tube, and resume ventilations (**Step 3**).
4. **Monitor the capnographer** or capnometer for appropriate reading (appropriate color change or digital reading) (**Step 4**).

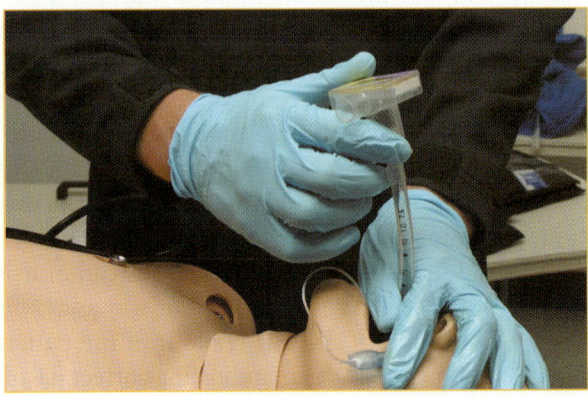

Figure 9-42 End-tidal carbon dioxide detector.

The final determination of correct tube placement is BVM ventilation compliance. The bag should be easy to compress with corresponding chest expansion. Increased resistance to BVM compliance may indicate gastric distention, esophageal placement, or tension pneumothorax.

Evidence of a misplaced tube, regardless of when it was last checked, must be reconfirmed. Confirmation of tube placement must be performed by multiple methods immediately after tube placement. Reconfirmation should be performed after any major move and after any manipulation of the neck. Manipulation of the neck may displace the tube up to 5 cm.

Table 9-21 lists indications, contraindications, advantages, disadvantages, and complications of orotracheal intubation by direct laryngoscopy.

Corrective Measures

If the ET tube is confirmed to be in the esophagus, it must be removed immediately. Be ready to vigorously suction as needed. The likelihood of emesis is increased, especially if gastric distention is present. Ideally, you should preoxygenate the patient before reintubation. The misplaced tube may be removed before or after proper tracheal placement is confirmed. Leaving the first tube in place may serve as a guide or block for the second tube. If the tube is removed before reintubation, make sure diligent and vigorous airway suctioning is ready.

If breath sounds are heard only on the right side, the tube may be advanced too far into the right mainstem bronchus. Follow these steps to reposition the tube:

- Loosen or remove the securing device.
- Deflate the balloon cuff.
- While ventilation continues, SLOWLY retract the tube while simultaneously listening for breath sounds over the left side of the chest.
- STOP as soon as breath sounds are heard in the left side of the chest.
- Note the tube depth.
- Reinflate the balloon cuff.
- Secure the tube.
- Resume ventilations.

Misplacement of an ET tube can be fatal if not corrected. It is imperative that you frequently check tube placement and quickly remedy any misplacement.

Securing the Tube

The last, and very important step, is to secure the tube. Inadvertent extubation caused by the patient or someone else is common and very traumatic to the patient. A second intubation would not be as easy as the first because of swelling and possible bleeding. It is disheartening to accomplish a difficult intubation and then find that the tube has been accidentally dislodged. Be sure to secure the tube well to prevent this from happening.

Many commercial tube holders are available that have varying degrees of efficiency. If one is available in your facility, become familiar with its use. Every EMT-I should know how to secure a tube using tape, because it is almost always available Figure 9-43.

TABLE 9-21	Orotracheal Intubation by Direct Laryngoscopy

Indications
- Apnea
- Hypoxia
- Poor respiratory effort
- Suppression or absence of gag reflex

Contraindication
- Caution in unsuppressed gag reflex

Advantages
- Direct visualization of anatomy and tube placement
- Ideal method for confirming placement
- May be performed in breathing or apneic patients

Disadvantage
- Requires special equipment

Complications
- Dental trauma
- Laryngeal trauma
- Misplacement
  - Right mainstem
  - Esophagus

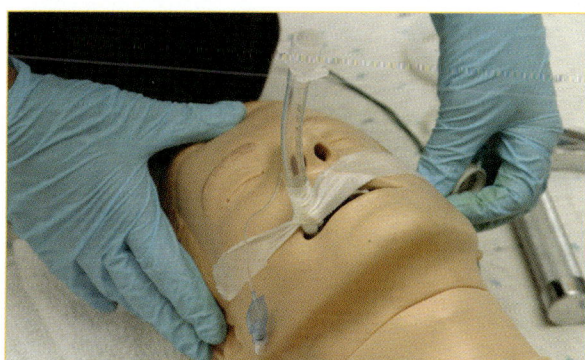

Figure 9-43 Every EMT-I should know how to secure a tube using tape, because it is almost always available.

Securing an Endotracheal Tube With Tape

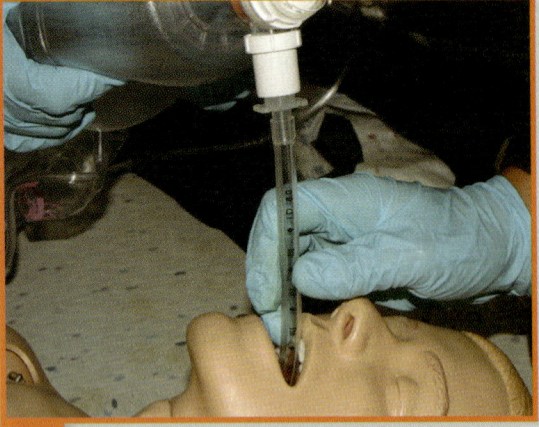
1 Note the centimeter marking on the tube at the level of the patient's teeth.

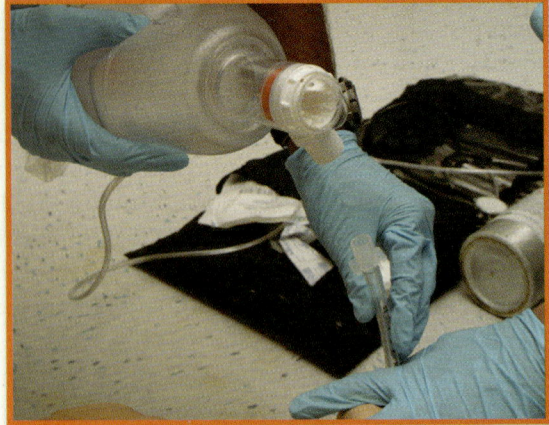
2 Remove the bag-valve device from the ET tube.

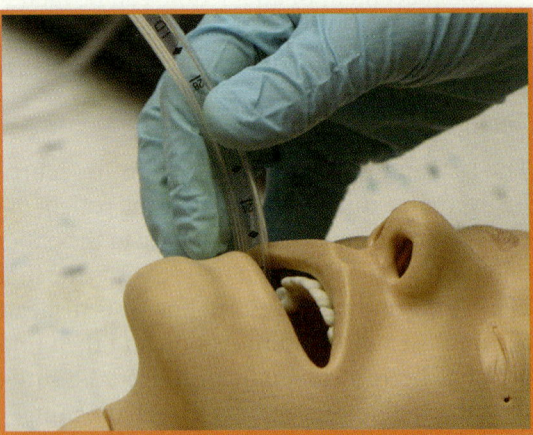
3 Move the ET tube to the corner of the patient's mouth.

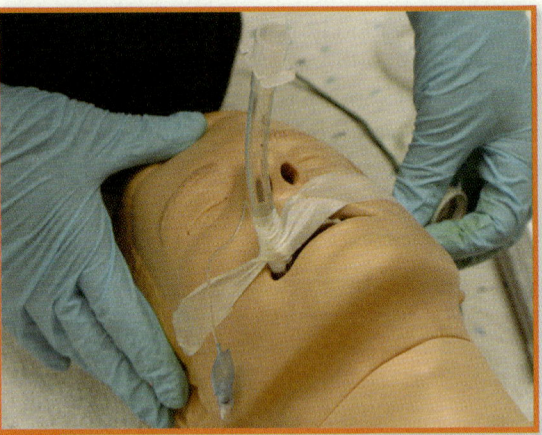
4 Encircle the ET tube with tape, and secure the tape to the patient's maxilla (using tincture of benzoin to facilitate tape adhesion).

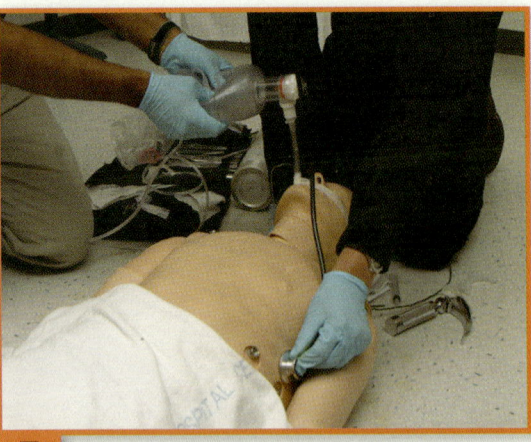
5 Reattach the bag-valve device, and auscultate again over the apices and bases of the lungs and over the epigastrium.

The steps for securing an ET tube with tape are listed here and shown in (Skill Drill 9-25 ◀):
1. **Note the centimeter marking** on the tube at the level of the patient's teeth (**Step 1**).
2. **Remove the bag-valve device** from the endotracheal (ET) tube (**Step 2**).
3. **Move the ET tube** to the corner of the patient's mouth (**Step 3**).
4. **Encircle the ET tube** with tape, and secure the tape to the patient's maxilla (using tincture of benzoin to facilitate tape adhesion) (**Step 4**).
5. **Reattach the bag-valve device**, and auscultate again over the apices and bases of the lungs and over the epigastrium (**Step 5**).

The steps for securing an ET tube with a commercial device are listed here and shown in (Skill Drill 9-26 ▶):
1. **Note the centimeter marking** on the tube at the level of the patient's teeth (**Step 1**).
2. **Remove the bag-valve device** from the ET tube (**Step 2**).
3. **Position the ET tube** in the center of the patient's mouth (**Step 3**).
4. **Place the commercial device** over the ET tube and secure (**Step 4**).
5. **Reattach the bag-valve device**, and auscultate again over the apices and bases of the lungs and over the epigastrium (**Step 5**).

After the tube is secured, be sure that a bite block or oral airway is inserted into the patient's mouth. If the patient bites the tube or has a seizure, there is a risk of occluding the airway. A rigid device that will not damage the teeth but that is hard enough to prevent biting the tube should be placed in the mouth. Finally, it is important to limit head movement in the intubated patient. With a firmly secured tube, the tip can move as much as 5 cm during head flexion and extension. If you are going to move the patient, consider placing the patient on a rigid board and using a cervical collar and/or head immobilization device to reduce the likelihood of tube dislodgment during head movement.

Tracheobronchial Suctioning

Following endotracheal intubation, thick pulmonary secretions may occlude the ET tube, preventing effective ventilation. In this case, you must pass a suction catheter into the ET tube to remove the secretions. Use a sterile technique if possible when performing tracheobronchial suctioning. Preoxygenation is essential before suctioning. Prelubricate a soft-tip catheter, and hyperoxygenate for 30 seconds to 1 minute. It may be necessary to inject 3 to 5 mL of sterile water down the ET tube to loosen secretions. Gently insert the catheter until resistance is felt. Apply suction as the catheter is extracted, taking care not to exceed 15 seconds in the adult patient. Continue to ventilate and oxygenate the patient.

Field Extubation

Extubation is the process of removing the tube from an intubated patient. In the critical care environment, the decision to extubate a patient is very complicated and depends on many factors. It may take days or weeks to

You are the Provider   Part 9

After preoxygenating the patient, you have successfully intubated her and confirmed proper placement of the ET tube. You attach the patient's ET tube to an automatic transport ventilator and set the ventilatory rate and tidal volume accordingly. After a few minutes, you reassess the patient's condition.

Reassessment	Recording Time: 15 Minutes After Patient Contact
Level of consciousness	Unconscious and unresponsive
Respirations	Absent (baseline); intubated with a 7.5-mm ET tube; ventilated with an automatic transport ventilator at a rate of 15 breaths/min
Pulse	100 beats/min, regular
Skin	Color is improving; quality is dry; cyanosis is resolving
Blood pressure	110/62 mm Hg
Sao$_2$	94% with ventilation and 100% O$_2$

12. What are the indications for intubation?

Securing an Endotracheal Tube With a Commercial Device

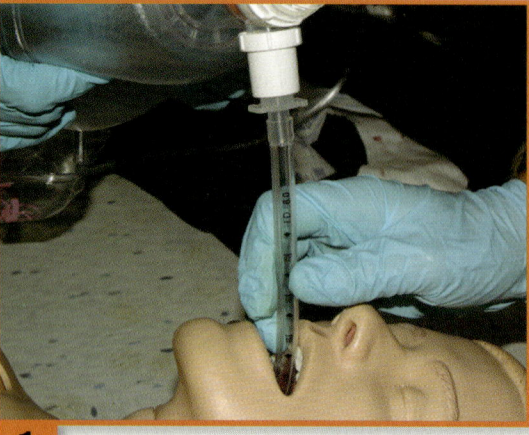

1 Note the centimeter marking on the tube at the level of the patient's teeth.

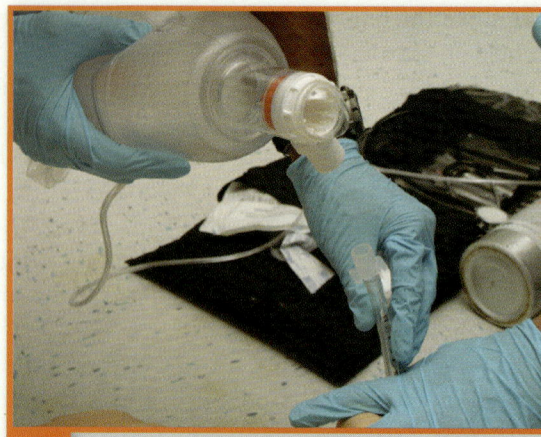

2 Remove the bag-valve device from the ET tube.

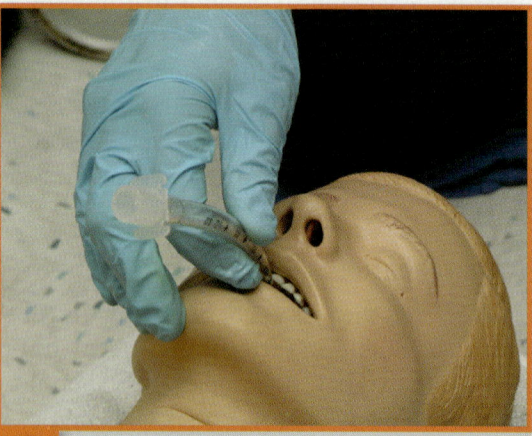

3 Position the ET tube in the center of the patient's mouth.

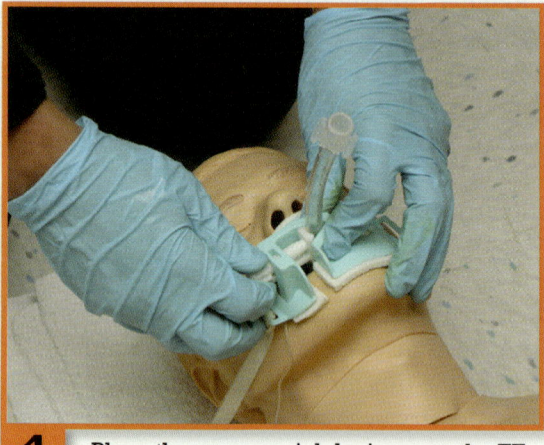

4 Place the commercial device over the ET tube and secure.

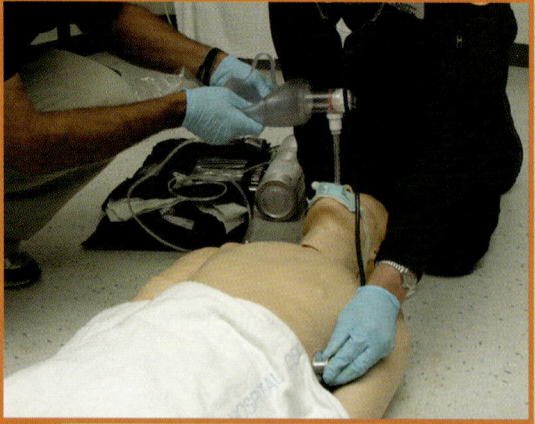

5 Reattach the bag-valve device, and auscultate again over the apices and bases of the lungs and over the epigastrium.

wean a patient off of a ventilator and be confident that the person will be able to ventilate and maintain his or her own airway. The decision to extubate the critical care patient is beyond the scope of this book.

In emergency medicine, we rarely extubate patients. The major indication for extubation is when the patient's level of consciousness improves and he or she begins gagging on the tube. In general, it is better to sedate the patient than to remove the tube, but this may not be an option in some systems or in patients who are in hemodynamically unstable condition.

There are a number of risks in extubating patients in emergency situations. The most obvious is overestimating the ability of the patient to protect his or her own airway. Once you remove the tube, there is no guarantee that you will be able to replace it. Patients who are awake are at a high risk for laryngospasm on removal of an ET tube, and most patients experience some degree of upper airway swelling because of the trauma of having a tube in the throat. These two facts, complicated by the ever-present possibility of vomiting, make reintubation challenging and maybe impossible. These risks must be factored against the benefit of removing the tube.

Field extubation is indicated when the patient is able to protect and maintain the airway, the patient is not sedated, and you are confident that you will be able to ventilate and reintubate if necessary. Field extubation should never be performed if there is a risk of continued or recurrent respiratory failure. Keep in mind that post-extubation vomiting and laryngospasm are possible.

Field extubation is accomplished by first hyperoxygenating the patient. Discuss the procedure with the patient, and explain what you are going to do. If possible, it is best to have the patient sit up or lean slightly forward. Be sure to assemble and have available all equipment to suction, ventilate, and reintubate, if necessary. After you have confirmed that the patient remains responsive enough to protect his or her own airway, suction the oropharynx to remove any debris or secretions that may threaten the airway. Deflate the cuff on the ET tube at the beginning of an exhalation so that any accumulated secretions just above the cuff are not aspirated into the lungs. On the next exhalation, remove the tube in one steady motion, following the curvature of the airway. You may find it useful to hold a towel or emesis basin in front of the patient's mouth, in case the patient gags or vomits. The steps for performing extubation are summarized here and shown in **Skill Drill 9-27** :

1. **Hyperoxygenate** the patient (**Step 1**).
2. **Ensure** that ventilation and suction equipment are immediately available (**Step 2**).
3. **Confirm** patient responsiveness (**Step 3**).
4. **Lean the patient** forward (**Step 4**).
5. **Suction** the oropharynx (**Step 5**).
6. **Deflate the distal cuff** of the ET tube (**Step 6**).
7. **Remove the ET tube** during a cough or when the patient exhales (**Step 7**). Following extubation, provide 100% oxygen via nonrebreathing mask. Have suction immediately available. Monitor breathing and oxygenation carefully.

Pediatric Endotracheal Intubation

Although endotracheal intubation has been considered the "gold standard" for out-of-hospital airway management, recent studies have suggested that effective BVM ventilation in pediatric patients can be as effective as intubation for EMS systems with short transport times. Indications for pediatric endotracheal intubation are as follows:

- Cardiopulmonary arrest
- Respiratory arrest
- Respiratory failure
- Traumatic brain injury
- Unresponsiveness
- Inability to maintain a patent airway
- Need for prolonged ventilation

Pediatric Needs

Differences in the Pediatric Airway

- Infants have a larger, rounder occiput, which causes the head of an infant or young child who lies supine to be in a flexed position.
- In children, the tongue is proportionately larger than in adults and the mandible is smaller, increasing the child's propensity for airway obstruction.
- The epiglottis in a child is more floppy and omega-shaped, so it must be lifted, or positioned, out of the way to see the vocal cords.
- The trachea in a child is smaller, shorter, and narrower than in an adult, and it is positioned more anteriorly and superiorly.
- The narrowest portion of the airway in a child is the cricoid ring, which is below the vocal cords, and the anatomy below the vocal cords is more funnel-shaped as opposed to the straight tube in an adult. This makes a cuff less necessary for occluding the trachea, and, in addition, the developing cartilage of the cricoid ring could potentially be injured by inflation of a cuffed ET tube.

Performing Extubation

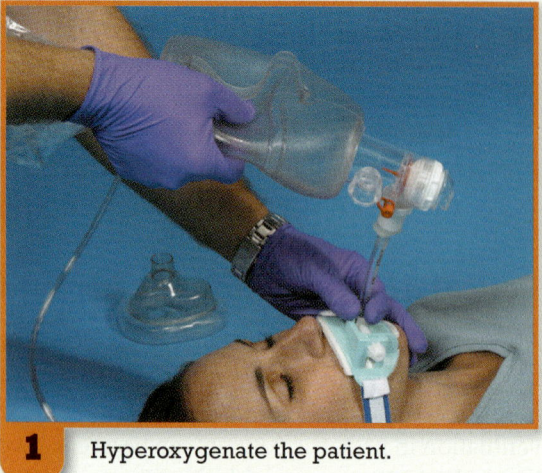
1. Hyperoxygenate the patient.

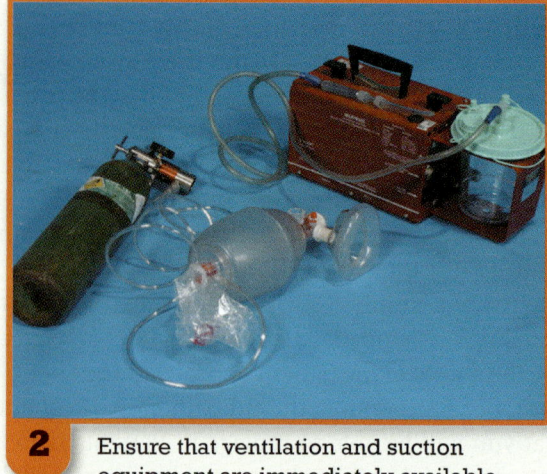
2. Ensure that ventilation and suction equipment are immediately available.

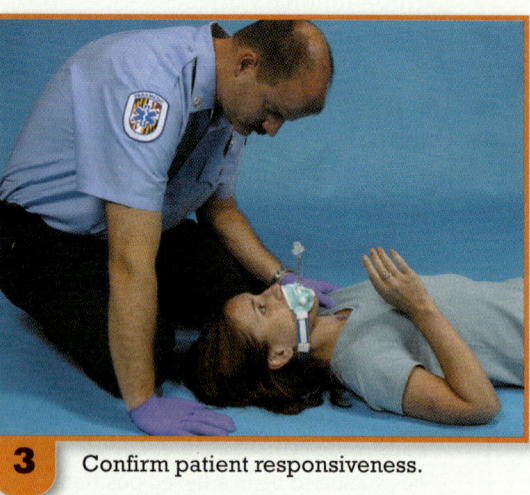
3. Confirm patient responsiveness.

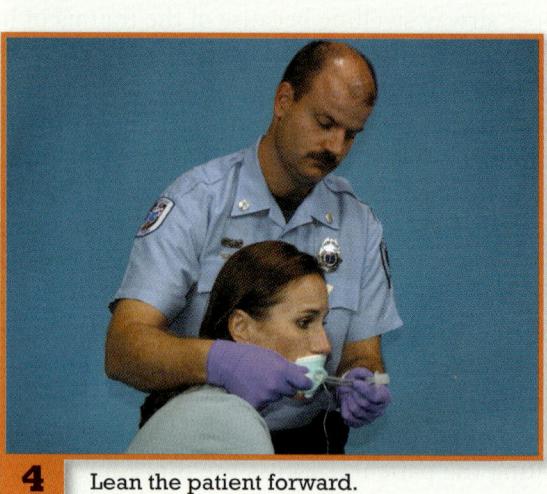
4. Lean the patient forward.

- Need for endotracheal administration of resuscitative medications

While some of these indications are similar to those for BVM ventilation, endotracheal intubation is indicated when BVM ventilation is ineffective. Once again, the most important part of pediatric endotracheal intubation is preparation and equipment selection. Some of the anatomic differences between children and adults have a role in performing a successful intubation, as proper airway position is critical.

Laryngoscope Handle and Blades

Any size laryngoscope handle can be used, although some prefer the thinner pediatric handles. Straight (Miller or Wis-Hipple) blades are preferred because they make it easy to lift the floppy epiglottis. If a curved (Macintosh) blade is used, the tip of the blade is positioned in the vallecula to lift the jaw and epiglottis to visualize the vocal cords.

The appropriately sized blade extends from the patient's mouth to the tragus of the ear. Acceptable means of measuring include using a length-based resuscitation tape or the following general guidelines:

- Premature newborn, size 0 straight blade
- Full-term newborn to 1 year, size 1 straight blade
- 2 years to adolescent, size 2 straight blade
- Adolescent and older, size 3 straight or curved blade

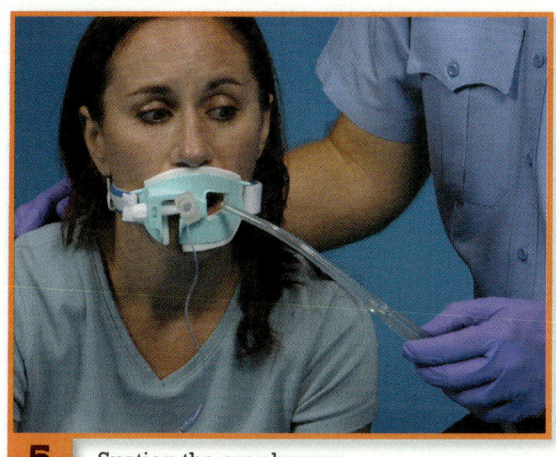

5 Suction the oropharynx.

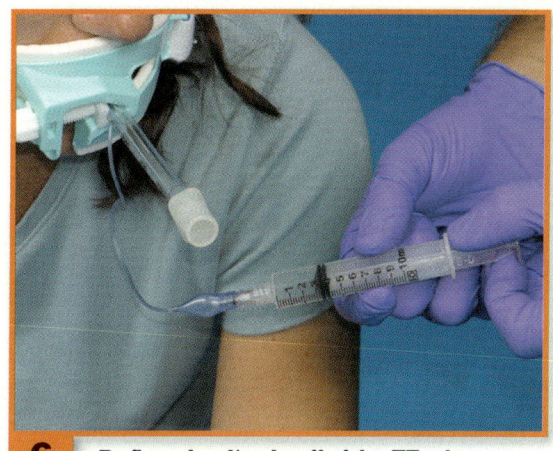

6 Deflate the distal cuff of the ET tube.

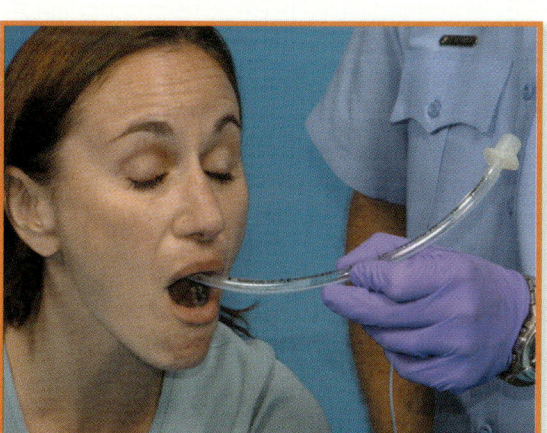

7 Remove the ET tube during a cough or when the patient exhales. Following extubation, provide 100% oxygen via nonrebreathing mask. Have suction immediately available. Monitor breathing and oxygenation carefully.

Endotracheal tube size can be selected by using a length-based resuscitation tape. For children older than 1 year, use this formula: age (in years) ÷ 4 + 4 (for example, a 4-year-old would need a 5.0 tube: [4 ÷ 4] + 4 = 5.0). In addition, anatomic clues, such as the size of the child's fifth digit or nares, or general guidelines can be used (Table 9-22).

One key point is to use uncuffed tubes in children under 8 years of age. A cuff at the cricoid ring is unnecessary to obtain a seal in young children. Furthermore, a cuff can cause <u>ischemia</u> and damage the mucosa of the trachea at this location. It is important to have a tube one size smaller and a tube one size larger than expected always available for situations in which there is variability in upper airway diameter.

The appropriate depth for insertion is 2 to 3 cm beyond the vocal cords. The tube should then be inserted an additional 2 to 3 cm. The depth should be recorded as the mark at the corner of the child's mouth. For uncuffed tubes, there is often a black glottic marker to use as a guide. When you see this line go through the vocal cords, stop. For cuffed tubes, when the cuff is just below the cords, stop. Another guideline is to insert the tube to a depth three times the inside diameter of the ET tube minus 1. For example, a 3.5-mm tube should be inserted to 9.5 cm (10.5 − 1 = 9.5 cm).

TABLE 9-22 | General Guidelines for Selecting Pediatric Endotracheal Tubes

Age	Endotracheal tube, mm	Insertion depth, cm
Premature infant	2.0-2.5 uncuffed	5.0-8.0
Newborn	3.0-3.5 uncuffed	8.0-9.5
Infant to 1 year	3.5-4.0 uncuffed	9.5-11.0
Toddler (2-4 years)	4.0-5.0 uncuffed	11.0-14.0
Preschool (5-6 years)	5.0-5.5 uncuffed	14.0-15.5
School age (6-8 years)	5.5-6.5 uncuffed	15.5-18.5
School age (8-10 years)	5.5-6.5 cuffed	15.5-18.5
School age (10-12 years)	6.5 cuffed	18.5
Adolescent	7.0-8.0 cuffed	20.0-23.0

The use of a stylet is based on personal preference. If you use a stylet, insert it into the ET tube, stopping at least 1 cm from the end of the tube. Pediatric stylets will fit into tubes sized 3.0 to 6.0 mm, whereas adult stylets are used for tubes sized 6.0 mm or larger. With the stylet in place, bend the ET tube into a gentle upward curve. In some cases, bending the tube into the shape of a hockey stick is beneficial.

Procedure

The steps for performing pediatric endotracheal intubation are listed here and shown in Skill Drill 9-28:

1. Take BSI precautions (gloves and face shield) (**Step 1**).
2. Check, prepare, and assemble your equipment (**Step 2**).
3. Manually open the patient's airway, and insert an adjunct if needed (**Step 3**).
4. Preoxygenate the child with a BVM device and 100% oxygen for at least 30 seconds (**Step 4**).
5. Insert the laryngoscope blade in the right side of the mouth, and sweep the tongue to the left (**Step 5**). Lift the tongue with firm, gentle pressure. Avoid using the teeth or gums as a fulcrum.
6. Identify the vocal cords (**Step 6**). If the cords are not visible, instruct your partner to apply cricoid pressure.
7. Introduce the ET tube in the right corner of the patient's mouth (**Step 7**).
8. Pass the ET tube through the vocal cords to approximately 2 to 3 cm below the vocal cords. Inflate the cuff if a cuffed tube is used (**Step 8**).
9. Attach an end-tidal carbon dioxide detector (**Step 9**).
10. Attach the BVM device, ventilate, and auscultate for equal breath sounds over each lateral chest wall high in the axillae. Ensure absence of breath sounds over the epigastrium (**Step 10**).
11. Secure the ET tube, noting the placement of the distance marker at the patient's teeth or gums, and reconfirm tube placement (**Step 11**).

Preoxygenation

The child should be adequately preoxygenated with a BVM device and 100% oxygen for at least 30 seconds before attempting intubation. Adequate preoxygenation cannot be overemphasized because respiratory failure or arrest is the most common cause of cardiac arrest in the pediatric population. During this time, you must also ensure that the child's head is in the proper position—the neutral position for those with suspected spinal trauma or the sniffing position for those without trauma. An airway adjunct can be inserted if needed to ensure adequate ventilation.

Additional Preparation

Stimulation of the parasympathetic nervous system and bradycardia can occur during intubation; therefore, a cardiac monitor should be applied if available. A pulse oximeter should be used before, during, and after the intubation attempt to monitor the patient's pulse rate and oxygen saturation.

In addition, suction apparatus should be readily available to clear oral secretions from the child's airway before, during, or after intubation.

Intubation Technique

Open the patient's mouth by applying thumb pressure on the chin. Some patients may require use of the cross-finger technique: Use your thumb and index finger or thumb and third finger to push the upper and lower teeth apart. If an oral airway has been inserted, remove it. If needed, suction the child's mouth and pharynx to clear any secretions.

Hold the laryngoscope handle in your left hand, using your thumb and second (index) and third (middle) finger to hold the handle (the "trigger finger" position). Insert the laryngoscope blade in the right side of the patient's mouth, sweeping the tongue to the left side and keeping the tongue under the blade. Advance the blade straight along the tongue, while applying gentle traction upward along the axis of the laryngoscope handle at a 45° angle. Never press the blade against the teeth or gums of a child. A child's teeth do not have the strong root system of an adult, so they could be loosened or cracked more easily during a traumatic intubation attempt.

When the blade passes the epiglottis, gently lift the epiglottis if you are using a straight blade. If you are using a curved blade, the tip of the blade should be placed in the vallecula and the jaw, tongue, and blade lifted gently at a 45° angle.

Identify the vocal cords and other normal anatomic landmarks. If they are not visible, have your partner apply gentle cricoid pressure. Additional gentle suctioning may be needed to clearly view the vocal cords.

Hold the tube in your right hand, and insert the tube from the right-hand corner of the patient's mouth. Do not pass the tube through the channel of the laryngoscope blade, because you will lose sight of the vocal cords. Guide the tube through the vocal cords, and advance the tube until the glottic/vocal cord mark is positioned just beyond the vocal cords (approximately 2 to 3 cm). Record the depth of the tube as measured at the right-hand corner of the patient's mouth, and remove the laryngoscope blade. Remove the stylet from the tube if one was used. Be sure to hold the tube securely at the level of the mouth while removing the stylet to avoid inadvertent extubation. Next, recheck the tube depth to be certain it did not displace during stylet removal. If you are using a cuffed tube, inflate the cuff until the pilot balloon is full. Suction the tracheal tube if there is fluid present. Attach the tube to a ventilation bag and 100% oxygen. Release cricoid pressure.

Confirm proper ET tube placement using one or more of several techniques. Look for bilateral chest rise during ventilation. Listen to the lungs bilaterally at the midaxillary line at the third intercostal space. You should listen for two breaths in each location. If breath sounds are decreased on the left side, the tracheal tube may be positioned too deep and aimed toward or in the right mainstem bronchus. To correct this, listen to the left side of the chest while ventilating and slowly withdrawing the tube, until breath sounds are equal on both sides. Re-record the depth of the tube.

Breath sounds travel easily in a child because of a child's small chest. It is important to listen over the patient's stomach to ensure that there are no bubbling or gurgling sounds in the epigastric region. These sounds indicate <u>esophageal intubation</u>. If noted, the tube should be removed, and the intubation procedure reattempted. Additional methods to confirm appropriate tracheal tube position include improvement in the child's skin color, pulse rate, oxygen saturation as measured by pulse oximetry, exhaled carbon dioxide level according to a carbon dioxide detector, and confirmation with esophageal detection devices. If the tube is properly positioned, hold the tracheal tube firmly in place and secure the tube with tape or a commercially available device.

Reconfirm tube placement by listening for bilateral breath sounds and for sounds in the epigastric region. It is important to reconfirm tube placement not only after securing the tube, but also after any patient movement (for example, onto the stretcher or into the ambulance), because tubes can easily become dislodged. Remember to record and frequently monitor the depth of the tube. Once tube position has been confirmed, resume assisted ventilation and oxygenation.

If during the intubation attempt you realize the tube is too large or the vocal cords and glottic landmarks cannot be identified, stop the intubation attempt and ventilate the patient with the BVM device and 100% oxygen. Modify your equipment selection appropriately, and start the procedure from the beginning. If intubation cannot be accomplished after two attempts, discontinue attempts, and resume BVM ventilation for the remainder of the transport.

Securing the ET Tube

Although there are several methods of using tape to secure ET tubes, no single method is fail-safe. One person should always hold the tube in place while another secures the device. The steps for securing an ET tube are listed here and shown in Skill Drill 9-29▶:

1. With the tube positioned at the corner of the mouth, **tear a strip of tape and anchor one end** to the side of the face. Wrap it around the tube several times and anchor the other end over the maxilla (**Step 1**).
2. **Wrap another piece of tape** around the tube, and anchor it over the mandible (**Step 2**).
3. **Reinforce the tape** around the child's neck (**Step 3**).
4. **Reconfirm tube placement** by auscultating over the lungs and at the epigastrium (**Step 4**).

Confirmation of ET Tube Position

Three methods to confirm the ET tube position include clinical assessment, use of end-tidal carbon dioxide devices, and use of esophageal aspiration bulbs or syringes. Most of the process of confirmation of ET

Performing Pediatric Endotracheal Intubation

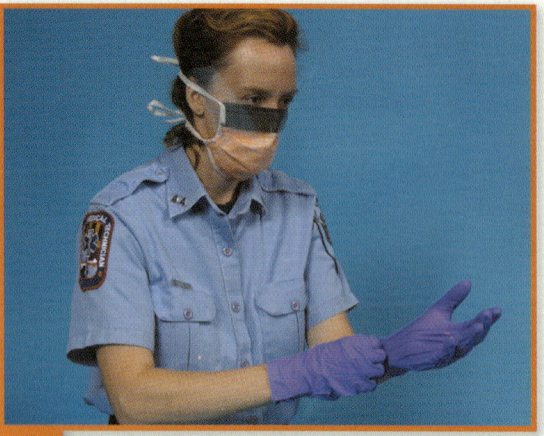

1 Take BSI precautions (gloves and face shield).

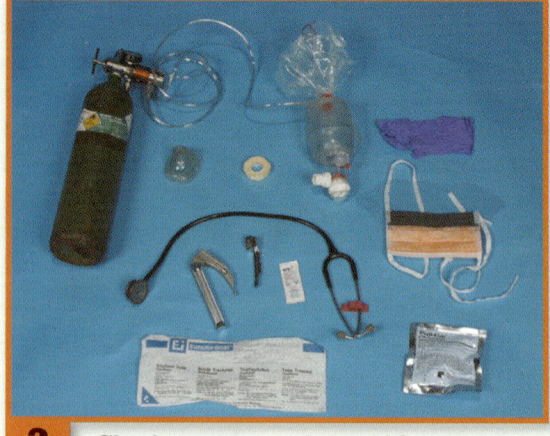

2 Check, prepare, and assemble your equipment.

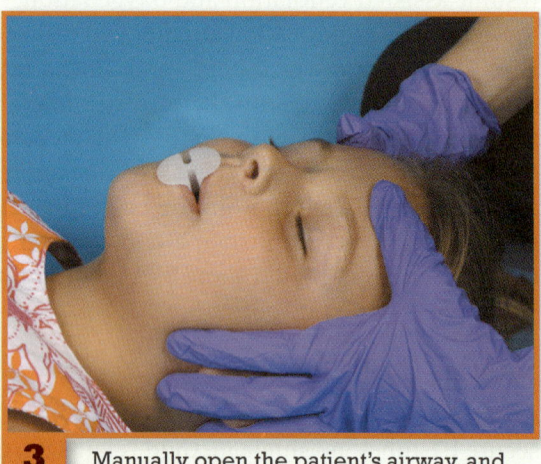

3 Manually open the patient's airway, and insert an adjunct if needed.

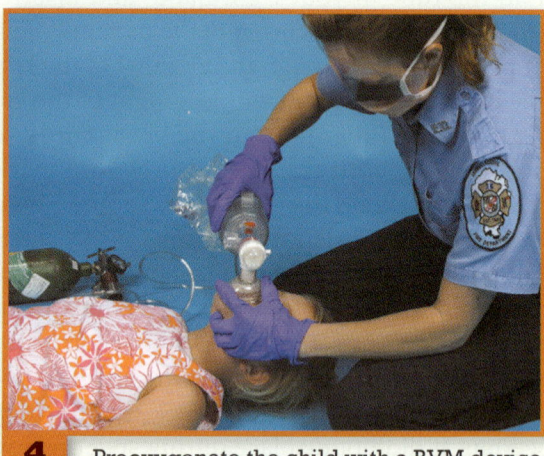

4 Preoxygenate the child with a BVM device and 100% oxygen for at least 30 seconds.

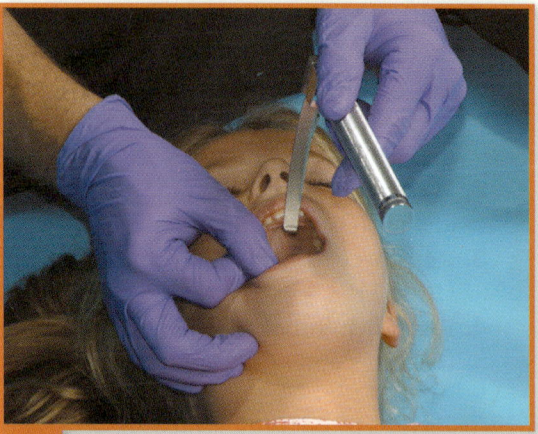

5 Insert the laryngoscope blade in the right side of the mouth, and sweep the tongue to the left. Lift the tongue with firm, gentle pressure. Avoid using the teeth or gums as a fulcrum.

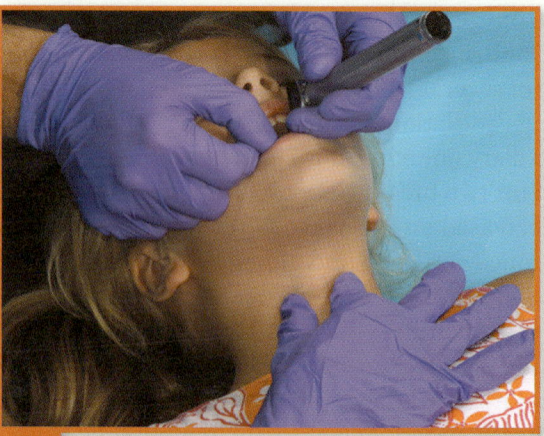

6 Identify the vocal cords. If the cords are not visible, instruct your partner to apply cricoid pressure.

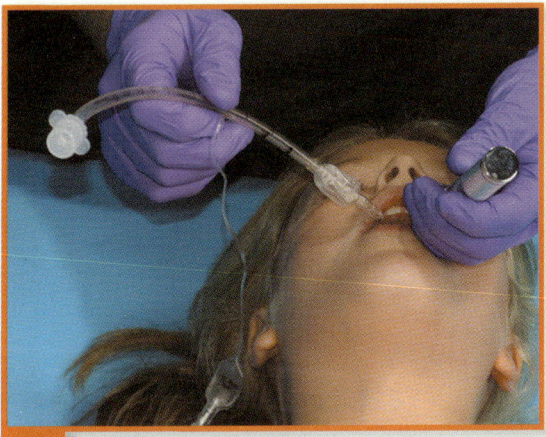

7 Introduce the ET tube in the right corner of the patient's mouth.

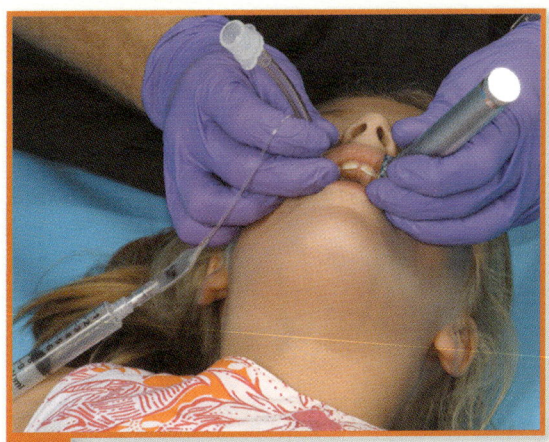

8 Pass the ET tube through the vocal cords to approximately 2 to 3 cm below the vocal cords. Inflate the cuff if a cuffed tube is used.

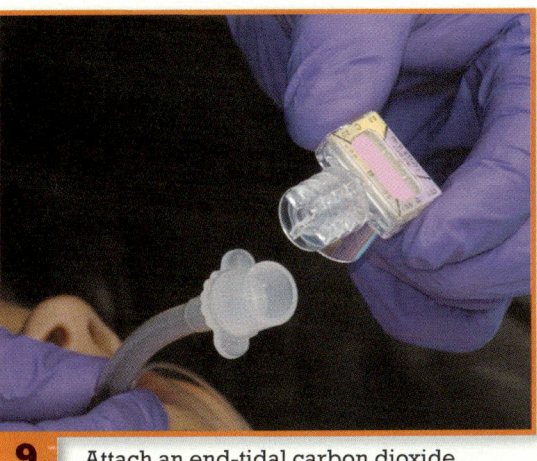

9 Attach an end-tidal carbon dioxide detector.

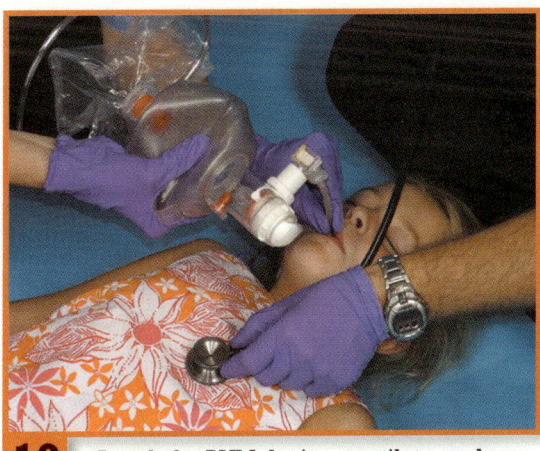

10 Attach the BVM device, ventilate, and auscultate for equal breath sounds over each lateral chest wall high in the axillae. Ensure absence of breath sounds over the epigastrium.

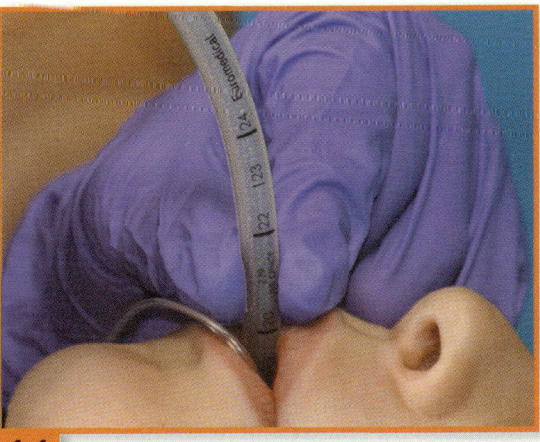

11 Secure the ET tube, noting the placement of the distance marker at the patient's teeth or gums, and reconfirm tube placement.

Securing an Endotracheal Tube

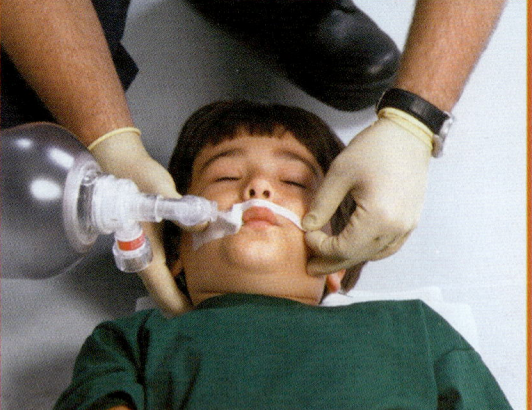

1 With the tube positioned at the corner of the mouth, tear a strip of tape and anchor one end to the side of the face. Wrap it around the tube several times and anchor the other end over the maxilla.

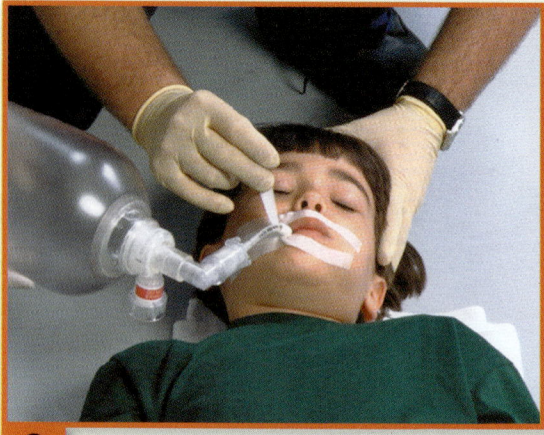

2 Wrap another piece of tape around the tube, and anchor it over the mandible.

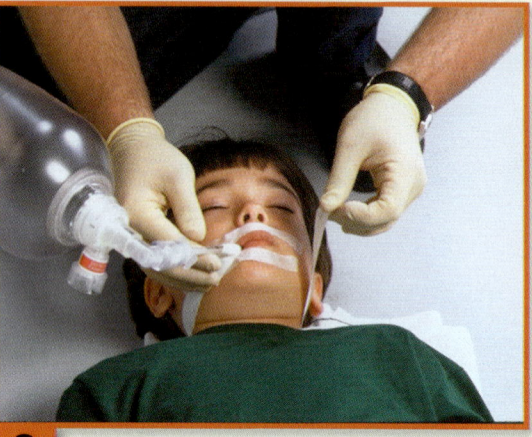

3 Reinforce the tape around the child's neck.

4 Reconfirm tube placement by auscultating over the lungs and at the epigastrium.

---

tube placement is identical to that used in adults. However, there are several important factors that must be remembered when using some of these devices in children.

- The adult colorimetric end-tidal carbon dioxide detector cannot be used in children weighing less than 15 kg. (The pediatric detector can be used in any infant or child.)
- The esophageal bulb or syringe cannot be used in children younger than 5 years who weigh less than 20 kg.
- The carbon dioxide detector must be removed from the ET tube before endotracheal drug administration.

Indications for Immediate Tracheal Tube Removal

- No chest rise with ventilation
- Presence of epigastric gurgling sounds or vomitus in tracheal tube
- Failure to confirm proper tube position with detection devices

Complications of Endotracheal Intubation

- Unrecognized esophageal intubation
- Induction of emesis and aspiration
- Hypoxia resulting from prolonged intubation attempts
- Damage to teeth, soft tissues, and intraoral structures

Esophageal Obturator Airway (EOA)

Esophageal airways were initially introduced in 1968 and became popular as a primary method of airway management for prehospital care providers during the early 1970s. The <u>esophageal obturator airway (EOA)</u> was endorsed by the American Heart Association in 1974 and has been used in prehospital settings. The effectiveness of esophageal airways is extremely controversial, and the issue is complicated by conflicting research findings. One of the main contributions of esophageal airways has been the continual refinement of design that has led to improved devices. Although they are not commonly used today, esophageal airways are available and have some advantages in specific situations.

The concept of an esophageal airway is simple. If you occlude the esophagus completely, all of the gas delivered under pressure to the patient will go into the lungs. In addition, by placing an <u>obturator</u> in the esophagus, you effectively eliminate the risk of regurgitation and subsequent aspiration. The common characteristic of esophageal airways is a long tube attached to a ventilation mask. The tube has a large inflatable balloon at its distal end, which serves as a cuff. The tube is inserted blindly into the esophagus, the mask is sealed to the patient's face, and the balloon is inflated. Ventilation is accomplished by positive pressure generated within the mask by a bag-valve device (Figure 9-44 ▶). Esophageal airways are a misnomer because they do not provide a patent airway. Although the theoretical advantage of the esophageal obturator is clear, in practice it does not ensure a patent airway, and you cannot control ventilation well with an EOA.

Advantages and Disadvantages of Esophageal Airways

There are a number of advantages of esophageal airways over intubation. First, they require less technical skill than intubation. In theory, they can be properly used with less practice and continual skill maintenance. This may be particularly advantageous in rural settings where there is an infrequent need for airway management. Esophageal airways also provide excellent protection against vomiting.

Unfortunately, there are also numerous disadvantages of esophageal airways. The most significant is the fact that the device still requires a mask seal to ventilate the patient. Second, the esophageal airway does little to maintain a patent airway. Although the device prevents gastric insufflation and regurgitation, the EMT-I must still maintain the airway manually.

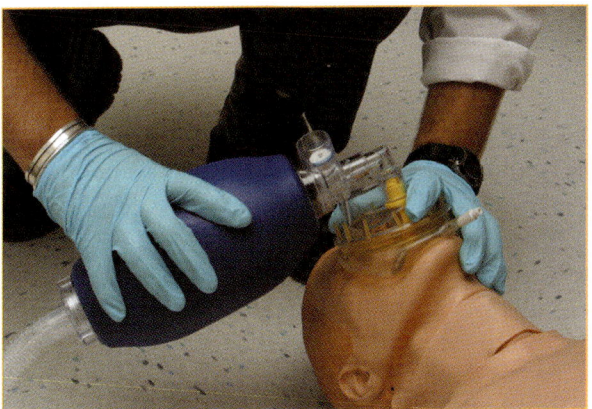

Figure 9-44 Esophageal airways prevent gastric inflation and regurgitation by obstruction of the esophagus.

Poor mask seal and difficulty in manually opening the airway are two of the major reasons for hypoventilation when the airway is unprotected and are major technical problems associated with using esophageal airways.

Indications for Esophageal Airways

The esophageal airway can be used only in deeply unconscious apneic patients without a gag reflex. In general, the indication for the use of an esophageal airway is an inability to intubate. Esophageal airways are considered temporary airway devices and should be removed within 2 hours.

Contraindications to Use of Esophageal Airways

Esophageal airways should not be used in patients younger than 16 years. Because the cuff has to come to rest in the esophagus above the cardiac sphincter but below the carina, the airway can be used only in patients between 5 and 7 feet tall. In a shorter person, the cuff may come to rest in the sphincter itself or in the stomach. In a taller person, the cuff may come to rest in the esophagus above the level of the carina. When inflated, it may cause a partial obstruction in the trachea because the open end of the tracheal rings faces the esophagus.

No airway that is intended to be inserted into the esophagus should ever be used if the patient has any history of esophageal disease (such as esophageal varices, strictures, or diverticula) or has ingested a caustic substance, because of the increased risk of esophageal rupture. The trachea must be protected before removal of an esophageal airway because regurgitation occurs in almost all patients. Intubation with an esophageal airway in place can be challenging.

Complications of Esophageal Airways

The most significant complication of esophageal airway insertion is inadvertent tracheal intubation. If tracheal placement goes unrecognized, the patient will receive no pulmonary ventilation. Confirmation of tube placement is just as important following esophageal airway placement as it is following endotracheal intubation, and the consequences of unrecognized misplacement are just as disastrous.

In addition to misplacement, the complication rate of esophageal airways is quite high. Hypoventilation due to poor mask seal and airway control is common. Esophageal rupture, while uncommon, is life threatening. Laryngospasm caused by excessive upper airway stimulation, as well as vomiting and aspiration, can occur during insertion or in failed attempts. If the cuff is left in place too long or inflated with too much air, it can cause localized tissue necrosis.

Equipment for Esophageal Airways

The original esophageal airway was called the esophageal obturator airway (EOA) Figure 9-45. The EOA is no longer manufactured, and very few are still in circulation. EOAs should not be used because of the inability to decompress the stomach before removal.

The esophageal gastric tube airway (EGTA) is a modification of the EOA. It consists of a mask attached to a plastic tube that is 34 cm long and 13 mm in diameter. The tube has a 35-mL balloon at its distal end. The EGTA has an opening at the distal tip of the esophageal tube, enabling a 16F gastric tube to be inserted for decompression of the stomach before removal of the esophageal airway. The mask has a 15/22-mm ventilation port enabling ventilation Figure 9-46.

Technique for Esophageal Airway Placement and Placement Confirmation

Remember that the goal of an EGTA is to occlude the esophagus. Therefore, the technique is intended to facilitate entry of the tube into the esophagus, not the trachea. If the procedure is followed correctly, esophageal placement occurs in most cases, but its position must be confirmed.

All of the alternative airway procedures before and after insertion are similar to the procedures discussed in the previous sections of this chapter. Therefore, only the differences from those procedures will be discussed here.

Procedures Before Insertion As with every airway procedure, all equipment is checked and assembled before you start the technique. In particular, check the cuff of the esophageal airway and ensure that it holds 35 mL of air. The tube must be inserted into the mask before being inserted into the patient to prevent the tube from migrating too far into the airway. It should snap firmly in place, with the curvature of the tube following the natural contour of the airway.

The patient should be preoxygenated before insertion. Ventilation should not be interrupted longer than 30 seconds to accomplish airway placement. This is rarely a problem because the procedure is blind and generally faster than endotracheal intubation.

Finally, patient positioning is extremely important. In contrast with endotracheal intubation, in which the goal of preintubation positioning is to align the axes of the airway, you want this tube to go into the esopha-

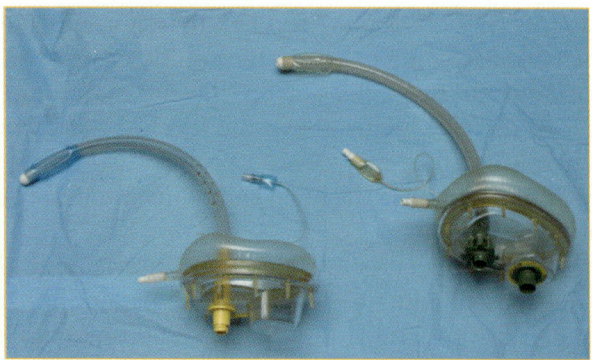

Figure 9-45 Esophageal obturator airway and esophageal gastric tube airway.

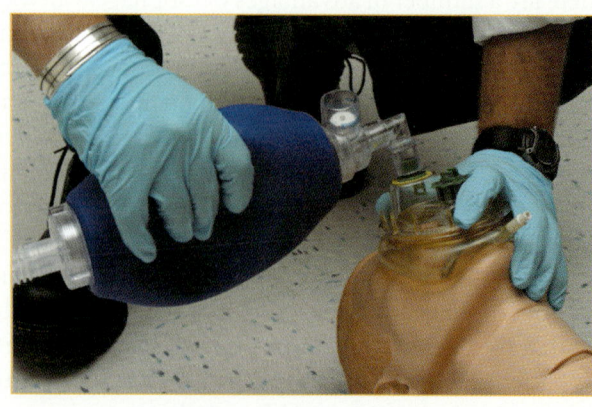

Figure 9-46 Ventilation with an EGTA in place.

gus. Therefore, the patient's head should be placed in the neutral or slightly flexed position.

- **Displace the jaw forward.** With the head in the neutral or flexed position, insert the thumb of your gloved, nondominant hand into the patient's mouth and lift the jaw. This action lifts the hyoid bone, pulling the base of the tongue off the posterior pharyngeal wall.
- **Insert the esophageal tube.** Following the curvature of the tube, insert the device blindly into the posterior pharynx and (presumably) into the esophagus. Be gentle, and stop advancing the tube if you meet resistance. Continue to advance it until you are able to seal the mask to the patient's face.
- **Inflate the cuff.** The device is inserted completely when the mask contacts the patient's face. Inflate the balloon with 35 mL of air. Do not inflate with additional air because this would significantly increase the risk of esophageal rupture and necrosis. Be sure to remove the syringe. If it remains attached, it will cause the balloon to deflate.

Procedures After Insertion Following inflation of the balloon, obtain a mask seal, perform a head tilt–chin lift or jaw-thrust maneuver, and begin to ventilate the patient. Confirm the presence of breath sounds. Use other clinical indicators to continuously monitor the location of the tube. There are no specific requirements to secure the esophageal airway in place, but be careful with it. Inadvertent removal can be quite traumatic to the esophagus and can result in extensive regurgitation.

Esophageal airways, although not frequently used anymore, can be very useful in prehospital emergency medicine. The EGTA is an excellent way to stop vomiting that may be making intubation impossible. Insert the EGTA and suction out any vomit in the mouth. Ventilate the patient through the EGTA for preintubation oxygenation. Remove the mask (but keep the tube in place), and intubate around the tube inserted in the esophagus.

The Laryngeal Mask Airway

The laryngeal mask airway (LMA) is a relatively new airway management device that has become popular with anesthesiologists (Figure 9-47 ▶). The LMA was invented by Dr. A. I. J. Brain at the London Hospital in 1981 and became commercially available in 1988. The device was originally developed as an alternative to face-mask ventilation (as is commonly used during short surgical procedures) and endotracheal intubation (used for longer periods of anesthesia) in the operating room. Before the development of the LMA, no device provided a viable option for cases of intermediate length that required more airway support than mask ventilation but did not require intubation.

The LMA was not designed for emergency use. Although it is not a replacement for endotracheal intubation, the LMA may have a role in emergencies if

You are the Provider — Part 10

The patient's condition improves following intubation and ventilation with 100% O_2. Shortly before arriving at the emergency department, you reassess the patient and note the following:

Reassessment	Recording Time: 18 Minutes After Patient Contact
Level of consciousness	Occasional movement; not resisting the ET tube
Respirations	Occasional respirations (baseline); intubated and ventilated with an automatic transport ventilator and 100% O_2
Pulse	92 beats/min, regular
Skin	Pink, warm, and dry
Blood pressure	118/70 mm Hg
Sao_2	98% with ventilation and 100% O_2

13. What is the definition of ventilation?

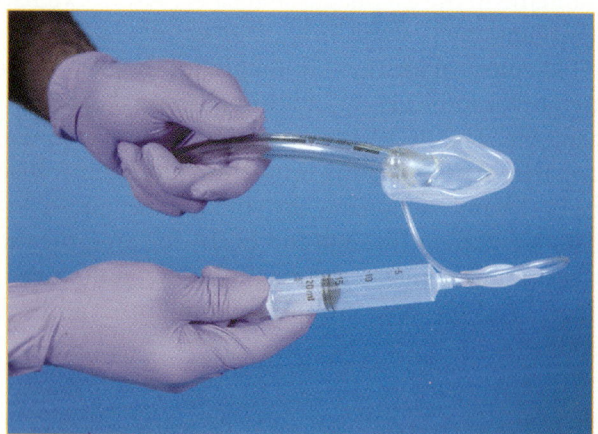

Figure 9-47 The laryngeal mask airway.

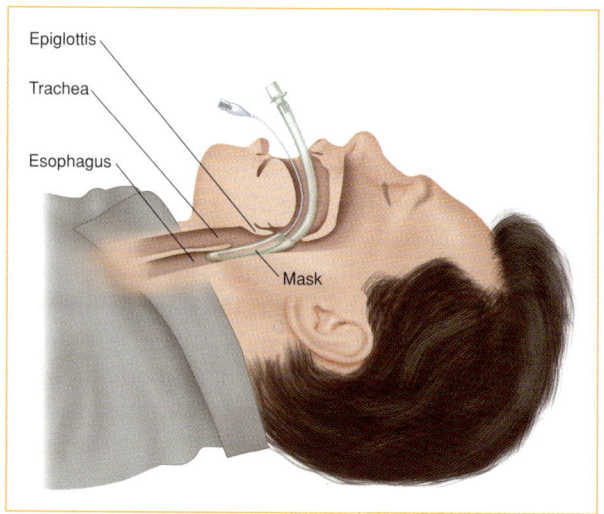

Figure 9-48 When properly positioned, the opening of the LMA is at the glottic opening, the tip is at the entrance of the esophagus, the lateral portions in the pyriform fossae, and the upper border at the base of the tongue.

intubation is not possible and the only option is mask ventilation. Because of the newness of the LMA, very few studies have been conducted on the use of the device in emergency situations. Emergency care practitioners are encouraged to be cautious about the use of the LMA until more studies have been conducted. Nevertheless, the positive experience with the LMA in the operating room suggests that the LMA has some potential in emergency medicine. In emergency medicine, the LMA should be considered better than mask ventilation but inferior to endotracheal intubation.

The LMA is designed to provide a conduit from the glottic opening to the ventilation device. This is achieved by surrounding the opening of the larynx with an inflatable silicone cuff positioned in the hypopharynx. When properly inserted, the opening of the LMA is positioned right at the glottic opening. The tip of the device is inserted into the proximal esophagus, the lateral portions in the pyriform fossae, and the upper border at the base of the tongue. The inflatable cuff conforms to the contours of the airway and makes a relatively airtight seal Figure 9-48 ▶.

A to Z Terminology Tips

On the lateral side of the glottic opening are two pockets of tissue known as the *pyriform fossae*. Airway devices are occasionally inadvertently inserted into these pockets, resulting in "tenting" of the skin under the jaw.

Advantages and Disadvantages of the LMA

The LMA has many advantages compared with ventilating the unprotected airway with a mask. The LMA has been shown to provide better oxygenation than mask ventilation with an oral airway, and ventilation with an LMA does not require the continual maintenance of a mask seal. Compared with an ET tube, LMA insertion is easier and does not require laryngoscopy. There is significantly less risk of soft tissue, vocal cord, tracheal wall, and dental trauma than with endotracheal intubation and other forms of intubation that rely on esophageal obturation. The LMA provides protection from upper airway secretions, and the tip of the LMA wedged into the proximal esophagus probably provides some obturation.

The main disadvantage of the LMA, especially in emergencies, is that it does not provide protection against aspiration. In fact, the LMA actually increases the risk of aspiration if the patient regurgitates because the patient's stomach contents would most likely be directed into the trachea. Experience in the operating room may not accurately predict the risk of aspiration in emergency situations because patients undergoing surgery have fasted before receiving anesthesia.

During prolonged LMA ventilation, some air may be insufflated into the stomach because the seal made in the airway is not airtight. Because of the risk of aspiration, it is unlikely that the LMA will ever replace endotracheal intubation in prehospital emergency care. The

LMA should not be considered a primary airway for emergency patients, but it may have a role. For a patient who cannot be intubated, the LMA should be considered superior to mask ventilation.

Indications for the LMA

The LMA should be considered as one possible alternative to mask ventilation only when the patient cannot be intubated.

Contraindications for the LMA

The product literature for the LMA states that it should be used only in "fasting" patients. Unfortunately, this would eliminate all emergency patients. It could conceivably be considered a potential alternative to mask ventilation in the prehospital emergency setting but not as a replacement for intubation. You must weigh the risk of aspiration against the risk of hypoventilation with mask ventilation in the context of a given clinical scenario.

The LMA is less effective in obese patients and should not be used in patients with morbid obesity. Patients who are pregnant or have a hiatal hernia are at an increased risk for regurgitation and must be evaluated carefully if LMA use is considered. The LMA is ineffective for the ventilation of patients requiring high pulmonary pressures.

Complications of Using the LMA

The biggest complications involve regurgitation and subsequent aspiration. The incidence of misplacement in the operating room is relatively low (1% to 5%) and seems to decrease with experience. Nevertheless, the EMT-I should observe the patient for clinical indications of adequate ventilation (chest rise, breath sounds) during LMA ventilation. Hypoventilation of patients who require high ventilatory pressures can also occur. A few cases of upper airway swelling have been reported.

Equipment for the LMA

The LMA comes in five sizes and is sized based on the patient's weight. The device consists of an inflatable cuff attached to an obliquely cut tube. The cuff provides a collar that is designed to position the opening of the tube at the glottic opening when inflated. Two vertical bars are present at the opening of the tube to prevent occlusion. The proximal end of the tube is fitted with a standard 15/22-mm adapter. The cuff has a one-way valve assembly and should be inflated with a predetermined volume of air (based on the size of the airway) (Figure 9-49 ▶).

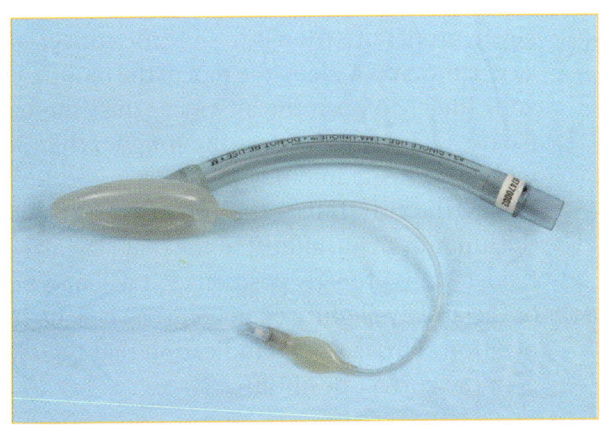

Figure 9-49 The LMA.

Technique for LMA Insertion

Procedures Before Insertion Check and prepare all equipment. Check the cuff of the LMA by inflating it with 50% more air than is required for that size airway. The cuff should then be completely deflated so that no folds appear near the tip. Deflation is best accomplished by pressing the device, cuff down, on a flat surface (Figure 9-50 ▼). Lubricate the base of the device. The patient should be preoxygenated before it is inserted. Ventilation should not be interrupted for more than 30 seconds to accomplish airway placement. Place the patient in the sniffing position.

- **Insert your finger between the cuff and the tube.** Proper insertion of the LMA depends on holding the device properly. Place the index finger of your dominant hand in the notch between the tube and the cuff. Open the patient's mouth.

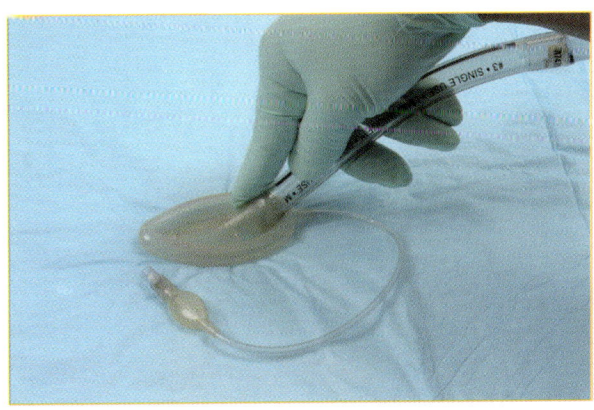

Figure 9-50 Press the LMA against a flat surface to remove all wrinkles from the cuff.

- **Insert the LMA along the roof of the mouth.** The key to proper insertion is to slide the convex surface of the airway along the roof of the mouth. Use your finger to push the airway against the hard palate. Once it slides past the tongue, the LMA will move easily into position.
- **Inflate the cuff.** Inflate the cuff of the LMA with the amount of air indicated for that size airway. If the LMA is properly positioned, it will move out of the airway slightly (1 to 2 cm) as it seats into position. This is a good indication that the LMA is in the correct position.

Procedures After Insertion Following inflation of the cuff, begin to ventilate the patient. Confirm chest rise and the presence of breath sounds. Continuously and carefully monitor for regurgitation in the tube. The LMA can be easily dislodged because it was not designed for patients who are being transported. Carefully attend to the airway during any patient movement, and be prepared to mask ventilate if the LMA becomes dislodged.

One of the design features of the LMA is the fact that you can intubate through it. A 6.0-mm ET tube can be passed through a size 3 or 4 LMA. The vertical bars are designed to allow a well-lubricated tube to pass straight through, and research in the operating room found a 90% success rate of endotracheal intubation following this technique. The Fasttrach LMA is actually designed to guide an ET tube into the trachea and may prove to be an alternative to direct laryngoscopy (Figure 9-51).

The steps for using an LMA are summarized here and in (Skill Drill 9-30):

1. **Check the cuff** of the LMA by inflating it with 50% more air than is required for that size airway. Then deflate the cuff completely (**Step 1**).
2. **Lubricate the base** of the device (**Step 2**).
3. **Preoxygenate the patient** before insertion. Ventilation should not be interrupted for more than 30 seconds to accomplish airway placement. Place the patient in the sniffing position (**Step 3**).
4. **Insert your finger between the cuff and the tube.** Place the index finger of your dominant hand in the notch between the tube and the cuff. Open the patient's mouth (**Step 4**).
5. **Insert the LMA along the roof of the mouth.** Use your finger to push the airway against the hard palate (**Step 5**).
6. **Inflate the cuff** with the amount of air indicated for that size airway (**Step 6**).
7. **Begin to ventilate the patient.** Confirm chest rise and the presence of breath sounds. Continuously and carefully monitor the patient (**Step 7**).

(Table 9-23) compares endotracheal intubation to other nonsurgical alternative airway management techniques.

Tracheostomy, Stoma, and Tracheostomy Tubes

A tracheostomy is a surgical opening into the trachea. The procedure is performed in an operating room under controlled conditions. A stoma is the resultant orifice connecting the trachea to the outside air. The stoma is located just superior to the suprasternal notch. The patient now breathes through this surgical opening. A tracheostomy tube is a plastic tube placed within the tracheostomy site (Figure 9-52). It requires a 15-mm connector to be compatible with a ventilatory device, such as a mechanical ventilator or BVM device. A patient may receive supplemental oxygen using tubing designed to fit over the stoma or by placing an oxygen mask over the tube. Ventilation is accomplished by simply attaching the BVM to the tracheostomy tube.

BVM device ventilation may be needed for patients who have had a laryngectomy (surgical removal of the larynx). These patients have a permanent tracheal stoma. It may be seen as an opening at the center, at the front and base of the neck. Some patients may have other openings in the neck from unrelated surgical procedures. You should ignore any opening other than the midline tra-

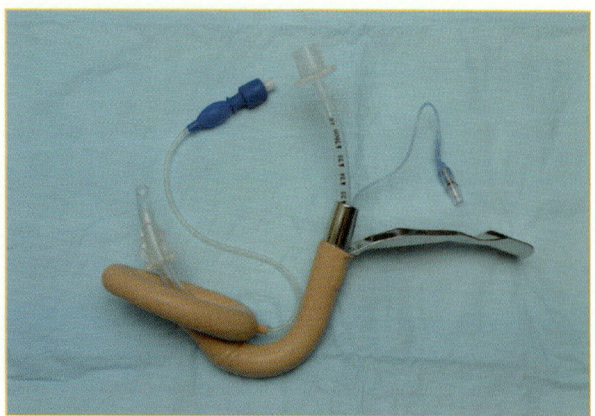

Figure 9-51 The Fasttrach LMA with a 6.0-mm ET tube.

TABLE 9-23	Comparison of Endotracheal Intubation With Nonsurgical Alternative Airway Procedures*						
	Ease of Placement	Overcoming Obstruction	Prevention of Aspiration	Oxygenation	Ventilation	Complications
Endotracheal intubation	Difficult	Excellent	Excellent	Excellent	Excellent	High
Esophageal airways (EOA/EGTA)	Moderate	Poor	Good	Good	Good	High; can be done only in deeply unconscious patients
PtL	Moderate	Poor	Good	Good	Very good	Low
Combitube	Easy	Poor	Good	Good	Very good	Low
LMA	Moderate	Poor	Poor	Very good	Excellent	Moderate

* EOA indicates esophageal obturator airway; EGTA, esophageal gastric tube airway; PtL, pharyngeotracheal lumen airway; and LMA, laryngeal mask airway.

cheal stoma. The midline opening is the only one that can be used to deliver air into the patient's lungs.

Neither the head tilt–chin lift nor the jaw-thrust maneuver is required for ventilating a patient with a stoma. If the patient has a tracheostomy tube, you should ventilate through the tube with a BVM device and 100% oxygen. If the patient has a stoma and no tube is in place, use an infant or child mask with the BVM device to make a seal over the stoma. Seal the patient's mouth and nose with one hand to prevent a leak of air up the trachea when you ventilate through a stoma. Release the seal of the patient's mouth and nose following each ventilation, allowing exhalation to occur through the upper airway.

If you are unable to ventilate a patient who has a stoma, try suctioning the stoma and the mouth with a French or soft-tip catheter before providing artificial ventilation through the mouth and nose. If you seal the stoma during ventilation, the ability to artificially ventilate the patient in this way may be improved, or it may help to clear any obstructions.

Ventilation of Stoma Patients

Mouth-to-Stoma Ventilation (Using a Resuscitation Mask)

When ventilating via mouth-to-stoma, perform the following steps (Skill Drill 9-31 ▶):

1. **Position the patient's head** in a neutral position with the shoulders slightly elevated (**Step 1**).
2. **Locate and expose the stoma site** (**Step 2**). Use of a pocket mask is preferential to protect the rescuer from blood and other body fluids.
3. **Place the resuscitation mask** (pediatric mask preferred) over the stoma, and ensure an adequate seal (**Step 3**).
4. **Maintain the patient's neutral head position**, and ventilate the patient by exhaling directly into the resuscitation mask.
5. **Assess the patient** for adequate ventilation by observing his or her chest rise and feeling for air leaks around the mask (**Step 4**).
6. **If air leakage is evident**, seal the patient's mouth and nose and ventilate (**Step 5**).

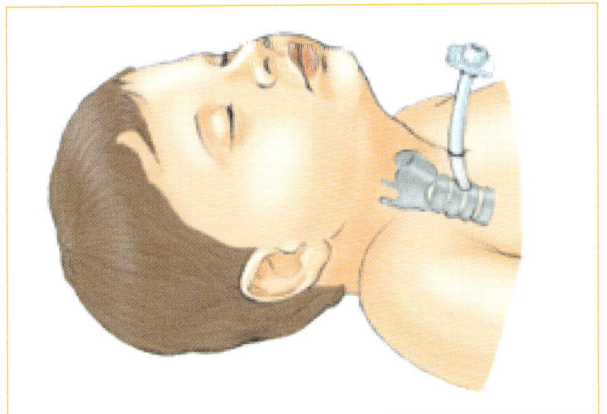

Figure 9-52 A tracheostomy tube.

Skill Drill 9-30: LMA Insertion

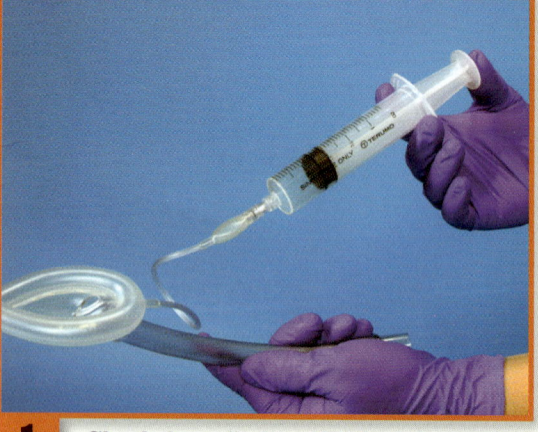

1 Check the cuff of the LMA by inflating it with 50% more air than is required for that size airway. Then deflate the cuff completely.

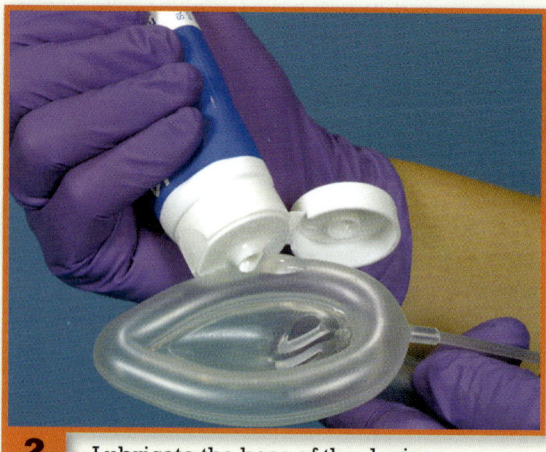

2 Lubricate the base of the device.

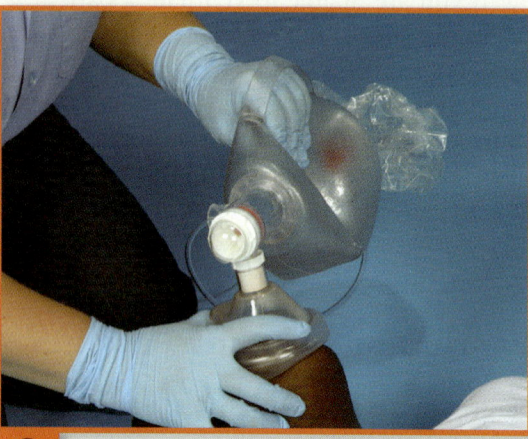

3 Preoxygenate the patient before insertion. Ventilation should not be interrupted for more than 30 seconds to accomplish airway placement. Place the patient in the sniffing position.

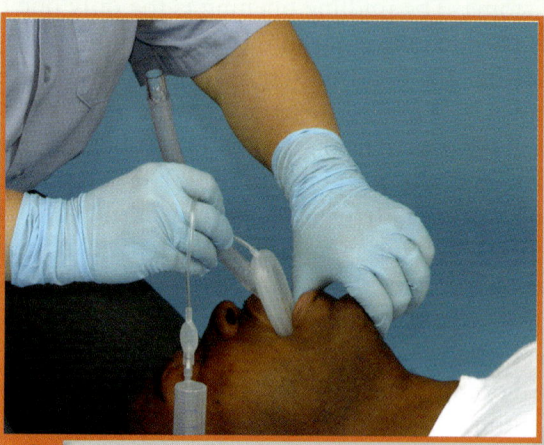

4 Lift the jaw with one hand and begin to insert the device with the other hand.

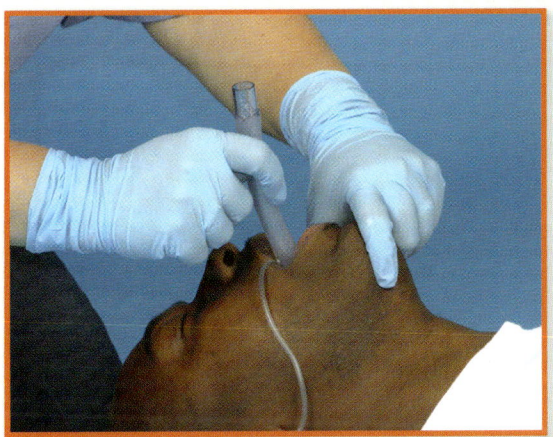

5 Insert the LMA along the roof of the mouth. Use your finger to push the airway against the hard palate.

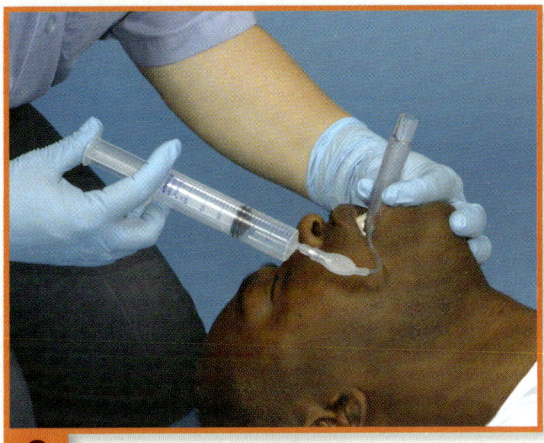

6 Inflate the cuff with the amount of air indicated for that size airway.

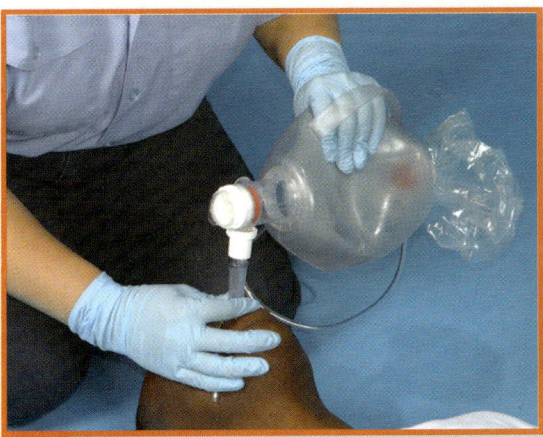

7 Begin to ventilate the patient. Confirm chest rise and the presence of breath sounds. Continuously and carefully monitor the patient.

Mouth-to-Stoma Ventilation (Using a Resuscitation Mask)

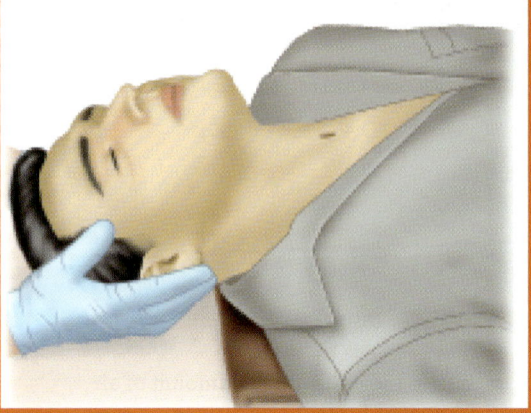

1 Position the patient's head in a neutral position with the shoulders slightly elevated.

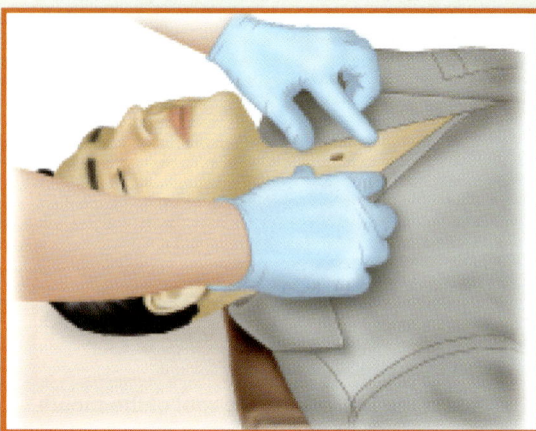

2 Locate and expose the stoma site.

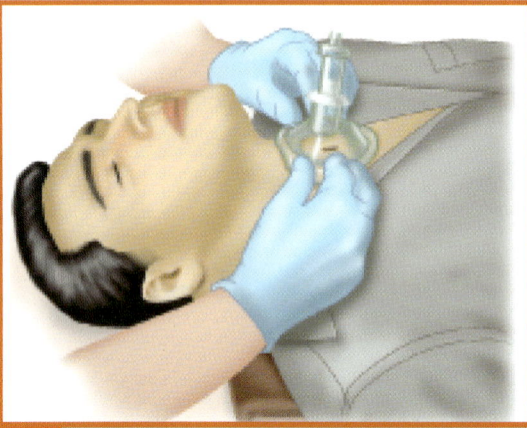

3 Place the resuscitation mask (pediatric mask preferred) over the stoma, and ensure an adequate seal.

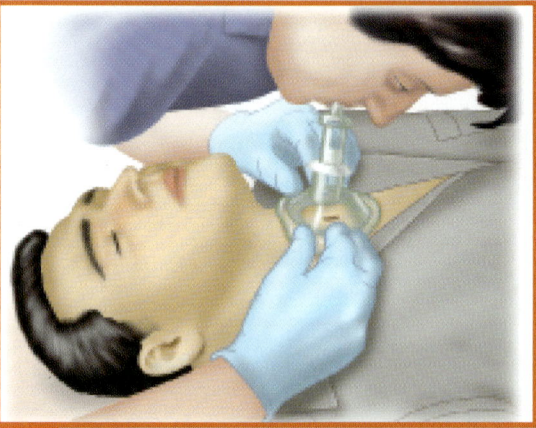

4 Maintain the patient's neutral head position, and ventilate the patient by exhaling directly into the resuscitation mask.

Assess the patient for adequate ventilation by observing his or her chest rise.

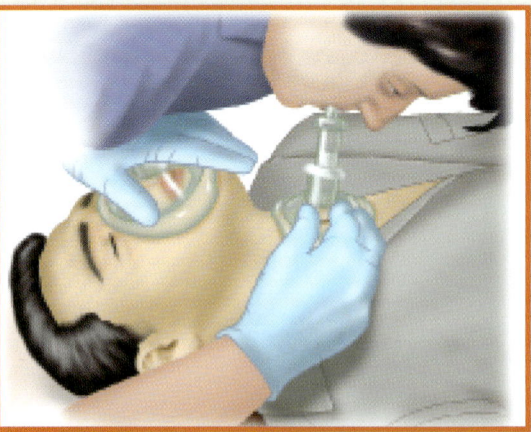

5 If air leakage is evident, seal the patient's mouth and nose and ventilate.

BVM to Stoma Ventilation

Skill Drill 9-32

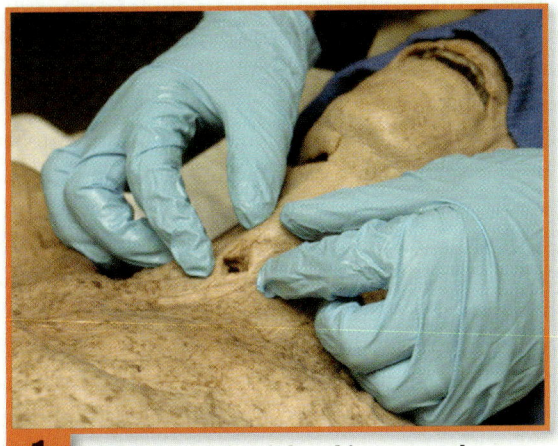

1 With the patient's head in a neutral position, locate and expose the stoma.

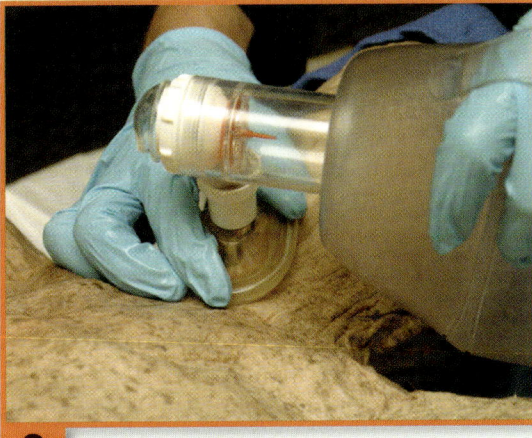

2 Place the BVM device over the stoma, and ensure an adequate seal.

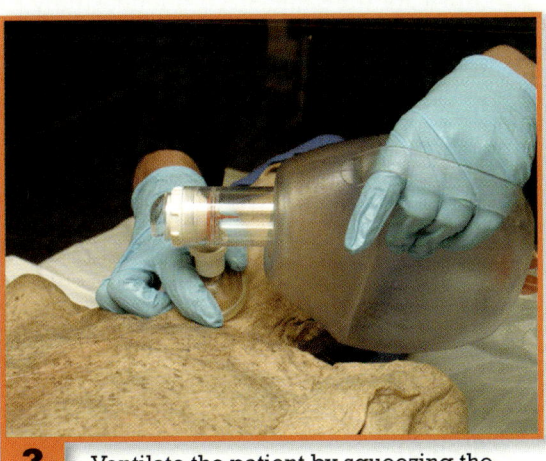

3 Ventilate the patient by squeezing the BVM device, and assess for adequate ventilation by observing chest rise.

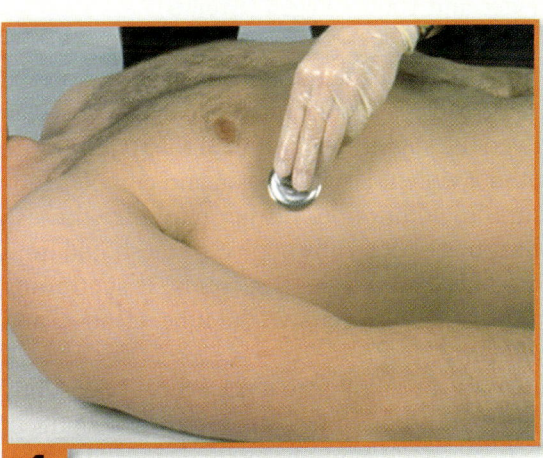

4 Auscultate over the lungs to confirm adequate ventilation.

BVM to Stoma

To perform BVM to stoma ventilation, follow the steps in (Skill Drill 9-32 ▲):

1. With the patient's head in a neutral position, **locate and expose the stoma** (**Step 1**).
2. **Place the BVM device over the stoma**, and ensure an adequate seal (**Step 2**).
3. **Ventilate the patient** by squeezing the BVM device, and assess for adequate ventilation by observing chest rise and feeling for air leaks when using a mask. Seal the mouth and nose if an air leak is evident from the upper airway (**Step 3**).
4. **Auscultate over the lungs** to confirm adequate ventilation (**Step 4**).

Special Patient Considerations

A <u>laryngectomy</u> is a surgical procedure in which the entire larynx (complete or total laryngectomy) or a portion of the larynx (partial laryngectomy) is removed, most commonly as part of the treatment for laryngeal cancer. Patients with laryngectomies have a stoma in the front of the neck, through which they breathe. Stomas affect the delivery of supplemental oxygen and airway management.

You may encounter patients who require suctioning of thick secretions from the stoma. Failure to recognize and identify these patients could result in hypoxia to the patient. It is not uncommon for the patient's stoma to become occluded with mucous plugs. Because patients with laryngectomies possess a less efficient cough, they will clearly have difficulty in spontaneously clearing the stoma themselves. Steps for suctioning a stoma are listed here and shown in (Skill Drill 9-33 ▶):

1. **Take BSI precautions** (gloves and face mask) (**Step 1**).
2. **Preoxygenate the patient** with a BVM device and 100% oxygen (**Step 2**).
3. **Inject 3 mL of sterile saline** through the stoma and into the trachea (**Step 3**).
4. **Instruct the patient to exhale**, and insert the catheter (without providing suction) until resistance is felt (no more than 12 cm) (**Step 4**).
5. **Suction** while withdrawing the catheter as you instruct the patient to cough or exhale (**Step 5**).
6. **Resume oxygenating the patient** with a BVM device and 100% oxygen (**Step 6**).

Suctioning of the patient's stoma must be performed with extreme care, especially if laryngeal edema is suspected. Even the slightest irritation of the tracheal wall can result in a violent laryngospasm and complete airway closure. In addition, to further minimize the risk of complications, specifically hypoxia, you should limit suctioning of the stoma to 10 seconds. If suctioning does not clear the tube, remove the tube, clean it, and replace it.

You may also be called on to replace the tracheostomy tube in a patient if it becomes inadvertently dislodged. When the tracheostomy tube becomes dislodged, stenosis (narrowing) of the stoma occurs, which can significantly impair the patient's ventilatory ability. Stenosis is potentially life threatening because soft tissue swelling decreases the stoma diameter. In such cases, you may not be able to replace the tracheostomy tube itself and may have to insert an ET tube into the stoma before it becomes totally occluded. Regardless of whether the stoma requires suctioning or the tracheostomy tube needs to be reinserted, the EMT-I must be prepared to take immediate action to minimize further compromise of oxygenation and ventilation. You must also consider the fact that the patient with the stoma has the device because of a significant medical problem (such as brain injury, chronic respiratory insufficiency), which means that the patient may be less tolerant of even brief periods of hypoxia. Steps for replacing a dislodged tracheostomy tube are listed here and shown in (Skill Drill 9-34 ▶):

1. **Take BSI precautions** (gloves and face mask) (**Step 1**).
2. **Lubricate** the same-sized tracheostomy tube or an ET tube (at least 5.0 mm) (**Step 2**).
3. **Instruct the patient to exhale**, and gently insert the tube approximately 1 to 2 cm beyond the balloon cuff (**Step 3**).
4. **Inflate the balloon cuff** (**Step 4**).
5. **Ensure that the patient is comfortable**, and confirm patency and proper placement of the tube by listening for air movement from the tube and noting the patient's clinical status. Ensure that a false lumen was not created (**Step 5**).
6. **Auscultate the lungs** to confirm tube placement (**Step 6**).

Suctioning of a Stoma

Skill Drill 9-33

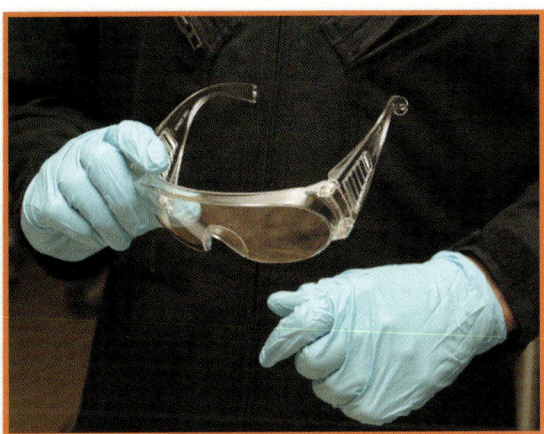
1 Take BSI precautions (gloves and face mask).

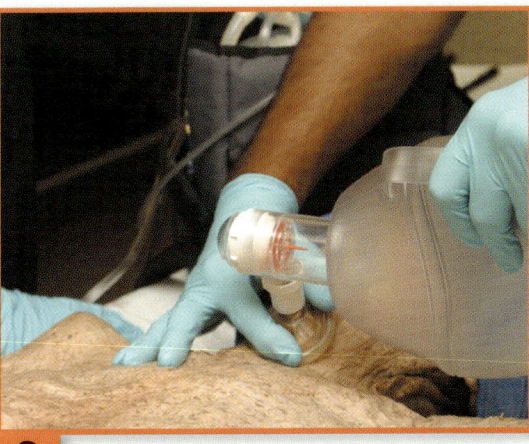
2 Preoxygenate the patient with a BVM device and 100% oxygen.

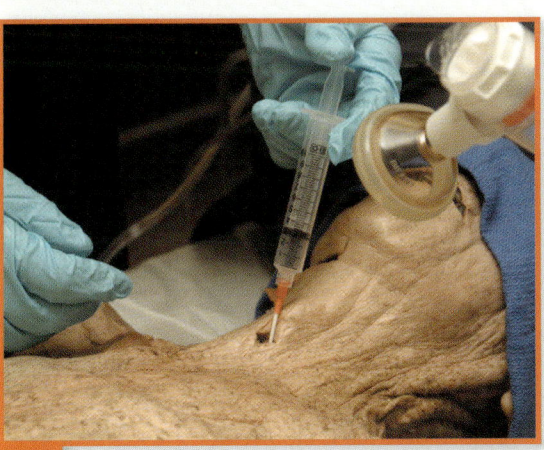
3 Inject 3 mL of sterile saline through the stoma and into the trachea.

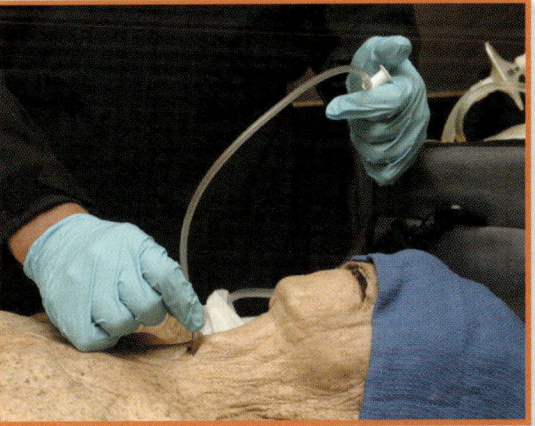
4 Instruct the patient to exhale, and insert the catheter (without providing suction) until resistance is felt (no more than 12 cm).

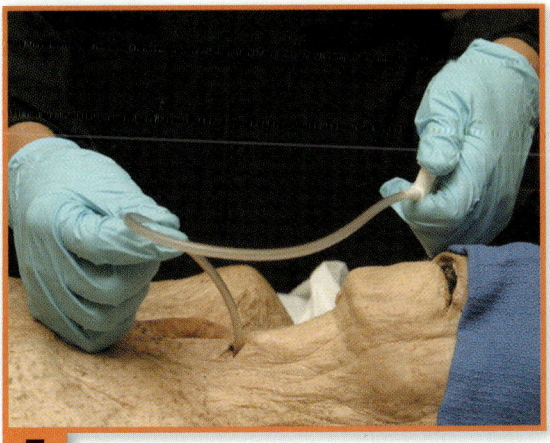
5 Suction while withdrawing the catheter as you instruct the patient to cough or exhale.

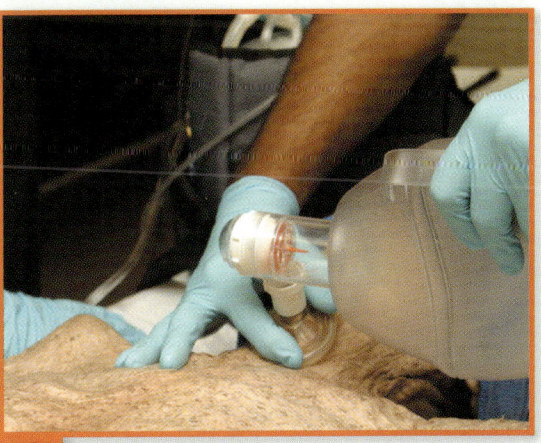
6 Resume oxygenating the patient with a BVM device and 100% oxygen.

Replacing a Dislodged Tracheostomy Tube

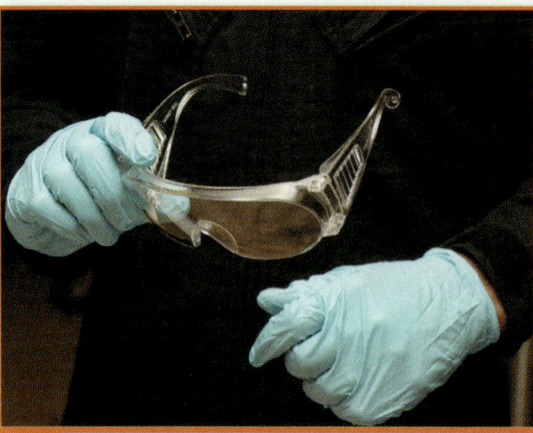

1 Take BSI precautions (gloves and face mask).

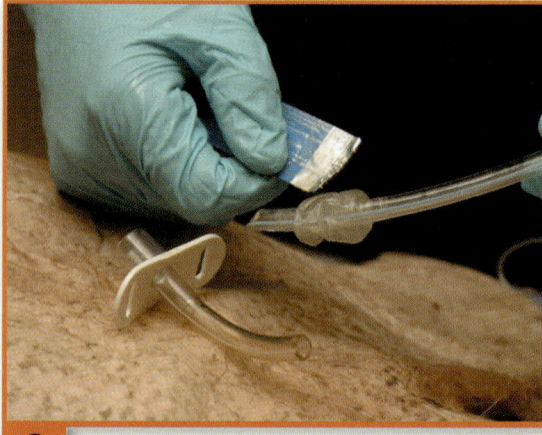

2 Lubricate the same-sized tracheostomy tube or an ET tube (at least 5.0 mm).

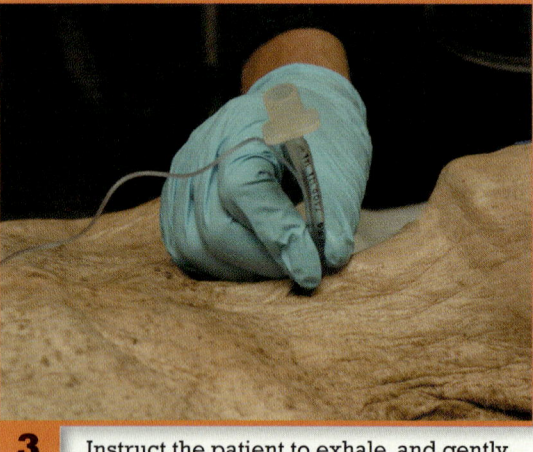

3 Instruct the patient to exhale, and gently insert the tube approximately 1 to 2 cm beyond the balloon cuff.

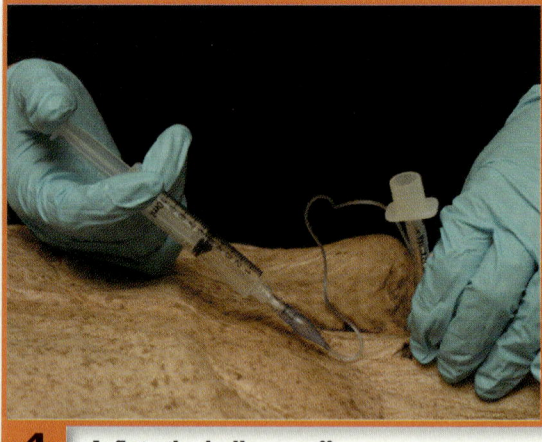

4 Inflate the balloon cuff.

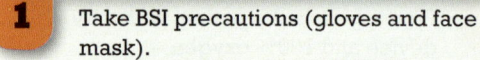

5 Ensure that the patient is comfortable, and confirm patency and proper placement of the tube by listening for air movement from the tube and noting the patient's clinical status. Ensure that a false lumen was not created.

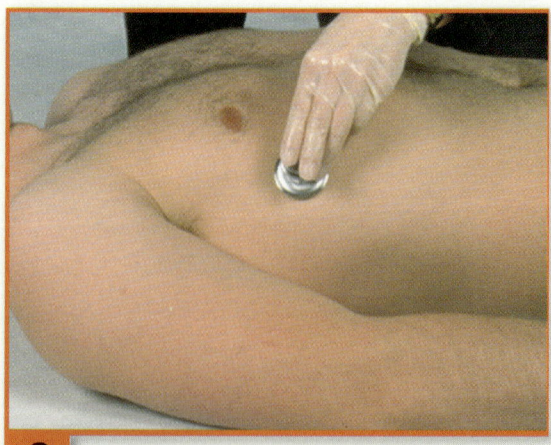

6 Auscultate the lungs to confirm tube placement.

You are the Provider

1. Why do airway and breathing assessment and care have such a prominent position in the realm of an EMT-I's scope of practice?

Because the single most important steps in caring for any patient are to ensure a patent airway and that the patient is breathing adequately. Without an airway, the patient will die. All organs, body tissues, and cells require a constant supply of oxygen to survive. Within seconds of being deprived of oxygen, vital body organs may not function normally.

2. Why is it necessary that you be familiar with all the airway equipment on your ambulance?

The use of artificial airway equipment can cause harm to the patient if not used properly by the EMT-I. Airway skills are often the most neglected skills. Poor technique on the part of the EMT-I can result in ineffective ventilation and inadequate care.

3. What is your priority of care for this patient? Why?

After ensuring a patent airway, you must administer 100% oxygen to the patient, who has signs and symptoms of significant hypoxemia. Oxygen should be administered as soon as possible to any patient with respiratory distress.

4. This patient is in obvious respiratory distress. What are some of the causes of respiratory distress that must be considered by the EMT-I?

Respiratory distress may be the result of upper and/or lower airway obstruction, inadequate ventilation, impairment of the respiratory muscles, or impairment of the nervous system.

Summary

5. What signs of respiratory distress should the EMT-I look for?

How is the patient positioned?
Is he or she in a tripod position?
Does breathing appear to be orthopneic (positional)?
Is there adequate rise and fall of the chest?
Do you note any gasping?
What is the color of the skin?
Is there any flaring of the nares?
Are the lips pursed?
Do you note any retractions?

- Intercostal
- Suprasternal notch
- Supraclavicular fossa
- Subcostal

Next, auscultate breathing with and without a stethoscope. Is air movement noted at the mouth and nose? Can equal and bilateral breath sounds be heard over all lung fields?

Finally, feel for air movement at the mouth and nose. Palpate the chest for symmetry and paradoxical motion.

6. What is your rationale for administering 100% oxygen to a COPD patient?

With COPD, the rising carbon dioxide levels no longer stimulate the patient to breathe; the stimulus to breathe is now based on low arterial oxygen levels. In rare cases, the administration of high-flow oxygen may suppress the patient's respiratory drive. Nevertheless, you must always administer 100% oxygen to any patient—whether or not the patient has COPD—who presents with respiratory distress and signs of hypoxemia. If the COPD patient's respirations become depressed or cease altogether, simply provide positive-pressure ventilation with a BVM device and 100% oxygen.

Continued

You are the Provider continued   Summary

7. What intervention should the EMT-I consider next?

Patients who are not breathing need artificial ventilation and supplemental oxygen. The same is true of patients who are breathing inadequately; that is, fewer than 12 breaths/min or more than 20 breaths/min with poor tidal volume or an irregular pattern of breathing. Keep in mind that fast, shallow breathing can be as dangerous as very slow breathing. Fast, shallow breathing moves air primarily in the larger airway passages (dead air space) and does not allow for adequate exchange of oxygen and carbon dioxide in the alveoli. Patients with inadequate breathing require assisted ventilation. Once you determine that a patient is not breathing or needs assisted ventilation, you should begin artificial ventilation immediately. With a patient who is not breathing, there are several ways to do this, some of which require equipment. The methods that an EMT-I may use to provide artificial ventilation include the one- or two-person BVM device; mouth-to-mouth, mouth-to-nose, and mouth-to-mask ventilation; and the flow-restricted, oxygen-powered ventilation device.

8. What must the EMT-I do next to maintain airway patency?

You must keep the airway clear so that you can ventilate the patient properly. If the airway is not clear, you will force secretions and other material (such as blood) into the lungs, further compromising oxygenation and ventilation. Therefore, suctioning is your next priority. If you have any doubt about the situation, remember this rule: If you hear gurgling, the patient needs suctioning!

9. What is the method you should use to determine the appropriate size of suction catheter?

Before you insert a suction catheter into the patient's mouth, you must make sure to measure for the proper size. This is accomplished by measuring from the corner of the mouth to the earlobe or angle of the jaw.

10. How long should you suction?

Suctioning Time Limits:
Adult   15 seconds
Child   10 seconds
Infant   5 seconds

11. What is the next step to be considered in managing the airway of this patient?

Because the patient is now unconscious and apneic, her airway must be secured definitively to prevent aspiration and to ensure the delivery of 100% oxygen directly into the lungs. Therefore, endotracheal intubation is indicated.

12. What are the indications for intubation?

- Present or impending respiratory failure
- Apnea
- Failure to protect own airway

13. What is the definition of ventilation?

Ventilation is the movement of air into and out of the lungs, either spontaneously by the patient (negative pressure ventilation) or with assistance from an EMT-I (positive pressure ventilation).

Prep Kit

Ready for Review

- The respiratory system includes the diaphragm, the muscles of the chest wall, and the accessory muscles of breathing.
- The term "airway" usually means the upper airway, which includes the respiratory structures above the vocal cords.
- Clearing the airway means removing obstructing material; maintaining the airway means keeping it open.
- Patients who are breathing inadequately show signs of hypoxia, a dangerous condition in which the body's tissues and cells do not have enough oxygen.
- Adequate breathing features a normal rate of 12 to 20 breaths/min, a regular pattern of inhalation and exhalation, bilateral clear and equal lung sounds, regular and equal chest rise and fall, and adequate tidal volume.
- Patients with inadequate breathing need to be treated immediately. Emergency medical care includes airway management, supplemental oxygen, and ventilatory support.
- Basic techniques for opening the airway include the head tilt–chin lift maneuver and the jaw-thrust maneuver.
- One basic airway adjunct is the oropharyngeal or oral airway, which keeps the tongue from blocking the airway in unresponsive patients with no gag reflex. If the oral airway is not the proper size or is inserted incorrectly, it can actually push the tongue back into the pharynx, causing an obstruction.
- Another basic airway adjunct is the nasopharyngeal or nasal airway, which is usually used with patients who have a gag reflex.
- Suctioning is the next priority after opening the airway. Rigid tonsil tips are the best catheters to use when suctioning the pharynx; soft, plastic catheters are used to suction the nose and liquid secretions in the back of the mouth.
- The recovery position is used to help maintain the airway in patients without traumatic injuries who are breathing adequately on their own.
- You should always give supplemental oxygen to patients who are not breathing on their own or who have inadequate breathing. Handle compressed gas cylinders very carefully; their contents are under pressure.
- Always make sure the correct pressure regulator is firmly attached before transporting a cylinder.
- The pin-indexing safety system features a series of pins on a yoke that must be matched with the holes on the valve stem of the gas cylinder.
- Pressure regulators reduce the pressure of gas in an oxygen cylinder to between 40 and 70 psi. Pressure-compensated flowmeters and Bourdon-gauge flowmeters permit the regulated release of gas measured in liters per minute.
- When oxygen therapy is complete, disconnect the tubing from the flowmeter nipple and turn off the cylinder valve, then turn off the flowmeter. As long as there is a pressure reading on the regulator gauge, it is not safe to remove the regulator from the valve stem.
- Keep any possible source of fire away from the area while oxygen is in use.
- Nasal cannulas and the far more effective nonrebreathing masks are used most often to deliver oxygen in the field; always try to use the latter with patients you suspect may have hypoxia. Nonrebreathing masks can provide more than 90% inspired oxygen.
- Pulse oximetry, an assessment tool to evaluate the effectiveness of oxygenation, does not take the place of a good assessment. This measurement depends on adequate perfusion to the capillary beds and is inaccurate when the patient is cold or in shock or has been exposed to carbon monoxide.

Technology

- Interactivities
- Vocabulary Explorer
- Anatomy Review
- Web Links
- Online Review Manual

www.EMSzone.com/EMTT

Prep Kit Continued...

- The methods of providing artificial ventilation include a one-, two-, and three-person BVM device, mouth-to-mask ventilation, and a flow-restricted, oxygen-powered ventilation device. The flow-restricted, oxygen-powered ventilation device, however, is not a recommended ventilation device by many standards.
- Combined with your own exhaled breath, mouth-to-mask ventilation with supplemental oxygen attached will give your patient up to 55% oxygen; a BVM device with an oxygen reservoir can deliver nearly 100% oxygen.
- Patients with altered mental status or those who are unable to maintain their own airway should be considered candidates for definitive airway management. These devices include esophageal airways, multilumen airways, and endotracheal tubes.
- It is imperative to be familiar with indications, contraindications, advantages, disadvantages, and special considerations when choosing the appropriate device. This is especially important when dealing with pediatric patients. Regardless of the method, aggressive airway management is essential to a positive patient outcome.
- When you are providing artificial ventilation, remember that ventilating too forcefully can cause gastric distention. Delivering each breath over 1 second and using cricoid pressure can help to prevent gastric distention.
- Also consider patients who have a tracheal stoma or a tracheostomy tube. You will need to ventilate these patients through the tube or the stoma.
- Foreign body airway obstruction usually occurs during a meal in an adult or while a child is eating, playing with small objects, or crawling about the house.
- The earlier you recognize any airway obstruction, the better. You must learn to recognize the difference between airway obstruction caused by a foreign object and that caused by a medical condition.
- The Heimlich maneuver should be performed to remove a severe airway obstruction in a conscious child or adult.
- Treat patients with a severe airway obstruction by alternating between chest compressions and attempts to ventilate. Patients with mild airway obstruction should be closely monitored.
- Check for loose dental appliances in a patient before assisting ventilation. Loose appliances should be removed to prevent them from obstructing the airway.

Vital Vocabulary

acid Any molecule that gives up a hydrogen ion; often referred to as H^+.

agonal respirations Occasional, gasping breaths that occur after the heart has stopped.

airway The upper airway tract or the passage above the larynx, which includes the nose, mouth, and throat. Also used to refer to devices used to open and maintain a patient's airway.

alcoholic ketoacidosis The metabolic acidotic state that manifests from the poor nutritional habits of chronic alcohol abuse. Both the liver and the body experience inadequate fuel reserves of glycogen and, thus, have to switch to fatty acid metabolism.

alveolar air The amount of gas that reaches the alveoli with each breath.

American Standard System A safety system for oxygen cylinders larger than size E, designed to prevent the accidental attachment of a regulator to a cylinder containing the wrong type of gas.

apnea Absence of breathing; periods of not breathing.

aspiration The introduction of vomit or other foreign material into the lungs.

atelectasis A condition of airless or collapsed alveoli that causes pulmonary shunting, ventilation-perfusion mismatching, and possibly hypoxemia.

atlanto-occipital joint The joint formed at the articulation of the atlas of the vertebral column and the occipital bone of the skull.

automatic transport ventilator (ATV) A mechanical ventilator that is used to ventilate the intubated patient during transport; has settings for the tidal volume and ventilatory rate.

bag-valve-mask (BVM) device A device with a face mask attached to a ventilation bag containing a reservoir and connected to oxygen; delivers more than 90% supplemental oxygen.

barrier device A protective item, such as a pocket mask with a valve, that limits exposure to a patient's body fluids.

base Any molecule that can accept a hydrogen ion; often referred to as OH⁻.

bilateral A body part or condition that appears on both sides of the midline.

bradypnea Slow respiratory rate.

bronchioles Small airways made of smooth muscle that lead to the alveoli.

BURP maneuver Acronym for **B**ackward, **U**pward, and **R**ightward **P**ressure.

capnographer A device used to confirm ET tube placement that contains colorimetric paper, which should turn yellow during exhalation, indicating proper tube placement.

capnometer A device used to confirm ET tube placement that provides an LED readout of the patient's exhaled carbon dioxide, indicating proper tube placement.

cardiac dysrhythmia An abnormal cardiac rhythm.

central nervous system (CNS) depression The slowing of the nervous system function of the brain secondary to delays in nerve cell transmission. Several factors can influence CNS depression, including nerve cell permeability, hypoxia, drugs, and injury.

cerebral perfusion The ability of fluid to move from cerebral circulation to cerebral tissue, carrying oxygen and nutrients to the cells.

cerebral vasodilation Enlargement of cerebral blood vessels.

chemoreceptors Peripheral and central receptors that monitor the levels of chemicals in the blood.

Combitube A dual-lumen airway device that is inserted blindly. You can ventilate the patient whether the tube is placed in the esophagus or the trachea.

cricoid pressure Application of pressure on the cricoid cartilage to inhibit gastric distention and aspiration of vomitus in an unresponsive patient.

dead space The amount of inhaled air that does not participate in respiration.

diffusion A process in which molecules move from an area of higher concentration of molecules to an area of lower concentration.

direct laryngoscopy A technique to accomplish endotracheal intubation by visualizing the glottic opening with the aid of a laryngoscope.

dissociate To lose a hydrogen atom in the presence of water. Acids are classified as strong or weak, depending on how completely they dissociate in water.

dyspnea Shortness of breath or difficulty breathing.

endotracheal intubation Placement of a tube into the trachea.

endotracheal tube A tube designed to be placed into the trachea for the purpose of airway management, ventilatory control, and/or medication delivery.

esophageal gastric tube airway (EGTA) An esophageal airway device that is designed to occlude the esophagus, thus preventing regurgitation; allows for gastric decompression.

esophageal intubation The placement of a tube into the esophagus. When discussed in the context of airway management, this usually refers to the misplacement of a tube intended for the trachea into the esophagus.

esophageal obturator airway (EOA) The original esophageal airway that is no longer manufactured or used because it does not allow for decompression of the stomach before the EOA is removed; replaced by the esophageal gastric tube airway (EGTA).

exhalation The part of the breathing process in which the diaphragm and the intercostal muscles relax, forcing air out of the lungs.

expiration The process of moving air out of the lungs.

expiratory reserve volume The amount of air that can be exhaled following normal exhalation.

extubation The process of removing the tube from an intubated patient.

flow-restricted, oxygen-powered ventilation device (FROPVD) A manually triggered ventilation device that can be used for apneic patients and breathing patients; delivers a high volume and concentration of oxygen at 40 L/min.

functional reserve capacity The amount of air that can be forced from the lungs in a single forced exhalation.

gag reflex A normal reflex mechanism that causes retching; activated by touching the soft palate or the back of the throat.

gastric decompression The removal of air and other contents from the stomach.

Prep Kit Continued...

gastric distention A condition in which air fills the stomach as a result of high volume and pressure during artificial ventilation.

gastric tube A tube placed into the stomach.

glottic opening The narrowest portion of the adult's airway; space between the vocal cords.

gum bougie A device that is placed between the vocal cords under direct laryngoscopy. The endotracheal tube is then advanced over the gum bougie and into the trachea. This device is useful when you are unable to obtain a full view of the glottic opening.

head tilt–chin lift maneuver A combination of two movements to open the airway by tilting the forehead back and lifting the chin; used for nontrauma patients.

heat cramps Painful muscle spasms usually associated with vigorous activity in a hot environment.

Hering-Breuer reflex The nervous system mechanism that terminates inhalation and prevents lung overexpansion.

hyperventilation An increased amount of air entering the alveoli, which lowers blood carbon dioxide levels and usually is a result of rapid or deep breathing.

hypoperfusion A condition that develops when the circulatory system is not able to deliver sufficient blood and oxygen to body organs, resulting in organ failure and eventual death if untreated.

hypoxemia A deficiency of oxygen in arterial blood.

hypoxia A dangerous condition in which the body's tissues and cells do not have enough oxygen.

hypoxic drive A backup system to control respirations when oxygen levels fall.

inhalation The active, muscular part of breathing that draws air into the airway and lungs.

inspiration The process of moving air into the lungs.

inspiratory reserve volume The maximum amount of air that can be forcefully inhaled following a full inhalation.

ischemia A lack of oxygen that deprives tissues of necessary nutrients.

jaw-thrust maneuver Technique to open the airway by placing the fingers behind the angle of the jaw and bringing the jaw forward; used when a patient may have a cervical spine injury.

ketoacidosis An acidotic state created by the production of ketones via fat metabolism.

ketones The by-products of fat metabolism secondary to the use of fatty acids rather than glucose by body cells. An excess of ketones can lead to ketoacidosis.

lactic acidosis The metabolic acidotic state resulting from the accumulation of lactic acid secondary to anaerobic cellular metabolism.

laryngeal mask airway (LMA) An airway device that is inserted into the mouth blindly and comes to rest at the glottic opening. A flexible cuff is inflated, creating an almost airtight seal.

laryngectomy A surgical procedure in which all of the larynx (complete or total laryngectomy) or a portion of the larynx (partial laryngectomy) is removed.

laryngospasm The spasmodic contraction of the vocal cords, accompanied by an enfolding of the arytenoid and aryepiglottic folds.

larynx A complex structure formed by the epiglottis, thyroid cartilage, the cricoid cartilage, the arytenoid cartilage, the corniculate cartilage, and the cuneiform cartilage.

lung compliance The ability of the alveoli to fully expand when air is drawn in on inhalation.

metabolic acidosis A metabolic state of acidosis resulting from retention of H^+ or other positively charged ions not related to respiratory compromise.

metabolism The chemical processes that provide the cells with energy from nutrients.

mild airway obstruction A condition in which an obstruction leaves the patient able to exchange some air, but also causes some degree of respiratory distress.

minute volume The amount of air moved in and out of the respiratory tract per minute, which is determined by the tidal volume multiplied by the respiratory rate.

multilumen airways Airway devices with a single long tube that can be used for esophageal obturation or endotracheal tube ventilation, depending on where it comes to rest following blind positioning.

Murphy's eye The opening on the side of the endotracheal tube at its distal end; prevents occlusion of the tube with secretions.

nasal cannula An oxygen-delivery device in which oxygen flows through two small, tubelike prongs that fit into the patient's nostrils.

nasogastric (NG) tube A tube placed into the stomach through the nose.

nasopharyngeal (nasal) airway An airway adjunct inserted into the nostril of a conscious patient who is not able to maintain a natural airway.

neural permeability The rate at which a nerve cell permits calcium to cross its cell membrane. Accelerated rates of calcium absorption lead to rapid, continual nerve impulse transmission, whereas decelerated rates of calcium absorption lead to decreased nerve impulse transmission.

neural transmission The speed at which an impulse travels through the nerve cell. The rate of transmission is directly related to neural permeability.

nonrebreathing mask A combination mask and reservoir bag system that is the preferred way to give oxygen in the prehospital setting; delivers up to 90% inspired oxygen.

obturator A device that closes or blocks an opening.

orogastric (OG) tube A tube placed into the stomach through the mouth.

oropharyngeal (oral) airway An airway adjunct inserted into the mouth to keep the tongue from blocking the upper airway and to make suctioning the airway easier.

pH A measure of acidity of a solution.

pharyngotracheal lumen airway (PtL) A dual-lumen airway device that is inserted blindly into the mouth. The patient can be ventilated whether the tube is placed in the esophagus or into the trachea.

pin-indexing system A system established for portable cylinders to ensure that a regulator is not connected to a cylinder containing the wrong type of gas.

pneumothorax A partial or complete accumulation of air in the pleural space.

pulmonary edema A buildup of fluid in the lungs, usually as a result of congestive heart failure.

pulse oximetry An assessment method that measures the oxygen saturation of hemoglobin in the capillary beds.

recovery position A side-lying position used to maintain a clear airway in patients without injuries.

residual volume The air that remains in the lungs after a maximal expiration.

respiration The process of exchanging oxygen and carbon dioxide.

respiratory alkalosis A metabolic state of alkalosis resulting from excessive losses of carbon dioxide secondary to hyperventilation.

respiratory rate The number of ventilatory cycles in a unit of time, usually 1 minute; also known as the ventilation rate.

retractions Movements in which the skin pulls in around the ribs during inspiration.

Sellick maneuver A technique that is used to prevent gastric distention in which pressure is applied on the cricoid cartilage.

severe airway obstruction Occurs when a foreign body completely obstructs the patient's airway. Patients cannot breathe, talk, or cough.

stenosis Abnormal narrowing of a structure, such as a stoma.

stoma A surgical opening in the body that connects an internal structure to the skin, such as a stoma in the neck that connects the trachea directly to the skin.

suction catheter A hollow, cylindrical device used to remove fluids and secretions from the airway.

surfactant The proteinaceous substance that lines the inside of the alveoli and allows for easy expansion and recoil of the alveoli.

tidal volume The amount of air moved during one breath.

tongue-jaw lift maneuver A method of opening the airway for suctioning or placing an oral airway; involves grasping the incisors or gums and lifting the jaw.

Prep Kit Continued...

tonsil tips Large, semirigid suction tips recommended for suctioning the pharynx; also called Yankauer tips.

tracheostomy Surgical creation of a hole in the trachea.

tracheostomy tube A tube that goes through the hole created by a tracheostomy.

turbinates Bony shelves that extend from the lateral walls of the nose into the nasal passageway; increases the surface area of the nasal mucosa, improving filtration, warming, and humidification of inhaled air.

vallecula The anatomic space between the base of the tongue and the epiglottis. An important landmark for endotracheal intubation.

ventilation The exchange of air between the lungs and the air of the environment, spontaneously by the patient or with assistance from an EMT-I.

Assessment in Action

You are dispatched to an "unconscious female" at an office building. About 7 minutes later, you pull up in front of the office building and are escorted to the patient.

You arrive at the patient's side, and you determine she is unresponsive. You hear snoring respirations and notice that her skin is cyanotic. You open the patient's airway and assess her breathing. You also note that she has a strong, bounding pulse. Your partner is trying to obtain a history, but her coworkers state they just found her on the floor next to her desk.

1. The structure(s) of the upper airway that often causes snoring respirations in the unresponsive patient is (are) the:
   A. larynx.
   B. tongue.
   C. uvula.
   D. vocal cords.

2. What part of the nasal passage is responsible for the filtering of air that is inhaled?
   A. Cilia
   B. Turbinates
   C. Nasopharynx
   D. Adenoids

3. All of the following are poor techniques for effective ventilation, EXCEPT:
   A. unproductive seal.
   B. improper positioning of airway.
   C. use of two or three providers to ventilate a patient.
   D. failure to reassess the patient frequently.

4. The stimulus to breathe comes from the respiratory center, located in the:
   A. heart.
   B. spinal cord.
   C. brainstem.
   D. diaphragm.

5. The normal breathing rate in an adult patient is:
   A. 6 to 10 times per minute.
   B. 10 to 12 times per minute.
   C. 12 to 20 times per minute.
   D. 20 to 26 times per minute.

6. The normal pH for the body to function is:
   A. 6.25–6.45.
   B. 7.10–7.20.
   C. 7.35–7.45.
   D. 7.55–8.10.

7. A patient with respiratory difficulty may rapidly develop:
   A. respiratory alkalosis.
   B. respiratory acidosis.
   C. metabolic acidosis.
   D. metabolic alkalosis.

8. The most common cause of respiratory alkalosis is:
   A. hypoventilation.
   B. apnea.
   C. hypoxia.
   D. hyperventilation.

9. The chemoreceptors in the brain sense the rising levels of _____ and signal the respiratory center to increase ventilations.
   A. H^+
   B. CO_2
   C. carbonic acid
   D. H_2O

10. The term hypoxemia means:
    A. lack of oxygen.
    B. too little oxygen in the blood.
    C. lack of carbon dioxide.
    D. too much oxygen in the blood.

11. The appropriate oxygen-delivery device for a patient with poor chest excursion is the:
    A. nasal cannula.
    B. simple face mask.
    C. nonrebreathing mask.
    D. BVM device with reservoir.

Assessment in Action

12. When delivering oxygen to a pediatric patient, the minimum tidal volume to be used for full-term neonates and infants is:
    A. 200 mL.
    B. 450 mL.
    C. 500 mL.
    D. 800 mL.

13. The exchange of gases between a living organism and its environment is called:
    A. inspiration.
    B. respiration.
    C. ventilation.
    D. expiration.

14. A condition that reduces the surface area for gas exchange owing to air inside the pleural cavity is called:
    A. hemothorax.
    B. COPD.
    C. pneumothorax.
    D. hemopneumothorax.

15. Two major components of air include 79% nitrogen and:
    A. 16% oxygen.
    B. 4% oxygen.
    C. 21% oxygen.
    D. 24% oxygen

16. The most common cause of airway obstruction in an unresponsive patient is:
    A. epiglottis.
    B. tongue.
    C. food.
    D. fluids.

17. When performing the Sellick maneuver, you are compressing the:
    A. thyroid.
    B. hyoid.
    C. cricoid.
    D. epiglottis.

18. The alveoli in the lungs are lined with a substance known as:
    A. surfactant.
    B. synovial fluid.
    C. sebaceous fluid.
    D. cerebrospinal fluid.

19. A condition that results when the alveoli collapse is known as:
    A. pneumothorax.
    B. atelectasis.
    C. effusion.
    D. diffusion.

20. The primary objective of emergency care is to:
    A. assess and provide definitive care.
    B. ensure optimal ventilation to facilitate the delivery of oxygen and elimination of carbon dioxide.
    C. perform endotracheal intubation to assure direct access for ventilation.
    D. ensure optimal ventilation to facilitate the delivery of carbon dioxide and the elimination of oxygen.

21. The air that remains in the lungs after maximal expiration is called:
    A. expiratory reserve volume.
    B. inspiratory reserve volume.
    C. functional reserve capacity.
    D. residual volume.

22. A form of respiratory breathing in which there is an irregular pattern, rate, and volume with intermittent periods of apnea resulting from increased intracranial pressure is called:
    A. Cheyne-Stokes.
    B. Kussmaul.
    C. Biot.
    D. agonal.

23. All of the following are major components of the buffer systems found in the body, EXCEPT:

    A. bicarbonate.
    B. metabolic.
    C. respiratory.
    D. renal.

24. An invasive gastric decompression involves inserting a tube called:

    A. Combitube.
    B. esophageal obturator airway.
    C. a nasal or oral gastric tube.
    D. French tip catheter.

25. A condition in which the systolic blood pressure drops more than 10 mm Hg with inspiration is called:

    A. pulse pressure.
    B. pulsus paradoxus.
    C. cardiac tamponade.
    D. paradoxical hypotension.

Points to Ponder

You are dispatched to a motor vehicle collision. On arrival you find a patient lying next to a vehicle. According to bystanders, the driver had gotten out of the car and then collapsed. You assess the patient and determine that he is breathing and has a pulse. You administer high-flow oxygen and continue to evaluate him. As you prepare to position the patient on a long board, your partner tells you the patient is turning blue. While placing the patient on the backboard, you notice that he has shallow respirations. Also, despite the high-flow oxygen, the patient's oxygen saturation reads 90%. What is the problem with this patient's condition?

Issues: Maintaining Adequate Oxygenation and Ventilation; High-flow Oxygen Needs and Adequate Tidal Volume; Letting the Patient's Condition, Not the Pulse Oximeter Reading, Guide Your Treatment

Patient Assessment

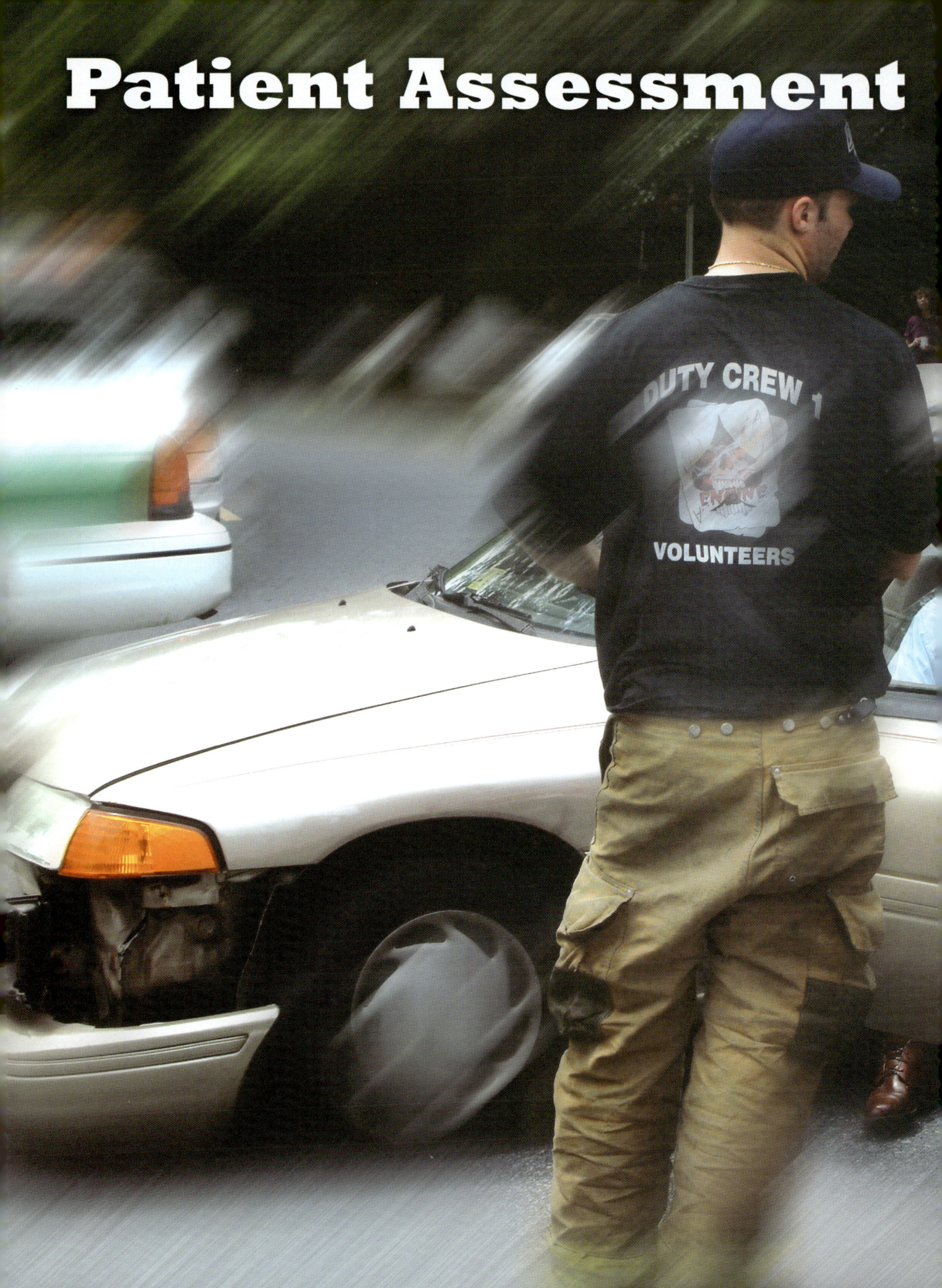

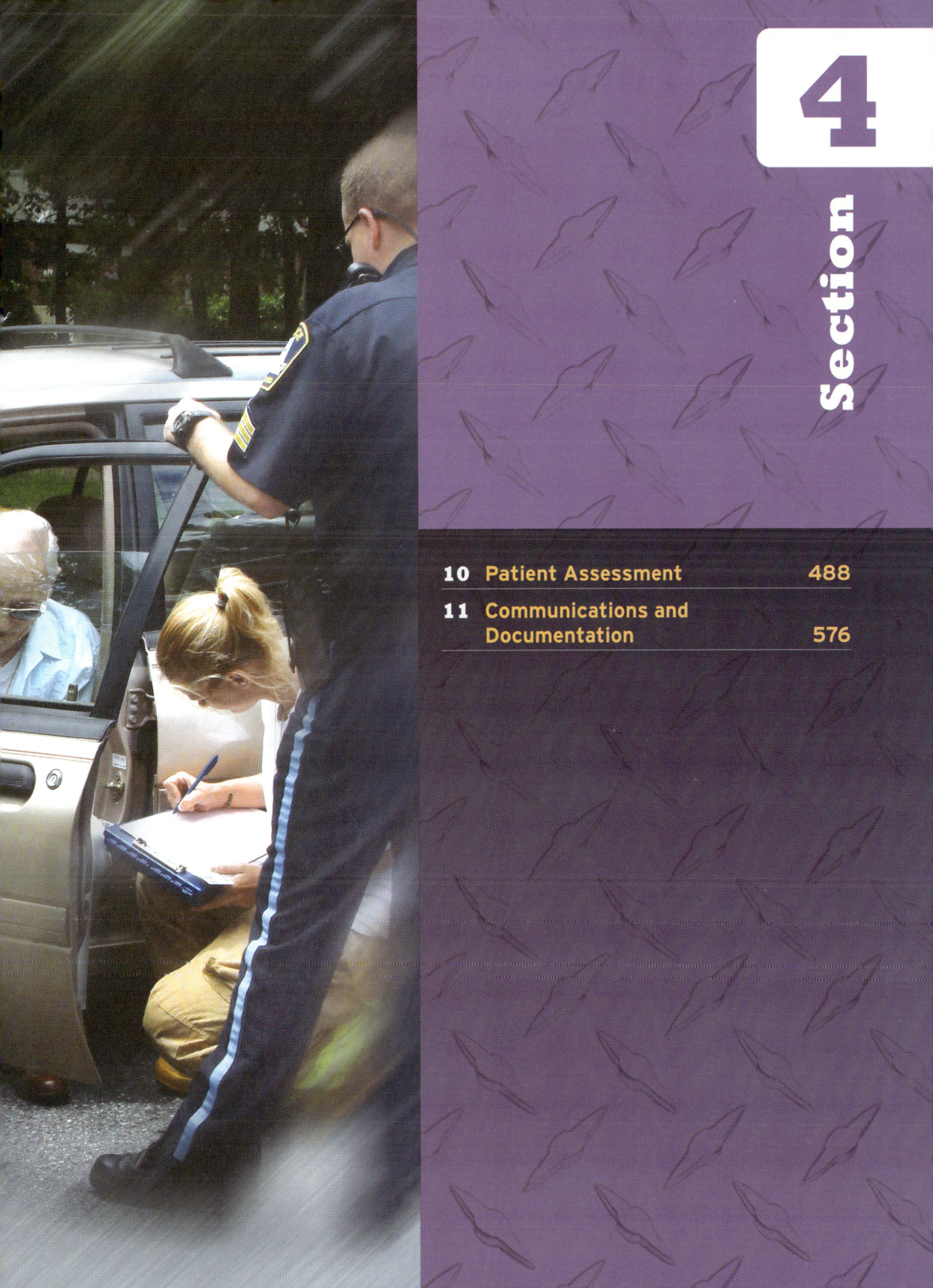

Section 4

| 10 | Patient Assessment | 488 |
| 11 | Communications and Documentation | 576 |

Patient Assessment

1999 Objectives

Scene Size-up
Cognitive

- 3-3.1 Recognize hazards/potential hazards. (p 497)
- 3-3.2 Describe common hazards found at the scene of a trauma and a medical patient. (p 497)
- 3-3.3 Determine hazards found at the scene of a medical or trauma patient. (p 497)
- 3-3.4 Differentiate safe from unsafe scenes. (p 498)
- 3-3.5 Describe methods to making an unsafe scene safe. (p 498)
- 3-3.6 Discuss common mechanisms of injury/nature of illness. (p 500)
- 3-3.7 Recognize the importance of determining the mechanism of injury. (p 499)
- 3-3.8 Discuss the reason for identifying the total number of patients at the scene. (p 502)
- 3-3.9 Organize the management of a scene following size-up. (p 503)
- 3-3.10 Explain the reasons for identifying the need for additional help or assistance. (p 499)

Affective

- 3-3.45 Explain the rationale for crew members to evaluate scene safety prior to entering. (p 498)
- 3-3.46 Serve as a model for others explaining how patient situations affect your evaluation of mechanism of injury or illness. (p 498)

Initial Assessment
Cognitive

- 3-2.3 Review the procedure for taking and significance of vital signs (pulse, respiration, and blood pressure). (p 525)
- 3-2.4 Describe the evaluation of mental status. (p 509)
- 3-2.5 Evaluate the importance of a general survey. (p 562)
- 3-2.6 Describe the examination of skin and nails. (p 513)
- 3-2.7 Differentiate normal and abnormal findings of the assessment of the skin. (p 513)
- 3-2.8 Distinguish the importance of abnormal findings of the assessment of the skin. (p 513)
- 3-3.11 Summarize the reasons for forming a general impression of the patient. (p 505)
- 3-3.12 Discuss methods of assessing mental status. (p 509)
- 3-3.13 Categorize levels of consciousness. (p 509)
- 3-3.14 Discuss methods of assessing the airway. (p 509)
- 3-3.15 Describe why the cervical spine is immobilized during the assessment of the trauma patient. (p 511)
- 3-3.16 Analyze a scene to determine if spinal precautions are required. (p 505)
- 3-3.17 Describe methods used for assessing if a patient is breathing. (p 511)
- 3-3.18 Differentiate between a patient with adequate and inadequate minute ventilation. (p 510)
- 3-3.19 Discuss the need for assessing the patient for external bleeding. (p 512)
- 3-3.20 Describe normal and abnormal findings when assessing skin color. (p 513)
- 3-3.21 Describe normal and abnormal findings when assessing skin temperature. (p 513)
- 3-3.22 Describe normal and abnormal findings when assessing skin condition. (p 513)
- 3-3.23 Explain the reason for prioritizing a patient for care and transport. (p 514)
- 3-3.24 Identify patients who require expeditious transport. (p 515)
- 3-3.25 Describe orthostatic vital signs and evaluate their usefulness in assessing a patient in shock. (p 662)

Affective

- 3-3.47 Explain the importance of forming a general impression of the patient. (p 505)
- 3-3.48 Explain the value of performing an initial assessment. (p 505)
- 3-3.49 Demonstrate a caring attitude when performing an initial assessment. (p 507)
- 3-3.50 Attend to the feelings that patients with medical conditions might be experiencing. (p 507)

Psychomotor

- 3-3.57 Demonstrate the techniques for assessing mental status. (p 509)
- 3-3.58 Demonstrate the techniques for assessing the airway. (p 510)
- 3-3.59 Demonstrate the techniques for determining if the patient is breathing. (p 511)
- 3-3.60 Demonstrate the techniques for determining if the patient has a pulse. (p 512)
- 3-3.61 Demonstrate the techniques for determining the patient for external bleeding. (p 512)
- 3-3.62 Demonstrate the techniques for determining the patient's skin color, temperature, and condition. (p 513)

10

Focused History and Physical Exam

Cognitive

- **3-1.1** Describe the factors that influence the EMT-Intermediate's ability to collect medical history. (p 531)
- **3-1.2** Describe the techniques of history taking. (p 525)
- **3-1.3** Discuss the importance of using open and closed ended questions. (p 532)
- **3-1.4** Describe the use of facilitation, reflection, clarification, empathetic responses, confrontation, and interpretation. (p 18)
- **3-1.5** Differentiate between facilitation, reflection, clarification, sympathetic responses, confrontation, and interpretation. (p 18)
- **3-1.6** Describe the structure and purpose of a health history. (p 525)
- **3-1.7** Describe how to obtain a health history. (p 525)
- **3-1.8** List the components of a history of an adult patient. (p 525)
- **3-1.9** List and describe strategies to overcome situations that represent special challenges in obtaining a medical history. (p 535)
- **3-2.1** Define the terms inspection, palpation, percussion, auscultation. (p 521)
- **3-2.2** Describe the techniques of inspection, palpation, percussion, and auscultation. (p 521)
- **3-3.26** Apply the techniques of physical examination to the medical patient. (p 535)
- **3-3.27** Differentiate between the assessment that is performed for a patient who has an altered mental status and other medical patients. (p 536)
- **3-3.28** Discuss the reasons for reconsidering the mechanism of injury. (p 518)
- **3-3.29** State the reasons for performing a rapid trauma assessment. (p 520)
- **3-3.30** Recite examples and explain why patients should receive a rapid trauma assessment. (p 520)
- **3-3.31** Apply the techniques of physical examination to the trauma patient. (p 520)
- **3-3.32** Describe the areas included in the rapid trauma assessment and discuss what should be evaluated. (p 520)
- **3-3.33** Differentiate cases when the rapid assessment may be altered in order to provide patient care. (p 520)
- **3-3.34** Discuss the reason for performing a focused history and physical exam. (p 517)
- **3-3.44** Discuss medical identification devices/systems. (p 91)

Affective

- **3-1.10** Demonstrate the importance of empathy when obtaining a health history. (p 531)
- **3-1.11** Demonstrate the importance of confidentiality when obtaining a health history. (p 19, 88)
- **3-2.49** Demonstrate a caring attitude when performing physical examination skills. (p 531)
- **3-2.50** Discuss the importance of a professional appearance and demeanor when performing physical examination skills. (p 18)
- **3-2.51** Appreciate the limitations of conducting a physical exam in the out-of-hospital environment. (p 517, 546)
- **3-3.51** Value the need for maintaining a professional caring attitude when performing a focused history and physical examination. (p 531)
- **3-3.52** Explain the rationale for the feelings that these patients might be experiencing. (p 31, 33-34)
- **3-3.55** Recognize and respect the feelings that patients might experience during assessment. (p 31, 33-34)

Psychomotor

- **3-3.63** Using the techniques of examination, demonstrate the assessment of a medical patient. (p 535)
- **3-3.64** Demonstrate the techniques for assessing a patient who is responsive with no known history. (p 535)
- **3-3.65** Demonstrate the techniques for assessing a patient who has an altered mental status. (p 537)
- **3-3.66** Perform a rapid medical assessment. (p 537)
- **3-3.67** Perform a focused history and physical exam of the medical patient. (p 531)
- **3-3.68** Using the techniques of physical examination, demonstrate the assessment of a trauma patient. (p 520)
- **3-3.69** Demonstrate the rapid trauma assessment used to assess a patient based on mechanism of injury. (p 520)
- **3-3.70** Perform a focused history and physical exam on a non-critically injured patient. (p 526)
- **3-3.71** Perform a focused history and physical exam on a patient with life-threatening injuries. (p 520)

Patient Assessment

Detailed Physical Exam

Cognitive

3-2.9 Describe the normal and abnormal assessment findings of the head (including the scalp, skull, face, and skin). (p 542)

3-2.10 Describe the examination of the head (including the scalp, skull, face, and skin). (p 542)

3-2.11 Describe the examination of the eyes. (p 542)

3-2.12 Distinguish between normal and abnormal assessment findings of the eyes. (p 546)

3-2.13 Describe the examination of the ears. (p 542)

3-2.14 Differentiate normal and abnormal assessment findings of the ears. (p 542)

3-2.15 Describe the examination of the nose. (p 546)

3-2.16 Differentiate normal and abnormal assessment findings of the nose. (p 546)

3-2.17 Describe the examination of the mouth and pharynx. (p 546)

3-2.18 Differentiate normal and abnormal assessment findings of the mouth and pharynx. (p 546)

3-2.19 Describe the examination of the neck and cervical spine. (p 546)

3-2.20 Differentiate normal and abnormal assessment findings of the neck and cervical spine. (p 546)

3-2.21 Describe the inspection, palpation, percussion, and auscultation of the chest. (p 547)

3-2.22 Describe the examination of the thorax and ventilation. (p 542, 545)

3-2.23 Describe the examination of the anterior and posterior chest. (p 542)

3-2.24 Differentiate the percussion sounds and their characteristics. (p 547)

3-2.25 Differentiate the characteristics of breath sounds. (p 547)

3-2.26 Differentiate normal and abnormal assessment findings of the chest examination. (p 542)

3-2.27 Describe the examination of the arterial pulse including rate, rhythm, and amplitude. (p 549)

3-2.28 Distinguish normal and abnormal findings of the arterial pulse. (p 548)

3-2.29 Describe the assessment of jugular venous pressure and pulsations. (p 546)

3-2.30 Distinguish normal and abnormal examination findings of jugular venous pressure and pulsations. (p 542)

3-2.31 Describe the examination of the heart. (p 548)

3-2.32 Differentiate normal and abnormal assessment findings of the heart. (p 548)

3-2.33 Describe the auscultation of the heart. (p 548)

3-2.34 Differentiate the characteristics of normal and abnormal findings associated with the auscultation of the heart. (p 548)

3-2.35 Describe the examination of the abdomen. (p 548)

3-2.36 Differentiate normal and abnormal assessment findings of the abdomen. (p 548)

3-2.37 Describe the examination of the female external genitalia. (p 548)

3-2.38 Differentiate normal and abnormal assessment findings of the female external genitalia. (p 549)

3-2.39 Describe the examination of the male genitalia. (p 549)

3-2.40 Differentiate normal and abnormal findings of the male genitalia. (p 549)

3-2.41 Describe the examination of the extremities. (p 549)

3-2.42 Differentiate normal and abnormal findings of the extremities. (p 549)

3-2.43 Describe the examination of the peripheral vascular system. (p 549)

3-2.44 Differentiate normal and abnormal findings of the peripheral vascular system. (p 549)

3-2.45 Describe the examination of the nervous system. (p 550)

3-2.46 Differentiate normal and abnormal findings of the nervous system. (p 550)

3-2.47 Discuss the considerations of examination of an infant or child. (p 542)

3-3.35 Describe when and why a detailed physical examination is necessary. (p 541)

3-3.36 Discuss the components of the detailed physical exam in relation to the techniques of examination. (p 541)

3-3.37 State the areas of the body that are evaluated during the detailed physical exam. (p 542)

3-3.38 Explain what additional care should be provided while performing the detailed physical exam. (p 542)

3-3.39 Distinguish between the detailed physical exam that is performed on a trauma patient and that of the medical patient. (p 541)

3-3.40 Differentiate between patients requiring a detailed physical exam from those who do not. (p 541)

Affective

3-3.53 Demonstrate a caring attitude when performing a detailed physical examination. (p 531)

Psychomotor

- **3-2.52** Demonstrate the examination of skin and nails. (p 549)
- **3-2.53** Demonstrate the examination of the head and neck. (p 543)
- **3-2.54** Demonstrate the examination of the eyes. (p 546)
- **3-2.55** Demonstrate the examination of the ears. (p 542)
- **3-2.56** Demonstrate the examination of the nose. (p 546)
- **3-2.57** Demonstrate the examination of the mouth. (p 546)
- **3-2.58** Demonstrate the examination of the neck. (p 546)
- **3-2.59** Demonstrate the examination of the thorax and ventilation. (p 546)
- **3-2.60** Demonstrate the examination of the anterior and posterior chest. (p 546)
- **3-2.61** Demonstrate auscultation of the chest. (p 548)
- **3-2.62** Demonstrate percussion of the chest. (p 547)
- **3-2.63** Demonstrate the examination of the arterial pulse including location, rate, rhythm, and amplitude. (p 543, 545)
- **3-2.64** Demonstrate the assessment of jugular venous pressure and pulsations. (p 542, 545)
- **3-2.65** Demonstrate the examination of the heart. (p 548)
- **3-2.66** Demonstrate the examination of the abdomen. (p 548)
- **3-2.67** Demonstrate auscultation of the abdomen. (p 542-543, 545)
- **3-2.68** Demonstrate the external visual examination of the female external genitalia. (p 549)
- **3-2.69** Demonstrate the examination of the male genitalia. (p 549)
- **3-2.70** Demonstrate the examination of the peripheral vascular system. (p 549)
- **3-2.71** Demonstrate the examination of the extremities. (p 549)
- **3-2.72** Demonstrate the examination of the nervous system. (p 550)
- **3-3.72** Perform a detailed physical examination. (p 542)

Ongoing Assessment

Cognitive

- **3-2.48** Describe the general guidelines of recording examination information. (p 554)
- **3-3.41** Discuss the reasons for repeating the initial assessment as part of the on-going assessment. (p 554)
- **3-3.42** Describe the components of the on-going assessment. (p 553)
- **3-3.43** Describe the trending of assessment components. (p 553)

Affective

- **3-3.54** Explain the value of performing an on-going assessment. (p 553)
- **3-3.56** Explain the value of trending assessment components to other health professionals who assume care of the patient. (p 553)

Psychomotor

- **3-3.73** Demonstrate the skills involved in performing the on-going assessment. (p 559)

Clinical Decision Making

Cognitive

- **3-4.1** Compare the factors influencing medical care in the out-of-hospital environment to other medical settings. (p 557)
- **3-4.2** Differentiate between critical life-threatening, potentially life-threatening, and non life-threatening patient presentations. (p 558)
- **3-4.3** Evaluate the benefits and shortfalls of protocols, standing orders, and patient care algorithms. (p 559)
- **3-4.4** Define the components, stages, and sequences of the critical thinking process for EMT-Intermediates. (p 561)
- **3-4.5** Apply the fundamental elements of critical thinking for EMT-Intermediates. (p 561)
- **3-4.6** Describe the effects of the "fight or flight" response and the positive and negative effects on an EMT-Intermediate's decision making. (p 562)
- **3-4.7** Develop strategies for effective thinking under pressure. (p 562)
- **3-4.8** Summarize the "six Rs" of putting it all together: Read the patient, Read the scene, React, Reevaluate, Revise the management plan, Review performance. (p 563)

Affective

- **3-4.9** Defend the position that clinical decision making is the cornerstone of effective EMT-Intermediate practice. (p 557)

Patient Assessment

3-4.10   Practice facilitating behaviors when thinking under pressure. (p 562)

1985 Objectives

Scene Size-up

1.2.18   Discuss the EMT-I's initial responsibilities when arriving on the scene. (p 497)
1.2.20   Discuss the varying philosophies between the management of medical patients and trauma patients, prehospital. (p 498)
1.6.2   Describe the four phases of patient assessment. (p 495)
1.6.3   Discuss the possible environmental hazards that the EMT-I may encounter and the means of protecting him in this environment. (p 497)
1.6.4   Describe the environmental hazards which a patient might encounter. (p 497)
1.6.5   Describe the problems an EMT-I might encounter in a hostile situation and describe mechanisms of management. (p 498)
1.6.6   Describe the various types of protective equipment available to the EMT-I for self-protection and patient protection. (p 498)
1.6.7   Discuss the appropriate methods of patient protection in each situation. (p 497)
1.6.8   Discuss backup personnel, transportation, and equipment. (p 498)
1.6.9   Define and describe the various classifications of emergencies which an EMT-I will encounter. Base this on medical needs. (p 498)

Initial Assessment

1.2.3   Define stabilization of patients. (p 513-514)
1.6.1   Establish priorities of care based on threat to life conditions. (p 508)
1.6.10   Describe the primary survey and what areas are critical to evaluate. (p 505)
1.6.31   Describe the mechanisms of evaluating the effectiveness of perfusion, including pulse, skin color, capillary refill. (p 513)
1.6.37   Define a mini-neurological examination (level of consciousness). (p 509)

Focused History and Physical Exam

1.6.38   Describe exposing the patient's body for total evaluation. (p 520)
1.6.39   Discuss when this should and should not be carried out. (p 529)
1.6.41   Describe the reasons for and mechanisms of patient reassessment in the resuscitation phase. (p 509-514)
1.6.42   Define the components of secondary survey and its benefits for patient evaluation. (p 517)
1.6.43   Describe the assessment of the head, neck, thorax, abdomen, extremities, and nervous system. (p 520)
1.6.44   Describe the trauma score, define its usefulness and how it is accomplished. (p 526)
1.6.45   Discuss the important components that must be identified in taking an appropriate history from a patient. (p 525)
1.6.47   Define the definitive care phase. (p 517)
1.6.48   Describe how a patient is packaged and stabilized for transportation to the hospital, including airway ventilation, IV fluids, pneumatic anti-shock garment, fracture stabilization, bandaging. (p 553)
S1.6.58   Perform a rapid assessment of the patient to identify priorities for care. (p 520)
S1.6.59   Demonstrate the assessment of the head, neck, thorax, abdomen, extremities, and neurological system. (p 520)

Detailed Physical Exam

There are no 1985 objectives for this section.

Ongoing Assessment

1.6.52   Describe how the patient is monitored en route to the hospital. (p 553)
1.6.53   Describe how the hospitals are selected for receipt of patients based on patient need and hospital capability. (p 555)
1.6.57   Describe the mechanisms of continued evaluation of the patient en route to the hospital. (p 554)

Clinical Decision Making

There are no 1985 objectives for this section.

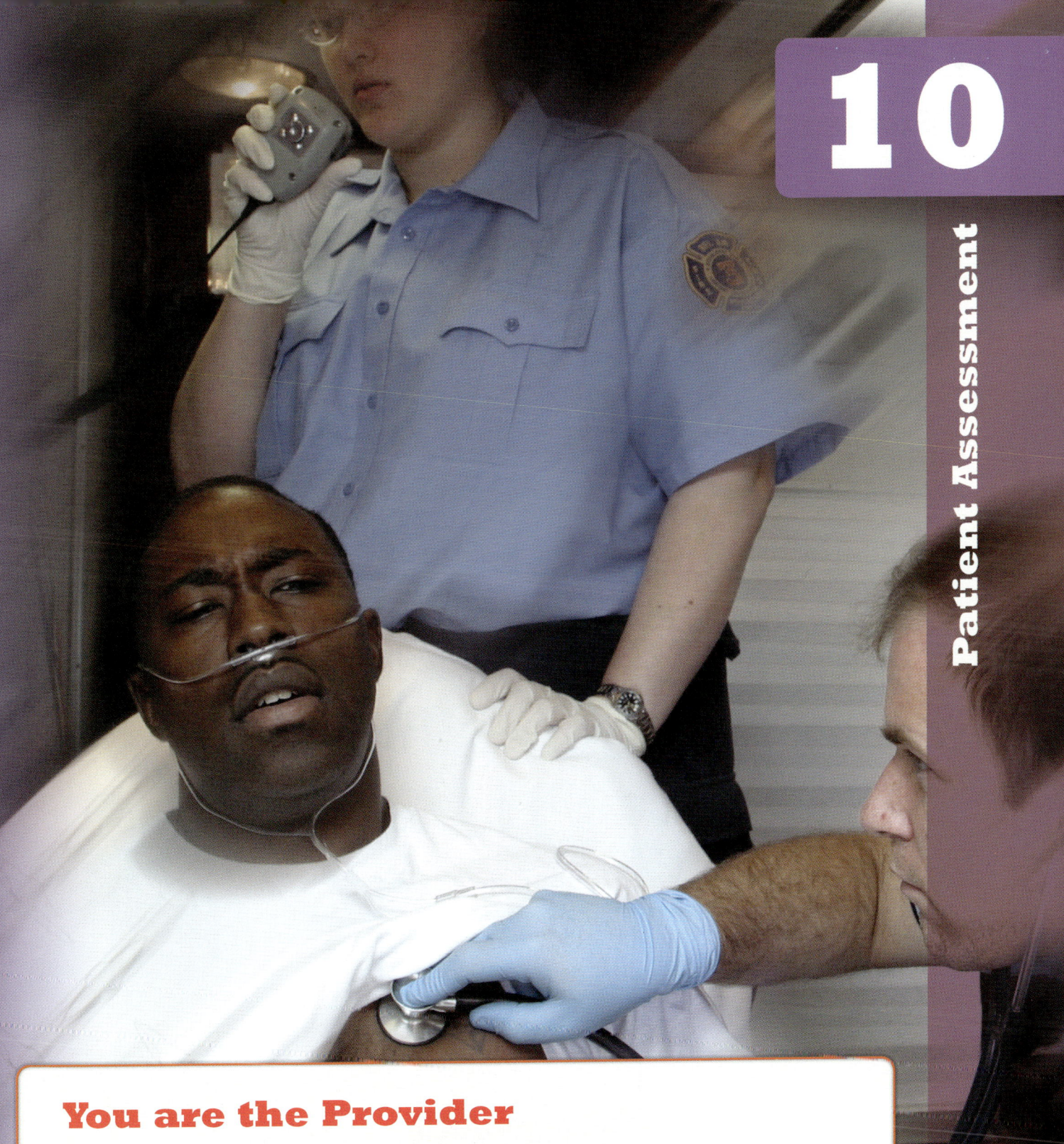

10

Patient Assessment

You are the Provider

You are called to an assisted-living facility where two elderly patients are complaining of feeling ill.
  This chapter will teach you the steps involved in patient assessment and how to apply the information to the care of your patient, in addition to answering the following questions.

1. What are the steps involved in performing patient assessment?
2. Why is it important for the EMT-I to conduct a scene size-up?
3. What is involved in a scene size-up?

Patient Assessment

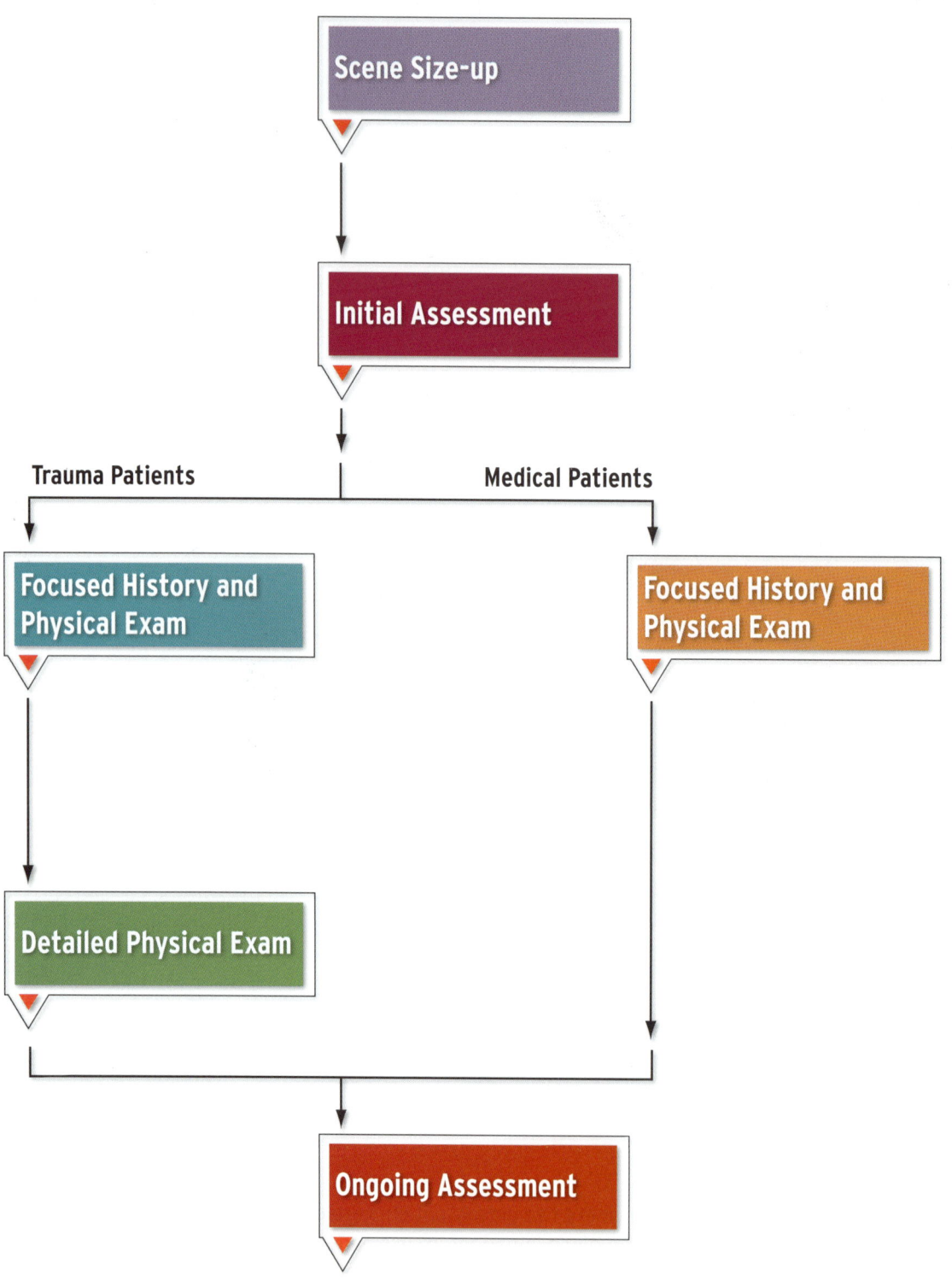

About This Chapter

This chapter will provide a clear and comprehensive approach to patient assessment. A flowchart has been developed to provide a quick, visual reference to guide you through the patient assessment process. The chapter has been divided into six sections. Every section is color coded and numbered for easy reference. The Patient Assessment Flowchart is repeated at every section to show you "at a glance" where you are in the patient assessment process.

Special care has been taken to reflect the EMT-Intermediate National Standard Curriculum, but enhancement information will prepare you for your work in the field.

Patient Assessment

Patient assessment is the cornerstone of prehospital care. The very basis of patient care is centered on a solid, systematic approach to assessing the patient. Rather than reacting to what is seen in the field, the successful EMT-I is able to think his or her way through a call, using intellect to control and direct emotional response. Throughout this chapter, you will be given the tools necessary to accomplish such a task. Consider the adage, "You cannot treat what you did not find."

Although every call is as unique as the individual you will be assisting, the steps of the patient assessment are always the same:

- Perform the scene size-up.
- Perform an initial assessment.
- Perform a focused history and physical exam.
- Perform a detailed physical exam.
- Perform ongoing assessment.

Patient Assessment

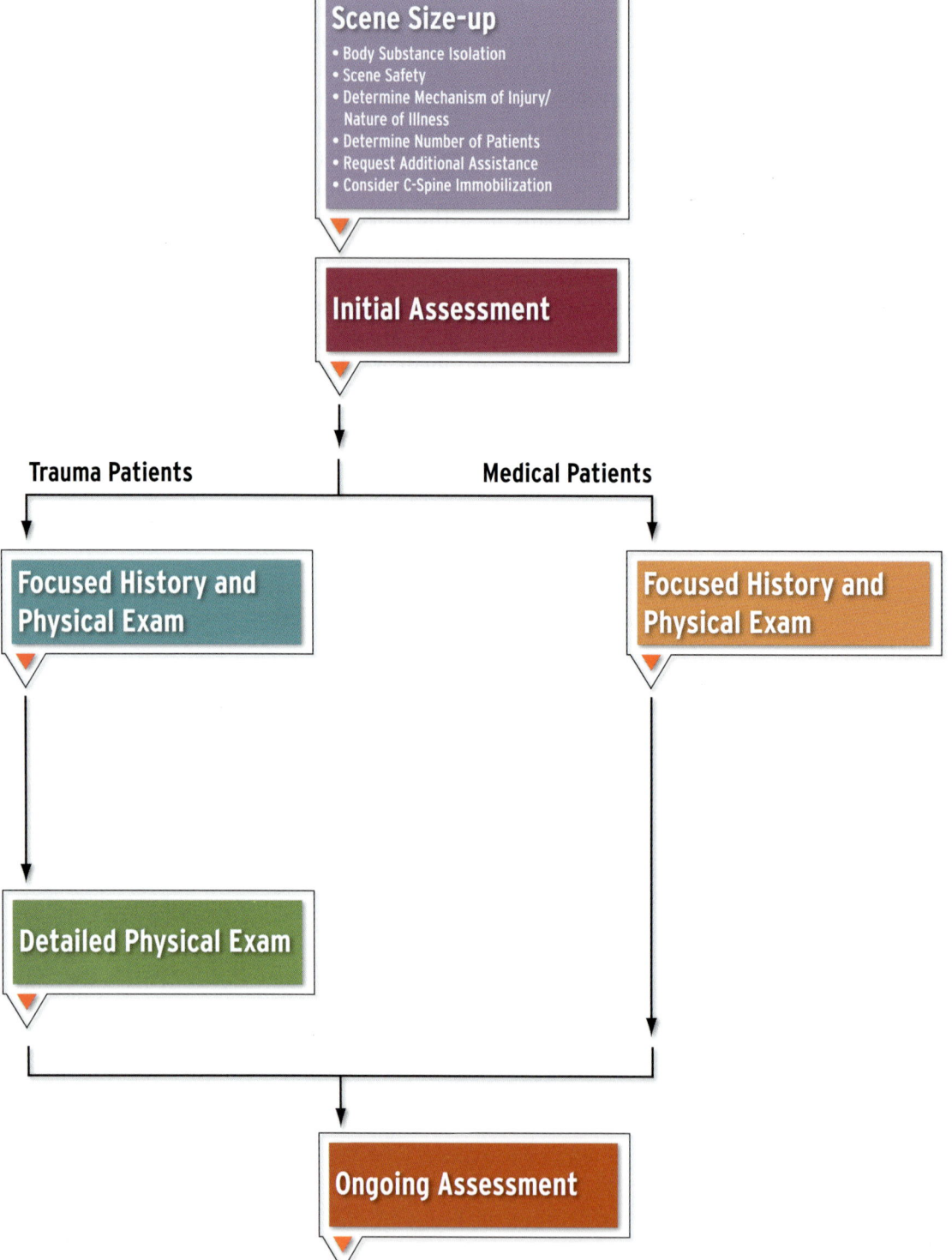

Scene Size-up

Scene size-up begins as you approach the scene and is considered throughout the entire call. The scene size-up is a quick assessment of the scene and the surroundings that will provide you and your partner with as much information as possible about the safety of the scene, any mechanism of injury and/or nature of illness, the number of patients involved, and the need for additional resources before you enter the scene and begin patient care. Table 10-1 lists the components of the scene size-up.

TABLE 10-1	Scene Size-up
■ Body substance isolation	
■ Scene safety	
■ Determine mechanism of injury/nature of illness	
■ Determine number of patients	
■ Request additional assistance	
■ Consider cervical spine immobilization	

Body Substance Isolation

On every emergency call, you need to be sure to wear the proper protective equipment because this equipment will reduce your risk of exposure to a communicable disease. The best way to reduce your risk of exposure is to follow <u>body substance isolation (BSI)</u> precautions. The concept of BSI assumes that all body fluids present a possible risk for infection.

Before you step out of the unit, you and your partner must be wearing the proper protective equipment. Protective gloves are always indicated. Eye protection, masks, and gowns may also be indicated if there is blood, other body fluids, or risk of respiratory exposure in the patient area Figure 10-1. Eye protection is needed when there may be a risk that blood, other body fluids, or secretions will splatter or become airborne. In some situations, for example childbirth, you should put on a mask and gown, if needed and dictated by your protocol, before you enter the area immediately around the patient. If the scene involves hazardous materials or fire, wear the appropriate gear for the situation or do not enter the scene unless you are properly trained to do so.

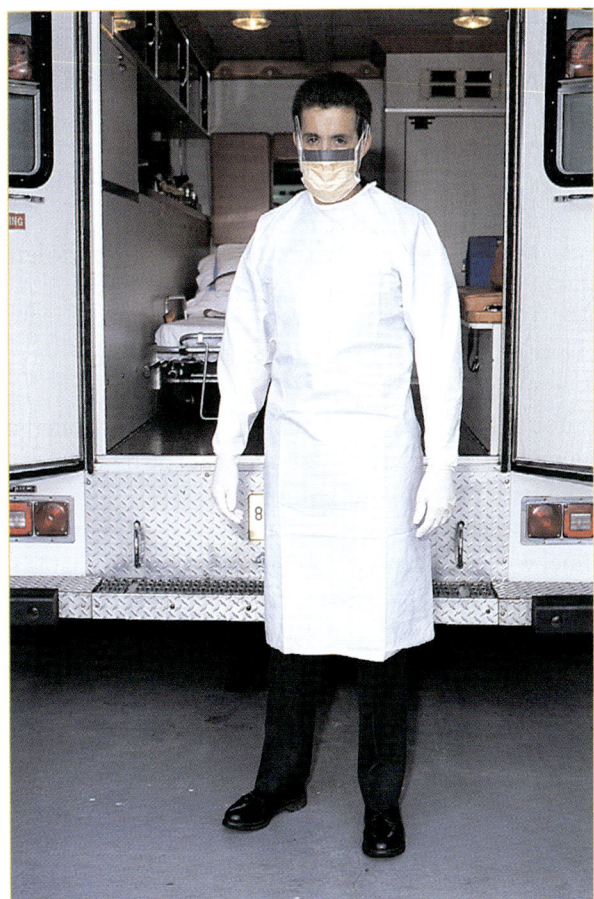

Figure 10-1 Proper protective equipment is vital when you are called to a scene where there is a lot of blood or other body fluids.

Scene Safety

Scene safety is an assessment focused on ensuring the well-being of the EMT-I, his or her partner, and bystanders. It is ongoing and considered throughout the entire call. If at anytime the scene becomes unsafe, leave the area and call for help. An EMT-I will not be found guilty of abandonment when fleeing from danger. You cannot help your patient if you, your partner, or bystanders become injured.

Personal Protection

Look for the following possible dangers before you step out of the unit Figure 10-2:

- Oncoming traffic
- Unstable surfaces (for example, wet or icy patches, loose gravel, slopes)
- Leaking gasoline or diesel fuel
- Downed electrical lines

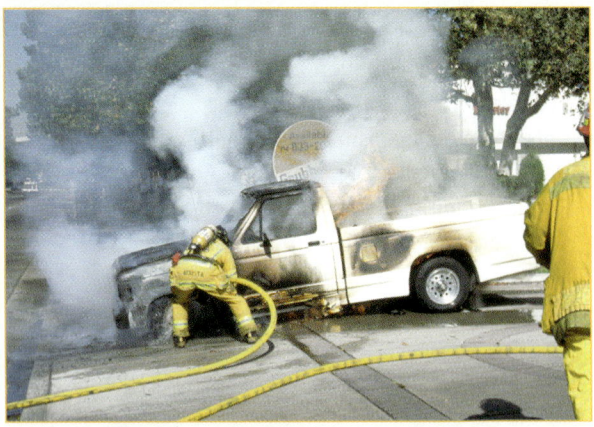

Figure 10-2 Before you step out of your unit, be sure to evaluate the scene for any hazards.

- Hostile bystanders or the potential for violence
- Fire or smoke
- Possible hazardous or toxic materials
- Other dangers at crash or rescue scenes
- Crime scenes

You should park your unit in a place that will offer you and your partner the greatest safety but also rapid access to the patient and your equipment (Figure 10-3). In many instances involving trauma, law enforcement personnel will be at the scene before you arrive. If that is the case, you should talk with them before entering the scene. Make sure to follow local protocol if the scene is a crime scene. Also be sure to have law enforcement personnel accompany you if the patient is a suspect in the crime. Consider your unit a safe haven. You are no help to the patient if you enter the scene without first protecting yourself and your partner.

Your next concern is the safety of the patient(s) and bystanders. This is not an easy task. Bystanders can become a problem when they try to help with or direct your care. Protect yourself and bystanders alike by moving them to a safe area or assigning them a specific task.

Making the Unsafe Scene Safe

Occasionally you and your partner will not be able to enter a scene safely. This may be due to the need for extrication, possible hazardous conditions, or the presence of multiple patients that you cannot handle alone. These situations seem very difficult when you want to provide medical care to sick or injured patients. However, your safety and that of your partner are the priority. If you need more help in staging the scene, do not hesitate to ask for it. Be as specific as possible about the type of help you need. Remember that it takes time for additional resources, such as an extrication team, law enforcement personnel, or other EMS units, to arrive at the scene.

> **EMT-I Safety**
>
> Assessing the safety of a scene before entering may be the single most important way in which emergency responders can attend to their own well-being. Subtle signs of danger not recognized and neutralized—or avoided—at this point can grow much more threatening without being noticed once you shift your attention to patient assessment and care. Initial scene assessment usually makes the difference between a manageably safe scene and one that could spin dangerously out of control without further warning.

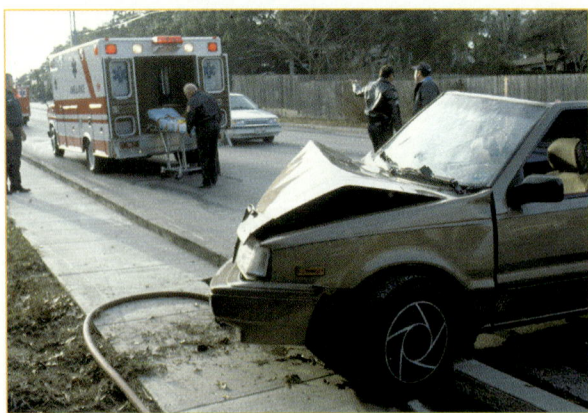

Figure 10-3 Park your unit in a place that is safe, yet allows for rapid access to the patient and your equipment. If law enforcement personnel are already on the scene, make sure to check in with them first.

Determine the Mechanism of Injury or Nature of the Illness

One of the great dangers in performing the prehospital assessment is giving in to the temptation to categorize your patient immediately as a trauma patient or a medical patient. Remember, the fundamentals of good patient assessment do not change, despite the unique aspects of trauma and medical care. Careful evaluation of the scene, including the possible mechanism of injury and/or the nature of illness, along with the other information that you gather will help you to lean in one direction or the other. Family members, bystanders, and law enforcement personnel can often tell you what prompted the call to 9-1-1. After you have completed your assessment, you will come to a conclusion as to whether the origin of your patient's main problem is medical, traumatic, or both.

Determine from the patient why EMS was activated. You might also need to rely on information provided by family or bystanders.

Determine how many patients are involved. If there are more patients than you and your partner can effectively handle, request additional assistance. Call for additional help before making contact with patients or beginning triage. You are less likely to call for help once you are involved in patient care. Consider the need for law enforcement personnel, utility crews, lifting assistance, or other specialized services.

Mechanism of Injury

The mechanism of injury (MOI) is how the patient became injured. Determining the MOI will provide many clues to finding hidden injuries and should be your first clue of a potentially critically injured patient. Furthermore, it contributes to your decision about whether to perform a rapid assessment or focused physical exam on your patient. With a traumatic injury, the body has been exposed to some force or energy that has resulted in a temporary injury, permanent damage, or even death Figure 10-4.

As you might expect, certain parts of the body are more easily injured than others. The brain and the spinal cord are very fragile and easy to injure. Fortunately, they are protected by the skull, the vertebrae, and several layers of soft tissues. The eyes are also easily injured. Even small forces to the eye may result in serious injury. The bones and certain organs are stronger and can absorb small forces without sustaining serious injury. The net result of this information is that you can use the MOI as a kind of guide to predict the potential for a serious injury by evaluating three factors: the amount of force applied to the body, the length of time the force was applied, and the areas of the body involved. Keep in mind two principles of physics. The first principle—force travels in a straight line until acted on by an outside force—relates to the human body when impact occurs. The outside force takes the form of automobiles, the ground, or even body organs impacting internal body structures. The second principle of physics—energy cannot be created or destroyed but can change form—relates to force or energy translating into body damage. When force or energy comes into contact with the body, it continues in a straight line until it is forced to deviate. In other words, energy impacts a body structure. It is at that point that energy translates into body injury such as fractures or injury to internal organs.

You will commonly hear the terms blunt trauma and penetrating trauma. With blunt trauma, the force of the injury occurs over a broad area, and the skin is usually not broken Figure 10-5. However, the

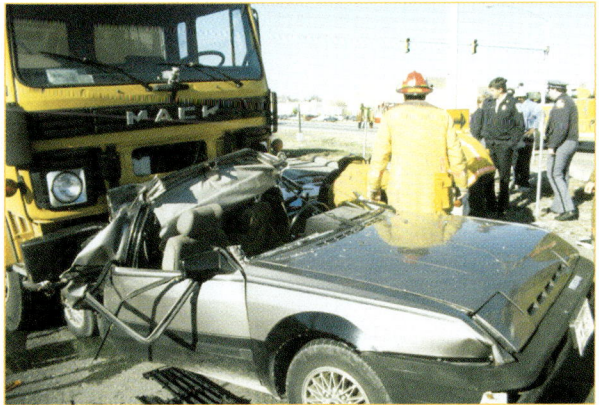

Figure 10-4 With traumatic injuries, the patient has been exposed to some force or energy that has resulted in injury or possibly even death. You can learn a great deal about that force by simply evaluating the MOI.

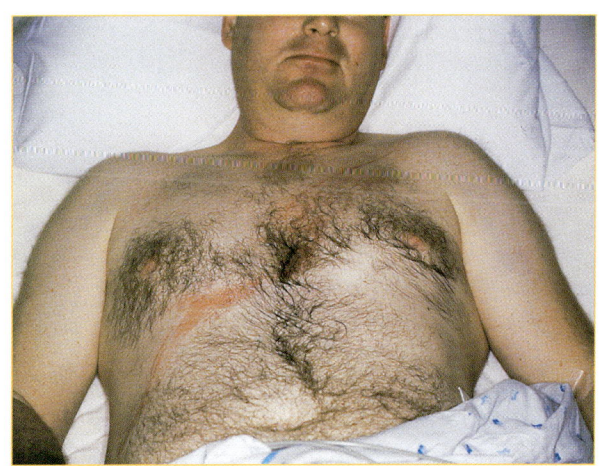

Figure 10-5 With blunt trauma, the force of the injury occurs over a broad area and the skin is not broken.

tissues and organs under the area of impact may be damaged. With <u>penetrating trauma</u>, the force of the injury occurs at a small point of contact between the skin and the object. The object pierces the skin and creates an open wound that carries a high potential for damage to the organs directly under the penetration and for infection Figure 10-6 ◀ . The severity of injury depends on the characteristics of the penetrating object, the amount of force or energy, and the part of the body affected.

Motor Vehicle Crashes

In a motor vehicle crash (MVC), the amount of force that is applied to the body is directly related to the speed of the crash. As the speed of a crash increases, the forces that are exerted on the patient increase as well. Therefore, patients should be assessed according to the area of the body that was most likely injured. Your evaluation should also be based, to some extent, on the patient's position in the car, the use of seat belts, and how the patient's body shifted during the crash Figure 10-7 ▼ . Drivers are typically at higher risk for serious injury than passengers because of the potential for striking the steering wheel with the chest, abdomen, or head. Front seat passengers may also be injured by striking the dashboard or windshield.

Risk for serious injury also varies depending on whether seat belts are used, what type they are, and whether they are worn properly. Unbelted victims are at much

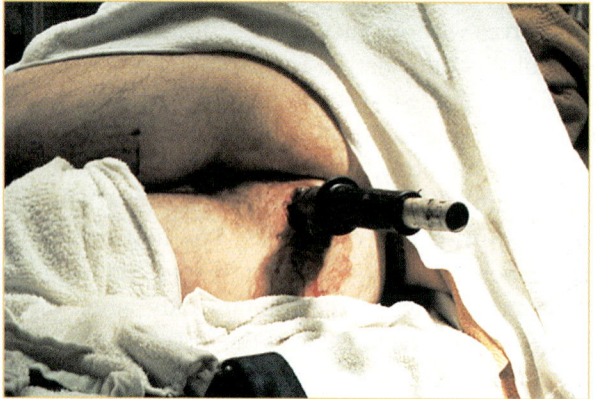

Figure 10-6 With penetrating trauma, an object pierces the skin and creates an open wound.

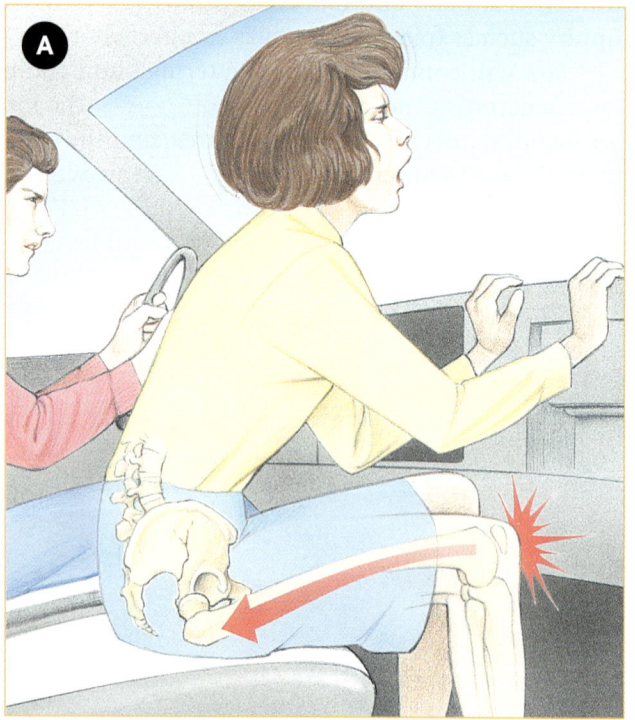
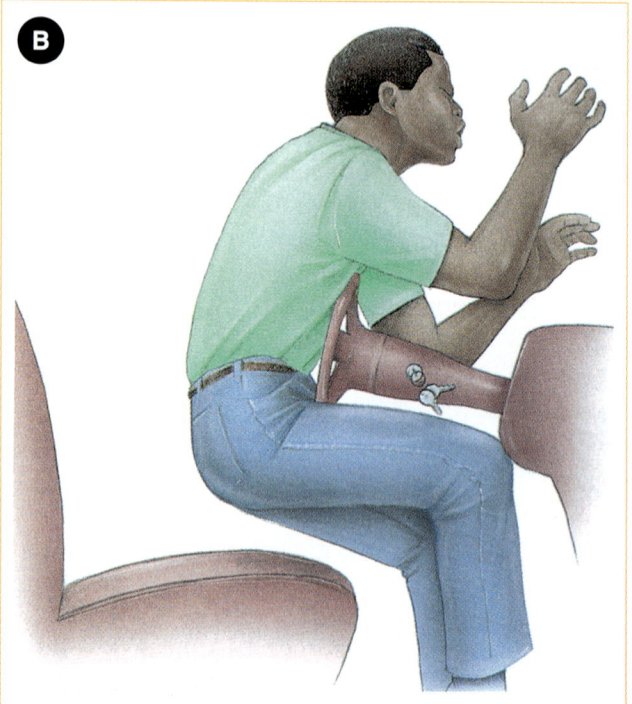

Figure 10-7 A. Injury to the lower extremity, hip, or pelvis can occur when the knee strikes the dashboard. **B.** Injury to the chest and abdomen occurs when the patient's chest and/or abdomen strike the steering wheel.

higher risk for a number of injuries because they may be catapulted throughout the car. As they go "up and over" or "down and under," they may strike the sides, roof, floor, dashboard, steering wheel, or windshield. Even worse, the unrestrained victim may be ejected from the vehicle, dramatically increasing the risk of head injury, spinal cord injury, and death.

> **EMT-I Tips**
>
> A patient's chances of death are 25 times greater if the patient is ejected from the vehicle.

Falls

In falls, the amount of force that is applied to the body is directly related to the distance fallen, the type of surface the patient lands on, and the area of the body that impacts first. However, the area of the body injured is very hard to predict. Falls from significant heights are high-energy force falls, and patients should be evaluated accordingly. Any patient who has fallen more than three times his or her own height, or greater than 15′ to 20′, should be considered at risk for multiple systems injury. With children, a fall of two to three times their height, or approximately 10′ or more, is potentially serious.

If the patient's condition is stable, you should attempt to determine exactly what happened to cause the fall; did the person simply slip and fall or pass out and then fall? When possible, you should also identify what type of surface the patient landed on and how he or she landed. This information, which may be gleaned from the environment, the patient, and/or bystanders, may help you to predict what areas of the body might be the most seriously injured.

Gunshot and Stab Wounds

Penetrating trauma, often the result of a gunshot or stab injury, is also very difficult to assess because there is often little external evidence of the actual damage. The amount of force that is applied to the body in a gunshot wound is most directly related to the caliber of the weapon and the distance of the weapon from the patient when it was fired. Point-blank or high-caliber gunshot wounds are high-velocity injuries. By comparison, the force that is exerted on the patient in stab injuries is minimal, even though these injuries can still be lethal.

The area of the body that is actually involved in penetrating trauma may be very difficult to predict. In gunshot wounds, the internal organs that are injured may have no relationship to the entrance wound and the exit wound, if one exists (Figure 10-8 ▼). It is important to remember that bullets may bounce off bones or dense organs in the body, making the exact path almost impossible to determine. Some bullets are designed to tumble, break apart, or "mushroom" after they enter the body. Therefore, take spinal precautions with any gunshot wound to the head, neck, or thorax.

In other penetrating wounds, such as stab wounds, the body area that is involved can be estimated by looking at the location of entrance and the length of the weapon, if known. Remember that you can only estimate the extent of the injury. In some cases of assault, an assailant may have moved the weapon in a back-and-forth motion after it entered the patient.

Nature of the Illness

As an EMT-I, you are likely to care for more medical patients than trauma patients. For trauma patients, you examine the MOI as part of your scene size-up. For medical patients, you must examine the nature of the illness (NOI). There are similarities between the MOI and the NOI. Both require you to search for clues regarding how the incident occurred. You must make an effort to determine the general type of illness, or NOI. This is often best described by the patient's chief complaint, the reason EMS was called, and by the patient's medical history. To quickly determine the NOI, talk with the patient, family, or bystanders about the problem. But at

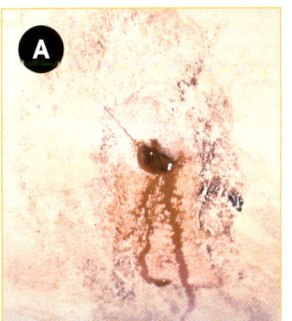 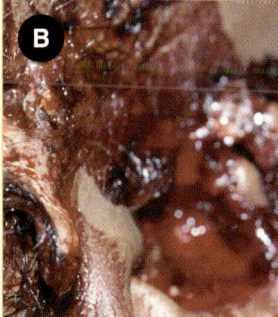

Figure 10-8 **A.** Entrance wound from a gunshot. **B.** Exit wound from a gunshot.

the same time, use your senses to check the scene for clues to the possible problem. You may see open or spilled medicine containers, poisonous substances, unsanitary living conditions, open food on the counter, oxygen tanks, or home nebulizers. You may smell an unusual or strong odor, such as the odor of fresh paint in a closed room, the odor of acetone, or the nauseating odor associated with gastrointestinal bleeding. You may hear crowing or stridor when the patient attempts to breathe, or you may hear audible wheezes. Keep these observations of the scene in mind as you begin to assess the patient.

Determine the Number of Patients

As part of your scene size-up, it is essential that you accurately determine the number of patients. This determination is critical for your estimate of the need for additional resources, such as the HazMat (hazardous materials) team or a specialized rescue group. You should ask yourself the following questions when considering the need for additional resources:

- Does the scene pose a threat to you or your patient's safety?
- How many patients are there?
- What is the nature of their condition?
- Who contacted EMS?
- Is this a possible crime scene in which evidence may need to be preserved?
- Are hazardous materials, such as chemicals or leaking fuel, involved?

When there are multiple patients, consider the environment. If they are all in an enclosed space, consider the possibility of a hazardous scene such as carbon monoxide. Immediately remove the patients and your crew from the scene and contact the appropriate authorities. In the case of a traumatic incident, such as a multiple vehicular crash or a school bus crash, you should call for additional units immediately and then begin triage (Figure 10-9). Triage is a process of sorting patients based on the severity of each patient's condition. Once that is accomplished, you can begin to establish treatment and transport priorities. One care provider, experienced in triage, should be assigned to perform triage. This process will help you to provide care and allocate your personnel and equipment resources most effectively and efficiently in a multiple-patient situation. If there is a large number of patients or if patient needs are greater than the available resources, put your local multiple-patient incident or mass-casualty plan into action.

In these situations, you should always call for additional resources, such as law enforcement, the fire department, rescue units, a paramedic crew, and even a utility crew, as soon as possible. It is never wrong to call for backup, even if the extra units are sent back. Remember, by nature, you are less likely to ask for help after you begin patient care because at that point, you are part of the scene, particularly at an MVC in which patients require spinal immobilization.

You are the Provider Part 2

It has been determined that the scene is safe and that there is no threat to emergency personnel. Your first patient is a 78-year-old woman. As you approach her, you notice the following:

Initial Assessment	Recording Time: Zero Minutes
Appearance	In pain; moaning and holding her abdomen; pale
Level of consciousness	Responsive verbally
Airway	Open and clear
Breathing	Respiratory rate, normal; depth, adequate
Circulation	Skin, pale; radial pulse, rapid

4. What is the goal of the initial assessment?
5. What information should the EMT-I use to form his or her general impression of the patient's condition?

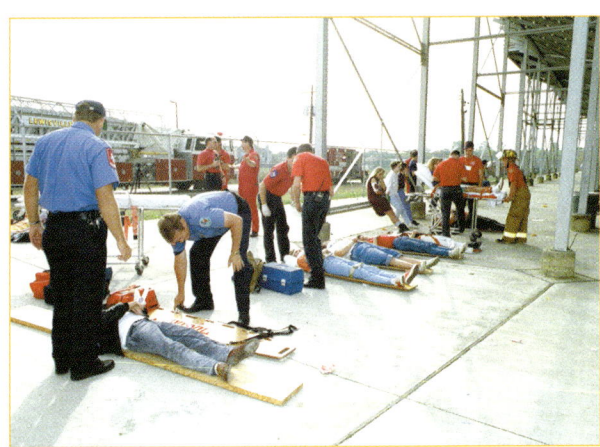

Figure 10-9 With multiple patients, you should call for additional resources and then begin triage.

> **Terminology Tips**
>
> The purpose of *triage* is to do the most good for the greatest number of patients.

Patient Assessment

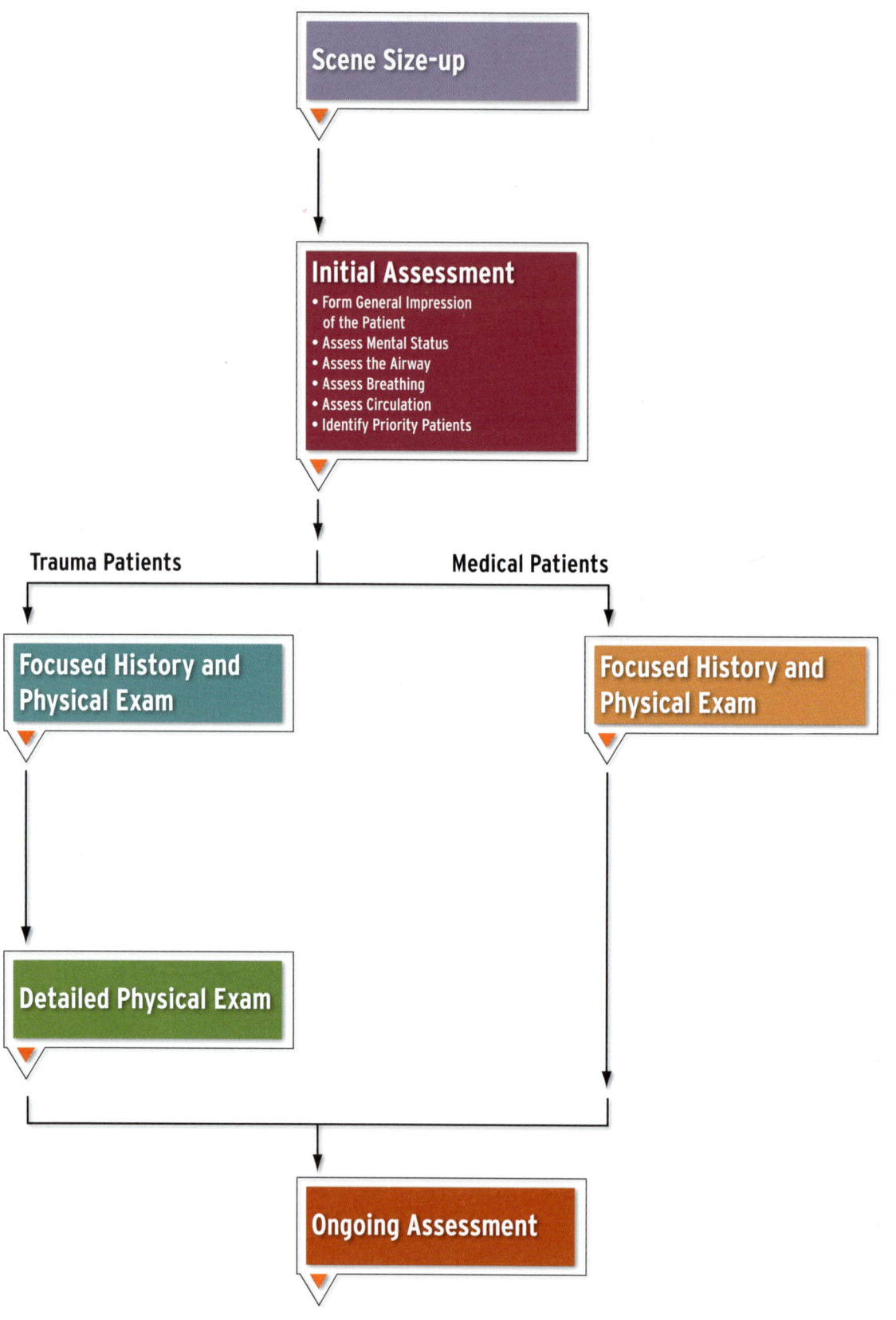

Initial Assessment

During the scene size-up, you speculated about the patient's condition, based on dispatch information, and asked and answered questions about scene safety. These steps are critically important, particularly in light of their role in ensuring your safety. However, patient assessment actually begins when you come into contact with the patient.

The initial assessment (formerly called the primary survey) has a single, critical, all-important goal: to identify and initiate treatment of immediate or potential life threats. Information concerning life-threatening conditions comes from a variety of sources, such as the visual appearance of the patient, the patient's chief complaint, and the MOI when trauma is involved. As you approach the scene and, ultimately, the patient, you will form a general impression of the patient's condition. The general impression is based on your immediate assessment of the environment, the presenting signs and symptoms, the MOI in a trauma patient, and the patient's chief complaint. Table 10-2 lists the components of the initial assessment.

Form a General Impression of the Patient's Condition

The general impression is important, because it helps you to determine the priorities of care, identify the MOI (if trauma was involved), assess the potential for life-threatening conditions, and determine the reliability of the information the patient is providing Figure 10-10.

As you approach the scene, note the patient's position, check to see whether the patient is moving or still, awake or unresponsive, bleeding or not. Look for the MOI or the NOI. Listen to what the patient and bystanders have to say. Make note of odors that suggest chemical hazards, smoke, or alcohol on the patient's breath. You can feel for pulses, pain, and deformities when you reach the patient. If the patient is responsive, try to learn as much as possible about what is wrong before you begin your examination. At this time, you should tell the patient your name, identify yourself as an EMT-I, and explain that you are there to help. You should determine the patient's age and chief complaint and continue to ask questions and talk to the patient throughout the entire assessment.

You must answer the following questions to begin to form your general impression:

- Does the patient appear to have a life-threatening condition? Clues include unresponsiveness, obvious difficulty breathing, severe external bleeding, and cyanotic (blue) or very pale skin color. If you suspect a life-threatening condition, provide immediate care and transport.
- Was the patient injured? If so, what was the MOI? On the basis of the MOI, would you expect the patient to be severely injured? If so, assume the worst and begin treatment, including spinal immobilization.
- Does the patient seem coherent and able to answer questions? If not, you need to rely more heavily on your physical assessment skills and/or the information that you can obtain from others.

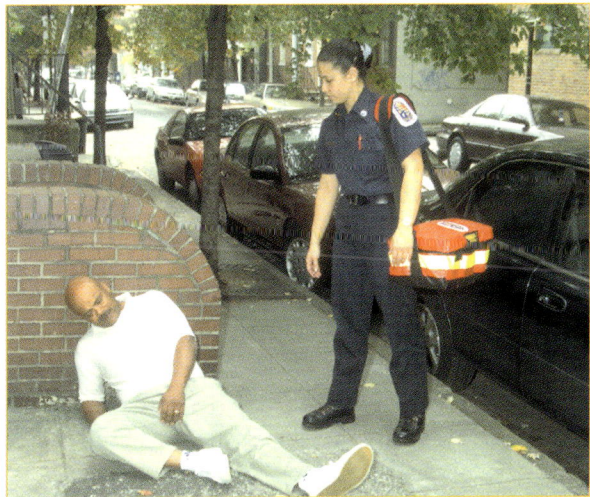

Figure 10-10 As you approach the patient, form a general impression of his or her overall condition.

TABLE 10-2	Initial Assessment

- Form general impression of the patient's condition
- Assess mental status
- Assess the airway
- Assess breathing
- Assess circulation
- Identify priority patients

Distinguishing Between Medical and Trauma Patients

Remember that as an EMT-I, you will be called to treat an almost infinite number of different patient problems. Some patients will have a problem that is not related to trauma; these patients are typically referred to as medical patients (for example, those with chest pain or having difficulty breathing). Others will have been injured in an incident such as a fall, an MVC, or a shooting. These patients are usually considered trauma patients. In some situations, this distinction will be obvious. If the primary problem appears to be traumatic in origin, you will want to assume the worst and begin treatment, including spinal immobilization. However, quite frequently, it will not. For instance, a patient who falls at a long-term care facility could simply be treated as a trauma patient; however, it is also possible that the fall was caused by a medical condition such as a syncopal episode (fainting), a cerebrovascular accident (stroke), or even a myocardial infarction (heart attack). You will learn that it is not usually easy or prudent to label patients as medical or trauma until you have finished your assessment. In many cases, medical emergencies and trauma go hand in hand.

For this reason, the assessment process does not encourage you to differentiate immediately between medical and trauma patients. Rather, the assessment process begins by assuming that all patients may have both medical and trauma aspects to their condition. Through the assessment process, you will develop an understanding of the patient's problems, both medical and traumatic, and will begin treatment on the basis of that understanding. As each call unfolds, your patient's primary problem will become apparent.

This rather general assessment is your opportunity to evaluate "the big picture" before you focus on the patient's specific needs, so use all of your senses in observing the scene and patient.

The first steps in caring for any patient focus on finding and treating the most life-threatening illnesses and injuries Figure 10-11 ▼. Through all of the avenues

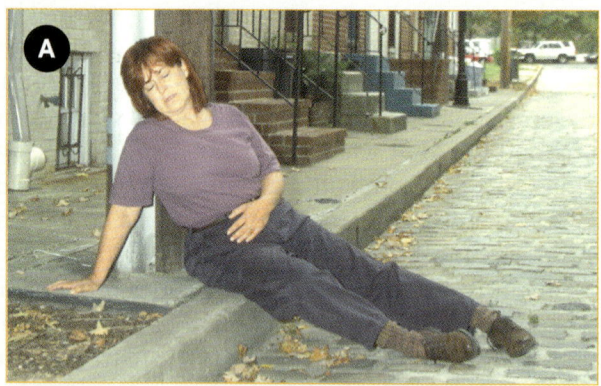

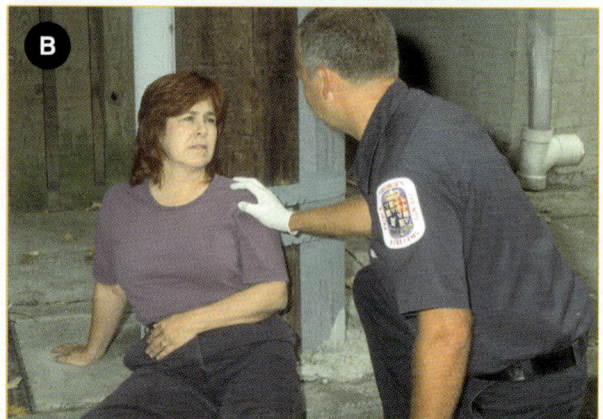

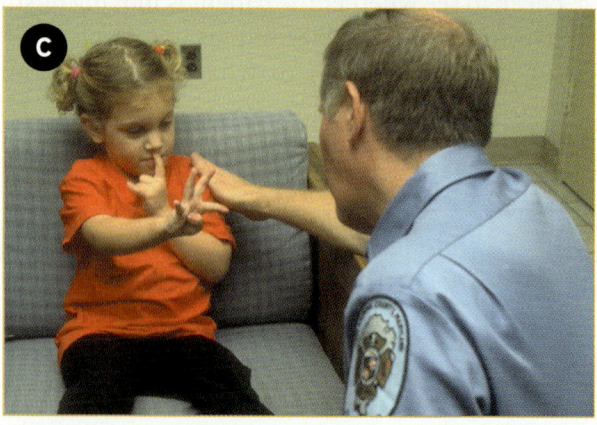

Figure 10-11 Performing the initial assessment. **A.** Observe the patient to form a general impression. **B.** Assess the patient's mental status. **C.** Assess the mental status of a child.

> **In the Field**
>
> Whether the patient is a medical or trauma patient has nothing to do with the severity of the patient's condition. Not every trauma patient is in critical condition, nor is every medical patient in stable condition. A patient who falls over a tree root and breaks two toes is a trauma patient, and a patient experiencing a myocardial infarction is a medical patient. Categorize "load and go" patients by the severity of their condition, not whether they are a trauma patient or a medical patient.

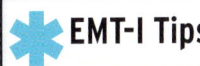
EMT-I Tips

People call 9-1-1 during some of the most difficult times of their lives. In some cases, they call because of a serious illness or injury. In others, they call because the patient or family is frightened, overwhelmed, or unable to cope with a more minor problem any longer. The patient is often fatigued, sick, frightened, angry, or sad, and the family often shares some or all of these feelings. Regardless of the exact nature of the call, the patient, family, and bystanders expect you to bring comfort, control, and resolution of these problems—emotional and physical.

In many ways, good communication skills are as important as technical proficiency, if not more so. Each step in the assessment process can be impeded by poor communication and each can be enhanced by a good connection between you and the patient and family. Here are five tips that can vastly improve your communication skills during the assessment process:

1. **Do whatever you can, quickly, to make yourself and the patient comfortable.** Patients are uncomfortable communicating with someone who is standing over them, pacing, or looking away. When time permits, sit down and/or position yourself near the patient, introduce yourself, and ask the patient's name **Figure 10-12**. This simple action signals the patient that you have time to talk; it opens the channels of communication as nothing else will. At the same time, be conscious of the patient's personal space. Do not move in too quickly. Ask the patient whether there is something you can do to make him or her more comfortable. Caring gestures and good body language are visible demonstrations of your care and concern.

2. **Actively listen to the patient.** In many cases, patients will be able to tell you what is wrong with them if you are paying attention and are truly listening. You can use several skills to actively listen, including leaning in toward the patient, taking selective notes, and periodically repeating back important points to the patient to ensure that you understood correctly. Active listening is often more difficult than it might seem, because scenes are often noisy and chaotic, and you will be receiving information from the patient, the family, your partner, and other EMS, fire, or law enforcement individuals on the scene. Try to screen them out for a few minutes so that you can truly listen to the patient; it will prove beneficial.

3. **Make eye contact with the person with whom you are speaking.** Eye contact signals that you are listening, so the patient is more likely to open up. An added benefit is that you will see facial expressions that, in some cases, communicate more clearly than the patient's words. For instance, you might see a facial grimace of pain or averted eyes possibly indicating embarrassment. Note that some cultures are uncomfortable with or offended by direct eye contact. Be sure to be familiar with the cultural background of citizens in your area.

4. **Base your initial questions on the patient's complaints.** No one likes to think that he or she is "just another patient," but that is what you communicate if you always ask the same questions of every patient, regardless of their complaints. If you ask questions about the Medicare number while the patient is trying to tell you about his or her pain, you are communicating that you are not really interested in the patient's problem. Talk about the patient's problem first; obtain demographic information after tending to the patient's needs.

5. **Before you start treatment, stop for a moment and mentally summarize** what you have learned and what you are going to do, then tell the patient. By providing necessary information to the patient and family, you help to relieve their anxiety and fear. This will also give them an opportunity to give you additional information if you have missed something.

You should spend your entire EMS career fine-tuning your patient assessment skills, as they are the cornerstone of high-quality prehospital care. A poor assessment almost always results in substandard patient care. Therefore, each patient should be approached with the same thorough assessment. Unless you take a systematic approach to patient assessment, you will systematically fail to find and treat life threats.

Be sure to focus some of your energy on improving the communication process. You will make it easier for patients to feel comfortable around you, which will help them to give honest, direct answers to your questions. As a result, you will get better assessment information in less time.

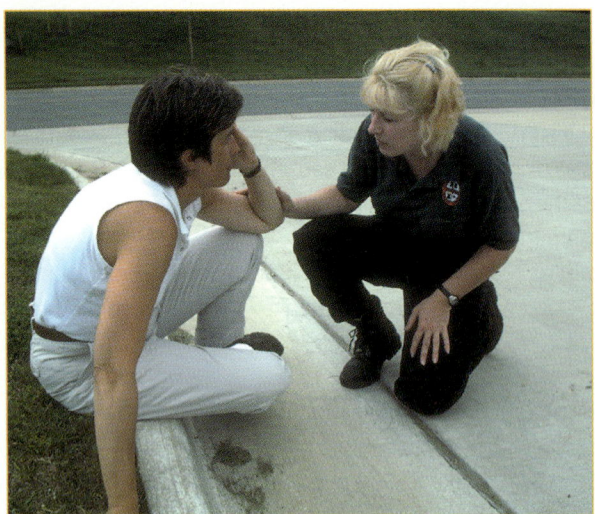

Figure 10-12 Position yourself near the patient, at eye level when possible, to begin to establish a relationship with the patient.

Approach to the Assessment Process

Remember, after developing a general impression of the patient's condition, you should begin your assessment and care in this order of importance:

- **A** = Airway
- **B** = Breathing
- **C** = Circulation

In all cases, your assessment of the patient's airway, breathing, and circulation (ABCs) will govern the extent of your treatment at the scene. As you approach you patient, attempt to make eye contact, and see if the patient can track your movement. This will help to determine the patient's level of consciousness. Next, look at the rise and fall of the chest. What is the patient's work of breathing? Does it appear adequate? Introduce yourself to the patient and ask how you can help (gaining consent). If the patient is able to speak, the airway is patent. Is the patient alert and oriented? Look for signs of poor <u>perfusion</u> (circulation). Is the skin pink, warm, and dry? Pale, cool, and <u>diaphoretic</u> (sweaty) skin is a telltale sign of hypoperfusion (shock).

Always give priority to emergency care of the ABCs to ensure life- and limb-saving treatment. Remember to assess the NOI or the MOI as part of the assessment process.

available to you, you need to ask and get answers to the following questions:

- Does the patient have an altered level of consciousness?
- Does the patient have an obstructed airway?
- Does the patient have inadequate breathing?
- Does the patient have inadequate circulation?
- Does the patient have the potential to develop any of these problems?
- Does the patient have the potential for a spinal cord injury?

If the answer to any of these questions is "yes," you need to take immediate action to treat or prevent the life-threatening condition by performing one or more of the following: opening the airway, assisting ventilation, giving supplemental oxygen, controlling severe bleeding, performing spinal immobilization, providing transport, or calling for a paramedic unit to assist or assume responsibility for patient care.

 Pediatric Needs

Mental status may be difficult to evaluate in children. First, determine whether the child is alert. Even infants should be alert to your presence and should follow you with their eyes (a process called "tracking"). Ask the parent whether the child is behaving normally, particularly in regard to alertness. Most children older than 2 years should know their own name and the names of their parents and siblings. Evaluate mental status in school-age children by asking about holidays, recent school activities, or teachers' names.

 EMT-I Tips

The quality of care that you provide to your patient is only as good as the assessment that you perform.

Assess Mental Status

Evaluating a patient's mental status is important because it reflects the functioning of the brain. Remember to maintain spinal immobilization if there is an MOI that

> **A to Z Terminology Tips**
>
> The terms *obtunded* and *stuporous* may also be used when describing mental status.
> - **Obtunded**—The patient does not perceive the environment fully and responds to stimuli appropriately but slowly.
> - **Stuporous**—The patient is aroused by intense stimuli only. Motor response and reflex reactions are usually intact unless the patient is paralyzed.

suggests trauma or the MOI is unclear. Many conditions may alter brain function and, hence, the level of consciousness. You will learn about many of these conditions as you progress through the EMT-I course.

Mental status and level of consciousness can be evaluated in just a few seconds by using two separate tests: responsiveness and orientation. The test for <u>responsiveness</u> assesses how well a patient responds to external stimuli, including verbal stimuli (sound) and painful stimuli (touch, such as pinching the patient's earlobe). For a patient who is alert and responding to verbal stimuli, you should next evaluate orientation. <u>Orientation</u> tests assess mental status by checking the patient's memory of person (his or her name), place (the current location), time (the current year, month, and approximate date), and event (what happened). These four questions were not selected at random. They evaluate long-term memory (name and place if the patient is at home), intermediate-term memory (place and time), and short-term memory (event). If the patient answers these questions appropriately, he or she is said to be "alert and fully oriented." If a patient is not able to answer one or more of your questions appropriately, he or she is considered disoriented. Loss of intermediate- and long-term memory (person and place) is thought to be related to more severe problems than loss of short-term memory. Collectively, your evaluation of the patient's responsiveness and orientation will paint a picture of the patient's overall mental status.

Responsiveness can be evaluated by using the <u>AVPU</u> scale:

- **Alert.** The patient's eyes open spontaneously as you approach, and the patient appears aware of and responsive to the environment. The patient appears to follow commands, and the eyes visually track people and objects.
- **Responsive to Verbal Stimuli.** The patient's eyes do not open spontaneously. However, the patient's eyes do open to verbal stimuli, and the patient is able to respond in some meaningful way when spoken to.
- **Responsive to Pain.** The patient does not respond to your questions but moves or cries out in response to a painful stimulus. This response is tested by gently but firmly pinching the patient's earlobe (Figure 10-13A▶), by pressing down on the bone above the eye (Figure 10-13B▶), or by pinching the muscles of the neck (Figure 10-13C▶). The sternal rub, although advocated in CPR training, is not recommended because it may be inaccurate in patients with cervical spine injuries because of the loss of sensation in that area. The use of ammonia inhalants (smelling salts) is not recommended. The patient may respond to painful stimuli by moaning, pushing your hand away, or withdrawing from the pain. Use of extremely painful stimuli is never appropriate.
- **Unresponsive.** The patient does not respond to any stimuli. If you are in doubt about whether a patient is truly unresponsive, assume the worst and treat appropriately.

An <u>altered mental status</u> (patient is less than alert and fully oriented) may be caused by a wide variety of conditions, including head trauma, hypoxemia, hypoglycemia, stroke, cardiac problems, or drug use. If the patient has altered mental status, you should rapidly complete the initial assessment and give high-flow supplemental oxygen. If the patient is breathing inadequately (that is, fast or slow respirations, reduced tidal volume [shallow breathing]), assist ventilations as needed. Perform spinal immobilization if trauma is suspected or cannot be ruled out, and initiate transport as soon as possible. Support the ABCs as required, and continually reassess for changes in the patient's condition.

Assess the Airway

As you move through the steps of assessment, you must always be alert for signs of respiratory compromise or airway obstruction. Regardless of the cause, airway obstruction may result in inadequate or absent air flow into and out of the lungs, which may cause permanent damage to the brain, heart, and lungs or may result in death. Proceeding with the assessment of a patient whose airway is not patent is futile; no airway, no patient!

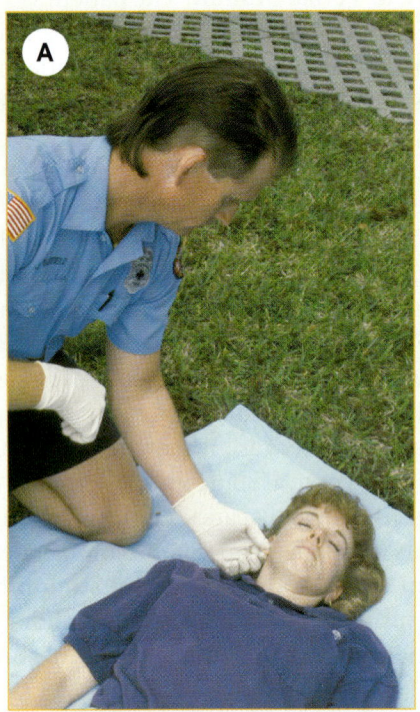 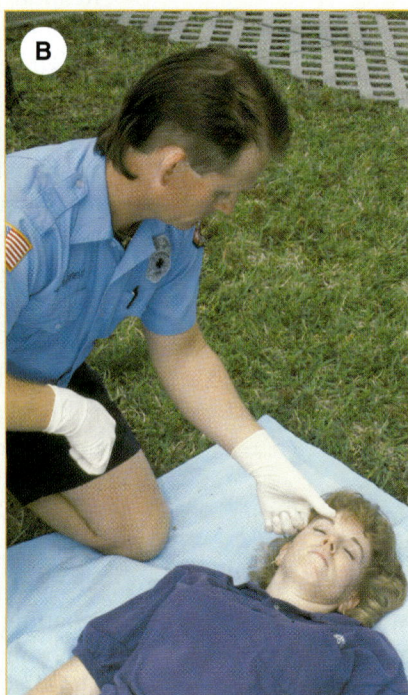 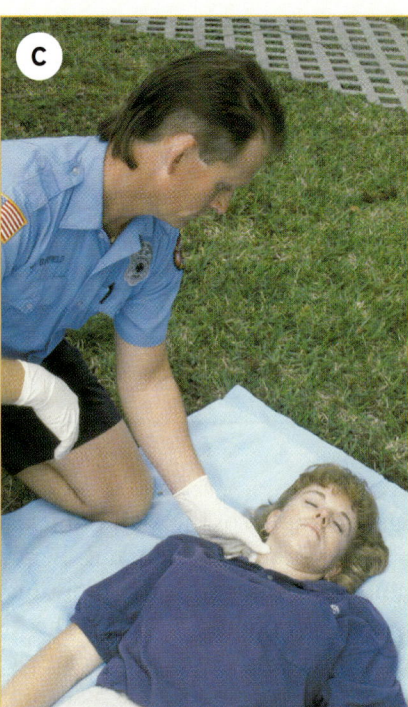

Figure 10-13 **A.** Gently but firmly pinch the patient's earlobe. **B.** Press down on the bone above the eye. **C.** Pinch the muscles of the neck.

Responsive Patients

Patients of any age who are responsive and are talking or crying have a patent airway. However, watching and listening to how patients speak, particularly those with respiratory problems, may provide important clues about the adequacy of their breathing status.

If you identify an airway problem, stop the assessment process, and open the airway using the head tilt–chin lift or, if trauma is suspected, the jaw-thrust maneuver. Although airway and breathing problems are not the same, their signs and symptoms often overlap. A patient who can speak only two to three words without pausing to take a breath, a condition known as <u>two-</u>

You are the Provider — Part 3

Your second patient is an 82-year-old man. He is complaining of nausea, vomiting, and diarrhea. As you approach him, you notice the following:

Initial Assessment	Recording Time: Zero Minutes
Appearance	In pain
Level of consciousness	Responsive verbally
Airway	Open and clear
Breathing	Respiratory rate, normal; depth, adequate
Circulation	Skin, pale and clammy; radial pulse, normal

6. What questions can the EMT-I ask to assess for potential life-threatening injuries or illnesses?
7. What method should the EMT-I use to evaluate the responsiveness of this patient?

to three-word dyspnea, has a severe breathing problem. The presence of retractions or the use of the accessory muscles (secondary muscles) of respiration is also a sign of inadequate breathing. Nasal flaring and use of the accessory muscles indicate that a child has inadequate breathing. Finally, obviously labored breathing is also a sign of airway or breathing difficulties.

Any of these signs may signal an immediate or pending airway and/or breathing problem. You should administer supplemental oxygen, be prepared to assist ventilations, and initiate transport.

Unresponsive Patients

With an unresponsive patient or one with a decreased level of consciousness, you should immediately assess the patency of the airway. If it is clear, you can continue your assessment. If the airway is not clear, your next priority is to open it using the head tilt–chin lift or jaw-thrust maneuver. Airway obstruction in an unresponsive patient is most commonly due to relaxation of the tongue, which falls back and occludes the posterior pharynx. Dentures, blood clots, vomitus, mucus, food, and other foreign objects may also create a blockage. Signs of airway compromise in an unresponsive patient include the following:

- Obvious trauma, blood, or other obstruction
- Noisy breathing, such as bubbling, gurgling, crowing, or other abnormal sounds (normal breathing is quiet)
- Extremely shallow (reduced tidal volume) or absent breathing

To open the airway, positioning depends on the nature of the problem. For medical patients, perform the head tilt–chin lift maneuver. For trauma patients or those whose condition is of an unknown cause, manually stabilize the cervical spine in a neutral, in-line position, and open the airway with the jaw-thrust maneuver.

Assess Breathing

As you assess the patient's breathing, look at how much work it takes for the patient to breathe. Normal respirations are not unusually shallow or excessively deep, and their rate varies widely in adults, anywhere from 12 to 20 breaths/min. Shallow respirations, which can be identified by minimal movement of the chest wall, indicate a reduction in tidal volume. Conversely, deep respirations cause a great deal of chest wall rise and fall and often can be heard as large volumes of air moving into and out of the patient's lungs. As you assess the patient, ask yourself the following questions:

- Are the patient's respirations shallow or deep?
- Does the patient appear to be choking?
- Is the patient cyanotic (blue)?
- Does the patient have adequate air movement from the nose and mouth?

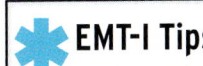

EMT-I Tips

Normal (eupneic) breathing should be quiet and not grossly evident to you. If you can see or hear the patient breathe, there is a problem.

If a patient is having difficulty breathing, you should immediately administer high-flow oxygen with a non-rebreathing mask. If the patient's breathing effort is inadequate, begin positive-pressure ventilatory assistance with a bag-valve-mask device and 100% oxygen.

Any patient with a decreased level of consciousness, respiratory distress, or poor skin color should also receive high-flow oxygen. If there is no risk of spinal injury, the patient should remain in a comfortable position that supports breathing; this is typically sitting up at a 45° angle (semi-Fowler's position) or a 90° angle (full Fowler's position). In any patient who has a possible risk for spinal injury, you should immobilize the cervical spine, ensuring that respirations are not compromised. Never withhold oxygen from a patient who needs it!

Use the look, listen, and feel technique to evaluate the adequacy of an unresponsive patient's breathing. If the patient is not breathing or is breathing inadequately, begin immediate positive pressure ventilations. The look, listen, and feel technique may be more difficult in infants and small children because they have so little chest wall movement during respirations; they are typically referred to as "belly breathers."

A spinal injury should be considered a possibility for any unresponsive trauma patient. These patients must immediately be rolled or moved as a single unit onto a flat surface or backboard to assess and manage the ABCs. Remember, you must move the head, neck, torso, and legs as a unit without any unnecessary bending or twisting.

Once the patient is properly positioned and the airway is open and clear, you should begin to treat and support the patient's breathing. For patients with adequate breathing, provide high-flow oxygen with a nonrebreathing mask; begin ventilations with a bag-valve-mask device and 100% oxygen if the patient is not breathing or is breathing inadequately.

Assess Circulation

Assessing circulation helps you evaluate how well blood is circulating to the major organs, including the brain, lungs, heart, and kidneys and to the rest of the body. A variety of problems can impair circulation, including blood loss, shock, and conditions that affect the heart and major blood vessels. Circulation is evaluated by assessing the presence and quality of the pulse, identifying external bleeding, and evaluating skin condition.

If the patient has a pulse but is not breathing, continue providing ventilations at a rate of 12 breaths/min for an adult and 20 breaths/min for an infant or child. Continue to monitor the pulse to evaluate the effectiveness of your ventilations. If at any time the pulse is lost, start CPR immediately and apply the automatic external defibrillator (AED) as soon as possible.

TABLE 10-3 Normal Pulse Rates in Infants and Children

Age	Range (beats/min)
Neonate: birth to 1 month	120 to 160
Infant: 1 month to 1 year	100 to 160
Toddler: 1 to 3 years	90 to 150
Preschool-age: 3 to 5 years	80 to 140
School-age: 6 to 12 years	70 to 120
Adolescent: 12 to 18 years	60 to 100
Older than 18 years: Adult normal range	60 to 100

Once a medical patient has been assessed to be in cardiac arrest, attach a cardiac monitor as soon as possible, interpret the cardiac rhythm, and perform immediate defibrillation if indicated.

Assess and Control External Bleeding

The next step is to identify any major external bleeding. In some instances, blood loss can be very rapid and can quickly result in shock and even death. Therefore, this step demands your immediate attention as soon as the patient's airway is secured and breathing is stabilized. Signs of blood loss include active bleeding from wounds and/or evidence of bleeding such as blood on the clothes or near the patient. Serious bleeding from a large vein may be characterized by steady flow of dark red blood. Bleeding from an artery is characterized by a spurting flow of bright red blood. When you evaluate an unresponsive patient, do a sweep for blood by quickly and lightly running your gloved hands from head to toe, pausing periodically to see whether your gloves are bloody.

Controlling external bleeding is often very simple. In almost all cases, direct pressure with your gloved hand and a sterile bandage over the wound will control bleeding. This pressure stops the flow of blood and helps the blood to **coagulate**, or clot naturally. Remember to take the appropriate BSI precautions whenever you are assessing any patient.

Most often, bleeding can be adequately controlled by using direct pressure, along with elevating the extremity if bleeding is from the arms or legs. When direct

Pediatric Needs

You can feel the pulse of a child at the carotid artery, as in an adult. However, palpating this pulse in an infant may present a problem. Because an infant's neck is often very short and fat and an infant's pulse is often quite fast, you may have a hard time finding the carotid pulse. Therefore, in children younger than 1 year, you should palpate the brachial artery to assess the pulse. Normal pulse rates for children are shown in Table 10-3 ▶.

Assess the Pulse

The rate, rhythm, and strength of the patient's pulse will give you a rough idea of the overall status of the patient's cardiac function. The pulse is one of the vital signs that you should reassess often in most patients, even en route to the hospital.

If you cannot **palpate** a pulse in an unresponsive patient, begin CPR. The AED should be used on medical (nontrauma) patients who are at least 1 year old and who have been assessed to be unresponsive, apneic, and pulseless.

pressure and elevation are not successful, you may apply pressure directly over arterial pressure points.

Evaluate Skin Color, Temperature, and Condition

Assessing the skin is one of the most important and most readily accessible ways of evaluating circulation. You should assess the patient's skin color, temperature, and condition.

Color

Skin color depends on pigmentation and blood oxygen levels and on the amount of blood circulating through the vessels of the skin. For this reason, skin color is a valuable assessment tool. The normal skin color of lightly pigmented people is pinkish. Abnormal skin color in people with deeply pigmented skin may be difficult to assess. Therefore, you should look for changes in color in areas of the skin that have less pigment: the fingernail beds, the <u>sclera</u> (white of the eyes), the <u>conjunctiva</u> (lining of the eyelid), and the mucous membranes of the mouth. Normal skin color, particularly of the conjunctivae and mucous membranes, is pinkish. Skin colors that should alert you to possible problems include blue (<u>cyanosis</u>), red (flushed), white (pale), and yellow (<u>jaundice</u>).

Temperature

The skin is actually an organ, and like all other organs, it has many functions. It helps maintain the water content of the body, acts as insulation and protection from infection, and also has a role in regulation of body temperature. Generally speaking, normal body temperature is 98.6°F (37°C); however, this varies from person to person. Body temperature can also change as a result of illness or injury. When assessing temperature, lift the shirt and touch the trunk of the body, comparing the temperature to the temperature of the extremities, which may be much cooler. Abnormally cool skin could indicate shock or hypothermia and abnormally warm skin could indicate fever or hyperthermia (such as in heatstroke). Assess the skin temperature by touching the patient's skin with your wrist or the back of your hand (Figure 10-14 ▶).

Condition

Finally, determine whether the patient's skin is dry or moist. The skin is normally warm and dry. Cool or cold, moist, clammy skin suggests shock. Hot skin may indicate an abnormally elevated body temperature or fever.

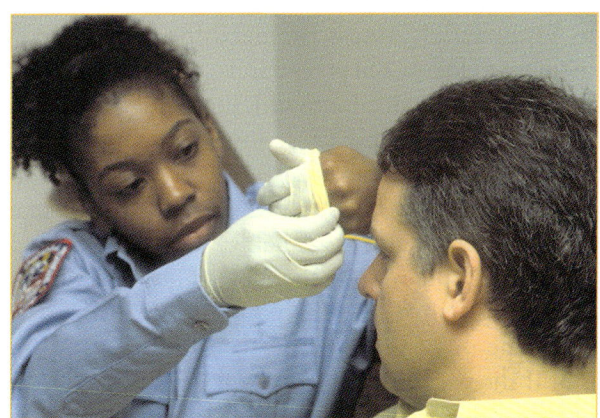

Figure 10-14 Assess skin temperature by touching the patient's skin with the back of your ungloved hand.

Capillary Refill

Another way to assess circulation is to check capillary refill, especially in children younger than 6 years. <u>Capillary refill</u> is the ability of the circulatory system to restore blood to the capillaries after circulation has been interrupted. Test capillary refill by squeezing the patient's fingernail bed until the area blanches (turns white). Next, release the fingernail bed, and watch for it to return to a normal color. The area should return to its normal color within 2 seconds. If the area remains white or becomes blue, you know that circulation is inadequate, at least in the area being tested.

Capillary refill can be checked in children by squeezing the entire arm or leg at a distal point and observing the return to normal color. Although capillary refill is a quick and very general way to evaluate circulation, it is important to remember that other conditions, not related to the body's circulation, may also slow capillary refill. These conditions include the patient's age and sex, exposure to a cold environment (which can result in <u>hypothermia</u>), frozen tissue (<u>frostbite</u>), and injuries to bones or muscles that cause local circulatory compromise.

Restoring Circulation

If a patient has inadequate circulation, you must take immediate action to restore or improve circulation, control severe bleeding, and improve oxygen delivery to the tissues. The apparent absence of a palpable pulse in a responsive patient is indicative of a low cardiac output state—not cardiac arrest. However, if you cannot feel a pulse in an unresponsive adult, you should begin CPR if an AED or manual defibrillator is not readily available. Once an AED or manual defibrillator is available, immediately assess the need for defibrillation. Remember to follow BSI precautions, which may include use of a barrier device for ventilation, gloves, and protective eyewear. Follow these four steps for a patient who has no pulse and is unresponsive:

1. **Immediately begin CPR** until an AED or manual defibrillator is available.
2. **Apply and operate the AED** as quickly as possible. Defibrillation is your first priority if the patient is 1 year or older.
3. **If the cardiac arrest is associated** with an obvious, apparently catastrophic traumatic event, perform CPR. Traumatic cardiac arrest is usually the result of massive blood loss and typically does not respond to defibrillation; therefore, an AED is generally not indicated for these patients. Treatment should include airway management, bleeding control, and chest compressions, followed by rapid transport to the hospital. Immediate transport to a trauma center is the most valuable therapy for the patient in traumatic cardiac arrest.
4. **Initiate use of the AED** in association with CPR, if in doubt about a traumatic origin of the arrest.

Although the AED is not indicated for patients with traumatic cardiac arrest or for patients younger than 1 year, you must evaluate the cardiac rhythm of *any* patient in cardiac arrest with a manual cardiac monitor/defibrillator, trauma and age notwithstanding. Identifying the patient's cardiac rhythm will enable you to administer the most appropriate medication therapy. Although patients with traumatic cardiac arrest will likely require intravenous (IV) fluid therapy for blood loss, certain medications will be needed to treat the cardiac arrest itself.

Continued impaired circulation is devastating to the body's cells because it deprives the cells of vital oxygen, which is necessary for cell function. CPR and bleeding control are intended to maintain circulation. Oxygen delivery is improved through the administration of 100% supplemental oxygen. Any patient with impaired circulation should receive high-flow oxygen via a nonrebreathing mask or assisted ventilation to improve oxygen delivery at the cellular level.

Identify Priority Patients

Once you have completed the initial assessment, you have to make some decisions about patient care. You should have already addressed all life-threatening injuries and/or illnesses immediately on discovery. Next, you must identify priority patients, or those who need other interventions and/or immediate transport Figure 10-15 ▶. It is crucial to recognize which patients require further care before transport as opposed to those who need immediate transport with other interventions performed en route. Prehospital care providers, regardless of their level of certification, cannot provide definitive care in the field; they

---

You are the Provider — Part 4

You and your partner work together, and you continue to assess the first patient, which reveals the following:

Vital Signs	Recording Time: 2 Minutes After Patient Contact
Respirations	20 breaths/min; unlabored
Pulse	124 beats/min; slightly irregular
Skin	Pale
Blood pressure	112/68 mm Hg
SaO_2	90% while breathing room air

8. What conditions should the EMT-I consider high priority or consider for paramedic backup?
9. What are three goals of the focused history and physical exam?

can only recognize the patient's problem, attempt to stabilize the patient's condition, and provide transport to an appropriate medical facility.

For example, a trauma patient with signs of intra-abdominal bleeding could have a lacerated liver or spleen. Definitive care of these types of injuries can only be provided in an operating room. Therefore, the EMT-I's role is limited to improving oxygenation, maintaining perfusion, and providing prompt transport to a trauma center.

Patients with one of the following conditions are considered high priority and should be transported immediately, while considering the need for paramedic backup:

- A serious MOI
- Poor general impression
- Unresponsive with no gag or cough reflexes
- Responsive but unable to follow commands
- Difficulty breathing
- Pale skin or other signs of poor perfusion
- Complicated childbirth
- Uncontrolled bleeding
- Severe pain in any area of the body
- Chest pain, especially when the systolic blood pressure is less than 100 mm Hg
- Inability to move any part of the body

Correct identification of high-priority patients is an essential aspect of the initial assessment and helps to improve patient outcome.

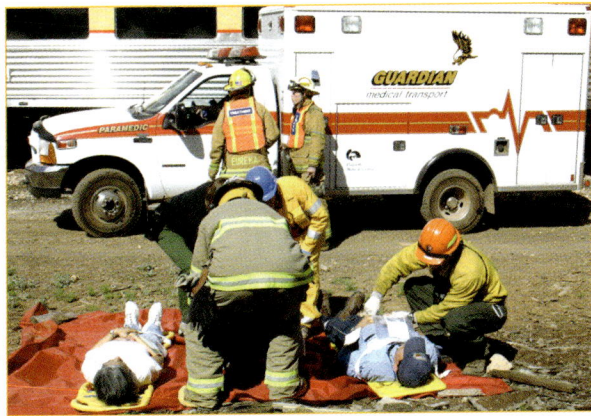

Figure 10-15 Identifying priority patients.

While initial treatment is important, it is essential to remember that immediate transport is one of the keys to the survival of any high-priority patient. Transport should be initiated as soon as practical and possible. Once you have completed the initial assessment and made a transport decision, you can turn to the focused history and physical exam. The appropriate focused history and physical exam is based on your current assessment of whether the cause of the patient's problem is trauma, a medical emergency, or both.

Patient Assessment

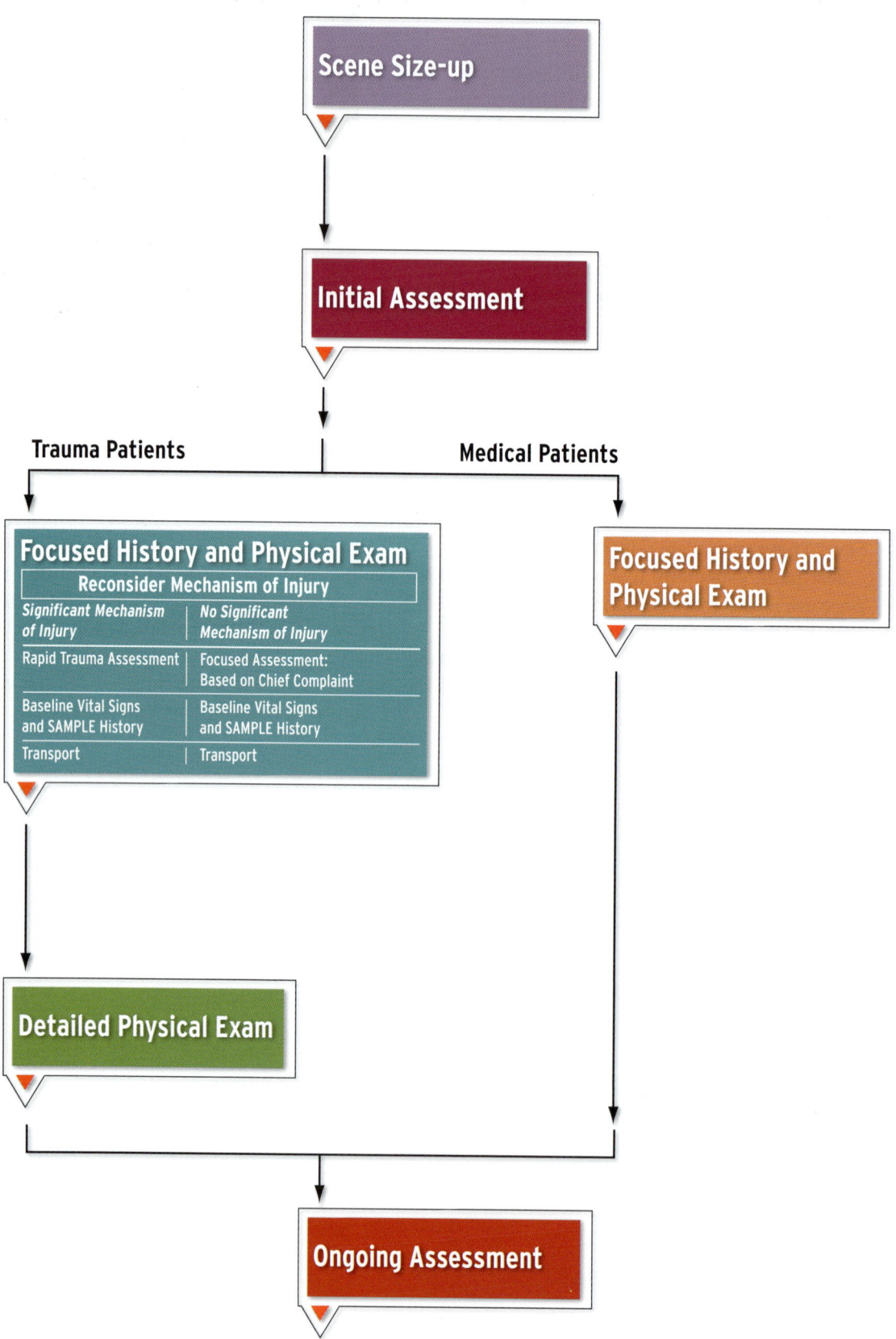

Focused History and Physical Exam: Trauma Patients

As a rule, all prehospital emergency calls are divided into two categories: medical calls and trauma calls. However, it is vitally important that we do not categorize the patients as medical patients or trauma patients until we have sufficient evidence. To prematurely label a patient can cause one to miss possible life threats. For example, if you were to arrive on scene where a man had fallen from a ladder, was unresponsive, and had bilateral femur fractures, it would be easy to label him as a trauma patient and care for his injuries. If he was hypoglycemic, however, which caused him to fall off the ladder, the diabetic life threat might be missed. Although this section examines the specifics of trauma and medical patients, you should avoid approaching any call with the preconceived notion that the patient's problem is exclusively traumatic or medical in origin. A careful, systematic assessment will be required to determine the patient's primary problem.

Goals of the Focused History and Physical Exam

The focused history and physical exam (formerly called the secondary survey) helps you to focus on specific problems. There are three goals:

1. Identify the patient's chief complaint.
   - What happened to this patient?
2. Understand the specific circumstances surrounding the chief complaint.
   - What circumstances were associated with the event?
   - Is the MOI a high risk for serious injuries?
3. Direct further physical examination.
   - What problems can be identified through the physical exam?

The focused history and physical exam, like the entire assessment process, guides you to take actions that will stabilize the patient's problems. Depending on the answers to these questions, you should be prepared to return to the initial assessment and treat potentially life-threatening conditions immediately on identification, perform spinal immobilization, and provide immediate transport while considering the need to coordinate a rendezvous with a paramedic unit.

Patients who call 9-1-1 following an emergency may have any number of problems—medical, traumatic, or a combination of both. Assess and manage all patients in the same systematic manner. Once you have identified that a patient has sustained a traumatic injury, you need to rapidly make some important treatment and transport decisions. This is because some traumatic injuries are life threatening and cannot be treated definitively in the field. These patients have the best chance for survival if they arrive at an appropriate hospital, usually a trauma center if available, for definitive care within 60 minutes of the time of injury. Definitive care is defined as the care that the patient requires in order to survive, whether it be surgery, hospitalization, or other care. You will often hear this period called the Golden Hour. The Golden Hour is the time interval between injury and definitive care, after which survival from shock or traumatic injuries decreases (Figure 10-16). After the first 60 minutes, the body has increasing difficulty compensating for traumatic injuries. For this reason, you should spend as little time as possible on the scene with patients who have sustained severe trauma. Aim to assess, treat immediate life threats, package, and begin transporting the patient no more than 10 minutes after arrival on the scene (that is, the Platinum Ten Minutes). This may not be possible in cases of a difficult or lengthy extrication or in other extenuating circumstances. Table 10-4 lists the components of the focused history and physical exam for the trauma patient.

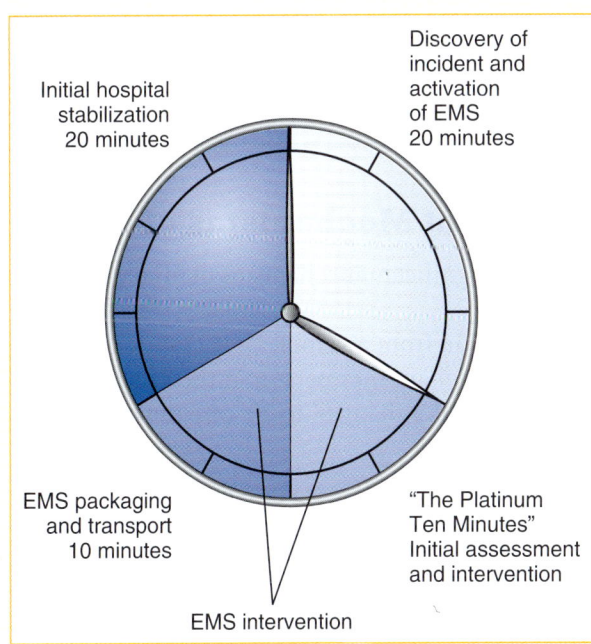

Figure 10-16 The Golden Hour is the time after which survival from shock or traumatic injuries decreases.

TABLE 10-4 Focused History and Physical Exam: Trauma Patients

Reconsider the MOI	
Trauma Patients With Significant MOI	**Trauma Patients With No Significant MOI**
Rapid trauma assessment	Focused assessment: based on chief complaint
Baseline vital signs and SAMPLE history	Baseline vital signs and SAMPLE history
Transport	Transport

Reconsider the MOI

As part of the scene size-up, you evaluated the MOI before you began treatment. At this point in the assessment process, you should look at the mechanism again to ensure that you have not missed important information. Understanding the MOI helps you to understand the potential severity of the patient's problem and provide valuable information to hospital staff as well. Some patients have experienced a significant MOI; others clearly have not. The MOI will also serve as a guide in choosing the focused assessment or the rapid trauma assessment.

EMT-I Tips

When reconsidering the MOI, do not let your guard down and reclassify the patient at a lower level of severity. Human instinct is your most effective tool when assessing a patient with potentially critical injuries. When in doubt, assume that a potentially life-threatening injury exists and treat the patient accordingly.

Significant Mechanisms of Injury

Recall that significant mechanisms of injury include the following:

- Ejection from a vehicle
- Death of another person in the same vehicle
- Fall greater than 15′ to 20′ or 3 times the patient's height
- Vehicle rollover
- High-speed (≥35 mph) vehicle collision
- Vehicle-pedestrian collision
- Motorcycle crash
- Unresponsiveness or altered mental status following trauma
- Penetrating trauma to the head, chest, or abdomen

Infant and Child Considerations

Significant mechanisms of injury for children include those in the preceding list with the following additions or modifications:

- Fall greater than 10′ or two to three times the child's height
- Bicycle crash

Hidden Injuries

Seat belts and airbags have significantly reduced the death and disability associated with MVCs. However, you should be aware that seat belts and airbags can also cause injuries. When evaluating a patient who was involved in an MVC, you should look for and ask questions to determine whether seat belts and/or an airbag were involved.

A to Z Terminology Tips

When assessing a patient, always consider *occult* injuries. Think of the *occult* as things we cannot visibly see (for example, poltergeists, ghosts). Occult injuries are those that are not visible to the eye. This includes damage to internal organs such as a lacerated liver from impact with the steering wheel.

Seat Belts

Seat belts have prevented many thousands of injuries and have saved countless numbers of lives. Patients who otherwise would have been ejected from their vehicle owe their lives to seat belts. However, if the force of a crash is great enough, patients can sustain internal injuries under the seat belts, although these injuries are less severe than the injuries the patients would have sustained if they had not been wearing seat belts. Seat

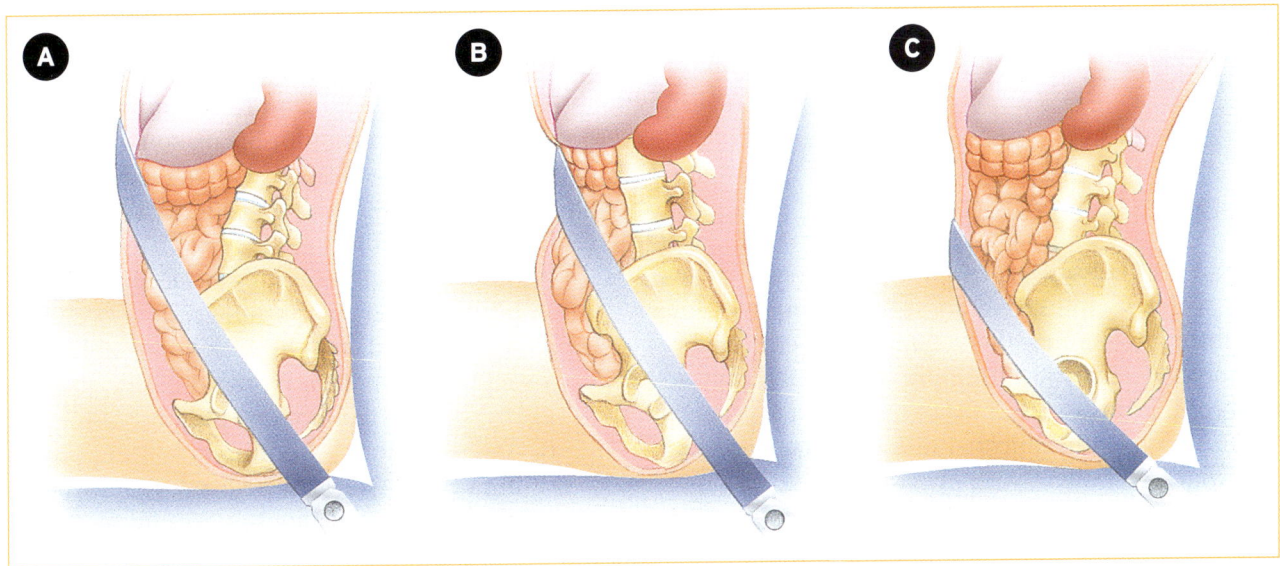

Figure 10-17 **A.** Injury may occur if the seat belt is placed too far above the iliac crest. **B.** A sudden stop could cause compression of the organs between the belt and the spine. **C.** The proper location of the seat belt is below the iliac crests.

belts that are worn improperly across the abdomen rather than across the pelvic bones increase the potential for internal injuries Figure 10-17 ▲. Lap seat belts must be worn so that they lie below the iliac crests, snugly up against the hip joints. If the seat belt is worn too high, sudden slowing or an abrupt stop (deceleration) may result in abdominal injuries. Occasionally, injuries of the lumbar spine can occur, even if the patient is wearing the seat belt properly.

Lap belts and shoulder belts are now commonly combined into a single unit. Some cars still have separate lap and shoulder belts. Used alone, shoulder belts can cause injuries to the head, chest, ribs, and liver.

Airbags

Airbags represent a great advance in automotive safety. Before airbags were common, individuals in head-on crashes would typically have significant facial injuries and bleeding—clear, visible signs that they had been injured. With airbags, patients occasionally have facial burns or respiratory problems from the chemical process that causes the airbag to expand, or they may have abrasions from the airbag itself. However, with airbags and seat belts, patients may or may not have visible injuries. Remember, patients who have been involved in serious crashes may initially look uninjured but still may have internal injuries.

When an airbag deploys, a patient who is not wearing a seat belt can still go up and over or down and under the steering column. You should always look under a deployed airbag to see whether the steering wheel is bent or deformed in any way Figure 10-18 ▼. Remove the patient from the car, using spinal precautions. If the steering wheel is bent or deformed, you should suspect possible internal injuries. Injuries, however, are still possible if the steering wheel is not bent or deformed. The general health of the patient, the patient's age, and other factors can also affect the likelihood of severe injuries.

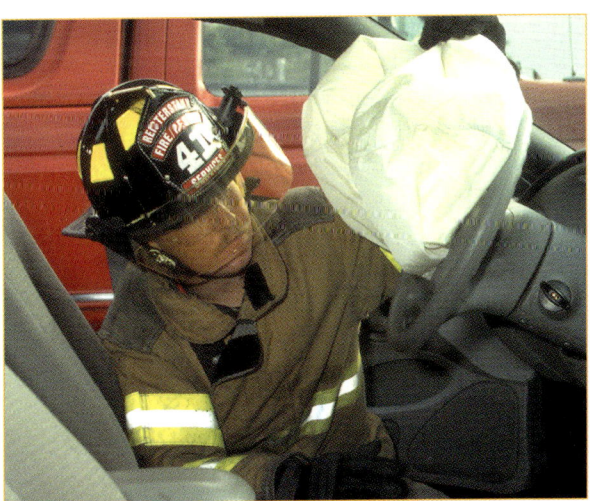

Figure 10-18 If an airbag has deployed, you should lift the airbag and check the steering wheel to see whether it is bent.

During your hand-off report at the hospital, make sure that you tell hospital personnel whether seat belts were worn and whether the airbag deployed.

Trauma Patients With a Significant MOI

The rapid trauma assessment should be performed on any patient with a significant MOI to identify and treat any life-threatening injuries; it should also be performed if any abnormalities are identified in the initial assessment. The purpose of this assessment is to zero in on the patient's problems and identify potentially life-threatening conditions, which will direct your physical exam. The rapid trauma assessment should be performed on responsive patients with a significant MOI and unresponsive patients who cannot tell you what happened. Remember, you can use a responsive patient as a resource; you should ask him or her about symptoms throughout your assessment.

An integral part of this assessment is evaluation using the simple mnemonic "DCAP-BTLS." For each area of the body, you should quickly look and feel for Deformities, Contusions, Abrasions, Punctures/Penetrations, Burns, Tenderness, Lacerations, and Swelling (DCAP-BTLS). Remember, you should treat any immediately or potentially life-threatening conditions encountered during the rapid trauma assessment. Once these conditions have been treated, you should continue with your assessment.

Rapid Trauma Assessment

As you prepare for the rapid trauma assessment, consider your transport decision and request paramedic backup if appropriate. The rapid trauma assessment is indicated for any patient with a significant MOI or abnormal findings in the initial assessment and for unresponsive patients. The goal of the rapid assessment is to find and treat any immediate life threats and is usually accomplished on scene before transport. Follow the steps in (Skill Drill 10-1 ▶):

1. **Continue spinal immobilization** while you check the patient's ABCs for any changes in status since the initial assessment, and evaluate mental status.
2. **Assess the head**, looking and feeling for DCAP-BTLS and crepitus (**Step 1**).
3. **Assess the neck**, looking and feeling for DCAP-BTLS, tracheal deviation, jugular venous distention (JVD), and crepitus (**Step 2**).
4. **Apply a cervical spinal immobilization collar** (**Step 3**).
5. **Assess the chest**, looking and feeling for DCAP-BTLS, paradoxical motion, and crepitus. You should also assess for breath sounds (**Step 4**).
6. **Assess the abdomen**, looking and feeling for DCAP-BTLS, rigidity, tenderness, and distention (**Step 5**).
7. **Assess the pelvis**, looking and feeling for DCAP-BTLS. If there is no pain, gently compress the pelvis inward and downward to determine tenderness or instability; never assess the pelvis using a rocking motion (**Step 6**).
8. **Assess all four extremities**, looking and feeling for DCAP-BTLS. Also assess and compare bilaterally for distal pulses, motor function, and sensation (**Step 7**).
9. **Log roll the patient using spinal precautions**, and assess the posterior aspect of the body, looking and feeling for DCAP-BTLS (**Step 8**).
10. **Fully immobilize the spine**, and assess baseline vital signs and SAMPLE history (**Step 9**).

Recognizing a possible spinal injury is one of your principal responsibilities as an EMT-I. You should assume a spinal injury in any patient who has a mechanism that reflects or suggests a significant history of trauma, is intoxicated and may have been traumatized, is unresponsive, received trauma above the clavicles, complains of neck or back pain following a traumatic event, or cannot move or feel in any or all four extremities following a traumatic event. Immediately begin manual immobilization of the spine. Consider requesting paramedic backup or transporting the patient with priority status. Also reevaluate the patient's mental status. Finally, be sure to expose covered or closed areas in significant trauma patients so you can completely assess and treat the patient. You cannot treat what you cannot see.

Head, Neck, and Cervical Spine

Look for abnormalities of the head, neck, and cervical spine. Gently palpate the head and the back of the neck for deformity, tenderness, or crepitus, also checking as you feel for any bleeding. Crepitus is the grating or grinding sensation that is often felt or heard when two ends of a broken bone rub together. Ask a responsive patient if he or she feels any pain or tenderness. Next, check the neck for signs of trauma, swelling, or bleeding. Feel the skin of the neck for air under the skin, known as subcutaneous emphysema, and for any abnormal lumps or masses. It is particularly important to evaluate the neck before covering it with a cervical collar. Also look for pronounced or distended jugular veins. This is normal in a patient who is lying down; however, their presence in a patient who is sitting up suggests some problem with blood returning to the heart. Also note whether the trachea is in the midline position or is deviated away from the midline. Report and record your findings carefully. Do not move on to the next step until you are sure that the airway is secure, the patient is breathing adequately, and you have initiated or continued spinal immobilization.

Chest

Next, look at and feel over the chest area for injury or signs of trauma, including bruising, tenderness, or swelling. Watch the chest rise and fall with breathing. Normal breathing should be symmetrical, in which both sides of the chest rise and fall together. Look for abnormal breathing signs, including retractions (when the skin pulls in around the ribs during inspiration) or paradoxical motion (when one section falls on inspiration while the remainder of the chest rises).

Retractions indicate that the patient has some condition that is impairing the flow of air into and out of the lungs. Paradoxical motion is associated with a fracture of several ribs (flail chest), causing the affected section to move independently from the rest of the chest. When palpating the chest, note if there is any crepitus, which is indicative of fractured ribs. Do not purposely elicit for crepitus, as this may cause further injury to the patient. Palpate the chest for subcutaneous emphysema, especially in cases of severe blunt chest trauma.

If the patient reports difficulty breathing or has evidence of trauma to the chest, auscultate for breath sounds. This helps you to evaluate air movement in and out of the lungs and to determine the presence of unilaterally diminished or absent breath sounds Figure 10-19 ▶.

Here's how and where to auscultate breath sounds:
- First, remember that you can almost always hear breath sounds better from the patient's back. So if the patient's back is accessible, listen there. If you have immobilized the patient or if the patient is in a supine position, auscultate over the anterior part of the chest.
- Auscultate all lung fields and compare side to side. Listen over the upper lungs (apices), the lower lungs (bases), and over the major airways (midclavicular and midaxillary lines).
- Lift the clothing, or slide the stethoscope under the clothing. When you listen over clothing, you are hearing primarily the sound of the stethoscope sliding over the fabric, which will generate an inaccurate sound.
- Place the diaphragm of the stethoscope firmly against the chest to most effectively hear the breath sounds.

What are you auscultating for? Besides normal breath sounds, you may hear adventitious (abnormal) sounds such as rales (crackles), rhonchi, stridor, wheezing, and pleural friction rubs. Rales (also known as crackles) are sounds that are produced by oxygen passing through moisture in the bronchoalveolar system, or from closed alveoli opening abruptly. The sound can be likened to rubbing two pieces of hair together. It can be associated with heart failure or chronic bronchitis, as the smaller airways in the lungs begin to fill with fluid. Rales are often difficult to hear, especially in the back of a moving ambulance.

Rhonchi are continuous sounds with a lower pitch and a rattling quality and are indicative of fluid in the larger airways in the lungs. Rhonchi are commonly heard

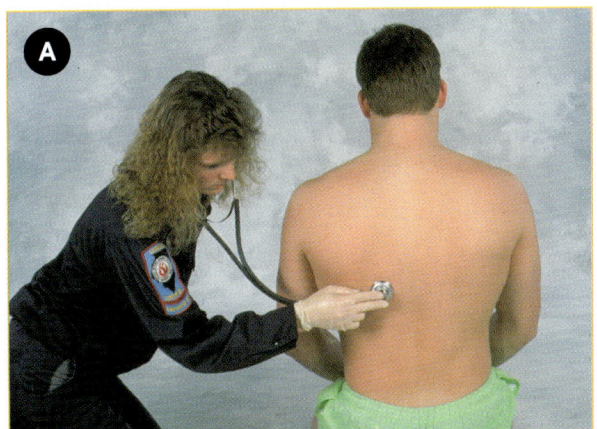

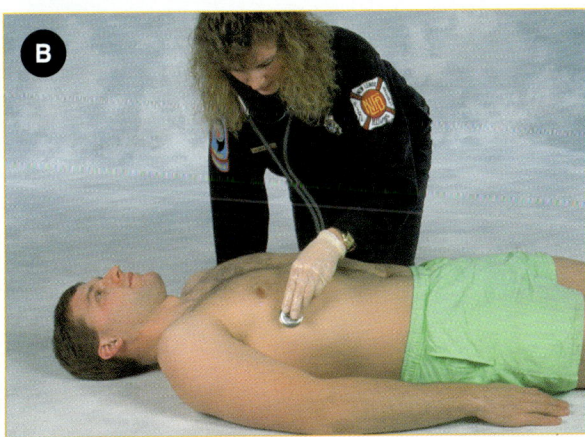

Figure 10-19 A. Listen to breath sounds from the patient's back if possible, over the apices, the bases, and the major airways. **B.** If the patient is immobilized or in a supine position, listen from the front.

Skill Drill 10-1: Performing a Rapid Trauma Assessment

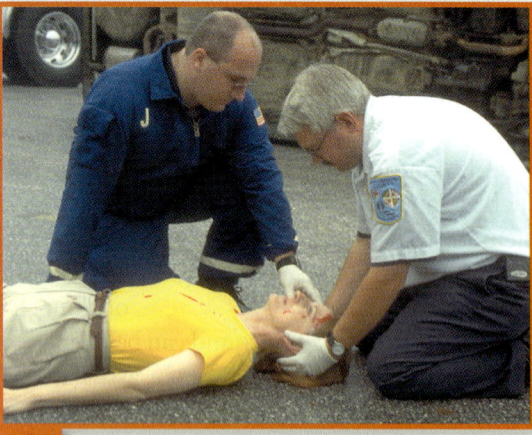

1. Check the ABCs, continue spinal immobilization, and assess mental status. Assess the head.

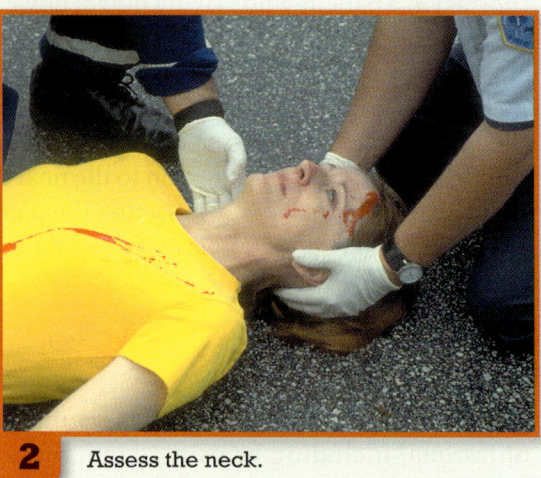

2. Assess the neck.

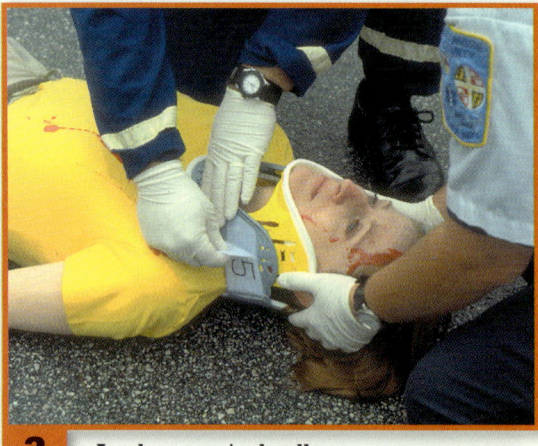

3. Apply a cervical collar.

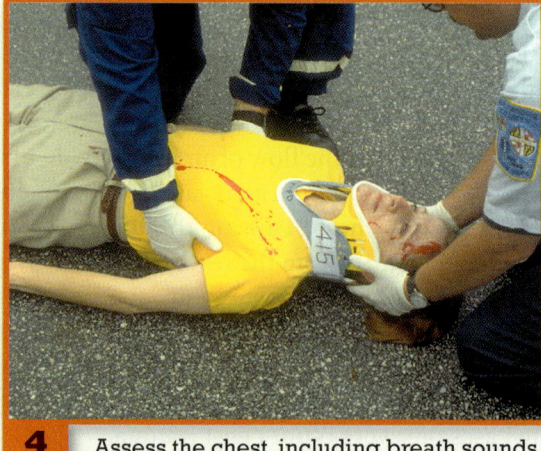

4. Assess the chest, including breath sounds.

5. Assess the abdomen.

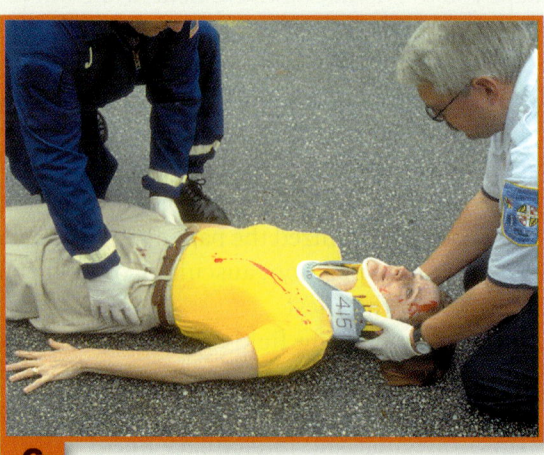

6. Assess the pelvis.

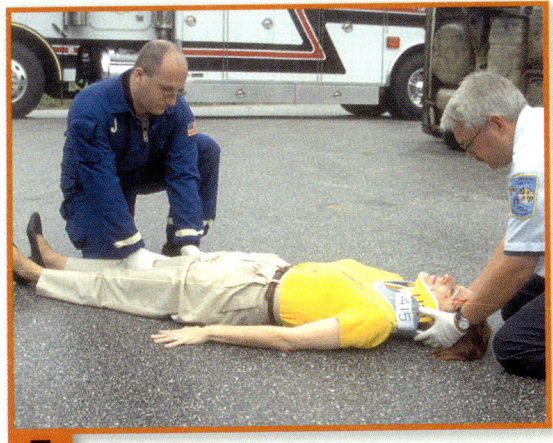
7 Assess the extremities.

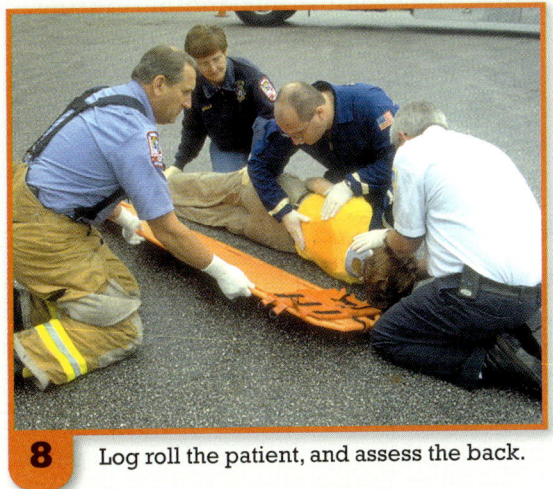
8 Log roll the patient, and assess the back.

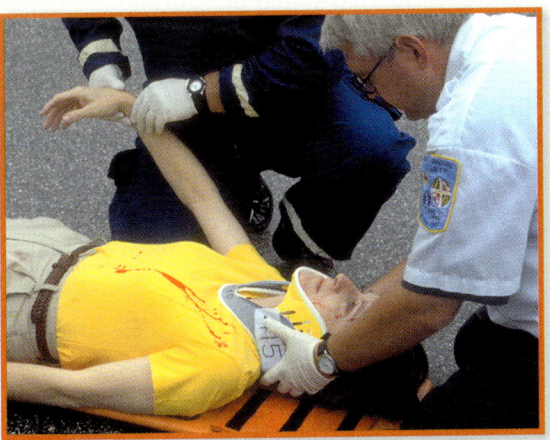
9 Fully immobilize the spine and assess baseline vital signs and obtain a SAMPLE history.

in cases of severe congestive heart failure, pulmonary edema, bronchitis, and pneumonia. They are usually heard during exhalation, but may be heard during inhalation as well. In severe cases, rhonchi are often audible without a stethoscope. **Aspiration** of fluid may also result in rhonchi.

Stridor is usually heard during inspiration, even without a stethoscope. It is a crowing-type sound caused by the narrowing, swelling, or obstruction of the upper airway. Stridor may be caused by bacterial **epiglottitis**, viral **croup**, swelling from upper airway burns, or a partial foreign-body airway obstruction. Stridor often indicates a life-threatening problem, especially in children, and requires astute observation for hypoxia and respiratory failure.

Wheezing is a high-pitched, whistling noise that is usually more prominent during expiration. It is caused by air being forced through narrowed airways and is often associated with asthma, bronchitis, and other disease processes that cause constriction of the bronchioles (**bronchospasm**). Wheezes are classified as mild, moderate, and severe. Mild wheezing is typically noted on expiration; moderate wheezing is typically heard during inspiration and expiration; and severe wheezing is often faint or difficult to hear, indicating severe bronchospasm.

Pleural friction rub is a low-pitched, dry, rubbing sound caused by the movement of inflamed pleural surfaces as they slide against one another during breathing. It is usually the loudest over the lower anterolateral surface of the chest wall and may indicate pleurisy, viral infection, tuberculosis, or a pulmonary embolism.

Abdomen

Visually inspect the abdomen for bruising or other discoloration, bleeding, swelling, masses and aortic pulsations. Palpate all four quadrants, beginning with the quadrant that is farthest from any pain, if present. Use the terms "firm," "soft," "tender," or "distended" (swollen) to report your abdominal exam findings. If the patient is conscious and alert, ask him or her to describe the pain. Do not palpate obvious soft-tissue injuries, and be careful not to palpate too hard.

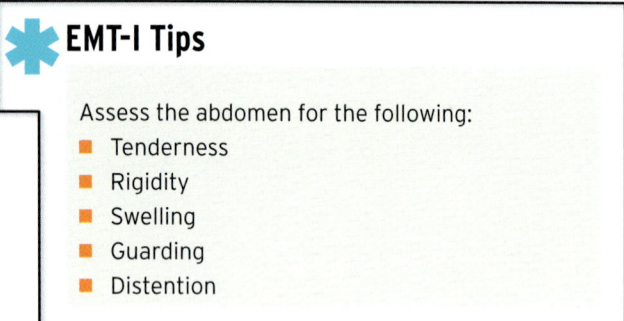

EMT-I Tips

Assess the abdomen for the following:
- Tenderness
- Rigidity
- Swelling
- Guarding
- Distention

Pelvis

Look for any signs of obvious injury, bleeding, or deformity. If the patient reports no pain, gently press inward and downward on the pelvic bones. Do not rock the pelvis because this motion may move an unstable spine. Use the heel of your hand to press down gently over the pubic symphysis to check for stability. If you feel any deformities or crepitus or the patient reports pain or tenderness to palpation, there may be a severe injury. If the pelvis is unstable or is painful to palpation, do not log roll the patient when placing him or her onto the backboard. Instead, use an orthopaedic (scoop) stretcher to place the patient onto the backboard.

Injuries to the pelvis and abdomen may result in severe internal bleeding, so continue to monitor the patient carefully and administer 100% oxygen. Once en route to the hospital, at least one large-bore IV line should be inserted in case fluid resuscitation is needed.

Extremities

Look for lacerations, ecchymosis, swelling, obvious injuries, and bleeding. Next, feel along each extremity for deformities. Ask the patient about any tenderness or pain. As you evaluate the extremities, check for circulation and motor and sensory function:

- **Circulation**: Check the distal pulses on the foot (dorsalis pedis or posterior tibial) and wrist (radial). Evaluate the skin color in the hands or feet. Is it normal? How does it compare with the skin color of the other extremities? Pale or cyanotic skin may indicate poor circulation in the extremity.
- **Motor function**: Ask the patient to wiggle his or her fingers or toes. An inability to move a single extremity can be the result of a bone, muscle, or nerve injury. Inability to move several extremities may be a sign of a brain abnormality or spinal cord injury. Verify that spinal precautions are in place.
- **Sensory function**: Evaluate normal feeling in the extremity by asking the patient to close his or her eyes. Gently squeeze or pinch a finger or toe, and ask the patient to identify what you are doing. The inability to feel sensation in an extremity may indicate a local nerve injury. Inability to feel in several extremities may be a sign of spinal cord injury. Recheck to be sure that you have begun and/or are maintaining spinal immobilization.

In the Field

A Babinski test may be used to check for sensation in an unresponsive patient. This is accomplished by stimulating the sole of the foot by rubbing your pen or other object along the sole of the foot. A normal reaction in young children and infants is for the great toe to flex toward the top of the foot and the other toes to fan out. However, this is an abnormal reaction in older children or adults. **DO NOT** perform a Babinski test on a patient who has injuries to the lower extremities. This could cause the patient to pull the leg back, causing pain.

Back

Inspect the back for discoloration or open wounds, and palpate for tenderness or deformity. When placing the patient onto a backboard, it is particularly important that you check the back as you log roll the patient. Ensure that you keep the spine in line at all times as you log roll the patient onto his or her side. **Do not remove the hand that is supporting the shoulder because this could cause the spine to torque and create further injury.** Carefully palpate the spine from the neck to the pelvis with the other hand, examining for tenderness or deformity, and look for obvious injuries, including bruising and bleeding. In addition, assess for the presence of rectal bleeding.

Baseline Vital Signs and SAMPLE History

After you have completed the rapid trauma assessment, it is time to obtain baseline vital signs and a SAMPLE history.

The baseline vital signs provide useful information about the overall functions of the patient's heart and lungs. They also provide a starting point by which we begin to trend and monitor the patient. Trending is the process of determining, following several sets of vital signs, whether the severely injured patient's condition has stabilized or is deteriorating. If the patient's condition is stable, you should reassess the vital signs every 15 minutes until you reach the emergency department. If the patient's condition is unstable, you should reassess at a minimum of every 5 minutes, or as often as the situation permits. Table 10-5 through Table 10-10 provide more information on baseline vital signs.

Do not be falsely reassured by apparently normal vital signs. The body has amazing abilities to compensate for severe injury or illness, especially in children and young adults. Even patients with severe medical or traumatic conditions may initially present with relatively normal vital signs. However, the body eventually loses its ability to compensate, and the vital signs may deteriorate rapidly, especially in children. This underscores the importance of frequently monitoring and recording the patient's vital signs.

For many EMT-Is, obtaining the patient's history seems to be a bewildering series of questions that seem to bear little or no relationship to the patient's need for help. Do not fall into this trap. Crucial information can be gained from patients while they're still conscious or while family members/bystanders are available. For example, you'll need to know whether the patient has any allergies or takes any medications that could contraindicate prehospital interventions and the patient's weight for drug calculations. Remember that the mnemonic SAMPLE includes the following elements:

- **S**igns and Symptoms of the episode
- **A**llergies, particularly to medications
- **M**edications, including prescription, over-the-counter, and recreational (illicit) drugs
- **P**ertinent past history, particularly involving similar episodes in the past
- **L**ast oral intake, including food and/or drinks. This is particularly important if the patient may need surgery or is diabetic.
- **E**vents leading up to the episode, which may include precipitating factors

TABLE 10-5	Determining the Quality of Breathing
Normal	■ Neither shallow nor deep ■ Adequate and symmetrical chest wall motion ■ No use of accessory muscles
Shallow	■ Minimal chest or abdominal wall motion
Labored	■ Increased breathing effort ■ Grunting, stridor ■ Use of accessory muscles ■ Gasping for air ■ Nasal flaring, supraclavicular and intercostal retractions
Noisy	■ Increase in sound of breathing, including snoring, wheezing, gurgling, and stridor

TABLE 10-6	Normal Respiratory Rates (breaths/min)
Adults	12 to 20
Children	15 to 30
Infants	25 to 50

Note: These ranges are per the 2002 Airway Management supplement to the US DOT 1994 EMT-Basic National Standard Curriculum. Ranges presented in other courses or texts may vary. Also, these rates are only adequate if the patient has a sufficient tidal volume.

TABLE 10-7	Average Pulse Rates (beats/min)
Adults	60 to 100
Children	70 to 140
Toddlers	90 to 150
Infants	100 to 160

TABLE 10-8	Assessing the Skin			
Color	Possible Cause		Temperature/Moisture	Possible Cause
Pink	- Normal color		Warm	- Normal condition
Ashen or pale	- Hypovolemia - Hypoxia		Hot	- Significant fever - Sunburn - Hyperthermia - Heavy exercise or sweating
Gray-blue (cyanotic)	- Insufficient air exchange - Low blood oxygen level (hypoxia)		Cool	- Early shock - Heat exhaustion
Red (flushed)	- High blood pressure - Carbon monoxide poisoning (late) - Significant fever - Heatstroke - Sunburn - Allergic reaction		Cold	- Profound shock - Hypothermia (late finding) - Frostbite
Yellow (jaundice)	- Liver disease or dysfunction		Dry Clammy or moist	- Normal condition - Shock

TABLE 10-9	Systolic Blood Pressure Readings	
Age/Gender	Readings	Critically Low Readings
Adult men	Add 100 to the patient's age, up to 150 mm Hg	Male adults and adolescents: 90 mm Hg or less
Adult women	Add 90 to the patient's age, up to 150 mm Hg	Female adults and adolescents: 80 mm Hg or less
Children	Age (in years) × 2 + 70 (lower limit of normal)	Children: 70 mm Hg or less

In addition to history, the Glasgow Coma Scale, covered in Chapter 24, can be used to assess a patient's neurologic status. In most parts of the country, this has replaced other types of trauma scoring. If your area uses trauma scoring, check local protocol for specifics on its use.

Transport

Your next steps are to provide the necessary emergency medical care and then to provide transport to the facility that is most appropriate for the patient's condition (for example, a trauma center). For critically injured patients, time-consuming interventions (such as IV therapy) should be performed en route to the emergency department.

Trauma Patients With No Significant MOI

You will not need to perform such a complete exam on most of your patients. After you have completed the initial assessment and care for any actual or potentially life-threatening conditions, you should focus on anything associated with the patient's chief complaint.

Focused Assessment: Chief Complaint

Once you are sure that the ABCs are stable, move to the patient's specific injury site or chief complaint: the patient's description of "what is wrong." In many cases, especially with trauma, this is logical. For example, if

TABLE 10-10 Pupillary Reactions

Appearance	Possible Cause
Round and equal size	Normal condition
Fixed with no reaction to light	Depressed brain function (head injury or stroke)
Fully dilated and fixed (blown pupil)	Increased intracranial pressure
Dilate with bright light, constrict with low light	Depressed brain function
Constricted	Drugs (opiates) or bright light
Dilated	Drugs (barbiturates) or dim lighting
Sluggish reaction	Severe increase in ICP
Unequal size	Depressed brain function Medication placed in eye Injury or condition of the eye Congenital anisocoria*

*Approximately 20% of the population has normally unequal pupils, a condition called anisocoria. In such patients, the pupils usually differ in size by less than 1 mm.

---

the patient reports ankle pain, you should check the ankle. Note, though, that nontraumatic complaints may be a little less obvious. Here are specific items to assess with some common chief complaints:

- **Chest pain**: Evaluate the skin, pulse, and blood pressure Figure 10-20 ▶. Look for injuries to the chest, assess the external jugular veins, and listen to the breath sounds.
- **Shortness of breath**: Evaluate the skin, pulse, blood pressure, and rate and depth of respirations. Look for signs of airway obstruction and for trauma to the neck and chest. Listen carefully to the breath sounds, and assess for hypoxemia (that is, use pulse oximetry).
- **Abdominal pain**: Evaluate the skin, pulse, and blood pressure. Look for trauma to the abdomen,

---

You are the Provider — Part 5

Your partner continues to assess your second patient. This assessment reveals the following:

Vital Signs	Recording Time: 2 Minutes After Patient Contact
Respirations	20 breaths/min; adequate depth
Pulse	88 beats/min; strong and regular
Skin	Pale and clammy
Blood pressure	154/96 mm Hg
SaO_2	90% while breathing room air

10. What useful information is provided by the patient's baseline vital signs?
11. What does the mnemonic SAMPLE stand for?

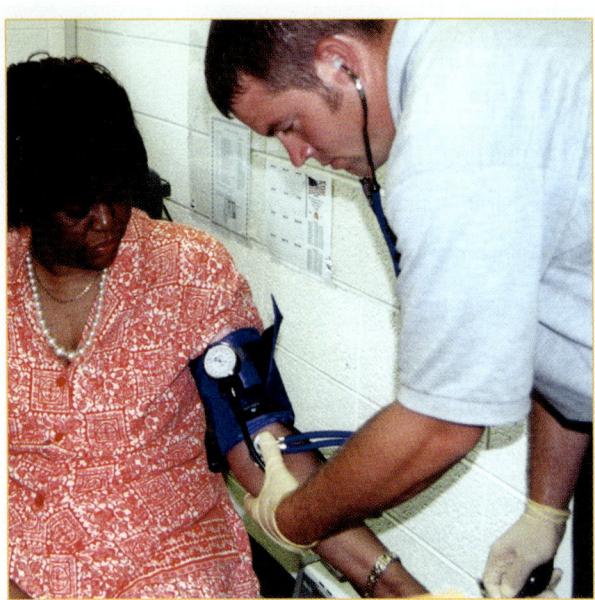

Figure 10-20 Use an approximately sized blood pressure cuff to ensure an accurate reading.

and palpate the abdomen to identify any tenderness or rigidity.
- **Any pain associated with bones or joints**: Evaluate the skin, movement, and sensation adjacent to and below the affected area. Expose the injury site.
- **Dizziness**: Evaluate the skin, pulse, blood pressure, and rate and quality of respirations. Monitor the level of consciousness and orientation carefully. Check the head for signs of trauma. Assess for signs of dehydration.

Next, examine any noticeable abnormalities. This could be something you noticed during the initial assessment and focused history, such as a laceration, a deformed bone, unilateral weakness, or abnormal pupils. Avoid being distracted by these conditions while caring for life threats; it is easy to let big lacerations or deformities draw your attention away from more important, potentially life-threatening problems. In many cases, it is the most obvious that is the least life-threatening.

However, once you have evaluated and treated life-threatening conditions and have examined the area associated with the chief complaint, you can come back to any minor problems you previously found. Be sure to ask the patient questions about the abnormality while you are evaluating it. In some cases, deformities or abnormalities may be long-term and unrelated to the patient's present condition. For example, a patient who has had a stroke may have a weakness on one side of the body for months following the stroke; it is not a new problem and is not likely to be related to the patient's chief complaint.

Once you have assessed for problems that are potentially life threatening or related to the chief complaint or specific injury site and have evaluated abnormalities, you may begin to perform the focused assessment. As we have noted before, use the appropriate BSI precautions; be sure your gloves are on before you begin the focused examination.

Baseline Vital Signs and SAMPLE History

As you know, baseline vital signs provide useful information about the overall functions of the patient's heart and lungs. Remember, if the patient's condition is stable, you should reassess the vital signs every 15 minutes until you reach the emergency department. If the patient's condition is unstable, you should reassess at a minimum of every 5 minutes, or as often as the situation permits. Also obtain a SAMPLE history if possible.

Transport

Your next steps are to provide the necessary emergency medical care addressing the chief complaint and then to provide transport to the emergency department. Remember, the patient's spine should be immobilized if you suspect significant trauma or if there is an MOI that would make you suspect a spinal injury.

Documentation

Accurately document all pertinent assessment findings, the treatment that you provided, and the patient's response to your treatment. For all trauma patients, regardless of whether the MOI is significant, your written report should include documentation of the following:
- Initial assessment findings
- Focused physical exam findings
- Treatment given and the patient's response to the treatment
- Baseline vital signs, subsequent vital signs, and SAMPLE history
- Circulation, sensory, and motor function in all extremities

- Breath sounds; skin color, condition, and temperature
- Any changes in the patient's condition that occurred during transport—good or bad

Other Considerations

Remember, for many patients, you will need to assess the entire body because of the potential severity of their condition. The following patients require a complete rapid trauma assessment, coupled with short scene time and immediate transport to the hospital:

- Any patients who experienced a significant MOI
- Any patients who are unresponsive or disoriented, because they cannot contribute to the focused history or exam
- Any patients with altered mental status (for example, intoxicated from drugs or alcohol and cannot reliably contribute to the focused history or exam)
- Any patients with a complaint that cannot be identified or clearly understood by using a focused exam (These patients should receive a more complete exam.)

Patient Assessment

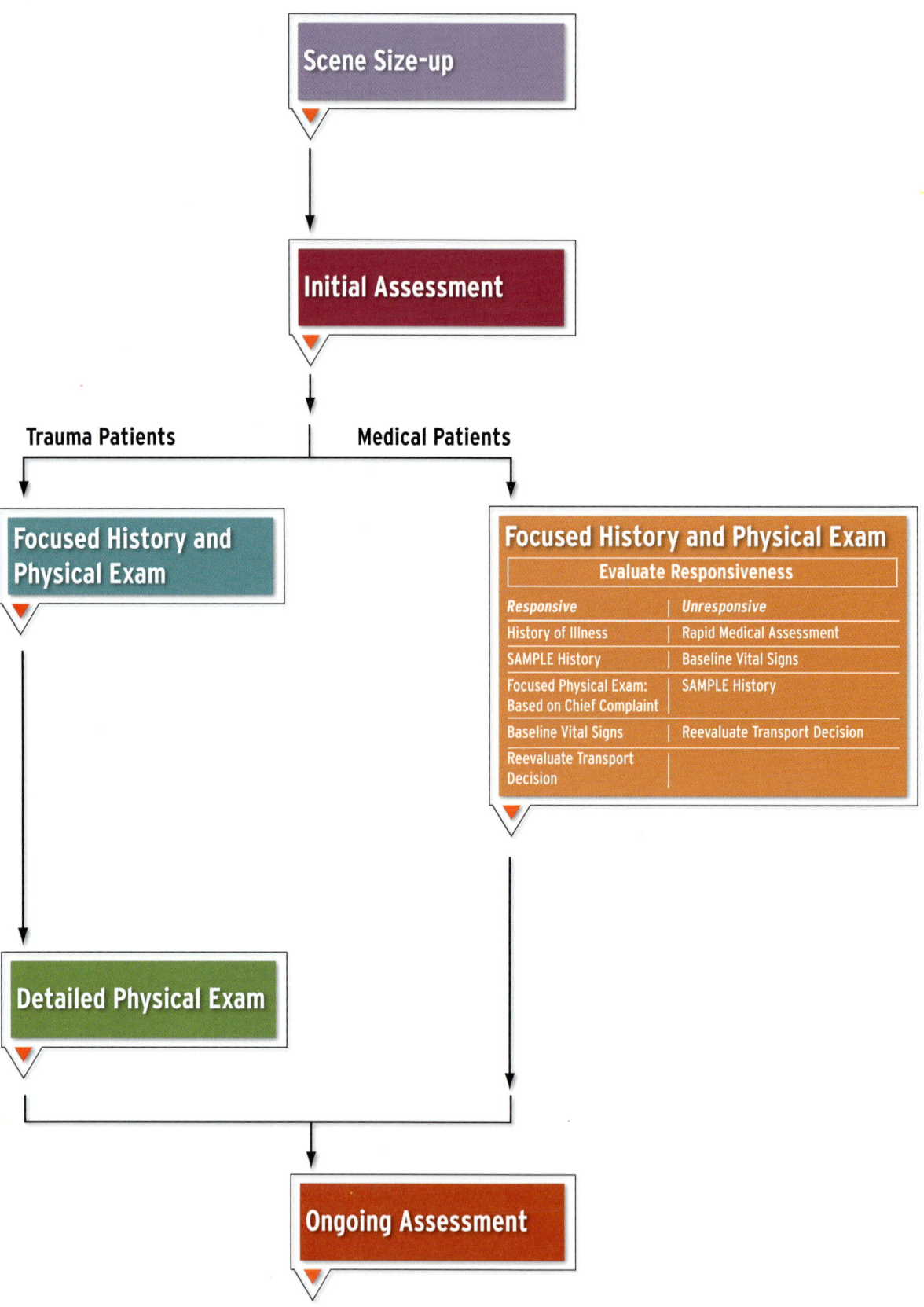

Focused History and Physical Exam: Medical Patients

Evaluate Responsiveness

Early in the assessment process, you need to begin evaluating the patient's problem. In most cases, the patient is alert and able to discuss the problem with you. However, in some cases, the patient may be confused, intoxicated, unable to speak your language, or unresponsive. After ruling out trauma, you should immediately proceed to the rapid medical assessment. Table 10-11 ▼ lists the components of the focused history and physical exam for the medical patient.

History of Present Illness

The patient's response to general questions such as "What's wrong?" or "What happened today?" is the chief complaint Figure 10-21 ▶. This response is what drives your assessment of the history of the present illness (focused history) and the physical exam of the medical patient. The chief complaint is the problem that is bothering the patient the most, prompting the call to 9-1-1.

If possible, take the time to sit down and help the patient to get comfortable. Now is the time to listen, as you develop an increased understanding of the patient's condition. Be careful not to jump to conclusions regarding the chief complaint because of what you have seen or heard about the patient. Treat patients who use EMS frequently as if you are seeing them for the first time. In many cases, the chief complaint will not be obvious; it may even be different from what the dispatcher received from the caller or reported to you. When this occurs, treat the patient's problem rather than simply reacting to the dispatch report. Nevertheless, the chief complaint represents what is bothering the patient and will help you to focus your history and physical exam. If the patient cannot tell you what is wrong, perhaps because of a language barrier, altered mental status, or severe respiratory difficulty, you may learn the chief complaint from a family member or bystander or from your observations of the scene and patient actions. However, remember that information directly from the patient is far more valuable. You should try, whenever possible, to speak directly to the patient.

As you listen to the patient, you might want to make some brief notes to aid your memory and assist with documentation after the call. You should attempt to record the chief complaint in the patient's own words, using appropriate quotation marks. Be sure to note if your information comes from someone other than the patient.

> **A to Z Terminology Tips**
>
> The *chief complaint* is what you were called for, and the *primary problem* is what is actually wrong with the patient.
> For example:
> **Chief complaint**—(dyspnea) The call is for a patient experiencing difficulty breathing.
> **Primary problem**—(congestive heart failure with pulmonary edema) The patient has an exacerbation of congestive heart failure and the pulmonary edema is creating the dyspnea.

TABLE 10-11	Focused History and Physical Exam: Medical Patients
Evaluate Responsiveness	
Responsive Patient	**Unresponsive Patient**
History of present illness: OPQRST-I	Rapid medical assessment
SAMPLE history	Baseline vital signs
Focused physical exam: based on chief complaint	SAMPLE history
Baseline vital signs	Reevaluate transport decision
Reevaluate transport decision	

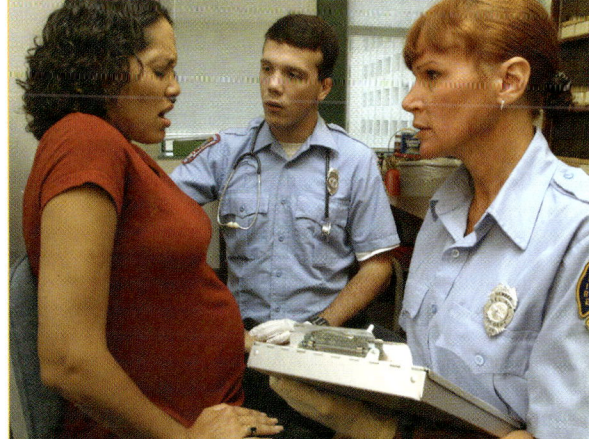

Figure 10-21 The patient's initial response to the question, "What's wrong?" is the chief complaint.

OPQRST-I

As you learn about the chief complaint, you should broaden your knowledge to include the circumstances surrounding the complaint. You can remember the seven most important circumstances by using the letters OPQRST-I, which stand for Onset, Provoking/palliating factors, Quality, Radiation/referred pain, Severity, Time, and any Interventions performed before your arrival.

Onset

The onset refers to when the patient's problem began. You should ask the patient when the problem started or when the incident occurred and how long ago the patient first noticed the problem. If the patient reports that the problem started a long time ago (days or weeks), you should also ask, "What prompted you to call now?" In most cases, the patient will note a sudden worsening of the problem or an additional problem that compounded the first one. For example, a patient who has experienced shortness of breath for the past 3 days may have called because of an onset of chest pain an hour ago. You often will not learn about this second problem unless you ask.

For patients with traumatic problems, there may be a delay between when they were hurt and when they called. Again, ask them why they delayed and what prompted them to call today. The information they give may be valuable to you and the hospital staff.

Provoking/Palliating Factors

Learning about provoking and palliating factors can be extremely helpful in determining the cause and severity of the patient's problem. Provoking factors include anything that seems to bring on the problem or that seems to makes the problem worse, such as increased shortness of breath during exertion. Palliating factors include anything that brings the patient relief from the problem, such as taking a nitroglycerin tablet for chest pain.

The answer to these questions often helps you to appreciate the potential cause. For example, shortness of breath that started when the patient climbed a set of stairs may be respiratory or cardiac in origin. However, shortness of breath that started after the patient was struck in the chest by a baseball might be the result of fractured ribs or internal injury. These questions are often the clues to hidden medical problems in traumatic incidents, such as the patient who reports that he or she fell down the stairs following an episode of dizziness.

Quality of Pain

The patient's description of the pain may be very useful to hospital staff who are trying to determine the cause of the problem. For example, patients who are having a heart attack classically describe their chest pain as "squeezing" or "pressure," although they may also say things like, "My chest feels funny," for lack of having a better description. To learn about the quality of the pain, ask the patient to describe the pain or explain what the pain feels like. Avoid asking the patient leading questions when possible, such as those that can be simply answered yes or no; this may not give you an accurate description of what the patient is actually feeling.

Patients will often initially say, "I don't know," or "It's hard to describe." Once again, the key is for you to be patient. If you wait, most patients will ultimately describe the quality of their pain. Carefully document in the patient's own words; these may be very significant to other providers who become involved in the patient's care. Some patients have limited vocabulary when it comes to their bodies; it may be best to let them simply point to their pain, rather than describe it. Ask patients to point to the area of pain, describe the area of pain, or describe pain anywhere else associated with the problem. If the patient still cannot describe the pain or if the patient cannot speak, you might consider offering several descriptions of pain and letting the patient choose. For example, you might ask, "Which of these words best describes your pain: Sharp or dull? Burning, stabbing, crushing, or throbbing?"

You can learn a great deal about the patient's problem through these questions. For example, a patient who points to a single place for his or her pain has what is known as focal pain (Figure 10-22A ▶). Many problems, such as fractures or areas of inflammation, commonly cause focal pain. However, some patients cannot point to a single location. Instead, they often move their finger around in a circle as they are asked to point to their pain. These patients are experiencing diffuse pain (Figure 10-22B ▶). A number of conditions, including heart attack and internal bleeding, typically cause diffuse pain.

Radiation/Referred Pain or Discomfort

Patients can often provide clues about the cause of their problems by describing the region or location of any pain or discomfort. Radiation refers to an area of the body from which the origin of pain or discomfort may travel (Figure 10-22C ▶). The presence of radiating pain will not alter your treatment very much; however, physicians and nurses caring for the patient in the hospital may be very interested in hearing about areas of radiation. For example, a patient who is having a heart attack may report chest pain that radiates to the left arm and jaw. Document carefully what you learn.

Be careful how you ask about radiation of pain. Most patients will not understand if you ask, "Does your pain radiate anywhere else?" And asking, "Does your pain

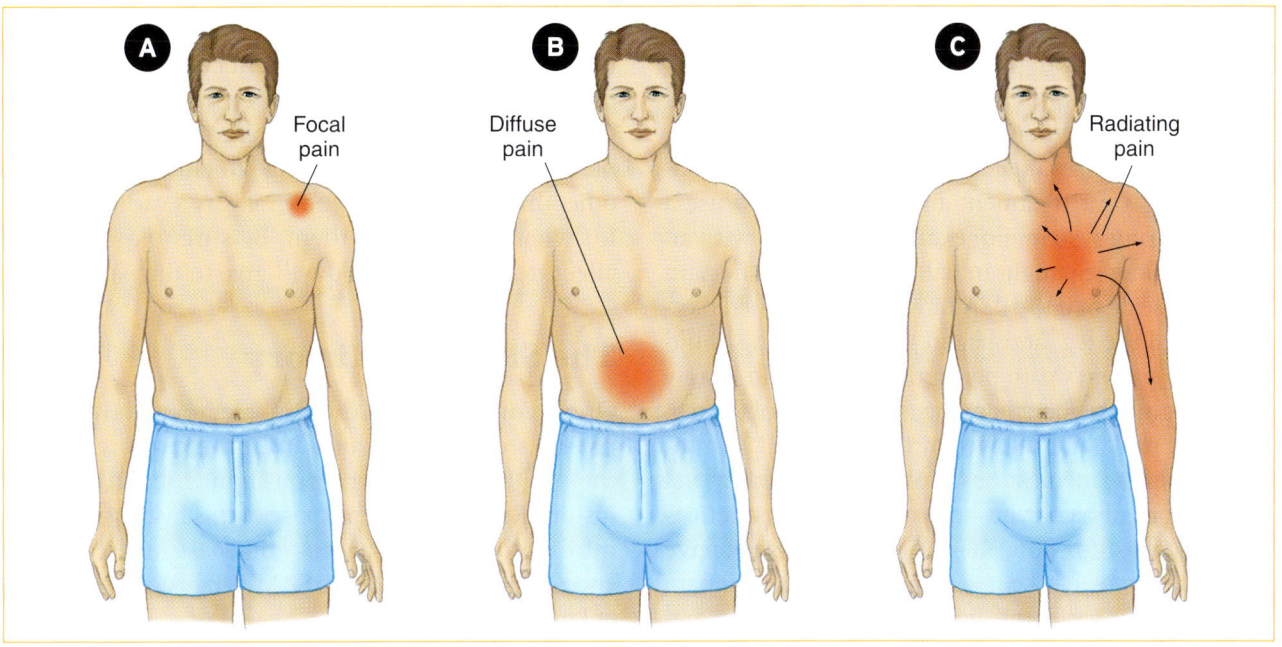

Figure 10-22 **A.** Focal pain. **B.** Diffuse pain. **C.** Radiating pain.

> 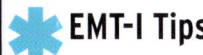 **EMT-I Tips**
>
> Your documentation of any pain complaint should include a description in the patient's words and your findings from the other OPQRST-I questions. Record all pain complaints in detail. Not all pain symptoms are "classic"; the exact description may help hospital personnel make the correct diagnosis in a case that is not typical.

go (or travel) anywhere else?" might confuse the patient. After all, who ever heard of pain "traveling"? The best way to ask patients about radiation is to ask, "Do you have pain or discomfort anywhere else?" or, "Does it feel like the pain moves around?"

Referred pain is pain that exists in more than one place, without a "trail" of pain in between. For example, it is common for a patient with gallbladder disease to complain of pain in the right upper quadrant of the abdomen and in the right shoulder. However, there is no pain in between the right upper quadrant and right shoulder.

Severity

Severity refers to the patient's perception of "how bad" the current incident is in comparison with others. In some cases, particularly when the patient has experienced the problem before, his or her perception provides extremely useful information. For example, a patient with asthma may be very helpful by comparing this episode with previous asthma attacks. However, if the problem has never occurred, the patient's perception may not be very useful except as a guide to whether it is getting worse or better during transport.

To assess severity, you may ask the following questions:

- "How bad is this episode in comparison with previous ones?" (if the problem is chronic or recurring)
- "What happened the last time you had an episode this bad?" (if the problem is chronic or recurring)
- "How would you rate this problem in numbers, if 0 is normal (that is, pain-free) and 10 is the worst pain or discomfort you can imagine?"

For patients with chronic problems, obtaining the answer to the question "What happened the last time you had an episode this bad?" is invaluable. In most cases, patients have been very accurate in their self-assessments of severity. For example, a patient with asthma might tell you that the last time he had an attack this bad, he was intubated and spent 2 weeks in the intensive care unit. The patient's comments tell you that this episode is extremely serious and that you should complete your assessment and provide immediate transport. At the other extreme, the patient might tell you that he was kept in the emergency department for about an hour and then discharged. Obviously, these two episodes are very different in urgency, and you can adjust your plans for treatment and transport accordingly. Bear in mind, however, that there may be no relationship between the severity of previous incidents and the current one; treat the patient as he or she presents, and keep past information in mind.

Another way to evaluate changes in the patient's condition during your treatment and transport is to use a numeric scoring system. For example, a patient with an apparent broken leg might initially tell you that the pain is an 8 on a scale of 0 to 10. After you have applied oxygen, splinted the leg, and begun transport, you should recheck the patient's pain perception. If the pain is now a 9, you might consider changing the position of the leg, using an ice pack, or, if allowed by local protocol, administering analgesic medications. However, if the pain level is now reportedly a 5, you know that the treatment is effective, at least for now. Remember, patients perceive pain in different ways, so it is inappropriate to compare one patient's numeric score with another patient's score.

Time

The questions related to time provide information about when the problem began and whether the patient has experienced the problem on other occasions. You might want to find out whether the problem has been constant or intermittent. If the patient states that the problem is intermittent, ask what seemed to make it better or worse.

The answers to these questions will further help you and other health care professionals involved with the patient's care to understand the nature of the problem. Some conditions, such as those involving abdominal organs, have classically intermittent pain. Other problems, such as fractures, typically have constant pain.

Interventions

Some patients may self-treat or self-medicate before calling 9-1-1. For example, a patient complaining of chest pain may have taken his or her (or someone else's) nitroglycerin or aspirin before your arrival. It is even feasible that the patient was being "doctored" by someone other than a physician. People may try a variety of "cures" for whatever is ailing them. Be sure to ask; this may affect treatment that you will give to the patient.

The SAMPLE History

Once you have obtained a clearer picture of the patient's chief complaint and have explored it using the OPQRST-I questions, you should obtain a SAMPLE history. Recall that the purpose of this history is to obtain information about the patient's past medical experiences. The elements of the SAMPLE history are repeated below for your review.

- Signs and Symptoms of the episode
- Allergies, particularly to medications
- Medications, including prescription, over-the-counter, and recreational (illicit) drugs
- Past medical history, particularly involving similar episodes in the past
- Last oral intake, including food and/or drinks. This is particularly important if the patient may need surgery or is diabetic. Last menstrual cycle. This is particularly important in the female of childbearing age complaining of abdominal or pelvic pain.
- Events leading up to the episode.

Be sure to ask whether the patient has any other problems that you should know about. This question is

---

You are the Provider — Part 6

You are continuing to care for your first patient as you conduct the focused history and physical exam and prepare for transport. Your reassessment reveals the following:

Reassessment	Recording Time: 5 Minutes After Patient Contact
Respirations	20 breaths/min; adequate depth
Pulse	122 beats/min, slightly irregular
Skin	Pale
Blood pressure	124/68 mm Hg
Sao_2	97% with 15 L oxygen via nonrebreathing mask

12. What are the seven most important factors to help the EMT-I learn more about a patient's chief complaint?

EMT-I Tips

Common Chief Complaints and Focused Physical Exams

- **Chest pain.** Evaluate skin, pulse, and blood pressure. Look for trauma to the chest, assess the external jugular veins, and listen to breath sounds.
- **Abdominal pain.** Evaluate skin, pulse, and blood pressure. Look for trauma to the abdomen, and palpate the abdomen for tenderness or rigidity.
- **Shortness of breath.** Evaluate skin, pulse, blood pressure, and rate and depth of respirations. Assess for airway obstruction. Listen carefully to breath sounds, and assess for hypoxemia (that is, use pulse oximetry).
- **Dizziness.** Evaluate skin, pulse, blood pressure, and adequacy of respirations. Monitor the level of consciousness and orientation carefully. Check the head for signs of trauma.
- **Any pain associated with bones or joints.** Evaluate skin, pulse, movement, and sensation adjacent and distal to the affected area.

In the Field

When questioning a patient about medical history it is helpful to ask, "What problems do you take medications for?" Otherwise, you may find that the patient denies any history but has multiple prescriptions. For example, when asked about having seizures, a patient may deny having them even though there are prescriptions in the patient's name for antiseizure medications. The typical answer when asked about the medication is, "No, I don't have seizures as long as I take my medicine."

useful because it provides the patient with an opportunity to tell you something about apparently unrelated previous medical problems. In most cases, this will serve as useful background information. Occasionally, it will provide you and hospital staff with essential information, such as when you discovered that the patient who fell for no apparent reason has a history of diabetes. This information suggests the possibility that the fall was caused by a complication of the diabetes.

No matter what you have learned about the patient's history, you need to be aware of certain medical problems that the patient may have forgotten to mention. These conditions might help to explain the current episode or could affect your treatment decisions or those made at the hospital. As you conclude the SAMPLE history, ask the patient the following questions:

1. "Have you ever been told that you have a heart condition?"
2. "Have you ever been told that you have asthma, emphysema, or any other problems with your lungs?"
3. "Have you ever been told that you have seizures?"

These three questions will prevent you from missing important, potentially life-threatening cardiac, respiratory, or neurologic conditions. If the patient answers "yes" to any of these three questions, reevaluate the chief complaint in light of this new information. If you have time, return to the history questions to learn more about the nature of the problem.

The Focused Physical Exam

Now that you have learned about the chief complaint, using OPQRST-I, and have obtained a thorough history, you should perform a focused exam.

The key to this examination is to emphasize the priorities that you learned during the history. Be logical, and investigate problems that you identified during the initial assessment and focused history.

Chief Complaint

Once you know that the ABCs are stable, move to the patient's chief complaint. Remember to assess the following chief complaints carefully, as described previously:

- **Chest pain.** Evaluate the skin color, pulse, and blood pressure. Look for trauma to the chest, assess the external jugular veins, and listen to the breath sounds.
- **Shortness of breath.** Apply oxygen if you haven't already done so. Evaluate the skin color, pulse, blood pressure, and rate and depth of respirations. Look for airway obstruction and for trauma to the neck and chest. Listen carefully to the breath sounds and assess for hypoxemia (that is, use pulse oximetry).
- **Abdominal pain.** Evaluate the skin color, pulse, and blood pressure. Look for trauma to the abdomen, and palpate the abdomen to identify tenderness or rigidity.
- **Any pain associated with bones or joints.** Evaluate the skin color, movement, and sensation adjacent to and below the affected area.

- **Dizziness**. Evaluate the skin color, pulse, blood pressure, and adequacy of respirations. Monitor the level of consciousness and orientation carefully. Check the head for signs of trauma. Assess for signs of dehydration.

Abnormalities

Next, examine anything that has a noticeable abnormality. Sometimes, during the initial assessment and focused history, you will see something that is obviously abnormal. It may be a laceration, a deformed bone, unilateral weakness, abnormal pupils, or some other abnormality. Avoid being distracted by these conditions; it is easy to let large lacerations or deformities draw your attention away from more important, potentially life-threatening problems.

However, once you have evaluated and treated life-threatening conditions and have examined the area associated with the chief complaint, you can come back to the abnormalities you noted. Be sure to ask the patient questions about the abnormality while you are evaluating it. Remember that deformities or abnormalities may be long-term and unrelated to the patient's present condition. For example, a patient who has had a stroke may have a weakness on one side for months after the stroke; it is not a new problem, and it is not likely related to the patient's current call for EMS.

Baseline Vital Signs

As you know, baseline vital signs provide useful information about the overall functions of the patient's heart and lungs. Remember that if the patient's condition is stable, you should reassess the vital signs every 15 minutes until you reach the emergency department. If the patient's condition is unstable, you should reassess at a minimum of every 5 minutes, or as often as the situation permits.

Reevaluate the Transport Decision

Your next steps are to provide the necessary emergency medical care addressing the chief complaint and then to reevaluate your transport decision.

Documentation

Documenting your assessment findings helps identify and track trends in the patient's condition and helps hospital staff provide definitive treatment. Your report for the responsive medical patient should include documentation of the following:
- Initial assessment findings
- Focused physical exam findings
- Treatment given and the patient's response to the treatment
- Baseline vital signs, subsequent vital signs, and SAMPLE history
- Circulation, sensory, and motor function in all extremities
- Breath sounds; skin color, condition, and temperature
- Any changes in the patient's condition that occurred during transport—good or bad

Evaluating the Unresponsive Patient

Sometimes, new EMT-Is ask how to assess the chief complaint and history in an unresponsive patient (Figure 10-23 ▼). The answer is simple: In many cases, you cannot.

With unresponsive patients, you may never get to that part of the focused history and physical exam. Instead, you should focus your attention on opening and maintaining the airway, immobilizing the spine, administering supplemental oxygen or ventilatory assistance if needed, controlling bleeding, providing CPR if necessary, and providing immediate transport to an appropriate facility. These priorities reflect the importance of the ABC approach to the initial assessment.

If you have successfully stabilized the ABCs, you should ask chief complaint and SAMPLE history questions of a family member or bystander, if available, en route to the hospital. Never delay transport of a critically

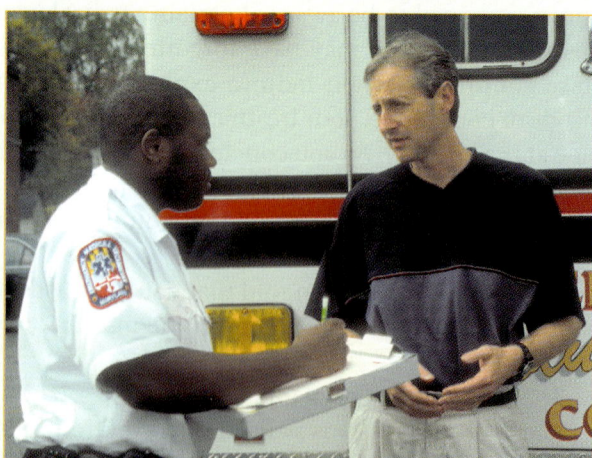

Figure 10-23 If the patient is unresponsive, obtain the chief complaint and any pertinent history from family members or bystanders.

ill patient to obtain a history from family members (or from the patient, for that matter) at the scene.

Rapid Medical Assessment

If you have successfully stabilized the ABCs for any patient who is unresponsive, confused, or unable to relate the chief complaint adequately, you should perform a rapid assessment, using the mnemonic DCAP-BTLS and following the order of the rapid trauma assessment. The purpose of the rapid medical assessment is to identify existing or potentially life-threatening conditions quickly. Follow the brief sequence of assessment steps shown in **Skill Drill 10-2** ▶ :

1. **Assess the head** for DCAP-BTLS and crepitus (**Step 1**).
2. **Assess the neck** for DCAP-BTLS, JVD, and crepitus (**Step 2**).
3. **Assess the chest** for DCAP-BTLS, paradoxical motion, and crepitus (**Step 3**).
4. **Assess the abdomen** for DCAP-BTLS, rigidity, and distention (**Step 4**).
5. **Assess the pelvis** for DCAP-BTLS (**Step 5**).
6. **Assess all four extremities** for DCAP-BTLS (**Step 6**).
7. **Assess the back** for DCAP-BTLS (**Step 7**).

Baseline Vital Signs

Baseline vital signs should be obtained after the rapid medical exam to provide information for assessing trends in the patient's condition. Remember, if the patient's condition is stable, you should reassess the vital signs every 15 minutes until you reach the emergency department. If the patient's condition is unstable, you should reassess at a minimum of every 5 minutes, or as often as the situation permits.

History of Present Illness/ SAMPLE History

As previously stated, determining the history of the present illness and the SAMPLE history is not easy with an unresponsive patient, because your best source of information—the patient—cannot respond adequately. But you can still rely somewhat on witnesses, such as family members who were present at the time the patient became unresponsive.

Family members are normally aware of medical conditions such as diabetes, seizures, stroke, heart disease, and respiratory disease. Family members may also be able to provide information relative to the SAMPLE history. For example, they may be able to describe the signs and symptoms the patient had before becoming unresponsive. A family member is also likely to know whether the patient has any allergies, is using any medication, or has experienced previous similar incidents. A family member caring for an elderly person can identify the last time the patient had a meal and the events leading up to the loss of consciousness or altered mental status.

Bystanders, especially family members, who were with the patient before the time that he or she became unresponsive can provide some valuable information. For example, a family member may be able to tell you that the patient has insulin-dependent diabetes (type 1 diabetes mellitus) and has taken his or her insulin, but has also

You are the Provider — Part 7

Your partner reports that the second patient is now complaining of increased abdominal pain. He is completing the focused history and physical exam and is preparing to transport. Reassessment of this patient at this time reveals the following:

Reassessment	Recording Time: 5 Minutes After Patient Contact
Respirations	24 breaths/min; shallow
Pulse	92 beats/min and regular
Skin	Pale and slightly clammy
Blood pressure	168/94 mm Hg
SaO_2	96% with 15 L oxygen via nonrebreathing mask

13. What information should be included in the EMT-I's report on this responsive medical patient?

Skill Drill 10-2

Performing a Rapid Medical Assessment: Unresponsive Patient

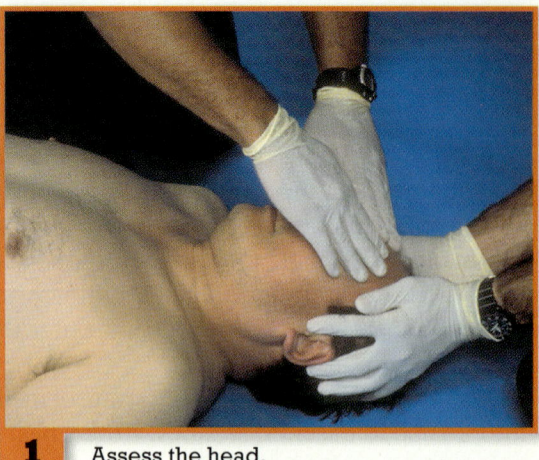
1. Assess the head.

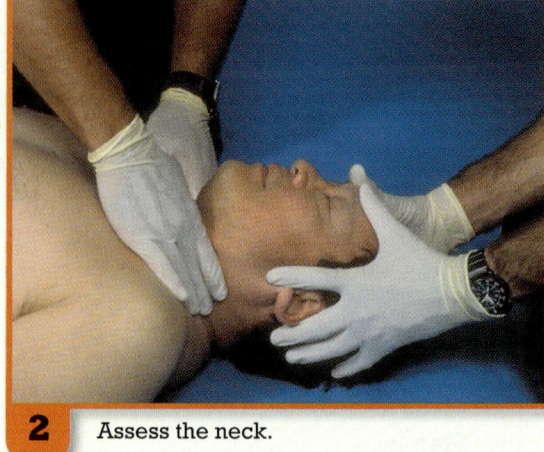
2. Assess the neck.

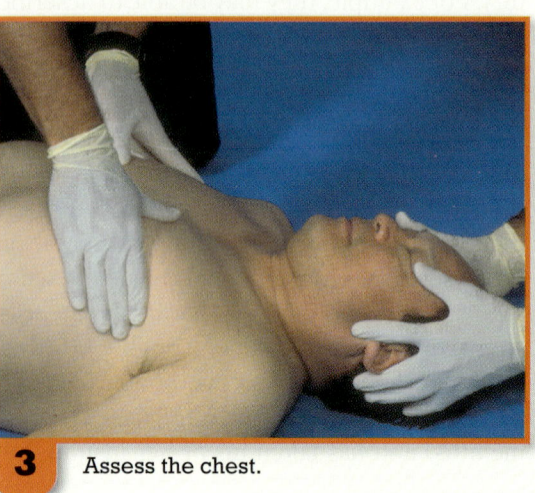
3. Assess the chest.

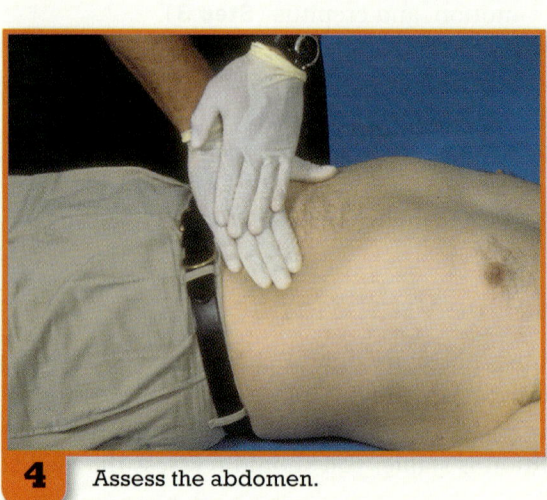
4. Assess the abdomen.

been ill for the past 24 hours, has vomited, and has not eaten normally. The family member may also be able to describe signs of lethargy and confusion and pale, moist skin that the patient exhibited before losing consciousness.

Reevaluate the Transport Decision

Your next steps are to provide the necessary emergency medical care and then to provide transport to the emergency department. Remember, the patient's spine should be immobilized if you suspect significant trauma or if there is an MOI that would make you suspect a spinal injury. For a critically ill patient, transport rapidly to the closest, *most appropriate* facility.

Documentation

Documenting your baseline findings during this examination is important to track trends in the patient's condition and to help hospital staff provide definitive

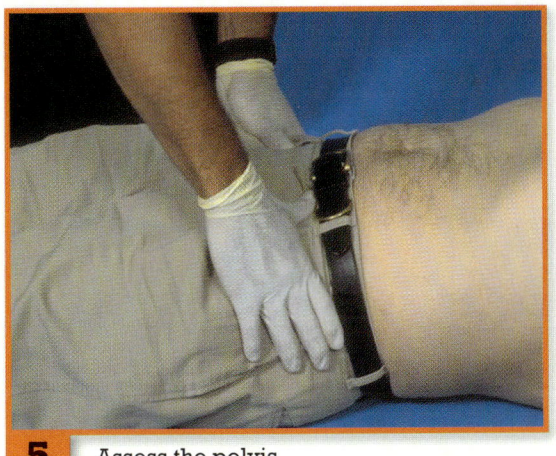

5 Assess the pelvis.

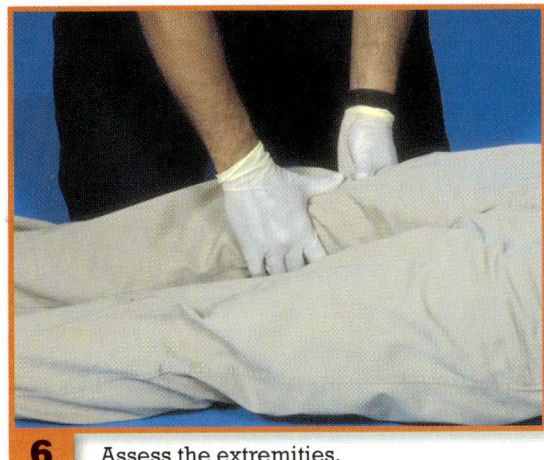

6 Assess the extremities.

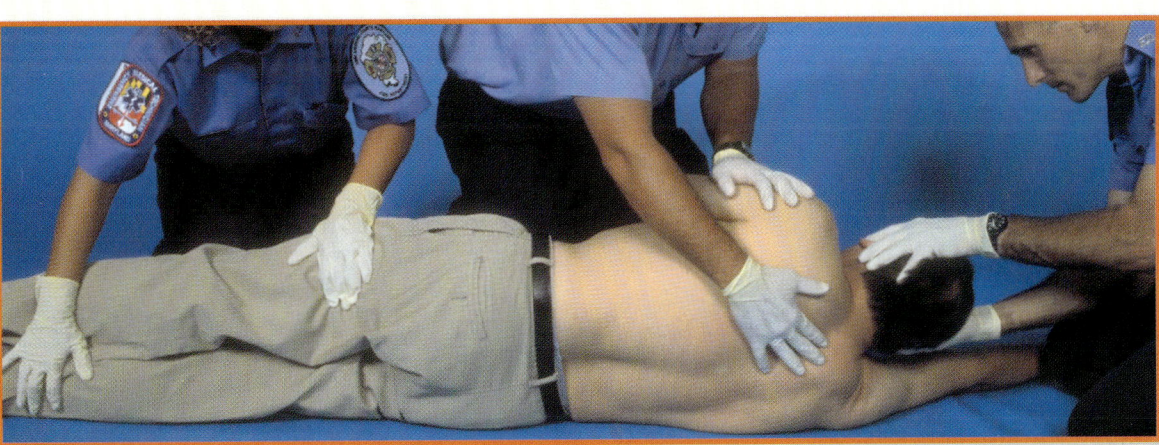

7 Assess the back.

treatment. Your report for the unresponsive medical patient should include documentation of the following:

- Initial assessment findings
- Focused physical exam findings
- Treatment given and the patient's response to the treatment
- Baseline vital signs, subsequent vital signs, and SAMPLE history
- Circulation, sensory, and motor function in all extremities
- Breath sounds; skin color, condition, and temperature
- Any changes in the patient's condition that occurred during transport—good or bad

Patient Assessment

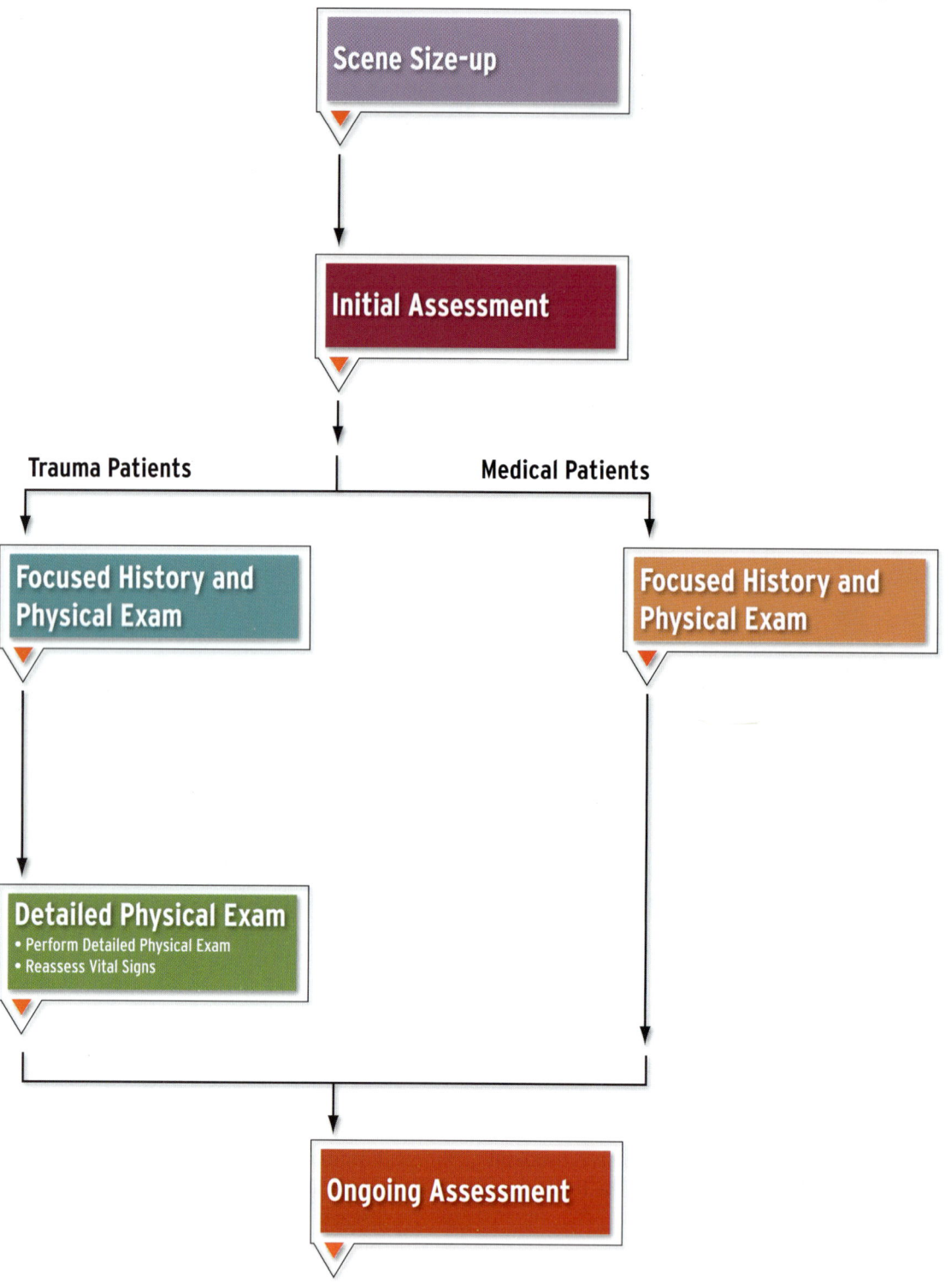

Detailed Physical Exam

Recall that the assessment process began with anticipation and hazard preparation when you received the dispatch information and performed the scene size-up. Then you performed the initial assessment, in which you identified and treated potential and/or immediate life-threatening conditions. If trauma was a factor in your patient's situation, you also initiated spinal immobilization. When indicated, you followed up on the initial assessment by performing a focused history and physical exam or a rapid assessment. You also provided immediate transport if your patient had an obvious life-threatening condition. On the basis of what you learned from the history, you assessed selected areas of the body or assessed body systems, such as the respiratory system, taking into account how those body systems relate to the patient's complaint and how those systems also interrelate with one other. You have also taken at least one set of vital signs.

At this point, in most cases you are already en route to the hospital. If you are still on the scene, it is because the patient does not have any life-threatening conditions and you have not found the cause for the patient's complaints. In the case of a trauma patient with a significant MOI, you are en route but may still have unanswered questions. In the case of the medical patient, you may be trying to determine the best course of treatment or a probable cause for the complaint. Depending on the acuity of the situation and the need for immediate treatment, you may be at the scene or already en route. In either case, this is the time to perform the detailed physical exam. Table 10-12 lists the components of the detailed physical exam. The goals of this exam are to further explore problems that were identified during the focused history and physical exam and to possibly identify the cause of complaints that were not identified during previous assessments. In most cases, it is the trauma patient with a significant MOI or an unresponsive medical patient with no readily identifiable cause for the chief complaint who receives the detailed exam. In these cases, getting the patient to a hospital takes priority over performing a detailed exam at the scene.

To achieve the goals of the detailed physical exam, you must simply ask and answer two questions: "What additional problems can be identified through a detailed physical exam?" and "How will these findings change my treatment choices?" The detailed physical exam will provide you with additional information that will enable you to recognize patterns of response, particularly compensatory mechanisms, and help you understand more about the nature of the patient's problem. Depending on what is learned, you should be prepared to do the following:

- Return to the initial assessment if a potentially life-threatening condition is identified. This is unlikely this late in the exam, but it is always possible. Compensatory mechanisms may temporarily mask the seriousness of a situation. Recognition may not occur until decompensation begins. If something doesn't look right or feel right, return to the initial assessment and vital signs. Remember, stay focused on the ABCs.
- Perform spinal immobilization if neck or back pain or abnormality in sensation or movement is identified in relationship to trauma. (Again, this is unlikely this late in the exam, but it may occur, especially in the case of spinal cord contusion in a pediatric or geriatric patient.) In a medical emergency, abnormality in sensation or movement is most likely related to a problem with the central nervous system (CNS; for example, a stroke); immobilization may or may not be indicated, depending on the situation. Remember, patients with degenerative diseases may have orthopaedic trauma through seemingly insignificant movement such as turning of the head.
- Modify any treatment that is underway on the basis of any new information.
- Initiate treatment for additional problems identified during the exam.
- Modify transport decisions to a more appropriate facility, if the patient's condition deteriorates or potential life threats are discovered.

The detailed physical exam is a more in-depth examination that builds on the focused physical exam, using the focused physical exam as a baseline for comparison. The techniques include observation, palpation, auscultation, and percussion. You have already learned about and performed observation, palpation, and auscultation but percussion is a technique that is not commonly performed in the field. Percussion will be discussed during assessment of the chest wall.

The patient situation, the NOI, and/or the particular injury will determine the need for this exam.

TABLE 10-12	Detailed Physical Exam

- Detailed head-to-toe exam using DCAP-BTLS
- Reassess vital signs

Many of your patients will not receive a detailed physical exam because it will be irrelevant or unnecessary or because it is not possible given the time constraints.

Most patients have isolated problems that can be adequately evaluated earlier in the assessment process. You will identify the problem and treat it, making a more detailed physical exam of the entire body unnecessary. If you do perform a detailed physical exam, it will be to further explore what you learned during previous assessments.

A few patients will have life-threatening conditions that were identified during the initial assessment. You may spend all of your time stabilizing ABCs, which means you will never have a chance to perform a detailed assessment.

In addition to performing a detailed exam on critically injured or unresponsive patients, you should perform a detailed exam on patients in stable condition with problems that cannot be identified earlier in the patient assessment process. In most cases, these patients have extremely minor, obscure, or isolated problems, which is why you did not identify them earlier. Regardless of the exact situation, the detailed physical exam is usually performed en route to the hospital and is rarely totally completed because you could literally spend hours on the scene performing every step. Instead, the patient's problem and related body systems determine the focus of the detailed assessment. In the case of trauma, the detailed assessment looks at every body area for any outward signs of trauma, using the DCAP-BTLS mnemonic. In the case of a medical problem, the detailed assessment looks at body areas, prioritizing them by systems, such as including assessment for pedal edema (vascular system) after assessment of JVD (vascular system) and lung sounds (respiratory system), followed by assessing the patient's electrocardiogram (ECG; cardiac system), if applicable to your level of certification.

Regarding the pediatric patient, the basic steps of the detailed physical examination remain the same with few exceptions. The exceptions are related to the physique of the pediatric patient and the developmental stage the patient has achieved. These will be more fully explained in the pediatric emergencies chapter.

Steps of the Detailed Physical Exam

Here, organized by body region, are some additional assessments that you should consider performing during the detailed exam. As you evaluate each region, visualize and palpate to find evidence of signs of injury or the NOI, again using the mnemonic DCAP-BTLS with the addition of observation for symmetry, edema and pitting edema, rash, and petechiae. Follow the steps in Skill Drill 10-3 ▶:

1. **Look at the face** for obvious lacerations, bruises, deformities, edema, rash, and petechiae (**Step 1**).
2. **Inspect the area around the eyes and eyelids** for swelling, nodules, and discharge (**Step 2**).
3. **Examine the sclera and conjunctiva of the eyes** for color, contact lenses, and discharge. Assess the pupils for size, equality, and reactivity (**Step 3**).
4. **Pull the patient's ear forward** to assess for bruising (Battle's sign) (**Step 4**).
5. **Use the penlight to look for drainage**, discharge, and blood in the ears (**Step 5**).
6. **Look for bruising and lacerations to the head**. Palpate for tenderness, depressions of the skull, and deformities (**Step 6**).
7. **Palpate the zygomas** for tenderness or instability and for normal or abnormal sensation (**Step 7**).
8. **Palpate the maxillae** (**Step 8**).
9. **Palpate the mandible** (**Step 9**).
10. **Assess the mouth for obstructions**, foreign bodies (including loose teeth or dentures), bleeding, lacerations, deformities, pallor, and cyanosis (**Step 10**).
11. **Check for unusual odors** on the patient's breath (**Step 11**).
12. **Look at the neck** for accessory muscle use, obvious lacerations, bruises, deformities, swelling, rash, and petechiae (**Step 12**).
13. **Palpate the front and the back of the neck** for tenderness, deformity, and crepitus (**Step 13**).
14. **Look for distended or pulsating jugular veins**. Note that distended neck veins are not necessarily significant in a patient who is lying down (**Step 14**).
15. **Look at the chest** for pallor, rash, petechiae, intercostal retractions, and obvious signs of injury before you begin palpation. Be sure to watch for movement and symmetry of the chest with respirations (**Step 15**).
16. **Gently palpate over the ribs** to elicit tenderness and note any crepitus. Avoid pressing over obvious bruises or suspected rib fractures (**Step 16**).
17. **Listen for breath sounds** using an orderly, sequential approach, comparing one side with

the other as you go. Listen (A) anteriorly in the apices at the midclavicular line, (B) centrally at the fourth intercostal space lateral to the sternum, (C) at the fifth intercostal space, midclavicular line, and (D) at the midaxillary space at the anterior bases (**Step 17**).

18. **In the medical patient, listen for posterior breath sounds** in the same manner using an orderly, sequential approach starting at the apices, working around the scapula for sounds central and in the bases, ending in the lower midaxillary space. In the trauma patient, assessing posterior lung sounds may not be possible because he or she will usually be immobilized on a long board (**Step 18**).
19. **Look at the abdomen and pelvis** for obvious lacerations, bruises, deformities, rash, and petechiae (**Step 19**).
20. **Gently palpate the abdomen** for tenderness and unusual findings such as masses or pulsations. If the abdomen is unusually tense, you should describe the abdomen as rigid (**Step 20**).
21. **Gently compress the pelvis** from the sides, pressing inward to assess for tenderness. Do not reassess the pelvis if it was previously found to be unstable or the patient complained of pain (**Step 21**).
22. **Gently press downward on the iliac crest** on both sides simultaneously to assess for instability and tenderness and to note any crepitus. Again, avoid reassessment of the pelvis if it was previously found to be unstable or the patient complained of pain (**Step 22**).
23. **Inspect all four extremities** for DCAP-BTLS and for medical alert anklets or bracelets. Also assess the presence, equality, and character of distal pulses and motor and sensory function in all extremities. Assess for the presence of edema and pitting edema (**Step 23**).
24. **Assess the back for tenderness, deformities**, presence of edema in the sacral area, rash, and petechiae. In a trauma patient, reassessment of the back may not be possible because the patient usually is immobilized on a backboard (**Step 24**). Complete assessment of the respiratory and circulatory systems.

The following is designed to provide a brief explanation of the detailed assessment. More definitive descriptions of specific body area assessments will be discussed as specific injury or disease entities are explained. As pattern recognition and an intuitive grasp of pathophysiology and the interrelationship of body systems is incorporated into decision making, you will learn which assessment steps are most appropriate for your patient's situation and your priorities.

Head, Neck, and Cervical Spine

A more detailed exam of these areas should include a careful check of the head, face, scalp, ears, eyes, nose, and mouth for puncture wounds, including insect bites, rash, petechiae, abrasions, lacerations, and contusions. Examine the eyes and eyelids, checking for swelling; nodules; discharge; color of the lids, sclera, and conjunctiva (such as redness, jaundice), and for contact lenses. Use a penlight to check whether the pupils are

You are the Provider   Part 8

You have completed the focused history and physical exam on your 78-year-old female patient. You have initiated treatment and are preparing to transport.

Reassessment	Recording Time: 7 Minutes After Patient Contact
Respirations	20 breaths/min; adequate depth
Pulse	122 beats/min; slightly irregular
Skin	Pale
Blood pressure	124/68 mm Hg
Sao$_2$	97% with 15 L oxygen via nonrebreathing mask

14. What are the components of a focused history and physical exam for this medical patient that should be performed by the EMT-I?

Performing the Detailed Physical Exam

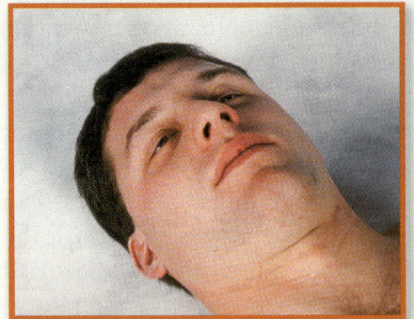
1 Observe the face.

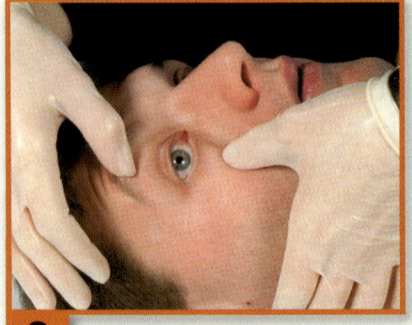
2 Inspect the area around the eyes and eyelids.

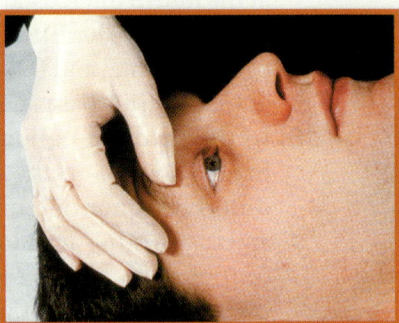
3 Examine the sclera and conjunctiva of the eyes.

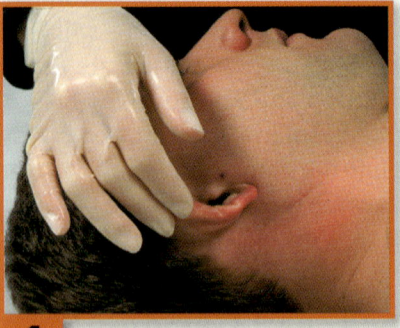
4 Look behind the ears for Battle's sign.

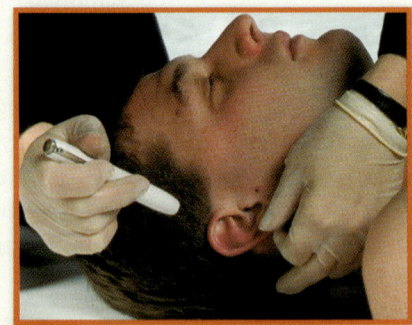
5 Check the ears.

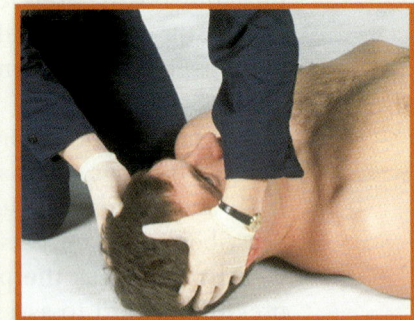
6 Observe and palpate the head.

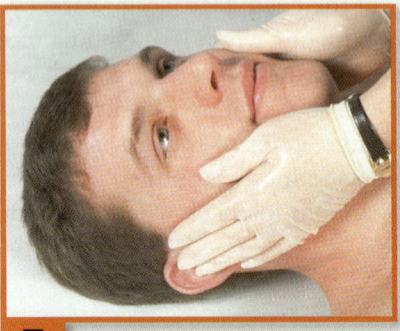
7 Palpate the zygomas.

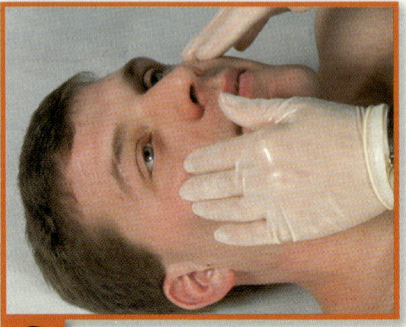
8 Palpate the maxillae.

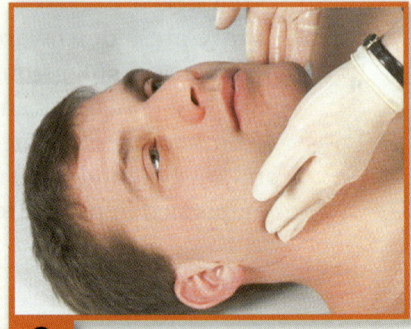
9 Palpate the mandible.

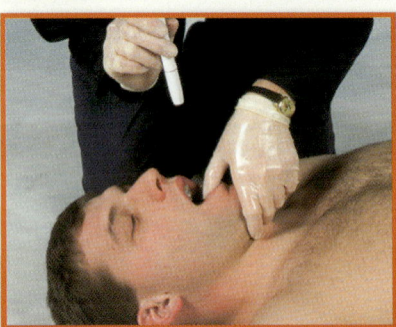
10 Assess the mouth.

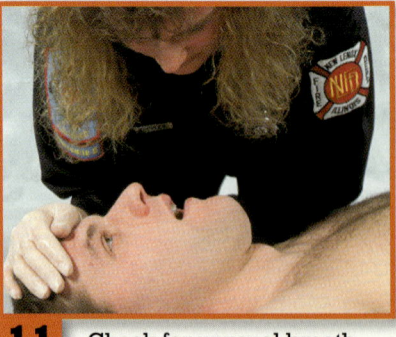
11 Check for unusual breath odors.

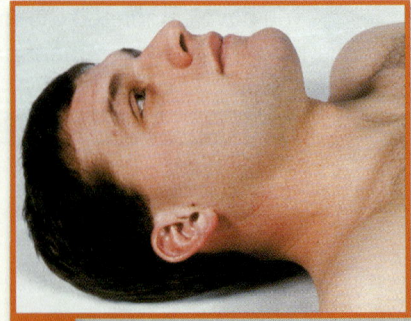
12 Inspect the neck.

Chapter 10 Patient Assessment 545

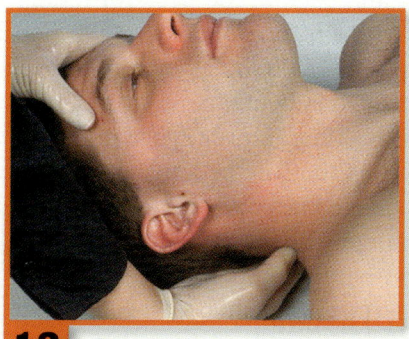
13 Palpate the neck, front and back.

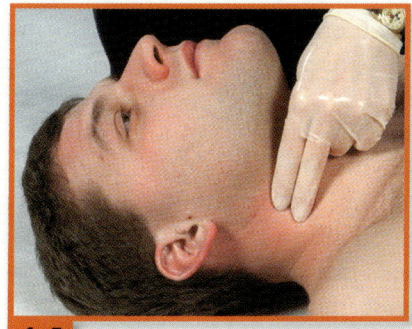
14 Observe for distended or pulsating jugular veins.

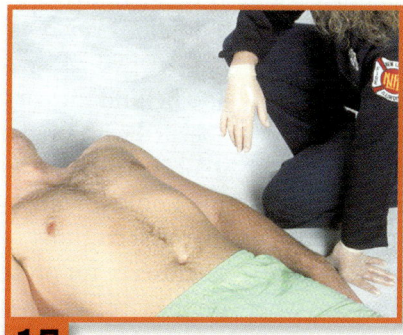
15 Inspect the chest.

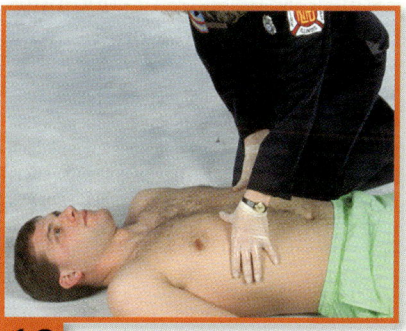
16 Gently palpate the ribs.

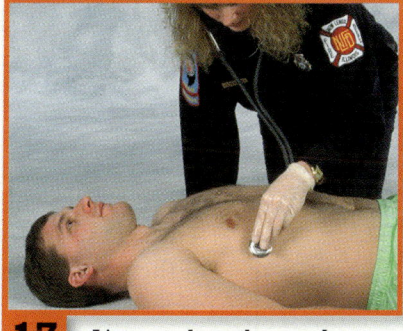
17 Listen to breath sounds.

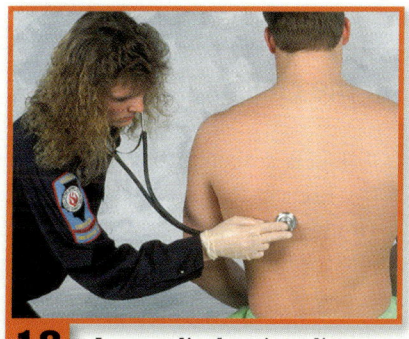
18 In a medical patient, listen for posterior breath sounds.

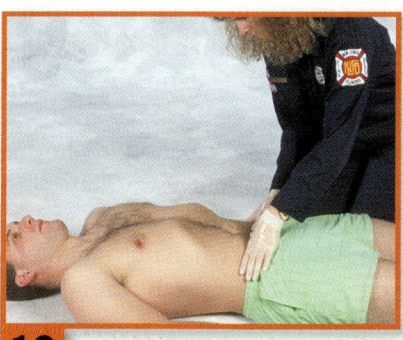
19 Observe the abdomen and pelvis.

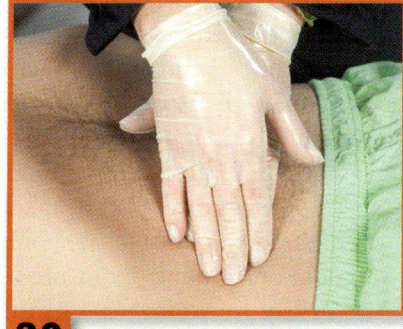
20 Gently palpate the abdomen.

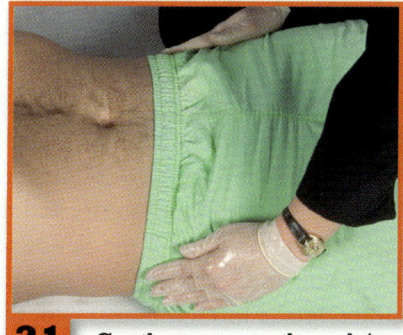
21 Gently compress the pelvis.

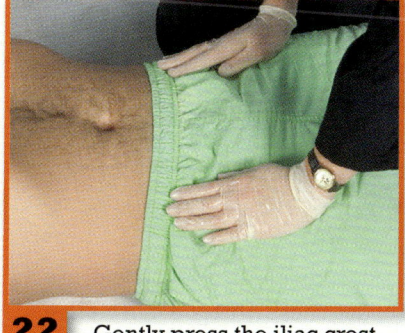
22 Gently press the iliac crest.

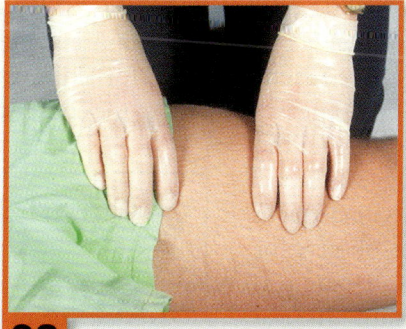
23 Inspect all four extremities; assess distal circulation and motor and sensory function. Assess for the presence of edema and pitting edema.

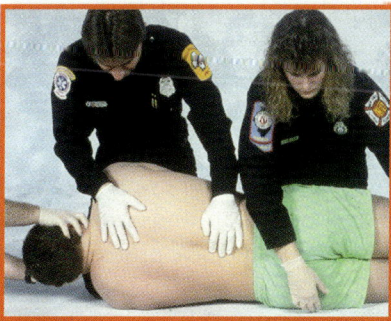
24 Assess the back, unless the patient is immobilized. Complete assessment of the respiratory system. Complete assessment of the cardiovascular system.

equal and reactive or have evidence of surgery (for example, oblong pupils, nicks in the iris). Also check for foreign objects and/or blood in the anterior chamber of the eye (hyphema). Look for bruising or discoloration around the eyes (raccoon eyes), also referred to as periorbital ecchymosis, and behind the ears (Battle's sign); these signs may be associated with head trauma. Swelling of the eyes may be associated with edema, which may be medical in origin. Look for any swelling, fluid drainage, and crusting of secretions or blood around the ears and nose. Also observe for presence of rash and petechiae anywhere on the face, which suggest an infectious process and should alert you to the necessity for a mask and goggles.

> 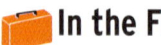 **In the Field**
>
> If fluid is draining from the ears, perform a *halo* test to check for the presence of cerebrospinal fluid. Wrap a 4″ × 4″ gauze around your finger and dip it into the fluid. If cerebrospinal fluid is present it will separate from the blood and form a ring, or *halo*, around it.

Next, gently but firmly palpate around the face, scalp, eyes, ears, and nose for tenderness, altered sensation, deformity, and instability. Altered sensation may suggest a CNS problem such as a stroke or a cranial nerve problem. Tenderness or abnormal movement of bones often signals a serious injury and may cause upper airway obstruction. Monitor the airway carefully in these patients. Look and feel inside the mouth next. Loose or broken teeth or a foreign object may block the airway. Remember to be cautious when inserting your fingers into a patient's mouth. It is much safer if a bite block is used. You should also look for lacerations, swelling, and bleeding. Presence of a bruised or lacerated tongue in an unresponsive patient or a patient with altered mental status in the absence of any known trauma suggests a seizure. Note any discoloration in the mouth and the tongue such as pallor or cyanosis. Pallor suggests blood loss or hypoperfusion, and cyanosis suggests inadequate oxygenation. If a medical problem is present, observe for white, gray, or strawberry-colored spots or patches. These are significant and suggest certain disease processes. Smell the patient's breath. Any unusual odors should be reported and documented. Odors such as a strong alcohol odor or fruity breath odor suggest the need to check the blood glucose level.

Palpate the front and back of the neck for tenderness and deformity. The sensation of crackling or popping, not unlike palpating the bubbles in bubble-pack packing material, is called subcutaneous emphysema. It indicates that air is leaking into the space under the skin. Usually this means that the patient has a pneumothorax or has a damaged larynx. Also look for JVD. This is normal in a patient who is lying down; however, JVD in a patient who is sitting up may suggest a condition related to the heart or lungs such as severe hypertension, tension pneumothorax, cardiac tamponade, or ventricular tachycardia. Observe for the presence of rash and petechiae. In some disease states or conditions, a rash or petechiae are more easily noted on the neck.

Chest

A thorough assessment of the chest includes assessment of the chest wall, breath sounds, percussion, and listening to heart sounds, which is part of the assessment of the cardiovascular system.

Chest: Chest Wall

A detailed assessment of the chest wall cannot be completed unless the entire chest wall is visualized. In some circumstances, such as when an isolated extremity fracture is suspected, exposure of the chest wall is not warranted. In other circumstances, such as exacerbation of chronic obstructive pulmonary disease, exposure is warranted but care must be taken to preserve the patient's privacy. Circumstances should dictate how and when that should be done. Exposure to find bullet holes or stab wounds in a young male is vastly different from exposure to assess lung sounds or place ECG chest leads in a female patient.

When the chest wall is visualized, look for DCAP-BTLS, accessory muscle use, symmetry of chest wall expansion, and the presence of rash and petechiae. Assessment for skin turgor may also be done on the sternal area of the chest wall rather than on the hands. Long-term

> **Geriatric Needs**
>
> When assessing skin turgor in an older patient, use the skin of the upper chest. This is a much more reliable indicator than the extremities.

exposure to the sun on the hands and/or arms predisposes to premature loss of elasticity of the skin, leading to a possible inaccurate conclusion that the patient is dehydrated.

Chest: Breath Sounds

Throughout the patient assessment process, you should monitor the patient's breathing. If you have not already done so, you should carefully palpate the patient's chest. Feel for subcutaneous emphysema, because this occurs with a ruptured trachea or mainstem bronchus and with pneumothorax. Also evaluate the movement of the chest wall during breathing. Paradoxical motion of the chest wall suggests that your patient has a flail chest and will need supplemental oxygen or, if breathing is inadequate, assisted ventilation. You might also want to perform a more detailed evaluation of the patient's breath sounds. Instructing the patient to take a deep breath with his or her mouth open, listening during inspiration and expiration, and using an orderly, sequential method as described will be your best approach to obtain an accurate assessment of breath sounds. During your assessment you may be able to identify one of the following:

- **Normal breath sounds.** These are clear and quiet on inspiration and expiration. Tracheal sounds (noted over the trachea) are very loud and harsh. The loud, high pitch and hollow sounds noted over the manubrium (over the mainstem bronchus) are known as bronchial sounds. The soft, breezy, and lower pitch sounds found at the midclavicular line are known as bronchovesicular sounds. The finer and somewhat fainter breath sounds noted in the lateral wall of the chest are from the smaller bronchioles and alveoli and are known as vesicular sounds.
- **Wheezing breath sounds.** These suggest an obstruction of the lower airways, usually by bronchoconstriction. Wheezing is a high-pitched squeal that is most prominent on expiration. If wheezing is unilateral, an aspirated foreign body or infection should be suspected. If wheezing is bilateral, an inhaled irritant such as chlorine or disease states such as reactive airway disease, asthma, or other less common lung diseases such as asbestosis may be the problem.
- **Wet breath sounds.** These may indicate cardiac failure or infection, especially in a very young child. A moist crackling may be heard on inspiration and expiration and is termed rales, or crackles. The presence of rales or crackles is documented as localized or diffuse, unilateral or bilateral, and basilar or apical (or both).
- **Congested breath sounds.** These may suggest the presence of mucus in the lungs, which suggests the presence of an infection (such as pneumonia) or inflammation (for example, bronchitis). Expect to hear low-pitched, noisy sounds most prominent on expiration, which may be referred to as rhonchi. The patient often reports a productive cough associated with these sounds. Bilateral rhonchi suggest bronchitis, while localized rhonchi suggest pneumonia. Documentation is the same as for rales.
- **A crowing sound.** This sound may also be referred to as stridor. Early onset is heard on inhalation and is typically very faint. As the problem worsens, crowing is often heard without a stethoscope and suggests that the patient has an airway obstruction in or around the larynx. The sudden onset of crowing or stridor suggests an inhaled foreign body. Onset of crowing or stridor in the presence of fever or upper respiratory infection suggests swelling of the epiglottis, laryngeal folds, or vocal cords and should be recognized as a potential threat to life. Expect to hear a brassy, crowing sound that is most audibly prominent on expiration.
- **Pleural friction rubs.** These sounds are squeaking or grating sounds that occur when the pleural linings rub together (as may happen in pleurisy [inflammation of the pleura]). If this occurs, the pleural layers have lost their lubrication, most commonly due to inflammation. This condition is usually associated with pain on inspiration. The sounds may be heard any time the chest wall moves; therefore, they can be heard on inspiration, expiration, or both.

Percussion is a method of assessing the presence of air trapping (as in asthma or chronic obstructive pulmonary disease) or consolidation (as with pneumonia). Percussion is not a method commonly used in the field because it requires full access to the bare chest wall, a quiet atmosphere, and practice. However, you will encounter medical professionals who use this technique, so familiarity with it may be useful. Percussion is tapping on areas of the chest wall to determine whether normal resonance or a hollow sound is present. Tympany, or a drumlike sound (hyperresonance), suggests air trapping, such as that seen with pneumothorax or asthma, whereas a dull thud (hyporesonance) suggests an area of consolidation, infection, or a hemothorax (blood within the pleural space). The tapping is produced by placing the middle finger of the nondominant hand on the area of the chest wall to be assessed and using the middle finger of the dominant hand to strike the bone of the middle finger of the nondominant hand, listening for the quality of the sound produced.

Assessment of the respiratory system also includes monitoring pulse oximetry and/or capnography. Pulse oximetry may alert you to changes in oxygenation but is inaccurate in states of hypoperfusion. Capnography may alert you to changes in carbon dioxide retention (for example, hypoventilation) and perfusion and aids in monitoring of endotracheal tube placement.

Chest: Heart Sounds

The normal heart sounds include S_1 and S_2, also known as the "lub-dub" of the heart; there should be no other sounds. The best way to listen for heart sounds is to use the diaphragm of your stethoscope. The best place to listen for heart sounds is to first locate the point of maximal impulse (PMI). Normally it is found at the fifth intercostal space, just medial to the midclavicular line. This is the location of the mitral valve. Listen for S_1 at the fifth intercostal space at the left sternal border (tricuspid valve) and at the PMI. Listen for S_2 at the second intercostal space at the right sternal border (aortic valve) and at the second intercostal space at the left sternal border (pulmonic valve) (Figure 10-24▼). Any sounds noted in addition to lub-dub are abnormal and may suggest the presence of a murmur (incompetent valve, inflammation, or decreased ventricular compliance). Accurate heart sound assessment also requires a quiet environment. The field is not a quiet place, so assessment of heart sounds is not always practical.

As mentioned before, heart sounds are only part of the assessment needed for the cardiovascular system. The rest of this assessment includes assessing for carotid bruits (listening over the carotid artery with your stethoscope for the abnormal presence of bruits, a harsh, gurgling sound that suggests plaque formation), vital signs, trending vital signs, and ECG monitoring.

Abdomen

During the detailed physical exam, you should perform a more complete examination of the abdomen. Observe the abdomen for symmetry, distention, rash, petechiae, and bruising in or around the navel (Cullen's sign) and along the sides of the abdomen (Grey-Turner's sign). Bruising in these areas suggests blood collecting in the retroperitoneal space and may occur from trauma or from a ruptured or "leaking" organ such as the aorta or a kidney. Abnormal symmetry may suggest a swollen organ immediately under that area. The most frequently noted asymmetry is due to an inflamed liver in cases of cirrhosis or hepatitis. Gentle pressure in that area often results in JVD. Distention may not be readily apparent. If it is suspected, ask the patient or a family member if the abdomen seems larger and, if so, when this was noticed and how it has progressed. How rapidly the distention has occurred is important for the receiving hospital to know. Severe distention may be due to fluid in the peritoneal space, as in ascites; blood, as in a slow leak from a rupture; obstruction, as in a bowel blockage; or infection, as in some cases of sepsis. Percussion is sometimes used to assess the abdomen to help differentiate between a dull thud, which indicates a solid organ, and tympany, which is normal over the stomach but suggests accumulated gas if found over the rest of the abdomen.

Some disease processes, such as chickenpox, start with a rash over the trunk of the body. Some allergic reactions result in urticaria (hives) that may occur first on the abdomen, particularly around the waist. Also observe for distended veins spreading upward from the navel, analogous to varicose veins. This is termed caput medusa and suggests severe, ongoing backup of pressure in the hepatic portal system. The presence of caput medusa should alert you to the possibility of esophageal varices.

As you palpate around the abdomen, using the four-quadrant approach, use the terms firm, soft, tender, or

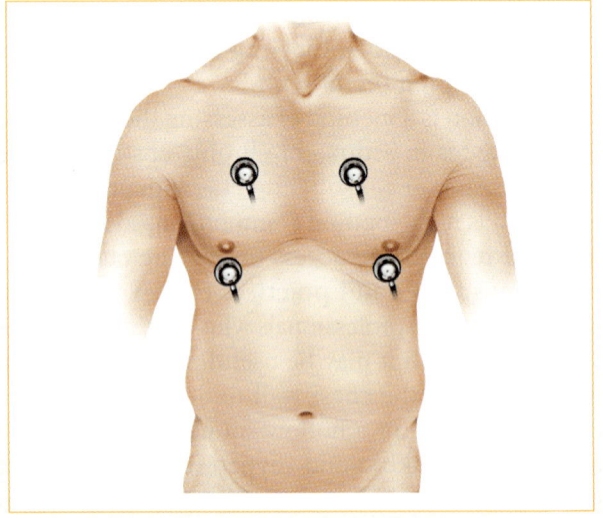

Figure 10-24 Listening to heart sounds.

distended (swollen) to report your findings. Some patients may tense the abdomen as you touch it. This is termed guarding. If the patient is complaining of abdominal pain, start your palpation at the most distal point, working toward the area of tenderness last. Assessing for rebound tenderness can be done by gentle, steady pressure on the abdomen, then releasing quickly. However, this often produces severe pain and is not encouraged. The same assessment can be accomplished by determining whether abdominal pain is produced by having the patient cough or tapping the heel of the patient's foot on the affected side. The significance of noting the position in which the patient is most comfortable lies in determining whether visceral (organ) pain or parietal (peritoneal irritation) pain is present. This will be further explained later in the text.

Pelvis

If you have not previously identified any pelvic injury, recheck the pelvis to identify pain, tenderness, instability, and crepitus; all may indicate a fractured pelvis and the potential for severe internal hemorrhage and shock. Inspection of the pelvic area, including the genitalia, is not often done in cases of medical emergencies with several notable exceptions: pain and bleeding. The pelvic area is the area that is below an imaginary line drawn from one iliac crest to the other. When the abdomen is palpated, the area below the navel should also be palpated. When abdominal pain is due to a bladder infection, that area will be tender to palpation. There is often an associated complaint of burning during urination, or dysuria. The complaint by a male patient of severe, excruciating pain in the groin or in one testicle, as occurs in testicular torsion, warrants examination of the testicular area. The affected testicle is often discolored and/or swollen. Testicular torsion is a serious emergency that requires immediate transport.

The other exception is in the case of bleeding in the groin or pelvic area. In females it is important to determine whether the bleeding is coming from the vaginal opening, female external genitalia, or the rectum. In males, it is important to determine whether bleeding is coming from the urethra or the rectum.

Extremities

If you have not already done so, you should carefully evaluate the extremities for any signs of trauma, again using the DCAP-BTLS mnemonic. You should also evaluate the distal circulation, sensation, and movement; areas of edema and pitting edema; and for rash and petechiae. If you have already identified an injury, regular evaluation of the circulation, sensation, and movement below the injury will allow you to be sure that the injury has not compromised neurovascular status. Assessment of the hands and feet, particularly the nail beds, can give you clues to adequacy of perfusion and oxygenation. Note the color of the fingers and nail beds. Cyanosis may be noted; an early onset of cyanosis may cause the nail beds to darken and appear gray. This is sometimes termed a "dusky" appearance. In cases of Raynaud's syndrome, one or more fingers or toes may be strikingly pale or cyanotic and cold to the touch.

Pay close attention to the color of the hands and arms in comparison with one another. A ruddy color in one arm suggests obstruction of venous return, whereas edema suggests blockage of the lymphatic system.

Assessment for distal pulses is also an important detail for assessing peripheral circulation. Pulses should be assessed in comparison with one another in terms of location (radial, femoral, and pedal pulses compared), strength of pulsation, rate, and regularity. A difference from one side to the other suggests unilateral impairment of arterial blood flow.

Assessment for pitting edema in the ankles and shins is an important indicator of cardiac involvement and may be your only sign of that problem. Looking for ulcer formation is particularly important for diabetic patients, although any patient with compromised peripheral circulation is at risk. Infection may be noted by looking for redness, swelling, and heat around an open wound or puncture site. Red streaks migrating up an extremity, even in the absence of a visible wound, suggest infection and/or phlebitis.

A detailed examination for sensation and movement is usually not warranted unless the patient has had an unexplained episode of syncope or loss of memory of an event or has an unusual presentation of altered movement and/or sensation and you suspect a CNS problem.

The Cincinnati Stroke Scale is a quick field assessment tool designed to look for signs of a stroke Table 10-13 ▶ . This tool includes assessment of three things: facial symmetry, clarity of speech, and pronator drift. Facial symmetry is assessed by having the patient grin and show his or her teeth. Clarity of speech is assessed by giving the patient a sentence to say with consonants, such as "the sky is blue in Cincinnati" or a similar sentence. Pronator drift is assessed by having the patient sit or stand with arms outstretched, palms up, and eyes closed. Observe for the hand to pronate (turn down) and/or drift in one direction or another. If

TABLE 10-13	Cincinnati Stroke Scale	
Test	Normal	Abnormal
Facial droop (Ask patient to show teeth or smile.)	Both sides of face move equally well.	One side of face does not move as well as the other.
Arm drift (Ask patient to close eyes and hold both arms out with palms up.)	Both arms move the same, or both arms do not move.	One arm does not move, or one arm drifts down compared with the other side.
Speech (Ask patient to say, "The sky is blue in Cincinnati.")	Patient uses correct words with no slurring.	Patient slurs words, uses inappropriate words, or is unable to speak.

the patient is standing, you must be close by for support in case the patient loses balance.

Cranial Nerve Assessment

In cases of assessment for a suspected head or spine injury or a more detailed nervous system assessment for a more subtle medical condition, you may do a quick field assessment of 11 of the 12 cranial nerves (CNs) and/or a gross assessment of the neural areas of the spine.

Because CN I is the olfactory nerve, the sense of smell is not commonly tested in the field. However, the rest of the cranial nerves can be rapidly assessed as follows:

- CN II, III—Check pupil response to light
- CN III, IV, VI—Test for extraocular movement using the "H" method. This test, often performed at regular eye checkups in the optometrist's office, involves holding a finger in front of the patient's face and moving it in the shape of an H. Starting at the middle of an imaginary "H," move your finger horizontally to one side, then up and down, then to the other side, then up and down, and finally returning to the middle. The patient's eyes should follow your finger.
- CN V—Have the patient clench his or her teeth, and palpate the masseter muscles; check sensation to the forehead, cheek, and chin
- CN VII—Have the patient smile wide and show the teeth
- CN IX, X—While the patient says "ah-h-h," watch the uvula for movement; check for the gag reflex
- CN XI—Have the patient shrug the shoulders and turn the head against resistance
- CN VIII—Test by checking for the ability to maintain an upright position (for 15 to 20 seconds) with eyes closed and for pronator drift (described above); assess for hearing by moving your fingers together about 2″ to 3″ away from the patient's ears and ask the patient what is heard.

Usually, the need for a spinal nerve assessment occurs when the patient complains of neck or back pain following trauma. The first step in this assessment procedure is to palpate down the spine to determine the area where pain occurs. Assess for equality and strength of hand grip, then for abduction and adduction against an opposing force of the hands, forearms, thighs, and feet. The final assessment step is to assess for the presence, character, and normalcy of sensation on the hands and feet, little finger and toe to thumb and big toe, comparing reactions on one side of the body with those on the other. This is only a gross assessment designed to determine a general location of the problem, not a specific spinal nerve root.

Back

During the rapid assessment, if performed, you should have visualized and palpated the patient's back for signs of trauma, especially near the spine. You must use spinal precautions when log rolling the patient for assessment of back injuries. The presence of a significant MOI or spinal deformity or pain suggests the need for spinal immobilization, if you have not already done so. Look for and document any other conditions that you find on the back.

Cardiovascular System

Assessment of the cardiovascular system includes vital signs; assessment of perfusion, including mental status; and assessment of the heart, including heart sounds and the ECG. A full set of vital signs is necessary to identify trends, such as rising or falling blood pressure; certain compensatory mechanisms, such as hypotension with tachycardia in some states of shock; hypertension; bradycardia and irregular respirations in the case of increased intracranial pressure; and certain disease states, such as irregular heart rate despite a regular ECG tracing in the case of a paradoxical pulse. The assessment of heart sounds is not always practical in the field, but assessment of the cardiac rhythm is an important assessment tool because it may help determine the course of your treatment. Recognition of the ECG rhythm will be discussed in a later chapter.

Baseline Vital Signs

Sometimes you will be so busy establishing and maintaining the ABCs that you will not have a chance to obtain the patient's vital signs. That is as it should be. Nothing should take priority over the airway, breathing, and circulation. However, whenever possible, it is important to get a set of baseline vital signs following completion of the initial assessment and rapid assessment, if performed. If you have not assessed the vital signs before the detailed assessment, a complete set of vital signs should be obtained by completion of the detailed assessment.

Mental Status

All during your assessment process you should be taking note of the patient's mental status. Changes in mental status will be your best indicator for improvement or deterioration in your patient's condition. As stated earlier, the AVPU method of determining response is very useful for your initial assessment. As you continue to interact with your patient, you will be determining orientation to person, place, time, and event and obtaining as much of a history as you can. During your conversation, you will be noting your patient's appearance (for example, clean and neat, indicators of trauma) and behavior (for example, anxious, depressed); posture (for example, upright or slumped, favoring a body part) and motor activity (for example, smooth muscle tone, jittery and nervous); and ease of speech and language (for example, slurring speech, using inappropriate words, perseverating). Memory function, perceptions, and judgment are all indicators of mental status that take time to determine and can be done during history taking. Assessment of mental status and function is ongoing throughout your entire time spent with the patient. If at any time changes in mental status or function occur, your immediate attention is required and the severity of your patient's condition should be upgraded. More information regarding mental status changes, potential causes, and treatment will be explained later in this text.

You are the Provider — Part 9

Both patients are now being transported to the closest appropriate emergency department. While en route, the ongoing assessment of your 82-year-old patient reveals the following:

Reassessment	Recording Time: 8 Minutes After Patient Contact
Respirations	22 breaths/min, adequate depth
Pulse	88 beats/min and regular
Skin	Pale
Blood pressure	152/88 mm Hg
SaO_2	97% with 15 L oxygen via nonrebreathing mask

15. What is the purpose of the ongoing assessment?
16. What is the procedure for the ongoing assessment?

Patient Assessment

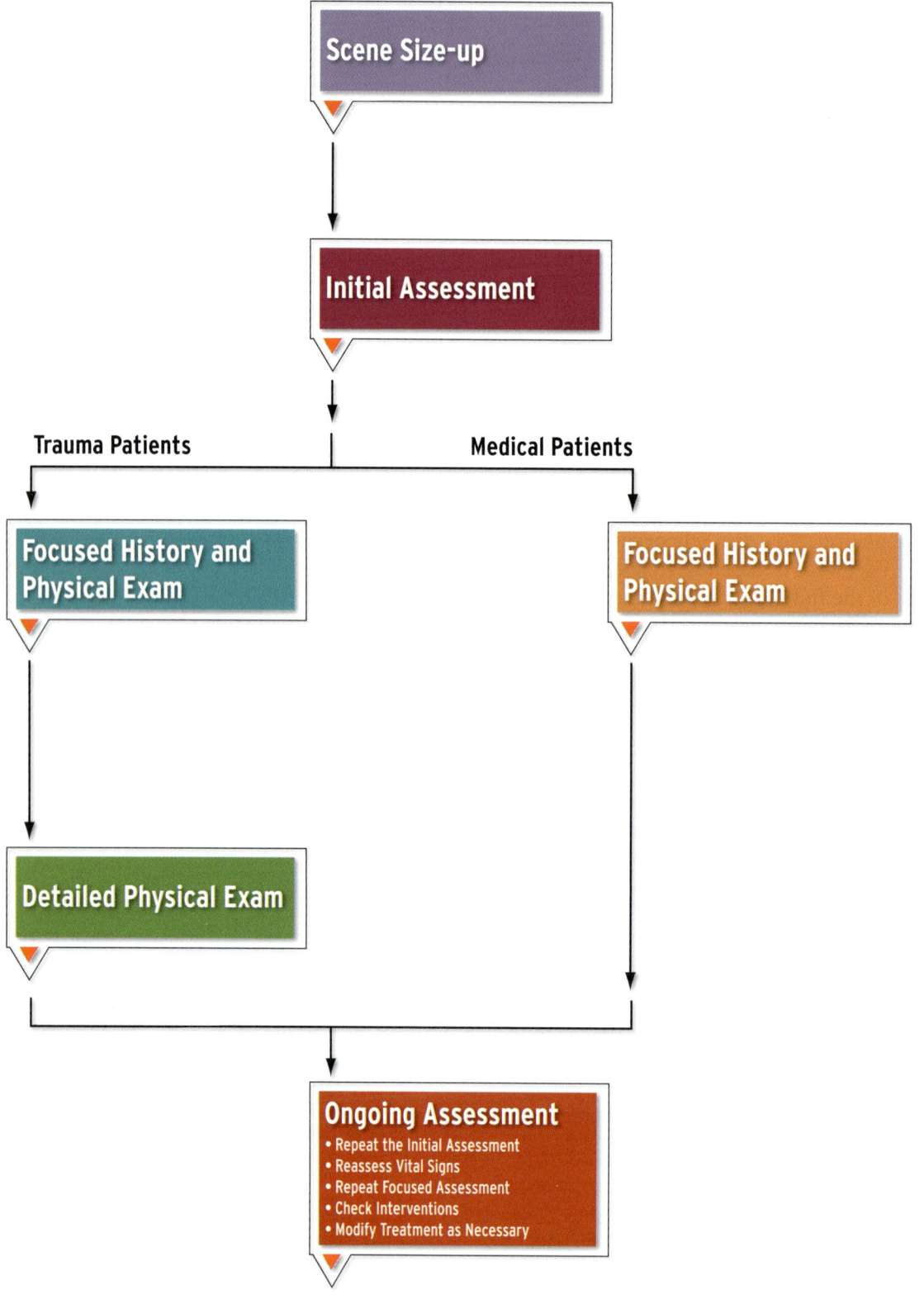

Ongoing Assessment

Unlike the detailed physical exam, the <u>ongoing assessment</u> is performed on all patients during transport. Its purpose is to ask and answer the following questions:

- Is treatment improving the patient's condition?
- Has an already identified problem improved? Or has the patient's condition deteriorated?
- What is the nature of any newly identified problems?
- How do I need to modify treatment to address changes found in the patient's condition?

The ongoing assessment helps you to monitor treatment modalities, track trends, and monitor changes in the patient's condition. The monitoring of treatment modalities includes constant monitoring of the airway, airway management, and any other treatment you have given. For example, you must monitor the security of splints and the integrity of any bandages that have been applied. If per local protocol you have used a pneumatic anti-shock garment, this must be monitored as well. Tracking trends refers to evaluating assessment findings and comparing the findings with initial findings. In this manner, you can determine whether assessed areas such as mental status, vital signs, and lung sounds are improving, remaining the same, or deteriorating. If the changes are improvements, you may decide to continue whatever treatment you are providing, such as maintaining oxygenation for a patient whose mental status is improving, or administering an additional IV fluid bolus for a trauma patient whose last measurement of systolic pressure had increased only 6 mm Hg after a total of 800 mL of an isotonic crystalloid solution, or you might modify treatment, such as refraining from administering additional dextrose to a hypoglycemic patient who is now conscious and verbally responsive.

In some cases, the patient's condition will deteriorate. When this happens, you should immediately repeat the initial assessment and be prepared to modify and implement treatment as appropriate on the basis of the problem identified.

Consider this example: You have a patient with a stab wound to the right anterior portion of the chest about 4″ below the clavicle. He is unresponsive and has poor skin color and a rapid carotid pulse. The patient has been intubated and is being ventilated (treatment has begun). However, his skin color is worsening and his tachycardia increasing, despite adequate ventilation and 100% oxygen (the patient's condition deteriorates). Endotracheal tube placement is visually checked and verified, and lung sounds are evaluated for equality (the patient is reassessed). They are unequal with no sounds on the left. A left-sided chest needle decompression is performed to relieve a tension pneumothorax (treatment is modified based on reassessment findings, and a new treatment plan is implemented).

Table 10-14 ▼ lists the components of the ongoing assessment.

Steps of the Ongoing Assessment

The procedure for the ongoing assessment is simply to repeat the initial assessment, vital signs, and the focused assessment and to check the intervention steps that pertain to the problems you are treating. These steps should be repeated and recorded every 15 minutes for a patient in stable condition and every 5 minutes for a patient in unstable condition Figure 10-25 ▼). Remember to use your judgment when timing the ongoing assessments. Some patients may require more frequent assessments.

TABLE 10-14	Ongoing Assessment

- Repeat the initial assessment
- Reassess vital signs
- Repeat the focused assessment
- Check interventions
- Modify treatment as necessary

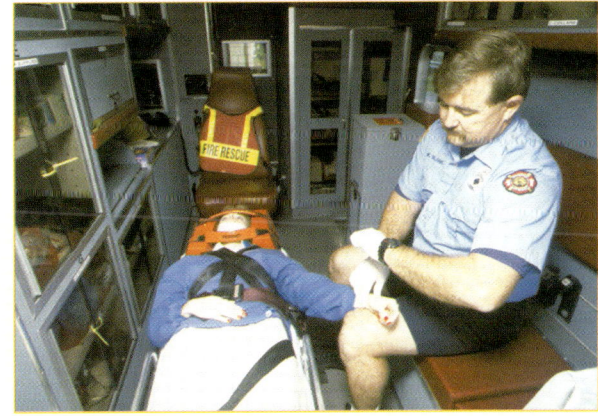

Figure 10-25 During the ongoing assessment, repeat your initial assessment, recheck vital signs, and recheck interventions every 5 minutes if the patient is unstable and every 15 minutes if the patient is stable.

The steps of the ongoing assessment are as follows:
1. Repeat the initial assessment.
   - Reassess mental status.
   - Maintain an open airway.
   - Monitor the patient's breathing.
   - Reassess pulse rate and quality.
   - Monitor skin color and temperature.
   - Reestablish patient priorities.
2. Reassess and record vital signs.
3. Repeat your focused assessment regarding patient complaint or injuries, including questions about the patient's history.
4. Identify patterns of improvement, maintenance, or deterioration.
5. Check interventions.
   - Ensure adequacy of oxygen delivery or artificial ventilation.
   - Ensure management of bleeding.
   - Ensure adequacy of other interventions.
6. Modify and implement treatment as necessary.

Repeat the Initial Assessment

The first step in the ongoing assessment is to repeat the initial assessment. If you have been treating the ABCs, you need to continue monitoring these essential functions. It is particularly important to reassess mental status; changes can be initially subtle, and the patient's status can then rapidly decline.

Reassess Vital Signs

Be sure that the patent's vital signs have not changed. Record these so that your documentation is accurate and complete. If the vital signs have changed, evaluate what may have happened and what you should do about it. Include pulse oximetry in this assessment of vital signs. Reassessment of vital signs will help you determine a trend. Trending of vital signs is very important. Pulse rates may increase but only gradually, so serial pulse rates will help you identify a trend of increasing or decreasing rates. The same can be said for blood pressure. Identifying trends will help you to recognize patterns and make treatment decisions, such as when to administer a fluid bolus or when to administer another nebulizer treatment. Trending will also help you identify whether a patient's condition is improving, staying the same, or deteriorating.

Repeat the Focused Assessment

A repeated focused assessment is designed to reevaluate all other signs and symptoms not covered by vital signs, especially the things for which you administered treatment. If the chief complaint is difficulty breathing, is breathing getting better or worse? Is there any change in ease of breathing? Is there any pain or discomfort associated with breathing that has changed? If the chief complaint is pain or discomfort, reassess palliating and provoking factors (whether the pain is getting better or worse), the quality (does it differ?), radiation (present or absent), and the severity based on the 0 to 10 scale (do a repeated scale).

Pay particular attention to mental status and any changes that might have occurred and to any changes in behavior, such as agitation or drowsiness, and document what time(s) the changes occurred. Changes in respiratory pattern or speech will alert you to worsening or improvement in the patient's condition. For example, a patient with asthma who is initially unable to talk may start to audibly wheeze and verbalize one-word phrases after treatment has been initiated. In contrast, the patient with syncope who suddenly seems to fall asleep is the patient whose condition is probably getting worse and needs reassessment of airway, breathing, and circulation.

Pay attention to the cardiac monitor, and be alert for dysrhythmias.

Together with trending vital signs, noting these changes will help you determine whether your treatment is improving the patient's condition or maintaining the patient's status or whether you need to adjust your treatment steps because of lack of improvement.

Check Interventions

Reevaluate any interventions you performed. Take a moment to make certain that the oxygen is still flowing, the backboard straps are still tight, the bleeding has been controlled, the airway is still open, pulse oximetry is still functioning, the leads on the ECG are still securely attached, and the IV line is patent and running. Things often change in the uncontrolled prehospital environment, so this is a good time to be sure that your treatments and equipment are still working the way you expect.

Transportation Considerations

Once you are ready to transport the patient, choosing a hospital is your next task. Choosing one hospital over another depends on proximity, specialized care, local protocols, and even patient requests. Typically, patients with special needs will go to a specialty care facility (ie, burn injuries will go to a burn center, trauma calls will go to a trauma center, etc.). There are, however, exceptions to every rule. Be sure to familiarize yourself with the policies of the agency for whom you are transporting.

The patient assessment process is shown in its entirety in a flowchart on the next page.

Patient Assessment

Scene Size-up
- Body Substance Isolation
- Scene Safety
- Determine Mechanism of Injury/Nature of Illness
- Determine Number of Patients
- Request Additional Assistance
- Consider C-Spine Immobilization

Initial Assessment
- Form General Impression of the Patient
- Assess Mental Status
- Assess the Airway
- Assess Breathing
- Assess Circulation
- Identify Priority Patients

Trauma Patients

Focused History and Physical Exam
Reconsider Mechanism of Injury

Significant Mechanism of Injury	No Significant Mechanism of Injury
Rapid Trauma Assessment	Focused Assessment: Based on Chief Complaint
Baseline Vital Signs and SAMPLE History	Baseline Vital Signs and SAMPLE History
Transport	Transport

Medical Patients

Focused History and Physical Exam
Evaluate Responsiveness

Responsive	Unresponsive
History of Illness	Rapid Medical Assessment
SAMPLE History	Baseline Vital Signs
Focused Physical Exam: Based on Chief Complaint	SAMPLE History
Baseline Vital Signs	Reevaluate Transport Decision
Reevaluate Transport Decision	

Detailed Physical Exam
- Perform Detailed Physical Exam
- Reassess Vital Signs

Ongoing Assessment
- Repeat the Initial Assessment
- Reassess Vital Signs
- Repeat Focused Assessment
- Check Interventions
- Modify Treatment as Necessary

Clinical Decision Making

Effective clinical decision making is dependent on the EMT-I's ability to gather and evaluate patient information, develop a <u>differential diagnosis</u> based on gathered information and the patient's presentation, and formulate a <u>field impression</u>, on which an appropriate patient treatment plan will be based.

The prehospital setting is one of controlled chaos, at best; your sources of information can be overwhelming or severely limited. You must be able to "mentally triage" this information in a very short time, separate relevant from irrelevant data, and provide the most appropriate care for the patient. These are the cornerstones of being an effective EMT-I.

The performance of your duties will constantly be challenged by the environment in which you must function. Time is perhaps your biggest challenge, especially when managing a critically ill or injured patient; split-second decisions regarding treatment and transport must be made to save the patient's life.

Although you, your partner, and other prehospital care providers must work together as a team, you must each be able to:

- Think and work effectively under pressure
- Make independent decisions
- Exercise sound judgment

Basing your treatment or transport decisions on an incomplete assessment and/or disregarding important information can lead to inadequate care and potential harm to the patient.

The Prehospital Environment

The nature of emergency medicine requires critical decisions to be made that will affect the outcome of the patient, whether those decisions are made by an EMT-I in the back of an ambulance or a physician in the emergency department. The prehospital environment, however, poses unique challenges to EMS personnel that are not encountered in a clinical setting.

Invasive procedures (such as IV therapy) that you will routinely perform in the field were intended to be performed in a controlled setting, not the chaotic, unpredictable nature of the prehospital environment. Nevertheless, you must still make the same critical decisions, perform many of the same invasive procedures, and provide the same quality patient care that is expected from a nurse or physician, working conditions notwithstanding.

Factors that can hamper your ability to perform patient care—crowds of people, volatile scenes, poor lighting, weather extremes, bumpy ambulances—do not exist in other medical settings (Figure 10-26 ▶). Your ability to improvise, adapt, and overcome these unique obstacles—and still provide appropriate patient care—

You are the Provider — Part 10

Both patients are now being transported to the closest appropriate emergency department. While en route, the ongoing assessment of your 78-year-old female patient reveals the following:

Reassessment	Recording Time: 8 Minutes After Patient Contact
Respirations	20 breaths/min, adequate depth
Pulse	112 beats/min, slightly irregular
Skin	Pale and warm and dry to touch
Blood pressure	142/72 mm Hg
SaO_2	96% with 15 L oxygen via nonrebreathing mask

17. What is the process of critical thinking, and how can it help the EMT-I care for patients in the prehospital setting?

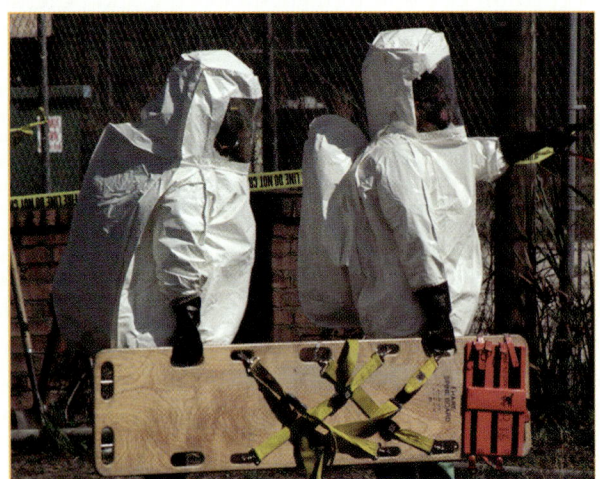

Figure 10-26 The prehospital environment poses unique challenges to the EMT-I that are not encountered in other medical settings.

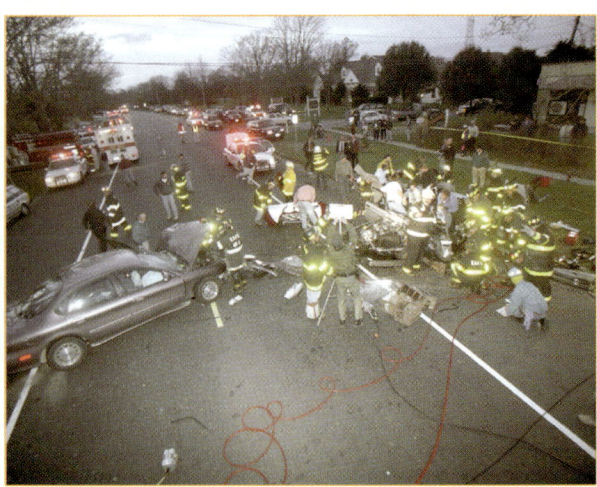

Figure 10-27 Multiple patient situations challenge the EMT-I's ability to think under pressure and practice effective clinical decision-making skills.

will make you an effective clinical decision maker and a true prehospital professional.

The Spectrum of Prehospital Patients

As an EMT-I, you will be exposed to a variety of patients who can be categorized by their levels of <u>acuity</u>: obviously critical, potentially critical, and non–life threatening.

Most of the time, you are exposed to only one patient at a time, allowing you to devote all of your attention to that one patient. However, situations such as mass casualty incidents, in which there are multiple patients with varying levels of acuity, challenge the EMT-I's ability to think under pressure and practice effective clinical decision-making skills (**Figure 10-27** ▶).

Levels of Patient Acuity

When arriving at the scene and encountering a patient with a gunshot wound to the chest, it is obvious that you will be assessing and treating a critically injured patient. The same is true when walking into a residence and finding the patient slumped over in a chair, cyanotic, and apneic. Patients with obviously critical illnesses or injuries clearly have a higher rate of mortality and morbidity. However, because the treatment is often as straightforward as the condition itself, some providers are more comfortable treating such patients as opposed to patients with potentially critical or non–life-threatening conditions. For example, you know that a patient who is apneic will require ventilation; a profusely bleeding patient in shock will require immediate bleeding control, oxygen, IV therapy, and rapid transport.

Potentially critical patients are perhaps the most challenging to manage; they require the greatest amount of scrutiny and careful assessment skills. Many times, your only indicator of the potential for severe injuries is the mechanism by which the patient was injured. The condition of a patient with blunt head trauma may seem fine initially, only to deteriorate later due to an intracranial hemorrhage. Other patients may have multiple, chronic disease processes that could exacerbate, or be exacerbated by, an acute condition. It is in these situations that you must maintain the highest <u>index of suspicion</u>.

Some injuries and illnesses, although unpleasant and painful for the patient, are clearly not life threatening. Examples include isolated distal extremity injuries and healthy patients with acute gastritis and vomiting.

Unfortunately, patients do not read EMS textbooks; you will not always encounter the "classic" patient. Clinical presentations often vary from what one would expect to see for a given condition. Because all patients present differently, even if only slightly, there is no definite way to be prepared for every type of patient encounter. However, by following a careful, systematic approach to every patient and using your knowledge of common

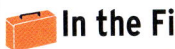

> **In the Field**
>
> If you think that the patient is sick or injured, but the clinical presentation suggests otherwise, go with your gut instinct and assume that at a minimum, a potential life-threatening condition exists and treat the patient accordingly.

medical conditions and traumatic injuries, your ability to care for patients with a wide variety of conditions will be enhanced.

Protocols, Standing Orders, and Algorithms

Tools, developed by the medical director or other entity, exist to guide and assist the EMT-I in performing his or her job. Protocols are predefined written treatment guidelines that provide general guidance to the EMT-I when caring for the most commonly encountered medical and trauma emergencies. They are intended to be followed in case medical control is unable to be contacted.

Standing orders, a type of protocol, are written orders that delineate functions to be carried out by the EMT-I. Unlike protocols, however, standing orders usually provide a specific list of tasks or functions that the EMT-I should carry out before contacting medical control. For example, attaching an AED to a potentially viable patient in cardiac arrest is a common standing order, as is oxygen administration to a hypoxic patient.

Patient care algorithms, such as those developed by the American Heart Association for advanced cardiac life support (or ACLS), provide step-by-step approaches to the care of patients with a variety of cardiac and respiratory emergencies. Although most of the common treatment algorithms are universal, the medical director can alter them, as he or she sees fit, for a given patient situation.

Protocols, standing orders, and patient care algorithms are valuable because they provide a standardized approach to patients with common medical or trauma emergencies. If written clearly, they can also define and outline performance parameters.

Unfortunately, however, the EMT-I will not always encounter the most common patient presentations; patients often present in a not-so-classic manner. These situations, because they require the EMT-I to follow a different treatment path, limit the value of predefined treatment guidelines. Other limitations of such guidelines include the following:

- They do not address multiple disease causes.
- They do not address multiple treatment modalities.
  - Some patient conditions require the integration and implementation of more than one treatment algorithm or protocol.
- The EMT-I follows the protocol or algorithm without an adequate knowledge of the condition being treated (cookbook medicine).

Medical ambiguity occurs when an EMT-I focuses on a specific complaint, which may be vague; however, because the patient neglected to inform the EMT-I of other important symptoms, the focus of treatment may be directed away from the patient's primary problem.

> **EMT-I Tips**
>
> Not only must you know what you are treating, you must understand why you are treating the patient and how the patient may respond to your treatment. Without adequate knowledge of anatomy, physiology, and pathophysiology, predefined treatment guidelines are of minimal value to you and of no value to the patient.

Critical Thinking and the EMT-I

Gathering, analyzing, and correctly synthesizing patient information will culminate in an appropriate treatment plan. This process requires an understanding of the patient's injury or illness and the impact that your care will have on it. Formulation of a general impression and subsequent treatment plan requires an understanding of certain critical thinking concepts: concept formation, data interpretation, application of principles, evaluation, and reflection on action.

Concept Formation

Concept formation, a pattern of understanding based on initially obtained information, begins when you receive a call. You should be able to form an initial impression, the accuracy of which depends on the quality and quantity of information that the caller provides to the dispatcher. While en route to the scene, additional information may be provided to you by the dispatcher; this will further enhance the accuracy of your initial impression.

While approaching the scene, but before making contact with the patient, a thorough scene assessment, such as safety issues, MOI or NOI, and the number of patients, will also influence the decision-making process. From this information, you will be able to develop a general impression of the situation and the potential severity of the patient's illness or injury.

After making contact with the patient, you will obtain important information based on the patient's chief complaint (if the patient is conscious) and initial assessment findings. These data will further your ability to determine whether the patient's condition is critical, potentially critical, or non–life threatening. Further examination of the patient will pinpoint the body system(s) involved.

In conscious patients, overall affect (behavior and appearance) can provide key information about mental status, which can be affected by conditions such as hypoxia, alcohol or drug intoxication, electrolyte derangements, and psychiatric disorders.

Ancillary assessment tools, such as pulse oximeters and glucometers, can aid in your impression of the patient's condition, if used correctly. You must realize that these tools have limitations, which underscores the importance of focusing your attention on the patient and taking the readings from these ancillary tools into consideration.

> **In the Field**
>
> Focus your attention on the patient and treat based on signs, symptoms, and hemodynamic status. Do not rely solely on assessment adjuncts, such as pulse oximeters and glucometers.

Data Interpretation

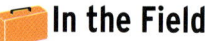 is the process of formulating a conclusion based on comparing the patient's condition with information from your training, education, and past experiences. All of the data gathered about the patient—dispatch information, chief complaint, history, and physical assessment findings—will integrate with your base knowledge of normal anatomy, physiology, and pathophysiology. How you use this information to treat the patient depends on your attitude, the reliability of the information obtained, and past experiences with similar patients. Remember, however, that no two patients present the same.

Application of Principles

As you analyze and synthesize the information obtained, you will be able to form a working field impression of the patient's condition, that is, what body systems are in dysfunction. It is the field impression on which you will base your treatment of the patient. While providing initial care, you may also reflect on patients that you have cared for in the past who had the same or similar problems.

Evaluation

It is crucial to constantly reassess the patient to determine whether changes in condition warrant modifications in your treatment strategies. For example, during a 30-minute transport to the hospital with a critically ill or injured patient, you should reassess (perform an ongoing assessment) at least six times; a 15-minute transport time with a patient in stable condition would require at least one reassessment. All treatment must not be based on a single assessment of the patient. Patient's conditions are often dynamic, requiring frequent assessments and modifications in treatment.

Reflection on Action

To constantly improve the quality of care you provide to your patients, you should frequently reflect on or critique your performance following an EMS call, especially if the call was challenging or out of the ordinary. This practice will posture you to care for future patients with similar problems.

It is common practice for an EMT-I and his or her partner to discuss the events of the call after delivering the patient to the hospital. This informal discussion is not only valuable to you as an individual, but also can enhance the ability of you and your partner to work effectively as a team.

Fundamental Elements of Critical Thinking

Critical thinking cannot be taught in a classroom; its concepts can only be studied and practiced. Through field experience in dealing with multiple patients with varying problems, your critical thinking skills will evolve. The following seven essential elements form the foundation of critical thinking for the EMT-I:

- **Adequate fund of knowledge.** This means your knowledge and understanding of how injuries and illnesses will affect the patient. Knowledge is acquired from three primary sources: initial training, continuing education, and past experiences.
- **Ability to focus on specific and multiple elements of data.** Multiple amounts of specific, crucial data, often from multiple sources, must be obtained to direct your assessment and subsequent treatment.
- **Ability to identify and organize data and form concepts.** Your overall understanding of the situation and the treatment that you provide to the patient are only as good as the quality and quantity of data that you obtain.
- **Ability to differentiate between relevant and irrelevant data.** As previously discussed, your sources of information can be overwhelming or severely limited. You must be able to determine which data are relevant to your assessment and care of the patient. Irrelevant or extraneous data can skew your interpretation of the overall situation, potentially leading to inappropriate care.
- **Ability to analyze and compare similar situations.** Although no two patients present in the exact same manner, you must be able to integrate the information obtained regarding the current incident with similar situations and experiences. This will enhance your overall understanding of the current situation and will prepare you to deal with future situations.
- **Ability to recall contrary situations.** Recalling and learning from bad experiences enhances your ability to manage the current situation.
- **Ability to articulate assessment-based decisions and construct arguments.** You must be able to defend your actions and justify the decisions on which you based your treatment.

> **Documentation Tips**
>
> You must be prepared to justify and defend your actions for any assessment and treatment that you give to the patient, whether to the medical director or in a court of law. It is therefore critical to accurately and thoroughly document the event.

Field Application of Assessment-Based Management

The Spectrum of Patient Acuity

The varying range of patients' conditions—critical, potentially critical, non–life threatening—that the EMT-I will encounter is referred to as the spectrum of acuity. Because of the vast interpretations of the definition of "emergency," EMS is activated for countless reasons. Relative to the EMS system's total call volume, true life-threatening emergencies constitute only a small percentage. Most patients fall into the categories of obviously critical and non–life threatening, the treatment of which is rather straightforward and requires minimal critical thinking on the part of the EMT-I.

The greatest challenge for the EMT-I is to assess and implement a treatment plan for a patient with potentially critical injuries; these patients' clinical presentations are often vague or obscure. Therefore, it is paramount to perform a careful, systematic assessment and maintain a high index of suspicion when managing this patient population.

During a true life-threatening emergency, patient survival is dependent on the EMT-I's ability to efficiently and expeditiously perform the appropriate interventions and rapidly transport the patient to the appropriate medical facility.

Thinking Under Pressure

Because of the unpredictable nature of the prehospital environment, the EMT-I must be able to think and work effectively under pressure. A multitude of factors may affect your ability to do this: upset or hostile family members, patient acuity, an inexperienced partner, and your own stress reaction to the situation.

Hormonal Influence

The sympathetic nervous system (SNS), a component of the autonomic nervous system, prepares your body to handle stressful events, good or bad. The fight-or-flight response of the SNS is mediated by the hormone adrenaline. It is important to note that the surge of adrenaline can impact the EMT-I's decision-making abilities both negatively and positively.

Activation of the SNS can enhance your visual and auditory acuity and improve your reflexes and muscle strength. However, this same response can impair your critical thinking skills and concentration and your ability to perform an accurate patient assessment. New EMT-Is often fall victim to the negative effects of the SNS during an emergency; however, experience will facilitate the ability to think and work under pressure.

Mental Conditioning

Mental conditioning is the key to effective performance while under pressure. The development of certain habits that are applied to every call (regardless of acuity) will lead to an approach that is second nature to the EMT-I. While not everyone develops and practices the same habits, they are usually acquired during the initial training program and in repeated exposure to patients with a variety of injuries and illnesses.

Mental Checklist for Thinking Under Pressure

To effectively think and work under pressure, the habits that the EMT-I must develop center around a variety of actions that occur and overlap during an EMS call. They include the following:
- Stop and think
- Scan the situation
- Decide and act
- Maintain clear, concise control
- Regularly and continually reevaluate the patient

Facilitating Behaviors

With each EMS call that you respond to, you will become more experienced and more efficient at patient assessment and management. Facilitating behaviors will pave the way to efficient patient care; therefore, they should be emphasized to the EMT-I student early in the initial educational process.

First and foremost, *you must stay calm; don't panic.* An anxious provider can precipitate or exacerbate anxiety in the patient. Although a patient may be critically ill or injured, he or she may still notice your actions and behaviors. Approaching the patient with confidence will gain trust, allowing you to proceed with your assessment and management. Patient care can suffer if your assessment and/or management skills are haphazard, sloppy, or otherwise disorganized. In addition, critical elements of information, some of which may have a profound impact on the care and outcome of the patient, may be missed.

A mainstay of prehospital emergency care is to err on the side of the patient; treat for the worst and hope for the best. When forming a differential diagnosis based on the patient's chief complaint, assume the worst-case scenario. For example, a patient complaining of chest pressure or pain should be treated for a heart attack, in hopes that it is merely a musculoskeletal issue. This is the only logical approach, considering that definitive diagnosis and care cannot occur in the field.

Maintain a systematic patient assessment pattern and practice it routinely during every patient encounter. This will facilitate a reflex approach to the assessment of all patients you assess, even under the most stressful situations.

Although the patient may appear clinically stable, you must anticipate changes in the patient's condition. This will prepare you psychologically and logistically if additional, unexpected treatment is required.

Analysis, Data Processing, and Decision-Making Styles

Different patient encounters require a variety of clinical decision-making styles. Adapting the appropriate style to each patient you encounter will ensure that the patient receives the best possible care. The styles of information management and clinical decision making are shown in (Table 10-15▶).

Situational Awareness

Situational awareness is the consideration of all aspects of the scene and patient, resulting in your ability to look at the "big picture." Before arriving at the scene, you routinely perform a scene size-up, which consists of a variety of factors: safety, MOI, number of patients, and the need for additional help.

This gross scene assessment should occur repeatedly throughout the entire call, not just on arriving at the scene. Like patients, scenes are dynamic; you must read the scene to determine whether a new situation

TABLE 10-15	Clinical Decision-Making Styles and Information Management
Situation analysis	■ *Reflective:* Promotes and facilitates a thorough assessment of the patient before initiating treatment; appropriate for patients in stable condition with no immediate life threats ■ *Impulsive:* Acting instinctively to address an immediate life threat, such as a patient who is bleeding profusely
Data processing	■ *Divergent:* Considering all aspects of the situation before taking further action; useful when managing a patient in stable condition who has multiple medical problems ■ *Convergent:* Focusing narrowly on the most significant aspects of the patient's problem; for example, proceeding immediately with ventilations to a patient who is not breathing
Decision making	■ *Anticipatory:* Anticipating a problem and taking deliberate actions to prevent it ■ *Reactive:* Waiting for a problem to occur before addressing it

has arisen that puts you, your partner, or the patient in jeopardy. You must also read the patient, which will allow you to detect changes in condition and adjust your treatment accordingly.

Putting It All Together: "The Six Rs"

During your initial training as an EMT-I and the experiences that follow, you are constantly honing your skills in preparation for all aspects of an EMS call. Through the same training and the same experiences, you are also learning to apply the skills of the clinical decision-making process. The "six Rs" of clinical decision making, each of which will be discussed individually, emphasize the critical points in that process:

- Read the patient
- Read the scene
- React
- Reevaluate
- Revise the management plan
- Review performance at the run critique

Read the Patient

After experience in dealing with different types of patients, you will develop a "knack" for being able to look at a patient and say, "This patient is sick!" This observation is typically made when you form a general impression of the patient's condition. Key elements to reading a patient include the following:

1. **Observe the patient.** Is the patient conscious, semiconscious, or unresponsive? If he or she is conscious, what is the reaction to your presence or the presence of family members or bystanders? What is the color of the patient's skin (pale, flushed, cyanotic)? In what position did you find the patient (prone, supine, ambulatory, sitting)? Are there any obvious deformities or bleeding?
2. **Talk to the patient.** Is the airway patent? Is the patient able to speak? What is the chief complaint? Is this a new problem or an exacerbation of a preexisting one?
3. **Touch the patient.** Note the condition and temperature of the skin (moist, dry, warm, cool). What are the rate, quality, and regularity of the patient's pulse?
4. **Auscultate the patient's airway.** Are there any abnormal upper airway sounds (such as stridor, crowing, snoring)? Are there any abnormal lower airway sounds (such as wheezing, rales, rhonchi)?

At this point, you have gathered information regarding the patient's ABCs and have corrected immediate life threats. As you determine which assessment technique is appropriate (rapid assessment, focused exam), your partner should obtain a set of vital signs, which, in combination with your additional assessment, will help to determine the severity of the patient's condition.

EMT-I Tips

Be aware that the patient's age, underlying physical and medical conditions, and current medications can affect the patient's vital signs. Like any other assessment tool, consider the vital signs, but devote your attention to the patient.

Read the Scene

Your scene size-up begins by determining whether the scene is safe for you and your partner to enter. Remember that the scene may be safe initially, only to become unsafe with alarming unpredictability.

Other scene observations include notation of the MOI, the number of patients involved in the incident, and the need for additional assistance. Determine whether there are any environmental factors (such as rain, lightning, cold) that could affect the patient's condition.

React

To save a patient's life, you must be able to rapidly identify life-threatening conditions and react immediately to correct them. Following the correction of any immediate life threats, determine the most common and probable cause of the patient's problem based on the clinical presentation.

As previously discussed, you should treat for the worst and hope for the best; consider the most serious condition that correlates with the patient's presentation. If a clear medical problem is not evident, treat the patient based on the signs and symptoms.

Reevaluate

After formulating a field impression of the patient and initiating treatment, you must reevaluate the patient's condition to assess the effectiveness of your treatment, which may require modification. If time permits, perform a detailed physical examination to detect less serious or less obvious conditions.

Revise the Management Plan

On an as-needed basis, revise or modify your treatment plan for the patient. This is based on the response to your initial treatment and the findings of your ongoing assessment. Repeatedly check vital signs as needed to determine trends in the patient's condition. If the patient's condition deteriorates, immediately repeat an initial assessment to correct newly developed life threats.

Review Performance at the Run Critique

Reviewing your performance or having your performance reviewed is the key to constantly improving the quality of care provided to your patients. There are several ways to review or critique a call: a formal review, informal discussion with your partner following the call, and personal reflection. Regardless of the venue in which you review the call, it is important to understand that the purpose is not to humiliate, insult, or embarrass any of the providers involved in the call. Instead, you should identify certain practices or habits that proved effective and those that did not. Remember, every call is a learning experience.

You are the Provider   Summary

1. What are the steps involved in performing patient assessment?

Although every EMS call is unique, the steps of the patient assessment are always the same:
- Perform the scene size-up.
- Perform an initial assessment.
- Perform a focused history and physical exam.
- Perform a detailed physical exam.
- Perform ongoing assessments.

2. Why is it important for the EMT-I to conduct a scene size-up?

Scene size-up begins as you approach the scene and is considered throughout the entire call. The scene size-up is a quick assessment of the scene and the surroundings that will provide you and your partner with as much information as possible about the safety of the scene, the MOI, and/or the NOI before you enter the scene and begin patient care.

3. What is involved in a scene size-up?

The following are components of sizing up a scene: BSI, scene safety, determining the MOI or NOI, determining the number of patients, requesting additional assistance, and considering c-spine immobilization.

4. What is the goal of the initial assessment?

The initial assessment has a single, critical, all-important goal: to identify and initiate treatment of immediate or potential life threats.

5. What information should the EMT-I use to form his or her general impression of the patient's condition?

The general impression is based on your immediate assessment of the environment, the presenting signs and symptoms, MOI in a trauma patient, and the patient's chief complaint.

6. What questions can the EMT-I ask to assess for potential life-threatening injuries or illnesses?

To focus on finding and treating the most life-threatening illnesses and injuries, you need to ask and get answers to the following questions:
- Does the patient have an altered level of consciousness?
- Does the patient have an obstructed airway?
- Does the patient have inadequate breathing?
- Does the patient have inadequate circulation?
- Does the patient have the potential to develop any of these problems?
- Does the patient have the potential for a spinal cord injury?

If the answer to any of these questions is "yes," you need to take immediate action to resolve or prevent the life-threatening condition.

7. What method should the EMT-I use to evaluate the responsiveness of this patient?

Responsiveness can be evaluated by using the AVPU scale:
- **A**lert. The patient's eyes open spontaneously as you approach, and the patient appears aware of and responsive to the environment. The patient appears to follow commands, and the eyes visually track people and objects.
- Responsive to **V**erbal stimuli. The patient's eyes do not open spontaneously. However, the patient's eyes do open to verbal stimuli, and the patient is able to respond in some meaningful way when spoken to.
- Responsive to **P**ain. The patient does not respond to your questions but moves or cries out in response to a painful stimulus. This response is tested by gently but firmly pinching the patient's earlobe, by pressing down on the bone above the eye, or by pinching the muscles of the neck. Use of extremely painful stimuli is never appropriate.
- **U**nresponsive. The patient does not respond to any stimuli.

Continued

You are the Provider continued   Summary

8. What conditions should the EMT-I consider high priority or consider for paramedic backup?

Patients with one of the following conditions are considered high priority and should be transported immediately or be considered for paramedic backup:

- Poor general impression
- Unresponsive with no gag or cough reflexes
- Responsive but unable to follow commands
- Difficulty breathing
- Pale skin or other signs of poor perfusion
- Complicated childbirth
- Uncontrolled bleeding
- Severe pain in any area of the body
- Chest pain, especially when the systolic blood pressure is less than 100 mm Hg
- Inability to move any part of the body

9. What are three goals of the focused history and physical exam?

The focused history and physical exam help the EMT-I to "focus in" on specific problems. They have three goals:

- Identify the patient's chief complaint—What happened to this patient?
- Understand the specific circumstances surrounding the chief complaint—What circumstances were associated with the event? Is the MOI a high risk for serious injuries?
- Direct further physical examination—What problems can be identified through the physical exam?

10. What useful information is provided by the patient's baseline vital signs?

The baseline vital signs provide the EMT-I useful information about the overall functions of the patient's heart and lungs. The baseline vital signs also provide a starting point by which we begin to trend findings and monitor the patient's condition.

11. What does the mnemonic SAMPLE stand for?

The mnemonic SAMPLE includes the following elements:

- **S**igns and Symptoms of the episode
- **A**llergies, particularly to medications
- **M**edications, including prescription, over-the-counter, and recreational (illicit) drugs
- **P**ertinent past history, particularly involving similar episodes in the past
- **L**ast oral intake, including food and/or drinks. This is particularly important if the patient may need surgery or is diabetic.
- **E**vents leading up to the episode, which may include precipitating factors

12. What are the seven most important factors to help the EMT-I learn more about a patient's chief complaint?

You can remember the seven most important circumstances by using the letters OPQRST-I, which stand for Onset, Provoking/Palliating factors, Quality, Radiation/Referred, Severity, Time, and any Interventions performed before your arrival.

13. What information should be included in the EMT-I's report on this responsive medical patient?

Your report for the responsive medical patient should include documentation of the following:
- The skin color, temperature, and moisture
- Findings from the initial assessment
- Baseline vital signs (pulse, blood pressure, respirations, temperature) and SAMPLE history
- The sensation and movement in all extremities
- Breath sounds

14. What are the components of a focused history and physical exam for this medical patient that should be performed by the EMT-I?

The components of a focused history and physical exam for medical patients are to evaluate responsiveness and then perform the following depending on whether the patient is responsive:
- Responsive: Obtain a history of the present illness (OPQRST-I), obtain a sample history, perform a focused physical exam based on the chief complaint, obtain baseline vital signs, and reevaluate your transport decision.
- Unresponsive: Perform a rapid medical assessment, obtain baseline vital signs, obtain a SAMPLE history, and reevaluate your transport decision.

15. What is the purpose of the ongoing assessment?

The ongoing assessment is performed on all patients during transport. Its purpose is to ask and answer the following questions:
- Is treatment improving the patient's condition?
- Has an already identified problem improved? Or has the patient's condition deteriorated?
- What is the nature of any newly identified problems?
- How do I need to modify treatment to address changes found in the patient's condition?

16. What is the procedure for the ongoing assessment?

The procedure for the ongoing assessment is simply to repeat the initial assessment, vital signs, and the focused assessment and to check the intervention steps that pertain to the problems you are treating. These steps should be repeated and recorded every 15 minutes for a patient in stable condition and every 5 minutes for a patient in unstable condition.

17. What is the process of critical thinking, and how can it help the EMT-I care for patients in the prehospital setting?

By gathering, analyzing, and correctly synthesizing patient information, the EMT-I will be able to develop an appropriate treatment plan for the patient.

Prep Kit

Ready for Review

- The assessment process begins with the scene size-up, which identifies actual or potential hazards.
- The patient should not be approached until these hazards have been dealt with in a way that eliminates or minimizes risk to the EMT-Is and the patient(s).
- After the scene size-up, you need to determine the MOI or the NOI.
- The initial assessment is performed on all patients. By forming a general impression of the patient's condition, you can identify any life-threatening conditions to the airway, breathing, and circulation (ABCs). Any life threats identified must be treated before moving to the next step of the assessment.
- The rapid assessment is performed quickly on any patient who is unresponsive or unable to articulate the nature of the problem to identify injuries or illnesses. When injuries and conditions are found, they should be prioritized and treated as appropriate.
- The focused history and physical exam are performed on all patients once their ABCs are stabilized.
- The focused history and physical exam identify potentially life-threatening conditions and help you to identify and explore the patient's chief complaint.
- In most cases, the focused history and physical exam will provide adequate information to enable you to initiate treatment.
- The detailed physical exam is performed on a select group of patients; those with a significant MOI and those who are unconscious.
- The detailed physical exam helps you to further understand problems that were identified during the focused exam and may also be used to evaluate problems that cannot be identified using the focused exam.
- The detailed physical exam is usually performed en route to the hospital.
- The ongoing assessment is performed on all patients during transport. It gives you an opportunity to reevaluate problems that are being treated and to recheck treatments to be sure that they are still being delivered correctly.
- Information from the ongoing assessment may be used to change treatment plans.
- Effective clinical decision making is dependent on your ability to gather and evaluate patient information, develop a differential diagnosis, and form a field impression on which a treatment plan is based. And you must do this in the pressure of the unpredictable field.

Vital Vocabulary

accessory muscles The secondary muscles of respiration.

acuity The severity of the patient's illness or injury.

adventitious Abnormal; as in adventitious breath sounds (for example, stridor, rhonchi).

air trapping An accumulation of air in the lungs that is unable to escape because of bronchoconstriction or other causes.

algorithms Predetermined guidelines that provide a step-by-step approach to the care of common illnesses or injuries (for example, ACLS [advanced cardiac life support] algorithms).

altered mental status A change in the way a person thinks and behaves that may signal disease in the central nervous system.

anisocoria A state of normally unequal pupils; present in approximately 20% of the population; pupil size difference is usually less than 1 mm.

aortic pulsations Pulsations of the aorta. In this chapter it is referring to a pulsating mass in the abdomen due to an aortic aneurysm.

ascites The accumulation of serous fluid in the peritoneal cavity.

Technology

- Interactivities
- Vocabulary Explorer
- Anatomy Review
- Web Links
- Online Review Manual

www.EMSzone.com/EMTI

aspiration Drawing in or out by suction. This may occur in the lungs when the patient is unable to maintain his or her own airway and there is blood or fluid in the mouth.

auscultate To listen to, as with a stethoscope.

AVPU A method of assessing a patient's level of consciousness by determining whether a patient is Awake and alert, responsive to Verbal stimuli or Pain, or Unresponsive; used principally in the initial assessment.

Battle's sign Bruising behind an ear.

blunt trauma A mechanism of injury in which force occurs over a broad area and the skin is not usually broken.

body substance isolation (BSI) An infection control concept and practice that assumes that all body fluids are potentially infectious.

breath sounds An indication of air movement in the lungs, usually assessed with a stethoscope.

bronchoalveolar system The system concerning the bronchi and the alveoli.

bronchoconstriction Constriction of the bronchial tubes.

bronchospasm Constriction or contraction of the bronchioles in the lungs; synonymous with bronchoconstriction.

bronchovesicular sounds Pertaining to the bronchial tubes and the alveoli with special reference to sounds intermediate between bronchial or tracheal sounds and alveolar sounds.

capillary refill The return of blood in an area such as a nail bed after pressure (caused by squeezing to blanch) is released; observing the time to refill and the color of the skin helps evaluate the function of the distal circulatory system function.

capnography Continuous recording of the carbon dioxide level in expired air in mechanically ventilated patients.

caput medusa A plexus of dilated veins about the umbilicus seen in one form of cirrhosis of the liver.

cardiac tamponade A life-threatening state of cardiac compression that develops as a result of a large pericardial effusion.

cerebrovascular accident Stroke.

chief complaint The reason a patient called for help; also, the patient's response to general questions such as "What's wrong?" or "What happened?"

Cincinnati Stroke Scale A quick field assessment tool designed to look for signs of a stroke; includes assessment for three things: facial symmetry, clarity of speech, and pronator drift.

coagulate To form a clot to plug an opening in an injured blood vessel and stop blood flow.

concept formation Pattern of understanding based on initially obtained information.

conjunctiva The delicate membrane that lines the eyelids and covers the exposed surface of the eye.

consolidation The process of becoming solid, especially in the lungs.

cookbook medicine Treating a patient based on a protocol or algorithm without adequate knowledge of the condition being treated.

crepitus A grating or grinding sensation caused by fractured bone ends or joints rubbing together; also air bubbles under the skin that produce a crackling sound or crinkly feeling.

croup An infectious disease of the upper respiratory system that may cause partial airway obstruction and is characterized by a barking cough; usually seen in children.

Cullen's sign Bluish discoloration of the periumbilical skin caused by intraperitoneal hemorrhage.

cyanosis Bluish-gray skin caused by reduced oxygen levels in the blood.

data interpretation The process of formulating a conclusion based on comparing the patient's condition with information from your training, education, and past experiences.

DCAP-BTLS A mnemonic for assessment in which each area of the body is evaluated for Deformities, Contusions, Abrasions, Punctures/Penetrations, Burns, Tenderness, Lacerations, and Swelling.

detailed physical exam The part of the assessment process in which a detailed area-by-area exam is performed on patients whose problems cannot be readily identified or when more specific information is needed about problems identified in the focused history and physical exam.

diaphoretic Sweaty.

differential diagnosis A list of possible causes of the patient's condition, based on clinical presentation.

Prep Kit continued...

diffuse pain Pain that is not identified as being specific to a single location.

dynamic Ever changing; not staying the same.

dysuria Difficult or painful urination.

ecchymosis Bruising or discoloration associated with bleeding within or under the skin.

edema The presence of abnormally large amounts of fluid between cells in the body tissues, causing swelling of affected areas.

entrance wound The area of the body where a penetrating trauma occurs. In knife or gunshot wounds, this would be the area where the bullet or blade entered; also seen in serious electrical injuries.

epiglottitis An inflammation of the soft tissue in the area above the vocal cords.

esophageal varices A tortuous dilatation of an esophageal vein, especially in the distal portion; frequently associated with cirrhosis of the liver.

exit wound The area of the body where a penetrating trauma exited. In gunshot wounds, this would be the area where the bullet exited.

facilitating behaviors In the context of this chapter, practices or habits that enhance the efficiency of patient care.

field impression A field conclusion of the patient's problem based on the clinical presentation and the exclusion of other possible causes through considering the differential diagnoses.

focal pain Pain that is easily identified as being specific to a single location.

focused history and physical exam The part of the assessment process in which the patient's major complaints or any problems that are immediately evident are further and more specifically evaluated.

frostbite Damage to tissues as the result of exposure to cold; frozen or partially frozen body parts.

general impression The overall initial impression that determines the priority for patient care; based on the patient's surroundings, the mechanism of injury, signs and symptoms, and the chief complaint.

golden hour The time interval between injury and definitive care, after which survival from shock or traumatic injuries decreases.

Grey-Turner's sign Bruising along the sides of the abdomen.

guarding Involuntary muscle contractions (spasm) of the abdominal wall; an effort to protect an inflamed or painful abdomen; a sign of peritonitis.

hyphema Blood in the anterior chamber of the eye.

hypothermia A condition in which the internal body temperature falls below 95°F (35°C) after exposure to a cold environment.

index of suspicion A heightened awareness of the potential for serious illness or injury.

initial assessment The part of the assessment process that helps you to identify any immediately or potentially life-threatening conditions so that you can initiate lifesaving care.

jaundice Yellow skin that is seen in patients with liver disease or dysfunction.

JVD Abbreviation for jugular venous distention.

left sternal border The left side of the sternum.

manubrium The upper quarter of the sternum.

mechanism of injury (MOI) The way in which traumatic injuries occur; the forces that act on the body to cause damage.

medical ambiguity Focusing on a specific complaint, which may be vague, and being distracted from the real problem; commonly the result of the patient's neglect to inform the EMT-I of all of his or her symptoms.

mitral valve The valve in the heart that separates the left atrium from the left ventricle.

myocardial infarction Blockage of the arteries that supply oxygen to the heart, resulting in death to a portion of the myocardium; heart attack.

nasal flaring Flaring out of the nostrils, indicating that there is an airway obstruction.

nature of the illness (NOI) The general type of illness.

ongoing assessment The part of the assessment process in which problems are reevaluated and responses to treatment are assessed.

OPQRST-I The six pain questions: Onset, Provoking/Palliating factors, Quality, Radiation/Referred pain, Severity, Time, and any Interventions performed before EMS arrival.

orientation The mental status of a patient as measured by memory of person (name), place (current location), time (current year, month, and approximate date), and event (what happened).

palpate Examine by touch.

paradoxical motion The motion of the chest wall that is detached in a flail chest; the motion is exactly the opposite of normal motion during breathing: in during inhalation, out during exhalation.

patency The state of being freely open.

pedal edema Swelling of the feet and ankles caused by collection of fluid in the tissues; a possible sign of congestive heart failure (CHF).

penetrating trauma A mechanism of injury in which force occurs in a small point of contact between the skin and the object. The skin is broken and the potential for infection is high.

perfusion Circulation.

petechiae Small, purplish, hemorrhagic spots on the skin; indicates severe sepsis.

pitting edema Edema that is severe enough to leave pits or indentations when touched.

pleural friction rub Contact of the inflamed pleura with the internal chest wall, causing friction as the patient breathes.

pleurisy Inflammation of the pleura.

point of maximal impulse (PMI) The point on the chest wall over the heart at which the contraction of the heart is best seen or felt.

pronator drift The arm on the affected side drifts when the patient is asked to hold both arms out; a portion of the Cincinnati Stroke Scale.

protocols Predefined patient care guidelines that are designed to be carried out in case medical control is unobtainable.

pulmonary embolism A blood clot that breaks off from a large vein and travels to the blood vessels of the lung, causing obstruction of blood flow.

pulse oximetry An assessment method that measures the oxygen saturation of hemoglobin in the capillary beds.

raccoon eyes Bruising under the eyes that may indicate skull fracture.

radiation A continuation of an area of pain or discomfort distal to the site of the origin of the pain; gives the sensation that the pain is moving (radiating) away from the origin.

rales Crackling, rattling breath sounds that signal fluid in the air spaces of the lungs; also called crackles.

Raynaud's syndrome A peripheral vascular disease marked by abnormal vasoconstriction of the extremities on exposure to cold or emotional stress.

referred pain Pain in two separate locations of the body, without a "trail" of pain between the two locations.

responsiveness The way in which a patient responds to external stimuli, including verbal stimuli (sound), tactile stimuli (touch), and painful stimuli.

retractions Movements in which the skin pulls in around the ribs during inspiration.

rhonchi Coarse, low-pitched breath sounds heard in patients with chronic mucus in the airways.

right sternal border The right side of the sternum.

SAMPLE history A key brief history of a patient's condition to determine Signs and Symptoms, Allergies, Medications, Pertinent past history, Last oral intake, and Events leading to the illness or injury.

sclera The white portion of the eye; the tough outer coat that gives protection to the delicate, light-sensitive, inner layer.

sepsis The spread of an infection from its initial site into the bloodstream.

situational awareness Consideration of all aspects of the scene and patient, resulting in your ability to look at the "big picture."

spectrum of acuity The varying severity of illnesses and injuries that the EMT-I will encounter.

standing orders Specific tasks or duties that the EMT-I should perform before contacting medical control; a form of protocol.

stridor A harsh, high-pitched inspiratory sound that is often heard in acute laryngeal (upper airway) obstruction; may sound like crowing and be audible without a stethoscope.

subcutaneous emphysema The presence of air in soft tissues, causing a characteristic crackling sensation on palpation.

Prep Kit continued...

sympathetic nervous system (SNS) The portion of the autonomic nervous system that prepares your body to handle stress; mediated by the hormone adrenaline; referred to as the fight-or-flight response.

syncopal episode Fainting spell or transient loss of consciousness, often caused by an interruption of blood flow to the brain.

tension pneumothorax An accumulation of air or gas in the pleural cavity that progressively increases the pressure in the chest, with potentially fatal results.

trending Determining a pattern of the patient's condition following serial assessments.

triage The process of establishing treatment and transportation priorities according to severity of injury and medical need.

tuberculosis A chronic bacterial disease, caused by *Mycobacterium tuberculosis,* that usually affects the lungs but can also affect other organs such as the brain or kidneys.

turgor Fullness; assessment of this in the skin provides clues to the state of hydration.

two- to three-word dyspnea A severe breathing problem in which a patient can speak only two or three words at a time without pausing to take a breath.

tympany Tympanic resonance on percussion; a clear hollow note like that of a drum.

urticaria Small spots of generalized itching and/or burning that appear as multiple raised areas on the skin; hives.

ventricular tachycardia Rapid heart rhythm in which the electrical impulse begins in the ventricle (instead of the atrium), which may result in inadequate blood flow and eventually deteriorate into cardiac arrest.

vesicular sounds The sounds heard over the normal lung.

wheezing A whistling breath sound caused by air traveling through narrowed air passages within the bronchioles; a sign of lower airway obstruction.

Assessment in Action

It's a cold winter day, and it has been snowing all day. You and your partner are dispatched to an auto collision with several injuries. The roads are beginning to get icy, so you are careful in your approach. The collision is in the middle of a busy street.

One vehicle slid into a utility pole, and there are wires on the ground. You notice that a total of four cars are involved. The passengers of two cars are walking around; there was one person in the car that slid into the utility pole who has been removed from the vehicle by a couple of bystanders; and there are three passengers in the other vehicle. As you get out of your unit, bystanders tell you that the patient who was in the car that hit the pole appeared to be driving erratically and was out of control as he hit the other cars.

1. On the basis of seeing the number of potential patients that you have, what should you do?
   A. Cancel all additional units that may be en route.
   B. Request at least one additional ambulance.
   C. Ask for law enforcement assistance.
   D. Do not begin patient care until additional EMS units arrive.

2. As you approach the patient who was removed from the vehicle that hit the pole, you should:
   A. open the airway using the head tilt–chin lift maneuver.
   B. determine the patient's chief complaint.
   C. open the airway using the jaw-thrust maneuver while maintaining cervical spine stabilization.
   D. conduct a focused assessment.

3. What assessment acronym should be used when trying to learn more about a patient's pain?
   A. DCAP-BTLS
   B. SAMPLE
   C. AVPU
   D. OPQRST-I

4. One patient who was sitting in a car was wearing a seatbelt and is complaining of abdominal pain. You should assess the patient's abdomen during what part of the patient assessment?
   A. Initial assessment
   B. General impression
   C. Detailed physical exam
   D. Focused history and physical exam

5. Which of the following are evaluated during the detailed physical exam?
   A. Airway
   B. Pulse
   C. Heart sounds
   D. Skin color

6. How often should you check vital signs on a patient who is in stable condition?
   A. Every 3 minutes
   B. Every 5 minutes
   C. Every 10 minutes
   D. Every 15 minutes

7. Your ability to respond promptly and proficiently during an emergency even in bad weather and other potential hazards is due to release of what inside the body?
   A. Glucose
   B. Adrenaline
   C. Glycogen
   D. Cholesterol

www.EMSzone.com/EMTI

Assessment in Action

8. What hazards should you be aware of as you approach the scene of the collision?
   - A. Fires
   - B. Power lines
   - C. Inclement weather
   - D. All of the above

9. During the initial assessment, which of the following is evaluated?
   - A. History
   - B. Breathing
   - C. Blood pressure
   - D. Vital signs

10. When conducting a focused history and physical exam, you should:
    - A. make sure you do not expose the patient.
    - B. expose the patient to properly evaluate the patient's condition.
    - C. check the patient's airway.
    - D. perform the exam every 5 minutes.

Points to Ponder

You are providing care for a patient who was struck by a car. The patient is alert and complaining of severe pain to the lower extremities. At the same time the patient's wife arrives on the scene. The patient is very upset and is getting belligerent because of his pain. The patient's wife comes up to you and asks, "What are you going to do for my husband who is in so much pain?"

What should you say?

Issues: Caring Attitude, Professional Appearance and Demeanor, Recognize and Respect the Feelings That Patients May Experience

Communications and Documentation

1999 Objectives

Cognitive

3-5.1 Identify the importance of communications when providing EMS. (p 580)
3-5.2 Identify the role of verbal, written, and electronic communications in the provision of EMS. (p 580)
3-5.3 Describe the phases of communications necessary to complete a typical EMS event. (p 580)
3-5.4 Identify the importance of proper terminology when communicating during an EMS event. (p 580)
3-5.5 Identify the importance of proper verbal communications during an EMS event. (p 593)
3-5.6 List factors that impede effective verbal communications. (p 594)
3-5.7 List factors that enhance verbal communications. (p 594)
3-5.8 Identify the importance of proper written communications during an EMS event. (p 600)
3-5.9 List factors that impede effective written communications. (p 600)
3-5.10 List factors that enhance written communications. (p 600)
3-5.11 Recognize the legal status of written communications related to an EMS event. (p 600)
3-5.12 State the importance of data collection during an EMS event. (p 600)
3-5.13 Identify technology used to collect and exchange patient and/or scene information electronically. (p 580)
3-5.14 Recognize the legal status of patient medical information exchanged electronically. (p 589)
3-5.15 Identify and differentiate among the following communications systems:
   a. Simplex
   b. Multiplex
   c. Duplex
   d. Trunked
   e. Digital communications
   f. Cellular telephone
   g. Facsimile
   h. Computer (p 584, 585)
3-5.16 Identify the components of the local dispatch communications system and describe their function and use. (p 584)
3-5.17 Describe the functions and responsibilities of the Federal Communications Commission. (p 586)
3-5.18 Describe how the Emergency Medical Dispatcher functions as an integral part of the EMS team. (p 586)
3-5.19 List appropriate information to be gathered by the Emergency Medical Dispatcher. (p 580)
3-5.20 Identify the role of Emergency Medical Dispatch in a typical EMS event. (p 580)
3-5.21 Identify the importance of pre-arrival instructions in a typical EMS event. (p 587)
3-5.22 Describe the procedure of verbal communication of patient information to the hospital. (p 588)
3-5.23 Describe information that should be included in patient assessment information verbally reported to medical direction. (p 588)
3-5.24 Diagram a basic model of communications. (p 594)
3-5.25 Organize a list of patient assessment information in the correct order for electronic transmission to medical direction according to the format used locally. (p 588)
3-6.1 Identify the general principles regarding the importance of EMS documentation and ways in which documents are used. (p 600)
3-6.2 Identify and use medical terminology correctly. (p 602)
3-6.3 Recite appropriate and accurate medical abbreviations and acronyms. (p 602)
3-6.4 Record all pertinent administrative information. (p 600)
3-6.5 Explain the role of documentation in agency reimbursement. (p 601)
3-6.6 Analyze the documentation for accuracy and completeness, including spelling. (p 603)
3-6.7 Identify and eliminate extraneous or nonprofessional information. (p 602, 603)
3-6.8 Describe the differences between subjective and objective elements of documentation. (p 602)
3-6.9 Evaluate a finished document for errors and omissions. (p 604)

11

3-6.10 Evaluate a finished document for proper use and spelling of abbreviations and acronyms. (p 604)

3-6.11 Evaluate the confidential nature of an EMS report. (p 602)

3-6.12 Describe the potential consequences of illegible, incomplete, or inaccurate documentation. (p 606)

3-6.13 Describe the special considerations concerning patient refusal of transport. (p 604)

3-6.14 Record pertinent information using a consistent narrative format. (p 604)

3-6.15 Explain how to properly record direct patient or bystander comments. (p 602)

3-6.16 Describe the special considerations concerning mass casualty incident documentation. (p 606)

3-6.17 Apply the principles of documentation to computer charting, as access to this technology becomes available. (p 594)

3-6.18 Identify and record the pertinent, reportable clinical data of each patient interaction. (p 594)

3-6.19 Note and record "pertinent negative" clinical findings. (p 602)

3-6.20 Correct errors and omissions using proper procedures as defined under local protocol. (p 604)

3-6.21 Revise documents, when necessary, using locally-approved procedures. (p 604)

3-6.22 Assume responsibility for self-assessment of all documentation. (p 604)

3-6.23 Demonstrate proper completion of an EMS event record used locally. (p 603)

Affective

3-5.26 Show appreciation for proper terminology when describing a patient or patient condition. (p 603)

3-6.24 Advocate among peers the relevance and importance of properly completed documentation. (p 606)

3-6.25 Resolve the common negative attitudes toward the task of documentation. (p 606)

Psychomotor

3-5.27 Demonstrate the ability to use the local dispatch communications system. (p 584)

3-5.28 Demonstrate the ability to use a radio. (p 580)

3-5.29 Demonstrate the ability to use the biotelemetry equipment used locally. (p 582)

1985 Objectives

1.5-1 Describe the phases of communications necessary to complete a typical EMS event. (p 580)

1.5-2 Name the possible components of an EMS communications system and explain the function of each. (p 580)

1.5-3 Describe maintenance procedures for field radio equipment. (p 591)

1.5-4 Describe the position of the antenna on a portable transmitter/receiver that will deliver maximum coverage. (p 582)

1.5-5 Describe an advantage of a repeater system over a nonrepeater system. (p 582)

1.5-6 Describe basic functions and responsibilities of the Federal Communications Commission. (p 586)

1.5-7 Describe the responsibilities of an EMS dispatcher. (p 586)

1.5-8 Name information items that *must* be gathered from a caller by the dispatcher. (p 586)

*1.5-9 Describe the ten-code used in the local community. (p 588)

1.5-10 Describe three communications techniques that influence the clarity of radio transmissions. (p 590)

1.5-11 Describe three communications techniques that influence the content of radio transmissions. (p 590)

1.5-12 Describe the importance of written medical protocols. (p 591)

1.5-13 Describe two purposes of verbal communication of patient information to the hospital. (p 593)

1.5-14 Describe information that should be included in patient assessment information verbally reported to the physician. (p 594)

1.5-15 Organize a list of patient assessment information in the correct order for radio transmission to the physician according to the format used locally. (p 588)

Communications and Documentation

1.5-16 Name five uses of the written EMS run form. (p 584)

S1.5-17 Demonstrate the proper use of a mobile transmitter/receiver to receive and transmit information. (p 581)

S1.5-18 Demonstrate the proper use of a portable transmitter/receiver to receive and transmit information. (p 581)

S1.5-19 Demonstrate the proper use of a digital encoder. (p 582)

S1.5-20 Demonstrate the proper use of a mobile or portable transmitter in a real or simulated patient situation to:
   a. Organize and transmit patient assessment information, using a standardized format (p 581)

S1.5-21 Properly complete a written EMS form based on a real or simulated patient situation. (p 602)

1.6-55 Describe the interaction between the EMT-I and Medical Command authority in regard to: receiving hospital, family physician on the scene, bystander physician on the scene, orders for patient care, needs of the family, and needs of the patient. (p 588, 593)

1.6-56 Describe the usefulness of a run report. (p 591)

*This is an optional objective.

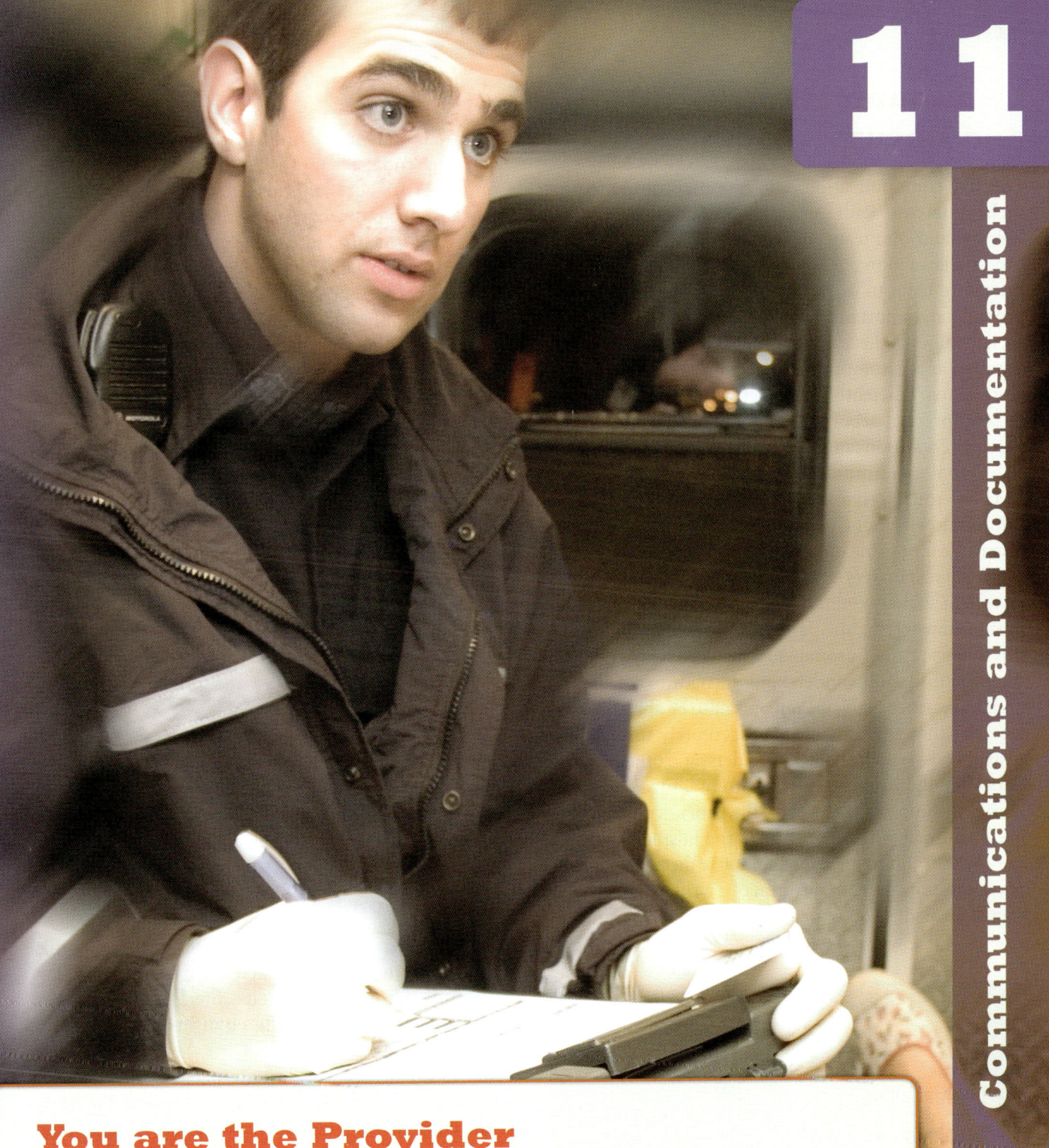

11

Communications and Documentation

You are the Provider

You receive a call for a man who has fallen off a cliff. You are familiar with the area and know it to be remote and heavily wooded. You and your partner assemble all the necessary specialized rescue equipment and proceed to the scene.

This chapter will help demonstrate the important role that communications play in the provision of care to patients in the prehospital setting and will also help you answer the following questions:

1. What aspects of communications should every EMT-I know?
2. Why is it important to know what communication system your service uses?

Communications and Documentation

Effective communication is an essential component of prehospital care. Radio and telephone communications link you and your team with other members of the EMS, fire, and law enforcement communities. This link helps the entire team to work together more effectively and provides an important layer of safety and protection for each member of the team. You must know what your system can and cannot do, and you must be able to use your system efficiently and effectively. You must be able to send precise, accurate reports about the scene, the patient's condition, and the treatment that you provide.

Verbal communications are also a vital skill for EMT-Is. Your verbal skills will enable you to gather information from the patient and bystanders. They will also make it possible for you to effectively coordinate the variety of responders who are often present at the scene. Excellent verbal communications are also an integral part of transferring the patient's care to the nurses and physicians at the hospital. You must possess good listening skills to fully understand the nature of the scene and the patient's problem. You must also be able to organize your thoughts quickly and accurately to verbalize instructions to the patient, bystanders, and other responders. Finally, you must be able to organize and summarize the important aspects of the patient's presentation and treatment when reporting to the hospital staff.

Written communications complete the process. Written communication, in the form of a written patient care report, provides you with an opportunity to communicate the patient's story to others who may participate in the patient's care in the future. Adequate reporting and accurate records ensure the continuity of patient care. Complete patient records also guarantee proper transfer of responsibility, comply with the requirements of health departments and law enforcement agencies, and fulfill your organization's administrative policies. Reporting and record keeping duties are an essential aspect of patient care, although they are performed only after the patient's condition has been stabilized.

This chapter describes the skills you need to be an effective communicator. It begins by identifying the kinds of equipment that are used, along with standard radio operating procedures and protocols. Next, the roles of the Federal Communications Commission (FCC) in EMS are described. The chapter concludes with a discussion of a variety of effective methods of verbal communications and guidelines for appropriate written documentation of patient care.

Communications Systems and Equipment

As an EMT-I, you must be familiar with two-way radio communications and have working knowledge of the mobile and handheld portable radios that are used in your unit. You must also know when to use them and what to say when you are transmitting.

Base Station Radios

The dispatcher usually communicates with field units by transmitting through a fixed radio base station that is controlled from the dispatch center. A base station is any radio hardware containing a transmitter and receiver that is located in a fixed place Figure 11-1. The base station may be used in a single place by an operator speaking into a microphone that is connected directly to the equipment. It also works remotely through telephone lines or by radio from a communications center. Base stations may include dispatch centers, fire stations, ambulance bases, or hospitals.

A two-way radio consists of two units: a transmitter and a receiver. Some base stations may have more than one transmitter and/or more than one receiver. They may also be equipped with one multi-channel transmitter and several-single channel receivers. A channel is an assigned frequency or frequencies that are used to carry voice and/or data communications. Regardless of the number of transmitters and receivers, they are com-

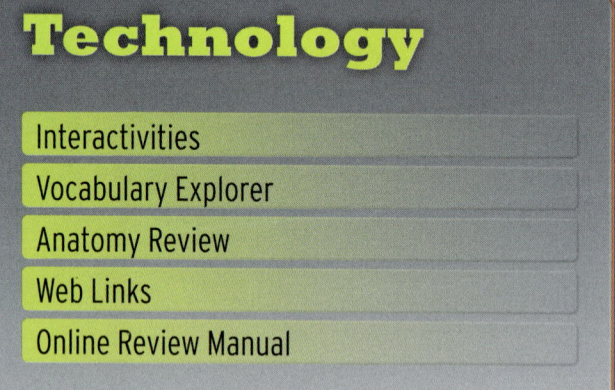

Technology

- Interactivities
- Vocabulary Explorer
- Anatomy Review
- Web Links
- Online Review Manual

www.EMSzone.com/EMTI

monly called base radios or stations. Base stations usually have more power (often 100 watts or more) and higher, more efficient antenna systems than mobile or portable radios. This increased broadcasting range allows the base station operator to communicate with field units and other stations at much greater distances.

The base radio must be physically close to its antenna. Therefore, the actual base station cabinet and hardware are commonly found on the roof of a tall building or at the bottom of an antenna tower. The base station operator may be miles away in a dispatch center or hospital, communicating with the base station radio by dedicated lines or special radio links. A <u>dedicated line</u>, also known as a hot line, is always open or under the control of the individuals at each end. This type of line is immediately "on" as soon as you lift the receiver and cannot be accessed by outside users.

Mobile and Portable Radios

In the ambulance, you will use both mobile and portable radios to communicate with the dispatcher and/or medical control. An ambulance will often have more than one mobile radio, each on a different frequency (Figure 11-2 ▶). One radio may be used to communicate with the dispatcher or other public safety agencies. A second radio is often used for communicating patient information to medical control.

Radios used for EMS communications typically use one of the four major frequency bands: VHF low band, VHF high band, UHF band, or 800 MHz. Radio frequencies are designated by cycles per seconds called *megahertz* (MHz).

The frequencies are assigned by the Federal Communications Commission (FCC), and each frequency has characteristics that make it more useful in various applications.

A mobile radio is installed in a vehicle and usually operates at lower power than a base station. Most <u>VHF (very high frequency)</u> mobile radios operate at 100 watts of power. VHF low band operates between 32 to 50 MHz and offers the greatest distance. Because the transmissions will bend and follow the curvature of the earth, it is excellent for open areas. It does not work well in metropolitan areas due to poor penetration. It can also be interrupted by mountains, weather disturbances, and electrical equipment. VHF high band operates between 150 to 174 MHz. These signals are transmitted in a straight line and are less susceptible to weather and electrical disturbances. It is better in metropolitan areas than the VHF low band but does not transmit well inside concrete buildings or other solid structures.

<u>UHF (ultra-high frequency)</u> mobile radios usually have only 40 watts of power. They operate on a frequency band between 450 to 470 MHz. Like the VHF high band, the UHF radios transmit in a straight line but have excellent penetration. It is the least susceptible to interference and works very well in metropolitan areas.

Radios that operate at 800 MHz are common in EMS systems. This frequency offers excellent penetration of buildings, has minimal interference, and reduced channel noise. Because of this it works quite well in metropolitan areas; 800 MHz also allows for <u>trunking</u>, multiple agencies or systems that can share frequencies. It can also be linked to a computer system to transmit voiceless communications.

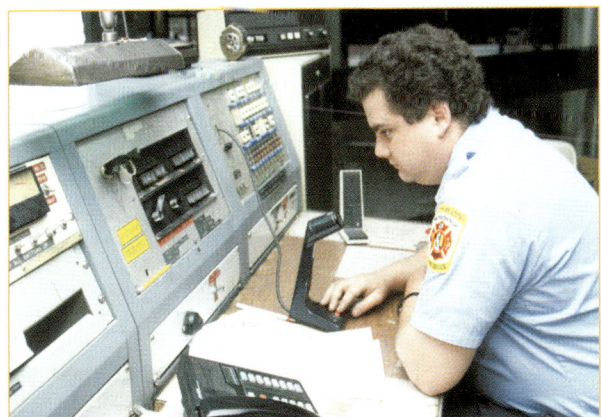

Figure 11-1 A base station consists of radio hardware containing a transmitter and a receiver that is located in a fixed place. Some have more than one transmitter and/or more than one receiver.

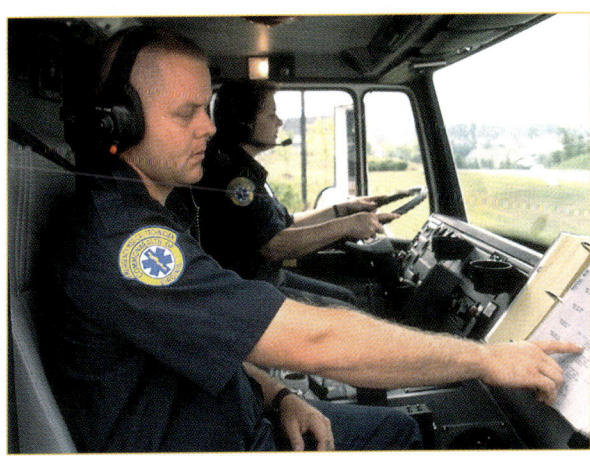

Figure 11-2 Some ambulances have more than one mobile radio to allow communications with mutual aid agencies and other jurisdictions.

Cellular telephones operate on 3 watts of power or less. Mobile antennas are much closer to the ground than base station antennas, so communications from the unit are typically limited to 10 to 15 miles over average terrain. Base station antennas are usually located on high sites to increase the coverage area.

Portable radios are hand-carried or handheld devices that operate at 1 to 5 watts of power Figure 11-3 . Because the entire radio can be held in your hand when in use, the antenna is often no higher than the EMT-I who is using the radio. The transmission range of a portable radio is more limited than that of mobile or base station radios. Portable radios are essential in helping to coordinate EMS activities at the scene of a multiple-casualty incident. They are also helpful when you are away from the ambulance and need to communicate with dispatch, another unit, or medical control.

Repeater-Based Systems

A <u>repeater</u> is a special base station radio that receives messages and signals on one frequency and then automatically retransmits them on a second frequency. Because a repeater is a base station (with a large antenna), it is able to receive lower power signals, such as those from a portable radio, from a long distance away. The signal is then rebroadcast with all the power of the base station Figure 11-4 . EMS systems that use repeaters usually have outstanding systemwide communications and are able to receive the best signal from portable radios. There are also mobile repeaters that may be found in ambulances or placed in various areas around an EMS system area.

Digital Equipment

Although most people think of voice communications when they think of two-way radios, digital signals are also a part of EMS communications. Some EMS systems use telemetry to send electrocardiograms from the unit to the hospital. With <u>telemetry</u>, electronic signals are con-

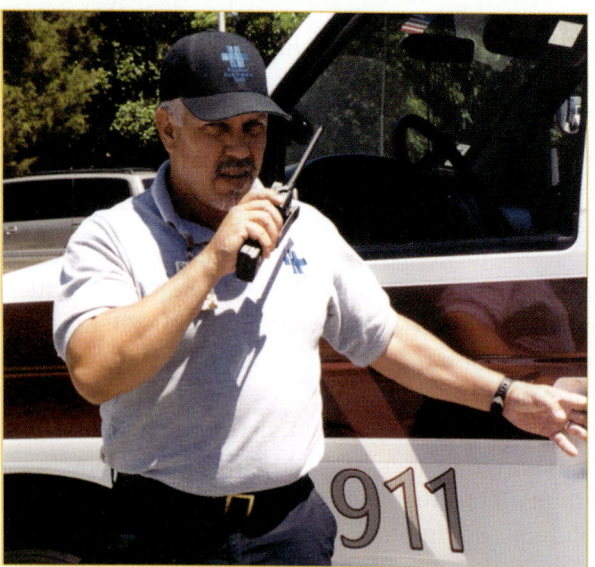

Figure 11-3 A portable radio is essential if you need to communicate with the dispatcher or medical control when you are away from the ambulance.

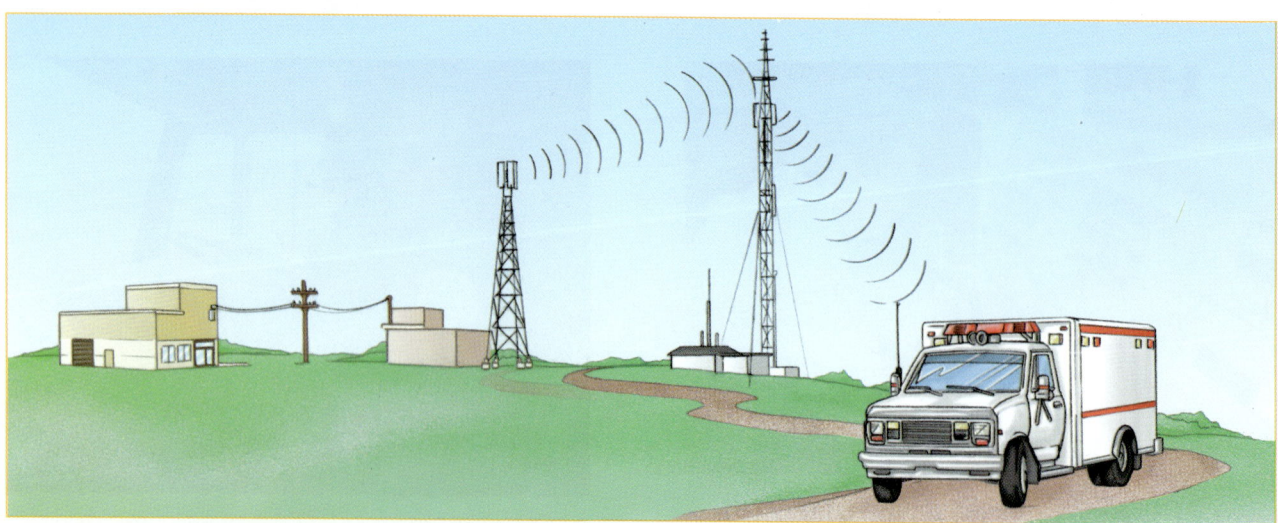

Figure 11-4 A message is sent from the control center by a land line to the transmitter. The radio carrier wave is picked up by the repeater for rebroadcast to outlying units. Return radio traffic is picked up by the repeater and rebroadcast to the control center.

verted into coded, audible signals. These signals can then be transmitted by radio or telephone to a receiver at the hospital with a decoder. The decoder converts the signals back into electronic impulses that can be displayed on a screen or printed. Another example of telemetry is a fax message.

Digital signals are also used in some kinds of paging and tone-alerting systems because they transmit faster than spoken words and allow more choices and flexibility.

Cellular Telephones

<u>Cellular telephones</u> are becoming more common in EMS communications systems (Figure 11-5 ▶). These telephones are simply low-power portable radios that communicate through a series of interconnected repeater stations called "cells" (hence the name "cellular"). Cells are linked by a sophisticated computer system and connected to the telephone network. Cellular telephones are also popular with other public safety agencies, particularly as more cell sites are constructed in rural areas.

Unlike typical two-way mobile communications, which have free access, a cellular system charges fees for its use. Your system can buy portable or mobile radios on the local EMS frequency and use them at no cost. However, buying a cellular telephone is only half of the process of being able to use it. A cellular telephone cannot simply access the telephone network. The user must be assigned a specially coded number that the cellular system's computers will recognize. It is that access and

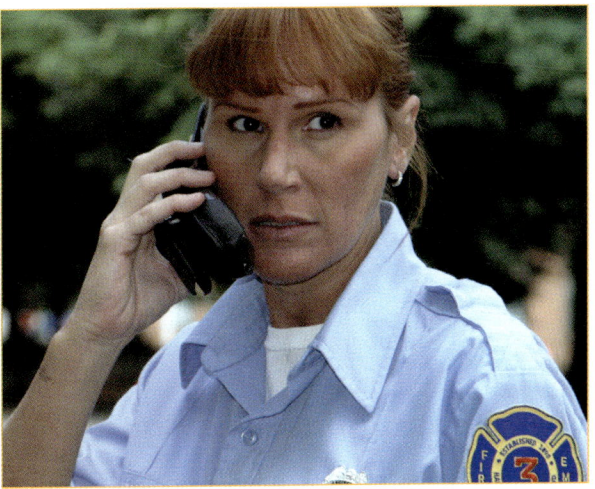

Figure 11-5 Use of cellular phones is becoming more common in EMS communications systems.

the amount of time a user spends on the telephone for which the cellular system charges. However, once you are connected to the network, you can call any other telephone in the world and can send voice, data, and telemetry signals.

Many cellular systems make equipment and air time available to EMS services at little or no cost as a public service. The public is often able to call 9-1-1 or other emergency numbers on a cellular telephone free of charge. However, this easy access may result in overloading and jamming of cellular systems in multiple-casualty and disaster situations.

You are the Provider   Part 2

You and your partner have successfully reached your patient. He is at the bottom of a 30' cliff. You begin your initial assessment.

Initial Assessment	Recording Time: Zero Minutes
Appearance	Severe pain; pale and diaphoretic
Level of consciousness	Moaning and crying out that his chest and right leg hurt
Airway	Open and clear
Breathing	Respiratory rate, increased and labored
Circulation	Skin, pale and clammy; radial pulse, rapid

3. Why are verbal communication skills so vital for EMT-Is?
4. The portable radio you are carrying is essential for what reasons?

As with all repeater-based systems, a cellular telephone is useless if the equipment fails, loses power, or is damaged by severe weather or other circumstances. Like all voice radio communications systems, cellular telephones can be easily overheard on scanners. A <u>scanner</u> is a radio receiver that searches or "scans" across several frequencies until the message is received. Although cellular telephones are more private than most other forms of radio communications, they can still be overheard. Therefore, you must always speak in a professional manner every time you use any form of an EMS communications system.

Other Communications Equipment

Ambulances and other field units are usually equipped with an external public address (PA) system. This system may be a part of the siren or the mobile radio. The intercom between the cab and the patient compartment may also be a part of the mobile radio. These components do not involve radio wave transmission, but you must understand how they work and practice using them before you really need them.

EMS systems may use a variety of two-way radio hardware. Some systems operate VHF equipment in the <u>simplex</u> (push to talk, release to listen) mode. In this mode, radio transmissions can occur in either direction but not simultaneously. When one party transmits, the other can only receive and then wait for the other party to finish before he or she can reply. Other systems conduct <u>duplex</u> (simultaneous talk-listen) communications on UHF frequencies and also use cellular telephones. In the full duplex mode, radios can transmit and receive communications simultaneously on one channel. This is sometimes called "a pair of frequencies." Some base station hospitals provide online medical direction that employs a multiplex system. <u>Multiplex</u> communications can simultaneously transmit two or more different types of information, such as voice and telemetry, in either or both directions over the same frequency. A number of VHF and UHF channels, commonly called <u>MED channels</u>, are reserved exclusively for EMS use. However, hundreds of other commercial, local government, and fire services frequencies are also used for EMS communications.

Some EMS systems rely on dedicated lines (hot lines) as control links for their remotely located base stations and antennas. Other systems are more simply configured and require no off-site control links. No matter what type of equipment is used, all EMS communications systems have some basic limitations. Therefore, you must know what your equipment can and cannot do.

The ability for you to communicate effectively with other units or medical control depends on how well the weaker radio can "talk back." Base and repeater station radios often have much greater power and higher antennas than mobile or portable units do. This increased power affects your communications in two ways. First, their signals are generally heard and understood from a much greater distance than the signal produced from a mobile unit. Second, their signals are received clearly from a much greater distance than is possible with a mobile or portable unit. Remember, when you are at the scene, you may be able to clearly hear the dispatcher or hospital on your radio, but you may be poorly heard or understood when you transmit.

Even small changes in your location can significantly affect the quality of your transmission. Also remember that the location of the antenna is critically important for clear transmission. Commercial aircraft flying at 37,000' can transmit and receive signals over hundreds of miles, yet their radios have only a few watts of power. The "power" comes from their 37,000'-high antenna.

At times, you may be able to communicate with a base station radio but you will not be able to hear or transmit to another mobile unit that is also communicating with that base. Repeater base stations eliminate such problems. They allow two mobile or portable units that cannot reach each other directly to communicate through the repeater, using its greater power and antenna.

The success of communications depends on the efficiency of your equipment. A damaged antenna or microphone often prevents high-quality communications. Check the condition and status of your equipment at the start of each shift, and then correct or report any problems. 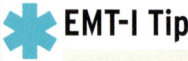 lists advantages and disadvantages of various systems.

> **✳ EMT-I Tips**
>
> You must always speak in a professional manner every time you use the EMS communications system.

Components of the Local Dispatch Communications System and Function

Most areas of the country now offer easy access to emergency help through the use of a universal number. The 9-1-1 and E 9-1-1 systems offer access to any public safety assistance and may be called toll-free from any phone. By dialing 9-1-1, the caller is immediately routed

TABLE 11-1 Advantages and Disadvantages of Various Systems

	Advantage	Disadvantage
Simplex	Allows speaker to get the message out without interruption	Slows process, takes away the ability to discuss the case
Multiplex	Either party can interrupt, facilitates discussion	Each end has a tendency to interrupt the other, voice interferes with data transmission
Duplex	Either party can interrupt, facilitates discussion	Each end has a tendency to interrupt the other
Cellular telephone	Less formal, promotes discussion, can reduce online times, physician can speak directly with the patient	Geography can interfere with signal, cell site may be unavailable, external antenna necessary, costly
Facsimile	Provides earlier notification, produces another piece of medical documentation	Must have access to a fax machine at each end
Computer	Potential to save retrospective data, can document in real-time, sort on many categories, create multiple reporting formats, provide system data quickly	Subject to limitation of the computer and the operator, lose flexibility

to a central dispatcher who takes the information and relays it appropriately. The E 9-1-1 system, or *enhanced 9-1-1*, utilizes computers tied into the phone lines to display caller information on the screen as the dispatcher speaks with the caller. Because the address of the phone is displayed automatically, the dispatcher is able to send help to that location even if the caller is unfamiliar with the address or is disconnected. This is especially helpful with small children who are taught through school, the media, and public safety agencies to call 9-1-1 for help almost from the time they can talk. E 9-1-1 has been instrumental in saving countless lives in instances where the caller was very young.

The emergency medical dispatcher (EMD) is trained to take and route calls, and may go through an emergency medical dispatchers course to learn to use the card system for routing calls and giving pre-arrival instructions. Pre-arrival instructions include explaining to the caller how to perform procedures such as bleeding control and CPR until help arrives. The dispatcher may also provide emotional support for the caller until someone arrives on scene.

You are the Provider — Part 3

Due to the patient's location, you know that this will be a prolonged extrication and will take a while to get him to the top of the cliff. Your continued assessment of your patient reveals the following:

Vital Signs	Recording Time: 2 Minutes After Patient Contact
Respirations	26 breaths/min, adequate depth
Pulse	114 beats/min, irregular
Skin	Pale and diaphoretic
Blood pressure	90/62 mm Hg
Sao_2	95% on 15 L/min O_2 via nonrebreathing mask

5. What is the principal reason for radio communications?
6. What reasons are there for contacting medical direction in this situation?

Radio Communications

All radio operations in the United States, including those used in EMS systems, are regulated by the Federal Communications Commission (FCC). The FCC has jurisdiction over interstate and international telephone and telegraph services and satellite communications—all of which may involve EMS activity.

The FCC has five principal EMS-related responsibilities:

1. **Allocating specific radio frequencies for use by EMS providers.** Modern EMS communications began in 1974. At that time, the FCC assigned 10 MED channels in the 460- to 470-MHz (UHF) band to be used by EMS providers. These UHF channels were added to the several VHF frequencies that were already available for EMS systems. However, these VHF frequencies had to be shared with other "special emergencies" uses, including school buses and veterinarians. In 1993, the FCC created an EMS-only block of frequencies in the 220-MHz portion of the radio spectrum.
2. **Licensing base stations and assigning appropriate radio call signs for those stations.** An FCC license is usually issued for 5 years, after which time it must be renewed. Each FCC license is granted only for a specific operating group. Often, the longitude and latitude (locations) of the antenna and the address of the base station determine the call signs.
3. **Establishing licensing standards and operating specifications for radio equipment used by EMS providers.** Before it can be licensed, each piece of radio equipment must be submitted by its manufacturer to the FCC for type acceptance, based on established operating specifications and regulations.
4. **Establishing limitations for transmitter power output.** The FCC regulates broadcasting power to reduce radio interference between neighboring communications systems.
5. **Monitoring radio operations.** This includes making spot field checks to help ensure compliance with FCC rules and regulations.

The FCC's rules and regulations fill many volumes and are written in technical and legal language. Only a small section (part 90, subpart C) deals with EMS communication issues. You are not responsible for reading these detailed and often confusing documents. For appropriate guidance on technical issues, contact your EMS system supervisor. In fact, many EMS systems look to radio and telephone communications experts for advice on technical issues.

Responding to the Scene

Communications must exist between the party requesting help and the dispatcher, the dispatcher and the EMT-I, the EMT-I and the receiving hospital and/or medical direction physician, and with the receiving hospital personnel on arrival at the hospital. EMS communication systems may operate on several different frequencies and may use different frequency bands. Some EMS systems may even use different radios for different purposes. However, all EMS systems depend on the skill of the dispatcher. The dispatcher receives the first call to 9-1-1 (Figure 11-6). You are part of the team that responds to calls once the dispatcher notifies your unit of an emergency.

The dispatcher has several important responsibilities during the alert and dispatch phase of EMS communications. The dispatcher must do all of the following:

- Properly screen and assign priority to each call (according to predetermined protocols).
- Select and alert the appropriate EMS response unit(s).
- Dispatch and direct EMS response unit(s) to the correct location.
- Coordinate EMS response unit(s) with other public safety services until the incident is over.
- Provide emergency medical instructions, pre-arrival instructions, to the telephone caller so that essential care (eg, CPR) may begin before the EMT-Is arrive (according to predetermined protocols).
- Maintain a record of the incident.

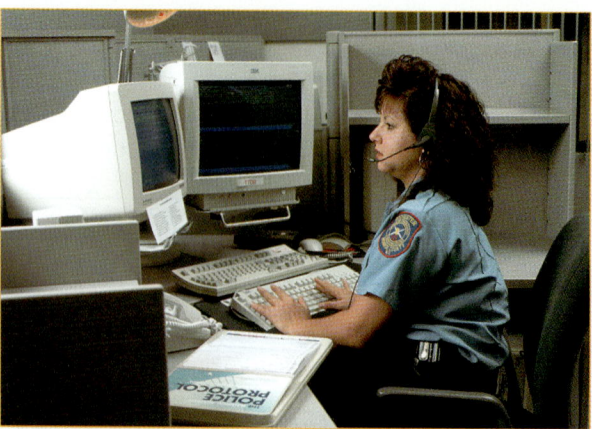

Figure 11-6 The dispatcher receives the first call to 9-1-1.

When the first call to 9-1-1 comes in, the dispatcher must determine its relative importance to begin the appropriate EMS response using emergency medical dispatch protocols. First, the dispatcher must find out the exact location of the patient and the nature and severity of the problem. The dispatcher asks for the caller's telephone number, the patient's age and name, and other information, as directed by local protocol. Next, some description of the scene, such as the number of patients or special environmental hazards, is needed. However, the dispatcher has to rely on the accuracy of the person calling. Callers can be upset, anxious, unable to communicate and even unreliable, which makes the dispatcher's task difficult. Therefore, from time to time the dispatch information may be different from what you actually encounter on the scene.

From this information, the dispatcher will assign the appropriate EMS response unit(s) on the basis of local protocols to determine the level and type of response and the following:

- The dispatcher's perception of the nature and severity of the problem
- The anticipated response time to the scene
- The level of training (first responder, BLS, ALS) of available EMS response unit(s)
- The need for additional EMS units, fire suppression, rescue, a HazMat team, air medical support, or law enforcement

The dispatcher's next step is to alert the appropriate EMS response unit(s) (Figure 11-7). Alerting these units may be done in a variety of ways. The dispatch radio system may be used to contact units that are already in service and monitoring the channel. Dedicated lines (hot lines) between the control center and the EMS station may also be used.

The dispatcher may also page EMS personnel. Pagers are commonly used in EMS operations to alert on-duty and off-duty personnel. Paging involves the use of a coded tone or digital radio signal and a voice or display message that is transmitted to pagers (beepers) or desktop monitor radios. Paging signals may be sent to alert only certain personnel or may be blanket signals that will activate all the pagers in the EMS service. Pagers and monitor radios are convenient because they are usually silent until their specific paging code is received. Alerted personnel contact the dispatcher to confirm the message and receive details of their assignments.

While dispatching the appropriate unit(s), the dispatcher may also be providing pre-arrival instructions to the caller. These may include talking the caller through a procedure for controlling bleeding, performing CPR, or other procedures. Pre-arrival instructions provide immediate assistance for the patient and may be a crucial step for saving a life in a critical situation. In addition to helping the patient, it also helps to provide emotional support for the caller and provides updated information to the responding units.

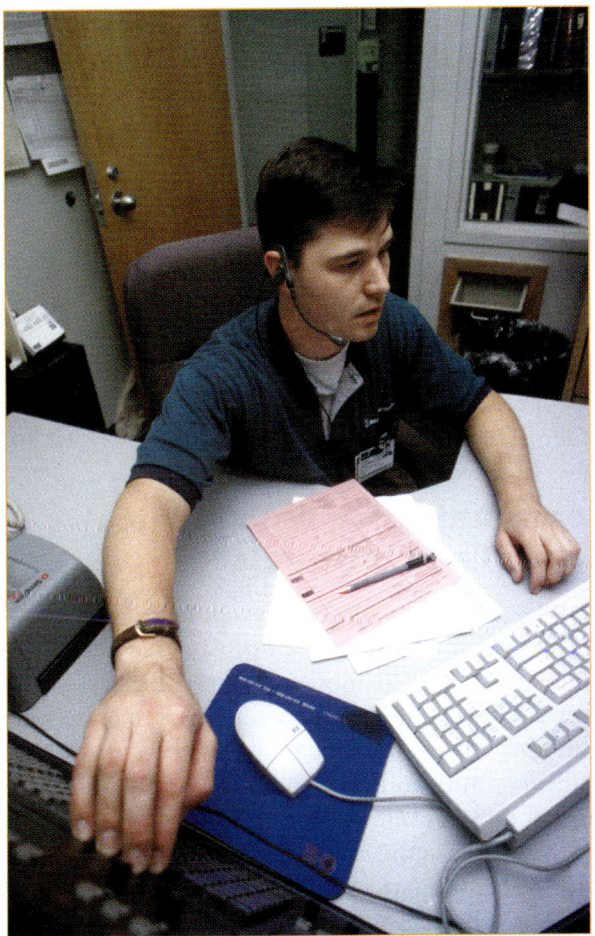

Figure 11-7 You will be directed to a scene by the dispatcher.

EMT-I Tips

Some agencies use a tiered response system. Initially a basic unit responds to a scene and makes the determination of what resources are needed. If a higher level of training is required, the dispatcher then sends the appropriate unit(s). This frees up resources and ensures that advanced units only respond to ALS calls.

Once EMS personnel have been alerted, they must be properly dispatched and sent to the incident. Every EMS system should use a standard dispatching procedure. The dispatcher will give the responding unit(s) the following information as available:

- The nature and severity of the injury, illness, or incident
- The exact location of the incident
- The number of patients
- Responses by other public safety agencies
- Special directions or advisories, such as adverse road or traffic conditions or severe weather reports
- The time at which the unit or units are dispatched

Your unit must confirm to the dispatcher that you have received the information and that you are en route to the scene. Local protocol will dictate whether it is the job of the dispatcher or your unit to notify other public safety agencies that you are responding to an emergency. In some areas, the emergency department is also notified whenever an ambulance responds to an emergency.

You should report any problems during your response to the dispatcher. You should also inform the dispatcher that you have arrived at the scene. The arrival report to the dispatcher should include any obvious details that you see during scene size-up. For example, you might say, "Dispatcher, Medic One is on scene at Main Street with a two-vehicle collision."

All radio communications during dispatch, as well as other phases of operations, must be brief and easily understood. Although speaking in plain English is best, many areas find that 10 codes are shorter and simpler for routine communications. The development and use of such codes require strict discipline. When used improperly or not understood, codes create confusion rather than clarity.

Communicating With Medical Control and Hospitals

The principal reason for radio communication is to facilitate communication between you and medical control (and the hospital). Medical control may be located at the receiving hospital, another facility, or sometimes even in another city or state. You must, however, consult with medical control to notify the hospital of an incoming patient, to request advice or orders from medical control, or to advise the hospital of special situations.

It is important to plan and organize your radio communication before you push the transmit button. Remember, a concise, well-organized report demonstrates your competence and professionalism in the eyes of all who hear your report. Well-organized radio communications with the hospital will engender confidence in the receiving facility's physicians and nurses, as well as others who are listening. In addition, the patient and family will be comforted by your organization and ability to communicate clearly. A well-delivered radio report puts you in control of the information, which is where you need to be.

Hospital notification is the most common type of communication between you and the hospital. The purpose of these calls is to notify the receiving facility of the patient's complaint and condition Figure 11-8. On the basis of this information, the hospital is able to prepare staff and equipment appropriately to receive the patient.

Giving the Patient Report

The patient report should follow a standard format established by your EMS system. The patient report commonly includes the following eight elements:

1. **The receiving hospital, your unit identification, level of certification, and status of transport.** Example: "Columbus Community Hospital, this is Med 2, Paramedic Smythe and EMT-I Jennings, en route to you emergency status."
2. **The patient's age, gender, and approximate weight (if needed for drug orders).** Example:

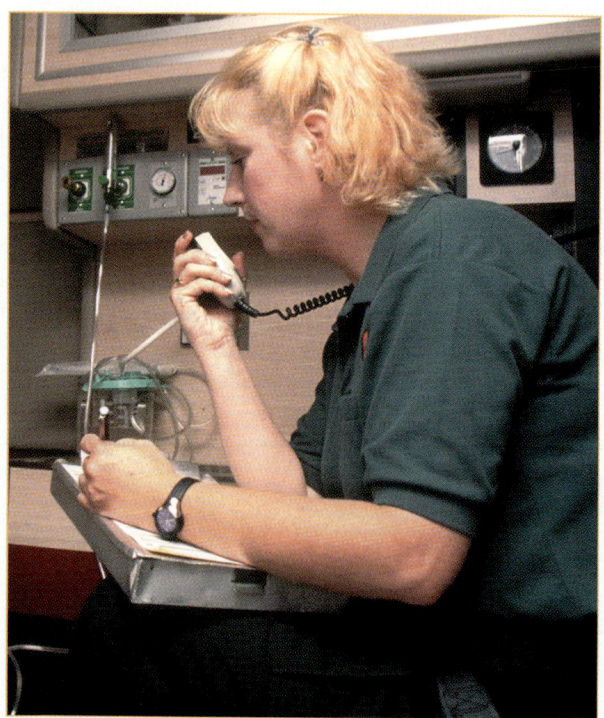

Figure 11-8 Giving the patient report should be done in an objective, accurate, professional manner.

"We are en route to your facility with a 15-year-old male, approximately 50 kg." The patient's name should not be given over the radio because it may be overheard. This is a violation of the patient's confidentiality.

3. **Description of the scene.** Example: "Patient was playing on a neighbor's trampoline when he jumped off the one-story garage onto the trampoline. From there he bounced off and landed on his head and shoulders."
4. **The patient's chief complaint or your perception of the problem and its severity and associated symptoms.** Example: "The patient denies any loss of consciousness, but stated he had the wind knocked out of him. Complains of numbness and tingling in all four extremities.
5. **A brief, pertinent history of the patient's present illness or injury.** Example: "The patient has a history of epilepsy and takes Dilantin. He says he takes it daily, but has forgotten to take it today."
6. **A brief report of physical findings.** This report should include level of consciousness, the patient's general appearance, pertinent abnormalities noted, and vital signs. Example: "The patient is alert and oriented, pale, cool, and diaphoretic. Complains of numbness and tingling in all four extremities. B/P is 78/32, pulse is 116, and respirations of 20."
7. **A brief summary of the care given and any patient response.** Example: "We have immobilized him to the spine board, PMS (Pulse, Motor, and Sensory) in the extremities are intact. We initiated an IV of normal saline and patient is showing a normal sinus rhythm on the cardiac monitor."
8. **Any other pertinent information and the estimated time of arrival.** Example: "Patient physician is Kip Anderson. ETA is four minutes."

Be sure that you report all patient information in an objective, accurate, and professional manner. People with scanners are listening. You could be successfully sued for slander if you describe a patient in a way that injures his or her reputation.

The Role of Medical Control

The delivery of EMS involves an impressive array of assessments, stabilization, and treatments. Intermediate and advanced EMTs may initiate medication therapy based on the patient's presenting signs. For logical, ethical, and legal reasons, the delivery of such sophisticated care must be done in association with physicians. For this reason, every EMS system needs input and involvement from physicians. One or more physicians, including your system or department medical director, will provide medical direction (medical control) for your EMS system. Medical control is either off-line (indirect) or online (direct), as authorized by the medical director. Medical control guides the treatment of patients in the system through protocols, direct orders and advice, and post-call review.

Depending on how the protocols are written, you may need to call medical control for direct orders (permission) to administer certain treatments, to determine the transport destination of patients, or to be allowed to stop treatment and/or transport of a patient. In these cases, the radio or cellular phone provides a vital link between you and the expertise available through the base physician.

To maintain this link 24 hours a day, 7 days a week, medical control must be readily available on the radio at the hospital or on a mobile or portable unit when you call (Figure 11-9 ▼). In most areas, medical control is provided by the physicians who work at the receiving hospital. However, many variations have developed across the country. For example, some EMS units receive medical direction from one hospital even though they are taking the patient to another hospital. In other areas, medical direction may come from a free-standing center or even from an individual physician. Regardless of your system's design, your link to medical control is vital to maintain the high quality of care that your patient requires and deserves.

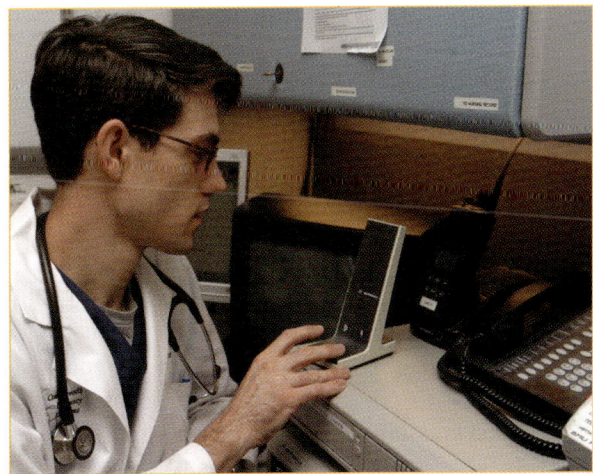

Figure 11-9 Medical control must be readily available on the radio at the hospital.

> **In the Field**
>
> When contacting medical control for orders, always "echo" the orders back to the online physician to avoid misunderstandings. If an order is not clear or seems inappropriate, ask for clarification, repeating vital signs and other information as needed.

Calling Medical Control

You can use the radio in your unit or a portable radio to call medical control. A cellular telephone can also be used. Regardless of the type of communication, you should use a channel that is relatively free of other radio traffic and interference. There are a number of ways to control access on ambulance-to-hospital channels. In some EMS systems, the dispatcher monitors and assigns appropriate, clear medical control channels. Other EMS systems rely on special communications operations, such as a CMED (Centralized Medical Emergency Dispatch) or resource coordination centers, to monitor and allocate the medical control channels.

Because of the large number of EMS calls to medical control, your radio report must be well organized, precise, and contain only important information. In addition, because you need specific directions on patient care, the information that you provide to medical control must be accurate. Remember, the physician on the other end bases his or her instructions on the information that you provide.

You should never use codes when communicating with medical control unless you are directed by local protocol to do so. You should use proper medical terminology when giving your report. Never assume that medical control will know what a "10-50" or "Signal 70" means. Most medical control systems handle many different EMS agencies and will most likely not know your unit's special codes or signals.

To ensure complete understanding, once you receive an order from medical control, you must repeat the order back, word for word, and then receive confirmation. Whether the physician gives an order for medication or a specific treatment or denies a request for a particular treatment, you must repeat the order back word for word. This "echo" exchange helps to eliminate confusion and the possibility of poor patient care. Orders that are unclear or seem inappropriate or incorrect should be questioned. Do not blindly follow an order that does not make sense to you. The physician may have misunderstood or may have missed part of your report. In that case, he or she may not be able to respond appropriately to the patient's needs.

Information About Special Situations

Depending on your system's procedures, you may initiate communication with one or more hospitals to advise them of an extraordinary call or situation. For instance, a small rural hospital may be better able to respond to multiple victims of a highway crash if it is notified when the ambulance is first responding. At the other extreme, an entire hospital system must be notified of any disaster, such as a plane or train crash, as early as possible

You are the Provider   Part 4

Using rope rescue techniques, you are preparing to send your patient up the side of the cliff in the Stokes basket. You contacted medical control earlier to advise them of your situation. Your patient's condition is unchanged and you are preparing to call in a report.

Reassessment	Recording Time: 5 Minutes After Patient Contact
Respirations	36 breaths/min, shallow
Pulse	114 beats/min, irregular
Skin	Pale and diaphoretic
Blood pressure	90/62 mm Hg
Sao_2	92% on 15 L/min o_2 via nonrebreathing mask

7. What elements should be included in your verbal patient report to the receiving facility?

TABLE 11-2	Phases of Communications Necessary to Complete a Typical EMS Event

1. Occurrence
2. Detection
3. Notification and response
   - Pre-arrival instructions
4. Treatment and preparation for transport
   - Communication on scene among other providers and with patient
5. Preparation for next event

to enable activation of its staff call-in system. These special situations might also include HazMat situations, rescues in progress, multiple-casualty incidents, or any other situation that might require special preparation on the part of the hospital. In some areas, mutual aid frequencies may be designated in multiple-casualty incidents so that responding agencies can communicate with one another on a common frequency.

When notifying the hospital(s) of any special situations, keep the following in mind: The earlier the notification, the better. You should ask to speak to the charge nurse or physician in charge, as he or she is best able to mobilize the resources necessary to respond. Also, whenever possible, provide an estimate of the number of individuals who may be transported to the facility. Be sure to identify any conditions the patient(s) might have that require special needs, such as burns or hazardous materials exposure, to assist the hospital in preparation. In many cases, hospital notification is part of a larger disaster or HazMat plan. Follow the plan for your system.

The phases of communication in a typical EMS event are listed in Table 11-2.

Standard Procedures and Protocols

You must use your radio communications system effectively from the time you acknowledge a call until you complete your run. Standard radio operating procedures are designed to reduce the number of misunderstood messages, to keep transmissions brief, and to develop effective radio discipline. Standard radio communications protocols help both you and the dispatcher to communicate properly Table 11-3. Protocols should include guidelines specifying a preferred format for transmitting messages, definitions of key words and phrases, and procedures for troubleshooting common radio communications problems.

The "call up" from one unit to another begins by identifying the called unit first, followed by the unit calling, such as "Dispatch, this is Medic One." This exchange alerts the dispatcher to listen for both the identity of the unit calling and the message.

Reporting Requirements

Proper use of the EMS communications system will help you to do your job more effectively. From acknowledgment of the call until you are cleared from the medical emergency, you will use radio communications. You must report in to dispatch at least six times during your run:

1. **To acknowledge the dispatch information** and to confirm that you are responding to the scene.
2. **To announce your arrival at the scene.**
3. **To announce that you are leaving** the scene and are en route to the receiving hospital. (At this point, you typically should also state the number of patients being transported, your estimated arrival time at the hospital, and the run status.)
4. **To announce your arrival at the hospital** or facility.
5. **To announce that you are clear of the incident** or hospital and available for another assignment.
6. **To announce your arrival back at quarters** or other off-the-air location.

While en route to and from the scene, you should report to the dispatcher any special hazards or road conditions that might affect other responding units. Report any unusual delay, such as roadblocks, traffic, or construction. Once you are at the scene, you may request additional EMS or other public safety assistance and then help to coordinate their response.

During transport, you must periodically reassess the patient's overall condition, vital signs, and response to care provided. You should immediately report any significant changes in the patient's condition, especially if the patient seems worse. Medical control can then give new orders and prepare to receive the patient.

Maintenance of Radio Equipment

Like all other EMS equipment, radio equipment must be serviced by properly trained and equipped personnel. Remember that the radio is your lifeline to other public safety agencies (who function to protect you), as well as medical control, and it must perform under emergency conditions. Radio equipment that is operating properly should be serviced at least once a year. Any equipment that is not working properly should be immediately removed from service and sent for repair.

TABLE 11-3 Guidelines for Effective Radio Communication

1. **Monitor the channel before transmitting** to avoid interfering with other radio traffic.
2. **Plan your message before pushing the transmit button.** This will keep your transmissions brief and precise. You should use a standard format for your transmissions.
3. **Press the push-to-talk (PTT) button on the radio**, then wait for 1 second before starting your message. Otherwise, you might cut off the first part of your message before the transmitter is working at full power.
4. **Hold the microphone 2" to 3" from your mouth.** Speak clearly, but never shout into the microphone. Speak at a moderate, understandable rate, preferably in a clear, even voice.
5. **Identify the person or unit you are calling** first, then identify your unit as the sender. You will rarely work alone, so say "we" instead of "I" when describing yourself.
6. **Acknowledge a transmission as soon as you can** by saying, "Go ahead," or whatever is commonly used in your area. You should say, "Clear, over and out," or whatever is commonly used in your area, when you are finished. If you cannot take a long message, simply say, "Stand by" until you are ready.
7. **Use plain English.** Avoid meaningless phrases ("Be advised"), slang, or complex codes. Avoid words that are difficult to hear, such as "yes" and "no." Use "affirmative" and "negative."
8. **Keep your message brief.** If your message takes more than 30 seconds to send, pause after 30 seconds and say, "Are you clear?" The other party can then ask for clarification if needed. Also, someone else with emergency traffic can break through if necessary.
9. **Avoid voicing negative emotions**, such as anger or irritation, when transmitting. Courtesy is assumed, making it unnecessary to say "please" or "thank you," which wastes air time. Listen to other communications in your system to get a good idea of the common phrases and their uses.
10. **When transmitting a number with two or more digits, say the entire number first** and then each digit separately. For example, say, "sixty-seven," followed by "six-seven."
11. **Do not use profanity on the radio.** It is a violation of FCC rules and can result in substantial fines and even loss of your organization's radio license.
12. **Use EMS frequencies for EMS communications.** Do not use these frequencies for any other type of communications.
13. **Reduce background noise as much as possible.** Move away from wind, noisy motors, or tools. Close the window if you are in a moving ambulance. When possible, shut off the siren during radio transmissions if you are in transit.
14. **Be sure other radios on the same frequency are turned down** to avoid feedback.

Sometimes, radio equipment will stop working during a run. Your EMS system must have several backup plans and options. The goal of a backup plan is to make sure that you can maintain contact when the usual procedures do not work. There are quite a few options.

The simplest backup plan relies on written standing orders. <u>Standing orders</u> are written documents that have been signed by the EMS system's medical director. These orders outline specific directions, permissions, and sometimes prohibitions regarding patient care. By their very nature, standing orders do not require prior communication with medical control. When properly followed, standing orders or formal protocols have the same authority and legal status as orders given over the radio. They exist to one extent or another in every EMS system and can be applied to all levels of EMS providers.

Maintaining radio equipment will also help to ensure efficient, effective communication. If possible, do not subject radio equipment to harsh environments. Dusty conditions, damp or wet conditions, and even dropping radio equipment are among the most frequent causes of equipment failure. Check your equipment at the beginning of each shift. When malfunctioning, radio equipment must be referred to a licensed technician.

Frequent cleaning of radio equipment will improve its appearance as well as life expectancy. Use only a slightly damp rag with very mild detergent (no cleaning solvents on the exterior surfaces of radio equipment).

Properly used, rechargeable batteries in portable equipment (including monitor/defibrillators) will maximize life and power output. Certain rechargeable batteries must be properly "exercised" for best results. Be sure to familiarize yourself with the manufacturer's instructions for each piece of equipment you're using.

Verbal Communications

As an EMT-I, you must master many communication skills, including radio operations and written communications. Verbal communications with the patient, the family, and the rest of the health care team are an essential part of high-quality patient care. And as an EMT-I, you must be able to find out what the patient needs and then tell others. The EMT-I functions as one part of a team. You must effectively communicate patient information and scene assessment to medical direction. Never forget that you are the vital link between the patient and the remainder of the health care team.

Communicating With Other Health Care Professionals

EMS is the first step in what is often a long and involved series of treatment phases. Effective communication between the EMT-I and health care professionals in the receiving facility is an essential cornerstone of efficient, effective, and appropriate patient care.

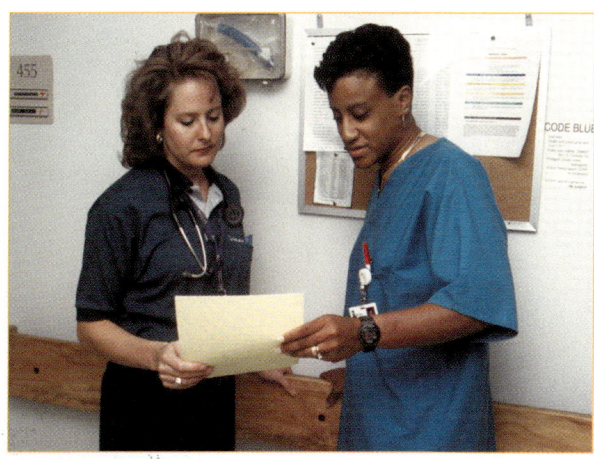

Figure 11-10 Once you arrive at the hospital, a staff member will take responsibility for the patient from you.

Your reporting responsibilities do not end when you arrive at the hospital. In fact, they have just begun. The transfer of care officially occurs during your oral report at the hospital, not during your radio report en route. Once you arrive at the hospital, a hospital staff member will take responsibility of the patient from you (Figure 11-10 ▲). Depending on the hospital and the condition of the patient, the training of the person who takes over the care of the patient varies. However, you may transfer the care of your patient only to someone with at least your level of training. Once a hospital staff member is ready to take responsibility for the patient, you must provide that person with a formal oral report of the patient's condition (Figure 11-11 ▶).

You are the Provider — Part 5

Your rescue team has successfully extricated the patient and he is now on the top of the cliff. You load him into the back of your ambulance and, following standing orders, you continue to care for your patient. Prior to leaving for the hospital, your reassessment reveals the following:

Reassessment	Recording Time: 10 Minutes After Patient Contact
Respirations	24 breaths/min, adequate depth
Pulse	120 beats/min, irregular
Skin	Remains pale and diaphoretic
Blood pressure	90/62 mm Hg
Sao_2	97% on 15 L/min o_2 via nonrebreathing mask

8. What are standing orders and what is their purpose?

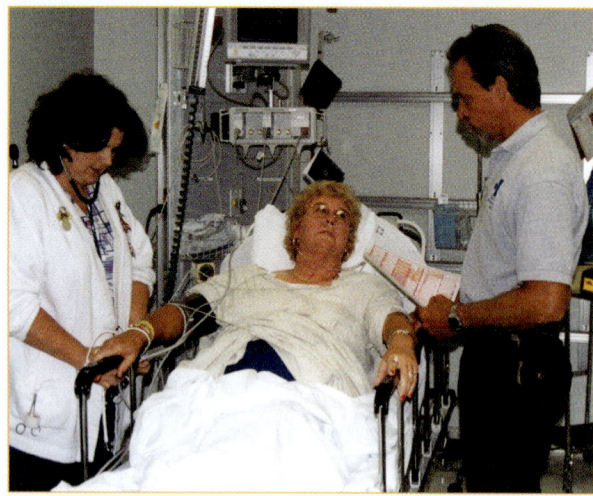

Figure 11-11 Providing a detailed report for hospital personnel will ensure quality continuity of care for the patient.

Giving a report is a longstanding and well-documented part of transferring the patient's care from one provider to another. Your oral report is usually given at the same time that the staff member is doing something for the patient. For example, a nurse or physician may be looking at the patient, beginning assessment, or helping you to move the patient from the stretcher to an examination table. Therefore, you must report important information in a complete, precise way. The following six components must be included in the oral report:

1. **The patient's name (if you know it) and the chief complaint, nature of illness, or mechanism of injury.** Example: "This is Kory Michaels. He had been jumping on a trampoline when he decided to try jumping off the one-story garage onto the trampoline. He bounced off the trampoline and landed on his head and shoulders. He denies losing consciousness."
2. **A summary of the information** that you gave in your radio report. Example: "He has a history of epilepsy and takes Dilantin, but forgot to take it today."
3. **Any important history** that was not given already. Example: "Kory is complaining of numbness and tingling in all four extremities, but has intact pulse, motor, and sensory function to his hands and feet. Pupils are equal and reactive."
4. **The patient's response to treatment** given en route. It is especially important to report any changes in the patient or the treatment provided since your radio report. Example: "We started oxygen by nonrebreathing face mask at 15 L/min. This seems to have helped his numbness and slowed his heart rate from 116 to 104."
5. **The vital signs assessed** during transport and after the radio report. Example: "His vitals prior to transport were blood pressure 78/32, pulse 116, respirations 20. Currently, he has a B/P of 100/62, heart rate of 104, and respirations of 18."
6. **Any other information** that you may have gathered that was not important enough to report sooner. Information that was gathered during transport, any patient medications you have brought with you, and any other details about the patient that was provided by family members or friends may be included. Example: "Kory's father was contacted and should be meeting us here at the hospital soon."

Communicating With Patients

Your communication skills will be put to the test when you communicate with patients and/or families in emergency situations. Remember that someone who is sick or injured is scared and might not understand what you are doing and saying. Therefore, your gestures, body movements, and attitude toward the patient are critically important in gaining the trust of both patient and family. These Ten Golden Rules will help you to calm and reassure your patients:

1. **Make and keep eye contact** with your patient at all times Figure 11-12 ▶. Give the patient your undivided attention. This will let the patient know that he or she is your top priority. Look the patient straight in the eye to establish rapport. Establishing <u>rapport</u> is building a trusting relationship with your patient. This will make the job of caring for the patient much easier for both you and the patient.
2. **Use the patient's proper name** when you know it. Ask the patient what he or she wishes to be called. Never use terms such as "Honey" or "Dear." Avoid using a patient's first name unless the patient is a child or the patient asks you to use his or her first name. Rather, use a courtesy title, such as "Mr. Peters," "Mrs. Smith," or "Ms. Butler." If you do not know the patient's name, refer to him or her as "sir" or "ma'am."
3. **Tell the patient the truth.** Even if you have to say something very unpleasant, telling the truth is better than lying. Lying will destroy the patient's trust in you and decrease your own

confidence. You might not always tell the patient everything, but if the patient or a family member asks a specific question, you should answer truthfully. A direct question deserves a direct answer. If you do not know the answer to the patient's question, say so. For example, a patient may ask, "Am I having a heart attack?" "I don't know" is an adequate answer.

4. **Use language that the patient can understand.** Do not talk up or down to the patient in any way. Avoid technical medical terms that the patient might not understand. For example, ask the patient whether he or she has a history of "heart problems." This will usually result in more accurate information than if you ask about "previous episodes of myocardial infarction" or a "history of cardiomyopathy."

5. **Be careful of what you say about the patient to others.** A patient might hear only part of what is said. As a result, the patient might seriously misinterpret (and remember for a long time) what was said. Therefore, assume that the patient can hear every word you say, even if you are speaking to others and even if the patient appears to be unconscious or unresponsive.

6. **Be aware of your body language** Figure 11-13 . Nonverbal communication is extremely important in dealing with patients. In stressful situations, patients may misinterpret your gestures and movements. Be particularly careful not to appear threatening. Instead, position yourself at a lower level than the patient when practical. Remember that you should always, always conduct yourself in a calm, professional manner.

7. **Always speak slowly, clearly, and distinctly.** Pay close attention to your tone of voice.

8. **If the patient is hearing impaired, speak clearly,** and face the person so that he or she can read your lips. Do not shout at a person who is hearing

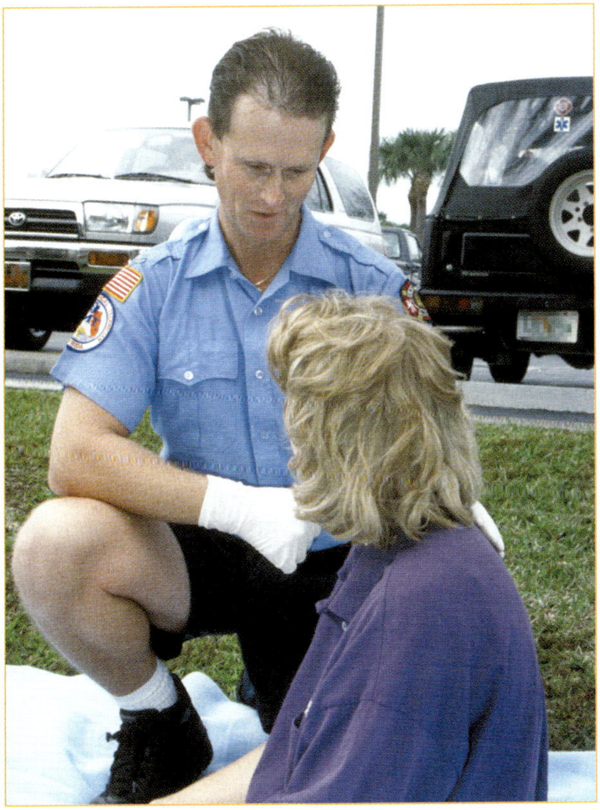

Figure 11-12 Maintaining eye contact with your patient builds trust and lets the patient know that he or she is your first priority.

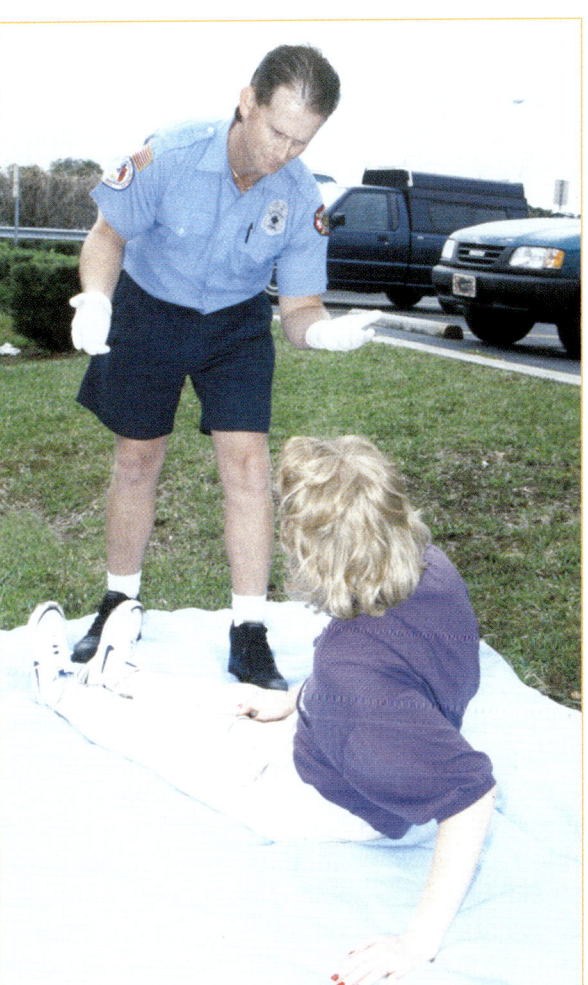

Figure 11-13 Watch your body language, as patients may misinterpret your gestures, movements, and stance.

impaired. Shouting will not make it any easier for the patient to understand you. Instead, it may frighten the patient and make it even more difficult for the patient to understand you. Never assume that an elderly patient is hearing impaired or otherwise unable to understand you. Also, never use baby talk with elderly patients or with anyone but babies.

9. **Allow time for the patient to answer** or respond to your questions. Do not rush a patient unless there is immediate danger. Sick and injured people may not be thinking clearly and may need time to answer even simple questions. This is especially true in treating elderly patients.

10. **Act and speak in a calm, confident manner** while caring for the patient. Make sure that you attend to the patient's needs. Try to make the patient physically comfortable and relaxed. Find out whether the patient is more comfortable sitting or lying down. Is the patient cold or hot? Does the patient want a friend or relative nearby?

Patients literally place their lives in your hands. They deserve to know that you can provide medical care and that you are concerned about their well-being.

Communicating With Older Patients

Approximately 34% of calls (3.4 million responses) for emergency medical services involve patients older than 60 years. It is important for prehospital providers to have a solid understanding of geriatric patients to be successful in providing emergency medical care.

As an EMS provider, when you step onto a scene to care for an older patient, you are being asked to take control. People called you because they needed help. Whether that call was for emergent or nonemergent care, they called you to do something they could not do themselves. What you say and how you say it will have an impact on the patient's perception of the call. You should present yourself as competent, confident, and concerned. You must take charge of the situation, but do so with compassion. You are there to listen, then act on what you learn. Don't limit your assessment to the obvious problem. Oftentimes older patients who express that they are not well or who are overly concerned about their health or general condition are at risk for a serious decline in their physical, emotional, or psychological state. **Table 11-4** provides guidelines for interviewing an older patient.

TABLE 11-4 | **Interviewing an Older Patient**

In general, when interviewing the older patient, the following techniques should be employed:

- Identify yourself. Do not assume the older patient knows who you are.
- Be aware of how you present yourself. Frustration and impatience can be portrayed through body language.
- Look directly at the patient.
- Speak slowly and distinctly.
- Explain what you are going to do before you do it. Use simple terms to explain the use of medical equipment and procedures, avoiding medical jargon or slang.
- Listen to the answer the patient gives you.
- Show the patient respect. Refer to the patient as Mr., Mrs., or Miss.
- Do not talk about the patient in front of him or her; to do so gives the impression that the patient has no choice in his or her medical care. This is easy to forget when the patient has impaired cognitive (thought) processes or has difficulty communicating.
- Be patient!

Most older people think clearly, can give you a clear medical history, and can answer your questions **Figure 11-14**. Do not assume that an older patient is senile or confused. Remember, though, that communicating with some older patients is extremely difficult. Some may be hostile, irritable, and/or confused. Do not assume this is normal behavior for an older patient. These signs may be caused by a lack of oxygen (hypoxia), brain injury including a cerebrovascular accident (CVA), unintentional drug overdose, or even hypovolemia. Never attribute altered mental status simply to "old age." Others may have difficulty hearing or seeing you. You need great patience and compassion when you are called upon to care for such a patient. Think of the patient as someone's grandmother or grandfather—or even as yourself when you reach that age.

Approach an older patient slowly and calmly. Allow plenty of time for the patient to respond to your questions. Watch for signs of confusion, anxiety, or impaired hearing or vision. The patient should feel confident that you are in charge and that everything possible is being done for him or her.

Older patients often do not feel much pain. An older person who has fallen or been injured may report no pain. In addition, older patients might not be fully aware of important changes in other body systems. As a result, be especially vigilant for objective changes—no matter how subtle—in their condition. Even minor changes in breathing or mental state may signal major problems.

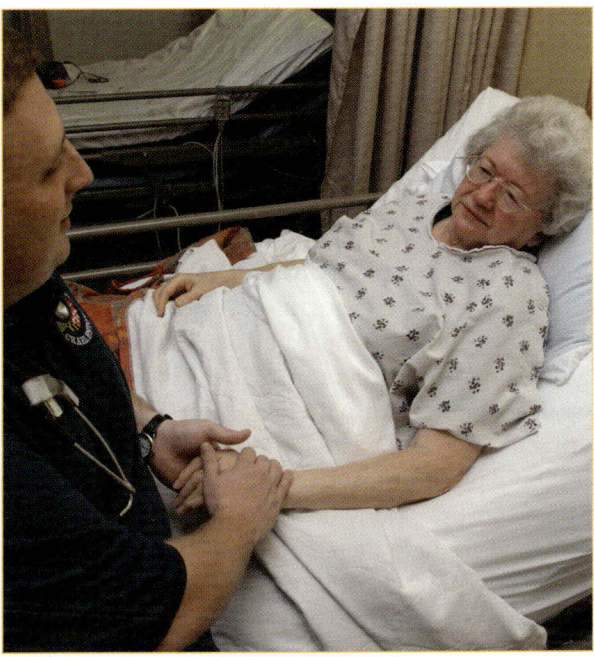

Figure 11-14 You need a great deal of compassion and patience when caring for older patients, but do not assume that the patient is senile or confused.

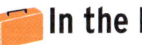

> **In the Field**
>
> Patients deserve to know that you can provide medical care and that you are concerned about their well-being.

to get any hearing aids, glasses, or dentures packed before departure; it will make the patient's hospital stay much more pleasant. You should document on the pre-hospital care report that these items accompanied the patient to the hospital and were given to a specific staff person in the emergency department.

Communicating With Children

Everyone who is thrust into an emergency situation becomes frightened to some degree. However, fear is probably most severe and most obvious in children. Children may be frightened by your uniform, the ambulance, and the number of people who have suddenly gathered around. Even a child who says little may be very much aware of all that is going on.

Familiar objects and faces will help to reduce this fright. Let a child keep a favorite toy, doll, or security blanket to give the child some sense of control and comfort. Having a family member or friend nearby is also helpful. It is often helpful to let the parent or an adult friend hold the child during your evaluation and treatment if it is not contraindicated due to the child's condition. Make sure that this person will not upset the child. Sometimes adult family members are not helpful

Remember to attend to an older patient's family members and friends. Seeing a loved one taken away in an ambulance can be a particularly frightening experience. Take a few minutes to explain to an older patient's spouse or family what is being done and why such action is being taken. When possible (which is more often than you'd think), give the patient some time to pack a few personal items before leaving for the hospital. Be sure

You are the Provider   Part 6

You have arrived at the closest appropriate hospital and are preparing to turn over care of your patient to the nurse in the Emergency Department.

Reassessment	Recording Time: 14 Minutes After Patient Contact
Respirations	22 breaths/min, adequate depth
Pulse	110 beats/min, irregular
Skin	Remains pale and diaphoretic
Blood pressure	100/62 mm Hg
Sao_2	98% on 15 L/min o_2 via nonrebreathing mask

9. What components should be included in your oral report to the Emergency Department nurse?

because they become too upset by what has happened. An overly anxious parent or relative can make things worse. Be careful about selecting the proper adult for this role.

Children can easily see through lies or deceptions, so you must always be honest with them. Make sure that you explain to the child over and over again what and why certain things are happening. If treatment is going to hurt, such as applying a splint, tell the child only when you are ready to apply the splint. You do not need to announce 10 minutes in advance that the child will experience pain. Tell the child that it will not hurt for long and that it will help "make it better." For example, when initiating an IV, have your materials out and ready to go. Tell the child to count to 5 after the pinch and it will be over. Then begin the IV.

Respect a child's modesty. Both little girls and boys are often embarrassed if they have to undress or be undressed in front of strangers. This anxiety often intensifies during adolescence. When a wound or site of injury has to be exposed, try to do so out of sight of strangers. Again, it is extremely important to tell the child what you are doing and why you are doing it.

You should speak to a child in a professional yet friendly way. A child should feel reassured that you are there to help in every way possible. Maintain eye contact with a child, as you would with an adult, to let the child know that you are helping and that you can be trusted Figure 11-15. It is helpful to position yourself at their level so that you do not appear to tower above them.

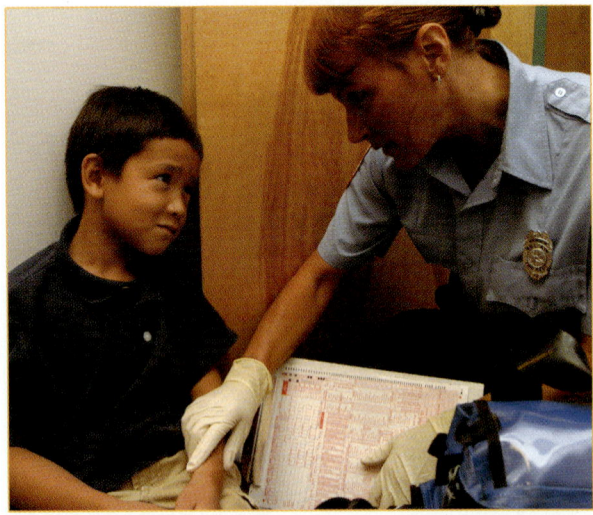

Figure 11-15 Maintain eye contact with a child to let the child know that you are there to help and that you can be trusted.

Communicating With Hearing-Impaired Patients

Patients who are hearing impaired or deaf are usually not ashamed or embarrassed by their disability. Often, it is the people around a deaf or hearing-impaired person who have the problem coping. Remember that you must be able to communicate with hearing-impaired patients so that you can provide necessary or even lifesaving care.

Hearing-impaired patients have normal intelligence. Hearing-impaired patients can usually understand what is going on around them, provided that you can successfully communicate with them. Most patients who are hearing impaired can read lips to some extent. Therefore, you should place yourself in a position so that the patient can see your lips. Many hearing-impaired patients have hearing aids to help them communicate. Be careful that hearing aids are not lost during an accident or fall. Not only are they extremely expensive, hearing aids will often make it easier to communicate. Hearing aids may also be forgotten if the patient is confused or ill. Look around, or ask the patient or the family about a hearing aid.

Remember the following five steps to help you efficiently communicate with patients who are hearing impaired:

1. **Have paper and a pen available.** This way, you can write down questions and the patient can write down answers, if necessary. Be sure to print so that your handwriting is not a communications barrier.
2. **If the patient can read lips**, you should face the patient and speak slowly and distinctly. Do not cover your mouth or mumble. If it is night or dark, consider shining a light on your face.
3. **Never shout.**
4. **Be sure to listen carefully**, ask short questions, and give short answers. Remember that although many hearing-impaired patients can speak distinctly, some cannot.
5. **Learn some simple phrases in sign language.** For example, knowing the signs for "sick," "hurt," and "help" may be useful if you cannot communicate in any other way Figure 11-16.

Communicating With Visually Impaired Patients

Like hearing-impaired patients, visually impaired and blind patients have usually accepted and learned to deal with their disability. Of course, not all visually impaired patients are completely blind. Many can perceive light and dark or can see shadows or movement. Ask the patient whether he or she can see at all. Also remember that, as with other patients who have disabilities, you should expect that visually impaired patients have normal intelligence.

As you begin caring for a visually impaired patient, explain everything that you are doing in detail as you are doing it. Be sure to stay in physical contact with the patient as you begin your care. Hold your hand lightly on the patient's shoulder or arm. Try to avoid sudden movements. If the patient can walk to the ambulance, place his or her hand on your arm, taking care not to rush. Transport any mobility aids, such as a cane, with the patient to the hospital. A visually impaired person may have a guide dog. Guide dogs are easily identified by their special harnesses. They are trained not to leave their masters and not to respond to strangers Figure 11-17 ▼. A visually impaired patient who is conscious can tell you about the dog and give instructions for its care. If circumstances permit, bring the guide dog to the hospital with the patient. If the dog has to be left behind, you should arrange for its care.

In the Field

If at all possible, allow a guide dog to accompany the visually impaired patient to the hospital. In a critical situation, be sure to leave the dog in the care of law enforcement or a family member.

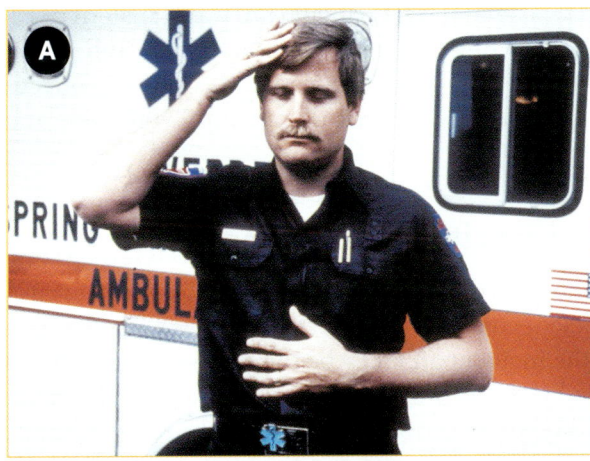
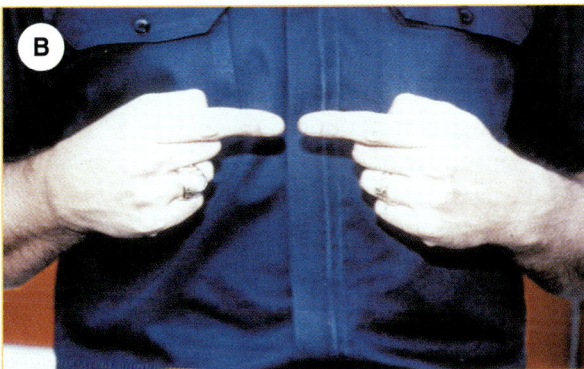
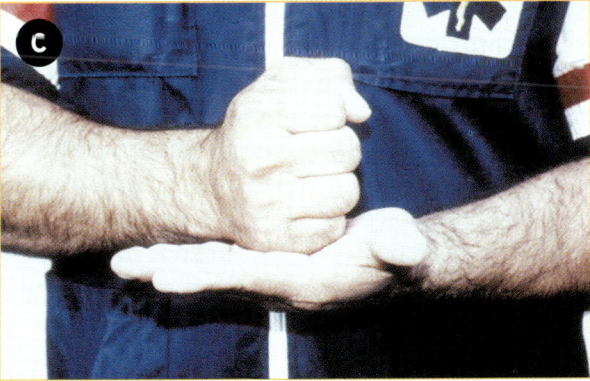

Figure 11-16 Learn simple phrases in sign language. **A.** Sick. **B.** Hurt. **C.** Help.

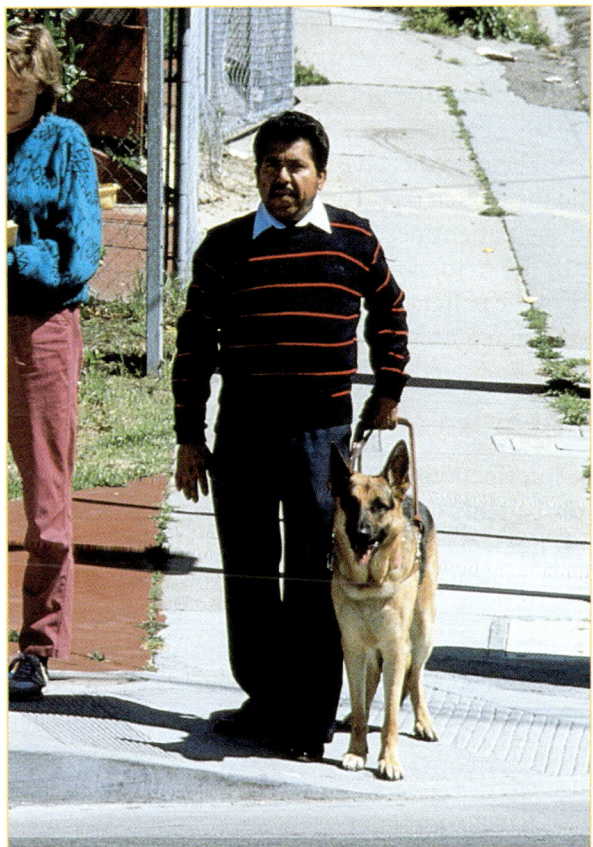

Figure 11-17 A guide dog is easily identified by its special harness.

Communicating With Non-English-Speaking Patients

As part of the focused history and physical exam, you must obtain a medical history from the patient. You cannot skip this step simply because the patient does not speak English. Most patients who do not speak English fluently will still know certain important words or phrases.

Your first step is to find out how much English the patient can speak. Use short, simple questions and simple words whenever possible. Avoid difficult medical terms. You can help patients to better understand if you point to specific parts of the body as you ask questions.

In many areas, particularly large urban centers, major segments of the population do not speak English. Your job will be much easier if you learn some common words and phrases in their language, especially common medical terms. Pocket cards are available that show the pronunciation of these terms. If the patient does not speak any English, find a family member or friend to act as an interpreter.

Written Communications and Documentation

Along with your radio report and verbal report, you must also complete a formal written report about the patient before you leave the hospital. You might be able to do the written report en route if the trip is long enough and the patient needs minimal care. Usually, you will finish the written report after you have transferred the care of the patient to a hospital staff member. Be sure to leave the report at the hospital before you leave.

Minimum Data Set

The information you collect during a call becomes part of the patient's medical record. The National EMS Information System (NEMSIS) has been collecting prehospital care information for research purposes since the early 1970s. NEMSIS has identified specific data points needed to enable communication and comparison of EMS runs between agencies, regions, and states. The minimum data set includes both narrative components and check-off boxes (Figure 11-18). An example of information collected on a prehospital care report (PCR) includes:

- Chief complaint
- Level of consciousness (AVPU) or mental status
- Systolic blood pressure for patients older than 3 years
- Capillary refill for patients younger than 6 years
- Skin color and temperature
- Pulse
- Respirations and effort

Examples of administrative information gathered in a patient care report:

- The time that the incident was reported
- The time that the EMS unit was notified
- The time that the EMS unit arrived at the scene
- The time that the EMS unit left the scene
- The time that the EMS unit arrived at the receiving facility
- The time that patient care was transferred

You will begin gathering the patient information as soon as you reach the patient. Continue collecting information as you provide care until you arrive at the hospital.

Prehospital Care Report

Prehospital care reports (known as PCRs) help to ensure efficient continuity of patient care. It is a written record of the incident and may be the only source of information for persons who subsequently care for the patient. This report describes the nature of the patient's injuries or illness at the scene and the treatment you provide. Although this report might not be read immediately at the hospital, it may very well be referred to later for important information. The prehospital care report serves the following six functions:

1. Continuity of care
2. Legal documentation
3. Education
4. Administrative
5. Research
6. Evaluation and continuous quality improvement

A good prehospital care report documents the patient's condition on arrival at the scene and the care that was provided. It also documents any changes in the patient's condition en route and upon arrival at the hospital. The information in the report is proof of the care you have provided. In some instances, it also shows that you have properly handled unusual or uncommon situations. Both objective and subjective information is included in this report. DO NOT include personal opinions. It is critical that you document everything in the clearest manner possible. The patient care report is a legal record of the incident and may be brought into court as evidence in the event of legal proceedings.

These reports also provide valuable administrative information. For example, the report provides infor-

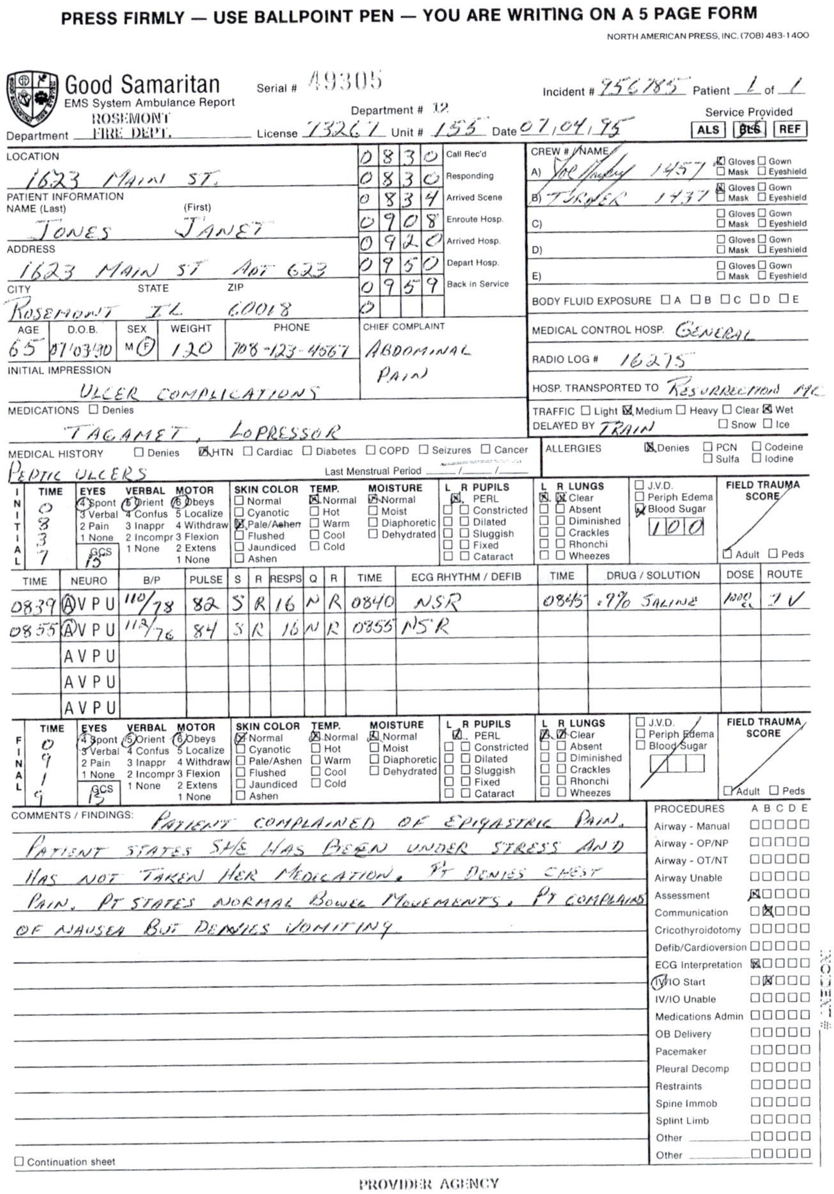

Figure 11-18 The minimum data set includes both patient information and administrative information.

mation for patient billing. It can also be used to evaluate response times, equipment usage, and other areas of administrative responsibility.

Data may be obtained from the prehospital care forms to analyze causes, severity, and types of illness or injury requiring emergency medical care. These reports may also be used in an ongoing program for evaluation of the quality of patient care. All records are reviewed periodically by your system's medical director. The purpose of this review is to make sure that trauma triage and/or other prehospital care criteria have been met. They may also be used to review an individual's performance. Finally, the administrative data may be used by the billing department to complete the billing process.

There are many requirements on a prehospital care report (Table 11-5 ▶). Often, these requirements vary from jurisdiction to jurisdiction, mainly because so many agencies obtain information from them. There is no universally accepted form.

| TABLE 11-5 | Components of Prehospital Care Report |

- Patient's name, gender, date of birth, and address
- Nature of call
- Chief complaint
- Location of the patient when first seen (including specific details, especially if the incident is a car crash or criminal activity is suspected)
- Rescue and treatment given before your arrival
- Signs and symptoms found during your patient assessment
- Care and treatment given on scene and during transport
- Baseline vital signs
- SAMPLE history
- Changes in vital signs and condition
- Date of the call
- Time of the call
- Location of the call
- Time of dispatch
- Time of arrival at the scene
- Time of leaving the scene
- Time of arrival at the hospital
- Patient's insurance information
- Names and/or certification numbers of the EMT-Is who responded to the call
- Name of the base hospital involved in the run
- Type of response to the scene: emergency or routine

Types of Forms

You will most likely use one of two types of forms. The first type is the traditional written form with check boxes and a narrative section. The second type is a computerized version in which you fill in information using an electronic clipboard or similar device.

If your service uses written forms, be sure to fill in the boxes completely, and avoid making stray marks on the sheet. Make sure that you are familiar with the specific procedures for collecting, recording, and reporting the information in your area.

If you must complete a narrative section, be sure to describe what you see and what you do. Be sure to include pertinent negative findings and important observations about the scene. Do not record your conclusions or opinions about the incident. For example, you may write, "The patient admits to taking cocaine today." This is a clear description that does not make any judgments about the patient's condition. However, a report that says "The patient was high" makes a conclusion about the patient's condition. Also avoid radio codes, and use only standard abbreviations. When information is of a sensitive nature, note the source of the information. Be sure to spell words correctly, especially medical terms. If you do not know how to spell a particular word, find out how to spell it, or use another word. Also be sure to record the time with all assessment findings. Record medical direction's advice and orders and the results of implementing such advice or orders. Upon arrival at the hospital, you should have the physician who gave the orders sign your patient care report.

Terminology Tips

Pertinent negatives include those findings that warrant no medical care or intervention, but which, by seeking them, show evidence of the thoroughness of the EMT-Is examination and history of the event.

For example, when you are examining a patient complaining of abdominal pain, the fact that the abdomen is soft and nontender would be pertinent negatives. The absence of nausea/vomiting in a patient complaining of chest pain would also be a pertinent negative. These are signs or symptoms you expect to find but are not there.

Documentation Tips

If you are unsure of an abbreviation, always spell the word out completely.

Remember that the report form itself and all the information on it are considered confidential documents. Be sure that you are familiar with state and local laws concerning confidentiality. All prehospital forms must be handled with care and stored in an appropriate manner once you have completed them. After you have completed a report, distribute the copies to the appropriate locations, according to state and local protocol. In most instances, a copy of the report will remain at the hospital and will become a part of the patient's record.

General Considerations

When completing a patient care report it is imperative to include all vital information as well as any supporting information gained from bystanders or family members. Record any statements that may have an impact on subsequent patient care or resolution of the situation including reports of mechanism of injury, patient's behavior, first aid intervention attempted prior to the arrival of EMS personnel, safety-related information (this also includes disposition of weapons), information of interest to crime scene investigators, and disposition of valuable personal property. You should put into quotation marks any statements by patients or others when documenting their information verbatim. Document the use of any support services, such as helicopter or rescue services, and also the use of any mutual aid services.

> **Documentation Tips**
>
> When quoting a patient, place quotation marks around the exact words stated. For example: Patient states his chest pain "feels like an elephant sitting on my chest."

Elements of a Properly Written EMS Document

A properly written report is accurate, legible, timely, unaltered, and free of any nonprofessional or extraneous information. Document accuracy depends on all information provided, both in the narrative section and any checkboxes, being both precise and comprehensive. All checkbox sections must show that the EMT-I attended to them, even if a given section was unused on a call. All medical terms, abbreviations, and acronyms should be properly used and correctly spelled.

Legibility means that handwriting, especially in the narrative portion, can be read by others without difficulty. If your handwriting is poor, be sure to print. The checkbox markings should be clear and consistent from the top page of the document to all underlying pages. Each report should also be completed in a timely fashion, preferably before leaving the emergency department or destination of the patient. Occasionally call volume will interfere with prompt completion of reports, but you should complete your report and distribute copies as soon as time permits.

Should you find it necessary to alter your documentation, there are certain procedures to follow. These are covered in the next section. And finally, make sure that a professional demeanor is maintained throughout your report. Avoid the use of jargon, slang, bias, or irrelevant

---

You are the Provider — Part 7

You have transferred care of your patient over to the Emergency Department nurse and now sit down and prepare to complete your prehospital care report.

Reassessment	Recording Time: 18 Minutes After Patient Contact
Respirations	22 breaths/min, adequate depth
Pulse	100 beats/min, irregular
Skin	Remains pale and diaphoretic
Blood pressure	110/68 mm Hg
SaO_2	98% on 15 L/min O_2 via nonrebreathing mask

10. What components of the prehospital care report must be completed by the EMT-I?

opinions or impressions. Only document those things that can be tangibly measured or things that the patient tells you. It is alright to say that a patient states he "has had two beers." Stating that the patient is drunk is not appropriate. There is no way to determine a patient's blood or breath alcohol level in an ambulance. Therefore, making such an accusation may result in a lawsuit for libel or slander. You may document that the patient had slurred speech or an unsteady gait, but remember to avoid judgment.

Reporting Errors

Everyone makes mistakes. If you leave something out of a report, or record information incorrectly, do not try to cover it up. Rather, write down what did or did not happen and the steps that were taken to correct the situation. Falsifying information on the prehospital report may result in suspension and/or revocation of your certification/license. More important, falsifying information results in poor patient care, because other health care providers have a false impression of assessment findings or the treatment given. Document only the vital signs that were actually taken. If you did not give the patient oxygen, do not chart that the patient was given oxygen.

If you discover an error as you are writing your report, draw a single horizontal line through the error, initial it, and write the correct information next to it (Figure 11-19 ▼). Do not try to erase or cover the error with correction fluid. This may be interpreted as an attempt to cover up a mistake.

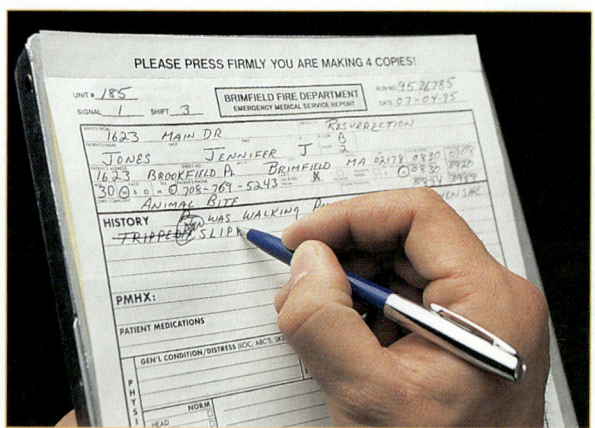

Figure 11-19 If you make a mistake in writing your report, the proper way to correct it is to draw a single horizontal line through the error, initial it, and write the correct information next to it.

If an error is discovered after you submit your report, draw a single line through the error, preferably in a different color ink, initial it, and date it. Make sure to add a note with the correct information. If you left out information accidentally, add a note with the correct information, the date, and your initials.

When you do not have enough time to complete your report before the next call, you will need to fill it out later.

Documenting Refusal of Care

Competent adult patients have the right to refuse treatment (Figure 11-20 ▶). If you are faced with this situation, you must inform medical control immediately. Before you leave the scene, try to persuade the patient to go to the hospital, and consult medical direction as directed by local protocol. Also make sure that the patient is able to make a rational, informed decision and is not under the influence of alcohol or other drugs or the effects of an illness or injury. Explain to the patient why it is important to be examined by a physician at the hospital. Also explain what may happen if the patient is not examined by a physician. If the patient still refuses, suggest other means for the patient to obtain proper care. Explain that you are willing to return. If the patient still refuses, document any assessment findings and emergency medical care given, then have the patient sign a refusal form. You should also have a family member, police officer, or bystander sign the form as a witness. If the patient refuses to sign the refusal form, have a family member, police officer, or bystander sign the form verifying that the patient refused to sign.

Be sure to complete the prehospital report, including the patient assessment findings. You must also include a statement explaining any advice rendered by medical direction and that you informed the patient of the possible consequences of failure to accept care, including potential death, and alternative methods of obtaining the care that you suggested.

Systems of Narrative Writing

When you are completing the narrative portion of your patient care report, there are numerous ways to document your findings. Regardless of the method you choose, it is always a good idea to be consistent. Not only does it help to remind you of what you may have omitted, but it may help your case in a lawsuit. You may

RELEASE FROM RESPONSIBILITY WHEN PATIENT REFUSES IV THERAPY

This is to certify that I, _____, am refusing IV treatment. I acknowledge
   patient's name
that I have been informed of the risk involved and hereby release the emergency medical services provider(s), the physician consultant, and the consulting hospital from all responsibility for any ill effects which may result from this action.

Witness _____   Signed _____
                                                                           patient name or nearest relative
Witness _____   _____
                                                                           relationship

---

RELEASE FROM RESPONSIBILITY WHEN PATIENT REFUSES SERVICE

This is to certify that I, _____, am refusing the services offered by the
   patient's name
emergency medical services provider(s). I acknowledge that I have been informed of the risk involved and hereby release the emergency medical services provider(s), the physician consultant, and the consulting hospital from all responsibility for any ill effects which may result from this action.

Witness _____   Signed _____
                                                                           patient name or nearest relative
Witness _____   _____
                                                                           relationship

---

RELEASE FROM RESPONSIBILITY WHEN PATIENT REFUSES SERVICES BUT ACCEPTS TRANSPORT

This is to certify that I, _____, am refusing _____
   patient's name
_____. I acknowledge that I have been informed of the risk involved and hereby release the emergency medical services provider(s), the physician consultant, and the consulting hospital from all responsibility for any ill effects which may result from this action. However, I do accept transportation to a medical facility.

Witness _____   Signed _____
                                                                           patient name or nearest relative
Witness _____   _____
                                                                           relationship

Figure 11-20 A competent adult patient has the right to refuse medical treatment and must sign a refusal form.

choose to use a head-to-toe approach, which is a comprehensive, consistent physical approach documenting your findings from head to toe. The body systems approach is another method in which you would list findings according to body systems.

Some EMT-Is prefer a simple paragraph form, while others like a set format. Your service may even dictate the method used. Table 11-6 ▼ shows another alternative to documenting the narrative portion of your report. The format chosen is not as important as knowing how to differentiate subjective from objective information, and not making a diagnosis or adding personal opinion.

Data Collection

Include the information from the minimum data set, discussed above. Table 11-7 ▶ provides guidelines on how to write the narrative portion of your report. Whether you completed a medical or trauma assessment, the assessment-based approach follows each step of the assessment(s) as a guideline to narrative writing.

Special Reporting Situations

In some instances, you may be required to file special reports with appropriate authorities. These may include incidents involving gunshot wounds, dog bites, certain infectious diseases, or suspected physical, sexual, or substance abuse. Learn your local requirements for reporting these incidents. Failure to report them may have legal consequences. It is important that the report is accurate, objective, and submitted in a timely manner.

Another special reporting situation is a multiple-casualty incident (MCI). The local MCI plan should have some means of recording important medical information temporarily (such as a triage tag that can be used later to complete the form). The standard for completing the form in an MCI is not the same as for a typical call. In some areas, one trip report may be completed for the entire incident instead of individual reports for each patient. Your local protocols should have specific guidelines.

Consequences of Errors, Omissions, and Inappropriate Documentation

An incomplete, inaccurate, or illegible report may cause subsequent care givers to provide inappropriate care to a patient. If patients are unable to speak for themselves, the patient care report may be the only link to their history or chain of events that led to seeking medical treatment. A lawyer considering the merits of an impending lawsuit may be dissuaded from a case when the documentation is done correctly. The converse is true if the documentation is anything less. Your best protection, and the patient's best opportunity for proper treatment, depend on a patient care report that is accurate, detailed, and completed in a timely manner.

TABLE 11-6 Documentation Shortcuts

SOAP and CHART are two common formats used in EMS. The information is entered in the narrative portion using the letters as a guideline for your findings.

S - Subjective information	C - Chief complaint
O - Objective information	H - History
A - Assessment	A - Assessment
P - Plan	R (Rx) - Treatment
	T - Transport

In the Field

CHART also works well for organizing your radio report. It can be used to give patient information in the following manner after giving your unit, status, and level of certification:

- C - Give the age, sex, chief complaint, where the patient was found, how he or she got there, and any pertinent scene information (damage to vehicle, distance of fall, etc.)
- H - Any **PERTINENT** history, medications, or allergies
- A - All assessment findings, including pertinent negatives
- R - Any treatment given and response to that treatment; any requested orders
- T - Estimated time of arrival (ETA) and any other pertinent information not given previously

TABLE 11-7	How to Write a Narrative
BSI	Did you have to take extraordinary BSI precautions? If so, state what precautions you took, and why.
Scene safety	Did you have to make your scene safe? If so, what was happening and why, and was there a delay of patient care?
NOI/MOI	Simply state.
Number of patients	Only need to record when more than one patient is present. "This is patient 2 of 3."
Additional help	Did you call for help? If so, state why, at what time, and what time the help arrived. Did it delay transport?
C-spine	State what C-spine precautions were initiated. You may want to include why. "Due to the significant MOI . . ."
General impression	Simply record, if not already documented on the PCR.
Level of consciousness	Be sure to report LOC found, any changes in LOC, and at what time.
Chief complaint	Note and quote pertinent statements made by patient/and or bystanders. This includes any pertinent denials, "Pt. denies chest pain . . ."
Life threats	List any and all interventions you took, and how the patient responded, "Assisted ventilations with O_2 (15 LPM) at 20 BPM with no change in LOC."
ABCs	Document what you found and any interventions performed.
Oxygen	Record if you used O_2, how it was applied and how much was administered.
Focused, rapid, or detailed assessment	State what assessment you used and any pertinent findings. "Detailed physical exam revealed unequal pupils, crepitus to right ribs, and deformity of left tibia."
SAMPLE/OPQRST-I	Note and quote any pertinent answers.
Baseline vitals	Your service may want you to record vitals in the narrative as well as other places on the PCR.
Medical direction	Quote any orders given to you by medical control and who gave them.
Management of secondary injuries/treat for shock	Report any and all interventions you completed, at what time, and how the patient responded—even if it is negatively.

Reprinted with permission. Courtesy of Jay C. Keefauver.

You are the Provider — Summary

1. What aspects of communications should every EMT-I know?

Radio and telephone communications link you and your team with other members of the EMS, fire, and law enforcement communities. This link helps the entire team to work together more effectively and provides an important layer of safety and protection for each member of the team. You must know what your system can and cannot do, and you must be able to use your system efficiently and effectively. You must be able to send precise, accurate reports about the scene, the patient's condition, and the treatment that you provide.

2. Why is it important to know what communication system your service uses?

You must know what your system can and cannot do, and you must be able to use your system efficiently and effectively. You must be able to send precise, accurate reports about the scene, the patient's condition, and the treatment that you provide.

3. Why are verbal communication skills so vital for EMT-Is?

Verbal skills will enable the EMT-I to gather information from the patient and bystanders. It will also make it possible to effectively coordinate the variety of responders who are often present at the scene. Excellent verbal communications are also an integral part of transferring the patient's care to the nurses and physicians at the hospital. Finally, the EMT-I must be able to organize and summarize the important aspects of the patient's presentation and treatment when reporting to the hospital staff.

4. The portable radio you are carrying is essential for what reasons?

A portable radio is essential if you need to communicate with the dispatcher or medical control when you are away from the ambulance.

5. What is the principal reason for radio communications?

The principal reason for radio communication is to facilitate communication between you and medical control (and the hospital).

6. What reasons are there for contacting medical control in this situation?

To consult with medical control, to notify the hospital of this patient's arrival, to request advice or orders from medical control, or to advise the hospital of special situations (ie, the prolonged extrication).

7. What elements should be included in your verbal patient report to the receiving facility?

The patient report commonly includes the following eight elements:

- The receiving hospital, your unit identification and level of certification
- The patient's age, gender, and approximate weight (if needed for drug orders)
- Description of the scene
- The patient's chief complaint or your perception of the problem and its severity and associated symptoms
- A brief, pertinent history of the patient's present illness or injury
- A brief report of physical findings
- A brief summary of the care given and any patient response
- Any other pertinent information and the estimated time of arrival at the hospital

8. What are standing orders and what is their purpose?

Sometimes radio equipment will stop working during a call. EMS systems must have a backup plan and options. The goal of a backup plan is to make sure that you can maintain contact when the usual procedures do not work. The simplest backup plan relies on written standing orders. Standing orders are written documents that have been signed by the EMS system's medical director. These orders outline specific directions, permissions, and sometimes prohibitions regarding patient care. By their very nature, standing orders do not require prior communication with medical control. When properly followed, standing orders or formal protocols have the same authority and legal status as orders given over the radio.

9. What components should be included in your oral report to the Emergency Department nurse?

The following six components must be included in the oral report:
- The patient's name (if you know it) and the chief complaint, nature of illness, or mechanism of injury
- A summary of the information that you gave in your radio report
- Any important history that was not given already
- The patient's response to treatment given en route. It is especially important to report any changes in the patient or the treatment provided since your radio report.
- The vital signs assessed during transport and after the radio report
- Any other information that you may have gathered that was not important enough to report sooner. Information that was gathered during transport, any patient medications you have brought with you, and any other details about the patient that was provided by family members or friends may be included.

10. What components of the prehospital care report must be completed by the EMT-I?

- Patient's name, gender, date of birth, and address
- Nature of call
- Chief complaint
- Location of the patient when first seen (including specific details, especially if the incident is a car crash or criminal activity is suspected)
- Rescue and treatment given before your arrival
- Signs and symptoms found during your patient assessment
- Care and treatment given on scene and during transport
- Baseline vital signs
- SAMPLE history
- Changes in vital signs and condition
- Date of the call
- Time of the call
- Location of the call
- Time of dispatch
- Time of arrival at the scene
- Time of leaving the scene
- Time of arrival at the hospital
- Patient's insurance information
- Names and/or certification numbers of the EMT-Is who responded to the call
- Name of the base hospital involved in the run
- Type of response to the scene: emergency or routine

Prep Kit

Ready for Review

- Excellent communication skills are crucial in relaying pertinent information to the hospital before arrival.
- Radio and telephone communication links you and your team to other members of the EMS, fire, and law enforcement communities. This enables your entire team to work together more effectively.
- It is your job to know what your communication system can and cannot handle. You must be able to communicate effectively by sending precise, accurate reports about the scene, the patient's condition, and the treatment that you provide.
- There are many different forms of communication that an EMT-I must understand and be able to use.
  - First, you must be familiar with two-way radio communications and have a working knowledge of mobile and handheld portable radios.
  - You must know when to use them and what type of information you can transmit.
- Remember, the lines of communication are not always exclusive; therefore, you should speak in a professional manner at all times.
- In addition to radio and oral communications with hospital personnel, EMT-Is must have excellent person-to-person communication skills. You should be able to interact with the patient and any family members, friends, or bystanders.
- It is important for you to remember that people who are sick or injured may not understand what you are doing or saying. Therefore, your body language and attitude are very important in gaining the trust of both the patient and family.
- You must also take special care of individuals such as children, the elderly, and hearing-impaired, visually impaired, and non-English-speaking patients.
- Along with your radio report and oral report, you must also complete a formal written report about the patient before you leave the hospital. This is a vital part of providing emergency medical care and ensuring the continuity of patient care. This information guarantees the proper transfer of responsibility, complies with the requirements of health departments and law enforcement agencies, and fulfills your administrative needs.
- Reporting and record-keeping duties are essential, but they should never come before the care of a patient.

Vital Vocabulary

base station Any radio hardware containing a transmitter and receiver that is located in a fixed place.

cellular telephone A low-power portable radio that communicates through an interconnected series of repeater stations called "cells."

channel An assigned frequency or frequencies that are used to carry voice and/or data communications.

dedicated line A special telephone line that is used for specific point-to-point communications; also known as a "hot line."

duplex The ability to transmit and receive simultaneously.

Federal Communications Commission (FCC) The federal agency that has jurisdiction over interstate and international telephone and telegraph services and satellite communications, all of which may involve EMS activity.

MED channels VHF and UHF channels that the FCC has designated exclusively for EMS use.

multiplex Communications can simultaneously transmit two or more different types of information, such as voice and telemetry, in either or both directions over the same frequency.

paging The use of a radio signal and a voice or digital message that is transmitted to pagers ("beepers") or desktop monitor radios.

Technology

- Interactivities
- Vocabulary Explorer
- Anatomy Review
- Web Links
- Online Review Manual

prehospital care report (PCR) A written record of the incident that describes the nature of the patient's injuries or illness at the scene and the treatment you provide.

rapport A trusting relationship that you build with your patient.

repeater A special base station radio that receives messages and signals on one frequency and then automatically retransmits them on a second frequency.

scanner A radio receiver that searches or "scans" across several frequencies until the message is completed; the process is then repeated.

simplex Single-frequency radio; transmissions can occur in either direction but not simultaneously in both; when one party transmits, the other can only receive, and the party that is transmitting is unable to receive.

standing orders Written documents, signed by the EMS system's medical director, that outline specific directions, permissions, and sometimes prohibitions regarding patient care; also called protocols.

telemetry A process in which electronic signals are converted into coded, audible signals; these signals can then be transmitted by radio or telephone to a receiver at the hospital with a decoder.

trunking Sharing of radio frequencies by multiple agencies or systems.

UHF (ultra-high frequency) Radio frequencies between 300 and 3,000 MHz.

VHF (very-high frequency) Radio frequencies between 30 and 300 MHz; the VHF spectrum is further divided into "high" and "low" bands.

Points to Ponder

You and your partner are dispatched for a patient with a general illness. Upon your arrival the patient states that he is not feeling right. He feels tired, fatigued, and has pain to the extremities. You tell the patient that you will be transporting him to the hospital to receive a full check up. The patient tells you that he does not want to go to the hospital and just wants you to tell him if he is okay. You explain to him some of the signs that you find and you tell him what care you would like to give and the potential of him having a serious underlying condition. The patient refuses your care. You do not want to get into an argument with the patient so your partner writes the patient refused care on the prehospital run report and asks the patient to sign it. You both agree that because the patient refused there is no need for further documentation. You then leave the scene. About 2 hours later you receive a call to the same address, this time for a patient in cardiac arrest. The patient is treated and transported and survives. The patient's family is concerned that the ambulance was there earlier and did not transport him. They are considering filing charges. Your medical director pulls the chart and wants to talk to you about the earlier refusal.

Issues: Relevance and Importance of Proper Documentation, Importance of Complete Documentation

Assessment in Action

Your crew responds to a call on the outskirts of town. You arrive on the scene, assess your patient, and prepare to transport. You attempt to make contact with the online physician while en route to the hospital using your 800-MHz radio.

Unable to get through, you attempt to use your cell phone but there is no reception. You are very frustrated because you cannot get through to the hospital. Your dispatcher advises you that a repeater at a tower near your location is out of service. There is also a big storm approaching the area. Your driver asks if you wish to use the low band to try and make contact.

1. A base station can be defined as:
   A. any radio hardware containing a transmitter and receiver that are located in a fixed place.
   B. transmission that is done from a fixed location.
   C. the place from which all communications takes place.
   D. the location where ambulances are kept when not responding to calls.

2. A special base station radio that receives messages and signals on one frequency and then automatically retransmits them on a second frequency is called a:
   A. trunk.
   B. repeater.
   C. retransmitter.
   D. receiver.

3. A low-powered portable radio that communicates through a series of interconnected repeater stations is called a:
   A. repeater.
   B. scanner.
   C. cellular phone.
   D. portable.

4. When using a simplex communication system, how do communications occur?
   A. Both units can transmit and receive at the same time.
   B. Radio transmissions can occur in either direction but not simultaneously.
   C. Two or more types of information may be transmitted.
   D. All of the above

5. Allocating specific radio frequencies, licensing base stations, establishing licensing standards, and establishing limitations for transmitter power are functions of which federal agency?
   A. DOT
   B. OSHA
   C. FCC
   D. FDA

6. To achieve proper transmission, once you key the mike on the radio, you should:
   A. begin speaking right away.
   B. wait one to two seconds before starting to speak.
   C. begin speaking before the mike is keyed.
   D. wait until you hear something.

7. When providing an oral report all of the following should be included, EXCEPT:
   A. chief complaint.
   B. relevant medical history.
   C. patient's response to treatment.
   D. patient's billing address.

8. All of the following are important rules to remember when communicating with patients, EXCEPT:
   A. make and keep eye contact.
   B. show authority and an unemotional approach.
   C. use language the patient can understand.
   D. act and speak in a calm, confident manner.

9. Which of the following is not a function of a prehospital care report?
   A. Research
   B. Continuity of care
   C. Evaluation and continuous quality improvement
   D. Determining a patient's insurance eligibility

10. If an error is made on the prehospital care report, what should you do?
    A. Draw a single horizontal line through the error, initial it, and write the correct information next to it.
    B. Make sure to completely black out what was written, initial it, and write the correct information next to it.
    C. Put the error inside parentheses and write the correct information after it.
    D. You are not allowed to make any errors on a prehospital care report.

11. When documenting a "patient refusal," you should:
    A. document very little because the patient refused care.
    B. document your patient's findings, attempt of care, explanation given to patient, and advice rendered by medical direction.
    C. patients are allowed to refuse care and providers are not allowed to encourage them or insist on providing care.
    D. immediately contact law enforcement and place patient in protective custody.

12. Two common formats used for documentation in EMS are:
    A. SAMPLE and OPQRST-I.
    B. BTLS and PHTLS.
    C. SOAP and CHART.
    D. RICE and DOTS.

13. A frequency band that is used for EMS communications, which allows for trunking, is called a(n):
    A. VHF low band.
    B. VHF high band.
    C. UHF band.
    D. 800 MHz.

14. A number of VHF and UHF channels reserved exclusively for EMS use are known as:
    A. priority channels.
    B. MED channels.
    C. MEDCOM channels.
    D. emergency channels.

15. How often should radio equipment be serviced?
    A. Monthly
    B. Semiannually
    C. Annually
    D. Daily

16. In order to be most effective, a base station needs to be located where in relation to the antenna?
    A. As far as possible to ensure the most coverage.
    B. Physically close to the antenna.
    C. A base station does not need to have an antenna.
    D. Within a mile of the antenna.

17. All of the following are responsibilities of a dispatcher, EXCEPT:
    A. properly screening and assigning priority to each call.
    B. dispatching and directing EMS response unit(s) to the correct location.
    C. determining which hospital the patient needs to be transported to.
    D. maintaining a record of the incident.

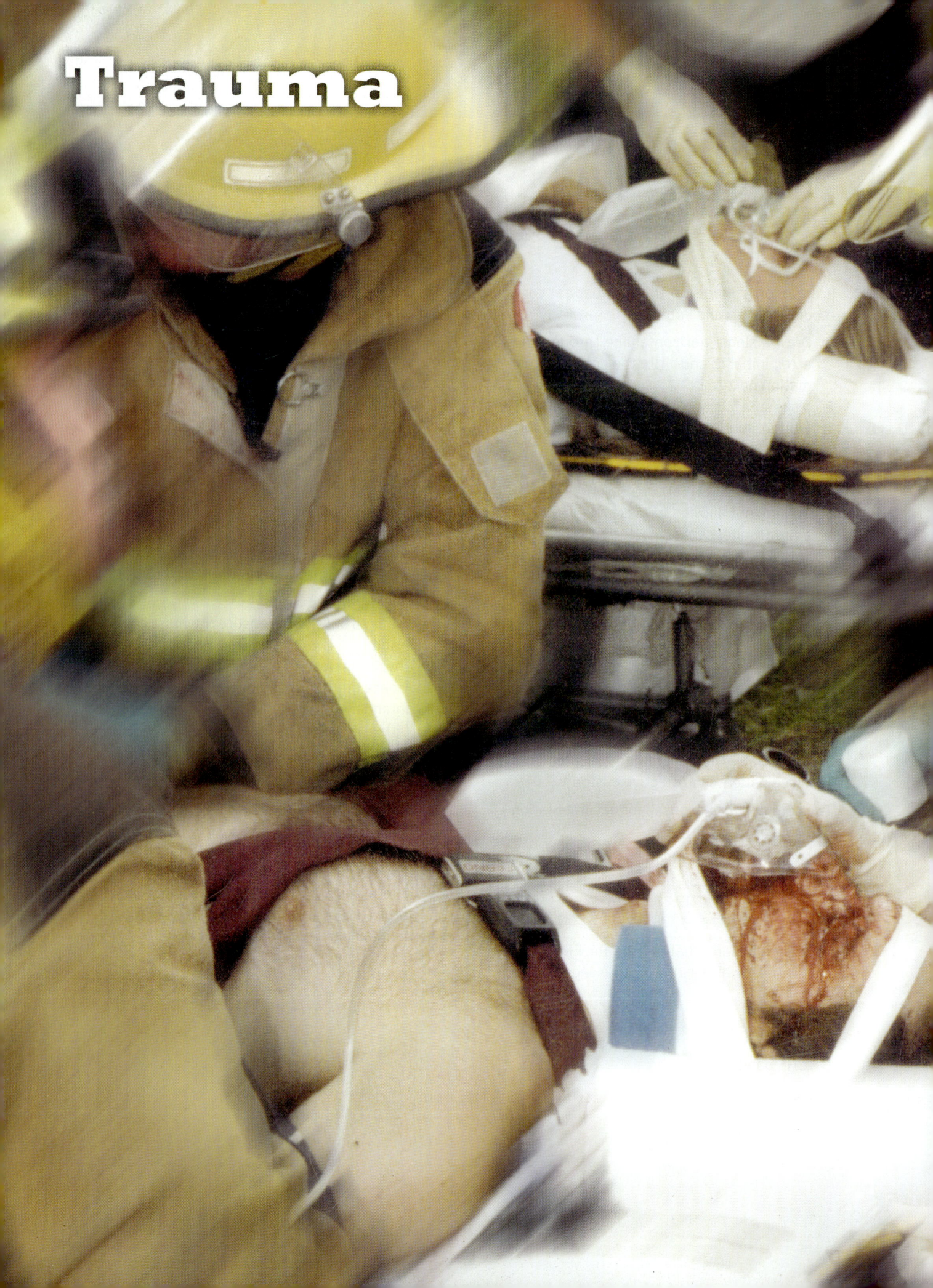

Trauma

Section 5

12	Trauma Systems and Mechanism of Injury	616
13	Hemorrhage and Shock	642
14	Burns and Soft-Tissue Injuries	674
15	Thoracic Trauma	712
16	Abdomen and Genitalia Injuries	742
17	Head and Spine Injuries	758
18	Musculoskeletal Care	798

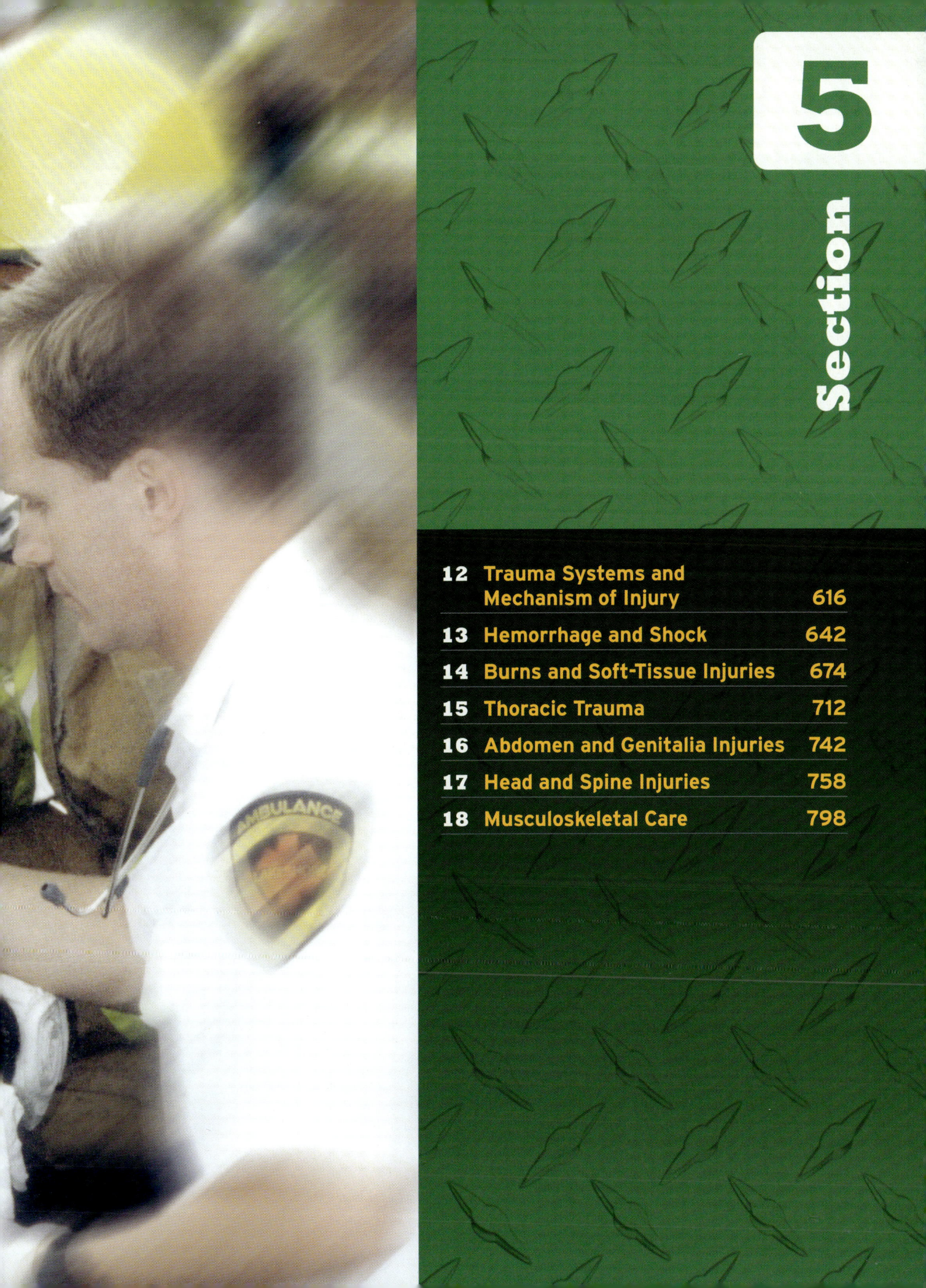

Trauma Systems and Mechanism of Injury

1999 Objectives

Cognitive

4-1.1 List and describe the components of a comprehensive trauma system. (p 618)
4-1.2 Describe the role of and differences between levels of trauma centers. (p 619)
4-1.3 Describe the criteria for transport to a trauma center. (p 619)
4-1.4 Describe the criteria and procedure for air medical transport. (p 619)
4-1.5 Define energy and force as they relate to trauma. (p 620)
4-1.6 Define laws of motion and energy and understand the role that increased speed has on injuries. (p 620)
4-1.7 Describe each type of impact and its effect on unrestrained victims (eg, frontal impacts, lateral impacts, rear impacts, rotational impacts, rollover). (p 623)
4-1.8 Describe the pathophysiology of the head, spine, thorax, and abdomen that results from the above forces. (p 626)
4-1.9 Describe the organ collisions that occur in blunt trauma and vehicular collisions. (p 623)
4-1.10 Describe the effects that restraint systems (including seat belts, airbags, and child safety seats) have on the injury patterns found in motor vehicle crashes. (p 627)
4-1.11 List specific injuries and their causes as related to interior and exterior vehicle damage. (p 624)
4-1.12 Describe the kinematics of penetrating injuries. (p 636)
4-1.13 List the motion and energy considerations of mechanisms other than motor vehicle crashes. (p 635)
4-1.14 Define the role of kinematics as an additional tool for patient assessment. (p 637)

Affective
None

Psychomotor
None

1985 Objectives

There are no 1985 objectives for this chapter.

12

Trauma Systems and Mechanism of Injury

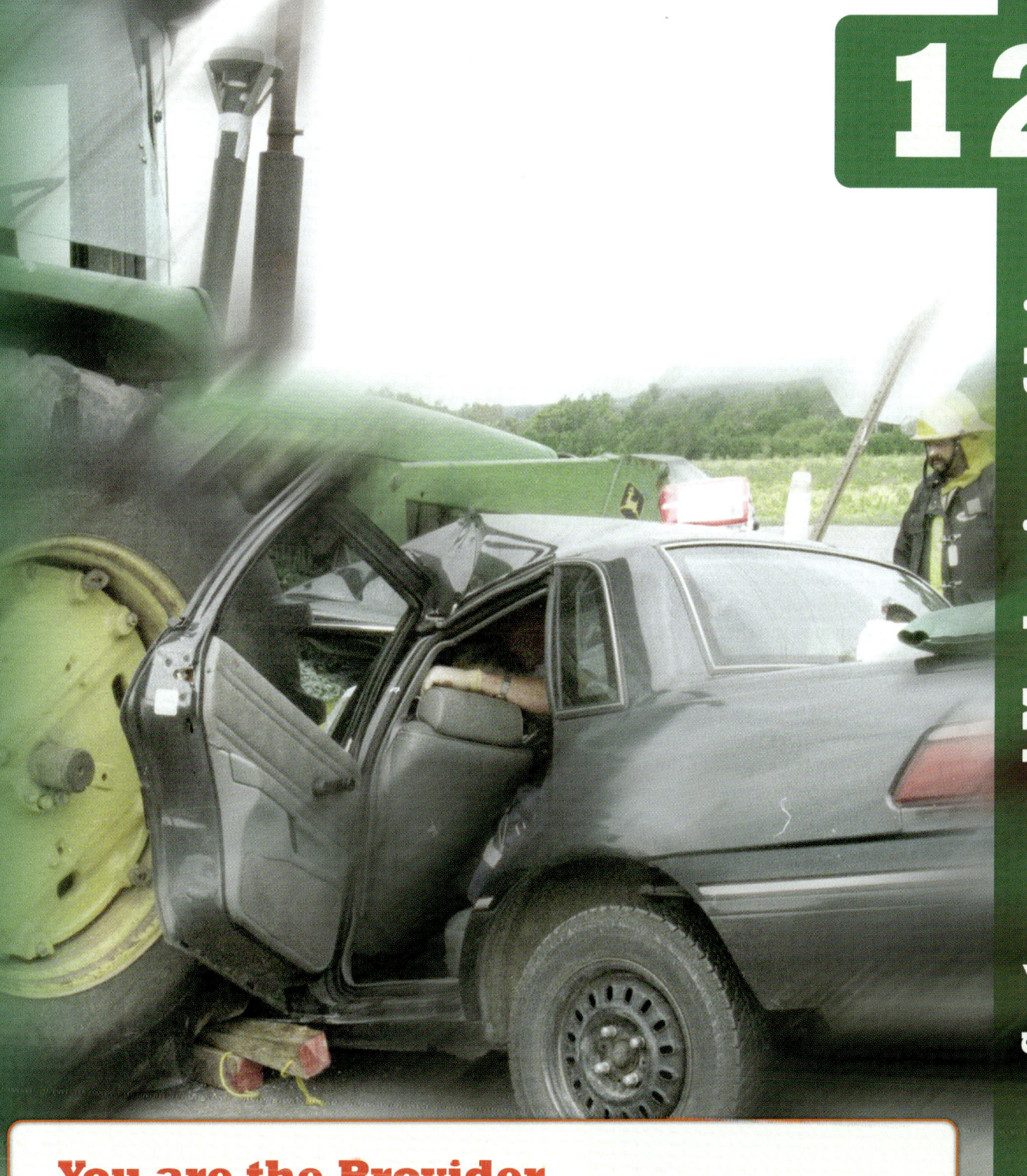

You are the Provider

You are dispatched to the scene of a rollover motor vehicle crash. Upon arrival, you note that a single vehicle is involved. The single occupant of the vehicle was unrestrained and has been ejected from the vehicle. Law enforcement officers at the scene estimate that the vehicle was traveling at high speed at the time of the crash.

Trauma takes many lives each year, often young people with their whole lives ahead of them. This chapter will help you understand what events occur during common traumatic situations, focusing primarily on your assessment skills. It will also help you answer the following questions:

1. How does a basic understanding of physics as it relates to kinetic energy contribute to improving the care you provide to trauma patients?
2. What are the so-called three collisions that occur during a motor vehicle crash?

Kinematics of Trauma

Injuries are the leading cause of death and disability in the United States among children and young adults (ages 1 to 44 years), claiming 140,000 lives annually—more than all diseases combined. There are more than 40,000 automobile-related deaths per year. Penetrating trauma is also on the rise and, in the near future, may exceed blunt trauma in the number of deaths caused. Each year, one person in three sustains an injury that requires medical treatment. Proper prehospital evaluation and care can do much to minimize suffering, long-term disability, and death from trauma.

This chapter introduces the basic physical concepts that dictate how injuries occur and affect the human body. When you understand these concepts, you will be better able to size up a crash scene and use that information as a vital part of patient assessment. The chapter begins with a basic discussion of energy and trauma. Next, different types of crashes and their impact on the body are explained. A complete and accurate history of the incident will identify the possibility for 95% of the injuries present. By assessing the body of a vehicle that has crashed and the incident site, you can often determine what happened to the passengers at the time of impact, which may allow you to predict what injuries and the severity of the injuries the passengers sustained at the time of impact. Evaluation of the mechanism of injury for the trauma patient will provide the EMT-I with an index of suspicion for serious underlying injuries. The index of suspicion is the EMT-I's concern for potentially serious underlying and unseen injuries. Certain injury patterns occur with certain types of injury events. The amount of energy exchanged also has a major role in the severity of injuries, along with the anatomic structures potentially involved. Answers to simple questions will provide you with information on how to identify life-threatening and other serious injuries. The chapter concludes with a brief discussion of falls and penetrating trauma. A brief section on Newton's laws is also presented.

Trauma Systems

Components

Injury prevention is the first component of a trauma system. Effective education may prevent the need for EMS is many situations. In the event of EMS activation, there are three considerations of prehospital care: treatment, transport, and trauma triage guidelines. Treatment is initiated at the scene and continued en route to definitive care. This may be as simple as bandaging minor wounds or as complex as attempting to resuscitate a patient in cardiac arrest. Patient presentation and status should dictate the mode of transport. Trauma triage guidelines help to decide where to transport the patient. A local emergency department may be sufficient, or the patient may require care in a trauma center.

Once the patient is delivered to the emergency department, care is continued. It may be necessary to transport to a local emergency department for stabilization and then to provide interfacility transport to another hospital for the definitive care needed. Trauma critical care may not be available at local facilities, and transport to a trauma center will be required.

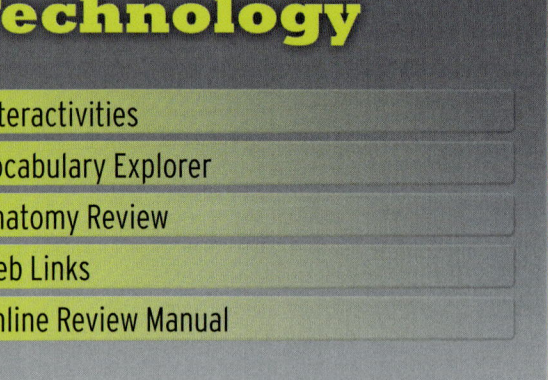

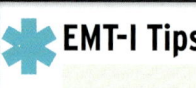

EMT-I Tips

Remember that the goal of the "golden hour" concept is for the patient to receive definitive care within 1 hour of the accident or injury.

Aside from prehospital and in-hospital care, rehabilitation is also an important component of a trauma system. Rehabilitation may be accomplished through outpatient therapy or may require a stay in a rehabilitation facility. Data collection and trauma registry help to determine needs in a specific demographic area as well as needs in public education. By educating the general public in first aid, CPR, and the use of safety devices to prevent injuries, many lives may be saved.

Trauma Centers

Trauma centers are designated by various agencies (for example, American College of Surgeons, individual states) according to levels based on the availability of staff and technology. There are typically four designated levels, with a Level I trauma center providing the greatest range of care. There are also centers with specialties such as burn care or pediatric care. Many Level I facilities are designated as adult Level I trauma centers with a "pediatric commitment." This is especially valuable in areas where access to a pediatric center is limited. **Table 12-1** lists some typical criteria for trauma center designation according to level.

Transport Considerations

When making the decision to transport a patient, several options must be considered. What are the needs of the patient? What is the level of the receiving facility? The patient should be transported to the closest, most appropriate facility to receive optimal care. You must also decide on the mode of transport that will offer the greatest benefit. Should you call for air transport or is ground transport sufficient?

When making the decision to transport by ground, several factors should be taken into consideration. Can the appropriate facility be reached within a reasonable time frame by ground? What is the extent of injuries? If in a congested area, can the patient be transported to a more accessible landing zone for air medical transport?

Air transport is a viable option in several situations: (1) when there is extended transport time by ground, (2) when there are mass casualties, (3) when extrication times are prolonged with critically injured patients, and (4) for long distances to an appropriate facility as opposed to the closest emergency department. There also may be other times that air transport is appropriate. If the patient can be transported to definitive care within a reasonable amount of time by ground, there is no need to call for air transport. Take into consideration the time it will take for the aircraft to lift off, travel, and land, just to reach the scene. By weighing the time frame against transport by ground, you will be able to make an informed decision. Also take into account the terrain. Is there an adequate area for landing? If not, how far will the patient need to be transported to reach a landing zone? If there is a great distance, ground transport may be a more reasonable option. Once the decision is made to call for

---

TABLE 12-1 | Trauma Center Levels

Level I:
- Level I facilities should be a regional resource center and will generally serve large cities or population-dense areas.
- A Level I facility will usually serve as the lead hospital for a system.
- The facility is expected to admit at least 1,200 trauma patients yearly.
- 24-hour in-house availability of a qualified attending surgeon is required.
- The attending surgeon's participation in the major decisions, presence in the emergency department for major resuscitations, and presence at operative procedures are mandatory.
- The facility is expected to conduct trauma research and be a leader in education, prevention, and outreach activities.

Level II:
- In one environment, the Level II institution may be in a population-dense area and may supplement the Level I facility. The two work together to optimize resources expended to care for all injured patients in their area.
- The second Level II environment involves less population-dense areas.
- The facility serves as the lead trauma facility for a geographic area, because a Level I institution is not likely to be geographically close.
- Local conditions may allow the surgeons to be rapidly available on short notice.
- A Level II hospital is expected to have an outreach program that incorporates smaller institutions in its service area.

Level III:
- Level III facilities will have continuous general surgical coverage.
- A Level III facility must have the capability to manage the initial care of the majority of injured patients and have transfer agreements with other trauma centers.
- The hospital must be involved with prevention and must have an active outreach program for referring communities.
- Level III facilities will conduct education programs for nurses, physicians, and allied health care workers involved with the management of trauma.

Level IV:
- Level IV hospitals are usually located in rural areas and supplement care within a larger network of hospitals.
- These facilities provide initial evaluation and assessment of injured patients. (Most patients will require transport to larger facilities for optimal care.)
- Facilities must have 24-hour emergency coverage by a physician.
- The hospitals have operative capabilities when the surgeon is available.
- Specialty coverage may or may not be available.
- Level IV facilities should be involved in prevention, outreach, and education.

EMT-I Tips

Newton's First Law

Newton's first law states that objects at rest tend to stay at rest and objects in motion tend to stay in motion unless acted on by some outside force. The first part of the law is fairly clear. An object such as an empty soda can will not move spontaneously unless some force, such as a gust of wind, acts on it. An example will help to illustrate the second part. In a car going 50 mph, the passengers and the car are moving at 50 mph. The passengers do not feel as though they are moving because they are not moving relative to the car. However, when the car strikes a concrete barrier and comes to a sudden stop, the passengers continue to travel at 50 mph. They stay in motion until they are acted on by an external force—most likely the seat belt, windshield, steering wheel, or dashboard. To appreciate the severity of the impact, think of the driver as sitting motionless while a steering wheel rams into his or her chest at 50 mph. Now consider that the same thing happens to the driver's internal organs. They also are in motion, traveling at 50 mph relative to the ground, until they are acted on by an external force, in this case the sternum, rib cage, or other body structure. This scenario illustrates the three collisions that are associated with blunt trauma.

Newton's Second Law

Newton's second law states that force (F) equals mass (M) times acceleration (A), that is, $F = M \times A$, in which acceleration is the change in velocity (speed) that occurs over time. Therefore, it is not so much that "speed kills," but that the change in velocity with respect to time generates the forces that cause injury. Simply put, it is not the fall, but the sudden stop at the bottom that hurts.

In the example of a car traveling at 30 mph, it takes about 3 seconds for the car to decrease its speed from 30 to 0 mph when the driver applies the brakes smoothly. If he or she is properly restrained by well-adjusted seat belts, the driver slows, or decelerates, at the same rate as the car. But if the car is stopped by hitting a large tree and the driver is not restrained, his or her body will continue to stay in motion at 30 mph until it is stopped by an external force—in this case, the steering wheel. Although the change in the body's velocity is the same as when the car was braking smoothly during 3 seconds (30 to 0 mph), that change now takes place in about 0.01 second. Because the period of deceleration is 300 times less, the average force of impact is 300 times greater. This means that the force is approximately 150 times the force of gravity. Imagine a force 150 times your body weight slamming into your chest. Therefore, Force = Mass × Deceleration.

Now consider the same car striking the same tree, but this time, the driver is restrained with a shoulder and lap belt. The driver is essentially tied to the car and stops during the same period the car stops. It takes some time, although brief, to crush the front of the car and bring it to a halt. The car comes to a stop in approximately

air medical transport, contact your dispatcher to request a unit or follow local protocols regarding contacting air support.

EMT-I Tips

Energy Law Summary
- Motion is created by force (energy exchange)
- Force (energy exchange) must stop this motion
- If such energy exchange occurs inside the body tissue, damage is produced
- For every action, there is an equal and opposite reaction

Energy and Trauma

Traumatic injury occurs to the body when the body's tissues are exposed to energy levels beyond their tolerance. Three concepts of energy are typically associated with injury (not including thermal energy, which causes burns): potential energy, kinetic energy, and work. In considering the effects of energy on the human body, it is important to remember that energy can be neither created nor destroyed, but can only be converted or transformed. This is known as the Law of Conservation of Energy. It is not the objective of this section to help you to reconstruct the scene of a motor vehicle crash. Rather, you should have a sense of the effects of work on the body and understand, in a broad sense, how that

0.05 second. The change in the driver's velocity is the same (30 to 0 mph), but the longer period of deceleration results in a *g*-force of only 30 times that of gravity. This is still a substantial force, but it is much less than the force that is experienced by the unrestrained driver. More to the point, it is survivable.

In a final example, the car and driver, as before, are traveling at 30 mph, and the driver is properly restrained with a 3-point belt. In this case, however, the car is also equipped with an air bag. When the car hits the tree and suddenly stops, the driver's upper body initially continues forward at 30 mph. The body is partially slowed by the lap and shoulder belts but is finally brought to rest by the air bag. The upper body compresses the air bag, which stops the body's forward motion in about 0.1 second. Thus, the air bag stretches the duration of impact by 0.05 second, buying the body even more time, and the force on the upper body drops to approximately 15 times that of gravity.

Mass × Acceleration = Force = Mass × Deceleration. A gunshot wound is another example of this law. To accelerate a bullet from the muzzle of a weapon requires the force from the explosion of the gunpowder. Once the bullet is set in motion by this explosion, an equal amount of tissue destruction must occur inside the body to stop the motion as was used to start it.

The air bag has another advantage. The force of its impact is applied over a much larger area than the area that is affected by the steering wheel or the shoulder belt, shrinking the force per unit area. This point can be illustrated by an analogy. A person standing on one toe on a sheet of ice applies a concentrated load in a very small area, thus breaking the ice and falling through. If the person lies flat on the ice, he or she greatly expands the contact area and reduces the stress on the ice, which, depending on certain conditions (for example, thickness of the ice), should not break. The dual action of the air bag (distributing the force of impact over a greater area and increasing the duration of impact) results in less severe injuries.

Newton's Third Law

Newton's third law states that for every action, there is an equal and opposite reaction. Therefore, if you push on a door, the door pushes back (reacts) with an equal force but in the opposite direction. In the case of a dented A-pillar, the force of the driver's head was sufficient to dent the strong metal. But in terms of patient assessment, the more important point is the reaction force of the pillar on the head. Newton's third law states that the two forces are equal but occur in opposite directions. In other words, the head was essentially hit by an A-pillar traveling at 30 mph. Similarly, it takes a substantial force to collapse a steering wheel. When you notice a collapsed steering wheel during scene size-up, you should suspect serious chest injuries, even if the driver initially has no visible signs of chest injury. Often, reading the scene and understanding the basic principles of energy transfer will give you as clear a picture of the patient's potential injuries and injury severity as the actual physical patient assessment.

work is related to potential and kinetic energy. For example, when you are assessing a patient who fell, you need not calculate the speed at which the person hit the ground. However, it is important to estimate the height from which he or she fell and to appreciate the injury potential of the fall.

Work is defined as *force* acting over a distance. For example, the force needed to bend metal multiplied by the distance over which the metal is bent is the work that crushes the front end of an automobile involved in a frontal impact. Similarly, forces that bend, pull, or compress tissues beyond their inherent limits result in the work that causes injury.

The energy contained in a moving object is called <u>kinetic energy (KE)</u> and is calculated as follows: KE = half the mass times the velocity squared (v^2), that is, $1/2mv^2$, where m = mass (weight) and v = velocity (speed). Therefore, velocity influences KE more than mass. Remember that energy cannot be created or destroyed, only converted. The greater speed means more energy is generated. In the case of a motor vehicle crash, the KE of the speeding car is converted into the work of stopping the car, usually by crushing the car's exterior (Figure 12-1 ▶). Similarly, the passengers of the car have KE because they were traveling at the same speed as the car. Their KE is converted to the work of bringing them to a stop. It is this work on the passengers that results in injury. Notice that, according to the equation for KE, the energy that is available to cause injury doubles when an object's weight doubles but

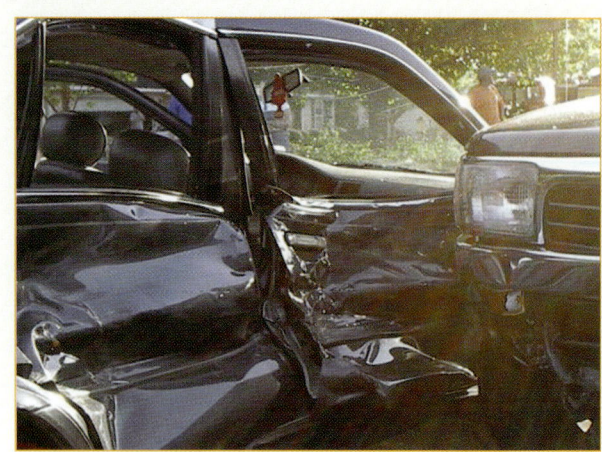

Figure 12-1 In a motor vehicle crash, the kinetic energy of the speeding car is converted, crushing the car's exterior.

quadruples when its speed doubles. Consider the debate over raising the speed limit. Increasing a car's speed from 50 to 70 mph doubles the energy that is available to cause injury. This point will be even clearer in considering gunshot wounds. The speed of the bullet (high-velocity compared with low-velocity) has a greater impact on producing injury than the mass (size) of the bullet. This is why it is so important to report to the hospital the type of firearm that was used in a shooting. The amount of KE that is converted to do work on the body dictates the severity of the injury. Energy can be absorbed, producing deformation of substance. High-energy injuries often produce such severe damage that patients can be saved only by immediate transport to an appropriate facility.

Potential energy is the product of mass (weight), force of gravity, and height and is mostly associated with the energy of falling objects. A worker on a scaffold has some potential energy because he or she is some height above the ground. When the worker falls, potential energy is converted into KE. As the worker hits the ground, the KE is converted into work, that is, the work of bringing the body to a stop and thereby breaking bones and damaging tissues.

> **EMT-I Tips**
>
> The Law of Conservation of Energy states that energy can be neither created nor destroyed, it can only change form. Think of it as being "conserved."

Energy Exchange

Cavitation occurs as the energy exchange produces particle motion. There is a temporary cavity that is short-lived and produced by stretching of the tissue surrounding the point of impact. The size of the cavity is dependent on the elasticity of the object involved. The energy exchange produces particle compression at the limits of the cavity. A permanent cavity may be produced by compression and destruction. It is visible when the energy exchange has been completed and the tissue does not return to its normal state. For energy exchange to occur, there must be an interaction between two bodies. At least one must be in motion, but both can be in motion. The exchange is dependent on the number of particles involved in the interface of the interaction. The amount of energy exchange is based on the density of the interacting bodies. Structures are classified according to three density categories: air, water, and solid. Those with air density have fewer particles, resulting in less damage. Examples include the lungs and intestinal tract. Water density structures consist of the vascular system, liver, spleen, and muscles. There are more particles, resulting in more significant injuries. Solid density structures, such as bones, have thick particles similar to asphalt and steel. In an energy exchange, they are more likely to splinter and fragment.

Another consideration of energy exchange is the area of interaction. The larger the area of impact, the greater the region of damage. The shape and position of the object affect the energy exchange and influence whether the object fragments.

Finally, the energy exchange of trauma is based on ingress. In blunt trauma, the tissue is not penetrated. Cavitation is away from the site of impact and in the direction of the impact. With penetrating trauma, the tissue is penetrated and cavitation is at a 90° angle to the bullet pathway. Tissue in line with the penetration is crushed. The extent of injury depends on the area impacted and structures located in that section.

Blunt and Penetrating Trauma

Traumatic injuries can be described in two separate categories: blunt trauma and penetrating trauma. Either type of trauma may occur from a variety of MOIs. It is important for the EMT-I to consider unseen as well as visible, obvious injuries with either type of trauma. Blunt trauma is the result of force (or energy transmission) to the body

> **EMT-I Tips**
>
> Do a "vehicle assessment" if circumstances at the scene allow it. There may be time for one EMT-I to circle the vehicle and assess for damage while the other EMT-I begins patient assessment.

that causes injury primarily without penetrating the soft tissues or internal organs and cavities. Penetrating trauma causes injury by objects that primarily pierce and penetrate the surface of the body and cause damage to soft tissues, internal organs, and body cavities.

Mechanism of Injury Profiles

Different types of MOI will produce many types of injuries. Some will involve an isolated body system; many will result in injury to more than one body system. Whether one body system or more than one system is involved, the EMT-I should maintain a high index of suspicion for serious unseen injuries. Injuries to trauma patients may be the result of falls, motor vehicle collisions, car versus pedestrian (or bicycle), gunshot wounds, and stabbings. These are a few of the common types of MOI patterns to which the EMT-I will respond to provide care and treatment to patients.

Blunt Trauma

Blunt force trauma results from an object making contact with the body. Motor vehicle crashes and falls are two of the most common MOIs for blunt trauma. Any object, for example a baseball bat, can cause blunt trauma if it is moving fast enough. The EMT-I should be alert to signs of skin discoloration or complaints of pain, as these may be the only signs of blunt trauma. The EMT-I should maintain a high index of suspicion during patient assessment for hidden injuries in the patient with blunt trauma.

Blunt Trauma: Vehicular Collisions

Motor vehicle crashes are classified traditionally as frontal (head-on), lateral (T-bone), rear-end, rotational (spins), and rollovers. The principal difference among these collision types is the direction of the force of impact; also, with spins and rollovers, there is the possibility of multiple impacts. Motor vehicle crashes typically consist of a series of three collisions. Understanding the events that occur during each collision will help you be alert for certain types of injury patterns. The three collisions in a frontal impact are as follows:

1. The collision of the car against another car, a tree, or some other object. Damage to the car is perhaps the most dramatic part of the collision, but it does not directly affect patient care, except possibly to make extrication difficult (Figure 12-2). However, it does provide information about the severity of the collision and, therefore, has an indirect effect on patient care. The greater the damage to the car, the greater the energy that was involved and, therefore, the greater the potential to cause injury to the patient. By assessing the body of a vehicle that has crashed, you can often determine the <u>mechanism of injury (MOI)</u>, which may allow you to predict what injuries may have happened to the passengers at the time of impact according to forces that acted on their bodies. When you arrive at the crash scene and perform your scene size up, quickly inspect the severity of damage to the vehicle(s). If there is significant damage to a vehicle, your index of suspicion for the presence of life-threatening injuries should automatically increase. A great amount of force is required to crush and deform a vehicle, cause intrusion into the passenger compartment, tear seats from their mountings, and collapse steering wheels. Such

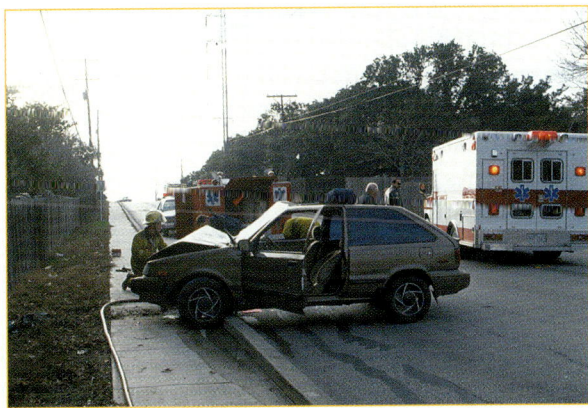

Figure 12-2 The first collision in a frontal impact is that of the car against another object (in this case, a utility pole). The appearance of the car can provide you with critical information about the severity of the crash. The greater the damage to the car, the greater the energy that was involved.

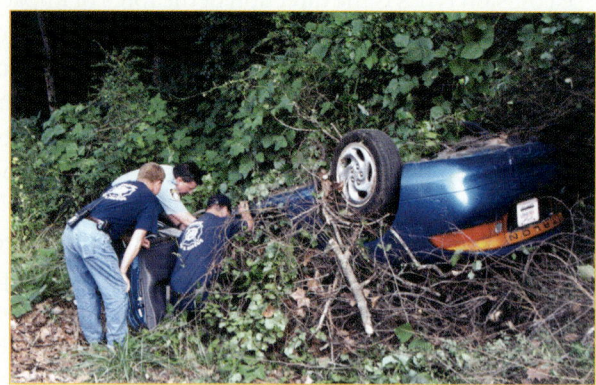

Figure 12-3 The second collision in a frontal impact is that of the passenger against the interior of the car. Examining the interior of the vehicle may give you clues to hidden injuries.

damage suggests the presence of high-energy trauma.

2. **The collision of the passenger against the interior of the car.** Just as the KE produced by the car's mass and velocity is converted into the work of bringing the car to a stop, the kinetic energy produced by the passenger's mass and velocity is converted into the work of stopping his or her body Figure 12-3. Just like the obvious damage to the exterior of the car, the injuries that result are often dramatic and usually immediately apparent during your initial assessment. Common injuries include lower extremity fractures (knees into the dashboard), flail chest (rib cage into the steering wheel), and head trauma (head into the windshield). Such injuries occur more frequently if the passenger is not restrained. But even when the passenger is restrained with a properly adjusted seat belt, injuries can occur, especially in lateral and rollover impacts.

3. **The collision of the passenger's internal organs against the solid structures of the body.** The injuries that occur during the third collision may not be as obvious as external injuries, but they are often the most life threatening. There are two types of organ injuries from blunt trauma: compression and changes in velocity. Compression injuries occur as the organs strike the interior of the body during the initial impact. Change-in-velocity injuries occur during acceleration as the organs move forward for the first impact and during deceleration as the organs pull against their attachments, risking separation and tearing. Injuries may be due to shearing as the organs pull against vessels and supporting structures, or organs may be avulsed. For example, as the passenger's head hits the windshield, the brain continues to move forward until it comes to rest by striking the inside of the skull. This results in compression injury (or bruising) to the anterior portion of the brain and stretching (or tearing) of the posterior portion of the brain Figure 12-4. Remember that for every action, there is an equal and opposite reaction. As the brain strikes the front of the skull, the body begins its path of moving backward. The head falls back against the headrest and/or seat, and the brain slams into the rear of the skull. Damage is produced to both the front and rear of the brain. This type of injury is known as a coup-contrecoup injury. The same type of injury may occur on opposite sides of the brain in a lateral collision. Similarly, in the thoracic cage, the heart may slam into the sternum, occasionally rupturing the aorta and causing fatal bleeding.

Understanding the relationship among the three collisions will help you to make the connections between the amount of damage to the exterior of the car and potential injury to the passenger. For example, in a high-speed collision that results in massive damage to the car, you should suspect serious injuries to the passengers,

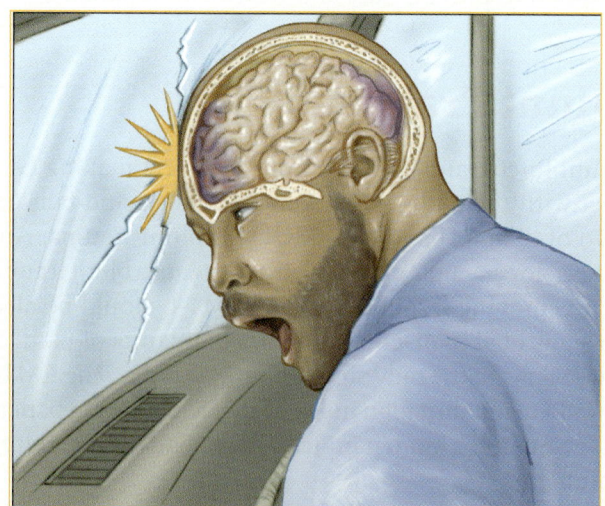

Figure 12-4 The third collision in a frontal impact is that of the passenger's internal organs against the solid structures of the body. In this illustration, the brain continues its forward motion and strikes the inside of the skull, resulting in a compression injury to the anterior portion of the brain and stretching of the posterior portion.

even if the injuries are not readily apparent. A number of potential physical problems may develop as a result of traumatic injuries. Your quick initial assessment of the patient and the evaluation of the mechanism of injury can help to direct lifesaving care and provide critical information to the hospital staff (Table 12-2 ▼). Therefore, if you see a contusion on the patient's forehead and the windshield is cracked and pushed out, you should strongly suspect an injury to the brain. After you inform medical control about the windshield, hospital staff can prepare the patient by ordering a computed tomographic (CT) scan of the brain. Without your input, the physician might have found the brain injury anyway, but it might not have been detected until the brain had swollen sufficiently to cause clinical signs of the injury. It is essential to report vehicle damage to hospital staff. This helps to assure that the patient receives optimal care for occult injuries that may not present until it is too late.

TABLE 12-2	Recognizing Developing Problems in Trauma Patients
Problem	**Signs and Symptoms or Mechanism of Injury**
Airway Obstruction	Noisy or labored respirations may indicate one or more of the following:
	Significant bleeding into the mouth, back of the throat, or nose
	Swelling or bleeding following blunt or penetrating trauma to the face
	Swelling about the neck (may compress the airway) following blunt or penetrating trauma to the neck
	Inability to swallow, resulting in possible choking on secretions
	Partial airway obstruction secondary to teeth or blood clots
Breathing Problems	Significant chest pain following blunt trauma
	Any penetrating trauma to the chest, unless it is a superficial cut (Remember to check the back too.)
	Bent or crushed steering wheel or deployed air bag, indicating blunt trauma to the chest
Hidden Blood Loss	Bruising, redness, abrasions, or obvious trauma to the upper abdomen
	Abdominal distention or rigidity
	Significant mechanism of injury, including blunt and penetrating trauma
	Obvious bruising, redness, or abrasions in the area of the pelvis
	Tenderness on gentle palpation of the pelvis
Damage to Major Vessels	Blunt or penetrating trauma to the neck, chest, or groin area (which could tear the major vessels in these areas)
	Bent or crushed steering wheel, indicating blunt trauma to the chest
Damage to the Heart	Bent or crushed steering wheel, indicating blunt trauma to the chest
Brain Injury	History of losing consciousness, inability to recall what happened, dazed appearance, confusion, disorientation, combativeness after the traumatic incident
	Slurred speech
	Difficulty moving the extremities
	Severe headache, especially if accompanied by nausea and vomiting
	Obvious blunt or penetrating trauma to the head, other than superficial cuts
	Appearance of intoxication; signs and symptoms (especially head trauma) may be masked by the effects of alcohol
	Cracked windshield, indicating that the patient's head flexed forward and struck the windshield with significant force
Possible Spinal Injury	Severe neck or back pain
	Difficulty moving or feeling the extremities
	Starred windshield, indicating that the patient's head flexed forward and struck the windshield with significant force

> **Documentation Tips**
>
> In trauma, mechanism of injury is a crucial element of patient history. Combine your knowledge of kinematics with observations at the scene to paint a verbal picture for later caregivers in the "History" section of your written report.

> **In the Field**
>
> Any death in the passenger compartment resulting from a collision is an indication of a significant mechanism of injury.

The amount of damage that is considered significant varies, depending on the type of collision, but any substantial deformity of the vehicle should be enough cause for you to consider transporting the patient to a trauma center. Significant mechanisms of injury include the following:

- Severe deformities of the frontal part of a vehicle, with or without intrusion into the passenger compartment
- Moderate intrusions from a lateral (T-bone) type of accident
- Severe damage from the rear
- Collisions in which rotation is involved (rollovers and spins)

Damage to the vehicle that was involved and information obtained from patient assessment are not the only clues to crash severity. Clearly, if one or more of the passengers are dead, you should suspect that the other passengers have sustained serious injuries, even if the injuries are not obvious. Therefore, you should focus on assessing for and treating life-threatening injuries and providing transport to a trauma center, because these passengers have likely experienced the same amount of force that caused the death of the other passenger(s). Photographs of the crash scene may provide valuable information to the staff and treating physicians of the trauma center.

Frontal Collisions

Occupant Collisions

Understanding the mechanism of injury after a frontal collision first involves evaluation of the supplemental restraint system, including seat belts and air bags. You should determine whether the passenger was restrained by a full and properly applied three-point restraint. In addition, you should determine whether the air bag was deployed. Identifying the types of restraints used and whether air bags were deployed will help you identify

You are the Provider 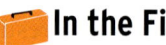 Part 2

The scene has been determined to be safe, and there is only the one victim, a woman. You approach the patient, and your partner assumes manual stabilization of the patient's cervical spine. Your initial assessment reveals the following findings:

Initial Assessment	Recording Time: Zero Minutes
Appearance	Pale and diaphoretic; obvious bleeding from a scalp laceration
Level of consciousness	Responds to pain by moaning
Airway	Open and clear
Breathing	Respirations, increased and shallow
Circulation	Skin, clammy; radial pulse, rapid and weak

After controlling the bleeding from the patient's head and rapidly removing her from the car, your partner begins immediate airway management as you perform a rapid trauma assessment.

3. What should you consider when determining the most appropriate facility to transport this patient to?
4. Why are rollover crashes particularly dangerous for restrained and unrestrained passengers?

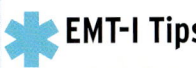

EMT-I Tips

Never place yourself or your patient in front of an undeployed airbag. Even if the battery cables are disconnected, a charge can be held in the line allowing the airbag to deploy at a later time, causing potentially severe injuries.

injury patterns that occur related to the supplemental restraint systems.

When properly applied, seat belts are successful in restraining the passengers in a vehicle and preventing a second collision inside the motor vehicle. In addition, they may decrease the severity of the third collision, that of the passenger's organs with the chest or abdominal wall. The very presence of air bags allows seat belts to provide even more "ride down," or the gentle cushioning of the occupant as the body slows, or decelerates. Air bags provide the final capture point of the passengers and again decrease the severity of deceleration injuries by allowing seat belts to be more compliant and by cushioning the occupant as he or she moves forward.

Remember that air bags decrease injury to the chest, face, and head very effectively. However, you should still suspect that other serious injuries to the extremities (resulting from the second collision) and to internal organs (resulting from the third collision) have occurred.

Most new motor vehicles are manufactured with airbag safety systems. These safety devices enhance the safety and survival of forward-facing occupants inside the vehicle during a collision. In an emergency braking event, or collision, the airbag inflates very quickly. Because a rear-facing car seat is in close proximity to the dashboard, rapid inflation of the airbag could cause serious injury or death to an infant. The National Highway Traffic Safety Administration (NHTSA) recommends children under the age of 1 year or less than 20 pounds should not ride in the front passenger seat of a vehicle when passenger-side air safety systems are present. In fact, NHTSA recommends that all children should ride in a rear-facing seat if a passenger-side airbag safety system is present to reduce the chance of serious injury.

When you are rendering care to an occupant inside a motor vehicle, it is important to remember that if the airbag system did not inflate, it may deploy during extrication. If this occurs, you may be seriously injured or even killed. Extreme caution must be used when extricating a patient in a vehicle with an airbag that has not deployed. You should also remember that supplemental restraint systems could cause harm whether they are used properly or improperly. For example, some older models have seat belts that buckle automatically at the shoulder but require the passengers to buckle the lap portion; these can result in the body "submarining" forward underneath the shoulder restraint when the lap portion is not attached. This movement of the body can cause the lower extremities and the pelvis to crash into the dashboard, as that part of the body is unrestrained. The feet may impact the floor pan, and the knees may impact the dash. Injuries sustained as the tibia impacts the dash can include knee dislocation, popliteal artery disruption, and knee support disruption. Femur impact may result in femur fractures or acetabular posterior fracture disruption. As the torso rotates, the body may impact the steering column, dash, or windshield. In addition, individuals of short stature can sustain significant neck and facial injuries, including decapitation, caused by the belting systems when their lower torso is unrestrained.

If the patient is unrestrained and involved in a frontal collision, he or she may be thrown up and over the steering wheel, resulting in the head impacting the windshield, roof, or rearview mirror. The chest may impact the steering column or dash, and the abdomen may also strike the steering column or dash. If the patient is driving, the femurs or pelvis may sustain significant injury as contact is made with the bottom of the steering wheel. See Table 12-3 ▶ for more injury patterns.

When passengers are riding in vehicles equipped with air bags but are not restrained by seat belts, they are often thrown forward in the act of emergency braking. As a result, they come into contact with the air bag and/or the doors at the time of deployment. This mechanism of injury is also responsible for some severe injuries to children who are riding unrestrained in the front seats of vehicles. In addition, some passengers may pass out before impact, and you may find them lying against the air bag when it deploys. You should look for abrasions and/or traction-type injuries on the face, lower part of the neck, and chest Figure 12-5 ▶.

Contact points are often obvious from a simple, quick evaluation of the interior of the vehicle. If there is no intrusion, you might see that an unrestrained front-seat passenger in a frontal collision will come into contact with the dashboard or instrument panel at the knees and transfer energy from the knees through the femur

TABLE 12-3 Frontal Collision Injury Patterns

Up-and-Over Pathway Injuries
- Head injuries
- Spine injuries
- Chest injuries
  - Rib fractures or flail chest
  - Pneumothorax
  - Hemothorax
  - Contusions
  - Great vessel injury
    - Vena cava
    - Aorta
- Abdominal injuries
  - Solid organs
  - Hollow organs
  - Diaphragm
- Fractured pelvis

Down-and-Under Pathway Injuries
- Posterior knee and hip dislocations
- Femur fractures
- Lower extremity fractures
- Pelvic and acetabular fractures

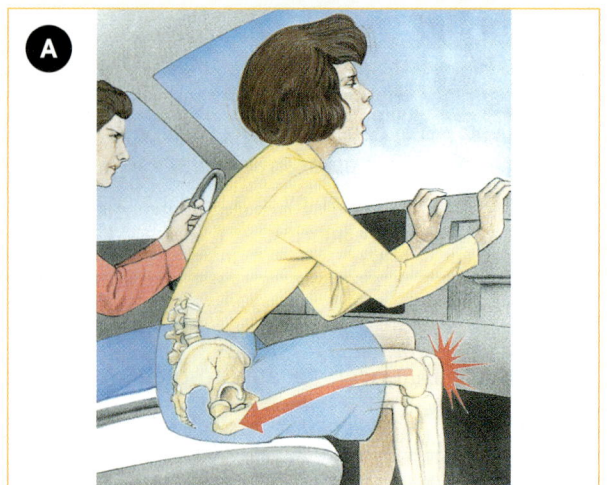

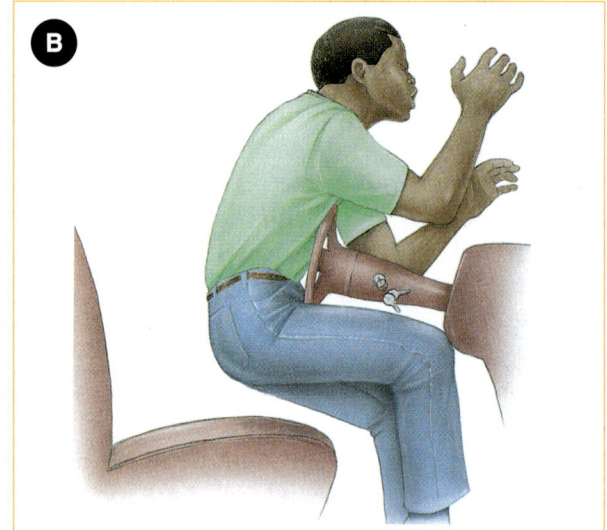

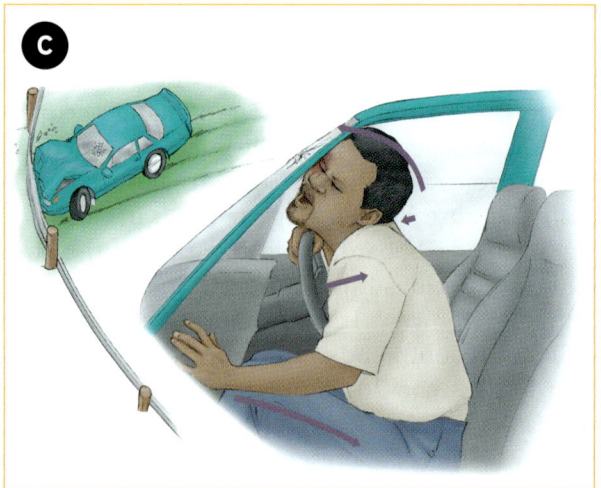

to the pelvis and hip joint (Figure 12-6A). The chest and/or abdomen may also hit the steering wheel (Figure 12-6B). In addition, the passenger's face often hits the steering wheel or may launch forward and up, hitting the windshield and/or the roof header in the area of the visors (Figure 12-6C). Signs of most of these injuries can be found by simply inspecting the interior of the vehicle during extrication of the patient.

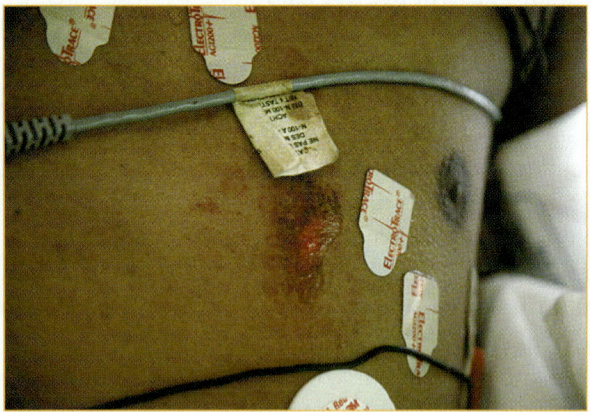

Figure 12-5 Air bags can cause injury in frontal collisions, specifically, abrasions and traction-type injuries to the face, neck, and chest.

Figure 12-6 Mechanism of injury and condition of the vehicle interior suggest likely areas of injury. **A.** The knee can strike the dashboard, resulting in a hip fracture or dislocation. **B.** Serious chest and abdominal injuries can result from striking the steering wheel. **C.** Head and spinal injuries can result when the face and head strike the windshield.

Organ Collisions

Compression injuries to the head in a frontal collision can result in skull fractures and cerebral contusions as the brain impacts the skull. On the opposite side of the skull, the brain may separate from the supporting structures, causing hemorrhage and stretching of the brain stem. The neck can sustain compression fractures, hyperextension injuries, or hyperflexion injuries. Hyperextension can cause posterior element compression and/or anterior body separation as the head is thrown excessively backward. Hyperflexion may cause anterior body compression and/or posterior element separation as the head is thrown excessively forward. Shearing injuries are not significant in the neck since it does not contain organs.

> **A to Z Terminology Tips**
>
> Remember, <u>hyper</u> = high or excessive; hyperextension = excessive extension (The head is bent backward as the neck hyperextends.); hyperflexion = excessive flexing (The chin is bent forward onto the chest as the neck is hyperflexed.)

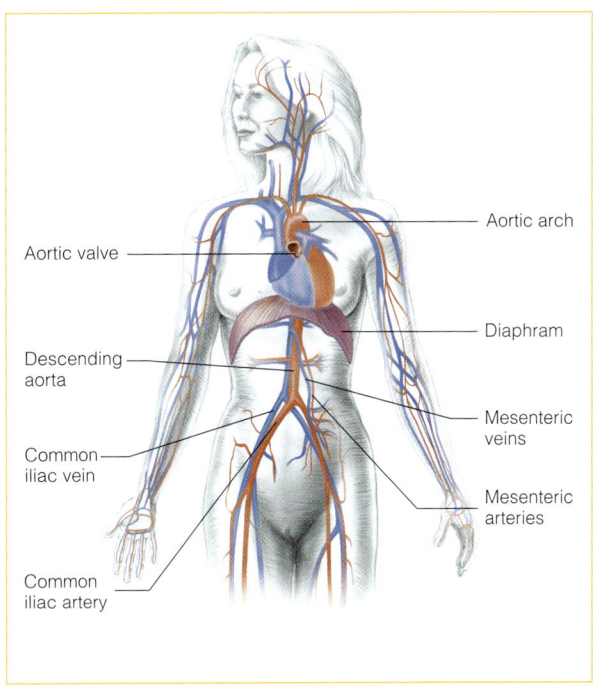

Figure 12-7 Areas that may stretch or tear include the origin of the aorta at the aortic valve, the junction between the arch and descending portions, and the level of the diaphragm.

Any serious injury to the chest or thorax has the potential to be fatal. As the body moves forward and impacts the airbag, steering wheel, or dash, compression may result in rib fracture(s), flail chest, pneumothorax, myocardial contusion or rupture, and possible puncture of the lung due to rib penetration. A pneumothorax may be the consequence of lung puncture by a fractured rib or the "paper bag effect." Aside from injuries caused by the actual impact, shearing injuries occur as structures are stretched. The thoracic spine may be fractured, or the aorta may tear. Because the aorta originates from the left ventricle of the heart and travels down through the midline of the abdomen, there are several areas that may stretch or tear. Less protected or weak areas include the origin of the aorta at the aortic valve, the junction arch and descending portions, and the level of the diaphragm **Figure 12-7 ▲**.

The abdominal cavity begins with the diaphragm as the superior border. The diaphragm, along with the abdominal wall, may sustain compression tears. Neither the diaphragm nor the abdominal wall present with significant shearing injuries. The solid organs, the liver and spleen, may burst, causing severe bleeding, and the hollow organs, the gall bladder and intestines, may rupture on impact, spilling their contents into the abdominal cavity. Shearing may cause tears from the ligamentum teres hepatis, which extends from the liver, or an avulsion of the liver from the inferior vena cava at the hepatic veins. There may be an avulsion of the pedicle, or stem, of the spleen. Avulsion of mesenteric vessels from the aorta or vena cava, tears along the mesenteric vessels, or avulsion of vessels from the intestines may also occur, as may avulsion of the gallbladder from the liver or avulsion of a cystic duct.

> **✳ EMT-I Tips**
>
> The "paper bag effect" occurs when the patient sees a crash about to happen and gasps, drawing a great deal of air into the lungs. On impact, the lungs "pop," as if you blew up a paper bag and smashed it against your hand.

> **A to Z Terminology Tips**
>
> The <u>mesentery</u> is the peritoneal fold that surrounds the small intestine and connects it to the posterior abdominal wall. Other abdominal organs also have a mesentery.

Rear-End Collisions

Occupant Collisions

Rear-end impacts are known to cause whiplash-type injuries, particularly when the head and/or neck is not restrained by an appropriately placed headrest (Figure 12-8 ▼). On impact, the vehicle seat pushes the body and torso forward. All body parts in contact with the seat move, and those that are not in contact with the seat are dragged along with the torso. As the body is propelled forward, the head and neck are left behind because a headrest does not restrain them, and they appear to be whipped back relative to the torso. As the vehicle comes to rest, the unrestrained passenger moves forward, striking the dashboard. In this type of collision, the cervical spine and surrounding area may be injured. The cervical spine is less tolerant of damage when it is extended. Other parts of the spine and the pelvis may also be at risk for injury. In addition, the patient may sustain an acceleration-type injury to the brain, that is, the third collision of the brain within the skull. Passengers in the back seat wearing only a lap belt might have a higher incidence of injuries to the thoracic and lumbar spine. If there is a secondary impact of the vehicle striking another object in front of it, look for injuries similar to those from a frontal impact.

Organ Collisions

The energy (velocity) imparted to the rear of the vehicle moves all of the attached parts of the vehicle in the same direction of travel. Occupants in direct contact with the vehicle move as well. The parts of the occupants not in direct contact with the vehicle do not move until pulled along. This is based on Newton's first law of motion. Unrestricted body parts will be separated or at least stretched by this differential velocity. The force of the energy exchange depends on the differential energy of the two vehicles and the exchange of energy between the two.

As the head is forced into structures behind the seat, compression injuries may occur to the occipital portion of the brain and skull. The energy of compression depends on the force of the change of energy between the vehicle and the impact into the head. Shearing forces may cause the separation of the brain and skull in the frontal portion. Compression injuries of the neck may occur as the unrestrained occupant is thrown into the top of the passenger compartment or into the rear of the seat. If the head restraint is not in the correct position to move the head forward with the motion of the vehicle, shearing injuries occur as the neck is hyperextended over the malpositioned head restraint. Usually ligaments and tendons stretch, without any resulting fractures.

Because most of the torso is in contact with the seat and springs of the seat, only minimal differential energy is exchanged onto the body parts. Unless there is rebound when the vehicle hits another vehicle, there is little injury to the torso. The extremities move with the torso and receive very little differential exchange.

Lateral Collisions

Occupant Collisions

Lateral impacts are probably now the number one cause of death associated with motor vehicle crashes. When a vehicle is struck from the side, it is typically struck above its center of gravity and begins to rock away from the side of the impact. The vehicle moves into the body. This results in a lateral whiplash injury (Figure 12-9 ▶). The movement is to the side, and the passenger's shoulders and head whip toward the intruding vehicle. This

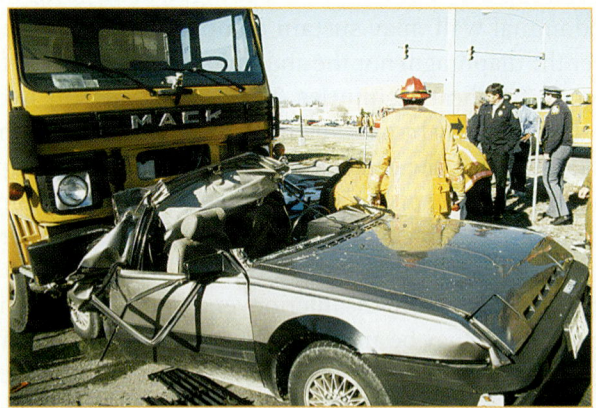

Figure 12-8 Rear-end impacts often cause whiplash-type injuries, particularly when the head and/or neck are not restrained by a headrest.

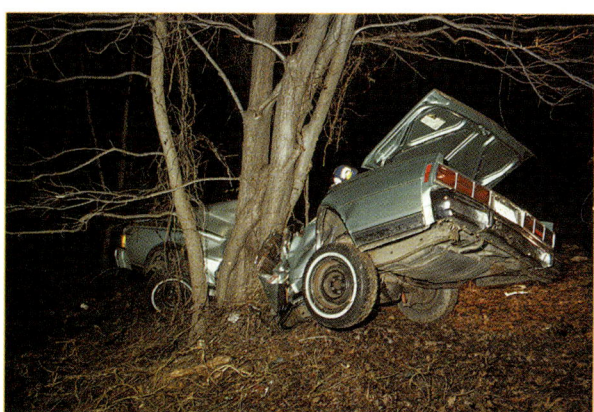

Figure 12-9 In a lateral collision, the car is typically struck above its center of gravity and begins to rock away from the side of impact. This causes a type of lateral whiplash in which the passenger's shoulders and head whip toward the intruding vehicle.

action may thrust the shoulder, thorax, upper extremity, and, more important, the skull, against the doorpost or the window. The patient could experience rotation of the neck, lateral flexion, or a combination of both. Because the cervical spine is relatively unstable, it has little tolerance for lateral bending.

If there is substantial intrusion into the passenger compartment, you should suspect lateral chest and abdominal injuries on the side of the impact, as well as possible fractures of the lower extremities, pelvis, and ribs. In addition, the organs within the abdomen are at risk because of a possible third collision. Approximately 25% of all severe injuries to the aorta that occur in motor vehicle crashes are a result of lateral collisions.

Organ Collisions

Compression injuries to the head in a lateral collision are similar to those in a frontal impact. The difference involves the side-to-side instead of front-to-rear motion. A coup-contrecoup injury occurs, but the parietal portions of the brain are injured. Shearing of the brain and vessels opposite the side of the impact occurs as the brain shifts. The cervical spine is at great risk in lateral collisions. Compression injury is minimal unless the head hits the top of the passenger compartment or the support for the windows. Shearing injuries are highly likely because the cervical spine is the weakest portion of the spinal column, allowing for excessive movement. The center of gravity of the head is anterior to the pivot point of the head and the spine at the odontoid process, the toothlike process that extends upward from the axis (C2) and about which the atlas (C1) rotates. As lateral impact occurs, the torso and then the cervical spine are forced under the head, out of normal alignment. The head rotates in relative position to the body, toward the impact. The center of gravity of the head is also superior to the point of support at the cervical spine. As the lateral forces push the torso away from the point of impact, the motion of the head produces lateral flexion of the head. The combination of these two forces is lateral flexion of the neck, opening the facets opposite the side of impact and rotating the vertebral bodies in relation to each other. If the force is great enough, significant torsion (twisting) of the spinal cord occurs.

Impact of the door into the thorax can cause compression of the lateral ribs, resulting in fractures and flail chest, a punctured lung resulting in pneumothorax, and spleen or liver lacerations, resulting in hemorrhage. With the lateral motion of the thoracic spine, the torso is pushed away from the impact. The thoracic aorta moves with the spine. The aortic arch and heart do not move until traction is pulled on the arch. Shearing forces tear the aorta at the junction of the movable arch and the descending aorta that is attached to the thoracic spine.

Depending on the side of the impact, the liver, spleen, or kidneys may be compressed, causing rupture or avulsion. Compression injuries of the diaphragm are similar to those sustained in a frontal impact. The abdominal aorta moves with the lumbar spine, producing shearing of the renal and splenic vessels. Impact on the femur may result in the femoral head being driven through the acetabulum or fracture of the ileum, sacroiliac joint, or other bones of the pelvis. Lateral force may also result in the clavicle being compressed between the humerus and sternum and/or lateral compression of the humerus on the side of the impact. There are no significant shearing injuries of the pelvis or extremities.

Rollover Crashes

Certain vehicles, such as large trucks and some sport utility vehicles, are more prone to rollover crashes due to their high center of gravity. Injury patterns that are commonly associated with rollover crashes differ, depending on whether the passenger was restrained. Body impacts are difficult to predict. An unrestrained passenger may have sustained multiple strikes within the interior of the vehicle as it rolled one or more times **Figure 12-10**. The pattern of injuries is very difficult to predict because the unrestrained occupant can hit all parts of the vehicle. The most common life-threatening

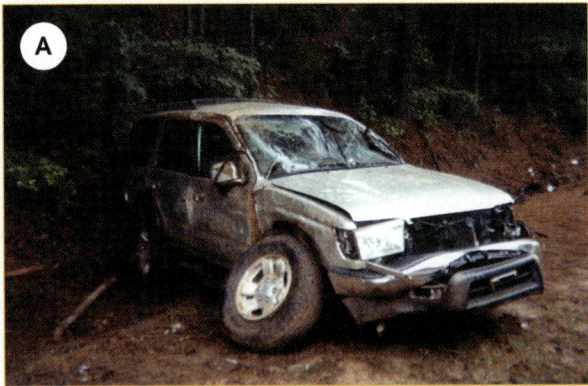

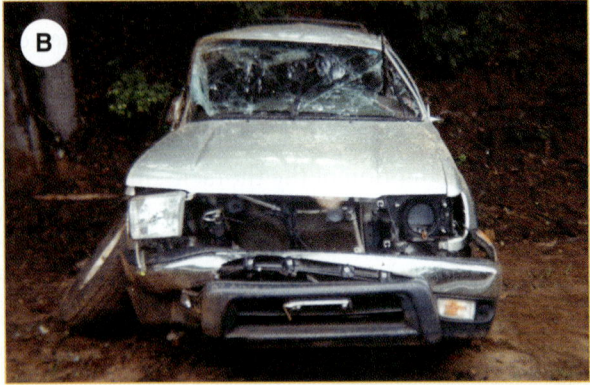

Figure 12-10 Expect multiple injury patterns in rollovers because of the various points of impact. **A.** Side view. **B.** Front view.

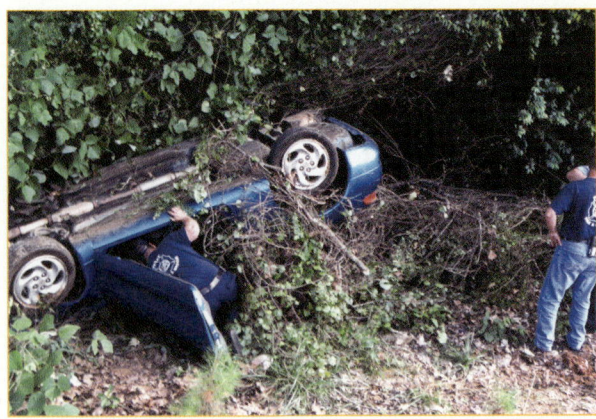

Figure 12-11 Look for clues, such as purses or car seats, that may indicate that there were other passengers who were ejected or wandered away.

event in a rollover is ejection or partial ejection of the passenger from the vehicle. Passengers who have been ejected may have struck the interior of the vehicle many times before ejection. The passenger may also have struck several objects, such as trees, a guardrail, or the vehicle's exterior, before landing. Passengers who have been partially ejected may have struck both the interior and exterior of the vehicle and may have been sandwiched between the exterior of the vehicle and the ground as the vehicle rolled. Ejection and partial ejection are significant mechanisms of injury; in these instances, you should prepare to care for life-threatening injuries **Figure 12-11**.

Even when restrained, passengers can sustain severe injuries during a rollover crash, although the patterns of injury tend to be more predictable, and when properly used, the restraint system will prevent ejection from the vehicle. A passenger on the outboard side of a vehicle that rolls over is at high risk for injury because of the centrifugal force (the patient is pinned against the door of the vehicle). When the roof hits the ground during a rollover, a passenger who is restrained can still move far enough toward the roof to make contact and sustain a spinal cord injury.

If the force is such in a rollover and the occupant is unrestrained, then ejection is possible. The major injuries occur inside the vehicle and on the way out rather than afterward on impact with the ground or some other object. Because the major part of the injuries occur on the way out, the EMT-I can better predict injuries by focusing on the first part of the collision rather than the latter portion. Therefore, rollover crashes are particularly dangerous for both restrained and, to a greater degree, unrestrained passengers because these crashes provide multiple opportunities for second and third collisions. In addition, the risk of death is 25 times greater if the occupant is ejected from the vehicle.

Rotational Impacts

Spins are conceptually similar to rollovers. The rotation of the vehicle as it spins provides opportunities for the vehicle to strike objects such as utility poles. Part of the vehicle stops, while the rest remains in motion. Injuries are the result of a combination of frontal and lateral impacts. For example, as a vehicle spins and strikes a pole, the passengers experience not only the rotational motion, but also a lateral impact.

In the pure rotational impact, one part of the vehicle hits an immovable object, while the rest continues in motion. This is an example of Newton's first law of motion: An object in motion will remain in motion until acted on by an outside force. As one part of the vehicle stops and the rest of the vehicle continues to move, the vehicle moves around the fixed point. The motion to the occupant is a combination of two motions: frontal and lateral, and rear and lateral. The injuries are combinations of the two motions with emphasis on the initial impact motion.

Restraints

Restraints are systems for absorbing the energy of the impact before the occupant hits something hard and for limiting the distance the body has to travel, thus helping to decrease velocity (speed). Common restraint systems include belt restraints, shoulder restraints, air bags, and child safety seats Figure 12-12 ▼.

Lap Belts

Contrary to popular belief, the belt restraint works in lateral impacts as well as in frontal impacts. However, they are not quite as effective in lateral impacts because the more solid parts of the passenger compartment are closer on the sides than in the front. Therefore, the belt systems do not have as much distance to be effective. The benefit of the belt restraint can be seen at any automobile racetrack. Lap belts are attached to the floor behind the occupant at a 45° angle to the floor.

Lap belts hold the lower torso close to the seat and away from the dash or steering column. They prevent forward motion of the lower torso in frontal collisions. Lap belts hold the torso in place and move the torso with the vehicle and away from the impact in lateral collisions. Wearing lap belts helps to avoid multiple impacts in rollover collisions and holds the occupant inside the vehicle, preventing ejection. Forward motion of the pelvis is held in check by the belt supporting the anterior part of the pelvis. Also, if the lap belt is worn properly, there is no impingement on the soft intra-abdominal contents.

There are, however, limitations with lap belts. Without shoulder belts, the upper torso is not supported. The pelvis is held in place, but the upper body is still thrown forward. If the lap belt is positioned above the anterior iliac spine, the belt stops the forward motion of the body against the lumbar spine with the intra-abdominal organs crushed between the belt and the spine. A high lap belt position can fracture or dislocate the lumbar spine, and increased intra-abdominal pressure can rupture the diaphragm.

Shoulder Restraints

Shoulder belts prevent forward motion of the upper torso in frontal impact collisions. They also prevent hyperflexion of the upper torso around the lap belts, thus preventing spinal injuries. In lateral impacts, the shoulder restraints move the upper torso with the vehicle, restricting multiple collisions. If shoulder restraints are worn without the lap belt, neck injuries can occur. The benefits are also lessened if the seat is very close to the dash or steering column.

Air Bags

Air bags provide supplemental protection with properly positioned shoulder restraints and lap belts. Protection is based on where the air bags are located and what type of impact is sustained. Frontal bags provide frontal protection only. However, automobile manufacturers today are placing air bags throughout vehicles, such as within the doors to protect the patient from lateral collisions.

Unfortunately, air bags alone are minimally effective. They are designed to be used in conjunction with properly positioned lap and shoulder restraints and can produce significant injuries if too close to the occupant. There is no room for bag expansion and no protective cover for the face or chest. If children are standing, they may be thrown into the seat, producing cervical spine fractures. Facial and forearm abrasions are common as well.

When assessing a vehicle in which an air bag has deployed, it is imperative to check underneath the bag for any structural damage to the vehicle. A bent steering wheel should create a high index of suspicion that

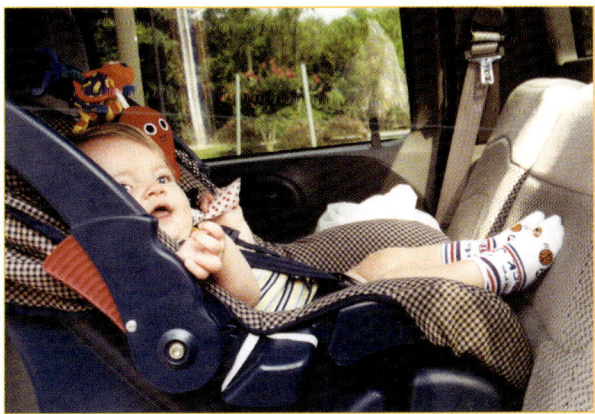

Figure 12-12 Secure infants in rear-facing car seats in the center of the back seat to protect from airbags.

the patient may have significant trauma to the thorax, even if it does not present externally. The deployed air bag can hide damage that may aid in assessment of the patient.

Child Safety Seats

There are various types of child safety seats on the market. The appropriate seat should be purchased based on the age and size of the child. Proper use is also imperative. A child in an unrestrained seat is no better off than one not in a safety seat at all. It is also important to place safety seats in the rear of the vehicle and as close to the center of the vehicle as possible. With proper use, injuries are limited. Infants should be placed with the safety seat facing the rear. *Never* place a child or infant in the front seat of a vehicle with air bags. If the child is not injured by the deployment of the air bag itself, he or she may suffocate underneath the air bag.

Motorcycle Collisions

Motorcycle collisions are especially dangerous because the rider has no surrounding structures to help protect him or her. In a frontal impact, the bike stops but the occupant continues forward. The initial impact is with the bike itself. The face, chest, abdomen, and femurs may be thrown into the handlebars and other parts of the motorcycle, creating various injuries. Because there are no restraints on a motorcycle, the rider is ejected over the handlebars of the bike. He or she may be thrown into the vehicle it collided with, onto the ground, or into objects in the path of travel. Injuries depend on how the occupant lands and on what type of surface. Cervical spine fractures are common, as are compound tibia-fibula fractures. Compression injuries of the torso may result in the crushing of solid organs and/or rupture of hollow organs. There may also be deceleration injuries of the aorta and organs with pedicles (stems).

If there is an angular impact, the patient may be trapped between the vehicle and bike. Trapped legs may be fractured and/or dislocated. There is lateral motion of the torso as it is thrown into the vehicle. Cervical spine injuries will be similar to those in a lateral impact. The torso may sustain compression injuries to the lateral chest and lateral abdomen and deceleration injuries of the aorta and pedicled organs.

Even though there are no restraints, there are measures riders can take for some protection. There is a 300% increase in brain injury in those who do not wear helmets. Helmets also provide a small amount of protection for the spine. Leather chaps and clothing are very protective during slides on asphalt, and strong boots help to protect the ankles and feet. The best protection for any rider is to stay alert for potential dangers and always ride in a safe manner.

You are the Provider — Part 3

After identifying and treating all immediately life-threatening injuries, you obtain the following set of vital signs:

Vital Signs	Recording Time: 2 Minutes
Respirations	32 breaths/min, shallow and labored (baseline); ventilation is being assisted by your partner
Pulse	124 beats/min, regular; radial pulses are weak
Skin	Pale, cool, diaphoretic
Blood pressure	88/52 mm Hg
SaO_2	95% with assisted ventilation and 100% oxygen

After the patient's spine is fully immobilized, she is quickly loaded into the ambulance and transported to a local trauma center. Additional treatment interventions are performed en route.

5. What are some of the potential problems that may develop in this patient that the EMT-I must be able to recognize and treat?

Pedestrian Versus Motor Vehicle

In accidents involving pedestrians, there are three phases of impact. Initially the vehicle-pedestrian impact occurs, the pedestrian rotates onto the hood, and then the pedestrian rolls off onto the ground. The injury pattern depends on the height of the pedestrian and the body area facing the impact.

In the first phase of the vehicle-pedestrian impact, the bumper typically strikes the legs. The feet tend to stay in place on the asphalt or ground while the bumper pushes the legs, with the torso moving after the legs. The torso and pelvis are crushed by the front of the vehicle. There may be lateral or posterior angulation with lumbar and/or thoracic fractures.

In the second phase, the pedestrian rotates onto the hood. Here, the impact is onto the torso. It is not uncommon to find compression injuries and shearing injuries in the torso. The cervical spine may experience severe anterior or lateral flexion, torsion, or fractures and dislocations.

In the third phase, the pedestrian rolls off of the vehicle and onto the ground or asphalt. If the pedestrian lands beside the vehicle, the impact into the ground will be the same as a fall from height. If the pedestrian falls in front of the vehicle, there is the potential to be run over or dragged by the vehicle. In either event, the pedestrian may experience any number of severe injuries.

Pediatric Needs

To evaluate the mechanism of injury when your patient is a child, remember this: Falls greater than three times the child's height indicate a significant mechanism of injury. Also note that small children are top heavy so they tend to land on their head even from small falls of a minimal height.

Geriatric Needs

Many geriatric patients are seriously injured from falls. Completely assess the older patient for all possible injuries, even from low-impact falls.

Patients who fall and land on their feet may have less severe internal injuries because their legs may have absorbed much of the energy of the fall Figure 12-13 ▼. Of course, as a result, they may have very serious injuries to the lower extremities, as well as pelvic and spinal injuries from energy that the legs do not absorb. The

Falls

The injury potential of a fall is related to the height from which the patient fell, the surface of the impact, objects struck during the fall, and the body part of first impact. The greater the height of the fall, the greater the potential for injury. A fall from more than 15′ or three times the patient's height is considered significant. The patient lands on the surface just as an unrestrained passenger smashes into the interior of a vehicle. The internal organs travel at the speed of the patient's body before it hits the ground and stop by smashing into the interior of the body. Again, as in a motor vehicle crash, it is these internal injuries that are the least obvious on assessment but pose the gravest threat to life. Therefore, you should suspect internal injuries in a patient who has fallen from a significant height, just as you would in a patient who has been in a high-speed motor vehicle crash. Always consider syncope or other underlying medical causes of the fall.

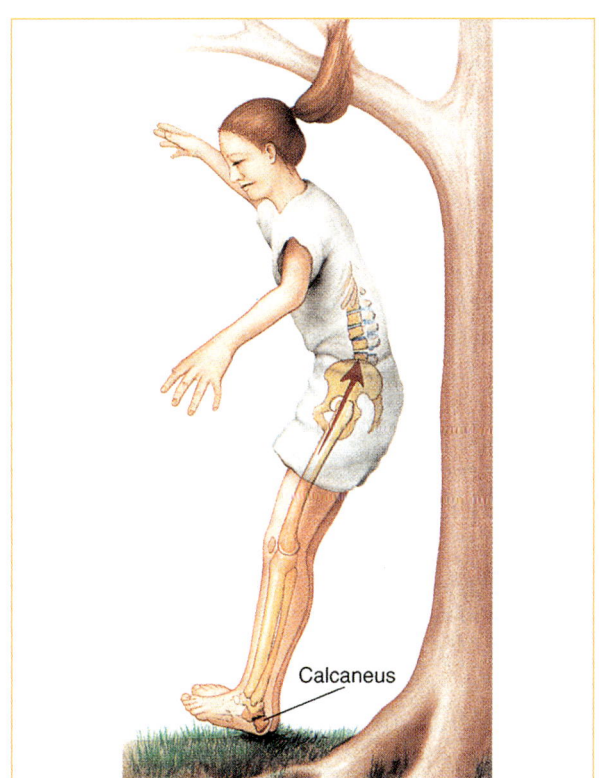

Figure 12-13 When a patient falls and lands on his or her feet, the energy is transmitted to the spine, sometimes producing a spine injury, as well as injuries to the legs and pelvis.

impact is initially on the calcaneus. The continued motion of the torso causes the energy to travel up through the ankles, knees, femur, acetabulum, pelvis, and spine. This can result in fractures and compression injuries of the spine. There may also be deceleration injuries to the liver, kidney, spleen, and aorta, similar to those seen in crashes.

Patients who fall onto their heads, as do children or victims of diving accidents, will likely have serious head and/or spinal injuries. In either case, a fall from a significant height is a serious event with great injury potential, and the patient should be evaluated thoroughly. Take the following factors into account:

- The height of the fall
- The surface struck
- Any object struck during the fall
- The part of the body that hit first, followed by the path of energy displacement

Head-first impact (or axial loading) may result in skull fractures from compression along with contusions or lacerations of the brain. There may also be compression injuries of the spine. The aorta, kidneys, and other organs may also sustain deceleration injuries if the fall is from a significant height. If the individual falls parallel to the ground, there may be compression injuries to all parts of the impact.

Some texts list falls as the most common form of trauma. Many falls, especially those by elderly people, are not considered "true" trauma, even though bones may be broken. Often, these falls occur as a result of a pathologic fracture. Elderly people often have osteoporosis, a condition in which the musculoskeletal system can fail under relatively low stress. Because of this condition, an elderly patient can sustain a fracture while in a standing position and then fall as a result. Therefore, an elderly patient may have actually sustained a fracture before the fall. These instances do not constitute true high-energy trauma unless the patient fell from a significant height.

EMT-I Tips

The nature and severity of injuries from falls are related to the height of the fall and the surface on which the individual lands.

Impact surface:
- Harder surface = greater injury

Height:
- Greater height = greater injury

Falls from a distance of more than three times the patient's height can produce critical injuries.

Penetrating Trauma

Penetrating trauma is the second leading cause of death in the United States after blunt trauma. It is classified as low energy, medium energy, or high energy (Table 12-4). Low-energy penetrating trauma may be caused accidentally by impalement or intentionally by a knife, ice pick, or other weapon (Figure 12-14). Many times it is difficult to determine entrance and exit wounds from projectiles in a prehospital setting (unless you can determine an obvious exit wound). Determine the number of penetrating injuries and combine that with the important things you already know about the potential pathway of penetrating projectiles to form an index of suspicion about unseen life-threatening injuries. With low-energy penetrations, injuries are caused by the sharp edges of the object moving through the body and are, therefore, close to the object's path. Weapons such as knives, however, may have been deliberately moved around internally, causing more damage than the external wound might suggest.

In medium-velocity and high-velocity penetrating trauma, the path of the object (usually a bullet) may not be as easy to predict. This is because the bullet may flatten out, tumble, or even ricochet within the body before exiting. In addition, because of its speed, pressure waves emanate from the bullet, causing damage remote from its path. This phenomenon, called cavitation, can result in serious injury to internal organs dis-

TABLE 12-4	Energy
Level of Energy	**Description**
Low energy	Hand-driven weapons such as knives, scissors, and ice picks. There is minimal cavitation, and the damage is only by the cutting edge.
Medium energy	Low-velocity weapons such as handguns and low-powered firearms (such as .38 special, .45 ATC [authorization to carry]) in which the muzzle velocity is less than 1,500' per second. The projectile is small, and cavitation is 6 to 10 times the bullet's frontal area.
High energy	High-velocity weapons such as high-powered rifles and military high-velocity, small-caliber weapons such as M16 or AK47. These have a muzzle velocity greater than 1,500' per second. Cavitation is 20 to 30 times the frontal area of the missile.

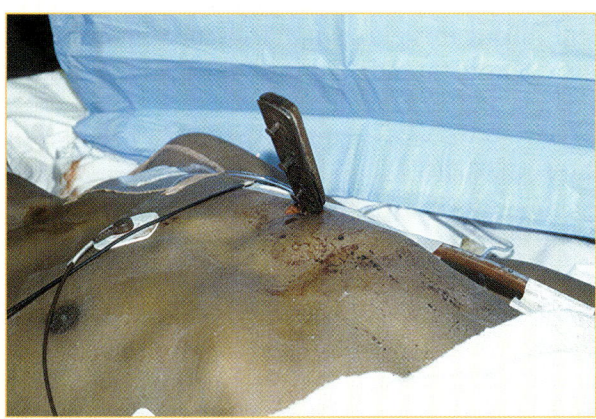

Figure 12-14 Injuries from low-energy penetrations, such as stab wounds, are caused by the sharp edges of the object moving through the body.

tant to the actual path of the bullet. Much like a boat moving through water, the bullet disrupts not only the tissues that are directly in its path, but also those in its wake. Temporarily, there is a compression wave of tissue particles away from the pathway of the bullet. It lasts only a few microseconds, and tissue damage is produced by stretching. Permanent damage occurs as tissue is crushed and is visible when examined. Therefore, the area that is damaged by medium- and high-velocity projectiles can be many times larger than the diameter of the projectile itself (Figure 12-15 ▼). This is one reason that exit wounds are often much larger than entrance wounds. As with motor vehicle crashes, the energy available for a bullet to cause damage is more a function of its speed than its mass (weight). If the mass of the bullet is doubled, the energy that is available to cause injury is doubled. If the speed (velocity) of the bullet is doubled, the energy that is available to cause injury is quadrupled. For this reason, it is important for you to try to determine the type of weapon that was used. Although it is not necessary (or always possible) for you to distinguish between medium- and high-velocity injuries, any information regarding the type of weapon that was used should be relayed to medical control. Police at the scene may be a useful source of information regarding the caliber of weapon.

Remember that $KE = \frac{1}{2} m \times v^2$. The velocity of the weapon is more important than the mass. The energy used to place the mass in motion must be completely exchanged into the body tissues to stop the mass (Mass × Acceleration = Force = Mass × Deceleration). Therefore, the greater the energy, the greater the force applied to the tissues, and, thus, the greater the injury.

The energy exchange is based on the number of particles involved or the density of tissue and the area of interaction. The more dense the tissue, the more damage that is done. Gas-filled organs such as the lungs and gastrointestinal tract sustain less injury than liquid-filled and solid organs. The blood vessels, muscles, and solid organs such as the spleen, liver, and kidneys are denser, resulting in greater tissue damage from penetrating injuries and a potential for massive hemorrhage. Bones are also very dense and have a tendency to fragment, creating more extensive trauma. Bones may splinter and penetrate other organs, tissues, or vessels.

The area of interaction has to do with the deformation of the bullet, tumbling, and fragmentation. As the bullet changes shape, it increases the area of damage. Tumbling projectiles, such as those from a rifle barrel, cause a larger area of cavitation as they rotate through the tissue. Fragmenting ammunition intensifies the damage by acting in the same manner as shrapnel from a grenade. All of these amplify the area of injury and increase the potential for damage to vital organs.

Organs injured in a gunshot wound vary depending on the pathway of the projectile. There is an entrance wound, and, if the bullet goes completely through, an exit wound as well. The entrance wound is characterized by a round or oval hole that is crushed inward. The rim is usually 1 to 2 mm wide and dark because of the grease or other substance on the bullet. There may be an abrasion produced by the spinning of the bullet. The size of the abrasion depends on the contact with the skin. It will be larger when the impact is at an angle. If the end of the weapon is within 4 to 6 inches from the skin, there may also be burns from the flame emitted from the barrel. In contrast, the exit wound is pushed

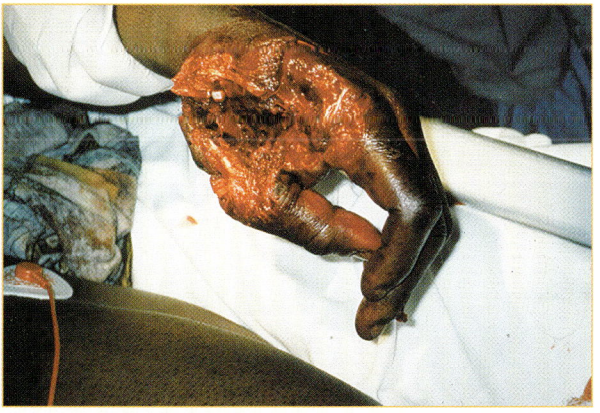

Figure 12-15 The zone of injury that results from high-velocity projectiles, such as bullets, can be many times larger than the diameter of the projectile itself.

outward and, rather than being round, may be stellate (star-shaped) or a slit.

Blast Injuries

The blast effect is broken down into three phases according to the type of force that occurs during that phase. Each phase has a different energy pattern. Injuries tend to be in direct proportion to the force of the explosion.

The primary phase is the pressure wave of the blast. This causes tearing or rupturing of gas-containing organs. The lungs and intestinal tract are typically affected during this phase. Aside from rupture of the organs, pulmonary bleeding and air emboli may also occur. The heat wave produced may cause burns on unprotected parts of the body, such as the skin and eyes. Death may occur during this phase in the absence of any outward signs; causes include rupture of organs, pulmonary bleeding, and air emboli.

During the secondary phase, flying debris causes injury. Affected areas are the body surface and skeletal system. As the body is struck by flying particles of glass, bricks, wood, metal, or other objects, lacerations, fractures, and compression injuries result.

The third phase, or tertiary phase, occurs as the patient becomes the flying object. As the victim is thrown against other objects, the area of the body affected depends on the area of impact. Injuries are similar to falls or those sustained in a vehicle ejection. Any or a combination of phases of a blast may contribute to serious injury or death.

You are the Provider   Summary

1. How does a basic understanding of physics as it relates to kinetic energy contribute to improving the care you provide to trauma patients?

There are certain basic physical concepts that dictate how injuries occur and how they can affect the human body. Understanding these concepts will facilitate the EMT-I's ability to size up a crash scene and use that information as a vital part of the patient assessment process. Obtaining a complete and accurate history of the incident will help identify up to 95% of the injuries present. In addition, assessing vehicular damage and the incident site will help the EMT-I determine what happened to the victim at the time of impact. This careful observation of the incident will assist the EMT-I in predicting the type and severity of injuries sustained at the time of impact.

2. What are the so-called three collisions that occur during a motor vehicle crash?

- Vehicle collision—vehicle collides with object (such as a tree)
- Body collision—body impacts with interior of the vehicle
- Organ collision—internal organs receive energy that is transmitted internally

3. What should you consider when determining the most appropriate facility to transport this patient to?

Several factors must be considered. What are the needs of the patient? What are the capabilities of the receiving facility? The patient should be transported to the closest, most appropriate facility in order to receive optimal care. The EMT-I must also determine which transport mode will be of most benefit to the patient.

4. Why are rollover crashes particularly dangerous for restrained and unrestrained passengers?

The injury patterns that occur during a rollover crash are very difficult to predict. Because the unrestrained occupant can hit all parts of the vehicle, impact to multiple parts of the body can occur. If ejected from the vehicle, the occupant has a 25 times greater chance of death. Even restrained occupants can sustain multiple impacts, especially when objects within the vehicle become projectiles during the crash.

5. What are some of the potential problems that may develop in this patient that the EMT-I must be able to recognize and treat?

- Airway obstruction
- Breathing problems
- Hidden blood loss
- Damage to major vessels
- Damage to the heart
- Brain injury
- Spinal injury

Prep Kit

Ready for Review

- Obtaining information about the mechanism of injury—that is, how the injuries occurred and what forces were likely involved—can be just as important as obtaining vital signs in assessing the patient. This information can help hospital staff to focus their attention on damage that may not be immediately obvious.
- Motor vehicle crashes are the leading cause of unintentional injury.
- In every crash, there are actually three collisions: the collision of the car against another car or some other object, the collision of the passenger against the interior of the car, and the collision of the passenger's internal organs against the solid structures of the body.
- You should suspect serious injuries in passengers who have been involved in a high-speed collision that results in massive damage to the car. The same is true of a patient who has fallen from a significant height, sustained a high-velocity penetrating injury, or is the victim of an explosion or blast.

Vital Vocabulary

blunt trauma Impact on the body by objects that cause injury without penetrating soft tissues or internal organs and cavities.

cavitation Formation of a temporary cavity occurs as energy exchange produces particle motion and stretches the tissue surrounding the point of impact, for example when speed causes a bullet to generate pressure waves, which cause damage distant from the bullet's path.

coup-contrecoup Damage is done to both sides of an organ as the body moves first in one direction and then in the opposite direction.

deceleration The slowing of an object.

index of suspicion The EMT-I's awareness that unseen life-threatening injuries may exist when determining the MOI.

kinetic energy (KE) The energy of a moving object.

mechanism of injury (MOI) The way in which traumatic injuries occur; the forces that act on the body to cause damage.

mesentery The peritoneal fold that surrounds the small intestine and connects it to the posterior abdominal wall; also the membranous fold that attaches other organs to a body wall.

penetrating trauma Injury caused by objects that pierce the surface of the body, such as knives and bullets, and damage internal tissues and organs.

potential energy The product of mass, gravity, and height, which is converted into kinetic energy and results in injury, such as from a fall.

Points to Ponder

You arrive at the scene of a car versus tree motor vehicle collision. As you approach the vehicle, you notice that the bumper is only scratched, the windshield is intact, and the airbag did not deploy. The driver is properly restrained in the vehicle. He is pale, diaphoretic, and unresponsive.

What may be causing the patient's condition? What is the LEAST likely cause of the patient's condition? What will your assessment of the patient consist of? What will your treatment of the patient consist of?

Issues: Importance of Using Mechanism of Injury as an Assessment Tool, Realizing That Mechanism of Injury Is Only One Piece of the Puzzle, Remembering to Consider the Possibility That an Underlying Medical Condition May Have Resulted in the Traumatic Injury

Technology

- Interactivities
- Vocabulary Explorer
- Anatomy Review
- Web Links
- Online Review Manual

Assessment in Action

You are dispatched to a multivehicle accident on an interstate highway. You arrive at the scene to discover that a minivan crossed the median, struck a motorcycle, and was then struck on the passenger side by a tractor-trailer.

The minivan has extensive damage to the passenger side of the vehicle, its windshield is caved in, both airbags were deployed, and its two occupants were unrestrained. The passenger is dead; and the driver, who is conscious and alert, is lying across the floorboard. The motorcyclist is lying in the roadway 50′ away from his mangled motorcycle. He is unconscious and is not wearing a helmet.

1. Which of the following mechanisms of injury MOST likely resulted in the death of the passenger?
   A. Frontal impact with the motorcycle
   B. Lateral impact by the tractor trailer
   C. Deployment of the airbag
   D. Failure to use his seatbelt

2. Why is the death of the passenger significant with regard to your care of the driver?
   A. There is no significance because the driver is conscious.
   B. It may indicate that the driver is seriously injured.
   C. It means that the driver will likely die of his injuries.
   D. It means that you should perform a focused exam of the driver.

3. Which of the following is a mechanism of injury?
   A. Femur, pelvic, and abdominal injuries
   B. Striking the dashboard on impact
   C. MVC versus pedestrian collision
   D. Chest and airway injuries

4. What injuries are you MOST likely to find when assessing the driver of the minivan?
   A. Chest injuries
   B. Head injuries
   C. Lower extremity injuries
   D. Upper extremity injuries

5. What effect does the proper use of restraints have on occupants involved in a motor vehicle crash?
   A. Restraints would decrease injury severity.
   B. Restraints would prevent serious injury and death.
   C. Restraints would cause serious injuries or death.
   D. Restraints would not make a difference in injury severity.

6. The motorcyclist is MOST likely unconscious because of:
   A. internal bleeding.
   B. spinal cord injury.
   C. airway obstruction.
   D. head trauma.

7. How will your knowledge of the motorcyclist's mechanism of injury affect your assessment?
   A. Cervical spine immobilization will not be needed.
   B. A focused physical exam of the head is all that is needed.
   C. Aggressive airway and breathing management will be needed.
   D. Vital signs will need to be monitored every 15 minutes.

8. Which of the following is NOT a reason for evaluating mechanism of injury?
   A. It guides the assessment and treatment process.
   B. It allows you to rule out medical conditions.
   C. It prepares you for symptom progression.
   D. It guides the transport priority.

Hemorrhage and Shock

1999 Objectives

Cognitive

4-2.1 Describe the epidemiology, including the morbidity, mortality, and prevention strategies for shock and hemorrhage. (p 646)
4-2.2 Discuss the various types and degrees of hemorrhage and shock. (p 663)
4-2.3 Discuss the pathophysiology of hemorrhage and shock. (p 649)
4-2.4 Discuss the assessment findings associated with hemorrhage and shock. (p 651)
4-2.5 Identify the need for intervention and transport of the patient with hemorrhage or shock. (p 653)
4-2.6 Discuss the treatment plan and management of hemorrhage and shock. (p 651)
4-2.7 Discuss the management of external and internal hemorrhage. (p 651)
4-2.8 Differentiate between controlled and uncontrolled hemorrhage. (p 649)
4-2.9 Differentiate between the administration rate and amount of IV fluid in a patient with controlled versus uncontrolled hemorrhage. (p 668)
4-2.10 Relate internal hemorrhage to the pathophysiology of compensated and decompensated hypovolemic shock. (p 663)
4-2.11 Relate internal hemorrhage to the assessment findings of compensated and decompensated hypovolemic shock. (p 663)
4-2.12 Describe the body's physiologic response to changes in perfusion. (p 647)
4-2.13 Describe the effects of decreased perfusion at the capillary level. (p 660)
4-2.14 Discuss the cellular ischemic phase related to hemorrhagic shock. (p 660)
4-2.15 Discuss the capillary stagnation phase related to hypovolemic shock. (p 660)
4-2.16 Discuss the capillary washout phase related to hypovolemic shock. (p 663)
4-2.17 Discuss the assessment findings of hypovolemic shock. (p 663)
4-2.18 Relate pulse pressure changes to perfusion status. (p 660)
4-2.19 Define compensated and decompensated shock. (p 661)
4-2.20 Discuss the pathophysiological changes associated with compensated shock. (p 659)
4-2.21 Discuss the assessment findings associated with compensated shock. (p 662)
4-2.22 Identify the need for intervention and transport of the patient with compensated shock. (p 661)
4-2.23 Discuss the treatment plan and management of compensated shock. (p 666)
4-2.24 Discuss the pathophysiological changes associated with decompensated shock. (p 662)
4-2.25 Discuss the assessment findings associated with decompensated shock. (p 662)
4-2.26 Identify the need for intervention and transport of the patient with decompensated shock. (p 663)
4-2.27 Discuss the treatment plan and management of the patient with decompensated shock. (p 668)
4-2.28 Differentiate between compensated and decompensated shock. (p 651)
4-2.29 Relate external hemorrhage to the pathophysiology of compensated and decompensated hypovolemic shock. (p 649)
4-2.30 Relate external hemorrhage to the assessment findings of compensated and decompensated hypovolemic shock. (p 649)
4-2.31 Differentiate between the normotensive, hypotensive, and profoundly hypotensive patient. (p 661)
4-2.32 Differentiate between the administration of fluid in the normotensive, hypotensive, and profoundly hypotensive patient. (p 668)
4-2.33 Discuss the physiologic changes associated with the pneumatic anti-shock garment (PASG). (p 654)
4-2.34 Discuss the indications and contraindications for the application and inflation of the PASG. (p 654)
4-2.35 Apply epidemiology to develop prevention strategies for hemorrhage and shock. (p 661)
4-2.36 Integrate the pathophysiological principles to the assessment of a patient with hemorrhage or shock. (p 651)
4-2.37 Synthesize assessment findings and patient history information to form a field impression for the patient with hemorrhage or shock. (p 651)
4-2.38 Develop, execute, and evaluate a treatment plan based on the field impression for the hemorrhage or shock patient. (p 666)

4-2.39 Differentiate between the management of compensated and decompensated shock. (p 666)

Affective

None

Psychomotor

4-2.40 Demonstrate the assessment of a patient with signs and symptoms of hypovolemic shock. (Objective 4-5.1) (p 662)

4-2.41 Demonstrate the management of a patient with signs and symptoms of hypovolemic shock. (Objective 4-5.2) (p 668)

4-2.42 Demonstrate the assessment of a patient with signs and symptoms of compensated hypovolemic shock. (Objective 4-5.3) (p 661)

4-2.43 Demonstrate the management of a patient with signs and symptoms of compensated hypovolemic shock. (Objective 4-5.4) (p 666)

4-2.44 Demonstrate the assessment of a patient with signs and symptoms of decompensated hypovolemic shock. (Objective 4-5.5) (p 662)

4-2.45 Demonstrate the management of a patient with signs and symptoms of decompensated hypovolemic shock. (Objective 4-5.6) (p 662)

4-2.46 Demonstrate the assessment of a patient with signs and symptoms of external hemorrhage. (Objective 4-5.7) (p 651)

4-2.47 Demonstrate the management of a patient with signs and symptoms of external hemorrhage. (Objective 4-5.8) (p 651)

4-2.48 Demonstrate the assessment of a patient with signs and symptoms of internal hemorrhage. (Objective 4-5.9) (p 651)

4-2.49 Demonstrate the management of a patient with signs and symptoms of internal hemorrhage. (Objective 4-5.10) (p 668)

1985 Objectives

Cognitive

1.6.35 Describe the anatomy of the skin, bones, vessels, and subcutaneous tissue as it relates to hemorrhage control. (p 647-648)

1.6.40 Define shock. (p 647)

1.6.36 Discuss the benefits and complications of hemorrhage control by the following means: (p 651, 654, 656)
   a. Direct pressure
   b. Tourniquets
   c. Hemostats

1.8.1 Define shock based on aerobic and anaerobic metabolism. (p 660)

1.8.2 Discuss the prevention of anaerobic metabolism. (p 661)

1.8.3 Discuss red blood cell oxygenation in the lungs based on alveolar O_2 levels and transportation across the alveolar capillary wall. (p 659)

1.8.4 Discuss tissue oxygenation based on tissue perfusion and release of oxygen. (p 659)

1.8.5 Discuss the role played by respiration, inadequate ventilation in the management of shock. (p 666)

1.8.6 Describe perfusion and the mechanisms of improvement of cardiac output based on the strength and rate of contractions. (p 659)

1.8.7 Discuss the fluid component of the cardiovascular system and the relationship between the volume of the fluid and the size of the container. (p 659)

1.8.8 Discuss the systemic vascular resistance, the relationship of diastolic pressure to the SVR and the effect of diastolic pressure on coronary circulation. (p 660)

1.8.9 Discuss the container size in its relationship to the fluid volume and the effect on blood returning to the heart. (p 664)

1.8.21 Describe the mechanism of the body response to perfusion change. (p 660)

1.8.22 Identify the role of the baroreceptor. (p 660)

1.8.23 Describe how the actions of the baroreceptor affect blood pressure and perfusion. (p 660)

1.8.24 Describe compensated shock. (p 661)

1.8.25 Describe uncompensated shock, both cardiac and peripheral effects. (p 662)

Hemorrhage and Shock

1.8.26 Discuss the assessment of the patient's perfusion status, based on physical observations within the primary survey, including pulse, skin, temperature, and capillary refill. (p 662)

1.8.27 Discuss the relationship of the neurological exam to assessment of hypoperfusion and oxygenation. (p 647)

1.8.28 Describe the information provided by the following in physical examination: pulse, blood pressure, diastolic pressure, systolic pressure, skin color, appearance, temperature, and respiration. (p 662)

1.8.29 Discuss management of a shocky patient. Include red cell oxygenation, tissue ischemic sensitivity, IV fluids, and the pneumatic antishock garment. (p 666)

1.8.30 Describe the beneficial and detrimental effects of the pneumatic antishock garment. (p 654)

1.8.31 Describe the indications and contraindications for the pneumatic antishock garment. (p 654)

Affective

None

Psychomotor

S1.8.35 Demonstrate in order of priority the steps of shock resuscitation. (p 666)

S1.8.36 Demonstrate the use of the pneumatic antishock garment (PASG). (p 655)

13

Hemorrhage and Shock

You are the Provider

You and your partner respond to a motor vehicle crash. The only patient is a 28-year-old woman who was unrestrained when her car struck a tree. There is moderate damage to the front of the vehicle. Upon your arrival, the patient is ambulatory at the scene. Blunt or penetrating trauma can produce injuries ranging from minor soft-tissue wounds to death, either of which can occur despite few visible outward signs indicating the severity of the injury.

This chapter will provide information on the methods recommended to control bleeding and assess and manage patients in shock, and it will help you answer the following questions:

1. Why does internal bleeding often go unnoticed until the patient "crashes"?
2. Under what circumstances might the rarely used tourniquet be the best choice for bleeding control?

Hemorrhage and Shock

After managing the airway, recognizing bleeding and understanding how it affects the body are perhaps the most important skills you will learn as an EMT-I. Bleeding can be external and obvious or internal and hidden. Either way, it is potentially dangerous, first causing weakness and, if left uncontrolled, eventually shock and death. The most common cause of shock after trauma is bleeding.

Shock has a number of meanings. In this chapter, shock describes a state of collapse and failure of the cardiovascular system in which blood circulation slows and eventually ceases. If not treated promptly, shock can be fatal. Shock often accompanies such events as heart attacks and automobile crashes to which you will respond as an EMT-I. Therefore, you must always be able to anticipate, recognize, and treat shock in order to manage patients effectively.

This chapter begins with bleeding control and recognition of internal bleeding, along with a close-up look at perfusion, the function that fails in shock. Next it looks at the physiologic causes of shock, describing each of its major forms. Finally, it discusses the emergency treatment of shock in general and of each kind of shock in particular.

Physiology and Perfusion

<u>Perfusion</u> is the circulation of blood within an organ or tissue in adequate amounts to meet the cells' current needs for oxygen, nutrients, and waste removal. Blood enters an organ or tissue first through the arteries,

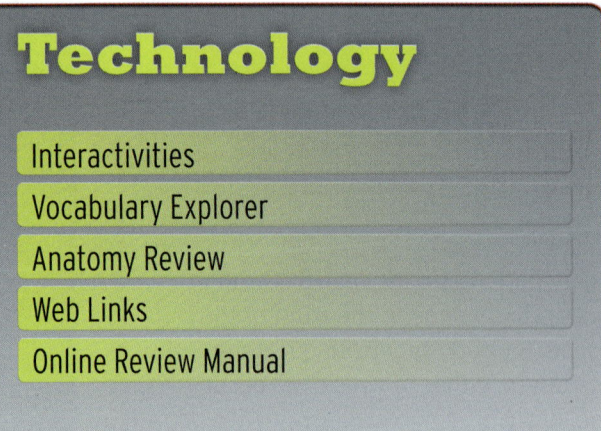

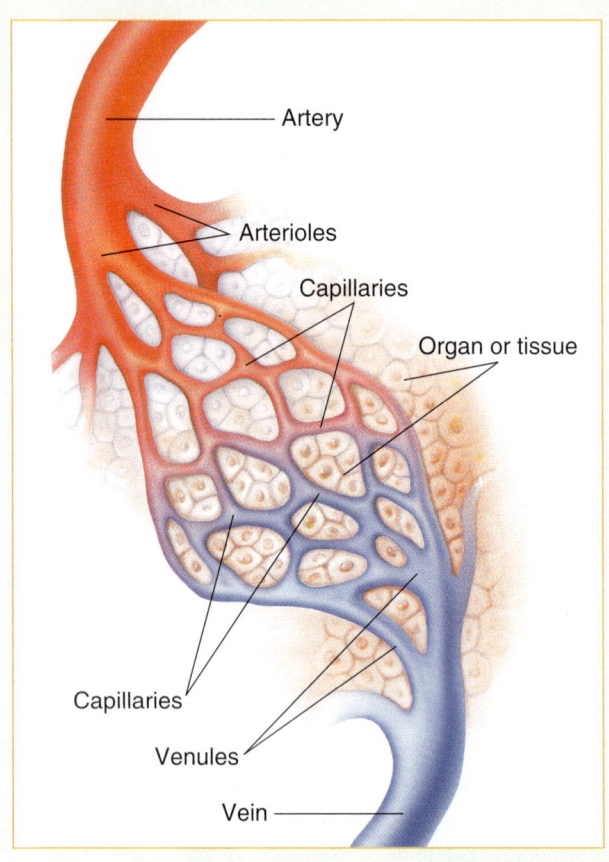

Figure 13-1 Perfusion occurs when blood circulates through tissues or an organ to provide the necessary oxygen and nutrients and remove waste products.

then the arterioles, and finally the capillary beds **Figure 13-1**. While passing through the capillaries, the blood delivers nutrients and oxygen to the surrounding cells and picks up the wastes they have generated. Then the blood leaves the capillary beds through the venules and finally reaches the veins, which take the blood back to the heart. Oxygen and carbon dioxide exchange takes place in the lungs.

Blood must pass through the cardiovascular system at a speed that is fast enough to maintain adequate circulation throughout the body and slow enough to allow each cell time to exchange oxygen and nutrients for carbon dioxide and other waste products. While some tissues, such as the lungs and kidneys, never rest and require a constant blood supply, most require circulating blood only intermittently, especially when active. Muscles are a good example. When you sleep, they are at rest and require a minimal blood supply. However, during exercise, they need a very large blood supply. The gastrointestinal tract requires a high flow of blood after a meal. After digestion is completed, it can do quite well with a small fraction of that flow.

The autonomic nervous system monitors the body's needs from moment to moment and adjusts the blood flow as required. During emergencies, the autonomic nervous system automatically redirects blood away from other organs to the heart, brain, lungs, and kidneys. Thus, the cardiovascular system is dynamic, constantly adapting to changing conditions. At times, the system fails to provide sufficient circulation for every body part to perform its function. This condition is called hypoperfusion, or shock.

Knowing which organs need adequate perfusion is the foundation on which your treatment of patients is based. Emergency medical care is designed to support the following systems:

- The heart (cardiovascular system)
- The brain and spinal cord (central nervous system)
- The lungs (respiratory system)
- The kidneys (renal system)

The heart requires constant perfusion, or it will not function properly. The brain and spinal cord cannot go for more than 4 to 6 minutes without perfusion, or the nerve cells will be permanently damaged. It is important to remember that cells of the central nervous system do not have the capacity to regenerate. The kidneys will be permanently damaged after 45 minutes of inadequate perfusion. Skeletal muscles cannot tolerate more than 2 hours of inadequate perfusion. The gastrointestinal tract can exist with limited (but not absent) perfusion for several hours. These times are based on a normal body temperature (98.6°F [37.0°C]). An organ or tissue that is considerably colder is much better able

>
> ### EMT-I Safety
>
> When dealing with a bleeding patient, be sure to take necessary precautions to protect yourself from splashing or splattering. Wear appropriate protective equipment, including gloves, gown, mask, and eye protection (Figure 13-2 ▼). This is especially essential when arterial bleeding is present. Also remember that frequent, thorough hand washing between patients and after every run is a simple yet important protective measure.

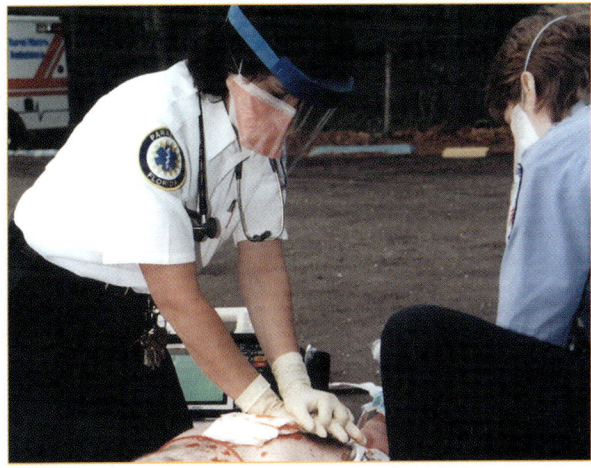

Figure 13-2 Your safety is paramount; therefore, you should always wear proper protective equipment when caring for a patient who is bleeding.

You are the Provider — Part 2

You approach the patient who is very upset about her car. She is crying and tells you her insurance was cancelled and she will have no way to get to work. She states that she is not injured and does not need an ambulance. After convincing her of the need for care, she allows you to assess her.

Initial Assessment	Recording Time: Zero Minutes
Appearance	Conscious, crying
Level of consciousness	Alert to person, place, and time
Airway	Open and clear
Breathing	Respiratory rate is slightly increased; adequate depth
Circulation	Radial pulses, increased and strong; small amount of bleeding above the left eye

3. What is your first step in the management of this patient?
4. Is there a significant mechanism of injury?

to resist damage from hypoperfusion because of the slowing of the metabolism. As metabolism decreases, so does the need for oxygen and nutrients. This also decreases the production of waste products that can be damaging if not promptly removed.

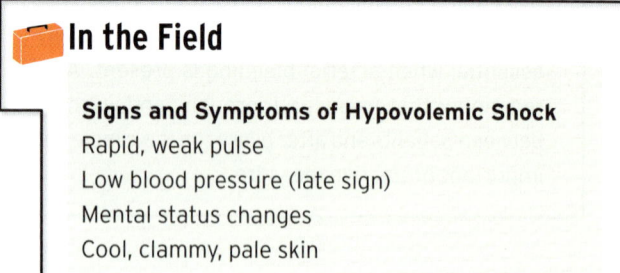

In the Field

Signs and Symptoms of Hypovolemic Shock
Rapid, weak pulse
Low blood pressure (late sign)
Mental status changes
Cool, clammy, pale skin

A to Z Terminology Tips

hypo = low; *vol* = volume; *emia* = blood
Hypovolemia is a low volume of blood, and *hypovolemic shock* is the result of inadequate perfusion due to low blood volume.

Hemorrhage

Hemorrhage means bleeding. External bleeding is a visible hemorrhage and may be controlled or uncontrolled. Likewise, internal bleeding may be controlled or uncontrolled and can lead to shock just as easily as external bleeding. Because internal bleeding is not visible, you must rely on signs and symptoms to determine the extent and severity of the hemorrhage. Internal bleeding as a result of trauma may appear in any portion of the body. An isolated fracture of a small bone (for example, humerus, ankle, tibia) produces a somewhat controlled environment, in which a relatively small amount of bleeding can occur, whereas bleeding into the trunk (for example, thorax, abdomen, pelvis), because of its much larger space, tends to be severe and uncontrolled. Nontraumatic internal hemorrhage usually occurs in cases of gastrointestinal (GI) bleeding from the upper or lower GI tract, ruptured ectopic pregnancies, ruptured aneurysms, or other conditions. Regardless of the cause, any internal bleeding is a serious emergency and must be treated promptly to ensure the optimum outcome.

The Significance of Bleeding

When patients suffer from serious external blood loss, it is often difficult to determine the amount of blood that is present. This is a difficult task since blood will look different on different surfaces; such as when it is absorbed in clothing or when it has been diluted when mixed in water. Always attempt to determine the amount of external blood loss, but the presentation and assessment of the patient will direct the care and treatment the patient will receive from you as an EMT-I.

The body will not tolerate an acute blood loss of greater than 20% of blood volume Figure 13-3. The typical adult has approximately 70 mL of blood per kilogram of body weight, or 6 L (10 to 12 pints) in a body

You are the Provider — Part 3

You talk to the patient and get her to sit down. She appears a little calmer. You dress and bandage her lacerations as she explains what happened. Your partner obtains the following vital signs:

Vital Signs	Recording Time: 2 Minutes After Patient Contact
Respirations	24 breaths/min, regular and unlabored
Pulse	114 beats/min, strong and regular
Blood pressure	102/68 mm Hg
Sao$_2$	97% on room air

5. What are your concerns for this patient?
6. Are her vital sign values clinically significant?

> **In the Field**
>
> Consider any patient exhibiting signs and symptoms of shock without obvious external injury to have probable internal bleeding, usually in the abdominal cavity.

weighing 80 kg (175 lb). If the typical adult loses more than 1 L of blood (about 2 pints), significant changes in vital signs will occur, including increasing heart and respiratory rates and decreasing blood pressure. An isolated femur fracture can easily result in the loss of 1 L or more of blood in the soft tissues of the thigh. Because infants and children have less blood volume to begin with, the same effect is seen with smaller amounts of blood loss. For example, a 1-year-old child has a total blood volume of about 800 mL. Significant symptoms of blood loss will occur after only 100 to 200 mL of blood loss. To put this in perspective, remember that a soft drink can holds roughly 345 mL of liquid.

How well people compensate for blood loss is related to how rapidly they bleed. A normal, healthy adult can comfortably donate 1 unit (500 mL) of blood over a period of 15 to 20 minutes, and can adapt well to this decrease in blood volume. However, if a similar blood loss occurs in a much shorter period, the person may rapidly develop <u>hypovolemic shock</u>, a condition in which low blood volume results in inadequate perfusion and even death. The body simply cannot compensate for such a rapid blood loss.

You should consider bleeding to be serious if the following conditions are present:
- A significant mechanism of injury, especially when the MOI suggests that severe forces affected the abdomen, chest, or both
- Poor general appearance of the patient
- Signs and symptoms of shock (hypoperfusion)
- Significant amount of blood loss
- Rapid blood loss
- Uncontrollable bleeding

In any situation, blood loss is an extremely serious problem. It demands your immediate attention as soon as you have cleared the airway and managed the patient's breathing.

Physiologic Response to Hemorrhage

Injuries and some illnesses can disrupt blood vessels and cause bleeding. Typically, bleeding from an open artery is bright red (high in oxygen) and spurts in time with the pulse. The pressure that causes the blood to spurt also makes this type of bleeding difficult to control. As the amount of blood circulating in the body drops, so does the patient's blood pressure and, eventually, the arterial spurting.

Blood from an open vein is much darker (low in oxygen) and flows steadily. Because it is under less pressure, most venous blood does not spurt and is easier to manage. Bleeding from damaged capillary vessels is dark red and oozes from a wound steadily but slowly. Venous and capillary bleeding is more likely to clot spontaneously than arterial blood **Figure 13-4**.

On its own, bleeding tends to stop rather quickly, within about 10 minutes, in response to internal mechanisms and exposure to air. When vessels are lacerated, blood flows rapidly from the open vessel. In response, the open ends of the vessel begin to narrow, or vasoconstrict. This reduces the amount of bleeding. Platelets aggregate at the site, plugging the hole and sealing the injured portions of the vessel. This process is called <u>hemostasis</u>. Bleeding will never stop if a clot does not form, unless the injured vessel is completely cut off from the main blood supply. Direct contact with body tissues and fluids or the external environment commonly triggers the blood's clotting factors.

Despite the efficiency of this system, it may fail in certain situations. A number of medications, including anticoagulants such as aspirin and prescription blood thinners, interfere with normal clotting. With a severe injury, the damage to the vessel may be so

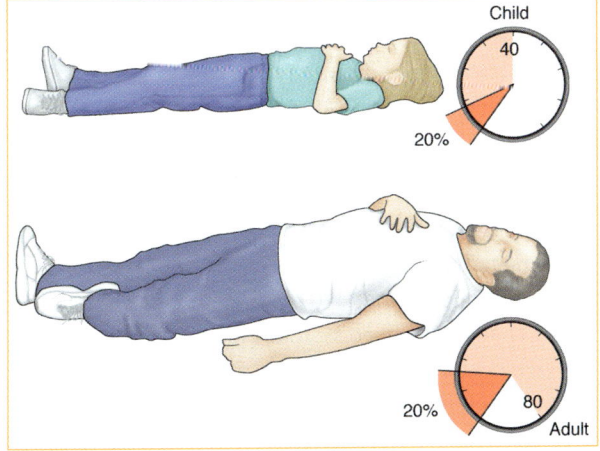

Figure 13-3 Loss of approximately 1 L of blood will cause significant changes in an adult; a much smaller blood loss will result in shock in a child or an infant.

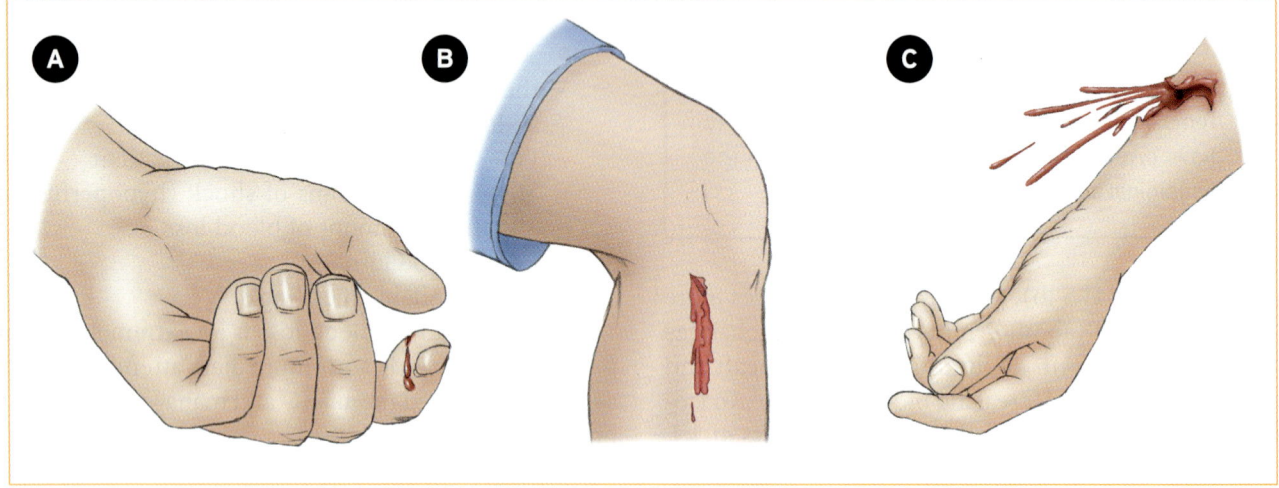

Figure 13-4 **A.** Bleeding from capillary vessels is dark red and oozes from the wound slowly but steadily. **B.** Venous bleeding is darker red and flows steadily. **C.** Arterial bleeding is characteristically bright red and spurts in a pulsatile manner.

large that a clot cannot completely block the hole. Sometimes, only part of the vessel wall is cut, preventing it from constricting. In these cases, bleeding will continue unless it is stopped by external means. Occasionally, blood loss occurs very rapidly. In these cases of acute blood loss, the patient might die before the body's hemostatic defenses of vasoconstriction and of clotting can help. Table 13-1 shows the stages of hemorrhage.

A very small portion of the population lacks one or more of the blood's clotting factors. This condition is called hemophilia. There are several forms of hemo-

TABLE 13-1 Stages of Hemorrhage

Stage 1
- Up to 15% intravascular loss
- Compensated by constriction of vascular bed
- Blood pressure maintained
- Normal pulse pressure, respiratory rate, and renal output
- Pallor of the skin
- Central venous pressure low to normal

Stage 2
- 15%–25% intravascular loss
- Cardiac output cannot be maintained by arteriolar constriction
- Reflex tachycardia
- Increased respiratory rate
- Blood pressure maintained
- Catecholamines increase peripheral resistance
- Increased diastolic pressure
- Narrow pulse pressure
- Diaphoresis from sympathetic stimulation
- Renal output near normal

Stage 3
- 25%–35% intravascular loss
- Classic signs of hypovolemic shock
  – Marked tachycardia
  – Marked tachypnea
  – Decreased systolic pressure
  – Decreased urine output
  – Alteration in mental status
  – Diaphoresis with cool, pale skin

Stage 4
- Loss greater than 35%
- Extreme tachycardia
- Pronounced tachypnea
- Significantly decreased systolic blood pressure
- Confusion and lethargy
- Skin is diaphoretic, cool, and extremely pale

Geriatric Needs

In older patients, dizziness, syncope, or weakness may be the first sign of nontraumatic internal hemorrhage.

philia, most of which are hereditary and some of which are severe. Sometimes, bleeding may occur spontaneously in hemophilia. Because the patient's blood does not clot, all injuries, no matter how trivial, are potentially serious. A patient with hemophilia should be transported immediately.

Assessment

Ensure an open and patent airway. If bleeding is from the mouth or facial areas, be sure to have suction readily available. Note the color of bleeding and try to determine the source. Bright red blood from a wound, mouth, rectum, or other orifice indicates fresh arterial bleeding. Coffee-ground emesis is a sign of upper GI bleeding. The blood is old and has the appearance of used coffee grounds. <u>Melena</u>, the passage of dark, tarry stools, is indicative of upper GI bleeding. <u>Hematochezia</u>, unlike the dark stools associated with melena, is the passage of stools containing bright red blood and may indicate bleeding close to the external opening of the colon. Hemorrhoids in the lower colon tend to cause hematochezia. <u>Hematuria</u>, or blood in the urine, may suggest serious renal injury or illness. Nonmenstrual vaginal bleeding is always significant as well.

Obtain a history of the present illness. Is there any dizziness or syncope on sitting or standing? This, along with orthostatic hypotension that may be determined by assessing blood pressure with changing positions, is an indication of hypovolemia. Are there any signs and symptoms of hypovolemic shock? Be sure to ask the patient about current medications that may thin the blood and about any history of clotting insufficiency. Is there any pain, tenderness, bruising, guarding, or swelling? These signs and symptoms may indicate internal bleeding.

Management

Always take BSI precautions. As with all patient care, ensure that the patient has an open airway and is breathing adequately. Provide high-flow oxygen and assist ventilation if needed with attention to c-spine control in trauma patients. You may then concentrate on controlling the bleeding. Follow the steps in **Skill Drill 13-1▶** to control external bleeding:

1. Almost all instances of external bleeding can be controlled simply by **applying direct local pressure to the bleeding site**. This method is by far the most effective way to control external bleeding. Pressure stops the flow of blood and permits normal coagulation to occur. You may apply pressure with your gloved fingertip or hand, over the top of a sterile dressing if one is immediately available. If there is an object protruding from the wound, apply bulky dressing to stabilize the object in place, and apply pressure as best you can. Never remove an impaled object from a wound. Hold *uninterrupted pressure* until the bleeding is controlled.

2. **Elevating a bleeding extremity** by as little as 6" often stops venous bleeding. Whenever possible, use both techniques: direct pressure and elevation. In most cases, this will stop the bleeding. However, if it does not, you still have several options. Remember to never elevate an open fracture to control bleeding. Fractures can be elevated after splinting and splinting helps control bleeding (**Step 1**).

3. Once you have applied a dressing and controlled the bleeding, you can **create a pressure dressing** to maintain the pressure by firmly wrapping a sterile, self-adhering roller bandage around the entire wound. Use 4" × 4" or 4" × 8" sterile gauze pads for small wounds and sterile universal dressings for larger wounds.

   Cover the entire dressing, above and below the wound. Stretch the bandage tight enough to control bleeding but not so tight as to decrease blood flow to the extremity. If you were able to palpate a distal pulse before applying the dressing, you should still be able to palpate a distal pulse on the injured extremity after applying the pressure dressing. If bleeding continues, the dressing is probably not tight enough. Do not remove a dressing until a physician has evaluated the patient. Instead, apply additional manual pressure through the dressing. Then add more gauze pads over the first dressing, and secure them both with a second, tighter, roller bandage.

   Bleeding will almost always stop when the pressure of the dressing exceeds arterial pressure.

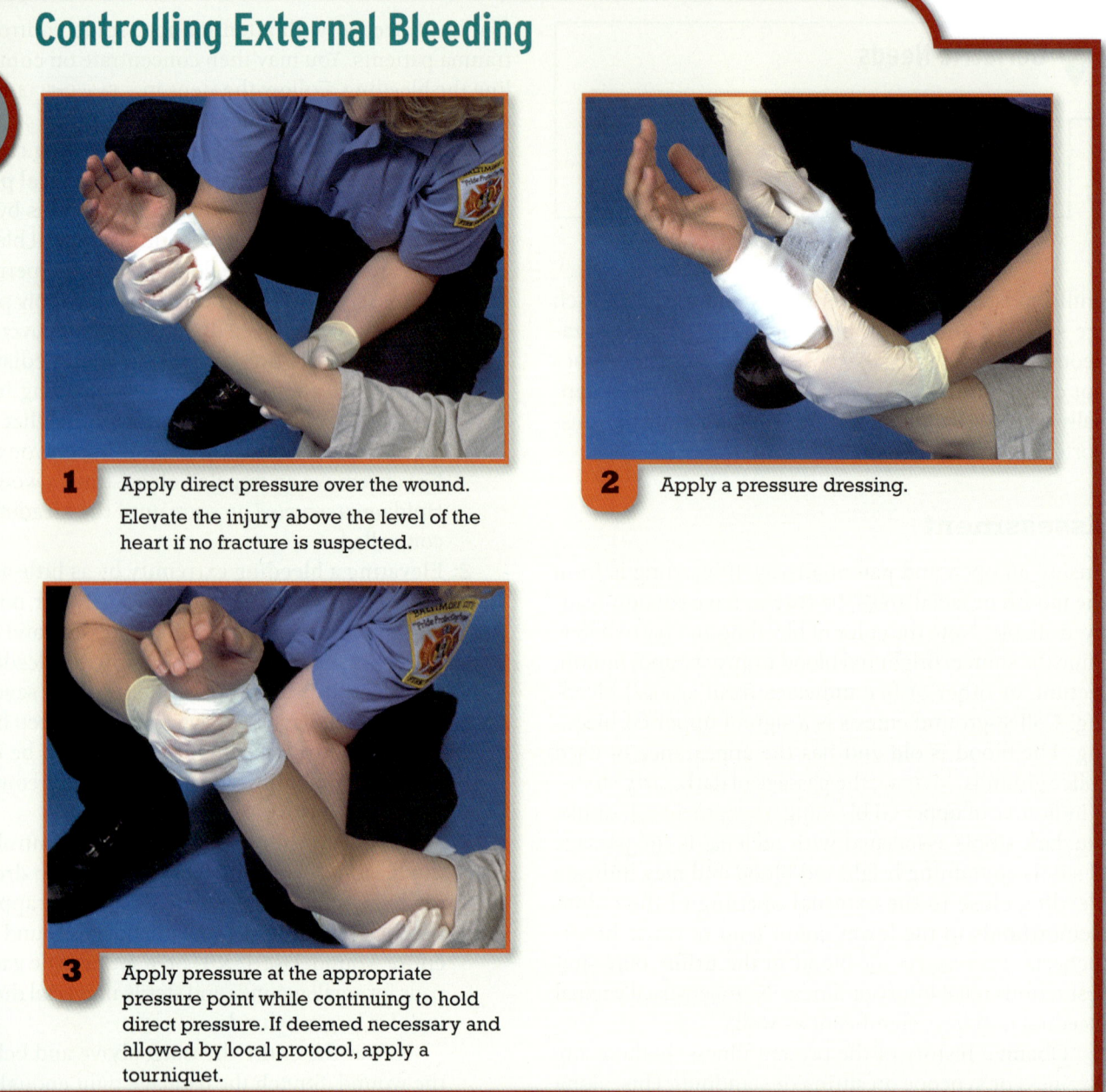

Skill Drill 13-1: Controlling External Bleeding

1. Apply direct pressure over the wound. Elevate the injury above the level of the heart if no fracture is suspected.

2. Apply a pressure dressing.

3. Apply pressure at the appropriate pressure point while continuing to hold direct pressure. If deemed necessary and allowed by local protocol, apply a tourniquet.

This will assist in controlling bleeding and helping blood to clot (**Step 2**).

4. **If a wound continues to bleed** despite use of direct pressure, elevate the extremity and try placing additional pressure over a proximal pressure point, or pulse point. A <u>pressure point</u> is a spot where a blood vessel lies near a bone. This technique is also useful if you have no material on hand to use for a dressing. Because a wound usually draws blood from more than one major artery, proximal compression of a major artery rarely stops bleeding completely, but it helps to slow the loss of blood. You must be thoroughly familiar with the location of the pulse points for this to work (**Figure 13-5**) (**Step 3**). If you suspect spinal injury, do not elevate the patient's legs. Instead, elevate the foot end of the backboard and do not cause movement of the spinal column. If the patient has an open fracture of an extremity, use direct pressure to control bleeding. However, do not apply so much pressure as to increase pain or injury.

Recent studies have called into question the effectiveness of using pressure points in severe hemorrhage. It is acceptable, if allowed by protocol and local policy, to move directly to the use of a tourniquet without attempting pressure point control.

If bleeding is from the nose or ears after head trauma, refrain from applying pressure. Instead, apply loose sterile dressings to protect from infection. With bleeding from other areas, control bleeding through use of the following:

- Direct pressure
- Elevation if appropriate
- Pressure dressings
- Pressure points (for upper and lower extremities)
- Ice or cold packs (especially for <u>epistaxis</u>, or nosebleed)
- Splints, air splints
- Packing of large gaping wounds with sterile dressings
- Consider applying a pneumatic antishock garment (PASG)
- Constricting band
- Tourniquets

Once bleeding is controlled and a sterile dressing and pressure bandage have been applied, keep the patient warm and in the appropriate position. Allow the patient's condition to dictate the mode of transport. If the patient is showing any signs of hypoperfusion, transport rapidly while providing aggressive management en route. Because the patient in shock is usually emotionally upset, psychological support should be provided as well.

Special Techniques

Much of the bleeding associated with broken bones occurs because the sharp ends of the bones lacerate vessels, muscles, and other tissues. As long as a fracture remains unstable, the bone ends will move and continue to cause damage to tissues and vessels. This may also include breaking up clots that have partially formed, resulting in ongoing bleeding. Therefore, stabilizing a fracture and decreasing movement is a high priority in the prompt control of bleeding. Often, simple splints will quickly control bleeding associated with a fracture (Figure 13-6 ▼). If not, you may need to use another splinting device.

- **Air splints.** Air splints can control the bleeding associated with severe soft-tissue injuries, such as massive or complex lacerations, or fractures

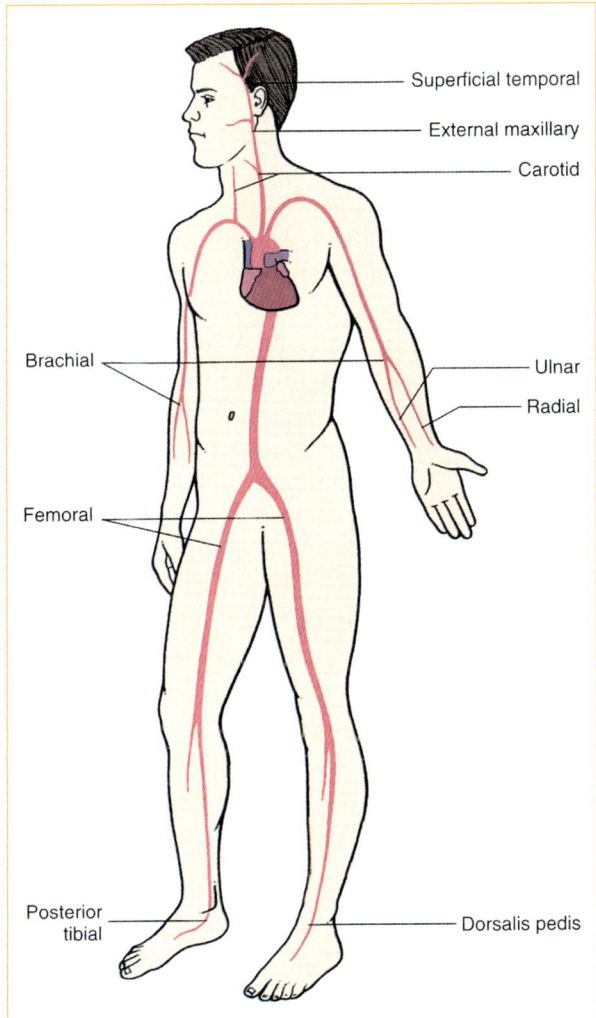

Figure 13-5 Locations of arterial pressure points.

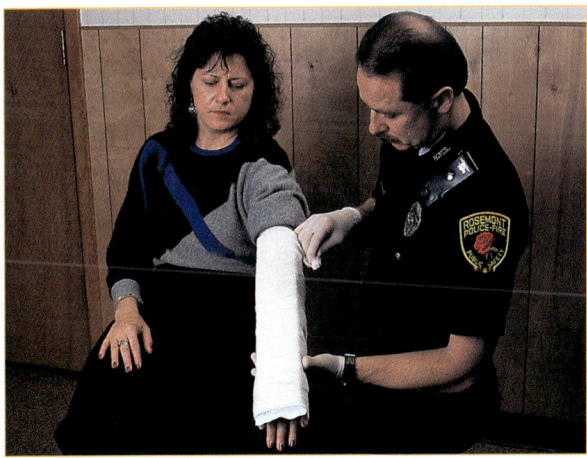

Figure 13-6 Use of a simple splint will often quickly control bleeding associated with a fracture. As long as a fracture is not immobilized, the bone ends are free to move and may continue to injure partially clotted vessels.

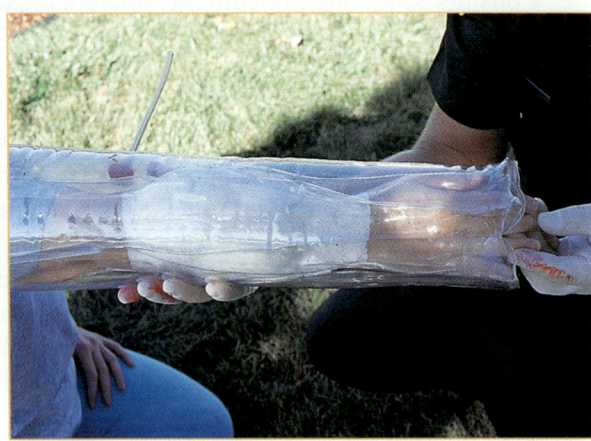

Figure 13-7 Air splints can also be used to control bleeding because they act as a pressure bandage for the entire extremity.

Figure 13-7 ▲). They also stabilize the fracture itself. An air splint acts like a pressure dressing applied to an entire extremity rather than to a small, local area. Once you have applied an air splint, be sure to monitor circulation in the distal extremity. Use only BSI-approved, clean, or disposable valve stems when orally inflating air splints.

- **Hemostats.** Hemostats may be helpful when a vessel has been severed, especially if it has retracted into the surrounding tissue. Simply apply hemostats to the ends of the vessel.
- **Pneumatic antishock garment (PASG).** The primary use of PASGs is for stabilization of an unstable pelvis, especially when the patient is exhibiting signs of hypoperfusion. If a patient has injuries to the lower extremities and/or pelvis, you may be able to use a PASG as a splinting device, if local protocol allows. Situations in which use of a PASG is allowed vary widely by locale. Be sure to check with medical control in every case.

> **In the Field**
>
> Some areas of the country use the mnemonic *MAST* instead of PASG. MAST stands for military antishock trousers.

Following are the few, very specific instances in which a PASG may be effective:

- To stabilize fractures of the pelvis and bilateral femurs
- To control significant internal bleeding associated with fractures of the pelvis and bilateral femurs
- To control massive soft-tissue bleeding of the lower extremities when direct pressure is not effective

Pulmonary edema is the only true contraindication to the use of the PASG. Following is a list of relative contraindications in which use may cause more harm to the patient:

- Pregnancy (leg sections may be used)
- Penetrating abdominal injuries or evisceration
- Penetrating chest injuries
- Groin injuries
- Major head injuries
- A transport time of less than 30 minutes

In these situations, the PASG may worsen or complicate the patient's condition. Consult with medical control if you think prolonged use or use in unusual circumstances may be necessary. The PASG works by compressing the abdomen and lower extremities, increasing peripheral resistance in the circulatory system. Contrary to popular belief, blood is not forced from the lower extremities back into central circulation. In actuality, only about 250 mL of blood is displaced from the portion covered by the PASG. Instead, the size of the container is decreased. This increases the amount of blood that is available to perfuse the vital organs.

In applying the PASG, you should carefully inflate the device in increments. Auscultate for pulmonary edema before inflation of each section. The legs should be inflated simultaneously before inflating the abdominal compartment. Auscultate breath sounds again before beginning inflation of the abdominal section. You may inflate only the leg sections to stabilize femur fractures. If you are using the device to stabilize a possible pelvic fracture, you must inflate all compartments. Always document all obvious injuries or deformities before application of the PASG, and pad any sharp bone ends to prevent puncture of the garment. Follow these steps to apply the PASG for bleeding control (Skill Drill 13-2 ▶):

1. Rapidly expose and examine the areas to be covered by the PASG. Pad any exposed bone ends to prevent puncture of the garment as it is inflated.

Applying a Pneumatic Antishock Garment (PASG)

Skill Drill 13-2

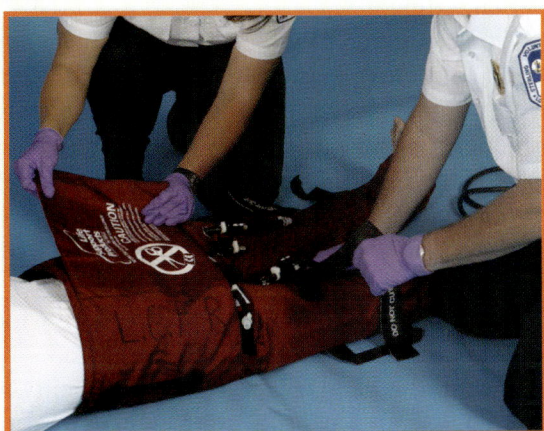

1 Rapidly expose and examine the areas to be covered by the PASG. Pad any exposed bone ends.

Apply the garment so that the top is below the lowest rib.

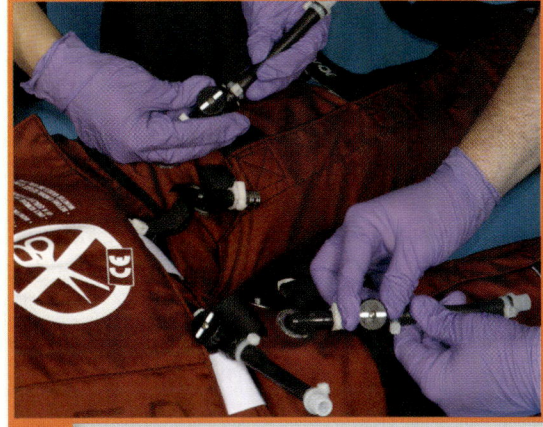

2 Close and fasten both leg compartments and the abdominal compartment.

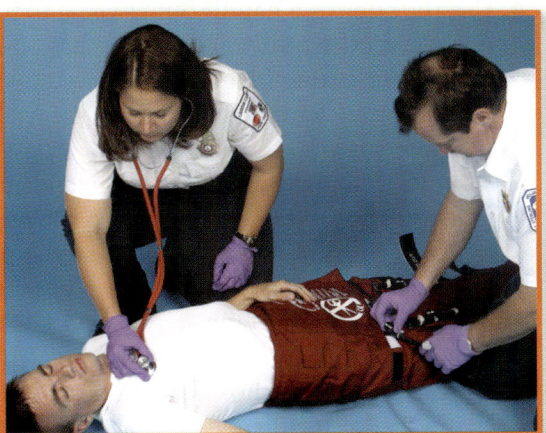

3 Open the stopcocks.

Auscultate breath sounds for pulmonary edema before inflation of any compartment.

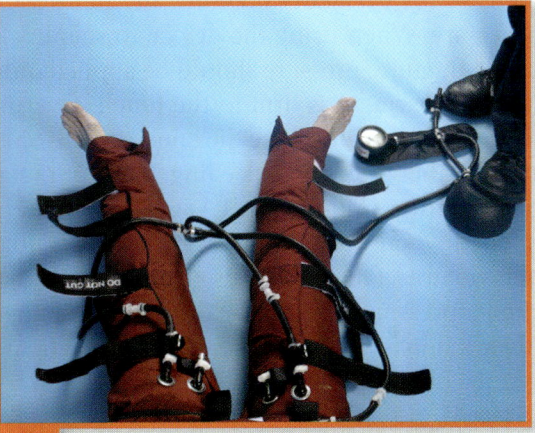

4 Inflate with the foot pump until the patient's blood pressure reaches 90 to 100 mm Hg or the Velcro crackles. Monitor radial pulses.

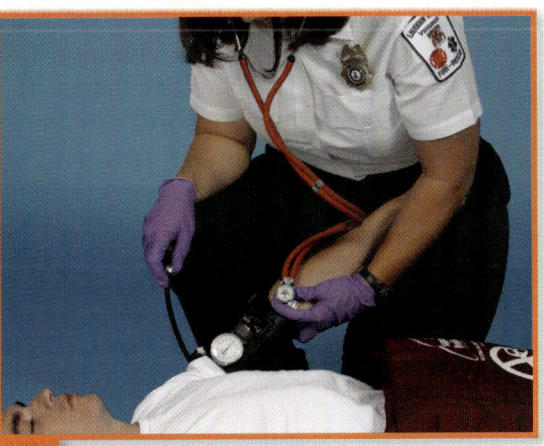

5 Check the patient's blood pressure again. Monitor vital signs.

2. **Apply the garment.** If you will immobilize or move the patient on a backboard, lay the PASG out on the board before rolling the patient onto it. Position the top of the abdominal section of the PASG below the lowest rib to ensure that it does not compromise chest expansion (**Step 1**).
3. **Close and fasten both leg compartments** and the abdominal compartment (**Step 2**).
4. **Open the stopcocks** (valves) to the compartments you are preparing to inflate, ensuring that the other compartments are closed off. You will inflate both legs (lower extremity bleeding) or all three compartments (internal pelvic or abdominal bleeding) (**Step 3**).
5. **Auscultate breath sounds** for pulmonary edema before inflation of any compartment.
6. **Inflate the compartments** with the foot pump. Be sure to turn off compartment valves after inflation to maintain pressure in the garment. Do not increase the garment's pressure any more than necessary. When using the device to stabilize a pelvic fracture, pressure should be applied only until the garment is firm to the touch. Overinflation may actually cause the bones to shift, creating further injury and bleeding. Monitor radial pulses while inflating. A PASG is adequately inflated when the Velcro crackles or the radial pulse returns if the PASG is used for hypovolemia. Higher pressures may cause local tissue damage. Always stop inflating the PASG once the patient's systolic blood pressure reaches 90 to 100 mm Hg (**Step 4**).
7. **Check the patient's blood pressure** during inflation, and continue to monitor vital signs at least every 5 minutes afterward. Remember that the pressure gauges of the PASG measure the air pressure in the device. They do not reflect the patient's blood pressure. Be aware of temperature extremes or external pressure changes that can significantly affect the pressure exerted by the PASG, thus requiring frequent monitoring and adjustment (**Step 5**).

Do not remove a PASG in the field. A physician must deflate it gradually in the hospital under careful supervision and only after appropriate IV solutions and medications have been given.

- **Tourniquets.** A tourniquet may be used to control severe hemorrhage. If a tourniquet is deemed necessary and allowed by local protocol, it should be applied quickly and not released in the prehospital setting.

If you cannot control bleeding from the major vessel in an extremity in *any other way*, a properly applied tourniquet may save a patient's life. Specifically, the tourniquet is useful if a patient is bleeding severely from a partial or complete amputation and no other method will control the bleeding.

Follow these steps to apply a tourniquet (**Skill Drill 13-3**):

1. **Fold a triangular bandage** until it is 4″ wide and six to eight layers thick.
2. **Wrap the bandage** around the extremity twice. Choose an area only slightly proximal to the bleeding to reduce the amount of tissue damage to the extremity (**Step 1**).
3. **Tie one knot** in the bandage. Then place a stick or rod on top of the knot, and tie the ends of the bandage over the stick in a square knot (**Step 2**).
4. **Use the stick as a handle**, and twist it to tighten the tourniquet until the bleeding has stopped; then stop twisting (**Step 3**).
5. **Secure the stick in place**, and make the wrapping neat and smooth.
6. **Write "TK" and the exact time** (hour and minute) that you applied the tourniquet on the patient's forehead, preferably in red ink. Use the phrase "time applied." You may use adhesive tape, but be aware that the tape may fall off. This is especially true of patients in shock who are diaphoretic. Notify hospital personnel on your arrival that your patient has a tourniquet in place. Record this same information in your documentation (**Step 4**).
7. **As an alternative method**, you can use a blood pressure cuff as an effective tourniquet. Position the cuff proximal to the bleeding point, and inflate it just enough to stop the bleeding. Leave the cuff inflated. If you use a blood pressure cuff, monitor the gauge continuously to make sure that the pressure is not gradually dropping. You may have to clamp the tube with a hemostat leading from the cuff to the inflating bulb to prevent loss of pressure (**Step 5**).

Chapter 13 Hemorrhage and Shock 657

Applying a Tourniquet

Skill Drill 13-3

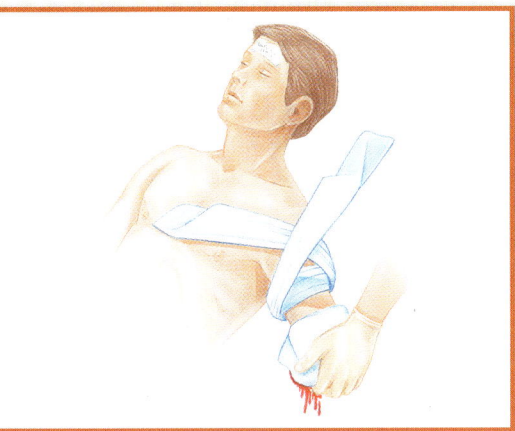

1 Create a 4"-wide, multilayered bandage. Wrap the bandage twice around the extremity, just above the bleeding site.

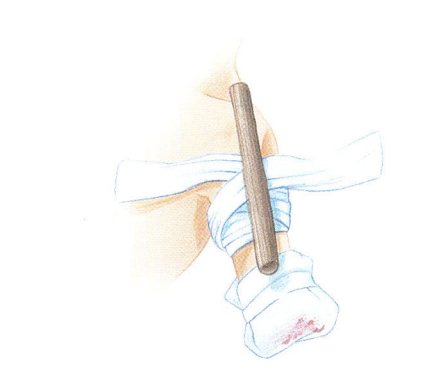

2 Tie a single knot, and place a stick on the top of it.

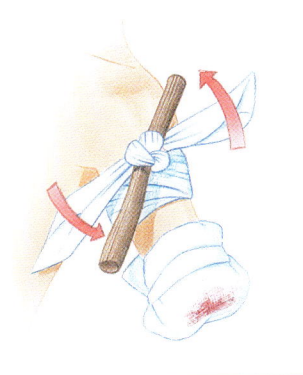

3 Tie a square knot over the stick, and then twist the stick until the bleeding stops.

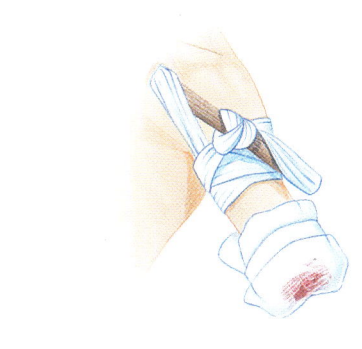

4 Secure the stick so that it will not unwind. Write "TK" and the exact time you applied the tourniquet on the patient's forehead, and notify hospital personnel on arrival.

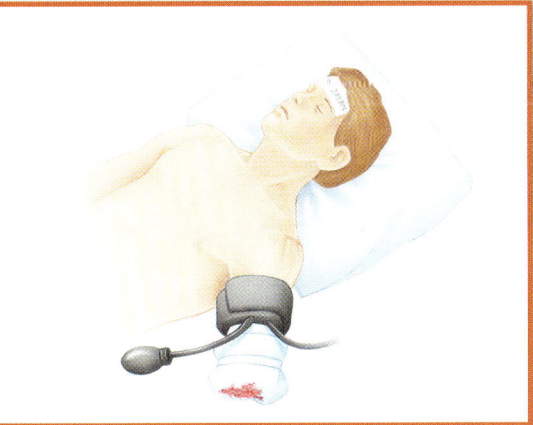

5 You can also use a blood pressure cuff as an effective tourniquet.

Whenever applying a tourniquet, make sure you observe the following precautions:

- Do not apply a tourniquet directly over any joint. Keep it as close to the injury as possible.
- Use the widest bandage possible. Make sure that it is tightened securely.
- Never use wire, rope, a belt, or any other narrow material. It could cut into the skin.
- Use wide padding under the tourniquet if possible. This will protect the tissues and help with arterial compression.
- Never cover a tourniquet with a bandage. Leave it open and in full view.
- Do not loosen the tourniquet after you have applied it. Hospital personnel will loosen it once they are prepared to manage the bleeding.

Bleeding from the Nose, Ears, and Mouth

Bleeding from the nose, which is known as epistaxis, or ears following a head injury may indicate a skull fracture. In these cases, you should not attempt to stop the blood flow. Second, applying excessive pressure to the injury may force the blood leaking through the ear or nose to collect within the head. This could increase intracranial pressure and possibly cause permanent damage. If you suspect a skull fracture, loosely cover the bleeding site with a sterile gauze pad to collect the blood and help keep contaminants away from the site. There is always a risk of infection to the brain. Apply light compression by wrapping the dressing loosely around the head (Figure 13-8 ▶). If blood or drainage contains cerebrospinal fluid, a characteristic staining of the dressing, much like a target, will occur.

> **In the Field**
>
> Wrap a 4" × 4" piece of gauze around your gloved finger and dip it into blood from the ears or nose to test for the presence of cerebrospinal fluid. This is called a *halo test* because when opened up the gauze will have the blood surrounded by a lighter ring of fluid (Figure 13-9 ▶).

You are the Provider Part 4

Initially the patient refuses transport but finally concedes when you explain the possible complications. She allows you and your partner to immobilize her on a long spine board. She is loaded into the ambulance, and your partner reassesses her vital signs while you inspect the damage to the vehicle. You note that the lower portion of the steering wheel is bent and the windshield is cracked in a spider web appearance.

Vital Signs	Recording Time: 6 Minutes After Patient Contact
Level of consciousness	Agitated
Respirations	28 breaths/min, slightly shallow
Pulse	Radial pulses, 124 beats/min, weak and thready
Blood pressure	94/62 mm Hg
Sao_2	93% on room air

7. What is your next step in the treatment of this patient?
8. What are your assessment concerns?

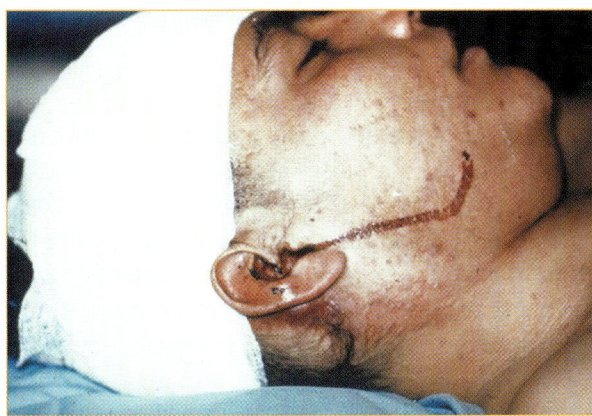

Figure 13-8 Bleeding from the ear after a head injury may indicate a skull fracture. Loosely cover the bleeding site with a sterile gauze pad, and apply light compression by wrapping the dressing loosely around the head.

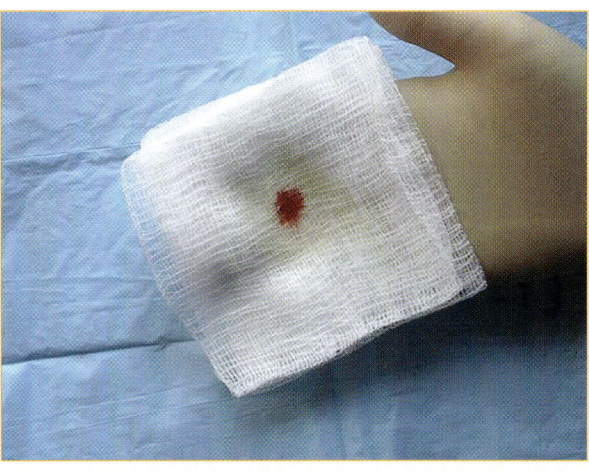

Figure 13-9 A "halo" on a piece of gauze dipped in blood from the ears or nose indicates the presence of cerebrospinal fluid.

Shock

Pathophysiology of Shock

Shock, or hypoperfusion, refers to a state of collapse and failure of the cardiovascular system that leads to inadequate circulation, creating inadequate tissue perfusion. Like internal bleeding, shock cannot be seen. It is not a specific disease or injury. However, it is a dangerous condition that results in the inadequate flow of blood to the body's cells and failure to rid the body of metabolic wastes. As perfusion decreases, the body attempts to compensate by redirecting blood flow from nonessential organs (skin and intestines) to essential organs (heart, lungs, and brain). If the conditions causing shock are not promptly addressed, the patient will soon die.

The cardiovascular system consists of three parts: a pump (heart), a container (vessels), and the fluid (blood) **Figure 13-10**. Blood is the vehicle for carrying oxygen and nutrients through the vessels to the capillary beds, where these supplies are exchanged for waste products. The blood keeps moving as a result of pressure that is generated by the contractions of the heart and affected by the dilating and constricting of the vessels. The body usually carefully controls this pressure, which is called blood pressure, so that there is always sufficient circulation, or perfusion, in the various tissues and organs. Blood pressure is, in fact, a rough measurement of perfusion. It tells us how well the body's oxygen, nutrient, and waste removal needs are being met.

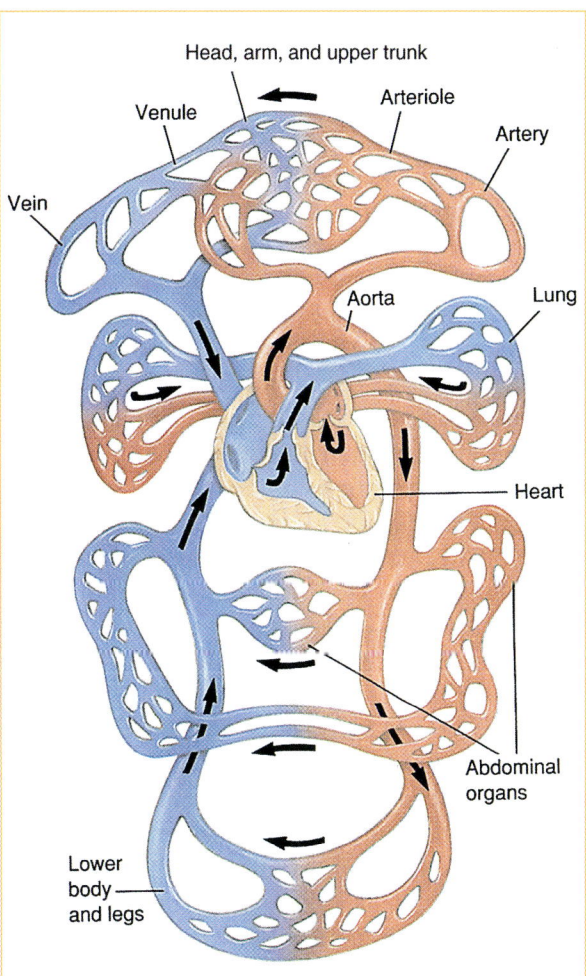

Figure 13-10 The cardiovascular system consists of three parts: the pump (heart), the container (vessels), and the contents (blood). The blood carries oxygen and nutrients through the vessels to the capillary beds, where they are exchanged for waste products.

Perfusion depends on cardiac output (CO), systemic vascular resistance (SVR), and transport of oxygen.

CO = HR × SV

Cardiac Output = Heart Rate × Stroke Volume

BP = CO × SVR

Blood Pressure = Cardiac Output × Systemic Vascular Resistance

Because the heart cannot pump out what is not in its holding chambers, blood pressure varies directly with cardiac output, SVR, and blood volume. Hypoperfusion can result from inadequate cardiac output, decreased SVR, or the inability of red blood cells to deliver oxygen to tissues.

Compensation for Decreased Perfusion

Central among the homeostatic mechanisms that regulate cardiovascular dynamics are those that maintain blood pressure. In any event that results in decreased perfusion, such as blood loss, myocardial infarction, loss of vasomotor tone, or tension pneumothorax, the body must respond immediately in an attempt to preserve the vital organs. Baroreceptors located in the aortic arch and carotid sinuses (as well as in most of the large arteries of the neck and thorax) sense the decreased flow and activate the vasomotor center, which oversees changes in the diameter of blood vessels, to begin constriction of the vessels and, therefore, increase blood pressure.

Normally stimulation occurs when the systolic pressure is between 60 and 80 mm Hg and even lower in children. A decrease in systolic pressure to less than 80 mm Hg stimulates the vasomotor center to increase arterial pressure by constricting vessels. The drop in arterial pressure decreases the stretching of the arterial walls, thereby decreasing baroreceptor stimulation. Normally baroreceptor stimulation inhibits the vasoconstrictor center of the medulla and excites the vagal center, leading to vasodilation in the peripheral circulatory system and a decrease in heart rate and contractility, causing a decrease in arterial pressure. The sympathetic nervous system is also stimulated at this time as the body recognizes a potential catastrophic event.

Short-term control of blood pressure is mediated by the nervous system and bloodborne chemicals to counteract fluctuations in blood pressure by altering systemic resistance. Chemoreceptors located in the carotid and aortic bodies are stimulated by decreases in PaO_2 and increases in $PaCO_2$ and are more important in regulating respiration than blood pressure. However, they also contribute to controlling blood pressure on a smaller scale. When the pH of the blood drops sharply as the carbon dioxide level rises, impulses are sent to the cardioacceleratory center to increase cardiac output and to the vasomotor center to stimulate vasoconstriction. Long-term control of blood pressure is regulated by the slower acting renal system, which helps regulate blood volume.

As perfusion decreases, the sympathetic nervous system is stimulated, initiating the "fight-or-flight" response. The adrenal medulla secretes two catecholamines, epinephrine and norepinephrine. The $alpha_1$ response to the release of epinephrine includes vasoconstriction, increased peripheral vascular resistance, and an increased afterload from the arteriolar constriction. $Alpha_2$ effects ensure a regulated release of $alpha_1$. Beta responses from the release of epinephrine primarily affect the heart and lungs. Increases in heart rate, contractility, conductivity, and automaticity occur in tandem with bronchodilation. Effects of norepinephrine are primarily $alpha_1$ and $alpha_2$ and are centered on vasoconstriction and increasing peripheral vascular resistance. See Table 13-2 for the alpha and beta effects of epinephrine and norepinephrine.

Failure of compensatory mechanisms to preserve perfusion leads to decreases in preload and cardiac output. Myocardial blood supply and oxygenation decrease, reducing myocardial perfusion. As cardiac output further decreases, coronary artery perfusion also decreases, leading to myocardial ischemia.

> **A to Z Terminology Tips**
>
> *Chronotropic* influencing heart rate
> *Inotropic* influencing contractility
> *Dromotropic* influencing conductivity
> Positive effects = increase; negative effects = decrease

Capillary and Cellular Changes

Cellular ischemia occurs as perfusion decreases. There is minimal blood flow through the capillaries, causing the cells to go from aerobic metabolism to anaerobic metabolism, which can quickly lead to metabolic acidosis. With less circulation in the capillaries, the blood

TABLE 13-2	Effects of Epinephrine and Norepinephrine
Epinephrine	
Alpha$_1$	Vasoconstriction
	Increase in peripheral vascular resistance
	Increased afterload from arteriolar constriction
Alpha$_2$	Regulated release of alpha$_1$
Beta$_1$	Positive chronotropic effects
	Positive inotropic effects
	Positive dromotropic effects
Beta$_2$	Bronchodilation
	Gastrointestinal smooth muscle dilation
Norepinephrine	
Alpha$_1$ and alpha$_2$	Vasoconstriction
	Increase in peripheral vascular resistance
	Increased afterload from arteriolar constriction

stagnates there. The precapillary sphincter relaxes in response to the buildup of lactic acid, vasomotor center failure, and increased amounts of carbon dioxide. The postcapillary sphincters remain constricted, causing the capillaries to engorge with fluid.

The capillary sphincters, circular muscular walls that constrict and dilate, regulate blood flow through the capillary beds. These sphincters are under the control of the autonomic nervous system, which regulates involuntary functions such as sweating and digestion. Capillary sphincters also respond to other stimuli such as heat, cold, the need for oxygen, and the need for waste removal. Thus, regulation of blood flow is determined by cellular need and is accomplished by vessel constriction or dilation, together with sphincter constriction or dilation.

As anaerobic metabolism continues, increasing lactic acid production causes the pH of the blood to significantly fall. Because arteries deprived of oxygenated blood cannot remain constricted, more vasodilation occurs. There is an aggregation, or accumulation, of red blood cells and formation of microemboli. Because the capillary walls are stretched, they lose their ability to retain large molecules, allowing leaking into the surrounding interstitial spaces. Hydrostatic pressure forces plasma into the interstitial spaces, further increasing the distance from the capillaries to the cells, and, as a result, oxygen transport decreases, increasing cellular hypoxia.

The continuing buildup of lactic acid and carbon dioxide acts as a potent vasodilator, leading to relaxation of the postcapillary sphincters. The accumulated hydrogen, potassium, carbon dioxide, and thrombosed (clotted) red blood cells wash out into the venous circulation, increasing the metabolic acidosis. The result is an even further drop in cardiac output.

Stages of Shock

Shock occurs in three successive stages. Your goal as an EMT-I is to recognize the signs of the early stages of shock and begin immediate treatment before permanent damage occurs. To accomplish this, you must be aware of the subtle signs exhibited in compensated shock and treat the patient aggressively. Anticipate the potential for shock from the scene survey. Recognize the signs of poor perfusion that precede hypotension, and do not rely on any one sign or symptom to determine the degree of shock. Always err on the side of caution when treating a potential shock patient. Rapid assessment and immediate transportation are essential to preserve any chance of patient survival.

Compensated (Nonprogressive) Shock

Although you cannot see shock, you can see its signs and symptoms Table 13-3. The earliest stage of shock, while the body can still compensate for blood loss, is called compensated shock, or nonprogressive shock. Signs and symptoms of early shock characterize it. Level of responsiveness is a better indicator of tissue perfusion than most other vital signs. Release of chemical mediators by the autonomic nervous system as it recognizes a potential catastrophic event causes the arterial blood pressure to remain normal or slightly elevated. There is an increase in the rate and depth of respirations to bring in more oxygen and remove more carbon dioxide. This helps to maintain the acid-base balance by creating respiratory alkalosis to offset the metabolic acidosis.

At this stage, the blood pressure is maintained. There is a narrowing of the pulse pressure, which is the difference between the systolic and diastolic pressures.

Pulse Pressure = Systolic Pressure − Diastolic Pressure

TABLE 13-3 Progression of Shock

Compensated (Nonprogressive) Shock

- Agitation
- Anxiety
- Feeling of impending doom
- Altered mental status, usually restlessness
- Tachypnea
- Tachycardia
- Weak, thready, or absent radial pulse
- Clammy, diaphoretic, cool skin
- Pallor, with cyanosis about the lips
- Dry mucosa
- Air hunger (shortness of breath), especially if there is a chest injury
- Nausea or vomiting
- Capillary refill in infants and children of longer than 2 seconds
- Marked thirst
- Weakness

Decompensated (Progressive) Shock

- Additional increases in pulse and respirations
- Significant decrease in level of consciousness
- Hypotension (systolic blood pressure of 90 mm Hg or lower in an adult)
- Labored or irregular breathing
- Cyanosis with white, waxy-looking skin
- Diaphoresis
- Thready or absent peripheral pulses
- Decreased capillary refill time
- Narrowing of the pulse pressure, indicating impairment of circulation
- Dull eyes, dilated pupils
- Dry mucosa
- Thirst (the body's call for increased volume)
- Nausea and vomiting (caused by shunting of blood from abdominal organs)
- Poor urinary output

Irreversible Shock

- Marked decrease in level of responsiveness (Glasgow Coma Scale score <7)
- Decreased respiratory rate and effort
- Inability to palpate a pulse
- Decrease in pulse rate
- Profound hypotension
- Death

The pulse pressure reflects the tone of the arterial system and is more sensitive to changes in perfusion than the systolic or diastolic blood pressure alone. Patients in the compensated stage will also have a positive orthostatic tilt test result. Treatment at this stage will typically result in recovery.

> **Terminology Tips**
>
> An *orthostatic tilt test* is used to determine dehydration or hypovolemia. The term *orthostatic* has to do with positioning. Orthostatic hypotension, for example, is a drop in systolic blood pressure when moving from a sitting to a standing position. Blood pressure and pulse are measured as patients are lying, seated, and standing. A positive tilt test result occurs if the patient becomes dizzy, has a pulse increase of at least 20 beats per minute, or has a systolic blood pressure decrease of at least 20 mm Hg.

> **In the Field**
>
> Shock can result from any illness or injury and can present in a variety of ways. Shock may also be hidden by compensatory mechanisms. Classic indicators of shock include:
> - Restlessness
> - Tachycardia
> - Tachypnea
> - Pallor
> - Diaphoresis
> - Thirst
> - Weakness

Decompensated (Progressive) Shock

The next stage, when blood pressure is falling, is called decompensated shock, also called uncompensated shock or progressive shock. It occurs when blood volume drops more than 15% to 25%. The compensatory mechanisms are beginning to fail, and signs and symptoms are much more obvious. Cardiac output falls dramatically, leading to further reductions in blood pressure and cardiac function. The signs and symptoms become more obvious as blood is shunted to the brain, heart, and kidneys. At this point, vasoconstriction can have a disastrous effect if allowed to continue. Cells in the nonperfused tissues become hypoxic, leading to anaerobic metabolism. Treatment at this stage will sometimes result in recovery.

Irreversible Shock

The last stage, when shock has progressed to a terminal stage, is called <u>irreversible shock</u>. Arterial blood pressure is abnormally low. There is a rapid deterioration of the cardiovascular system that cannot be reversed by compensatory mechanisms or medical interventions. There are life-threatening reductions in cardiac output, blood pressure, and tissue perfusion. Blood is shunted away from the liver, kidneys, and lungs to keep the heart and brain perfused. Cells begin to die, and, even if the cause of shock is treated and reversed, vital organ damage cannot be repaired, and the patient will eventually die. Even aggressive treatment at this stage does not usually result in recovery.

> **In the Field**
>
> Remember that blood pressure may be the last measurable factor to change in shock. The body has several automatic mechanisms to compensate for initial blood loss and to help maintain blood pressure. Thus, by the time you detect a drop in blood pressure, shock is well developed. This is particularly true in infants and children, who can maintain their blood pressure until they have lost more than half of their blood volume.

> **Documentation Tips**
>
> Just as they make for thorough written reporting, taking and recording frequent vital signs—and observing perfusion indicators such as skin condition and mental status—will give you a window into the progression of shock. Use your documentation to remind you to suspect shock early and treat it aggressively.

Etiologic Classifications

Hypovolemic Shock

Following injury, shock is often a result of fluid or blood loss. This type of shock is called hypovolemic (low-volume) shock or, when caused by blood loss specifically, hemorrhagic shock. The loss may be due to external bleeding, which is common in patients who have severe lacerations or fractures, or it may be due to internal bleeding, which follows a variety of injuries or diseases such as rupture of the liver or the spleen, lacerations of the great vessels within the abdomen or the chest, bleeding peptic ulcers, and tumors. Regardless of the event, the result is the same: significant loss of body fluids (for example, blood, water, electrolytes).

Hypovolemic shock also occurs with severe thermal burns. In this case, it is intravascular plasma (the colorless part of the blood) that is lost because it leaks

You are the Provider — Part 5

As you palpate the patient's abdomen, she moans and tells you it is very tender around the umbilicus. The abdomen is tense and slightly distended. You initiate transport to a trauma center and perform a reassessment en route.

Reassessment	Recording Time: 8 Minutes After Patient Contact
Level of consciousness	Confused
Skin	Pale and diaphoretic
Respirations	32 breaths/min, shallow
Pulse	Carotid, 142 beats/min, absent radial pulses
Blood pressure	88/60 mm Hg
Sao_2	94% on 100% oxygen via nonrebreathing mask

9. What might explain this patient's deterioration?
10. What is your next treatment option?

> **EMT-I Tips**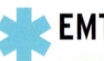
>
> Shock is a complex physiologic process that gives subtle signs to its presence before it becomes severe. These early signs relate very closely to the events that lead to more severe shock, so it is even more important than usual to know the underlying processes thoroughly. If you understand what causes shock, you will be able to recognize it in many patients before it gets out of control.

from the circulatory system into the burned tissues that lie adjacent to the injury. Likewise, crushing injuries may result in the loss of blood and plasma from damaged vessels into injured tissues. Dehydration, the loss of water from body tissues, aggravates shock. In these circumstances, the common factor is an insufficient volume of blood within the vascular system to provide adequate circulation to the organs of the body. This triggers a response by the endocrine system to release hormones and initiate compensation.

Distributive (Vasogenic) Shock

In some patients who have severe bacterial infections, toxins (poisons) generated by the bacteria or by infected body tissues produce a condition called <u>septic shock</u>. In this condition, the toxins damage the vessel walls, causing them to become leaky and unable to contract well, increasing venous capacitance and decreasing cardiac output. Widespread dilation of vessels, in combination with plasma loss through the injured vessel walls, results in distributive shock.

Septic shock is a complex problem. First, there is an insufficient volume of fluid in the container, because much of the blood has leaked out of the vascular system (hypovolemia). Second, the fluid that has leaked out often collects in the respiratory system, interfering with ventilation. Third, there is a larger-than-normal vascular bed to contain the smaller-than-normal volume of intravascular fluid.

<u>Anaphylaxis</u> is another cause of distributive shock. It occurs when a person reacts violently to a substance to which he or she has been sensitized. <u>Sensitization</u> means becoming sensitive (allergic) to a substance. An allergic reaction typically does not occur, or occurs in a milder form, during sensitization. Do not be misled by a patient who reports no history of allergic reaction to a substance following a first or second exposure. Each subsequent exposure after sensitization tends to produce a more severe reaction.

In anaphylactic shock, there is no loss of blood, no vascular damage, and only a slight possibility of direct cardiac muscular injury. Instead, there is widespread vascular dilation, resulting in relative hypovolemia. In other words, relative to the now larger container, the normal blood volume is less. Additionally, immune system chemicals result in severe broncoconstriction. The combination of poor oxygenation and poor perfusion in anaphylactic shock may easily prove fatal. Chapter 26 covers anaphylaxis in detail.

Cardiogenic Shock

<u>Cardiogenic shock</u> is caused by myocardial insufficiency, or pump failure. Circulation of blood throughout the vascular system requires the constant pumping action of a normal and vigorous heart muscle. Many diseases can cause destruction or inflammation of this muscle. Within certain limits, the heart can adapt to these problems. If too much muscular damage occurs, however, as sometimes happens after a myocardial infarction, the heart no longer functions effectively. Cardiogenic shock develops when the heart muscle can no longer generate enough pressure to circulate the blood to all organs or when the regularity of the heartbeat is so disrupted that the volume of blood within the system can no longer be circulated efficiently. Filling is impaired because of a lack of pressure to return blood to the heart (preload), or outflow is obstructed by lack of pumping function. In either case, direct pump failure is the cause of shock. The same process occurs as a result of a cardiac tamponade or tension pneumothorax in which the heart is physically obstructed and cannot pump effectively (obstructed shock).

Spinal Shock

Damage to the spinal cord, particularly at the upper cervical levels, may cause significant injury to the autonomic nervous system which controls the size and muscular tone of the blood vessels. <u>Neurogenic shock</u>, or spinal vascular shock, is usually the result. Although not as common, there are medical causes as well. These include brain conditions, tumors, pressure on the spinal cord, and spina bifida. In neurogenic shock, the muscles in the walls of the blood vessels are cut off from the nerve impulses that cause them to contract. Therefore, all vessels below the level of the spinal injury dilate widely, increasing the size and capacity of the vascular system Figure 13-11 and causing blood to pool. The available 5 to 6 L of blood in the body can no longer fill the enlarged vascular system. Even though no blood or fluid has been lost, perfusion of organs and tissues becomes inadequate, and shock occurs; therefore, the patient experiences relative hypovolemia. This produces hypotension with a systolic pressure usually between 80 and 100 mm Hg. In addition, relative bradycardia occurs because the sympathetic nervous system is not stimulated to release catecholamines. The skin is pink, warm, and dry because of cutaneous vasodilation. There is no release of the chemical mediators, epinephrine and norepinephrine, to produce the classic pale, cool, diaphoretic skin. A characteristic sign of this type of shock is the absence of sweating below the level of injury.

With an injury that results in spinal shock, many other functions that are under the control of the sympathetic nervous system are also lost. The most important of them, in an acute injury setting, is the ability to control body temperature. Body temperature in a patient with neurogenic shock can rapidly fall to match that of the environment. In many situations, significant hypothermia occurs, severely complicating the situation. Hypothermia is a condition in which the internal body temperature falls below 95°F (35°C), usually after prolonged exposure to cool or freezing temperatures. Maintenance of body temperature is always an important element of treatment for a patient in shock.

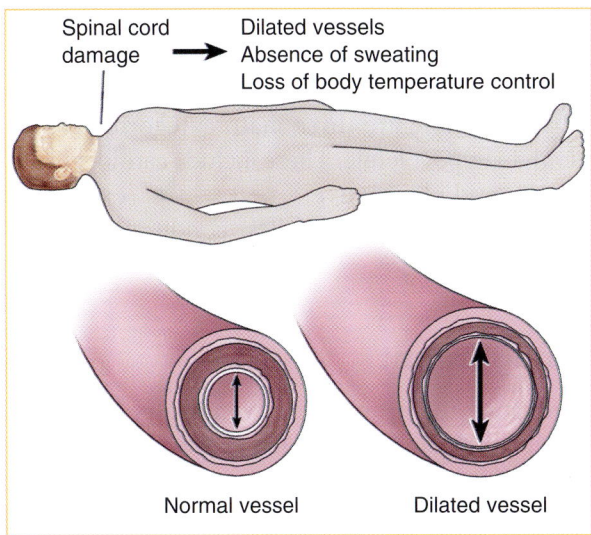

Figure 13-11 Damage to the spinal cord can cause significant injury to the autonomic nervous system which controls the size and muscle tone of blood vessels. If the muscles in the blood vessels are cut off from their impulses to contract, the vessels dilate widely, increasing the size and capacity of the vascular system. The blood in the body can no longer fill the enlarged vessels, resulting in inadequate perfusion.

Occurrence of spinal shock is rare. Shock is usually the result of hidden loss of blood volume from a chest injury, abdominal injury, or other violent injury. Treatment for spinal shock focuses primarily on volume replacement.

You are the Provider Part 6

You initiate an IV of normal saline with a 16-gauge catheter and administer a 20-mL/kg fluid bolus. The patient is now unresponsive, so you determine that a definitive airway must be obtained and insert a Combitube.

Insert an endotracheal tube.

Reassessment	Recording Time: 11 Minutes After Patient Contact
Level of consciousness	Unresponsive
Skin	Pale, cool, and diaphoretic
Respirations	Ventilation with 100% oxygen at a rate of 15 breaths/min
Pulse	Carotid, 154 beats/min
Blood pressure	84/56 mm Hg
Sao_2	97% (ventilated with 100% oxygen)

11. Would you apply the PASG? Why? Why not?
12. What stage of shock is this patient in?

Differential Shock Assessment Findings

Shock is considered to be hypovolemic until proven otherwise. There are three main categories of shock other than hypovolemic. These include cardiogenic, distributive, and obstructive. Table 13-4 explains the differences between each of these conditions and hypovolemic shock.

Management

As with any patient, airway and ventilatory support take top priority. Maintain an open airway, and suction as needed. Give high-flow oxygen via nonrebreathing mask or assist ventilation with a BVM device. Consider early definitive management in patients who are unable to maintain their own airway. If the patient is showing signs of tension pneumothorax, early decompression is critical to survival.

Skill Drill 13-4 provides a review of shock management:

1. As always, begin by following BSI precautions, **making sure the patient has an open airway and checking breathing and pulse**. In general, keep the patient in a supine position. Patients who have had a severe heart attack or who have lung disease may find it easier to breathe in a sitting or semi-sitting position. Remember that inadequate ventilation may be the primary cause of shock or a major factor in its development. Always provide oxygen, assist with ventilations as needed, and continue to monitor the patient's breathing (**Step 1**).
2. Next, **control all obvious external bleeding**. Place dry, sterile dressings over the bleeding sites, and secure with bandages (**Step 2**).
3. **Splint any bone or joint injuries**. This minimizes pain, bleeding, and discomfort, all of which can aggravate shock. It also prevents the ends of the broken bone from further damaging adjacent soft tissue. In general, splinting also makes it easier to move the patient. Handle the patient gently and no more than is necessary (**Step 3**). Consider the use of PASG only with the approval of medical control or established local protocols.
4. To prevent the loss of body heat, **place blankets under and over the patient**. Be careful not to overload the patient with covers or attempt to warm the body too much; it is best for the patient to maintain a normal body temperature. Do not use any external heat sources, such as hot water bottles or heating pads. They may harm a patient in shock by causing vasodilation and decreasing blood pressure even more (**Step 4**).
5. Once you have positioned the patient on a backboard or a stretcher, **place the patient in the Trendelenburg position**. This technique is easily accomplished by raising the foot of the backboard or stretcher about six to twelve inches. If the patient is not on a backboard, and no lower extremity fractures are suspected, place the patient in the shock position. This is accomplished by elevating the patient's legs 6 to 12 inches by propping them up on several blankets or other stable objects. These positions help to return blood from the extremities back to the core of the body where it is needed most. Patients with respiratory distress may benefit from a Trendelenburg position, but the lower extremities should only be raised 6 to 8 inches. Raising the lower extremities any higher may aggravate a patient's breathing because the abdominal organs push against the diaphragm (**Step 5**).

Circulatory Support

Control any external hemorrhage, and try to estimate the amount of blood lost. Look for signs of internal hemorrhage, and consider the potential for loss in the area of suspected hemorrhage. For example, a patient may lose up

---

TABLE 13-4 Differentiating Types of Shock

Cardiogenic Shock

Differentiated from hypovolemic shock by the presence of one or more of the following:
- Chief complaint: chest pain, dyspnea, tachycardia
- Heart rate: bradycardia or excessive tachycardia
- Signs of congestive heart failure: jugular vein distention, rales
- Dysrhythmias

Distributive Shock

Differentiated from hypovolemic shock by the presence of one or more of the following:
- Mechanism that suggests vasodilation: spinal cord injury, drug overdose, sepsis, anaphylaxis
- Warm, flushed skin, especially in dependent areas
- Lack of tachycardic response: This is not reliable though, because a significant number of hypovolemic patients never have tachycardia.

Obstructive Shock

Differentiated from hypovolemic shock by the presence of signs and symptoms suggestive of:
- Cardiac tamponade
- Tension pneumothorax

Chapter 13 Hemorrhage and Shock

Treating Shock

Skill Drill 13-4

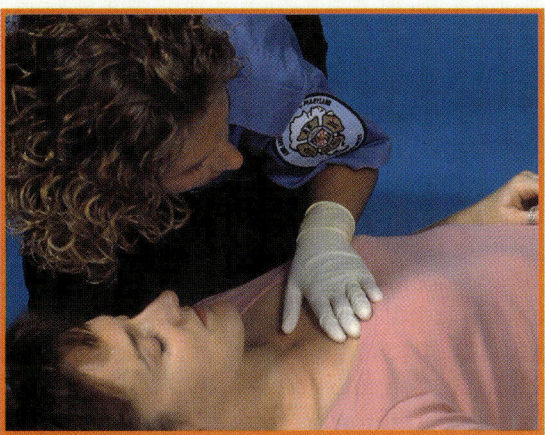
1 Keep the patient supine, open the airway, and check breathing and pulse.
Give high-flow oxygen and assist ventilations if needed.

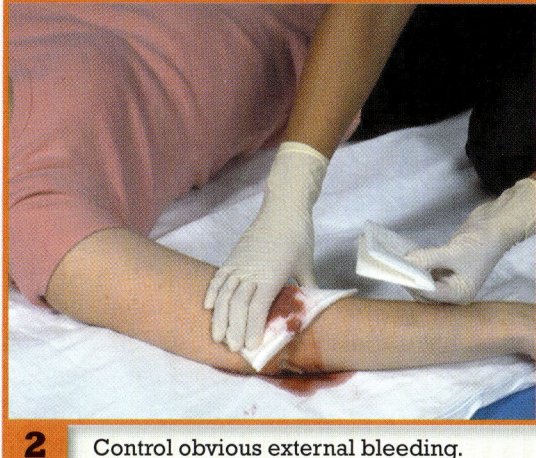
2 Control obvious external bleeding.

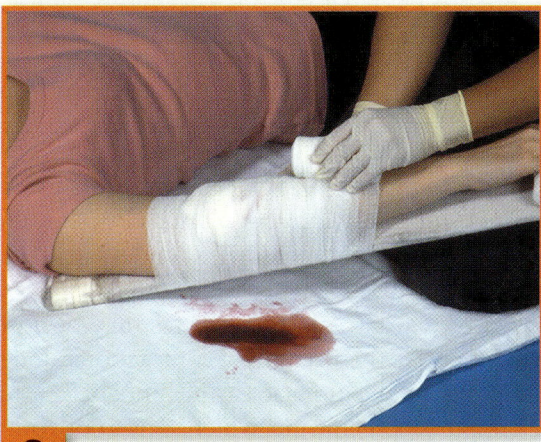
3 Splint any broken bones or joint injuries.

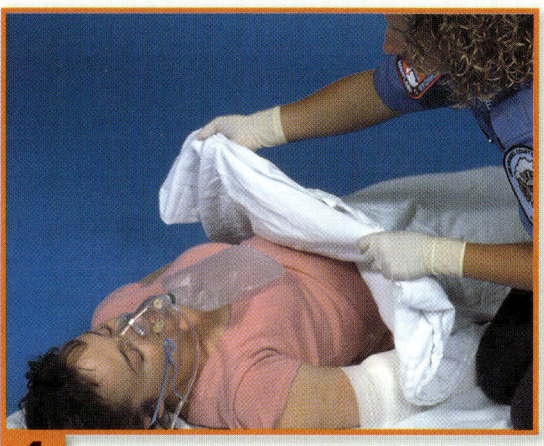
4 Place blankets under and over the patient.

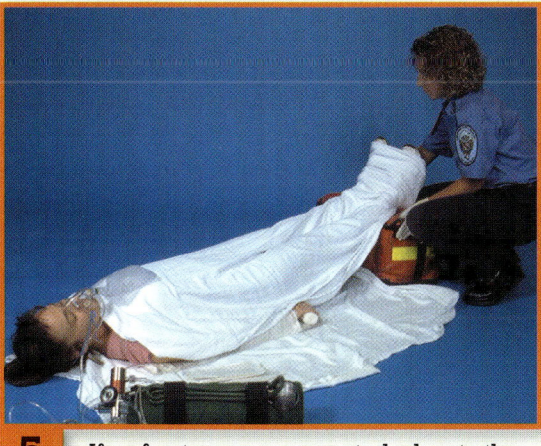
5 If no fractures are suspected, elevate the legs 6″ to 12″.
Start an IV and administer fluid.

to 1 L of blood in the tissues of the thigh in a closed femur fracture. Internal hemorrhage may be the result of blunt or penetrating trauma. It is important to always consider the mechanism of injury and to maintain a high index of suspicion for occult injuries, especially when the patient is exhibiting signs of shock with no obvious cause.

Establish IV access with two large bore catheters, (14 or 16 gauge) and administer IV volume expanders to replace blood loss. Isotonic crystalloids, such as normal saline or lactated Ringer's, should be used (synthetic solutions may also be used). The goal of volume replacement is to maintain perfusion without increasing internal or uncontrollable external hemorrhage. For this reason, most protocols advise administration of IV fluid in boluses of 20 mL/kg until there is a return of radial pulses. The presence of radial pulses equates to a systolic blood pressure of 80 to 90 mm Hg, which, in the majority of the population, is sufficient to perfuse the brain and other vital organs.

Effects resulting from inflation of the PASG include an increased arterial blood pressure above the garment, increased SVR, immobilization of the pelvis and possibly the lower extremities, and increased intraabdominal pressure. The increased SVR is accomplished through direct compression of tissues and blood vessels. As discussed earlier in this chapter, the actual autotransfusion effect is negligible. Increased resistance is the result of the decreased container size.

Hypoperfusion with an unstable pelvis is the primary indication for use of the PASG. Conditions of decreased SVR not corrected by other means, such as increasing fluid volume in cases of neurogenic shock, may also benefit from use of the PASG. Because use of the PASG is widely controversial, it is imperative that you always follow local protocols. As approved locally, other conditions characterized by hypoperfusion with hypotension are also indications.

As previously mentioned, the only true contraindication for inflation of the PASG is pulmonary edema. All other conditions are relative and should be addressed by local protocols and communication with medical control. In the event of advanced pregnancy, the abdominal section should not be inflated. Impaled objects in the abdomen or evisceration are also contraindications for inflating the abdominal compartment. In these situations, the patient may benefit from inflation of the leg sections only. In a patient with a ruptured diaphragm, inflation of the PASG will most likely exacerbate the problem by forcing the abdominal contents up into the thoracic cavity and preventing expansion of the lungs. Likewise, in cardiogenic shock, the increase in intrathoracic pressure increases the workload on the heart, causing further failure of the pump.

For the patient exhibiting signs of a tension pneumothorax, needle chest decompression is necessary to improve cardiac output. In cases of suspected cardiac tamponade, you must recognize the need for expeditious transport for pericardiocentesis at the emergency department. Either of these conditions further impairs circulation by compression of the heart and decreasing cardiac output.

Place the patient on the cardiac monitor and be alert for possible dysrhythmias.

Pharmacologic Interventions

Hypovolemic shock should be treated with volume expanders to replace what has been lost or to "fill the container" in relative hypovolemia. For cardiogenic shock, cautious use of volume expanders may increase preload and, subsequently, cardiac output.

Positive cardiac inotropic drugs may be administered to increase the strength of contractions along with rate-altering medications to further enhance perfusion. An example is epinephrine, which serves both purposes with its beta$_1$ effects.

The vasodilation that accompanies distributive shock creates relative hypovolemia. Regardless of the cause, the problem is still a lack of fluid for the size of the container. Treatment involves volume expanders, positive cardiac inotropic drugs, and consideration of the use of PASG. Volume expanders are also indicated for obstructive shock and spinal shock.

Nonpharmacologic interventions include proper positioning of the patient, preventing hypothermia, and rapid transport. When making your transport decision,

---

You are the Provider Part 7

You arrive at the emergency department and transfer care of the patient to the trauma team.

13. Is there anything else you could have considered?
14. What else could you have done to treat this patient's shock?

consider the need for a trauma center. If travel time is lengthy, air medical transportation may be the best option. Provide psychological support en route. Even unresponsive patients can sometimes hear and understand. Remember to speak calmly and reassuringly to the patient throughout assessment, care, and transport.

> **In the Field**
>
> Positioning the patient is an important part of treatment. Remember the following:
> If the face is *red*, raise the *head*. If the face is *pale*, raise the *tail*.

You are the Provider — Summary

1. Why does internal bleeding often go unnoticed until the patient "crashes"?

Unlike external bleeding, which is visibly obvious and can be promptly controlled, internal bleeding is not visibly evident and usually does not result in hemodynamic compromise until a significant amount of blood has been lost. This underscores the importance of maintaining a high index of suspicion when the mechanism of injury suggests the potential for internal bleeding.

2. Under what circumstances might the rarely used tourniquet be the best choice for bleeding control?

The tourniquet should only be used when all other methods to control bleeding have failed. Situations that may require the use of a tourniquet include amputated extremities or lacerations of a large artery (ie, femoral), in which blood loss is rapid and will result in death within a matter of minutes if not immediately controlled.

3. What is your first step in the management of this patient?

Calm the patient and obtain more information about the mechanism of injury.

4. Is there is a significant mechanism of injury?

Yes. There is moderate damage to the vehicle and the patient was unrestrained at the time of impact.

5. What are your concerns for this patient?

On the basis of the mechanism of injury, you should be concerned about the possibility of trauma to multiple organs; liver, diaphragm, chest, and cervical spine.

6. Are her vital sign values clinically significant?

Yes. Her pulse should decrease as she relaxes. Tachycardia following trauma should be assumed to be an early sign of shock.

7. What is your next step in the treatment of this patient?

Apply 100% supplemental oxygen with a nonrebreathing mask.

8. What are your assessment concerns?

Because of the significant mechanism of injury, a rapid trauma assessment should be performed.

9. What might explain this patient's deterioration?

Because there are no external signs of trauma, except the laceration above the eye, you should assume that the patient has internal bleeding, possibly into the abdomen.

10. What is your next treatment option?

Initiate at least one large-bore IV of an isotonic crystalloid and administer a bolus of 20 mL/kg. This may need to be repeated to maintain adequate perfusion (ie, radial pulses return, SBP of at least 90 mm Hg). Follow local protocols regarding IV fluid administration for trauma patients.

11. Would you apply the PASG? Why or why not?

The PASG are generally contraindicated in cases of internal bleeding. They function by increasing systemic vascular resistance, which could interfere with the body's hemostatic process and exacerbate the bleeding. Follow local protocols regarding the use of the PASG.

12. What stage of shock is this patient in?

Due to the absence of radial pulses, hypotension, and the patient's unresponsiveness, she is in decompensated shock.

13. Is there anything else you could have considered?

Obtain a SAMPLE history to identify a possible medical cause that led to the accident. Because of her altered mental status, her blood sugar should have been assessed as well.

Apply a cardiac monitor to any critically injured patient.

14. What else could you have done to treat this patient's shock?

As advanced skills are learned, basic skills seem to be taken for granted. Because the patient was immobilized on a long spine board, you should have placed her in the Trendelenburg position (legs elevated, head lowered), which may improve perfusion to vital organs such as the brain, heart, liver, and kidneys. Additionally, a blanket should have been placed on her to prevent hypothermia.

Section 5 Trauma

Prep Kit

Ready for Review

- Perfusion is the circulation of blood in adequate amounts to meet each cell's current needs for oxygen, nutrients, and waste removal.
- Hypoperfusion, or shock, occurs when the cardiovascular system fails to provide adequate perfusion.
- Both internal and external bleeding can cause shock. You must know how to recognize and control both.
- In the order of preference, the seven methods for controlling external bleeding are direct local pressure and elevation, pressure dressings, application of pressure to pressure points, splints, air splints, PASG, and tourniquets.
- Do not remove a dressing until a physician has evaluated the patient's condition; instead, apply additional dressings as needed. If bleeding continues, locate and apply pressure to the appropriate pressure point.
- Stabilizing a serious fracture has a high priority in the control of bleeding.
- Use a PASG to prevent or minimize hypovolemic shock only when there is massive soft-tissue bleeding of the lower extremities that cannot be otherwise controlled, or bleeding associated with fractures of the pelvis and bilateral femurs. Always follow local protocols and consult medical control for advice regarding the PASG.
- Tourniquets may be used in cases of severe, uncontrolled bleeding.
- You should assess and promptly transport any patient who may have internal bleeding, particularly if the mechanism of injury is severe and has affected the abdomen, the chest, or both.
- Signs of internal bleeding include hematemesis, melena, hemoptysis, broken ribs, bruised chest, distended abdomen, and referred pain.
- Signs of shock that suggest internal bleeding include change in mental status, pallor, weakness and dizziness, tachycardia, thirst, nausea and vomiting, and shallow, rapid breathing.
- If you suspect that a patient is bleeding internally, maintain the airway, administer 100% supplemental oxygen and be prepared to assist ventilation, keep the patient still and warm, apply a splint to any affected extremity, monitor vital signs at least every 5 minutes, and, in nontrauma patients, elevate the legs.
- Shock (hypoperfusion) is the collapse and failure of the cardiovascular system in which blood circulation slows and eventually ceases.
- Perfusion requires a cardiovascular system with all three parts (the pump, container, and fluid) working, but it also requires a functioning respiratory system.
- The signs and symptoms of shock are caused by the actions of the autonomic nervous system and of hormones (catecholamines) responding to the need for additional perfusion.
- Signs of compensated shock include agitation or anxiety; a weak, rapid pulse; clammy skin; air hunger; nausea or vomiting; slow capillary refill in children and infants; and marked thirst.
- Signs of decompensated shock include labored or irregular breathing, ashen or cyanotic skin, thready or absent peripheral pulses, dilated pupils, poor urinary output, and, finally, a falling blood pressure. By the time you detect a drop in blood pressure, shock is well developed.
- Expect shock in cases of massive internal or external bleeding, multiple severe fractures, abdominal or chest injury, spinal injury, severe infection, massive myocardial infarction, and anaphylaxis.
- Treat patients with shock by (1) opening and maintaining the airway; (2) providing 100% oxygen and, if necessary, assisting ventilations; (3) controlling all obvious external bleeding; (4) conserving body heat with blankets; (5) properly positioning the patient; (6) IV fluid replacement; and (7) transporting promptly.

Technology

- Interactivities
- Vocabulary Explorer
- Anatomy Review
- Web Links
- Online Review Manual

Vital Vocabulary

anaphylaxis An unusual or exaggerated allergic reaction to foreign protein or other substances.

autonomic nervous system The part of the nervous system that regulates involuntary functions, such as digestion and sweating.

cardiogenic shock Shock caused by inadequate function of the heart, or pump failure.

compensated shock The early stage of shock, in which the body can still compensate for blood loss.

decompensated shock The late stage of shock, when blood pressure is falling.

epistaxis Nosebleed.

hematochezia Passage of stools containing bright red blood, indicating lower GI bleeding.

hematuria Presence of blood in the urine.

hemophilia A congenital condition in which the patient lacks one or more of the blood's normal clotting factors.

hemorrhage Bleeding.

hemostasis Formation of clots to plug openings in injured blood vessels and stop blood flow.

hypothermia A condition in which the internal body temperature falls below 95°F (35°C), usually as a result of prolonged exposure to cool or freezing temperatures.

hypovolemic shock A condition in which low blood volume, due to massive internal or external bleeding or extensive loss of body water, results in inadequate perfusion.

irreversible shock The final stage of shock, resulting in death.

melena The passage of dark, tarry, foul-smelling stool, indicative of upper GI bleeding.

neurogenic shock Circulatory failure caused by paralysis of the nerves that control the size of the blood vessels, leading to widespread dilation; seen in spinal cord injuries.

nonprogressive shock A synonym for compensated shock.

orthostatic hypotension A drop in systolic blood pressure when moving from a sitting to a standing position.

perfusion Circulation of blood within an organ or tissue in amounts adequate to meet the cells' current needs.

pneumatic antishock garment (PASG) An inflatable device that covers the legs and abdomen; used to splint the lower extremities or pelvis, or to control bleeding in the lower extremities or pelvis.

pressure point A point where a blood vessel lies near a bone; useful when direct pressure and elevation do not control bleeding.

pulse pressure Difference between the systolic and diastolic pressures.

sensitization Developing sensitivity to a substance that initially caused no allergic reaction.

septic shock Shock caused by severe bacterial infection.

shock A condition in which the circulatory system fails to provide sufficient circulation to enable every body part to perform its function; also called hypoperfusion.

sphincters Circular muscles that encircle and, by contracting, constrict a duct, tube, or opening.

tourniquet The bleeding control method of last resort that occludes arterial flow; used only when all other methods have failed and the patient's life is in danger.

Assessment in Action

You are dispatched to a private residence because someone has fallen. You arrive at the scene to find a 45-year-old man lying supine on the front lawn. Bystanders state that the patient fell 12 feet from the roof of his house.

You note that he is unconscious and unresponsive, is bleeding from the back of the head, has pale skin, and is gurgling when he breathes. You also note deformity of both femurs.

Your physical exam reveals a large laceration to the back of the head and bilateral femoral swelling and deformity. The patient's respirations are 26 breaths/min, pulse is 122 beats/min and weak, and BP is 110/90 mm Hg.

1. The MOST immediate life threat to this patient's life is/are:
   A. external bleeding.
   B. femur fractures.
   C. airway compromise.
   D. severe internal bleeding.

2. Airway management for this patient should include all of the following EXCEPT:
   A. oral airway.
   B. nasal airway.
   C. supplemental oxygen.
   D. oropharyngeal suction.

3. You note a steady, heavy flow of dark red blood from the back of the patient's head. This is most likely due to lacerated:
   A. veins.
   B. arteries.
   C. capillaries.
   D. venules.

4. To control this patient's external bleeding, you should FIRST:
   A. apply direct pressure.
   B. place a pressure dressing.
   C. apply pressure to the temporal artery.
   D. elevate his head 45°.

5. The patient's altered LOC may be due to:
   A. head injury.
   B. hypovolemia.
   C. insulin shock.
   D. any of the above.

6. This patient's vital signs are consistent with:
   A. compensated shock.
   B. decompensated shock.
   C. irreversible shock.
   D. neurogenic shock.

7. Which of the following questions would be LEAST pertinent to ask the witnesses?
   A. Did the patient have chest pain before falling?
   B. Does the patient have any medical problems?
   C. How long have you known the patient?
   D. Did the patient slip before falling off the roof?

8. The most likely cause of the patient's condition is:
   A. septic shock.
   B. cardiogenic shock.
   C. hypovolemic shock.
   D. distributive shock.

9. The MOST significant source of significant blood loss in this patient is likely from:
   A. the femur fractures.
   B. external bleeding.
   C. the head laceration.
   D. closed head trauma.

10. Your treatment for this patient will include:
    A. immobilization with KED.
    B. maintaining body heat.
    C. oxygen by nasal cannula.
    D. restricting IV fluids.

Points to Ponder

It is the middle of the night when you are dispatched to treat a man down in a light industrial park south of town. You arrive at the scene to find an elderly man, dressed in pajamas, lying in the roadway. He was found by a police officer patrolling the area. There are no witnesses. He is unresponsive, pale, and diaphoretic. His respirations are 28 breaths/min, radial pulses are absent, and you are unable to detect a blood pressure. It appears that the patient may have vomited, so you suction his airway. The emesis is dark brown and has a coffee-ground appearance. Your physical exam reveals a large bump on his forehead.

What might have happened to the patient? What might be wrong with the patient? What is the significance of his being in pajamas? What is the significance of the emesis? Is he in shock? What will your treatment consist of?

Issues: Considering Both Trauma and Medical Causes of Shock, Relying on Signs and Symptoms of Shock to Guide Your Treatment

Burns and Soft-Tissue Injuries

1999 Objectives

Cognitive

4-3.1 Describe the anatomy and physiology pertinent to burn injuries. (p 678)

4-3.2 Describe the epidemiology, including incidence, morbidity/mortality, risk factors, and prevention strategies for the patient with a burn injury. (p 691)

4-3.3 Describe the pathophysiologic complications and systemic complications of a burn injury. (p 691)

4-3.4 Identify and describe types of burn injuries, including a thermal burn, an inhalation burn, a chemical burn, an electrical burn, and a radiation exposure. (p 679)

4-3.5 Identify and describe the depth classifications of burn injuries, including a superficial burn, a partial-thickness burn, a full-thickness burn, and other depth classifications described by local protocol. (p 693)

4-3.6 Identify and describe methods for determining body surface area percentage of a burn injury including the "rules of nines," the "rules of palms," and other methods described by local protocol. (p 694)

4-3.7 Identify and describe the severity of a burn including a minor burn, a moderate burn, a severe burn, and other severity classifications described by local protocol. (p 692)

4-3.8 Differentiate criteria for determining the severity of a burn injury between a pediatric patient and an adult patient. (p 694)

4-3.9 Describe special considerations for a pediatric patient with a burn injury. (p 695)

4-3.10 Discuss considerations which impact management and prognosis of the burn injured patient. (p 694)

4-3.11 Discuss mechanisms of burn injuries. (p 694)

4-3.12 Discuss conditions associated with burn injuries, including trauma, blast injuries, airway compromise, respiratory compromise, and child abuse. (p 694)

4-3.13 Describe the management of a burn injury, including airway and ventilation, circulation, pharmacologic, non-pharmacologic, transport considerations, psychological support/communication strategies, and other management described by local protocol. (p 695)

4-3.14 Describe the epidemiology of a thermal burn injury. (p 691)

4-3.15 Describe the specific anatomy and physiology pertinent to a thermal burn injury. (p 692)

4-3.16 Describe the pathophysiology of a thermal burn injury. (p 691)

4-3.17 Identify and describe the depth classifications of a thermal burn injury. (p 693)

4-3.18 Identify and describe the severity of a thermal burn injury. (p 692)

4-3.19 Describe considerations which impact management and prognosis of the patient with a thermal burn injury. (p 695)

4-3.20 Discuss mechanisms of burn injury and conditions associated with a thermal burn injury. (p 694)

4-3.21 Describe the management of a thermal burn injury, including airway and ventilation, circulation, pharmacologic, non-pharmacologic, transport considerations, and psychological support/communication strategies. (p 695)

4-3.22 Describe the epidemiology of an inhalation burn injury. (p 698)

4-3.23 Describe the specific anatomy and physiology pertinent to an inhalation burn injury. (p 698)

4-3.24 Describe the pathophysiology of an inhalation burn injury. (p 698)

4-3.25 Differentiate between supraglottic and infraglottic inhalation injuries. (p 698)

4-3.26 Identify and describe the severity of an inhalation burn injury. (p 698)

4-3.27 Describe considerations which impact management and prognosis of the patient with an inhalation burn injury. (p 699)

4-3.28 Discuss mechanisms of burn injury and conditions associated with an inhalation burn injury. (p 698)

4-3.29 Describe the management of an inhalation burn injury, including airway and ventilation, circulation, pharmacologic, non-pharmacologic, transport considerations, and psychological support/communication strategies. (p 699)

4-3.30 Describe the epidemiology of a chemical burn injury and a chemical burn injury to the eye. (p 700)

4-3.31 Describe the specific anatomy and physiology pertinent to a chemical burn injury and a chemical burn injury to the eye. (p 700)

4-3.32 Describe the pathophysiology of a chemical burn injury, including types of chemicals and their burning processes and a chemical burn injury to the eye. (p 700)

4-3.33 Identify and describe the depth classifications of a chemical burn injury. (p 699)

4-3.34 Identify and describe the severity of a chemical burn injury. (p 699)

4-3.35 Describe considerations which impact management and prognosis of the patient with a chemical burn injury and a chemical burn injury to the eye. (p 700)

4-3.36 Discuss mechanisms of burn injury and conditions associated with a chemical burn injury. (p 699)

4-3.37 Describe the management of a chemical burn injury and a chemical burn injury to the eye, including airway and ventilation, circulation, pharmacologic, non-pharmacologic, transport considerations, and psychological support/ communication strategies. (p 700)

4-3.38 Describe the epidemiology of an electrical burn injury. (p 703)

4-3.39 Describe the specific anatomy and physiology pertinent to an electrical burn injury. (p 703)

4-3.40 Describe the pathophysiology of an electrical burn injury. (p 703)

4-3.41 Identify and describe the depth classifications of an electrical burn injury. (p 703)

4-3.42 Identify and describe the severity of an electrical burn injury. (p 703)

4-3.43 Describe considerations which impact management and prognosis of the patient with an electrical burn injury. (p 703)

4-3.44 Discuss mechanisms of burn injury and conditions associated with an electrical burn injury. (p 703)

4-3.45 Describe the management of an electrical burn injury, including airway and ventilation, circulation, pharmacologic, non-pharmacologic, transport considerations, and psychological support/communication strategies. (p 704)

4-3.46 Describe the epidemiology of a radiation exposure. (p 705)

4-3.47 Describe the specific anatomy and physiology pertinent to a radiation exposure. (p 706)

4-3.48 Describe the pathophysiology of a radiation exposure, including the types and characteristics of ionizing radiation. (p 705)

4-3.49 Identify and describe the depth classifications of a radiation exposure. (p 706)

4-3.50 Identify and describe the severity of a radiation exposure. (p 706)

4-3.51 Describe considerations which impact management and prognosis of the patient with a radiation exposure. (p 706)

4-3.52 Discuss mechanisms of burn injury associated with a radiation exposure. (p 706)

4-3.53 Describe the management of a radiation exposure, including airway and ventilation, circulation, pharmacologic, non-pharmacologic, transport considerations, and psychological support/communication strategies. (p 707)

4-3.54 Formulate a field impression and implement the management plan for a thermal burn injury. (p 695)

4-3.55 Formulate a field impression and implement the management plan for an inhalation burn injury. (p 699)

4-3.56 Formulate a field impression and implement the management plan for a chemical burn injury. (p 700)

4-3.57 Formulate a field impression and implement the management plan for an electrical burn injury. (p 704)

4-3.58 Formulate a field impression and implement the management plan for a radiation exposure. (p 707)

Burns and Soft-Tissue Injuries

Affective

4-3.59 Value the changes of a patient's self-image associated with a burn injury. (p 678)
4-3.60 Value the impact of managing a burn injured patient. (p 691)
4-3.61 Advocate empathy for a burn injured patient. (p 678)
4-3.62 Value and defend the sense of urgency in burn injuries. (p 691)

Psychomotor

4-3.63 Take body substance isolation procedures during assessment and management of patients with a burn injury. (p 695)
4-3.64 Perform assessment of a patient with a burn injury. (p 695)
4-5.15 Demonstrate the assessment and management of a patient with signs and symptoms of soft tissue injury, including:
   a. Contusion
   b. Hematoma
   c. Crushing
   d. Abrasion
   d. Laceration
   e. Avulsion
   g. Amputation
   h. Impaled object
   f. Penetration/puncture
   g. Blast (p 681, 684-690)

1985 Objectives

There are no 1985 objectives for this chapter.

14

Burns and Soft-Tissue Injuries

You are the Provider

You receive a call to a residence for an unknown emergency. On arrival, you find a man with an electrical burn to his entire right arm. The patient tells you that he was attempting to rewire an electrical outlet in his kitchen and failed to shut off the power.

This chapter will help prepare you to properly care for soft-tissue injuries and burns and help you answer the following questions:

1. What is the difference between a dressing and a bandage?
2. Is there a difference in the care for chemical burns and electrical burns?

Burns and Soft-Tissue Injuries

The skin is our first line of defense against external forces, and, although it is relatively tough, skin is still quite susceptible to injury. Injuries to soft tissues range from simple bruises and abrasions to serious lacerations and amputations. Injury may result in loss of soft tissue, exposing deep structures such as blood vessels, nerves, and bones. In all cases, you must control bleeding, prevent further contamination, and protect the wound from further damage. Therefore, you must know how to apply dressings and bandages to various parts of the body.

The Anatomy and Function of the Skin

The skin is the largest organ in the body. It varies in thickness, depending on age and its location. The skin of very young and very old people is thinner than the skin of a young adult. The skin covering your scalp, your back, and the soles of your feet is quite thick, while the skin of your eyelids, lips, and ears is very thin. Obviously, thin skin is more easily damaged than thick skin.

Anatomy of the Skin

The skin has two principal layers: the epidermis and the dermis Figure 14-1 ▶ . The epidermis is the tough, external layer that forms a watertight covering for the body. The epidermis itself is composed of several layers. The cells on the surface layer of the epidermis are constantly worn away. They are replaced by cells that are pushed to the surface when new cells form in the germinal layer at the base of the epidermis. Deeper cells in the germinal layer contain pigment (melanin) granules. Along with blood vessels in the dermis, these granules produce skin color.

The dermis is the inner layer of the skin that lies below the germinal cells of the epidermis. The dermis contains the structures that give the skin its characteristic appearance: hair follicles, sweat glands, and sebaceous glands. The sweat glands help to cool the body. They discharge sweat onto the surface of the skin through small pores, or ducts, that pass through the epidermis. Sebaceous glands produce *sebum*, the oily material that waterproofs the skin and keeps it supple. Sebum travels to the skin's surface along the shaft of adjacent hair follicles. Hair follicles are small organs that produce hair. There is one follicle for each hair, each connected with a sebaceous gland and a tiny muscle, the erector pili, which pulls the hair erect whenever you are cold or frightened.

Blood vessels in the dermis provide the skin with nutrients and oxygen. Small branches reach up to the germinal cells, but no blood vessels penetrate farther into the epidermis. There are also specialized nerve endings within the dermis.

The skin covers all external surfaces of the body. The various orifices in our body, including the mouth, nose, anus, and vagina, are not covered by skin. Instead, these openings are lined with mucous membranes. These membranes are similar to skin in that they, too, provide a protective barrier against invasion of harmful

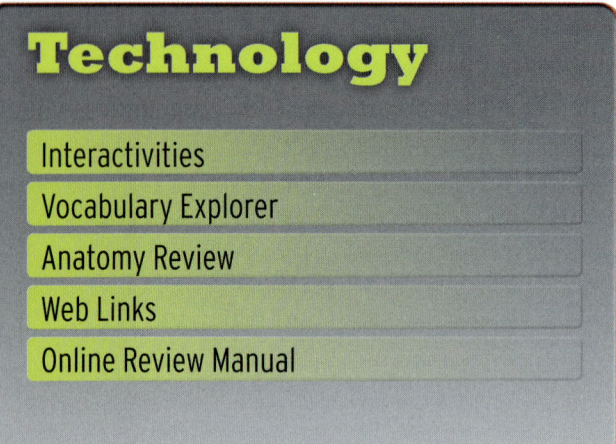

 EMT-I Tips

Although it may be tempting to think of skin injuries as unimportant, the skin has several crucial protective and regulatory roles. When dealing with skin injuries, remember the importance of this organ in protecting against infection and maintaining internal temperature and fluid balance. The skin can also be very important emotionally to the patient; concerns about how bruising and scarring will look later may require psychological support to patients with injuries to the skin.

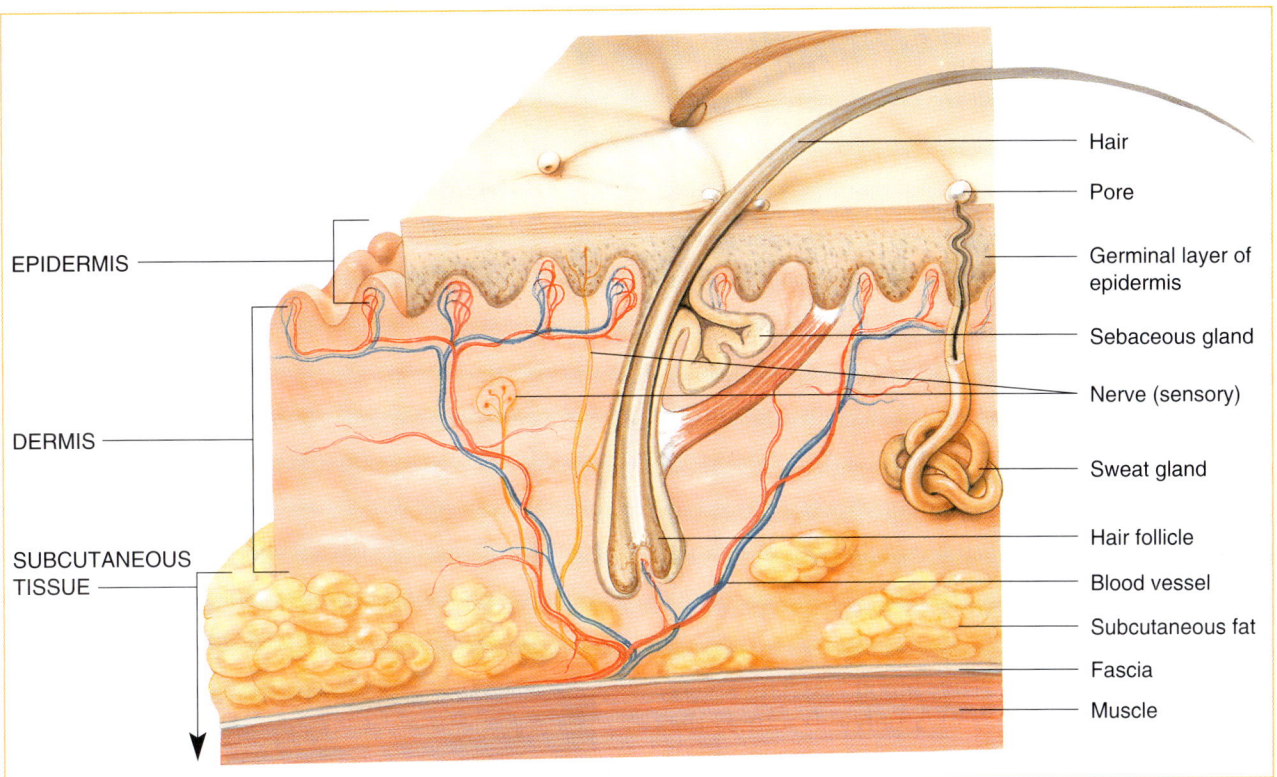

Figure 14-1 The skin is composed of a tough external layer called the epidermis and a vascular inner layer called the dermis.

agents. But mucous membranes differ from skin because they secrete a watery substance that lubricates the openings. Therefore, mucous membranes are moist, while skin is dry.

Functions of the Skin

The skin serves many functions. It protects the body by keeping harmful agents out and water in. The nerves in the skin report to the brain on the environment and on many sensations.

The skin is also the body's major organ for regulating temperature. In a cold environment, the blood vessels in the skin constrict, diverting blood away from the skin and decreasing the amount of heat that is radiated from the body's surface. In hot environments, the vessels in the skin dilate. The skin becomes flushed or red, and heat radiates from the body's surface. Also, sweat glands secrete sweat. As the sweat evaporates from the skin's surface, your body temperature drops, and you begin to cool down.

Any break in the skin allows potentially infectious agents to enter and raises the possibilities of infection, fluid loss, and loss of temperature control. Any one of these problems can cause serious illness and even death.

Types of Soft-Tissue Injuries

Soft tissues are often injured because they are exposed to the environment. There are three types of soft-tissue injuries:

- Closed injury, in which soft-tissue damage occurs beneath the skin or mucous membrane but the surface remains intact.
- Open injury, in which there is a break in the surface of the skin or the mucous membrane, exposing deeper tissue to potential contamination.
- Burns, in which the soft tissue receives more energy than it can absorb without injury. The source of this energy can be thermal heat, frictional heat, toxic chemicals, electricity, or nuclear radiation.

Closed Injuries

Closed soft-tissue injuries are characterized by a history of blunt trauma, pain at the site of injury, swelling beneath the skin, and discoloration. Such injuries can vary from mild to quite severe.

A contusion, or bruise, results from blunt force striking the body. The epidermis remains intact, but cells within the dermis are damaged, and small blood vessels are usually torn. The depth of the injury varies, depending on the amount of energy absorbed. As fluid and blood leak into the damaged area, the patient may have swelling and pain. The buildup of blood produces a characteristic blue or black discoloration called ecchymosis (Figure 14-2).

A hematoma is a pool of blood that has collected within damaged tissue or in a body cavity. It occurs whenever a large blood vessel is damaged and bleeds rapidly. It is usually associated with extensive tissue damage. A hematoma can result from a soft-tissue injury, a fracture, or any injury to a large blood vessel. In severe cases, such as a torn aorta or a pelvic fracture, the hematoma may contain more than a liter of blood (Figure 14-3).

A crushing injury occurs when a great amount of force is applied to the body for a long period of time (Figure 14-4). The extent of the damage depends on

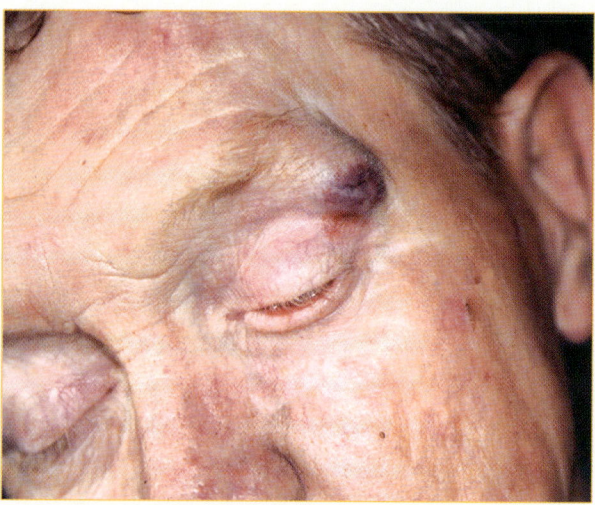

Figure 14-3 A hematoma develops whenever a blood vessel is damaged and bleeds substantially.

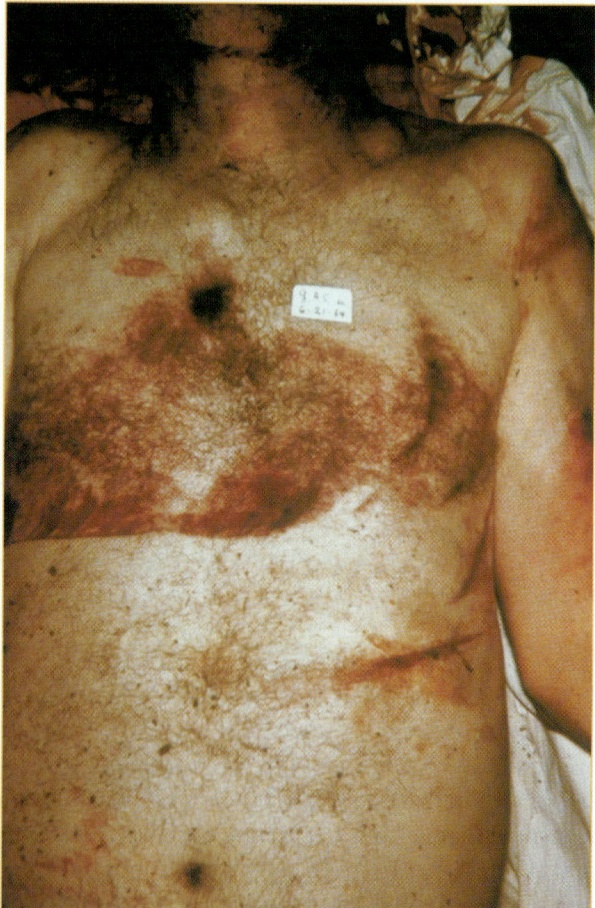

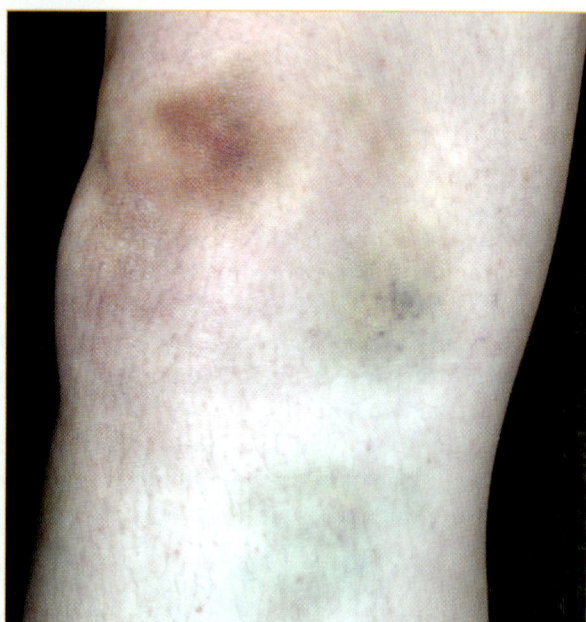

Figure 14-2 Contusions, more commonly known as bruises, occur as a result of a blunt force striking the body. The buildup of blood produces a characteristic blue or black discoloration (ecchymosis).

Figure 14-4 The damage associated with a crush or compression injury varies depending on the direct damage to the soft tissues and on how long the tissue was cut off from circulation.

just how long that period is. In addition to causing some direct soft-tissue damage, continued compression of the soft tissues will cut off their circulation, producing further tissue destruction. For example, if a patient's legs are trapped under a collapsed pile of rocks, damage to the leg tissues will continue until the rocks are removed.

Another form of compression can result from the swelling that occurs whenever tissues are injured. The cells that are injured leak watery fluid into the spaces between the cells. If swelling is excessive or occurs in a confined space such as the skull, the tissue pressure will increase to dangerous levels. The pressure of the fluid may become great enough to compress the tissue and cause further damage. This is especially true if the blood vessels become compressed, cutting off blood flow to the tissue. This condition is called compartment syndrome. Excessive swelling often follows injury of the brain, the spinal cord, and the extremities.

Severe closed injuries can also damage internal organs. The greater the amount of energy absorbed from the blunt force, the greater the risk of injury to deeper structures. Therefore, you must assess all patients with closed injuries for more serious hidden injuries. Remain alert for signs of shock or internal bleeding, and begin treatment of these conditions if necessary.

Emergency Medical Care

Small contusions require no special emergency medical care. More extensive closed injuries may involve significant swelling and bleeding beneath the skin, which could lead to hypovolemic shock. Before treating a closed injury, make sure to follow body substance isolation (BSI) precautions. Wear gloves as you work with the patient.

Soft-tissue injuries may look rather dramatic. However, you must still focus on airway and breathing first. Always provide oxygen to patients who need it, and maintain the airway in all patients. If the patient has difficulty breathing or is otherwise breathing inadequately, you may have to assist ventilation.

Treat a closed soft-tissue injury by applying the acronym ICES:

- **Ice** (or a cold pack) slows bleeding by causing blood vessels to constrict, and it also reduces pain.
- **Compression** over the injury site slows bleeding by compressing the blood vessels.
- **Elevation** of the injured part above the level of the patient's heart decreases swelling.

- **Splinting** decreases bleeding and also reduces pain by immobilizing a soft-tissue injury or an injured extremity.

In addition to using these measures to control bleeding and swelling, you should also be alert for signs of developing shock, including tachycardia, tachypnea, cool and/or clammy skin, and a later sign, hypotension. Any or all of these signs may indicate internal bleeding resulting from injuries to internal organs. If the patient appears to be in shock, you should elevate his or her legs 6″ to 12″, initiate intravenous (IV) therapy, give high-flow oxygen, and provide prompt transport to the hospital.

Open Injuries

Open injuries differ from closed injuries in that the protective layer of skin is damaged. This can produce more extensive bleeding. More important, however, a break in the protective skin layer or mucous membrane means that the wound is contaminated and may become infected. Contamination means that infective organisms or foreign bodies, such as dirt, gravel, or metal, are present. You must address these two problems in your treatment of open soft-tissue wounds. There are four types of open soft-tissue wounds that you must be prepared to manage: abrasions, lacerations, avulsions, and penetrating wounds.

An abrasion is a wound of the superficial layer of the skin caused by friction when a body part rubs or scrapes across a rough or hard surface. An abrasion usually does not penetrate completely through the dermis, but blood may ooze from the injured capillaries in the dermis. Known by a variety of names, including road rash, road burn, strawberry, and mat burn, abrasions can be extremely painful (Figure 14-5 ▶). Even though abrasions are usually superficial, their locations may indicate possible underlying injuries. You should maintain a high index of suspicion that injuries over the flank areas may be the only sign of potential kidney damage (Figure 14-6 ▶).

A laceration is a smooth or jagged cut caused by a sharp object or a blunt force that tears the tissue. The depth of the injury can vary, extending through the skin and subcutaneous tissue even into the underlying muscles and adjacent nerves and blood vessels (Figure 14-7 ▶). A laceration may appear linear (regular) or stellate (star-shaped) and may occur along with other types of soft-tissue injury. Lacerations that involve damaged arteries or veins may result in severe bleeding.

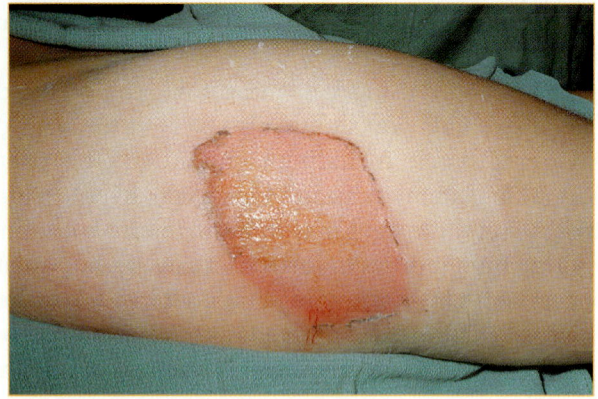

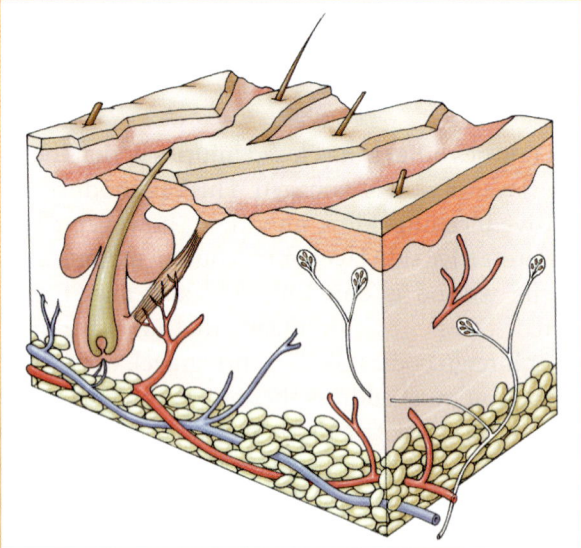

Figure 14-5 Abrasions usually do not penetrate completely through the dermis, but blood may ooze from the capillary beds. These wounds are typically superficial and result from rubbing or scraping across a hard surface.

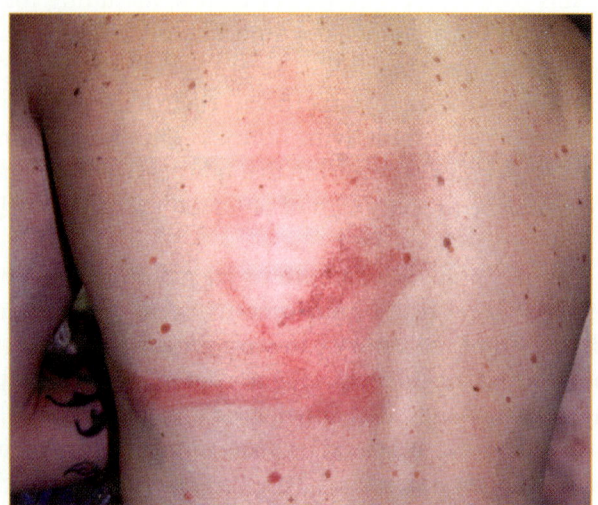

Figure 14-6 Injuries over the flank areas may be a sign of kidney damage.

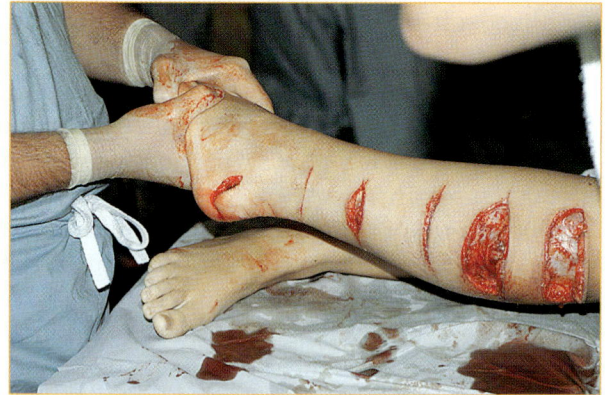

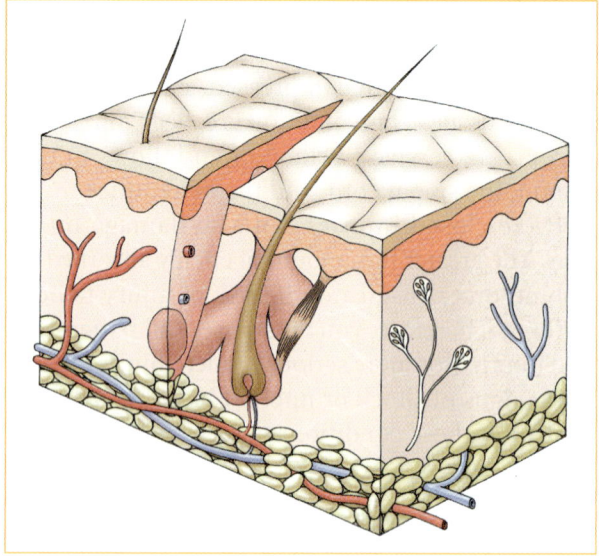

Figure 14-7 Lacerations vary in depth and can extend through the skin and subcutaneous tissue to the underlying muscles, nerves, and blood vessels. These wounds can be smooth or jagged as a result of a cut by a sharp object or a blunt force that tears the tissue.

An <u>avulsion</u> is an injury that separates various layers of soft tissue (usually between the subcutaneous layer and fascia) so that they are completely unattached or hanging as a flap (Figure 14-8 ▶). Usually, there is significant bleeding. If the avulsed tissue is hanging from a small piece of skin, the circulation through the flap may be at risk. If you can, replace the avulsed flap in its original position. If an avulsion is complete, you should wrap the separated tissue in sterile gauze and take it with you to the emergency department.

We usually think of amputations as involving the upper and lower extremities. But other body parts, such as the scalp, ear, nose, penis, or lips, may also be totally avulsed, or amputated. You can easily control the bleed-

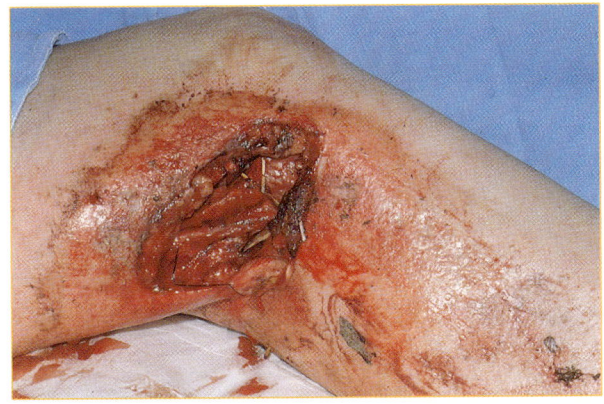
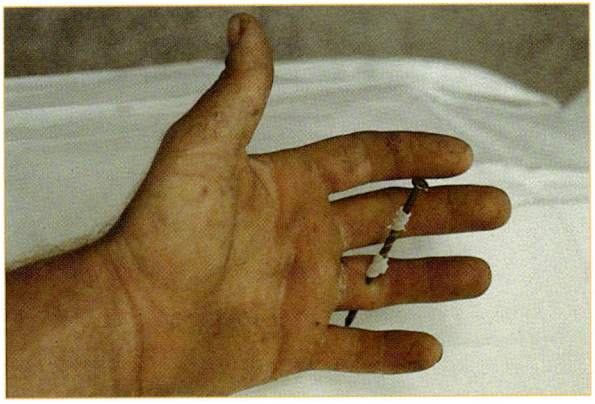
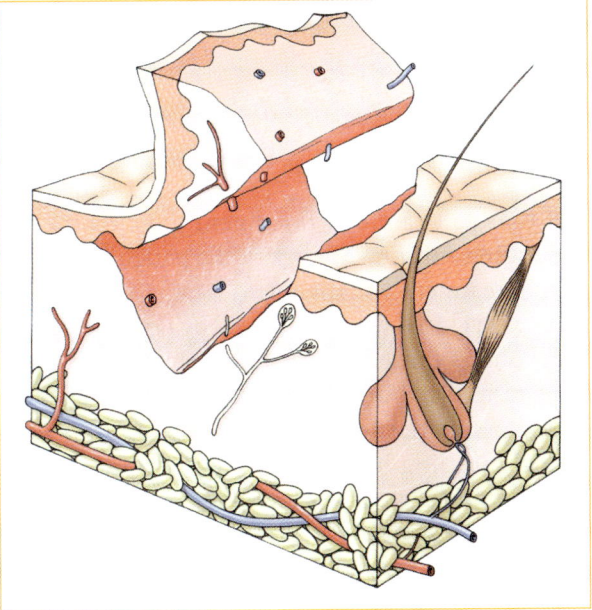
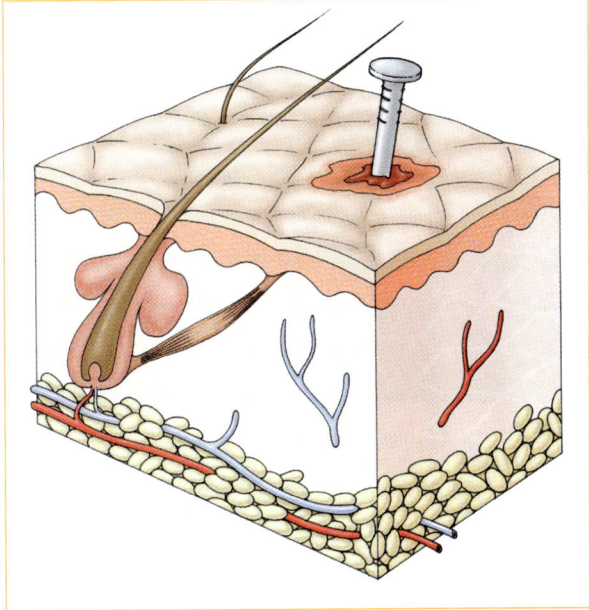

Figure 14-8 Avulsions are injuries characterized by complete separation of tissue or tissue hanging as a flap. Significant bleeding is common.

Figure 14-9 Penetrating wounds often cause very little external bleeding but can damage structures deep within the body.

ing from some amputations, such as the fingers, with pressure dressings. But if an avulsion involves a large area of muscle mass, such as a thigh, there may be massive bleeding. In this situation, you need to treat the patient for hypovolemic shock. The use of pressure points may also be necessary to control bleeding that is not controlled with a pressure dressing. Application and inflation of the pneumatic antishock garment (abbreviated PASG and also known as MAST, for military [or medical] antishock trousers) may also be considered for bleeding control (see Skill Drill 13-2 in Chapter 13).

A <u>penetrating wound</u> is an injury resulting from a sharp, pointed object, such as a knife, an ice pick, a splinter, or a bullet. Such objects leave relatively small entrance wounds, so there may be little external bleeding (Figure 14-9 ▲). However, these objects can damage structures deep within the body. If the wound is in the chest or abdomen, the injury can cause rapid, fatal bleeding. Assessing the amount of damage a puncture wound has created is very difficult and is reserved for the physician at the hospital.

Stabbings and shootings often result in multiple penetrating injuries. You must assess the patients carefully to identify all wounds. Because a penetrating object can pass completely through the body, always count the number of penetrating injuries (or holes), especially with gunshot wounds. Entrance wounds and exit

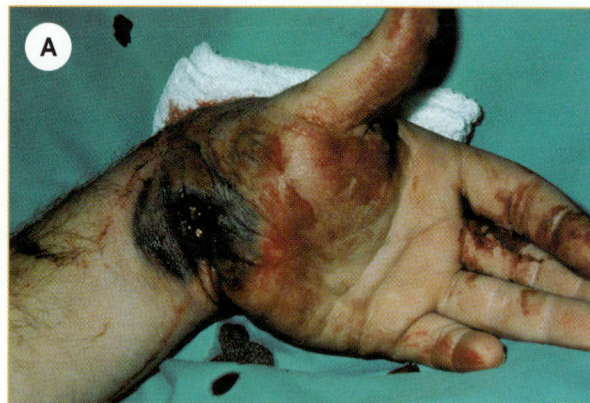
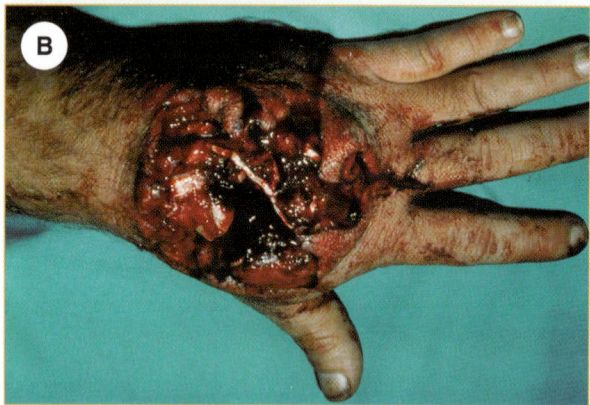

Figure 14-10 **A.** An entrance wound from a gunshot may have burns around the edges. **B.** An exit wound is often larger and associated with greater damage to surrounding skin.

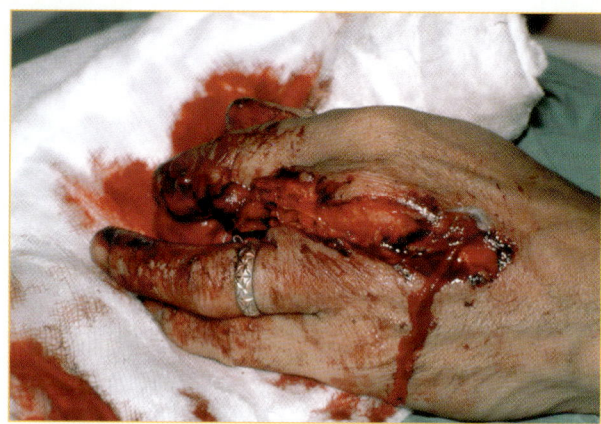

Figure 14-11 A crushing open wound is characterized by extensive tissue damage and deformity that is often accompanied by swelling and extreme pain.

wounds are difficult to tell apart in a prehospital setting, especially with the different types of ammunition; it is better to count the amount of penetrating injuries, and leave the distinguishing of entrance and exit to the physician who is working in a more controlled environment (Figure 14-10 ▲).

Gunshot wounds have some unique characteristics that require special care. The amount of damage from a gunshot wound is directly related to the speed of the bullet. Thus, it is important to find out the caliber of gun that was used in the shooting. Sometimes the patient or bystanders can tell you how many rounds were fired. This information can help hospital personnel to better care for the patient. Shotgun wounds create multiple paths of missiles (shot) and create a larger surface area of tissue damage. However, you should not waste valuable time trying to determine the caliber of weapon. Patient care is the first priority.

Most people charged with shooting another person end up in court at some point, and you may be called to testify. For this reason, it is even more than usual that you carefully document the circumstances surrounding any gunshot injury, the patient's condition, and the treatment you give.

As with closed wounds caused by crushing injuries, open wounds caused by crushing injuries may involve damaged internal organs or broken bones, as well as extensive soft-tissue damage (Figure 14-11 ▲). While external bleeding may be minimal, internal bleeding may be severe, even life threatening. The crushing force damages soft tissues, as well as vessels and nerves. This frequently results in a painful, swollen, deformed area.

Documentation Tips

Most people charged with shooting another person end up in court at some point, and you may be called to testify. Therefore, it is even more important than usual that you carefully document the circumstances surrounding the scene, the injury, the patient's condition, and the treatment you give.

Emergency Medical Care

Before you begin caring for a patient with an open wound, you should be sure to protect yourself by following BSI precautions. Wear gloves, eye protection, and a gown if necessary. Remember that you must be sure the patient has an open airway; administer high-flow oxygen as necessary. If life-threatening bleeding is observed, assign a team member to apply direct pressure to control the bleeding. Then assess the severity of the wound. If the wound is in the chest or upper abdomen, place an occlusive dressing on the wound.

Your treatment priority is the initial assessment, including controlling the bleeding, which can be extensive and severe. Then follow the steps in **Skill Drill 14-1** ▶ :

1. **Apply a dry, sterile dressing** over the entire wound. Apply pressure to the dressing with your gloved hand (**Step 1**).
2. **Maintain the pressure** and secure the dressing with a roller bandage (**Step 2**).
3. **If bleeding continues or recurs, leave the original dressing in place.** Apply a second dressing on top of the first, and secure it with another roller bandage (**Step 3**).
4. **Splint the extremity** to stabilize the injury even if there is no suspected fracture, help minimize movement, further control the bleeding, and keep the dressing in place (**Step 4**).

Assessment of the patient for further signs of injury follows the DCAP-BTLS method: inspect and palpate for Deformities, Contusions, Abrasions, Punctures/Penetrations/Paradoxical Movement, Burns, Tenderness, Lacerations, and Swelling. It is important not to focus all of your attention on the obvious open wound and neglect a systematic evaluation of the entire patient. If you follow this systematic approach, you are less likely to miss other significant injuries that the patient may have sustained.

All open wounds are assumed to be contaminated and present a risk of infection. By applying a sterile dressing, you are reducing the risk of further contamination. This keeps foreign material, such as hair, clothing, and dirt, out of the wound and decreases the risk of secondary infection. However, do not try to remove material from an open wound, no matter how dirty the wound is. Rubbing, brushing, or washing an open wound will only cause additional bleeding and unnecessary pain. The wound will be appropriately cleaned at the hospital. To prevent the wound from drying, you may apply moistened sterile dressings with sterile saline solution, if possible, and then cover the wound with a dry, sterile dressing.

Often, you can better control bleeding from open soft-tissue wounds by splinting the extremity, even if there is no fracture. Splinting can also help you to keep the patient calm and quiet, because it typically reduces pain. In addition, splinting keeps sterile dressings in place, minimizes damage to an already injured extremity, and makes moving the patient easier.

Keep in mind that a patient who is bleeding significantly from an open wound is at risk for hypovolemic shock. You must be alert for this possibility and provide treatment, as needed.

You are the Provider — Part 2

The scene is now safe, and the power to the outlet has been shut off. You perform an Initial assessment of the patient, and note the following:

Initial Assessment	Recording Time: Zero Minutes
Appearance	Pale and clammy
Level of consciousness	Alert and oriented and in severe pain
Airway	Open and clear
Breathing	Respirations, increased but have adequate depth
Circulation	Skin, clammy; radial pulses, rapid and bilaterally present

3. What is your first consideration in treating this patient?
4. Why is it difficult to accurately assess the severity of damage caused by an electrical burn?

Skill Drill 14-1

Controlling Bleeding From an Extremity Soft-Tissue Injury

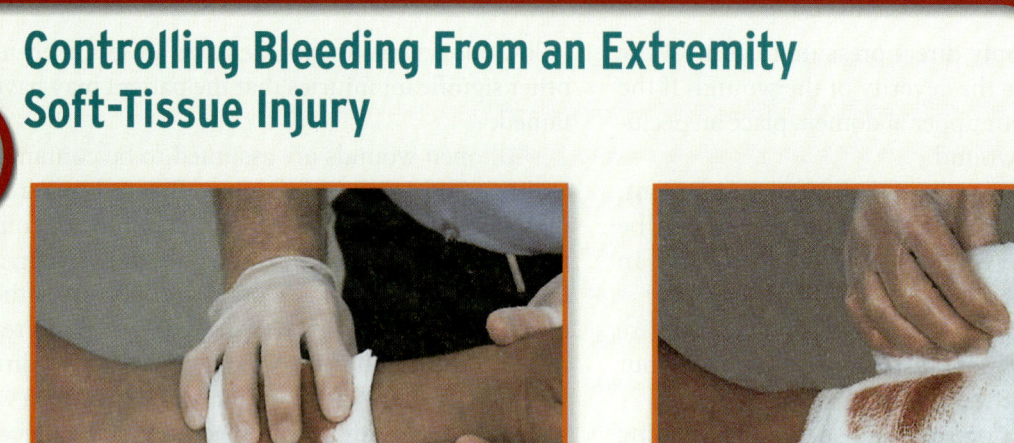

1. Apply direct pressure with a sterile dressing.

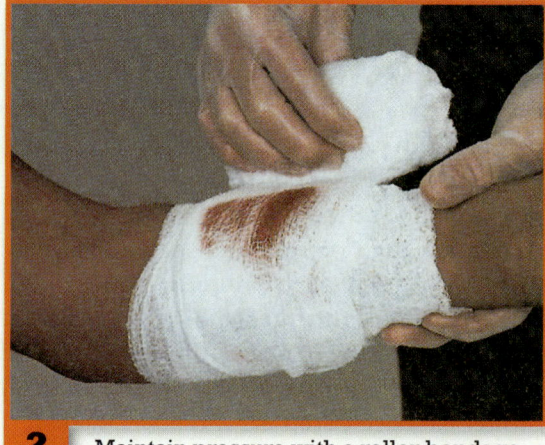

2. Maintain pressure with a roller bandage.

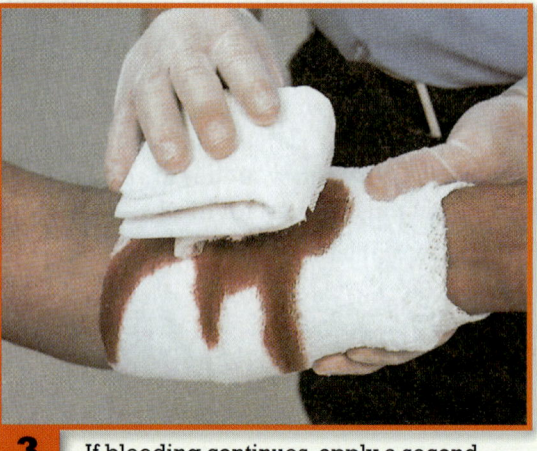

3. If bleeding continues, apply a second dressing and roller bandage over the first.

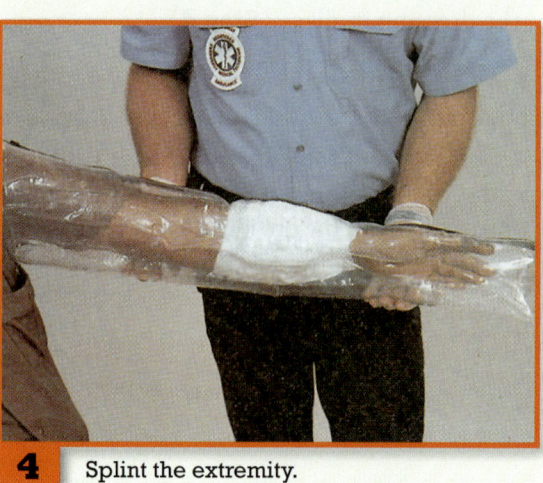

4. Splint the extremity.

Chest Wounds

A penetrating wound to the chest may cause air to enter the pleural space (**pneumothorax**) or blood to collect in the pleural space (**hemothorax**) (Figure 14-12 ▶). Ordinarily, the pressure inside the chest cavity is slightly lower than the pressure of the atmosphere. Inhalation further reduces this pressure, so air will move through a wound just as easily as it moves through the nose and mouth during normal breathing. The air that enters through the wound remains in the pleural space, and the lung does not expand; when the patient exhales, air passes back through the wound. Such "sucking chest wounds" reduce the ability of the lungs to provide fresh oxygen to the blood.

Initial emergency care should include giving supplemental oxygen, sealing the wound, and transporting the patient promptly to the nearest hospital. Follow the steps in (Skill Drill 14-2 ▶):

Sealing a Sucking Chest Wound

Skill Drill 14-2

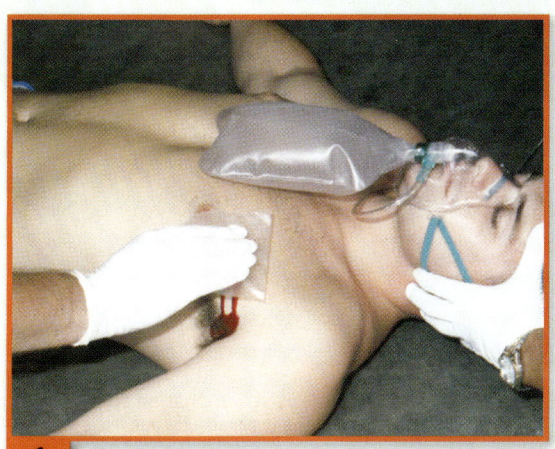

1 Keep the patient supine and give high-flow oxygen.

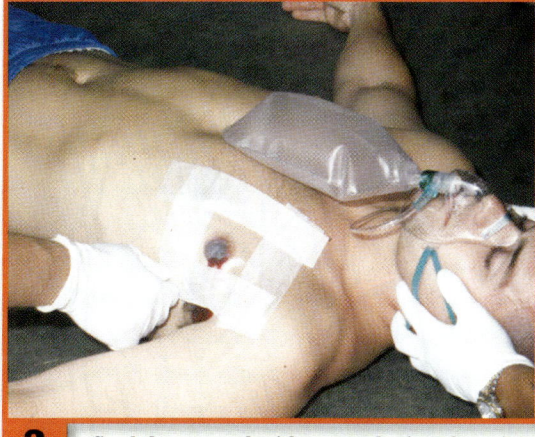

2 Seal the wound with an occlusive dressing.

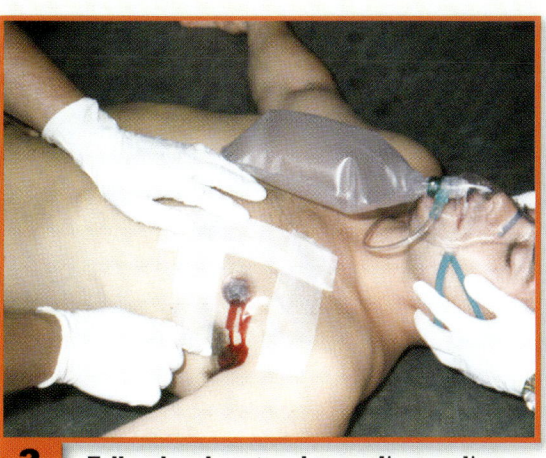

3 Follow local protocol regarding sealing or leaving open the dressing's fourth side.

1. **Keep the patient supine and administer high-flow oxygen.** The buildup of blood in the chest can result in difficulty breathing and shock. The patient may be placed in a position of comfort if no spinal injury is suspected (**Step 1**).
2. **Seal the wound** with an <u>occlusive dressing</u> large enough that it is not pulled or sucked into the chest cavity. An occlusive dressing prevents air from being sucked into the chest through the wound. Several sterile materials, including aluminum foil, Vaseline gauze, or a folded universal dressing, may be used for this purpose (**Step 2**).
3. **Depending on your local protocol, you may seal the dressing on all four sides**, or you may seal only three sides to create a flutter valve, which is a one-way valve that allows air to leave the chest cavity but not return (**Step 3**).

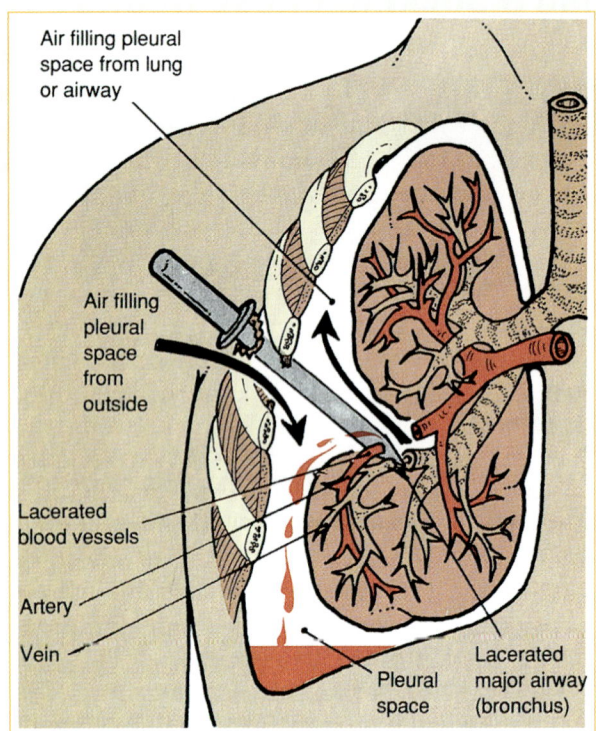

Figure 14-12 Penetrating wounds can cause air or blood to enter and collect in the pleural space, located between the parietal pleura and the visceral pleura.

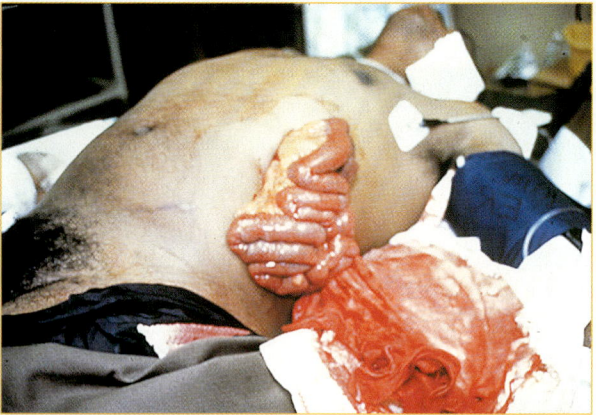

Figure 14-13 An abdominal evisceration is an open wound to the abdomen in which organs protrude through the wound.

Abdominal Wounds

An open wound in the abdominal cavity may expose internal organs. In some cases, the organs may even protrude through the wound, an injury called an evisceration (Figure 14-13 ▶). Do not touch or move the exposed organs. Cover the wound with sterile gauze compresses moistened with sterile saline solution, and secure the moist compresses in place with a dry, sterile dressing (Figure 14-14 ▶). Because the open abdomen radiates body heat very effectively and because exposed organs lose fluid rapidly, you must keep the organs moist and warm. If you do not have gauze compresses, you may use moist sterile dressings, covered and secured in place with a dry bandage and tape. Do not use any material that is adherent or loses its substance when wet, such as toilet paper, facial tissue, paper towels, or absorbent cotton. If the patient's legs and knees are uninjured, flex them to relieve pressure on the abdomen. Most patients with abdominal wounds require immediate transport to a trauma center, depending on the local protocol.

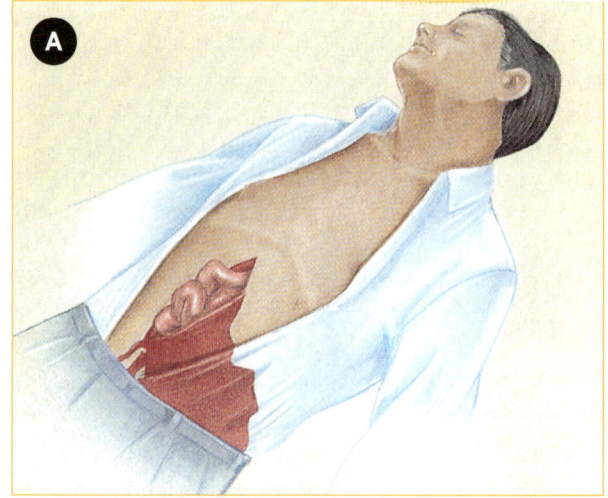
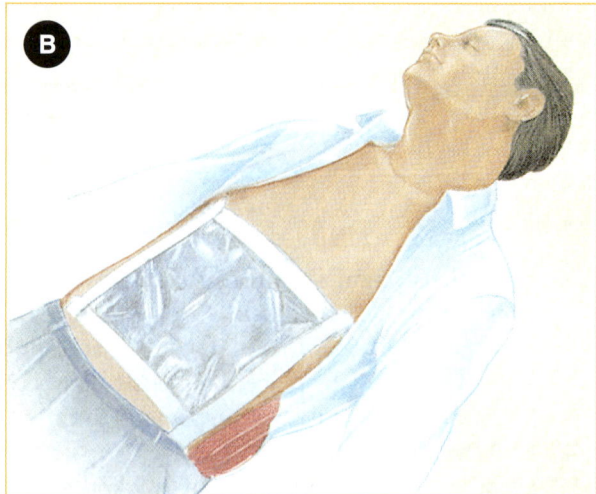

Figure 14-14 A. Cover exposed organs with sterile gauze compresses moistened with sterile saline solution. **B.** Place a dry dressing over the compresses, and secure it in place by taping all four sides.

Skill Drill 14-3: Stabilizing an Impaled Object

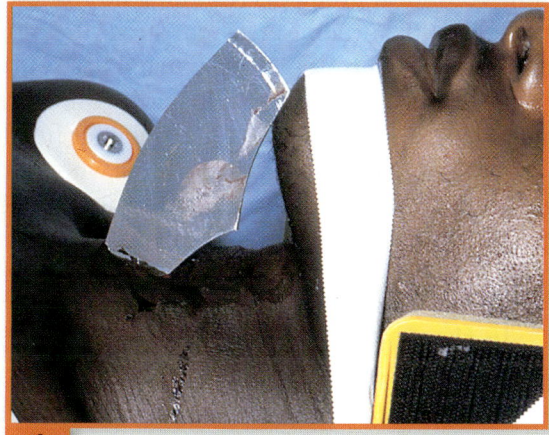

1 Do not attempt to move or remove the object.

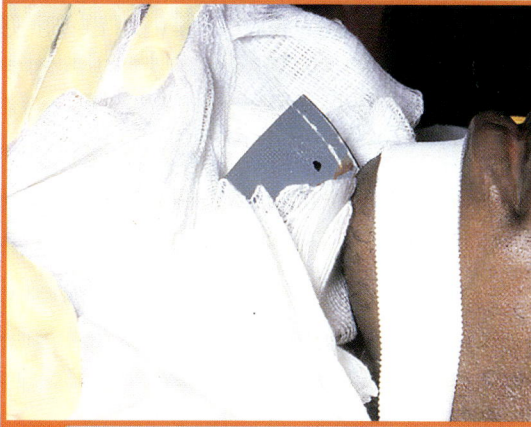

2 Control bleeding and stabilize the object in place using soft dressings, gauze, and/or tape.

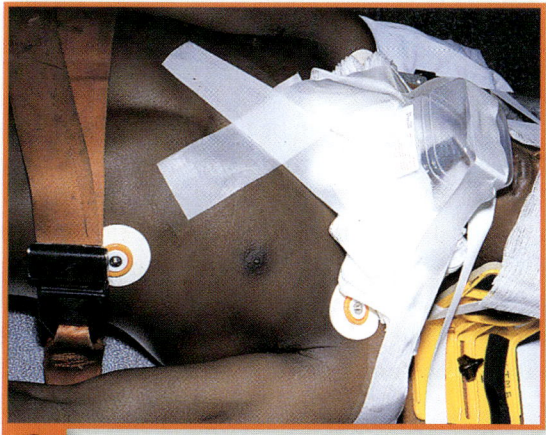

3 Tape a rigid item over the stabilized object to protect it from movement during transport.

Impaled Objects

Occasionally, a patient will have an object, such as a knife, fishhook, wood splinter, or piece of glass, impaled in his or her body. To treat this, follow the steps in Skill Drill 14-3:

1. **Do not attempt to move or remove the object** unless it is impaled through the cheek causing airway obstruction, or if the object is in the chest and interferes with CPR. In most cases, a surgeon will have to remove the object; removing it in the field may cause more bleeding, or damage nerves, blood vessels, or muscles within the wound (**Step 1**).

2. **Remove any clothing covering the injury.** Control bleeding, and apply a bulky dressing to stabilize the object. Some combination of soft dressings, gauze, and tape may be effective, depending on the location and size of the object. To prevent further injury, manually secure the object by incorporating it into the dressing (**Step 2**).

3. **Protect the impaled object** from being bumped or moved during transport by taping a rigid item such as a plastic cup, a section of a plastic water bottle, or a supply container over the stabilized object and its bandaging (**Step 3**).

The only exception to the rule of not removing an impaled object is an object in the cheek that obstructs breathing or in the chest that interferes with CPR. In this situation, restoring the airway takes priority. If the object is very long, cut off (shorten) the exposed portion, first securing it to minimize motion and thus internal damage and pain. Once the object is secured and the bleeding is under control, provide prompt transport.

Exercise great care when shortening an impaled object. A small amount of movement on the proximal end of the object will cause a significant amount of movement on the distal end, which is impaled in the person's body. This excessive distal movement may cause or worsen internal injuries and bleeding.

> **EMT-I Tips**
>
> There are only two exceptions to removing an impaled object: if it is through the cheek and interferes with the airway or through the chest and interferes with chest compressions.

Amputations

Surgeons today can often reimplant an amputated part 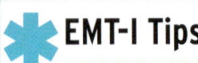. However, correct prehospital care of the amputated part is vital to successful reattachment. With partial amputations, make sure to immobilize the part with bulky compression dressings and a splint to prevent further injury. Do not detach any partial amputations because this may make it impossible to reimplant the part.

With a complete amputation, make sure to wrap the part in a sterile dressing and place it in a plastic bag. Follow your local protocols regarding how to preserve amputated parts. In some areas, dry sterile dressings are recommended for wrapping amputated parts; in other areas, dressings moistened with sterile saline are recommended. Put the bag in a cool container filled with ice water. The goal is to keep the part cool without allowing it to freeze or develop frostbite. The amputated part should be transported with the patient.

> **In the Field**
>
> Never place an amputated part directly on ice because this may cause frostbite and prevent reattachment.

Neck Injuries

An open neck injury can be life threatening. If the veins of the neck are open to the environment, they may suck in air 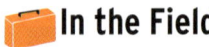. If enough air is sucked into a blood vessel, it can actually block the flow of blood in the lungs, sending the patient into cardiac arrest. This condition is called air embolism. To control bleeding and prevent the possibility of air embolism, cover the wound with an occlusive dressing. Apply manual pressure, but do not compress both carotid arteries at the same time; if you do, this will impair circulation to the brain Figure 14-17. Secure a pressure dressing over the wound by wrapping roller gauze loosely around the neck and then firmly through the opposite axilla.

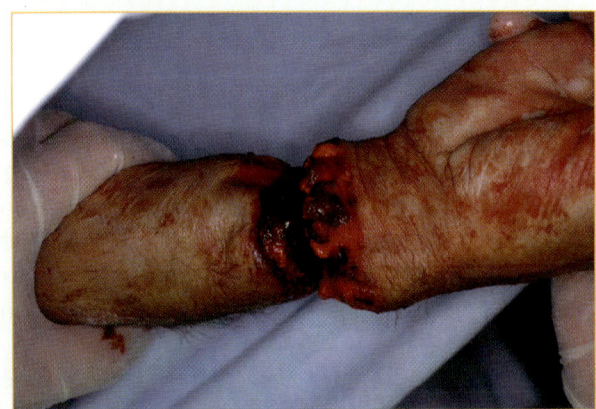

Figure 14-15 Amputated parts can often be reimplanted, so you should make every attempt to find the part and transport it to the emergency department along with the patient.

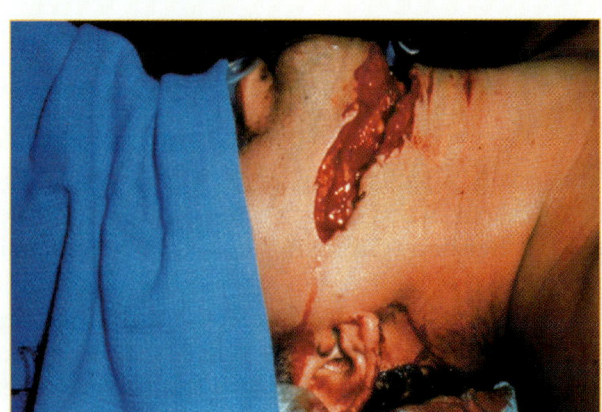

Figure 14-16 Open injuries to the neck can be very dangerous. If veins are open to the environment, they can suck in air, resulting in a potentially fatal condition called air embolism.

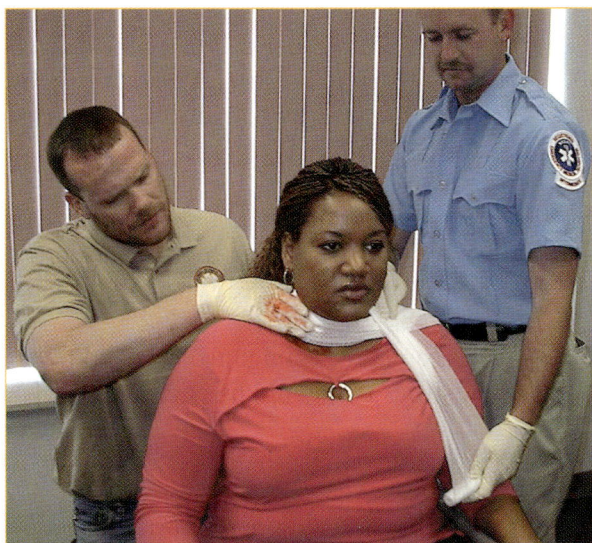

Figure 14-17 Cover neck wounds with an airtight dressing, and apply manual pressure. Be sure that you do not compress both carotid arteries at the same time, because this will impair circulation to the brain.

Burns

As an EMT-I, you will often provide care to patients who have been burned. Burns account for more than 10,000 deaths per year. Burns are also among the most serious and painful of all injuries. A <u>burn</u> occurs when the body, or a body part, receives more energy than it can absorb without injury. Potential sources of this energy include thermal, inhalation, toxic chemicals, radiation exposure, and electricity (including lightning). Mechanisms of burn injury include scalding, steam, flame, flash, retained heat, and other trauma. The proper emergency care of a burn may increase a patient's chances of survival and decrease the risk or duration of long-term disability. Although a burn may be the patient's most obvious injury, you should always perform a complete assessment to determine whether there are other, more serious injuries.

Pathophysiology

Any time there are large surface areas burned, the risk of shock increases. These risks come from local and systemic responses. Initially, during the emergent phase, there is a release of catecholamines (that is, epinephrine and norepinephrine) in response to the pain and stress of the situation. Because of the overall vasoconstriction, there is a decrease in blood flow to the injured area. During the next several hours there follows a fluid shift phase that is usually not seen in the prehospital setting. Damaged cells in the area release vasoactive substances, creating an inflammatory response and increasing capillary permeability. Massive edema is the result of fluid shifting from the intravascular space into the extravascular space. Sodium moves into the injured cells, creating even more fluid loss as osmotic pressure increases. This also causes a loss of electrolytes and may lead to hypovolemia.

Tissue damage reduces the ability of the body to regulate its core temperature. Fluid seeps into the damaged area where it is exposed to surface air, causing evaporation and loss of heat. In severe burns, this can rapidly lead to hypothermia.

As fluid volume decreases, there is less oxygen transported to the tissues and organs, leading to hypoxia, acidosis, and possibly anoxia. Hypovolemia causes a decrease in cardiac output, resulting in hypotension. In an attempt to maintain homeostasis, the body responds with vasoconstriction in an effort to elevate blood pressure and increase perfusion to vital organs and with tachypnea to offset the metabolic acidosis and hypoxia.

The burn process also releases myoglobin from dead or dying cells into the bloodstream that may plug tubules in the kidneys leading to renal failure. Myoglobin, along with the hypovolemia, can lead to liver failure, and excessive potassium released from the cells can create dysrhythmias and heart failure.

As the burn destroys skin, a tough leathery substance known as <u>eschar</u> is produced. Eschar is not pliable like normal skin. As edema increases, pressure is exerted on the underlying structures. Circulatory compromise secondary to circumferential eschar around an extremity may require an escharotomy, or surgical incision to relieve the pressure and restore circulation, once the patient arrives at the emergency department. A circumferential burn may result in compartment syndrome. The skin is unable to stretch, leading to eventual compression and decreased or absent circulation in the tissues below. If the burn is around the thorax, tidal volume and chest excursion may be drastically reduced by the eschar formation, thus resulting in ventilatory insufficiency.

Inhalation injury is present in 60% to 70% of all burn patients who die. This is generally the result of carbon monoxide or cyanide toxicity. If the patient survives the initial injury, death is usually the result of secondary infection. The barrier of protection offered by intact skin is breeched, which results in an invasion of various types of infectious agents. Pathogens invade the wound shortly after the burn and may do so until the area is healed. The best protection for the patient is the use of sterile dressings and avoidance of any preventable contamination of the site.

Management

After ensuring your own safety, management begins by removing the patient to a safe area and stopping the burning process. Treatment for a major burn injury is aimed at supportive care for hypovolemic shock. Aggressive fluid resuscitation and general wound care may significantly increase chances of survival. Apply high-flow oxygen and assist ventilation as needed. Consider early definitive airway management (for example, endotracheal intubation) if the patient has an altered mental status. Keep the patient warm to prevent hypothermia. Follow local protocols for thermal burn injury management. Transport to the closest, most appropriate facility for definitive care. Topical applications along with tetanus prophylaxis and antibiotic therapy are administered once the patient reaches the emergency department.

Remember to apply a cardiac monitor and follow advanced cardiac life support (ACLS) and local protocols for dysrhythmias that may present. Consider early intubation if signs of rapid airway swelling are present.

Geriatric Needs

When treating geriatric patients with burns, it is important to be vigilant for the possibility of elder abuse. Geriatric patients who are institutionalized, disoriented, or incapable of clear communication are particularly susceptible to abuse.

Signs of abuse in geriatric patients include evidence of multiple injuries in various stages of healing (for example, multiple bruises of different colors, new and old fractures involving more than one extremity), injuries that do not seem to correspond to the history provided by caregivers, and burns with a suspicious history of the incident.

Burns that appear in a "pattern" raise suspicion for intentional injuries. Multiple, small circular burns may be indicative of cigarette or cigar injuries. Other patterns may indicate irons, stovetops, or other hot surfaces not easily encountered accidentally. Scalding injuries to the hands or feet may also be indicative of abuse. It is important to remember that these injuries are often inflicted in areas not readily seen. If the situation raises suspicion of elder abuse, be sure to fully examine the patient under his or her clothing for signs of abuse. As always, appropriate support and transport of the patient in a timely manner remain a priority.

Burn Severity

The seriousness of a burn may influence medical control's choice of a treatment facility. Five factors will help you to determine the severity of a burn:

1. What is the depth of the burn?
2. What is the extent of the burn?

These first two factors are the most important. After gauging these, ask yourself the remaining questions:

3. Are any critical areas (face, upper airway, hands, feet, genitalia) involved?
4. Are there any preexisting medical conditions or other injuries that could be complicated by the burn injury?
5. Is the patient younger than 5 years or older than 55 years?

If the answer to any of these last three questions is yes, you should upgrade the burn's classification **Table 14-1**. Age, preexisting medical conditions, and trauma are all considerations that influence management and prognosis of the burn-injured patient.

TABLE 14-1 Classification of Burns in Adults

Critical (Severe) Burns
- Full-thickness burns involving the hands, feet, face, upper airway, or genitalia
- Full-thickness burns covering more than 10% of the body's total surface area
- Partial-thickness burns covering more than 30% of the body's total surface area
- Burns associated with respiratory injury (smoke inhalation)
- Burns complicated by fractures
- Burns on patients younger than 5 years or older than 55 years that would be classified as "moderate" burns in young adults

Moderate Burns
- Full-thickness burns involving 2% to 10% of the body's total surface area (except burns of the hands, feet, face, genitalia, or upper airway, which are classified as critical)
- Partial-thickness burns covering 15% to 30% of the body's total surface area
- Superficial burns covering more than 50% of the body's total surface area

Minor Burns
- Full-thickness burns covering less than 2% of the body's total surface area
- Partial-thickness burns covering less than 15% of the body's total surface area
- Superficial burns covering less than 50% of the body's total surface area

Depth

Burns are first classified according to their depth Figure 14-18 ▼. You must be able to identify the following three types of burns:

- <u>Superficial (first-degree) burns</u> involve only the top layer of skin, the epidermis. The skin turns red but does not blister or actually burn through to the dermis. The burn site is painful. Sunburn is a good example of a superficial burn.
- <u>Partial-thickness (second-degree) burns</u> involve the epidermis and some portion of the dermis. These burns do not destroy the entire thickness of the skin, and the subcutaneous tissue is not injured. Typically, the skin is moist, mottled, and white to red. Blisters are common. Partial-thickness burns cause intense pain.
- <u>Full-thickness (third-degree) burns</u> extend through all skin layers and may involve subcutaneous layers, muscle, bone, or internal organs. The burned area is dry and leathery and may appear white, dark brown, or even charred. This rough area is known as eschar. Some full-thickness burns feel hard to the touch. Clotted blood vessels or subcutaneous tissue may be visible under the burned skin. If the nerve endings have been destroyed, a severely burned area may have no feeling. However, the surrounding, less severely burned areas may be extremely painful.

A pure full-thickness burn is unusual. Severe burns are typically a combination of superficial, partial-thickness, and full-thickness burns. Superficial burns heal well without scarring. Small

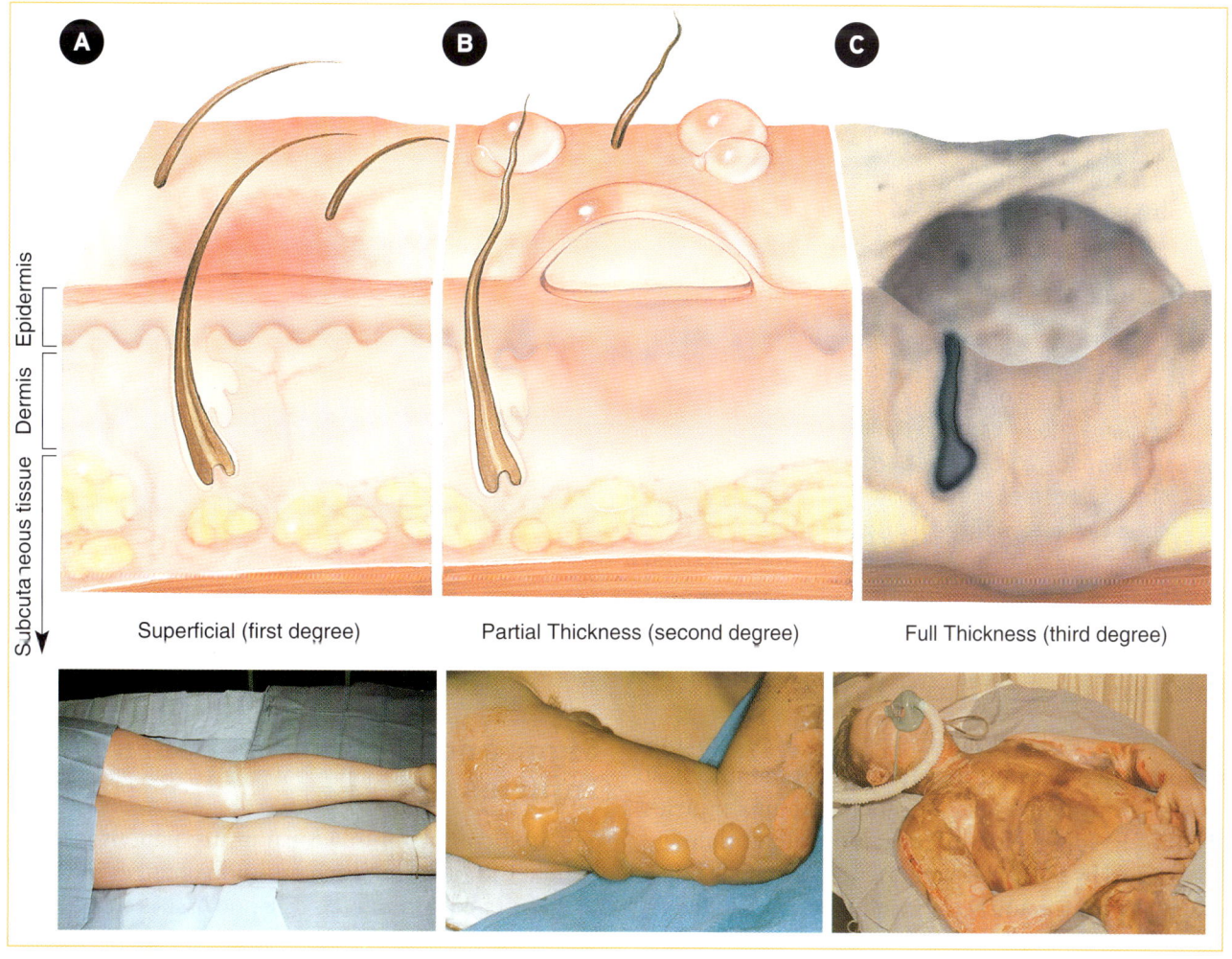

Figure 14-18 Classification of burns. **A.** Superficial or first-degree burns involve only the epidermis. The skin turns red but does not blister or actually burn through to the dermis. **B.** Partial-thickness or second-degree burns involve some of the dermis, but they do not destroy the entire thickness of the skin. The skin is mottled, white to red, and often blistered. **C.** Full-thickness or third-degree burns extend through all layers of the skin and may involve subcutaneous tissue and muscle. The skin is dry, leathery, and often white or charred.

partial-thickness burns also heal without scarring. However, deep partial-thickness burns and all full-thickness burns are best managed surgically and frequently require skin grafting.

Suspect significant airway burns if there is singed hair within the nostrils, soot around the nose and mouth, hoarseness, or hypoxia.

It may be impossible to accurately estimate the depth of a particular burn. Even experienced burn specialists sometimes underestimate or, more commonly, overestimate the extent of a particular burn.

Extent

One quick way to estimate the surface area that has been burned is to compare it with the size of the patient's palm, which is roughly equal to 1% of the patient's total body surface area. This is known as the rule of palms, sometimes called the "palmar method." This method is especially useful with irregularly shaped burns. Another useful measurement system is the rule of nines, which divides the body into sections, each of which is approximately 9% of the total surface area Figure 14-19 ▶. Remember that the head of an infant or child is relatively larger than the head of an adult, and the legs are relatively smaller.

> **Documentation Tips**
>
> Burn patterns often require description beyond calculating the amount of body surface involved. If you find written description difficult or too lengthy, try drawing in the affected areas on two outlines of the body, front and back. Your report form may include an area with the outlines provided; if not, do not hesitate to draw them in yourself. One picture can be worth many words.

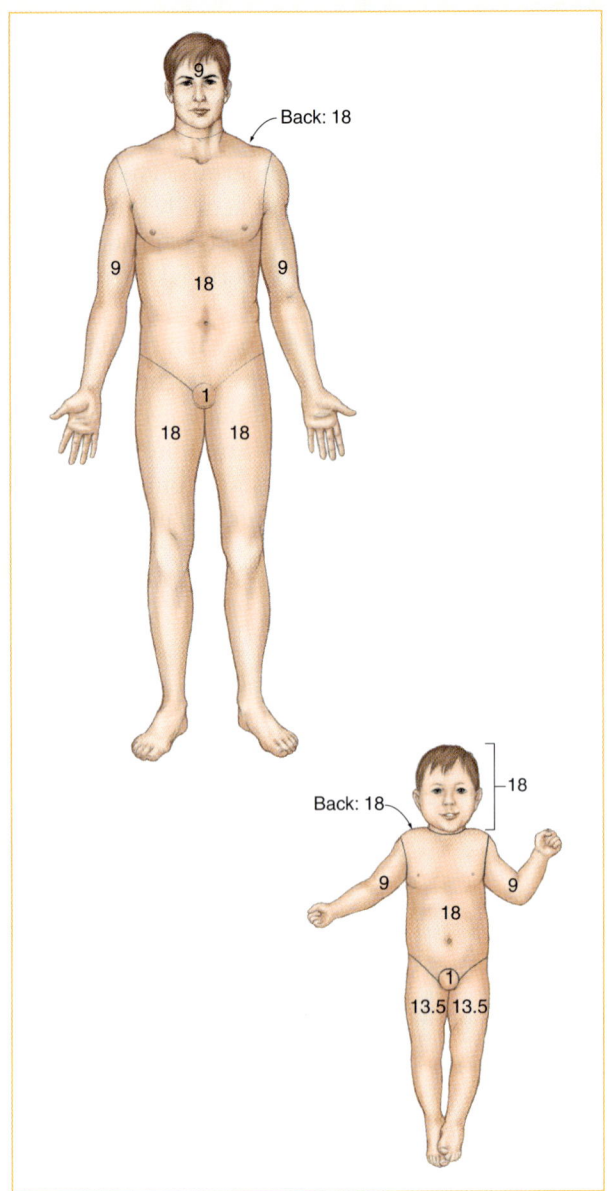

Figure 14-19 The rule of nines is a quick way to estimate the amount of surface area that has been burned. It divides the body into sections, each approximately 9% of the total body surface area.

Mechanisms of Burn Injuries

Burns may be isolated injuries or may occur in conjunction with other injuries such as burn trauma, blast or explosion trauma, falls, or others. Trauma injuries can include soft-tissue or musculoskeletal damage accompanied by burns. Blast injuries often include internal damage that is unseen. Burns around the face or exposure to superheated air tend to result in airway and respiratory compromise. Burns can also be indicative of child abuse and point to other potential areas of injury. Any hint of child abuse gained from burn patterns should raise suspicion of possible occult injuries and should be evaluated thoroughly.

Signs and Symptoms of Burn Injuries

The first complaint in a burn injury patient is usually pain at the site. The skin condition changes in relation to the affected burn site. As cells and tissues are destroyed, they slough off. Other soft tissue injuries may occur depending on the extent of the burn. If the burn is the result of a fall, blast, or other trauma, the patient might also present with musculoskeletal injuries. In severe burns, the musculoskeletal system sustains significant damage in the absence of actual musculoskeletal trauma.

Pediatric Needs

Burns to children are generally considered more serious than burns to adults (Table 14-2). This is because infants and children have more surface area relative to total body mass, which means greater fluid and heat loss. In addition, children do not tolerate burns as well as adults do. Children are also more likely to experience shock, hypothermia, and airway problems because of the unique differences of their ages and anatomy.

Some burns in infants and children result from child abuse. The classic burn resulting from deliberate immersion involves the hands and wrists, as well as the feet, lower legs, and buttocks. Similarly, burns around the genitals and multiple cigarette burns should be viewed as possible abuse. You should report all suspected cases of abuse to the proper authorities (Chapter 31).

TABLE 14-2 Classification of Burns in Infants and Children

Critical Burns
- Full-thickness or partial-thickness burns covering more than 20% of the body's total surface area
- Burns involving the hands, feet, face, airway, or genitalia

Moderate Burns
- Partial-thickness burns covering 10% to 20% of the body's total surface area

Minor Burns
- Partial-thickness burns covering less than 10% of the body's total surface area

Any burns near the face expose the airway to potential damage. Expect to hear adventitious (abnormal) sounds as the airway swells and narrows. Hoarseness, dyspnea, dysphagia, and dysphasia are common.

Other signs and symptoms associated with burns include burned hair, nausea and vomiting, altered levels of consciousness, edema, paresthesia, possible hemorrhage, and chest pain.

Terminology Tips

Remember that the prefix *dys-* means *difficulty*. Dyspnea = difficulty breathing; dysphagia = difficulty swallowing; dysphasia = difficult speaking

Emergency Medical Care

Your first responsibility in caring for a patient with a burn is to stop the burning process and prevent additional injury. Skill Drill 14-4 presents the steps in caring for a burn patient:

1. **Follow BSI precautions.** Because a burn destroys the patient's protective skin layer, always wear gloves and eye protection and use sterile technique when treating a burn patient.
2. **Move the patient away from the burning area.** If any clothing is on fire, wrap the patient in a blanket or follow specific guidelines outlined by your local fire department protocol to put out the flames, and then remove any smoldering clothing and/or jewelry.
3. **Immerse the area in cool, sterile water or saline solution**, or cover with a clean, wet, cool dressing, if the skin or clothing is hot. This not only stops the burning, it also relieves pain. However, immersion increases the risk of infection and hypothermia. For this reason, you should not keep the affected part under water for more than 10 minutes. If the burning has stopped before you arrive, *do not immerse it at all*. As an alternative to immersion, irrigation of the burned area until the burning stops may also be used, followed by the application of a sterile dressing (**Step 1**).
4. **Provide high-flow oxygen.** Provide airway and ventilatory support as needed and constantly reassess the patient's airway. Remember that more fire victims die of smoke inhalation than of skin burns. A patient who has burns about the face or has inhaled smoke or fumes may develop respiratory distress. Therefore, you should provide high-flow oxygen to these patients. Keep in mind that a patient who appears to be breathing well at first may suddenly develop severe respiratory distress. Therefore, you must continually assess the airway for possible problems (**Step 2**).

In the Field

Separate burned fingers and toes with dry sterile gauze to prevent them from sticking together.

Section 5 Trauma

Skill Drill 14-4

Caring for Burns

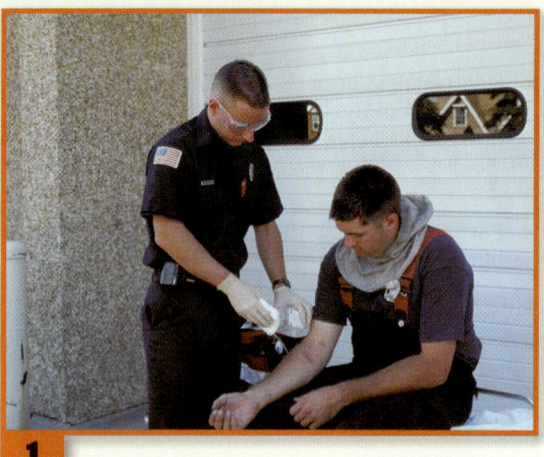

1

Follow BSI precautions and use sterile technique to help prevent infection.

Remove the patient from the burning area; extinguish or remove hot clothing and jewelry as needed.

If the wound(s) is still burning or hot, immerse the hot area in cool, sterile water, or cover with a wet, cool dressing.

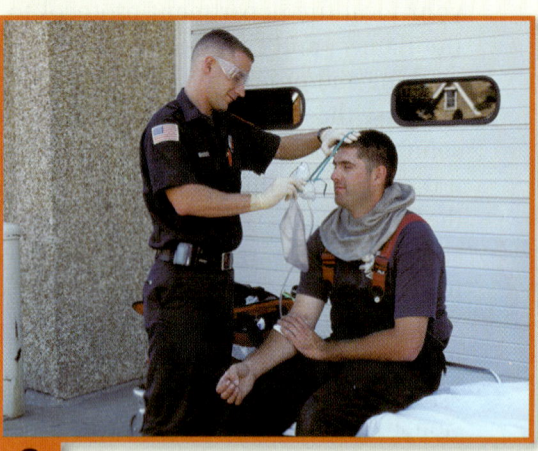

2 Provide high-flow oxygen and continue to assess the airway.

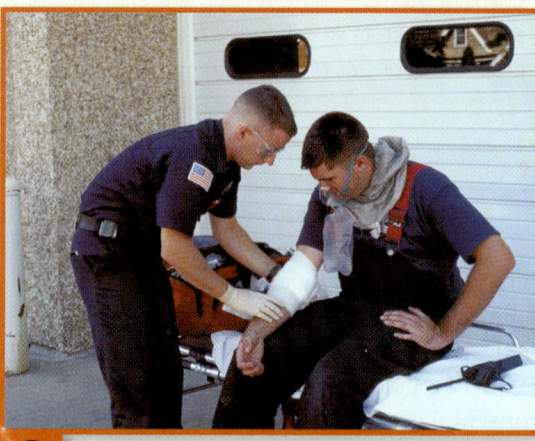

3 Estimate the severity of the burn, then cover the area with a dry, sterile dressing or clean sheet.

Assess and treat the patient for any other injuries.

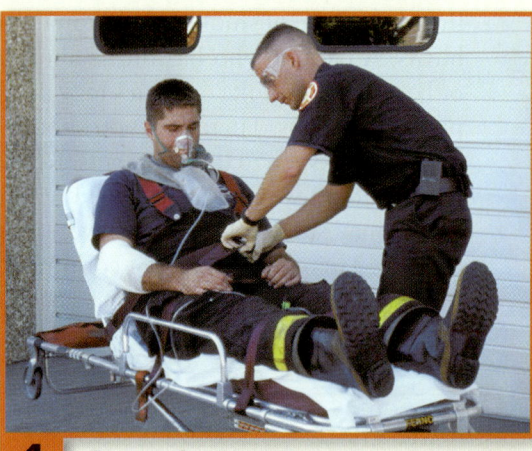

4 Prepare for transport.
Treat for shock if needed.

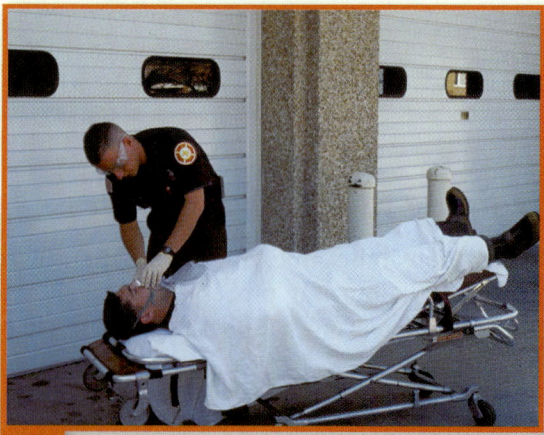

5 Cover the patient with blankets to prevent loss of body heat.

Transport promptly.

5. **Rapidly estimate the burn's severity.** Then cover the burned area with a dry, sterile dressing to prevent further contamination. Sterile gauze is best if the area is not too large. You may cover larger areas with a clean, white sheet. Most important, do not put anything else on the burned area. Use only a dry, sterile dressing, sterile burn sheet, or clean, white sheet. **Never** use ointments, lotions, or antiseptics of any kind, because these only increase the risk of infection and will have to be removed at the hospital. In addition, do not intentionally break any blisters.
6. **Check for traumatic injuries** or other medical conditions that may be more immediately life threatening. Most patients who have been burned have normal vital signs and can communicate at first, which will make your assessment easier (**Step 3**).
7. **Treat the patient for shock if necessary.** Provide circulatory support, including establishing IV access using an isotonic crystalloid solution, proper positioning, and keeping the patient warm (**Step 4**).
8. **An extensive burn can produce hypothermia** (loss of body heat). Prevent further heat loss by covering the patient with warm blankets.
9. **Provide prompt transport** by local protocol. Do not delay transport to do a prolonged assessment or to apply coverings to burns in a critically burned or injured patient. Transport to the closest, most appropriate facility in the proper mode based on the patient's condition. Provide psychological support en route (**Step 5**).

> **In the Field**
>
> To help prevent hypothermia, never apply moist dressings to any patient with more than 10% of the body surface area burned unless the burning process has not been stopped.

During lengthy transport times (greater than 1 hour), medical control may order you to administer IV fluids to the burned patient based on the Parkland formula. The Parkland formula recommends giving 4 mL of normal saline for each kilogram of body weight, multiplied by the percentage of body surface area (BSA) burned:

4 mL × patient's weight (kg) × BSA burned = Total fluid in 24 hours

Thus, for a 75-kg patient with 45% BSA burned, the calculation is as follows:

4 (mL) × 75 (kg) × 45 (BSA) = 13,500 mL during the first 24 hours

The Parkland formula further states that the patient should receive half of this amount of fluid in the first 8 hours following the burn; therefore, using the above example, the patient would receive 6,750 mL during the first 8 hours (approximately 850 mL per hour).

It should be noted, however, that the burn patient with signs of inadequate perfusion (ie, shock) should receive 20-mL/kg boluses of an isotonic crystalloid as needed to maintain adequate perfusion.

You are the Provider — Part 3

After giving the patient 100% oxygen and caring for his burn injury, you obtain the following vital signs:

Vital Signs	Recording Time: 2 Minutes After Patient Contact
Respirations	22 breaths/min, unlabored
Pulse	94 beats/min, and regular
Skin	Pale and clammy
Blood pressure	170/88 mm Hg
Sao_2	96% while receiving 100% oxygen

You load the patient into the ambulance and transport him to the closest emergency department.

5. Which body system is most commonly affected by electrical injuries?

> **EMT-I Tips**
>
> **General Emergency Medical Care of Burns**
> 1. Follow BSI precautions.
> 2. Move the patient away from the burning area.
> 3. Immerse the burning skin in cool sterile water.
> 4. Administer 100% oxygen, and be prepared to assist ventilation.
> 5. An extensive burn can produce hypothermia. Keep the patient warm.
> 6. Rapidly estimate the burn's severity.
> 7. Check for traumatic injuries.
> 8. Treat the patient for shock.
> 9. Provide prompt transport.

Consider providing an analgesic for pain relief. Always follow local protocols. Consider early intubation, if indicated, because inhalation injuries may cause airway edema, restricting placement of a definitive airway at a later time. Apply a cardiac monitor, and treat dysrhythmias based on ACLS and local protocols.

Inhalation Burns

Fire has been associated with three types of inhalation injuries. Toxins in the smoke greatly increase the risk of morbidity and mortality when inhalation injuries are combined with external burns. The three types of inhalation injuries from fire include damage from heat inhalation, damage from systemic toxins, and damage from smoke inhalation. Approximately 20% to 35% of patients admitted to burn centers have an inhalation injury, and chemical inhalation injuries are more frequent than thermal inhalation injuries.

A patient exposed to a burn environment is at increased risk of inhalation injury. As the fire uses up the oxygen in an enclosed space, the patient is left to breathe toxins such as carbon monoxide. Because carbon monoxide will bind to hemoglobin 200 times more readily than oxygen, signs of hypoxia can rapidly develop in the patient. Permanent damage to organs, including the brain, may occur if the patient is not rescued and treated promptly. Carbon monoxide is only one of numerous toxic gases released during a fire.

It is normal for a patient to try to escape from a burning environment. Unfortunately, this usually involves the patient standing up to try and run out. This is especially true if the patient was sleeping and is disoriented on awakening. Because the smoke and superheated air rise, the oxygen-rich air is near the ground. As soon as the patient stands and takes a breath, he or she breathes in the superheated air and smoke. The same thing occurs if the patient screams. If the temperature inside the environment is high enough, immediate death may be the result. Children should be taught from a young age to crawl out of a burning environment, and this should be practiced on a regular basis to ensure that they, as well as adults, remember what to do instinctively.

Supraglottic Inhalation Injury

Because of the location of supraglottic structures, they are very susceptible to inhalation injuries. The upper airway is very vascular and has a large surface area. Inhaling superheated steam or air can damage tissues, resulting in irritation and edema. This can quickly lead to partial or complete airway obstruction. Upper airway edema is the earliest consequence of inhalation injury. The tissue damage from inhaling hot air is not immediately reversible by introducing fresh, cool air. Signs and symptoms may include the following:

- Altered mental status
- Fire or smoke present in an enclosed area
- Evidence of respiratory distress or upper airway obstruction
- Soot around the mouth or nose
- Singed nasal hairs, eyebrows, or eyelashes
- Burns around the face or neck
- Carbonaceous sputum
- Hoarseness
- Stridor
- Cough

Early recognition and treatment for these patients is the key to survival. Consider early definitive airway management before edema makes it virtually impossible.

Infraglottic Inhalation Injury

Because of the location, thermal injury to the lower airway is rare. However, inhalation of toxins and smoke is just as hazardous. Systemic toxins affect the ability of the blood to absorb oxygen. Because carbon monoxide is colorless, odorless, and tasteless, your only clue may be the environment in which the patient is found.

> **A to Z Terminology Tips**
>
> Supra = above, so supraglottic = above the glottis
> Infra = below, so infraglottic = below the glottis

Burning materials also give off toxins that damage the lung parenchyma. This is especially true of petroleum-based products, such as wool, rubber, and polyurethane foam.

Smoke intoxication is frequently hidden by more visible injuries such as burns. The condition of a patient who appears unharmed may later deteriorate as a result of smoke inhalation. Approximately 60% to 80% of deaths resulting from burn injuries can be attributed to smoke inhalation. Most of the smoke at a fire is a suspension of small particles of carbon and tar, but there is also some ordinary dust floating in a combination of heated gases. Some of the suspended particles in smoke are merely irritating, but others may be lethal. The size of the particle determines how deeply into the lungs it will be inhaled. Signs and symptoms of infraglottic inhalation injury include the following:

- Hypoxemia
- Rales or rhonchi
- Wheezing
- Bronchospasm
- Productive cough
- Pulmonary edema

Signs and symptoms of lower airway injury are usually seen later than those of the upper airway. The patient may appear unharmed only to die several hours later of pulmonary complications. It is important to maintain a high index of suspicion for any patient exposed to a burning environment.

Management

Prehospital care of the inhalation injury patient is the same as for any other burn patient, with specific attention to the airway. Consider early definitive airway treatment for the patient with an altered mental status. Prompt transport to the closest, most appropriate facility is imperative. This may include transport to a facility with access to a hyperbaric chamber for patients with suspected carbon monoxide poisoning. Patients who are hypoxic may be anxious or agitated. Provide psychological support en route.

Apply a cardiac monitor, and consider early intubation. Follow local and ACLS protocols for cardiac dysrhythmias.

Chemical Burns

A chemical burn can occur whenever a toxic substance contacts the body. Strong acids or strong alkalis (bases) cause most chemical burns. Both acids and alkalis are defined as caustic and cause significant tissue damage on contact. The eyes are particularly vulnerable to chemical burns Figure 14-20 . Caustic chemicals introduced into the eyes will produce burns similar to those of thermal burns. If not removed quickly, the burning process will continue through the various layers of the eye. Treat chemical burns to the eyes by flushing with copious amounts of water.

Sometimes simply the fumes of strong chemicals can cause burns, especially to the respiratory tract. In the United States, more than 100,000 exposures to acid- or alkaline-type products occur every year, the majority of which involve household cleaning products. Of approximately 25,500 exposures to acid and alkaline chemicals in 1996, there were 128 cases of major toxicity and 7 deaths. Of 52,750 exposures to bleach, there were 43 cases of major toxicity and no deaths. Among 5,100 reported exposures to drain cleaners, 59 cases resulted in major toxicity, and 7 cases resulted in death. Overall, there were 19 reported fatalities in 1996.

The severity of a chemical burn is related to a number of factors. What is the pH of the agent? What is the concentration? What was the length of time the patient was exposed to the agent? What was the volume of the agent? And finally, what was the physical form of the agent? Ingestion of solid agents, such as pills, results in a longer exposure time as the offending substance travels through the digestive system. In addition, concentrated forms of some acids and alkalis generate significant heat when diluted, resulting in thermal and caustic injury. Because industrial accidents are the most frequent types of chemical exposure, consider the mechanism of injury as well.

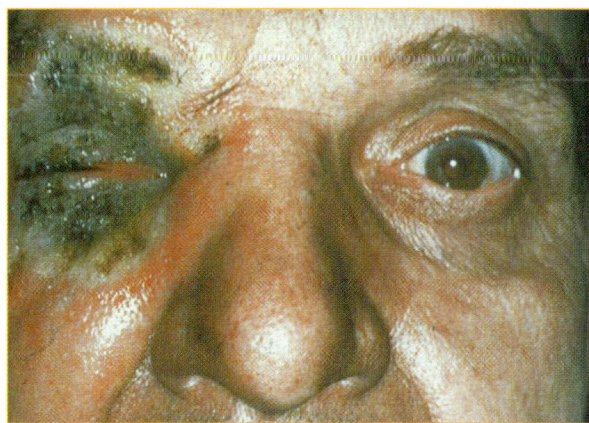

Figure 14-20 The eyes are particularly vulnerable to chemical burns.

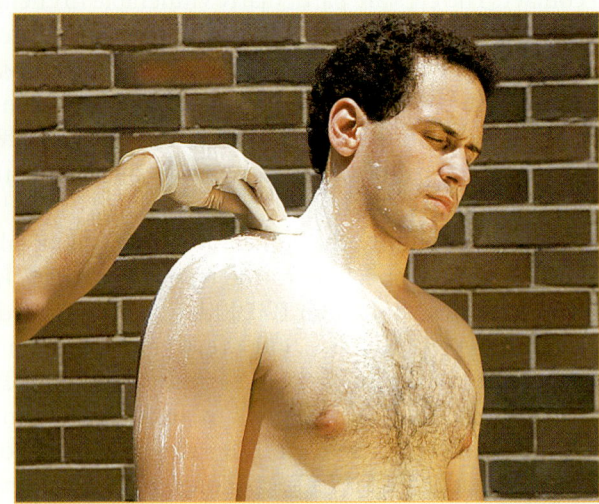

Figure 14-21 Brush dry chemicals off the patient before you flush the burned area with water.

To prevent exposure to hazardous materials, you must wear the appropriate personal protective equipment (such as gloves, eye protection) whenever you are caring for a patient with a chemical burn. Be particularly careful not to get any chemical, dry or liquid, on yourself or on your uniform; consider wearing a protective gown when this is a possibility. Remember that exposure risk is also present when you are cleaning up after the call. In cases of severe chemical burns or exposure, consider mobilization of the HazMat (hazardous materials) team, if appropriate.

The emergency care of a chemical burn is basically the same as that for a thermal burn. To stop the burning process, remove any chemical from the patient. *A dry chemical that is activated by contact with water may damage the skin more when it is wet than when it is dry.* Therefore, always brush dry chemicals off the skin and clothing before flushing the patient with water Figure 14-21. Remove the patient's clothing, including shoes, stockings, and gloves, because there may be small amounts of chemicals in the creases. Chemical burns are evaluated in the same manner as thermal burns when classifying depth or body surface area.

> **In the Field**
>
> For a patient who has had a chemical exposure, *never* pull the patient's shirt over his or her head. This could result in chemicals being rubbed into the mouth, nose, or eyes.

Immediately begin to flush the burned area with large amounts of water Figure 14-22, taking care not to contaminate uninjured areas or make the patient hypothermic. This should be integrated with your initial assessment of the patient. Never direct a forceful stream of water from a hose at the patient; the extreme water pressure may mechanically injure the burned skin. Continue flooding the area with copious amounts of water for 15 to 20 minutes after the patient says the burning pain has stopped. Continue flushing the contaminated area on the way to the hospital. Do not use any antidote or neutralizing agent. More damage may be caused by the chemical reaction of the antidote or neutralizing agent with the contaminant. Treat all chemical exposures according to local protocols. Table 14-3 lists specific information regarding various chemical exposures.

Determine the patient's mental status. Assess the airway and provide ventilatory support as needed. Consider early definitive airway management because the airway may constrict, making the airway more difficult to maintain. Assess circulation, and obtain IV access. Many chemicals, such as organophosphates, may affect the heart. If the ABCs are intact, continue with the rapid trauma assessment. Use the rule of nines or the rule of palms to determine the extent of the burn injury. Be sure to use the age-appropriate scale when calculating using the rule of nines. Provide reassurance to the patient, and transport promptly to the closest, most appropriate facility. The patient's status and local protocols should dictate mode of transport.

Consider electrocardiographic monitoring and follow ACLS and local protocols for pharmacologic interventions. Medications have a limited role in the treatment of most chemical burns. Pain medications may be indicated for burns, and steroids may be helpful in treating upper airway inflammation.

Chemical Burn Injury of the Eye

When treating chemical burns, pay particular attention to the eyes. Chemical injuries to the eyes may be the result of acids, alkalis, mace, pepper spray, or other irritants. Chemical burns require immediate emergency care, which consists of flushing the eye with water or a sterile saline irrigation solution. If sterile saline is not available, use any clean water. Industrial accidents are the most frequent cause of chemical eye injuries. Consider the possibility that if a chemical has been splashed or sprayed into the eyes, it may also have entered the respiratory tract. Always assess the airway as part of your initial assessment.

If an eye has been burned, hold the eyelid open while flooding the eye with a gentle stream of water Figure 14-23. Take care to avoid contamination of

TABLE 14-3 Characteristics of Specific Chemicals

Acids

Most acids produce a coagulation necrosis by denaturing (changing the nature) proteins. This forms a coagulum, or eschar, that limits the penetration of the acid.

Common Sources of Acids:

- Sulfuric acid—toilet bowl cleaners, drain cleaners, metal cleaners, automobile battery fluid, munitions, and fertilizer manufacturing
- Nitric acid—engraving, metal refining, and fertilizer manufacturing
- Hydrofluoric acid—rust removers, tire cleaners, tile cleaners, glass etching, dental work, tanning, semiconductors, refrigerant and fertilizer manufacturing, and petroleum refining
- Hydrochloric acid—toilet bowl cleaners, metal cleaners, soldering fluxes, dye manufacturing, metal refining, plumbing applications, and laboratory chemicals
- Phosphoric acid—metal cleaners, rustproofing, disinfectants, detergents, and fertilizer manufacturing
- Acetic acid—printing, dyes, rayon and hat manufacturing, disinfectants, and hair wave neutralizers; Vinegar is dilute acetic acid.
- Formic acid—airplane glue, tanning, and cellulose manufacturing

Alkalis (Bases)

Alkalis typically produce a more severe injury known as liquefaction necrosis. Not only are the proteins denatured, but fats are also broken down, which does not limit tissue penetration.

Common Sources of Bases:

- Cement (lime [calcium oxide])—lime, calcium oxide, is an ingredient of cement and mortar. Heat is produced when lime is mixed with water. Route of exposure and whether the lime is wet or dry determines the extent of illness or injury
- Sodium hydroxide and potassium hydroxide—drain cleaners, oven cleaners, and denture cleaners
- Calcium hydroxide—mortar, plaster, and cement (also known as slaked lime); not as caustic as calcium oxide
- Sodium and calcium hypochlorite—household bleach and pool chlorinating solution
- Ammonia—cleaners and detergents
- Anhydrous ammonia—industrial applications, particularly fertilizer manufacturing
- Phosphates—many types of household detergents and cleaners
- Silicates—used to replace phosphates in detergents
- Sodium carbonate—used in detergents

Phenols

Phenol, carbolic acid, is derived from the distillation of coal tar. It is corrosive to the eyes, skin, and respiratory tract, and also the digestive tract if ingested. It is found in disinfectants, cleaning agents, and in the manufacture of plastics, dyes, fertilizers, and explosives.

Source: www.cdc.gov/niosh Accessed October 12, 2003.

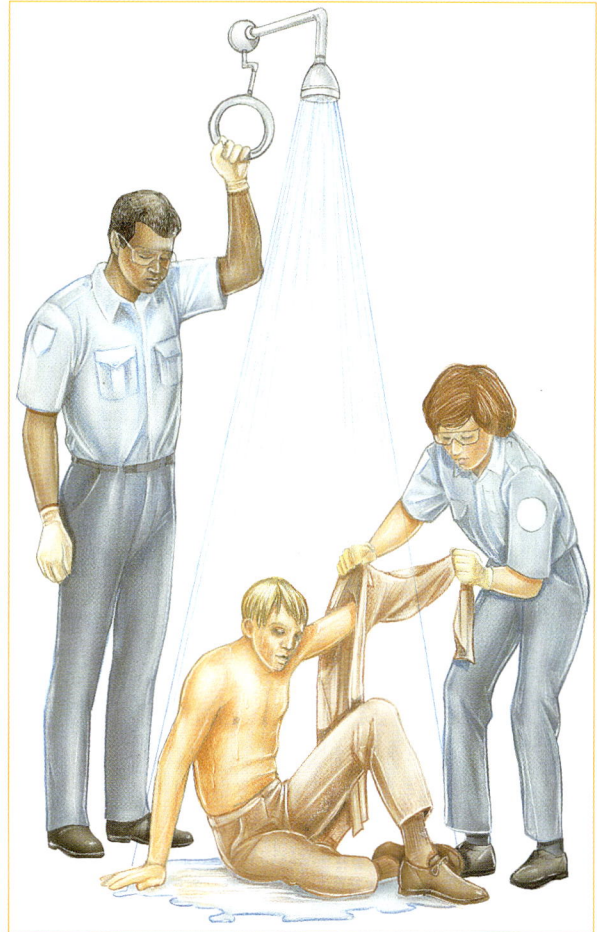

Figure 14-22 Flush the burned area with large amounts of water for 15 to 20 minutes after the patient says that the burning pain has stopped. Be careful to avoid contaminating uninjured areas.

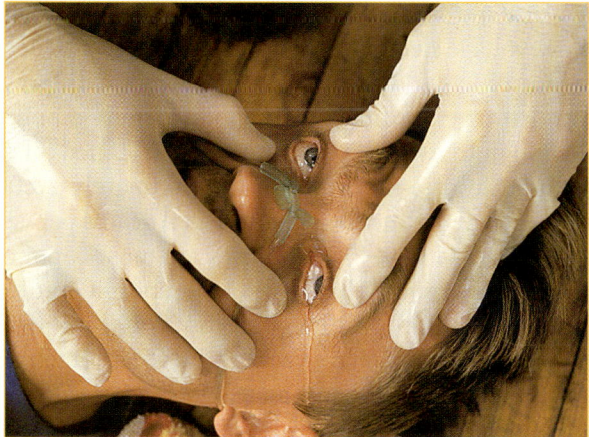

Figure 14-23 One method of irrigation is to direct saline into the injured eye using a round nasal airway or cannula. Always flush from the nose side of the eye toward the outside to avoid flushing material into the other eye.

the ears, mouth, and other areas of the face and head by runoff. When both eyes are affected, a nasal cannula attached to IV tubing provides a constant stream of irrigation that is easily adjusted and allows for simultaneous irrigation of both eyes. Place a clean towel around the patient's head and over the ears to catch runoff. The idea is to direct the greatest amount of solution or water into the eye as gently as possible. Because opening the eye spontaneously may cause the patient pain, you may have to force the lids open to irrigate the eye adequately. In some circumstances, you may have to resort to pouring water into the eye by holding the patient's head under a gently running faucet. You can even have the patient immerse his or her face in a large pan or basin of water and rapidly blink the affected eyelid. If only one eye is affected, care must be taken to avoid contaminated water from getting into the unaffected eye. This is accomplished by flushing the material laterally, away from the unaffected eye.

Irrigate the eye for at least 5 minutes. If an alkali or a strong acid caused the burn, you should irrigate the eye for 20 minutes. Strong acids and all alkaline solutions can penetrate deeply, requiring prolonged irrigation. Again, always take care to protect the uninjured eye and prevent irrigation fluid from running into it.

After you have completed irrigation, apply a clean, dry dressing to cover the eye and transport the patient promptly to the hospital for further care. If the irrigation can be carried out satisfactorily in the ambulance, it should be done during transport to save time. Care for other chemical burn injuries as explained in the previous section.

Electrical Burns

Electrical burns may be the result of contact with high- or low-voltage electricity. High-voltage burns may occur when utility workers make direct contact with power lines. However, ordinary household current is powerful enough to cause severe burns. In the United States, electrical injuries account for approximately 20,000 emergency department visits and 1,000 deaths per year. Low-voltage (110–440 V) injuries are most common, accounting for more than 60% of all reported injuries. Children account for 20% of all low-voltage injuries. Low-voltage injuries have very low morbidity and mortality. Both morbidity and mortality increase proportionately as voltage increases. However, at the same voltage, AC (alternating current) injuries have three times the morbidity and mortality rate as DC (direct current) injuries. Because the major risk factors for electrical injury include improper supervision of children and failure to make a child's environment safe, prevention is aimed at better control and attention to surroundings. Electricity involves the flow of energy along the path of least resistance toward a natural ground. For electricity to flow, there must be a complete circuit between the electrical source and the ground. Any substance that prevents this circuit from being completed, such as rubber, is called an insulator. Any substance that allows a current to flow through it is called a conductor. The human body, which is primarily water, is a good conductor. Thus, electrical burns occur when the body, or a part of it, completes a circuit connecting a power source to the ground (Figure 14-24).

Standard household current in the United States is 110 V AC with a frequency of 60 Hz. Skeletal muscle is stimulated into **tetany** (tonic muscle spasm) by currents with frequencies of 40 to 110 Hz. Most low- and high-tension electrical current is AC, which produces tetany and the locked-on phenomenon. Although tetany occurs in all muscles that are stimulated, flexor groups are usually stronger and predominate. As a result, an individual's grasp is uncontrollably locked onto the object, which can increase the length of time the current passes through the body and may result in greater injury. In contrast, DC tends to produce a single large muscular contraction that often throws the patient away from the source.

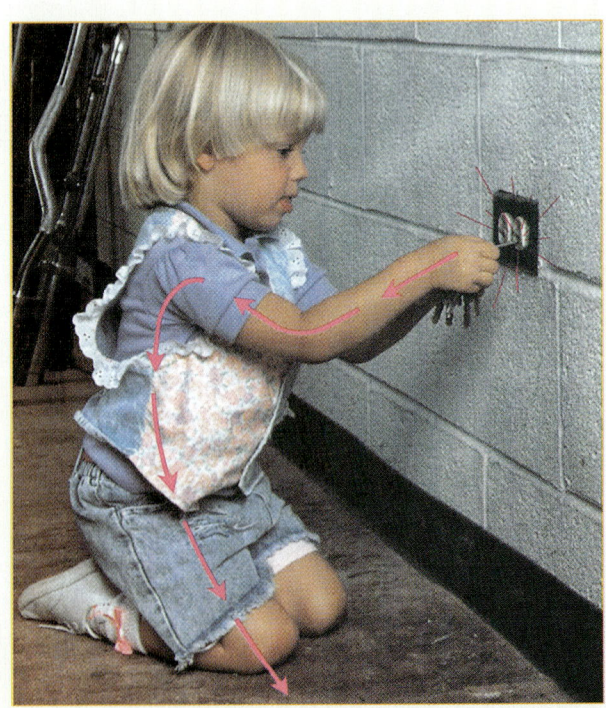

Figure 14-24 The human body is a good conductor of electricity. An electrical burn usually occurs when the body, acting as a conductor, completes a circuit.

Mechanism of Injury

There are four basic classifications of burn injuries: contact burn injuries, arc injuries, flame or flash burn injuries, and lightning injuries. Contact injuries occur from direct contact with an electrical source. Hands and wrists are common entrance sites, and the feet are common exit sites with this type of injury. Arc injuries occur when the patient is close enough to two contact points of a high-voltage (440–1,000 V) source that the current flows through the patient. Arc burns have a characteristic white center with a rim of congestion or erythema. Arc burns commonly are associated with significant internal transfer of energy and related injury. Flame or flash burn injuries are the result of an electrical source igniting a combustible material, resulting in fire. This may include clothing and other objects in the surroundings. Common sites of injury include the face and eyes along with other local tissue injuries depending on the area affected. This type of injury is common in welding. The final classification, lightning, may cause full cardiac arrest by inducing asystole or apnea. Massive depolarization of the heart leads to asystole. However, the heart's automaticity usually restarts the heart in a normal sinus rhythm. Massive depolarization of the brain is believed to stun the respiratory center, causing a much longer duration of apnea. If prompt artificial respiration is provided, many patients can survive.

Lightning usually is not associated with severe burns because the impulse is instantaneous. A direct strike occurs when the lightning bolt of energy directly strikes the individual, whereas in a contact injury, the individual is in contact with the object that is struck. A side-flash injury is a thermal flash burn that occurs as a result of proximity to a strike.

Pathophysiology

Electrical injury may cause disruption of the body's normal electrical activities. The neurologic system is affected most commonly. Neurologic dysfunction is present in some form, even if only temporarily, in virtually all patients. Transient nerve injuries resulting in temporary numbness and tingling are most common. Mass depolarization of the brain may lead to a loss of consciousness, amnesia, and coma. Spinal cord involvement may result in transverse myelitis (inflammation of the spinal cord), which may have a delayed onset and is associated with a poor prognosis for recovery.

Electrical injuries may also affect the heart, resulting in cardiac dysrhythmias. Some may be transient, but others may result in cardiac arrest. Sudden death from an AC electrical injury is usually the result of ventricular fibrillation, although asystole and other dysrhythmias are common. Ventricular fibrillation is three times more likely to occur if the flow of current is arm to arm, because the electrical current flows directly across the heart.

Heat is also generated by the flow of electrical current through body tissues, resulting in direct thermal injury. At higher voltages, higher temperatures are achieved, resulting in greater injury. High-tension voltages cause devastating injuries from huge amounts of internal thermal damage.

Vascular injury occurs as the result of vascular spasm. Heat generated by the injury can also cause coagulation and vascular occlusion. Damage to the vascular wall may produce delayed thrombosis and bleeding. Compartment syndrome may develop as a result of acute ischemic insult to the musculature.

Renal injuries may occur as a result of rhabdomyolysis. Rhabdomyolysis causes myoglobinuria from massive release of myoglobin. Myoglobin crystallization in the kidney tubules may cause acute renal failure.

History

Not all electrical or lightning injuries are the same. A detailed history, including all of the specific information associated with the event, is essential. Determine the voltage and type of current if possible. Identify whether the injury was brief or sustained and an approximate time of contact. Determine conditions associated with the injury that may have influenced the amount of energy transferred. These may include conditions such as wet skin or a puddle of water. If possible, determine the mechanism of injury. Was this a direct contact? Arc? Flash burn? Also ask about any loss of consciousness and any preexisting medical conditions that may exacerbate the problem and hinder effective resuscitation.

Safety

Your safety is of particular importance when you are called to the scene of an emergency involving electricity. Obviously, coming into direct contact with power lines can fatally injure you. In addition, touching a patient who is still in contact with a live power line or any other electrical source can be fatal to you as well. For this reason, you must never attempt to remove someone from an electrical source unless you are specially trained to do so. Likewise, you should never move a downed power line unless you have the special training and equipment necessary for the job or unless you are absolutely certain that the line is not live. Notify your dispatcher to send the power company for assistance. Before even approaching someone who may still be in contact with a power line or an electrical appliance, make certain that the power is turned off. Always assume that any downed power line is live.

Management

There is always a burn injury where the electricity entered the body (an entrance wound) and another where it exited (an exit wound). The entrance wound may be quite small (Figure 14-25A ▼), but the exit wound can be extensive and deep (Figure 14-25B ▼). Always look for both entrance and exit wounds. There are two dangers specifically associated with electrical burns. First, there may be a large amount of deep tissue injury. Electrical burns are always more severe than the external signs indicate. The patient may have only a small burn to the skin but massive damage to the deeper tissues (Figure 14-26 ▶). Second, the patient may go into cardiac arrest from the electric shock. When the path of electricity travels from hand to hand, it generally flows through the heart, disrupting normal functioning of the cardiac conduction system.

Assess the level of consciousness and ABCs. Provide high-flow oxygen, and assist ventilation as needed. As with thermal burns, consider early definitive care of the airway if the patient is unable to maintain his or her own. When assessing circulation, look for signs of hypoperfusion and assess the heart rate, specifically for regularity to detect potentially life-threatening dysrhythmias. Cardiac dysrhythmias are common with electrical burns. Patients with electrical burns may be at risk for hypothermia, which is associated with increased morbidity and mortality rates. Remove any wet clothing, and keep the patient warm and dry.

Consider cervical spine immobilization if there was a mechanism of injury indicating potential trauma. Look for any trauma associated with the injury that may be the result of a fall or explosion. Categorize burns according to the rule of nines or rule of palms using the same classifications used for thermal burns. Accurately estimating the body surface area involved is very difficult because the internal depth and degree of injury may be greater than would be assumed from external appearances.

If indicated, begin CPR and apply the automatic external defibrillator (abbreviated AED). Although CPR may need to be quite prolonged in electrical burn cases, it has a high success rate if started promptly. You should be prepared to defibrillate if necessary. If neither CPR nor defibrillation is indicated, give high-flow supplemental oxygen, and monitor the patient closely for respiratory and cardiac arrest. Establish IV access using an isotonic crystalloid solution, and administer a bolus of 20 mL/kg or according to local protocols. This will help to maintain an adequate urine output of 1 mL/kg per hour and adequate renal perfusion.

Treat external burns as you would thermal burns. Treat the soft-tissue injuries by placing dry, sterile dressings on all burn wounds and splinting suspected fractures. Provide prompt transport to the closest, most appropriate facility; all electrical burns are potentially severe injuries that require further treatment in the hospital. Remember that very old and very young patients, as well as those with preexisting conditions, are at greater risk for severe morbidity and mortality.

Consider early intubation for patients unable to maintain their own airway. Monitor the electrocardiogram, and consider analgesics for pain relief according to local protocols. For cardiac or respiratory arrests associated with electrical injuries, follow ACLS or local protocols.

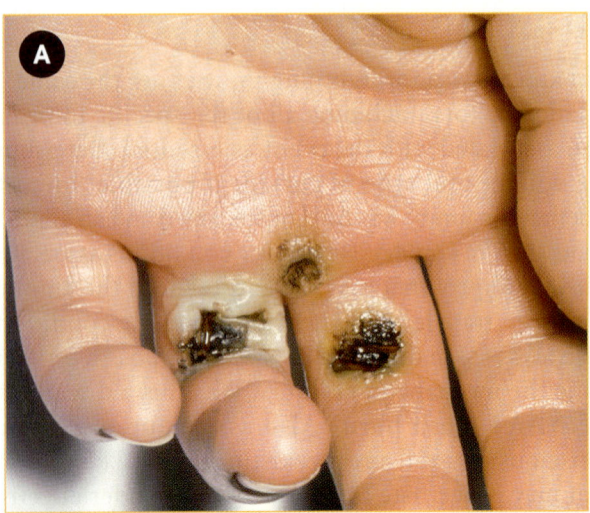

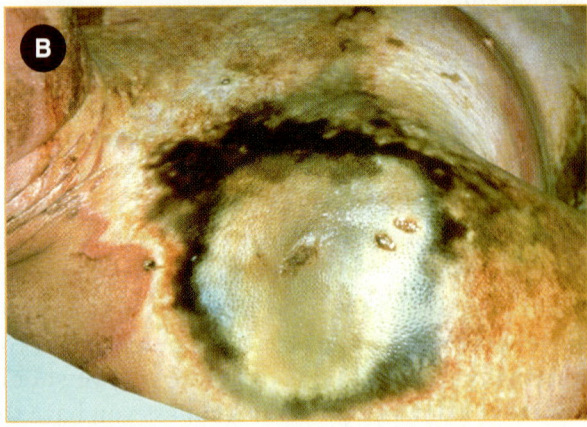

Figure 14-25 Electrical burns, like gunshot wounds, have entrance and exit wounds. **A.** An entrance wound is often quite small. **B.** The exit wound is typically more extensive.

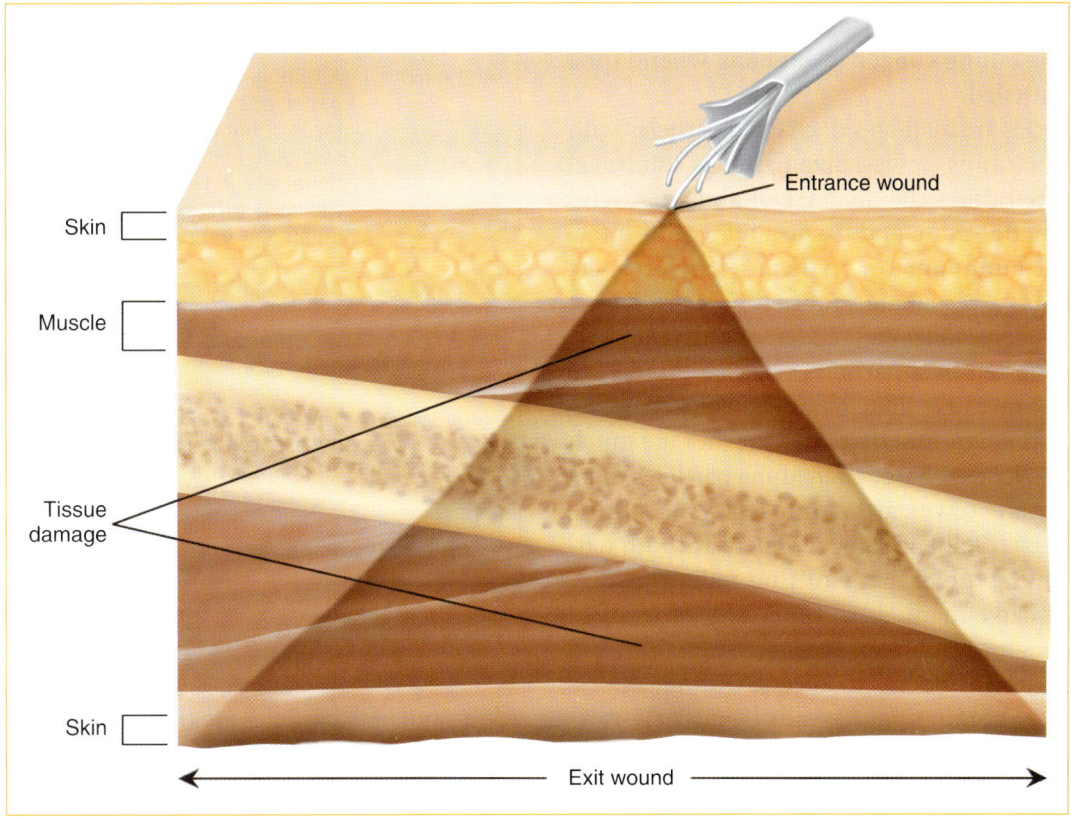

Figure 14-26 External signs of an electrical burn may be deceiving. The entrance wound may be a small burn, but the damage to deeper tissue may be massive.

> ### EMT-I Safety
>
> Your safety is the first priority when an electrical hazard may be involved. Do not try to remove someone from an electrical source or move a downed power line unless you are specially trained and equipped to do so. Before approaching someone who may still be in contact with a power line or electrical appliance, ensure that all power is turned off.

Radiation Exposure

Radiation injuries are caused by ionizing radiation emitted by sources such as the sun, x-ray and other diagnostic machines, tanning beds, and radioactive elements released in nuclear power plant accidents and detonation of nuclear weapons during war and acts of terrorism. Ionizing radiation is made up of unstable atoms that contain an excess amount of energy. In an attempt to stabilize, the atoms emit the excess energy into the atmosphere, creating radiation. These charged particles (ions) can cause damage to molecules, cells, and tissues. Any amount of ionizing radiation will produce some damage. Radiation can be found everywhere; however, the Earth's atmosphere protects us from most of the sun's radiation.

The three most common types of ionizing radiation are *alpha particles*, *beta particles*, and *gamma rays*. Inhalation, ingestion, and direct exposure are the three basic pathways by which people are exposed. The amount and duration of exposure affects the severity or type of health effect.

Most alpha emitters occur naturally in the environment. Human activity, such as uranium mining wastes, create or worsen the potential for exposure and contamination by bringing high concentrations of uranium and radium to the surface. Once brought to the surface, they can become airborne or enter surface water as runoff. Alpha particles are the least penetrating of the three types of ionizing radiation. They do not penetrate the skin and can be stopped by thin paper or clothing. A health hazard may occur when alpha-emitting materials are inhaled, swallowed, or enter the body through a wound. For this reason, they are an internal hazard only. Biologic damage from exposure to alpha particles increases the risk of cancer. Alpha radiation is known to cause lung cancer in humans when alpha emitters are inhaled.

Beta particles are high-speed, charged particles with moderate penetrating power. Beta particles can travel several hundred times the distance of alpha particles in air, can penetrate skin and tissue, and require a few millimeters of aluminum to stop them. Therefore, beta particles can be external and internal hazards. Direct exposure to beta particles can redden or burn the skin. Inhaled or ingested beta particles released directly to living tissue can cause damage at the cellular level, which can disrupt cell function. Because they are much smaller and have less charge than alpha particles, beta particles generally travel farther into tissues, resulting in more dispersed cellular damage. There are both natural and manufactured beta-emitting radionuclides. Beta emitters have many uses, especially in medical diagnosis, imaging, and treatment. Beta radiation can cause chronic and acute health effects. Chronic effects are much more common and result from fairly low-level exposures over a long period of time. The main chronic effect from radiation is cancer. When taken internally, beta emitters can cause tissue damage and increase the risk of cancer. This risk increases with increasing doses.

Gamma rays are the most energetic and most penetrating type of radiation and can travel many meters in air and many centimeters in tissue. Gamma photons have no mass and no electrical charge; they are pure electromagnetic energy. Both external and internal exposure to gamma rays or x-rays are of concern. Gamma rays can travel much farther than alpha or beta particles and have enough energy to pass entirely through the body, potentially exposing all organs. Because of the gamma ray's penetrating power and ability to travel great distances, it is considered the primary hazard to the general population during most radiologic emergencies.

Aspects of Exposure

Three basic concepts affect a person's exposure to radiation: time, distance, and shielding. The amount of radiation exposure depends on the time people spend near the source of radiation. Gamma and x-rays are the primary concern for external exposure. However, if radioactive material gets inside your body, you cannot move away from it. You have to wait until it decays or until your body can eliminate it. When this happens, the biologic half-life of the agent controls the time of exposure.

TABLE 14-4 Shielding Requirements

Alpha (α)	A thin piece of light material, such as paper, or even the dead cells in the outer layer of human skin, provides adequate shielding because alpha particles cannot penetrate it. However, living tissue inside the body offers no protection against inhaled or ingested alpha emitters.
Beta (β)	Additional covering, heavy clothing for example, is necessary to protect against beta emitters. Some beta particles can penetrate and burn skin.
Gamma (γ)	Thick, dense shielding, such as lead, is necessary to protect against gamma rays. The higher the energy of the gamma ray, the thicker the lead must be. X-rays pose a similar challenge, so radiologic technicians often give patients receiving medical or dental radiographs a lead apron to cover other parts of their body.

Alpha and beta particles are the main concern for internal exposure.

Distance is a prime concern when dealing with gamma rays, because they can travel long distances. Alpha and beta particles do not have enough energy to travel very far. The farther the person is from a source of exposure, the less the exposure.

Shielding means having something that will absorb the radiation between the person and the source of radiation. The amount of shielding required to protect against different kinds of radiation depends on how much energy they have. Table 14-4 shows the amount of shielding required for different kinds of radiation.

Assessment

Any living tissue in the human body can be damaged by ionizing radiation. The body attempts to repair the damage, but sometimes the damage is too severe or widespread or abnormalities occur in the natural repair process. Cancer is considered to be the primary health effect from chronic exposure. Unlike cancer, which is a slow process, in an acute exposure, health effects appear quickly. These include burns and radiation sickness or radiation poisoning.

Radiation sickness can cause premature aging or even death. If the dose is fatal, death usually occurs within 2 months. The symptoms of radiation sickness include nausea, weakness, hair loss, skin burns, or diminished organ function.

Management

The first concern when dealing with a radiation exposure is personal safety. Never approach a scene until it has been declared safe. It may be necessary to set up a staging area and wait for decontaminated patients to be brought to the ambulance.

ABCs are always primary in patient care. Open and assess the airway. Apply high-flow oxygen, and provide ventilatory support for those who are breathing inadequately. As with inhalation burns, consider early definitive treatment if there are any signs of airway irritation. Assess circulation and provide circulatory support. Treat for shock as needed.

Treat any burns in the same manner as thermal burns. Classify body surface area burned using the same scale. Follow local protocols. Establish IV access, and give fluid based on patient presentation. If there are signs of shock, give a 20-mL/kg bolus of an isotonic crystalloid solution and reassess. Provide reassurance, and transport promptly to the closest, most appropriate facility.

Consider early intubation for unresponsive patients. Follow local protocols for pain relief with analgesics. Monitor cardiac rhythm, and treat dysrhythmias according to ACLS protocols.

Dressing and Bandaging

All wounds require bandaging. In most cases, splints help to control bleeding and provide firm support for the dressing. There are many different types of dressings and bandages (Figure 14-27). You should be familiar with the function and proper application of each.

In general, dressings and bandages have three primary functions:
- To control bleeding
- To protect the wound from further damage
- To prevent further contamination and infection

Sterile Dressings

Universal dressings, conventional 4" × 4" and 4" × 8" gauze pads, and assorted small adhesive-type dressings and soft self-adherent roller dressings will cover most wounds.

Measuring 9" × 36" and made of thick, absorbent material, the universal dressing is ideal for covering large open wounds. It also makes an efficient pad for rigid splints. These dressings are available in compact, commercially sterilized packages.

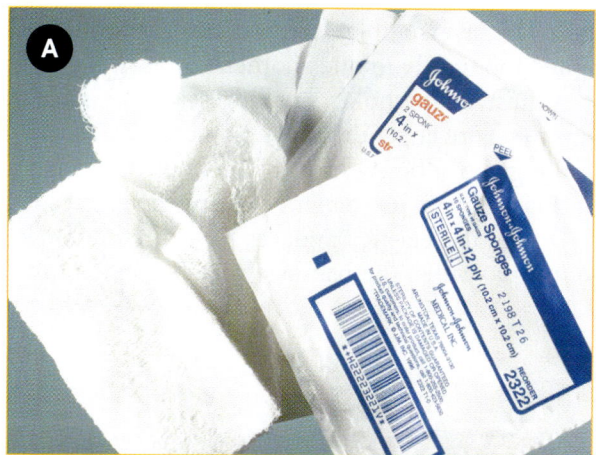
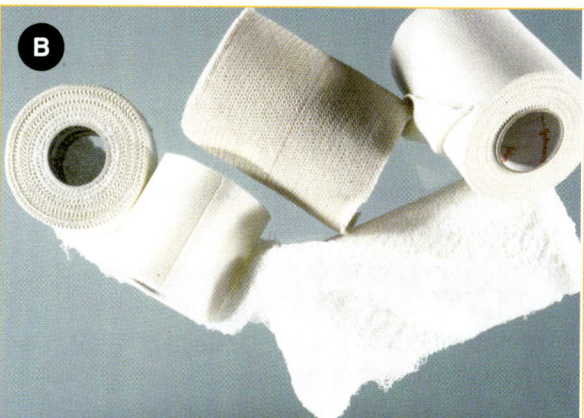

Figure 14-27 **A.** Many types of sterile dressings are used for covering open wounds, including universal dressings, gauze pads, adhesive dressings, and occlusive dressings. **B.** Bandages keep dressings in place and include soft roller bandages, triangular bandages, and adhesive tape. Splints may also be used to hold dressings in place.

Gauze pads are appropriate for smaller wounds, and adhesive-type dressings are useful for minor wounds. Occlusive dressings, made of Vaseline gauze, aluminum foil, or plastic, prevent air and liquids from entering (or exiting) the wound. They are used to cover sucking chest wounds, abdominal eviscerations, and open neck injuries.

Bandages

To keep dressings in place during transport, you can use soft roller bandages, rolls of gauze, triangular bandages, or adhesive tape. The self-adherent, soft roller bandages are probably easiest to use. They are slightly elastic, which makes them easy to apply, and you can tuck the end of the roll into a deeper layer to secure it in place. The layers adhere somewhat but should not be applied too tightly to one another.

Adhesive tape holds small dressings in place and helps to secure larger dressings. Some people, however, are allergic to adhesive tape. If you know that a patient has this problem, use paper or plastic tape instead.

Do not use elastic bandages to secure dressings. If the injury swells, the bandage may become a tourniquet and cause further damage. Any improperly applied bandage that impairs circulation can result in additional tissue damage or even the loss of a limb. For this reason, you should always check a limb distal to a bandage for signs of impaired circulation or loss of sensation, before, during, and after application of the bandage. Air splints are useful for stabilizing broken extremities, and they can be used with dressings to help control bleeding from soft-tissue injuries.

You are the Provider

Summary

1. What is the difference between a dressing and a bandage?

A dressing is placed directly over a wound to control bleeding and prevent further contamination, and a bandage is used to hold the dressing in place.

2. Is there a difference in the care for chemical burns and electrical burns?

The emergency care of a chemical burn is basically the same as that for a thermal burn. To stop the burning process, immediately remove any chemical from the patient. *A dry chemical that is activated by contact with water may damage the skin more when it is wet than when it is dry.* Therefore, always brush dry chemicals off the skin and clothing before flushing the affected area(s) with water. Electrical burns are like gunshot wounds because they have both an entrance wound and an exit wound. Other complications associated with electrical burns include interference with the cardiac conduction system, which can cause arrhythmias, and tetanic muscle spasms, which can result in fractures. Therefore, care for the patient with an electrical burn consists of covering the entry and exit wounds with sterile dressings, cardiac monitoring, and splinting suspected fractures.

3. What is your first consideration in treating this patient?

After completing an initial assessment, your first consideration is to administer 100% oxygen. If the patient is breathing adequately, use a nonrebreathing mask. If the patient is breathing inadequately, assist ventilation with a bag-valve-mask (BVM) device.

4. Why is it difficult to accurately assess the severity of damage caused by an electrical burn?

During an electrical burn, the majority of damage occurs to the internal structures of the body, such as the nerves, blood vessels, and muscles. This can make assessing the severity of the patient's injury difficult, especially when the only external visible signs of trauma are small entrance and exit wounds.

5. Which body system is most commonly affected by electrical injuries?

The nervous system is affected most commonly by electrical injuries. Neurologic dysfunction is present in some form, even if only temporarily, in virtually all patients. Transient nerve injuries, resulting in temporary numbness and tingling, are most common. However, interference with the cardiac conduction system can result in cardiac arrhythmias, and mass depolarization of the neurons in the brain may lead to seizures.

Prep Kit

Ready for Review

- The skin has two principal layers: the tough outer layer, called the epidermis, and the inner layer, called the dermis, which contains the hair follicles, sweat glands, and sebaceous glands.
- The functions of the skin are to keep bacteria out and water in, to report to the brain on the environment, and to regulate body temperature.
- There are three types of soft-tissue injuries: closed injuries, open injuries, and burns.
- Closed injuries include contusions, hematomas, and crushing injuries. They can be treated by applying ICES (ice, compression, elevation of the injured part, and splinting).
- Open injuries produce more extensive bleeding and may become infected. There are four types of open injuries: abrasions, lacerations, avulsions, and penetrating wounds.
- In treating these injuries, you must first control bleeding. Use a dry, sterile dressing, covered by a roller bandage, a second pressure dressing (if necessary), and a splint. Do not try to clean out an open wound.
- Burns are one of the most serious and painful of soft-tissue injuries. They can occur from heat (thermal), chemicals, electricity, and radiation.
- Burns are classified primarily by the depth and extent of the burn and the body area involved; they are superficial, partial-thickness, or full-thickness.
- Treatment for burns includes personal safety, BSI precautions, stopping the burning process, caring for the burn wounds, and treating the patient for shock (oxygen, IV therapy, and prevention of further heat loss). Always follow local protocols for invasive and pharmacologic interventions.
- Dressings and bandages are designed to control bleeding, protect the wound from further damage, and prevent further contamination and infection.
- Use universal dressings for large open wounds, gauze pads for smaller wounds, adhesive-type dressings for minor wounds, and occlusive dressings for sucking chest wounds and abdominal eviscerations. Use soft roller bandages, rolls of gauze, triangular bandages, or adhesive tape to keep dressings in place. Do not use elastic bandages. Always check a limb distal to a bandage for signs of impaired circulation.

Vital Vocabulary

abrasion Loss or damage of the superficial layer of skin as a result of a body part rubbing or scraping across a rough or hard surface.

avulsion An injury in which soft tissue is torn completely loose or is hanging as a flap.

burns An injury in which the soft tissue receives more energy than it can absorb without injury, from thermal heat, frictional heat, toxic chemicals, electricity, or nuclear radiation.

closed injury An injury in which damage occurs beneath the skin or mucous membrane but the surface remains intact.

compartment syndrome Swelling in a confined space that produces dangerous pressure; may cut off blood flow or damage sensitive tissue.

contamination The presence of infective organisms or foreign bodies such as dirt, gravel, or metal in a wound.

contusion A bruise without a break in the skin.

dermis The inner layer of the skin, containing hair follicles, sweat glands, nerve endings, and blood vessels.

ecchymosis Discoloration associated with a closed wound; signifies bleeding.

epidermis The outer layer of skin that acts as a watertight protective covering.

eschar Thick, coagulated crust or slough of leathery skin that develops following a burn.

evisceration The displacement of organs outside the body.

Technology

- Interactivities
- Vocabulary Explorer
- Anatomy Review
- Web Links
- Online Review Manual

www.EMSzone.com/EMTI

Prep Kit continued...

full-thickness (third-degree) burns Burns that affect all skin layers and may affect the subcutaneous layers, muscle, bone, and internal organs, leaving the area dry, leathery, and white, dark brown, or charred.

hematoma Blood collected within the body's tissues or in a body cavity.

hemothorax Collection of blood in the chest.

laceration A smooth or jagged open wound.

mucous membranes The linings of body cavities and passages that are in direct contact with the outside environment.

occlusive dressing A dressing made of Vaseline gauze, aluminum foil, or plastic that prevents air and liquids from entering or exiting a wound.

open injury An injury in which there is a break in the surface of the skin or the mucous membrane, exposing deeper tissue to potential contamination.

Parkland formula A formula that recommends giving 4 mL of normal saline for each kilogram of body weight, multiplied by the percentage of body surface area burned; sometimes used during lengthy transport times.

partial-thickness (second-degree) burns Burns affecting the epidermis and some portion of the dermis but not the subcutaneous tissue, characterized by blisters and skin that is white to red, moist, and mottled.

penetrating wound An injury that penetrates the skin, resulting from a sharp, pointed object or a bullet.

pneumothorax Entry of air into the pleural space.

Rule of nines A system that assigns percentages to sections of the body, allowing calculation of the amount of skin surface involved in the burn area.

Rule of palms A system that estimates total body surface area burned by comparing the affected area with the size of the patient's palm, which is roughly equal to 1% of the patient's total body surface area.

superficial (first-degree) burns Burns affecting only the epidermis, characterized by skin that is red but not blistered or actually burned through.

tetany Intermittent tonic spasms that involve the extremities.

Points to Ponder

You are dispatched to a house fire. On arrival, you find the owner of the home standing in the street watching the firefighters work. She is holding her dog, Fluffy. She tells you that she had been at a neighbor's home when the neighbor's son ran in and told her that there was smoke coming from her house. She said the house was smoke-filled, but she didn't see a fire at first. She ran in for a few seconds to rescue Fluffy and then exited the house. She has no complaints, her skin is pink, vital signs are normal, and lung sounds are clear. She refuses treatment and transport. You continue talking with her as you watch the firefighters extinguish the fire. Suddenly, she becomes pale, diaphoretic, and dyspneic. You run to get your equipment; however, by the time you return, she is lying on the ground with firefighters performing rescue breathing. Why is your previously stable patient now apneic? What should you have done differently?

Issues: Understanding the Importance of Transporting a Burn Patient Quickly, Appreciating the Incidence of Rapid Airway Swelling and Airway Compromise

Assessment in Action

You are dispatched to stand by at the scene of a house fire. When you arrive at the scene, you learn that the owner of the home is still in the house and firefighters are in the process of searching for him. A few minutes later, firefighters carry the man from the house.

On assessment, you note that he is unconscious, his respirations are rapid and shallow, and there is carbonaceous sputum in his nose and mouth. Further assessment reveals a large laceration to the side of his neck with heavy dark red bleeding and partial-thickness (second-degree) burns to his chest and the front of both of his arms. Firefighters tell you that the fire appears to have started in the kitchen due to an explosion. The patient was found unresponsive in the kitchen.

1. Immediate care for this patient should include suction, BVM ventilation, and:
   A. endotracheal intubation.
   B. bleeding control.
   C. cooling of the burns with water.
   D. large-bore IV therapy.

2. How should you manage the patient's neck laceration?
   A. Turn his head to the side and apply ice
   B. Apply pressure to the carotid artery
   C. Cover the wound with an occlusive dressing
   D. Wrap roller gauze tightly around his neck

3. Routine assessment and management of partial-thickness (second-degree) and full-thickness (third-degree) burns includes all of the following, EXCEPT:
   A. determining the extent of the burn.
   B. assessing lung sounds.
   C. IV fluid resuscitation.
   D. placing moist dressings.

4. According to the rule of nines, the extent of the patient's body surface area that is burned is:
   A. 9%.
   B. 18%.
   C. 27%.
   D. 36%.

5. The patient's burns are critical because:
   A. they are partial thickness and involve the chest.
   B. the burns cover less than 10% of the patient's body surface area.
   C. the burns are associated with smoke inhalation.
   D. the patient is likely unconscious due to hypoglycemia.

6. Based on your assessment findings you should treat this patient for his severe burns, as well as:
   A. respiratory compromise, shock, and abdominal injury.
   B. spinal injury, shock, and respiratory compromise.
   C. chest injury, shock, and closed head injury.
   D. shock, abdominal injury, and extremity fractures.

7. Additional treatment for this patient should include:
   A. maintaining body heat.
   B. irrigating the burns with water.
   C. keeping the patient cool.
   D. applying burn ointment.

8. Immediate death caused by burns is often the result of:
   A. the burn injury itself.
   B. massive infection.
   C. inhalation injury.
   D. associated trauma.

Thoracic Trauma

1999 Objectives

Cognitive

4-4.1 Describe the incidence, morbidity, and mortality of thoracic injuries in the trauma patient. (p 724)

4-4.2 Discuss the anatomy and physiology of the organs and structures related to thoracic injuries. (p 716)

4-4.3 Predict thoracic injuries based on mechanism of injury. (p 719)

4-4.4 Discuss the types of thoracic injuries. (p 719)

4-4.5 Discuss the pathophysiology of thoracic injuries. (p 720)

4-4.6 Discuss the assessment findings associated with thoracic injuries. (p 721)

4-4.7 Discuss the management of thoracic injuries. (p 722)

4-4.8 Identify the need for rapid intervention and transport of the patient with thoracic injuries. (p 722)

4-4.9 Discuss the epidemiology and pathophysiology of specific chest wall injuries, including:
   a. Rib fracture
   b. Flail segment
   c. Sternal fracture (p 723-725)

4-4.10 Discuss the assessment findings associated with chest wall injuries. (p 735)

4-4.11 Identify the need for rapid intervention and transport of the patient with chest wall injuries. (p 735)

4-4.12 Discuss the management of chest wall injuries. (p 724)

4-4.13 Discuss the pathophysiology of injury to the lung, including:
   a. Simple pneumothorax
   b. Open pneumothorax
   c. Tension pneumothorax
   d. Hemothorax
   e. Hemopneumothorax
   f. Pulmonary contusion (p 725-727, 730, 731)

4-4.14 Discuss the assessment findings associated with lung injuries. (p 726)

4-4.15 Discuss the management of lung injuries. (p 735)

4-4.16 Identify the need for rapid intervention and transport of the patient with lung injuries. (p 735)

4-4.17 Discuss the pathophysiology of myocardial injuries, including:
   a. Pericardial tamponade
   b. Myocardial contusion (p 732, 733)

4-4.18 Discuss the assessment findings associated with myocardial injuries. (p 733)

4-4.19 Discuss the management of myocardial injuries. (p 735)

4-4.20 Identify the need for rapid intervention and transport of the patient with myocardial injuries. (p 735)

4-4.21 Discuss the pathophysiology of vascular injuries, including injuries to:
   a. Aorta dissection/rupture
   b. Vena cava
   c. Pulmonary arteries/veins (p 733)

4-4.22 Discuss the assessment findings associated with vascular injuries. (p 733)

4-4.23 Discuss the management of vascular injuries. (p 735)

4-4.24 Discuss the pathophysiology of diaphragmatic injuries. (p 734)

4-4.25 Discuss the assessment findings associated with diaphragmatic injuries. (p 734)

4-4.26 Discuss the management of diaphragmatic injuries. (p 737)

4-4.27 Discuss the pathophysiology of esophageal injuries. (p 734)

4-4.28 Discuss the assessment findings associated with esophageal injuries. (p 734)

4-4.29 Discuss the management of esophageal injuries. (p 737)

4-4.30 Discuss the pathophysiology of tracheo-bronchial injuries. (p 734)

4-4.31 Discuss the assessment findings associated with tracheo-bronchial injuries. (p 734)

4-4.32 Discuss the management of tracheo-bronchial injuries. (p 737)

4-4.33 Discuss the pathophysiology of traumatic asphyxia. (p 734)

4-4.34 Discuss the assessment findings associated with traumatic asphyxia. (p 735)

4-4.35 Discuss the management of traumatic asphyxia. (p 737)

4-4.36 Differentiate between thoracic injuries based on the assessment and history. (p 721)

4-4.37 Formulate a field impression based on the assessment findings. (p 721)

4-4.38 Develop a patient management plan based on the field impression. (p 722)

Affective

4-4.39 Advocate the use of a thorough assessment to determine a differential diagnosis and treatment plan for thoracic trauma. (p 721)
4-4.40 Advocate the use of a thorough scene survey to determine the forces involved in thoracic trauma. (p 719)
4-4.41 Value the implications of failing to properly diagnose thoracic trauma. (p 722)
4-4.42 Value the implications of failing to initiate timely interventions to patients with thoracic trauma. (p 720)

Psychomotor

4-4.43 Demonstrate a clinical assessment for a patient with suspected thoracic trauma. (Objective 4-5.11) (p 721)
4-4.44 Demonstrate the following techniques of management for thoracic injuries:
   a. Needle decompression
   b. Fracture stabilization
   c. ECG monitoring
   d. Oxygenation and ventilation
   (Objective 4-5.12) (p 722, 723)

1985 Objectives

There are no 1985 objectives for this chapter.

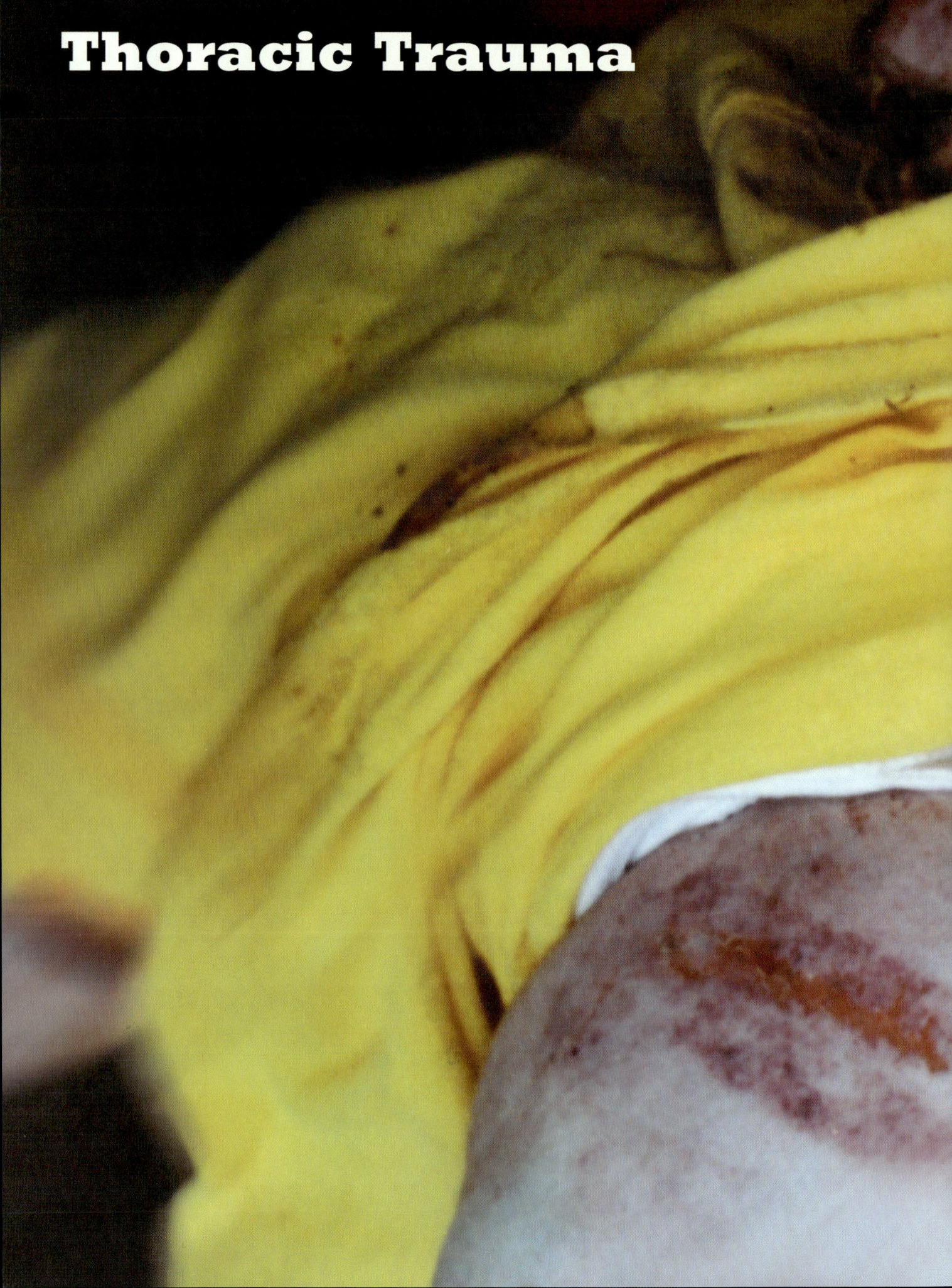
Thoracic Trauma

15

Thoracic Trauma

You are the Provider

You are called to a one-vehicle motor vehicle crash, where a car has hit a tree. On arrival, you find a 42-year-old man clutching the right side of his chest and gasping for air. The patient was unrestrained, and you note serious deformity to the steering wheel.

Many of the organs essential for life itself are found in the thoracic cavity. Injuries to this area of the body are, therefore, challenging to treat. This chapter will provide you with the knowledge you'll need to care for these injuries and will help you answer the following questions:

1. Why is it important to seal open chest wounds as quickly as possible? Stabilize flail segments?
2. What are some of the possible consequences of a blunt injury to the heart? A penetrating injury?

Thoracic Injuries

Thoracic injuries are very common and, given the likelihood of damage to the heart, lungs, or great blood vessels, potentially very serious. Any injury that interferes with normal breathing must be treated without delay to prevent permanent damage to tissues that depend on a continuous supply of oxygen. Another major problem with chest injuries may be internal bleeding. Blood from lacerations of the thoracic organs or major blood vessels can collect in the chest cavity, compressing the lungs. Also, air can collect in the chest and prevent the lungs from expanding. Your ability to act quickly to care for patients with these injuries can make the difference between survival and death. Prevention strategies include gun safety education, sports training, seat belts, and other protective measures.

This chapter begins with a review of the anatomy of the chest and the physiology of respiration. It then describes the common signs and symptoms of thoracic injuries and the proper emergency medical treatment for specific injuries.

Anatomy and Physiology Review of the Thorax

Anatomy

To understand and evaluate chest injuries in the prehospital setting, you must first understand the anatomy of the chest and the mechanism by which gases are exchanged during breathing. A quick review will help

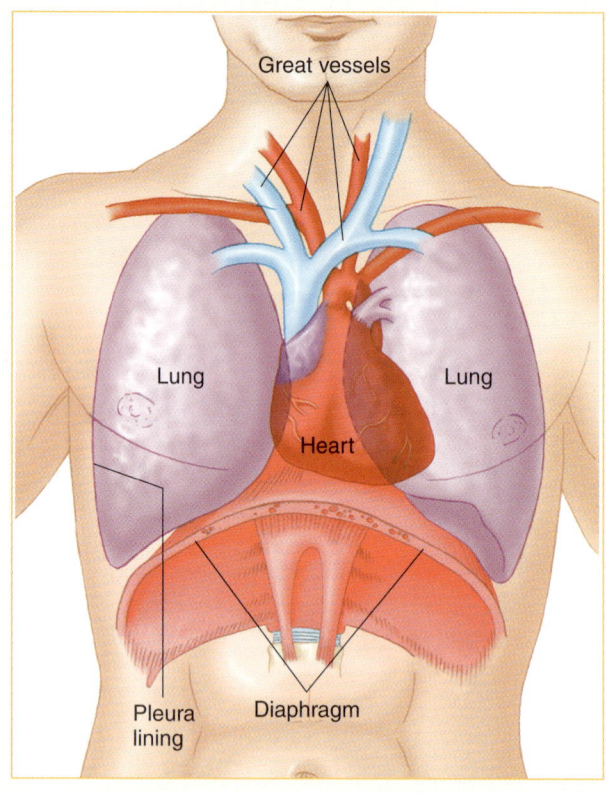

Figure 15-1 A view of the anterior aspect of the thoracic cavity shows the major organs beneath the surface.

you to appreciate the logic in the emergency treatment of chest injuries and the potential complications of that treatment.

The thoracic cavity extends from the lower end of the neck to the diaphragm (Figure 15-1 ▲). In an individual who is lying down or who has just completed exhalation, the diaphragm may rise as high as the nipple line. Thus, a penetrating injury to the chest, such as a gunshot or stab wound, may penetrate the lung and diaphragm and injure the liver or stomach. For this reason, any injury at the nipple line should be considered a thoracic injury and an abdominal injury.

The contents of the thorax are partially protected by the ribs, which are connected in the back to the 12 thoracic vertebrae and in the front, through the costal cartilages, to the sternum (Figure 15-2 ▶). The muscles of the thorax help protect the underlying organs and provide the necessary movement for breathing. The intercostal muscles (located between the ribs) and the diaphragm are the primary muscles of respiration. The sternocleidomastoid muscles that provide support and movement in the neck are accessory muscles of respiration. The trapezius, rhomboids, and latissimus dorsi muscles provide the covering for the framework of the

Technology

- Interactivities
- Vocabulary Explorer
- Anatomy Review
- Web Links
- Online Review Manual

www.EMSzone.com/EMTI

chioles and, finally, terminate in the alveoli. The pulmonary capillaries surround the alveoli, creating an interface for gas exchange. The lungs occupy the entire thoracic cavity except the mediastinum. The lung parenchyma is composed of two lobes on the left and three lobes on the right. It is surrounded by the pleurae. The parietal pleura covers the thoracic wall and superior face of the diaphragm, and the visceral pleura covers the external surface of the lungs. The pleurae produce a pleural or serous fluid that fills the pleural cavity, allowing the lungs to glide easily over the intrathoracic wall during breathing.

The thoracic cage also contains the heart, which is composed of the two upper chambers, or atria, and the two lower chambers, or ventricles. The chambers of the heart are connected by the tricuspid valve on the right and the bicuspid (or mitral) valve on the left. The pericardium is a membranous sac that surrounds the heart and the bases of the great vessels. The aorta exits the left ventricle, immediately branching into the coronary arteries. The right innominate and left subclavian arteries and their branches, the internal thoracic (also known as the mammary) arteries, the carotid arteries, and the anterior and posterior intercostal arteries, branch off of the aorta and provide the thoracic cavity with its blood supply. The superior and inferior venae cavae join together just before entering the right atria. The subclavian veins, internal jugular veins, and others return blood to the venae cavae. The pulmonary arteries transport blood to the lungs from the right ventricle and return it to the left atrium via the pulmonary vein.

The esophagus enters the thorax via the thoracic inlet and travels through the posterior of the chest, exiting through the esophageal foramen through the

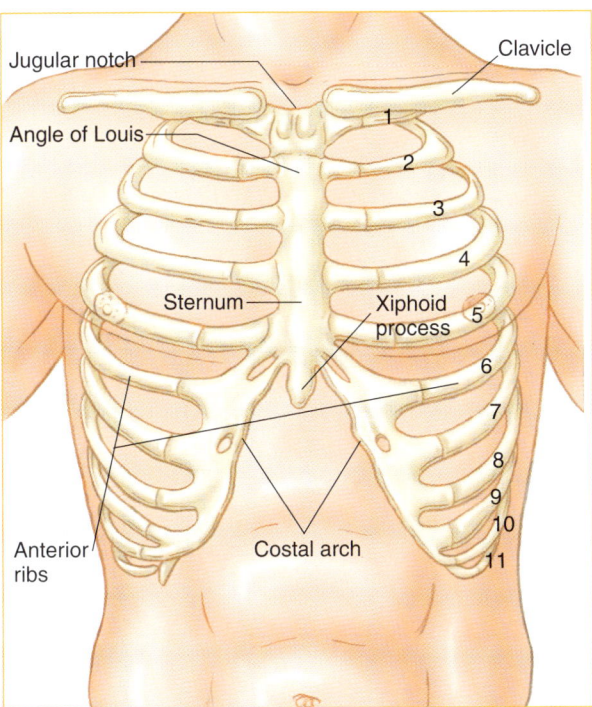

Figure 15-2 The organs within the thoracic cavity are protected by the ribs, which are connected in back by the vertebrae and in the front, through the costal cartilages, to the sternum.

posterior thorax, and the pectoralis major surrounds the rib cage in the front.

The trachea, which is in the middle of the neck, divides at the carina (the last tracheal cartilage) into the left and right mainstem bronchi, which supply air to the lungs. The bronchi divide into the smaller bron-

You are the Provider   Part 2

You approach the patient with your jump kit while your partner checks for other patients. Your patient was the only one involved, and your partner returns to assist you.

Initial Assessment	Recording Time: Zero Minutes
Appearance	In severe pain, pale, diaphoretic
Level of consciousness	Responsive, slightly confused
Airway	Open and clear
Breathing	Shallow, rapid, moderate distress
Circulation	Pale, cool, clammy skin with weak, rapid radial pulses

3. What do you think caused his injury?
4. What is your first consideration in treating this patient?

diaphragm. It connects the pharynx superiorly with the stomach and the abdomen. The diaphragm forms the inferior border of the thoracic cavity and the superior border of the abdominal cavity.

The mediastinum encompasses all of the structures located in the center of the chest, excluding the lungs. This includes the heart, trachea, venae cavae, aorta, and the esophagus.

Physiology

Ventilation occurs through expansion and contraction of the thoracic cage. Through a bellows system, the intercostal muscles between the ribs contract, elevating the rib cage and pulling the sternum forward on inhalation. At the same time, the diaphragm contracts and descends, pushing the contents of the abdomen down. The pressure inside the chest decreases, and air enters the lungs through the nose and mouth. On exhalation, the intercostal muscles and diaphragm relax, and the tissues move back to their normal positions. Because of their elasticity, the lungs assume the smallest size possible at any given time, allowing air to be exhaled. Use of the accessory muscles may be noted if the patient is dyspneic. The sternocleidomastoid muscles of the neck may be prominent, along with intercostal, supraclavicular, and subclavicular retractions. Air enters and leaves the lungs due to the changes in intrathoracic pressure.

Note that the nerves supplying the diaphragm (the phrenic nerves) exit the spinal cord at C3, C4, and C5. A patient whose spinal cord is injured at the C5 level or below may lose the power to move his or her intercostal muscles, but the diaphragm will still contract. The patient will still be able to breathe because the phrenic nerves remain intact. Patients with spinal cord injuries at C3 or above can completely lose their ability to breathe spontaneously (Figure 15-3 ▶).

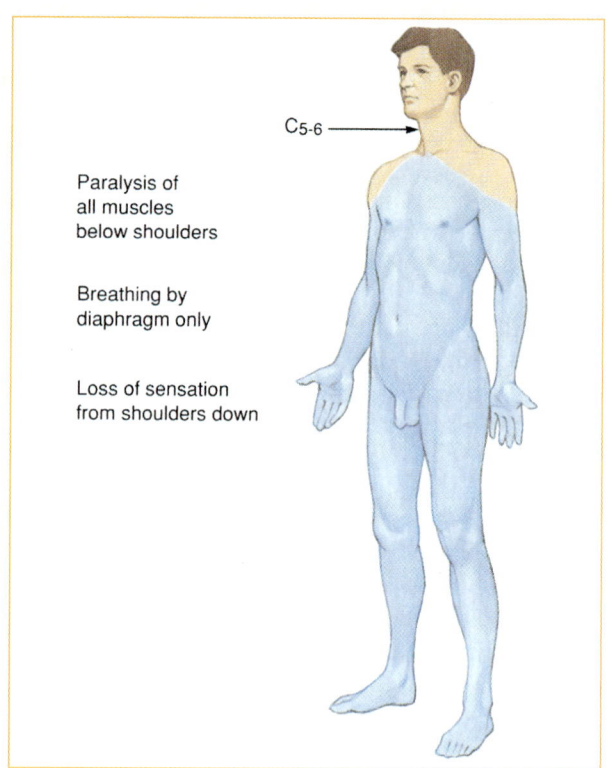

Figure 15-3 A patient who sustains a spinal cord injury at the level of C5 or below and is paralyzed can still breathe spontaneously because the phrenic nerves (which control the diaphragm) originate at the C3, C4, and C5 levels.

Even though the respiratory centers in the pons and medulla have a major role in regulating breathing, chemical changes are among the most important factors that influence the rate and depth of breathing. These include changing levels of carbon dioxide (CO_2), oxygen (O_2), and hydrogen ions in arterial blood. In respiratory physiology, <u>chemoreceptors</u> are sensors that respond to such chemical fluctuations and are located in two major body locations. Central chemoreceptors are found in the medulla, and peripheral chemoreceptors are located in the carotid and aortic bodies.

Inspired air enters the lungs and fills the alveoli that are surrounded by a network of capillaries transporting deoxygenated blood and waste products from the body. Through diffusion, CO_2 molecules move from the capillaries into the alveoli, and O_2 moves from the alveoli into the capillaries. The CO_2 is exhaled, while the O_2 is returned to the left atrium of the heart via the pulmonary vein. The oxygenated blood is then circulated throughout the body. Diffusion occurs in the opposite direction at the cellular level. Oxygen moves into the cells, while CO_2 moves into the capillaries. Chemoreceptors closely monitor changes in CO_2 levels and stimulate breathing accordingly.

Because peripheral chemoreceptors are only weakly responsive to changing levels of CO_2, rising levels are mediated mainly through influence on the central chemoreceptors of the brain stem. Carbon dioxide diffuses from the blood into the cerebrospinal fluid where it is hydrated and forms carbonic acid. It then dissociates, freeing hydrogen and decreasing the pH of the cerebrospinal fluid. This excites the central chemoreceptors to increase the rate and depth of respirations.

$$\uparrow CO_2 + H_2O = \uparrow H_2CO_3 = \uparrow H^+ + HCO_3^-$$

(Increased carbon dioxide combines with water to make carbonic acid. Carbonic acid is weak and easily dissociates, liberating hydrogen ions and decreasing the pH of the cerebrospinal fluid.)

Even though the increase in CO_2 is the initial stimulus, it is the rising hydrogen ion levels that incite the central chemoreceptors into action in an attempt to maintain homeostasis by regulating hydrogen ion concentrations in the brain.

Respiratory alkalosis is the result of hyperventilation, regardless of the cause. As CO_2 levels fall, there is a reduction in circulating carbonic acid. Treatment for the classic hyperventilation syndrome focuses on restoring the normal respiratory rate to increase levels of carbon dioxide. If the hyperventilation is caused by a serious medical condition, reducing the respiratory rate may seriously aggravate the problem.

$$\uparrow \text{Breathing} = \downarrow CO_2 = \downarrow H_2CO_3 = \uparrow pH$$

Respiratory acidosis is always related to hypoventilation. Chest trauma is a common cause of respiratory acidosis. A buildup of CO_2 and an inability of the respiratory system to excrete it causes the body to rely on the much slower renal system for compensation. This is a serious, life-threatening condition. The acidosis that results is quick, overwhelming, and usually fatal, making it impossible for the slower-acting renal system to compensate in time for the pH shift.

$$\downarrow \text{Breathing} = \uparrow CO_2 = \uparrow H_2CO_3 = \downarrow pH$$

Changes in arterial pH can modify respiratory rate and depth even when CO_2 and O_2 levels are normal. This occurs in metabolic imbalances. Because few hydrogen ions diffuse from the blood into the cerebrospinal fluid, there is little effect on central chemoreceptors. Ventilation changes occur in response to changes in pH detected by the peripheral chemoreceptors. A decrease in blood pH may be the result of CO_2 retention or a metabolic cause such as an increase in lactic acid. As the arterial pH falls, the respiratory system compensates by increasing the rate and depth of respirations in an attempt to eliminate CO_2 and, in turn, raise the pH level. The reverse occurs in metabolic alkalosis in which the respiratory rate and depth decrease in an attempt to retain CO_2 and lower pH levels.

Injuries of the Chest

There are two mechanisms of injury in thoracic trauma: blunt and penetrating. A thorough scene size-up will help you determine the forces involved. There are also two basic injury patterns of chest injuries as well: open and closed. As the name implies, a closed chest injury is one in which the skin overlying the injury remains intact. This type of injury is generally caused by blunt trauma, such as when a driver strikes a steering wheel in a motor vehicle crash or is struck by a falling object Figure 15-4. The force is distributed over a large area. Visceral injuries occur from deceleration, shearing forces, compression, or rupture. In an open chest injury, the chest wall itself is penetrated by some object, such as a knife, a bullet, or a piece of metal Figure 15-5. Penetrating injuries

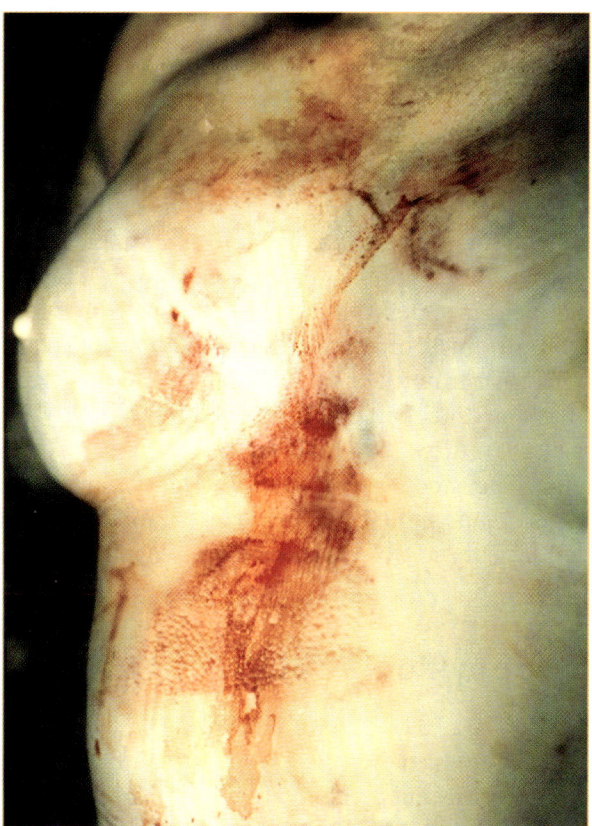

Figure 15-4 Closed injuries usually result from blunt trauma, such as when a patient strikes the steering wheel in a motor vehicle crash or is struck by a falling object.

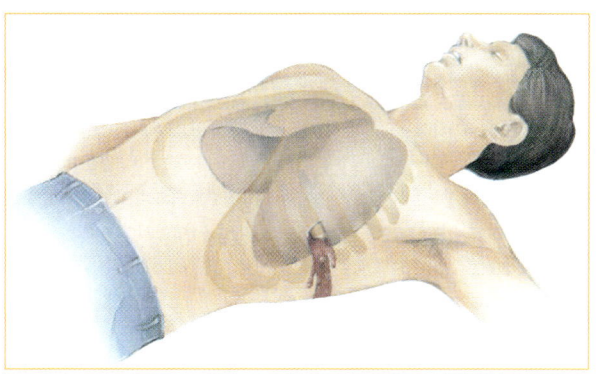

Figure 15-5 Open injuries occur when the chest wall is penetrated by some type of object.

distribute the forces of injury over a smaller area; however, the trajectory of a bullet is often unpredictable and all thoracic structures are at risk.

In blunt trauma, a blow to the chest may fracture the ribs, the sternum, or whole areas of the chest wall; bruise the lungs and the heart; and even damage the aorta. Almost one third of people who are killed immediately in car crashes die as a result of traumatic rupture of the aorta. Although the skin and chest wall are not penetrated in a closed injury, broken ribs may lacerate the intrathoracic organs. Indeed, vital organs can actually be torn from their attachment in the chest cavity without any break in the skin.

Blast injuries may be classified as blunt or penetrating. The shock wave during the primary blast compresses organs similar to blunt trauma, and, during the secondary phase, objects may be thrown and penetrate the body.

Pathophysiology of Thoracic Trauma

Thoracic trauma may impair cardiac output, decreasing blood pressure and perfusion to vital organs. Considering the contents, any injury to the chest has the potential to be lethal. Trauma may be blunt or penetrating and may result in blood loss, pressure changes, vital organ damage, or any combination thereof. Bleeding into the thoracic cavity significantly increases the chance of hypovolemia and hypoxia. Increased intrapleural pressures not only decrease lung volume and oxygenation, but also impair the heart's ability to pump effectively. Blood in the pericardial sac compresses the heart, eventually stopping it altogether. Myocardial valve damage from trauma to the heart can disrupt ventricular filling, allowing for backflow into the atria and further decreasing cardiac output. Vascular disruption may also occur as the result of blunt or penetrating trauma. A rupture of a major vessel can lead to fatal blood loss, and even a small tear or blockage can cause lack of oxygenation and tissue ischemia. A good understanding of underlying structures increases your assessment abilities and may increase the patient's chance of survival.

Aside from massive blood loss, impairments in ventilatory efficiency may also be rapidly fatal. Any injury that compromises the chest bellows action decreases air exchange and subsequent oxygenation. A patient experiencing severe chest pain tends to breathe shallowly in an attempt to decrease the discomfort created by movement. Air entering the pleural space as the result of open or closed pneumothorax, tracheal tear, or other damage compresses the lungs and decreases tidal volume. This also occurs as blood collects in the thoracic cavity and prevents full expansion of the lungs. Paradoxical motion resulting from interruption of the structural integrity of the rib cage lessens pressure changes and, therefore, air exchange. Ineffective diaphragmatic contraction can have the same effect as a flail segment. Because of minimal pressure changes, there is less movement of air in the process of equalizing, which further decreases the amount of oxygen available for gas exchange.

You are the Provider — Part 3

You ask other EMS personnel at the scene to bring the immobilization equipment. Your partner controls the cervical spine while you further assess the patient.

Vital Signs	Recording Time: 2 Minutes After Patient Contact
Respirations	32 breaths/min and shallow
Pulse	134 beats/min; regular, weak radial pulses
Skin	Pale, cool, diaphoretic; capillary refill time = 2.5 seconds
Blood pressure	104/72 mm Hg
Presentation	Contusion over the right lower chest and right upper quadrant of the abdomen. You feel crepitus, but no paradoxical motion is noted.

5. What is your next step in the management of this patient?
6. What type of oxygen-delivery device will you use? What flow rate?

Other complications are also capable of impairing gas exchange. Atelectasis significantly reduces the surface area available for gas exchange. The more alveoli that are damaged, the less gas exchange occurs. Contused lung tissue may produce marked hypoxemia as fluid accumulates and impairs gas exchange. Disruption of the respiratory tract occurring from rupture or tearing of any of the respiratory structures prevents oxygen from reaching the alveoli, further impairing gas exchange.

Assessment Findings

Important signs and symptoms of chest injury include the following:

- Pain at the site of injury
- Pain localized at the site of injury that is aggravated by or increased with breathing
- Dyspnea (difficulty breathing, shortness of breath)
- Hemoptysis (coughing up blood)
- Failure of one or both sides of the chest to expand normally with inspiration (asymmetric movement)
- Rapid, weak pulse and low blood pressure
- Cyanosis around the lips or fingernail beds

After a chest injury, any change in normal breathing is a particularly important sign. A healthy, uninjured adult usually breathes from 12 to 20 times per minute without difficulty and without pain. Respirations of fewer than 12 per minute or more than 20 per minute may indicate inadequate breathing, especially with poor tidal volume. Patients with chest injuries often have tachypnea (rapid respirations) and shallow respirations because it hurts to take a deep breath. They may also present with bradypnea (slow respirations) and labored respirations. Look for retractions around the ribs, neck, and clavicles, along with other evidence of respiratory distress.

As with any other injury, pain and tenderness are common at the point of impact as a result of a bruise or fracture. The normal process of breathing usually aggravates pain. Irritation of or damage to the pleural surfaces causes a characteristic sharp or stabbing pain with each breath when these normally smooth surfaces slide on one another. This sharp pain is called *pleuritic pain* or *pleurisy*.

In an injured patient, dyspnea (difficulty breathing) has many causes, including airway obstruction, damage to the chest wall, improper chest expansion due to the loss of normal control of breathing, or lung compression because of accumulated blood or air. Dyspnea in an injured patient indicates significant compromise of lung function; therefore, prompt, vigorous support and transport are required. Loss of muscle function may be the result of a direct injury to the chest wall, or it may be related to an injury of the nerves that control those muscles. Check also for paradoxical motion, an abnormality associated with multiple fractured ribs in which one segment of the chest wall moves opposite the remainder of the chest, for example, one part moves out with expiration and in with inspiration.

The presence or absence of a pulse in a particular location varies according to the nature and extent of injury. A rapid, weak pulse and hypotension are the principal signs of hypovolemic shock, which can result from extensive bleeding from lacerated structures within the chest cavity. Shock following a chest injury may also result from insufficient oxygenation of the blood by the poorly functioning lungs. An absence of radial pulses may indicate severe hypotension. Tachycardia may be indicative of compensatory shock or hypoxemia. Bradycardia is generally an ominous sign. It may be the result of spinal damage or the final stage of shock in which the body is no longer able to compensate.

Changes in blood pressure also vary with the nature and extent of injury. Hypertension may be the result of increased sympathetic discharge whereas hypotension is a sign of hypovolemia, relative hypovolemia (massive vasodilation), or late shock. Increased pressure on the myocardium decreases filling, resulting in a narrowed pulse pressure. Loss of the peripheral pulse during inspiration suggests pulsus paradoxus (the systolic blood pressure drops more than 10 mm Hg during inspiration compared with expiration) and the presence of cardiac tamponade. The patient may also present with hypothermia secondary to neurogenic shock if the injury involved the spinal cord.

Diaphoresis and pallor accompany peripheral vasoconstriction resulting from the sympathetic response of the autonomic nervous system to the injury. Cyanosis in a patient with a chest injury is a sign of inadequate respiration. The classic blue appearance around the lips and fingernail beds indicates that blood is not being oxygenated sufficiently. Patients with cyanosis are unable to provide a sufficient supply of oxygen to the blood through the lungs and require immediate respiratory support and high-flow supplemental oxygen. While assessing the skin, look for open wounds, ecchymosis, and other evidence of trauma.

Hemoptysis, the spitting or coughing up of blood, usually indicates that the lung parenchyma itself or the air passages leading to the lungs have been damaged. With a laceration of the lung, blood can enter the bronchial passages and is coughed up as the patient tries to clear the airway. Examine the neck for the presence of penetrating wounds, jugular venous distention, and the position of the trachea. Palpate and note the presence of any subcutaneous emphysema.

Examine the chest for blunt or penetrating trauma, impaled objects, open wounds, contusions, asymmetry, or paradoxical motion. Palpate for tenderness or crepitation. Auscultate for breath sounds, noting their location. Determine whether they are they absent or decreased in any area. Note whether the breath sounds are clear bilaterally or weak or absent on one side. Are bowel sounds heard in the lower hemithorax? If so, this could indicate possible diaphragmatic rupture. After auscultation, percuss the chest and note any abnormal findings. Hyperresonance may indicate the presence of air in the pleural space, whereas hyporesonance (dull percussion) may be due to the presence of blood in the pleural space. Determine whether heart tones are clear or muffled (indicating a possible cardiac tamponade) or whether there is a murmur indicating regurgitation (a sign of myocardial valve damage). Assess a shift of the apical pulse, which may indicate the heart has been displaced due to the trauma. Also note the presence of a scaphoid (hollow, boat-shaped) abdomen that would indicate the abdominal contents have shifted upward into the thoracic cavity as a result of a ruptured diaphragm.

Pay close attention to any changes in mental status. A decrease in level of consciousness may indicate worsening of the condition or increasing hypoxia. Obtain a history if the patient's mental status permits and include the following when applicable:

- Dyspnea
- Chest pain
- Associated symptoms
  - Other areas of pain or discomfort
  - Symptoms before the incident
- History of cardiorespiratory disease
- Use of restraint in motor vehicle crash

Apply the cardiac monitor and note the presence of any ST-segment elevation or depression, conduction disturbances, or dysrhythmias.

Many of these signs and symptoms occur simultaneously. When any one of them develops as a result of a chest injury, the patient requires prompt hospital care. Remember that the principal reason for concern about a patient who has a chest injury is that his or her body has no means of storing oxygen; it is supplied and used continuously, even during sleep. Any interruption in this supply can be rapidly lethal and must be treated aggressively.

Management

ABCs are primary management for any patient. Thoracic trauma is no exception. Evaluate the patient's airway and respiratory status while maintaining cervical spine control. Even if the patient is alert and oriented with no apparent distress, consider the mechanism of

---

You are the Provider — Part 4

You provide ventilatory assistance with a bag-valve-mask device and 100% oxygen. Your partner and the fire department assist in immobilizing the patient on a long backboard. Your partner has taken over ventilations and tells you the mental status of the patient is deteriorating.

Reassessment	Recording Time: 5 Minutes After Patient Contact
Level of consciousness	Voice responsive
Pulse	Very weak, rapid radial pulses
Skin	Increasing pallor and diaphoresis
Blood pressure	96/54 mm Hg
Other findings	Abdomen is slightly distended

7. Once the patient is loaded into the ambulance, what is the next step in treatment?
8. What condition do the vital signs and distended abdomen point to?
9. At what rate will you run intravenous (IV) fluids? Why?

injury and any area of complaint and treat aggressively with oxygen. Occlude any open wounds of the chest, and stabilize any flail segments. Use positive-pressure ventilation if indicated, and consider early definitive airway management.

Maintain circulation and gain IV access. Establish at least one large bore IV catheter, preferably two, and give a 20-mL/kg bolus of an isotonic crystalloid solution to maintain adequate perfusion. Always follow local protocols. Call for additional advanced life support, if available, in a timely manner if there is any suspicion of or impending cardiac arrest or a potential need for chest decompression. In-hospital management may include tube thoracostomy for a hemothorax or pericardiocentesis for cardiac tamponade. Early recognition of signs and symptoms and early transport drastically increases the chance of survival. Provide rapid transport to the closest, most appropriate facility, and offer reassurance en route.

In the Field

Remember that increasing the blood pressure may increase bleeding, causing a more rapid deterioration of the patient's condition. Adjust IV fluid rates to maintain perfusion without significantly raising the blood pressure.

Consider early endotracheal intubation. Manage any cardiac dysrhythmias, and give antiarrhythmics according to advanced cardiac life support (ACLS) and local protocols. Provide analgesics for pain according to local protocol. If the patient presents with signs of increasing pleural tension, obtain orders from medical control, and perform a needle thoracostomy on the affected side.

Chest Wall Injuries

Rib Fractures

Rib fractures are infrequent in children because of the pliability of their thoracic cage. Rib fractures occur most often in elderly patients who have lost pliability and whose bones may be very brittle (for example, because of osteoporosis). Because the upper four ribs are well protected by the bony girdle of the clavicle and scapula, a fracture of one of these upper ribs is a sign of a very severe mechanism of injury. A significant force is required to cause fractures and may be indicative of other injuries. The morbidity and mortality rates increase with age, number of fractures, and location of the fractures.

Be aware that a fractured rib may lacerate the surface of the lung, causing a pneumothorax, tension pneumothorax, hemothorax, or hemopneumothorax. One sign of this development can be a "crackly" feeling to the skin in the area (also called *subcutaneous emphysema*), which indicates that air escaping from a lacerated lung is leaking into the subcutaneous layer of the chest wall. Be sure to relay this finding to hospital personnel.

Rib fractures are most often caused by blunt trauma, with the fracture occurring at midshaft owing to the bowing effect of the ribs. Ribs four through nine are the most often fractured because they are thinner and poorly protected. The patient will usually present using an arm to splint the injury and with shallow respirations to decrease chest movement, thereby decreasing pain. Unfortunately, decreasing chest excursion also decreases tidal volume, minute volume, and the amount of oxygen available for gas exchange. Atelectasis, or collapse of the alveoli, due to trauma also decreases the surface area for gas exchange. The result is a ventilation/perfusion mismatch. The circulatory system is intact, but the amount of oxygen available for exchange has been greatly diminished. The mismatch may occur when inadequate perfusion is the culprit as well. An underlying pulmonary or cardiac contusion or an intercostal vessel injury may hinder perfusion, leading to hypoxemia that is just as severe.

When the first and second ribs are injured by severe trauma, the result may be a ruptured aorta, tracheobronchial tree injury, or vascular injury. The left lower rib may contribute to injury associated with splenic injury, and the right lower rib may result in hepatic injury. Multiple rib fractures may lead to diffuse atelectasis, hypoventilation, inadequate cough, and pneumonia. When there is an open rib fracture, the viscera are at risk for injury. With a posterior fracture, the fifth through the ninth ribs are the most frequently injured. Owing to their location in the thorax, lower rib fractures are associated with spleen and kidney injuries. The floating ribs, because they are well protected by the strong abdominal musculature, are rarely fractured; therefore, injury to these ribs suggests a severe mechanism of injury and a strong potential for other life-threatening injuries.

Regardless of the position, any rib fracture puts the patient at risk for multiple injuries. It is imperative to understand what underlying structures may be affected by trauma and to maintain a high index of suspicion, even if the patient appears to have no visible injury.

Assessment Findings

Patients with one or more fractured ribs will report localized tenderness and pain on breathing, typically during inspiration. This pain is the result of broken ends of the fracture rubbing against each other with each inspiration and expiration, deep breathing, and/or coughing. Patients will tend to avoid taking deep breaths, breathing rapidly and shallowly instead. They will often hold the affected portion of the rib cage in an effort to minimize the discomfort. On palpation, the patient may present with point tenderness over the site, crepitus or an audible crunch, and pain when anteroposterior pressure is applied.

Flail Chest

The most common cause of a flail segment is a vehicular crash. It may also be the result of falls from significant heights, industrial accidents, or assault. Significant chest trauma is required to cause a flail chest. Mortality rates increase 20% to 40% owing to associated injuries. Mortality also increases with advanced age, seven or more fractured ribs, three or more associated injuries, shock, and head injuries.

Ribs may be fractured in more than one place. If three or more ribs are fractured in two or more places or if the sternum is fractured along with several ribs, a segment of the chest wall may be detached from the rest of the thoracic cage, producing a free-floating segment Figure 15-6 ▶ . This condition is known as flail chest. In what is called paradoxical motion, the detached portion of the chest wall moves opposite of normal: in instead of out during inhalation, out instead of in during expiration. This occurs because of negative pressure that has built up in the thorax. Breathing with a flail chest can be extremely painful and often does not allow for adequate oxygenation. Paradoxical motion is usually minimal because of muscle spasm and must be extensive to actually compromise ventilation. Respiratory failure in a patient with a flail chest is generally due to an underlying pulmonary contusion, associated intrathoracic injury, or inadequate bellows action of the chest, resulting in a reduction in tidal volume. Pain also reduces thoracic expansion and decreases ventilation. The patient breathes as shallowly as possible to decrease movement of the thorax and, therefore, decrease pain.

A pulmonary contusion resulting from a flail segment may create a decrease in lung compliance. It may also

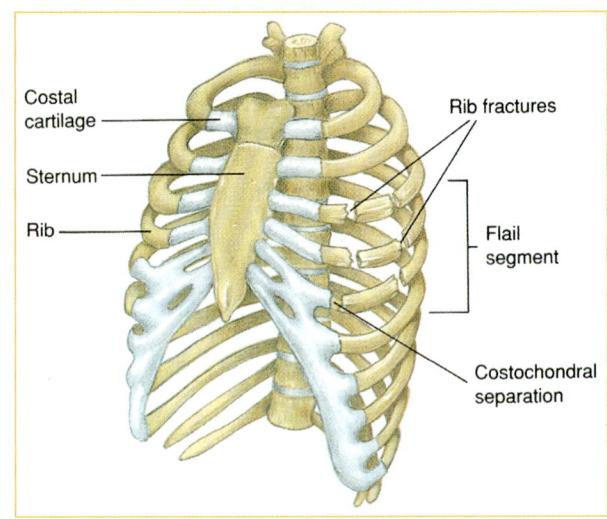

Figure 15-6 When three or more adjacent ribs are fractured in two or more places, a flail chest results. A flail segment will move paradoxically when the patient breathes.

produce an intra-alveolar–capillary or alveolar hemorrhage. Either way, gas exchange is impaired, leading to hypoxia and hypercapnia. Impaired gas exchange also results from decreased ventilation and impaired venous return with a resultant ventilation/perfusion mismatch.

Assessment Findings

Expose and examine the chest for DCAP-BTLS (**D**eformities, **C**ontusions, **A**brasions, **P**unctures/Penetrations/Paradoxical Movement, **B**urns, **T**enderness, **L**acerations, and **S**welling). Look for any chest wall contusions, signs of respiratory distress and accessory muscle use, and any paradoxical motion. The patient may also present with pleuritic chest pain, as well as pain and splinting of the affected side. Note any areas of crepitus on palpation of the thorax. Tachypnea and tachycardia may also be present and are signs of inadequate oxygenation.

Monitor the electrocardiogram, and be alert for cardiac dysrhythmias.

The patient may find it easier and less painful to breathe if the flail segment is immobilized. You can tape a bulky pad against that segment of the chest for this purpose, although taping too tightly will also prevent adequate ventilation Figure 15-7 ▶ . Never apply a bandage around the entire circumference of the chest. Avoid the use of sandbags or other heavy items, because these will decrease tidal volume. Keep in mind that while flail chest is itself a serious condition, it suggests force that

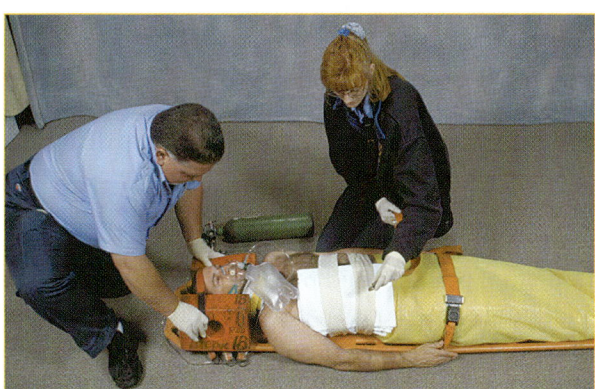

Figure 15-7 A flail anterior chest wall segment can be stabilized by securing (or having the patient hold) a pillow firmly against the chest wall. Never tape circumferentially or so tight that breathing is restricted.

was significant enough to also cause other serious internal damage.

Sternal Fracture

Sternal fracture occurs in 5% to 8% of patients experiencing blunt chest trauma. Deceleration compression of the sternum occurs as the patient strikes the steering wheel or dashboard. A blow significant enough to fracture the sternum causes severe hyperflexion of the thoracic cage. Fractures usually occur at or below the manubriosternal junction. There is a 25% to 45% mortality rate associated with sternal fracture and a high association with myocardial or lung injury. Myocardial and/or pulmonary contusion or myocardial rupture may occur with compression of the thorax.

Morbidity and mortality are generally the result of associated injuries. Enough force to fracture the sternum may also result in pulmonary and myocardial contusions, flail chest, vascular disruption of thoracic vessels, intra-abdominal injuries, and head injuries. It is rare for the fracture to be displaced posteriorly and directly impinge on the heart or vessels.

Assessment Findings

Expect to find localized pain and tenderness over the sternum, along with crepitus on palpation. The patient's clinical presentation or mechanism of injury should point to a history of blunt trauma to the chest. Tachypnea is a common finding, and there may be electrocardiographic (ECG) changes associated with a myocardial contusion.

Injury to the Lung

Simple Pneumothorax

In any chest injury, damage to the heart, lungs, great vessels, and other organs in the thorax can be complicated by the accumulation of air in the pleural space. This is a dangerous condition called a pneumothorax. In this condition, air enters through a hole in the chest wall or the surface of the lung as the patient attempts to breathe, causing the lung on that side to collapse Figure 15-8 ▼ as pressure continues to build in the pleural space. As a result, any blood that passes through the lung is not oxygenated, and hypoxia develops. Depending on the size of the hole and the rate at which air fills the cavity, the lung may collapse in a few seconds or a few hours.

Some individuals are born with or develop weak areas on the surface of the lungs. Occasionally, such a weak area will rupture spontaneously, allowing air to leak into the pleural space. Usually, this event, called spontaneous pneumothorax, is not related to trauma, but simply happens with normal breathing. The patient experiences sudden, sharp chest pain and increasing difficulty breathing. The affected lung collapses, losing its ability to expand normally. The amount of pneumothorax that develops varies, as does the amount of respiratory distress the patient experiences. You should suspect a spontaneous pneumothorax in a patient who experiences sudden sharp chest pain and shortness of breath without a specific known cause. Young males who are tall and thin seem to be at an increased risk for

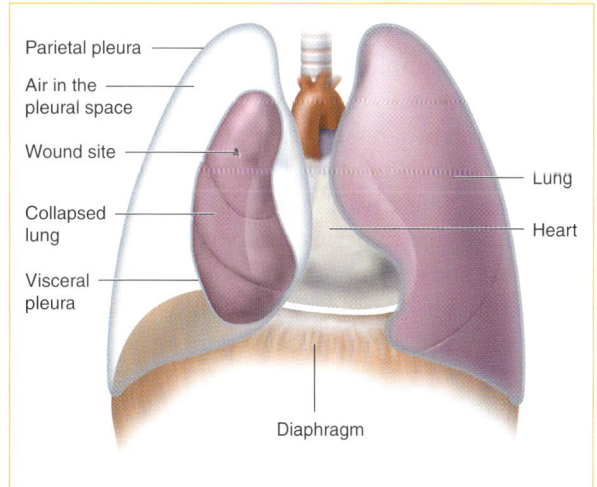

Figure 15-8 Pneumothorax occurs when air leaks into the space between the pleural surfaces from an opening in the chest wall or the surface of the lung. The lung collapses as air fills the pleural space.

a spontaneous pneumothorax, especially if they have recently engaged in air travel.

There is a 10% to 30% incidence of pneumothorax in blunt chest trauma and an almost 100% incidence with penetrating chest trauma. The extent of atelectasis and associated injuries dictate the rate of morbidity and mortality.

The lungs are situated in the thoracic cavity in such a manner that at any point they are only 1 to 3 cm away from the chest wall. In a simple pneumothorax, there may only be a small accumulation of air and pulmonary function may remain adequate. The internal wound allows air to enter the pleural space. Small tears may seal themselves, and the patient may experience only minor discomfort. However, larger tears may progress. A patient who takes a deep breath just before blunt trauma to the chest may experience what is known as the paper bag syndrome or paper bag effect. On impact, the lungs rupture in a manner similar to what happens when you blow up a paper bag and pop it with your hand.

If the patient is standing, air will accumulate in the apices. You should auscultate here first for diminished breath sounds. If the patient is supine, air accumulates in the anterior portion of the chest. As air accumulates, it forces the structures of the mediastinum toward the opposite side of the chest, dragging the trachea along. Although you may note the trachea tugging away from the affected side, tracheal deviation is a very late sign and is not seen in most cases. Compression of the lungs, myocardium, and great vessels cause a ventilation/perfusion mismatch because air is unable to enter the lungs and blood is unable to circulate.

Assessment Findings

Patients with a simple pneumothorax may present with tachypnea and tachycardia as a result of hypoxia. As their condition progresses, respiratory distress increases and breath sounds may be decreased or absent on the affected side. Chest wall movement decreases as pressure increases, and hyperresonance can be detected with percussion. The patient may also complain of dyspnea, chest pain that is referred to the shoulder or arm on the affected side, and pleuritic chest pain.

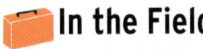
In the Field

Percussion of the chest produces hyperresonance when the thorax is full of air and hyporesonance, or dullness, when it is full of blood.

Open Pneumothorax

An open pneumothorax occurs with penetrating trauma to the chest. Profound hypoventilation could result, and death may occur quickly if management is delayed.

An open injury in the chest wall allows for communication between the pleural space and the atmosphere. This opening prevents development of negative intrapleural pressure and produces collapse of the ipsilateral lung. The increased thoracic pressure results in an inability to ventilate the affected lung. There is a ventilation/perfusion mismatch as blood is shunted to the unaffected side, hypoventilation results from the increased pressure, hypoxia occurs as less oxygen is available for gas exchange, and a large functional dead space is created.

> **A to Z Terminology Tips**
>
> Knowledge of prefixes is the key to understanding new terminology. The root word *lateral* means pertaining to a side. By adding prefixes, we can distinguish the particular side to which we are referring.
> Bi = two: bilateral = on both sides
> Uni = one: unilateral = on one side
> Ipsi = same: ipsilateral = on the same side
> Contra = opposite: contralateral = on the opposite side

Air enters the pleural space during the inspiratory phase. Negative pressure draws air into the lungs and through the opening in the chest wall. Air may exit during the exhalation phase or may remain trapped in the pleural space. Resistance to air flow through the respiratory tract may be greater than through the open wound, resulting in an ineffective respiratory effort. A one-way flap valve may let air in but not out, resulting in a buildup of pressure in the pleural space. Direct lung injury may be present if the lung parenchyma was penetrated. The vena cava may become kinked from swaying of the mediastinum as pressure builds, resulting in decreased preload and subsequently decreasing cardiac output.

Assessment Findings

The presence of a defect in the chest wall or penetrating injury that does not heal itself should be noted as the patient is exposed. To-and-fro air motion may be

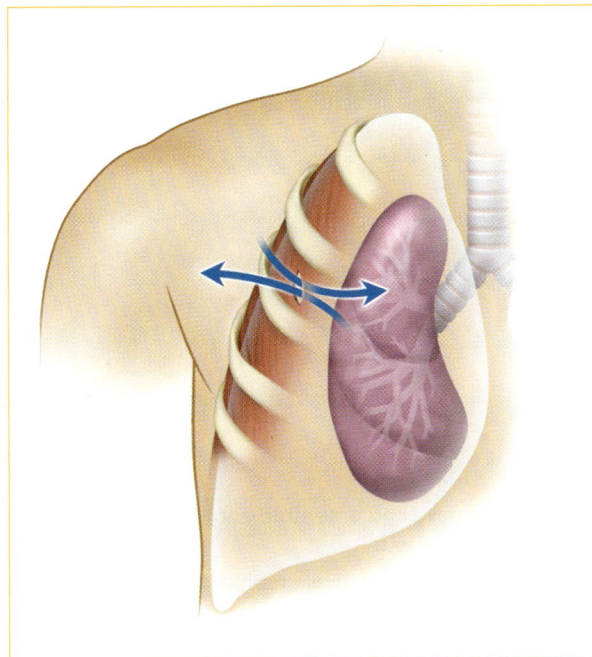

Figure 15-9 With a sucking chest wound, air passes from the outside into the pleural space and back out with each breath, creating the sucking sound.

detected out of the defect as the patient inhales and exhales. A sucking sound may be heard on inhalation as air is drawn into the thoracic cavity through the opening in the chest wall. For this reason, an open or penetrating wound to the chest wall is often called a sucking chest wound (Figure 15-9 ▲). Tachycardia and tachypnea increase in relation to the respiratory distress as intrathoracic pressure increases and oxygenation decreases. Subcutaneous emphysema may also be found, along with decreased breath sounds on the affected side.

Tension Pneumothorax

A tension pneumothorax may be the result of blunt or penetrating trauma and is an immediate life-threatening chest injury. Profound hypoventilation could result if treatment is not initiated quickly, and delayed management may rapidly result in death.

A defect in the airway allows for communication with the pleural space. This defect may be the result of blunt trauma in which a lung is penetrated by a fractured rib, a sudden increase in intrapulmonary pressure culminating in rupture of pulmonary structures, or bronchial disruption from shearing forces, allowing air to enter the pleural space and raise intrathoracic pressure. The pressure increase causes the lung to collapse on the affected side and the mediastinum to shift to the contralateral side. The lung collapse leads to right-to-left intrapulmonary shunting and hypoxia. There is an ensuing reduction in cardiac output as the increased intrathoracic pressure causes compression of the heart and vena cava, reducing preload by decreasing venous return to the heart.

Assessment Findings

Assessment findings in a patient experiencing a pneumothorax that is developing tension include the following:

- Unilaterally decreased or absent breath sounds
- Dyspnea
- Tachypnea
- Respiratory distress
- Extreme anxiety
- Cyanosis
- Bulging of the intercostal muscles
- Tachycardia
- Hypotension
- Narrowed pulse pressure
- Subcutaneous emphysema
- Jugular venous distention
- Tracheal deviation
- Hyperresonance

Remember that tracheal deviation is a late sign and should not be used as the determining factor for initiating invasive treatment.

Management

Decompression of a tension pneumothorax, or needle decompression, can be performed as described below (Skill Drill 15-1 ▶).

1. **Assess the patient** to ensure that the presentation is due to a tension pneumothorax (**Step 1**):
   - Difficult ventilation despite an open airway
   - Jugular venous distention (may not be present with associated hemorrhage)
   - Absent or decreased breath sounds on the affected side
   - Hyperresonance to percussion on the affected side
   - Tracheal deviation away from the affected side (remember that this a late sign and may not be present)

Decompression of a Tension Pneumothorax

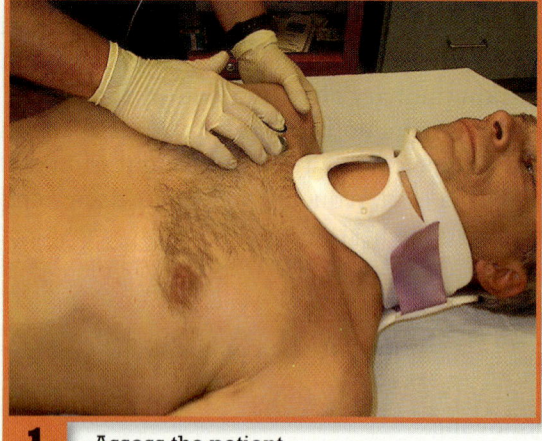
1. Assess the patient.

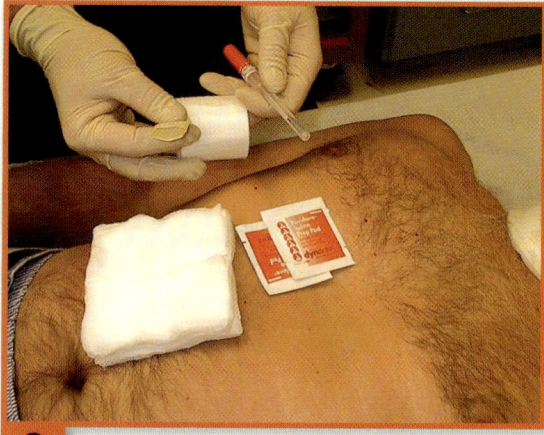
2. Prepare and assemble necessary equipment.
Obtain orders from medical control.

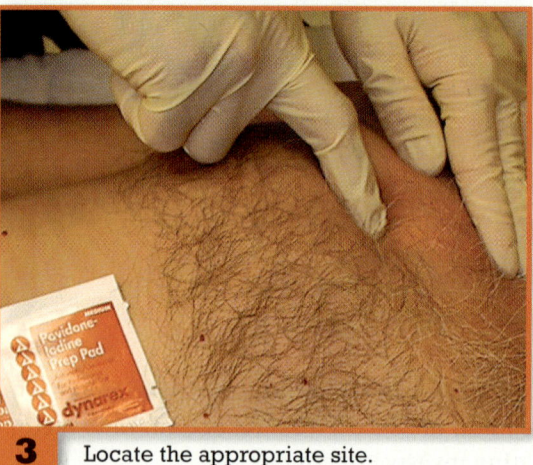
3. Locate the appropriate site.

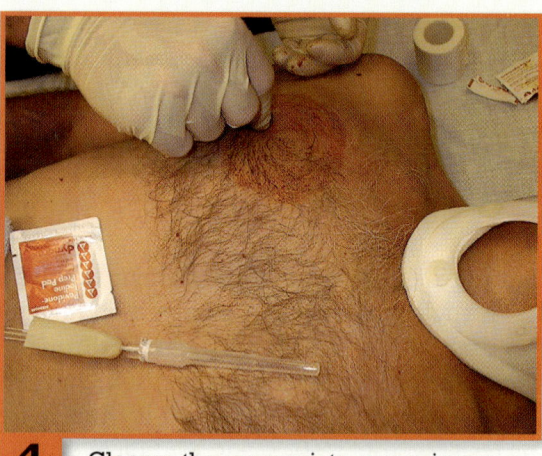
4. Cleanse the appropriate area using an aseptic technique.

2. **Prepare and assemble necessary equipment** (**Step 2**):
   - Large bore IV catheter, preferably 10- to 14-gauge at least 2 inches long
   - Alcohol or Betadine (povidone iodine) preps
   - Cut off one finger of a glove to use as a substitute if you do not have a commercial device or condom available.
   - Adhesive tape
3. **Obtain orders** from medical control.
4. **Locate the appropriate site** (Figure 15-10 ▶) (**Step 3**). Find the second or third intercostal space in the midclavicular line on the affected side. If there is significant trauma to the anterior portion of the chest, the fourth or fifth intercostal space in the midaxillary line on the affected side is preferable. However, the midclavicular line is generally easier to access with less chance of dislodging the needle.

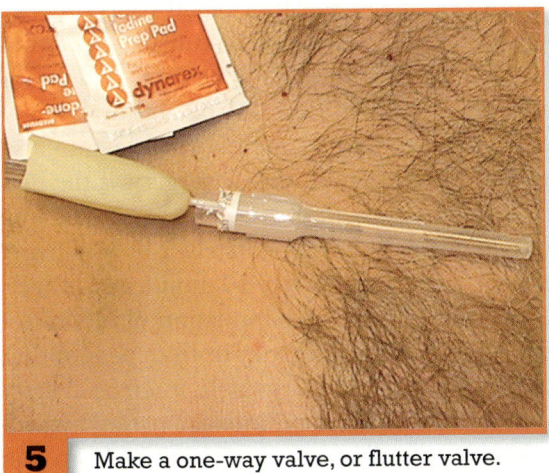

5 Make a one-way valve, or flutter valve.

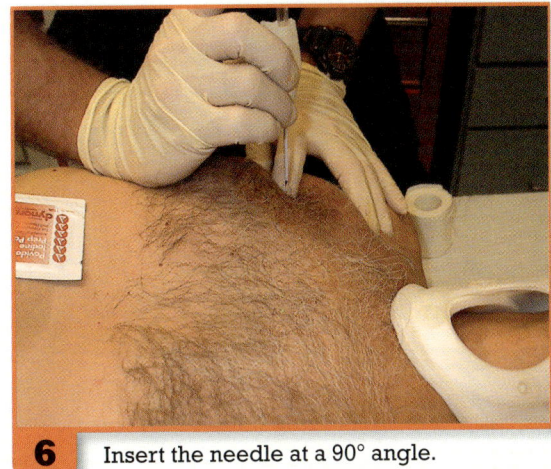

6 Insert the needle at a 90° angle.

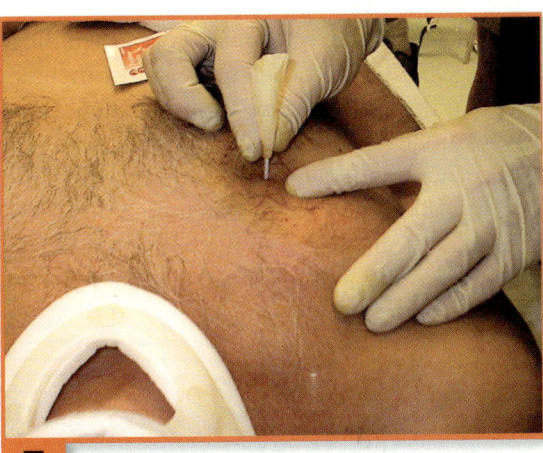

7 Remove the needle and listen for release of air. Properly dispose of the needle in the sharps container.

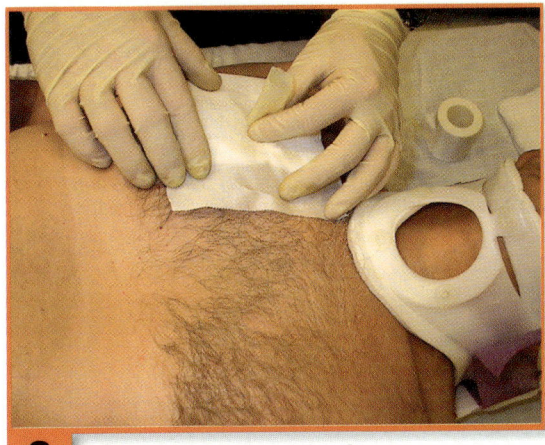

8 Secure the catheter in place. Monitor the patient closely for recurrence of the tension pneumothorax.

5. **Cleanse the appropriate** area using aseptic technique (**Step 4**).
6. **Make a one-way valve**, or <u>flutter valve</u>, by inserting the catheter through the end of a condom or use a commercially prepared device or the finger of a medical glove, cut off from the glove (**Step 5**).
7. **Insert the needle at a 90° angle**, and listen for the release of air (**Step 6**). Be sure to insert it just superior to the third rib, midclavicular, or just above the sixth rib, midaxillary. The nerves, arteries, and veins run along the inferior borders of each rib.
8. **Advance the catheter** over the needle, and place the needle in the sharps container (**Step 7**).
9. **Secure the catheter in place** in the same manner you would use to secure an impaled object (**Step 8**).
10. **Monitor the patient closely for recurrence of the tension pneumothorax**. This procedure may need to be repeated several times before arrival at the emergency department.

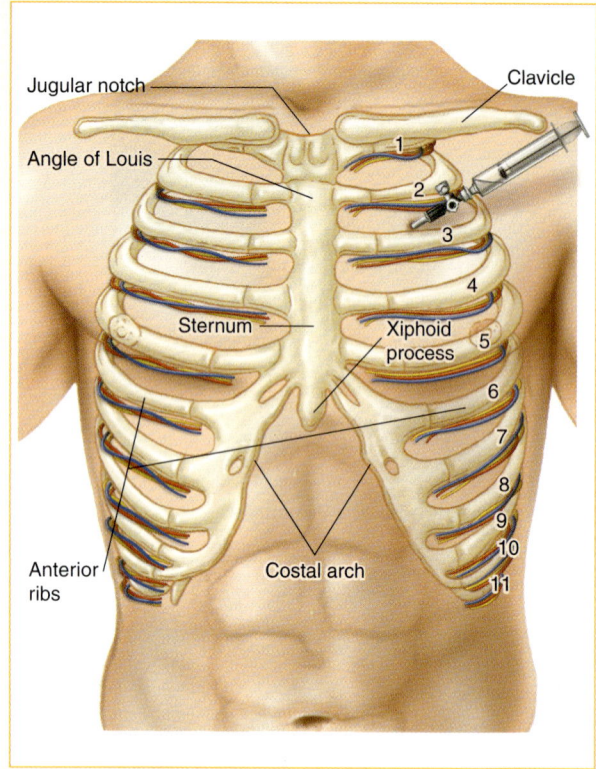

Figure 15-10 Correct placement of needle for decompression. The position of nerves, arteries, and veins are shown in relation to the ribs.

Hemothorax

A <u>hemothorax</u> (Figure 15-11▶), blood collecting in the pleural space, is often associated with a pneumothorax and may occur with blunt or penetrating trauma. Rib fractures are a frequent cause. A hemothorax is a life-threatening injury that frequently requires the urgent placement of a chest tube and/or surgery. If the hemothorax is associated with great vessel or cardiac injury, 50% of patients will die immediately, 25% will live 5 to 10 minutes, and 25% may live 30 minutes or longer.

A hemothorax is an accumulation of blood in the pleural space. The bleeding may be from penetrating or blunt lung injury, chest wall vessels, intercostal vessels, or the myocardium. The pulmonary parenchyma is a low-pressure vascular system. Bleeding from a pulmonary contusion can cause up to 1,500 mL of blood loss. A massive hemothorax indicates there is a great vessel or cardiac injury.

As blood accumulates, it causes collapse of the ipsilateral lung. The degree of respiratory insufficiency is dependent on the amount of blood in the pleural space. Hypoxia results from the decreased gas exchange, and hypotension and inadequate perfusion may result from the blood loss. The chest cavity can hold 2,000 to 3,000 mL of blood, and the extent of the hemothorax is classified by the amount of blood loss. An intercostal artery can easily bleed 50 mL per minute, rapidly leading to

You are the Provider Part 5

You have inserted IV catheters at two sites: a 16-gauge in the right antecubital fossa and a 14-gauge in the left antecubital fossa. You are providing a 20-mL/kg bolus of normal saline while monitoring vital signs. The airway is secured with a Combitube (endotracheal tube if following 1999 EMT-I curriculum), and the firefighter ventilating the patient tells you it is getting more difficult to squeeze the bag.

Reassessment	Recording Time: 9 Minutes After Patient Contact
Level of consciousness	Unresponsive
Respirations	Ventilating; circumoral cyanosis noted; decreased breath sounds on the right side of the chest
Pulse	Weak radial pulses; carotid pulse, 142 beats/min
Skin	Very pale, cool, diaphoretic
Blood pressure	Unable to palpate

10. What could cause the decreased breath sounds on the right side of the chest?
11. What are some other signs you should check for before making a treatment decision?

Pulmonary Contusion

In addition to fracturing ribs, any severe blunt trauma to the chest can also injure the lung. The pulmonary alveoli become filled with blood, and fluid accumulates in the injured area, leaving the patient hypoxic. Pulmonary contusion is the most common injury from blunt thoracic trauma. Of all patients with blunt trauma, 30% to 75% have a pulmonary contusion. It is commonly associated with rib fracture.

Severe <u>pulmonary contusion</u>, bruising of the lung, should always be suspected in patients with a flail chest and usually develops over a period of hours. Bruising of the lung parenchyma may also occur with high-energy shock waves from an explosion, high-velocity missile wounds, low-velocity weapons, and rapid deceleration. There is also a high incidence of extrathoracic injuries indicating underlying damage. Pulmonary contusions are often missed because of the high incidence of other associated injuries, resulting in a mortality rate of 14% to 20%.

There are three physical mechanisms for creating pulmonary contusions. The first is the implosion effect. Overexpansion of air in the lungs secondary to a positive-pressure concussive wave, blunt trauma, results in rapid, excessive stretching and tearing of the alveoli. The second, the inertial effect, strips the alveoli from the heavier bronchial structures when accelerated at varying rates by the concussive wave. The final mechanism is the Spalding effect. The liquid-gas interface, or exchange, is disrupted by the shock wave. The wave releases energy, and this differential transmission of energy causes disruption of the tissues.

Alveolar and capillary damage resulting from any of these mechanisms cause interstitial and intra-alveolar extravasation of blood. Interstitial edema occurs, and there is increased capillary membrane permeability, which worsens the edema. As fluid accumulates, gas exchange is greatly impaired. This results in hypoxemia and CO_2 retention. The hypoxia causes a reflex thickening of mucous secretions, which leads to bronchiolar obstruction and atelectasis. Blood is then shunted away from the unventilated alveoli, leading to further hypoxemia.

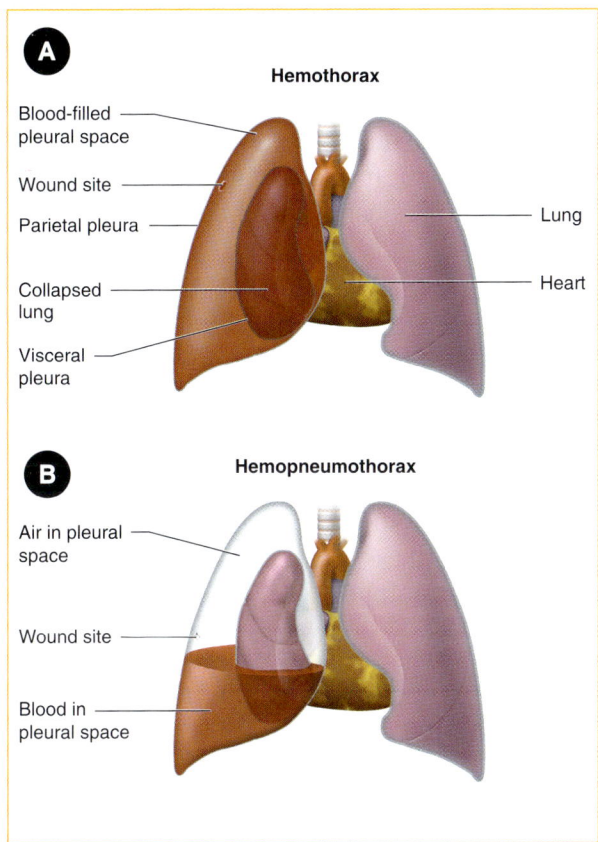

Figure 15-11 **A.** A hemothorax is a collection of blood in the pleural space produced by bleeding within the chest. **B.** When both blood and air are present, the condition is called a hemopneumothorax.

hypoxia and hypovolemic shock. Intrapulmonary hemorrhage comes from the bronchus or lung parenchyma.

Assessment Findings

Signs and symptoms of a massive hemothorax are produced by hypovolemia and respiratory compromise. You should suspect a hemothorax if the patient has signs and symptoms of shock or decreased breath sounds on the affected side, an indication that the lung is being compressed by the blood. Expect to find tachypnea; tachycardia; dyspnea; respiratory distress; hypotension; a narrowed pulse pressure; pleuritic chest pain; pale, cool, moist skin; dullness on percussion; and decreased breath sounds.

Hemopneumothorax. A pneumothorax with bleeding in the pleural space is known as a hemopneumothorax. Findings and management are the same as those for a hemothorax.

Assessment Findings

Signs and symptoms of a pulmonary contusion include tachypnea, tachycardia, cough, hemoptysis, apprehension, respiratory distress, dyspnea, evidence of blunt chest trauma, and cyanosis. Any or all of these may be present. The degree of respiratory compromise is directly related to the size of the contused area.

Myocardial Injuries

Pericardial Tamponade

In pericardial tamponade, blood or other fluid collects in the pericardium, the fibrous sac surrounding the heart (Figure 15-12). This prevents the heart from filling during the diastolic phase, causing a decrease in the amount of blood pumped to the body and decreased blood pressure. Ultimately, as blood accumulates within the pericardial sac, it compresses the heart until it can no longer function and cardiac arrest occurs. Pericardial tamponade is relatively uncommon and is seen more often with penetrating injuries to the heart itself than with blunt injuries to the chest. It occurs in fewer than 2% of chest trauma patients. Gunshot wounds carry a higher mortality rate than stab wounds, and the mortality rate is lower if only an isolated tamponade is present.

The pericardium is a tough fibrous sac that encloses the heart. It attaches to the great vessels at the base of the heart. There are two layers: the visceral pericardium, which forms the epicardium, and the parietal pericardium, which is regarded as the sac itself. The purpose of the pericardium is to anchor the heart, restricting excess movement and preventing kinking of the great vessels. The parietal layer cannot distend acutely but can slowly distend with as much as 1,000 to 1,500 mL of blood or other fluid. The space between the visceral and parietal layers is a potential space that is normally filled with 30 to 50 mL of a straw-colored fluid secreted by the visceral layer. It provides lubrication as the heart beats, lymphatic drainage, and immunologic protection for the heart.

Rapid accumulation of fluid over minutes to hours leads to increases in intrapericardial pressure. This increased intrapericardial pressure compresses the heart and decreases cardiac output owing to restricted diastolic expansion and filling. It also hampers venous return. Myocardial perfusion decreases owing to pressure effects on the walls of the heart and decreased diastolic pressures. Ischemic dysfunction may result in infarction. Removal of as little as 20 mL of blood may drastically improve cardiac output.

> **Terminology Tips**
>
> Intra = within; peri = around; cardi(o) = pertaining to the heart; centesis = puncture
> Therefore:
> Intrapericardial pressure = pressure within the sac surrounding the heart; pericardiocentesis = puncture of the sac surrounding the heart

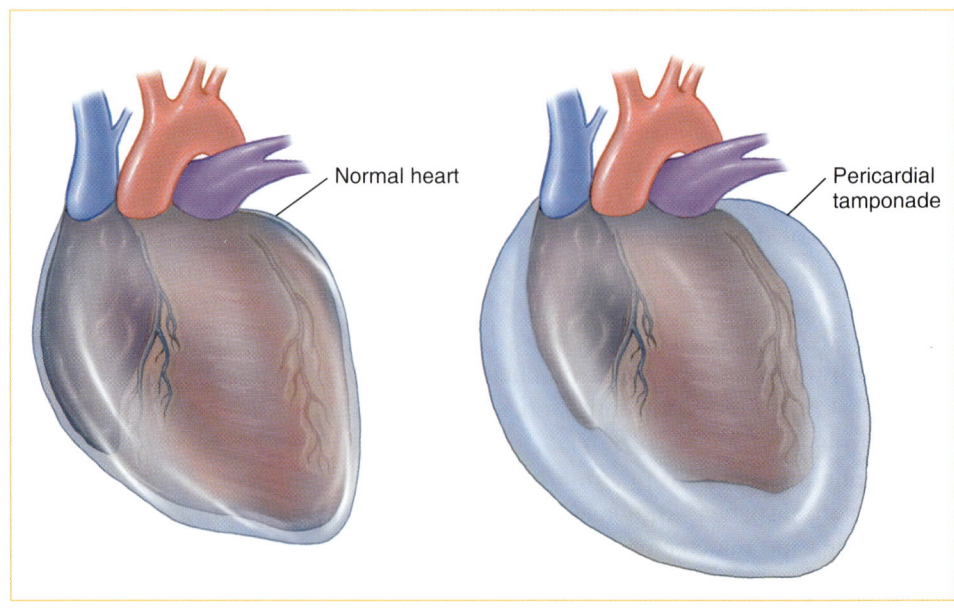

Figure 15-12 Pericardial tamponade is a potentially fatal condition in which fluid builds up within the pericardial sac, causing compression of the heart's chambers and dramatically impairing its ability to pump blood to the body.

Assessment Findings

Signs and symptoms of pericardial tamponade include tachycardia with a weak pulse, respiratory distress, very soft and faint heart tones, often called muffled heart sounds, low blood pressure, narrowed pulse pressure, and jugular vein distention. The patient may also present with pulsus paradoxus (also known as a paradoxical pulse), or a loss of peripheral pulses during inspiration, which corresponds with a 10- to 15-mm Hg drop in systolic blood pressure. Cyanosis may be present to the face, neck, and upper extremities. The Beck triad—composed of narrowing pulse pressure, neck vein distention, and muffled heart tones—makes up the classic signs for diagnosing a cardiac tamponade. However, these signs occur in the advanced stage and are only seen in 30% of patients.

Apply the cardiac monitor and be prepared to treat dysrhythmias.

Myocardial Contusion

There is a 16% to 76% incidence of myocardial contusion, or bruising of the heart muscle, in blunt trauma. It is a significant cause of morbidity and mortality in blunt trauma patients. Blunt myocardial injury results in hemorrhage with edema and fragmented myocardial fibers along with cellular injury. Vascular damage may occur, and hemopericardium may occur from a lacerated epicardium or endocardium. The fibrinous reaction at the contusion site may lead to delayed rupture and/or a ventricular aneurysm. The areas of damage are well demarcated, and conduction defects may occur.

Assessment Findings

Associated injuries include one to three rib fractures and/or a sternal fracture. The patient may also present with retrosternal chest pain. Often, the pulse rate is irregular, but dangerous rhythms such as ventricular tachycardia and ventricular fibrillation are uncommon. The patient may develop a new cardiac murmur, and, as the pressure builds, a pericardial friction rub may be heard; however, this is a very late sign.

ECG changes may involve any of the following:
- Persistent tachycardia
- ST-segment elevation, T-wave inversion
- Atrial flutter, fibrillation
- Premature ventricular contractions
- Premature atrial contractions

Vascular Injuries

Aortic Dissection and Rupture

Dissection or rupture of the aorta occurs most often in blunt trauma due to motor vehicle crashes and falls. It is also the cause of 15% of all blunt trauma deaths. Of patients with an aortic dissection or aortic rupture, 85% to 95% die instantaneously; 10% to 15% survive to arrive at the hospital. Of the survivors, one third die within 6 hours, one third die within 24 hours, and one third survive 3 days or longer.

Shearing injuries cause a separation of the aortic intima (inner layer or lumen) and media (middle layer). Blood enters the media through a small intimal tear. This tear is due to the effect of high-speed deceleration on portions of the aorta at points of relative fixation. Increased intraluminal pressure results from the impact, and the thin outer layer may rupture. The most common site of rupture is the ligamentum arteriosum, the part of the descending aorta at the isthmus just distal to the left subclavian artery. Ruptures of the ascending aorta are much less common.

Assessment Findings

Assessment findings associated with aortic dissection or rupture include retrosternal or interscapular pain, dyspnea, dysphagia, ischemic pain of the extremities, upper extremity hypertension with absent or decreased amplitude of femoral pulses, and a harsh systolic murmur over the precordium (the area on the anterior surface of the body that lies over the heart and lower thorax) or interscapular region.

Penetrating Wounds of the Great Vessels

Injuries to the great vessels usually are associated with injuries to the chest, abdomen, or neck. The chest contains several large blood vessels: the superior vena cava, the inferior vena cava, the pulmonary arteries, four main pulmonary veins, and the aorta, with its major branches distributing blood throughout the body. The abdominal aorta and inferior vena cava travel through the abdomen, and the carotid arteries and external jugular veins are located in the neck. Wounds to any of these vessels may be accompanied by massive hemothorax, hypovolemic shock, cardiac tamponade, and enlarging hematomas. Frequently, blood loss is not obvious, because it remains within the chest cavity. Hematomas may cause compression of any structure, including the vena cava, trachea, esophagus, great vessels, or heart. Here, particularly, immediate transport to the hospital is critical—a few minutes can mean the difference between life and death.

Other Thoracic Injuries

Diaphragmatic Injury

Injuries to the diaphragm may be the result of blunt or penetrating trauma. Diaphragmatic injury is a frequently encountered injury that could be life threatening. Injury occurs as high-pressure compression to the abdomen results in an increase in intra-abdominal pressure. Bowel obstruction and strangulation may also occur. As the diaphragm impinges on the thoracic cavity, lung expansion is restricted, causing hypoventilation and hypoxia. A mediastinal shift can result in cardiac and respiratory compromise.

Assessment Findings

Signs and symptoms may be very subtle. Findings include tachypnea, tachycardia, respiratory distress, dullness to percussion, scaphoid (hollow; boat-shaped) abdomen, bowel sounds in the affected hemithorax, and decreased breath sounds.

Esophageal Injury

Penetrating trauma is the most frequent cause of esophageal injury. It is rare in blunt trauma. However, it is an injury that could be life threatening if undetected. Missile and knife wounds may penetrate the esophagus, or it may perforate spontaneously in violent emesis, carcinoma (cancer), or anatomic distortions produced by diverticula or gastric reflux.

Assessment Findings

Patients typically present with pain, fever, hoarseness, dysphagia, respiratory distress, and shock. Signs of cervical esophageal perforation include local tenderness, subcutaneous emphysema, and resistance of the neck on passive motion. If the perforation is in the intrathoracic esophagus, signs may include mediastinal emphysema, mediastinitis, subcutaneous emphysema, mediastinal crunch, and splinting of the chest wall.

Tracheobronchial Injuries

Tracheobronchial injuries are rare, occurring in fewer than 3% of chest trauma cases. When they occur, they are usually the result of blunt or penetrating trauma and carry a high mortality rate of greater than 30%.

The majority of injuries occur within 3 cm of the carina. A tear can occur anywhere along the tracheobronchial tree and result in rapid movement of air into the pleural space. Tension pneumothorax is refractory to needle decompression, and there is a continuous flow of air from the needle of the decompressed chest. It also causes severe hypoxia.

Assessment Findings

Findings associated with tracheobronchial injuries include tachypnea, tachycardia, massive subcutaneous emphysema, dyspnea, respiratory distress, hemoptysis, and signs of tension pneumothorax that do not respond to needle decompression.

Traumatic Asphyxia

Sometimes a patient will experience a sudden, severe compression injury of the chest, which produces a rapid increase in intrathoracic pressure. This may occur in an unrestrained driver who hits a steering wheel or

You are the Provider   Part 6

You note distended jugular veins and increased cyanosis. Pulmonary compliance remains decreased when ventilating the patient.

12. What is your next course of action?

a pedestrian who is compressed between a vehicle and a wall. A sudden compressional force squeezes the chest, and blood backs up into the head and neck, causing the jugular veins to engorge and capillaries to rupture.

Assessment Findings

The sudden increase in intrathoracic pressure results in a very characteristic appearance, including distended neck veins, cyanosis in the face and upper neck, bulging eyes, and swelling or hemorrhage of the conjuctiva. The skin below the area of compression remains pink, and hypotension ensues when the pressure is released.

Management of Thoracic Injuries

Care for all thoracic injuries begins with assessment and management of the ABCs. Every patient should receive high-flow oxygen with positive-pressure ventilation as needed. Aggressive treatment of airway compromise and shock and rapid recognition of injuries, along with rapid transport to the closest, most appropriate facility, greatly increase the patient's chance for survival. Provide psychological support en route. Table 15-1 lists the guidelines for treating individual thoracic injuries based on your level of EMT-I training. Always follow local protocols.

TABLE 15-1 Guidelines for Treating Thoracic Injuries

Injury	1985 Treatment	1999 Treatment
Rib Fractures	Airway and ventilatory support	Airway and ventilatory support
	Positive-pressure ventilation (PPV) as needed	PPV as needed
	Encourage coughing and deep breathing	Encourage coughing and deep breathing
	Provide circulatory support	Provide circulatory support
	Splint, but avoid circumferential splinting	Splint, but avoid circumferential splinting
		Analgesics
Flail Segment	Airway and ventilatory support	Airway and ventilatory support
	PPV as needed; consider definitive airway (Combitube)	PPV as needed; consider definitive airway (endotracheal intubation)
	Stabilize flail segment per local protocols	Stabilize flail segment per local protocols
	Consider positive end expiratory pressure (PEEP)	Consider PEEP
	Restrict IV fluids	Restrict IV fluids
		Analgesics
	Position the patient for optimal respiratory support	Position the patient for optimal respiratory support
Sternal Fracture	Airway and ventilatory support	Airway and ventilatory support
	Restrict IV fluids if pulmonary contusion is suspected	Restrict IV fluids if pulmonary contusion is suspected
	Allow for chest wall self-splinting	Analgesics
		Allow for chest wall self-splinting
		Cardiac monitoring
Simple Pneumothorax	Airway and ventilatory support; PPV as needed	Airway and ventilatory support; PPV as needed
	Monitor for the development of tension	Monitor for the development of tension
	Circulatory support	Circulatory support
	Call for backup if needed	Call for backup if needed
		Needle thoracostomy (See Skill Drill 15-1)

Continued

TABLE 15-1	Guidelines for Treating Thoracic Injuries—cont'd	
Injury	**1985 Treatment**	**1999 Treatment**
Open Pneumothorax	Airway and ventilatory support; PPV as needed Monitor for the development of tension pneumothorax Circulatory support Cover the wound with an **occlusive dressing**	Airway and ventilatory support; PPV as needed Monitor for the development of tension pneumothorax Circulatory support Cover the wound with an occlusive dressing
Tension Pneumothorax	Airway and ventilatory support; PPV as needed Relieve tension to improve cardiac output Occlude open wounds Call for backup if needed	Airway and ventilatory support; PPV as needed Relieve tension to improve cardiac output Occlude open wounds Call for backup if needed Needle thoracentesis
Hemothorax	Airway and ventilatory support; PPV as needed Circulatory support Reexpand the affected lung to reduce bleeding Call for backup if needed	Airway and ventilatory support; PPV as needed Circulatory support Reexpand the affected lung to reduce bleeding Call for backup if needed
Pulmonary Contusion	Airway and ventilatory support; PPV as needed Restrict IV fluids (use caution when restricting fluids in hypovolemic patients—follow local protocols)	Airway and ventilatory support; PPV as needed Restrict IV fluids (use caution when restricting fluids in hypovolemic patients—follow local protocols)
Pericardial Tamponade	Airway and ventilatory support Circulatory support: fluid challenge of 20 mL/kg Pericardiocentesis: in-hospital management	Airway and ventilatory support Circulatory support: fluid challenge of 20 mL/kg Monitor ECG readings Pericardiocentesis: in-hospital management
Myocardial Contusion	Airway and ventilatory support Circulatory support: IV fluid for volume maintenance	Airway and ventilatory support Circulatory support: IV fluid for volume maintenance Monitor ECG readings Antiarrhythmics Inotropic drugs
Aortic Dissection or Rupture	Airway and ventilatory support Circulatory support; do not over hydrate	Airway and ventilatory support Circulatory support; do not over hydrate
Great Vessel Injuries	Airway and ventilatory support Manage hypovolemia Use of pneumatic antishock garment (PASG) **not** recommended Expeditious transport	Airway and ventilatory support Manage hypovolemia PASG **not** recommended Expeditious transport

TABLE 15-1 Guidelines for Treating Thoracic Injuries—cont'd

Injury	1985 Treatment	1999 Treatment
Diaphragmatic Injury	Airway and ventilatory support; PPV as needed (Caution: IPPB [intermittent positive-pressure breathing] may worsen the injury) Circulatory support **Do not** place patient in Trendelenburg position	Airway and ventilatory support, PPV as needed (Caution: IPPB may worsen the injury) Circulatory support **Do not** place patient in Trendelenburg position
Esophageal Injury	Airway and ventilatory support Circulatory support	Airway and ventilatory support Circulatory support
Tracheobronchial Injuries	Airway and ventilatory support Circulatory support	Airway and ventilatory support Circulatory support
Traumatic Asphyxia	Airway and ventilatory support Circulatory support; expect hypotension once compression is released	Airway and ventilatory support Circulatory support; expect hypotension once compression is released Use of sodium bicarbonate should be guided by arterial blood gas testing in the hospital

Documentation Tips

When you use an occlusive dressing to seal an open chest wound, record the type of material used, whether three or four sides were sealed, and any changes noted afterward: skin color, vital signs, breath sounds, and particularly the patient's level of respiratory distress.

In the Field

If a patient with an open chest wound sealed with an occlusive dressing shows signs of developing tension, simply raise one side of the dressing to allow the air to escape. This is known as "burping" the dressing.

You are the Provider Part 7

A chest decompression is performed on the affected side. On arrival at the emergency department, the patient is moaning and his skin color has improved. The firefighter is having no difficulty ventilating him.

Reassessment	Recording Time: 15 Minutes After Patient Contact
Level of consciousness	Pain responsive
Respirations	Ventilating well, decreased cyanosis
Pulse	128 beats/min with stronger radial pulses
Blood pressure	90/60 mm Hg
Skin	Pale, cool, less diaphoretic

You turn the patient over to the charge nurse and give a report.

13. Would PASG have been appropriate? Why or why not?

You are the Provider — Summary

1. Why is it important to seal open chest wounds as quickly as possible? Stabilize flail segments?

Open chest wounds, especially large wounds, and flail segments of the chest wall, impair ventilation. This results in decreased tidal volume during inspiration. Remember that if tidal volume is inadequate, minute volume will be as well. Overall, this will cause tissue hypoxia and eventual death.

2. What are some of the possible consequences of a blunt injury to the heart? A penetrating injury?

Myocardial contusion is perhaps the most significant consequence of blunt trauma to the heart. Additionally, if impact to the chest wall occurs during a certain period of the cardiac cycle, the patient can develop ventricular fibrillation (V-Fib). Penetrating injuries to the heart may result in pericardial tamponade, laceration of coronary arteries, or penetration of the myocardium itself. These conditions will be rapidly fatal if not treated promptly.

3. What do you think caused his injury?

There is a deformed steering wheel, indicating that his chest sustained a significant impact.

4. What is your first consideration in treating this patient?

Ensure a patent airway with simultaneous C-spine precautions.

5. What is your next step in the management of this patient?

Provide 100% oxygen.

6. What type of oxygen delivery device will you use? What flow rate?

Use a bag-valve-mask device for ventilation with 100% oxygen at 15 L/min. Ventilations are shallow and rapid, indicating poor tidal volume.

7. Once the patient is loaded into the ambulance, what is the next step in treatment?

Definitive airway treatment with a Combitube. Establish IV access.

Endotracheal intubation, IVs, cardiac monitor.

8. What condition do the vital signs and distended abdomen point to?

Hypovolemia; the patient appears to be bleeding into the abdomen.

9. At what rate will you run IVs? Why?

To maintain radial pulses and perfusion. Increasing the blood pressure excessively may increase internal bleeding.

10. What could cause the decreased breath sounds on the right side of the chest?

The patient has a pneumothorax that is developing tension.

11. What are some other signs you should check for before making a treatment decision?

Jugular venous distention, subcutaneous emphysema, signs of shock.

12. What is your next course of action?

Call for backup if needed to perform a needle thoracostomy.

Obtain orders from medical control and perform a needle thoracostomy.

13. Would PASG have been appropriate? Why or why not?

No. The PASG should not be used in patients with open or penetrating trauma to the chest. Increased intrathoracic pressure generated by the PASG may exacerbate internal bleeding and may also cause further reductions in pulmonary capacity.

Prep Kit

Ready for Review

- There are two types of chest injuries: penetrating, or open, injuries and blunt, or closed, injuries.

- In blunt trauma, a blow to the chest may fracture the ribs, the sternum, or whole areas of the chest wall. Compression of these structures creates other problems, including contusions of the lungs and the heart and possible damage to the aorta. Even if the skin and chest wall are in tact, the contents of the thorax may be injured.

- A sucking chest wound can be the result of an open pneumothorax, in which air entering through the wound accumulates in the pleural space, causing the lung to collapse.

- You should seal a sucking chest wound with an occlusive dressing, either taping it down on all four sides or creating a flutter valve by sealing only three sides. Sealing all four sides may create a tension pneumothorax, in which air leaking from a lacerated lung is unable to escape and the lung collapses. Eventually, this air may push the mediastinum into the opposite hemithorax and prevent blood from returning to the heart. Cardiac arrest may result. If tension begins to develop, simply "burp" the dressing to allow trapped air to escape.

- A tension pneumothorax can also occur in a closed, blunt injury of the chest in which a fractured rib lacerates the surface of the lung or as a result of the paper bag syndrome. Look for increasing respiratory distress, shock, jugular vein distention, and decreased breath sounds on the affected side. Remember, contralateral tracheal deviation is a late sign.

- The accumulation of blood in the pleural space is called a hemothorax; the collection of both blood and air is called a hemopneumothorax.

- Multiple rib fractures, with or without a fracture of the sternum, often result in a condition called flail chest, in which a portion of the chest wall is detached from the thoracic cage and moves paradoxically during respiration.

- A flail chest causes very painful breathing and requires respiratory support and supplemental high-flow oxygen. It may help to immobilize the flail segment with a bulky dressing. Remember to never tape around the entire circumference of the thorax because this may impede breathing. Do not use heavy objects such as sandbags.

- Other thoracic injuries include rupture or dissection of the aorta, diaphragmatic injuries, contusions of the lungs and heart, and traumatic asphyxia, in which a sudden, severe compression of the chest produces a rapid increase in intrathoracic pressure. Signs of this condition include distended neck veins, cyanosis to the face, bulging eyes, and hemorrhage in the sclera. Provide ventilatory support, monitor vital signs, and provide immediate transport.

- In pericardial tamponade, blood collects in the pericardium, preventing the heart from filling during the diastolic phase and eventually causing cardiac arrest. Signs include a weak pulse and the Beck triad: narrowing pulse pressure, distended neck veins, and muffled heart sounds. Definitive treatment includes a pericardiocentesis performed in the hospital. Here as well, you should provide vigorous respiratory support and immediate transport.

- Laceration of the large blood vessels in the chest can cause a fatal hemorrhage. Suspect such a wound in any patient with a chest wound who shows signs of shock, even if you see little blood; it may be collecting within the chest cavity. The thorax will sound dull (hyporessonant) to percussion. This person needs supplemental high-flow oxygen with possible positive-pressure ventilation, immediate transport, and CPR if cardiac arrest develops.

- Intravenous fluid therapy during thoracic trauma should be closely monitored and administered according to local protocol. The goal is to maintain adequate perfusion without causing a marked increase in blood pressure. Early recognition and prompt transport to the closest, most appropriate facility are vital to patient survival in thoracic trauma.

Technology

- Interactivities
- Vocabulary Explorer
- Anatomy Review
- Web Links
- Online Review Manual

Prep Kit continued...

- Any injury to the thoracic cavity may disrupt normal cardiac function. Always monitor ECG readings and treat the patient based on ACLS and local protocols. Consider aggressive airway management, including endotracheal intubation when indicated.
- A needle thoracostomy is the treatment of choice for a tension pneumothorax. Consider analgesics for pain relief according to local protocol, and consider sodium bicarbonate to offset metabolic acidosis in traumatic asphyxia. Follow local protocols or contact medical control as needed.

Vital Vocabulary

bradypnea Slow respirations.

chemoreceptors Sensors that respond to chemical fluctuations such as a decreased oxygen concentration in the bloodstream.

closed chest injury An injury to the chest in which the skin is not broken, usually due to blunt trauma.

dyspnea Difficulty with breathing.

flail chest A condition in which three or more ribs are fractured in two or more places or in association with a fracture of the sternum, so that a segment of chest wall is effectively detached from the rest of the thoracic cage.

flutter valve A one-way valve that allows air to leave the chest cavity but not return. Formed by taping three sides of an occlusive dressing to the chest wall, leaving the fourth side open as the valve.

hemoptysis The spitting or coughing up of blood.

hemothorax A collection of blood in the pleural cavity.

myocardial contusion A bruise of the heart muscle.

occlusive dressing A dressing made of Vaseline gauze, aluminum foil, or plastic that prevents air and liquids from entering or exiting a wound.

open chest injury An injury to the chest in which the chest wall itself is penetrated by some external object such as a knife or bullet.

paper bag syndrome Rupture of the lungs that occurs as the chest meets with blunt trauma after taking a deep breath, usually during a motor vehicle crash, similar to rupture of an air-filled paper bag.

paradoxical motion The motion of the portion of the chest wall that is detached in a flail chest; the motion—in during inhalation, out during exhalation—is exactly the opposite of normal chest wall motion during breathing.

pericardial tamponade Compression of the heart due to a buildup of blood or other fluid in the pericardial sac.

pericardium The fibrous sac that surrounds the heart.

pneumothorax An accumulation of air or gas in the pleural space.

pulmonary contusion A bruise of the lung.

spontaneous pneumothorax Pneumothorax that occurs when a weak area on the lung ruptures in the absence of major injury, allowing air to leak into the pleural space.

sucking chest wound An open or penetrating chest wall wound through which air passes during inspiration and expiration, creating a sucking sound.

tachypnea Rapid respirations.

tension pneumothorax An accumulation of air or gas in the pleural space that progressively collapses the lung with potentially fatal results.

Points to Ponder

You respond to a snowmobile accident in which a snowmobile struck a tree stump that was hidden by the snow. The driver was thrown a short distance from the snowmobile. You find the patient sitting in the snow, conscious and alert. He is in no obvious distress and complains of pain to his left leg only. You focus your assessment on the left lower leg, which reveals swelling and deformity. You take your time and splint the leg and then transport the patient to the hospital. When you assess his vital signs, you notice that his pulse is irregular but decide that this is probably normal for him. On arrival at the hospital, cardiac arrest occurs. When the patient's snowsuit is removed, you see a bruise to the left side of his chest. What happened to this patient? What should you have done differently?

Issues: Understanding the Importance of Conducting a Thorough Exam, Understanding the Meaning of Assessment Findings, Treating a Chest Injury as a Potentially Life-threatening Injury Regardless of the Patient's Presentation

Assessment in Action

Law enforcement requests your assistance at the scene of an attempted burglary, where the homeowner has shot an intruder. On arrival, you find a 32-year-old man lying supine on the kitchen floor in an impressive pool of blood.

A police officer is holding a kitchen towel to the man's chest. During your assessment, you note that he is conscious and restless, stating that he cannot breathe. His respirations are rapid and labored; pulse is weak and rapid; and his skin is pale and diaphoretic. Further assessment reveals an entrance wound to the right anterior portion of the chest, just lateral to the sternum. You also note blood bubbling from the wound when the patient exhales.

1. This patient most likely has a:
   A. pneumothorax.
   B. pulmonary contusion.
   C. flail chest.
   D. rib fracture.

2. As your partner begins to administer oxygen, you should:
   A. prepare for endotracheal intubation.
   B. insert a nasopharyngeal airway.
   C. apply an occlusive dressing.
   D. insert an IV catheter and give a fluid bolus.

3. The patient's chest injury is best described as a/an:
   A. open chest injury due to blunt force trauma.
   B. open chest injury due to penetrating trauma.
   C. closed chest injury due to blunt force trauma.
   D. closed chest injury due to penetrating trauma.

4. Complications of chest injury may include all of the following, EXCEPT:
   A. respiratory distress.
   B. obstructive shock.
   C. cardiac dysrhythmias.
   D. increased minute volume.

5. The patient's labored respirations are MOST likely due to:
   A. severe pain.
   B. severe hypoxia.
   C. lung compression.
   D. airway obstruction.

6. Your assessment of this patient will MOST likely reveal:
   A. symmetric chest expansion.
   B. jugular venous distention.
   C. diminished lung sounds on the right side.
   D. diminished lung sounds on the left side.

7. Shock that accompanies a chest injury may be due to:
   A. hypoxia.
   B. blood loss.
   C. impaired cardiac function.
   D. any of the above.

8. Signs of tension pneumothorax that differ from a simple pneumothorax include:
   A. widening pulse pressure.
   B. tracheal deviation toward the injured side.
   C. jugular vein distention.
   D. dull sounds with percussion of the chest wall.

9. Your treatment for this patient should include all of the following, EXCEPT:
   A. high-flow oxygen.
   B. large bore IV access.
   C. spinal immobilization.
   D. elevating the feet.

10. You notice that the patient's respiratory distress has worsened and his oxygen saturation is decreasing. You should FIRST:
    A. perform a needle thoracentesis.
    B. assess the patient for signs of hemothorax.
    C. lift one side of the occlusive dressing.
    D. insert an oropharyngeal airway.

Abdomen and Genitalia Injuries

Additional Objectives*

Cognitive
1. Describe how solid and hollow organs can be injured (p 744).
2. State the steps in the emergency medical care of a patient with a blunt or penetrating abdominal injury (p 746).
3. State the steps in the emergency medical care of a patient with an object impaled in the abdomen (p 749).
4. State the steps in the emergency medical care of a patient with an abdominal evisceration wound (p 750).
5. State the steps in the emergency medical care of the patient with a genitourinary injury (p 753).

Affective
None

Psychomotor
6. Demonstrate proper treatment of a patient who has an object impaled in the abdomen (p 749).
7. Demonstrate how to apply a dressing to an abdominal evisceration wound (p 758).

*All of the objectives in this chapter are noncurriculum objectives. There are no 1985 or 1999 objectives for this chapter.

16

Abdomen and Genitalia Injuries

You are the Provider

It's late on a Saturday night and you and your partner receive a call for the victim of an assault. Upon arrival, law enforcement advises you that the scene is safe and that the victim is a young male that was hit several times in the stomach with a baseball bat.

This chapter will help prepare you to properly assess and care for patients with abdominal injuries as well as help you answer the following questions:

1. What are the two types of abdominal injures likely to be encountered in the prehospital setting?
2. What is one principal complaint that patients with abdominal injuries generally have?

Abdomen and Genitalia Injuries

The abdomen is the lower of the two major body cavities, extending from the diaphragm to the pelvis. It contains several organs that make up the digestive, urinary, and genitourinary systems. Although any of these organs may be injured, some are better protected than others. You must know where these organs are located within the abdominal and pelvic cavities. You must also understand their functions so that when an illness or injury occurs, you can assess its seriousness.

This chapter begins with a brief review of the anatomy of the abdomen, followed by a discussion of common types of abdominal injuries. Next, patient assessment strategies are discussed, followed by a description of specific abdominal injuries that you are likely to encounter and how to treat each injury. The genitourinary system is then described, and common injuries and treatment are discussed.

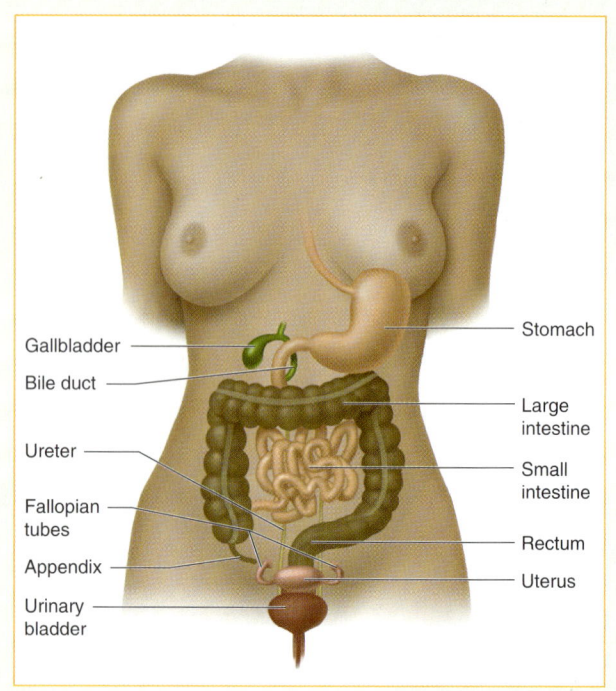

Figure 16-1 The hollow organs in the abdominal cavity are structures through which materials pass.

Anatomy of the Abdomen

The abdomen contains both hollow and solid organs, any of which may be damaged. Hollow organs, including the stomach, intestines, ureters, and bladder, are actually structures through which materials pass Figure 16-1▶. They usually contain food that is in the process of being digested, urine that is being passed to the bladder for release, or bile. When ruptured or lacerated, these organs spill their contents into the peritoneal cavity (the abdominal cavity), causing an intense inflammatory reaction called peritonitis. The first signs of peritonitis are severe abdominal pain, tenderness, and muscular spasm. Later, normal bowel sounds diminish or disappear as the bowel stops functioning. A patient may feel nauseous and may vomit; the abdomen may become distended and firm to the touch.

The solid organs, as their name suggests, are solid masses of tissue. They include the liver, spleen, pancreas, and kidneys Figure 16-2▶. It is here that much of the chemical work of the body—digestion, excretion, and energy production—takes place. Solid organs have a rich blood supply, so injury can cause severe hemorrhage. The same is true of the aorta and inferior vena cava, whether the injury is open or closed. Unlike gastric juices and bacteria, blood within the peritoneal cavity does not provoke an inflammatory response. Therefore, the absence of pain and tenderness does not necessarily mean the absence of major bleeding in the abdomen.

The bony landmarks in the abdomen include the pubic symphysis, the costal arch, the iliac crests, and

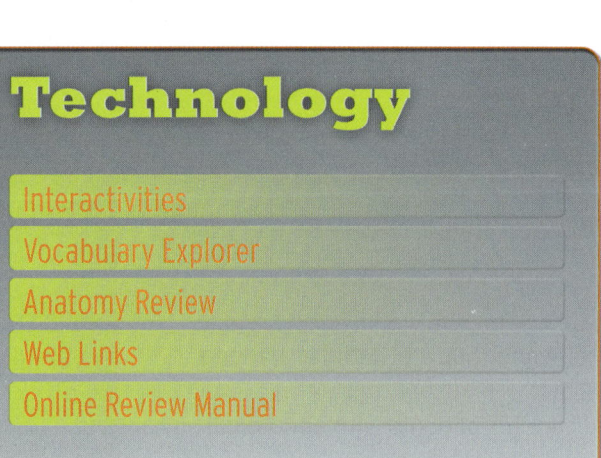

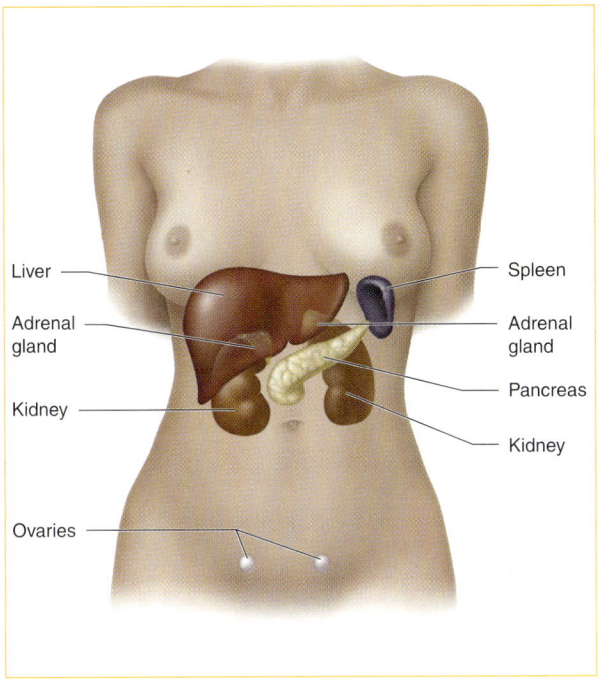

Figure 16-2 The solid organs are solid masses of tissue that do much of the chemical work in the body.

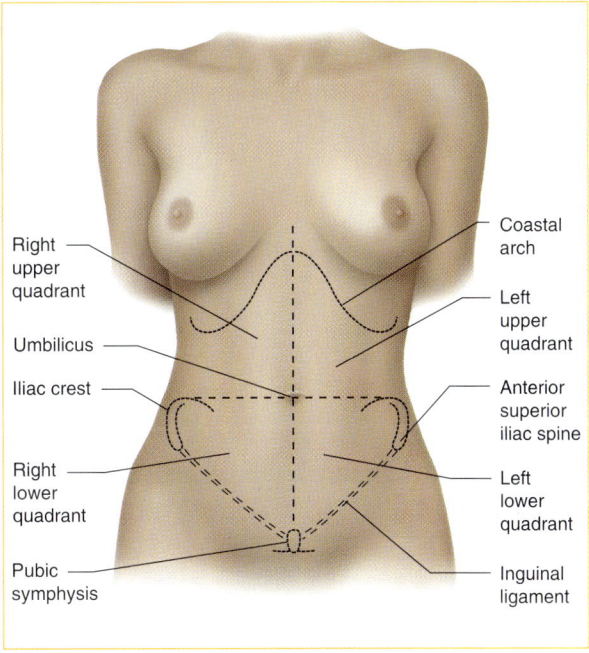

Figure 16-3 The abdominal cavity is divided into four quadrants, which serve as your means of identifying and reporting problems in the abdomen.

the anterior superior iliac spines. The major soft-tissue landmark is the umbilicus, which overlies the fourth lumbar vertebra. The abdomen is divided arbitrarily into quadrants by two perpendicular lines that intersect at the umbilicus Figure 16-3 ▶. These quadrants provide a frame of reference for identifying and reporting abdominal signs and symptoms.

Injuries to the Abdomen

Abdominal injuries may be as obvious as loops of intestines protruding from a stab wound or as subtle as a laceration to the liver or spleen. Remember to follow BSI precautions as you begin your initial assessment; these injuries often bleed profusely, and even if they do not, some blood or other body fluid is likely to be present. Injuries to the abdomen are considered open or closed and can involve hollow and solid organs. A <u>closed abdominal injury</u> is one in which a severe blow damages the abdomen without breaking the skin; closed abdominal injuries are also known as blunt injuries. Such a blow might come from the patient's striking the handlebar of a bicycle or the steering wheel of a car Figure 16-4 ▼. An <u>open abdominal injury</u> is one in which a foreign object enters the abdomen and opens the peritoneal cavity to the outside; open abdominal injuries are also known as penetrating injuries Figure 16-5 ▶.

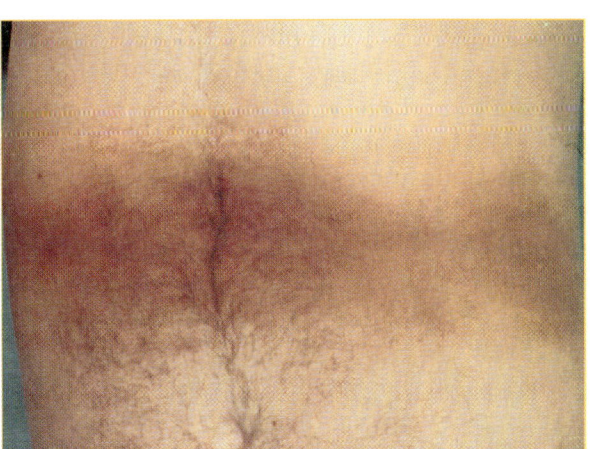

Figure 16-4 Blunt trauma to the abdomen can occur when a patient strikes the steering wheel of an automobile as a result of a crash.

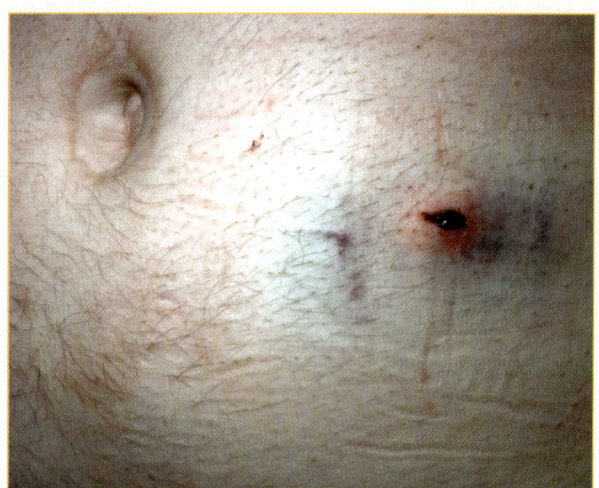

Figure 16-5 Because it is difficult to know how deep a penetrating injury is, assume organ damage and transport promptly.

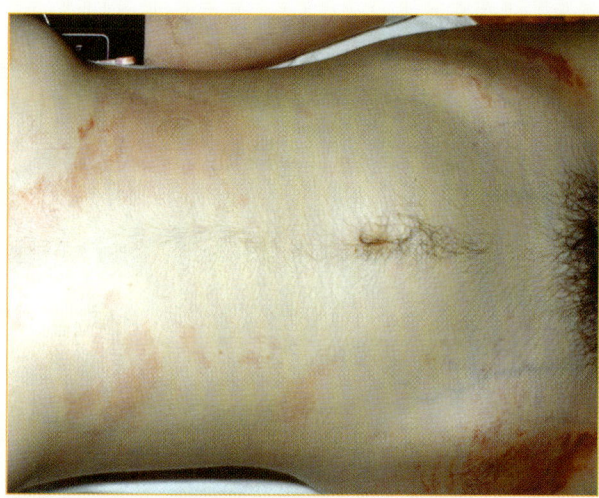

Figure 16-6 Bruising on the abdomen suggests possible injury to the underlying organs.

Open injuries might not go deeper than the wall of the abdomen, but this is difficult to determine. Therefore, you must assume the worst—that organs have been damaged—and provide prompt transport. Stab wounds and gunshot wounds are examples of open injuries.

Signs and Symptoms

Patients with abdominal injuries generally have one principal complaint: pain. But other significant injuries may mask the pain at first, and some patients may not be able to tell you about pain because they are unresponsive, such as after a head injury or drug or alcohol overdose. The most common sign of significant abdominal injury is tachycardia. Later signs are those of shock: decreased blood pressure and pale, cool, moist skin. In some cases, the abdomen may become distended from the accumulation of blood and fluid. As an EMT-I, you must look for other clues. Blunt injuries include bruises or other visible marks, whose location should guide your attention to underlying structures (Figure 16-6 ▶). For example, bruises in the right upper quadrant, left upper quadrant, or flank might suggest an injury to the liver, spleen, or kidney, respectively.

The signs of abdominal injury are usually more definite than the symptoms, including firmness on palpation of the abdomen, obvious entry and exit wounds, bruises, and altered vital signs such as increased pulse rate, increased respiratory rate, decreased blood pressure, and shallow respirations (although this might not appear until later). Common symptoms include abdominal tenderness, particularly localized tenderness, and difficulty with movement because of pain.

Evaluating Abdominal Injuries

Your goal during the initial assessment is to evaluate the patient's ABCs and then immediately care for any life threats. You should then begin the focused history and physical exam to determine the type of abdominal injury (open or closed), the extent of the injury, and the presence of shock. Note that patients may or may not be able to tell you about the severity and location of their pain. However, they may report that they feel nauseous, and they may vomit. Remember to keep the airway clear of vomitus so that it is not aspirated into the lungs, especially in a patient who is unresponsive or has an altered level of consciousness. Turn the patient to one side, using spinal precautions if necessary, and try to clear any material from the throat and mouth. Note the nature of the vomitus: undigested food, blood, mucus, or bile.

Normally, you will evaluate all patients with abdominal injuries in the same manner. First, you should place the patient in a supine position with the knees slightly flexed and supported (Figure 16-7 ▶). Remove or loosen clothes. Then, before you do anything else, assess and record baseline vital signs. Many abdominal emergencies, aside from those that cause severe bleeding, can cause a rapid pulse and low blood pressure. Your record of vital signs, made as early as possible and periodically thereafter, will be of tremendous help to physicians in evaluating the problem when the patient arrives in the emergency department.

Further assessment follows the DCAP-BTLS sequence: Inspect and palpate the abdomen for the presence of **Deformity**, which may be subtle in abdominal injuries. Look for the presence of **Contusions** and **Abrasions**, which can help localize focal points of impact and may indicate significant internal injury. Puncture wounds and other **Penetrating** injuries must not be overlooked, as the intra-abdominal extent of these injuries may be life threatening. The presence of **Burns** must be noted and managed appropriately. Palpate for **Tenderness** and attempt to localize to a specific quadrant of the abdomen. Identify and treat any **Lacerations** with appropriate dressings. Swelling may involve the abdomen globally and indicate significant intra-abdominal injury.

Quickly assess the patient's condition with a simple inspection, noting the manner in which he or she is lying. Movement of the body or the abdominal organs irritates the inflamed peritoneum, causing additional pain. To minimize this pain, patients will lie still, usually with the knees drawn up, and breathe using rapid and shallow breaths. For the same reason, they will contract their abdominal muscles, a sign called *guarding*.

Next, inspect the skin of the abdomen for holes through which bullets, knives, or other missile-type foreign bodies may have passed. Keep in mind that the size of the wound does not necessarily indicate the extent of underlying injuries. If you find an entry wound, you must always check for a corresponding exit wound in the patient's back or sides. If the injury was caused by a very high-velocity missile from a rifle, you may see a small, harmless-looking entrance wound with a large, gaping exit wound. Do not attempt to remove a knife or other object that is impaled in the patient. Instead, stabilize the object with bulky dressings and supportive bandaging. Bruises or other visible marks are important clues to the cause and severity of any blunt injury. Steering wheels and seat belts produce characteristic patterns of bruising on the abdomen or chest.

> **EMT-I Tips**
>
> Log rolling the patient onto a backboard is always a valuable chance to examine the back for signs of injury. Instruct and position assistants to ensure your ability to inspect and palpate the back briefly while the patient is rolled onto the side.

Types of Abdominal Injuries

Blunt Abdominal Wounds

A patient with a blunt abdominal wound may have one or some combination of the following:

- Severe bruises of the abdominal wall
- Laceration of the liver and spleen
- Rupture of the intestine
- Tears in the mesentery, membranous folds that attach the intestines to the walls of the body, and injury to blood vessels within them
- Rupture of the kidneys or tearing of the kidneys from their supporting structures
- Rupture of the bladder, especially in a patient who had been drinking and, therefore, had a full and distended bladder at the time of impact
- Severe intra-abdominal hemorrhage
- Peritoneal irritation and inflammation in response to the rupture of hollow organs

A patient who has sustained a blunt abdominal injury should be log rolled to a supine position on a backboard. Ensure that you protect the spine as you do so. If the patient vomits, turn him or her to one side and clear the mouth and throat of vomitus. Monitor the patient's vital signs for any indication of shock such as pallor; diaphoresis; rapid, thready pulse; or low blood pressure. If you see any of these signs, administer supplemental oxygen via nonrebreathing mask and take all

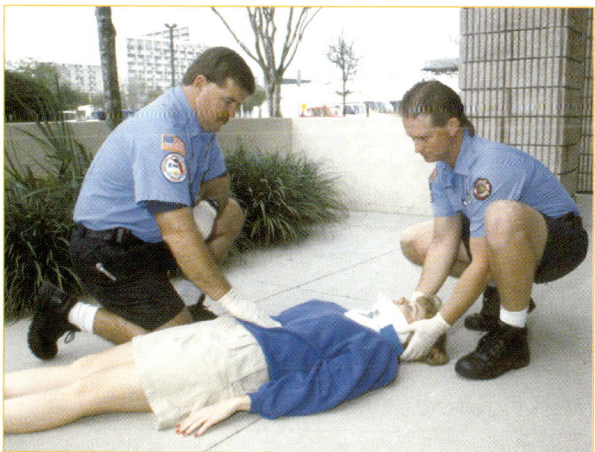

Figure 16-7 Patients with abdominal injuries may have firmness on palpation, wounds, bruises, or signs of shock on examination.

the appropriate measures to treat for shock. Keep the patient warm with blankets, and provide prompt transport to the emergency department.

Injuries From Seat Belts and Airbags

Seat belts have prevented many thousands of injuries and saved many lives, including those of people who otherwise would have been ejected from the vehicle. However, seat belts occasionally cause blunt injuries to the abdominal organs. When worn properly, a seat belt lies below the anterior superior iliac spines of the pelvis and against the hip joints. If the belt lies too high, it can squeeze abdominal organs or great vessels against the spine when the car suddenly decelerates or stops (Figure 16-8 ▶). Occasionally, fractures of the lumbar spine have been reported. If you are called to the scene of such an accident, keep in mind that the use of seat belts in many cases turns what could have been a fatal injury into a manageable one.

In all current-model automobiles, the lap and diagonal (shoulder) safety belts are combined into one so that they may not be used independently. Of course, people can still place the diagonal portion of the belt behind the back; however, this significantly reduces the effectiveness of this design. In some older cars, only lap belts or two separate belts are provided. Used alone, diagonal shoulder safety belts can cause injuries to the upper part of the trunk, such as thoracic bruising, fractured ribs, lacerated liver, or even decapitation. Far

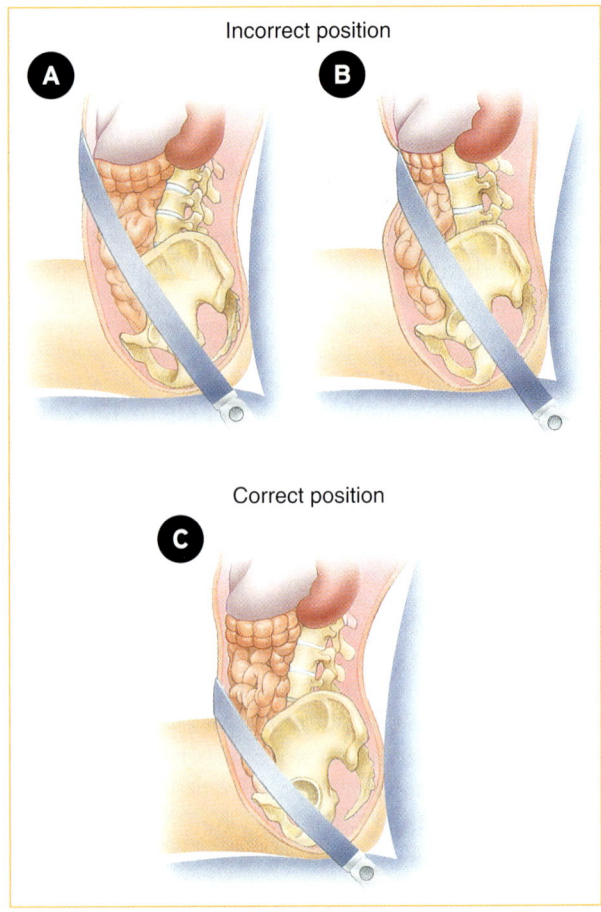

Figure 16-8 The proper position for a seat belt is below the anterior superior iliac spines of the pelvis and against the hip joints, as shown in diagram **C**. Diagrams **A** and **B** show improper positioning of seat belts.

You are the Provider — Part 2

As you begin your initial assessment, you note the following about your patient:

Initial Assessment	Recording Time: Zero Minutes
Appearance	Anxious, clutching his abdomen
Level of consciousness (LOC)	Alert to person, place, and time
Airway	Open and clear
Breathing	Respirations increased; adequate depth
Circulation	Radial pulses, present; rate is increased; no gross bleeding

3. What is your first step in the management of this patient?
4. What is the most common sign of significant abdominal injury?

fewer head and neck injuries are seen when this belt is used in combination with a lap belt and a properly positioned headrest.

The airbag, which is standard in today's vehicles, is a great advance in automotive safety. In head-on collisions, it can be a genuine lifesaver. However, because frontal airbags provide no protection in a side impact or rollover, they must be used in combination with properly worn safety belts. Small children and short individuals who are in the front seat of the automobile may be at risk of injury when the airbag is deployed. Special attention should be used in evaluating these patients when a deployed airbag is noted. Remember to inspect beneath the airbag for signs of damage to the steering wheel.

> **Documentation Tips**
>
> Hospital personnel will depend on you to record scene findings that explain the mechanism of injury. Be thorough, for instance, in documenting your observations about the vehicle in which a patient rode. Notes about deployment of airbags and the condition of the exterior and the steering wheel will help in the assessment of possible internal injuries.

Penetrating Abdominal Injuries

Patients with penetrating injuries generally have obvious wounds and external bleeding Figure 16-9A . A large wound may have bowel, fat, or a fold of peritoneum protruding from it. In addition to pain, these patients often report nausea and vomiting. Patients with peritonitis generally prefer to lie very still with their legs drawn up because it hurts to move or straighten their legs. They may complain about every bump in the road during transport.

Some penetrating injuries go no deeper than the abdominal wall, but the severity of the injury can be hard to determine. Only a surgeon can accurately assess the damage. Therefore, as you care for a patient with this type of wound, you should assume that the object has penetrated the peritoneum, entered the abdominal cavity, and possibly injured one or more organs, even if there are no immediate obvious signs.

If major blood vessels are cut or solid organs are lacerated, bleeding may be rapid and severe. Other signs of intra-abdominal injuries may develop slowly, particularly in penetrating wounds to hollow organs. Once such an organ is punctured and its contents are discharged into the abdominal cavity, peritonitis may develop, but this may take several hours.

In caring for a patient with a penetrating wound of the abdomen, follow the general procedures previously described for care of a blunt abdominal wound, as well as the following specific steps for the penetrating wound: Inspect the patient's back and sides for exit wounds, and apply a dry, sterile dressing to all open wounds. If the penetrating object is still in place, apply bulky dressings around it to control external bleeding and then secure the dressings in place with a stabilizing bandage, which will minimize movement of the object Figure 16-9B .

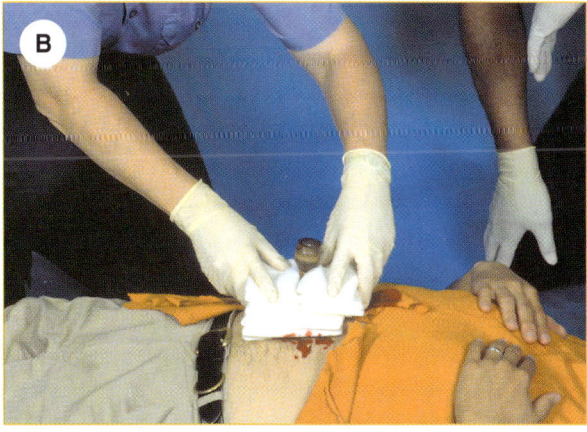

Figure 16-9 **A.** Penetrating injuries have obvious wounds and may also have external bleeding. **B.** If the penetrating object is still in place, use bulky dressings and a roller bandage to stabilize the object and to control bleeding.

Abdominal Evisceration

Severe lacerations of the abdominal wall may result in <u>evisceration</u>, in which internal organs protrude through the wound (Figure 16-10 ◀). Never try to replace an organ that is protruding from an abdominal laceration, whether it is a small fold of peritoneum or nearly all of the intestines. Instead, cover it with sterile gauze compresses moistened with sterile saline solution, and secure them with a dry, sterile dressing. (Protocols in some EMS systems call for an occlusive dressing over the organs, secured by trauma dressings.) Because the open abdomen radiates body heat very effectively and because exposed organs lose fluid rapidly, you must keep the organs moist and warm. If you do not have gauze compresses, you may use moist, sterile dressings, covered and secured in place with a bandage and tape (Figure 16-11 ▼). Do not use any mate-

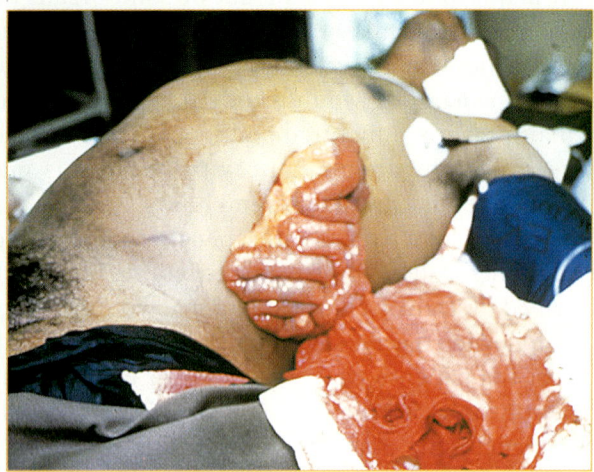

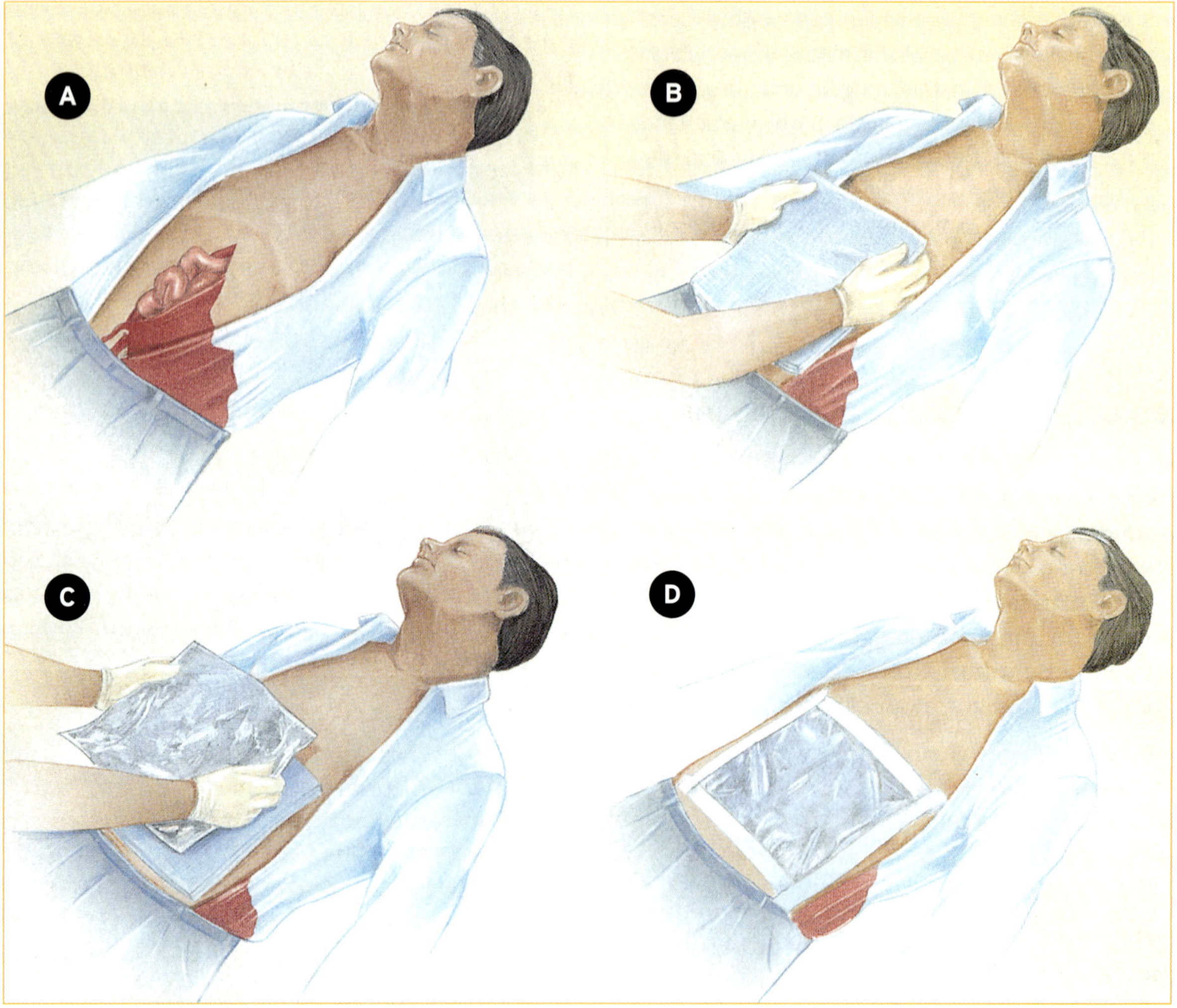

Figure 16-10 An abdominal evisceration is an open abdominal wound from which internal organs protrude.

Figure 16-11 **A.** The open abdomen radiates body heat rapidly and must be covered. **B.** Cover the wound with moistened sterile gauze or with an occlusive dressing, depending on local protocol. **C.** Secure the dressing with a bandage. **D.** Secure the bandage with tape.

rial that is adherent or loses its substance when wet, such as toilet paper, facial tissue, paper towels, or absorbent cotton.

Once you have covered the extruding organ, you should provide other emergency care as necessary and provide prompt transport to the emergency department.

Management of Abdominal Injuries

All patients presenting with trauma-related injuries should be completely immobilized. Tilt the backboard slightly for pregnant patients to take the pressure off of the inferior vena cava. The foot of the board may also be elevated to place the patient in a Trendelenburg position. If there is no suspected spinal trauma involved, the patient may be placed in a position of comfort. High-flow oxygen should also be administered.

Stabilize any impaled objects and cover eviscerations as previously described. Initiate two large-bore intravenous lines (14- or 16-gauge) or follow local protocol, and administer isotonic crystalloid solutions to deliver a 20-mL/kg bolus or the amount needed to maintain radial pulses. Increasing blood pressure can increase internal bleeding, so fluid should be given in a volume to maintain perfusion to vital organs.

Most abdominal trauma requires rapid transport to the closest most appropriate facility. Surgery is often the required definitive care for these patients. Provide emotional and psychological support en route.

Place the patient on the cardiac monitor and consider the use of analgesics for pain.

Anatomy of the Genitourinary System

The genitourinary system controls the reproductive functions and the waste discharge system, which are generally considered together.

The urinary system controls the discharge of certain waste materials filtered from the blood by the kidneys. In the urinary system, the kidneys are solid organs; the ureters, bladder, and urethra are hollow organs (Figure 16-12 ▶).

The genital system controls the reproductive processes from which life is created. The male genitalia, except for the prostate gland and the seminal

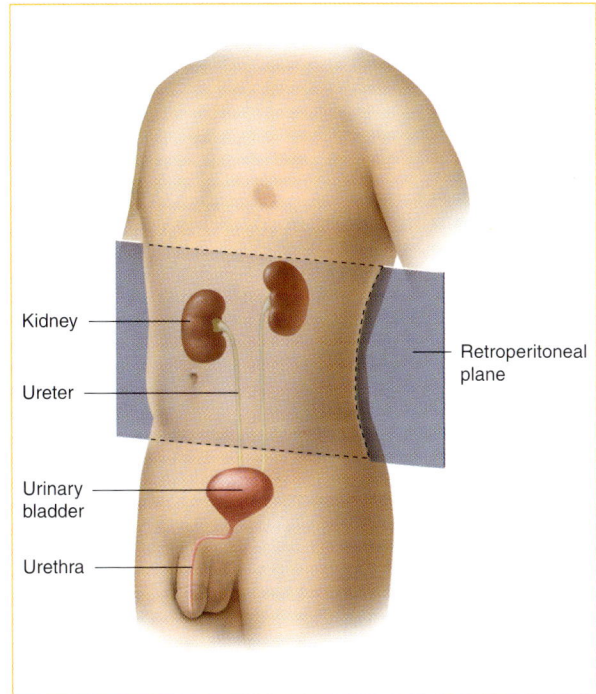

Figure 16-12 The urinary system lies in the retroperitoneal space behind the digestive tract. The kidneys are solid organs; the ureters, bladder, and urethra are hollow organs.

vesicles, lie outside the pelvic cavity (Figure 16-13 ▶). The female genitalia, except for the vulva, clitoris, and labia, are contained entirely within the pelvis (Figure 16-14 ▶). The male and female reproductive organs have certain similarities and, of course, basic differences. They allow for the production of sperm and egg cells and appropriate hormones, the act of intercourse, and, ultimately, reproduction.

Injuries to the Genitourinary System

Injuries to the Kidney

Injuries to the kidney are not unusual and rarely occur in isolation. This is because the kidneys lie in the well-protected retroperitoneal space, which is the area behind the true, or anterior, abdomen. A penetrating wound that reaches the kidneys almost always involves other organs. The same is true with blunt injuries. A blow that is forceful enough to cause significant kidney damage almost always damages other intra-abdominal organs, often fracturing ribs as well. Less significant injuries to the kidneys may result from a direct blow or even from

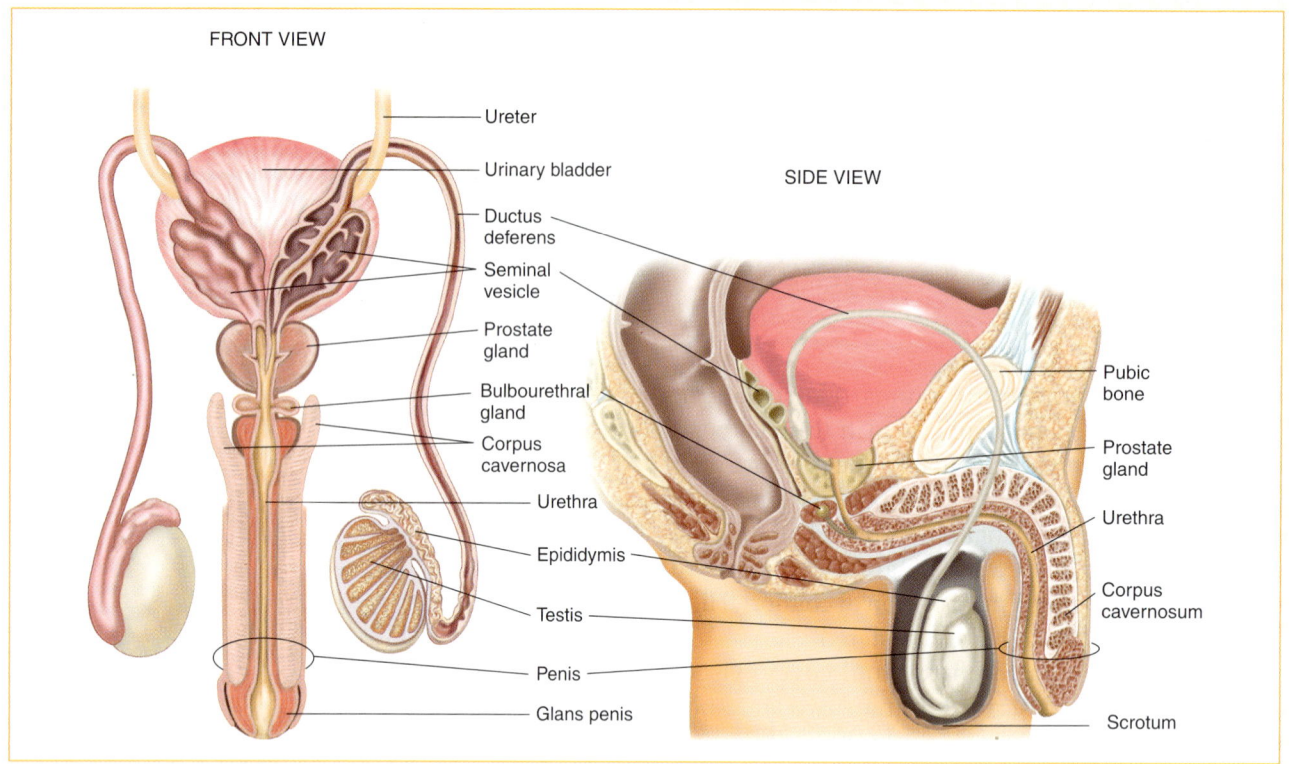

Figure 16-13 The male reproductive system includes the testicles, vas deferens, seminal vesicles, prostate gland, urethra, and penis.

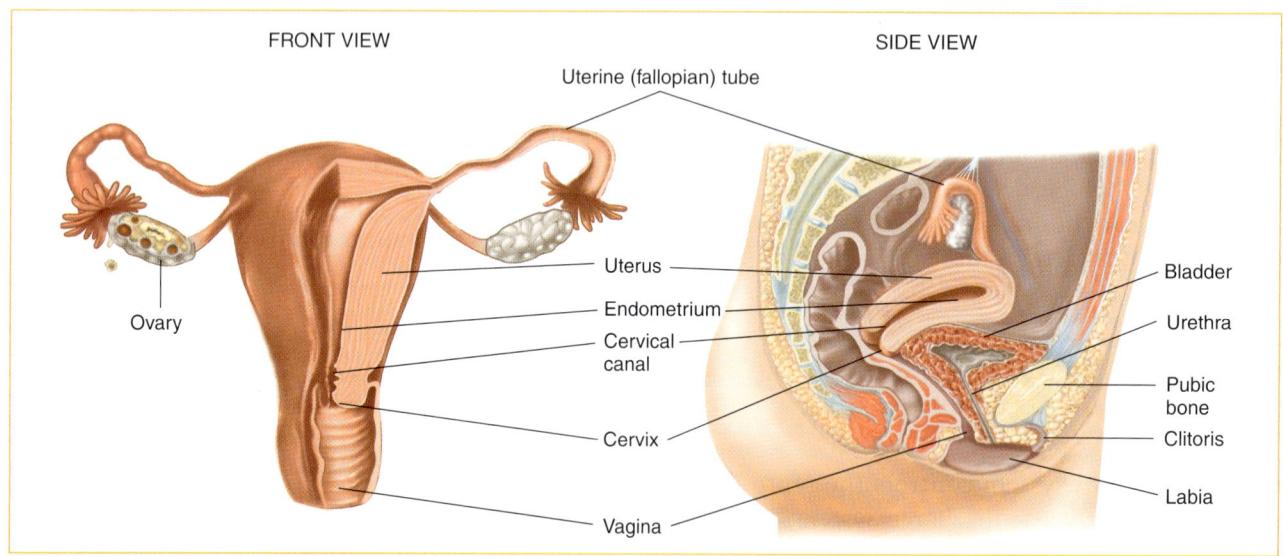

Figure 16-14 The female reproductive system includes the ovaries, fallopian tubes, uterus, cervix, and vagina.

a tackle in football **Figure 16-15** . Suspect kidney damage if the patient has a history or physical evidence of any of the following findings:

- An abrasion, laceration, or contusion to the flank
- A penetrating wound in the region of the lower rib cage (the flank) or the upper abdomen
- Fractures on either side of the lower rib cage or of the lower thoracic or upper lumbar vertebrae

Damage to the kidneys may not be obvious on inspection of the patient. You may or may not see bruises or lacerations on the overlying skin. However, you will see signs of shock if the injury is associated with sig-

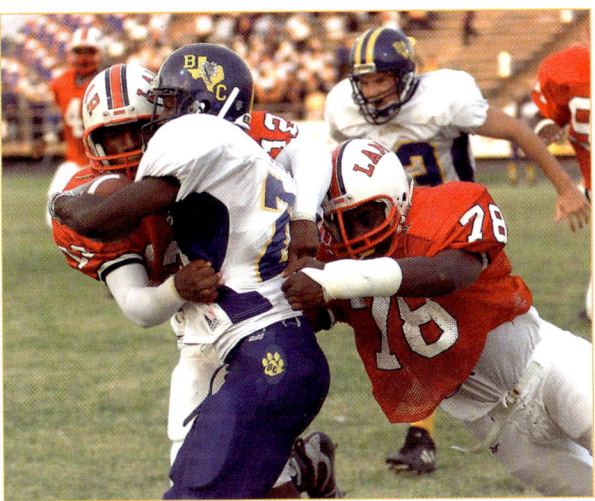

Figure 16-15 A tackle in football that results in blunt trauma to the lower rib cage or the flank can cause kidney injury.

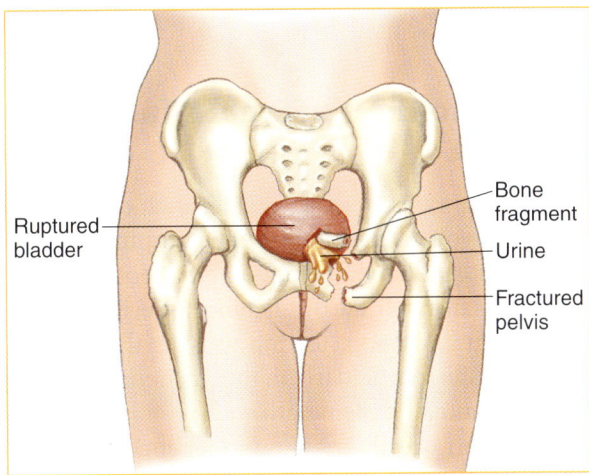

Figure 16-16 Fracture of the pelvis can result in a laceration of the bladder by the bony fragments. Urine then leaks into the pelvis.

nificant blood loss. Because one of the functions of the kidney is the formation of urine, another sign of kidney damage is blood in the urine, called hematuria. Treat shock and associated injuries in the appropriate manner. Provide prompt transport to the hospital, monitoring the patient's vital signs carefully en route.

Injuries to the Urinary Bladder

Injury to the urinary bladder, either blunt or penetrating, may result in its rupture. When this happens, urine spills into the surrounding tissues, and any urine that passes through the urethra is likely to be bloody. Blunt injuries to the lower abdomen or pelvis often cause rupture of the urinary bladder, particularly when the bladder is full and distended. Sharp, bony fragments from a fracture of the pelvis often perforate the urinary bladder Figure 16-16. Penetrating wounds of the lower midabdomen or the perineum (the pelvic floor and associated structures that occupy the pelvic outlet) can directly involve the bladder. In the male, sudden deceleration from a motor vehicle or motorcycle crash can literally shear the bladder from the urethra.

Suspect a possible injury to the urinary bladder if you see blood at the urethral opening or physical signs of trauma on the lower abdomen, pelvis, or perineum. There may be blood at the tip of the penis or a stain on the patient's underwear.

The presence of associated injuries or shock will dictate the urgency of transport. In most instances, pro-

You are the Provider   Part 3

During your rapid trauma assessment, you note tenderness and rigidity to the patient's abdomen. You prepare to transport your patient to the closest trauma center. Just prior to leaving, you obtain the following:

Vital Signs	Recording Time: 5 Minutes After Patient Contact
Respirations	24 breaths/min, regular with adequate depth
Pulse	128 beats/min, thready
Blood pressure	90/62 mm Hg
SaO_2	97% on 100% via nonrebreather mask

5. What are your concerns for this patient?

vide prompt transport, and monitor the patient's vital signs en route.

Injuries to the External Male Genitalia

Injuries to the external male genitalia include all types of soft-tissue wounds. Although these injuries are very painful and generally a source of great concern to the patient, they are rarely life threatening. Especially in industrial accidents, avulsion (tearing away) of the skin of the penis can occur, particularly in the uncircumcised male. If you encounter a patient with such an injury, wrap the penis in a soft, sterile dressing moistened with sterile saline solution, and transport the patient promptly. Use direct pressure to control any bleeding. You should try to save and preserve the avulsed skin, but do not delay treatment or transport for more than a few minutes to do so.

Managing blood loss is your top priority in amputation of the penile shaft, whether partial or complete. You should use local pressure with a sterile dressing on the remaining stump. Never apply a constricting device to the penis to control bleeding. Surgical reconstruction of even a completely amputated penis is possible if you can locate the amputated part. Wrap it in a moist, sterile dressing; place it in a plastic bag; and transport it in a cooled container without allowing it to come in direct contact with ice.

If the connective tissue surrounding the erectile tissue in the penis is severely damaged, the shaft of the penis can be fractured or severely angled, sometimes requiring surgical repair. The injury may occur during particularly active sexual intercourse. It is associated with intense pain, bleeding into the tissues, and fear. Provide prompt transport to the emergency department.

Accidental laceration of the skin about the head of the penis usually occurs when the penis is erect and is associated with heavy bleeding. The injury usually appears worse than it actually is; once the penis becomes flaccid, the size of the laceration decreases. Local pressure with a sterile dressing is usually sufficient to stop the hemorrhage.

It is not uncommon for the skin of the shaft of the penis or the foreskin to get caught in the zipper of pants. If a small segment of the zipper is involved (one or two teeth), you can try to unzip the pants. If a longer segment is involved or the patient is agitated, use heavy scissors to cut the zipper out of the pants to make the patient more comfortable during transport. Explain all procedures to alert patients. This reduces anxiety in an already stressful situation.

If the patient is hemodynamically stable, consider administering analgesia such as morphine sulfate.

Urethral injuries in the male are uncommon. Lacerations of the urethra can result from straddle injuries, pelvic fractures, or penetrating wounds of the perineum. These injuries may bleed quite severely, although this may not be evident externally. Direct pressure with a dry, sterile dressing usually controls any external hemorrhage. Because the urethra is the channel for urine, it is very important to know whether the patient can urinate and whether hematuria is present. For this reason, you should save any voided urine for later examination at the hospital. Any foreign bodies that may be protruding from the urethra will have to be removed in a surgical setting.

Avulsion of the skin of the scrotum may damage the scrotal contents. If possible, preserve the avulsed skin in a moist, sterile dressing for possible use in reconstruction. Wrap the scrotal contents or the perineal area with a sterile, moist compress, and use a local pressure dressing to control bleeding. Transport this patient promptly to the emergency department.

Direct blows to the scrotum can result in the rupture of a testicle or significant accumulation of blood around the testes. In either case, you should apply an ice pack to the scrotal area while transporting the patient.

A few general rules apply to the treatment of injuries involving the external male genitalia:

- These injuries are very painful. Make the patient as comfortable as possible.
- Use sterile, moist compresses to cover areas that have been stripped of skin.
- Apply direct pressure with dry, sterile gauze dressings to control bleeding.
- Never move or manipulate impaled instruments or foreign bodies in the urethra.
- If possible, always identify and take avulsed parts to the hospital with the patient.

Remember, these are rarely life-threatening injuries and should not be given priority over other, more severe wounds.

Injuries to the Female Genitalia

Internal Female Genitalia

The uterus, ovaries, and fallopian tubes are subject to the same kinds of injuries as any other internal organ. However, they are rarely damaged because they are small, deep in the pelvis, and well protected by the pelvic bones. Unlike the bladder, which lies adjacent to the bony pelvis, they are usually not injured in a pelvic fracture.

An exception is the pregnant uterus. As pregnancy progresses, the uterus enlarges substantially and rises out of the pelvis, becoming vulnerable to both penetrating and blunt injuries. These injuries can be particularly severe because the uterus has a rich blood supply during pregnancy. You must also keep in mind that another life—that of the unborn child—is at risk. You can expect to see the signs and symptoms of shock with these patients; be prepared to provide all necessary support and prompt transport. Note that contractions may begin as well. If possible, ask the patient when she is due, and report this information to the hospital.

In the last trimester of pregnancy, the uterus is large and may obstruct the inferior vena cava, decreasing the amount of blood returning to the heart, if the patient is placed in a supine position (supine hypotensive syndrome). As a result, blood pressure may decrease. The patient should be carefully placed on her left side so that the uterus will not lie on the vena cava. If the patient is secured to a backboard, tilt the board to the left.

External Female Genitalia

The external female genitalia include the vulva, the clitoris, and the major and minor labia (lips) at the entrance of the vagina. Injuries to the external female genitalia can include all types of soft-tissue injuries. Because these genital parts have a rich nerve supply, injuries are very painful. Lacerations, abrasions, and avulsions should be treated with moist, sterile compresses. Use local pressure to control bleeding and a diaper-type bandage to hold dressings in place. Under no circumstances should you pack or place dressings into the vagina. Leave any foreign bodies in place, and stabilize them with bandages.

If the patient is hemodynamically stable, consider administering analgesia such as morphine sulfate.

In general, although these injuries are painful, they are not life threatening. Bleeding may be heavy, but it can usually be controlled by local compression. Contusions and other blunt injuries all require careful in-hospital evaluation. However, the urgency of the need for transport will be determined by associated injuries, the amount of hemorrhage, and the presence of shock.

Remember that victims of sexual assault, whether they are male or female, need medical assistance. In these cases, you must treat the patient's injuries but also provide privacy, support, and reassurance.

You are the Provider — Summary

1. What are the two types of abdominal injuries likely to be encountered in the prehospital setting?

Closed abdominal injuries and open abdominal injuries are encountered. Closed abdominal injuries are those in which a severe blow damages the abdomen without breaking the skin; these are also known as blunt injuries. Open abdominal injuries are those in which a foreign object enters the abdomen and opens the peritoneal cavity to the outside; these are also known as penetrating injuries.

2. What is one principal complaint that patients with abdominal injuries generally have?

Pain is a principal complaint.

3. What is your first step in the management of this patient?

Administer 100% oxygen by nonrebreathing mask.

4. What is the most common sign of significant abdominal injury?

Tachycardia is the most common sign.

5. What are your concerns for this patient?

Many abdominal emergencies, aside from those that cause severe bleeding, can cause a rapid pulse and low blood pressure, leading to shock. Your record of vital signs, made as early as possible and periodically thereafter, will help physicians in evaluating the problem when the patient arrives in the emergency department. While en route to the hospital, initiate at least one large bore IV of an isotonic crystalloid and administer 20 mL/kg boluses as needed to maintain adequate perfusion.

Prep Kit

Ready for Review

- Abdominal injuries are classified as open (penetrating) or closed (blunt). Either type can damage hollow organs, such as the stomach and bladder, and solid organs, such as the liver, spleen, and kidneys.
- Penetrating injuries are most frequently caused by knives or handguns; blunt injuries are often the result of a collision with a steering wheel. Both types of injury cause pain, although this may be masked at first.
- These injuries are evaluated in a similar manner. Place the patient in a supine position, assess and record vital signs, and perform a visual inspection. Always assume that major damage has occurred to abdominal organs, even if there are no obvious signs.
- Look for bruises or other marks that may point you toward underlying damage: a firm abdomen, difficulty moving, abdominal tenderness and guarding, obvious entry and exit wounds, and altered vital signs.
- If hollow organs have spilled their contents into the peritoneal cavity, peritonitis will develop. In an effort to minimize the pain of this condition, patients will want to lie still with their knees drawn up.
- Treat for shock as necessary, keep the airway clear of vomitus, keep the patient warm, and promptly transport him or her to the emergency department.
- Never try to replace an eviscerated organ; keep it warm and moist with sterile gauze compresses.
- Establish intravenous access and administer fluid at a rate to maintain radial pulses. Do not attempt to increase the blood pressure above 90 mm Hg because it may increase internal bleeding.
- Injuries to the kidneys or bladder will not have obvious external signs, but there are usually more subtle clues such as lower rib pain or a possible pelvic fracture.
- The external genitalia in both males and females can sustain injuries that can be extremely painful, but these are rarely life threatening.

Vital Vocabulary

closed abdominal injury An injury to the abdomen caused by a nonpenetrating instrument or force, in which the skin remains intact; also called blunt abdominal injury.

evisceration The displacement of organs outside of the body.

guarding Contracting the stomach muscles to minimize the pain of abdominal movement; a sign of peritonitis.

hematuria The presence of blood in the urine.

hollow organs Structures through which materials pass, such as the stomach, small intestines, large intestines, ureters, and bladder.

open abdominal injury An injury to the abdomen caused by a penetrating or piercing instrument or force, in which the skin is lacerated or perforated and the cavity is opened to the atmosphere; also called penetrating injury.

peritoneal cavity The abdominal cavity.

peritonitis Inflammation of the peritoneum.

solid organs Solid masses of tissue where much of the chemical work of the body takes place (for example, the liver, spleen, pancreas, and kidneys).

supine hypotensive syndrome A drop in blood pressure caused when the heavy uterus of a supine, third-trimester pregnant patient obstructs the vena cava, lowering blood return to the heart.

Technology

- Interactivities
- Vocabulary Explorer
- Anatomy Review
- Web Links
- Online Review Manual

Assessment in Action

You are dispatched to an industrial site for a patient who is vomiting. You find a 30-year-old man on a bench in a lunchroom in the fetal position. A garbage can is positioned next to him.

You immediately notice that he is pale, diaphoretic, and lying very still. He tells you that his pain started about 30 minutes ago and that he has vomited twice. His airway is clear.

1. What treatment, if any, is indicated at this point?
   A. Administration of oxygen
   B. Suctioning of the airway
   C. Sitting him up in case he vomits again
   D. No treatment is needed

2. What may be causing this patient's symptoms?
   A. Abdominal injury
   B. Heat exhaustion
   C. Food poisoning
   D. All of the above

3. Which of the following would NOT be an important question to ask?
   A. Have you been in any accidents lately?
   B. What kind of environment have you been working in today?
   C. Have you ever had food poisoning?
   D. Do you have any medical problems?

When asked about recent trauma, the patient states: "No, nothing. Almost though. Luckily I had my safety belt on." When questioned further the patient explains that he slipped and fell off of a scaffolding earlier but was caught by his safety belt, which had a 4' safety line. He says nothing hurt at that time. Your assessment reveals a bruise to the lateral aspect of the right upper quadrant, slight abdominal distention, and pain on palpation of both upper quadrants of the abdomen.

4. On the basis of this new information, what is the most likely explanation for the patient's condition?
   A. Shock
   B. Pelvic fracture
   C. Head injury
   D. Kidney injury

5. The patient's injury can be described as:
   A. closed abdominal injury to a hollow organ.
   B. closed abdominal injury to a solid organ.
   C. open abdominal injury to a hollow organ.
   D. open abdominal injury to a solid organ.

6. The organs most likely to have been injured in the patient's fall are the:
   A. spleen, appendix, kidney.
   B. appendix, stomach, colon.
   C. intestines, gallbladder, bladder.
   D. liver, spleen, spinal cord.

7. Other shock-related signs and symptoms that the patient may display include:
   A. bradycardia.
   B. hypertension.
   C. elevated respirations.
   D. warm, moist skin.

8. Your assessment of the patient will include:
   A. palpating the abdomen.
   B. observing the patient's position.
   C. assessing vital signs frequently.
   D. all of the above.

9. Your treatment of the patient will include:
   A. spinal immobilization.
   B. applying ice to the bruise.
   C. initiating a small-bore IV.
   D. giving him water to drink.

Points to Ponder

You respond to a residence for a patient with abdominal pain. You find a 16-year-old girl lying in bed complaining of severe abdominal pain, nausea, and vomiting. She is somewhat pale and moist, pulse is weak and respirations are rapid and shallow. Her mother indicates that the patient has no medical history.

What questions will you ask the patient? What assessment procedures will you conduct? What are some possible explanations for the patient's symptoms?

Issues: Appropriate Questions for Female Patients with Abdominal Pain, Physical Exam Procedures for Abdominal Pain

Head and Spine Injuries

1999 Objectives

Cognitive

None

Affective

None

Psychomotor

4-5.16 Demonstrate a clinical assessment to determine the proper management modality for a patient with a suspected traumatic spinal injury. (p 768)

4-5.17 Demonstrate a clinical assessment to determine the proper management modality for a patient with a suspected non-traumatic spinal injury. (p 768)

4-5.18 Demonstrate immobilization of the urgent and non-urgent patient with assessment findings of spinal injury from the following presentations:
    a. Supine
    b. Prone
    c. Semi-prone
    d. Sitting
    e. Standing (p 771, 773, 774)

4-5.19 Demonstrate preferred methods for stabilization of a helmet from a potentially spine injured patient. (p 788)

4-5.20 Demonstrate helmet removal techniques. (p 790)

4-5.21 Demonstrate alternative methods for stabilization of a helmet from a potentially spine injured patient. (p 788)

4-5.22 Demonstrate documentation of assessment before spinal immobilization. (p 768)

4-5.23 Demonstrate documentation of assessment during spinal immobilization. (p 771)

4-5.24 Demonstrate documentation of assessment after spinal immobilization. (p 771)

1985 Objectives

1.6.49 Describe how the patient is immobilized on the backboard. (p 771-773)

17

Additional Objectives*

Cognitive

1. State the components of the nervous system (p 762).
2. List the functions of the central nervous system (p 762).
3. Define the structure of the skeletal system as it relates to the nervous system (p 766).
4. Relate mechanism of injury to potential injuries of the head and spine (p 767).
5. Describe the implications of not properly caring for potential spinal injuries (p 767).
6. State the signs and symptoms of a potential spinal injury (p 768).
7. Describe the method of determining if a responsive patient may have a spinal injury (p 768).
8. Relate the airway emergency medical care techniques to the patient with a suspected spinal injury (p 769).
9. Describe how to stabilize the cervical spine (p 770).
10. Discuss indications for sizing and using a cervical spine immobilization device (p 771).
11. Establish the relationship between airway management and the patient with head and spinal injuries (p 769).
12. Describe a method for sizing a cervical spine immobilization device (p 771).
13. Describe how to log roll a patient with a suspected spinal injury (p 771).
14. Describe how to secure a patient to a long spine board (p 771).
15. List instances when a short spine board should be used (p 773).
16. Describe how to immobilize a patient using a short spine board (p 774).
17. Describe the indications for the use of rapid extrication (p 774).
18. State the circumstance when a helmet should be left on the patient (p 788).
19. Discuss the circumstances when a helmet should be removed (p 788).
20. Identify different types of helmets (p 788).
21. Describe the unique characteristics of sports helmets (p 788).
22. Explain the preferred methods to remove a helmet (p 789).
23. Discuss alternative methods for removal of a helmet (p 788).
24. Describe how the patient's head is stabilized to remove the helmet (p 788).
25. Differentiate how the head is stabilized with a helmet compared to without a helmet (p 788).

Affective

26. Explain the rationale for immobilization of the entire spine when a cervical spine injury is suspected (p 767).
27. Explain the rationale for utilizing immobilization methods apart from the straps on the cots (p 767).
28. Explain the rationale for utilizing a short spine immobilization device when moving a patient from the sitting to the supine position (p 771).
29. Explain the rationale for utilizing rapid extrication approaches only when they indeed will make the difference between life and death (p 773).
30. Defend the reasons for leaving a helmet in place for transport of a patient (p 788).
31. Defend the reasons for removal of a helmet prior to transport of a patient (p 788).

*These are noncurriculum objectives.

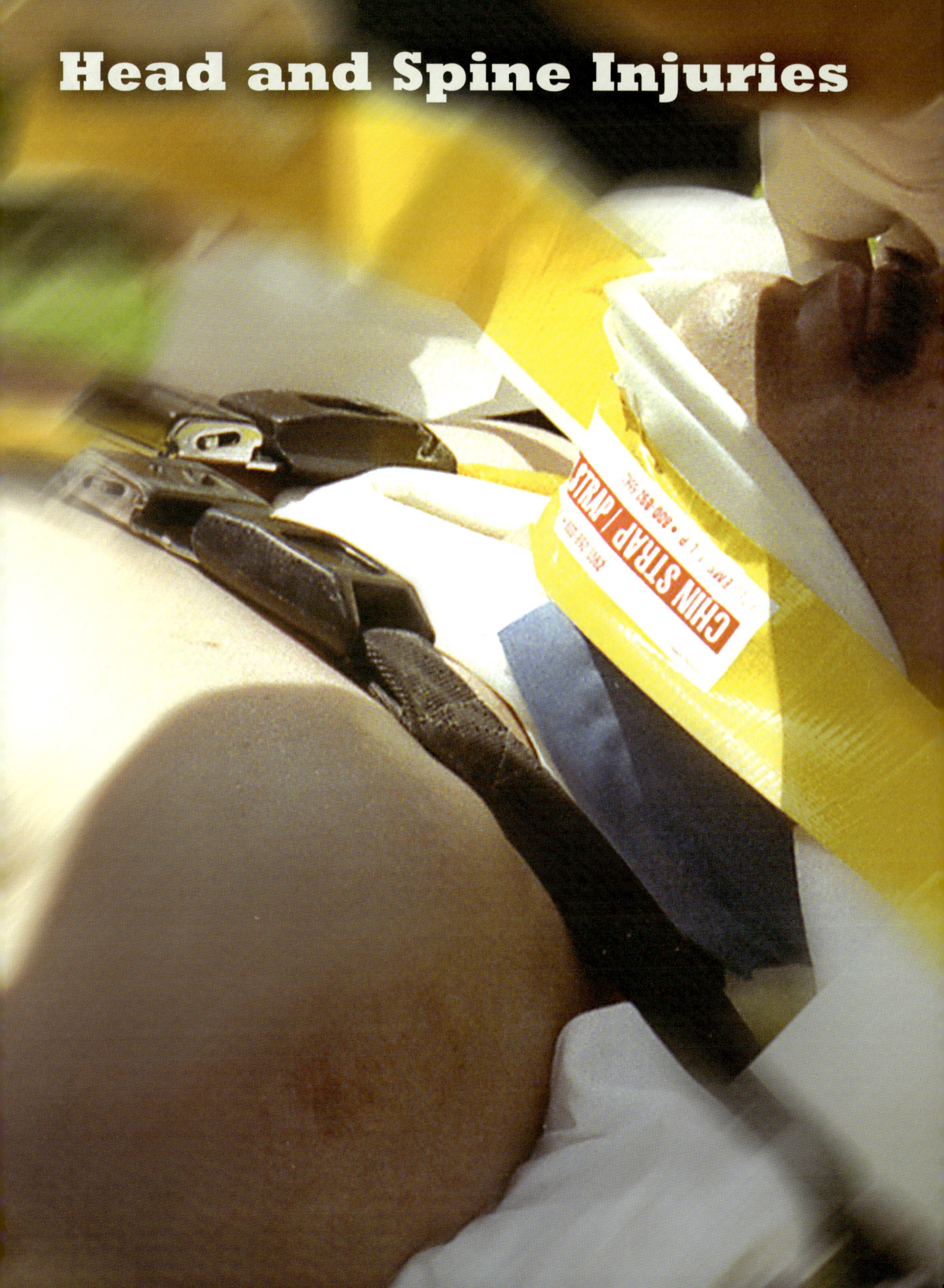

Head and Spine Injuries

17

Head and Spine Injuries

You are the Provider

You are dispatched for an injured person at a local park. On arrival you are met by an individual who tells you that a young man has crashed his all-terrain vehicle (ATV) into a tree about 25 yards down a gravel path. With body substance isolation (BSI) precautions in place, you and your partner gather your airway and trauma equipment and proceed to the patient. As you approach the patient, you see him lying supine on the gravel, not moving.

This chapter will help prepare you to properly care for patients with suspected head and spine injuries and help you answer the following questions:

1. What are the three major areas of the brain?
2. What mechanisms of injury are likely to cause head and spinal cord injuries?

Head and Spine Injuries

The nervous system is a complex network of nerve cells that enables all parts of the body to function. It includes the brain, spinal cord, and peripheral nervous system, which contains several billion nerve fibers that carry information to and from all parts of the body. Because the nervous system is so vital, it is well protected. The brain lies within the skull, and the spinal cord is inside the bony spinal canal. Despite this protection, serious blows can damage the nervous system.

This chapter first briefly reviews the anatomy and function of the central and peripheral nervous systems and of the skeletal system, information that you will need to make an accurate assessment of injuries to these systems. It then discusses specific head and spinal injuries, including signs, symptoms, and treatment. Extrication of patients with possible spinal injuries and removal of helmets are also described.

Anatomy and Physiology of the Nervous System

The nervous system is divided into two anatomic parts: the central nervous system and the peripheral nervous system (Figure 17-1 ▶). The central nervous system (CNS) consists of the parts of the nervous system that are covered and protected by bones: the brain and the spinal cord. Long fibers link the nerve cells to the body's various organs through openings in the bony coverings. These cables of nerve fibers make up the peripheral nervous system.

Central Nervous System

The CNS is composed of the brain and spinal cord. The brain is the organ that controls the body, the center of consciousness. It is divided into three major areas: the cerebrum, the cerebellum, and the brain stem (Figure 17-2 ▶).

The cerebrum, which comprises about 75% of the brain's total size, controls a wide variety of activities. Inferior and posterior to the cerebrum lies the cerebellum, which coordinates body movements. The most primitive part of the CNS, the brain stem, controls virtually all functions that are necessary for life, including the cardiac and respiratory systems. Deep within the cranium, the brain stem is the best-protected part of the CNS.

The spinal cord, the other major portion of the CNS, is made mostly of fibers that extend from the brain's nerve cells. The spinal cord carries messages between the brain and the body.

Protective Coverings

The cells of the brain and spinal cord are soft and easily injured. Once damaged, they cannot be regenerated or reproduced. Therefore, the entire CNS is contained within a protective framework.

The thick, bony structures of the skull and spinal canal withstand injury very well. The skull is covered by a layer of muscle fascia and, above that, the scalp (a thick vascular layer of skin). The spinal canal, too, is surrounded by a thick layer of skin and muscles.

The CNS is further protected by the meninges, three distinct layers of tissue that suspend the brain and the spinal cord within the skull and the spinal canal (Figure 17-3 ▶). The outer layer, the dura mater, is a tough, fibrous layer that closely resembles leather. This layer forms a sac to contain the CNS, with small openings through which the peripheral nerves exit along the spinal column.

The inner two layers of the meninges, called the arachnoid and the pia mater, are much thinner than the dura mater. They contain the blood vessels that nourish the brain and spinal cord. Both the arachnoid and the pia mater produce cerebrospinal fluid (CSF), which fills the spaces between them and acts as an excellent shock absorber. The brain and spinal cord essentially float in this fluid, buffered from injury.

Technology

- Interactivities
- Vocabulary Explorer
- Anatomy Review
- Web Links
- Online Review Manual

www.EMSzone.com/EMTI

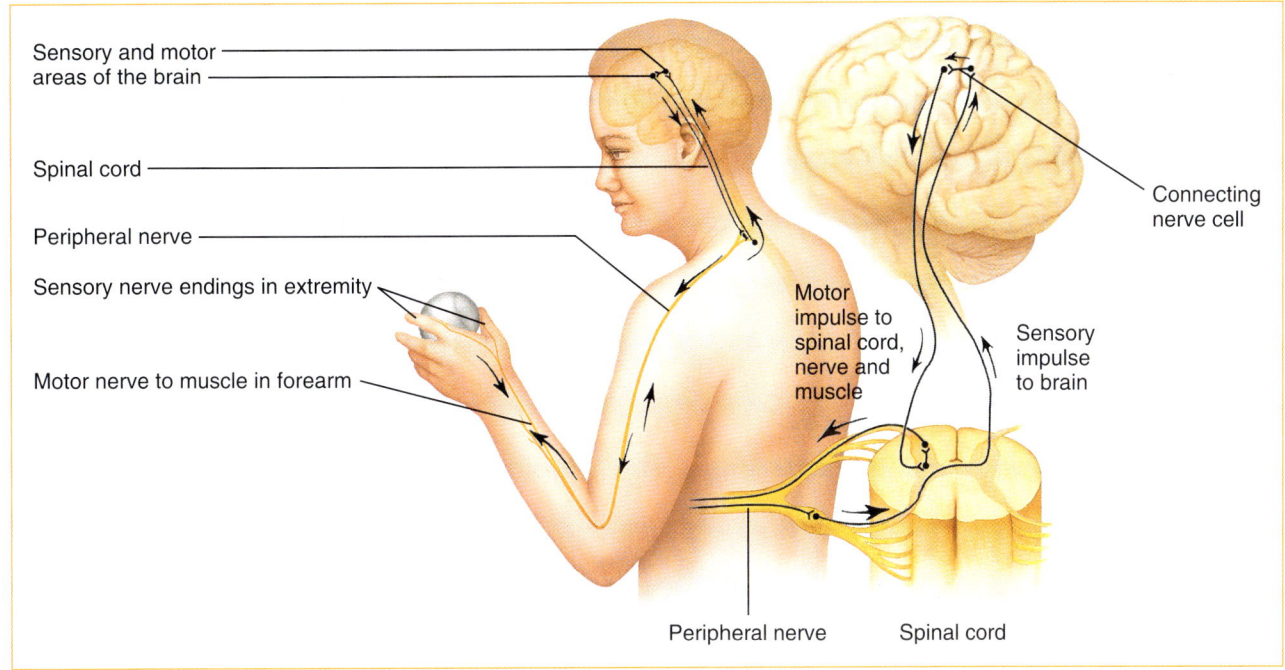

Figure 17-1 The nervous system has two anatomic components: the CNS and the peripheral nervous system. The CNS is composed of the brain and the spinal cord. The peripheral nervous system conducts sensory and motor impulses from the skin and other organs to the spinal cord.

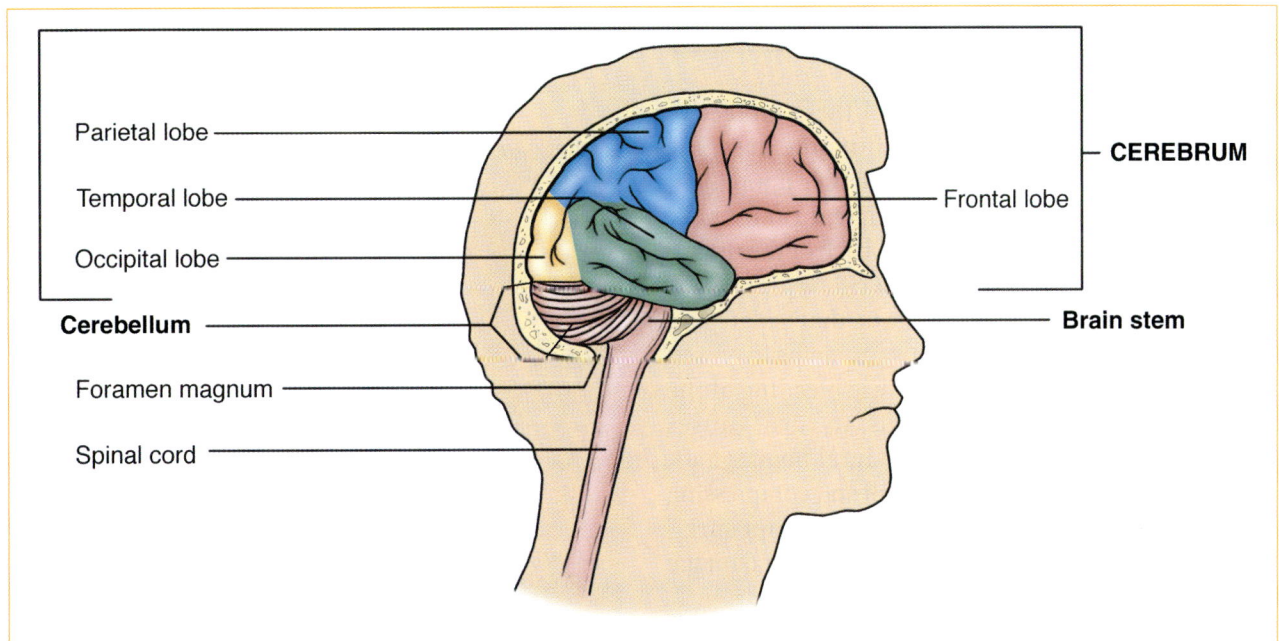

Figure 17-2 The brain is part of the CNS and is the organ that controls all functions of the body. It is divided into three major areas: the cerebrum, the cerebellum, and the brain stem.

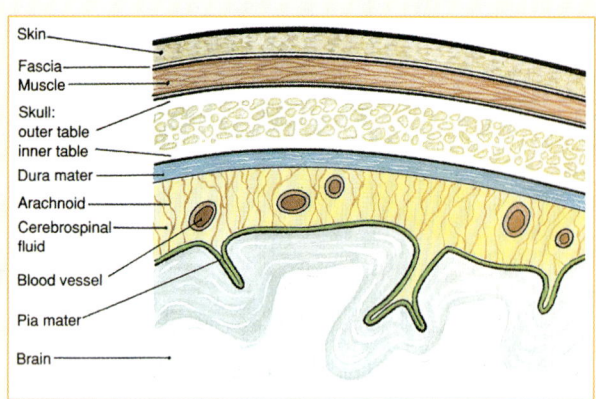

Figure 17-3 The CNS has several layers of protective coverings: the skin, muscles and their fascia, bone, and the meninges. The three layers of the meninges include the dura mater, the arachnoid, and the pia mater.

> **A to Z Terminology Tips**
>
> The tissue known as the *meninges* forms the covering of the brain and spinal cord.
> Remember: the suffix *itis* means "inflammation." Therefore, *meningitis* is an inflammation of the meninges that causes swelling around the brain and spinal cord.

The 31 pairs of spinal nerves conduct sensory impulses from the skin and other organs to the spinal cord. They also conduct motor impulses from the spinal cord to the muscles. Because the arms and legs have so many muscles, the spinal nerves serving the extremities are arranged in complex networks. The brachial plexus controls the arms, and the lumbosacral plexus controls the legs.

Cranial nerves are the 12 pairs of nerves that pass through openings in the skull and transmit sensations directly to or from the brain. For the most part, they perform special functions in the head and face, including sight, smell, taste, hearing, and facial expressions.

There are three major types of peripheral nerves. The <u>sensory nerves</u>, with endings that can perceive only one type of information each, carry information from the body to the brain via the spinal cord. The <u>motor nerves</u>, one for each muscle, carry information from the CNS to the muscles. The <u>connecting nerves</u>, found only in the brain and spinal cord, connect the sensory and motor nerves with short fibers, which allow the cells on either end to exchange messages.

When an injury penetrates all of these protective layers, clear, watery CSF may leak from the nose, the ears, or an open skull fracture. Therefore, if a patient with a head injury has what looks like a runny nose (rhinorrhea) or has a salty taste at the back of the throat, you should assume that the fluid is CSF.

Ironically, the very layers of tissue that isolate and protect the CNS can lead to serious problems in closed head injuries. Severe injury may cause bleeding of the vessels under the dura mater. This, in turn, causes blood to collect in this space (a subdural hematoma), increasing the pressure inside the skull and compressing softer brain tissue. In many cases, only prompt surgical intervention can prevent permanent brain damage or death.

Peripheral Nervous System

The peripheral nervous system has two anatomic parts: 31 pairs of spinal nerves and 12 pairs of cranial nerves ▶ Figure 17-4 ▶.

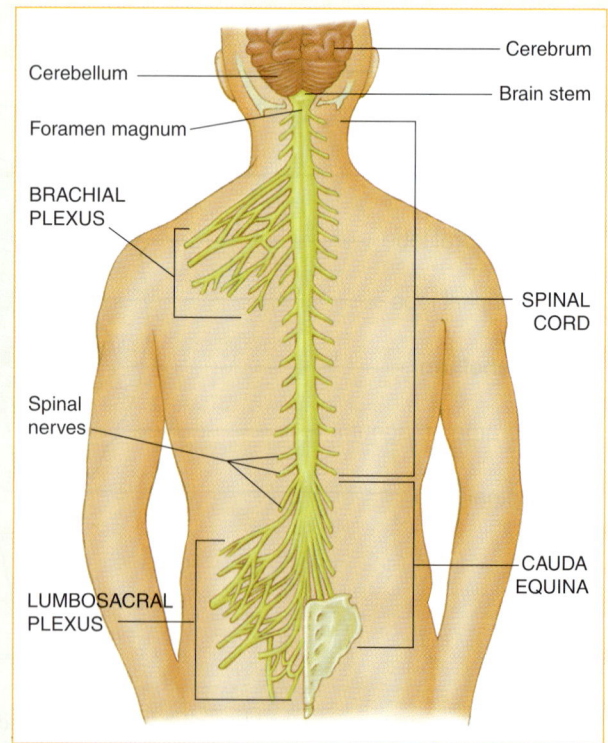

Figure 17-4 The peripheral nervous system is a complex network of motor and sensory nerves. The brachial plexus controls the arms, and the lumbosacral plexus controls the legs.

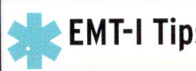

EMT-I Tips

CNS structures, with bony enclosures that protect them quite well, are also very fragile. Protecting them from further damage is vital to the patient's future ability to live a normal life. Lean toward caution and overprotection in assessing and treating possible brain and spinal cord injuries.

How the Nervous System Works

The nervous system controls virtually all of our body's activities, including reflex, voluntary, and involuntary activities.

By connecting the sensory and motor nerves of the limbs, the connecting nerves in the spinal cord form a reflex arc. If a sensory nerve in this arc detects an irritating stimulus, such as heat, it will bypass the brain and send a message directly to the motor nerve (Figure 17-5 ▼).

Voluntary activities are the actions that we consciously perform, in which sensory input determines the specific muscular activity—for example, reaching across the table for a salt shaker or to pass a dish. Involuntary activities are the actions that are not under conscious control, such as breathing; in most instances, we inhale and exhale without consciously thinking about it. Many of our body's functions occur independent of thought, or involuntarily.

The part of the nervous system that regulates or controls our voluntary activities, including almost all coordinated muscular activities, is called the somatic (voluntary) nervous system. The mechanism of the somatic nervous system is simple. The brain interprets the sensory information that it receives from the peripheral nerves and responds by sending signals to the voluntary muscles.

The body functions that occur without conscious effort are regulated by the much more primitive autonomic (involuntary) nervous system. The autonomic nervous system controls the functions of many of the body's vital organs, over which the brain has no voluntary control.

The autonomic nervous system, like so much in our nervous system, is composed of two parts: the sympathetic nervous system and the parasympathetic nervous system. Confronted with a threatening situation, the sympathetic nervous system reacts to the stress with the fight-or-flight response. The parasympathetic nervous system has the opposite effect on the body, causing blood vessels to dilate, slowing the heart rate, and relaxing the muscle sphincters. These two divisions of the autonomic nervous system tend to balance each other so that basic body functions remain stable and effective.

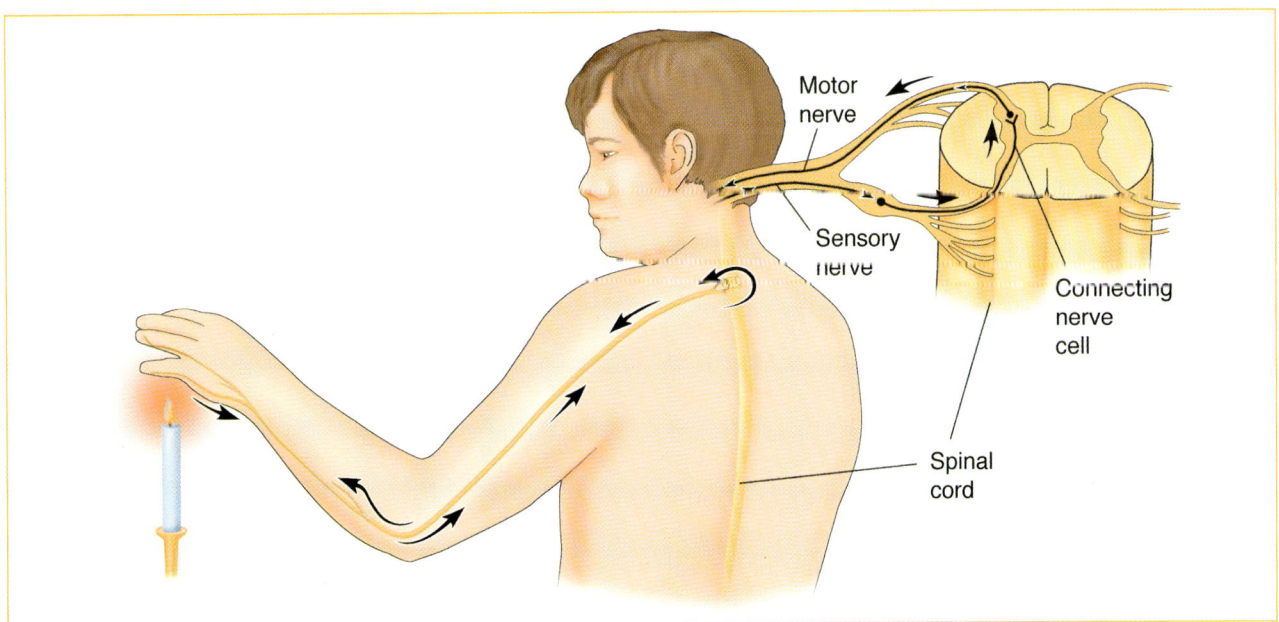

Figure 17-5 The connecting nerves in the spinal cord form a reflex arc. If a sensory nerve in this arc detects an irritating stimulus, it will bypass the brain and send a direct message to the motor nerve.

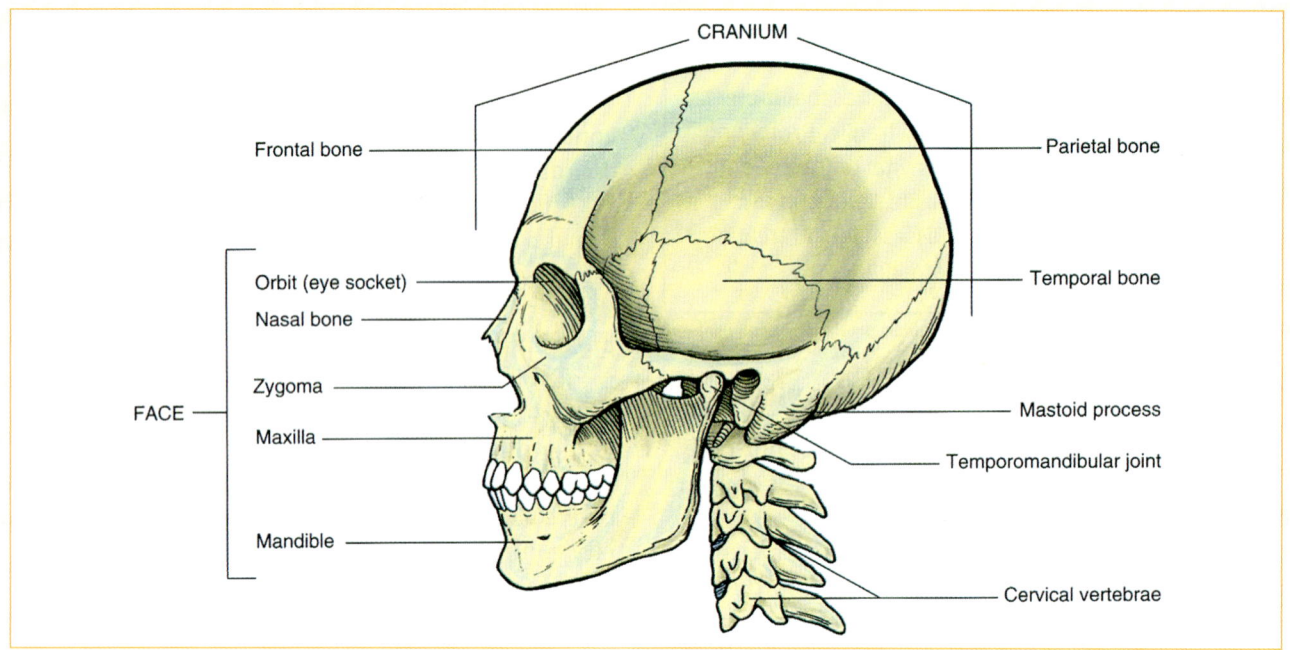

Figure 17-6 The skull has two large structures: the cranium and the face.

Anatomy and Physiology of the Skeletal System

The skull has two layers of bone, the outer and inner tables, which protect the brain. It is divided into two large structures: the cranium and the face Figure 17-6. The mandible (lower jaw), the only movable facial bone, is connected to the cranium by the temporomandibular joint in front of each ear.

The spinal column is the body's central supporting structure. It has 33 bones, called vertebrae, and is divided into five sections: cervical, thoracic, lumbar, sacral, and coccygeal Figure 17-7.

The front part of each vertebra consists of a round, solid block of bone called the "body"; the back part forms a bony arch. From one vertebra to the next, the series of arches forms a tunnel running the length of the spine. This is the spinal canal, which encases and protects the spinal cord Figure 17-8.

The vertebrae are connected by ligaments and separated by cushions, called intervertebral disks. While allowing the trunk to bend forward and back, these ligaments and disks also limit motion so that the spinal cord is not injured. When the spine is injured or fractured, the spinal cord and its nerves are left unprotected. Therefore, until the spine is stabilized, you must keep it aligned as best you can to prevent further injury to the spinal cord. Injury to the spinal cord, depending on the level at which the injury occurs, can result in paralysis.

The spinal column itself is almost entirely surrounded by muscles. However, you can palpate the posterior spinous process of each vertebra, which lies

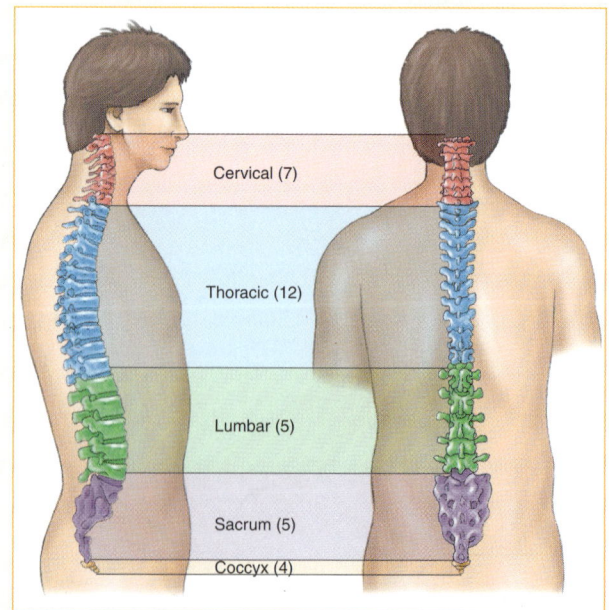

Figure 17-7 The spinal column is the body's central supporting system and consists of 33 bones divided into five sections. Injury to the spinal cord can cause paralysis.

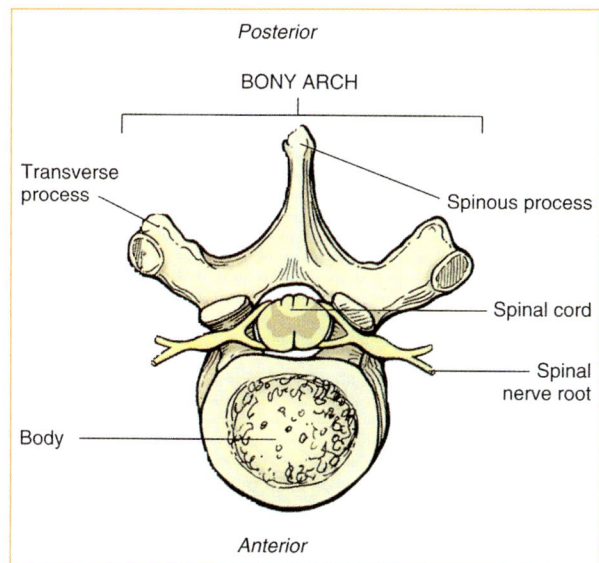

Figure 17-8 The spinal canal is formed by the vertebral body in the front (or anteriorly) and the bony arch in the back (or posteriorly).

just under the skin in the midline of the back. The most prominent and most easily palpable spinous process is at the seventh cervical vertebra at the base of the neck.

Injuries of the Spine

The cervical, thoracic, and lumbar portions of the spine can be injured in a variety of ways. Compression injuries can occur as a result of a fall, regardless of whether the patient landed on his or her feet, coccyx, or, as in diving accidents, the top of the head. Motor vehicle crashes or other types of trauma can overextend, flex, or rotate the spine. Any one of these unnatural motions, as well as excessive lateral bending, can result in fractures and neurologic deficits.

Any time the spine is **distracted**, or pulled along its length, you can expect to find serious injuries to the spine. For example, hangings typically fracture the vertebrae high up in the cervical spine.

Assessment of Spinal Injuries

You should always suspect a possible spinal injury any time you encounter one of the following mechanisms of injury:

- Motor vehicle crashes
- Pedestrian—motor vehicle collisions
- Falls
- Blunt trauma
- Penetrating trauma to the head, neck, or torso
- Motorcycle crashes
- Hangings
- Diving accidents
- Recreational accidents

If a trauma patient is unresponsive and you do not know the mechanism of injury, you should always assume that he or she has a spinal injury. Take great care to avoid any movement that could cause further injury.

In fact, this is the safest approach to any injured patient, responsive or unresponsive. The reason is that complications of spinal cord injuries are serious, often

You are the Provider Part 2

Your partner assumes manual stabilization of the patient's cervical spine as you perform an initial assessment:

Initial Assessment	Recording Time: Zero Minutes
Appearance	Pale and not moving; not wearing a helmet
Level of consciousness	Unresponsive
Airway	Open and clear
Breathing	Respiratory rate, increased; respirations, irregular and shallow
Circulation	Radial pulses, present and normal rate; skin, cool and clammy

3. What is your first consideration in treating this patient?
4. Following initial treatment of this patient, what is your next step?

leading to death or lifelong disability. Examples include respiratory failure resulting from direct injury to the brain stem or upper spinal cord and partial or complete paralysis below the point of injury.

> ### Documentation Tips
>
> Proper care of a patient with a possible spinal injury requires assessment of motor and sensory functions before and after immobilizing the patient. Likewise, careful observation of the level of consciousness at different stages of your care for a head-injured patient provides crucial information. Document your detailed findings of these repeated neurologic exams to help hospital personnel provide effective and timely care and to establish that your care has been thorough and appropriate.

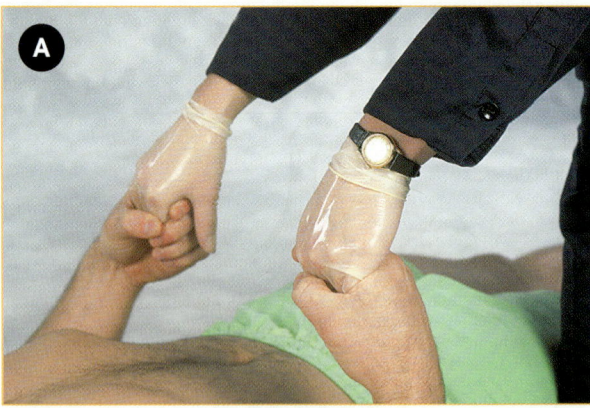

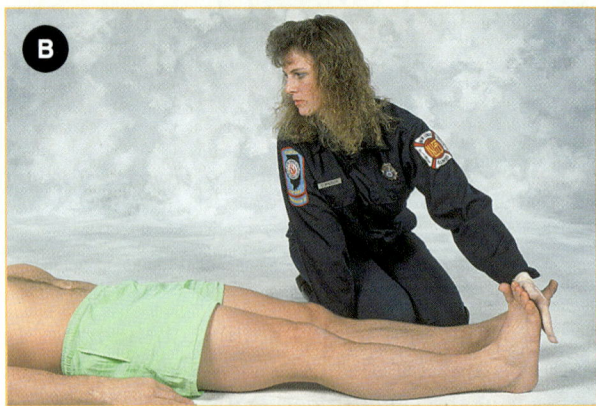

Figure 17-9 **A.** Assess the equality of strength of each extremity by asking the patient to squeeze your hands. **B.** Next, ask the patient to gently push each foot against your hands.

When assessing a patient for possible spinal injury, you should begin with an initial assessment, focusing on the ABCs. If the patient is responsive, make sure you ask about the mechanism of injury and about his or her symptoms, starting with these five questions:

1. Does your neck or back hurt?
2. What happened?
3. Where does it hurt?
4. Can you move your hands and feet?
5. Can you feel me touching your fingers? Your toes?

As part of your focused physical exam, inspect the spinal area for DCAP-BTLS: Deformities, Contusions, Abrasions, Punctures/Penetrations, Burns, Tenderness, Lacerations, and Swelling. Make sure that you do not move any body parts excessively. Determine whether the strength in each extremity is equal by asking the patient to squeeze your hands and to gently push each foot against your hands (Figure 17-9 ▶). Finally, assess the equality of strength of the extremities by comparing the strength in the right limb with that in the left limb.

With unresponsive patients, you should try to identify the mechanism of injury. As part of your assessment, inspect the patient for DCAP-BTLS. First responders, family members, or bystanders may provide helpful information, including when the patient lost consciousness or what his or her previous level of consciousness was.

Remember that the ability to walk, move the extremities, or feel sensation does not rule out a spinal cord injury, nor does an absence of pain. Do not ask patients with possible spinal injuries to move as a test for pain. Instead, instruct them to be still.

However, pain or tenderness when you palpate the spinal area is certainly a warning sign that a spinal injury may exist. Patients with spinal injuries may complain of constant or intermittent pain along the spinal column or in their extremities. A spinal cord injury may also produce pain independent of movement or palpation.

Other signs and symptoms of spinal injury include an obvious deformity as you palpate the spine; numbness, weakness, or tingling in the extremities; and soft-tissue injuries in the spinal region. Patients with severe spinal injury may lose sensation or experience paralysis below the suspected level of injury or be incontinent (Figure 17-10 ▶). Obvious injury to the head and neck may indicate injury to the cervical spine. Injury to the shoulders, back, or abdomen may indicate injury to the thoracic or lumbar spine. Injuries of the lower extremities may indicate associated injuries of the lumbar spine or sacrum.

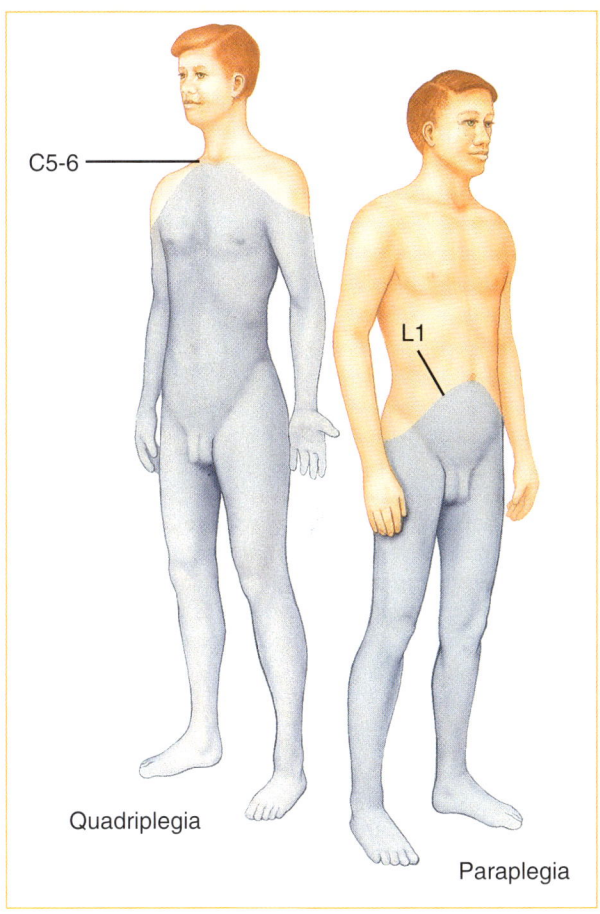

Figure 17-10 With severe spinal injuries, patients may lose sensation or experience paralysis below the suspected level of injury.

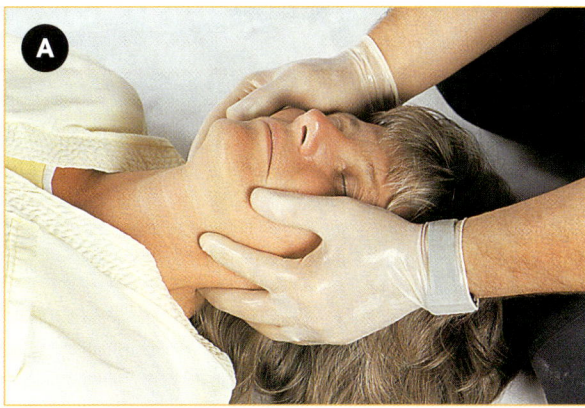
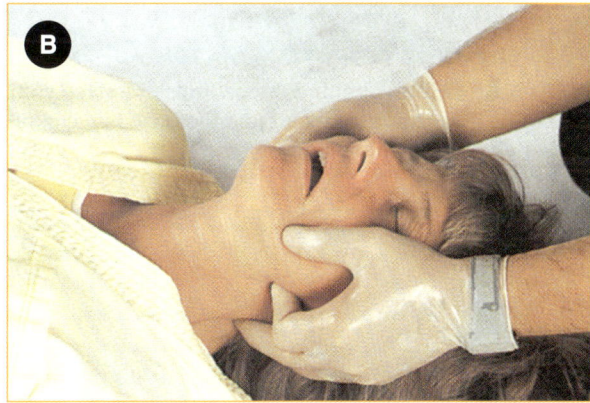

Figure 17-11 Jaw-thrust maneuver. **A.** Stabilize the neck in a neutral, in-line position. **B.** Push the angle of the lower jaw forward.

Emergency Medical Care

Emergency medical care of a patient with a possible spinal injury begins, as does all patient care, with your protection; therefore, you must remember to follow BSI precautions. Next, you must maintain the airway in the proper position, assess respirations, and provide supplemental oxygen or ventilatory support as needed.

Managing the Airway

Knowing that improper handling of a spinal injury can leave a patient permanently paralyzed should not paralyze you in the presence of an airway obstruction. Remember, all patients without a patent airway will die. If a patient with a spinal injury has an airway obstruction, you should perform the jaw-thrust maneuver to open the airway **Figure 17-11**. Do not use the head tilt–chin lift maneuver because it extends the neck and may further damage the cervical spine. If the patient is unresponsive, you can lift or pull the tongue forward so that you do not have to move the neck. Once the airway is open, hold the head still, in a neutral, in-line position, until it can be fully immobilized.

After you open the airway, consider inserting an oropharyngeal airway. If you do so, be sure to monitor the airway closely and have a suctioning unit available because you will often need to clear away blood, saliva, or vomitus. Give oxygen to any patient who is having trouble breathing or has altered mental status and be prepared to assist ventilation if the patient has an inadequate tidal volume.

If you cannot open the airway because of the position of the head, gently and carefully realign the neck. Firmly grasp the patient's head with both hands, pull the head gently and firmly away from the trunk, and turn the face toward the front. Maintain the head in this position while you or your partner repeats the jaw-thrust maneuver.

Skill Drill 17-1

Performing Manual In-Line Stabilization

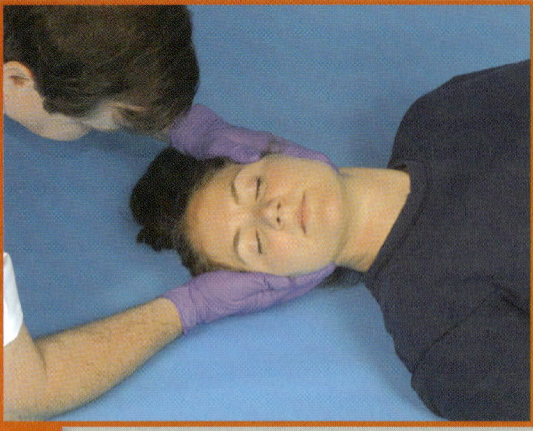

1 Kneel behind the patient, and place your hands firmly around the base of the skull on either side.

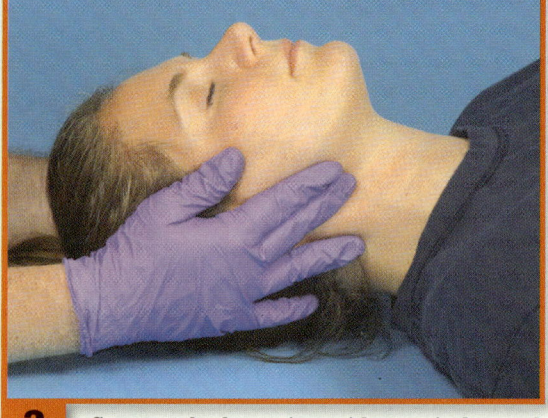

2 Support the lower jaw with your index and long fingers and the head with your palms. Gently move the head into a neutral position, aligned with the torso. Do not move the head or neck excessively.

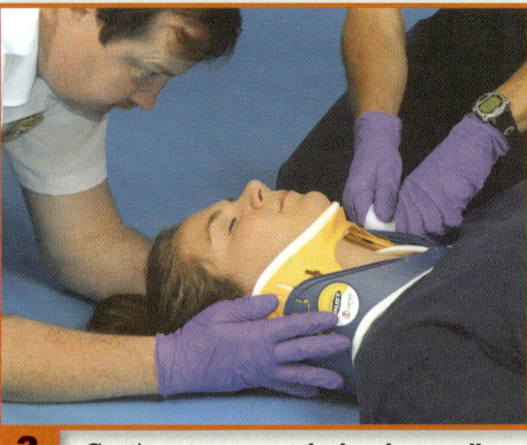

3 Continue to support the head manually while your partner places a rigid cervical collar around the neck. Maintain manual support until the patient is secured to a backboard.

Stabilization of the Cervical Spine

Stabilizing the airway is your first priority. You must then stabilize the head and trunk so that potentially fractured bone fragments of the spine do not cause further damage. Even small movements can significantly injure the spinal cord. Follow the steps in **Skill Drill 17-1**:

1. **Begin manual in-line stabilization** by holding the head firmly with both hands. Whenever possible, kneel behind the patient, and place your hands around the base of the skull on either side (**Step 1**).

2. **Support the lower jaw** with your index and long fingers, while you are supporting the head with your palms. Then gently move the head until the patient's eyes are looking straight ahead and the head and torso are in line. This neutral **eyes-forward position** makes stabilization easier. Align the nose with the navel. Never twist, flex, or extend the head or neck excessively (**Step 2**).

3. **Manually maintain this position** as you continue to maintain the airway. Have your partner place a rigid cervical collar around the neck

to provide more stability. Do not remove your hands from the patient's head until the patient is properly secured to a backboard and the head is immobilized. The patient must remain immobilized until he or she is examined at the hospital (**Step 3**).

Once the patient's head and neck are manually immobilized, assess the pulse, motor functions, and sensation in all extremities. Then assess the cervical spine area and neck. Keep in mind that the cervical collar (also called a c-collar) is used to provide increased stability to the neck. It is used in addition to, not instead of, manual cervical spine (also called c-spine) immobilization. An improperly fitting collar will do more harm than good. If you do not have the proper size, place a rolled towel around the head, and tape it to the backboard as you immobilize the patient on the board. In any case, maintain manual support until the patient is fully secured to a backboard.

There are some situations in which you should not force the head into a neutral, in-line position. Do not move the head if any of the following exist:

- Muscle spasms in the neck
- Increased pain with movement
- Numbness, tingling, or weakness
- Compromised airway or ventilation

In these situations, immobilize the patient in the position in which you found him or her.

Preparation for Transport

Supine Patients

A patient who is supine can be effectively immobilized by securing him or her to a long backboard. The ideal procedure for moving a patient from the ground to a backboard is the <u>four-person log roll</u>. This procedure is recommended any time you suspect a spinal injury. In other cases, you may choose instead to slide the patient onto a backboard or use a scoop stretcher. The patient's condition, the scene, and the available resources, will dictate the method you choose.

You should first take the necessary BSI precautions and then direct the team from a kneeling position by the patient's head so that you can maintain manual in-line immobilization. Your job is to ensure that the head, torso, and pelvis move as a unit, with your teammates controlling the movement of the body. If necessary, you may recruit bystanders to the team, but be sure to instruct them fully before moving the patient. To immobilize a patient on a backboard, follow the steps in **Skill Drill 17-2** ▶:

1. **Maintain in-line stabilization** from a kneeling position at the patient's head. This EMT-I directs all patient movement.
2. **Assess pulse, motor, and sensory function** in each extremity (**Step 1**).
3. **Apply an appropriately sized cervical collar** (**Step 2**).
4. **The other team members** should position the immobilization device (backboard) and place their hands on the far side of the patient to increase their leverage. Instruct them to use their body weight and their shoulder and back muscles to ensure a smooth, coordinated pull, concentrating their pull on the heavier portions of the patient's body (**Step 3**).
5. **On command** from the EMT-I at the head, the rescuers roll the patient toward themselves. One rescuer quickly examines the back while the patient is rolled on the side, then slides the backboard behind and under the patient. The team rolls the patient back onto the board, avoiding rotating the head, shoulders, and pelvis (**Step 4**).
6. **Ensure that the patient is centered** on the board (**Step 5**).
7. **Secure the upper torso** to the board once the patient is centered on the backboard (**Step 6**).
8. **Secure the pelvis and upper legs**, using padding as needed. For the pelvis, use straps over the iliac crests and/or groin loops (leg straps) (**Step 7**).
9. **Begin to immobilize the head to the board** by positioning a commercial immobilization device or towel rolls (**Step 8**).
10. **Secure the head by taping** the head-immobilization device, or towels, across the forehead. To prevent airway problems and leave access to the airway, do not tape over the throat or chin. Instead, tape across the cervical collar just under the chin without covering the opening, allowing visual access to the neck (**Step 9**).
11. **Check and readjust straps** as needed to ensure that the entire body is snugly secured and will not slide during movement of the board or patient transport.
12. **Reassess pulse, motor, and sensory function** in each extremity, and continue to do so periodically (**Step 10**).

Immobilizing a Patient to a Long Backboard

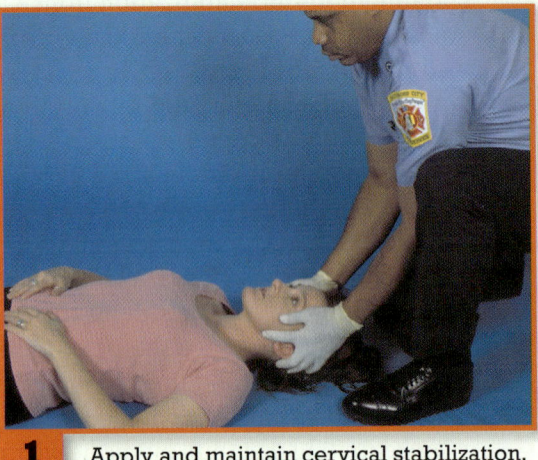

1 Apply and maintain cervical stabilization. Assess distal functions in all extremities.

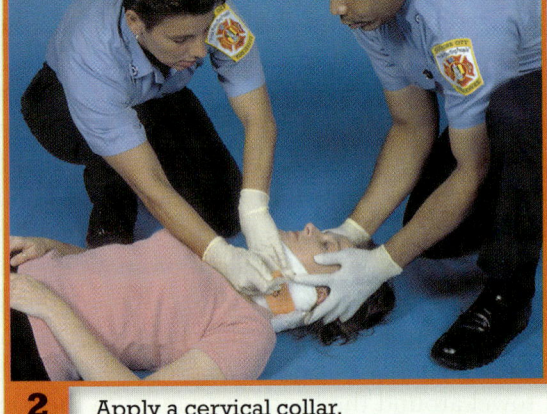

2 Apply a cervical collar.

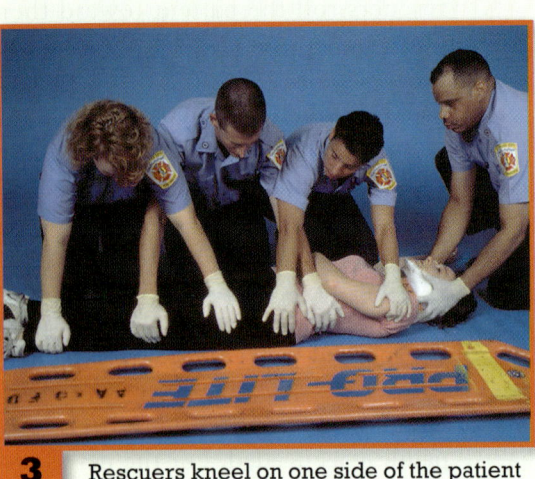

3 Rescuers kneel on one side of the patient and place hands on the far side of the patient.

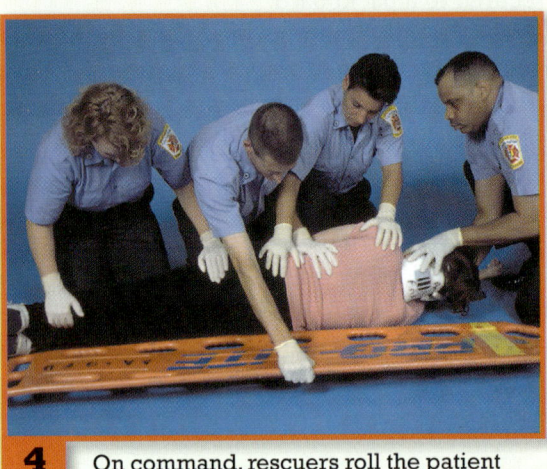

4 On command, rescuers roll the patient toward themselves, quickly examine the back, slide the backboard under the patient, and roll the patient onto the board.

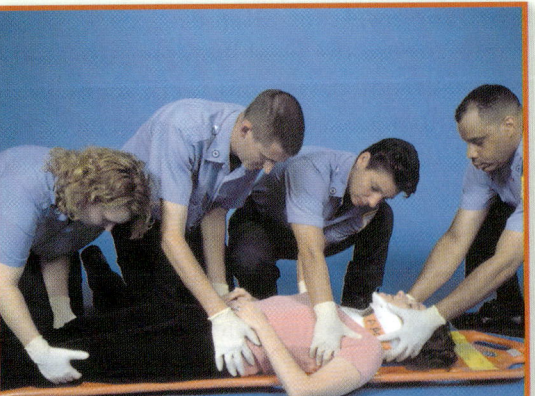

5 Center the patient on the board.

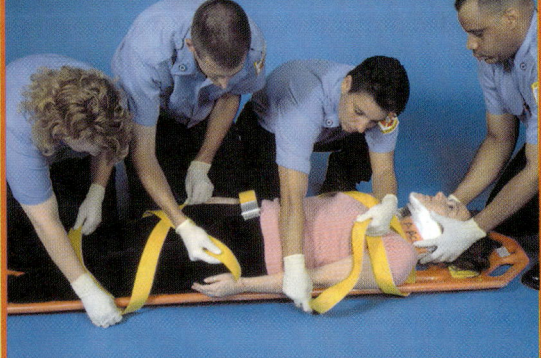

6 Secure the upper torso first.

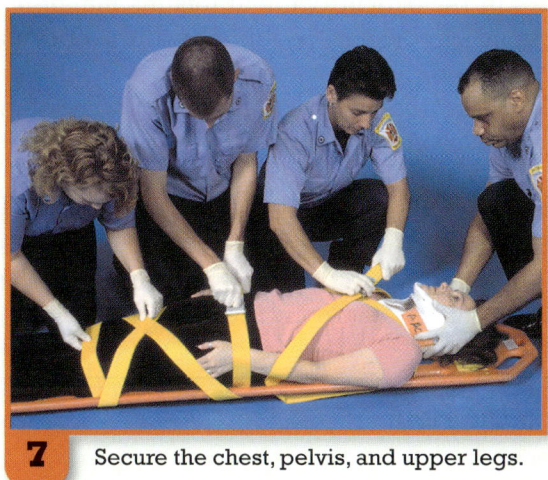
7 Secure the chest, pelvis, and upper legs.

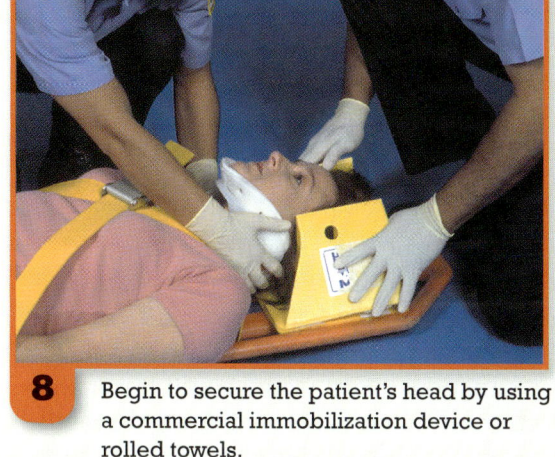
8 Begin to secure the patient's head by using a commercial immobilization device or rolled towels.

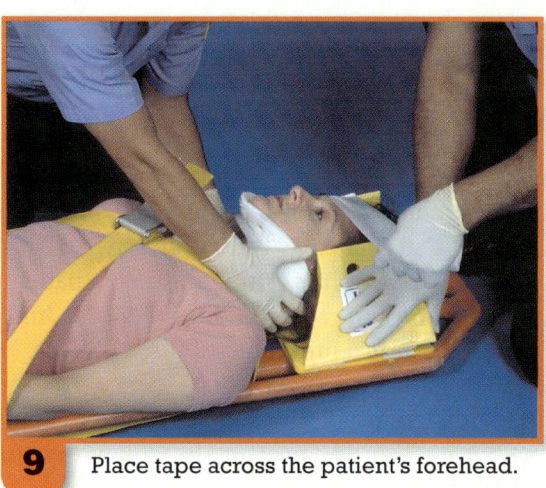
9 Place tape across the patient's forehead.

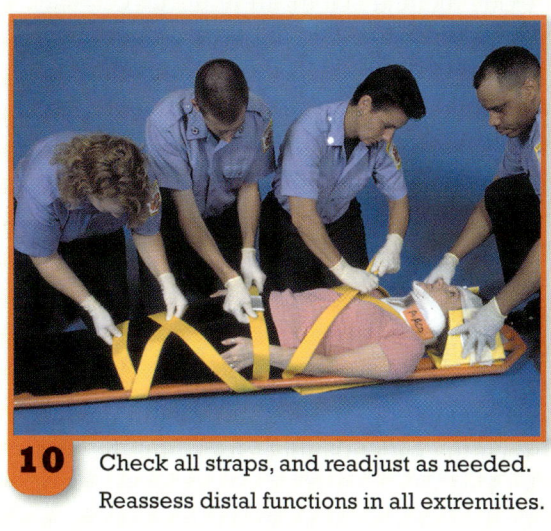
10 Check all straps, and readjust as needed. Reassess distal functions in all extremities.

Patients found in a prone or semiprone position must be placed in a supine position to assess airway, breathing, and circulation and to properly immobilize the spine. One rescuer should take control of the cervical spine using a crossed-hand position to roll the patient. The second rescuer should be positioned at the torso with any additional help at the pelvis and legs. The rescuer at the head counts, and the patient should be rolled as a unit into a supine position. Assessment and immobilization should then continue as usual.

If the patient is in a prone or semi-prone position, the patient should be log rolled into the supine position, and then immobilized as discussed and shown in Skill Drill 17-2.

Sitting Patients

Some patients with a possible spinal injury will be in a sitting position, such as after an automobile crash. With these patients, you should use a short backboard or a vest-style spinal extrication device to immobilize the cervical and thoracic spine. The short immobilization device is then secured to the long board.

> **EMT-I Tips**
>
> Make sure that everyone is clear on the count *before* moving a patient. Will the count be 1, 2, 3, roll, or will the roll be performed *on* 3?

> **EMT-I Tips**
>
> These short spine immobilization devices should be used only with patients in *stable* condition who do not need rapid extrication.

The exceptions to this rule are situations in which you do not have time to first secure the patient to the short board, including the following situations:

- You or the patient is in danger.
- You need to gain immediate access to other patients.
- The patient's injuries justify urgent removal.

In these situations, your team should lower the patient directly onto a long backboard, using the rapid extrication technique, discussed in Chapter 34. Be sure that you provide manual stabilization of the cervical spine as you move the patient. Rapid extrication is indicated only in cases of life- or limb-threatening injury. In all other cases, follow the steps in **Skill Drill 17-3** to immobilize a sitting patient:

1. As with the supine patient, you must **first stabilize the head** and then maintain manual in-line stabilization until the patient is secured to the long backboard.
2. **Assess pulse, motor, and sensory function** in each extremity.
3. Apply the cervical collar (**Step 1**).
4. **Insert a short spine immobilization device** between the patient's upper back and the seat back (**Step 2**).
5. Open the board's side flaps (if present), and position them around the patient's torso and snug to the armpits (**Step 3**).
6. Once the device is properly positioned, **secure the upper torso straps** (**Step 4**).
7. Position and fasten both groin loops (leg straps). Pad the groin as needed. Check all torso straps to make sure they are secure. Make any adjustments necessary without excessive movement of the patient (**Step 5**).
8. **Pad any space** between the patient's head and the device as necessary.
9. **Secure the forehead strap, or tape the head securely,** then fasten the lower head strap around the cervical collar (**Step 6**).
10. **Place the long backboard** next to the patient's buttocks, perpendicular to the trunk (**Step 7**).
11. **Turn the patient parallel** to the long board, and slowly lower him or her onto it.
12. **Lift the patient** (without rotating him or her), and slip the long board under the short device (**Step 8**).
13. **Release the leg straps and loosen the chest strap** to allow the legs to straighten and give the chest room to fully expand.
14. **Secure the short device and long board** together.
15. **Reassess the pulse, motor function, and sensation** in all four extremities. Note your findings, and prepare for transport (**Step 9**).

> **In the Field**
>
> Ask the patient to take a deep breath before tightening the torso straps. This will ensure that breathing is not impeded by the device.

Standing Patients

You may arrive at a scene in which you find a patient standing or wandering around after an accident or injury. If you suspect that there may be underlying head, neck, or spinal injuries, you should immobilize the patient to a long backboard before proceeding to assess him or her. This will require a minimum of three EMT-Is. Follow the steps in **Skill Drill 17-4**:

1. **Establish manual, in-line stabilization,** apply a cervical collar, and instruct the patient to remain still.
2. **Position the board upright** directly behind the patient (**Step 1**).
3. **Two EMT-Is stand on either side** of the patient, and the third is directly behind the patient, maintaining immobilization.
4. **The two EMT-Is grasp the handholds at shoulder level** or slightly above by reaching under the patient's arms while standing at either side (**Step 2**).
5. **Prepare to lower** the patient to the ground (**Step 3**).
6. **Carefully lower the patient** as a unit under the direction of the EMT-I at the head. The EMT-I at the head will have to make sure the head stays against the board and carefully rotate his or her hands while the patient is being lowered to maintain in-line stabilization (**Step 4**).

Head Injuries

All head injuries are potentially serious. If not properly treated, those that at first seem minor may end up being life threatening. On the other hand, severe lacerations of the scalp or fractures of the skull may occur with little or no brain injury and may produce minimal or no long-term deficits.

Scalp Lacerations

Scalp lacerations can be minor or very serious. Because both the face and the scalp have rich blood supplies, even small lacerations can quickly lead to significant blood loss Figure 17-12. Occasionally, this blood loss may be severe enough to cause hypovolemic shock, particularly in children. In any patient with multiple injuries, bleeding from scalp or facial lacerations contributes to hypovolemia. In addition, because scalp lacerations are usually the result of direct blows to the head, they often indicate deeper, more serious injuries.

You can almost always control bleeding from a scalp laceration by applying direct pressure over the wound. Remember to follow BSI techniques. Use a dry sterile dressing, and fold any avulsions (torn skin flaps) back down onto the skin bed before applying pressure Figure 17-13A. In some cases, you will have to apply firm compression for several minutes to control the bleeding Figure 17-13B. If you suspect a skull fracture, do not apply excessive pressure to the open wound. Otherwise, you may push bone fragments into the brain.

If the dressing becomes soaked, do not remove it. Instead, place a second dressing over the first. Continue applying manual pressure until the bleeding is controlled, then secure the dressing in place with a soft, self-adhering roller bandage Figure 17-13C.

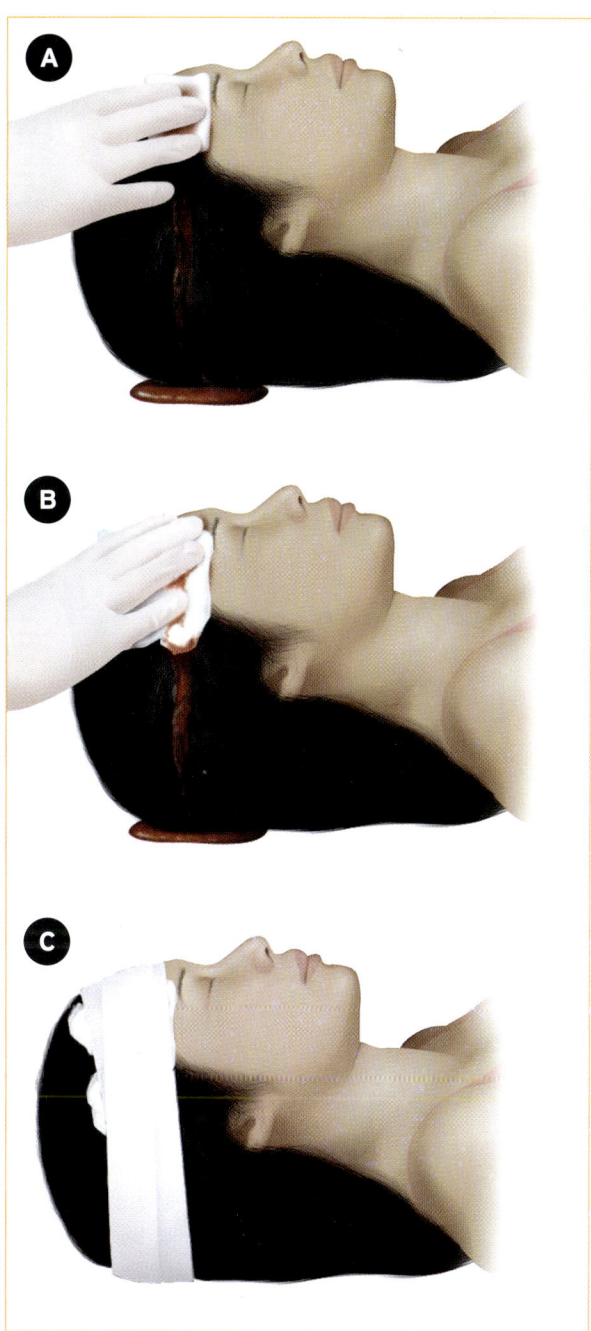

Figure 17-13 **A.** Apply pressure with a sterile dressing to fold any torn skin flaps back down onto the skin bed. **B.** Apply firm compression for several minutes to control the bleeding. **C.** Secure the compression dressing in place with a soft, self-adhering roller bandage.

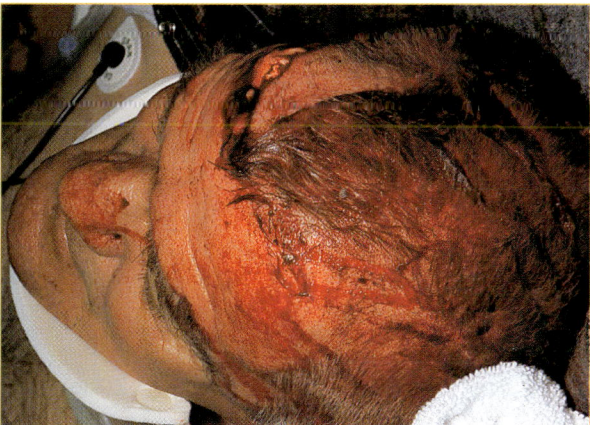

Figure 17-12 The scalp has a rich blood supply; therefore, even small lacerations can result in significant blood loss.

Skill Drill 17-3: Immobilizing a Patient Found in a Sitting Position

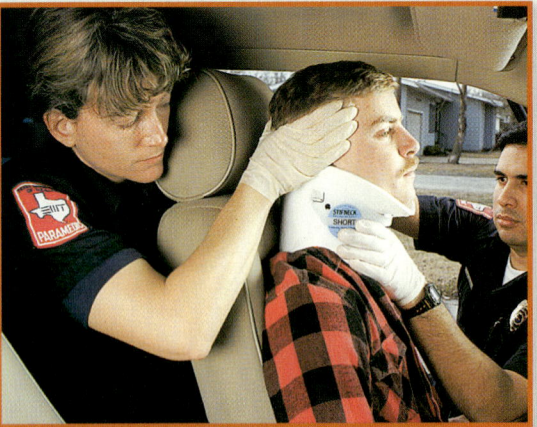

1 Stabilize the head and neck in a neutral, in-line position.

Assess pulse, motor, and sensory function in each extremity.

Apply a cervical collar.

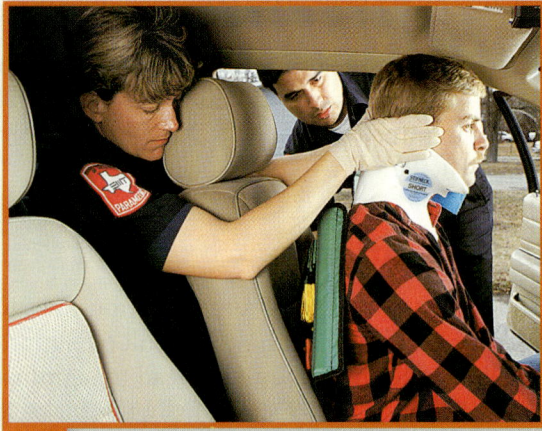

2 Insert a short spine immobilization device between the patient's upper back and the seat.

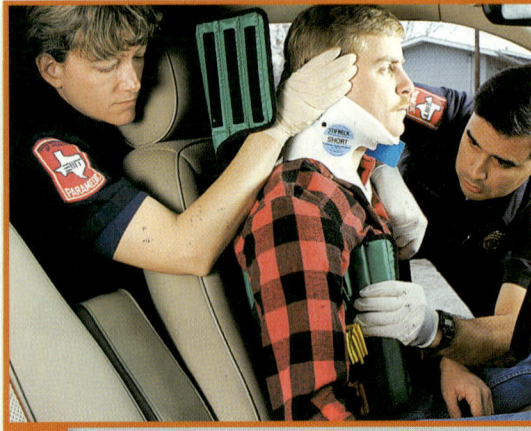

3 Open the side flaps and position them around the patient's torso, snug around the armpits.

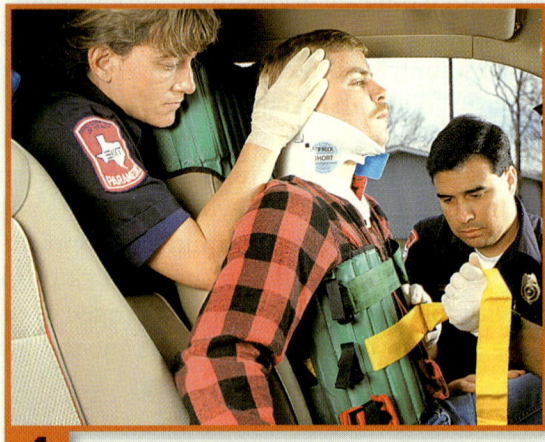

4 Secure the torso straps.

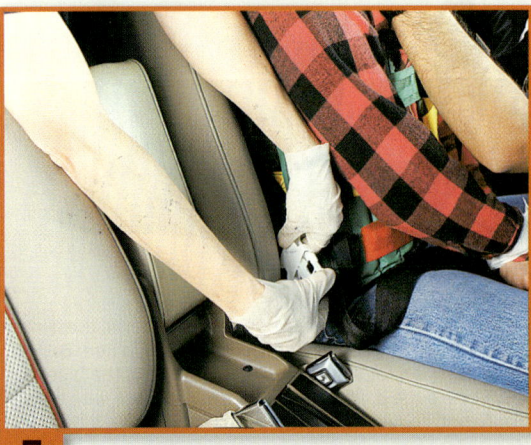

5 Secure the groin (leg) straps. Pad the groin as needed. Check and adjust torso straps.

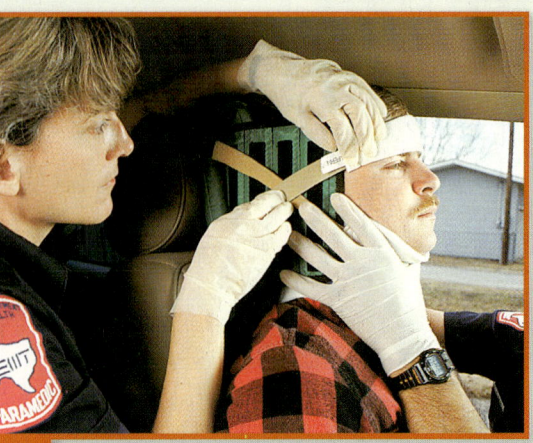

6 Pad between the head and the device as needed.

Secure the forehead strap, and fasten the lower head strap around the collar.

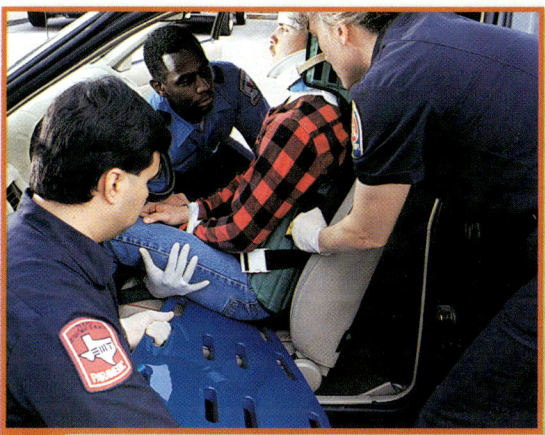

7 Wedge a long backboard next to the patient's buttocks.

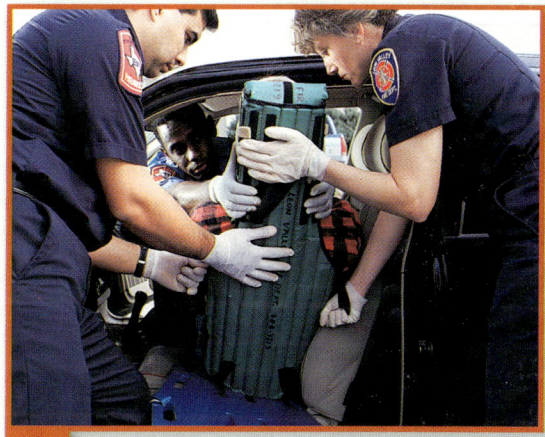

8 Turn and lower the patient onto the long board.

Lift the patient, and slip the long board under the spine device. Release the leg straps and loosen the chest strap.

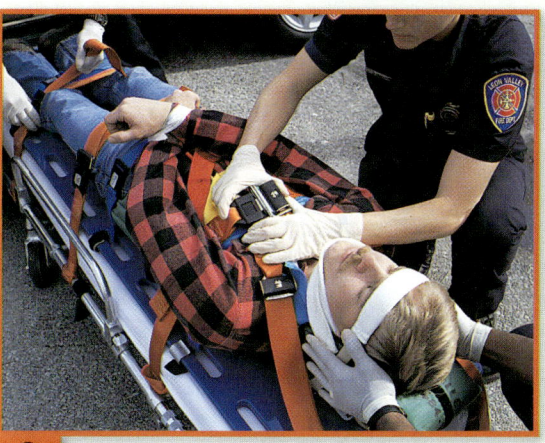

9 Secure the immobilization devices to each other.

Reassess pulse, motor, and sensory functions in each extremity.

Skull Fracture

Fracture of the skull is an indication that a significant force has been applied to the head. As with any fracture, a skull fracture may be open or closed, depending on whether there is an overlying laceration of the scalp. Injuries from bullets or other penetrating weapons frequently result in fractures of the skull. The diagnosis of a skull fracture is usually made in the hospital by radiographic examination, but you can conclude that a fracture is present if the patient's head appears deformed or if there is a visible crack in the skull within a scalp laceration. Another sign of skull fracture that you may see is ecchymosis (bruising) that develops under the eyes (raccoon eyes) Figure 17-14A ▶, known as periorbital ecchymosis, or behind the ear over the mastoid process (Battle's sign) Figure 17-14B ▶. Note, however, that raccoon eyes or Battle's sign are usually later signs of a skull fracture; therefore, their absence does not rule out a skull fracture.

Immobilizing a Patient Found in a Standing Position

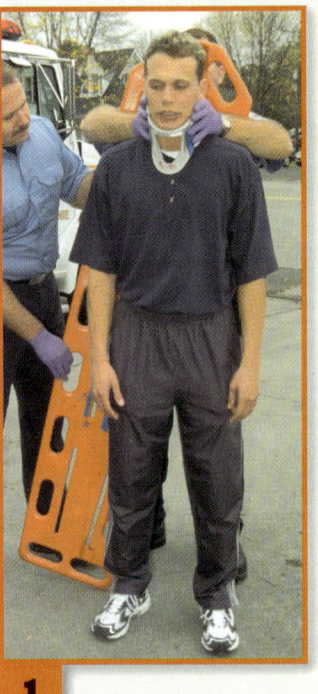

After manually stabilizing the head and neck, apply a cervical collar.

Position the board behind the patient.

1

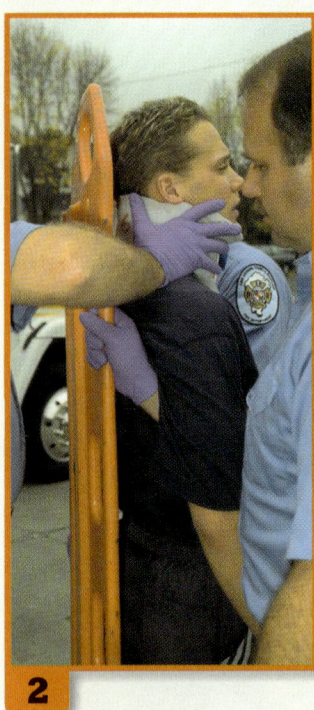

Position EMT-Is at the sides of and behind the patient.

The EMT-Is on the sides reach under patient's arms and grasp handholds at or slightly above shoulder level.

2

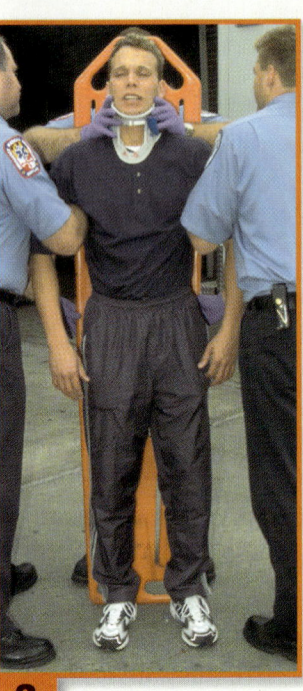

Prepare to lower the patient. EMT-Is on the sides should be facing the EMT-I at the head and wait for his or her direction.

3

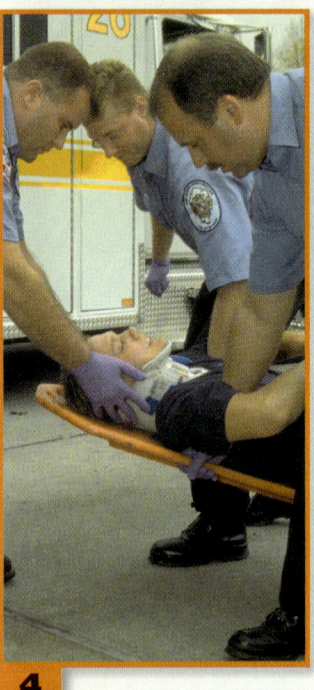

On command, lower the backboard to the ground.

4

> **A to Z Terminology Tips**
>
> Ecchymosis = bruising; peri = around; orbital = involving the orbits, or eye sockets
> Therefore, *periorbital ecchymosis* is bruising around the eyes, usually indicating a skull fracture.

Brain Injuries

Concussion

A blow to the head or face may cause concussion of the brain. There is no universal agreement on the exact definition of a concussion, but in general, it means a temporary loss or alteration of part or all of the brain's abilities to function without actual physical damage to the brain. For example, a person who "sees stars" after being struck in the head has had a concussion that affects the occipital portion of the brain. A concussion may result in unresponsiveness and even apnea for short periods.

A patient with a concussion may be confused or have amnesia (loss of memory). Occasionally, the patient can remember everything but the events leading up to the injury; this is called retrograde amnesia. Inability to remember events after the injury is called antegrade (posttraumatic) amnesia. Usually the effects of a concussion last only a short time. In fact, the symptoms have often resolved by the time you arrive at the scene. Nevertheless, you should ask about symptoms of concussion in any patient who has sustained an injury to the head; these symptoms include dizziness, weakness, visual changes, and loss of consciousness.

Contusion

Like any other soft tissue in the body, the brain can sustain a contusion, or bruise, when the skull is struck. A contusion is far more serious than a concussion because it involves physical injury to the brain tissue, which may sustain long-lasting or even permanent damage. As with contusions elsewhere, there is associated bleeding and swelling from injured blood vessels. Injury of brain tissue or bleeding inside the skull will cause an increase of pressure within the skull. A patient who has had a cerebral contusion may exhibit any or all of the signs of brain injury described later in this chapter.

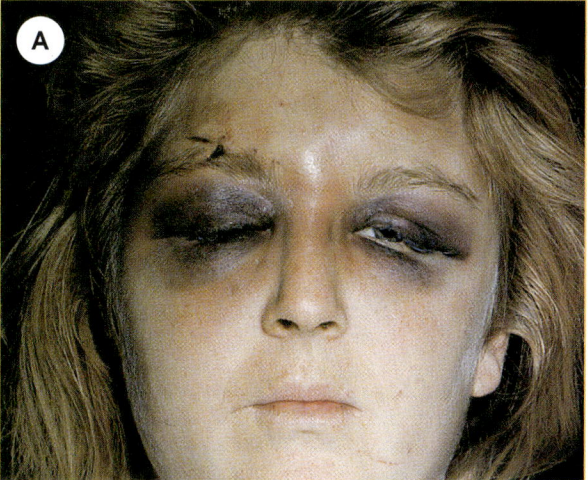
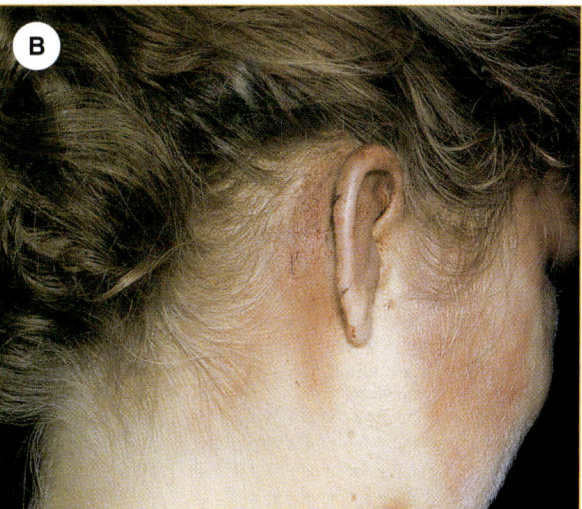

Figure 17-14 Skull fracture is a possibility if a patient has ecchymosis **A.** Under the eyes (raccoon eyes) or **B.** Behind the ear over the mastoid process (Battle's sign).

Intracranial Bleeding

Laceration or rupture of a blood vessel inside the brain or in the meninges that cover the brain will produce intracranial bleeding resulting in a hematoma in one of three areas (Figure 17-15 ▶):

- Beneath the dura but outside the brain: a subdural hematoma
- Within the parenchyma of the brain itself: an intracerebral hematoma
- Outside the dura and under the skull: an epidural hematoma

A hematoma may develop rapidly, usually because of arterial injury, as in an epidural hematoma; or it may

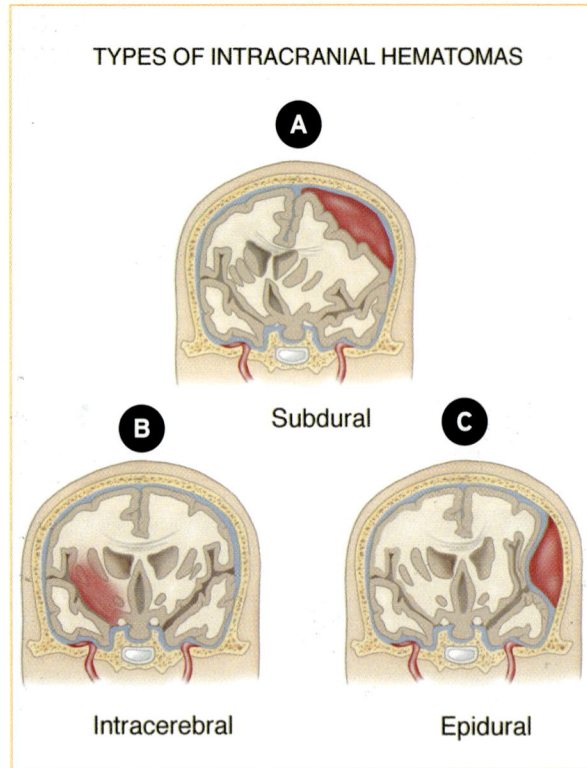

Figure 17-15 Intracranial bleeding can occur in one of three areas. **A.** Beneath the dura but outside the brain (subdural hematoma). **B.** Within the parenchyma of the brain (intracerebral hematoma). **C.** Outside the dura and under the skull (epidural hematoma).

develop very slowly, as with a subdural hematoma. In any case, because the brain occupies nearly the entire space inside the skull, the result is increased pressure inside the skull, leading to compression of the brain tissue. The expanding hematoma will cause progressive loss of brain function and, if not treated promptly and appropriately, death.

Rapid deterioration of neurologic signs following a head injury is a sign of intracranial pressure. You must act quickly to evaluate and treat patients with such signs. Provide oxygen or ventilatory assistance, monitor the airway and intubate if necessary (and if allowed by your local protocol), monitor oxygen saturation, and provide immediate transport.

Other Brain Injuries

Brain injuries are not always a result of trauma. Certain medical conditions, such as blood clots or hemorrhaging, can also cause brain injuries that produce significant bleeding or swelling. Vascular disease, high blood pressure, and any number of other causes may cause spontaneous bleeding in the brain, affecting the patient's level of consciousness or mental status. The signs and symptoms of nontraumatic injuries are the same as those of traumatic brain injuries, except that there is no obvious mechanism of injury or any evidence of trauma.

You are the Provider — Part 3

After completing your initial treatment of the patient, you perform a rapid trauma assessment. You note that the patient's right pupil is dilated and unresponsive. After fully immobilizing the patient's spine, you place him into the ambulance and obtain the following vital signs:

Vital Signs	Recording Time: 5 Minutes After Patient Contact
Respirations	26 breaths/min; irregular and shallow
Pulse	70 beats/min and regular
Skin	Pale and clammy
Blood pressure	170/90 mm Hg
Sao_2	96% with assisted ventilation and 100% oxygen

5. What do the patient's vital signs indicate to you?
6. What is one of the most common complications associated with head trauma?

Complications of Head Injury

Cerebral edema, or swelling of the brain, is one of the most common complications of any head injury. It is also one of the most serious because, as we have seen, swelling in the skull compresses the brain tissue, resulting in a loss of brain function.

Cerebral edema is aggravated by a low oxygen level in the blood and improved by a high level. For this reason, you must make sure that the airway is open and that adequate ventilation and high-flow oxygen are given to any patient with a head injury. This is especially true if the patient is unresponsive. Do not wait for cyanosis or other obvious signs of hypoxia to develop. Patients should be ventilated at a rate of 10 breaths/min or as dictated by local protocols. Hyperventilating a patient may cause vasoconstriction, further reducing oxygenation of the brain. Currently, the only indication for hyperventilation in a head-injured patient is evidence of cerebral herniation such as abnormal pupils (unilaterally or bilaterally fixed and dilated) or extensor posturing. Hyperventilation (20 breaths/min) should be initiated only after hypotension and hypoxemia have been addressed.

It is not uncommon for the patient with a head injury to have a seizure (also called convulsion). This is the result of excessive excitability of the brain, caused by direct injury or the accumulation of fluid within the brain (edema). You should be prepared to manage seizures in all patients who have had a head injury. Other effects of cerebral edema and increased intracranial pressure may be increased blood pressure, decreased pulse, and irregular respirations (these three effects are also known as the Cushing reflex or triad).

A common response to head injuries, especially among children with very slight head injuries, is vomiting. This is usually the result of increased intracranial pressure. In managing such vomiting, you should pay particular attention to protecting the airway.

As discussed earlier, the appearance of clear or pink watery CSF from the nose, the ear, or an open scalp wound indicates that the dura and the skull have both been penetrated. You should make no attempt to pack the wound, ear, or nose in this situation. Cover the scalp wound, if there is one, with sterile gauze to prevent further contamination, but do not bandage it tightly.

Assessing Head Injuries

Motor vehicle crashes, direct blows, falls from heights, assault, and sports injuries are common causes of head injury. A patient who has experienced any of these events should immediately arouse your suspicion and cause

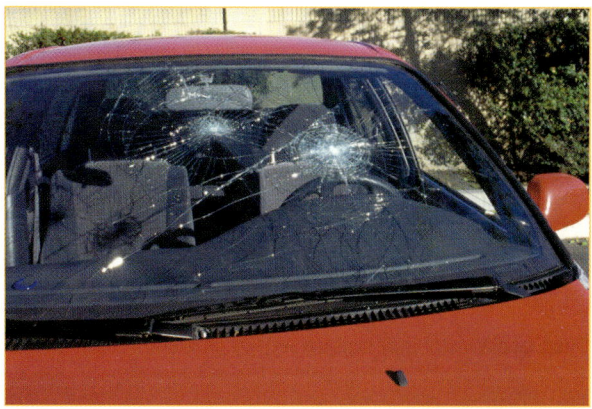

Figure 17-16 The classic "star" on the windshield after an automobile crash is a significant indicator of injury. Be alert for the signs and symptoms of head injury.

you to start looking for specific signs and symptoms of head injury. A deformed windshield or dented helmet may indicate a major blow to the head, which is likely to have caused injury Figure 17-16 ▲ . It is especially important to evaluate and monitor the level of consciousness in patients with suspected head injuries, paying particular attention to any changes that may occur.

Types of Head Injuries

A closed head injury, usually associated with trauma, is one in which the brain has been injured but the skin has not been broken and there is no obvious bleeding. In assessing a patient with a possible closed head injury, consider the mechanism of injury. Did the patient fall? Was he or she in an automobile crash or the victim of an assault? Was there deformity of the windshield or deformity of the helmet? Look for scalp lacerations, contusions, hematomas, or skull deformities. Sometimes, a segment of the skull will appear to have been pushed into the brain.

A decreased level of consciousness is the most reliable sign of closed head injury. Monitor the patient for changes in level of consciousness, including signs of confusion, disorientation, anxiety, combativeness, and deteriorating mental status. Is the patient unresponsive or repeating questions? Experiencing seizures? Nauseated or vomiting? Next, assess the patient for decreased movement and/or numbness and tingling in the extremities. Assess the vital signs carefully. People with head injuries may have irregular respirations, depending on which region of the brain has been affected. Look for blood or CSF leaking from the ears, nose, or mouth and for bruising around the eyes and behind the ears.

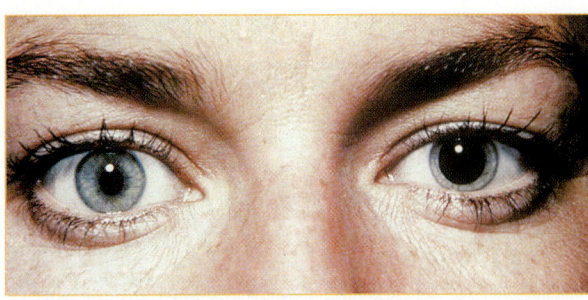

Figure 17-17 Assess pupil size if you suspect a head injury. Unequal pupil size may signal a serious problem.

You should also evaluate the patient's pupils, especially if he or she has a decreased level of consciousness. Often, unequal pupil size after a head injury signals a serious problem. Developing blood clots may be pressing on the oculomotor nerve (cranial nerve III), causing one pupil to dilate Figure 17-17.

The patient with severe brain trauma may also present with decorticate or decerebrate posturing, both of which indicate pressure on the brainstem. Decorticate (flexor) posturing is characterized by flexion of the arms and extension of the legs and decerebrate (extensor) posturing is characterized by extension of the arms and legs. When observed, posturing is an ominous sign and indicates significant intracranial pressure.

Scalp contusions, lacerations, hematomas, and obvious skull deformities are signs of an open head injury, which is often caused by a penetrating object. There may be bleeding and exposed brain tissue. Do not probe open scalp lacerations with your gloved finger, as this may push bone fragments into the brain. Do not remove an impaled object; stabilize it in place

Signs and Symptoms of Head Injury

Open and closed head injuries have essentially the same signs and symptoms.

Following an injury, any patient who exhibits one or more of these signs or symptoms should be evaluated promptly in the emergency department:

- Lacerations, contusions, or hematomas to the scalp
- Soft area or depression noted on palpation
- Visible fractures or deformities of the skull
- Ecchymosis around the eyes or behind the ear over the mastoid process
- Clear or pink CSF leakage from a scalp wound, the nose, or the ear
- Failure of the pupils to respond to light
- Unequal pupil size
- Loss of sensation and/or motor function
- A period of unresponsiveness
- Amnesia
- Seizures
- Numbness or tingling in the extremities
- Irregular respirations
- Dizziness
- Visual complaints
- Combative or other abnormal behavior
- Nausea or vomiting

Level of Consciousness

A change in the level of consciousness is the single most important observation that you can make in assessing the severity of brain injury. The level of consciousness usually corresponds to the extent of loss of brain function. As soon as you determine that a head injury is present, you should perform a baseline assessment using the AVPU scale (Alert; responsive to Verbal stimuli; responsive to Pain; Unresponsive), and record the time. Reevaluate the patient and record your observations every 15 minutes if the patient's condition is stable and at least every 5 minutes if the patient's condition is unstable, until you reach the hospital.

Frequently the level of consciousness will fluctuate, improving, deteriorating, and then improving again over time. On other occasions, there is a gradual, progressive deterioration in the patient's response to stimuli; this usually indicates serious brain damage that may need aggressive medical and/or surgical treatment. The physicians who treat the patient will need to know when the loss of consciousness occurred and for how long. They will want to compare their neurologic evaluation with the one you performed in the field.

Your EMS system may choose to use the more detailed Glasgow Coma Scale (GCS) instead of the AVPU scale to assess a patient's level of consciousness Figure 17-18. In either case, you should always use simple, easily understood terms when reporting the level of consciousness, such as "does not remember events immediately preceding injury" or "confused about date and time." Terms such as "dazed" have different meanings to different people and should not be used in written or verbal reports.

Perform frequent assessments of the patient's GCS. According to the Brain Trauma Foundation (BTF), a *single* drop in the patient's GCS score to less than 9, or a decrease in the GCS score of more than two points at any time, doubles the brain-injured patient's chance of death.

Consider endotracheal intubation in any brain-injured patient with a GCS score of less than 9.

GLASGOW COMA SCALE

Eye Opening	
Spontaneous	4
To Voice	3
To Pain	2
None	1
Verbal Response	
Oriented	5
Confused	4
Inappropriate Words	3
Incomprehensible Words	2
None	1
Motor Response	
Obeys Command	6
Localizes Pain	5
Withdraws (pain)	4
Flexion (pain)	3
Extension (pain)	2
None	1
Glasgow Coma Score Total	**15**

Figure 17-18 The Glasgow Coma Scale is one method of evaluating the level of consciousness. Note that the lower the score, the more severe the extent of brain injury.

Changes in Pupil Size

The nerves that control dilation and constriction of the pupils are very sensitive to pressure within the skull. When you shine a bright light into the eye, the pupil should briskly constrict. Failure to constrict is an early and important sign of increased intracranial pressure. Unequal pupil size may indicate increased pressure on one of the two oculomotor nerves.

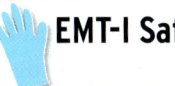

EMT-I Safety

Many mechanisms that cause head and spine injuries for the patient can also entail risk to emergency responders. Before you approach the patient, get the "big picture" of scene safety and take any actions necessary to ensure your own well-being. Do not rely entirely on assistance from fire or police personnel; maintain your own awareness of the scene from the beginning to the end of the call.

As soon as you have assessed the patient's level of consciousness, determine the reaction of each pupil to light. You may consider sketching the size of both pupils on the ambulance report to indicate any difference between the two eyes. Continue to monitor the pupils. Any change in their reactions over time may indicate progressive increases in intracranial pressure.

Emergency Medical Care

Patients with head injuries often have injuries to the cervical spine as well. Therefore, when treating a patient with a head injury, you must keep in mind the need to protect and stabilize the cervical spine at all times. Avoid moving the neck unnecessarily until the spine can be appropriately immobilized. An initial assessment with simultaneous spinal immobilization should be done on scene with a complete, detailed physical examination performed en route to the hospital.

Beyond this, you should treat the patient with a head injury according to three general principles, which are designed to protect and maintain the critical functions of the CNS:

1. **Establish an adequate airway.** If necessary, begin and maintain ventilation and always provide high-flow supplemental oxygen. Consult local protocols for the appropriate rate if ventilation via a bag-valve-mask (BVM) device is required.
2. **Control bleeding**, and provide adequate circulation to maintain cerebral perfusion. Begin CPR, if necessary. Be sure to follow BSI precautions.
3. Start a large bore IV of an isotonic crystalloid solution.
4. **Assess the patient's baseline** level of consciousness, and continuously monitor it.

As you continue to treat the patient, do not apply pressure to an open or depressed skull injury. In addition, you must assess and treat other injuries, dress and bandage open wounds as indicated in the treatment of soft-tissue injuries, splint fractures, anticipate and manage vomiting to prevent aspiration, be prepared for seizures and changes in the patient's condition, and transport the patient promptly and with extreme care.

Managing the Airway

The most important step in the treatment of patients with head injury, regardless of the severity, is to establish and maintain a patent airway. If the patient has an airway obstruction, you should perform the jaw-thrust maneuver to open the airway. Once the airway is open, maintain the head and cervical spine in a neutral, in-line position until the patient can be fully immobilized with a cervical collar Figure 17-19 ▼. Remove any foreign bodies, secretions, or vomitus from the airway. Make sure a suctioning unit is available, because you will often need to clear blood, saliva, or vomitus from the airway.

Once you have cleared the airway, assess the patient's ventilatory status. If the respiratory control center of the brain (pons, medulla) has been injured, the rate and/or depth of breathing may be ineffective. Ventilation may also be limited by concomitant chest injuries or, if the spinal cord is injured, by paralysis of some or all of the muscles of respiration. Give high-flow oxygen to any patient who is having trouble breathing. This reduces hypoxia and may minimize cerebral edema. An injured brain is even less tolerant of hypoxia than a healthy brain, and studies have shown that supplemental oxygen can reduce brain damage. However, to be effective, it must be administered as soon as possible. Do not wait until the patient becomes cyanotic. Continue to assist ventilation and administer supplemental oxygen until the patient reaches the hospital.

Closely monitor the patient's oxygen saturation (SaO_2) and maintain it at 95% or higher. According to the BTF, a *single* drop in the patient's SaO_2 to less than 90% doubles the brain-injured patient's chance of death. Insertion of a Combitube may be necessary to definitively protect the patient's airway and facilitate oxygenation.

Circulation

If the patient is pulseless, providing airway maintenance, ventilation, and oxygen accomplishes nothing. You must also begin CPR if the patient is in cardiac arrest.

Active blood loss aggravates hypoxia by reducing the available number of oxygen-carrying red blood cells. Although they rarely cause shock except in infants and children, scalp lacerations often cause the loss of large volumes of blood, which must be controlled. Bleeding inside the skull may cause intracranial pressure to rise to a life-threatening level, even though the actual volume of blood lost inside the skull is relatively small.

Shock that develops in a patient with a head injury may be due to hypovolemia caused by bleeding from other injuries. As with other trauma patients, shock indicates that the situation is critical. Such patients must be transported immediately, preferably to a trauma center. Maintain the airway while you protect the patient's cervical spine, ensure adequate ventilation, administer 100% oxygen, control obvious sites of bleeding with direct pressure, place the patient supine on a spine board, keep the patient warm, and provide immediate transport.

Hypotension in the brain-injured patient could also indicate a decrease in cerebral perfusion pressure (CPP), which if left untreated, will result in death of brain cells. If the patient's systolic BP falls below 90 mm Hg, infuse 20 mL/kg of an isotonic crystalloid as needed to maintain a systolic BP of at least 90 mm Hg. According to the BTF, a *single* drop in the systolic BP to less than 90 mm Hg doubles the brain-injured patient's chance of death.

Apply a cardiac monitor and observe the patient for dysrhythmias. If dysrhythmias occur, treat according to standard ACLS or local protocols.

If the patient has a medical condition or nontraumatic injury along with the head injury, place the patient on the left side to prevent aspiration if vomiting occurs. *Be sure to maintain the head in the neutral, in-line position* Figure 17-20 ▶, *with the cervical collar in place.* You should also have a suctioning unit available.

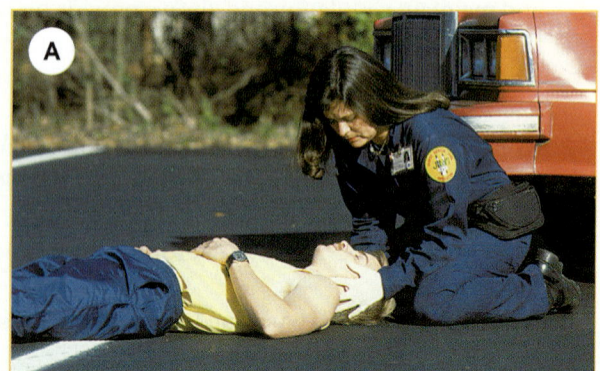
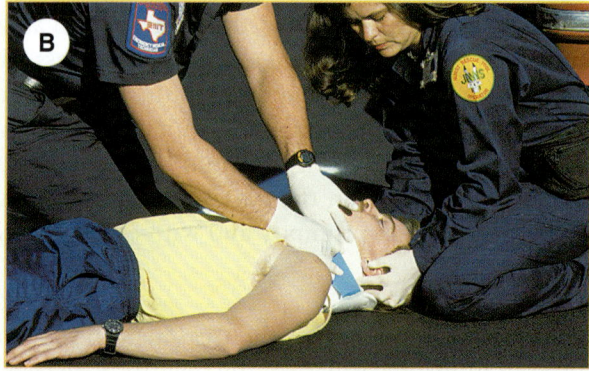

Figure 17-19 **A.** Maintain the head and cervical spine in a neutral, in-line position. **B.** Apply a cervical collar as you finish the initial assessment.

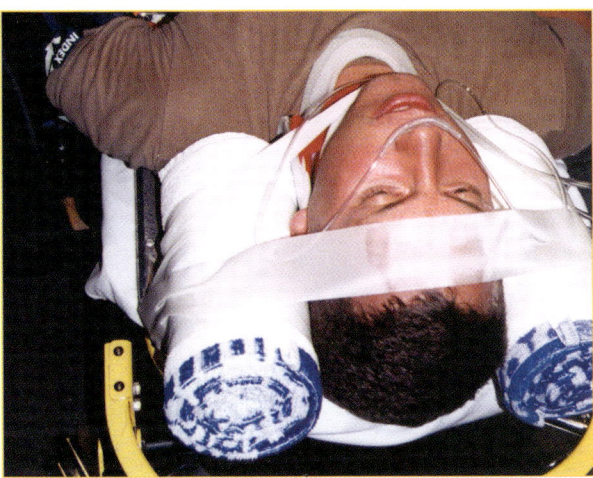

Figure 17-20 Maintain the head and cervical spine in a neutral, in-line position. Be sure to use an appropriately sized cervical collar for the patient.

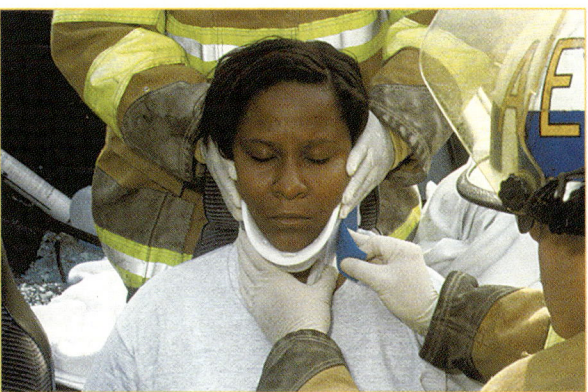

Figure 17-21 Proper fit is essential in applying a cervical collar. The collar should rest on the shoulder girdle and provide firm support under both sides of the mandible without obstructing the airway or any ventilation efforts.

Immobilization Devices

An injured spine is often very difficult to evaluate in a patient with a head injury. Sometimes there is no neurologic deficit. Pain in the spine may be missed because of shock or because the patient's attention is directed to more painful injuries. Evaluation is even more difficult if the patient is unresponsive. Because any manipulation of an unstable cervical spine may cause permanent damage to the spinal cord, you must assume the presence of spinal injury in all patients who have sustained head injuries. Fully immobilize the patient with a cervical collar and long backboard.

Cervical Collars

Rigid cervical immobilization devices, or cervical collars, provide preliminary, partial support. A cervical collar should be applied to every patient who has a possible spinal injury based on mechanism of injury, history, or signs and symptoms. Keep in mind, however, that cervical collars do not fully immobilize the cervical spine. Therefore, you must maintain manual support until the patient is completely secured to a spinal immobilization device, such as a long or a short backboard.

To be effective, a rigid cervical collar must be the correct size for the patient. It should rest on the shoulder girdle and provide firm support under both sides of the mandible, without obstructing the airway or ventilation efforts in any way (**Figure 17-21**). Follow the steps in (**Skill Drill 17-5**):

1. **One EMT-I** provides continuous, manual, in-line support of the head while the other prepares the collar (**Step 1**).
2. **Measure the proper size of the collar** according to the manufacturer's specifications. It is essential that the cervical collar fit properly. An improperly sized immobilization device could cause further injury. If you do not have the correct size, use a rolled towel; tape it to the backboard around the patient's head, and provide continuous manual support (**Figure 17-22**) (**Step 2**).
3. **Begin by placing the chin support** snugly underneath the chin (**Step 3**).
4. **While maintaining head stabilization** and neutral neck alignment, wrap the collar around the neck and secure the collar to the far side of the chin support (**Step 4**).
5. **Assure that the collar fits properly**, and recheck that the patient is in a neutral, in-line position. Maintain in-line stabilization until the patient is completely secured to the board (**Step 5**).

Short Backboards

There are several types of short-board immobilization devices. The most common are the vest-type device and the rigid short board (**Figure 17-23**). These devices are designed to stabilize and immobilize the head, neck, and torso. They are used to immobilize patients in

Application of a Cervical Collar

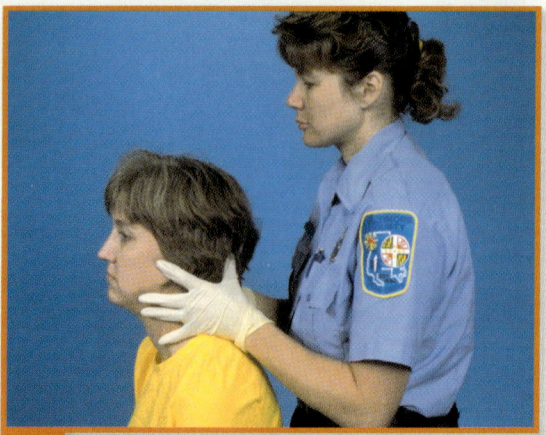

1. Apply in-line stabilization.

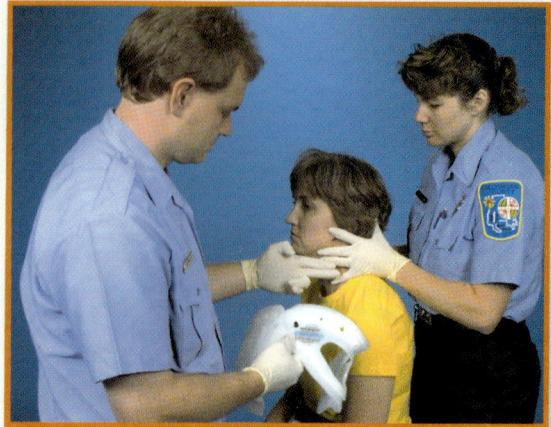

2. Measure the proper collar size.

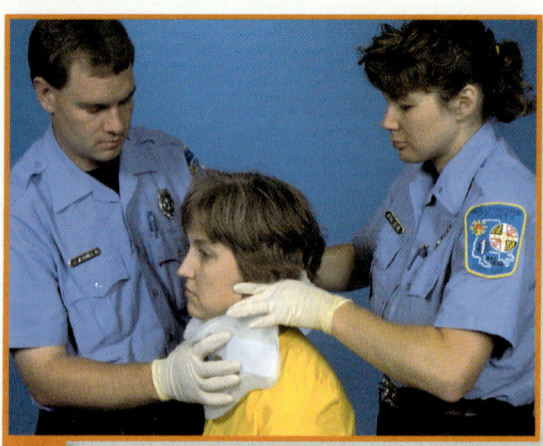

3. Place the chin support first.

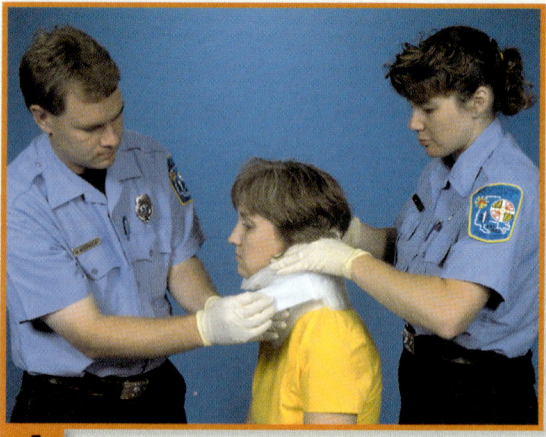

4. Wrap the collar around the neck, and secure the collar.

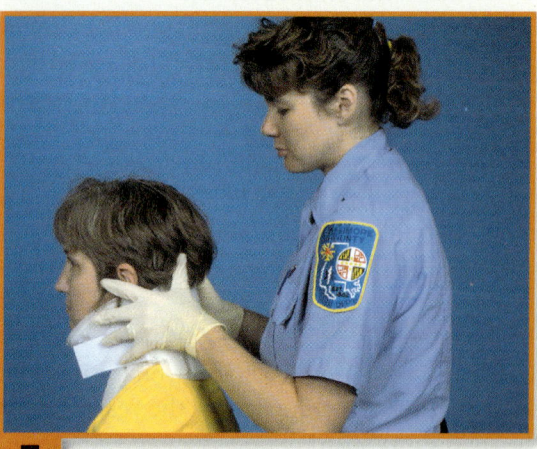

5. Assure proper fit, and maintain neutral, in-line stabilization.

Chapter 17 Head and Spine Injuries

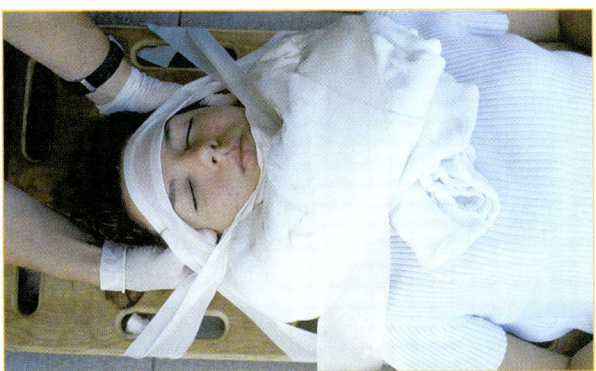

Figure 17-22 If you do not have an appropriately sized cervical collar, you may use a rolled towel. Tape it to the backboard around the patient's head, and provide continuous manual support.

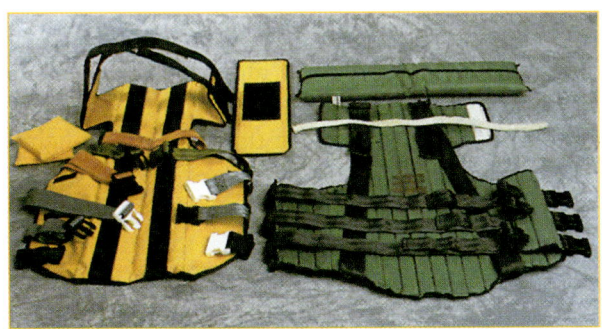

Figure 17-23 The most common types of short-board immobilization devices are vest-type devices.

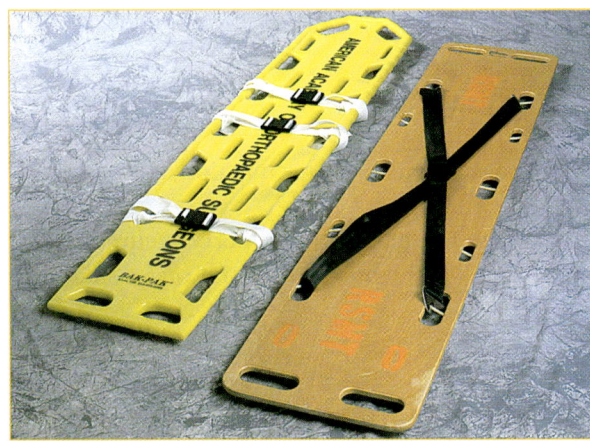

Figure 17-24 Long backboard immobilization devices allow for full body spinal immobilization, including stabilization of the head, neck and torso, pelvis, and extremities.

Long Backboards

There are several types of long backboard immobilization devices that provide full-body spinal immobilization **Figure 17-24 ▲**). They also provide stabilization and immobilization to the head, neck and torso, pelvis, and extremities. Long backboards are used to immobilize patients who are found in any position (standing, sitting, supine), sometimes in conjunction with short backboards.

Securing a patient to a long backboard was described in detail earlier in this chapter. Briefly, you should begin by providing manual, in-line support of the head. Assess pulse, motor function, and sensation in all extremities, and assess the cervical area. Then apply an appropriately sized cervical collar, and proceed as follows:

1. **Position the device.**
2. **Log roll the patient onto the device.** You may also move the patient onto the device by a suitable lift or slide or by scoop stretcher. As you maintain in-line support, your partner should kneel by the patient's head and direct the other two EMT-Is as you roll the patient. Your partner's job is to make sure that the head, torso, and pelvis move as a unit. As the patient's back comes into view, quickly assess its condition if you did not do so during the initial assessment. One EMT-I should position the device under the patient. Then, at your partner's command, roll the patient onto the board.
3. **If there are spaces** between the patient's head and torso and the board, fill them with padding. In an adult, these spaces are usually under the head and torso. In a child, place padding from the shoulders to the toes to establish a neutral position.

noncritical condition who are found in a sitting position and have possible spinal injuries.

As described earlier in this chapter, the first step in securing a patient to a short board or device is to provide manual, in-line support of the cervical spine. Assess the pulse, motor function, and sensation in all extremities, and then assess the cervical area. Then apply an appropriately sized cervical collar.

Position the device behind the patient, and secure it to the torso. Evaluate how well the torso and groin are secured, and make adjustments as necessary. Avoid excessive movement of the patient. Next, evaluate the position of the patient's head. Pad behind the head as needed to maintain neutral, in-line immobilization.

Now secure the patient's head to the device. Once you have done that, you may release manual support of the head. Rotate or lift the patient to the long backboard. At this point, you must reassess the pulses, motor function, and sensation in all four extremities to determine whether the change in position affected the patient's perfusion or neurologic status. Finally, you should immobilize the patient on the long backboard.

4. **Secure the torso to the device** by applying, at a minimum, three straps—one each across the chest, pelvis, and legs. Adjust these straps as needed. Then secure the patient's head to the board.
5. **Reassess pulse**, motor function, and sensation in all extremities.
6. **When the patient is properly secured**, you can safely lift the board or turn it on its side, if necessary.

Helmet Removal

As you plan your care of a patient wearing a helmet, ask yourself the following questions:

- Is the patient's airway clear?
- Is the patient breathing adequately?
- Can you maintain the airway and assist ventilation if the helmet remains in place?
- How well does the helmet fit?
- Can the patient's head move within the helmet?
- Can the spine be immobilized in a neutral position with the helmet on?

A helmet that fits well prevents the patient's head from moving and should be left on, as long as (1) there are no impending airway or breathing problems, (2) it does not interfere with assessment and treatment of airway or ventilation problems, and (3) you can properly immobilize the spine, which may involve padding underneath the shoulders. You should also leave the helmet on if there is any chance that removing it will further injure the patient.

Remove a helmet if (1) it makes assessing or managing airway problems difficult, (2) it prevents you from properly immobilizing the spine, or (3) it allows excessive head movement. Finally, always remove a helmet from a patient who is in cardiac arrest.

Sports helmets are typically open in the front and may or may not include an attached face mask. The mask can be removed without affecting helmet position or function by simply removing or cutting the straps that hold it to the helmet. In this way, sports helmets allow easy access to the airway Figure 17-25 . Motor-

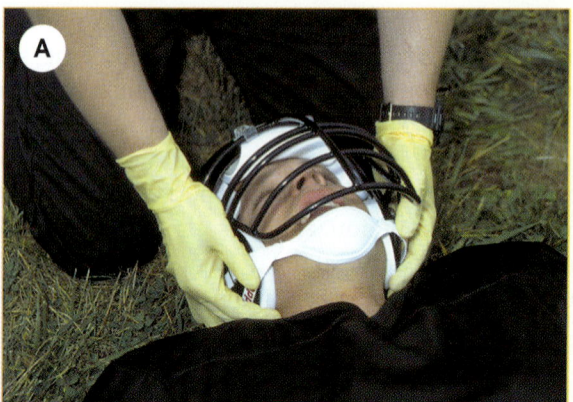
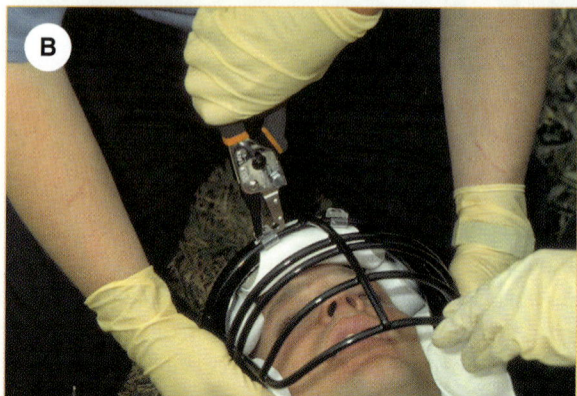
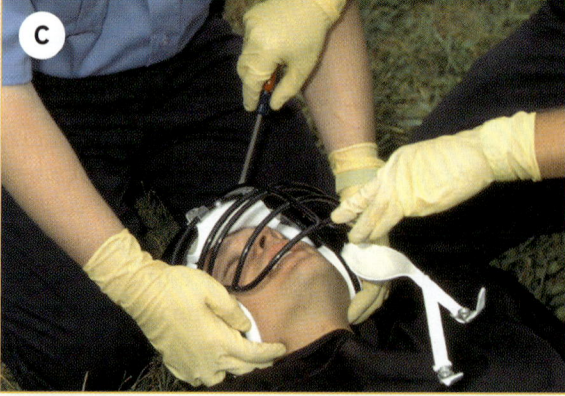
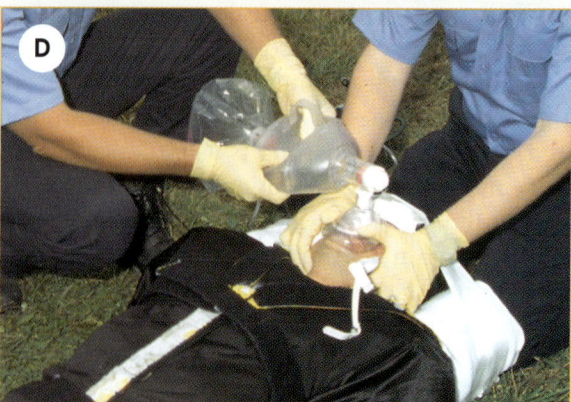

Figure 17-25 Removing the mask on a sports helmet can be done without affecting helmet position or function. **A.** Stabilize the patient's head and helmet. Then remove the face mask in one of two ways: **B.** Use a trainer's tool designed for cutting retaining clips, or **C.** Unscrew the retaining clips for the face mask. **D.** Once the face mask is removed, the helmet can be immobilized against the backboard and a BVM device can be used effectively.

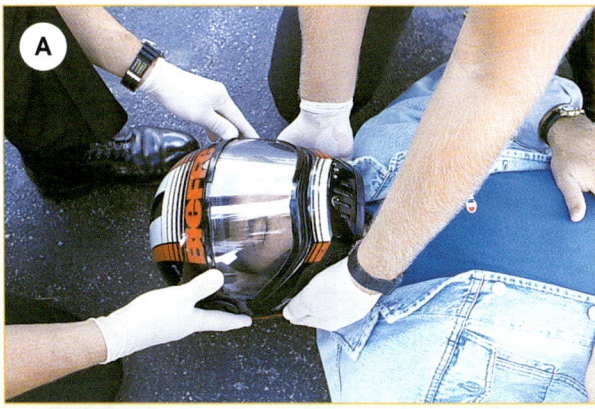

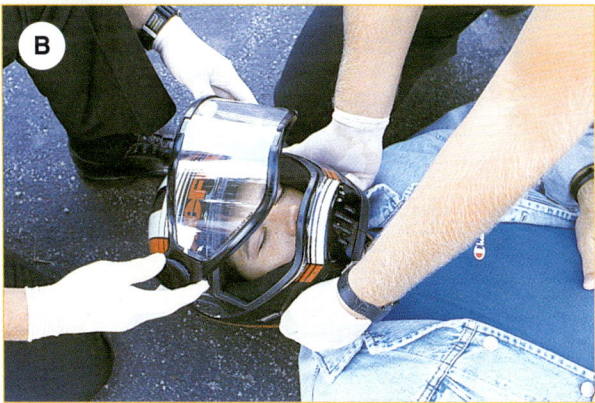

Figure 17-26 Motorcycle helmets often have a shield covering the face that can be removed. **A.** Stabilize the neck in a neutral, in-line position. **B.** Unbuckle or snap off the face shield to access the airway.

cycle helmets often have a shield covering the face. This, too, can be unbuckled to allow access to the airway (Figure 17-26 ▲). If a shield cannot be removed, the helmet must be removed.

Preferred Method

Removing a helmet is at least a two-person job; however, the technique for helmet removal depends on the actual type of helmet worn by the patient. One EMT-I provides constant in-line support as the other moves; you and your partner should not move at the same time. You should first consult with medical control, if possible, about your decision to remove a helmet. When you decide to do so, follow the steps in (Skill Drill 17-6 ▶):

1. **Begin by kneeling** at the patient's head. Your partner should kneel on one side of the patient, at the shoulder area.

2. **Open the face shield,** if there is one, and assess the patient's airway and breathing. Remove eyeglasses if the patient is wearing them (**Step 1**).
3. **Stabilize the helmet** by placing your hands on either side of it, with your fingers on the patient's lower jaw to prevent movement of the head. Once your hands are in position, your partner can loosen the face strap (**Step 2**).
4. **Once the strap is loosened,** your partner should place one hand on the patient's lower jaw at the angle of the jaw and the other behind the head at the back of the helmet. Once your partner's hands are in position, you may pull the sides of the helmet away from the patient's head (**Step 3**).
5. **Gently slip the helmet** halfway off the patient's head, stopping when the helmet reaches the halfway point (**Step 4**).
6. **Your partner then slides** his or her hand from the back of the helmet to the occiput. This will prevent the head from falling back once the helmet is completely removed (**Step 5**).
7. With your partner's hand in place, **remove the helmet,** and immobilize the cervical spine.
8. **Apply the cervical collar,** and then secure the patient to the backboard.
9. **With large helmets** or small patients, you may need to pad under the shoulders. This will prevent flexion of the neck. If shoulder pads or a heavy jacket is in place, you may need to pad behind the patient's head to prevent extension of the neck (**Step 6**).

Remember, you do not need to remove a helmet if you can access the patient's airway, if the head is snug inside the helmet, and if the helmet can be secured to an immobilization device.

Alternative Method

An alternative method for removal of football helmets is possible. The advantage of this method is that it allows the helmet to be removed with less force applied, therefore reducing the possibility of motion at the neck. The disadvantage of this method is that it is slightly more time-consuming. The first step involves removal of the chin strap. This can be cut or unsnapped carefully. Be careful during removal of the chin strap to avoid jarring the neck or head and causing excessive motion. Next, remove the face mask. The face mask is anchored to the helmet by plastic clips secured with screws. These can be removed with a screwdriver or, alternatively, cut with a knife (see Figure 17-25). After the face mask has

Skill Drill 17-6

Removing a Helmet

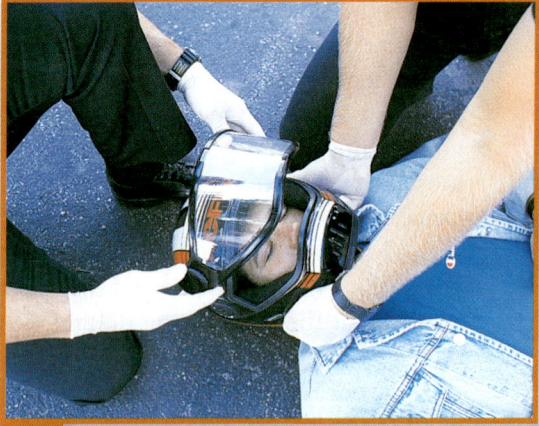

1 Kneel at the patient's head with your partner at one side.

Open the face shield to assess airway and breathing. Remove eyeglasses if present.

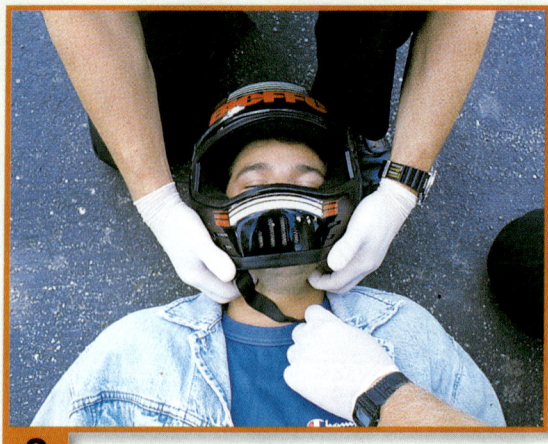

2 Prevent head movement by placing your hands on either side of the helmet and fingers on the lower jaw. Have your partner loosen the strap.

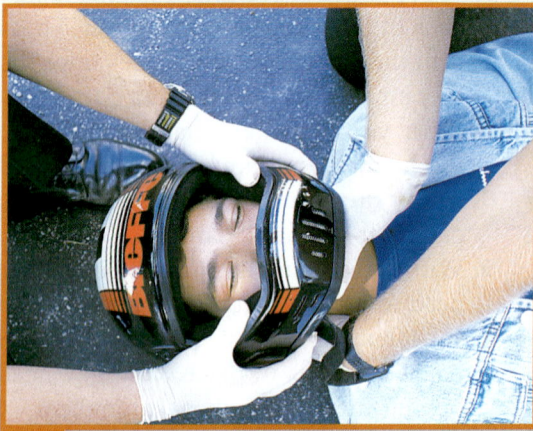

3 Have your partner place one hand at the angle of the lower jaw and the other at the back of the helmet.

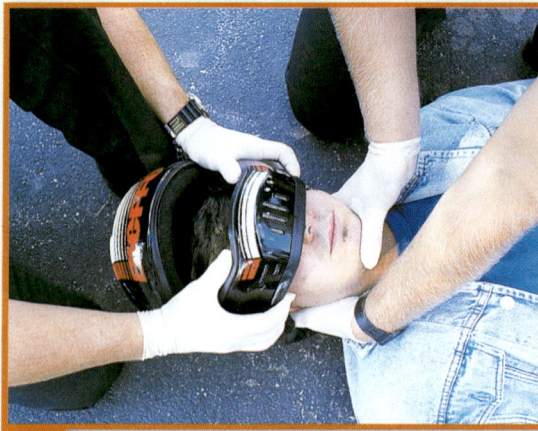

4 Gently slip the helmet about halfway off, then stop.

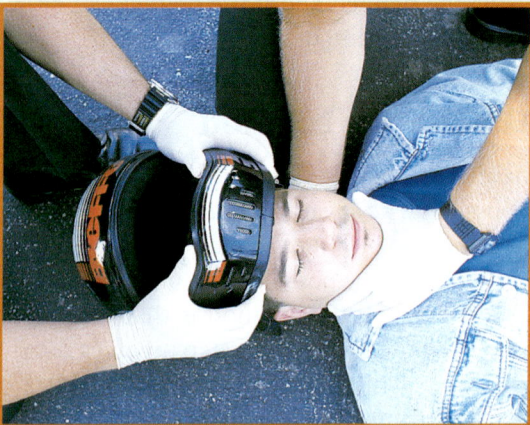

5 Have your partner slide the hand from the back of the helmet to the occiput to prevent the head from falling back.

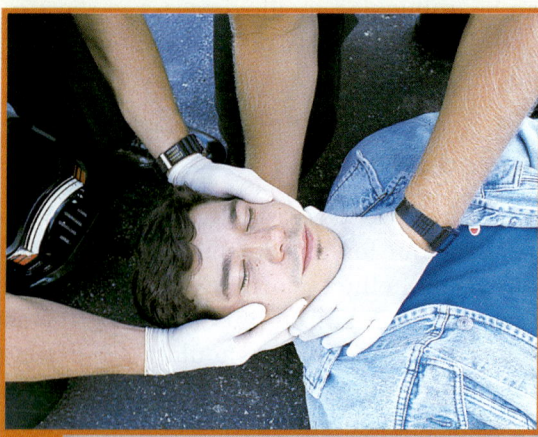

6 Remove the helmet, and stabilize the cervical spine.

Apply a cervical collar, and secure the patient to a long backboard.

Pad as needed to prevent neck flexion or extension.

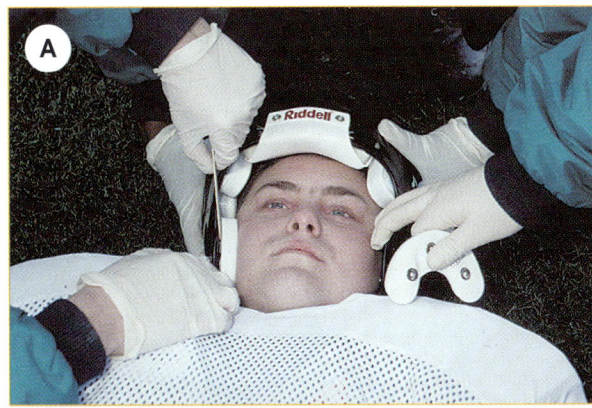

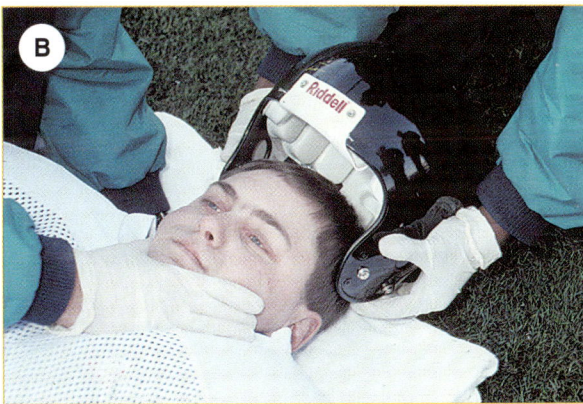

Figure 17-27 **A.** The jaw pads can be removed from the inside of the helmet with the aid of a tongue depressor. **B.** Place the fingers inside the helmet, and gently rock it out of place. The person at the foot controls the lower jaw with one hand and the occiput with the other. Insert padding behind the occiput to prevent neck extension.

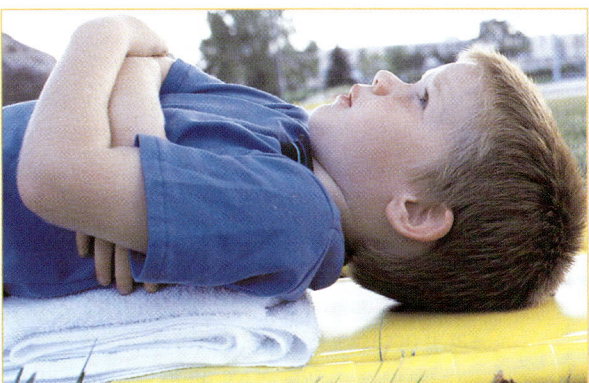

Figure 17-28 Children have proportionately larger heads than adults, so you may need to place padding under the shoulders to avoid excessive flexion of the neck.

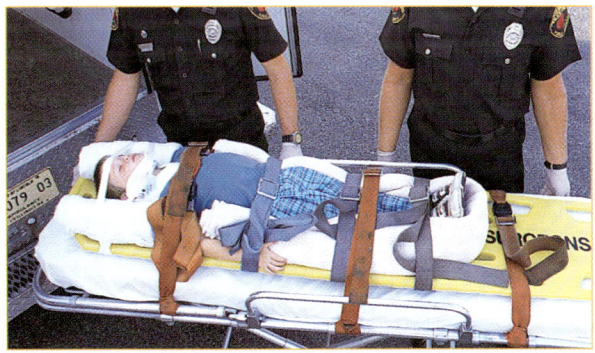

Figure 17-29 Place blanket rolls between the child and the sides of an adult-sized board to prevent the child from slipping to one side or the other.

been removed, the jaw pads can be popped out of place. This can be accomplished with the use of a tongue depressor **Figure 17-27A**. The fingers can be placed inside the helmet, allowing greater control of the helmet during removal as the helmet is gently rocked back off the top of the head. The person at the side of the patient controls the head by holding the jaw with one hand and the occiput with the other **Figure 17-27B**. Padding is inserted behind the occiput to prevent neck extension. If the shoulder pads are in place, appropriate padding must be applied behind the head to prevent hyperextension. Just as with the previously described method, the person at the patient's chest is responsible for making sure that the head and neck do not move during removal of the helmet.

Remember that small children may require additional padding to maintain the neutral, in-line position. Children are not small adults. They have smaller airways, so padding is important to maintain the airway. Pad under the shoulders to the toes, as needed, to avoid excessive neck flexion **Figure 17-28**. In addition, place blanket rolls between the child and the sides of an adult-sized board to prevent the child from slipping to one side or the other **Figure 17-29**. Appropriately sized backboards are available for children.

Pediatric Needs

You are likely to find infants and children who have been in automobile crashes still in their car seats. Your best course of action is to immobilize the child in the car seat if possible. Whenever you apply a cervical collar, make sure it is properly sized. If a properly fitting collar is not available, use a rolled towel and tape it to the car seat. Pad the sides of the car seat, if necessary, to prevent lateral movement Figure 17-30 ▶), and place additional padding in any spaces between the patient and the car seat. If the child is not in a car seat or was removed before your arrival, use an appropriately sized immobilization device. If the cervical immobilization device does not fit, use a rolled towel, and tape it to the board and manually support the head.

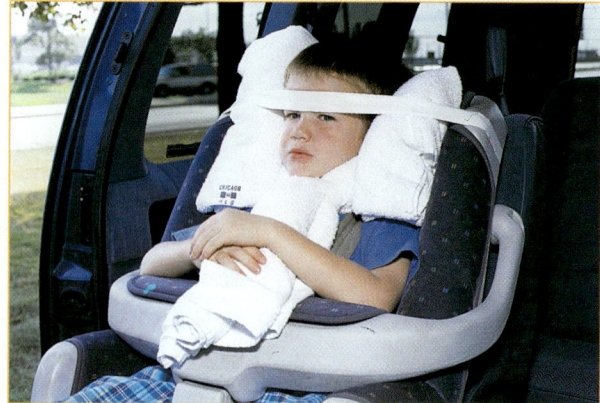

Figure 17-30 If you do not have an appropriately sized cervical collar for a child, you may use a rolled towel and tape it to the car seat. Pad the sides of the car seat, if needed, to prevent lateral movement.

You are the Provider: Summary

1. What are the three major areas of the brain?

The cerebrum, which comprises about 75% of the brain's total size, controls a wide variety of activities. Underneath the cerebrum lies the cerebellum, which coordinates body movements. The most primitive part of the brain, the brain stem, controls virtually all the functions that are necessary for life, including heart rate, blood pressure, and breathing.

2. What mechanisms of injury are likely to cause head and spinal cord injuries?

Motor vehicle crashes
Pedestrian-motor vehicle collisions
Falls
Blunt trauma
Penetrating trauma to the head, neck, or torso
Motorcycle crashes
Hangings
Diving accidents
Recreational accidents

3. What is your first consideration in treating this patient?

Following your initial assessment, you must immediately treat all life-threatening injuries. In this patient, you should assist ventilation with a BVM device and 100% oxygen. Further immediate care includes controlling any active bleeding.

4. Following initial treatment of this patient, what is your next step?

After treating all immediately life-threatening injuries or conditions identified in the initial assessment, your next step is to perform a rapid trauma assessment to identify and treat other, potentially life-threatening injuries.

5. What do the patient's vital signs indicate to you?

This patient's vital signs indicate increased intracranial pressure. The Cushing reflex, a progressive increase in blood pressure (especially systolic), indicates the body's attempt to maintain cerebral perfusion pressure. Bradycardia often occurs in response to hypertension and is caused by increased parasympathetic tone. The presence of abnormal respiratory patterns (for example, irregular, rapid) indicates pressure on the brain stem.

6. What is one of the most common complications associated with head trauma?

When the brain is significantly injured, the most common complication is swelling (cerebral edema). If left untreated, intracranial pressure will increase, resulting in severe brain dysfunction and eventual herniation (the brain, which is significantly compressed, is forced out of the cranial vault).

Prep Kit

Ready for Review

- The nervous system is divided into two parts: the CNS and the peripheral nervous system.
- The CNS consists of the brain and the spinal cord. The cables of nerve fibers linking nerve cells in the brain and spinal cord to the body's organs make up the peripheral nervous system.
- In addition to the skull and spinal canal, the CNS is protected by the meninges, which are three layers of tissue called the dura mater, arachnoid, and pia mater.
- The peripheral nervous system consists of 31 pairs of spinal nerves, which conduct sensory impulses from the skin and other organs to the spinal cord and conduct motor impulses from the spinal cord to the muscles, and 12 pairs of cranial nerves, which transmit sensations relating to sight, smell, taste, and hearing directly to the brain. The three major types of peripheral nerves are sensory nerves, motor nerves, and connecting nerves.
- The part of the nervous system that regulates our voluntary activities is called the somatic or voluntary nervous system.
- The much more primitive autonomic or involuntary nervous system regulates involuntary body functions. The autonomic nervous system is composed of the sympathetic and parasympathetic nervous systems, which balance each other.
- The skull is divided into two large bony structures that protect the brain: the cranium and the face.
- The spinal column has 33 bones, called vertebrae, in five sections: cervical, thoracic or dorsal, lumbar, sacral, and coccygeal.
- The cervical, thoracic, and lumbar portions of the spine can be injured through compression resulting from a fall; through unnatural motions such as overextension caused by motor vehicle crashes and other types of trauma; and through distraction (pulling) along the length of the spine, as in hanging.
- Start your assessment of a patient with a possible spinal injury by focusing on the ABCs and, if he or she is responsive, by asking five questions: Does your neck or back hurt? What happened? Where does it hurt? Can you move your hands and feet? Can you feel me touching your fingers and toes?
- Look for contusions, punctures, or skull deformities; test for strength in the extremities; ask about pain; and check for numbness, weakness, or tingling in the extremities. Patients with severe spinal injury may lose sensation or be paralyzed below the suspected injury.
- Keep the head in a neutral, in-line position while you open and maintain the airway, assess respirations, and give supplemental oxygen. Provide manual immobilization until the patient is properly secured to a backboard.
- A patient who is supine can be immobilized with a long backboard, using the four-person log roll.
- With sitting patients, you should use a short immobilization device, then secure the short device to a long board.
- If the patient is standing, immobilize him or her to a long backboard before starting your assessment; this requires three EMT-Is.
- Common head injuries include skull wounds (scalp lacerations and skull fracture) and brain injuries (concussion, contusion, intracranial bleeding), typically caused by direct blows, car crashes, falls from heights, assault, and sports injuries.
- Cerebral edema, seizures, vomiting, and leakage of CSF are common complications of open and closed head injuries.
- Signs and symptoms of head injuries include lacerations, visible deformities of the skull, ecchymosis around the eyes or behind the ear, unequal pupil size and failure of the pupils to respond to light, loss of sensation and/or motor function, visual disturbances, irregular respirations and posturing.
- The single most important observation that you can make in assessing a brain injury is of change in the level of consciousness. Use the AVPU scale or the Glasgow Coma Scale to assess consciousness immediately and every 15 minutes for a patient in stable condition and every 5 minutes for a patient in unstable condition, recording scores and times as you do so. Also monitor pupil size and reactions.

Technology

- Interactivities
- Vocabulary Explorer
- Anatomy Review
- Web Links
- Online Review Manual

- Patients with head injuries often have injuries to the cervical spine as well. Therefore, when treating a patient with a head injury, you must protect and stabilize the cervical spine at all times.
- Three principles govern treatment of head injuries: airway, ventilation, and high-flow supplemental oxygen; bleeding and circulation; and assessing and monitoring the level of consciousness.
- Immobilization devices include cervical collars, which must be the correct size; short backboards, including vest-type devices and rigid short boards; and long backboards.
- A helmet that fits well prevents the patient's head from moving and should be left on, as long as it does not interfere with assessment and treatment of airway or ventilation problems and you can properly immobilize the spine. Remove a helmet if it makes assessing or managing airway problems difficult, prevents you from immobilizing the spine, or allows excessive head movement.
- Never remove a helmet if doing so will further injure the patient. Always remove a helmet if the patient is in cardiac arrest.

Vital Vocabulary

antegrade (posttraumatic) amnesia Inability to remember events after an injury.

autonomic (involuntary) nervous system The part of the nervous system that regulates functions that are not controlled consciously, such as digestion and sweating.

Battle's sign Bruising behind an ear over the mastoid process that may indicate skull fracture.

brain stem The part of the central nervous system that controls virtually all functions that are necessary for life, including the cardiac and respiratory systems.

central nervous system (CNS) The brain and spinal cord.

cerebellum The part of the brain that coordinates body movements.

cerebral edema Swelling of the brain.

cerebrum The largest part of the brain, comprising about 75% of the brain's total size.

closed head injury An injury in which the brain has been injured but the skin has not been broken and there is no obvious bleeding.

concussion A temporary loss or alteration of part or all of the brain's abilities to function without actual physical damage to the brain.

connecting nerves The nerves in the brain and spinal cord that connect the motor and sensory nerves.

decerebrate (extensor) posturing A posture characterized by extension of the arms and legs; indicates pressure on the brainstem and may appear in patients with severe brain trauma

decorticate (flexor) posturing A posture characterized by flexion of the arms and extension of the legs; indicates pressure on the brainstem and may appear in patients with severe brain trauma.

distracted The action of pulling the spine along its length.

eyes-forward position A head position in which the patient's eyes are looking straight ahead and the head and torso are in line.

four-person log roll The recommended procedure for moving a patient with a suspected spinal injury from the ground to a long spine board.

Glasgow Coma Scale (GCS) A method of evaluating the level of consciousness that uses a scoring system for neurologic responses to specific stimuli.

intervertebral disks The cushions that lie between the vertebrae.

involuntary activities The actions that we do not consciously control.

meninges Three distinct layers of tissue that surround and protect the brain and the spinal cord within the skull and the spinal canal.

motor nerves The nerves that carry information from the central nervous system to the muscles.

open head injury An injury to the head often caused by a penetrating object in which there may be bleeding and exposed brain tissue.

peripheral nervous system The 31 pairs of spinal nerves and 12 pairs of cranial nerves that link the body's other organs to the central nervous system.

raccoon eyes (periorbital ecchymosis) Bruising under the eyes that may indicate skull fracture.

retrograde amnesia The inability to remember events leading up to a head injury.

sensory nerves The nerves that transmit sensory input, such as touch, taste, heat, cold, and pain, from the body to the central nervous system.

somatic (voluntary) nervous system The part of the nervous system that regulates our voluntary activities, such as walking, talking, and writing.

voluntary activities The actions that we consciously perform, in which sensory input determines the specific muscular activity.

Assessment in Action

You arrive at the scene of an ATV accident, in which a male patient was thrown from his ATV after he lost control on an incline. He was not wearing a helmet. You find the patient lying prone on the ground next to a tree.

After assuming manual cervical-spine stabilization, you and your partner log roll the patient to a supine position. Your initial assessment reveals that the patient is semiconscious. His airway is patent, and his respirations are slow and shallow. Further assessment reveals that his pulse is slow and bounding and his skin is cool and dry. He has multiple abrasions to his body and a large hematoma to his forehead.

1. Your initial treatment for this patient should include:
   A. insertion of an nasopharyngeal airway.
   B. 100% oxygen via nonrebreathing mask.
   C. two large-bore intravenous (IV) lines for normal saline.
   D. assisted ventilation with a BVM device.

2. The patient's blood pressure is 160/94 mm Hg, and his pulse is 60 beats per minute. These vital signs are MOST suggestive of:
   A. head injury.
   B. spinal injury.
   C. internal bleeding.
   D. compensated shock.

3. This patient's slow, shallow respirations are MOST likely the result of:
   A. cerebral edema.
   B. hypovolemia.
   C. severe pain.
   D. internal bleeding.

4. Assessment for spinal injury should include all of the following EXCEPT:
   A. having the patient squeeze your hands.
   B. manipulating the head to elicit a pain response.
   C. seeing if the patient feels you touching his finger.
   D. determining if the patient has neck or back pain.

5. Signs and symptoms of spinal injury include all of the following EXCEPT:
   A. pain.
   B. deformity.
   C. paralysis above the point of the injury.
   D. paralysis below the point of the injury.

6. Signs and symptoms of isolated brain injury with increased intracranial pressure include:
   A. tachycardia.
   B. hypotension.
   C. posturing.
   D. paraplegia.

7. The patient's eyes open in response to pain; he answers questions inappropriately, and he withdraws from painful stimuli. His Glasgow Coma Scale score is:
   A. 9.
   B. 10.
   C. 11.
   D. 12.

8. Which of the following treatment regimens is MOST appropriate for this patient?
   A. Immobilization with a Kendrick extrication device (KED), 500-mL bolus of normal saline, and elevation of the lower extremities.
   B. Immobilization with a long spine board, IV set to keep the vein open, and cardiac monitoring.
   C. Immobilization with a long spine board, two large-bore IVs running wide open, and cardiac monitoring.
   D. Immobilization with a KED, IV set to keep the vein open, and elevation of the lower extremities.

9. During transport, you must monitor this patient for the following complications:
   A. Respiratory arrest
   B. Shock
   C. Vomiting
   D. Any of the above

Points to Ponder

You arrive at the scene of a motor-vehicle accident. Your patient is a 50-year-old man who ran off the road and into a ditch to avoid a collision with another vehicle. You observe heavy front-end damage to his vehicle and note that the airbag deployed. The patient is ambulatory at the scene and states that he was wearing his seat belt. Your assessment reveals no obvious injury or neurologic deficits; therefore, you allow the patient to sit comfortably on the cot. On arrival at the emergency room, the patient states he cannot move his legs. What went wrong? What should you have done differently?

Issues: Understand the Relationship Between Signs and Symptoms and Spinal Injury, Restraint Does Not Necessarily Prevent Spinal Cord Injury

Musculoskeletal Care

1999 Objectives

Cognitive
None

Affective
None

Psychomotor

4-5.13 Demonstrate a clinical assessment to determine the proper treatment plan for a patient with a suspected musculoskeletal injury. (p 808)

4-5.14 Demonstrate the proper use of fixation, soft, and traction splints for a patient with a suspected fracture. (p 814, 815)

1985 Objectives

There are no 1985 objectives for this chapter.

Additional Objectives*

Cognitive

1. Describe the function of the muscular system. (p 800)
2. Describe the function of the skeletal system. (p 801)
3. List the major bones or bone groupings of the spinal column, the thorax, the upper extremities, and the lower extremities. (p 801)
4. Differentiate between an open and closed painful, swollen, deformed extremity (fracture). (p 804)
5. State the reasons for splinting. (p 813)
6. List the general rules of splinting. (p 814)
7. List the complications of splinting. (p 824)
8. List the emergency medical care for a patient with a swollen, painful, deformed extremity (fracture). (p 814)

Affective

9. Explain the rationale for splinting at the scene versus load and go. (p 809)
10. Explain the rationale for immobilization of the painful, swollen, deformed extremity (fracture). (p 813)

Psychomotor
None

*These are noncurriculum objectives.

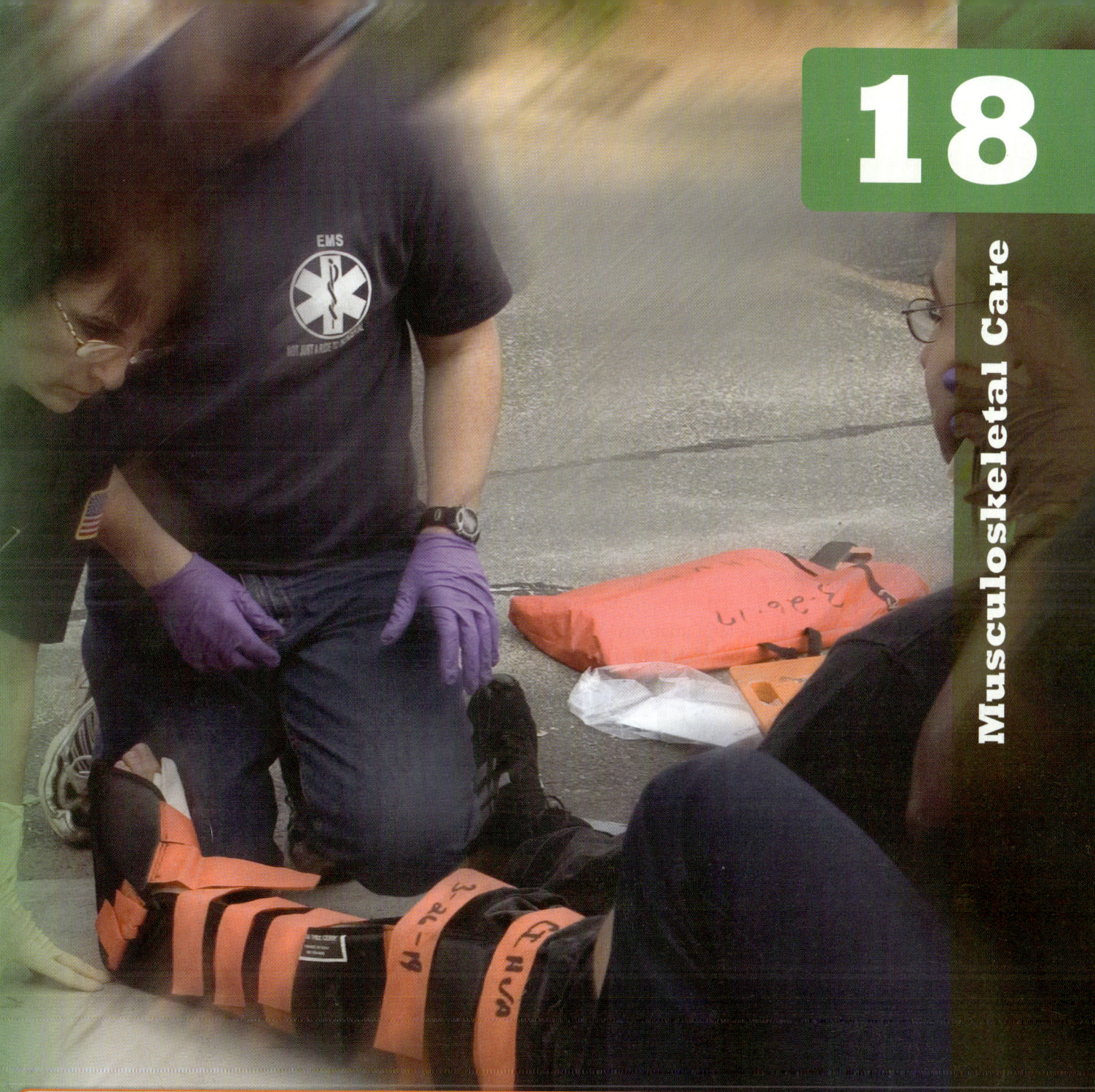

18

Musculoskeletal Care

You are the Provider

Your rescue squad is dispatched to the local high school for an injured baseball player. You arrive to find the player out on the field by second base. His coach tells you that he was attempting to steal, slid into the base, and heard a "snapping" sound in his lower leg.

This chapter will help prepare you to properly care for patients with musculoskeletal injuries and help you answer the following questions:

1. What common musculoskeletal injures are likely to be encountered by the EMT-I?
2. What are the two classifications of fractures?

Musculoskeletal Care

The human body is a well-designed system whose form, upright posture, and movement are provided by the musculoskeletal system, which also protects the vital internal organs of the body. As its combination form suggests, the term "musculoskeletal" refers to the bones and voluntary muscles of the body. However, the bones and muscles themselves are susceptible to external forces that can cause injury. Also at risk are the tendons that attach muscles to bones, the joints that form wherever two bones come into contact, and the ligaments that hold the bone ends of a joint together.

As an EMT-I, you must be familiar with the basic anatomy of the body's musculoskeletal system. Although muscles are technically soft tissue, they are discussed in this chapter because of their close relationship to the skeleton. Therefore, the chapter begins with a review of the musculoskeletal anatomy. Various types and causes of musculoskeletal injuries in general are identified, and the assessment and treatment process for each is explained, followed by a detailed discussion of splinting. The chapter then focuses on specific musculoskeletal injuries, beginning at the clavicle and ending at the feet.

Anatomy and Physiology of the Musculoskeletal System

Muscles

The musculoskeletal system is composed of three types of muscles: skeletal, smooth, and cardiac (Figure 18-1 ▼). Skeletal muscle, also called striated muscle because of its characteristic stripes, attaches to the bones and usually crosses at least one joint, forming the major muscle mass of the body. This type of muscle is also called voluntary muscle, because it is under direct voluntary control of the brain, responding to commands to move specific body parts. Usually, movement is the result of several muscles contracting and relaxing simultaneously.

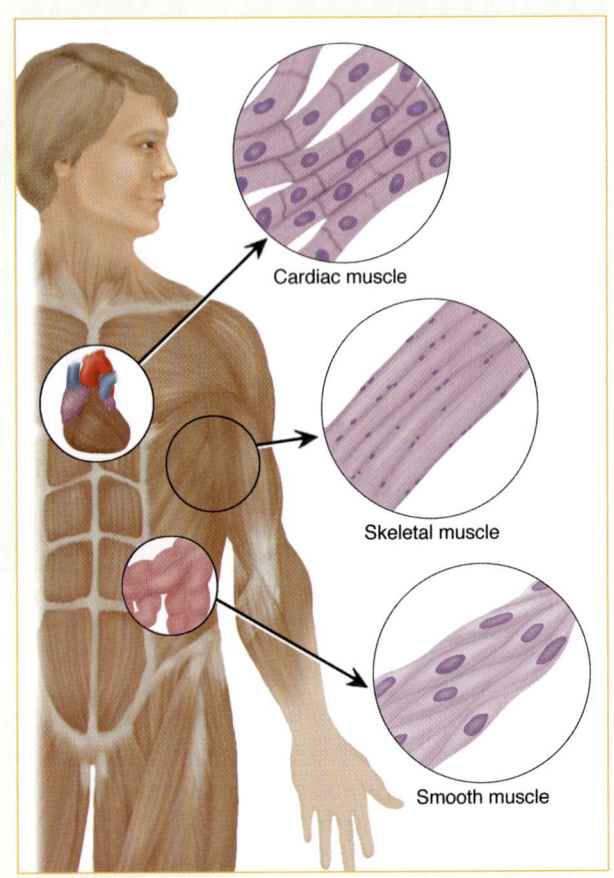

Figure 18-1 The musculoskeletal system includes three types of muscle: skeletal or voluntary muscles, smooth or involuntary muscles, and cardiac muscle.

Technology

- Interactivities
- Vocabulary Explorer
- Anatomy Review
- Web Links
- Online Review Manual

www.EMSzone.com/EMTI

All skeletal muscles are supplied with arteries, veins, and nerves. Blood from the arteries brings oxygen and nutrients to the muscles Figure 18-2 . Waste products, including carbon dioxide and lactic acid, are carried away in the veins. Either disease or trauma can result in the loss of a muscle's nervous energy; this, in turn, can lead to *atrophy,* or a wasting of the muscle. Muscle tissue is directly attached to the bone by tough, ropelike fibrous structures known as tendons, which are extensions of the fascia that covers all skeletal muscle.

Smooth muscle, also called involuntary muscle, performs much of the automatic work of the body. This type of muscle is found in the walls of most tubular structures of the body, such as the gastrointestinal tract and the blood vessels. Smooth muscle contracts and relaxes to control the movement of the contents of these structures Figure 18-3 .

Cardiac muscle, unlike skeletal or smooth muscle, is able to efficiently generate electrical impulses. It is a specially adapted involuntary muscle with its own regulatory system.

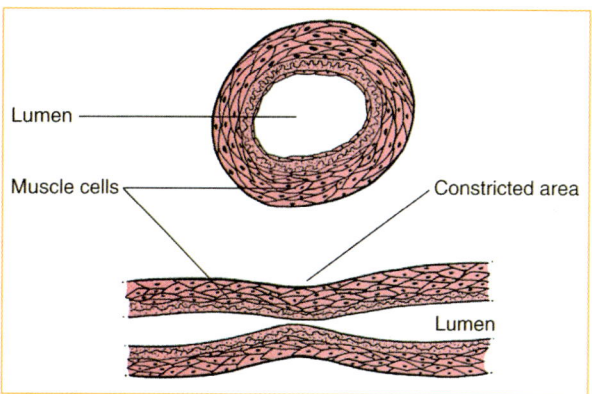

Figure 18-3 Smooth muscle is found in the walls of most tubular structures in the body. The autonomic nervous system generates impulses that cause these muscles to contract and relax to control the movement of the contents of these structures.

The remainder of this chapter is concerned exclusively with skeletal muscle.

The Skeleton

The skeleton, which gives us our recognizable human form, protects our vital internal organs, and allows us to move, is made up of approximately 206 bones Figure 18-4 . The bones in the skeleton also produce blood cells (in the bone marrow) and serve as a reservoir for important minerals and electrolytes.

The skull surrounds and protects the brain. The thoracic cage protects the heart, lungs, and great vessels; the lower ribs protect the liver and spleen. The bony spinal canal encases and protects the spinal cord. The upper extremity extends from the shoulder to the fingertips and is composed of the arm, elbow, forearm, wrist, hand, and fingers. The arm extends from the shoulder to the elbow. The pelvis supports the body's weight and protects the structures within the pelvis: the bladder, rectum, and female reproductive organs. The lower extremity consists of the thigh, leg, and foot. The joint between the pelvis and the thigh is the hip; the joint between the thigh and lower leg is the knee, and the joint between the lower leg and foot is the ankle.

The bones of the skeleton provide a framework to which the muscles and tendons are attached. Bone is a living tissue that contains nerves and receives oxygen and nutrients from the arterial system. Therefore, when a bone breaks, a patient typically experiences severe pain

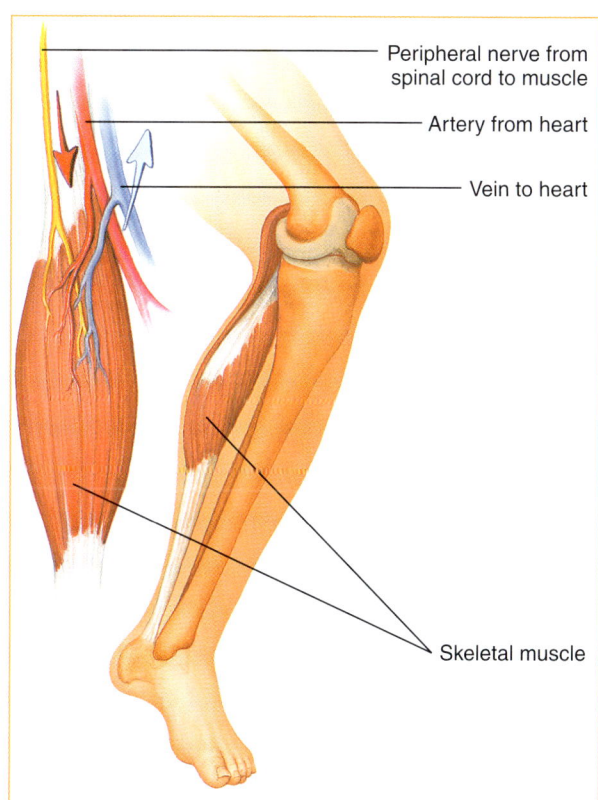

Figure 18-2 Skeletal muscles are supplied with arteries, veins, and nerves that bring oxygen and nutrients, carry away waste products, and supply nervous stimuli.

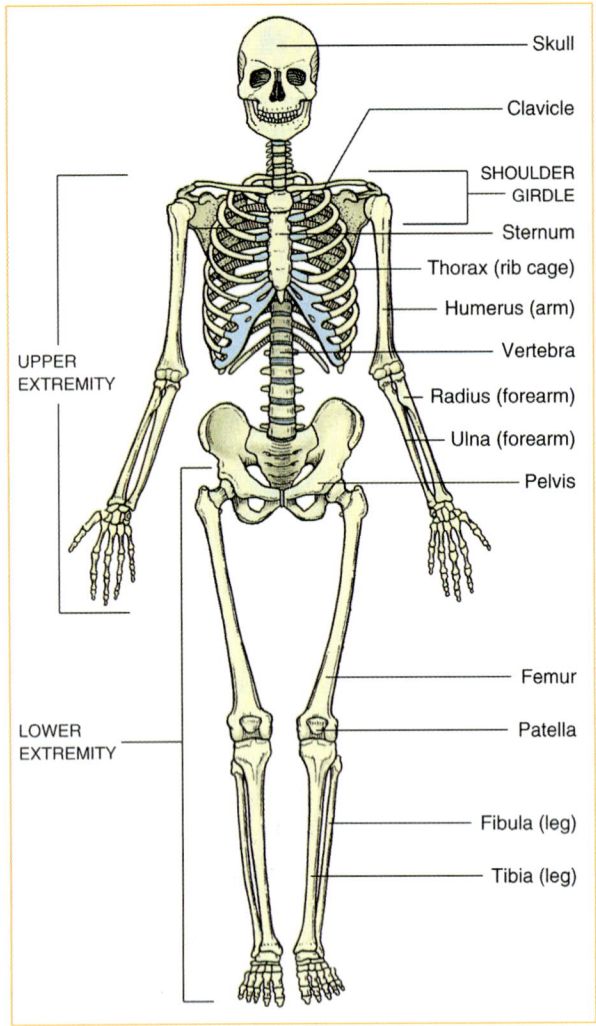

Figure 18-4 The human skeleton, consisting of approximately 206 bones, gives us our form and protects our vital organs.

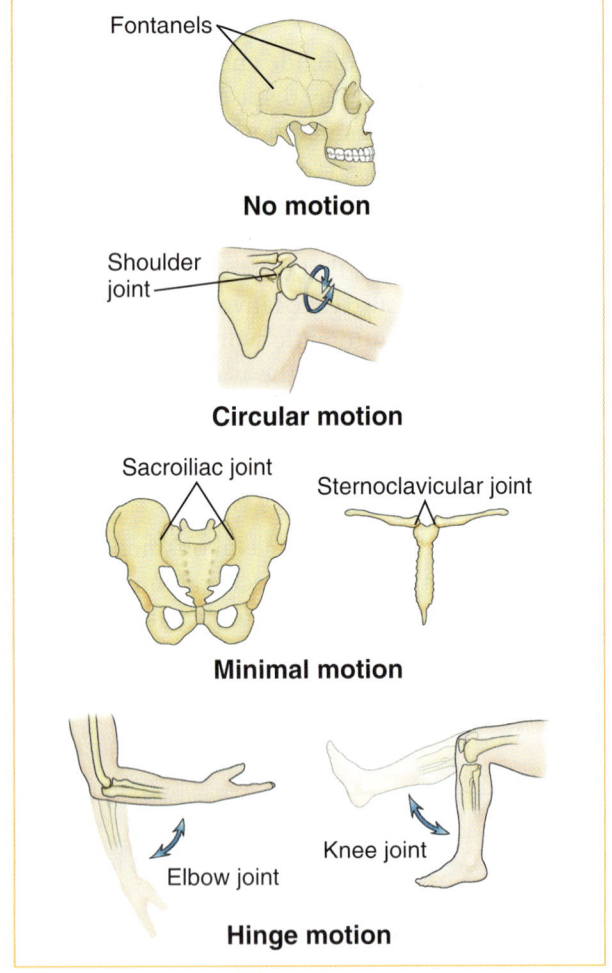

Figure 18-5 Joints have many functions. Some joints allow for motion to occur in a circular manner; others act as hinges. Still others allow only a minimum amount of motion or none at all.

and bleeding. Bone marrow, located in the center of each bone, is constantly producing red blood cells to provide oxygen and nourishment to the body and remove waste.

A joint is formed wherever two bones come into contact. The sternoclavicular joint, for example, is where the sternum and the clavicle join. Joints are held together in a tough fibrous structure known as a capsule, which is supported and strengthened in certain key areas by bands of fibrous tissue called ligaments. In moving joints, the ends of the bones are covered with a thin layer of cartilage known as articular cartilage. This cartilage is a pearly substance that allows the ends of the bones to glide easily. Joints are bathed and lubricated by synovial fluid.

Most joints, such as the shoulder, allow motion to occur in a circular manner. Other joints, such as the knee and elbow, act as hinges. Still other joints, including the sacroiliac joint in the lower back and the sternoclavicular joints, allow only a minimum amount of motion. Certain joints, such as the fontanels in the skull, fuse two bones together to create a solid, immobile, bony structure (Figure 18-5 ▲).

Musculoskeletal Injuries

A fracture is a broken bone. More precisely, it is a break in the continuity of the bone, often occurring as a result of an external force (Figure 18-6 ▶). The break can occur anywhere on the surface of the bone.

A dislocation is a disruption of a joint in which the bone ends are no longer in contact. The supporting

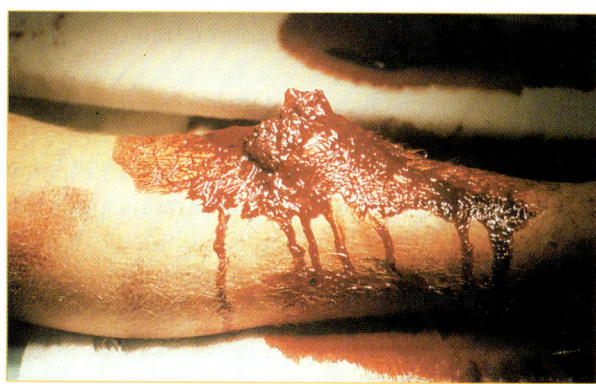

Figure 18-6 A fracture can occur anywhere on a bone and may or may not break the skin.

A sprain is a joint injury in which there is some partial or temporary dislocation of the bone ends and partial stretching or tearing of the supporting ligaments. After the injury, the joint surfaces generally fall back into alignment, so the joint is not significantly displaced. Sprains can range from mild to severe, depending on the amount of damage done to the supporting ligaments. The most severe sprains involve complete dislocation of the joint; mild sprains typically heal rather quickly.

A strain, or muscle pull, is a stretching or tearing of the muscle, causing pain, swelling, and bruising of the soft tissues in the area. Unlike a sprain, no ligament or joint damage occurs.

Injury to bones and joints is often associated with injury to the surrounding soft tissues, especially to the adjacent nerves and blood vessels. The entire area is known as the zone of injury Figure 18-8. Depending on the amount of kinetic energy the tissues absorb from forces acting on the body, the zone may extend to a distant point. For this reason, you should not focus on

ligaments are torn, usually completely, allowing the bone ends to separate completely from each other Figure 18-7. A fracture-dislocation is a combination injury at the joint in which the joint is dislocated and there is a fracture of the end of the bone.

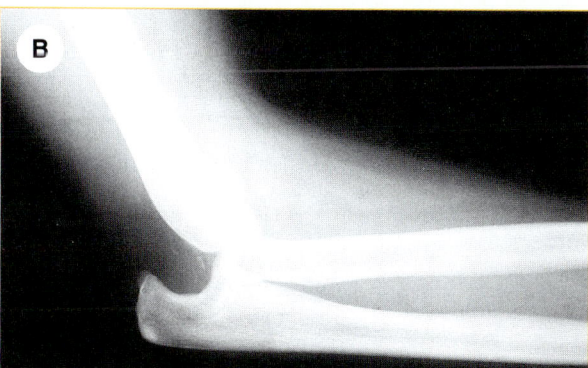

Figure 18-7 A dislocation is a disruption of a joint in which the bone ends are no longer in contact. **A.** The clinical appearance of an elbow dislocation. **B.** Radiographic appearance of the same elbow.

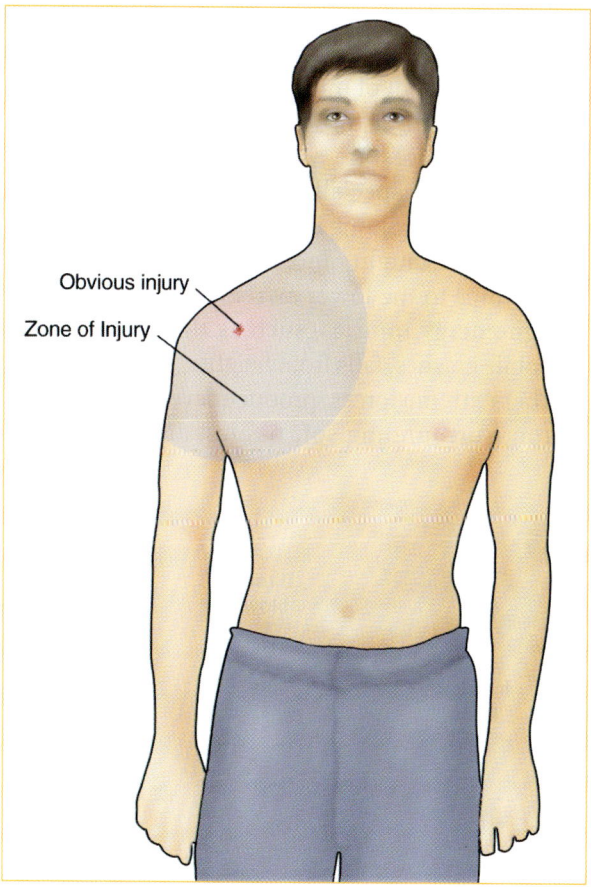

Figure 18-8 The zone of injury is the area of soft tissue, including the adjacent nerves and blood vessels, that surrounds the obvious injury of a bone or joint.

a patient's obvious injury without first completing an initial assessment to check for associated injuries, which may be even more serious. This is especially true in assessing damage from gunshots and falls from a height.

Mechanism of Injury

Significant force is generally required to cause fractures or dislocations. This force may be applied to the limb in any of the following ways (Figure 18-9):

- Direct blows
- Indirect forces
- Twisting forces
- High-energy injury

A direct blow fractures the bone at the point of impact. An example is the patella (kneecap) that fractures when it strikes the dashboard in an automobile crash.

Indirect force may cause a fracture or dislocation at a distant point, as when a person falls and lands on an outstretched hand. The direct impact may cause the wrist fracture, but the indirect force can cause dislocation of the elbow or a fracture of the forearm, humerus, or even clavicle. Therefore, when caring for patients who have fallen, you must identify the point of contact and the mechanism of injury so that you will not overlook associated injuries.

Twisting forces are a common cause of musculoskeletal injury, especially to the anterior cruciate ligament at the knee. Skiing injuries often happen this way. A ski becomes caught, and the skier falls, applying a twisting force to the lower extremity.

High-energy injuries, such as those that occur in automobile crashes, falls from heights, gunshot wounds, and other extreme forces, produce severe damage to the skeleton, surrounding soft tissues, and vital internal organs. A patient may have multiple injuries to many body parts, including more than one fracture or dislocation in a single limb.

A significant mechanism of injury (MOI) is not necessary to fracture a bone. A slight force can easily fracture a bone that is weakened by a tumor or *osteoporosis*, a generalized bone disease that is common among postmenopausal women. In elderly patients with osteoporosis, minor falls, simple twisting injuries, or even a muscle contraction can cause a fracture, most often of the wrist, spine, or hip. You should suspect the presence of a fracture in any older patient who has sustained even a mild injury.

Fractures

Fractures are classified as closed or open. In assessing and treating patients with possible fractures or dislocations, your first priority is to determine whether the overlying skin has been damaged. If it is not, the patient has a closed fracture. However, making this determination is not always as easy as it sounds. With an open fracture, there is an external wound, caused by the same blow that fractured the bone or by the broken bone ends lacerating the skin. The size of the wound may vary from a very small puncture to a gaping tear that exposes bone and soft tissue. Regardless of the extent and severity of the damage to the skin, you should treat any injury that breaks the skin as a possible open fracture. Greater blood loss and a higher likelihood of infection, possibilities that you must try to prevent, tend to occur with open fractures.

Fractures are also described by whether the bone is moved from its normal position. A nondisplaced fracture (also known as a hairline fracture) is a simple crack of the bone that may be difficult to distinguish from a

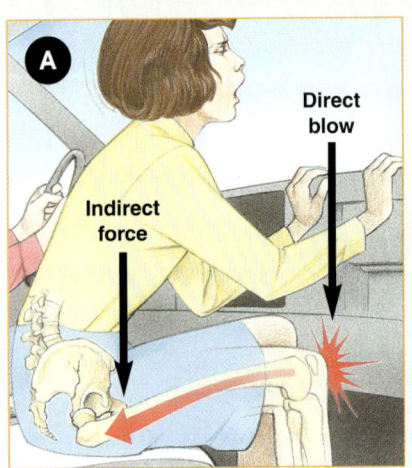
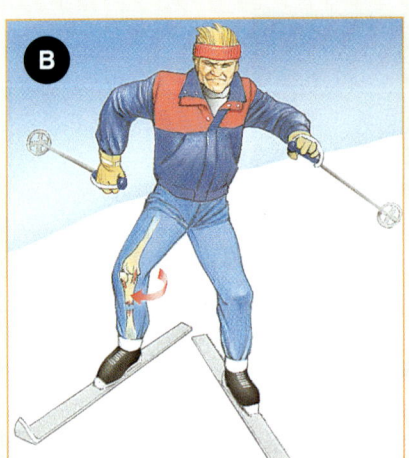
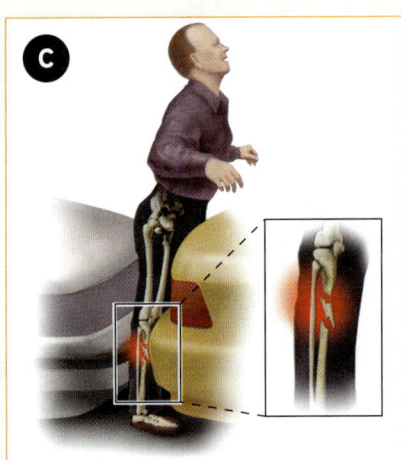

Figure 18-9 Significant force is required to cause fractures or dislocations. Among these are **A.** Direct blows and Indirect forces, **B.** Twisting forces, and **C.** High-energy injuries.

sprain or simple contusion. In fact, radiographs may be required for hospital personnel to diagnose a nondisplaced fracture. A displaced fracture produces actual deformity, or distortion, of the limb by shortening, rotating, or angulation. Often the deformity is obvious and can be associated with crepitus; however, in some cases, the deformity is minimal. Be sure to look for differences between the injured limb and the opposite uninjured limb in any patient with a fracture of an extremity Figure 18-10 ▼.

Medical personnel often use the following special terms to describe particular types of fractures Figure 18-11 ▶:

- **Greenstick fracture.** An incomplete fracture that passes only partway through the shaft of a bone but may still cause severe angulation; occurs in children
- **Comminuted fracture.** A fracture in which the bone is broken into more than two fragments
- **Pathologic fracture.** A fracture of weakened or diseased bone, seen in patients with osteoporosis or cancer; generally produced by minimal force
- **Epiphyseal fracture.** A fracture that occurs in the growth section of a child's bone and may prematurely stop growth of the bone if not properly treated

You should suspect a fracture if one or more of the following signs is present in any patient who has a history of injury and reports pain.

Deformity

The limb may appear to be shortened, rotated, or angulated at a point where there is no joint Figure 18-12 ▶. Always use the opposite limb as a mirror image for comparison.

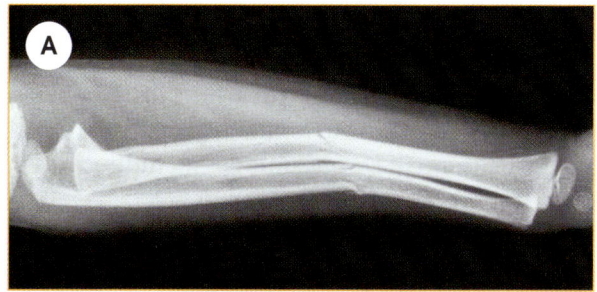
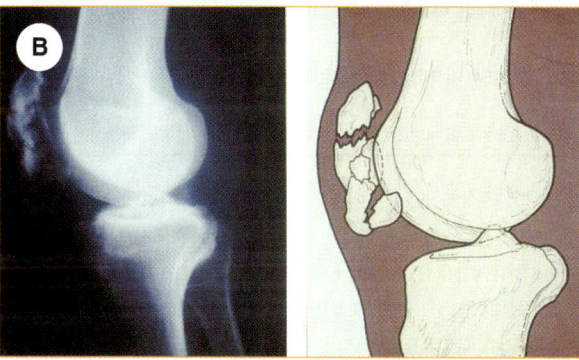
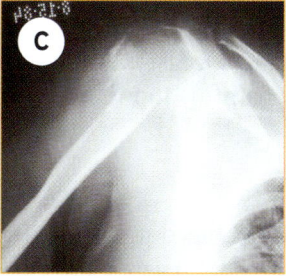
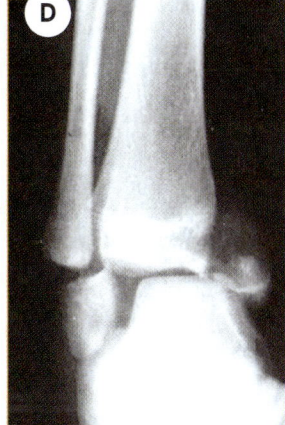

Figure 18-11 Special terms to describe fractures.
A. Greenstick fracture.
B. Comminuted fracture.
C. Pathologic fracture.
D. Epiphyseal fracture.

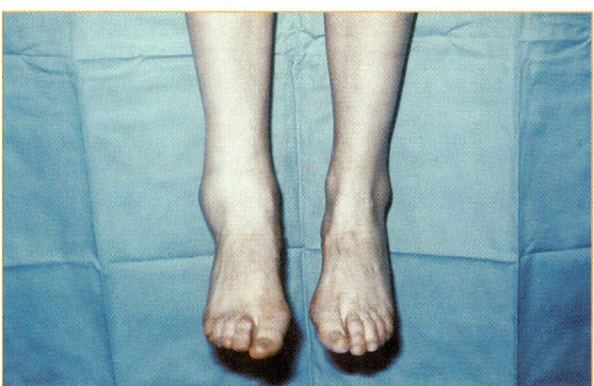

Figure 18-10 You should always compare the injured limb with the uninjured limb when checking for deformity.

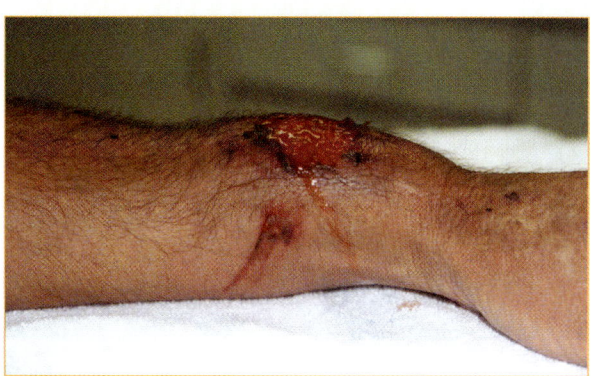

Figure 18-12 Obvious deformity, shortening, rotation, or angulation suggests a fracture. Remember to compare the injured limb with the opposite, uninjured limb.

Tenderness

Point tenderness on palpation in the zone of injury is the most reliable indicator of an underlying fracture, although it does not tell you the type of fracture (Figure 18-13 ▼). Be sure to follow appropriate body substance isolation (BSI) precautions, including wearing gloves, if there are any open wounds.

> 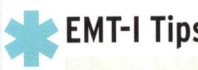 **EMT-I Tips**
>
> Point tenderness is the most reliable indicator of an underlying fracture.

Guarding

An inability to use the extremity is the patient's way of immobilizing it to minimize pain. The muscles around the fracture contract in an attempt to prevent any movement of the broken bone. Guarding does not occur with all fractures; some patients may continue to use the injured part for a period of time. Occasionally, nondisplaced fractures are not very painful, and there is minimal soft-tissue damage.

Swelling

Rapid swelling usually indicates bleeding from a fracture site and is typically followed by severe pain. Often, if the swelling is severe enough, it may mask deformity of the limb (Figure 18-14 ▼). Generalized swelling from fluid buildup may occur several hours after an injury.

Bruising

Fractures are almost always associated with ecchymosis (discoloration) of the surrounding soft tissues (Figure 18-15 ▼). Bruising may be present after almost any injury; it is not specific for bone or joint injuries.

Crepitus

A grating or grinding sensation known as crepitus can be felt and sometimes even heard when fractured bone ends rub together.

False Motion

Motion at a point in the limb where there is no joint is a positive indication of a fracture.

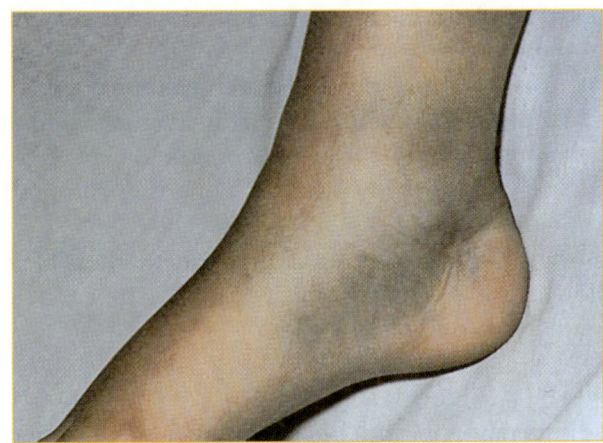

Figure 18-14 Swelling that occurs in association with a fracture can often mask deformity of the limb.

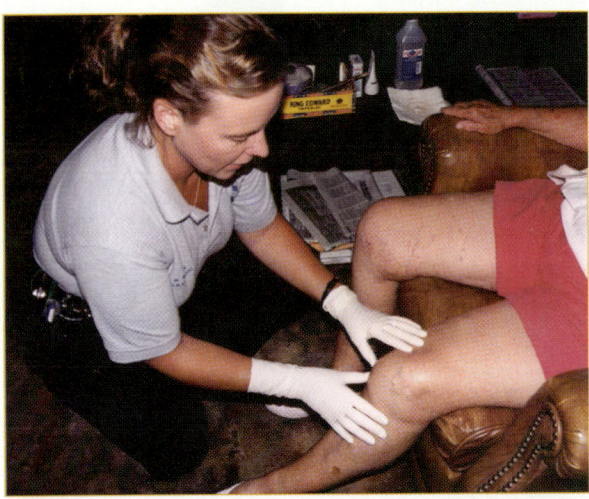

Figure 18-13 Gently palpate to determine point tenderness and compare with the uninjured side to determine the degree of swelling. Check for distal pulses before moving the patient.

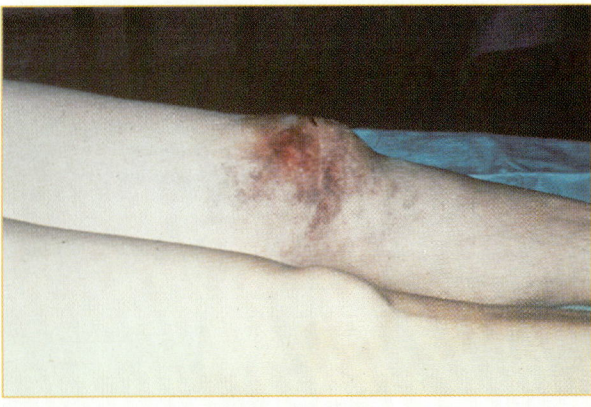

Figure 18-15 Fractures almost always have associated bruising into the surrounding soft tissue.

Exposed Fragments

In open fractures, bone ends may protrude through the skin or be visible within the wound Figure 18-16 ▼.

Pain

Pain, along with tenderness and bruising, commonly occurs in association with fractures and is the primary indicator of a fracture.

Locked Joint

When a joint is locked into position, any attempt to move the joint is difficult and painful.

Keep in mind that crepitus and false motion appear only when a limb is moved or manipulated and are associated with injuries that are extremely painful. Do not manipulate the limb excessively in an effort to elicit these signs.

Dislocations

A dislocated joint may spontaneously <u>reduce</u>, or return to its normal position, before your assessment. In this situation, you will be able to confirm the dislocation only by taking a patient history. Often, however, injury to the supporting ligaments and capsule is so severe that the joint surfaces remain completely separated from one another. A dislocation that does not spontaneously reduce is a serious problem. The ends of the bone can be locked in a displaced position, making any attempt at motion of the joint very difficult and very painful. The most commonly dislocated joints are the fingers, shoulders, elbows, hips, and ankles.

The signs and symptoms of a dislocated joint are similar to those of a fracture Figure 18-17 ▼:

- Marked deformity
- Swelling
- Pain that is aggravated by any attempt at movement
- Tenderness on palpation
- Virtually complete loss of normal joint motion (locked joint)
- Numbness or impaired circulation to the limb or digit

Sprains

A sprain occurs when a joint is twisted or stretched beyond its normal range of motion. As a result, the supporting capsule and ligaments are stretched or torn. A sprain should be considered a partial dislocation or subluxation. The alignment generally returns to a fairly normal position, although there may be some displacement. Note that severe deformity does not typically occur with a sprain. Sprains most often occur in the knee and the ankle, but a sprain can occur in any

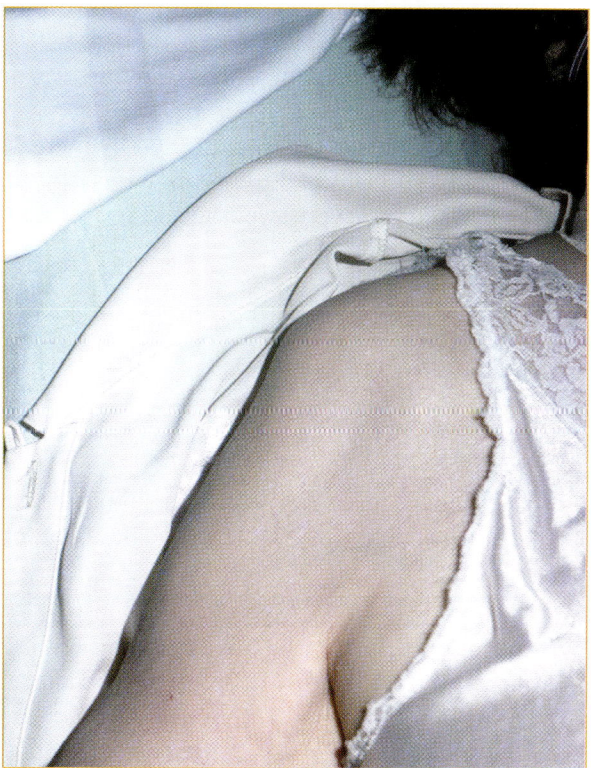

Figure 18-17 Joint dislocations, such as this shoulder, are characterized by deformity, swelling, pain with any movement, tenderness, locking, and impaired circulation.

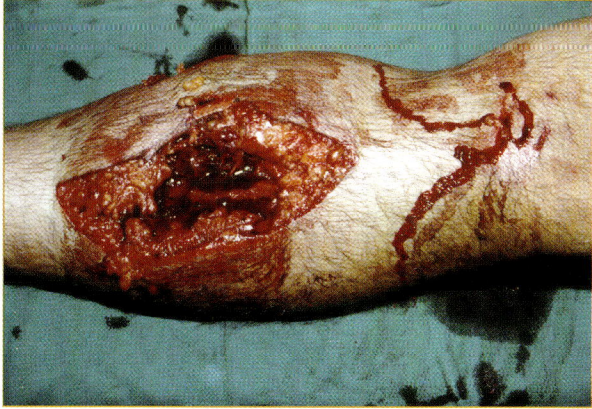

Figure 18-16 Bone ends may protrude through the skin or be visible within the wound of an open fracture.

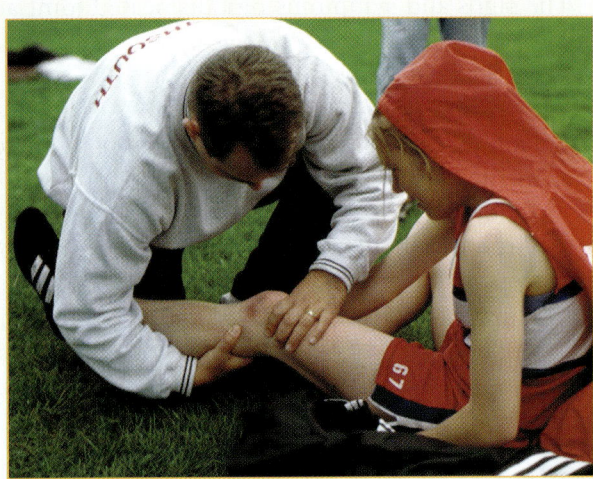

Figure 18-18 Sprains frequently occur in the knee or ankle and are characterized by swelling, bruising, point tenderness, pain, and joint instability.

joint. The following signs and symptoms often indicate that the patient may have a sprain (Figure 18-18):

- Point tenderness can be elicited over the injured ligaments.
- Swelling and ecchymosis appear at the point of injury to the ligament as a result of torn blood vessels.
- Pain prevents the patient from moving or using the limb normally.
- Instability of the joint is indicated by increased motion, especially at the knee; however, this may be masked by severe swelling and guarding.

A fracture can look like a sprain, and vice versa. You will not be able to distinguish a nondisplaced fracture from a sprain, especially at the ankle. Therefore, remember to document the mechanism of injury, as certain sprains and fractures occur more consistently with certain mechanisms. This is especially true at the ankle. In general, your approach should always be to treat the injury as though a fracture exists. The basic principles of field management for sprains, dislocations, and fractures are essentially the same, and radiographic evaluation will be needed for a definitive diagnosis.

Assessing Musculoskeletal Injuries

As an EMT-I, you are the point person in the team approach to the trauma patient. Therefore, your assessments, attempts to splint, and work to stabilize the patient are very important. Look at the big picture, evaluating the overall complexity of the situation. Always carefully assess the mechanism of injury to try to determine the amount of kinetic energy that an injured limb has absorbed.

Assessment of patients with musculoskeletal injuries must include an initial assessment of the patient, followed by a focused physical exam of the painful, swollen, deformed extremity, including evaluation of neurovascular function. Be sure to follow BSI precautions. If oxygen is indicated and you have not already applied it, be sure to do so.

You are the Provider Part 2

Your patient tells you that he caught his foot on the base and that he heard his left ankle "snap." You perform an initial assessment, and note the following:

Initial Assessment	Recording Time: Zero Minutes
Appearance	Skin, normal; severe pain present
Level of consciousness	Alert and oriented to person, place, and time
Airway	Open and clear
Breathing	Respirations, normal in rate and quality
Circulation	Skin, pink, warm, and dry to touch; radial pulses, present and of normal rate

3. What is the proper management of a patient with a musculoskeletal injury?
4. What additional assessment approach should be performed by the EMT-I?

For musculoskeletal trauma, use the DCAP-BTLS approach. Identify any extremity **D**eformities that likely represent significant musculoskeletal injury and stabilize appropriately. **C**ontusions and **A**brasions may overlie more subtle injuries and should prompt you to carefully evaluate the stability and neurovascular status of the limb. The presence of **P**uncture wounds or other signs of **P**enetrating injury should alert you to the possibility of an open fracture. Associated **B**urns must be identified and treated appropriately. Palpate for **T**enderness, which, like contusions or abrasions, may be the only significant sign of an underlying musculoskeletal injury. When **L**acerations are present on an injured extremity, an open fracture must be considered, bleeding controlled, and dressings applied. Careful inspection for **S**welling with attention to comparison with the opposite limb may also reveal occult musculoskeletal injury.

Because patients often have multiple injuries, you must assess their overall condition, stabilize the ABCs, and control any serious bleeding before further treating the injured extremity. In a critically injured patient, you should secure the patient to a long spine board to rapidly immobilize the spine, pelvis, and extremities and provide prompt transport to a trauma center. In this situation, extensive evaluation and splinting of limb injuries in the field are a waste of valuable time.

If the patient has no life-threatening injuries, you may take extra time at the scene to stabilize the patient's overall condition and more completely evaluate the injured extremity. During the focused physical exam, you can inspect and gently palpate the other extremities and the spine to identify areas of point tenderness that may indicate underlying fractures, dislocations, or sprains. Remember to compare the injured limb with the opposite, uninjured limb. If possible, gently and carefully remove the patient's clothing to look for open fractures or dislocations, severe deformity, swelling, and/or ecchymosis.

Again, it is not important to distinguish among fractures, dislocations, sprains, and contusions. In most instances, your assessment will be reported as an "injury to the limb." However, you must be able to distinguish mild injuries from severe injuries because some severe injuries may compromise neurovascular functioning.

If your assessment reveals no external signs of injury, ask the patient to move each limb carefully, stopping immediately if a movement causes pain. Skip this step in your evaluation if the patient reports neck or back pain; even the slightest motion could cause permanent damage to the spinal cord, potentially resulting in paralysis.

Be on the alert for compartment syndrome, which most commonly occurs in the fractured tibia or forearm of children and is often overlooked, especially in patients with an altered level of consciousness. The name <u>compartment syndrome</u> refers to elevated pressure in the fascial compartment, which is the fibrous tissue that surrounds and supports the muscles and neurovascular structures. Compartment syndrome occurs within 6 to 12 hours after injury, usually as a result of excessive bleeding, a severely crushed extremity, or the rapid return of blood to an ischemic limb. This syndrome is characterized by pain that is out of proportion to the injury, pallor, decreased sensation, and decreased power (ranging from decreased strength and movement of the limb to complete palsy). The patient with compartment syndrome may report a feeling of pressure or tension in the affected extremity.

If you suspect that a patient has compartment syndrome, splint the affected limb, keeping it at the level of the heart, and provide immediate transport, checking neurovascular status frequently during transport. Compartment syndrome must be managed surgically.

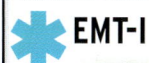

EMT-I Tips

Extremity injuries that impair circulation or nerve function in distal tissues are urgent situations. Patients with these need careful assessment, prompt transport, and frequent reassessment of distal functions. It is also crucial to report this information in your initial radio contact with the hospital, to let personnel prepare for a condition in which prompt surgery may be necessary to save the limb.

Assessing Pulse, Motor, and Sensory Function

Many important blood vessels and nerves lie close to the bone, especially around the major joints. Therefore, any injury or deformity of the bone may have associated vessel or nerve injury. For this reason, you must assess neurovascular function during the focused physical exam, repeating it every 5 to 10 minutes, depending on the patient's condition, until the patient is at the hospital. Always recheck the neurovascular function before and after you splint or otherwise manipulate the limb. Manipulation can cause a bone fragment to press against or impale a nerve or vessel. Failure to restore circulation in this situation can lead to death of the limb. Always give priority to patients with impaired circulation resulting from bone fragments.

Examination of the injured limb should include assessment of four major signs that are good indicators

Skill Drill 18-1

Assessing Neurovascular Pulse

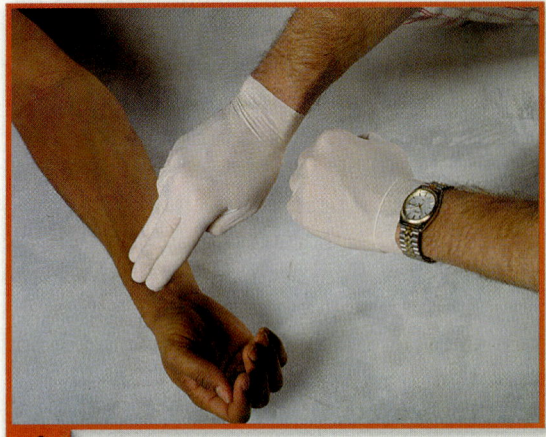

1 Palpate the radial pulse in the upper extremity.

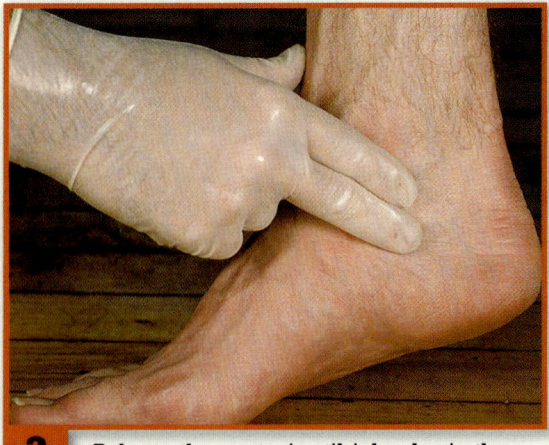

2 Palpate the posterior tibial pulse in the lower extremity.

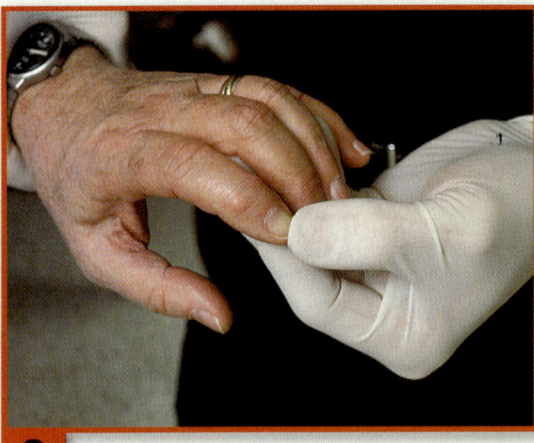

3 Assess capillary refill by blanching a fingernail or toenail.

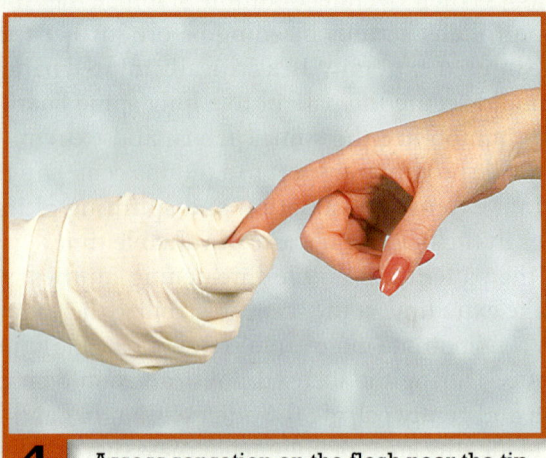

4 Assess sensation on the flesh near the tip of the index finger.

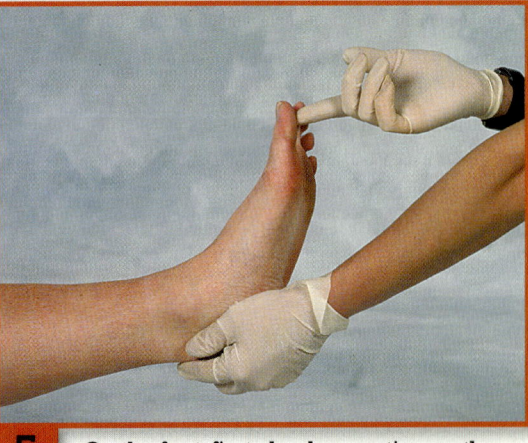

5 On the foot, first check sensation on the flesh near the tip of the great toe.

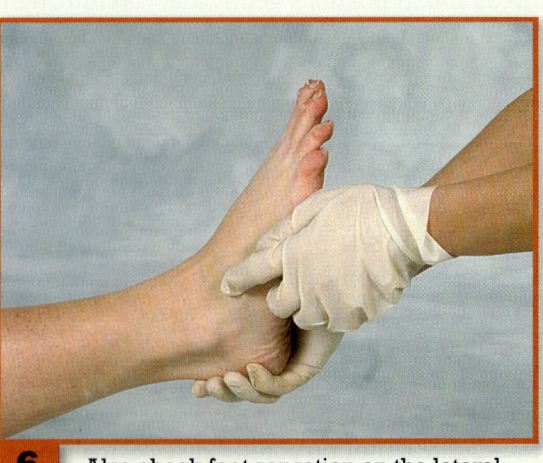

6 Also check foot sensation on the lateral side of the foot.

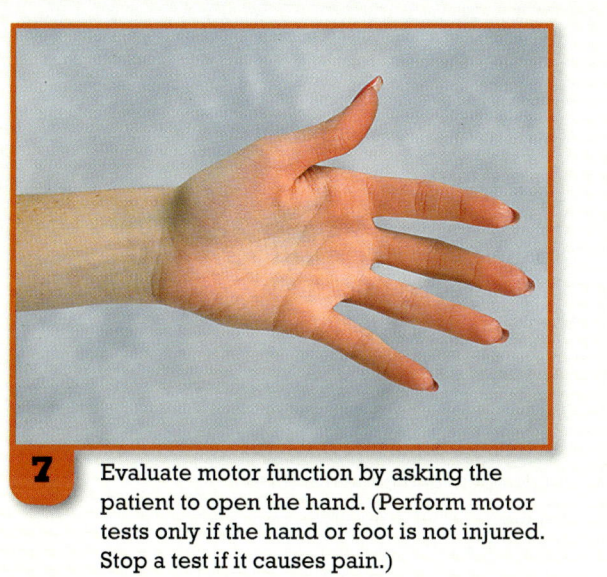
7 Evaluate motor function by asking the patient to open the hand. (Perform motor tests only if the hand or foot is not injured. Stop a test if it causes pain.)

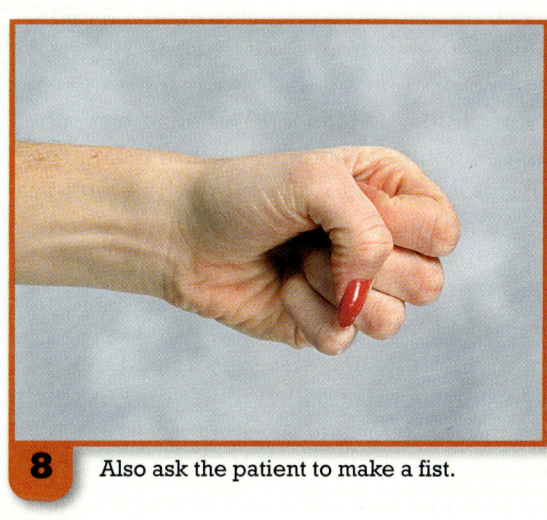
8 Also ask the patient to make a fist.

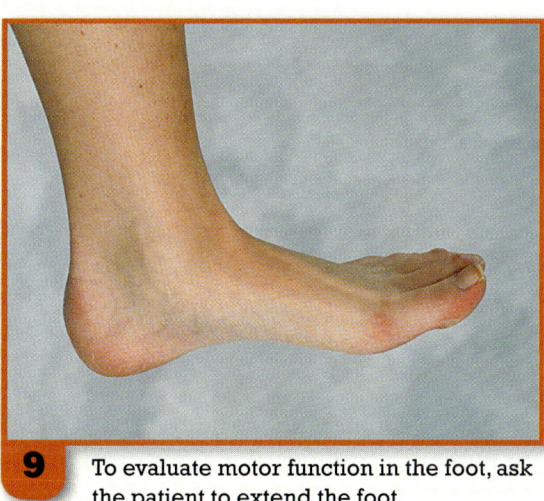
9 To evaluate motor function in the foot, ask the patient to extend the foot.

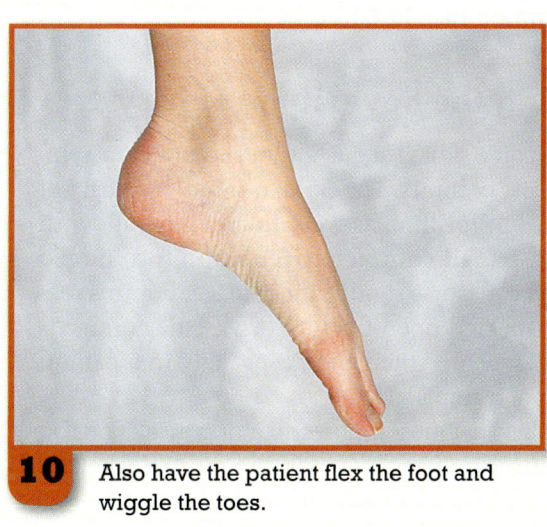
10 Also have the patient flex the foot and wiggle the toes.

of circulatory and nervous status distal to the injury: pulse, capillary refill, motor function, and sensory function. Follow the steps in Skill Drill 18-1:

1. **Pulse.** Palpate the pulse distal to the point of injury.
   - Palpate the radial pulse in the upper extremity (**Step 1**).
   - In the lower extremity, palpate the posterior tibial and dorsalis pedis pulses (**Step 2**).
2. **Capillary refill.** Note and record the skin color, identifying any pallor or cyanosis. Then apply firm pressure to the tip of the fingernail or toenail, which will cause the skin to blanch (turn white). If normal color does not return within 2 seconds after you release the nail, you can assume that circulation is impaired. This test is typically recommended for use in children, although it can be used in adults as well (**Step 3**).
3. **Sensation.** In the hand, check the feeling on the flesh near the tip of the index finger and thumb, as well as the little finger (**Step 4**). In the foot, check the feeling on the flesh of the big toe (**Step 5**) and on the lateral side of the foot (**Step 6**). The patient's ability to sense light touch in the fingers or toes distal to the site of a fracture is a good indication that the nerve function is intact.

4. **Motor function.** Evaluate muscular activity when the injury is proximal to the patient's hand or foot. Ask the patient to open and close a fist for an upper extremity injury and to wiggle the toes and move the foot up and down for a lower extremity injury (**Steps 7-10**). Sometimes, an attempt at motion will produce pain at the injury site. If this happens, do not continue this part of the examination. To avoid causing pain, do not perform this test at all if the injury involves the hand or foot itself.

Because many of the steps require patient cooperation, you will not be able to assess sensory and motor function in an unresponsive patient, but you can still evaluate the limb for deformity, swelling, ecchymosis, false motion, and crepitus. If a patient is unresponsive, first perform an initial assessment, addressing all life-threatening problems, and then examine the extremities. Assume that an unresponsive patient has a spinal fracture, and immobilize the spine.

Assessing the Severity of Injury

You must become skilled at quickly and accurately assessing the severity of injury. The Golden Hour is critical not just for life, but for limb as well. In an extremity with anything less than complete circulation, prolonged hypotension can cause significant damage. For this reason, any suspected open fracture or vascular injury is considered an acute emergency, especially in a patient with multiple trauma.

Remember that most injuries are not critical; you can identify critical injuries by using the musculoskeletal injury grading system shown in (**Table 18-1** ▶).

Emergency Medical Care

Your first steps in providing care for any patient are the initial assessment and stabilizing the patient's ABCs. After you have done so, you can focus on specific injuries. Remember to always follow BSI precautions.

Follow the steps in (**Skill Drill 18-2** ▶) when caring for patients with musculoskeletal injuries:

1. **Completely cover open wounds** with a dry, sterile dressing, and apply local pressure to control bleeding. Once you have applied a sterile dressing, treat an open fracture in the same way as a closed fracture (**Step 1**).
2. **Apply the appropriate splint**, and elevate the extremity. Patients with lower extremity injuries should lie supine with the limb elevated about 6″ to minimize swelling. For any patient, if possible, position the injured limb slightly above the level of the heart. Never allow the injured limb to flop about or dangle from the edge of the backboard. Always assess pulse and motor and sensory functions before and after the application of splints (**Step 2**).
3. **If swelling is present**, apply cold packs to the area; however, avoid placing cold packs directly on the skin or other exposed tissues. Placing a cold pack on top of an air splint or other thick, insulating material will not help to reduce swelling (**Step 3**).
4. **Prepare the patient for transport.** A patient with an isolated upper extremity injury for whom spinal precautions are not indicated will most likely be more comfortable in a semiseated position rather than lying flat; however, either position is acceptable. Ensure that the extremity is

TABLE 18-1	Musculoskeletal Injury Grading System

Minor Injuries
- Minor sprains
- Fractures or dislocations of digits

Moderate Injuries
- Open fractures of digits
- Nondisplaced long bone fractures
- Nondisplaced pelvic fractures
- Major sprains of a major joint

Serious Injuries
- Displaced long bone fractures
- Multiple hand and foot fractures
- Single open long bone fractures
- Displaced pelvic fractures
- Dislocations of major joints
- Multiple digit amputations
- Laceration of major nerves or blood vessels

Severe, Life-Threatening Injuries (survival is probable)
- Multiple closed fractures
- Limb amputations

Critical Injuries (survival is uncertain)
- Multiple open fractures of the limbs
- Pelvic fractures with hemodynamic instability

Skill Drill 18-2: Caring for Musculoskeletal Injuries

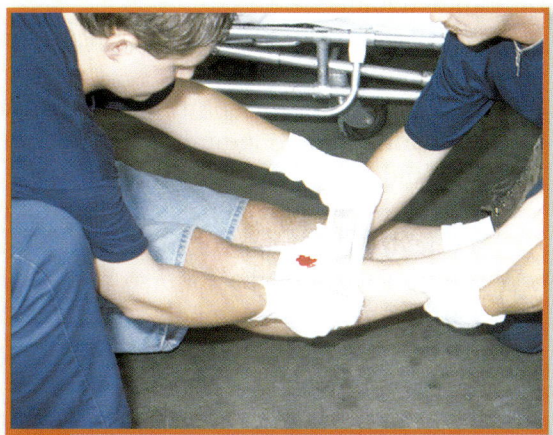

1 Cover open wounds with a dry, sterile dressing, and apply pressure to control bleeding.

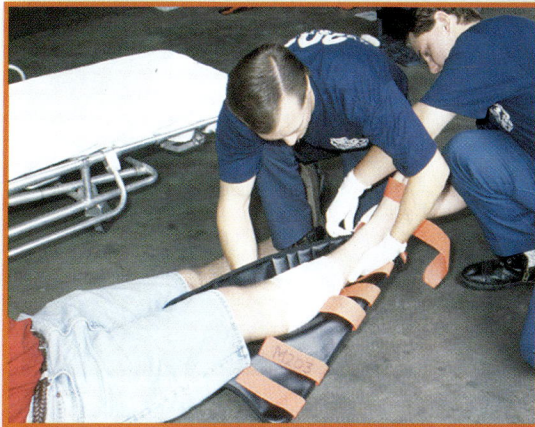

2 Assess pulse, motor, and sensory functions. Apply a splint, and elevate the extremity about 6″ (slightly above the level of the heart).

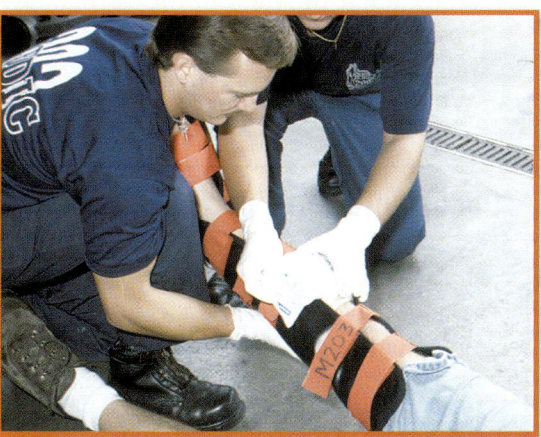

3 Apply cold packs if there is swelling, but do not place them directly on the skin.

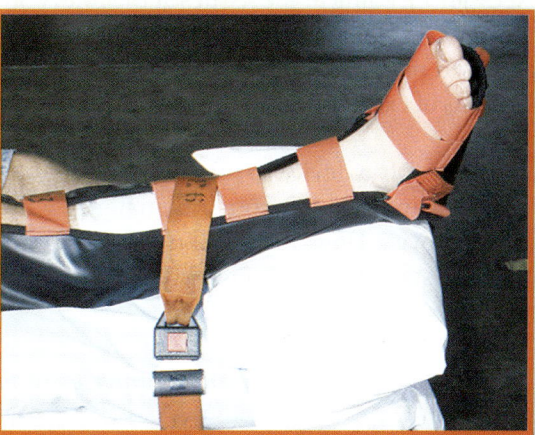

4 Position the patient for transport, and secure the injured area.

elevated above the level of the heart and secured so that it does not dangle from the edge of the backboard (**Step 4**).

5. **Always inform hospital personnel** about all wounds that have been dressed and splinted.

Splinting

A splint is a flexible or rigid device that is used to protect and maintain the position of an injured extremity Figure 18-19 ▶. Unless the patient's life is in immediate danger, you should splint all fractures, dislocations, and sprains before moving the patient. By preventing movement of fracture fragments, bone ends, a dislocated joint, or damaged soft tissues, splinting reduces pain and makes it easier to transfer and transport the patient. In addition, splinting will help to prevent the following:

- Further damage to muscles, the spinal cord, peripheral nerves, and blood vessels from broken bone ends
- Laceration of the skin by broken bone ends. One of the primary indications for splinting is to prevent a closed fracture from becoming an open fracture (conversion).
- Restriction of distal blood flow resulting from pressure of the bone ends on blood vessels

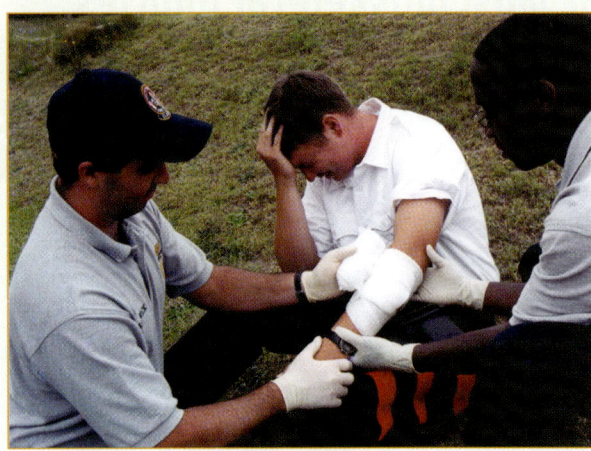

Figure 18-19 Splinting reduces pain and prevents additional damage to the injured extremity. Maintain manual support of the injured extremity during bandaging and splinting.

- Excessive bleeding of the tissues at the injury site caused by broken bone ends
- Increased pain from movement of bone ends
- Paralysis of extremities resulting from a damaged spine

A splint is simply a device to prevent motion of the injured part. It can be made from any material when you need to improvise. However, you should have an adequate supply of standard commercial splints on hand.

General Principles of Splinting

The following principles of splinting apply to most situations:

1. **Remove clothing from the area** of any suspected fracture or dislocation so that you can inspect the extremity for DCAP-BTLS.
2. **Note and record the patient's neurovascular status** distal to the site of the injury, including pulse, sensation, and movement. Continue to monitor the neurovascular status until the patient reaches the hospital.
3. **Cover all wounds with a dry, sterile dressing** before splinting. Be sure to follow BSI precautions. Do not intentionally replace protruding bones. Notify the receiving hospital of all open wounds.
4. **Do not move the patient before splinting** an extremity unless there is an immediate hazard to the patient or yourself.
5. In a suspected fracture of the shaft of any bone, be sure to **immobilize the joints** above and below the fracture.
6. With injuries in and around the joint, be sure to **immobilize the bones** above and below the injured joint.
7. **Pad all rigid splints** to prevent local pressure and discomfort to the patient.
8. While applying the splint, **maintain manual immobilization** to minimize movement of the limb and to support the injury site.
9. If fracture of a long bone shaft has resulted in severe deformity, **use constant, gentle manual traction** to align the limb so that it can be splinted. This is especially important if the distal part of the extremity is cyanotic or pulseless.
10. **If you encounter resistance** to limb alignment, splint the limb in its deformed position.
11. **Immobilize all suspected spinal injuries** in a neutral, in-line position on a long backboard.
12. **If the patient has signs of shock** (hypoperfusion), align the limb in the normal anatomic position and provide transport (total body immobilization).
13. **When in doubt, splint.**

Documentation Tips

Straightening or splinting an injured limb can compromise distal functions, just as the initial injury can. Record the status of distal circulation and nervous function (neurovascular status) before *and* after splinting. At a minimum, your written record should describe these functions before splinting and confirm that they were normal immediately after splinting and on arrival at the hospital. For any but the shortest transports, also indicate the results of reassessments en route.

General Principles of In-line Traction Splinting

In-line <u>traction</u> is the act of exerting a pulling force on a body structure in the direction of its normal alignment. It is the most effective way to realign a fracture of the shaft of a long bone so that the limb can be splinted more effectively. Excessive traction can be very harmful to an injured limb. When applied correctly, however, traction stabilizes the bone fragments and improves the overall alignment of the limb. You should not attempt to reduce the fracture or force all the bone fragments back into alignment. This is the physician's responsibility and is outside the EMT-I's scope of practice. In the field, the goals of in-line traction are as follows:

1. To **stabilize the fracture** fragments to prevent excessive movement
2. To **align the limb** sufficiently to allow it to be placed in a splint
3. To **avoid** potential neurovascular compromise

The amount of pull that is required to accomplish these objectives varies but rarely exceeds 15 lb. You should use the least amount of force necessary. Grasp the foot or hand at the end of the injured limb firmly; once you start pulling, you should not stop until the limb is fully splinted. When pulling traction for a possible femur fracture, one hand should be placed underneath the knee for support. The direction of traction pull is always along the long axis of the limb. Imagine where the normal, uninjured limb would lie, and pull gently along the line of that imaginary limb until the injured limb is in approximately that position (Figure 18-20). Grasping the foot or hand and the initial pull of traction usually causes some discomfort as the bone fragments move. It helps if a second person can support the injured limb directly under the site of the fracture. This initial discomfort quickly subsides, and you can then apply further, gentle traction. However, if the patient strongly resists the traction or if it causes more pain that persists, you must stop and splint the limb in the deformed position.

Remember that many different materials can be used as splints if necessary. When no splinting materials are available, the arm can be bound to the chest wall, and an injured leg can be bound to the uninjured leg to provide at least temporary stability. The three basic types of splints include rigid, formable, and traction splints.

Rigid Splints

Rigid (nonformable) splints are made from firm material and are applied to the sides, front, and/or back of an injured extremity to prevent motion at the injury site. Common examples of rigid splints include padded board splints, molded plastic and metal splints, padded wire ladder splints, and folded cardboard splints. As always, be sure to follow BSI precautions. It takes two EMT-Is to apply a rigid splint. Follow the steps in (Skill Drill 18-3 ▶):

1. **Assess pulse, motor, and sensory functions.** First EMT-I: **Gently support the limb** at the site of injury as others prepare and begin to position the equipment. Apply steady, in-line traction if necessary. Maintain this support until the splint is completely applied (**Step 1**).
2. Second EMT-I: **Place the rigid splint under or alongside the limb**.
3. Second EMT-I: **Place padding between the limb and the splint** to make sure there is even pressure and even contact. Look for bony prominences, and pad them (**Step 2**).
4. Second EMT-I: **Apply bindings** to hold the splint securely to the limb (**Step 3**).
5. Second EMT-I: **Check and record** the distal nervous and circulatory (neurovascular) function (**Step 4**).

There are two situations in which you must splint the limb in the position of deformity: when the deformity is severe, as is the case with many dislocations, or when you encounter resistance or extreme pain when applying gentle traction to the fracture of a shaft of a long bone. In either situation, you should apply padded board splints to each side of the limb and secure them with soft roller bandages (Figure 18-21 ▼).

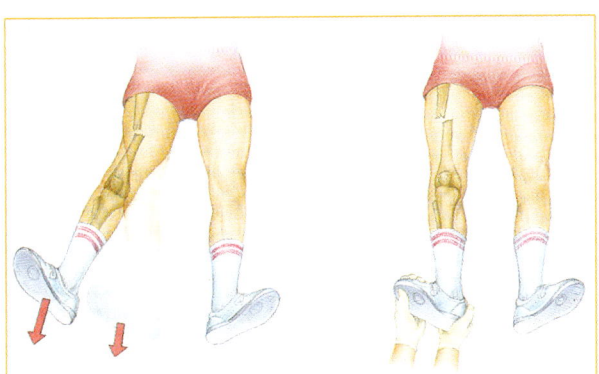

Figure 18-20 To apply traction, imagine the position where the normal uninjured limb would lie, then gently pull along that line until the injured limb is in that position. Do not release traction once you have applied it.

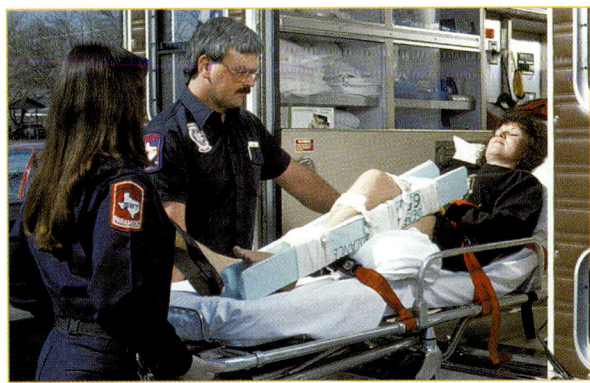

Figure 18-21 If you encounter resistance or extreme pain when applying traction to a long bone, apply padded board splints to each side of the limb, and secure them with soft roller bandages, immobilizing the limb in its deformed position.

Skill Drill 18-3: Applying a Rigid Splint

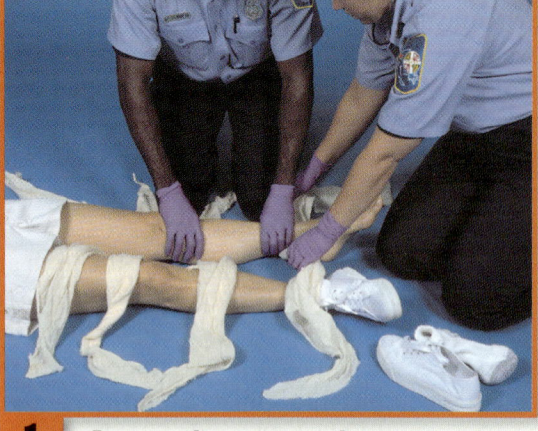

1. Assess pulse, motor, and sensory functions. Provide gentle support and in-line traction of the limb.

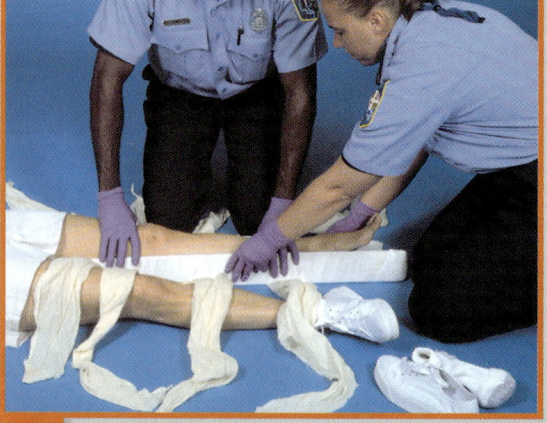

2. Second EMT-I places the splint alongside or under the limb.

Pad between the limb and the splint as needed to ensure even pressure and contact.

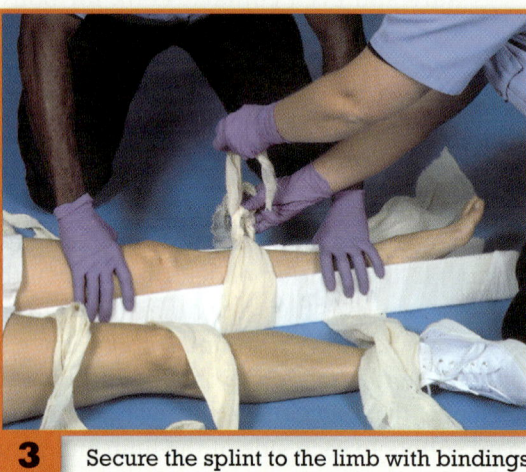

3. Secure the splint to the limb with bindings.

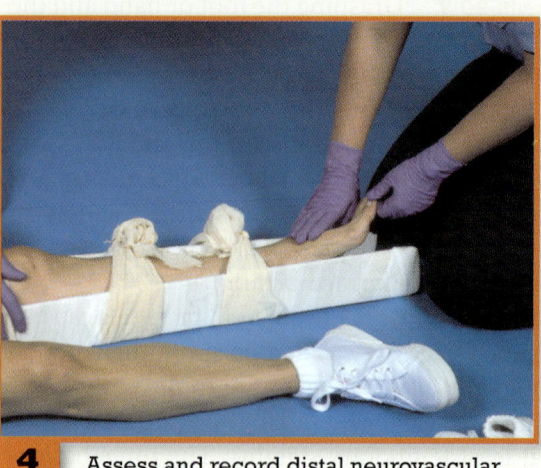

4. Assess and record distal neurovascular function.

Formable Splints

The most commonly used formable or soft splint is the precontoured, inflatable, clear plastic *air splint*. These are available in a variety of sizes and shapes, with or without a zipper that runs the length of the splint. Always inflate the splint after applying it. The air splint is comfortable, provides uniform contact, and has the added advantage of applying firm pressure to a bleeding wound. Air splints are used to immobilize injuries below the elbow or below the knee.

Air splints have some drawbacks, particularly in cold weather areas. The zipper can stick, clog with dirt, or freeze. Significant changes in the weather affect the pressure of the air in the splint, decreasing, as the environment grows colder and increasing as the environment grows warmer. The same thing happens when there are changes in altitude, which can be a problem with helicopter transport of patients. Therefore, you should carefully monitor the splint and let air out if the splint becomes overinflated.

Skill Drill 18-4: Applying a Zippered Air Splint

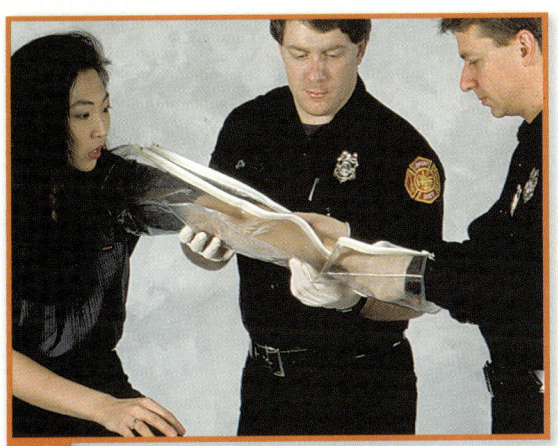

1 Assess pulse, motor, and sensory functions. Support the injured limb and apply gentle traction as your partner applies the open, deflated splint.

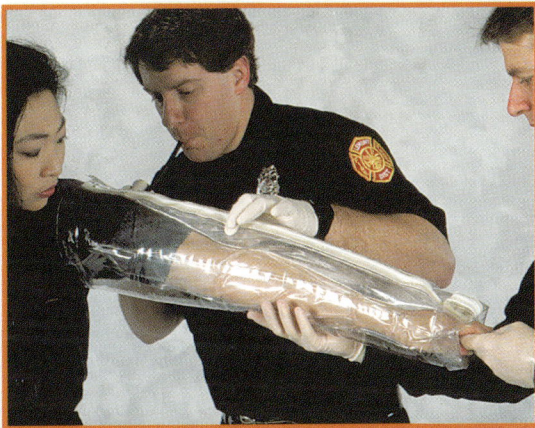

2 Zip up the splint, inflate it by pump or by mouth, and test the pressure.

Check and record distal neurovascular function.

The method of applying an air splint depends on whether it has a zipper. With either type, you must first cover all wounds with a dry, sterile dressing, making sure that you use BSI precautions. For a splint that has a zipper, follow the steps in **Skill Drill 18-4**:

1. **Assess pulse, motor, and sensory functions.**
2. **Hold the injured limb** slightly off the ground, applying gentle traction and supporting the site of injury. Have your partner place the open, deflated splint around the limb (**Step 1**).
3. **Zip the splint up and inflate it** by pump or by mouth. When this is done, test the pressure in the splint. With proper inflation, you should just be able to compress the walls of the splint together with a firm pinch between the thumb and index finger near the edge of the splint.
4. **Check and record pulse, motor, and sensory functions**, and monitor them periodically until the patient reaches the hospital (**Step 2**).

If you use an unzippered or partially zippered type of air splint, have another person help you follow the steps in **Skill Drill 18-5**:

1. **Assess pulse, motor, and sensory functions.**
2. First EMT-I: **Support the patient's injured limb** until splinting is accomplished.
3. Second EMT-I: **Place your arm through the splint.** Extend your hand beyond the splint, and grasp the hand or foot of the injured limb (**Step 1**).
4. Second EMT-I: **Apply gentle traction** to the hand or foot while sliding the splint onto the injured limb. The hand or foot of the injured limb should always be included in the splint (**Step 2**).
5. First EMT-I: **Inflate the splint** by pump or by mouth (**Step 3**).
6. Second EMT-I: **Test the pressure** in the splint. This is something that you must do with either type of air splint.

Skill Drill 18-5

Applying an Unzippered Air Splint

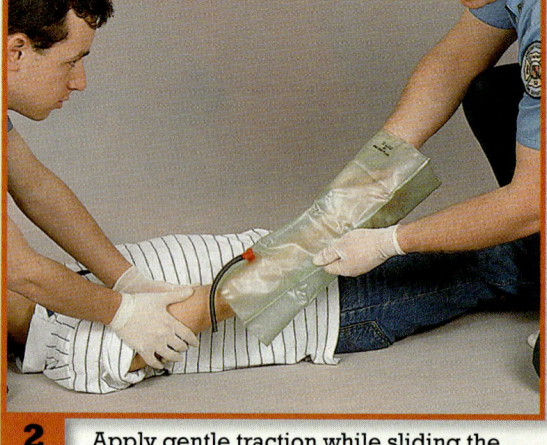

1. Assess pulse, motor, and sensory functions. Support the injured limb.

Have your partner place his or her arm through the splint to grasp the patient's hand or foot.

2. Apply gentle traction while sliding the splint onto the injured limb.

3. Inflate the splint.

---

7. Second EMT-I: **Check and record pulse, motor, and sensory functions**, and monitor them en route.

Other formable splints include vacuum splints, pillow splints, SAM splints, a sling and swathe, and the pneumatic antishock garment (PASG), also known as military antishock trousers (MAST), for pelvic fractures. Just like an air splint, a vacuum splint can be easily shaped to fit around a deformed limb. Instead of pumping air in, however, you can use a hand pump to pull the air out through a valve. Follow the steps in **Skill Drill 18-6** to apply a vacuum splint:

1. Assess pulse, motor, and sensory functions.
2. **Support and stabilize the injured limb**, applying traction if needed, while your partner applies the splint (**Step 1**).
3. Gently place the injured limb onto the **vacuum splint** and wrap the splint around the limb (**Step 2**).
4. **Draw the air out of the splint** through the suction valve, and then seal the valve. Once the valve is sealed, the vacuum splint becomes rigid, conforming to the shape of the deformed limb and immobilizing it (**Step 3**).
5. **Check distal circulation and nervous functions**, and monitor them en route.

Skill Drill 18-6: Applying a Vacuum Splint

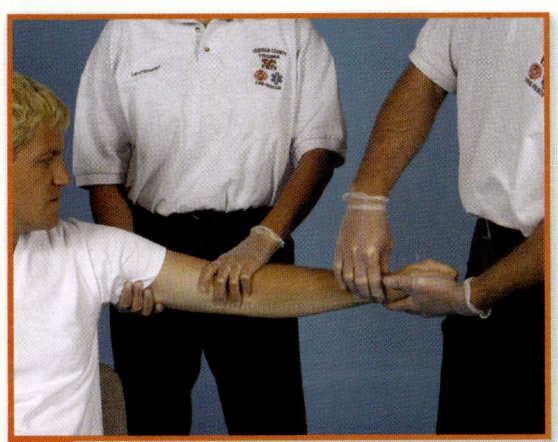
1. Assess pulse, motor, and sensory functions. Stabilize and support the injury.

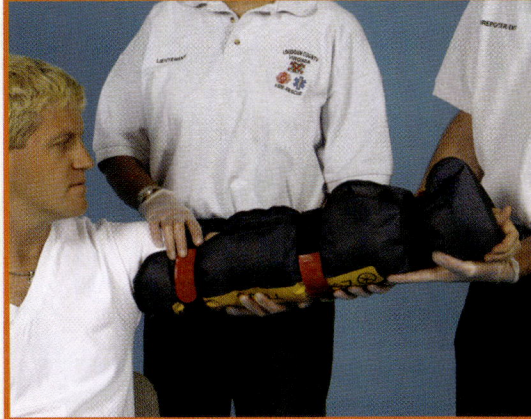
2. Place the splint and wrap it around the limb.

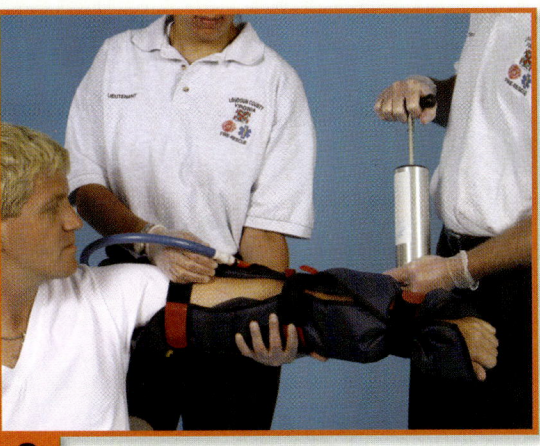
3. Draw the air out of the splint and seal the valve.

Traction Splints

Traction splints are used primarily to secure fractures of the midshaft of the femur, which are characterized by pain, swelling, and deformity of the midthigh. A traction splint should not be used if the patient has a joint or lower leg injury. Several different types of lower extremity traction splints are commercially available, such as the Hare traction splint, the Sager splint, and the Kendrick splint, each with its own unique method of application with which you must be familiar. The use of the Hare and Sager splints is described in this chapter.

The Hare traction splint uses a force called countertraction, which is applied by the upper end of the splint against the ischial tuberosity of the patient's pelvis. This splint is not suitable for use on the upper extremity because the major nerves and blood vessels in the patient's axilla cannot tolerate countertraction forces.

You should not use traction splints for any of the following conditions:

- Injuries of the upper extremity
- Injuries close to or involving the knee
- Injuries of the hip
- Injuries of the pelvis
- Partial amputations or avulsions with bone separation
- Lower leg or ankle injury

Skill Drill 18-7

Applying a Hare Traction Splint

1 Expose the injured limb and check pulse, motor, and sensory function.

Place the splint beside the uninjured limb, adjust the splint to the proper length, and prepare the straps.

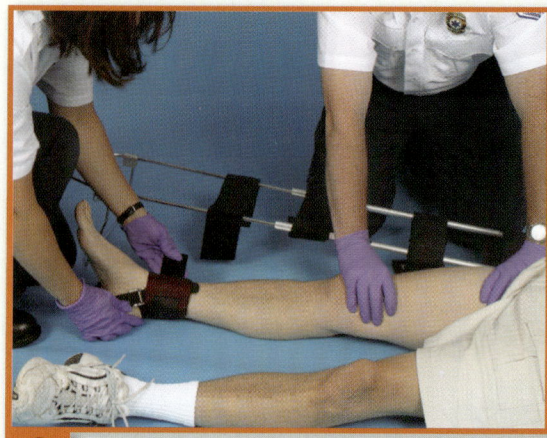

2 Support the injured limb as your partner fastens the ankle hitch about the foot and ankle.

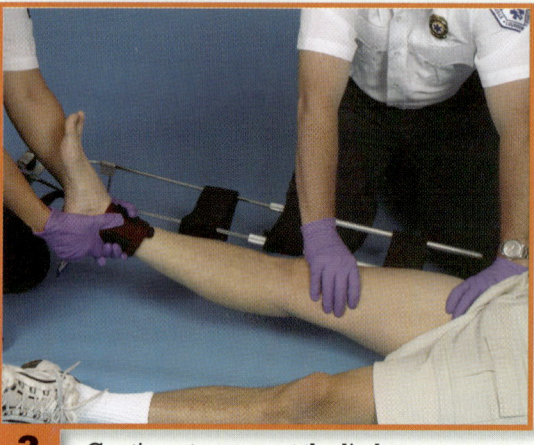

3 Continue to support the limb as your partner applies gentle in-line traction to the ankle hitch and foot.

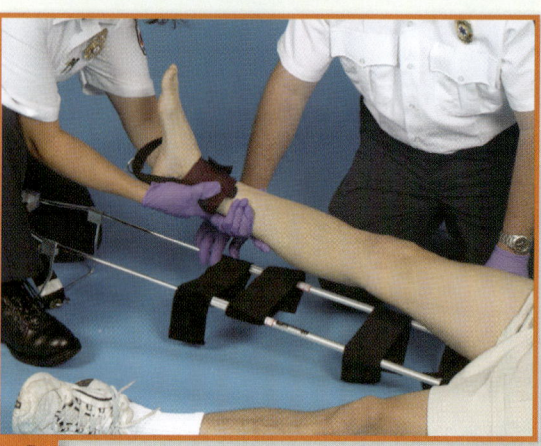

4 Slide the splint into position under the injured limb while your partner supports the heel and underneath the calf.

Proper application of a traction splint requires two well-trained providers working together. Practice the steps in Skill Drill 18-7 ▲ with your partner until the sequence and necessary teamwork have become routine:

1. **Cut open the patient's pants leg**, or otherwise expose the injured lower extremity. Follow BSI precautions as needed. Be sure to assess and record the pulse, motor function, and sensation distal to the injury.
2. **Place the splint beside the patient's uninjured leg**, and adjust it to the proper length, with the ring at the ischial tuberosity and the splint extending 6″ to 10″ beyond the foot. Open and adjust the four Velcro support straps, which should be positioned at the midthigh, above the knee, below the knee, and above the ankle. Be sure not to place a strap over the fracture site (**Step 1**).
3. First EMT-I: **Manually support and stabilize** the injured limb so that no motion will occur at the fracture site while the second EMT-I fastens the appropriately sized ankle hitch about the patient's ankle and foot. Usually, the patient's shoe is removed for this procedure (**Step 2**).
4. First EMT-I: **Support the leg at the site of the suspected injury** while the second EMT-I man-

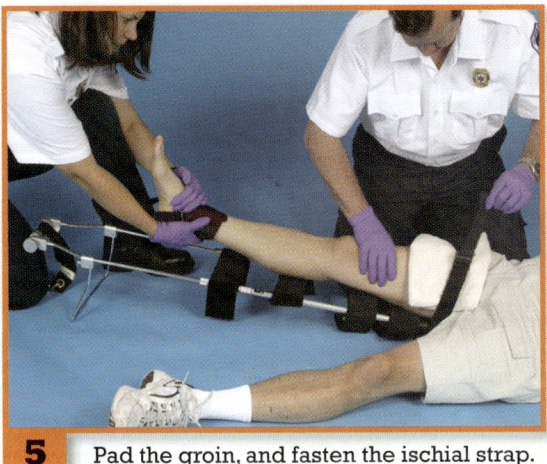

5 Pad the groin, and fasten the ischial strap.

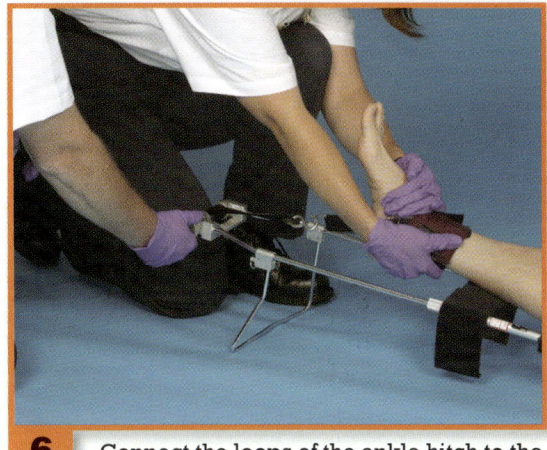

6 Connect the loops of the ankle hitch to the end of the splint as your partner continues to maintain traction. Carefully tighten the ratchet to the point that the splint holds adequate traction.

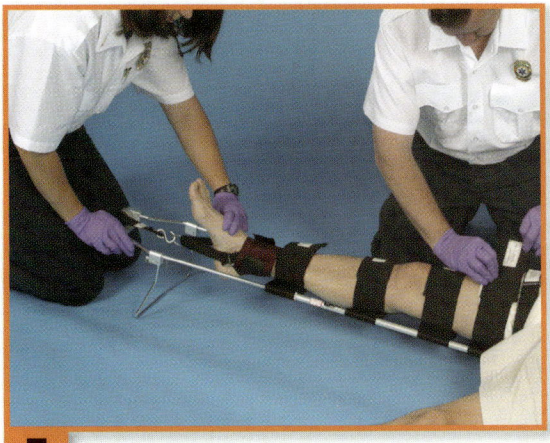

7 Secure and check support straps. Assess pulse, motor, and sensory functions.

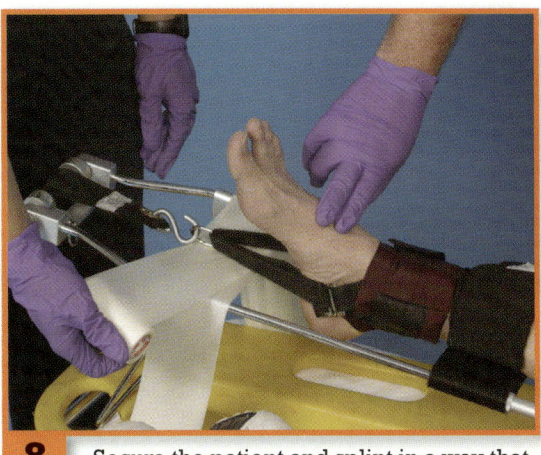

8 Secure the patient and splint in a way that will prevent movement of the splint during patient transfer and transport.

ually applies gentle longitudinal traction to the ankle hitch and foot. Place one hand underneath the heel and the second hand underneath the calf. Use only enough force to align (reposition) the limb so that it will fit into the splint; do not attempt to align the fracture fragments anatomically (**Step 3**).

5. First EMT-I: **Slide the splint into position** under the patient's injured limb, making certain that the ring is seated well on the ischial tuberosity (**Step 4**).
6. **Pad the groin area**, and gently apply the ischial strap (**Step 5**).
7. First EMT-I: While the second EMT-I continues to maintain traction, **connect the loops of the ankle hitch** to the end of the splint. Then apply gentle traction to the connecting strap between the ankle hitch and the splint, just strongly enough to maintain limb alignment. Use caution. This splint comes with a ratchet mechanism to tighten the strap, which can overstretch the limb and further injure the patient. Adequate traction has been applied when the leg is the same length as the other leg or the patient feels relief (**Step 6**).

Applying a Sager Traction Splint

1 After exposing the injured area, check the patient's pulse and motor and sensory function.

Adjust the thigh strap so that it lies anteriorly when secured.

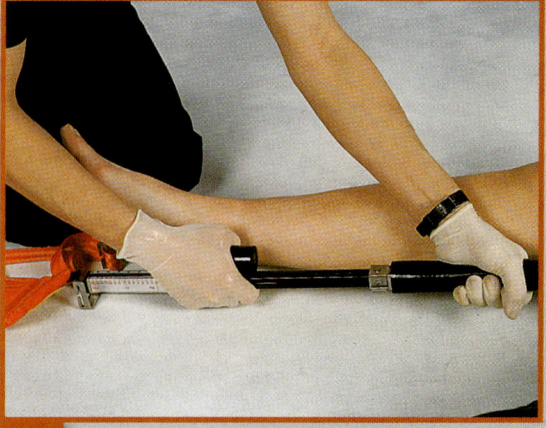

2 Estimate the proper length of the splint by placing it next to the injured limb.

Fit the ankle pads to the ankle.

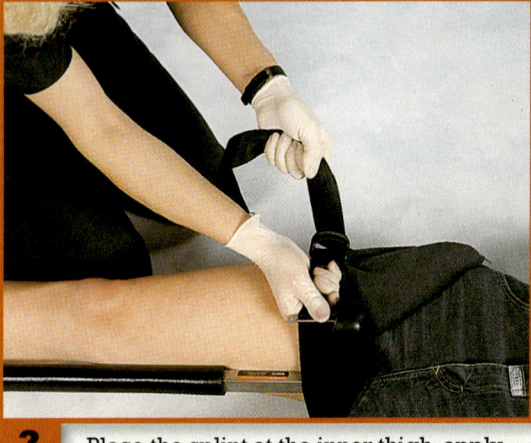

3 Place the splint at the inner thigh, apply the thigh strap at the upper thigh, and secure snugly.

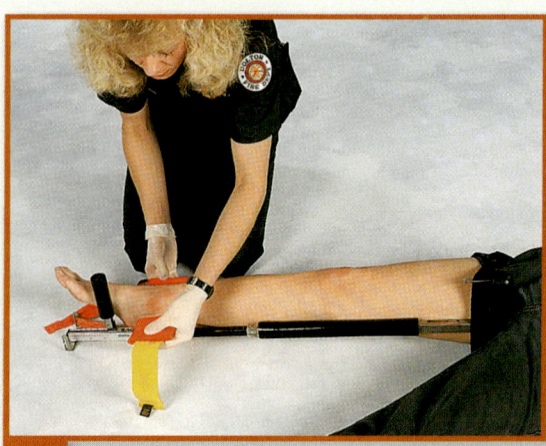

4 Tighten the ankle harness just above the malleoli.

Snug the cable ring against the bottom of the foot.

8. Once proper traction has been applied, **fasten the support straps** so that the limb is securely held in the splint. Check all proximal and distal support straps to make sure they are secure (**Step 7**).

9. At this point, **reassess distal pulses**, motor function, and sensation.

10. **Secure the patient and splint** in a way that will prevent movement of the splint during transport to the emergency department. You may need to load the patient feet first into the ambulance so that you do not shut the door against the splint (**Step 8**).

Because this traction splint immobilizes the limb by producing countertraction on the ischium and in the groin, you should use care to pad these areas well. You must avoid excessive pressure on the external genitalia. Always use commercially available padded ankle hitches rather than pieces of rope, cord, or tape. Such improvised hitches can sometimes be painful and can potentially obstruct circulation in the foot.

The Sager splint is lightweight, is easy to store, applies a measurable amount of traction, and can be used with a PASG. Best of all, you can apply it by yourself when necessary. As with any splint, in addition to knowing the precise sequence of steps to apply the splint

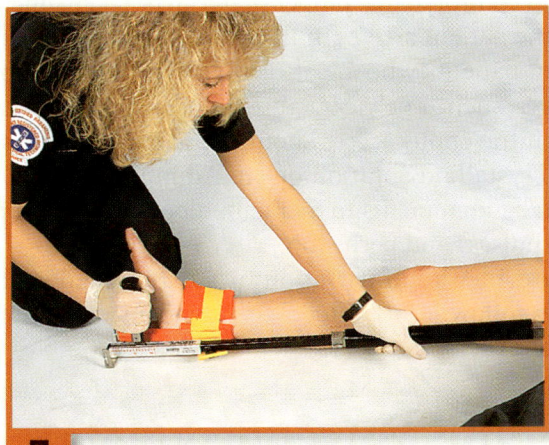

5 Extend the splint's inner shaft to apply traction of about 10% of body weight.

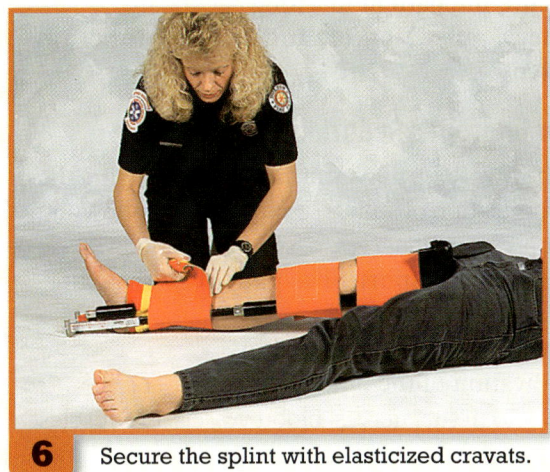

6 Secure the splint with elasticized cravats.

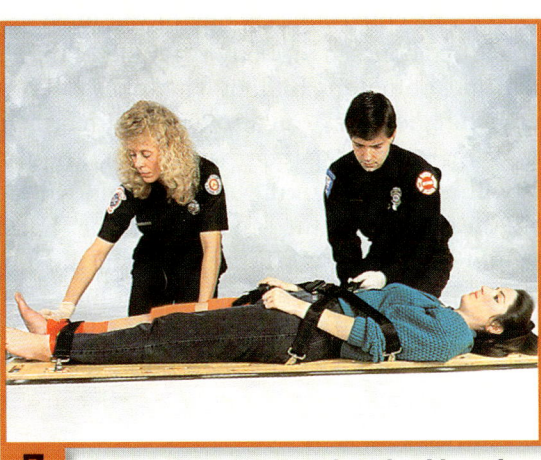

7 Secure the patient to a long backboard. Check pulse, motor, and sensory functions.

properly, you must practice the splinting technique frequently to maintain the necessary skills. Follow these steps to apply a Sager splint (Skill Drill 18-8 ◄):

1. **Expose the injured extremity.** Use BSI precautions as needed, and assess and record the pulse, motor function, and sensation distal to the injury.
2. Before applying the splint, **adjust the thigh strap** so that it will lie anteriorly when secured in place (**Step 1**).
3. **Estimate the proper splint length** by placing it alongside the injured limb, so that the wheel is at the level of the heel.
4. **Arrange the ankle pads** to fit the size of the patient's ankle (**Step 2**).
5. **Place the splint along the inner aspect of the limb**, and slide the thigh strap around the upper thigh so that the perineal cushion is snug against the groin and the ischial tuberosity. Tighten the thigh strap snugly (**Step 3**).
6. **Secure the ankle harness** tightly around the patient's ankle just above the malleoli.
7. **Pull the cable ring** snugly up against the bottom of the foot (**Step 4**).
8. **Pull out the inner shaft** of the splint to apply traction of approximately 10% of body weight, using a maximum of 15 lb (**Step 5**).

9. **Secure the limb** to the splint using elasticized cravats (**Step 6**).
10. **Secure the patient** to a long backboard.
11. **Check pulse, motor, and sensory function** (**Step 7**).

Hazards of Improper Splinting

You must be aware of the hazards associated with the improper application of splints, including the following:

- Compression of nerves, tissues, and blood vessels
- Delay in transport of a patient with a life-threatening injury
- Reduction of distal circulation
- Aggravation of the injury
- Injury to tissue, nerves, blood vessels, or muscles as a result of excessive movement of the bone or joint

Transportation

Once an injured limb is adequately splinted, the patient is ready to be transferred to a backboard or stretcher and transported.

Very few, if any, musculoskeletal injuries justify the use of excessive speed during transport. The limb will be stable once a dressing and splint have been applied. However, the patient with a pulseless limb must be given a higher priority. Still, if the hospital is only a few minutes away, speeding to the emergency department will make little or no difference to the patient's eventual outcome. If the treatment facility is an hour or more away, the patient with a pulseless limb should be transported by helicopter or immediate ground transportation. If circulation in the distal limb is impaired, always notify medical control so that proper steps can be taken quickly once the patient arrives in the emergency department.

For patients who are at risk for hypovolemia from fractures, such as pelvic fractures or bilateral femur fractures, intravenous access should be gained and an isotonic crystalloid solution given. Administer fluids in 20-mL/kg increments to maintain blood pressure (and radial pulses) and perfusion.

Consider administration of narcotic analgesics. Always follow local protocol or contact medical direction for orders.

Specific Musculoskeletal Injuries

Injuries of the Clavicle and Scapula

The <u>clavicle</u>, or collarbone, is one of the most commonly fractured bones in the body. Fractures of the clavicle occur most often in children when they fall on an outstretched hand. They can also occur with crushing injuries of the chest. A patient with a fracture of the clavicle will report pain in the shoulder and will usually hold the arm across the front of his or her body. A young child often reports pain throughout the entire arm and is unwilling to use any part of that limb. These complaints may make it difficult to localize the point of injury, but, generally, swelling and point tenderness occur over the clavicle (**Figure 18-22**). Because the

---

You are the Provider — Part 3

You have splinted your patient's leg and are preparing him for transport. Assessment of his vital signs reveals the following:

Vital Signs	Recording Time: 5 Minutes After Patient Contact
Respirations	20 breaths/min, unlabored
Pulse	84 beats/min, and regular
Skin	Pink, warm, and dry
Blood pressure	110/68 mm Hg
SaO_2	100% while breathing room air

5. What hazards are associated with the improper application of splints?

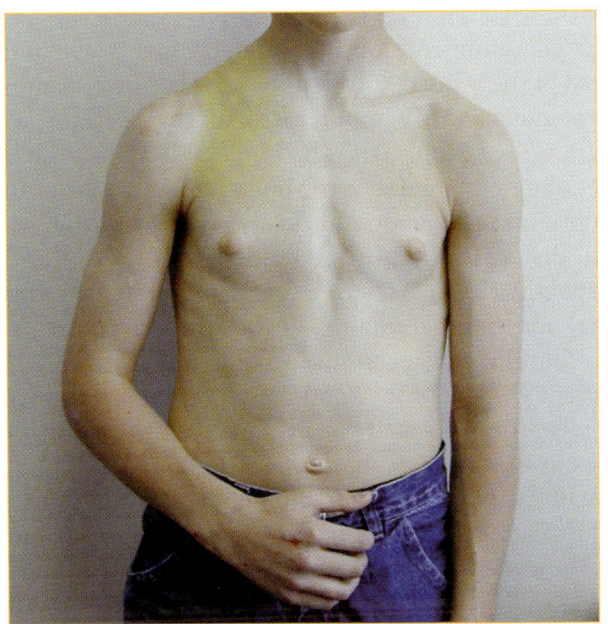

Figure 18-22 A clavicle injury is characterized by swelling, point tenderness, and "tenting" over the fracture fragment.

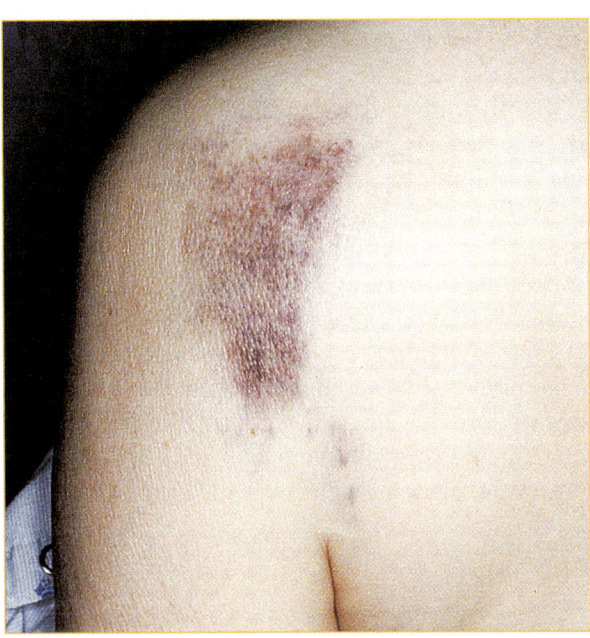

Figure 18-23 Contusions or abrasions over the scapular area may indicate a fracture.

clavicle is subcutaneous (just beneath the skin), the skin will occasionally "tent" over the fracture fragment. The clavicle lies directly over major arteries, veins, and nerves; therefore, fracture of the clavicle may lead to neurovascular compromise.

Fractures of the scapula, or shoulder blade, occur much less frequently because this bone is well protected by many large muscles. Fractures of the scapula are almost always the result of a forceful, direct blow to the back, directly over the scapula, which may also injure the thoracic cage, lungs, and heart. For this reason, you must carefully assess the patient for signs of breathing problems. Provide supplemental oxygen and prompt transport for patients who are having difficulty breathing. Remember, it is the associated chest injuries, not the fractured scapula, that pose the greatest threat of death.

Abrasions, contusions, and significant swelling may also occur, and the patient will often limit use of the arm because of pain at the fracture site (Figure 18-23). The scapula also has bony projections that may be fractured with a lesser degree of force.

The joint between the lateral aspect of the clavicle and the acromion process of the scapula is called the acromioclavicular (A/C) joint. This joint is frequently separated during football and hockey games when a player falls and lands on the point of the shoulder, driving the scapula away from the outer end of the clavicle. This dislocation is often called an A/C separation. The distal end of the clavicle will usually stick out, and the patient will complain of pain, including point tenderness over the A/C joint (Figure 18-24).

Fractures of the clavicle and scapula and A/C separations can all be splinted effectively with a sling and swathe. A sling is any bandage or material that helps support the weight of an injured upper extremity, relieving the downward pull of gravity on the injured site. To be effective, a sling must apply gentle upward support to the olecranon process of the ulna (at the elbow). The

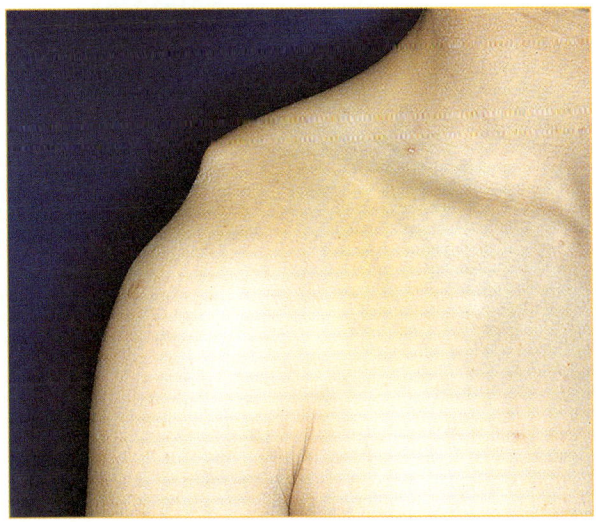

Figure 18-24 With A/C separations, the distal end of the clavicle usually sticks out.

knot of the sling should be tied to one side of the neck so that it does not press uncomfortably on the cervical spine Figure 18-25A ▼.

To fully immobilize the shoulder region, a swathe, a bandage that passes completely around the chest, must be used to bind the arm to the chest wall. The swathe should be tight enough to prevent the arm from swinging freely but not so tight as to compress the chest and compromise breathing. Leave the patient's fingers exposed so that you can assess neurovascular function at regular intervals Figure 18-25B ▼.

Commercially available shoulder immobilizers or slings will provide adequate splinting for injuries of the shoulder region, as will triangular bandage slings. When all else fails, place a T-shirt over the arm.

Dislocation of the Shoulder

The glenohumeral joint (shoulder joint) is where the head of the humerus, the supporting bone of the upper arm, meets the glenoid fossa of the scapula. The glenoid fossa joins with the humeral head to form the glenohumeral joint. It is the most commonly dislocated large joint in the body. Almost always, the humeral head will dislocate anteriorly, coming to lie in front of the scapula as a result of forced abduction (away from the midline) and external rotation of the arm Figure 18-26 ▼.

Shoulder dislocations are extremely painful. The patient will guard the shoulder and try to protect it by holding the dislocated arm in a fixed position away from the chest wall Figure 18-27 ▶. The shoulder joint will usually be locked, and the shoulder will appear squared off or flattened. The humeral head will protrude anteriorly underneath the pectoris major on the anterior chest wall. As a result, the axillary nerve may be compressed, causing a numb patch on the outer aspect of the shoulder. Be sure to document this finding. Some patients may also report some numbness in the hand because the nerves or the circulation is compromised.

Immobilizing an anterior shoulder dislocation is difficult, because any attempt to bring the arm in toward the chest will produce pain. You must splint the joint in whatever position is most comfortable for the patient. If necessary, place a pillow or rolled blankets or towels between the arm and chest to fill up the space between

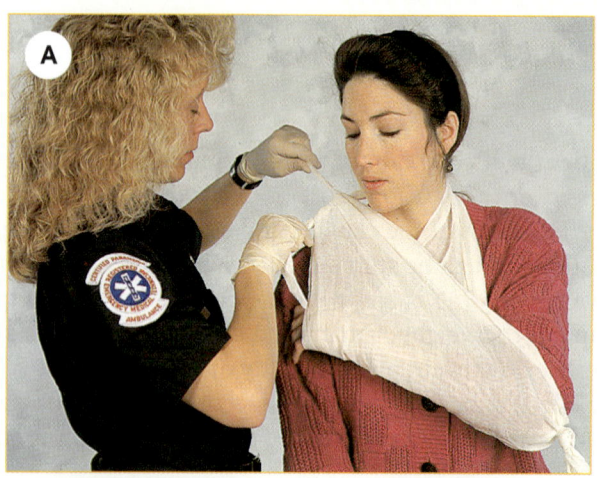

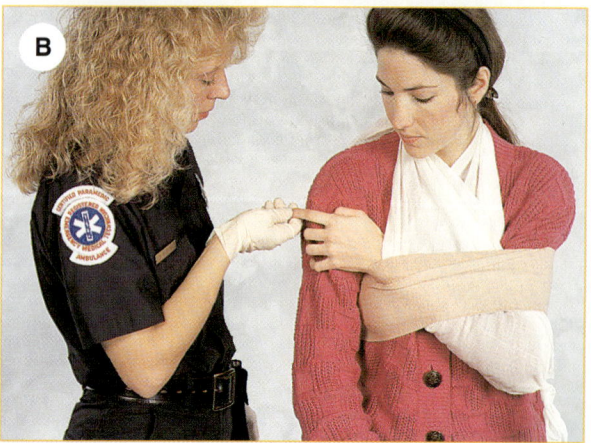

Figure 18-25 **A.** Apply the sling so that the knot is tied to one side of the neck. **B.** Bind the arm to the chest wall with a swathe so that the arm cannot swing freely. Leave the patient's fingers exposed so that you can assess distal circulation.

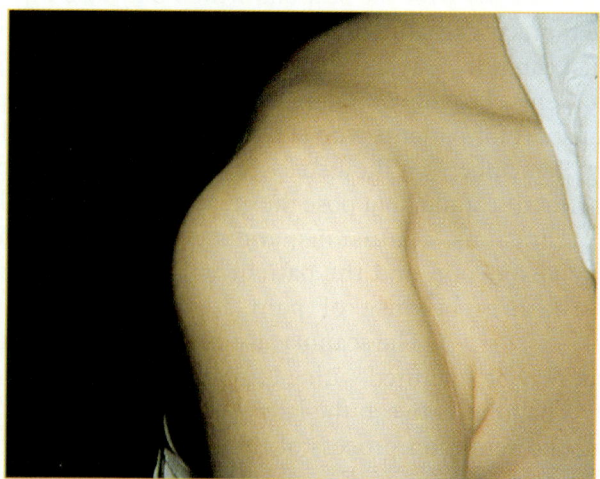

Figure 18-26 The shoulder most commonly dislocates anteriorly. Note the absence of the normal rounded appearance of the shoulder.

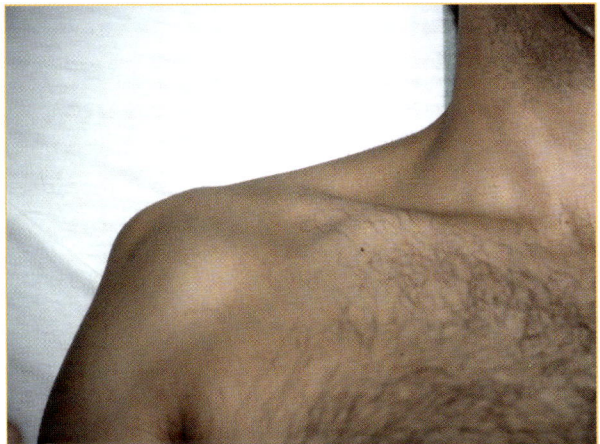

Figure 18-27 A patient with a dislocated shoulder will guard the shoulder, trying to protect it by holding the arm in a fixed position away from the chest wall.

compromise and joint injury. In certain cases, surgical repair may be required. Some patients are able to reduce (set) their own dislocated shoulders. Generally, however, this maneuver must be done in a hospital setting and only after radiographs have been obtained.

A shoulder will dislocate posteriorly instead of anteriorly about once in every 20 occurrences. Football players, especially linemen, are susceptible to this injury. The arm will often be locked in an adducted position (toward the midline), so it cannot be rotated. Reducing the dislocation usually requires a physician.

> **EMT-I Tips**
>
> When assessing a patient with a possible shoulder dislocation, position yourself behind the patient and compare the shoulders. The dislocated side is usually lower than the uninjured side.

them (Figure 18-28 ▼). Once the arm is stabilized in this way, the elbow can usually be flexed to 90° without causing further pain. At this point, you can apply a sling to the forearm and wrist to support the weight of the arm. Finally, secure the arm in the sling to the pillow and chest with a swathe. Transport the patient in a sitting or semiseated position.

Dislocation of the shoulder disrupts the supporting ligaments of the anterior aspect of the shoulder. Often these ligaments fail to heal properly, so dislocation recurs, each time causing further neurovascular

Fracture of the Humerus

Fractures of the humerus occur proximally, in the midshaft, or distally, at the elbow (Table 18-2 ▶). Fractures of the proximal humerus resulting from falls are common among elderly people. Fractures of the midshaft occur more often in young patients, usually as the result of a violent injury.

With any severely angulated fracture, you should consider applying traction to realign the fracture fragments before splinting them. Check your local protocols for indications and techniques for applying traction to a severely angulated fracture. Support the site of the fracture with one hand, and with the other hand, grasp the two humeral condyles (its lateral and medial protrusions) just above the elbow. Pull gently in line with the normal axis of the limb (Figure 18-29 ▶). Once you achieve gross alignment of the limb, splint the arm with a sling and swathe, supplemented by a padded board splint on the lateral aspect of the arm (Figure 18-30 ▶). If the patient reports significant pain or resists gentle traction, splint the fracture in the deformed position with a padded wire ladder or a padded board splint, using pillows to support the injured limb. Note that compartment syndrome can develop in the forearm in children with these fractures.

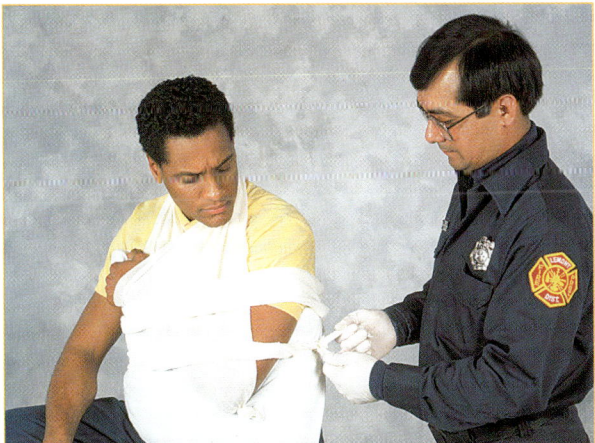

Figure 18-28 Splint the joint in a position of comfort, and place a pillow or towel between the arm and the chest wall to stabilize the arm, after which the elbow can be flexed to 90°. Apply a sling, and secure the arm to the chest with a swathe.

TABLE 18-2 | Characteristics and Treatment of Fractures of the Humerus

Type	Characteristics	Treatment
Proximal Humeral Fractures	■ Significant swelling, but no deformity, of the upper arm ■ Possible neurovascular compromise ■ Any or all of the brachial plexus affected, depending on the degree of displacement ■ Concurrent soft-tissue injuries ■ Possible rotator cuff injury (if radiographs show no fracture, a tear of the rotator cuff is possible, especially if the patient cannot move the arm toward the medial plane)	■ Immobilize in a sling and swathe or a shoulder immobilizer. ■ Use the chest wall as a splint, and secure the injured arm to the chest wall. ■ Place a short, padded board splint on the lateral side of the arm under the sling and swathe for additional support.
Midshaft Fractures	■ Gross angulation of the arm ■ Marked instability and crepitus of fracture fragments ■ Possible neurovascular compromise ■ Possible entrapment of the radial nerve (The patient cannot extend or dorsiflex the wrist or fingers and may report numbness on the dorsum of the hand; classic "wrist drop.")	■ Immobilize with a sling and swathe or a shoulder immobilizer. ■ Use the chest wall as a splint, and secure the injured arm to the chest wall. ■ Place a short, padded board splint on the lateral side of the arm under the sling and swathe for additional support.
Distal Humeral Fractures	■ Significant swelling at the elbow ■ Possible neurovascular compromise ■ Possible injury to the ulnar or median nerves (Document nerve status before and after splinting.)	■ Immobilize in a splint, in addition to a sling and swathe or a shoulder immobilizer.

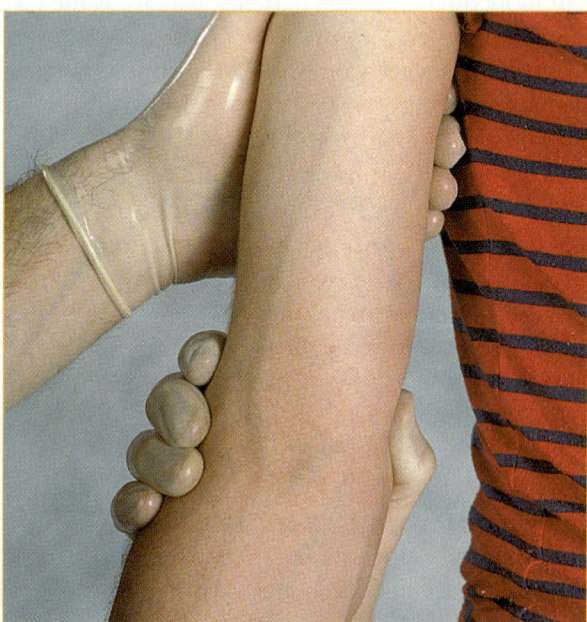

Figure 18-29 To align a severe deformity associated with a humeral shaft fracture, apply gentle pressure to the humeral condyles, as shown in this uninjured arm.

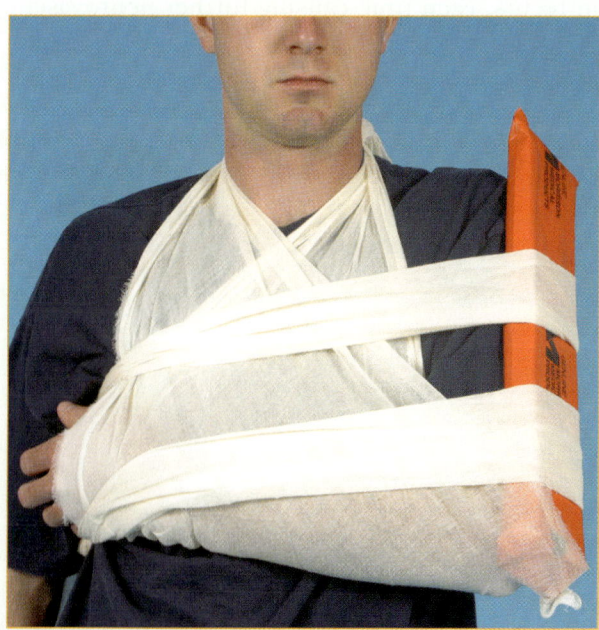

Figure 18-30 Splint a humeral shaft fracture with a sling and swathe supplemented by a padded board splint on the lateral aspect of the arm.

Elbow Injuries

Fractures and dislocations often occur around the elbow, and the different types of injuries are difficult to distinguish without radiographs. However, they all produce similar limb deformities and require the same emergency care. Injuries to nerves and blood vessels are quite common in this region. Such injuries can be caused or worsened by inappropriate emergency care, particularly by excessive manipulation of the injured joint.

Fracture of the Distal Humerus

This type of fracture, also known as a supracondylar or intercondylar fracture, is common in children. Frequently, the fracture fragments rotate significantly, producing deformity and causing injuries to nearby vessels and nerves. Swelling occurs rapidly and is often severe.

Dislocation of the Elbow

This type of injury typically occurs in athletes is rare in young children. The ulna and radius are most often displaced posteriorly. The ulna, the bone on the small finger (medial) side of the forearm, and the radius, the bone on the thumb (lateral) side of the forearm, both join the distal humerus. The posterior displacement makes the olecranon process of the ulna much more prominent (Figure 18-31). The joint is usually locked, making any attempt at motion extremely painful. Also, with a fracture of the distal humerus, there is swelling and significant potential for vessel or nerve injury.

Elbow Joint Sprain

This injury is rare and is usually diagnosed by radiograph. Often the real problem is a hard-to-detect fracture.

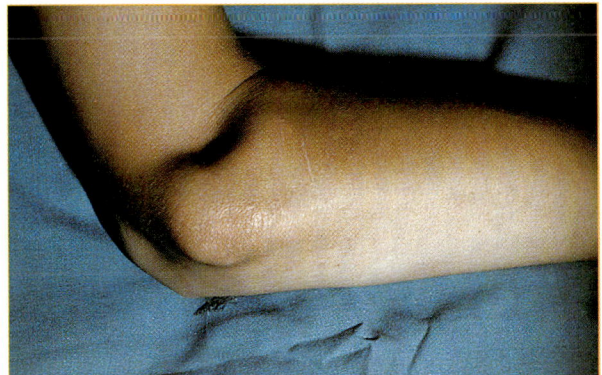

Figure 18-31 Posterior dislocation of the elbow makes the olecranon process of the ulna much more prominent.

Fracture of the Olecranon Process of the Ulna

This fracture is usually the result of a direct blow and is often characterized by lacerations and abrasions. Often, the patient will be unable to extend the elbow.

Fracture of the Radial Head

Often missed during diagnosis, this fracture generally occurs as a result of a fall on an outstretched arm or a direct blow to the lateral aspect of the elbow. Attempts to rotate the elbow and wrist cause severe discomfort.

Care of Elbow Injuries

As with any joint injury, elbow injuries are serious and require careful management. Always assess distal neurovascular functions periodically in patients with elbow injuries. If you find strong pulses and good capillary refill, splint the elbow in the position in which you found it, adding a wrist sling if this seems helpful. Two padded board splints, applied to each side of the limb and secured with soft roller bandages, usually are enough to stabilize the arm (Figure 18-32A). Make sure the board extends from the shoulder joint to the wrist joint, immobilizing the entire bone above and below the injured joint. Alternatively, you can mold a padded wire ladder splint or a SAM splint to the shape of the limb (Figure 18-32B). If necessary, you may add further support to the limb with a pillow.

A cold, pale hand or a weak or absent pulse and poor capillary refill indicate that the blood vessels have likely been injured. Further care of this patient must be dictated by a physician. Notify medical control immediately. If you are within 15 minutes of the hospital, splint the limb in the position in which you found it and provide prompt transport. Otherwise, medical control may direct you to try to realign the limb to improve circulation in the hand.

If the limb is pulseless and significantly deformed at the elbow, apply gentle manual traction in line with the long axis of the limb to decrease the deformity. This maneuver may restore the pulse. Be careful, because excessive manipulation will only worsen the vascular problem. If no pulse returns *after one attempt*, splint the limb in the most comfortable position for the patient. If the pulse is restored by gentle longitudinal traction, splint the limb in whatever position allows the strongest pulse. Provide prompt transport for all patients with impaired distal circulation.

Pediatric Needs

Epiphyseal (growth) plate injuries in children are common, especially around the wrist, elbow, knee, and ankle. Injuries tend to occur through these cartilaginous growth centers because they are inherently weaker than the surrounding bone. Because longitudinal growth of the limb is dependent on the function of the growth plate, it is extremely important to recognize the possibility of growth plate injuries, stabilize the injured limb, and transport the patient in a timely manner to an appropriate center with pediatric orthopaedic and surgical coverage. Proper functioning of the injured growth plate throughout the remainder of skeletal growth is dependent on urgent anatomic reduction of the fracture and close follow-up by an orthopaedist.

Any deformity in proximity to a joint in children younger than 16 years should be assumed to be a growth plate injury, and the child should be transported and treated appropriately.

Fractures of the Forearm

Fractures of the shaft of the radius and ulna are common in people of all age groups but are seen most often in children and elderly people. Usually, both bones break at the same time when the injury is the result of a fall on an outstretched hand Figure 18-33 ▼. An isolated fracture of the shaft of the ulna may occur as the result of a direct blow to it; this is known as a nightstick fracture.

Fractures of the distal radius, which are especially common in elderly patients with osteoporosis, are often known as Colles fractures. The term "silver fork deformity" is used to describe the distinctive appearance of the patient's arm Figure 18-34 ▶. In children, this fracture may occur through the growth plate Figure 18-35 ▶ and can have long-term consequences.

To immobilize fractures of the forearm or wrist, you can use a padded board, air, vacuum, or pillow splint. If the shaft of the bone has been fractured, be sure to include the elbow joint in the splint. Splinting of the elbow joint is not essential with fractures near the wrist; however, the patient will be more comfortable if you add a sling or pillow for more support.

Injuries of the Wrist and Hand

Injuries of the wrist, ranging from dislocations to sprains, must be confirmed by radiographs. Dislocations are usually associated with a fracture, resulting in a fracture-dislocation. Another common wrist injury is the isolated, nondisplaced fracture of a carpal bone, especially the scaphoid. Any questionable wrist sprain must be splinted and evaluated in the emergency department.

There are a great variety of hand injuries, some with potentially serious consequences. Industrial, recreational,

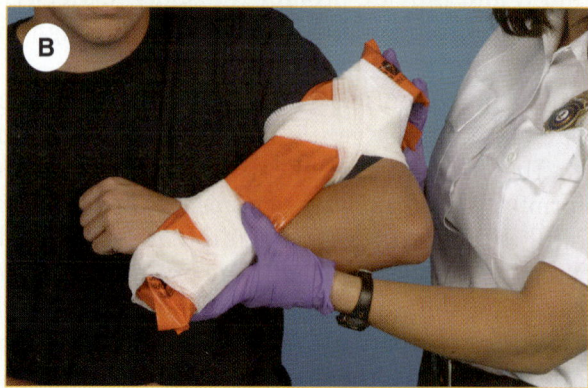

Figure 18-32 **A.** Two padded board splints provide adequate stabilization for an injured elbow. A wrist sling provides additional support. **B.** A SAM splint can be molded to the shape of the limb so that you can splint it in the position in which it was found.

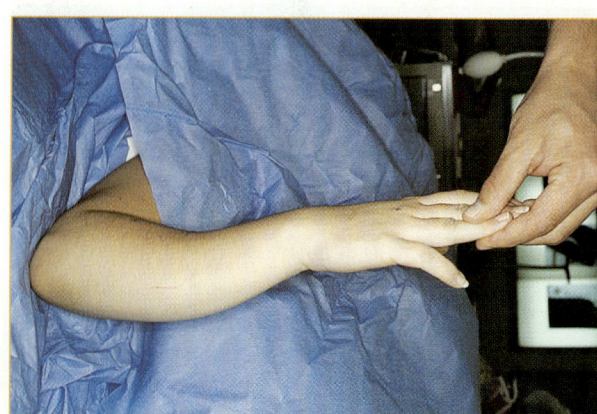

Figure 18-33 Fractures of the forearm often occur in children as a result of a fall on an outstretched hand.

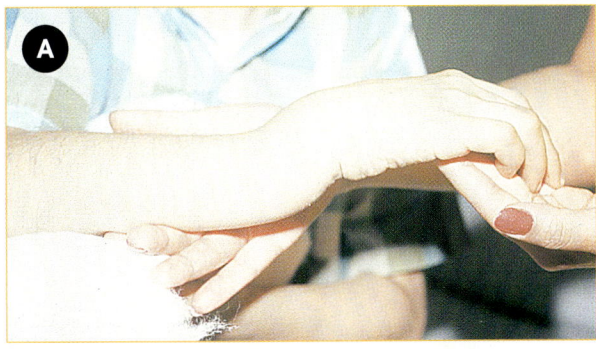

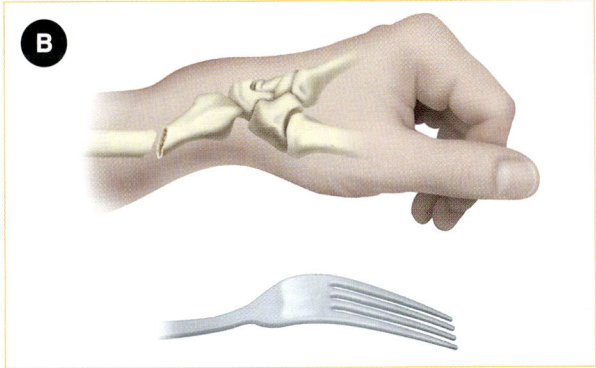

Figure 18-34 **A.** Fractures of the distal radius produce a characteristic silver fork deformity. **B.** An artist's illustration of same.

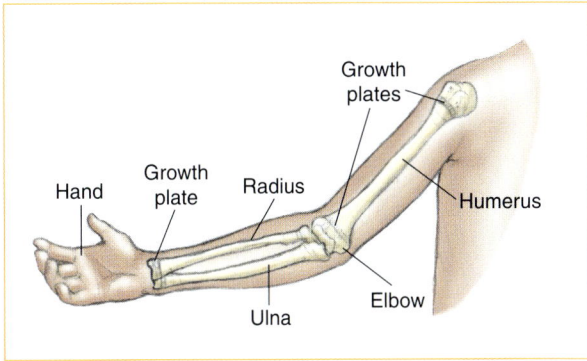

Figure 18-35 The growth plates at the ends of children's bones are easily fractured.

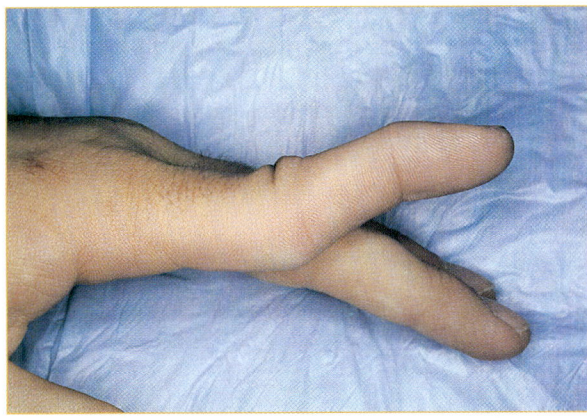

Figure 18-36 Dislocation of the finger joint. Do not be tempted to try to "pop" the joint back into place.

and home accidents often result in dislocations, fractures, lacerations, burns, and amputations. Because the fingers and hands are required to function in such intricate ways, any injury that is not treated properly may result in permanent disability, as well as deformity. For this reason, all injuries to the hand, including simple lacerations, must be evaluated promptly by a physician. For example, you should not attempt to "pop" a dislocated finger joint back in place (Figure 18-36 ▶). Always take any amputated parts to the hospital with the patient. Be sure to wrap the amputated part in a dry or moist sterile dressing, depending on your local protocol, and place it in a dry plastic bag. Put the bag in a cooled container; *do not soak the part in water or allow it to freeze.*

A bulky forearm dressing makes an effective splint for any hand or wrist injury. Follow the steps in (Skill Drill 18-9 ▶):

1. Follow BSI precautions.
2. **Cover all wounds** with a dry, sterile dressing.
3. **Assess pulse, motor, and sensory functions. Supporting the injured limb, form the injured hand into the** position of function, with the wrist slightly bent down and all finger joints moderately flexed. This is the position that is used to hold a can most comfortably.
4. **Place a soft roller bandage** into the palm of the hand (**Step 1**).
5. **Apply a padded board splint to the palmar side of the wrist**, leaving the fingers exposed (**Step 2**).
6. **Secure the entire length of the splint** with a soft roller bandage (**Step 3**).
7. **Apply a sling and swathe** or prop the splinted hand and wrist on a pillow or on the patient's chest during transport to the hospital.

Fractures of the Pelvis

Fracture of the pelvis is most often a result of direct compression in the form of a heavy blow that literally crushes the pelvis. The blow may be from a motor vehicle crash, a weapon used deliberately, a falling object, or a fall from a height. Indirect forces can also cause injuries to the pelvis. For example, when the knee strikes

Skill Drill 18-9

Splinting the Hand and Wrist

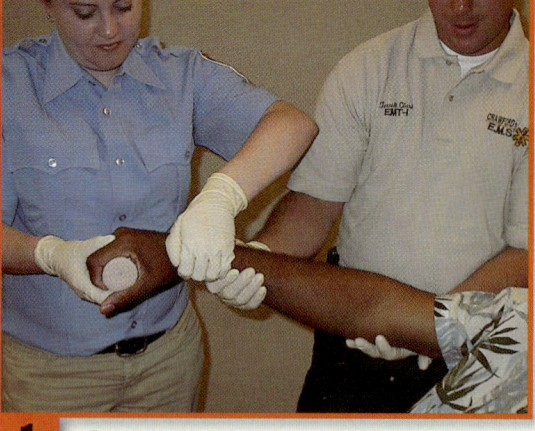

1. Assess pulse, motor, and sensory functions.
Move the hand into the position of function.
Place a soft roller bandage in the palm.

2. Apply a padded board splint on the palmar side with fingers exposed.

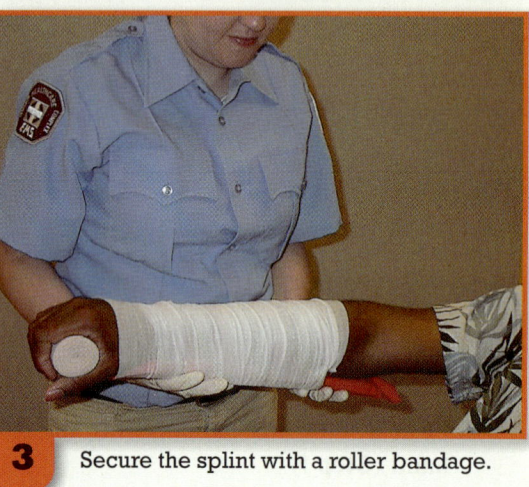

3. Secure the splint with a roller bandage.

the dashboard in an automobile crash, the impact of the force is transmitted along the line of the <u>femur</u>, or the thighbone, which is the longest and largest bone in the body. The head of the femur is driven into the pelvis, causing it to fracture. However, not all pelvic fractures result from violent trauma. Even a simple fall can produce a fracture of the pelvis, especially in elderly individuals with osteoporosis.

Fractures of the pelvis may be accompanied by life-threatening loss of blood from the laceration of blood vessels affixed to the pelvis at certain key points. Up to several liters of blood may drain into the pelvic space and the retroperitoneal space, which lies between the abdominal cavity and the posterior abdominal wall. The kidneys and pancreas are contained in the <u>retroperitoneal space</u>. The result is significant hypotension, shock, and sometimes death. For this reason, you must take immediate steps to treat shock, even if there is only minimal swelling. Often there are no visible signs of bleeding until severe blood loss has occurred. You should be prepared to resuscitate the patient rapidly if this becomes necessary. Start at least one large-bore IV and be prepared to administer isotonic crystalloids to maintain perfusion.

Because the pelvis is surrounded by heavy muscle, open fractures of the pelvis are quite uncommon. However, pelvis fracture fragments can lacerate the rectum and vagina, creating an open fracture that is often overlooked. Once the protective pelvic ring is broken, the structures it is designed to protect, including the urinary bladder, are open to injury. The bladder may be lacerated by pelvic bone fragments, but more often, it tears or ruptures as a result of tension on the bladder or the urethra.

You should suspect a fracture of the pelvis in any patient who has sustained a high-velocity injury and complains of discomfort in the lower back or abdomen. Because heavy muscles and other soft tissues cover the area, deformity or swelling may be very difficult to see. The most reliable sign of fracture of the pelvis is simple tenderness on firm compression and palpation. Firm compression on the two iliac crests will produce pain at a fracture site in the pelvic ring. Assess for tenderness by taking the following steps (Figure 18-37 ▼):

1. Place the palms of your hands over the lateral aspect of each iliac crest, and **apply firm but gentle inward pressure** on the pelvic ring.
2. With the patient lying supine, **place a palm over the anterior aspect of each iliac crest, and apply firm downward pressure**.
3. Use the palm of your hand to firmly but gently **palpate the <u>pubic symphysis</u>**, the firm cartilaginous joint between the two pubic bones. This area will be tender if there is injury to the anterior portion of the pelvic ring.

If there has been injury to the bladder or the urethra, the patient will have lower abdominal tenderness and may have evidence of <u>hematuria</u> (blood in the urine) or blood at the urethral opening.

Perform an initial assessment, and carefully monitor the general condition of any patient you suspect has a pelvic fracture, because he or she is at high risk for hypovolemic shock. Patients in stable condition can be secured to a long backboard or a scoop stretcher to immobilize isolated fractures of the pelvis. Because of the risk of causing nerve or vascular compromise, you should not log roll a patient with a potentially fractured pelvis. Place a PASG on the backboard or stretcher before transferring the patient to the backboard (Figure 18-38 ▼). The PASG will be ready to apply and inflate if the patient develops signs of shock. Remember,

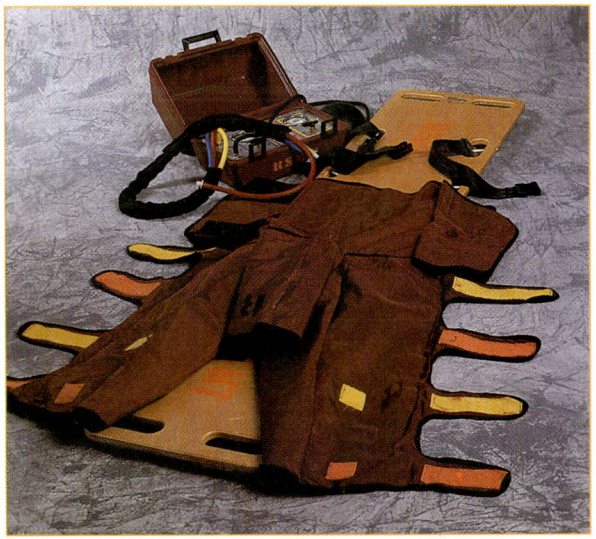

Figure 18-38 Place a PASG, or MAST, on the backboard before log rolling a patient with a suspected pelvic fracture.

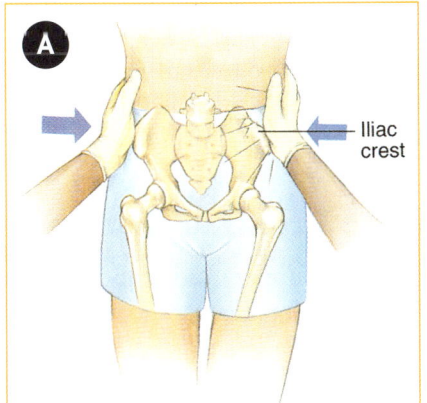
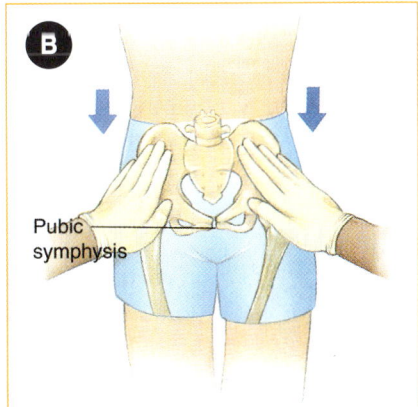
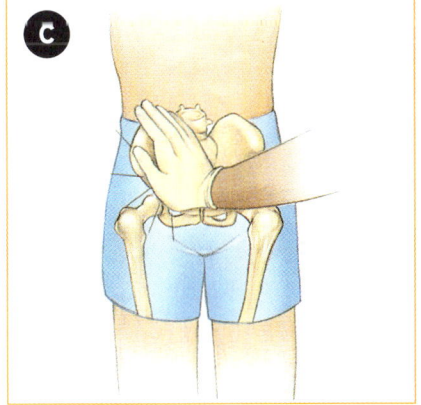

Figure 18-37 A. To assess for tenderness in the pelvic region, place your hands over the lateral aspect of each iliac crest, and gently compress the pelvis. **B.** With the patient in a supine position, place your palms over the anterior aspect of each iliac crest, and apply firm but gentle downward pressure. **C.** Palpate the pubic symphysis with the palm of your hand.

the PASG is only a temporary stabilization device and must be removed within 24 hours. Such a critically injured patient must be transferred to the hospital immediately.

Dislocation of the Hip

The hip joint is a very stable ball-and-socket joint that dislocates only after significant injury. Almost all dislocations of the hip are posterior. The femoral head is displaced posteriorly to lie in the muscles of the buttock. Posterior dislocation of the hip most commonly occurs during automobile crashes in which the knee meets with a direct force, such as the dashboard, and the entire femur is driven posteriorly, dislocating the joint (Figure 18-39). Thus, you should suspect a hip dislocation in any patient who has been in an automobile crash and has a contusion, laceration, or obvious fracture in the knee region. Very rarely does the femoral head dislocate anteriorly; in this circumstance, the legs are suddenly and forcibly spread wide apart and locked in this position.

Posterior dislocation of the hip is frequently complicated by injury to the sciatic nerve, which is located directly behind the hip joint. The <u>sciatic nerve</u> is the most important nerve in the lower extremity; it controls the activity of muscles in the thigh and below the knee, as well as sensation in the entire leg and foot. When the head of the femur is forced out of the hip socket, it may compress or stretch the sciatic nerve, leading to partial or complete paralysis of the nerve. The result is decreased sensation in the leg and foot and, frequently, weakness in the foot muscles. Generally, only the dorsiflexors, the muscles that raise the toes or foot, are involved, causing the "foot drop" that is characteristic of damage to the peroneal portion of the sciatic nerve.

Patients with a posterior dislocation of the hip typically lie with the hip joint flexed (the knee joint drawn up toward the chest) and the thigh rotated inward toward the midline of the body over the top of the opposite thigh (Figure 18-40A). With the rare anterior dislocation, the limb is in the opposite position, extended straight out, rotated, and pointing away from the midline of the body.

Dislocation of the hip is associated with very distinctive signs. The patient will have severe pain in the hip and will strongly resist any attempt to move the joint. The lateral and posterior aspects of the hip region will be tender on palpation. With some thin individuals, you can palpate the femoral head deep within the muscles of the buttock. Check for a sciatic nerve injury by carefully assessing sensation and motor function in the lower extremity. Occasionally, sciatic nerve function will be normal at first and then slowly diminish.

As with any other extremity injury, you should make no attempt to reduce the dislocated hip in the field. Splint the dislocation in the position of the deformity and place the patient supine on a scoop stretcher or long spine board. Support the affected limb with pillows and rolled blankets, particularly under the flexed knee (Figure 18-40B). Then secure the entire limb to the spine board with long straps so that the hip region will not move. Be sure to provide prompt transport.

Fractures of the Proximal Femur

Fractures of the proximal (upper) end of the femur are among the most common fractures, especially in elderly people. Although they are usually called hip fractures, they rarely involve the hip joint. Instead, the break goes through the neck of the femur, the intertrochanteric (middle) region, or across the proximal shaft of the femur (subtrochanteric fractures). Although these three fracture types occur most often in older patients, par-

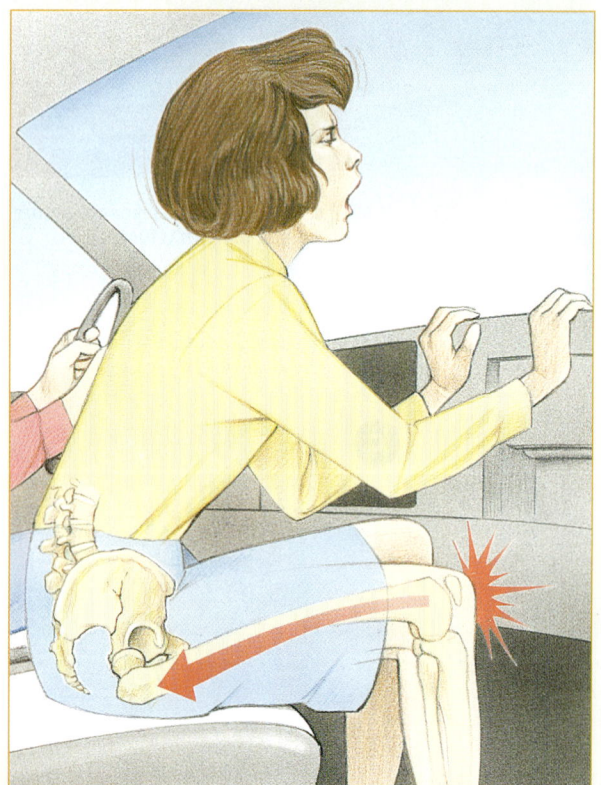

Figure 18-39 Posterior dislocation of the hip can occur as a result of the knee hitting the dashboard in an automobile crash. The impact drives the femur posteriorly (see arrow), dislocating the joint.

ticularly patients with osteoporosis, they may also be seen as a result of high-energy injuries in young adults.

All patients with displaced fractures of the proximal femur display a characteristic deformity. They lie with the leg externally rotated, and the injured leg is usually shorter than the opposite, uninjured limb. When the fracture is not displaced, this deformity is not present. With any kind of hip fracture, patients typically are unable to walk or move the leg because of pain in the hip region or in the groin or inner aspect of the thigh. The hip region is usually tender on palpation, and gentle rolling of the leg will cause pain but will not do further damage. On occasion, the pain is referred to the knee, and it is not uncommon for an elderly patient with a hip fracture to complain of knee pain after a fall. You should splint the lower extremity of an elderly patient who has fallen and complains of pain in the hip or the knee, even if there is no deformity, and then transport the patient to the emergency department.

The age of the patient and the severity of the injury will dictate how you splint the fracture. With young people, fractures of the hip resulting from violent injury are best immobilized with a traction splint or the combination of a PASG and a spine board. The PASG offers an added advantage: It will help to control bleeding in the region. Apply the traction splint as you would for a femoral shaft fracture, taking special care to protect the injured region from excessive pressure from the ring of a Hare traction splint.

An older patient with an isolated hip fracture does not require a traction splint **Figure 18-41A**. You can effectively immobilize such a fracture by placing the patient on a long spine board or scoop stretcher, using pillows or rolled blankets to support the injured limb in the deformed position. Then secure the injured limb carefully to the stretcher with long straps **Figure 18-41B**.

All patients with hip fractures may lose significant amounts of blood. Therefore, you should treat with

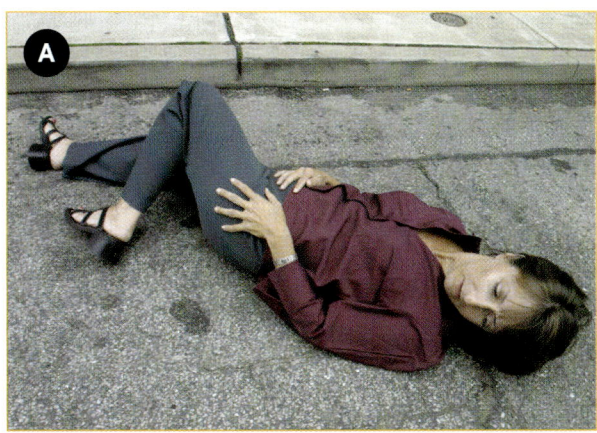

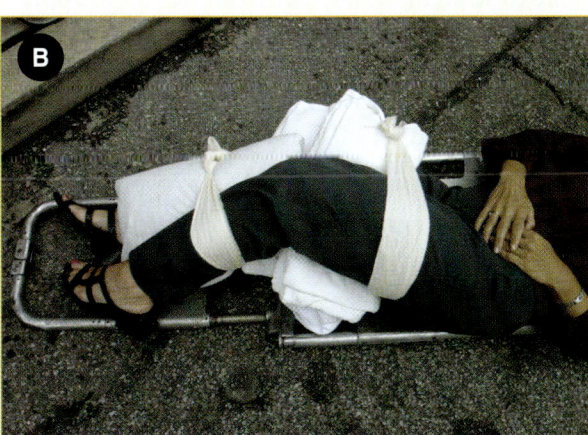

Figure 18-40 **A.** The usual position of a patient with a posterior dislocation of the hip. The hip joint is flexed, and the thigh is rotated inward and adducted across the midline of the body. **B.** Support the affected limb with pillows and blankets, particularly under the flexed knee. Secure the entire limb to a long board with long straps to prevent movement during transport.

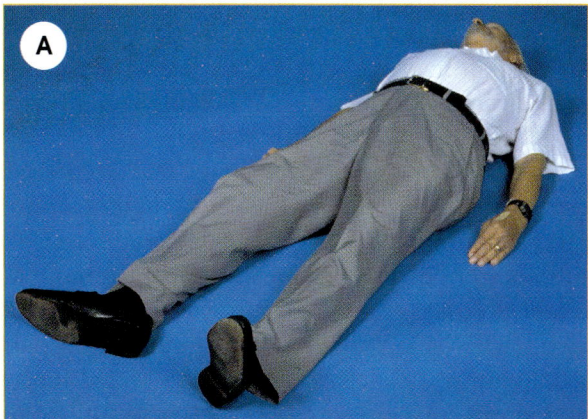

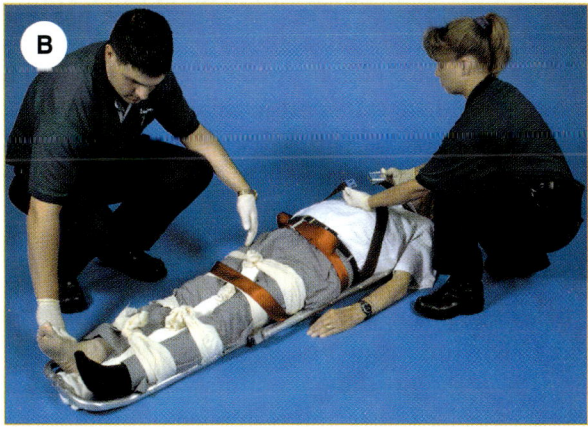

Figure 18-41 **A.** A patient with a fracture of the proximal femur will typically lie still with the extremity rotated, making the injured leg appear shorter than the other leg. **B.** Splint the injured leg to the uninjured leg, and secure the patient on a scoop stretcher or spine board.

high-flow oxygen and monitor vital signs frequently, being alert for signs of shock. Initiate intravenous therapy and give a 20-mL/kg bolus of an isotonic crystalloid solution, repeating as necessary.

Femoral Shaft Fractures

Fractures of the femur can occur in any part of the shaft, from the hip region to the femoral condyles just above the knee joint. Following a fracture, the large muscles of the thigh spasm in an attempt to "splint" the unstable limb. The muscle spasm often produces significant deformity of the limb, with severe angulation or external rotation at the fracture site. Usually the limb shortens significantly as well. Fractures of the femoral shaft are often open, and fragments of bone may protrude through the skin.

There may be a significant amount of blood loss, as much as 500 to 1,000 mL, after a fracture of the shaft of the femur. With open fractures, the amount of blood loss may be even greater. Thus, it is not unusual for hypovolemic shock to develop. Handle patients with femoral shaft fractures with extreme care, because any extra movement or fracture manipulation will increase internal bleeding, if present.

Because of the severe deformity that occurs with these fractures, bone fragments may penetrate or press on important nerves and vessels and produce significant damage. For this reason, you must carefully and periodically assess the distal neurovascular function in patients who have sustained a fracture of the femoral shaft. Remove the clothing from the affected limb so that you can adequately inspect the injury site for any open wounds. Remember to follow BSI precautions. Monitor the patient's vital signs closely, and continue to watch for the onset of hypovolemic shock. You must provide immediate transport in this situation.

Cover any wound with a dry sterile dressing. If the foot or leg below the level of the fracture shows signs of impaired circulation (is pale, cold, or pulseless), apply gentle longitudinal traction to the deformed limb in line with the long axis of the limb. Gradually turn the leg from the deformed position to restore the limb's overall alignment. Often, this restores or improves circulation to the foot. If it does not, the patient may have sustained a serious vascular injury and is in need of prompt medical attention.

A fracture of the femoral shaft is best immobilized with a traction splint, such as a Hare traction splint or a Sager splint (see Skill Drills 18-7 and 18-8).

Injuries of Knee Ligaments

The knee is very vulnerable to injury; therefore, many different types of injuries occur in this region. Ligament injuries, for example, range from mild sprains to complete dislocation of the joint. The patella can also dislocate. In addition, all the bony elements of the knee (distal femur, upper tibia, and patella) can fracture.

The knee is especially susceptible to ligament injuries, which occur when abnormal bending or twisting forces are applied to the joint. Such injuries are often seen in both recreational and competitive athletes. The ligaments on the medial side of the knee are the ones that are most frequently injured, typically when the foot is fixed to the ground and a heavy object strikes the lateral aspect of the knee, such as when a football player is clipped or tackled from the side.

Usually the patient with a knee ligament injury will report pain in the joint and be unable to use the extremity normally. When you examine the patient, you will generally find swelling, occasional ecchymosis, point tenderness at the injury site, and joint effusion (excess fluid in the joint).

You must splint all suspected knee ligament injuries. The splint should extend from the hip joint to the foot, immobilizing the bone above the injured joint (the femur) and the bone below it (the tibia). A variety of splints can be used, including a padded, rigid, long leg splint or two padded board splints securely applied to the medial and lateral aspects of the limb. A long spine board, a pillow splint, or simply binding the injured limb to its uninjured mate are acceptable but less effective splinting techniques. The patient may be able to straighten the knee to allow you to apply the splint. However, if you encounter resistance or pain when trying to straighten the knee, splint it in the flexed position. Then continue to monitor the distal neurovascular function until the patient reaches the hospital.

Dislocation of the Knee

Complete disruption of the ligaments supporting the knee may result in dislocation of the joint. When this happens, the proximal end of the tibia completely displaces from its juncture with the lower end of the femur, usually producing a significant deformity. Although substantial ligament damage always occurs with a knee dislocation, the more urgent injury is to the popliteal artery, which is often lacerated or compressed by the displaced tibia. When gross deformity, severe pain, and an inability to move the joint cause you to suspect a dislocation of the knee, always check the distal circulation carefully before taking any other step. If the distal pulses are absent, contact medical control immediately for further stabilization instructions.

If adequate distal pulses are present, splint the knee in the position in which you found it, and transport the patient promptly. Do not attempt to manipulate or straighten any severe knee injury if there are good distal pulses. If the limb is straight, apply leg splints to both sides of the limb to immobilize it (Figure 18-42A). If the knee is bent and the foot has a good pulse, splint the joint in the bent position, using parallel padded board splints secured at the hip and ankle joint to provide a stable A-frame (Figure 18-42B). Secure the limb to a spine board or stretcher with pillows and straps to eliminate any motion during transport.

On rare occasions, medical control may instruct you to realign a deformed, pulseless limb to reduce compression of the popliteal artery and, thus, restore distal circulation. You should make **only one** attempt to do this. First, straighten the limb by applying gentle longitudinal traction in the axis of the limb. Once you apply manual traction, maintain it until the limb is fully splinted; otherwise, the limb will return to its deformed position. If traction significantly increases the patient's pain, do not continue. As you apply traction, monitor the posterior tibial pulse to see whether it returns. Splint the limb in the position in which you feel the strongest pulse. If you are unable to restore the distal pulse, splint the limb in the position that is most comfortable for the patient, and then provide prompt transport to the hospital. Notify medical control of the status of the distal pulse so that arrangements to treat the patient can be made in advance.

Fractures About the Knee

Fractures about the knee may occur at the distal end of the femur, at the proximal end of the tibia, or in the patella. Because of local tenderness and swelling, it is easy to confuse a nondisplaced or minimally displaced fracture about the knee with a ligament injury. Likewise, a displaced fracture about the knee may produce significant deformity that makes it look like a dislocation. Management of the two types of injuries is as follows:
- If there is an adequate distal pulse and no significant deformity, splint the limb with the knee straight.

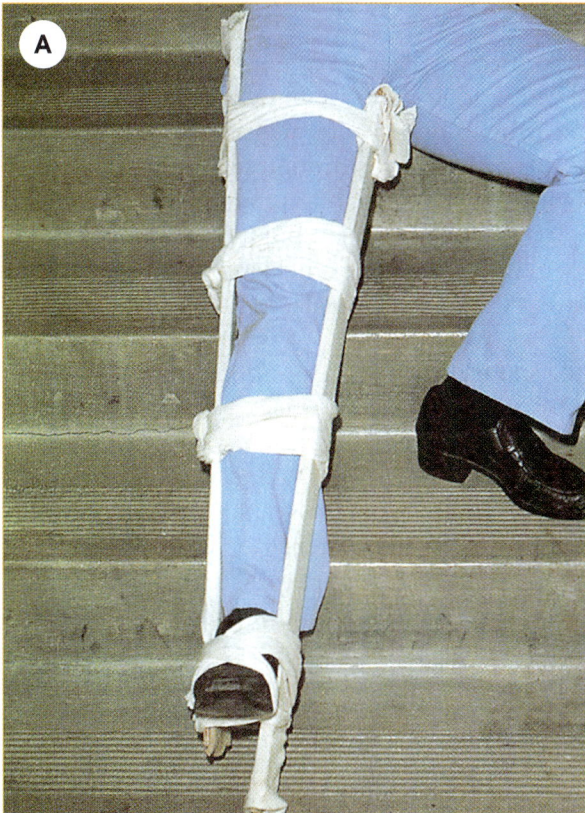

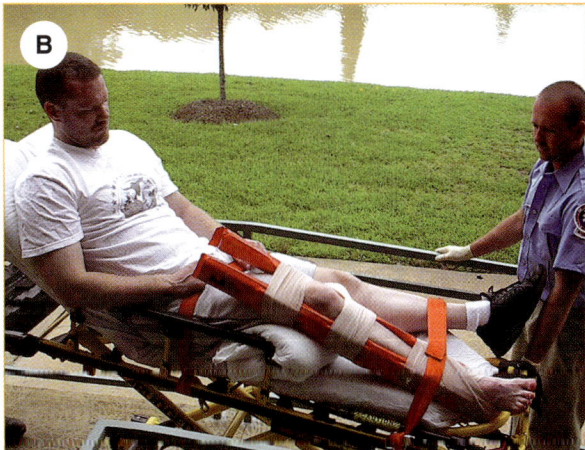

Figure 18-42 A. When the injured knee is straight, apply padded board splints extending from the hip to the ankle. **B.** If the knee is flexed and the foot has good pulses, apply padded board splints with the knee in the flexed position.

- If there is an adequate pulse and significant deformity, splint the joint in the position found.
- If the pulse is absent below the level of the injury, contact medical control immediately for further instructions.

Dislocation of the Patella

A dislocated patella most commonly occurs in teenagers and young adults who are engaged in athletic activities. Some patients have recurrent dislocations of the patella. As with recurrent dislocation of the shoulder, minor twisting may be enough to produce the problem. The displacement of the patella produces a significant deformity in which the knee is held in a slightly flexed position and the patella is displaced to the lateral side of the knee Figure 18-43.

Splint the knee in the position in which you found it. Most often, this is with the knee flexed to a moderate degree. To immobilize the knee, apply padded board splints to the medial and lateral aspects of the joint, extending from the hip to the ankle. Use pillows to support the limb on the stretcher.

Occasionally as you apply the splint, the patella will return to its normal position spontaneously. When this occurs, immobilize the limb as for a knee ligament injury, in a padded long leg splint. The patient still needs to be transported to the emergency department. Report the spontaneous reduction as soon as you arrive at the hospital so that the medical staff is aware of the severity of the injury.

Injuries of the Tibia and Fibula

The tibia (shinbone) is the larger of the two leg bones that are responsible for supporting the major weight-bearing surface of the knee and ankle; the fibula is the smaller of them. Fractures of the shaft of the tibia or the fibula may occur at any place between the knee joint and the ankle joint. Usually both bones fracture at the same time Figure 18-44. Even a single fracture may result in severe deformity, with significant angulation or rotation. Because the tibia is located just beneath the skin, open fractures of this bone are quite common Figure 18-45.

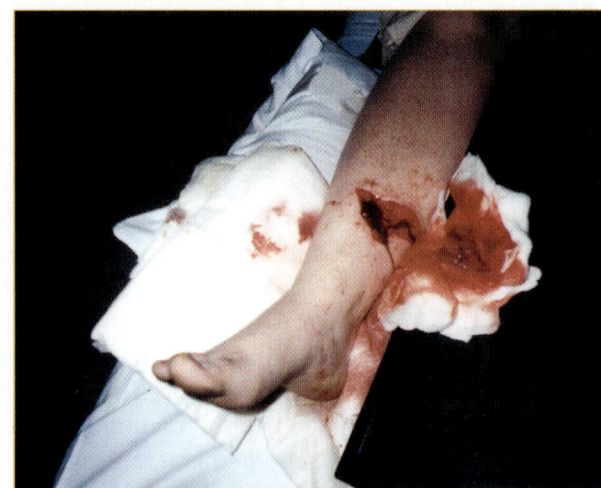

Figure 18-44 Open tibia and fibula fracture.

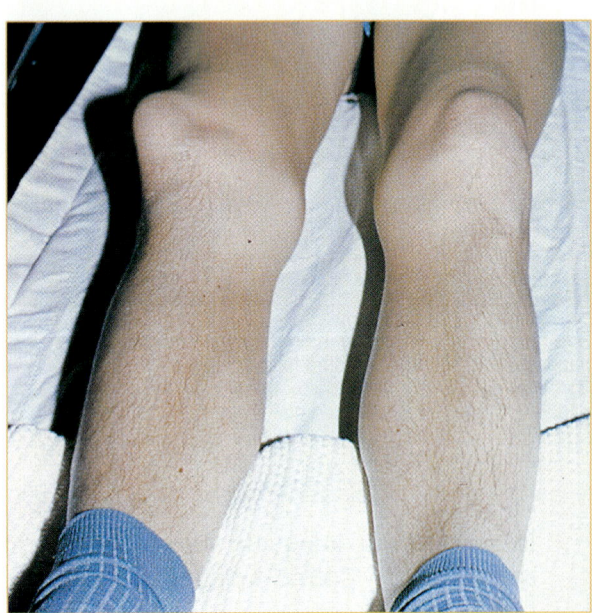

Figure 18-43 A dislocated patella will typically appear with the patella displaced lateral to the knee and with the knee slightly flexed.

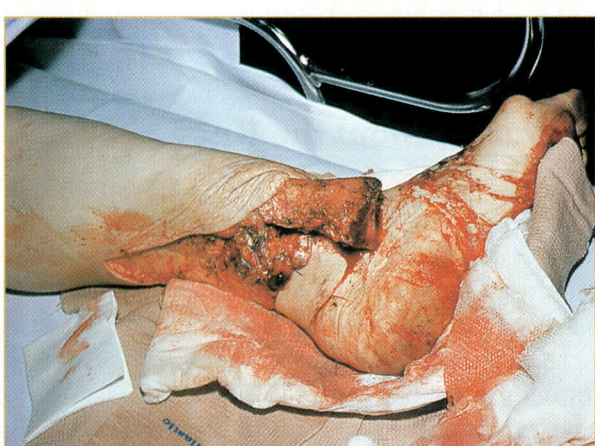

Figure 18-45 Because the tibia is so close to the skin, open fractures are quite common.

Fractures of the tibia and fibula should be immobilized with a padded, rigid long leg splint or an air splint that extends from the foot to the upper thigh. Traction splints are not indicated for isolated tibial fractures. As with most other fractures of the shaft of long bones, you should correct severe deformity before splinting by applying gentle longitudinal traction. The goal here is to restore a position that will take a standard splint; it is not necessary to replace the fracture fragments in their anatomic position.

Fractures of the tibia and fibula are often associated with vascular injury as a result of the distorted position of the limb following injury. Realigning the limb may restore adequate blood supply to the foot. If it does not, transport the patient promptly and notify medical control while you are en route.

Ankle Injuries

The ankle is the most commonly injured joint. Ankle injuries occur in individuals of all ages and range in severity from a simple sprain, which heals after a few days' rest, to severe fracture-dislocations. As with other joints, it is sometimes difficult to tell a nondisplaced ankle fracture from a simple sprain without radiographs Figure 18-46. Therefore, any ankle injury that produces pain, swelling, localized tenderness, or the inability to bear weight must be evaluated by a physician. The most frequent mechanism of ankle injury is twisting, which stretches or tears the supporting ligaments. A more extensive twisting force may result in fracture of one or both malleoli. Dislocation of the ankle is usually associated with fractures of both malleoli.

You can manage the wide spectrum of injuries to the ankle in the same way, as follows:

1. Dress all open wounds.
2. Assess distal neurovascular function.
3. Correct any gross deformity by applying gentle longitudinal traction to the heel.
4. Before releasing traction, apply a splint Figure 18-47.

You can use a padded rigid splint, an air splint, or a pillow splint. Just make sure it includes the entire foot and extends up the leg to the level of the knee joint.

Foot Injuries

Injuries to the foot can result in the fracture of one or more of the tarsals, metatarsals, or phalanges of the toes. Toe fractures are especially common.

Of the tarsal bones, the <u>calcaneus</u>, the heel bone, is the most frequently fractured. Injury usually occurs when the patient falls or jumps from a height and lands directly on the heel. The force of injury compresses the calcaneus, producing immediate swelling and ecchymosis. If the force of impact is great enough, as from a fall from a roof or tree, there may be other fractures as well.

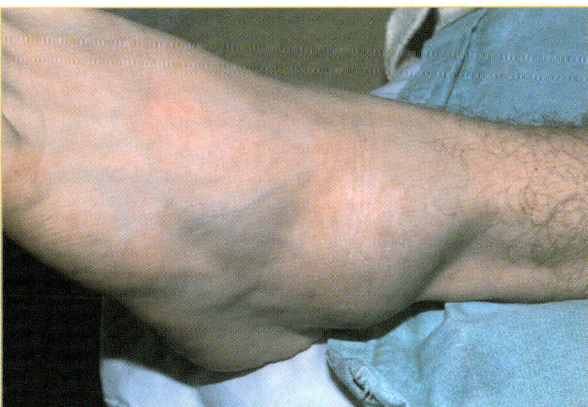

Figure 18-46 Swelling about the ankle is characteristic of both sprains and fractures.

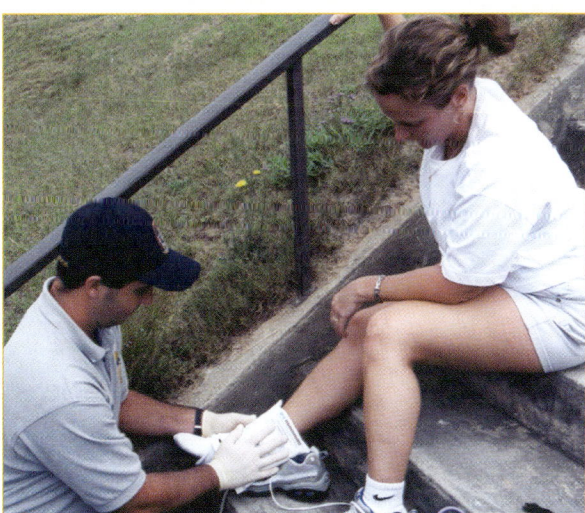

Figure 18-47 Apply ice packs to ankle injuries, and splint with the foot in the position of function. Remember to check the distal pulse.

Frequently, the force of injury is transmitted up the legs to the spine, producing a fracture of the lumbar spine (Figure 18-48 ▼). When a patient who has jumped or fallen from a height complains of heel pain, be sure to ask him or her about back pain and carefully check the spine for tenderness or deformity.

Injuries of the foot are associated with significant swelling but rarely with gross deformity. Vascular injuries are not common. As in the hand, lacerations about the ankle and foot may damage underlying nerves and tendons. Puncture wounds of the foot are common and may cause serious infection if not treated early. All of these injuries must be evaluated and treated by a physician.

To splint the foot, apply a rigid padded board splint, an air splint, or a pillow splint, immobilizing the ankle joint as well as the foot (Figure 18-49 ▼). Leave the toes exposed so that you can periodically assess neurovascular function.

When the patient is lying on the stretcher, elevate the foot approximately 6″ to minimize swelling. All patients with lower extremity injuries should be transported in the supine position to allow for elevation of the limb. Never allow the foot and leg to dangle off the stretcher onto the floor or ground.

If a patient has fallen from a height and complains of heel pain, use a long backboard to immobilize any possible spinal injury in addition to splinting the foot.

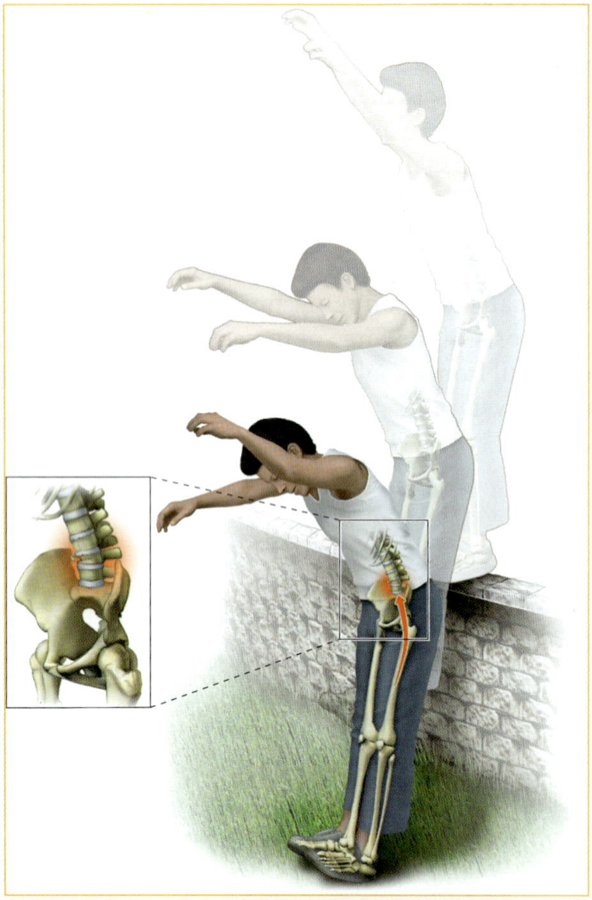

Figure 18-48 The force of injury is transmitted up the legs to the spine, often resulting in a fracture of the lumbar spine.

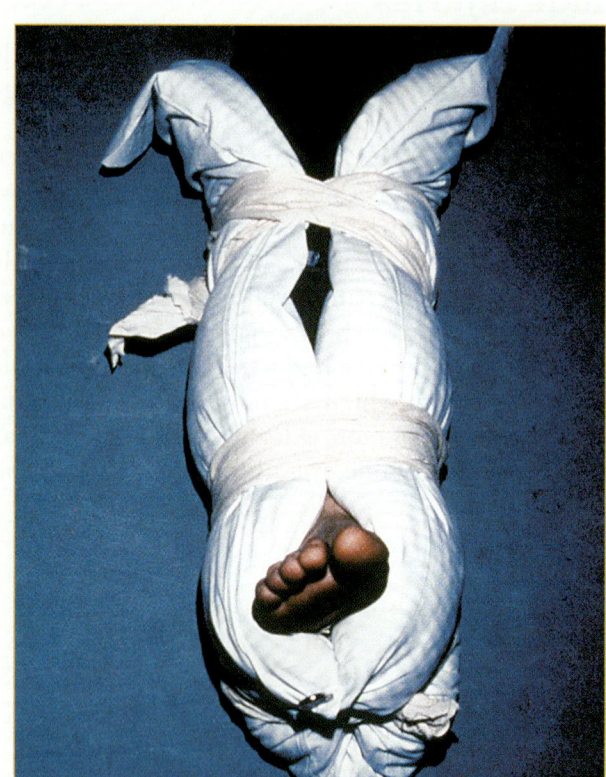

Figure 18-49 A pillow splint provides good immobilization of the foot and ankle.

You are the Provider — Summary

1. What common musculoskeletal injuries are likely to be encountered by the EMT-I?

The EMT-I will frequently encounter a variety of musculoskeletal injuries, including fractures, dislocations, sprains, and strains.

2. What are the two classifications of fractures?

Fractures are classified as closed or open. If the overlying skin has not been damaged, the patient has a closed fracture. With an open fracture, there is an external wound, caused by the same blow that fractured the bone or by the broken bone ends lacerating the skin.

3. What is the proper management of the patient with a musculoskeletal injury?

Your first steps in providing care for any patient are the initial assessment and stabilizing the patient's ABCs. After you have done so, you can focus on specific injuries. Remember to always follow BSI precautions.

- **Completely cover open wounds** with a dry, sterile dressing, and apply local pressure to control bleeding.
- **Apply the appropriate splint,** and elevate the extremity.
- **If swelling is present,** apply cold packs to the area; however, avoid placing cold packs directly on the skin or other exposed tissues.
- **Prepare the patient for transport.** A patient with an isolated upper extremity injury will most likely be more comfortable in a semiseated position rather than lying flat; however, either position is acceptable. If possible, elevate the injured extremity to help reduce swelling.

4. What additional assessment approach should be performed by the EMT-I?

For musculoskeletal trauma, use the DCAP-BTLS mnemonic. Identify any extremity **D**eformities that likely represent significant musculoskeletal injury and stabilize appropriately. **C**ontusions and **A**brasions may overlie more subtle injuries and should prompt you to carefully evaluate the stability and neurovascular status of the limb. The presence of **P**uncture wounds or other signs of **P**enetrating injury should alert you to the possibility of an open fracture. Associated **B**urns must be identified and treated appropriately. Palpate for **T**enderness, which, like contusions or abrasions, may be the only significant sign of an underlying musculoskeletal injury. When **L**acerations are present on an extremity, an open fracture must be considered, bleeding controlled, and dressings applied. Careful inspection for **S**welling with attention to comparison with the opposite limb may also reveal occult musculoskeletal injury.

5. What hazards are associated with the improper application of splints?

Hazards associated with the improper application of splints include:

- Compression of nerves, tissues, and blood vessels
- Delay in transport of a patient with a life-threatening injury
- Reduction of distal circulation
- Aggravation of the injury
- Injury to tissue, nerves, blood vessels, or muscles as a result of excessive movement of the bone or joint

Prep Kit

Ready for Review

- Skeletal or voluntary muscle, which attaches to bone and forms the major muscle mass of the body, is supplied with arteries, veins, and nerves. The 206 bones of the skeleton are living tissue that, when fractured, can bleed and cause severe pain.
- Wherever two bones come into contact, a joint is formed, strengthened in key areas by ligaments. A fracture is a broken bone; a dislocation is a disruption of a joint; a sprain is a joint injury that involves partial or temporary dislocation of bone ends and partial stretching or tearing of ligaments; and a strain is a muscle pull.
- Depending on the amount of kinetic energy absorbed by the tissues, the zone of injury may extend to a distant point, so you must always check for associated injuries beyond the obvious ones.
- Fractures are open or closed, displaced or nondisplaced.
- Signs of fracture and dislocation include pain, deformity, point tenderness, guarding, swelling, crepitus, and false motion.
- Signs of sprain include ecchymosis and instability of the joint.
- Your approach to patients with all painful, swollen, deformed extremities should include a rapid initial assessment, stabilization of vital functions and control of serious bleeding, focused physical exam of the injured body part, assessment of neurovascular function in the affected limb, splinting to immobilize the affected part, and prompt transport to the hospital.
- For each limb, your neurovascular examination should include pulse, sensation, and motor function. Repeat this exam every 5 to 10 minutes.
- The principles of splinting include the following: If you suspect a fracture of the shaft of any bone, make sure the splint immobilizes the joints above and below the fracture; with injuries in and around a joint, make sure the splint immobilizes the bones above and below the injured joint; where fracture of a long bone shaft has resulted in severe deformity, use constant, gentle, manual traction (pull) to align the limb so that it can be splinted, unless this is too painful.
- There are three types of splints: rigid splints and traction splints, which require two people to apply, and formable splints, including air splints. In addition, slings and swathes are used to help support the weight of an injured upper extremity and immobilize the shoulder region, respectively.
- Provide immediate transport to any patient if you are unable to restore a pulse to a pulseless limb by applying traction.
- The only life-threatening musculoskeletal injuries are multiple fractures, fractures with arterial injuries, severe open fractures, limb amputations, and pelvic fractures with hemodynamic instability.

Vital Vocabulary

acromioclavicular (A/C) joint A simple joint in which the bony projections of the scapula and the clavicle meet at the top of the shoulder.

articular cartilage A pearly layer of specialized cartilage covering the articular surfaces (contact surfaces on the ends) of bones in synovial joints.

calcaneus The heel bone.

clavicle The collarbone.

closed fracture A fracture in which the skin is not broken.

compartment syndrome An elevation of pressure within the fascial compartment, characterized by extreme pain, decreased pain sensation, pain on stretching of affected muscles, and decreased power; most frequently seen in fractures below the elbow or knee in children.

Technology

- Interactivities
- Vocabulary Explorer
- Anatomy Review
- Web Links
- Online Review Manual

www.EMSzone.com/EMTT

crepitus A grating or grinding sensation or sound caused by fractured bone ends or joints rubbing together.

dislocation Disruption of a joint in which ligaments are damaged and the bone ends are completely displaced.

displaced fracture A fracture in which bone fragments are separated from one another and not in anatomic alignment.

ecchymosis Bruising or discoloration associated with bleeding within or under the skin.

femur The thighbone, which extends from the pelvis to the knee and is responsible for formation of the hip; the longest and largest bone in the body.

fibula The outer and smaller bone of the two bones of the lower leg.

fracture A break in the continuity of a bone.

glenoid fossa The part of the scapula that joins with the humeral head to form the glenohumeral joint.

hematuria Blood in the urine.

humerus The supporting bone of the upper arm that joins with the scapula (at the glenoid fossa) to form the shoulder joint and with the ulna and radius to form the elbow joint.

joint The place where two bones come into contact.

ligaments Bands of fibrous tissue that connect bones to bones and support and strengthen the joints.

nondisplaced fracture A simple crack in the bone that has not caused the bone to move from its normal anatomic position; also called a hairline fracture.

open fracture Any break in a bone in which the overlying skin has been damaged.

patella The kneecap.

point tenderness Tenderness that is sharply localized at the site of the injury, found by gently palpating along the bone with the tip of one finger.

position of function A hand position in which the wrist is slightly dorsiflexed and all finger joints are moderately flexed.

pubic symphysis The firm cartilaginous joint between the two pubic bones.

radius The bone on the thumb side of the forearm; most important in wrist function.

reduce Return a dislocated joint or fractured bone to its normal position; set.

retroperitoneal space The space between the abdominal cavity and the posterior abdominal wall, containing the kidneys, certain large vessels, and parts of the gastrointestinal tract.

scapula Shoulder blade.

sciatic nerve The major nerve to the lower extremity; controls much of muscle function in the leg and sensation in the entire leg and foot.

skeletal muscle Striated muscles that are attached to bones and usually cross at least one joint.

sling A bandage or material that helps to support the weight of an injured upper extremity.

splint A flexible or rigid appliance used to protect and maintain the position of an injured extremity.

sprain A joint injury involving damage to supporting ligaments and partial or temporary dislocation of bone ends.

strain Stretching or tearing of a muscle; also called a muscle pull.

swathe A bandage that passes around the chest to secure an injured arm to the chest.

tendons Tough, ropelike cords of fibrous tissue that attach skeletal muscles to bones.

tibia The larger of the two lower leg bones responsible for supporting the major weight-bearing surface of the knee and the ankle; the shinbone.

traction The act of exerting a pulling force on a structure.

ulna The bone on the small finger side of the forearm; most important for elbow function.

Assessment in Action

You are on standby at a basketball tournament. Your job is to provide initial treatment in the event of an illness or injury and call in a transporting unit. You are observing the tournament when you see a player land hard on his extended arm.

As he gets up from the ground he is holding his left wrist against his body. You can tell by the look on his face that he is in pain. On exam you note swelling and deformity to his left forearm just above the wrist.

1. The description of this patient's injury is consistent with a:
   A. nondisplaced closed fracture.
   B. nondisplaced open fracture.
   C. displaced closed fracture.
   D. displaced open fracture.

2. Your treatment will include all of the following EXCEPT:
   A. application of a rigid splint.
   B. application of ice to the injury.
   C. assessment of pulse, motor ability, and sensation.
   D. positioning the hand flat on the splint.

You hand off your patient to an ambulance crew and plan to return to an uneventful competition when your next patient approaches you. He is being supported by two teammates and is not putting weight on his right leg.

3. Your assessment will include all of the following EXCEPT:
   A. assessing the patient's ability to put weight on the foot.
   B. assessing for pain, swelling, and deformity.
   C. comparing the injured extremity with the uninjured one.
   D. questioning the patient about mechanism of injury.

4. His ankle is slightly swollen and is painful. You will treat the patient for a:
   A. dislocation.
   B. fracture.
   C. sprain.
   D. strain.

Just when you thought it was safe to go back to the tournament.... You settle into your seat just in time to see a player land on the leg of a player who had fallen. The injured player cries out in pain. You rush over and observe bone ends protruding through his lower leg with heavy bleeding.

5. Your first action is to:
   A. use BSI precautions.
   B. control the bleeding.
   C. check ABCs.
   D. apply manual cervical immobilization.

6. Your treatment will for this patient will include:
   A. applying a traction splint.
   B. immobilizing the bones above and below the injury.
   C. applying a bulky dressing to control bleeding.
   D. immediately moving the patient to the ambulance.

7. The purpose of a splint is to:
   A. reduce pain.
   B. restrict blood flow.
   C. increase bleeding.
   D. prevent safe transport.

You are thinking that these people are not cut out for basketball when your next patient approaches. He has obvious deformity to his right shoulder after landing on his outstretched hand. You suspect a shoulder dislocation.

8. On assessment, you should expect to find:
   A. the injured shoulder to be higher than the uninjured shoulder.
   B. the patient to be unable to move the affected arm.
   C. the patient to be able to abduct the affected arm.
   D. the injured shoulder to have a rounded appearance.

Finally, the competition is over! No more injuries to deal with! As you are heading to your ambulance, you hear screeching tires. You turn in time to see one of the players get struck by a car. Your partner establishes manual cervical spine immobilization while you assess the patient. He is conscious and alert but in extreme pain. Your rapid assessment reveals deformity and swelling to the left thigh.

9. All of the following are true concerning femur fractures EXCEPT:
   A. They often present with shortening and external rotation.
   B. They are very painful due to muscle spasm.
   C. They can cause shock due to nerve damage.
   D. A traction splint should be applied if the patient is in stable condition.

10. Your treatment will include all of the following EXCEPT:
    A. Spinal immobilization
    B. Eliciting crepitus
    C. 100% oxygen
    D. Ice to reduce swelling

Points to Ponder

You are dispatched to a motor vehicle crash. Your patient was the driver of a midsize vehicle that was struck from behind by a semitrailer traveling at 30 mph. This impact in turn pushed him into a semitrailer stopped ahead of him. There is extensive damage to the vehicle. Your patient is conscious and alert, and his only complaint is pain to his right arm. On exam, you note swelling and deformity to his right forearm. No other obvious injuries are noted, and his vital signs are stable. Your partner has established manual cervical immobilization. You apply a KED and then splint the arm. As you are splinting his arm, you notice that he has become quiet and his skin has become pale and moist. You place him on a long spine board and begin transport. En route to the hospital, his condition deteriorates further and he develops cardiac arrest. What happened to your stable patient? What should you have done differently?

Issues: Understanding the Importance of Recognizing a Load-and-Go Situation and When Transport Takes Priority Over Immobilizing Extremity Fractures

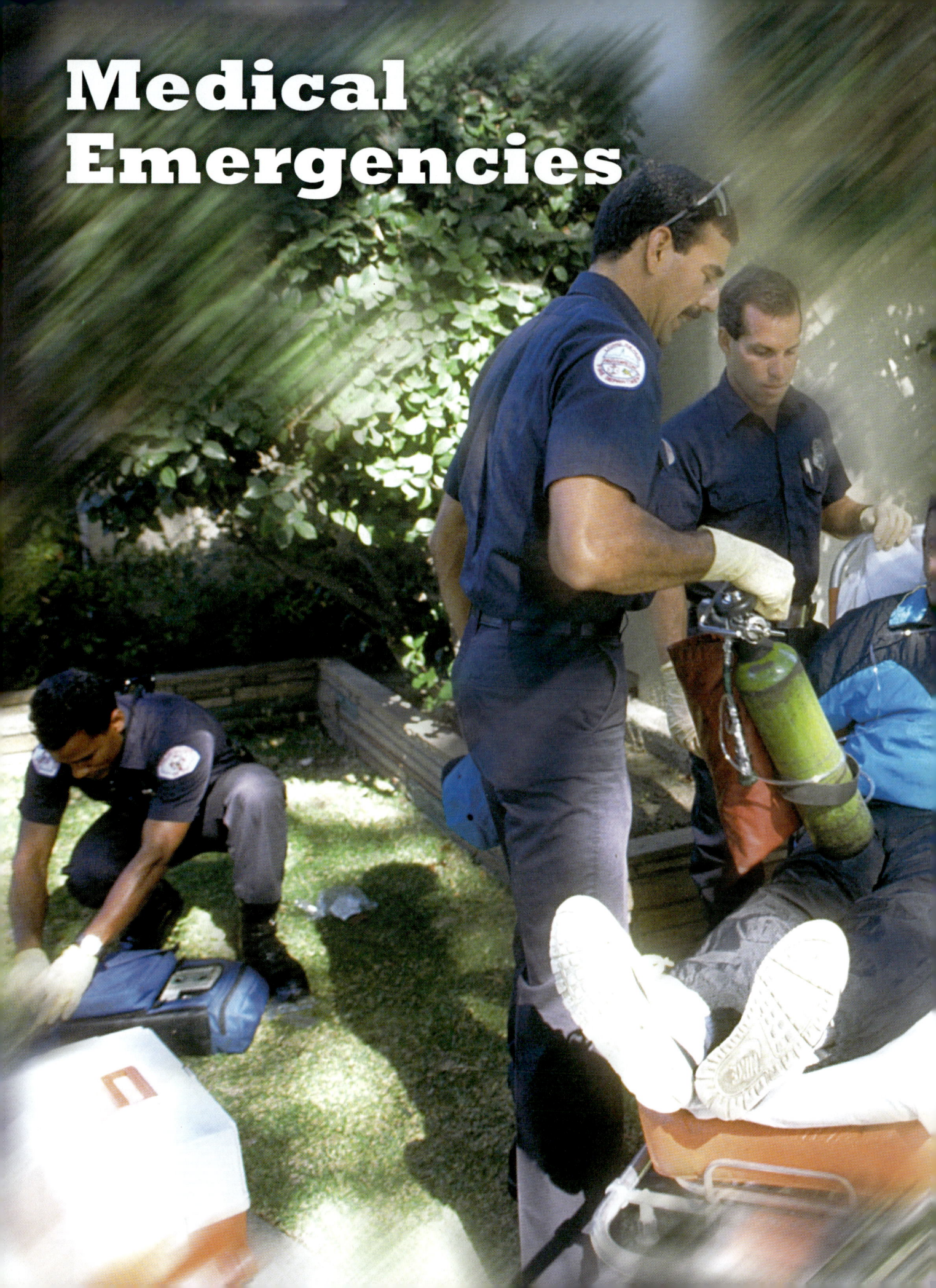

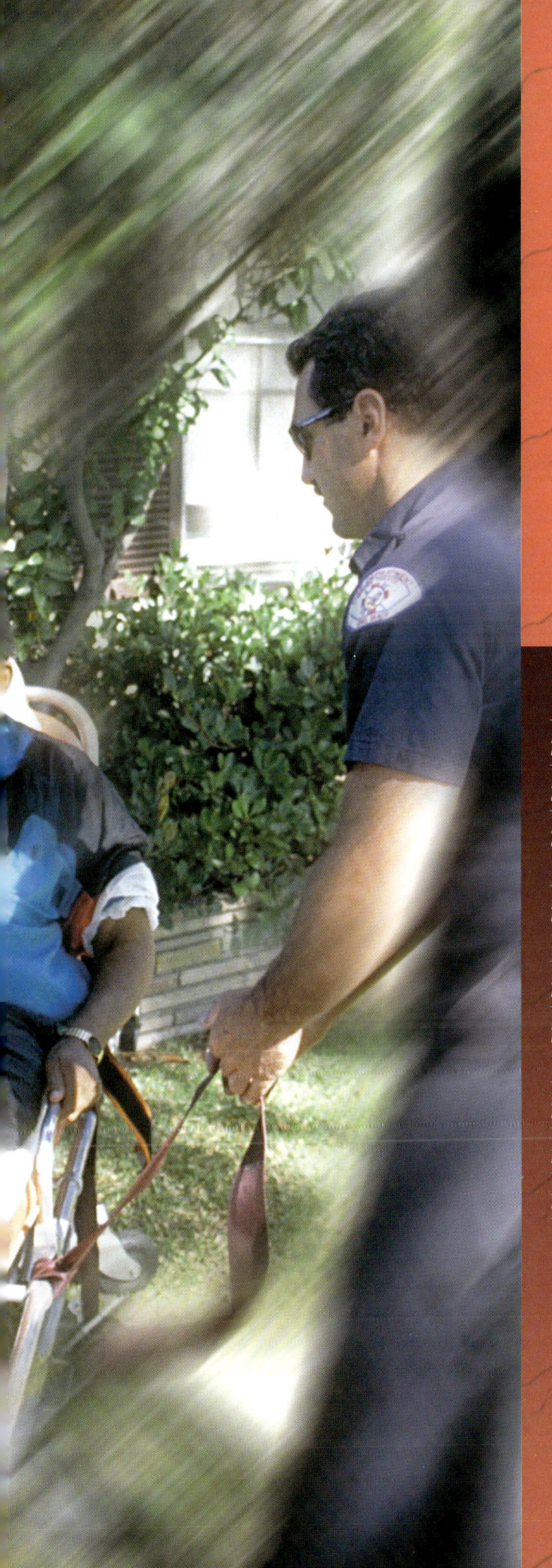

Section 6

19	Respiratory Emergencies	848
20	Cardiovascular Emergencies	880
21	Diabetic Emergencies	984
22	Allergic Reactions and Envenomations	1004
23	Poisonings and Overdose Emergencies	1032
24	Neurologic Emergencies	1058
25	Nontraumatic Abdominal Emergencies	1082
26	Environmental Emergencies	1098
27	Behavioral Emergencies	1130
28	Gynecologic Emergencies	1150

Respiratory Emergencies

1999 Objectives

Cognitive

5-1.1 Identify and describe the function of the structures located in the upper and lower airway. (p 851)

5-1.2 Discuss the physiology of ventilation and respiration. (p 851)

5-1.3 Identify common pathological events that affect the pulmonary system. (p 851)

5-1.4 Discuss abnormal assessment findings associated with pulmonary diseases and conditions. (p 853)

5-1.5 Compare various airway and ventilation techniques used in the management of pulmonary diseases. (p 870)

5-1.6 Review the pharmacological preparations that EMT-Intermediates use for management of respiratory diseases and conditions. (p 871)

5-1.7 Review the use of equipment used during the physical examination of patients with complaints associated with respiratory diseases and conditions. (p 870)

5-1.8 Describe the epidemiology, pathophysiology, assessment findings, and management for the following respiratory diseases and conditions:
   a. Bronchial asthma
   b. Chronic bronchitis
   c. Emphysema
   d. Pneumonia
   e. Pulmonary edema
   f. Spontaneous pneumothorax
   g. Hyperventilation syndrome
   h. Pulmonary thromboembolism (p 856)

Affective

5-1.9 Recognize and value the assessment and treatment of patients with respiratory diseases. (p 850)

5-1.10 Indicate appreciation for the critical nature of accurate field impressions of patients with respiratory diseases and conditions. (p 850)

Psychomotor

5-1.11 Demonstrate and record pertinent assessment findings associated with pulmonary diseases and conditions. (p 868)

5-1.12 Review proper use of airway and ventilation devices. (p 868)

5-1.13 Conduct a simulated history and patient assessment, record the findings, and report appropriate management of patients with pulmonary diseases and conditions. (p 868)

1985 Objectives

There are no 1985 objectives for this chapter.

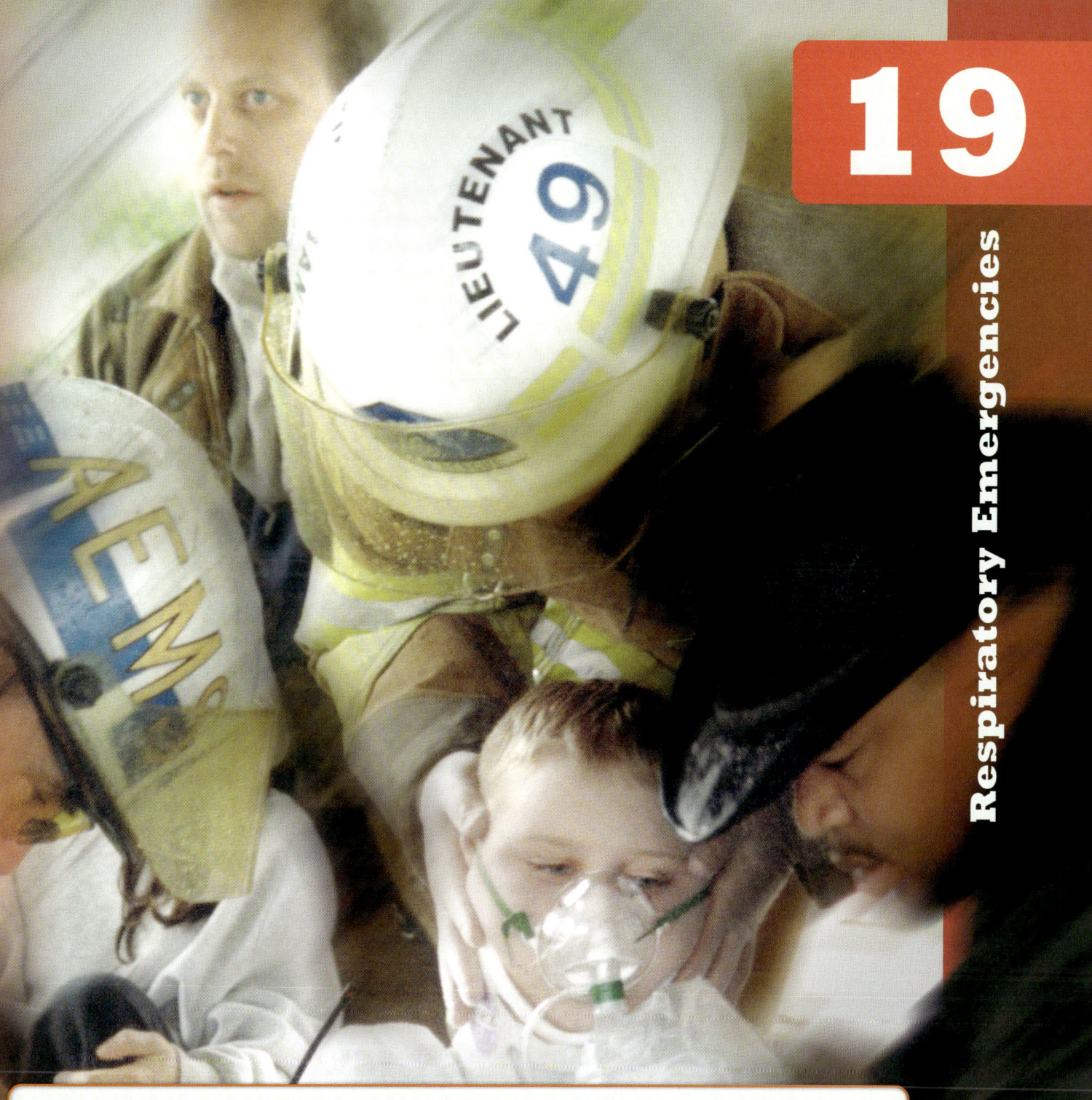

19

Respiratory Emergencies

You are the Provider

You are called to assist a 54-year-old man complaining of severe dyspnea. On arrival, you find the patient sitting in a chair leaning forward. His lips are pursed, and you can see signs of accessory muscle use. Given the frequency with which calls to EMS are related to breathing, it is paramount that an EMT-I be prepared to handle these calls. This chapter will prepare you to do that and to answer the following questions:

1. What are the most common signs and symptoms of difficulty breathing?
2. What is the relationship between airway management and breathing difficulty?

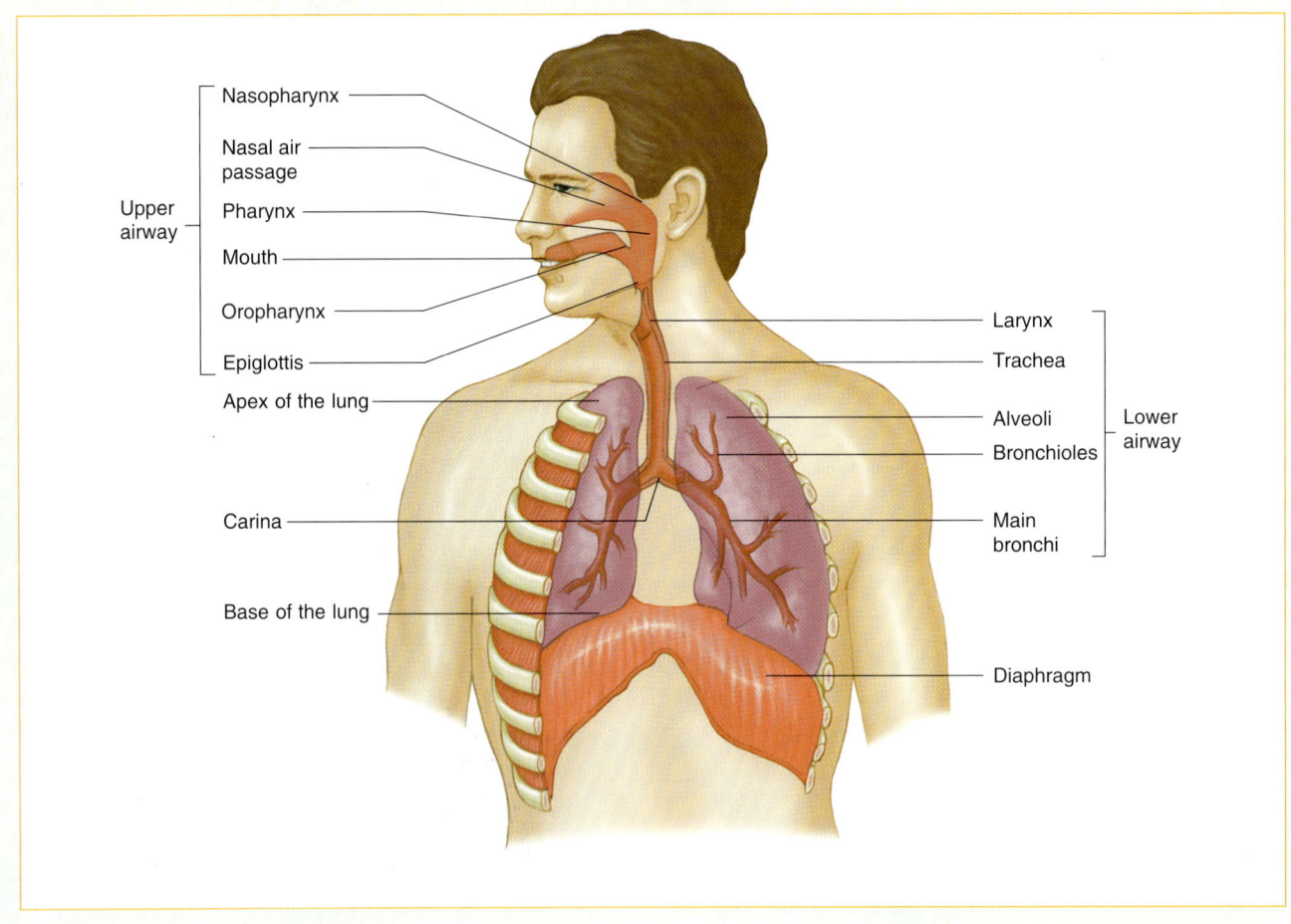

Figure 19-1 The upper airway includes the nasopharynx, nasal air passages, pharynx, mouth, oropharynx, and epiglottis. The lower airway includes the larynx, trachea, alveoli, bronchioles, and main bronchi.

Technology

www.EMSzone.com/EMTI

- Interactivities
- Vocabulary Explorer
- Anatomy Review
- Web Links
- Online Review Manual

Respiratory Emergencies

Dyspnea, or difficulty breathing, is a complaint that you will encounter often. It is a symptom of many different conditions, from the common cold and asthma to heart failure and pulmonary embolism. You may or may not be able to determine what is causing dyspnea in a particular patient; this can be difficult even for physicians in a hospital setting. Also, several different problems may contribute to a patient's dyspnea at the same time, including some that are serious or life threatening. Even without a definitive diagnosis, however, you may still be able to save a life.

This chapter begins with a basic explanation of how the lungs function. It then looks at common medical problems that can impede normal functioning and cause dyspnea, including acute pulmonary edema, chronic obstructive pulmonary disease (COPD), and asthma. You will learn the signs and symptoms of each condition. You should keep all of these possible medical problems in mind as you obtain the patient's medical history and perform a physical assessment, a process that this chapter describes in detail. The information that you obtain will help you determine the best treatment, which may differ based on the underlying cause of the dyspnea.

Remember, the sensation of not getting enough air can be terrifying, regardless of its cause. As an EMT-I, you must be prepared to treat not just the patient's symptoms and underlying problem, but the anxiety that it produces as well.

Anatomy and Function of the Lungs

The respiratory system consists of all the structures of the body that contribute to the breathing process. Important anatomic features include the upper and lower airways, the lungs, and the diaphragm (Figure 19-1 ◀). Air enters the trachea and moves through the bronchial tubes to the air spaces in the lungs, called alveoli, where oxygen and carbon dioxide are exchanged. Each day, 10,000 L of air are filtered, warmed, humidified, and exchanged in adults. Oxygen is diffused into the bloodstream for use in cellular metabolism by the body's 100 trillion cells. Wastes, including carbon dioxide, are excreted from the body via the respiratory system.

The principal function of the lungs is respiration, which is the exchange of oxygen and carbon dioxide. The two processes that occur during respiration are inspiration, the act of breathing in or inhaling, and expiration, the act of breathing out or exhaling. Ventilation is the process of moving air into and out of the lungs. During respiration, oxygen is provided to the blood, and carbon dioxide is removed from it. This exchange of gases takes place rapidly in normal lungs at the level of the alveoli. Alveoli are microscopic, thin-walled air sacs that lie against the pulmonary capillary vessels. Oxygen and carbon dioxide must be able to pass freely between the alveoli and the capillaries (Figure 19-2 ▶). Oxygen entering the alveoli from inhalation passes through tiny passages in the alveolar wall into the capillaries, which carry the oxygen to the heart. This is known as pulmonary respiration. The heart, in turn, pumps oxygenated blood throughout the body. Carbon dioxide produced by the body's cells (Figure 19-3A ▶) returns to the lungs in the blood that circulates through and around the alveolar air spaces. The exchange of gases that moves oxygen into the cells and carbon dioxide into the capillaries is known as cellular respiration. The carbon dioxide diffuses back into the alveoli and travels back up the bronchial tree and out the upper airways during exhalation (Figure 19-3B ▶). Again, carbon dioxide is "exchanged" for oxygen, which travels in exactly the opposite direction (during inhalation).

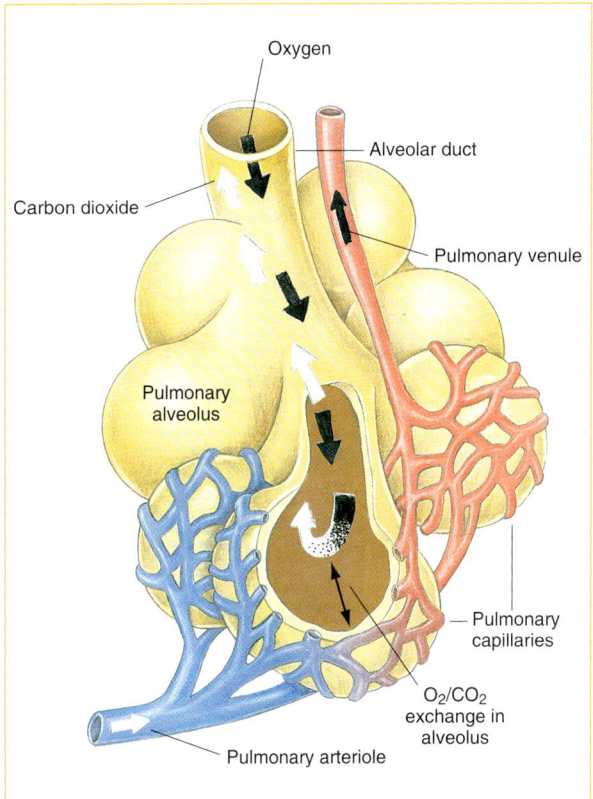

Figure 19-2 An enlarged view of a single alveolus (air sac) showing where the exchange of oxygen and carbon dioxide between air in the sac and blood in the pulmonary capillaries takes place.

For the body to receive the required nutrients and oxygen and to dispose of waste products, adequate ventilation, diffusion, and perfusion must occur. There are multiple complications that interfere with an ample intake of oxygen. These can be separated into four areas: (1) Upper airway obstruction may be from a foreign body obstruction, trauma, or an inflammation such as tonsillitis or epiglottitis. (2) Lower airway obstruction may be due to trauma. Obstructive lung disease and other complications, such as mucus accumulation, smooth muscle spasm, and airway edema, can also create narrowing and blockage of the lower airways. (3) Chest wall impairment is another cause of impaired ventilation. Trauma, hemothorax, pneumothorax, empyema (pleural effusion), pleural inflammation, and neuromuscular diseases such as multiple sclerosis or muscular dystrophy all prevent adequate chest wall excursion. (4) Problems in neurologic control can impair ventilation. These include brain stem malfunction from CNS depressant drugs, stroke or other medical neuro-

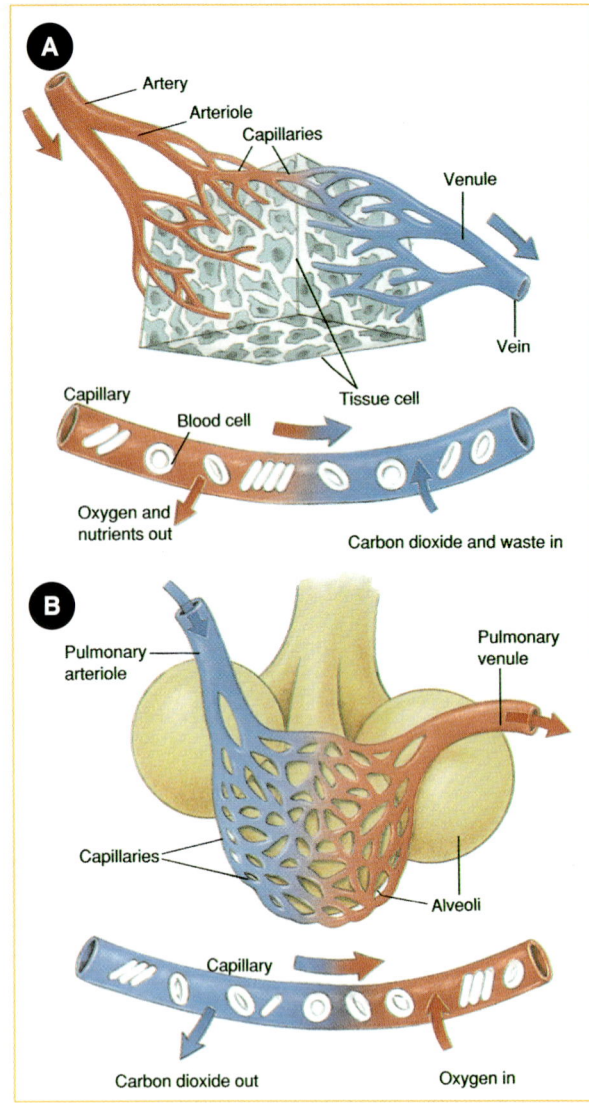

Figure 19-3 The exchange of oxygen and carbon dioxide during respiration. **A.** Oxygen passes from the blood through capillaries to tissue cells. Carbon dioxide passes from tissue cells through capillaries to the blood. **B.** In the lungs, oxygen is picked up by the blood and carbon dioxide is given off.

environmental lung diseases, blebs or bullae (blisters) associated with chronic obstructive lung disease, and inhalation injuries such as those from breathing poisonous gases or superheated air, all damage the alveoli and prevent sufficient gas exchange. Even with an ample amount of inspired oxygen and undamaged alveoli, there may still be problems related to diseases or injury affecting the interstitial space and preventing diffusion. Pulmonary edema also creates a barrier to diffusion. The fluid buildup occurs through two mechanisms, high pressure (cardiogenic) and high permeability (noncardiogenic). High pressure is the result of left-sided heart failure or idiopathic (of unknown cause) pulmonary hypertension. High permeability is caused by acute respiratory distress syndrome, environmental lung diseases, near drowning, and inhalation injuries, and it can occur after 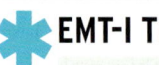.

Diffusion is the first step in supplying the body with the oxygen it needs. However, without an intact vascular system to transport the oxygen and other vital nutrients to the tissues and organs, the patient will not survive. Inadequate blood volume or hemoglobin levels present a perfusion hurdle. This may be due to hypovolemia or anemia (deficiency of red blood cells). Impaired circulatory blood flow from any cause also impairs perfusion. Adequate ventilation, diffusion, and perfusion describe what is commonly referred to as the Fick Principle discussed in the EMT-I Tips box below.

A variety of problems can affect the pulmonary system's ability to achieve its goal of gas exchange to provide for cellular needs and excretion of wastes.

> **EMT-I Tips**
>
> **Fick Principle**
> The movement and utilization of oxygen in the body is dependent on:
> 1. Adequate concentration of inspired oxygen (FIO_2 [fraction of inspired oxygen])
> 2. Appropriate movement of oxygen across the alveolar-capillary membrane into the arterial bloodstream
> 3. Adequate number of red blood cells to carry the oxygen
> 4. Proper tissue perfusion
> 5. Efficient off-loading of oxygen at the tissue level
>
> These elements are collectively known as the Fick Principle.

logic condition, or trauma. Trauma and neuromuscular diseases can also cause phrenic or spinal nerve dysfunction, preventing normal neurologic control. By rapidly assessing the patient and providing the necessary interventions, problems associated with oxygenation and ventilation can be minimized or avoided altogether.

Numerous obstacles may prevent diffusion. If there is an inadequate concentration of oxygen in the ambient air, such as in a smoke-filled environment, there will not be enough oxygen for adequate gas exchange. Alveolar disease also affects diffusion. Asbestosis or other

Understanding these problems can enable the EMT-I to quickly and effectively identify the underlying cause(s) and provide the necessary interventions. In most disorders of the lung, one or more of the following situations exists:

- The pulmonary vessels are prevented from absorbing oxygen or releasing carbon dioxide by fluid, infection, or collapsed air spaces.
- The alveoli are damaged and cannot transport gases properly across their own walls.
- The air passages are obstructed by muscle spasm, mucus, or weakened, floppy airway walls.
- Blood flow to the lungs is obstructed by blood clots.
- The pleural space is filled with air or excess fluid, so the lungs cannot expand properly.

All these conditions prevent the proper exchange of oxygen and carbon dioxide. In addition, the pulmonary blood vessels themselves may have abnormalities that interfere with blood flow and, thus, with the transfer of gases.

The brain stem senses the level of carbon dioxide in the arterial blood. The level of carbon dioxide bathing the brain stem is what stimulates a healthy person to breathe. If the level drops too low, the person automatically breathes at a slower rate and with less depth (tidal volume). As a result, less carbon dioxide is expired, allowing carbon dioxide levels in the blood to return to normal. Conversely, if the level of carbon dioxide in the arterial blood rises above normal, the patient breathes more rapidly and more deeply. When more fresh air (containing no carbon dioxide) is brought into the alveoli, more carbon dioxide diffuses out of the bloodstream, thereby lowering the level.

The following are the characteristics of adequate breathing:
- Normal rate and depth
- A regular pattern of inhalation and exhalation
- Good audible breath sounds on both sides of the chest
- Equal rise and fall on both sides of the chest (symmetrical)

In the Field

To differentiate between ventilation and respiration, ventilation is the act of air going into and out of the lungs. Respiration is the exchange of gases at the pulmonary or cellular level.

A to Z Terminology Tips

<u>Diffusion</u> is the movement of gases from a higher concentration to a lower concentration. <u>Perfusion</u> is supplying an organ or tissue with the nutrients and oxygen it needs. Perfusion requires the arterial system to be intact.

- Pink, warm, dry skin

The following are signs of inadequate breathing:
- A rate of breathing that is slower than 12 breaths/min or faster than 20 breaths/min in an adult
- Reduced flow of expired air at the nose and mouth
- Muscle retractions above the clavicles, between the ribs, and below the rib cage, especially in children
- Diminished, noisy, or absent breath sounds
- Unequal (asymmetrical) chest wall movement, which results in reduced tidal and minute volume
- Pale or cyanotic skin
- Cool, damp (clammy) skin
- Shallow respirations (reduced tidal volume)
- Irregular respirations, such as a patient taking a series of deep breaths followed by periods of apnea
- Pursed lips
- Nasal flaring

The level of carbon dioxide in the arterial blood can rise for a number of reasons. Various types of lung disease may impair the exhalation process. The body may also produce too much carbon dioxide, either temporarily or chronically, depending on the disease or abnormality.

If, over a period of years, arterial carbon dioxide levels rise slowly to an abnormally high level and remain there (as in late COPD), the respiratory center in the brain, which senses carbon dioxide levels and controls breathing, may work less efficiently. This is called chronic <u>carbon dioxide retention</u>. If the condition is severe, a secondary drive, called the <u>hypoxic drive</u>, stimulates the respiratory center. In these patients low blood oxygen levels cause the respiratory center to respond and stimulate respiration. If the arterial level of oxygen then is raised, as happens when the patient is given additional oxygen, there is no longer any stimulus to breathe; both the high carbon dioxide and low oxygen drives are lost. Patients with chronic lung diseases frequently have a chronically high level of blood carbon dioxide. Therefore, giving too much oxygen to these patients may actually depress, or completely stop, the respirations.

People older than 65 years are especially prone to problems with respiration, from occult (not obvious) stroke, lung disease, cardiovascular disease, liver disease, or certain medications.

Causes of Dyspnea

Dyspnea is shortness of breath or difficulty breathing. Many different medical problems may cause dyspnea. Be aware that if the problem is severe and the brain is deprived of oxygen, the patient may not be conscious and alert enough to complain of shortness of breath. More commonly, altered mental status is a sign of hypoxia of the brain.

Patients with the following medical conditions often develop breathing difficulty or hypoxia:
- Acute pulmonary edema
- Obstruction of the airway
- COPD
- Asthma or allergic reaction
- Rib fractures
- Spontaneous pneumothorax
- Upper or lower airway infection
- Pleural effusion
- Pulmonary thromboembolism
- Hyperventilation syndrome
- Prolonged seizures
- Use of CNS depressant drugs (for example, narcotics, barbiturates, or benzodiazepines)
- Neuromuscular disease (such as multiple sclerosis or muscular dystrophy)

> **EMT-I Tips**
>
> **Never** withhold oxygen from any patient exhibiting signs of distress. If a patient with COPD stops breathing spontaneously (rare) due to increased levels of oxygen, it is a simple matter to coach breathing or to ventilate the patient and continue oxygenating organs and tissues. Withholding oxygen may result in an insufficient amount of inspired oxygen, and due to the decreased rate, depth, or other obstructive problem, vital organ damage may occur.

> **EMT-I Safety**
>
> If you suspect that a patient has an airborne disease, place a surgical mask (or a nonrebreathing mask if needed) on the patient. When you have specific reason to suspect tuberculosis, do this and also wear a high-efficiency particulate air (HEPA) respirator yourself. See Chapter 2 for detailed discussion on disease transmission precautions.

Upper or Lower Airway Infection

Infectious diseases causing dyspnea may affect all parts of the airway. Some cause mild discomfort. Others obstruct the airway to the point that patients require total respiratory support. In general, the problem is always some form of obstruction, either to the flow of air in the major passages (colds, diphtheria, epiglottitis, and croup) or to the exchange of gases between the alveoli and the capillaries (pneumonia). Table 19-1 shows infectious diseases that are associated with some degree of dyspnea.

Acute Pulmonary Edema

Pulmonary edema is divided into two categories: high pressure or cardiogenic and high permeability or noncardiogenic. Although the pathophysiologic mechanisms are quite different, the resulting problems are the same. With an accumulation of fluid, there is a decrease in gas exchange causing severe dyspnea. Severe

You are the Provider — Part 2

As you approach the patient, you notice a full ashtray on a table beside his chair and an oxygen tank with a nasal cannula draped over it on the opposite side.

3. What questions should you ask the patient?
4. What is your general impression?

TABLE 19-1	Diseases Associated With Dyspnea		
Disease	**Characteristics**	**Disease**	**Characteristics**
Bronchitis	■ An acute or chronic inflammation of the lung that may damage lung tissue, usually associated with cough and production of sputum and, depending on its cause, sometimes fever. ■ Fluid also accumulates in the surrounding normal lung tissue, separating the alveoli from their capillaries. (Sometimes, fluid can also accumulate in the pleural space.) ■ The lung's ability to exchange oxygen and carbon dioxide is impaired. ■ The breathing pattern in bronchitis does not indicate major airway obstruction, but the patient may experience tachypnea, an increase in the breathing rate, which is an attempt to compensate for the reduced amount of normal lung tissue and for the buildup of fluid.	Pneumonia *continued*	■ The breathing pattern in pneumonia does not indicate major airway obstruction, but the patient may experience tachypnea, an increase in the breathing rate, which is an attempt to compensate for the reduced amount of normal lung tissue and for the buildup of fluid.
		Epiglottitis	■ A bacterial infection of the epiglottis that can produce severe swelling of the flap over the larynx (epiglottis). ■ In preschool and school-aged children especially, the epiglottis can swell to two or three times its normal size (Figure 19-4A ▼). ■ The airway may become almost completely obstructed, sometimes quite suddenly (Figure 19-4B ▼).
Common Cold	■ A viral infection usually associated with swollen nasal mucous membranes and the production of fluid from the sinuses and nose. ■ Patients complain of "stuffiness" or difficulty breathing through the nose.		
Diphtheria	■ Although well controlled during the past decade, it is still highly contagious and serious when it occurs. ■ The disease causes the formation of a diphtheritic membrane lining the pharynx that is composed of debris, inflammatory cells, and mucus. This membrane can rapidly and severely obstruct the passage of air into the larynx.		
Pneumonia	■ An acute bacterial or viral infection of the lung that damages lung tissue, usually associated with fever, cough, and production of sputum. ■ Fluid also accumulates in the surrounding normal lung tissue, separating the alveoli from their capillaries. (Sometimes, fluid can also accumulate in the pleural space.) ■ The lung's ability to exchange oxygen and carbon dioxide is impaired.		

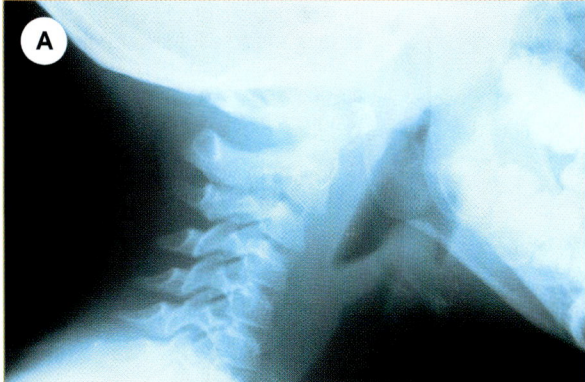

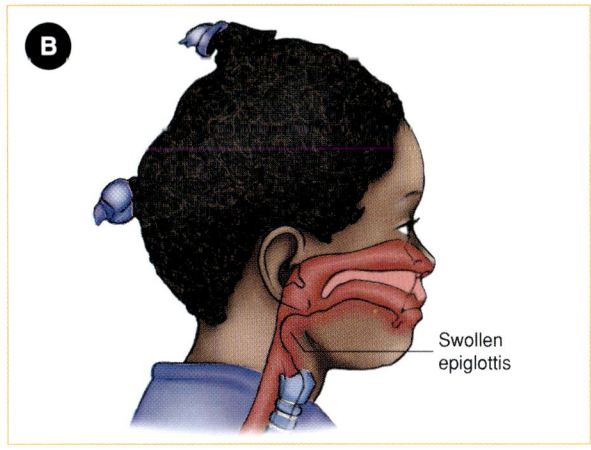

Figure 19-4 Acute epiglottitis. **A.** Epiglottitis is caused by a bacterial infection resulting in severe swelling of the epiglottis. **B.** The epiglottis is massively swollen and almost fully obstructs the airway.

Continued

TABLE 19-1 Diseases Associated With Dyspnea—cont'd

Disease	Characteristics	Disease	Characteristics
Epiglottitis *continued*	■ Stridor (harsh, high-pitched, rough, barking inspiratory sounds) may be heard late in the development of airway obstruction. ■ Acute epiglottitis in the adult is characterized by a severe sore throat. ■ The disease is now much less common in children than it was 20 years ago because of a vaccine that can help to prevent most cases. ■ Epiglottitis is also referred to as acute supraglottic laryngitis.	Severe Acute Respiratory Syndrome (SARS)	■ A virus that has caused significant concern. SARS is a serious, potentially life-threatening viral infection caused by a recently discovered family of viruses best known as the second most common cause of the common cold. SARS usually starts with flu-like symptoms, which may progress to pneumonia, respiratory failure, and, in some cases, death. SARS is thought to be transmitted primarily by close person-to-person contact.
Croup	■ A viral infection causing inflammation and swelling of the lining of the larynx, the narrowest point of the airway, typically seen in children between ages 6 months and 3 years (Figure 19-5). ■ The common signs of croup are stridor and a seal-bark cough, which signal a significant narrowing of the air passage of the larynx that may progress to significant obstruction. ■ Croup often responds well to the administration of humidified oxygen. ■ Croup is also referred to as laryngotracheobronchitis.		

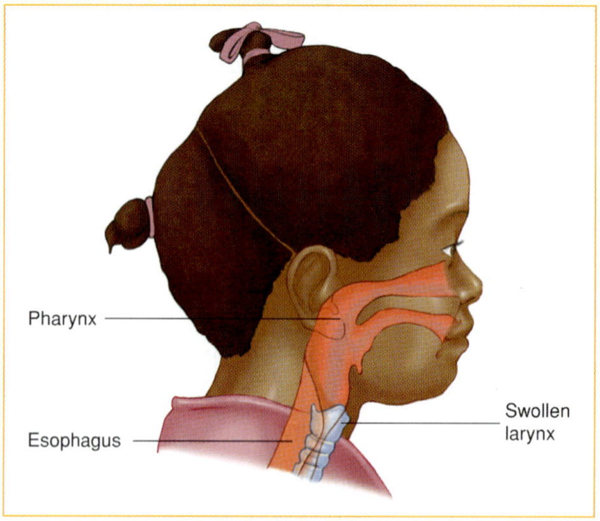

Figure 19-5 Croup swells the lining of the larynx, which is the narrowest point in a child's airway.

myocardial damage caused by an acute problem (such as acute myocardial infarction) or a chronic problem (such as cardiomyopathy) results in reduced contractile force of the myocardium. In these cases, the left side of the heart cannot remove blood from the lungs as fast as the right side delivers it. As a result, fluid eventually backs up into the alveoli and in the lung tissue between the alveoli and the pulmonary capillaries, creating a diffusion disorder. First, the pulmonary vasculature becomes engorged with fluid because of the increase in the pulmonary venous pressure and increase in hydrostatic pressure. Next, because of the failure of coughing and the lymphatic system to drain the excess fluids, there is an excessive buildup or widening in the interstitial space, impairing diffusion. In severe cases, fluid accumulates in the alveoli. This accumulation of fluid, called pulmonary edema, can develop quickly, especially following a major cardiovascular insult. By physically separating the alveoli from the pulmonary capillary vessels, the edema interferes with the exchange of carbon dioxide and oxygen (Figure 19-6). There is not enough room left in the lung for slow, deep breaths. The patient usually experiences dyspnea with rapid, shallow respirations. In the most severe instances, you will see frothy pink sputum at the nose and mouth.

In most high-pressure cases, patients have a long-standing history of chronic congestive heart failure, myocardial infarction, chronic hypertension, or myocarditis that can be controlled with medication. However, an acute exacerbation may occur if the patient stops taking medication, eats food that is too salty, or has a stressful illness, another myocardial infarction, or an abnormal heart rhythm (dysrhythmia). Pulmonary edema is one of the most common causes of hospital admission in the United States. It is not uncommon for a patient to have repeated episodes.

Some patients who experience pulmonary edema do not have an underlying cardiac history. The edema is a result of high permeability. Severe hypotension or hypoxemia, high altitude, environmental toxins, and septic shock may cause disruption of the alveolar-capillary membranes. Inhaling large amounts of smoke or toxic chemical fumes or other pulmonary irritants can produce pulmonary edema, as can traumatic injuries of the chest. In these cases, the disrupted membranes leak fluid into the interstitial space, and the widened interstitial space impairs diffusion. Other causes include acute hypoxemia, near drowning, high altitude exposure, and adult respiratory distress syndrome; after cardiac arrest and shock, patients also might experience pulmonary edema.

Regardless of the initial cause, the resulting assessment findings are similar. Patients with pulmonary edema that is cardiogenic in origin may present with signs and symptoms of a cardiac emergency. Patients with noncardiogenic pulmonary edema tend to have a history of associated factors such as a hypoxic episode, shock, chest trauma, recent acute inhalation of toxic gases or particles, or recent ascent to a high altitude without acclimatizing. In both cases, patients may also present with dyspnea, orthopnea, fatigue, reduced exercise capacity, and pulmonary rales.

The management of cardiogenic pulmonary edema is much the same as that of other cardiac emergencies. Place the patient in a position of comfort. Assess the airway, administer high-flow oxygen, and provide assisted ventilation as needed. Establish intravenous (IV) access.

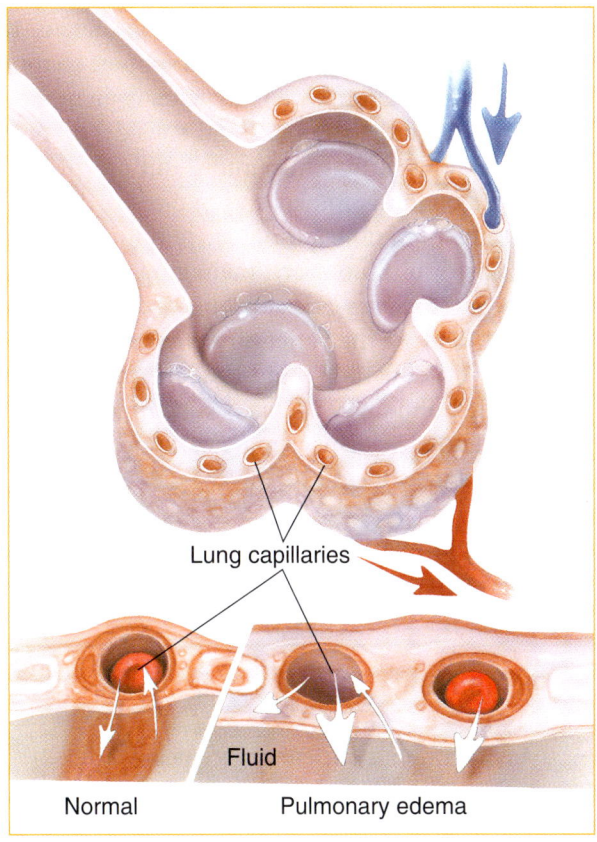

Figure 19-6 In pulmonary edema, fluid fills the alveoli and separates the capillaries from the alveolar wall, interfering with the exchange of oxygen and carbon dioxide.

Monitor flow rates carefully to avoid fluid excess, which will exacerbate the patient's pulmonary edema. For patients complaining of chest pain, consider the administration of nitroglycerin, provided the patient has his or her own prescription and the systolic blood pressure is greater

You are the Provider — Part 3

You kneel next to the patient and place a pulse oximeter on him while your partner checks his vital signs.

Vital Signs	Recording Time: 1 Minute After Patient Contact
Respirations	28 breaths/min, shallow
Pulse	124 beats/min
Blood pressure	150/100 mm Hg
Level of consciousness	Alert and oriented
Breath sounds, Sao_2	Expiratory wheezes, 88%

5. What type of oxygen delivery device should you use for this patient?
6. At what rate should you set the flowmeter?

than 100 mm Hg. Transport the patient to the closest appropriate facility; the patient's condition dictates the transport mode. Provide psychological support en route.

Consider intubation for airway management. Place the patient on a cardiac monitor and consider administration of nitroglycerin, furosemide, and morphine as needed based on local protocol and/or medical direction.

Management of noncardiogenic pulmonary edema includes position of comfort, managing the ABCs as with cardiogenic causes, and appropriate transport considerations. Remove the patient from any environmental toxins, and consider rapid descent in altitude if high-altitude pulmonary edema is suspected. Reassure the patient, and provide psychological support en route to definitive care.

Consider intubation and positive pressure ventilation for severe cases.

> **In the Field**
>
> Any nontrauma patient experiencing difficulty breathing should immediately be placed in a position of comfort.

Obstructive Airway Disease

Obstructive airway disease encompasses a spectrum of diseases that affect a substantial number of people worldwide. These diseases include asthma and COPD (which includes emphysema and chronic bronchitis). Factors that may exacerbate underlying conditions may be intrinsic (internal) or extrinsic (external). Intrinsic factors include stress, upper respiratory infection, and exercise. Intrinsic factors include tobacco smoke, allergens, drugs, and occupational hazards.

Obstruction occurs in the bronchioles and may be the result of smooth muscle spasm caused by beta-2 receptor stimulation in the lungs or mucus production from the goblet cells in the respiratory tract. The cilia are unable to remove the excess mucus, creating a buildup. The obstruction may be reversible or irreversible and is caused by air trapping secondary to the mucus and smooth muscle spasm. The bronchioles dilate naturally on inspiration, enabling air to enter the alveoli despite the presence of obstruction. The bronchioles naturally constrict on expiration, and air becomes trapped distal to the obstruction on exhalation.

Chronic obstructive pulmonary disease is a common lung condition, affecting some 10% to 20% of the entire adult population in the United States. It is the end of a slow process, which over several years results in disruption of the airways, the alveoli, and the pulmonary blood vessels. The process itself may be a result of genetic predisposition, direct lung and airway damage from repeated infections, or inhalation of toxic agents such as industrial gases, but most often it results from cigarette smoking. Although it is well known that cigarettes are a direct cause of lung cancer, their role in the development of COPD is far more significant and much less publicized.

Tobacco smoke itself is a bronchial irritant and can create <u>chronic bronchitis</u>, an ongoing irritation of the trachea and bronchi. Chronic bronchitis is not uncommon in adult men. The obstruction may be reversible or irreversible.

With bronchitis, excess mucus is constantly produced, obstructing small airways and alveoli. Protective cells and mechanisms in the lungs that remove foreign particles are destroyed, further weakening the airways. The mucus-producing glands enlarge, creating further problems. The clinical definition of chronic bronchitis is a productive cough for at least 3 months per year for 2 or more consecutive years. It is typically associated with cigarette smoking, but may also occur in nonsmokers. Chronic oxygenation problems can also lead to right-sided heart failure and fluid retention, such as edema in the lower extremities. Because these patients tend to have a bluish skin color and edema, they are sometimes called "blue bloaters."

Pneumonia develops easily when the passages are persistently obstructed. Ultimately, repeated episodes of irritation and pneumonia cause scarring in the lung and some dilation of the obstructed alveoli, leading to COPD (Figure 19-7 ▶).

Another type of COPD is called <u>emphysema</u>. Emphysema is a degenerative condition characterized by decreased alveolar surface tension (loss of elasticity) secondary to the destruction of pulmonary surfactant. Surfactant is a lubricant that lines the alveolar walls, allowing them to easily expand and recoil. Normally, lungs act like a spongy balloon that is inflated; once they are inflated, they naturally recoil because of their elastic nature, expelling gas rapidly. However, when they are constantly obstructed or when the "balloon's" elasticity is diminished, air is no longer expelled rapidly, and the walls of the alveoli eventually fall apart, leaving large "holes" in the lung that resemble a large air pocket or cavity.

Emphysema is an irreversible condition. A diffusion defect also exists because of the presence of blebs, or weak spots in the alveoli. Because blebs have extremely thin walls, the alveoli are prone to collapse (<u>atelectasis</u>). To prevent collapse, the patient often exhales through

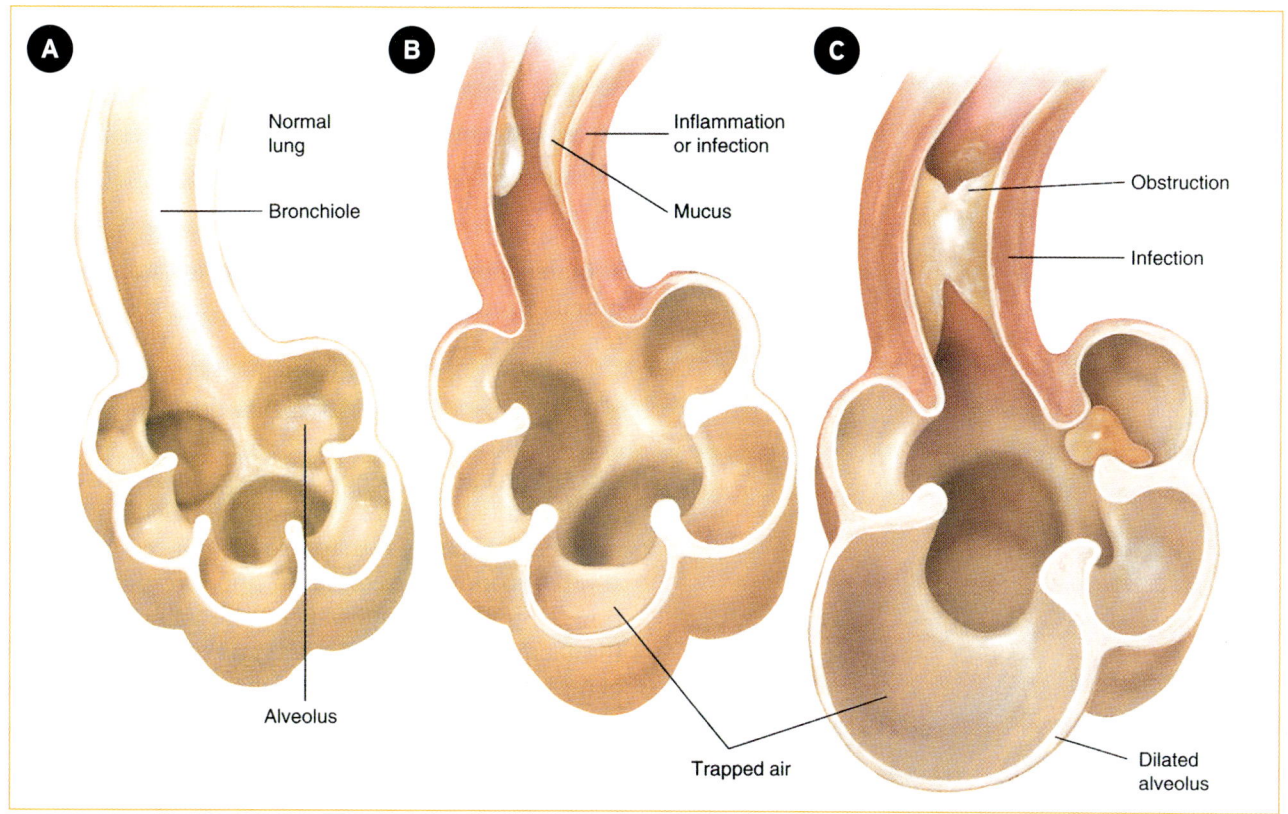

Figure 19-7 Repeated episodes of irritation and inflammation in the alveoli result in the obstruction, scarring, and some dilation of the alveolar sac characteristic of COPD. **A.** Normal alveolus. **B.** Infection produces mucus and swelling. **C.** A mucous plug creates an obstruction and further dilation of the alveolus.

pursed lips, effectively maintaining a constant positive airway pressure. Chronically low oxygen levels associated with emphysema stimulate the production of red blood cells, sometimes in excessive quantity (polycythemia). As a result, the patient's skin tends to remain pink. Because of the "pursed-lip" breathing and the maintenance of pink skin color, patients with emphysema are sometimes referred to as "pink puffers." Emphysema is almost always associated with cigarette smoking or significant exposure to environmental toxins.

Most patients with COPD have elements of both chronic bronchitis and emphysema. Some patients will have more elements of one condition than the other; few patients will have only emphysema or bronchitis. Therefore, most patients with COPD will consistently produce sputum, have a chronic cough, and have difficulty expelling air from their lungs, with long expiration phases and wheezing.

Patients with COPD cannot handle pulmonary infections well, because the existing airway damage makes them unable to expel the mucus or sputum produced by the infection. The chronic airway obstruction makes it difficult to breathe deeply enough to clear the lungs.

Gradually, the arterial oxygen level falls, and the carbon dioxide level rises. If a new infection of the lung occurs in a patient with COPD, the arterial oxygen level may fall rapidly. In a few patients, the carbon dioxide level may rise high enough to cause sleepiness. These patients require respiratory support and administration of oxygen.

Patients with COPD usually are older than 50 years. They always have a history of recurring lung problems and are almost always long-term cigarette smokers. Patients with COPD may complain of tightness in the chest and constant fatigue. Because air has been gradually and continuously trapped in their lungs in increasing amounts, their chests often have a barrel-like appearance (Figure 19-8 ▶). If you listen to the chest with a stethoscope, you will hear abnormal breath sounds. These may include rales, which are fine, crackling sounds that are usually associated with fluid in the lungs and are related to chronic scarring of small airways. Rhonchi, which are coarse, rattling sounds, are caused by mucus in the larger airways. Wheezing, which makes a whistling sound, is typically heard on expiration and is common in patients with asthma. Because of large emphysematous air pockets and diminished airflow, sounds of breathing are

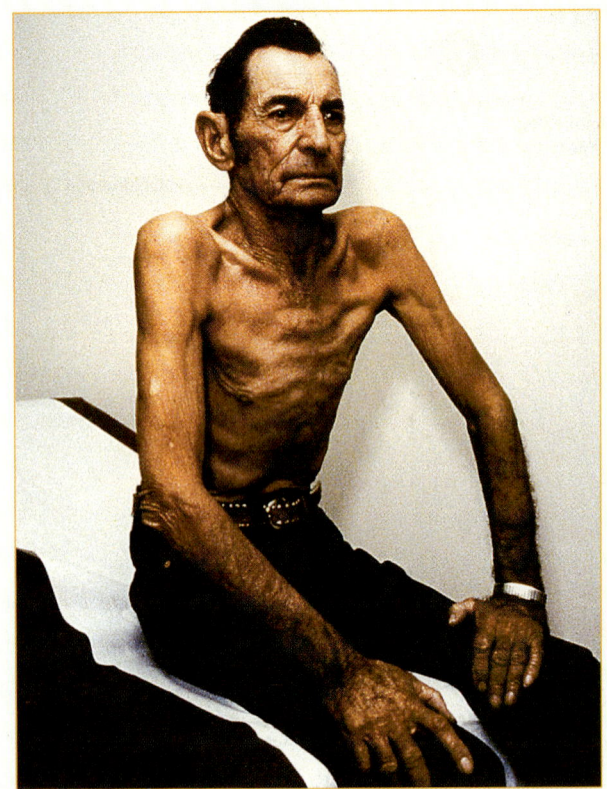

Figure 19-8 Typically, a patient with COPD has a barrel-shaped chest and uses accessory muscles and pursed lips for breathing. Notice also that the patient is sitting in the tripod position.

frequently difficult to hear and may be detected only high up on the posterior portion of the chest.

The patient with COPD usually presents with a long history of dyspnea with a sudden increase in shortness of breath. There is rarely a history of chest pain. More often, the patient will remember having had a recent "chest cold" with fever and either inability to cough up mucus or a sudden increase in sputum production. If the patient is able to cough up sputum, it will be thick and is often green or yellow. The blood pressure of patients with COPD is normal; however, the pulse is rapid and occasionally irregular. Pay particular attention to the respirations, which may be rapid or slow.

Asthma is an acute spasm of the smaller air passages called bronchioles that is associated with excessive mucus production and spasm of the bronchiolar muscles (Figure 19-9 ▶). It is a common but serious disease, affecting about 6 million Americans and killing some 4,000 to 5,000 Americans each year. Asthma produces a characteristic wheezing sound as patients attempt to exhale through partially obstructed air passages. These same air passages open easily during inspiration. In other words, when patients inhale, breathing appears relatively normal; the wheezing is heard only when they exhale. This wheezing may be so loud that you can hear it without a stethoscope. This is known as "audible wheezing." In other cases, the airways are so blocked that no air movement is heard. In severe cases, the actual work of exhaling is very tiring, and cyanosis, respiratory arrest, or both may develop.

Asthma is a reversible obstruction that is caused by a combination of smooth muscle spasm (bronchospasm), mucus production, and edema. Exacerbating factors tend to be extrinsic in children and intrinsic in adults. Status asthmaticus, a potentially life-threatening event, is a prolonged exacerbation that does not respond to conventional therapy.

Asthma affects people of all ages and is usually the result of an allergic reaction to an inhaled, ingested, or injected substance. It may also be induced by exercise, severe emotional stress, or an upper respiratory infection. Note that the substance itself is not the cause of the allergic reaction; rather, it is an exaggerated response of the body's immune system to that substance that causes the reaction. In some cases, however, there is no identifiable substance, or allergen, that triggers the body's immune system. Almost anything can be considered an allergen. An allergic response to certain foods or some other allergen may produce an acute asthma attack. Between attacks, patients may breathe normally. In its most severe form, an allergic reaction can produce anaphylactic shock. This, in turn, may cause respiratory distress that is severe enough to result in coma and death.

Most patients with asthma are familiar with their symptoms and know when an attack is imminent. Typically, they will have appropriate medication with them or at home. You should listen carefully to what these patients tell you; they often know exactly what they need.

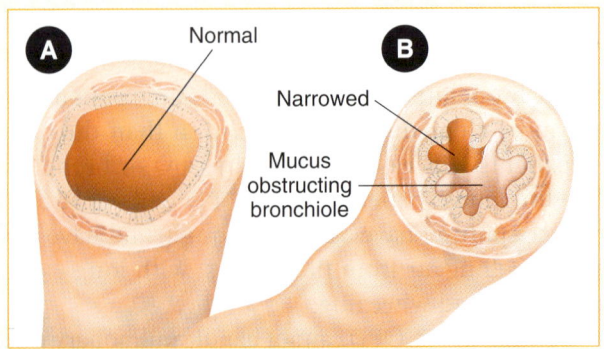

Figure 19-9 Asthma is an acute spasm of the bronchioles. **A.** Cross-section of a normal bronchiole. **B.** The bronchiole in spasm; a mucous plug has formed and partially obstructed the bronchiole.

Assessment Findings

Patients with obstructive airway disease typically present with signs of severe respiratory impairment. These may include two-to-three word dyspnea (able to say only two or three words between breaths), diminished or absent breath sounds, and altered mental status. The chief complaint is typically that of dyspnea, cough, or nocturnal dyspnea (awakens the person from sleep).

Obtain a thorough history, including any personal or family history of asthma and allergies. Determine whether the patient has had an acute exposure to any pulmonary irritant or any previous similar episodes. Ask the patient if he or she has ever been intubated. If so, the patient may require more aggressive treatment than one who has not.

Wheezing may be present in all types of obstructive lung disease. Look for retractions and the use of accessory muscles. Use a peak flow meter to establish the baseline expiratory airflow and a pulse oximeter to document the degree of hypoxemia and response to therapy. Remember that the pulse oximeter is designed to detect gross abnormalities, not subtle changes.

Begin management of obstructive airway disease by placing the patient in a position of comfort. Monitor the airway, apply high-flow oxygen, and assist ventilation if needed. Establish IV access and provide circulatory support. Intravenous therapy may be necessary to improve hydration and to thin and loosen mucus. Assist patients with their metered-dose inhalers as needed. Continue monitoring, and transport the patient to the closest appropriate facility. Contact medical control for further orders. Airway problems can be very frightening. Provide psychological support en route to the hospital.

Consider intubation to secure the airway. Place the patient on a cardiac monitor and consider the use of beta agonists such as albuterol or epinephrine based on local protocol and/or medical direction.

> ### EMT-I Tips
>
> When administering or assisting with a beta agonist, always place the patient on the cardiac monitor. Remember the side effects of beta agonists on the heart:
> - Increased automaticity
> - Increased contractility
> - Increased heart rate
> - Increased conductivity
>
> Also remember the vasoconstricting effects of epinephrine on the vessels and monitor blood pressure. Adjust intravenous flow rates accordingly.

> ### In the Field
>
> To determine the degree of nocturnal dyspnea, ask the patient how many pillows he or she sleeps on at night. The greater the number of pillows needed, the greater the degree of respiratory difficulty.

> ### Terminology Tips
>
> Nocturnal = night; dys- = difficulty; -pnea = related to breathing. Therefore, nocturnal dyspnea is difficulty breathing at night. Paroxysmal = characterized by sudden onset.

Asthma and Anaphylactic Reactions

Patients who do not have asthma may still have severe allergic reactions. The same allergens that cause asthma attacks may cause anaphylaxis, a reaction characterized by airway swelling and dilation of blood vessels all over the body, which may lower blood pressure significantly. Anaphylaxis may be associated with widespread itching and an asthma-like condition. The airway may swell so much that breathing problems can progress from extreme difficulty in breathing to total airway obstruction in a matter of a few minutes. Most anaphylactic reactions occur within 30 minutes of exposure to the allergen, which can be anything from certain nuts or other foods to a penicillin injection. Because this may be the first time such a reaction to the substance has occurred, some patients may not know what caused the swelling and allergic reaction. In other cases, the patient may know of the allergen but not be aware of exposure. In severe cases, epinephrine is the treatment of choice. Oxygen and antihistamines are also useful. As always, medical direction should guide appropriate therapy.

Hay Fever

A much milder and more common allergy problem is hay fever. This is caused by an allergic reaction to substances such as pollen, molds, grasses, weeds, and dust. In some areas of the country where these allergens are present in the air throughout the year, hay fever is almost a universal illness. Generally, it does not produce major emergency problems, but it does produce a number of

> **Terminology Tips**
>
> Pneumo- = air; thorax = thoracic cavity. Therefore, a pneumothorax is air inside the thoracic cavity, but outside the lung.

difficulties in the upper respiratory tract, such as a stuffy or runny nose (rhinorrhea) and sneezing.

Spontaneous Pneumothorax

Normally, the "vacuum" pressure in the pleural space keeps the lung inflated. When the surface of the lung is disrupted, however, air escapes into the pleural cavity, and the negative vacuum pressure is lost; the natural elasticity of the lung tissue causes the lung to collapse. The accumulation of air in the pleural space, which may be partial or complete, is called a pneumothorax (Figure 19-10). Pneumothorax is most often caused by trauma, but it also can be caused by some medical conditions without any injury. In these cases, the condition is called a "spontaneous" pneumothorax, and it occurs in approximately 18 of every 100,000 people. A 15% to 20% partial pneumothorax may be well tolerated in a healthy person.

Spontaneous pneumothorax may occur in patients with certain chronic lung infections or in young people born with weak areas of the lung. Patients with emphysema and asthma are at high risk for spontaneous pneumothorax when a weakened portion of lung ruptures, often during coughing. Young, thin males are also at higher risk for spontaneous pneumothorax. A patient with a spontaneous pneumothorax becomes acutely dyspneic (short of breath) and typically complains of pleuritic chest pain, a sharp, stabbing pain on one side that is worse during breathing or with certain movement of the chest wall. The patient may also present with subcutaneous emphysema, or air bubbles trapped under the skin in the subcutaneous tissue. By listening to the chest with a stethoscope, you may note that breath sounds are absent or decreased on the affected side. However, altered breath sounds are very difficult to detect in patients with severe emphysema. Spontaneous pneumothorax may be the cause of a sudden worsening of dyspnea in a patient with underlying emphysema. Patients experiencing minor problems may be pale, diaphoretic, and tachypneic. Severe findings include altered mental status, cyanosis, tachycardia, unilaterally decreased breath sounds, local hyperresonance to percussion, and subcutaneous emphysema. These patients require immediate care to survive.

Management of a spontaneous pneumothorax begins with the ABCs. Provide airway and ventilatory support, including high-flow oxygen and assisting ventilation as needed. Be alert for the signs of the development of a tension pneumothorax.

Consider IV initiation if severe symptoms are present. Pharmacological interventions are not typically necessary, because the patient is generally treated symptomatically. Place the patient in a position of comfort, and transport to the closest appropriate facility. The patient's condition should dictate the transport mode. Provide reassurance en route. Consider calling for a paramedic unit if the patient shows signs of developing a tension pneumothorax.

Consider intubation to maintain the airway if the patient loses consciousness. Place the patient on the cardiac monitor and be alert for rhythm disturbances that may result from pressure on the heart as tension develops. Perform a needle decompression if progression to a tension pneumothorax occurs, based on local protocol and/or medical direction.

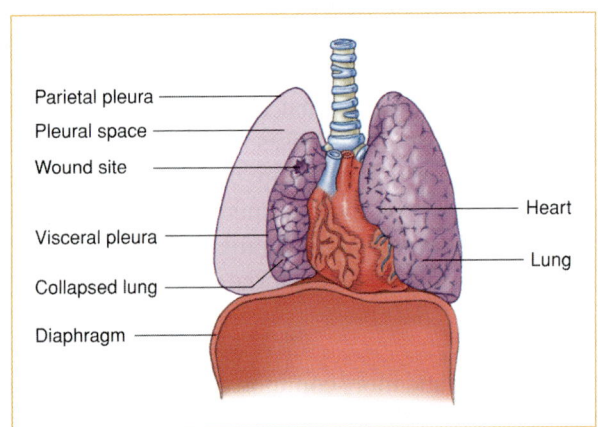

Figure 19-10 A pneumothorax occurs when air leaks into the pleural space from an opening in the chest wall or the surface of the lung. The lung collapses as air fills the pleural space and the two pleural surfaces are no longer in contact.

> **Terminology Tips**
>
> Tachy- = fast; -pnea = related to breathing; cardia = heart. Therefore, tachypnea is a fast respiratory rate, and tachycardia is a fast heart rate.

Pneumonia

Pneumonia is a ventilation disorder caused by an infection of the lung parenchyma, which is the tissue of the lung itself. It most commonly is bacterial, but it may be viral or fungal. It is the fifth leading cause of death in the United States and is not a single disease, but a group of specific infections. Risk factors for pneumonia include cigarette smoking, alcoholism, and exposure to cold. Very young children are at risk for pneumonia because of their immature immune systems. Elderly people are also at risk because of age-related weakening of the immune system.

Pneumonia presents as a localized infection in the lungs that may cause atelectasis, or alveolar collapse. If not treated promptly, the infection may become systemic, leading to sepsis and septic shock. Typical findings with pneumonia include an acute onset of fever and chills, productive cough with purulent (thick) sputum, pleuritic chest pain, and excessive mucus causing pulmonary consolidation that may be detected by auscultation in the form of rales or rhonchi. Atypical pneumonia may present with a nonproductive cough, headache, myalgias, fatigue, sore throat, nausea, vomiting, diarrhea, and fever and chills.

Management includes monitoring the ABCs and providing high-flow oxygen and ventilatory support as needed. Administration of IV fluids may improve hydration and thin and mobilize mucus. If a high fever is present, cool the patient. Transport to the closest appropriate facility while providing psychological support.

Consider intubation in severe cases. Beta agonists may be required if lower airway obstruction is severe or if the patient has accompanying obstructive lung disease, based on local protocol and/or medical direction.

> **A to Z Terminology Tips**
>
> My(o)- = muscle; -algia = ache or pain. Therefore, myalgias are muscle aches.

Pleural Effusions

A *pleural effusion* is a collection of fluid outside the lung on one or both sides of the chest. By compressing one or both lungs, it causes dyspnea (Figure 19-11). This fluid may collect in large volumes in response to any irritation, infection, or cancer. Although it can build up gradually over days or even weeks, patients often

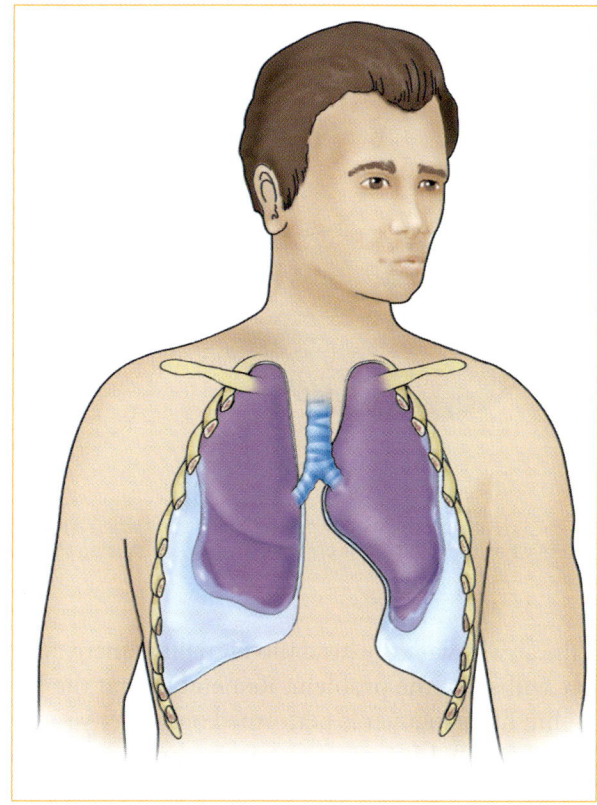

Figure 19-11 With a pleural effusion, fluid may accumulate in large volumes on one or both sides, compressing the lungs and causing dyspnea.

report that their dyspnea began suddenly. Pleural effusions should be considered a possibility in any patient with lung cancer and shortness of breath.

When you listen with a stethoscope to the chest of a patient with dyspnea resulting from pleural effusion, you will hear decreased breath sounds over the region of the chest where fluid has moved the lung away from the chest wall. These patients frequently feel better if they are sitting upright. Definitive care for the patient with a pleural effusion includes removing the fluid, a procedure that must be performed by a physician.

Mechanical Obstruction of the Airway

As an EMT-I, you should always be aware of the possibility that a patient with dyspnea may have a mechanical obstruction of the airway and be prepared to treat it quickly. In semiconscious and unconscious individuals, the obstruction may be the result of a foreign object (Figure 19-12A) or malpositioning of the head causing obstruction by the tongue (Figure 19-12B). Open-

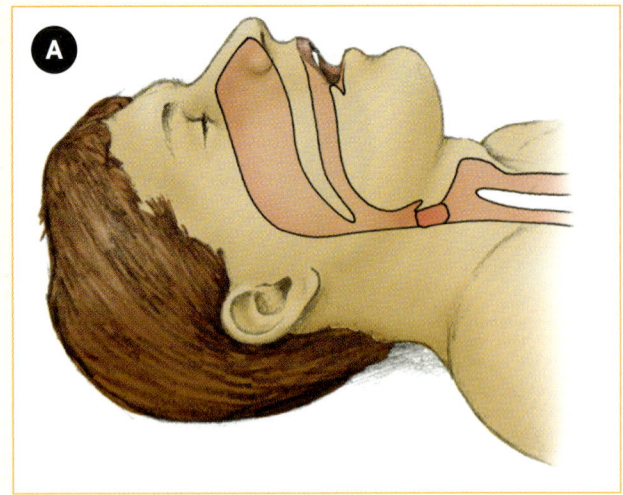 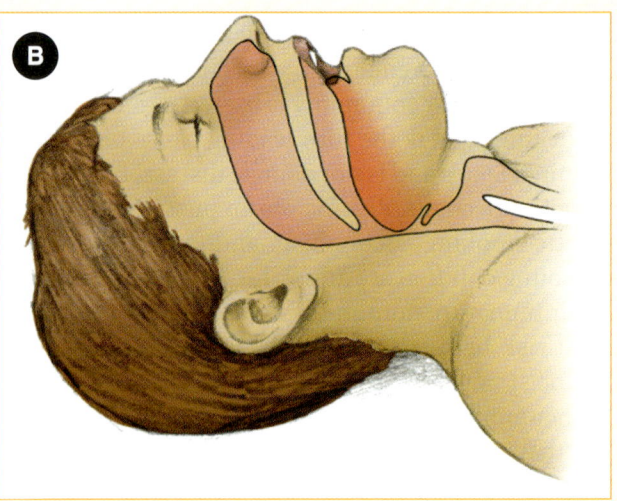

Figure 19-12 **A.** Foreign body obstruction occurs when an object, such as food, is lodged in the airway. **B.** Mechanical obstruction also occurs when the head is not properly positioned, causing the tongue to fall back into the throat.

ing the airway with the head tilt–chin lift maneuver typically will solve the problem. Remember that the head tilt–chin lift maneuver is performed only after you have ruled out spinal injury. If simply opening the airway does not correct the breathing problem, further assessment and management will be required (for example, abdominal thrusts).

Always consider upper airway obstruction from a foreign body first in patients who were eating just before becoming short of breath. The same is true of young children, especially crawling babies, who might have swallowed and choked on a small object. Inflammation of the tonsils may also partially occlude the airway, creating an obstruction.

The obstruction may be in the lower airway, below the vocal cords. Trauma to the trachea may result in a crushing injury, fractured larynx, or edema that obstructs the lower airway. Obstruction may also be in the form of obstructive lung disease, mucus accumulation, or smooth muscle spasm. Edema also may be present when a patient has been exposed to toxic chemicals or superheated air, as in a structural fire.

Pulmonary Thromboembolism

An <u>embolus</u> is anything in the circulatory system that travels to a distant site, where it lodges, creating a perfusion disorder by obstructing distal blood flow in that area. Beyond the point of obstruction, circulation can be markedly decreased or completely cut off, causing deep vein stasis or stagnation of blood, which, in turn, can result in a serious, life-threatening condition. Emboli can be fragments of blood clots in an artery or vein that break off and travel through the bloodstream. They also can be foreign bodies that enter the circulation, such as a bullet or a bubble of air. A <u>pulmonary thromboembolism</u> is the passage of a blood clot (thrombus) formed in a vein, usually in the legs or pelvis, that breaks off and circulates through the venous system. The large clot moves through the right side of the heart and into a pulmonary artery, where it becomes lodged, significantly decreasing or completely blocking blood flow (Figure 19-13 ▶). Even though the lung is actively involved in inhalation and exhalation of air, no exchange of oxygen or carbon dioxide takes place in the areas of blocked blood flow because there is no effective circulation. As a result of this "ventilation-perfusion mismatch," the level of arterial carbon dioxide rises, and the oxygen level may drop significantly, perhaps to a point at which cyanosis develops.

Pulmonary emboli may occur as a result of damage to the lining of vessels, causing platelet aggregation, a tendency for blood to clot unusually fast (hypercoagulability), or, most often, slow blood flow in a lower extremity. Slow blood flow in the legs can be caused by bed rest, which can lead to the collapse of veins. Patients whose legs are immobilized following a fracture or recent surgery are at risk for pulmonary emboli for days or weeks after the incident. Other risk factors include recent surgery, pregnancy, oral contraceptives, infection, cancer, sickle cell anemia, and prolonged inactivity; patients who are bedridden also are at risk. Only rarely do pulmonary emboli occur in active, healthy people. Other causes of pulmonary embolism include air, fat, foreign objects, sheared venous catheters, and amniotic fluid.

Although they are fairly common, pulmonary emboli can be difficult to diagnose. They occur about 650,000 times a year in the United States and are responsible for 50,000 deaths annually. Five percent are immediately fatal, but in many cases, the patient never notices them. Overall, up to 10% of pulmonary emboli result in death. Signs and symptoms, when they occur, include the following:
- Acute dyspnea
- Acute pleuritic chest pain
- Hemoptysis (coughing up blood)
- Cyanosis
- Tachypnea
- Varying degrees of hypoxia
- Tachycardia
- Normal breath sounds or localized wheezing
- Pleural friction rub
- Clinical evidence of thrombophlebitis (found in less than 50% of cases)

With a large enough embolus, complete, sudden obstruction of the blood flow from the right side of the heart can result in sudden death. Evidence of a significant life-threatening embolus in a proximal location includes the following:
- Altered mentation
- Severe cyanosis
- Profound hypotension
- Cardiac arrest

When a patient has a possible pulmonary embolus, the chief complaint is usually a sudden onset of chest pain, dyspnea, and nonproductive cough. Identifying possible risk factors may help to narrow the causes for the chief complaint.

Prevention plays a major role in the management of a pulmonary embolus. Again, signs and symptoms present based on the size and location of the embolus. Manage the airway and provide high-flow oxygen, assisting ventilation as needed. Initiate CPR if the patient is pulseless and apneic. Establish an IV of an isotonic crystalloid solution, and give fluid for hydration based on clinical symptoms. Other interventions are supportive, and the most severe cases will be managed as a cardiac arrest of unknown origin. Transport the patient in the appropriate mode to the most appropriate facility. Offer reassurance and psychological support en route.

Consider intubation, cardiac monitoring, and pharmacological interventions based on the patient's presentation and condition, and local protocol and/or medical direction.

Hyperventilation Syndrome

When acute dyspnea occurs in a patient with no known respiratory diseases, hyperventilation syndrome exists. <u>Hyperventilation</u> is defined as overbreathing to the point at which the level of arterial carbon dioxide falls below normal, and it may be an indicator of a major, life-threatening illness. For example, a patient with diabetes who has very high blood glucose levels, a patient who has overdosed with aspirin, or a patient with a severe infection is likely to hyperventilate. In these patients, rapid, deep breathing is the body's attempt to compensate for acidosis, the buildup of excess acid in the blood or body tissues, resulting from the primary illness. Because carbon dioxide mixed with water in the bloodstream can add to the blood's acidity, lowering the

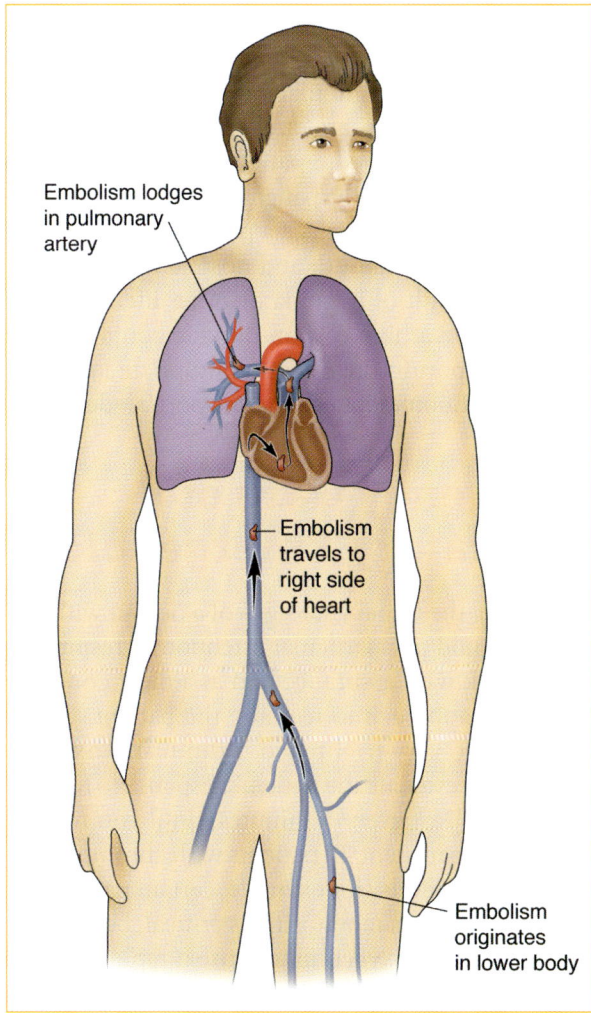

Figure 19-13 A pulmonary thromboembolism is a blood clot from the vein that breaks off, circulates through the venous system, and moves through the right side of the heart into a pulmonary artery. Here, it can become lodged and significantly obstruct blood flow.

TABLE 19-2	Causes of Tachypnea

- Hypoxia
- High altitude
- Pulmonary disorders
- Pneumonia
- Pulmonary emboli, vascular disease
- Bronchial asthma
- Cardiovascular disorders
- Congestive heart failure
- Hypotension and shock
- Metabolic disorders
- Acidosis
- Hepatic failure
- Neurologic disorders
- Central nervous system infection, tumors
- Drugs
- Fever, sepsis
- Pain
- Pregnancy

level of carbon dioxide helps to compensate for the other acids.

Similarly, in an otherwise healthy person, tachypnea without physiologic demand for increased oxygen causes respiratory alkalosis. The result is a relative lack of acids generally caused by anxiety. Carbon dioxide is washed out, and the level of carbonic acid is reduced. The shift in the acid-base balance moves toward the base end of the scale. The chief complaint is usually dyspnea or chest pain. Alkalosis is the cause of many of the symptoms associated with *hyperventilation syndrome*, including anxiety, dizziness, numbness, tingling of the hands and feet (which can progress to actual spasms of the phalanges known as carpopedal spasms), and even a sense of dyspnea and chest pain despite the rapid breathing. Although hyperventilation can be the body's response to illness and a buildup of acids, hyperventilation syndrome is not the same thing. Instead, this syndrome occurs in the absence of other physical problems. However, it is very common during psychological stress, affecting some 10% of the population at one time or another. The respirations of a person who is experiencing hyperventilation syndrome may be as high as 40 shallow breaths/min or as low as only 20 very deep breaths/min. Physical findings vary depending on the cause of the syndrome. Rapid breathing with a high minute volume and carpopedal spasms are most common.

The decision whether hyperventilation is caused by a life-threatening illness or a panic attack should not be made outside the hospital. All patients who are hyperventilating should be given supplemental oxygen and transported to the hospital, where physicians can make a definitive diagnosis.

There are multiple causes of tachypnea that are not related to hyperventilation syndrome but cause an increase in oxygen demand. These causes are listed in Table 19-2.

Management of hyperventilation syndrome depends on the cause of the syndrome. Oxygen should *never* be withheld from any patient complaining of dyspnea. The rate of oxygen administration is based on symptoms and pulse oximetry readings. Remember that factors such as carbon monoxide toxicity, which could also result in hyperventilation, may produce a falsely high oxygen saturation reading. If, through the patient's history, anxiety-related hyperventilation is confirmed, coached ventilation should be considered. When in doubt, always provide 100% oxygen.

Interventions for circulatory support and pharmacological interventions are rarely required. Provide psychological support for the patient with anxiety-related hyperventilation. Have the patient mimic your respiratory rate and volume. Never place a paper bag over a hyperventilating patient's mouth and nose; if the hyperventilation is the result of hypoxia or other life-threatening condition, rebreathing carbon dioxide could be lethal. Provide transport to the closest appropriate facility; the patient's condition dictates the transport mode.

Emergency Care of Respiratory Emergencies

When taking the initial vital signs of a person with dyspnea, you should pay particular attention to respirations. Always speak with assurance and assume a concerned, professional approach to reassure the patient, who, no doubt, will be very frightened. Administer oxygen as needed, and reevaluate the patient's response to treatment frequently, at least every 5 minutes, until you reach the emergency department. In patients with chronically high carbon dioxide levels (for example, certain patients with COPD), continuous monitoring is critical, because high concentrations of oxygen may cause a rapid rise in the arterial oxygen level, which, in turn, may abolish the secondary respiratory oxygen drive and cause respiratory depression. This is not a contraindication to oxygen, but rather a special consideration when managing such patients.

Never withhold oxygen from a patient who needs it for fear of depressing or stopping breathing, even in

Geriatric Needs

Normal aging processes alter the respiratory system and the ability to exchange oxygen and carbon dioxide. If the patient is a smoker, the disease processes of emphysema or chronic bronchitis can exacerbate these age-related changes.

Several changes occur as we age. The chest wall, including the muscles and ribs, become less resilient. In addition, the bronchi and bronchioles lose their muscle mass or tone, and the air sacs (alveoli) become stiffer and less able to recoil (relax and empty) during exhalation. If the chest wall, including muscles and ribs, is weaker or less flexible, the chest cavity cannot expand as easily, and the total amount of air that is allowed into the lungs will be reduced. With decreased recoil of the lungs, alveoli can become distended with air trapped inside. If you are required to ventilate an apneic (nonbreathing) geriatric patient, you will notice that it is more difficult because of increased resistance of the chest and airways and reduced compliance of the lungs.

The geriatric patient is at an increased risk of pneumonia or a worsening of asthma or COPD if the airways have lost muscle mass or tone. Secretions might not be expelled from the airways, allowing pneumonia to develop.

The results of normal changes with aging include a reduction of the total amount of air the lungs can hold, air becoming trapped in overstretched alveoli, and increased resistance to air flow into and out of the lungs. Ultimately, these changes cause decreased oxygen and carbon dioxide exchange in the respiratory system with reduced oxygen delivery to the cells. Consider changes in aging that affect the respiratory system, and provide adequate ventilation and oxygenation according to the patient's needs. Geriatric patients may need ventilatory support for conditions that, in younger adults, are easily accommodated by the respiratory system.

patients with COPD. Slowing of respirations after oxygen administration does not necessarily mean that the patient's condition is improving; it may be deteriorating. If respirations slow and perfusion diminishes after oxygen administration, simply assist breathing with a bag-valve-mask (BVM) device.

Scene Size-Up and Initial Assessment

Pulmonary complaints may be associated with exposure to a wide variety of toxins, including carbon monoxide, toxic products of combustion, or environments that have deficient ambient oxygen (such as silos and enclosed storage spaces). It is critical to assure a safe environment

You are the Provider — Part 4

You apply a nonrebreathing mask at 15 L/min and prepare to transport the patient. Your partner brings the stretcher in, and together you lift the patient onto it.

Reassessment	Recording Time: 3 Minutes After Patient Contact
Respirations	30 breaths/min, shallow
Pulse	124 beats/min, regular
Blood pressure	150/100 mm Hg
Level of consciousness	Becoming lethargic
Sao_2	87%

7. In what position should you transport the patient?
8. Why do you think the patient's condition is not improving?
9. How should you adjust your treatment?

for all EMS personnel before making patient contact. If necessary, individuals with specialized training and equipment should be utilized to remove the patient from a hazardous environment.

The major focus of the initial assessment is to recognize and treat life threats or potential life threats. A variety of pulmonary conditions pose a high risk for death. Recognition of life threats and the initiation of resuscitation take priority over performing a detailed assessment. Signs of life-threatening respiratory distress in adults, listed from most ominous to least severe, include the following:

- Alterations in mental status
- Severe cyanosis
- Absent breath sounds
- Audible stridor
- 1- to 2-word dyspnea
- Tachycardia of more than 130 beats/min
- Pallor and diaphoresis
- The presence of retractions or the use of the accessory muscles

Approach to the Patient in Respiratory Distress

Approach the patient while obtaining a general impression. What is the position of the patient? Sitting? Tripod? Feet dangling?

Your first questions are always the same: Is the patient responsive? Confusion is a sign of hypoxemia or hypercarbia. Restlessness and irritability may be signs of fear and hypoxemia. Severe lethargy or coma is a sign of hypercarbia.

Is the airway open and clear? Is the patient breathing? If not, you must take action. Assess the airway and give two ventilations. As you ventilate, you need to ask another series of questions, as follows:

1. **Is air going into the lungs?** Look for clues in the rise and fall of the chest, the respirations, and the heart rate.
2. **When you squeeze the BVM device, does the chest wall expand?**
3. **When you release the bag, does the chest fall?** If not, something is wrong. Try to reposition the patient and insert an airway adjunct to keep the tongue from blocking the airway. Reposition the head. Reassess your hand position and face mask seal.

Next, assess the rate at which you are assisting the patient's ventilation. You need to give breaths at roughly the same rate as the patient would if he or she were breathing spontaneously (that is, 12 to 20 breaths/min). Rescuers often get excited and ventilate the patient too rapidly. Breathing for the patient too rapidly can cause harm. With rapid squeezing of the bag, higher pressures force the air rapidly into the lungs. Higher pressures can fill the stomach, as well as the lungs, with air. If the air and fluid in the stomach are regurgitated from the esophagus, vomitus may enter the lungs, which can cause airway obstruction or pneumonia. Adults should be given one breath every 5-6 seconds. Infants and children need a smaller breath every 3-5 seconds. Use the appropriately sized BVM device for each age group.

If the patient is breathing, is he or she able to speak? Does the patient present with 1- to 2-word dyspnea, or is he or she able to speak freely? Rapid, rambling speech is a sign of anxiety and fear. What is the respiratory effort like? Hard work indicates an obstruction. Do you note any retractions or the use of accessory muscles? What is the patient's skin color? Is the patient diaphoretic? Is central or peripheral cyanosis present? If breathing rate and tidal volume are adequate, apply 100% supplemental oxygen with a nonrebreathing mask and continue with your assessment.

Finally, assess the pulse. If the patient has a pulse, continue to support respirations. If the pulse rate is too fast (more than 100 beats/min) or too slow (fewer than 60 beats/min), the patient may not be getting enough oxygen. Recheck everything. Is the oxygen bottle or tank hooked up to the mask? Is the oxygen turned on? Is the flow rate adequate (10 to 15 L/min)? Is there a good mask-to-face seal? Is the chest rising and falling adequately with each breath? Is the airway blocked by vomitus or the tongue?

Signs and Symptoms

If the patient is breathing, you need to decide whether the breathing is adequate. Table 19-3 and Table 19-4 list the clues that will help you decide whether breathing is adequate or inadequate.

Focused History and Physical Examination

After you form your general impression and have completed the initial assessment, ask the patient to describe the problem to determine the chief complaint. Is there any dyspnea or chest pain? Begin by asking an open-ended question: "What can you tell me about your breathing?" Pay close attention to "**OPQRST**": when the problem began (**O**nset), what makes the breathing difficulty worse or better (**P**rovocation or **P**alliation), how the breathing feels (**Q**uality), and whether the discomfort, if present, moves (**R**adiation). How much of a

TABLE 19-3	Signs and Symptoms of Difficulty Breathing

- The patient complains of difficulty breathing.
- **The patient appears anxious or restless.** This can happen if the brain is not getting enough oxygen for its needs. Check the vital signs.
- **The patient is using the accessory muscles in the neck to assist breathing.** Use of accessory muscles usually indicates that excess work is required to move air into and out of the lungs. This is usually caused by conditions that increase airway resistance such as asthma, severe bronchitis, or pneumonia.
- **The patient is coughing excessively,** which might mean that the patient has anything from mild upper respiratory infection or hay fever to pneumonia, asthma, or heart failure.
- **The patient is sitting up, leaning forward** with palms flat on the bed or the arms of the chair. This is called the tripod position, because the back and two arms are working together to support the upper body. This position allows the diaphragm the most room to function and helps the patient to use accessory muscles to assist breathing. You should allow the patient to stay in the most comfortable position.
- **The patient has an increased pulse rate** (heart rate more than 100 beats/min). Tachycardia indicates a sympathetic nervous system discharge in response to hypoxemia.

TABLE 19-4	Signs and Symptoms of Inadequate Breathing

- **The patient's respiratory rate is too slow or too fast** (respirations are fewer than 12 breaths/min or greater than 20 breaths/min with reduced tidal volume); you may need to assist ventilation with a BVM device.
- **The patient's skin is blue (cyanotic).** The tongue, nailbeds, and inside the lips are good places to look for cyanosis. These all have a large collection of blood vessels and thin skin, making cyanosis easy to detect.
- **The patient is wheezing, gurgling, snoring, or crowing or has stridor.** Common causes of stridor include a foreign body obstruction and infection.
- **The patient cannot speak more than a few words between breaths.** Ask the patient something such as "How are you doing?" If the patient cannot speak at all, he or she probably has a respiratory emergency that needs immediate attention.
- **The patient has an altered mental status associated with shallow breathing that is too fast or too slow.**
- **The patient's breathing rhythm is irregular.** Because the brain controls breathing, an irregular breathing rhythm may indicate a head injury. In this case, the patient probably will be unresponsive.

Note: The following may also be seen in patients with inadequate breathing:

- **The chest has a barrel shape.** In certain chronic lung diseases, air has been gradually and continuously trapped within the lung in increasing amounts. As a result, the anterior-posterior diameter of the chest increases, nearly equaling the side-to-side distance. A barrel chest may indicate a long history of breathing problems.
- **The mucous membranes are pale.** Perhaps the patient is short of breath because there are not enough red blood cells to carry oxygen to the tissues.

problem is the patient having (Severity)? Is the problem continuous or intermittent (Time)? If it is intermittent, how long does it last? Does the patient have a cough? Is it productive or nonproductive? If it is productive, what color is the sputum? Is there any hemoptysis? Wheezing? Fever? Chills? Any increased sputum production? Has there been any exposure to smoke or is there a smoking history?

Find out what the patient has already done for the breathing problem. Does the patient use a prescribed inhaler? If so, when was it used last? How many doses have been taken? Does the patient use more than one inhaler? When was the last time the patient saw a physician for this problem? Find out whether the patient has any allergies or history of medication reactions.

What are the patient's vital signs? What is the pulse rate? Tachycardia is a sign of hypoxemia or might be a result of sympathomimetic medications taken for respiratory difficulty. Bradycardia in a patient experiencing dyspnea is an ominous sign of severe hypoxemia and imminent cardiac arrest. What is the blood pressure? Hypertension may be associated with the use of sympathomimetic medication.

What is the respiratory status? The respiratory rate is not an accurate indicator of respiratory status unless it is very slow. However, respiratory trends are essential for evaluating chronically ill patients. A slowing respiratory rate in the face of an unimproved condition suggests physical exhaustion and impending respiratory failure. The patient's respiratory pattern should be noted as follows:

- Eupnea
  - Normal breathing pattern
- Tachypnea
  - Rapid respiratory rate
- Cheyne-Stokes respirations
  - A breathing pattern characterized by periods of rapid and slow respirations alternating with periods of apnea; commonly seen in patients with head injury

- Central neurogenic hyperventilation
  - Deep, rapid respirations commonly seen in patients with head injury
- Kussmaul respirations
  - Deep, rapid respirations accompanied by an acetone or fruity odor on the patient's breath; seen in patients with diabetic ketoacidosis
- Ataxic (Biot) respirations
  - Rapid, irregular respirations with periods of apnea
- Apneustic respirations
  - Impaired respirations with sustained inspiratory effort
- Apnea
  - Cessation of breathing

Diagnostic testing will provide baseline information and indicate the severity of respiratory difficulty. Pulse oximetry is used to evaluate or confirm the adequacy of oxygen saturation. However, pulse oximetry readings may be inaccurate in the presence of conditions that abnormally bind hemoglobin, including carbon monoxide poisoning. Using a peak flow meter provides a baseline assessment of expiratory airflow for patients with obstructive lung disease. Many patients with chronic asthma may already use a peak flow meter at home. Encourage these patients to take their records and medications with them to the hospital for evaluation of the progression of their illness.

Capnometry provides an ongoing assessment of endotracheal tube position. The end-tidal carbon dioxide drops immediately when the tube is displaced from the trachea. Capnometry can also be used to assess the level of expired carbon dioxide in spontaneously breathing patients.

In the Field

Always treat your patient, not diagnostic test results!

As you perform your head-to-toe assessment, look for signs of increased work of breathing. Are the lips pursed? Do you see any accessory muscle use in the neck? Does the patient have a productive cough? If so, what color is the sputum? Increasing amounts suggest infection. Thick, green, or brown sputum suggests infection (for example, pneumonia). Yellow or pale gray sputum may be related to allergic or inflammatory problems. Frank hemoptysis often accompanies severe tuberculosis or carcinoma (cancer). Pink, frothy sputum is associated with severe, late stages of pulmonary edema and is often seen in cases of severe left-sided congestive heart failure. Jugular venous distention may accompany right-sided heart failure, which may be caused by severe pulmonary arterial obstruction.

When examining the chest, are there any obvious signs of trauma? Any retractions? Is the chest symmetrical? A barrel chest indicates the presence of long-standing chronic obstructive pulmonary disease. Next, listen to the breath sounds. Are they normal or abnormal? Do you hear stridor, wheezing, rhonchi, or rales? Examine the extremities for skin color, condition, and temperature. Numbness, tingling, and carpopedal spasm may be associated with hypocapnia resulting from periods of rapid, deep respiration.

Management

If the patient complains of breathing difficulty, you should administer high-flow supplemental oxygen. If breathing difficulty is severe, put a nonrebreathing face mask on the patient and supply oxygen at a rate of 12 to 15 L/min (enough to keep the reservoir bag inflated).

If the patient has altered mental status, open the airway using manual maneuvers. Suction any secretions or blood from the airway. Insert an oropharyngeal or nasopharyngeal adjunct as needed to maintain airway patency. If the patient's tidal volume is inadequate (for example, shallow breathing), provide positive-pressure ventilation with a BVM device attached to 100% oxygen.

Consider insertion of a dual-lumen or other advanced airway device in unconscious patients. In some areas, oxygen-powered, manually triggered ventilators or an automatic transport ventilator may be used. Continue your assessment. Obtain a set of vital signs and document them.

Perform intubation in the unconscious patient. Use capnometry to confirm correct tube placement.

As stated previously, there is some concern about suppression of the "hypoxic" drive to breathe in some patients with COPD. Unless these patients have severe hypoxia, a more conservative approach is suggested. In stable patients who have longstanding COPD and probable carbon dioxide retention, administration of low-flow oxygen (2 L/min) is a good place to start, with adjustments to 3 L/min, then 4 L/min, and so on, until symptoms have improved (for example, the patient has less dyspnea or an improved mental status). When in doubt, err on the side of more oxygen, and monitor the patient closely.

Because chronically ill patients live with their condition every day, when they call EMS, something has changed for the worse. Obtain a thorough SAMPLE his-

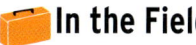

In the Field

The presence of corticosteroids or other steroids in the patient's daily medication regimen strongly suggests severe, chronic disease.

tory, including previous episodes, medication allergies, and current medications. The patient's subjective description of the problem is an accurate indicator of the acuity of this episode if the disease is chronic. Start by asking the patient "What happened the last time you had an attack this bad?" or "What did the doctor do then?" The answer provides an extremely useful predictor of the current episode's course. If you do not know the diagnosis, try to learn whether the problem is related primarily to ventilation, diffusion, perfusion, or a combination. Any history of intubation is an accurate indicator of severe pulmonary disease and suggests that intubation may be required again.

Pay close attention to the medications the patient is currently taking. Are there any pulmonary medicines, and if so, are they inhaled, oral, or parenteral? The patient probably has prescribed medications to use that are delivered by inhaler. Consult medical control. Remember to report the name of the medication, when the patient last took a puff, how many puffs were used at that time, and what the label states regarding dosage. If medical control permits, you may assist the patient in self-administering the medication. Be certain that the inhaler belongs to the patient, that it contains the correct medication, the expiration date has not passed, and the correct dose is being administered. Administer repeated doses of the medication if the maximum dose has not been exceeded and the patient is still experiencing shortness of breath.

If the patient does not have a prescribed inhaler, continue with the focused history and physical exam. Despite use of the inhaler, the patient's condition may continue to worsen. You need to reassess breathing frequently and be prepared to assist ventilation in severe cases. For a patient having an asthma attack, you must assist ventilation, using slow, gentle breaths. Remember, the problem in asthma is getting the air out of the lungs, not into them. Resist the temptation to squeeze the bag hard and fast. Assist with ventilation as a last resort, and then provide only 10 to 12 breaths/min.

Initiate an IV line, being careful to avoid fluid overload, especially in patients with pulmonary edema. In patients with excessive mucus buildup, IV rehydration may loosen pulmonary secretions, which, in combination with a productive cough, may facilitate their expulsion.

Prescribed Inhalers

Some of the most common medications used for shortness of breath are called inhaled beta-agonists, which, through stimulation of selective beta-2 receptors in the lungs, dilate the bronchioles. Typical trade names are Proventil, Ventolin, Alupent, Metaprel, and Brethine. The generic name for Proventil and Ventolin is albuterol; for Alupent and Metaprel, it is metaproterenol; and for Brethine, it is terbutaline. The action of most of these medications is to relax the smooth muscles within the bronchioles in the lungs, leading to enlargement (dilation) of the airways and easier passage of air. See Table 19-5 ▶ for a list of medications used for acute symptoms and medications used for chronic symptoms. Those used for acute symptoms are designed to give the

Documentation Tips

After assisting with the administration of an inhaler treatment, obtain another set of vital signs and note the patient's response to the treatment. Be sure to include lung sounds.

You are the Provider — Part 5

You and your partner place the patient in a position of comfort and quickly load him into the ambulance. You start an IV and draw blood while your partner assists his ventilations with a BVM device and 100% oxygen. A nasopharyngeal airway is inserted to assist in maintaining airway patency.

10. What IV fluid should you use?
11. At what rate will you run the IV?

TABLE 19-5 Respiratory Inhalation Medications

Medication		Indications			Usage: Acute vs Chronic	
Generic Drug Name	Trade Names	Asthma	Bronchitis	COPD	Acute	Chronic
Albuterol	Proventil, Ventolin, Volmax	Yes	Yes	Yes	Yes	No
Beclomethasone dipropionate	Beclovent	Yes	No	No	No	Yes
Cromolyn sodium	Intal	Yes	No	No	No	Yes
Fluticasone propionate	Flovent	Yes	No	No	No	Yes
Fluticasone propionate, salmeterol xinafoate	Advair Discus	Yes	No	No	No	Yes
Ipratropium bromide	Atrovent	Yes	Yes	Yes	Yes	No
Metaproterenol sulfate	Alupent	Yes	Yes	Yes	Yes	No
Montelukast sodium	Singulair	Yes	No	No	No	Yes
Salmeterol xinafoate	Serevent	Yes	Yes	Yes	No	Yes

> **In the Field**
>
> Positioning the patient in an upright position to loosen mucus and relieve buildup can be very effective in treating a patient with a respiratory emergency.

patient rapid relief from symptoms if the condition is reversible. Medications used for chronic symptoms are administered for preventative measures or as maintenance doses. The medications for chronic use will provide little relief of acute symptoms. Common side effects of inhalers used for acute shortness of breath include increased pulse rate, nervousness, and muscle tremors.

If the patient has a prescribed metered-dose inhaler, read the label carefully to make sure that the medication has, in fact, been prescribed to the patient by a physician 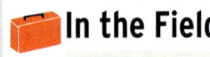. When in doubt, consult medical control.

Before helping a patient self-administer any metered-dose inhaler medication, make sure that the medication is indicated, that is, the patient has signs and symptoms of shortness of breath. Finally, ensure that there are no contraindications for its use, such as the following:

- The patient is unable to help coordinate inhalation with depression of the trigger, perhaps because the patient is too confused.
- The inhaler is not prescribed for this patient.
- You did not obtain permission from medical control or would be acting outside your local protocol.
- The patient had already met the maximum prescribed dose before your arrival (typically 2 to 4 puffs).

Consider the use of a sympathomimetic medication such as a beta-2 agonist or epinephrine based on local protocol and/or medical direction. Place the patient on the cardiac monitor, and be alert for cardiac dysrhythmias.

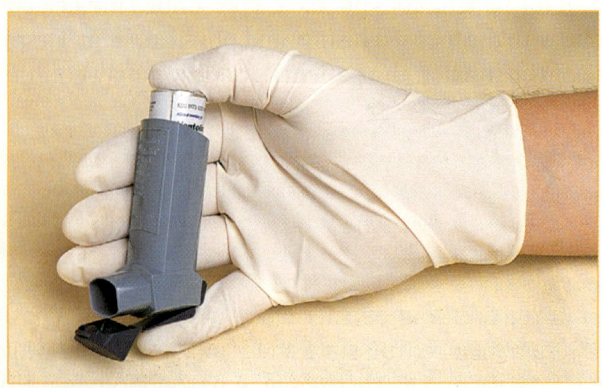

Figure 19-14 If the patient has a prescribed metered-dose inhaler, if possible, read the label to ensure that it was prescribed for this patient by a physician.

Assisting a Patient With a Metered-Dose Inhaler

Skill Drill 19-1

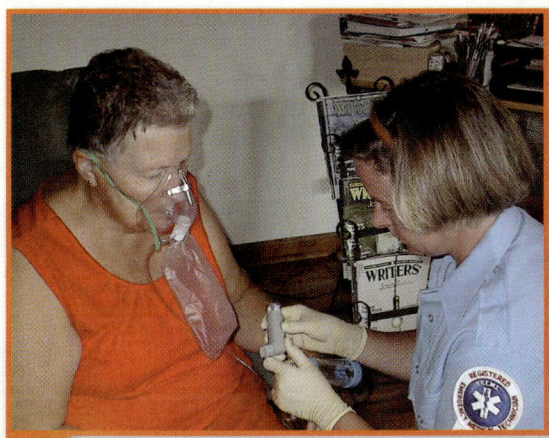

1 Ensure inhaler is at room temperature or warmer.

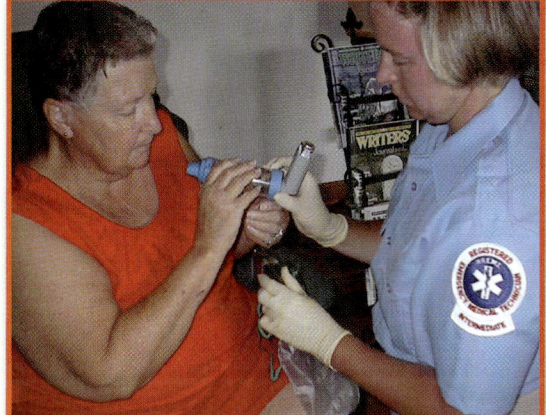

2 Remove oxygen mask.

Hand inhaler to patient. Instruct about breathing and lip seal.

Use a spacer if the patient has one.

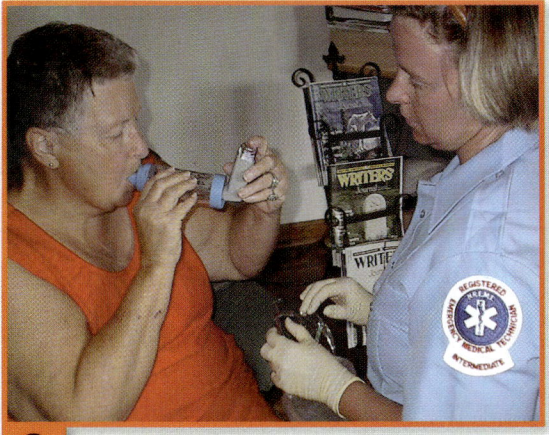

3 Instruct patient to press inhaler while inhaling deeply.

Instruct about breath holding.

4 Reapply oxygen. After a few breaths, have patient repeat dose if medical control or the local protocol allows and the patient's condition warrants it.

Administration of Metered-dose Inhaler Medication

To help a patient self-administer medication from an inhaler, follow these steps (Skill Drill 19-1 ▲):

1. **Obtain an order** from medical control or follow local protocol.
2. **Check that you have** the right medication, the right patient, and the right dose.
3. **Make sure that the patient is alert** enough to use the inhaler.
4. **Check the expiration date** of the inhaler.
5. **Check to see whether the patient** has already taken any doses.
6. **Make sure the inhaler** is at room temperature or warmer (**Step 1**).
7. **Shake the inhaler** vigorously several times.
8. **Remove the oxygen mask** from the patient's face.
9. **Ask the patient** to exhale deeply and, before inhaling, to put his or her lips around the opening of the inhaler.
10. **If the patient has a spacer**, attach it to allow more effective use of the medication (**Step 2**).
11. **Have the patient** depress the hand-held inhaler as he or she begins to inhale deeply.

Pediatric Needs

Asthma is a common childhood illness. When assessing a pediatric patient, look for retraction of the skin above the sternum and between the ribs. Retractions are typically easier to see in children than in adults. Cyanosis is a late finding in children. Keep in mind that a cough may not be a symptom of a cold; it could signal pneumonia or asthma. Even if you do not hear much wheezing, the presence of a cough can indicate some degree of reactive airway disease (for example, asthma or bronchiolitis).

The emergency care of a child with shortness of breath is the same as it is for an adult, including the use of supplemental oxygen. However, many small children will not tolerate (or may refuse to wear) a face mask. Rather than fighting with the child, hold the oxygen mask in front of the child's face or ask the parent to hold the mask (**Figure 19-15**). Many children with asthma also will have prescribed hand-held metered-dose inhalers. Assist with the use of these inhalers just as you would with an adult.

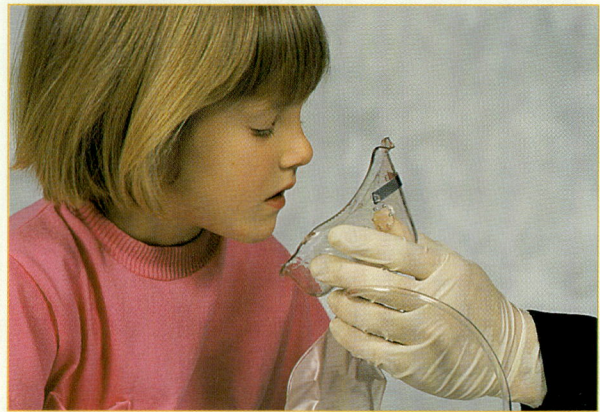

Figure 19-15 Because children may refuse to wear an oxygen mask, you may have to hold the mask in front of the child's face. If the child still refuses, enlist the parents' help.

12. **Instruct the patient** to hold his or her breath for as long as he or she comfortably can to help the lungs absorb the medication (**Step 3**).
13. **Replace the oxygen mask.**
14. **Allow the patient** to breathe a few times, then give the second dose per direction from medical control or according to local protocol (**Step 4**).

In the Field

While one EMT-I is getting oxygen ready, the second EMT-I should try to coach the patient with asthma or COPD to use pursed-lip breathing. This further opens the bronchioles to help air to escape.

You are the Provider — Part 6

The patient's color and mental status improve with the BVM ventilation, and his spontaneous respirations become deeper. You are able to reapply the nonrebreathing mask as your partner drives to the hospital.

Reassessment	Recording Time: 7 Minutes After Patient Contact
Respirations	22 breaths/min, regular, good tidal volume
Pulse	110 beats/min, regular
Blood pressure	148/88 mm Hg
Level of consciousness	Alert and oriented to person, place, and time
SaO_2	94% with oxygen via nonrebreathing mask

12. What should you do en route to the hospital?
13. Would a Combitube be appropriate for this patient?

Reassessment

You must carefully monitor patients with shortness of breath. About 5 minutes after the patient uses an inhaler, repeat the vital signs and the focused assessment. Ask the patient whether the treatment made any difference. Look at the patient's chest to see whether the patient is still using accessory muscles to breathe. Listen to the patient's speech pattern. Be prepared to assist ventilations with a BVM device if the patient deteriorates.

After helping the patient with the inhaler treatment, transport the patient to the emergency department. While en route, continue to assess the patient's breathing. Provide reassurance and continue to give supplemental oxygen. In cases of severe distress, do not delay transport. Metered-dose inhalers may be used en route.

You are the Provider — Summary

1. What are the most common signs and symptoms of difficulty breathing?

Dyspnea, accessory muscle use, tachycardia, possible cyanosis

2. What is the relationship between airway management and breathing difficulty?

Proper airway management should decrease the effort of breathing.

3. What questions should you ask the patient?

Medical history? Medications? Does he have a productive cough?

4. What is your general impression?

He is showing signs of respiratory distress and is noncompliant with his treatment as evidenced by the ashtray and the distress he is under when not using oxygen. He should be treated and transported promptly.

5. What type of oxygen delivery device should you use for this patient?

You should use a BVM device because he does not have an adequate tidal volume. If he does not tolerate it at this point, a nonrebreathing mask would be the next best choice.

6. At what rate should you set the flowmeter?

15 L/min

7. In what position should you transport the patient?

Position of comfort

8. Why do you think the patient's condition is not improving?

He is getting very tired from his effort to breathe, and his tidal volume is inadequate.

9. How should you adjust your treatment?

Assisted ventilations with a BVM device and 100% oxygen.

10. What IV fluid should you use?

An isotonic crystalloid, such as normal saline or lactated Ringer's.

11. At what rate will you run the IV?

The IV should be run at a keep-vein-open rate. More fluid would raise the blood pressure, which is already high.

12. What should you do en route to the hospital?

Constantly reassess the patient, and provide assistance with ventilations if needed.

13. Would a Combitube be appropriate for this patient?

No. He never lost his gag reflex or became unresponsive. Had his condition not improved, his level of consciousness most likely would have decreased. If he became completely unconscious, a Combitube would have been useful to secure his airway.

Prep Kit

Ready for Review

- Dyspnea is a common complaint that may be caused by numerous medical problems, including infections of the upper or lower airways, acute pulmonary edema, chronic obstructive pulmonary disease, spontaneous pneumothorax, asthma or allergic reactions, pleural effusions, mechanical obstruction of the airway, pulmonary embolism, and hyperventilation. Each of these lung disorders interferes in one way or another with the exchange of oxygen and carbon dioxide that takes place during respiration through problems with ventilation, diffusion, perfusion, or a combination. This interference may be in the form of damage to the alveoli, separation of the alveoli from the pulmonary vessels by fluid or infection, obstruction of the air passages, or air or excess fluid in the pleural space.

- Because carbon dioxide levels tend to be elevated and oxygen levels to be decreased in patients with chronic respiratory diseases, the administration of high concentrations of oxygen may suppress the respiratory drive. If this occurs coach breathing or provide positive-pressure ventilations as needed. Never withhold oxygen from a patient who needs it.

- Signs and symptoms of breathing difficulty include unusual breath sounds, including wheezing, stridor, rales, and rhonchi. Other signs may include nasal flaring; pursed-lip breathing; cyanosis; inability to talk; use of accessory muscles to breathe; and sitting in the tripod position, which allows the diaphragm the most room to function.

- In treating dyspnea, it is important to reassure the patient and provide supplemental oxygen. Remember to maintain the patient in a position that is comfortable for breathing, usually sitting upright. If the patient is not breathing or breathing inadequately, provide positive-pressure ventilations with a BVM device. Establish IV access and administer fluids as needed. Next, perform a focused history and physical exam, including vital signs. If the patient has a prescribed inhaler, or an epinephrine auto injector, consult medical control to assist with appropriate use of the inhaler or injector. Then transport the patient to the hospital, monitoring his or her condition en route. Talking with the patient is a good way to monitor some aspects of the patient's respiratory status.

- Remember, a patient who is breathing rapidly may be getting insufficient oxygen as a result of respiratory distress from a variety of problems, including pneumonia or a pulmonary embolism; trying to "blow off" more carbon dioxide to compensate for acidosis caused by a poison, a severe infection, or a high level of blood glucose; or having a stress reaction. In every case, prompt recognition of the problem, giving oxygen or providing ventilatory support, and prompt transport are essential.

Technology

- Interactivities
- Vocabulary Explorer
- Anatomy Review
- Web Links
- Online Review Manual

www.EMSzone.com/EMTI

Vital Vocabulary

allergen A substance that causes an allergic reaction.

asthma A disease of the lungs in which muscle spasm in the small air passageways and the production of large amounts of mucus result in airway obstruction.

atelectasis Collapse of the alveoli.

carbon dioxide retention A condition characterized by a chronically high blood level of carbon dioxide as the result of a respiratory disease.

carpopedal spasm Tingling and spasms of the phalanges resulting from hyperventilation.

chronic bronchitis Irritation and inflammation of the major lung passageways, from either infectious disease or irritants such as smoke.

chronic obstructive pulmonary disease (COPD) A slow, degenerative process that causes destructive changes in the alveoli and bronchioles in the lungs.

common cold A viral infection usually associated with swollen nasal mucous membranes and the production of fluid from the sinuses.

croup An infectious disease of the upper respiratory system that may cause partial airway obstruction and is characterized by a barking cough; usually seen in children. Croup is also referred to as laryngotracheobronchitis.

diffusion The movement of gases from a higher concentration to a lower concentration.

diphtheria An infectious disease in which a membrane lining the pharynx is formed that can severely obstruct passage of air into the larynx.

dyspnea A feeling of shortness of breath or difficulty breathing.

embolus A blood clot or other substance in the circulatory system that breaks free from its site of origin and obstructs blood flow in a distant blood vessel.

emphysema A disease of the lungs in which there is extreme dilation and eventual destruction of pulmonary alveoli with poor exchange of oxygen and carbon dioxide; it is one form of chronic obstructive pulmonary disease (COPD).

epiglottitis An infectious disease in which the epiglottis becomes inflamed and enlarged and may cause upper airway obstruction. Epiglottitis is also referred to as acute supraglottic laryngitis.

expiration The act of breathing out, or exhaling.

hyperventilation Rapid or deep breathing.

hypoxia A condition in which the body's cells and tissues do not have enough oxygen.

hypoxic drive Backup system to control respirations when oxygen levels fall dangerously low.

inspiration The act of breathing in, or inhaling.

perfusion Supplying an organ or tissue with required nutrients and oxygen.

pleural effusion A collection of fluid between the lung and chest wall that may compress the lung.

pleuritic chest pain Sharp, stabbing pain in the chest that is worsened by a deep breath or other chest wall movement; often caused by inflammation or irritation of the pleura.

pneumonia An infectious disease of the lung that damages lung tissue.

pneumothorax A partial or complete accumulation of air in the pleural space.

pulmonary edema A buildup of fluid in the lungs, usually as a result of left-sided congestive heart failure.

pulmonary thromboembolism A blood clot that breaks off from a large vein and travels to the blood vessels of the lung, causing obstruction of blood flow.

rales Crackling, moist breath sounds signaling fluid in the smaller air passages of the lungs.

respiration The exchange of gases that occurs at the pulmonary and cellular levels.

rhonchi Coarse, rattling breath sounds heard in patients with chronic mucus in the larger lower airways.

status asthmaticus A prolonged exacerbation of asthma that does not respond to conventional therapy.

stridor A harsh, high-pitched, barking inspiratory sound often heard in acute laryngeal (upper airway) obstruction.

subcutaneous emphysema Air bubbles trapped underneath the skin in the subcutaneous tissue.

ventilation The movement of air into and out of the lungs.

wheezing A high-pitched, whistling breath sound, characteristically heard on expiration in patients with asthma or COPD.

Assessment in Action

You respond to a 79-year-old man complaining of trouble breathing. He has a history of CHF and emphysema. Your assessment reveals that the patient's airway is open, and his respiratory rate is 36 breaths/min and labored. You auscultate the patient's lung sounds and hear bilateral basilar rales.

You notice that his condition is getting worse because he can only speak to you in one- or two-word sentences at a time. It is clear that this patient will require immediate ventilatory assistance.

1. The term ventilation is defined as the:
   A. principal function of the lungs.
   B. act of breathing in or inhaling.
   C. act of breathing out or exhaling.
   D. process of moving air into and out of the lungs.

2. The term respiration is defined as the:
   A. exchange of oxygen and carbon dioxide.
   B. act of breathing in or inhaling.
   C. act of breathing out or exhaling.
   D. process of moving air into and out of the lungs.

3. Air enters the _____ and moves through the bronchial tubes to the alveoli.
   A. Bloodstream
   B. Trachea
   C. Epiglottis
   D. Lungs

4. Which of the following will interfere with the body's ability to take in oxygen?
   A. Increased hemoglobin levels
   B. Increased tidal volume
   C. Chest wall impairment
   D. Increased red blood cell production

5. Adequate ventilation, diffusion, and perfusion describe the:
   A. Cushing's triad.
   B. Fick Principle.
   C. Boyle's law.
   D. Cushing's reflex.

6. The movement of gases from a higher molecular concentration to a lower molecular concentration is called:
   A. perfusion.
   B. ventilation.
   C. diffusion.
   D. hypoxia.

7. An acute bacterial or viral infection associated with fever, cough, and production of sputum is called:
   A. a common cold.
   B. diphtheria.
   C. pneumonia.
   D. epiglottis.

8. A bacterial infection that can produce acute, severe swelling of the epiglottis is called:
   A. croup.
   B. diphtheria.
   C. pneumonia.
   D. epiglottitis.

9. A condition in which the patient usually experiences dyspnea with rapid, shallow respirations and may even have a pink frothy sputum in the mouth and nose is called:
   A. asthma.
   B. emphysema.
   C. pulmonary edema.
   D. pulmonary contusion.

10. A chronic respiratory condition that results from the loss of the elastic material around the air spaces as a result of chronic stretching of the alveoli when damaged airways impede the easy expulsion of gases is called:
    A. bronchitis.
    B. pulmonary embolism.
    C. asthma.
    D. emphysema.

www.EMSzone.com/EMTI

Points to Ponder

You are dispatched to a private residence for a 60-year-old man complaining of trouble breathing. Upon your arrival you see a patient in obvious respiratory distress, speaking in two- to three-word sentences. He is receiving home oxygen at 2 L/min via nasal cannula. The patient's wife tells you that she tried to increase the flow of his oxygen but he would not let her. The patient, who has a history of chronic bronchitis, has a barrel-shaped chest and is sitting upright, laboring to breathe. You attach a pulse oximeter and it reads 85%. You attempt to place the patient on 100% oxygen with a nonrebreathing mask, but he will not allow you to do so because his doctor told him that high concentrations of oxygen would cause him to stop breathing.

How do you respond? Is the patient's concern with high-flow oxygen legitimate?

Issues: Recognizing Patients in Respiratory Distress; The Critical Nature of Accurate Field Impression of Respiratory Conditions

Cardiovascular Emergencies

1999 Objectives

Cognitive

5-2.1 Describe the incidence, morbidity, and mortality of cardiovascular disease. (p 884)

5-2.2 Review cardiovascular anatomy and physiology. (p 884)

5-2.3 Discuss prevention strategies that may reduce morbidity and mortality of cardiovascular disease. (p 884)

5-2.4 Identify the risk factors most predisposing to coronary artery disease. (p 884)

5-2.5 Identify and describe the components of assessment as it relates to the patient with cardiovascular compromise. (p 907)

5-2.6 Describe how ECG wave forms are produced. (p 925)

5-2.7 Correlate the electrophysiological and hemodynamic events occurring throughout the entire cardiac cycle with the various ECG wave forms, segments and intervals. (p 952)

5-2.8 Identify how heart rates may be determined from ECG recordings. (p 936)

5-2.9 List the limitations to the ECG. (p 937)

5-2.10 Describe a systematic approach to the analysis and interpretation of cardiac arrhythmias. (p 938)

5-2.11 Explain how to confirm asystole using more than one lead. (p 926)

5-2.12 List the clinical indications for defibrillation. (p 918)

5-2.13 Identify the specific mechanical, pharmacological and electrical therapeutic interventions for patients with arrhythmias causing compromise. (p 938)

5-2.14 List the clinical indications for an implanted defibrillation device. (p 912, 913)

5-2.15 Define angina pectoris and myocardial infarction. (p 900, 901)

5-2.16 List other clinical conditions that may mimic signs and symptoms of angina pectoris and myocardial infarction. (p 901)

5-2.17 List the mechanisms by which an MI may be produced by traumatic and non-traumatic events. (p 901)

5-2.18 List and describe the assessment parameters to be evaluated in a patient with chest pain. (p 901, 909)

5-2.19 Identify what is meant by the OPQRST of chest pain assessment. (p 909)

5-2.20 List and describe the initial assessment parameters to be evaluated in a patient with chest pain that may be myocardial in origin. (p 901, 902)

5-2.21 Identify the anticipated clinical presentation of a patient with chest pain that may be angina pectoris or myocardial infarction. (p 900)

5-2.22 Describe the pharmacological agents available to the EMT-Intermediate for use in the management of arrhythmias and cardiovascular emergencies. (p 909)

5-2.23 Develop, execute, and evaluate a treatment plan based on the field impression for the patient with chest pain that may be indicative of angina or myocardial infarction. (p 908)

5-2.24 Define the terms "congestive heart failure" and pulmonary edema." (p 904, 905)

5-2.25 Define the cardiac and non-cardiac causes and terminology associated with pulmonary edema. (p 906)

5-2.26 Describe the early and late signs and symptoms of pulmonary edema. (p 906)

5-2.27 Explain the clinical significance of paroxysmal nocturnal dyspnea. (p 912)

5-2.28 List and describe the pharmacological agents available to the EMT-Intermediate for use in the management of a patient with cardiac compromise. (p 909)

5-2.29 Define the term "hypertensive emergency." (p 906)

5-2.30 Describe the clinical features of the patient in a hypertensive emergency. (p 906)

5-2.31 List the interventions prescribed for the patient with a hypertensive emergency. (p 906)

5-2.32 Define the term "cardiogenic shock." (p 903)

5-2.33 Identify the clinical criteria for cardiogenic shock. (p 903)

5-2.34 Define the term "cardiac arrest." (p 915)

5-2.35 Define the term "resuscitation." (p 915)

5-2.36 Identify local protocol dictating circumstances and situations where resuscitation efforts would not be initiated. (p 915)

5-2.37 Identify local protocol dictating circumstances and situations where resuscitation efforts would be discontinued. (p 915)

5-2.38 Identify the critical actions necessary in caring for the patient in cardiac arrest. (p 915)
5-2.39 Synthesize patient history, assessment findings to form a field impression for the patient with chest pain and cardiac arrhythmias that may be indicative of a cardiac emergency. (p 907, 922)

Affective

5-2.40 Value the sense of urgency for initial assessment and intervention as it contributes to the treatment plan for the patient experiencing a cardiac emergency. (p 902)
5-2.41 Defend patient situations where ECG rhythm analysis is indicated. (p 915)
5-2.42 Value and defend the sense of urgency necessary to protect the window of opportunity for reperfusion in the patient with chest pain and arrhythmias that may be indicative of angina or myocardial infarction. (p 917)
5-2.43 Value and defend the urgency in rapid determination and rapid intervention of patients in cardiac arrest. (p 917)

Psychomotor

5-2.44 Demonstrate a working knowledge of various ECG lead systems. (p 925)
5-2.45 Set up and apply a transcutaneous pacing system. (p 925)
5-2.46 Given the model of a patient with signs and symptoms of pulmonary edema, position the patient to afford comfort and relief. (p 905)

1985 Objectives

1.6.28 Describe the anatomy of the heart and the cardiovascular system. (p 884)
1.6.29 Describe the problems that occur with decreased perfusion. (p 970)
1.6.30 Describe the pathophysiology of cardiac arrest. (p 915)
*1.9.1 Describe the size, shape, and location/orientation (in regard to other body structures) of the heart muscle. (p 884)

*1.9.2 Identify the location of the following structures on a diagram of the normal heart:
- Pericardium
- Myocardium
- Epicardium
- Right and left atria
- Interatrial septum
- Right and left ventricles
- Intraventricular septum
- Superior and inferior vena cava
- Aorta
- Pulmonary vessels
- Coronary arteries
- Tricuspid valve
- Mitral valve
- Aortic valve
- Pulmonic valve
- Papillary muscles
- Chordae tendinae (p 884-888)

*1.9.3 Describe the function of each structure listed in objective 1.9.2 (p 884)
*1.9.4 Describe the distribution of the coronary arteries and the parts of the heart supplied by each artery. (p 885)
*1.9.5 Differentiate the structural and functional aspects of arterial and venous blood vessels. (p 885)
*1.9.6 Define the following terms that refer to cardiac physiology:
- Stroke volume
- Starling's Law
- Preload
- Afterload
- Cardiac output
- Blood pressure (p 895, 896)

*1.9.7 Describe the electrical properties of the heart. (p 888)
*1.9.8 Describe the normal sequence of electrical conduction through the heart and state the purpose of this conduction system. (p 888)
*1.9.9 Describe the location and function of the following structures of the electrical conduction system:
- SA node
- Internodal and interatrial tracts
- AV node
- Bundle of His
- Bundle branches
- Purkinje fibers (p 889-891)

Cardiovascular Emergencies

*1.9.10 Define cardiac depolarization and repolarization and describe the major electrolyte changes that occur in each process. (p 892, 952)

*1.9.11 Describe an ECG. (p 925)

*1.9.12 Define the following terms as they relate to the electrical activity of the heart:
- Isoelectric line
- QRS complex
- P wave (p 926-929)

*1.9.13 Name the common chief complaints of cardiac patients. (p 902)

*1.9.14 Describe why the following occur in patients with cardiac problems:
- Chest pain or discomfort
- Shoulder, arm, neck, or jaw pain/discomfort
- Dyspnea
- Syncope
- Palpitations/abnormal heart beat (p 900-902)

*1.9.15 Describe those questions to be asked during history taking for each of the common cardiac chief complaints. (p 907)

*1.9.16 Describe the four most pertinent aspects of the past medical history in a patient with a suspected cardiac problem. (p 908, 909)

*1.9.17 Describe those aspects of the physical examination that should be given special attention in the patient with suspected cardiac problems. (p 903)

*1.9.18 Describe the significance of the following physical exam findings in a cardiac patient:
- Altered level of consciousness
- Peripheral edema
- Cyanosis
- Poor capillary refill
- Cool, clammy skin (p 903, 904)

*1.9.19 State the numerical values assigned to each small and each large box on the ECG graph paper for each axis. (p 933)

*1.9.20 Define ECG artifact and name the causes. (p 937)

*1.9.21 State the steps in the analysis format of ECG rhythm strips. (p 938)

*1.9.22 Describe two common methods for calculating heart rate on an ECG rhythm strip and the indications for using each method. (p 936)

*1.9.23 Name 8 causes of dysrhythmias. (p 940)

*S1.9.26 Demonstrate proper application of ECG chest electrodes and obtain a sample Lead II. (p 925)

*S1.9.27 Demonstrate the proper use of the defibrillator paddles electrodes to obtain a sample Lead II rhythm strip. (p 926)

*S1.9.28 Demonstrate how to properly assess the cause of poor ECG tracing. (p 937)

*S1.9.29 Demonstrate correct operation of a monitor-defibrillator to perform defibrillation on an adult and infant. (p 965)

*Indicates optional.

20

Cardiovascular Emergencies

You are the Provider

You receive a call for an older woman having chest pains. Dispatch tells you that the patient is conscious and has a pulse.

This chapter will help you to deal with cardiovascular emergencies, the leading cause of death, in addition to answering the following questions.

1. What are the risk factors for cardiovascular disease?
2. What causes a myocardial infarction?

Cardiovascular Emergencies

The American Heart Association reports that cardiovascular disease (CVD) claimed 931,108 lives in the United States in 2001. Cardiovascular disease accounted for 38.5% of all deaths, or 1 of every 2.6 deaths. Mortality due to CVD was about 60% of "total mortality." This means that of more than 2.4 million deaths due to all causes, CVD was listed as a primary or contributing cause on more than 1.4 million death certificates. Heart disease has been the leading killer of Americans since 1900. Thus, many of your calls will involve some type of cardiac emergency.

It is important for EMS providers to understand that many deaths caused by CVD occur from problems that may have been avoided by people living more prudent lifestyles, identifying and modifying certain risk factors (Table 20-1 ▶), and by access to improved medical technology. We can help to reduce these numbers of deaths with better public awareness, early access to EMS, increased numbers of laypeople trained in CPR, and with public access defibrillation.

This chapter begins with a brief description of the heart and how it works. It then discusses the relationship between chest pain and ischemic heart disease. It explains how to recognize and treat acute myocardial infarction (classic heart attack) and the complications of sudden death, cardiogenic shock, and congestive heart failure. The last part of the chapter is devoted to electrocardiogram (ECG) rhythm analysis and treatment of individual cardiac rhythms based on current American Heart Association ACLS (advanced cardiac life support) protocols.

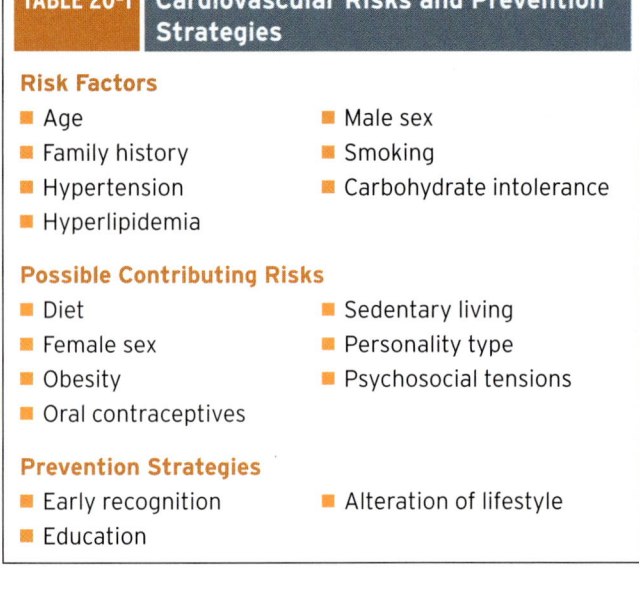

TABLE 20-1 Cardiovascular Risks and Prevention Strategies

Risk Factors
- Age
- Family history
- Hypertension
- Hyperlipidemia
- Male sex
- Smoking
- Carbohydrate intolerance

Possible Contributing Risks
- Diet
- Female sex
- Obesity
- Oral contraceptives
- Sedentary living
- Personality type
- Psychosocial tensions

Prevention Strategies
- Early recognition
- Education
- Alteration of lifestyle

Cardiovascular Anatomy and Physiology

The cardiovascular system consists of the heart, the blood vessels, and the blood. All components must interact effectively to maintain life.

The Heart

Location and Major Structures of the Heart

The heart is a muscular, cone-shaped organ whose function is to pump blood throughout the body. The heart is located behind the sternum and is about the size of the closed fist of the person it belongs to, roughly 5" long, 3" wide, and $2\frac{1}{2}$" thick. It weights 10 to 12 oz in men and 8 to 10 oz in women (Figure 20-1 ▶). Roughly two thirds of the heart lies in the left part of the mediastinum, the area between the lungs that also contains the great vessels (that is, the aorta and vena cavae) and other structures.

The heart muscle is referred to as the myocardium. The term "myo" means muscle and "cardium" means heart. The pericardium, also called the pericardial sac, is a thick fibrous membrane that surrounds the heart (Figure 20-2 ▶). The pericardium anchors the heart within the mediastinum and prevents overdistention of the heart. The inner membrane of the pericardium is the serous pericardium. This inner membrane contains

---

Technology
- Interactivities
- Vocabulary Explorer
- Anatomy Review
- Web Links
- Online Review Manual

www.EMSzone.com/EMTI

*This chapter and the illustrations contained therein are reprinted from *Arrhythmia Recognition: The Art of Interpretation* by Tomas B. Garcia, MD, FACEP and Geoffrey T. Miller, NREMT-P, © 2004 Jones and Bartlett Publishers, Inc.

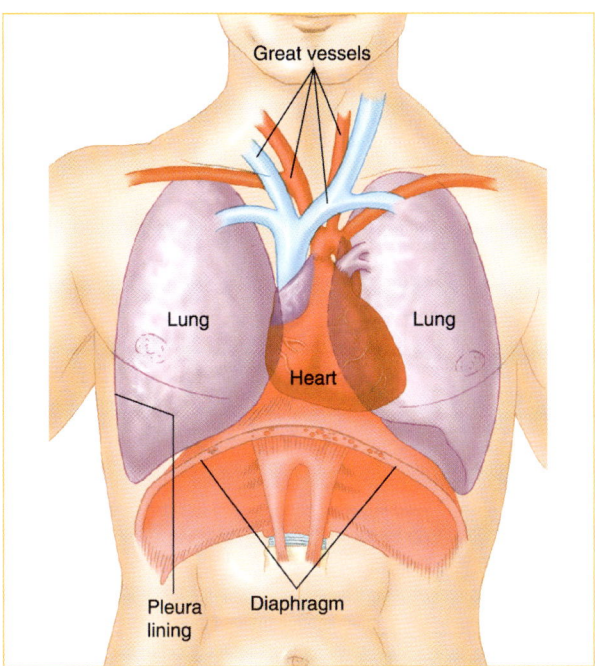

Figure 20-1 The anterior aspect of the thorax shows the relative position of the heart beneath the surface.

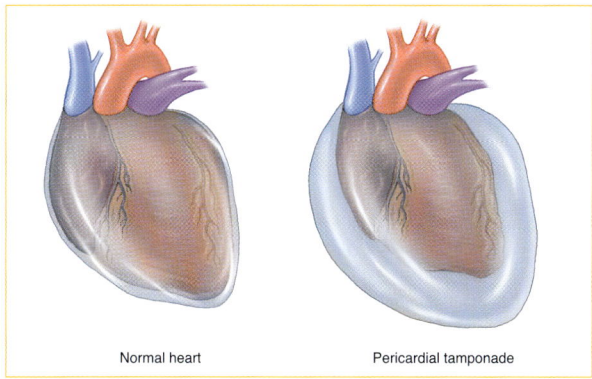

Figure 20-2 The pericardial sac surrounds the heart. When the pericardial sac fills with too much fluid (pericardial effusion), a life-threatening state of cardiac tamponade can develop. In this situation, the chambers of the heart are unable to expand and contract sufficiently. Death can rapidly result.

two layers: the visceral layer and the parietal layer. The visceral layer of the pericardium lies closely against the heart and is also called the epicardium. The second layer of the pericardium, the parietal layer, is separated from the visceral layer by a small amount of pericardial fluid that reduces friction within the pericardial sac.

The human heart consists of four chambers: two atria and two ventricles. The upper chambers are the atria, and the lower chambers are the ventricles. Each side of the heart contains one atrium and one ventricle. A membrane, the interatrial septum, separates the two atria; a thicker wall, the interventricular septum, separates the right and left ventricles. Each atrium receives blood that is returned to the heart from other parts of the body; each ventricle pumps blood out of the heart. The upper and lower portions of the heart are separated by the atrioventricular valves, which prevent backward flow of blood. Similar valves, the semilunar valves, are located between the ventricles and the arteries into which they pump blood (Figure 20-3▶).

Blood enters the right atrium via the superior and inferior venae cavae and the coronary sinus, which is the end of the great cardiac vein and collects blood returning from the walls of the heart. Blood from four pulmonary veins enters the left atrium. Between the right and left atria is a depression, the fossa ovalis, which represents the former location of the foramen ovale, an opening between the two atria that is present in the fetus.

Valves of the Heart

Blood passing from the atria to the ventricles flows through one of two atrioventricular valves. The tricuspid valve separates the right atrium from the right ventricle, and the mitral valve, a bicuspid valve, separates the left atrium from the left ventricle. The valves consist of flaps called cusps. Papillary muscles attach to the ventricles and send small muscular strands called chordae tendineae cordis to the cusps. When the papillary muscle contracts, these strands tighten, preventing regurgitation of blood through the valves from the ventricles to the atria.

Two semilunar valves, the aortic valve and the pulmonic valve, divide the heart from the aorta and the pulmonary artery. The pulmonic valve regulates blood flow from the right ventricle to the pulmonary artery. The aortic valve regulates blood flow from the left ventricle to the aorta. The semilunar valves are not attached to papillary muscles. When these valves close, they prevent backflow from the aorta and pulmonary artery into the left and right ventricles, respectively.

Blood Flow Within the Heart

Two large veins, the superior vena cava and the inferior vena cava, return deoxygenated blood from the body to the right atrium. Blood from the upper part of the body returns to the heart through the superior vena cava, and blood from the lower part of the body returns through the inferior vena cava. The inferior vena cava is the larger of the two veins. From the right atrium, blood passes through the tricuspid valve into the right ventricle. Blood is then pumped by the right ventricle through the pulmonic valve into the pulmonary artery

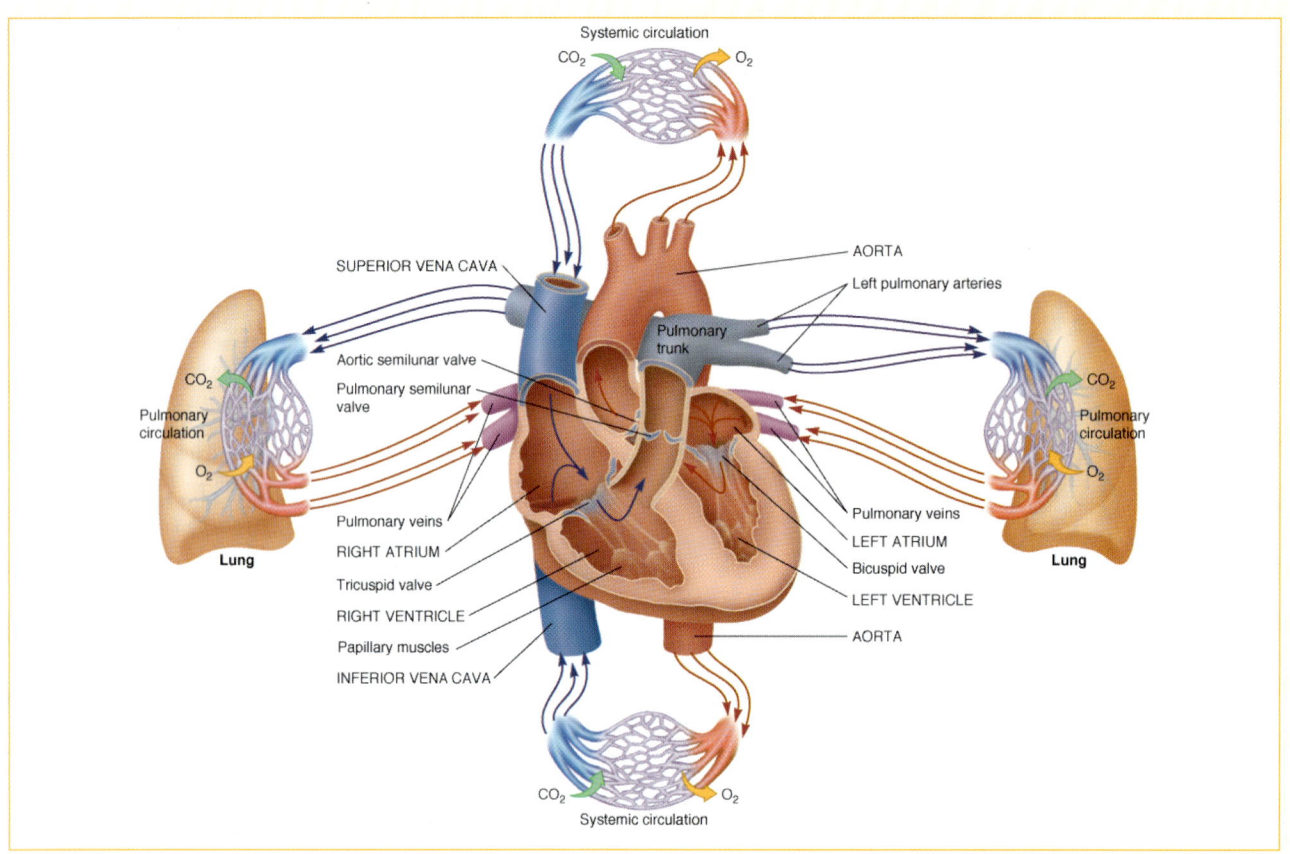

Figure 20-3 Blood flow through the heart.

and to the lungs. In the lungs, various processes take place that return oxygen to the blood and, at the same time, remove carbon dioxide and other waste products.

Freshly oxygenated blood is returned to the left atrium through the pulmonary veins. Blood then flows through the mitral valve into the left ventricle, which pumps the oxygenated blood through the aortic valve, into the aorta, the body's largest artery, and then to the entire body. The left ventricle is the strongest and largest of the four cardiac chambers because it is responsible for pumping blood through blood vessels throughout the body.

The contraction and relaxation of the heart, combined with the flow of blood, generate characteristic heart sounds during auscultation with a stethoscope. The normal pattern sounds much like "lub-DUB, lub-DUB, lub-DUB." The "lub" is referred to as the first heart sound or S1, and the "DUB" (emphasized because it is often louder) as the second heart sound or S2 Figure 20-4 ▶. Sound caused by the sudden closure of the mitral and tricuspid valves at the start of ventricular contraction results in the S1 sound, or the first heart sound. The S2, or second heart sound, results from the closure of both the aortic and pulmonic valves at the end of a ventricular contraction.

Two other heart sounds, S3 and S4, usually are not heard in individuals with normal heart sounds Figure 20-5 ▶. The S3, or third heart sound, is a soft, low-pitched heart sound that occurs about one third of the way through diastole (the period during which the ventricles are relaxed). When an S3 sound is present, the heartbeat cycle is described as sounding like "lub-DUB-da." This sound may represent a period of rapid ventricular filling associated with sound made by an inrush of blood. Although the S3 sound sometimes is present in healthy young individuals, it most commonly is associated with abnormally increased filling pressures in the atria secondary to moderate to severe heart failure.

The S4 heart sound is a moderately pitched sound that occurs immediately before the normal S1 sound. When an S4 sound is present, the heart contraction cycle sounds like "bla-lub-DUB." The S4 sound represents decreased stretching (compliance) of the left ventricle or increased pressure in the atria. An S4 heart sound almost always is abnormal.

Four other sounds, all abnormal, may be heard when auscultating the heart and great vessels. Some of these sounds are very easy to hear; others may require years of experience to identify. These additional abnormal

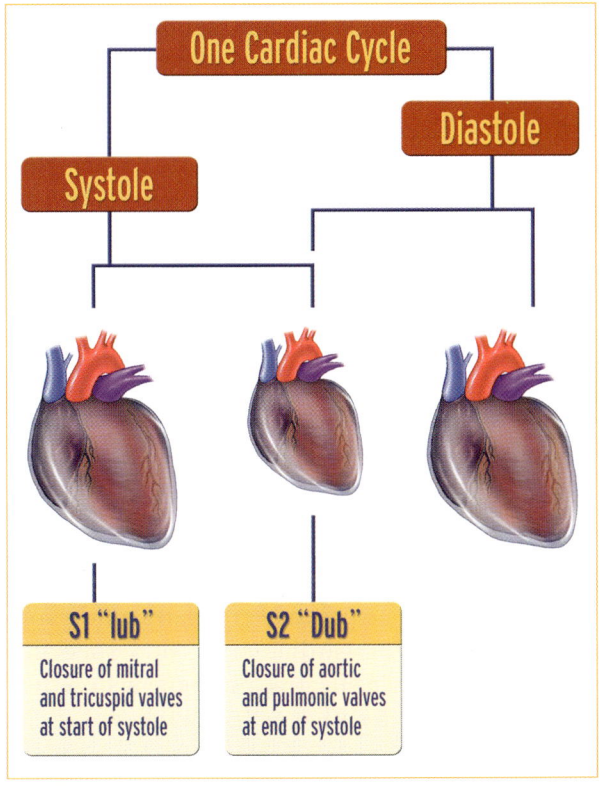

Figure 20-4 The normal S1 and S2 heart sounds.

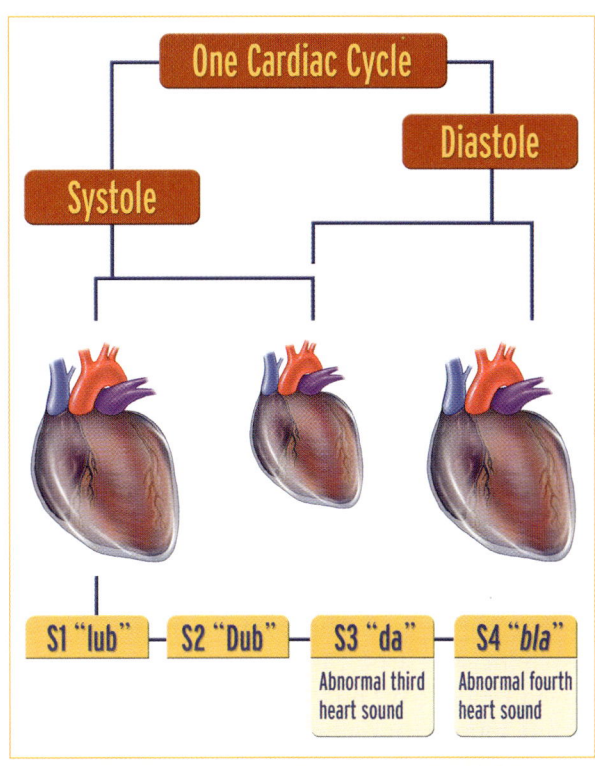

Figure 20-5 The abnormal S3 and S4 heart sounds.

sounds include murmurs, bruits, clicks, and snaps. A murmur is an abnormal "whooshing" sound heard over the heart that indicates turbulent blood flow within the heart. Although many murmurs are "functional" (benign) and often resolve spontaneously, several are characteristic of heart disease. A bruit is an abnormal whooshing sound heard over a main blood vessel that indicates turbulent blood flow within the blood vessel. A bruit often indicates localized arteriosclerotic disease (thickening or hardening of the arteries). Both clicks and snaps indicate abnormal cardiac valve function. They occur at different times in the cardiac cycle, depend-

You are the Provider — Part 2

As you approach the patient, you notice that she is clutching her chest and is in obvious respiratory distress.

Initial Assessment	Recording Time: Zero Minutes
Appearance	Appears to be in pain; pale and diaphoretic
Level of consciousness	Responsive verbally and appears to be fatigued
Airway	Open and clear
Breathing	Respiratory rate, increased and labored
Circulation	Skin, clammy; radial pulse, present and weak

3. What is the pacemaker function of the heart, and why do we need it?
4. What is the main pacemaker, and at what rate does it pace?

ing on which valve is diseased. Although these sounds are significant, most of these sounds are fleeting and difficult to hear.

Electrical Properties of the Heart and the Conduction System

The mechanical pumping action of the heart can occur only in response to an electrical stimulus. This impulse causes the heart to beat via a set of complex chemical changes within the myocardial cells. The brain partially controls the heart's rate and strength of contraction via the autonomic nervous system. Contractions of myocardial tissue, however, are initiated within the heart itself, in a group of complex electrical tissues that are part of a conduction system. The cardiac conduction system consists of six parts: the sinoatrial (SA) node, the atrioventricular (AV) node, the bundle of His, the right and left bundle branches, and the Purkinje fibers (Figure 20-6 ▼).

The sinoatrial (SA) node is located high in the right atrium and is the normal site of origin of the electrical impulse. It is the heart's natural pacemaker. Impulses originating in the SA node travel through the right and left atria, resulting in atrial contraction. The impulse then travels to the atrioventricular (AV) node, located in the right atrium adjacent to the septum, where it transiently slows. Electrical stimulation of the heart muscle then continues toward the bundle of His, which is a continuation of the AV node. From here, it proceeds rapidly to the right and left bundle branches, stimulating the interventricular septum. The impulse then spreads out, via the Purkinje fibers, to the left, then the right ventricular myocardium, resulting in ventricular contraction, or systole.

Pacemaker Function

What is the pacemaker function of the heart, and why do we need it? The pacemaker dictates the rate at which the heart will cycle through its pumping action to circulate the blood. The pacemaker creates an organized beating of all of the cardiac cells, in a specialized sequence, to produce effective pumping action. It sets the pace that all of the other cells will follow. Let's look at an analogy.

Imagine that each cell of the heart represents a single musician. When we have a few dozen of these musicians, we have an orchestra—the heart. Now, if each musician decides to play whenever he or she wants to, an unrecognizable jumble of sound would result. The musicians need a beat or signal to cue them when to start to play, direct them when to come into the piece and when to leave, and coordinate their actions to create a beautiful melody. In music, that pacemaker is the underlying beat kept by the drummer or the conductor. In sections that are swift, the beat increases. In sections that are slow and soft, the beat decreases. The same thing happens in the heart; during exercise the pace speeds up, and during rest it slows.

There are specialized cells whose function is to create an electrical impulse and act as the heart's pacemaker. The main area that fills this important function is the SA node, found in the muscle of the right atrium. This area responds to the needs of the body, controlling the beat based on information it receives from the nervous, circulatory, and endocrine systems. The main pacemaker paces at a rate of 60 to 100 beats/min, with an average of 70 beats/min.

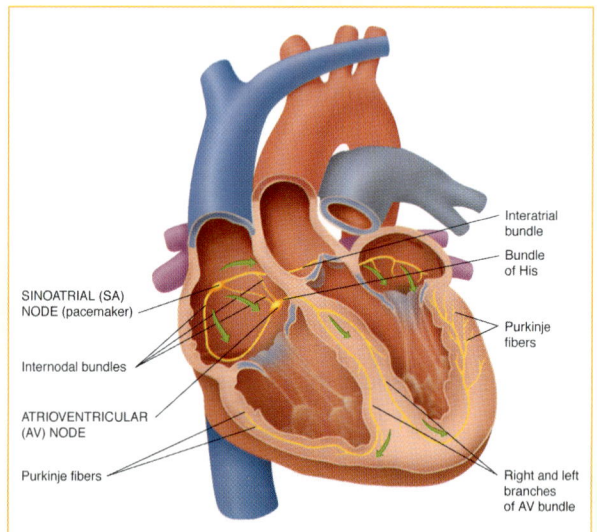

Figure 20-6 The cardiac conduction system. Specialized groups of cardiac muscle cells initiate an electrical impulse throughout the heart. The normal conduction pathway travels through the six parts of the cardiac conduction system. The impulse begins in the SA node and spreads through internodal bundles to the AV node. The AV node slows the impulse and initiates a signal that is conducted through the ventricles by way of the bundle of His, right and left bundle branches, and the Purkinje fibers.

Pacemaker Settings

One thing we know about the body is that everything has a backup. Every cell in the conduction system is capable of setting the pace (Figure 20-7 ▶). However, the intrinsic rate of each type of cell is slower than the cells that precede it. This means that the fastest pacer is the SA node, the next fastest is the AV node, and so on. The fastest pacer sets the pace because it causes all the ones that come after it to reset after each beat. In this way, the slower pacers will never fire. If the faster pacer does not fire for some reason, the next fastest will be there as a backup to ensure function that is as close to normal as possible.

The SA Node

The SA node, the heart's main pacemaker, is found in the wall of the right atrium at its junction with the superior vena cava Figure 20-8 . Its blood supply comes from the right coronary artery in 59% of cases. In 38%, the blood supply originates from the left coronary artery, and in the last 3%, it arises from both. The SA node is also referred to as the sinus node.

The Internodal Pathways

There are three internodal pathways: anterior, middle, and posterior Figure 20-9 . Their main purpose is to transmit the pacing impulse from the SA node to the AV node. In addition, there is a small tract of specialized cells known as the Bachman bundle that transmits the impulses through the interatrial septum. All of these pathways are found in the walls of the right atrium and the interatrial septum.

The AV Node

The AV node is located in the wall of the right atrium next to the opening of the coronary sinus, the largest vein of the heart, and the septal leaflet of the tricuspid valve Figure 20-10 . It is responsible for slowing

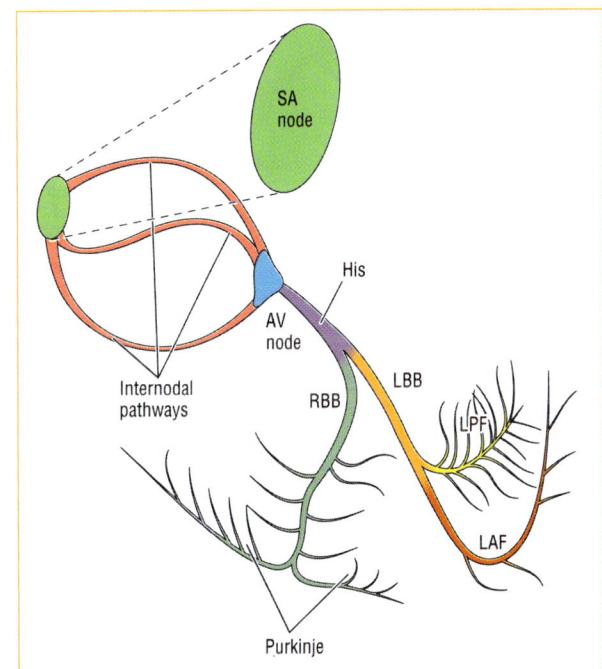

Figure 20-8 SA node.

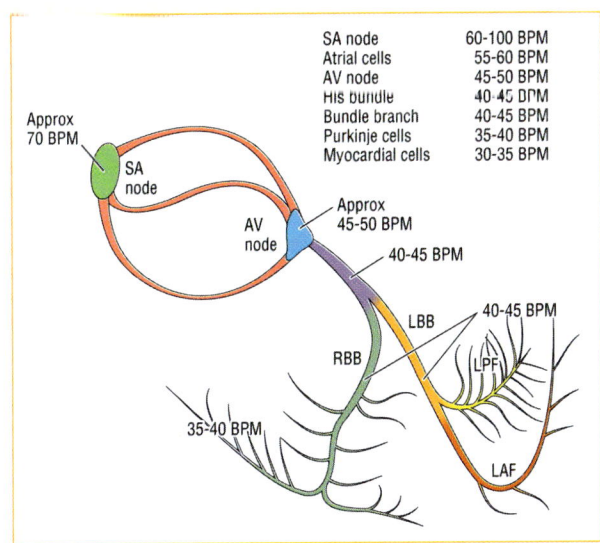

Figure 20-7 Intrinsic rates of pacing cells.

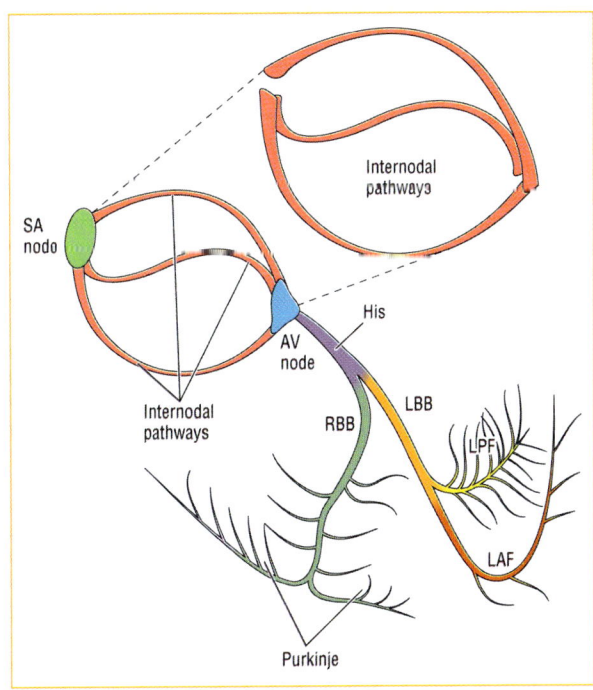

Figure 20-9 Internodal pathways.

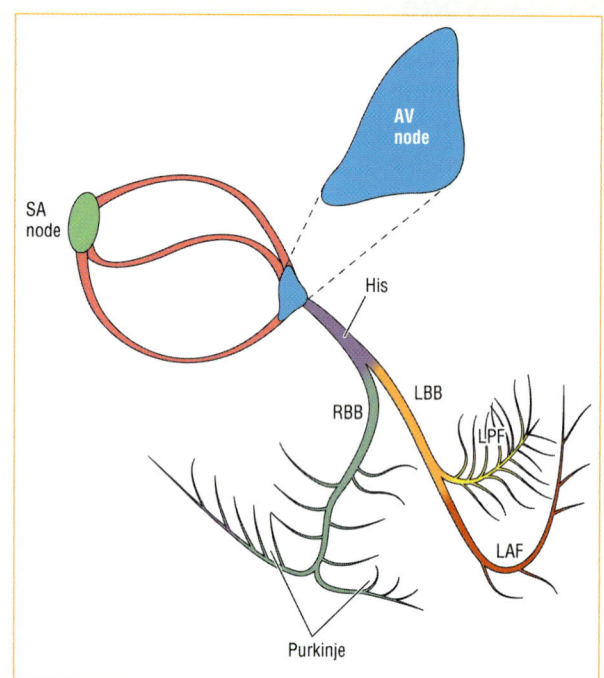

Figure 20-10 AV node.

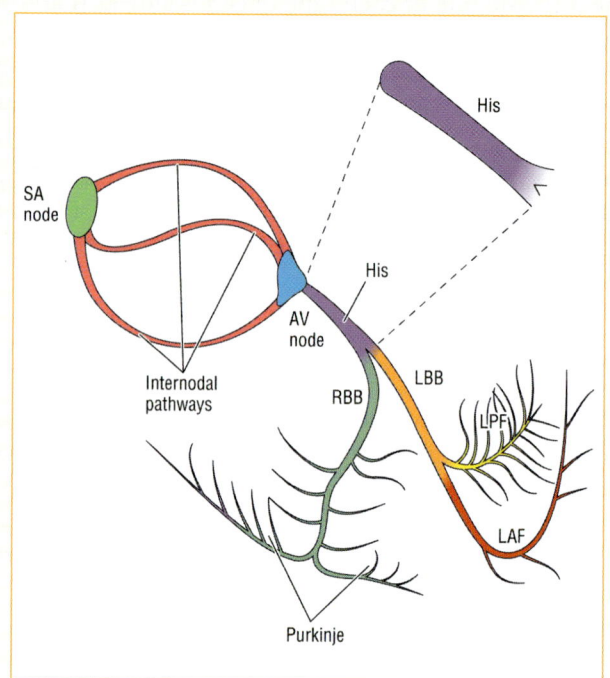

Figure 20-11 Bundle of His.

conduction from the atria to the ventricles just long enough for atrial contraction to occur. This slowing allows the atria to "overfill" the ventricles and helps maintain the output of the heart at a maximum level. The AV node is always supplied by the right coronary artery.

The Bundle of His

The bundle of His starts at the AV node and eventually gives rise to both the right and left bundle branches (Figure 20-11 ▶). It is found partially in the walls of the right atrium and in the interventricular septum. The bundle of His is the only route of communication between the atria and the ventricles.

The Left Bundle Branch (LBB)

The LBB begins at the end of the bundle of His and travels through the interventricular septum (Figure 20-12 ▶). The LBB gives rise to the fibers that will innervate the left ventricle and the left face of the interventricular septum. It first connects to a small set of fibers that innervate the upper segment of the interventricular septum. This will be the first area to depolarize, meaning that the heart's cells fire. The LBB ends at the beginning of the left anterior fascicle (LAF) and left posterior fascicle (LPF).

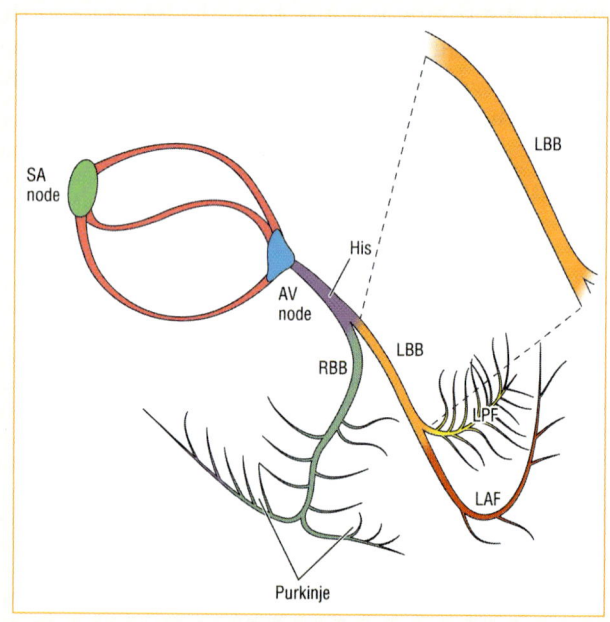

Figure 20-12 Left bundle branch.

The Right Bundle Branch (RBB)

The RBB, which starts at the bundle of His, gives rise to the fibers that will innervate the right ventricle and the right face of the interventricular septum (Figure 20-13 ▶). It terminates in the Purkinje fibers associated with it.

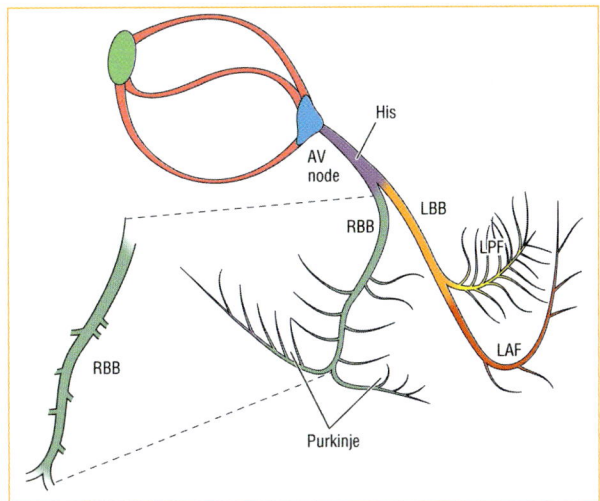

Figure 20-13 Right bundle branch.

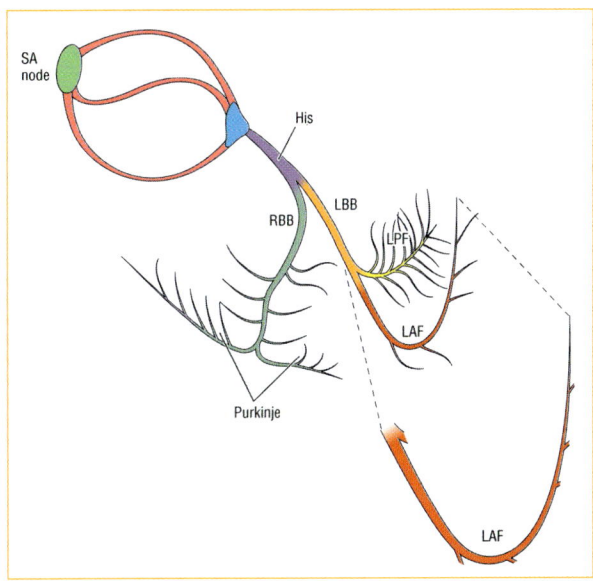

Figure 20-14 Left anterior fascicle.

The LAF

The LAF, also known as the left anterior superior fascicle, travels through the left ventricle to the Purkinje fibers that innervate the anterior and superior aspects of the left ventricle Figure 20-14 ▶. It is a single-stranded fascicle.

The LPF

The LPF is a fanlike structure leading to the Purkinje fibers that innervate the posterior and inferior aspects of the left ventricle Figure 20-15 ▶. It is very difficult to block this fascicle because it is so widely distributed, rather than being just one strand.

The Purkinje System

The Purkinje system is made up of individual cells just beneath the endocardium Figure 20-16 ▶. They are the cells that directly innervate the myocardial cells and initiate the ventricular depolarization cycle.

Special Electrical Properties of Cardiac Cells

The ability of cells to respond to electrical impulses is referred to as the property of excitability. The ability of the cells to conduct electrical impulses is referred to as the property of conductivity. Cardiac cells, unlike no other cells in the body, possess an ability to generate an impulse to contract even when there is no external nerve stimulus, a process called intrinsic automaticity.

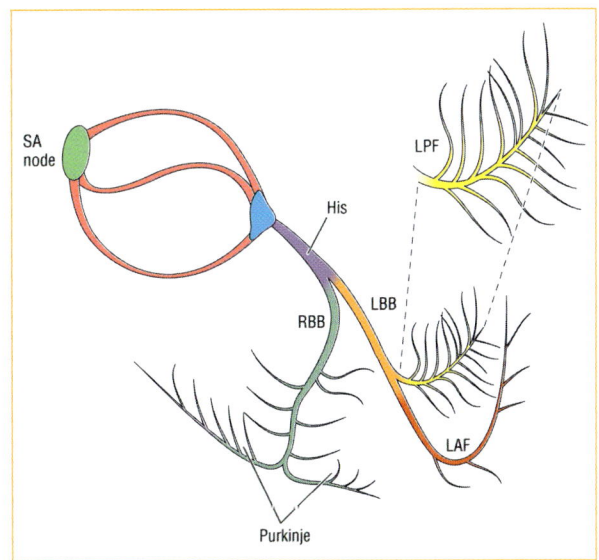

Figure 20-15 Left posterior fascicle.

Regulation of Heart Function

The heart's chronotropic state (control of the rate of contraction), dromotropic state (control of electrical conduction), and inotropic state (control of the strength of contraction) are provided by the brain, via the autonomic nervous system, the hormones of the endocrine system, and the heart tissue Table 20-2 ▶. Receptors in the blood vessels, kidneys, brain, and heart constantly monitor body functions to help maintain homeostasis. Baroreceptors respond to changes in pressure, usually within the heart or the main arteries. Chemoreceptors

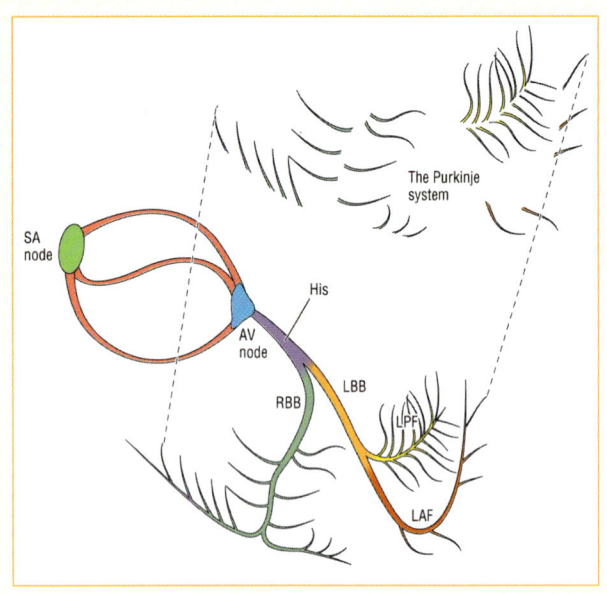

Figure 20-16 Purkinje system.

TABLE 20-2	Regulation of Heart Function

Chronotropic state refers to the heart's rate of contraction.
Dromotropic state refers to the heart's electrical conduction.
Inotropic state refers to the heart's strength of contraction.

sense changes in the chemical composition of the blood. If abnormalities are sensed, nerve signals are transmitted to the appropriate target organs, and hormones or neurotransmitters are released to correct the situation. Once conditions normalize, the receptors stop firing and the signals cease.

Often, stimulation of receptors causes activation of the parasympathetic or sympathetic branches of the autonomic nervous system, affecting both the heart rate and the strength of heart muscle contraction (contractility). Parasympathetic stimulation slows the heart rate, primarily by affecting the SA node. Sympathetic stimulation has two potential effects, alpha effects or beta effects, depending on which nerve receptor is stimulated (Figure 20-17 ▶). Alpha effects occur when alpha receptors are stimulated, resulting in vasoconstriction. Beta effects occur when beta receptors are stimulated, resulting in increased inotropic, dromotropic, and chronotropic states.

Epinephrine and norepinephrine are naturally occurring (endogenous) hormones that also may be given as cardiac drugs. Epinephrine has a greater stimulatory effect on beta receptors, and norepinephrine has predominant stimulatory actions on alpha receptors.

Electrolytes (Ions) and the Heart

Like all other cells in the body, myocardial cells are bathed in solutions of chemicals, or electrolytes (also called ions). Three positively charged ions, sodium (Na^+), potassium (K^+), and calcium (Ca^{++}), are responsible for initiating and conducting electrical signals in the heart. In the resting cell, the concentration of potassium is greater inside the cell, whereas the concentration of sodium is greater outside the cell. To maintain this difference, sodium is pumped out of the cell by a special ion-transporting mechanism called the sodium-potassium pump, and potassium is moved in. This process requires the expenditure of energy.

The Electrical Potential

The difference in sodium and potassium concentrations across a cell membrane at any given instant produces an electrical charge difference referred to as an electrical potential. An electrical potential is measured in millivolts. In a resting cell, the area outside the cell is more positively charged than the inside the cell. Hence, a negative electrical potential exists across the cell membrane. The resting cell normally has a net negative charge with respect to the outside of the cell. This is referred to as the polarized state (Figure 20-18 ▶).

Depolarization and Cardiac Contraction

When a myocardial cell receives a stimulus from the conduction system, the permeability of the cell wall changes and sodium rushes into the cell. This causes the inside of the cell to become more positive. Calcium also enters the cell, although its passage occurs more slowly. The resulting exchange of ions generates an electrical current. The rapid influx of sodium and the slow influx of calcium continue, causing the inside of the cell to continue to become more positively charged, eventually achieving a slightly positive electrical potential. The process of electrical discharge and flow of electrical activity is called depolarization (Figure 20-19 ▶).

The flow of electrical current is passed from cell to cell along the conduction pathway in a wavelike motion throughout the heart. As the myocardial cells are depolarized, calcium is released and comes into proximity with the actin and myosin filaments. This process causes

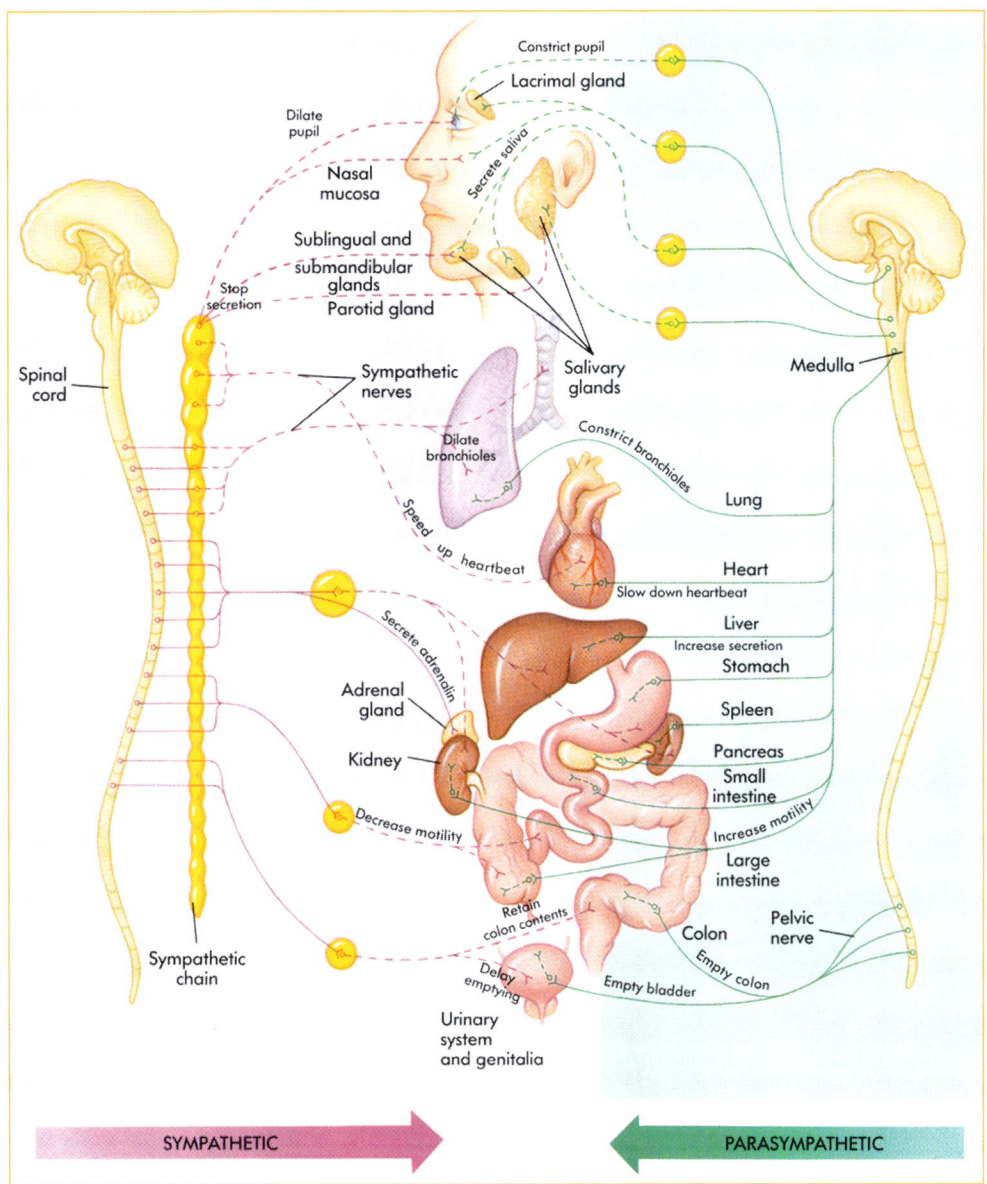

Figure 20-17 The autonomic receptors. Stimulation of the alpha receptors causes vasoconstriction of the organs they affect. Stimulation of beta receptors is split into beta-1, which causes increased heart rate and contractility, and beta-2, which causes bronchodilation.

the filaments to slide together, resulting in muscle contraction. Contraction of heart muscle squeezes blood out of the chambers. The combination of electrical stimulation and the resultant muscle contraction sometimes is referred to as excitation-contraction coupling.

Repolarization

Once the cardiac cells depolarize, they begin to return to their resting or polarized state, a process called repolarization (see Figure 20-19). At this time, the inside of the cell returns to its negative charge. Repolarization begins when the entry of sodium into the cells slows and positively charged potassium ions begin to flow out of the cells. Following the efflux of potassium, sodium is actively pumped out of the cells, and potassium is pumped back in. Calcium is returned to storage sites in the cells. As a result, the transmembrane potential returns to its baseline negative resting membrane potential and the cells regain their polarized state and resting length.

In the early phase of repolarization, the cell contains such a large concentration of ions that it cannot be stimulated to depolarize. This period is known as the absolute refractory period. In the latter phase of repolarization, the cells are able to respond to a stronger-than-normal stimulus. This period is known as the relative refractory period. It is important to note that if an electrical stimulus is strong enough, it could depolarize during the relative refractory period, potentially causing a life-threatening cardiac dysrhythmia.

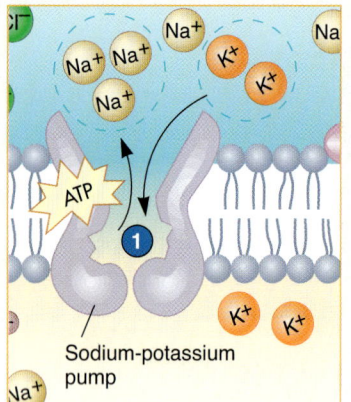
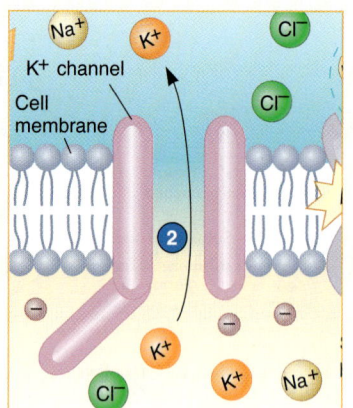
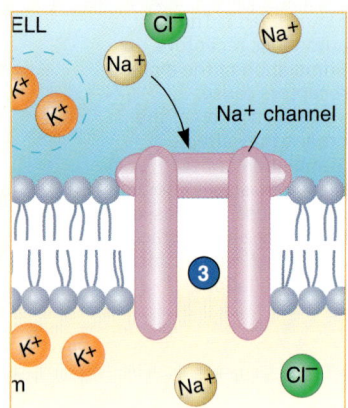
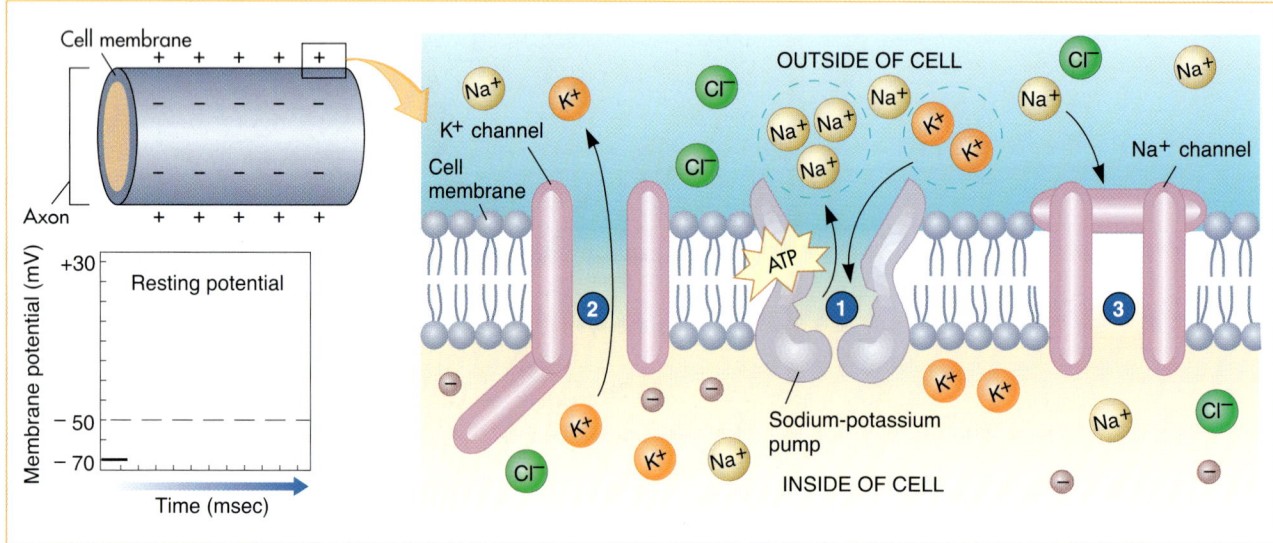

Figure 20-18 The difference in sodium and potassium concentrations across a cell membrane produces an electrical potential. During depolarization, sodium crosses the cell membrane through specific channels. Repolarization occurs with opening of potassium channels and through an ATP-dependent mechanism utilizing a sodium-potassium pump. The difference in charge across a cell membrane is the resting potential and is the basis for transmission of signals by nerves. ① indicates the sodium-potassium pump. ② indicates an open potassium channel. ③ indicates a closed sodium channel.

You are the Provider — Part 3

Your continued assessment of your patient reveals the following:

Vital Signs	Recording Time: 2 Minutes After Patient Contact
Respirations	24 breaths/min and labored
Pulse	72 beats/min and weak
Skin	Pale and diaphoretic
Blood pressure	112/68 mm Hg
Sao$_2$	90% while breathing room air

5. What are the causes of chest pain that you should consider in caring for this patient?

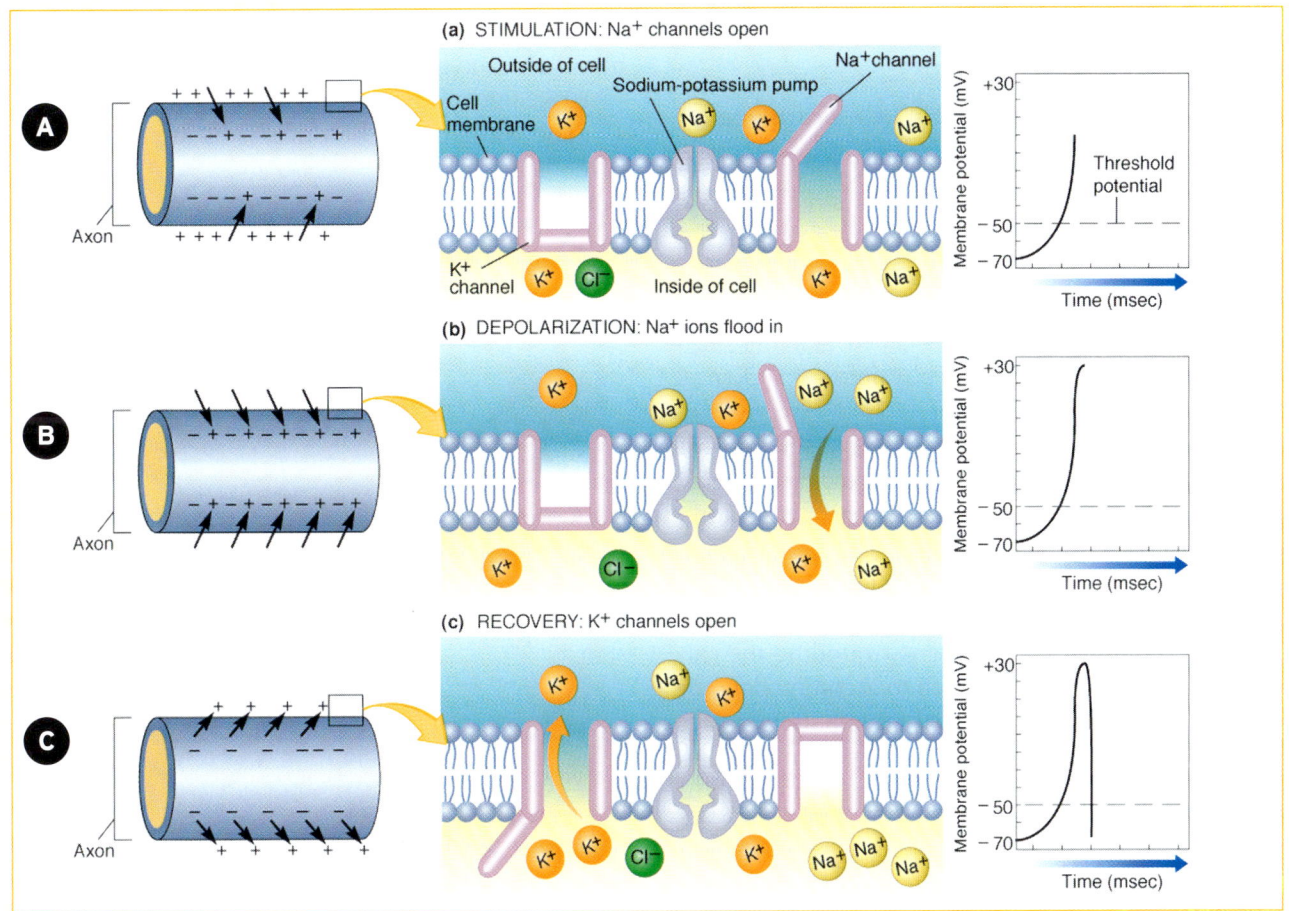

Figure 20-19 The action potential of the cell has three stages: **A.** Stimulation, **B.** Depolarization, and **C.** Recovery (repolarization, polarized state).

The Cardiac Cycle

The process that creates the pumping of the heart is known as the <u>cardiac cycle</u>. This cycle begins with myocardial contraction and concludes at the beginning of the next contraction. The heart's contraction results in pressure changes within the cardiac chambers, resulting in the movement of blood from areas of high pressure to areas of low pressure.

<u>Systole</u> is a term that refers to the contraction of the ventricular mass and the pumping of blood into the systemic circulation. During systole, a pressure is created within the arteries that can be recorded and is known as the systolic blood pressure. A normal systolic blood pressure in an adult is between 110 and 140 mm Hg. A pressure also exists in the vessels during <u>diastole</u>, the relaxation phase of the heart cycle, and is called the diastolic blood pressure. A normal diastolic blood pressure in an adult is between 70 and 90 mm Hg.

Blood pressure is noted as a fraction, and the systolic reading is placed above the diastolic reading (for example, a systolic reading of 140 and a diastolic reading of 70 would be noted as 140/70 mm Hg). The unit of measure mm Hg refers to millimeters of mercury and describes the height, in millimeters, to which the blood pressure elevates a column of liquid mercury in a glass tube. Although many blood pressure measurement devices now use dials, blood pressure is still described in millimeters of mercury.

The pressure in the aorta against which the left ventricle must pump blood is called the <u>afterload</u>. The greater the afterload, the harder it is for the ventricle to eject blood into the aorta, reducing the <u>stroke volume</u>, or the amount of blood ejected per contraction. To a large degree, afterload is governed by arterial blood pressure. Afterload is greater with vasoconstriction and less with vasodilation.

<u>Cardiac output</u> is the amount of blood pumped through the circulatory system in 1 minute. Cardiac

output is expressed in liters per minute (L/min). The cardiac output equals the heart rate multiplied by the stroke volume:

Cardiac Output = Stroke Volume × Heart Rate

Factors that influence the heart rate, the stroke volume, or both will affect cardiac output and, thus, oxygen delivery (<u>perfusion</u>) to the body's tissues.

Increased venous return to the heart stretches the ventricles to some extent, resulting in increased cardiac contractility. This relationship is called <u>Starling's law</u> of the heart, named after British physiologist Dr Ernest Henry Starling.

As discussed in Chapter 5, the heart has several ways of increasing stroke volume. According to Starling's law, the more cardiac muscle is stretched, the greater the force with which it contracts. If for any reason an increased volume of blood is returned from the systemic veins to the right side of the heart or from the pulmonary veins to the left side of the heart, the muscle surrounding the cardiac chambers will have to stretch to accommodate the larger volume. The more the cardiac muscle stretches, the greater will be the force of its contraction, the more completely it will empty, and, therefore, the greater will be the stroke volume. The amount of blood returning to the right atrium may vary somewhat from minute to minute, but the normal heart continues to pump out the same percentage of blood returned. This is called the <u>ejection fraction</u>. This allows the heart to function at the same capacity regardless of changes in the body's position or what the person is doing, whether sitting, moving, sneezing, or other activity.

The Blood Vessels

The General Scheme of Blood Circulation

Blood is transported through the body via the <u>arteries</u>, which carry blood away from the heart, and <u>veins</u>, which carry blood back to the heart. Arteries become smaller as they get farther from the heart. Eventually, they branch into many small arterioles that divide even further into <u>capillaries</u>, which are microscopic, thin-walled blood vessels. Oxygen and nutrients pass out of the capillaries into the cells, and carbon dioxide and waste products pass from the cells into the capillaries in a process called diffusion (Figure 20-20 ▶).

Once oxygenated blood has been delivered by the capillaries, deoxygenated blood is returned to the heart, starting from the capillaries. The capillaries eventually enlarge to form venules, which merge and form veins. Eventually the veins empty into the heart, where blood is reoxygenated and the process begins again (Figure 20-21 ▶).

The walls of the blood vessels are composed of three layers of tissue (Figure 20-22 ▶). The smooth, thin, inner lining is called the <u>tunica intima</u>, or endothe-

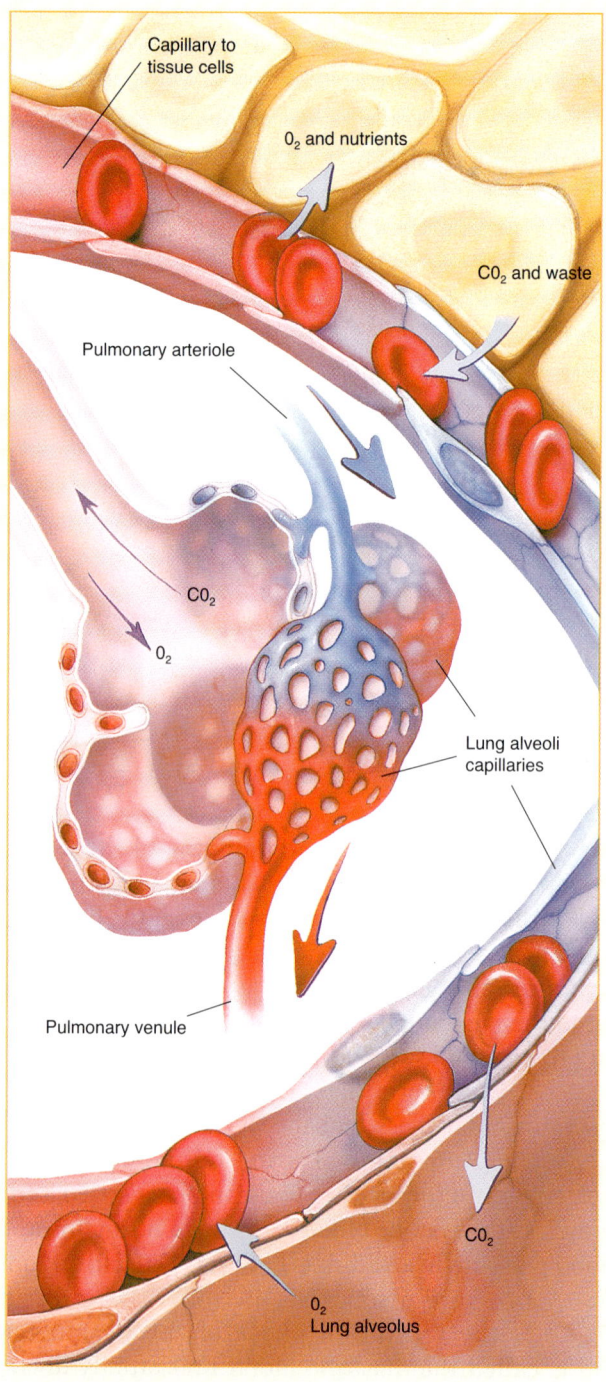

Figure 20-20 Diffusion. Oxygen and nutrients pass easily from the capillaries into the cells, and waste and carbon dioxide pass from the cells into the capillaries.

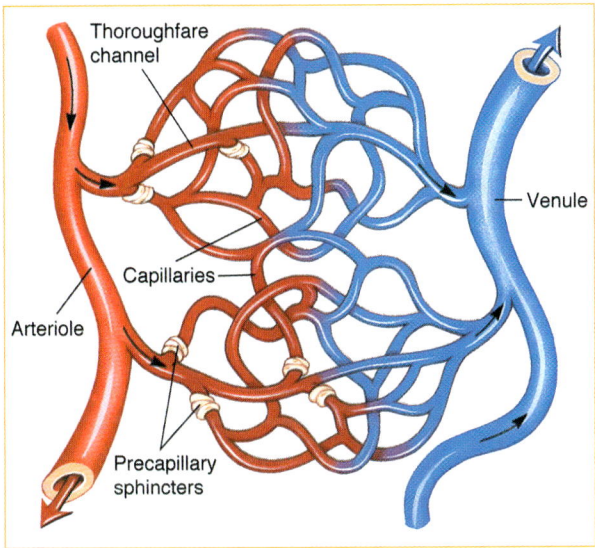

Figure 20-21 The scheme of circulation.

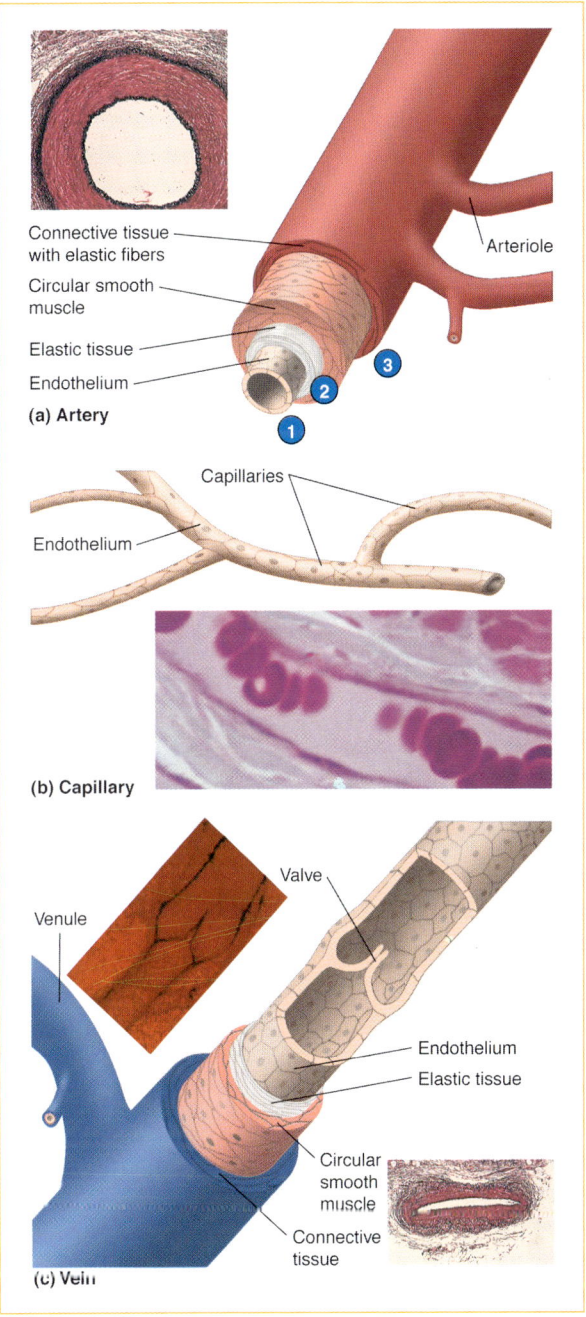

Figure 20-22 The walls of the blood vessels are composed of three layers of tissue: the endothelium, elastic tissue, and the connective tissue. **A.** Artery. **B.** Capillary. **C.** Vein.

lium. The middle layer, the <u>tunica media</u>, is composed of elastic tissue and smooth muscle cells that allow the vessels to expand or contract in response to the demands of the body. It is the thickest of the three tissue layers. The outer layer of tissue is called the <u>tunica adventitia</u> and consists of elastic and fibrous connective tissue.

Circulation to the Heart

The heart, like any other muscle, requires oxygen and nutrients. These are supplied via the <u>coronary arteries</u>, which arise from the aorta shortly after it leaves the left ventricle. The coronary circulation emanates from the left and right coronary arteries (Figure 20-23 ▶).

The right coronary artery divides into nine important branches: the conus branch, sinus node branch, right ventricular branch, atrial branch, acute marginal branch, atrioventricular node branch, posterior descending branch, left ventricular branch, and left atrial branch. Not all branches are always present in all people. These branches supply blood to the walls of the right atrium and ventricle, a portion of the inferior part of the left ventricle, and portions of the conduction system (the SA and AV nodes). When vessels to the conduction system fail to arise from the right coronary artery, they originate from the left side instead.

The left main coronary artery is the largest and shortest of the myocardial blood vessels. It rapidly divides into two branches, the <u>left anterior descending (LAD) artery</u> and the <u>circumflex coronary artery</u>. These arteries subdivide further, supplying blood to most of the left ventricle, the interventricular septum, and, at times, the AV node.

<u>Arteriosclerosis</u> is characterized by thickening of the arterial walls, which causes a loss of elasticity (thus, the term "hardening of the arteries") with a concomitant reduction in blood flow. Atherosclerosis is a type of arteriosclerosis in which plaque (made up of cholesterol and fatty substances) forms in the arteries, and

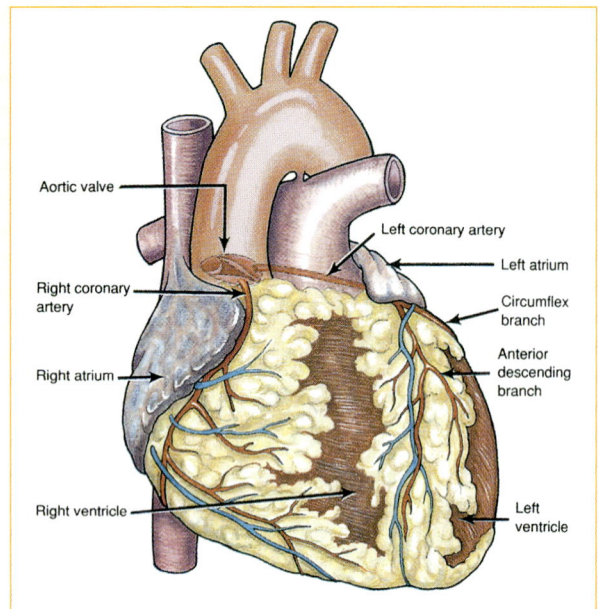

Figure 20-23 The coronary arteries supply oxygen and nutrients to the heart.

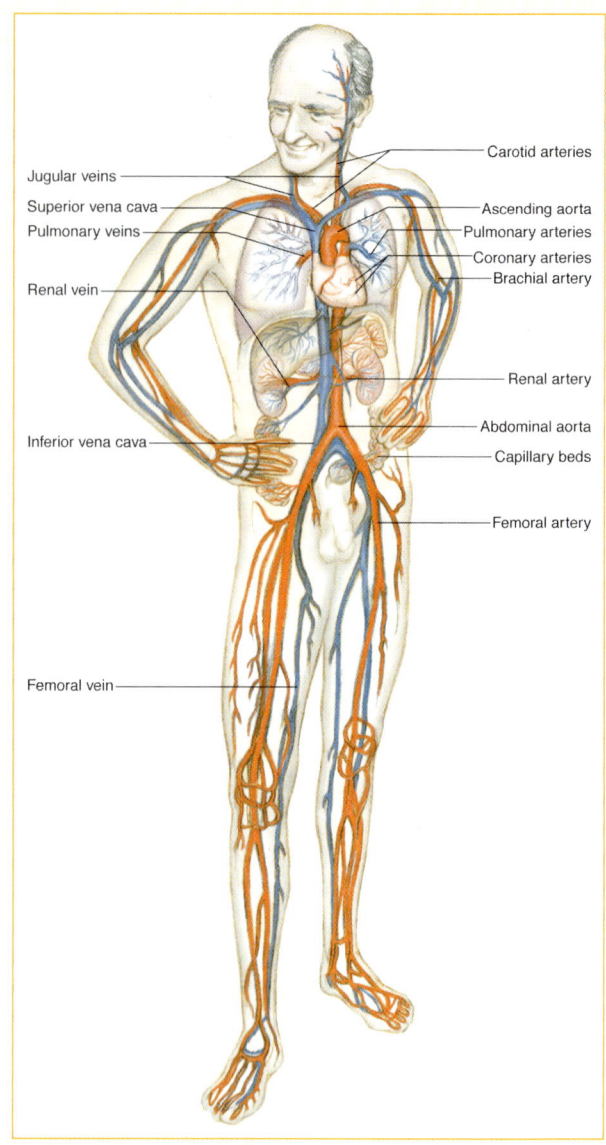

Figure 20-24 The cardiovascular system. The systemic arterial circulation is noted in red, and the systemic venous system is noted in blue.

the resulting condition is referred to as coronary artery disease (CAD).

The Pulmonary Circulation

Within the body, the pulmonary circulation carries blood from the right side of the heart to the lungs and back to the left side of the heart, and the systemic circulation is responsible for blood flow to the rest of the body. Deoxygenated blood from the right ventricle is pumped through the pulmonic valve into the pulmonary artery. This artery rapidly divides into the right and left pulmonary arteries. These arteries transport the blood to the lungs. Inside the lungs, the arteries branch, becoming smaller and smaller. At the level of the capillary, waste products are exchanged and the blood is reoxygenated. The reoxygenated blood travels through venules into the pulmonary veins. The four pulmonary veins empty into the left atrium, two from each lung (see Figure 20-3).

Systemic Arterial Circulation

Oxygenated blood leaves the heart through the aortic valve and passes into the aorta. From the aorta, blood is distributed to all parts of the body. All arteries of the body are derived from the aorta. The aorta is divided into three portions: the ascending aorta, the aortic arch, and the descending aorta.

The ascending aorta arises from the left ventricle and consists of only two branches, the right and left main coronary arteries (Figure 20-24 ▲). The aorta then arches posteriorly and to the left, forming the aortic arch. Three major arteries arise from the aortic arch: the brachiocephalic (innominate) artery, the left common carotid artery, and the left subclavian artery.

The descending aorta is the longest portion of the aorta and is subdivided into the thoracic aorta and the abdominal aorta. The descending aorta extends through the thorax and abdomen into the pelvis. In the pelvis, the descending aorta divides into the two common iliac arteries, which further divide into the internal and external iliac arteries.

Venous Return

Blood returns to the heart through the systemic venous system. The superior vena cava is the principal vein draining blood from the upper portion of the body. It is formed by the junction of the right and left brachiocephalic veins and empties into the right atrium. The inferior vena cava is the principal vein draining blood from the lower portion of the body. It is formed by the junction of the two common iliac veins and terminates in the right atrium.

Atherosclerosis

Most often, diminished blood flow to the myocardium is caused by coronary artery atherosclerosis. Atherosclerosis is a disorder in which a fatty material called cholesterol and other fatty substances build up and form a plaque inside the walls of blood vessels, obstructing flow and interfering with their ability to dilate or contract Figure 20-25 ▼. Eventually, atherosclerosis can cause complete occlusion, or blockage, of a coronary artery. Atherosclerosis usually involves other arteries of the body, as well.

The problem begins when the first deposit of cholesterol is laid down on the inside of an artery. This may happen during the teenage years. As a person ages, more of this fatty material is deposited; the lumen, or the inside diameter of the artery, narrows. As the cholesterol deposits grow, calcium deposits can form as well. The inner wall of the artery, which is normally smooth and elastic, becomes rough and brittle with these atherosclerotic plaques. Damage to the coronary arteries may become so extensive that they cannot accommodate increased blood flow at times of increased need.

For reasons that are still not completely understood, a brittle plaque will sometimes develop a crack, exposing the inside of the atherosclerotic wall. Acting like a torn blood vessel, the jagged edge of the crack activates the blood-clotting system, just as it does when an injury has caused bleeding. In this situation, however, the resulting blood clot will partially or completely block the lumen of the artery. Tissues downstream from the blood clot will experience a lack of oxygen (ischemia). If blood flow is resumed in a short time, the ischemic tissues will recover. However, if too much time goes by before blood flow is resumed, the tissues will die (undergo necrosis). This sequence of events results in an acute myocardial infarction (AMI), a classic heart attack Figure 20-26 ▼. Infarction means the death of tissue. The same sequence may also cause the death of cells in other organs, such as the brain. The death of heart muscle can lead to severe diminishment of the heart's ability to pump or to cardiac arrest.

In the United States, CAD is the number one cause of death for men and women. The peak incidence of heart disease occurs between the ages of 40 and 70 years, but it can also strike teens and individuals in their 90s. You must be alert to the possibility that, although less likely, a 26-year-old person with chest pain could actually be having a heart attack, especially if he or she has a higher than usual risk.

Factors that place a person at higher risk for a myocardial infarction are called risk factors. The major

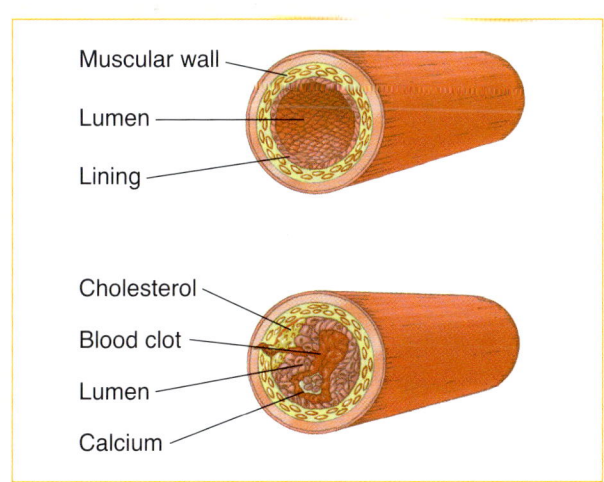

Figure 20-25 In atherosclerosis, cholesterol and other fatty substances build up inside the walls of the blood vessels, causing an obstruction in blood flow to the heart.

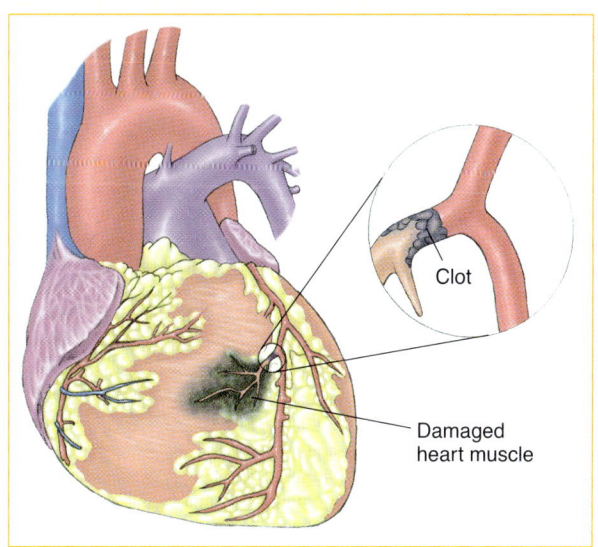

Figure 20-26 An acute myocardial infarction occurs when a blood clot prevents blood flow to an area of the heart muscle. If left untreated, this can result in death of heart tissue.

controllable factors are cigarette smoking, high blood pressure, elevated cholesterol levels, an elevated blood sugar level (diabetes), lack of exercise, and stress. The major risk factors that cannot be controlled are older age, family history of atherosclerotic CAD, and male sex.

> **EMT-I Tips**
>
> Various changes in the walls of coronary arteries can result in certain disease states. Atherosclerosis is a disorder characterized by the formation of plaques of material, mostly lipids and cholesterol, on the intima of the artery (Figure 20-27 ▼). This process gradually narrows the lumen (opening or hollow part of the artery), resulting in a reduction in arterial blood flow.

Angina Pectoris

Chest pain does not always mean that a person is having an AMI. When, for a brief period, heart tissues are not getting enough oxygen (ischemia), the pain is called angina pectoris, or angina. It is defined as a brief discomfort that has predictable characteristics and is relieved promptly. There is no change in the heart rhythm pattern with angina. Although it can result from a spasm of the artery, angina is most often a symptom of atherosclerotic CAD. Angina occurs when the heart's need for oxygen exceeds its supply, usually during periods of physical or emotional stress when the heart is working hard. A large meal or sudden fear may also trigger an attack. When the increased oxygen demand goes away (for example, the person stops exercising), the pain typically goes away.

Angina pain is typically described as crushing, squeezing, or "like somebody standing on my chest." It is usually felt in the midchest, under the sternum. However, it can radiate to the jaw, the arms (frequently the left arm), the midback, or the epigastrium (the upper-middle region of the abdomen). The pain usually lasts from 3 to 8 minutes, rarely longer than 15 minutes. It may be associated with shortness of breath, nausea, or sweating. It disappears promptly with rest, supplemental oxygen, or nitroglycerin, all of which increase the supply of oxygen to the heart. Although angina pectoris is frightening, it does not mean that heart cells are dying, nor does it usually lead to death or permanent heart damage. It is, however, a warning that you and the patient should both take seriously. A single episode may be a precursor to a myocardial infarction. Even with angina, because oxygen supply to the heart is diminished, the electrical system can be compromised and the person is at risk for significant cardiac rhythm problems. Even though chest pain may dissipate, myocardial ischemia and injury can continue.

The first episode of angina is called initial angina. Angina is generally classified as stable or unstable. Stable angina occurs at a relatively fixed frequency and is

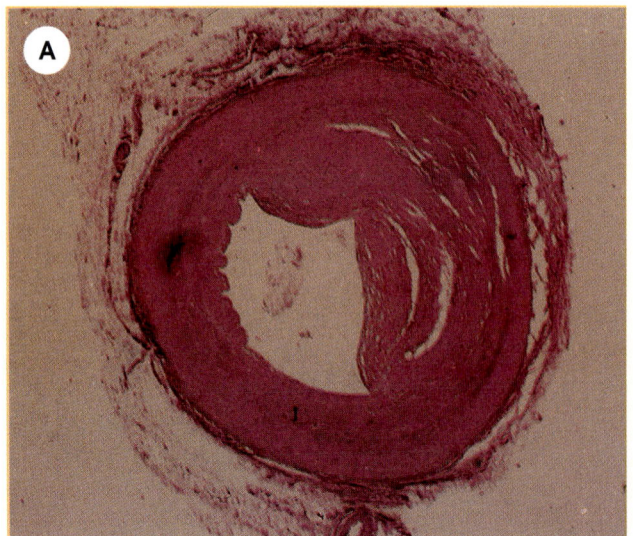
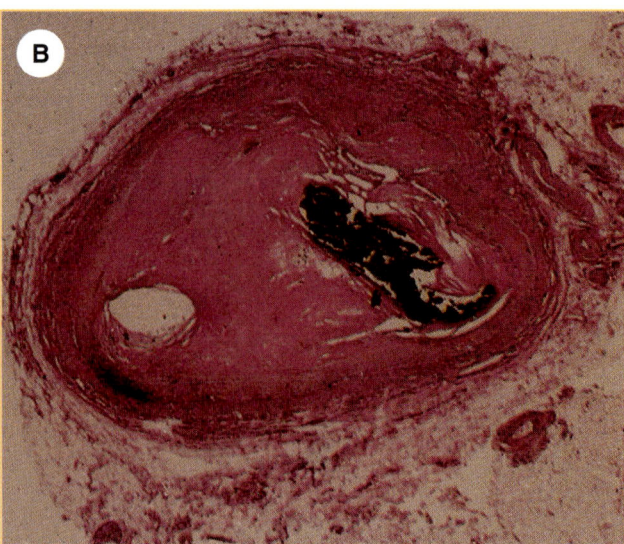

Figure 20-27 The formation of a plaque. **A.** The coronary artery exhibits severe atherosclerosis, and much of the passage of blood is blocked by buildup of cholesterol and other lipids on the intima of the artery, forming masses or plaques. **B.** The coronary artery is almost completely blocked. A blood clot blocks blood flow on the right side of the artery.

usually relieved by rest and/or medication. Unstable angina occurs without a fixed frequency and may or may not be relieved by rest and/or medication. Progressive angina is stable or unstable angina that is accelerating in frequency and duration. Preinfarction angina presents with pain that occurs at rest when the patient is sitting or lying down.

Keep in mind that it can be very difficult even for physicians in hospitals to distinguish between the pain of angina and the pain of a myocardial infarction. Table 20-3 ▶ lists possible causes of chest pain other than angina or a myocardial infarction.

Acute Myocardial Infarction

As we have seen, the pain of AMI signals the actual death of cells in the area of the heart where blood flow is obstructed. Once dead, the cells cannot be revived. Instead, they will eventually turn to scar tissue and become a burden to the beating heart. This is why fast action is so critical in treating a heart attack. The sooner the blockage can be cleared, the fewer the cells that may die. About 30 minutes after blood flow is cut off, some heart muscle cells begin to die. After about two hours, as many as half of the cells in the area can be dead; in most cases, after 4 to 6 hours, more than 90% of them will be dead. However, studies show that in many cases, opening the coronary artery with "clot-busting" medications, a class of medications called fibrinolytics, can prevent or minimize damage to the heart muscle if administered no later than 12 hours after the onset of symptoms. Angioplasty (mechanical clearing of the artery) can also prevent or minimize damage to the heart if performed promptly. Therefore, immediate treatment and transport to the emergency department is essential.

An AMI is more apt to occur in the larger, thick-walled left ventricle, which needs more blood and oxygen, than in the right ventricle.

Initial Assessment Findings

The pain of an AMI differs from the pain of angina in three ways:

- **It may or may not be caused by exertion** but can occur at any time, sometimes when a person is sitting quietly or even sleeping.

TABLE 20-3 | Other Possible Causes of Chest Pain

- Cholecystitis
- Aortic dissection or aneurysm
- Hiatal hernia
- Pleurisy
- Esophageal and gastrointestinal diseases
- Pulmonary embolism
- Pancreatitis
- Respiratory infections
- Pneumothorax
- Herpes zoster (shingles)
- Chest wall tumors
- Blunt trauma

You are the Provider — Part 4

You gave your patient 100% oxygen via nonrebreathing mask, applied a cardiac monitor, and initiated an intravenous (IV) line with normal saline to keep the vein open. You are preparing to transport, and your reassessment reveals the following:

Reassessment	Recording Time: 5 Minutes After Patient Contact
Respirations	24 breaths/min and labored
Pulse	72 beats/min and weak
Skin	Remains pale and diaphoretic
Blood pressure	112/68 mm Hg
Sao_2	96% with 100% O_2 via nonrebreathing mask

6. The pain of an AMI differs from the pain of angina in three ways. What are they?
7. What are three serious consequences of an AMI?

- **It does not resolve in a few minutes**; rather, it can last between 30 minutes and several hours.
- **It may or may not be relieved** by rest or nitroglycerin.

The most pertinent findings may vary from patient to patient. For example, while chest pain is a common finding of a patient experiencing an acute myocardial infarction, not all patients who are having an AMI experience pain or recognize it when it occurs. In fact, about a third of patients never seek medical attention. This can be attributed, in part, to the fact that people are afraid of dying and do not wish to face the possibility that their symptoms may be serious (cardiac denial). Middle-aged men, in particular, are likely to minimize their symptoms. However, a few patients, particularly elderly individuals and those with diabetes, do not experience any pain during an AMI. Others may feel only mild discomfort and may think it is "indigestion," or it may be referred to as "chest pressure."

Patients may present with anxiety or restlessness, near syncopal episodes, fatigue, or vertigo. Labored breathing may or may not be present. Rhythm and quality of peripheral pulses along with changes in skin color, temperature, and moisture are significant signs when treating a potential cardiac patient. Alterations in heart rate and rhythm may occur, although peripheral pulses are usually not affected. Blood pressure may be elevated during the episode and normalize afterwards.

Monitor the patient's ECG tracing. Note any abnormal cardiac rhythms, and, based on the patient's clinical presentation, treat per standard ACLS or local protocols.

Therefore, when you are called to a scene where the chief complaint is chest pain, complete a thorough assessment, no matter what the patient says. Ask the patient about recurring events along with any increase in frequency and/or duration of an event. Determine whether the patient has taken nitroglycerin, aspirin, or any other medications before your arrival. Any complaint of chest pain or discomfort or other symptoms suggestive of a cardiac etiology is a serious matter. In fact, the best thing you can do is to assume the worst.

It is imperative that you recognize a sense of urgency for reperfusion when the patient receives no relief with medications or presents with hypotension or signs of hypoperfusion. Provide emotional support for the patient and an explanation for the family or significant others.

Consequences of AMI

An AMI can have three serious consequences:
- Sudden death
- Cardiogenic shock
- Congestive heart failure

Sudden Death

Approximately 40% of all patients with AMI never reach the hospital. Sudden death is usually the result of cardiac arrest, in which the heart fails to generate an effective blood flow. Although you cannot feel a pulse in someone experiencing cardiac arrest, there may still be electrical activity, though chaotic. The heart is using up energy without pumping. Such an abnormality of heart rhythm is a ventricular dysrhythmia (also called an arrhythmia), known as ventricular fibrillation.

A variety of other lethal and nonlethal arrhythmias may follow AMI, usually within the first hour. In most cases, it is premature ventricular contractions (PVCs), or extra beats from the damaged ventricle. PVCs by themselves are harmless and are common among healthy people, as well as in sick individuals. Other dysrhythmias are much more dangerous (Figure 20-28 ▶). These include the following:

- Sinus tachycardia: Rapid beating of the heart, 100 beats/min or more.
- Sinus bradycardia: Unusually slow beating of the heart, 60 beats/min or fewer.
- Ventricular tachycardia (VT or V-tach): Rapid heart rhythm, usually at a rate of 150 to 200 beats/min. The electrical activity starts in the ventricle instead of the atrium. This rhythm usually does not allow adequate time between beats for the left ventricle to fill with blood. Therefore, the patient's blood pressure may fall. He or she may also feel weak or lightheaded or may even become unresponsive. In some cases, the patient may develop worsening chest pain or chest pain that was not there before onset of the dysrhythmia. A string of three or more PVCs, back to back, can be called a "run of V-tach." Most cases of VT will be more sustained and may deteriorate into ventricular fibrillation.
- Ventricular fibrillation (VF or V-fib): Disorganized, ineffective quivering of the ventricles due

Documentation Tips

Documenting exactly how a patient describes chest discomfort, in the patient's own words, is a valuable source of information for hospital staff. Remember—OPQRST (Onset, Provocation/Palliation, Quality, Radiation/Referred, Severity, Time).

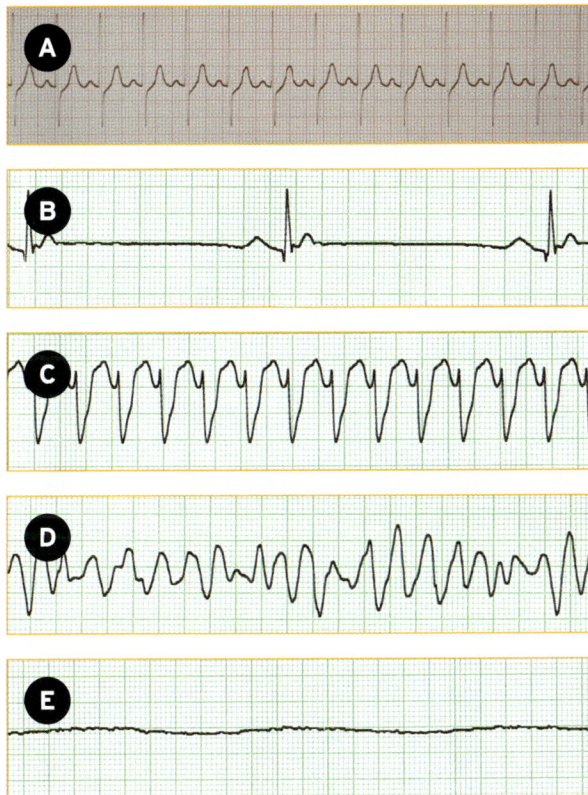

Figure 20-28 Common cardiac arrhythmias. **A.** Sinus tachycardia. **B.** Sinus bradycardia. **C.** Ventricular tachycardia (VT). **D.** Ventricular fibrillation (VF). **E.** Asystole.

to unorganized electrical activity. No blood gets to the body, and the patient usually becomes unresponsive within seconds. The only way to treat this dysrhythmia is to electrically defibrillate the heart. To **defibrillate** means to shock the heart with a specialized electrical current to stop all electrical activity in an attempt to restore a normal, rhythmic beat. By stopping the dysrhythmia, it gives the conduction system the chance to resume its normal activity. Defibrillation is highly successful in terms of saving a life if delivered within a minute or two. If a defibrillator is not immediately available, CPR must be initiated to buy a few more minutes for arrival of an automatic external defibrillator (AED) or manual defibrillator. Even if CPR is begun right at the time of collapse, chances of survival diminish each minute until defibrillation is accomplished.

If uncorrected, unstable ventricular tachycardia or ventricular fibrillation will eventually lead to **asystole**, the absence of all cardiac electrical and mechanical activity. Without CPR, this may occur within minutes. Because it reflects a long period of ischemia, nearly all patients you find in asystole will die.

Cardiogenic Shock

Shock is a simple concept but one that few people without medical training really understand. For that reason, Chapter 13 provides a more in-depth discussion of shock. The discussion of shock in this chapter is limited to that associated with cardiac problems.

For an EMT-I, shock is also a critical concept. Shock is present when body tissues do not get enough oxygen, causing body organs to malfunction. In **cardiogenic shock**, often caused by a myocardial infarction, the problem is that the heart lacks enough power to force the proper volume of blood through the circulatory system. Cardiogenic shock (also known as pump failure) can occur immediately or as late as 24 hours after the onset of an AMI. The improper functioning of the body's organs produces the various signs and symptoms of cardiogenic shock. The challenge for you is to recognize shock in its early stages, when treatment is likely to be more successful.

Cardiogenic shock may be differentiated from hypovolemic shock by one or more of the following:

- Chief complaint (chest pain, dyspnea, tachycardia)
- Heart rate (bradycardia or excessive tachycardia)
- Signs and symptoms of congestive heart failure
- Dysrhythmias

A patient with suspected cardiogenic shock should receive the same initial evaluation and treatment as any patient complaining of chest pain. Pay particular attention to respiratory effort and the presence of peripheral or pulmonary edema. It is imperative to recognize the urgency of transport and to make sure the patient is taken to the closest, most appropriate facility.

Patients with signs of cardiogenic shock may benefit from the use of inotropic drugs and antiarrhythmics as indicated. Follow local protocols, and contact medical control for direction.

Signs and Symptoms of Cardiogenic Shock

- One of the first signs of shock is anxiety or restlessness as the brain becomes relatively starved for oxygen. The patient may complain of "air hunger." Think of the possibility of shock when the patient is yelling, "I can't breathe." Obviously, the patient can breathe because he or she can talk. However, the patient's brain is sensing that it is not getting enough oxygen.
- As the shock continues, the body shunts blood to the most important organs, such as the brain

Skill Drill 20-1

Treating Cardiogenic Shock

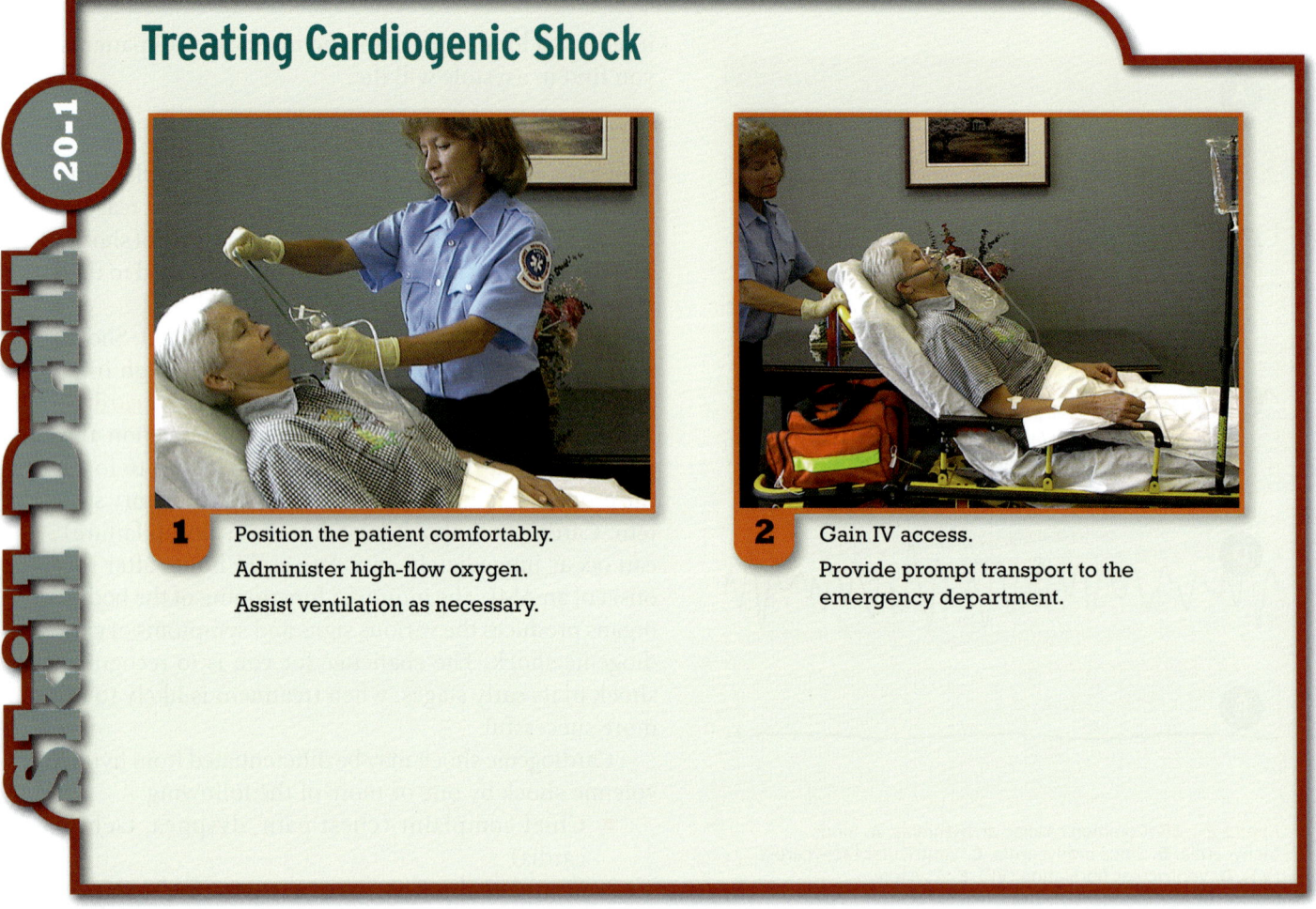

1. Position the patient comfortably. Administer high-flow oxygen. Assist ventilation as necessary.
2. Gain IV access. Provide prompt transport to the emergency department.

and heart, and away from less important organs, such as the skin. Therefore, you may see pale, clammy skin in patients with shock.

- As the shock gets worse, the body will attempt to compensate by increasing the amount of blood pumped through the heart. Therefore, the pulse rate will be higher than normal. In severe shock, the heart rate will usually, but not always, be more than 120 beats/min.
- Shock can also be characterized by rapid and shallow breathing, nausea and vomiting, and a decrease in body temperature.
- Finally, as the heart and other organs begin to malfunction, the blood pressure will fall below normal. A systolic blood pressure less than 90 mm Hg is easy to recognize, but it is a late finding that indicates decompensated shock. Do not assume that shock is not present just because the blood pressure is normal (compensated shock).

Treatment of Patients With Cardiogenic Shock. Follow the steps in Skill Drill 20-1 when treating patients with signs and symptoms of shock:

1. **Position the patient comfortably**. Most patients with heart failure will be more comfortable in the semi-Fowler's position; however, those with low blood pressure may not tolerate a semiupright position. These patients may be more comfortable and more alert in a supine position.
2. **Administer high-flow oxygen**.
3. **Assist ventilations as necessary** (**Step 1**).
4. Gain IV access, and give a fluid bolus of 20 mL/kg of an isotonic crystalloid solution if the patient is hypotensive.
5. **Provide prompt transport to the emergency department** (**Step 2**).

Consider pharmacologic interventions as dictated by local protocol. This may include dopamine, an inotropic drug, which increases myocardial contractility and may improve perfusion.

Congestive Heart Failure

Failure of the heart occurs when the ventricular myocardium is so damaged that it can no longer keep up with the return flow of blood from the atria. <u>Congestive heart failure (CHF)</u> can occur any time after a myocardial infarction, heart valve damage, or longstanding high blood pressure, but it usually happens between the first few hours and the first few days after an AMI.

Just as the pumping function of the left ventricle can be damaged by an AMI, diseased heart valves or chronic hypertension can also damage it. In any of these cases, when the myocardium can no longer contract effectively, the heart tries other ways to maintain an adequate cardiac output. Two specific changes in heart function occur: the heart rate increases, and the left ventricle enlarges in an effort to increase the amount of blood pumped each minute.

When these adaptations can no longer make up for the decreased heart function, CHF eventually develops. It is called "congestive" heart failure because the lungs become congested with fluid once the heart fails to pump the blood effectively. Blood tends to back up in the pulmonary veins, increasing the pressure in the capillaries of the lungs. When the pressure in the capillaries exceeds a certain level, fluid (mostly water) passes through the walls of the capillary vessels and into the alveoli. This condition is called pulmonary edema. It may occur suddenly, as in an AMI, or slowly over months, as in chronic CHF. Sometimes, patients with an acute onset of CHF will develop severe pulmonary edema, in which pink, frothy sputum and severe dyspnea are present.

Fluid also collects elsewhere in the body, usually in the feet and legs. This is called <u>pedal edema</u>. The swelling causes relatively few symptoms other than discomfort. However, chronic pedal edema may indicate underlying heart disease (right-sided heart failure) even in the absence of pain or other symptoms.

Signs and Symptoms of CHF. Watch for the following signs and symptoms in a patient you suspect has CHF:

- The patient finds it easier to breathe when sitting up. When the patient is lying down, more blood is returned to the right ventricle and lungs, causing further pulmonary congestion and shortness of breath.
- Often, the patient is mildly or severely agitated.
- Chest pain may or may not be present.
- The patient often has distended neck veins that do not collapse even when the patient is sitting at a 45° angle.
- The patient may have swollen ankles from pedal edema. If the patient is bedridden, the edema may be seen in the sacral area.
- The patient generally will have hypertension, tachycardia, and tachypnea.
- The patient will usually be using accessory breathing muscles of the neck and ribs, reflecting the additional hard work of breathing.
- The fluid surrounding small airways may produce rales, best heard by listening to either side of the patient's chest, about midway down the back. In severe CHF, these soft sounds can be heard even at the top (apex) of the lung.
- The patient may have a productive cough, or you may note the presence of pink, frothy sputum.
- The patient may have delayed capillary refill time. With damage to the myocardium, the pumping mechanism is effectively reduced; therefore, there is a lack of perfusion in the extremities, causing delayed capillary refill time.

Once CHF develops, it can be treated but not cured. Regular use of medications may alleviate the symptoms. However, these patients often become ill again and are frequently hospitalized. Approximately half will be dead within 5 years of the onset of symptoms.

Treatment of CHF. Treat a patient with CHF the same way as you would a patient with chest pain. Follow the steps in (Skill Drill 20-2 ▶):

1. **Take the vital signs, monitor heart rhythm, and give oxygen** by nonrebreathing face mask with an oxygen flow of 12 to 15 L/min. Assist ventilations as needed (**Step 1**).
2. **Allow the patient to remain sitting in an upright position with the legs down.**
3. **Gain IV access.** Before giving any medication, you need to gain IV access. You may also give fluid if the patient becomes hypotensive.
4. **Be reassuring;** many patients with CHF are quite anxious because they cannot breathe.
5. Patients who have had problems with CHF before will usually have specific medications for its treatment. **Gather these medications and take them along to the hospital.**
6. Nitroglycerin may be of value if the patient's systolic blood pressure is above 90 mm Hg. **If the patient has prescribed nitroglycerin, and medical control advises you to do so, you can administer it sublingually** (**Step 2**).
7. Prompt transport to the emergency department is essential.

Skill Drill 20-2

Treating CHF

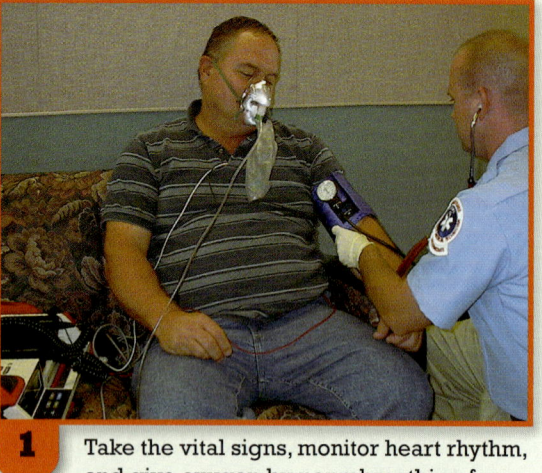

1. Take the vital signs, monitor heart rhythm, and give oxygen by nonrebreathing face mask.

Allow the patient to remain sitting in an upright position with the legs down.

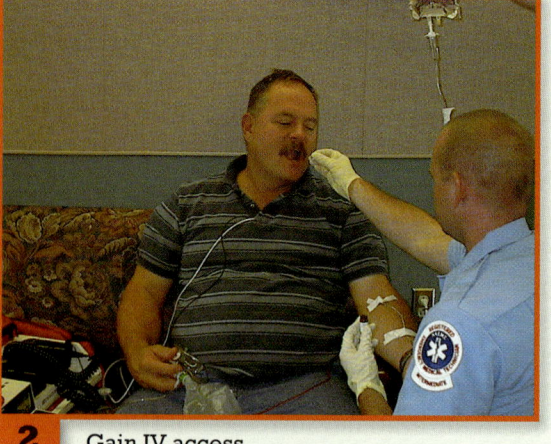

2. Gain IV access.

Reassure the patient.

Gather all medications, and take them along to the hospital.

If the patient has prescribed nitroglycerin, and medical control advises you to do so, you can administer it sublingually.

Consider the use of furosemide (Lasix) and morphine in conjunction with oxygen and nitroglycerin. Follow local protocols, and contact medical control for direction.

Pulmonary Edema

As stated earlier, pulmonary edema is a common complication of myocardial ischemia that may or may not be the result of an AMI. Without treatment, pulmonary edema can lead to acute respiratory failure and death. Precipitating causes include heart failure (left-sided and/or right-sided), myocardial infarction, pulmonary embolism, hypertension, and cardiomegaly (enlarged heart).

Preload and afterload can greatly influence the buildup of pulmonary edema. Preload is pressure on the ventricles at the end of the resting phase of the heart. It is influenced by blood returned to the heart from the body, the total volume of blood in the body, the distribution of the blood throughout the body, and the action of the atria. Afterload is the resistance the heart must pump against, or the systemic vascular resistance. As the left ventricle loses its ability to pump effectively, blood backs up into the pulmonary veins and, subsequently, into the lungs. This increased pressure causes fluid to leak from the capillaries into the interstitial tissue and the alveoli. This is common in CHF as the loss of contractile ability results in fluid overload. Pulmonary edema may be acute, as the result of an AMI, or may be chronic as a result of multiple events or chronic CHF.

Treatment is focused on maintaining ABCs and transporting the patient for definitive care. Obtain a thorough history from the patient, and provide psychological support en route. Administer 100% oxygen and be prepared to assist ventilations.

Hypertensive Emergencies

A hypertensive crisis exists when there is a severe elevation in diastolic blood pressure above 120 to 130 mm Hg. This is considered to be an emergency if there is evidence of rapid or progressive central nervous system, myocardial, hematologic, or renal deterioration. Blood pressure must be reduced without delay to prevent permanent damage or death.

Patients experiencing a hypertensive emergency typically have a history of hypertension and might not be taking their medications as prescribed. Toxemia of pregnancy (preeclampsia) is another precipitating cause. Continued hypertension can lead to hypertensive encephalopathy and/or stroke.

Initial assessment should focus on ABCs and obtaining a complete medical history, including compliance with medication prescriptions. Consider the general appearance of the patient along with the level of consciousness. Note the presence of any airway, breathing, or circulation compromise, and treat appropriately. Also pay attention to the signs that may directly relate to hypertension, such as vertigo, epistaxis, tinnitus (ringing in the ears), changes in visual acuity, nausea, vomiting, and/or seizures. A systolic blood pressure greater than 160 mm Hg or a diastolic pressure greater than 90 mm Hg is cause for concern and may require treatment.

Place the patient in a position of comfort, and apply oxygen via nonrebreathing mask at 12 to 15 L/min. Assist ventilations if needed. Transport the patient to the closest, most appropriate facility, and provide emotional support en route.

Initial Cardiovascular Assessment

All patient assessments begin by determining level of consciousness and ABCs. If the patient is responsive, is he or she experiencing any dizziness? Was there any loss of consciousness before EMS arrival? Is the airway patent? Is there any evidence of debris, blood, or frothy sputum in the airway? Is the patient breathing? Determine the rate, quality, and degree of distress. Auscultate breath sounds, and note any unusual characteristics.

Next, feel for the presence of bilateral radial pulses. If radial pulses are absent, assess the carotid artery. Determine the rate, rhythm, and quality of the pulse, and listen to heart tones. Note the color, temperature, and condition of the skin. Check skin turgor, and look for any edema, especially in dependent areas. Finally, assess blood pressure.

Follow the steps in (Skill Drill 20-3 ▶) when you are treating a conscious patient who complains of chest discomfort:

1. **Reassure the patient**, and perform the initial assessment. After confirming consciousness and the chief complaint of chest pain, reassure the patient as you prepare to apply oxygen. Act professionally; be calm. Speak to the patient in a normal voice that is neither too loud nor too soft. Let the patient know that trained individuals, including yourself, are present to provide care and that he or she will soon be taken to the hospital. Remember, some patients may act carefree, while others may be demanding. However, most are still frightened. Your professional attitude may be the single most important factor in winning the patient's cooperation and helping him or her through this event. Patients often have a good idea about what is happening, so do not lie and offer false reassurance. If asked, "Am I having a heart attack?" a suggested response would be, "I do not know for sure, but in case you are, we are taking care of you. We are going to help you now by giving oxygen, and we will be taking you to the hospital." Patients with an AMI sometimes

---

You are the Provider — Part 5

You are transporting your patient to the emergency department, and she tells you that she "feels funny." Cardiac monitor reveals a wide QRS complex tachycardic rhythm. Your reassessment of your patient reveals the following:

Reassessment	Recording Time: 7 Minutes After Patient Contact
Respirations	24 breaths/min, adequate depth
Pulse	180 beats/min, regular
Skin	Remains pale and diaphoretic
Blood pressure	96/62 mm Hg
Sao$_2$	94% with 100% O$_2$ via nonrebreathing mask

8. What rhythm is this patient in?
9. What should concern you about this rhythm?

experience an almost overwhelming feeling of impending doom. If a patient tells you, "I think I am going to die," pay attention.

2. **Apply oxygen.** If available, use pulse oximetry. Apply a nonrebreathing mask at 12 to 15 L/min. Be prepared to assist ventilations if the patient's breathing becomes inadequate (that is, shallow breathing) (**Step 1**).

3. **Apply the cardiac monitor**, and note the presence of any dysrhythmias. Treat symptomatic patients according to local and ACLS protocols (**Step 2**).

3. **Position the patient.** Place any patient complaining of chest pain in a comfortable position, usually sitting up and well supported. Make sure the patient has no difficulty breathing and has no airway obstruction. Try not to allow the patient to exert himself or herself, strain, or walk. If necessary, lift the patient, using care.

4. **Measure and record the patient's vital signs.** As your partner obtains the SAMPLE history, you should take baseline vital signs, including pulse, blood pressure, and the rate and depth of breathing. Document the time that each set of vital signs is taken. Vital signs should be reassessed according to the patient's condition—every 5 minutes if the patient is in unstable condition and every 15 minutes if the patient is in stable condition. It is essential to monitor the patient with a suspected AMI closely because sudden cardiac arrest is always a risk (especially within the first hour). If cardiac arrest occurs, you must be ready to perform automated defibrillation or CPR immediately. If an AED is immediately available, use it; if not, perform CPR until the AED is available.

5. **Gain IV access.** A saline lock is sufficient unless the patient is hypotensive. If so, consider a 20-mL/kg bolus of an isotonic crystalloid solution such as normal saline (**Step 3**).

   If cardiac arrest occurs, follow local protocols and ACLS guidelines.

6. **Obtain a focused history and physical exam.** Obtain a brief history from the patient. Friends or family members who are present often have helpful information. Ask them the following questions:

   - Has the patient ever had a heart attack before?
   - Has the patient been told about having previous heart problems?
   - Are there any risk factors for coronary artery disease?
   - Are there any signs of dyspnea, either continuous or intermittent?
   - Does the patient experience dyspnea on exertion, or are there no aggravating factors?
   - If the patient is dyspneic, is it orthopneic (does he or she have to be in an upright position to breathe)?
   - Has he or she had any episodes of paroxysmal nocturnal dyspnea?
   - Does the patient have a cough? If so, is it dry? Productive? Frothy? Bloody?
   - Is there any evidence of peripheral edema in the extremities or sacral area for patients who are bedridden? Is it pitting?

   Note any related signs and symptoms. Reassess the level of consciousness. Is the patient diaphoretic? Does he or she communicate restlessness, anxiety, or a feeling of impending doom? Is there nausea or vomiting, fatigue, or palpitations? Note the presence of edema in the extremities or sacral area. Has the patient had a headache or a syncopal episode? Has the patient's behavior changed? Note any anguished facial expressions or activity limitations. Inspect the neck, looking at the position of the trachea and the appearance of the neck veins. Inspect the thorax. Look for movement with respirations, and note the diameter of the chest. Examine the epigastrium for pulsation or distention. Auscultate breath sounds for depth, equality, and any adventitious sounds such as crackles or wheezing. Listen for gurgling, and look for blood-tinged or foamy froth from the mouth and/or nose. Palpate for any areas of crepitus or tenderness in the thorax and any pulsation or distention in the epigastrium. Finally, ask the patient or family members about any recent trauma.

7. **Ask specific questions** about the patient's chest discomfort. Use the OPQRST mnemonic to determine the type of pain (Table 20-4).

   In addition, ask whether the patient has had the same pain before. If so, ask "Do you take any medications for the pain?" and "Do you have any of the medication with you?" If the patient has had a heart attack or angina before, ask whether this is the same type of pain. Obtain a detailed medical history including the items listed in (Table 20-5) (**Step 4**).

8. **Prepare to assist with prescribed nitroglycerin: Check the medication and its expiration date.** Assess blood pressure if not done previously. The systolic blood pressure must be greater than

TABLE 20-4	OPQRST Mnemonic for Assessing Pain

- **Onset.** Determine what time the discomfort that motivated the call for help began.
- **Provocation/Palliation.** Ask if there is anything that makes the pain or discomfort better or worse. Is it positional? Does a deep breath or palpation of the chest make it worse? Is the pain steady?
- **Quality.** Ask what type of pain it is. Let the patient use his or her own words to describe what is happening. Try to avoid supplying the patient with only one option. Do not ask "Does it feel like an elephant is sitting on your chest?" Instead, say "Tell me what the pain feels like." If the patient cannot answer an open-ended question, then provide a list of alternatives. "There are lots of different kinds of pain. Is your pain more like a heaviness, pressure, burning, tearing, dull ache, stabbing, or needlelike?"
- **Radiation/Referred.** Ask whether the pain travels to another part of the body, such as the arms, back, or neck. Also, determine if the patient is experiencing pain to another part of the body.
- **Severity.** Ask the patient to rate the pain on a simple scale. Often, a scale ranging from 0 to 10 is used, in which 0 represents no pain at all and 10 represents the worst pain imaginable. Do not use the patient's answer to determine whether the pain has a serious cause. Instead, use it to check whether the pain is getting better or worse. After a few minutes of oxygen or administration of nitroglycerin, ask the patient to rate the pain again.
- **Time.** Find out how long the pain lasts when it is present and whether it has been intermittent or continuous. Ask whether it is worsening or improving and if it is associated with rest or activity.

TABLE 20-5	Medical History

Ask the patient or family members about all of the following:
- Coronary artery disease (CAD)
  - Angina
  - Previous myocardial infarction
  - Hypertension
  - Congestive heart failure (CHF)
- Valvular disease
- Aneurysm
- Pulmonary disease
- Diabetes
- Renal disease
- Vascular disease
- Inflammatory cardiac disease
- Previous cardiac surgery
- Congenital anomalies
- Current and past medications
  - Prescribed
    - Compliance
    - Noncompliance
  - Borrowed
  - Over-the-counter
  - Recreational
    - Cocaine
- Allergies
- Family history
  - Stroke, heart disease, diabetes, hypertension
  - Age at death of parents and siblings (if any are dead)
- Known cholesterol levels

90 mm Hg to support administration of nitroglycerin (**Step 5**).

9. **Help the patient administer prescribed nitroglycerin.** Nitroglycerin works in most patients within 5 minutes to relieve the pain of angina. Most patients who have been prescribed nitroglycerin carry a supply with them. Trade names of nitroglycerin include Nitrostat, Nitro-Dur, and others. Patients take one dose of nitroglycerin under the tongue whenever they have an episode of angina that does not immediately go away with rest. If the pain is still present after 5 minutes, patients are typically instructed by their doctors to take a second dose. If the second dose does not work, most patients are told to take a third dose and then call for EMS. If the patient has not taken all three doses, you can help to administer the medication, if you are allowed to do so by local protocol.

The mnemonic "MONA" is often used for pharmacologic interventions associated with suspected cardiac chest pain:

- M—Morphine
- O—Oxygen
- N—Nitroglycerin
- A—Aspirin

Note: This is a helpful mnemonic for remembering the appropriate medications to give a patient with a suspected AMI. However, it does not represent the most appropriate order in which to give the medications. The appropriate order is oxygen, aspirin, nitroglycerin, and morphine.

Nitroglycerin comes in several forms: as a small white pill, placed sublingually (under the tongue); as a spray, also taken sublingually; or as a skin patch applied to the chest (Figure 20-29). In any form, the effect is

Skill Drill 20-3

Treating a Conscious Patient for Chest Discomfort

1 Reassure the patient, and perform the initial assessment. Apply oxygen.

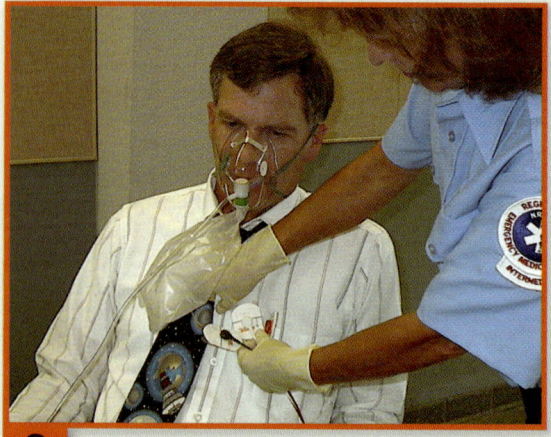

2 Apply a cardiac monitor, and note the presence of any dysrhythmias. Treat accordingly.

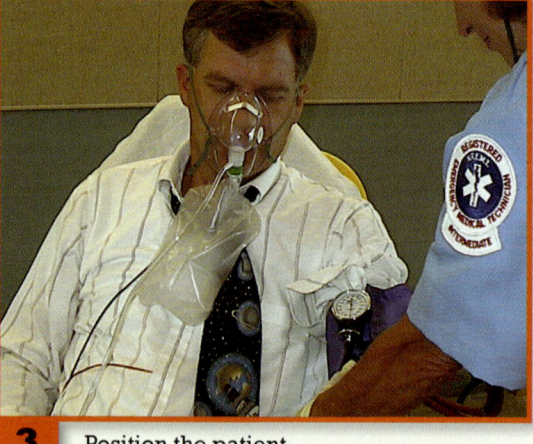

3 Position the patient. Measure and record the patient's vital signs. Gain IV access.

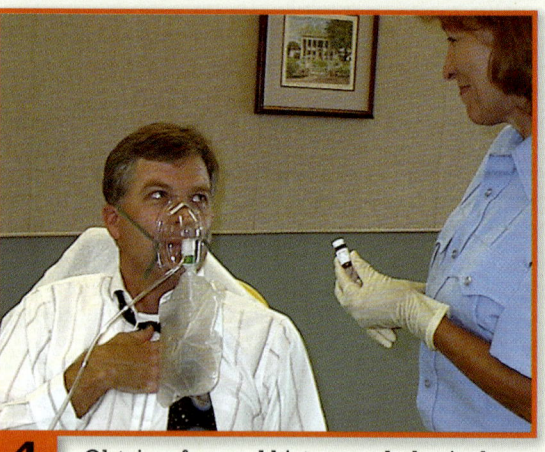

4 Obtain a focused history and physical exam. Ask specific questions about the patient's chest discomfort.

the same. Nitroglycerin relaxes the smooth muscle of blood vessel walls, dilates coronary arteries, increases blood flow and the supply of oxygen to the heart muscle, and decreases the workload of the heart. Nitroglycerin also dilates blood vessels in other parts of the body and can sometimes cause low blood pressure and/or a severe headache. Other side effects include changes in the patient's pulse rate, including tachycardia and bradycardia. For this reason, you should take the patient's blood pressure within 5 minutes after each dose. If the systolic blood pressure is less than 90 mm Hg, do not give any more nitroglycerin. Other contraindications include the presence of a head injury and that the maximum prescribed dose has already been given (usually three doses).

If the patient does not have prescribed nitroglycerin, continue with your focused assessment and prepare to transport. Be sure that this process does not consume too much time. Do not delay transport to assist with administration of nitroglycerin. The drug can be given en route. To safely assist the patient with nitroglycerin, follow the steps listed below.

- Obtain an order from medical direction, online or offline protocol.
- Take the patient's blood pressure. Continue with administration of nitroglycerin only if the systolic blood pressure is greater than 90 mm Hg.
- Check that you have the right medication, the right patient, and the right delivery route.
- Check the expiration date of the nitroglycerin.

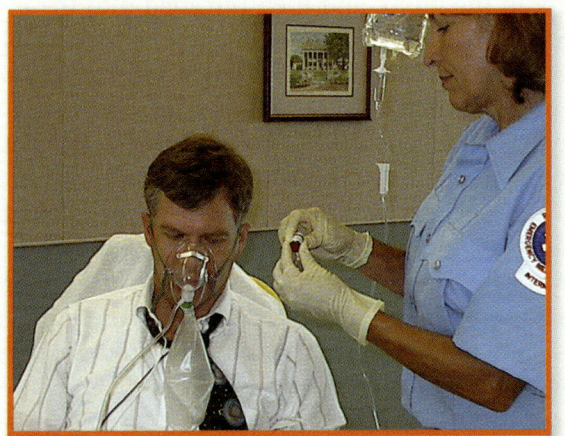

5 Prepare to assist with prescribed nitroglycerin; check the medication and its expiration date.

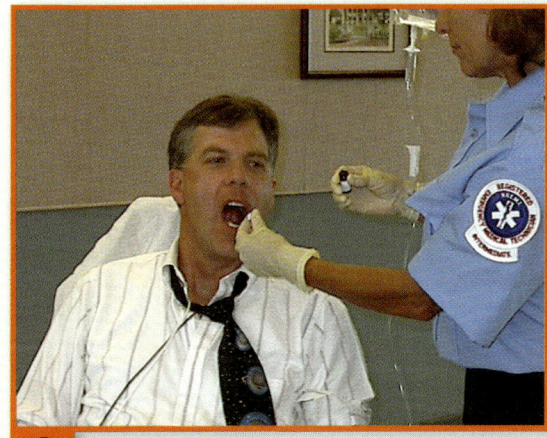

6 Help the patient administer prescribed nitroglycerin.

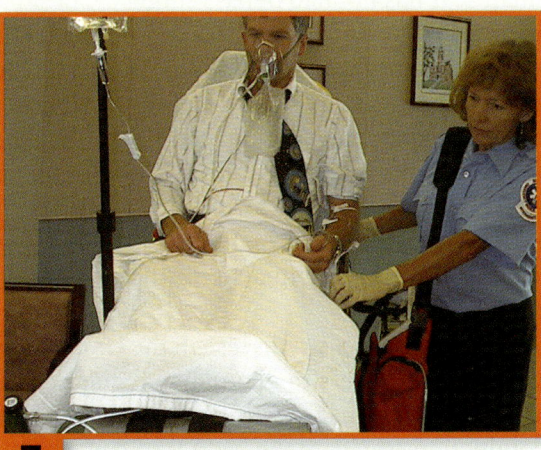

7 Transport the patient.

- Ask the patient about the last dose he or she took and its effects. Make sure that the patient understands the route of administration.
- When you give a patient nitroglycerin, you should be prepared to have the patient lie down to prevent fainting if the nitroglycerin substantially lowers the patient's blood pressure (the patient gets dizzy or feels faint).
- Ask the patient to lift his or her tongue. Place the tablet or spray the dose underneath the tongue (while wearing gloves), or have the patient do so.
- Have the patient keep his or her mouth closed with the tablet under the tongue until it is dissolved and absorbed. Caution the patient against chewing or swallowing the tablet.
- Recheck blood pressure within 5 minutes.
- Record each medication and the time of administration.
- Perform continued reassessment.

After giving nitroglycerin, reassess the patient and note the response to the medication. If the chest pain persists and the patient still has a systolic blood pressure greater than 90 mm Hg, repeat the dose as authorized by medical control. In general, a maximum of three doses of nitroglycerin are given for any one episode of chest pain (**Step 6**).

10. **Transport the patient.** Early, prompt transport to the emergency department is critical so that newer treatments, such as clot-busting (fibrinolytic) medications or angioplasty, can be initiated. To be most

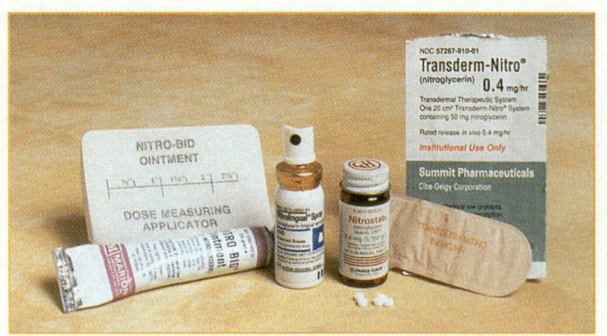

Figure 20-29 Nitroglycerin used to treat angina comes in many forms, including paste, spray, tablets, and skin patches.

effective, these treatments must be started as soon as possible after the onset of the attack. Therefore, alert the emergency department about the status of your patient and your estimated time of arrival. Report to medical control. Report to the hospital by radio or cellular telephone en route. Give the patient's history, vital signs, repeat vital signs, medications being taken, and the treatment you are giving. Follow the instructions of your medical control physician. Describe the patient's condition to the emergency department staff on arrival (**Step 7**).

Cardiac Surgery and Pacemakers

During the last 20 years, hundreds of thousands of open-heart operations were performed to bypass damaged segments of coronary arteries in the heart. In the coronary artery bypass graft operation, a blood vessel from the chest or leg is sewn directly from the aorta to a coronary artery beyond the point of the obstruction. Other patients may have had a procedure called percutaneous transluminal coronary angioplasty, which aims to dilate, rather than bypass, the coronary artery. In this procedure, usually called an angioplasty or balloon angioplasty, a tiny balloon is attached to the end of a long, thin tube. The tube is introduced through the skin into a large vein, usually in the groin, and then threaded into the narrowed coronary artery, with radiographs serving as a guide. Once the balloon is in position inside the coronary artery, it is inflated. The balloon is then deflated, and the tube is removed from the body. Sometimes, a metal mesh called a stent is placed inside the artery instead of or after the balloon. The stent is left in place permanently to help keep the artery from narrowing again.

You will almost certainly have a patient with previous AMI or angina who has had one of these procedures. Patients who have had a bypass graft will have a long surgical scar on their chest from the operation (**Figure 20-30**). Patients who have had an angioplasty or coronary artery stent usually will not. However, newer "keyhole" surgical techniques may not produce a large scar. You should not assume that a patient who has a small scar has not had bypass surgery. Chest pain in a patient who has had any of these procedures should be treated the same as chest pain in patients who have not had any heart surgery. Carry out all the described tasks, and transport the patient promptly to the emergency department of the closest most appropriate hospital. If CPR is required, perform it in the usual way, regardless of the scar on the patient's chest. Likewise, if indicated, an AED or manual defibrillator should be used as well.

Many people with heart disease in the United States have cardiac pacemakers to maintain a regular cardiac rhythm and rate. Pacemakers are inserted when the electrical conduction system of the heart is so damaged that it cannot function properly. These battery-powered devices deliver an electrical impulse through wires that are in direct contact with the myocardium. The generating unit is generally placed under a heavy muscle or a fold of skin; it typically resembles a small silver dollar under the skin in the left upper part of the chest (**Figure 20-31**). Pacemakers are constant, working con-

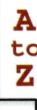 **Terminology Tips**

Paroxysmal nocturnal dyspnea: paroxysmal = sudden onset, nocturnal = night, and dyspnea = difficulty breathing. Paroxysmal nocturnal dyspnea is a sudden onset of difficulty breathing, usually occurring when the patient lies down for the night. It is generally the result of pulmonary edema.

In the Field

When assessing a patient with a complaint of chest pain or dyspnea, it is common to ask, "How many pillows do you sleep on at night?" Many patients with a history of CHF will tell you that they sleep on multiple pillows to keep their head up or are unable to sleep lying down and spend their nights in a recliner or similar position. The more upright the patient must sit, the more severe the condition.

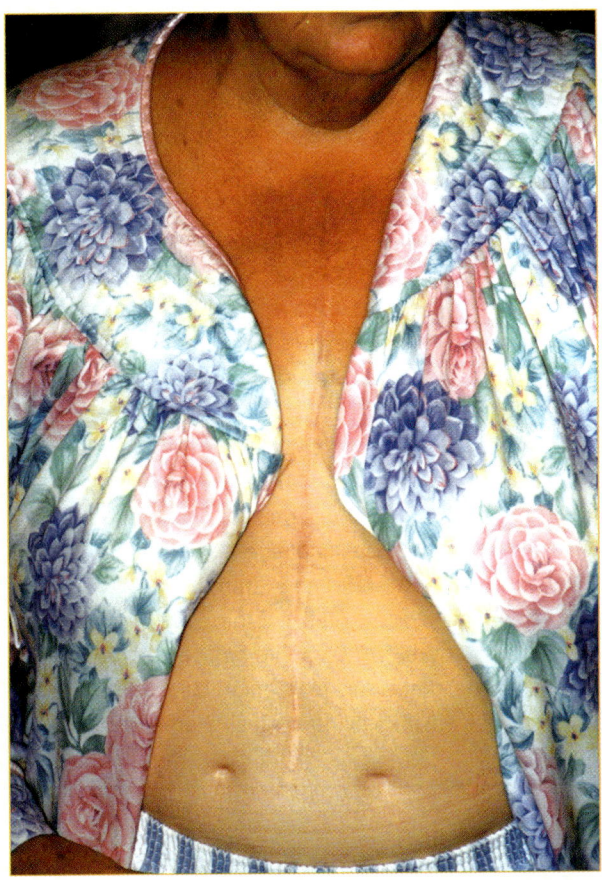

Figure 20-30 The surgical scar on a patient's chest suggests previous coronary artery bypass graft (CABG) surgery.

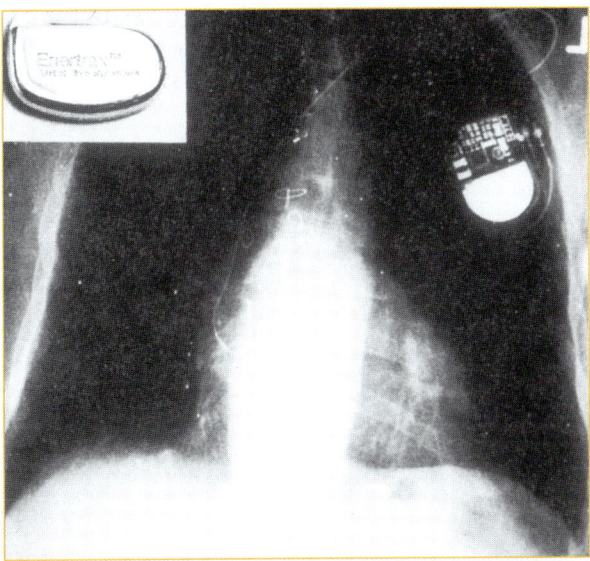

Figure 20-31 A pacemaker, which is typically inserted under the skin in the left upper part of the chest, delivers an electrical impulse to regulate heartbeat.

tinuously, or demand. Demand pacers only work when the patient's heart rate falls below the preset rate.

Normally, you do not need to be concerned about problems with pacemakers. Thanks to modern technology, an implanted unit will not require replacement or a battery charge for years. Wires are well protected and rarely broken. In the past, pacemakers sometimes malfunctioned when a patient got too close to an electrical radiation source, such as a microwave oven, but this is no longer the case. Every patient with a pacemaker still should be aware of the precautions, if any, which must be taken to maintain its proper functioning.

If a pacemaker does not function properly, as when the battery wears out, the patient may experience <u>syncope</u>, dizziness, or weakness because of an excessively slow heart rate. The pulse ordinarily will be less than 60 beats/min because the heart is beating without the stimulus of the pacemaker and without the regulation of its own electrical conduction system, which may be damaged. In these circumstances, the heart tends to assume a fixed slow rate that is not fast enough to allow the patient to function normally. A patient with a malfunctioning pacemaker should be promptly transported to the emergency department for evaluation and possible repair of the pacemaker. Use of a defibrillator should not be withheld if the patient has a pacemaker. Use caution when applying hands-free pads; do not place them directly over the pacemaker site. This will ensure a better flow of electricity through the patient's body. Defibrillation pads or paddles should be placed at least 1″ away from the pacemaker.

Automatic Implantable Cardiac Defibrillators

More and more patients who survive ventricular fibrillation cardiac arrests have a small automatic implantable cardiac defibrillator (AICD) implanted. Some patients who are at particularly high risk for a cardiac arrest have

In the Field

While your partner is getting the nitroglycerin ready, check to see if the patient's mucous membranes are moist. If not, a mouth rinse before using the pill form of the medication helps ensure that the pill dissolves and the patient gets its full benefit. This is not necessary if you are using the spray form.

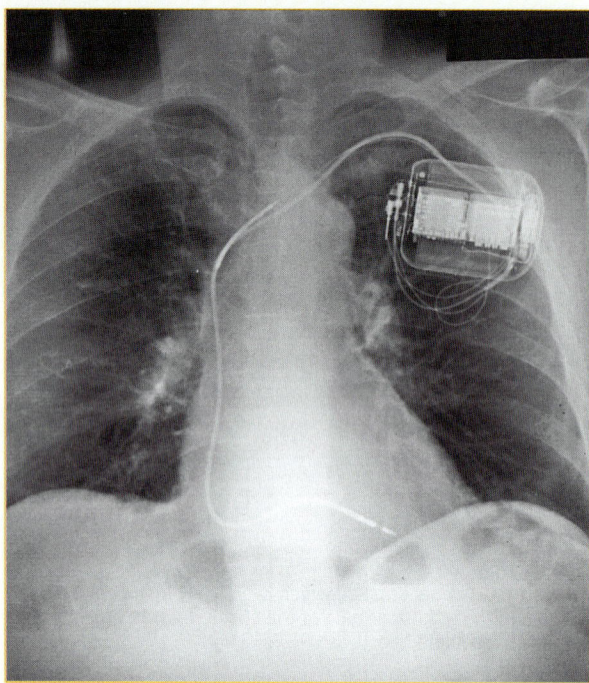

Figure 20-32 An AICD is attached directly to the heart and continuously monitors heart rhythm, delivering shocks as needed. The electricity from the AICD is so low that it has no effect on rescuers.

> ### Pediatric Needs
>
> Heart problems in childhood are uncommon and usually congenital, meaning that the patient was born with the problem. In general, your approach to these patients should be the same as that for an adult. You should attempt to reassure the patient. If possible, administer oxygen. If the patient will not wear a face mask, have the parent hold the oxygen in front of the child's face.
>
> Cardiac arrest in infants and children is usually the result of respiratory failure, not a primary cardiac event. However, the American Heart Association has determined that AEDs are safe to use in children older than 1 year of age. If the child is between 1 and 8 years of age, pediatric-sized pads and a dose-attenuating system (energy reducer) should be used. However, if these are unavailable, a regular adult AED should be used. At the present time, there is insufficient evidence to support the use of AEDs in infants less than 1 year of age.

them as well. These devices are attached directly to the heart and can prolong lives. They continuously monitor the heart rhythm, delivering shocks as needed **Figure 20-32**. Regardless of whether a patient having an AMI has an AICD, he or she should be treated like all other AMI patients. Treatment should include performing CPR and using an AED or manual defibrillator if the patient goes into cardiac arrest. Generally, the electricity from an AICD is so low that it will have no effect on rescuers and, therefore, should not be of concern to you. As with the implanted pacemaker, ensure that you place the defibrillation pads or paddles at least 1″ from the AICD.

You are the Provider — Part 6

You continue to monitor your patient en route to the emergency department. Your reassessment reveals the following:

Reassessment	Recording Time: 8 Minutes After Patient Contact
Respirations	24 breaths/min and labored
Pulse	180 beats/min, regular
Skin	Remains pale and diaphoretic
Blood pressure	96/62 mm Hg
Sao_2	94% with 100% O_2 via nonrebreathing mask

10. What steps should you take when treating a conscious patient complaining of chest discomfort?

Cardiac Arrest

Cardiac arrest may be the result of trauma or numerous medical conditions, such as end-stage renal disease, hyperkalemia with renal disease, or hypothermia, to name a few. Cardiac arrest in a pediatric patient is usually the result of respiratory failure unless the child has a congenital heart problem. Assisting ventilation may be all that is needed to avoid cardiac arrest in a pediatric patient. Geriatric patients, on the other hand, typically have a long history of multiple conditions, and cardiac arrest may result from any combination along with the normal aging process.

When called to the scene of a cardiac arrest, the first step is to verify that the patient is unresponsive, apneic, and pulseless. If a defibrillator is readily available, determine the ECG rhythm or attach an AED to verify whether the rhythm might respond to defibrillation. Because ventricular fibrillation is the rhythm seen most often in sudden cardiac arrest, defibrillation is the definitive treatment. If the defibrillator is available, it should be used immediately if the patient is in V-fib or pulseless V-tach.

If a defibrillator is not readily available, initiate CPR and try to obtain as much history as possible. In a witnessed event, a precordial thump works much like a defibrillator. However, this should only be used if you actually witness the arrest. Try to determine from bystanders how much time has lapsed from the time of discovery until CPR was initiated and EMS was called. Also try to obtain a pertinent medical history.

Indications for not initiating resuscitative techniques include rigor mortis, dependent lividity, and decapitation. Local protocols may also dictate other circumstances, such as advance directives (that is, living wills) and DNR orders.

> **A to Z Terminology Tips**
>
> *Resuscitation:* efforts to return spontaneous pulse and breathing to the patient in full cardiac arrest.
>
> *Survival:* patient is resuscitated and survives to hospital discharge.
>
> *Return of spontaneous circulation (ROSC):* patient is resuscitated to the point of having a pulse without CPR; may or may not have return of spontaneous respirations; patient may or may not survive to hospital discharge.

Once the patient has been defibrillated or determined to have a rhythm that will not respond to defibrillation, initiate airway and ventilatory support. Use an airway adjunct, or secure the airway with a Combitube based on local protocols. Ventilate using a bag-valve-mask (BVM) device connected to 100% oxygen at a rate of one breath every 3 to 5 seconds.

Continue ventilation and chest compression, alternating with defibrillation after 2 minutes of CPR assuming that the patient remains in a "shockable" rhythm. Gain IV access, and initiate fluid therapy based on patient status. Give a 20-mL/kg bolus of an isotonic crystalloid solution if hypovolemia is suspected.

Perform endotracheal intubation, and administer pharmacologic interventions based on local and ACLS protocols.

Prepare for transport as soon as possible. The patient should be taken to the closest, most appropriate facility. Provide psychological support for the family and significant others. On arrival at the emergency department, give a full report to the attending staff, including length of time since resuscitation efforts were initiated, how long the patient was "down" before EMS arrival, and any treatment given.

Termination of Resuscitation

Termination of efforts should be based on local protocol and direct communication with online medical direction. Although local protocols vary regarding when it is appropriate to terminate resuscitation, the following questions, which should be answered, are based on recommendations from the American Heart Association:

- What is the underlying medical condition of the patient?
- Are there any atypical features present (for example, young age)?
- Was appropriate CPR performed at all times?
- Was an advanced airway obtained and maintained?
- Was V-fib defibrillated to a nonshockable rhythm?
- Was IV access maintained?
- Were the appropriate medications administered to the patient?
- Are there any potentially reversible causes of the cardiac arrest?
- Has the family been informed of the situation? Is there any opposition from the family to your ceasing resuscitative efforts?

Maintain continuous documentation of the interventions that were performed, including all ECG strips.

Determine whether this case requires assignment of the patient to the medical examiner. On-scene law enforcement personnel should communicate with the attending physician for the death certificate. If there is any suspicion about the nature of the death or if the physician refuses or hesitates to sign the death certificate, the patient is turned over to the medical examiner. The patient will also be assigned to the medical examiner if there is no attending physician identified.

Automated External Defibrillation

In the late 1970s and early 1980s, scientists developed a small computer that could analyze electrical signals from the heart and determine when ventricular fibrillation was taking place. This development, along with improved battery technology, made possible the automated portable defibrillator, which can automatically administer an electrical shock to the heart when needed.

The AED machines come in models with different features (Figure 20-33 ▶). All of them require a certain degree of operator interaction, beginning with applying the pads and turning the machine on. The operator also has to push a button to deliver an electrical shock, depending on the model. Many AEDs use a computer voice synthesizer to advise the EMT-I or layperson which steps to take on the basis of the AED's analysis. Some have a button that tells the computer to analyze the heart's electrical rhythm; other models start doing this as soon as they are turned on. In the United States, the majority of the AEDs are semiautomated. Even though most defibrillators are now semiautomated, we are using the term automated external defibrillator (AED) as the general term to describe all of these machines. Fully automated AEDs were among the first AEDs made; however, unlike the semiautomated AED, they delivered the shock automatically; the operator had no control over when the shock was delivered. Because of the safety concerns generated by these devices, there are very few, if any, fully automated AEDs left; all manufacturers are producing only semiautomated external defibrillators.

AEDs also come equipped to give a monophasic shock or a biphasic shock. Monophasic means to send the energy in one direction, from negative to positive, and biphasic means to send the energy in two directions simultaneously. The advantage of biphasic shock is that it produces a more efficient defibrillation and may require a lower energy setting. The initial and subsequent energy setting for ventricular fibrillation and pulseless ventricular tachycardia on a monophasic machine is 360 joules. With the biphasic technology, the energy can be 120 joules for the first and all subsequent shocks or can start at 120 joules and then escalate. If the initial energy setting for a biphasic AED is unknown, a default setting of 200 joules should be used. The actual setting of the biphasic machines is still being studied, and no recommendation for either is currently supported in the literature.

The computer inside the AED is specially programmed to recognize rhythms that require defibrillation to correct, most commonly ventricular fibrillation and pulseless ventricular tachycardia. The current programs are extremely accurate. It would be rare for them to recommend a shock when a shock would not be indicated, and they rarely fail to recommend one when it would be indicated. Therefore, if the AED recommends a shock, you can believe that it is indicated.

When an error does occur, it is usually the result of operator error. The most common error is not having a charged battery. To avoid this problem, many defibrillator companies have built smarter machines that will

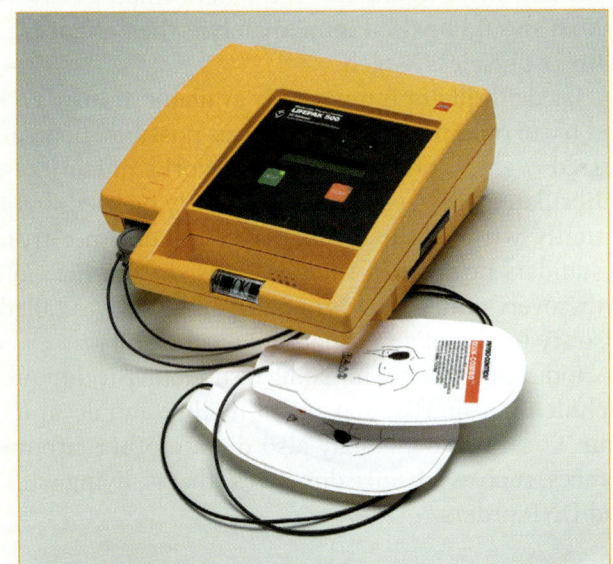

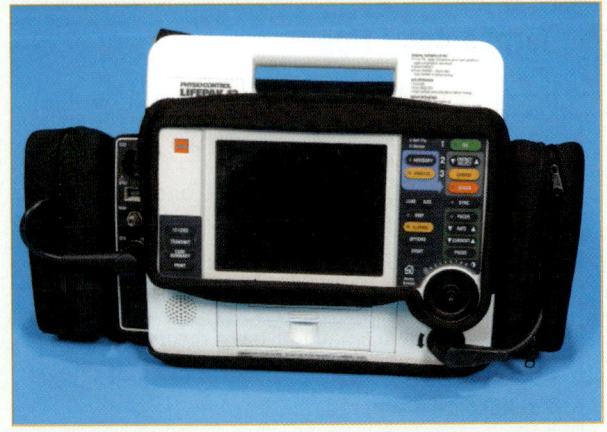

Figure 20-33 AEDs vary in their design, features, and operation.

warn the operator that the battery is unlikely to work. However, some of the older models do not have this feature. You should check the AED daily, and exercise the battery as often as the manufacturer recommends.

Another error occurs when the AED is applied to a patient who is moving. The computer may be unable to tell the difference between electrical signals from the heart and electrical signals from the arms and chest muscles that are moving. The way to avoid this error is to apply the AED only to pulseless, unresponsive patients and to stay clear of the patient (do not touch the patient) during analysis and shocking.

A third error can occur when the AED is applied to a responsive patient with a rapid heart rate. Most computers identify a regular rhythm faster than 150 or 180 beats/min as ventricular tachycardia, which, if pulseless, should be shocked. Sometimes, though, a patient has another heart rhythm that should not be shocked but that is fast enough to confuse the computer. Again, to avoid this problem, you should apply the AED only to unresponsive patients who are pulseless and apneic.

Automated external defibrillation offers the EMT-I a number of advantages. First, of course, the machine is fast, and it delivers the most important treatment for the patient in ventricular fibrillation or pulseless ventricular tachycardia: an electrical shock. It can be delivered within 1 minute of the EMT-I's arrival at the patient's side. Second, you will find that an AED is easy to operate. Paramedics do not have to be on the scene to provide this critical intervention.

Current AEDs offer two other advantages. The shock can be given through remote, adhesive defibrillator pads, which are safer for you than paddles. Also, the pad area is larger than paddles, which means that the transmission of electricity is more efficient. Usually, there are pictures on the pads to remind you where they go on the patient's chest.

Not all patients in cardiac arrest require an electrical shock. Although all patients in cardiac arrest should be analyzed with an AED, some do not have shockable rhythms (eg, pulseless electrical activity [PEA] and asystole). Asystole indicates that no electrical or mechanical activity is present, whereas PEA usually refers to a state of cardiac arrest despite an organized cardiac rhythm. In both cases, CPR should be initiated as soon as possible.

Rationale for Early Defibrillation

Few patients who experience sudden cardiac arrest outside of a hospital survive unless a rapid sequence of events takes place. The chain of survival is a way of describing the ideal sequence of events that should take place when out-of-hospital cardiac arrest occurs.

The four links in the chain of survival are as follows (Figure 20-34 ▼):

- Recognition of early warning signs and immediate activation of EMS
- Immediate bystander CPR
- Early defibrillation
- Early advanced cardiac life support

If any one of the links in the chain is absent or delayed, the patient's chances for survival diminish. For example, few patients benefit from defibrillation when more than 10 minutes elapse before administration of the first shock or if CPR is not performed in the first

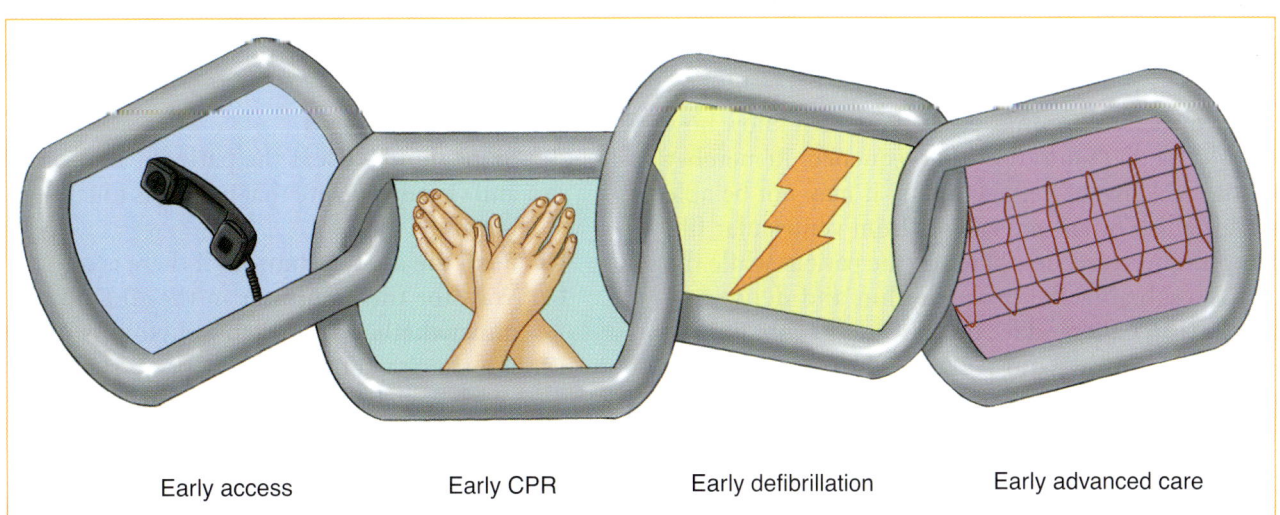

Early access   Early CPR   Early defibrillation   Early advanced care

Figure 20-34 The four links in the chain of survival.

2 to 3 minutes. If all links in the chain are strong, the patient has the best possible chance of survival. The link that is the greatest determinant for survival is the third link—early defibrillation. According to the American Heart Association, for each minute that a patient remains in V-fib, there is a 7% to 10% smaller likelihood of survival.

Giving CPR helps patients in cardiac arrest because it maintains myocardial and cerebral perfusion, thus prolonging the period of time during which defibrillation can be effective. Rapid defibrillation has successfully resuscitated many patients with cardiac arrest from ventricular fibrillation. However, defibrillation works best if it takes place within 2 minutes of the onset of the cardiac arrest. To try to achieve better survival rates among cardiac arrest victims, many communities are exploring the idea that nontraditional first responders should be trained to administer early defibrillation. These responders would include police officers, security personnel, lifeguards, maintenance workers, and flight attendants. As an EMT-I, you should support these efforts to shorten the time until defibrillation. Remember, seconds really do matter when the patient is in cardiac arrest.

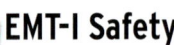

EMT-I Safety

When "clearing" the patient before an AED shock, ensure that no one is touching the patient and that no one is in contact with any object that is touching the patient, such as the stretcher, a BVM, etc.

Integrating the AED and CPR

Because most cardiac arrests occur in the home, a bystander at the scene may already have started CPR before you arrive. For this reason, you must know how to work the AED into the CPR sequence. Remember that the AED is not very complex; it may not be able to distinguish other movements from ventricular fibrillation. Therefore, do not touch the patient while the AED is analyzing the heart rhythm and delivering shocks. Stop CPR, and let the AED do its job. Follow directions given by your AED. Defibrillation is more important than CPR when ventricular fibrillation is present, especially if the patient's cardiac arrest was witnessed by you. However, if you did not witness the patient's cardiac arrest—especially if the call-to-arrival interval is greater than 5 minutes—you should perform 5 cycles (approximately 2 minutes) of CPR prior to analyzing the patient's cardiac rhythm. Research has shown that return of spontaneous circulation (ROSC) occurs more frequently if 2 minutes of CPR is performed before defibrillation in patients with unwitnessed cardiac arrest.

Prepare with body substance isolation precautions en route to the scene. On arrival at the scene, make sure that the scene is safe for you and your partner to enter. Ask any bystanders or first responders who are performing CPR to stop so that you can apply the AED and defibrillate the patient, if needed. Take the following steps to use the AED (**Skill Drill 20-4** ▶):

1. **Arrive on scene, and perform your initial assessment.** Stop CPR if it is in progress, and assess responsiveness. If the patient is responsive, do not apply the AED.
2. **Verify apnea and pulselessness.** Check for breathing and a pulse even if the patient appears to be breathing.
3. If the patient is unresponsive and not breathing or is breathing agonally (slow, gasping breaths), **give two ventilations** using a BVM device or a pocket mask (**Step 1**).
4. Have your partner start or resume CPR.
5. If an AED is close at hand, **prepare the AED pads.**
6. Turn on the machine (**Step 2**).
7. **Remove clothing from the patient's chest area.** Apply the pads to the chest: one just to the right of the breastbone (sternum) just below the collarbone (clavicle), the other on the left side of the chest with the top of the pad 2″ to 3″ below the armpit. Do not place the pads on top of breast tissue. If necessary, lift the breast out of the way and place the pad underneath. Ensure that the pads are attached to the patient cables (and that they are attached to the AED in some models).
8. Stop CPR (**Step 3**).
9. State aloud, "Clear the patient," and verbally and visually ensure that no one is touching the patient.
10. **Push the analyze button**, if there is one.
11. **Wait for the computer** in the AED to determine whether a shockable rhythm is present.
12. If a shock is not indicated, go to step 16. If a shock is advised, make sure that no one is touching the patient. When the area is clear, **push the shock button.**
13. **After the shock is delivered**, immediately begin five cycles of CPR beginning with chest compressions.

14. **After five cycles** (approximately 2 minutes) of CPR, reanalyze the patient's rhythm.
15. **If the machine advises a shock**, clear the patient and push the shock button (**Step 4**).
16. **If no shock is advised, check for a pulse.**
17. **If the patient has a pulse**, check the patient's breathing (at least 5 seconds but no more than 10 seconds) (**Step 5**).
18. **If the patient is breathing adequately**, give the patient oxygen via nonrebreathing mask and transport. If the patient is not breathing or is breathing inadequately, use necessary airway adjuncts and proper positioning of the head and jaw to ensure an open airway. Provide artificial ventilations with high-concentration oxygen and transport.
19. **If the patient has no pulse**, perform five cycles (approximately 2 minutes) of CPR.
20. **Gather additional information about the arrest event.**
21. **After 2 minutes of CPR**, make sure no one is touching the patient. Push the analyze button.
22. **If necessary, repeat Steps 14 and 15 until you reach definitive care.**
23. **Transport the patient, and contact medical control.**
24. **Continue to support the patient** as needed: ventilate the patient and continue CPR if needed (**Step 6**).

If, after any rhythm analysis, the AED advises no shock, check the patient's pulse. If the patient has a pulse, check the patient's breathing. If the patient is breathing adequately, give high-concentration oxygen via nonrebreathing mask and transport. If the patient is apneic or not breathing adequately, provide artificial ventilation with high-concentration oxygen via a BVM device and transport. Ensure that appropriate airway techniques are used at all times.

If the patient has no pulse, resume CPR for 2 minutes, then have the AED reanalyze the heart rhythm. If the AED advises a shock, deliver one shock followed by five cycles (approximately 2 minutes) of CPR beginning with chest compressions. Reanalyze the rhythm after 2 minutes. Repeat these steps if needed.

If the AED advises no shock and the patient has no pulse, resume CPR for five cycles (approximately 2 minutes), beginning with chest compressions. Stop and reanalyze the patient's rhythm. Shock if advised, followed by five cycles of CPR. If no shock is advised, continue CPR. Check with medical control and transport.

After AED Shocks

The care of the patient after the AED delivers its shock depends on your location and the EMS system; therefore, you should follow your local protocols. After the AED protocol is completed, the patient will have had one of the following occur:

- Regained a spontaneous pulse and adequate breathing
- Regained a pulse, but remains apneic or is breathing inadequately
- No pulse, and the AED indicates that no shock is advised
- No pulse, and the AED indicates that a shock is advised

If you reached the patient quickly and the patient started breathing adequately on his or her own, admin-

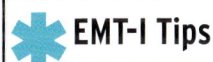

EMT-I Tips

AED operational tips
- One EMT-I operates the defibrillator while another performs CPR.
- Defibrillation comes first. Do not apply oxygen or do anything else that delays analysis of rhythm or defibrillation.
- Be familiar with the AED device used by your EMS system.
- Avoid all contact with the patient during analysis of the rhythm.
- State, "Clear the patient" before shocking. Another popular phrase is "I'm clear, you're clear, we're all clear" before delivering shocks.
- In applicable models of AEDs, check the batteries at the beginning of your shift; carry an extra charged battery with your AED.
- When using an AED for cardiac arrest in children younger than age 8 years or who weigh less than 55 lb (25 kg), use the pediatric pads with a dose-attenuating system designed for these patients, if available. If not, adult pads may be used on children age 1 year or older. Pads may need to be placed front and back to prevent them from touching.
- Unless indicated otherwise by local protocol, you do not need to perform pulse checks during rhythm analysis; the shock should be followed by immediate CPR for 2 minutes.
- Continued airway maintenance and artificial ventilation are of prime importance.

Skill Drill 20-4

AED and CPR

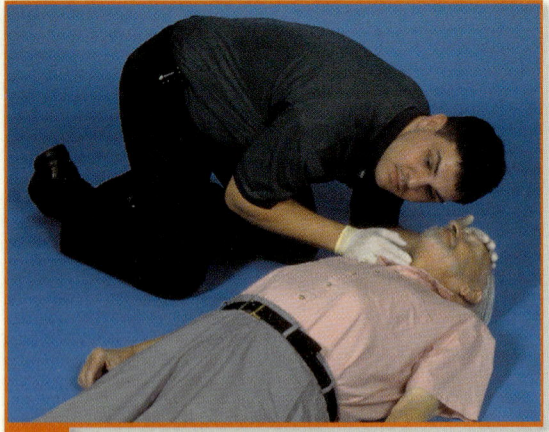

1 Stop CPR if in progress.
Assess responsiveness.
Check breathing and pulse.
If unresponsive, not breathing, or breathing inadequately, give two slow ventilations.

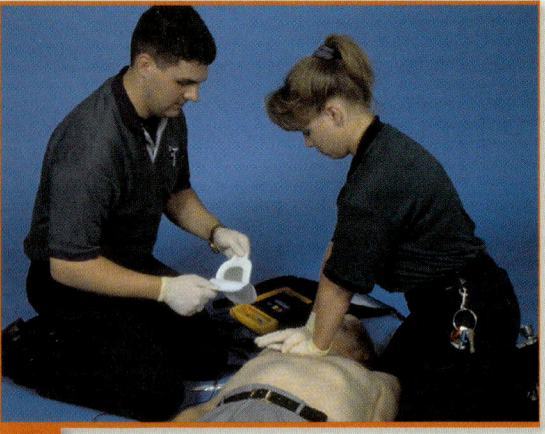

2 If pulseless, begin CPR.
Remove sufficient clothing to gain access to the patient's chest.
Prepare the AED pads.

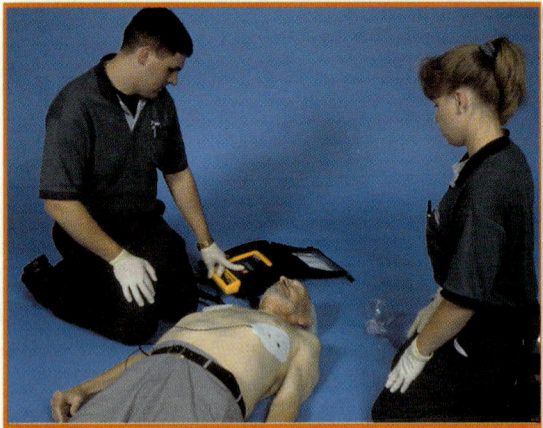

3 Turn on the AED; begin narrative if needed.
Apply AED pads.
Stop CPR.

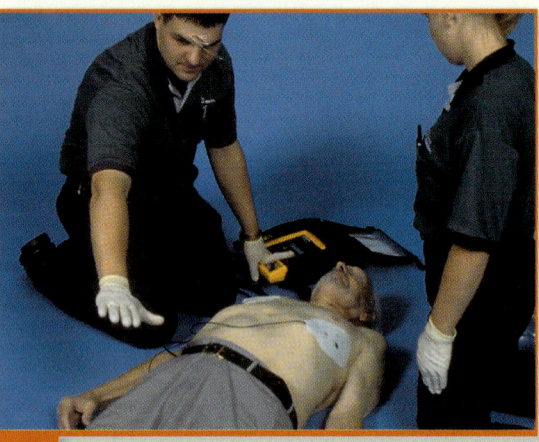

4 Verbally and visually clear the patient.
Push the analyze button if there is one.
Wait for the AED to analyze the rhythm.
If no shock is advised, perform five cycles (approximately 2 minutes) of CPR and reassess in two minutes.
If a shock is advised, recheck that all are clear, and push the shock button.
After the shock is delivered, immediately begin five cycles of CPR beginning with chest compressions.
After five cycles (approximately 2 minutes) of CPR, reanalyze the patient's rhythm.
If the machine advises a shock, clear the patient, push the shock button, and immediately resume CPR.

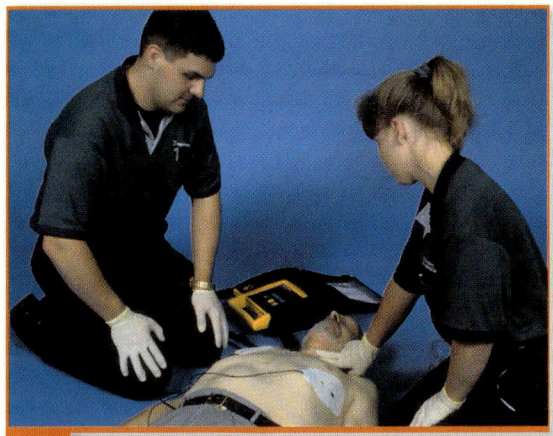

5 After 2 minutes of CPR, reanalyze the cardiac rhythm.

If no shock is advised, check the pulse.

If pulse is absent, continue CPR.

If pulse is present, check breathing.

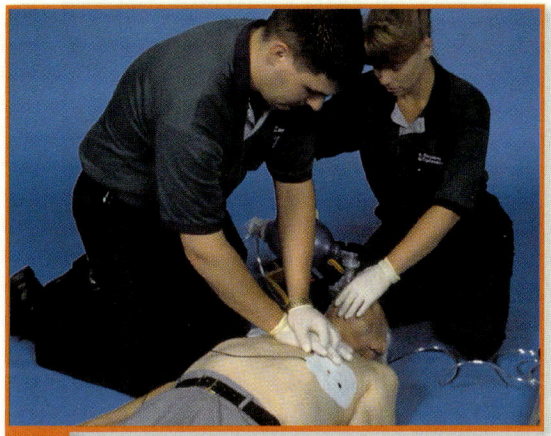

6 If breathing adequately, give 100% oxygen and transport. If apneic or breathing inadequately, continue rescue breathing at 10 to 12 breaths/min, and transport.

If no pulse, perform 5 cycles (approximately 2 minutes) of CPR.

Clear the patient, and analyze again.

If necessary, deliver another shock and immediately resume CPR. Repeat defibrillation every 2 minutes as needed.

Transport the patient, and contact medical control.

ister oxygen by nonrebreathing face mask with the oxygen flow set at 12 to 15 L/min. Check the patient's pulse. If the patient has a pulse but is apneic or not breathing adequately, assist ventilation using a BVM device with high-flow oxygen. Prepare for transport, keeping the AED attached to the patient. Recheck the pulse frequently, at least every 30 seconds. In applicable devices, push the analyze button on the AED if the pulse is lost. Commonly, patients who are successfully defibrillated by an AED will develop a normal heart rhythm for a while. However, because the heart still is not receiving optimal amounts of oxygen, ventricular fibrillation will often recur.

Patients who do not regain a pulse on the scene of the cardiac arrest usually do not survive. What you do with these patients will, again, depend on your EMS system's protocols. Whether you should transport the patient or wait for a paramedic unit to arrive should be in the local protocols established by medical direction. If paramedics are responding to the scene, the best option usually is to stay where you are and continue the sequence of shocks and CPR. Administering CPR while patients are being moved or transported is usually not effective. Patients have the best chance of survival if return of spontaneous circulation occurs at the scene. See Chapter 39 for a review of BLS for adults, children, and infants.

If paramedics are not responding to the scene and your local protocols agree, you should begin transport when one of the following occurs:

- The patient regains a pulse.
- Six to nine shocks delivered (or as directed by local protocol).
- The machine gives three consecutive messages (separated by 2 minutes of CPR) that no shock is advised (or as directed by local protocol).

If you transport a patient while performing CPR, you need a plan for managing the patient in the ambulance. Ideally, you should have two EMT-Is in the patient compartment while a third drives. You may deliver additional shocks at the scene or en route with the approval of medical control. *Keep in mind*

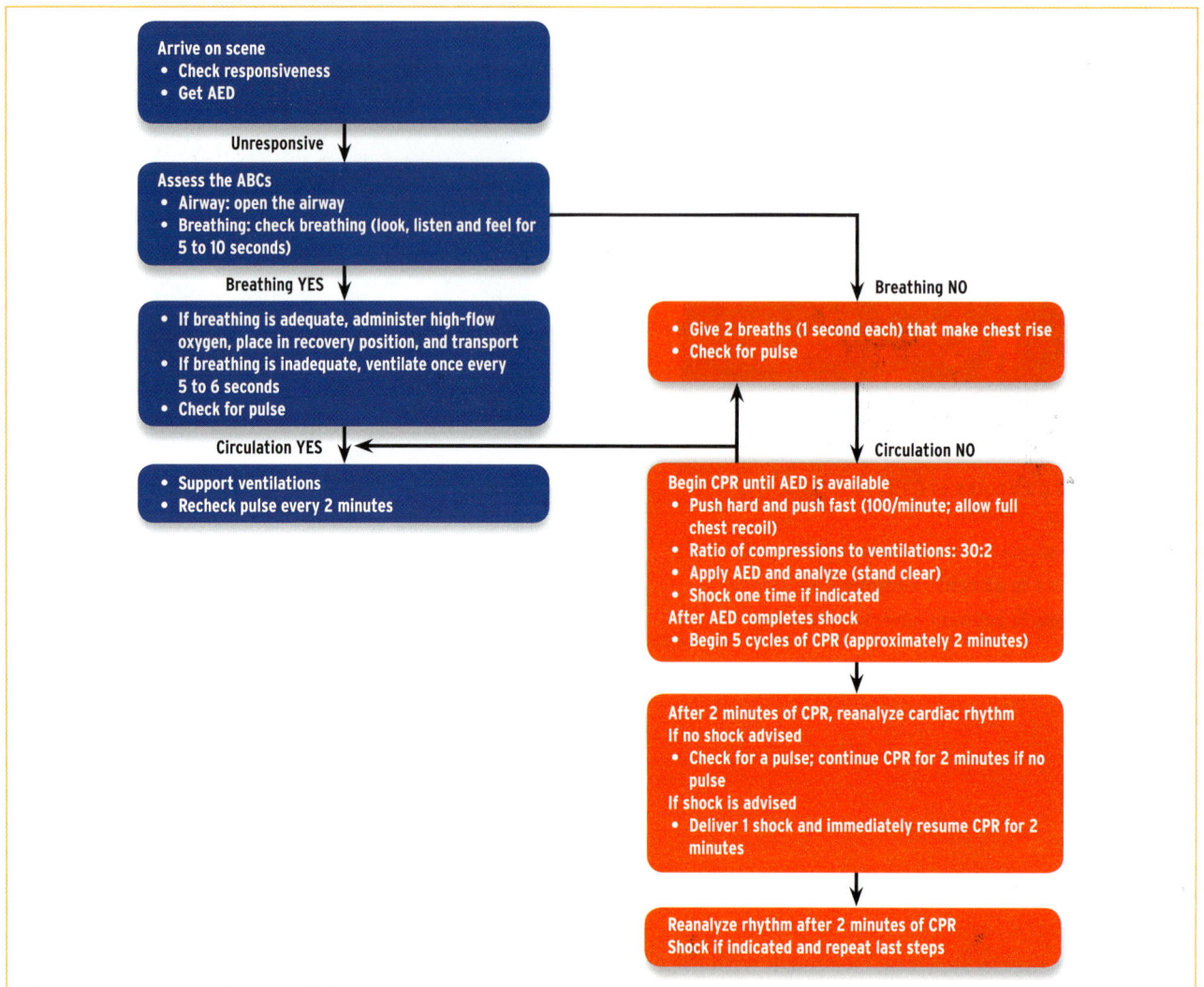

Figure 20-35 AED algorithm.

that AEDs cannot analyze rhythm while the vehicle is in motion; nor is it as safe to defibrillate in a moving ambulance. Therefore, you should come to a complete stop if more shocks are needed. Be sure to memorize the protocol of your EMS service so that you will know how to manage patients in this situation Figure 20-35 ▲).

Cardiac Arrest During Transport

If you are traveling to the hospital with an unresponsive patient, check the pulse at least every 30 seconds. If a pulse is not present, take the following steps:

1. Stop the vehicle.
2. If the AED is not immediately ready, perform CPR until it is available.
3. Analyze the rhythm.
4. Deliver a shock, if indicated, and immediately resume CPR.
5. Continue resuscitation according to your local protocol.

If you are en route with a conscious adult patient who is having chest pain and becomes unresponsive, take the following steps:

1. Check for a pulse.
2. Stop the vehicle.
3. If the AED is not immediately ready, perform CPR until it is ready.
4. Analyze the rhythm.
5. Deliver one shock, if indicated, and immediately begin CPR.
6. Continue resuscitation according to your local protocol. If a "no shock" message is given and

no pulse is present, you should start CPR, then continue transport.

Safety Considerations

As the operator of the AED, you are responsible for making sure that the electricity injures no one, including yourself. As long as you place the pads in the correct position and make sure no one is touching the patient, you should be safe. Do not defibrillate a patient who is in pooled water. While there is some danger to you if you are also in the water, there is another problem. Electricity follows the path of least resistance; instead of traveling between the pads and through the patient's heart, it will diffuse into the water. Therefore, the heart will not receive enough electricity to cause defibrillation. You can defibrillate a soaking wet patient, but try first to dry the patient's chest. Do not defibrillate someone who is touching metal that others are touching, and carefully remove a nitroglycerin patch with your gloved hands, or any other medication patch, from a patient's chest and wipe the area with a dry towel before defibrillation to prevent ignition of the patch.

AED Maintenance

One of your primary missions as an EMT-I is to deliver an electrical shock to a patient in ventricular fibrillation or pulseless ventricular tachycardia. To accomplish this mission, you need to have a functioning AED. You must become familiar with the maintenance procedures required for the brand of AED your service uses. Read the operator's manual. If your defibrillator does not work on the scene, someone will want to know what went wrong. That person may be your system's administrator, your medical director, the local newspaper reporter, or the family's attorney. You will be asked to show proof that you maintained the defibrillator properly and attended any mandatory in-service sessions.

The main legal risk in using the AED is failing to deliver a shock when one was indicated. The most common reason for this failure is that the battery did not work, usually because it was not properly maintained. Another problem is operator error. This means not pushing the analyze or shock buttons when the machine advises you to do so or failing to apply the AED to a patient in cardiac arrest. Of course, the AED is like any other manufactured item. It can fail, although this is rare. Ideally, you will encounter any such failure while doing routine maintenance, not while caring for a patient in cardiac arrest. Check your equipment, including your AED, at the beginning of each shift. Ask the manufacturer for a checklist **Figure 20-36** of items that should be checked daily, weekly, or less often.

Geriatric Needs

Like the other body systems, the cardiovascular system undergoes changes as we get older. The heart, like other major organs, will show the effects of aging. As the heart's muscle mass and tone decrease, the amount of blood pumped out of the heart per beat is decreased. The residual (reserve) capacity of the heart is also reduced; therefore, when the vital organs of the body need additional blood flow, the heart cannot meet the increased need. When blood flow to the tissues is decreased, the organs suffer. If blood flow to the brain is inadequate, the patient may complain of weakness, fatigue, or dizziness and may develop syncope.

The power to the heart muscle can fail. The heart runs on electricity and has its own electrical conduction system. Under normal conditions, electrical impulses travel throughout the heart, resulting in the contraction of the heart muscle and the pumping of blood from the heart's chambers. With aging, the electrical conduction system can deteriorate, causing the heart's contraction to weaken or, if blood flow to the heart muscle is affected, extra beats to form. With decreased strength of contraction, the heartbeat is weaker and blood flow to the tissues is reduced. If extra beats are produced, the patient's heart rhythm will be irregular. While some irregular heart rhythms are benign, others can be potentially lethal.

The arteries are also affected by aging. Arteriosclerosis (hardening of the arteries) can develop, affecting perfusion of the tissues. There is an increased chance of heart attack or stroke from decreased blood flow or plaque formation (atherosclerosis) in the narrowed arteries.

Patients with diabetes can experience reduced circulation to the hands and feet; this makes peripheral pulses harder to detect. It also puts the hands and feet at particular risk for developing infection or ulcerations.

In some older patients, particularly diabetics, chest pain is absent, and the clinical picture can be confused with other, noncardiac conditions.

The cardiovascular system is affected by aging. You should be aware of the changes, seeking to distinguish what is normal from what is chronic for the patient and from what is an acute condition. Sometimes the weakening of the heart muscle, the deterioration of its electrical conduction system, and the hardening of the arteries make the task of assessing and caring for elderly patients more difficult.

AUTOMATED EXTERNAL DEFIBRILLATOR
Daily/Shift Inspection Checklist

Serial # _____ Date _____ Time _____

Model # _____ Inspected by _____

Item	Pass	Fail
Exterior/Cables:		
Nothing stored on top of unit		
Carry case intact and clean		
Exterior/LCD screen clean and undamaged		
Cables/connectors clean and undamaged		
Cables securely attached to unit		
Batteries:		
Unit charger is plugged in and operational (if applicable)		
Fully charged battery in unit		
Fully charged spare battery		
Spare battery charger plugged in and operational (if applicable)		
Valid expiration date on both batteries		
Supplies:		
Two sets of electrodes		
Electrodes in sealed packages with valid expiration dates		
Razor		
Hand towel		
Alcohol wipes		
Memory/voice recording device–module, card, microcassette		
Manual override–module, key (if applicable)		
Printer paper (if applicable)		
Operation:		
Unit self-test per manufacturer's recommendation/instructions		
Display (if applicable)		
Visual indicators		
Verbal prompts		
Printer (if applicable)		
Attach AED to simulator/tester:		
Recognizes shockable rhythm		
Charges to correct energy level within manufacturer's specifications		
Delivers charge		
Recognizes nonshockable rhythm		
Manual override system in working order (if applicable)		

Signature:

Figure 20-36 A sample daily checklist for the AED.

If you do have an AED failure while caring for a patient, you must report the problem to your medical director, the manufacturer of the AED, and the US Food and Drug Administration. Be sure to follow the appropriate EMS procedures for notifying these organizations.

Medical Direction

Defibrillation of the heart is a medical procedure. While AEDs have made the process of delivering electricity much simpler, there is still a benefit in having a physician's involvement. The medical director of your service should help to teach you how to use the AED. At the very least, he or she should approve the written protocol that you will follow in caring for patients in cardiac arrest. In most states, AED training in an EMT-I course is not permitted without approval by state laws, rules, and local medical direction authority.

There should be a review of each incident in which the AED is used. After returning from the hospital or the scene, sit down with the rest of the team and critique the incident. This discussion will help all members of the team learn from the incident. Review such events by using the written report, any voice-ECG tape recorder, and the device's solid-state memory modules and magnetic tape recordings, if applicable.

There should also be a review of the incident by your service's medical director or quality improvement officer. Quality improvement involves individuals using AEDs and the responsible EMS system managers. This review should focus on speed of defibrillation, that is, the time from when the call was received until the first shock was delivered. Few systems will achieve the ultimate goal: shocking 100% of patients within 1 minute of the call. However, all systems should continuously work on improving patient care. Mandatory continuing education with skill competency review is generally required for EMS providers, with a continuing competency skill review every 3 to 6 months for the EMT-I.

The following section on electrocardiographic monitoring is required for users of the 1999 EMT-I curriculum but optional for users of the 1985 curriculum.

ECG Monitoring

The section is designed to give a brief overview of ECG rhythm analysis and to introduce ACLS algorithms for the treatment of various cardiac dysrhythmias. Remember that this is a guideline, and you should always follow local protocols or check with medical control for answers to any questions you may have while treating a patient.

Leads are like pictures of the heart. The electrodes (leads) pick up the electrical activity of the vectors, and the ECG machine converts them to waves.

The ECG monitor reads the positive and negative poles of the limb electrodes to produce leads I, II, and III. These are the only leads you will be able to monitor as an EMT-I. This is not as comprehensive as a 12-lead, but will allow you to see the basic rhythm, identify life-threatening dysrhythmias, and treat the patient appropriately. Typically, the negative white lead (RA) is placed on the right upper part of the chest, the positive red lead (LL) is placed over the left lower part of the chest, and the black lead (LA), or ground, is placed on the left upper part of the chest Figure 20-37 . Even

---

You are the Provider Part 7

Your patient suddenly becomes unresponsive, pulseless, and apneic. You look at the monitor and see that she is still in ventricular tachycardia.

Reassessment	Recording Time: 9 Minutes After Patient Contact
Respirations	0 breaths/min
Pulse	0 beats/min
Skin	Remains pale and diaphoretic
Blood pressure	N/A
SaO_2	N/A

11. What is your next step in the management of this patient?

if your leads are different colors, they should have labels indicating correct placement.

As electricity travels through the heart, it is shown on the ECG strip as a positive or negative deflection going away from the <u>isoelectric line</u>, or baseline. Electricity traveling toward the positive lead will be seen as an upright deflection, whereas electricity traveling away from the positive lead will be seen as a downward deflection.

Lead II is the most commonly used because the electricity flows toward the positive axis. This gives the best view of the ECG waves. Even though a single lead is adequate for detecting life-threatening dysrhythmias, as well as information about the heartbeat itself including rate and regularity, there is other information that cannot be obtained from a single lead. These include the presence or location of an infarct, the quality or presence of pumping action, axis deviation or chamber enlargement, and right-to-left differences in conduction or impulse formation.

To perform cardiac monitoring using the "quick look" technique, follow the steps in (Skill Drill 20-5 ▶):

1. **Set the lead select to "paddles," apply conductive gel to the paddles, and place the paddles on the chest in the same position as you would for defibrillation.** Place one paddle on the left lower part of the chest and one paddle on the right upper part of the chest, and apply 25 pounds of pressure to ensure a clear reading of the cardiac rhythm (**Step 1**).

2. **By holding the paddles in place you will be able to read the rhythm in lead II on the cardiac monitor** (**Step 2**).

3. **By swapping position of the paddles, you can see another lead or view.** This is especially helpful when verifying asystole. Rather than stopping to attach the lead wires and change the lead setting, simply reverse the position of the paddles.

> **EMT-I Tips**
>
> It is important to remember that you can only monitor through paddles when they are held against the patient's chest. For this reason, to free your hands, you should attach the lead wires as soon as possible after performing a "quick look" if defibrillation is not needed. Performing a "quick look" is only used for patients in cardiac arrest.

Introduction to Basic Components

Figure 20-38 ▼ shows the basic components of the ECG complex. Here are some basic definitions. A wave is a deflection from the baseline that represents some cardiac event. For instance, the P wave represents atrial depolarization. A segment is a specific portion of the complex as it is represented on the ECG. For example, the segment between the end of the P wave and the beginning of the Q wave is known as the P-R segment. An interval is the distance, measured as time, occurring between two cardiac events. The time interval between the beginning of the P wave and the beginning of the QRS complex is known as the P-R interval.

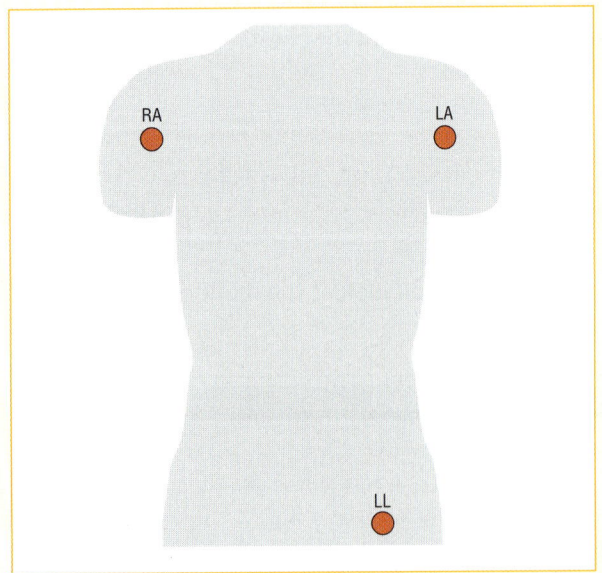

Figure 20-37 Lead placement.

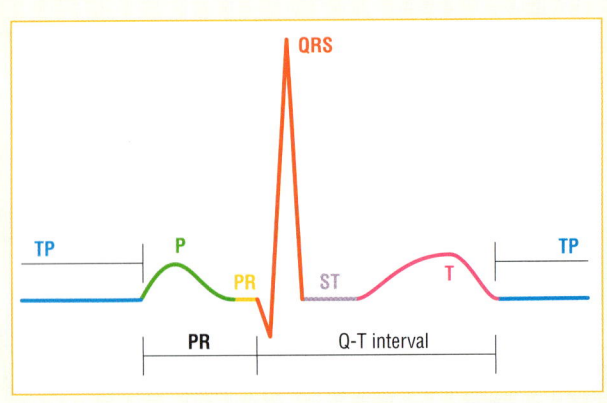

Figure 20-38 Basic components of the ECG complex.

Skill Drill 20-5: Using Paddles for Cardiac Monitoring

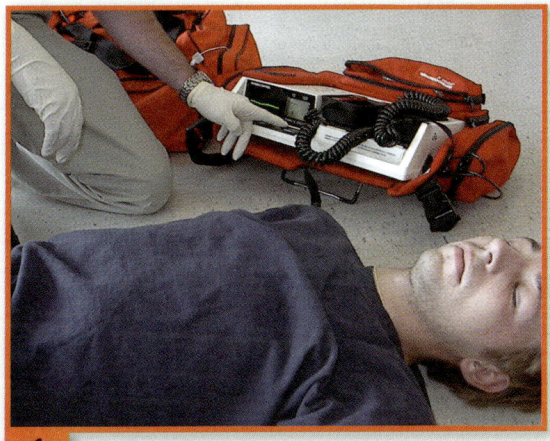

1 Set the lead select to "paddles," and place the paddles on the chest in the same position as you would for defibrillation.

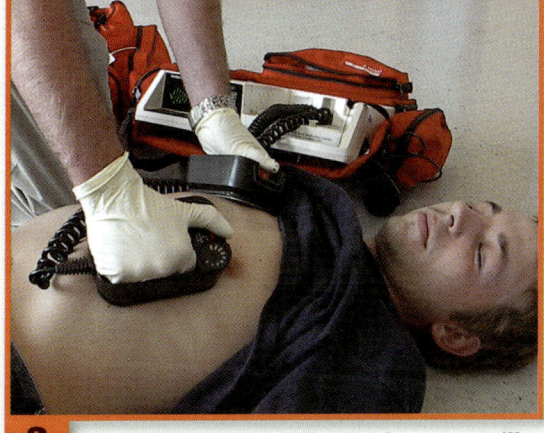

2 By holding the paddles in place, you will be able to read the rhythm in lead II on the cardiac monitor.

Note that there is a P-R interval and a P-R segment. In addition to the waves shown in Figure 20-38, there are a few others not mentioned, such as the R′ (R prime) wave and the U wave, which we will talk about individually. There are also other intervals that we are going to cover, such as the R-R interval and the P-P interval. Making sure that you understand the definitions of the basic terms will help prevent confusion. In Figure 20-38, we have labeled the waves and segments with colored letters and the intervals with black letters for easier identification.

Wave Nomenclature

A wave represents an electrical event in the heart, such as atrial depolarization, atrial repolarization, ventricular depolarization, ventricular repolarization, or transmission through the bundle of His, and so on. Waves can be single, isolated, positive, or negative deflections; biphasic deflections with both positive and negative components; or combinations that have multiple positive and negative components. Waves are deflections from the baseline. What is the baseline? It is a line from one T-P segment to the next.

Let's look at what that means in **Figure 20-39**. Note that the QRS complex is a combination of two or more waves. To be completely correct, these waves should be named according to size, location, and direction of deflection. Tall or deep waves in the QRS complex are given capital letters: Q, R, S, R′. Small waves are given small letters: q, r, s, r′. This is why the example in Figure 20-39 is called a qRs wave. This standard is unfortunately not followed as rigorously as you might expect. Many authors simply use all capital letters. In this book, we will follow the standard nomenclature with capital and small letters.

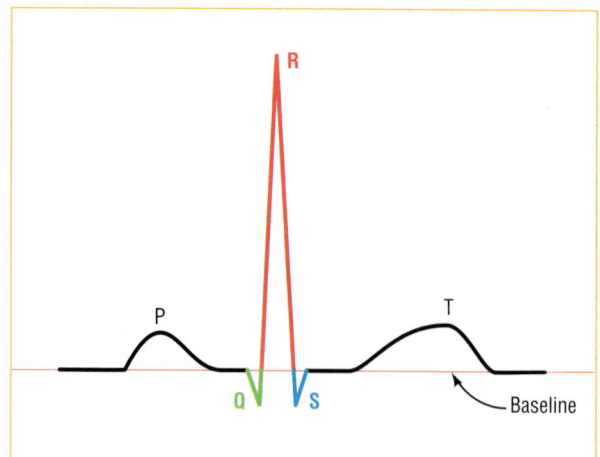

Figure 20-39 A QRS complex.

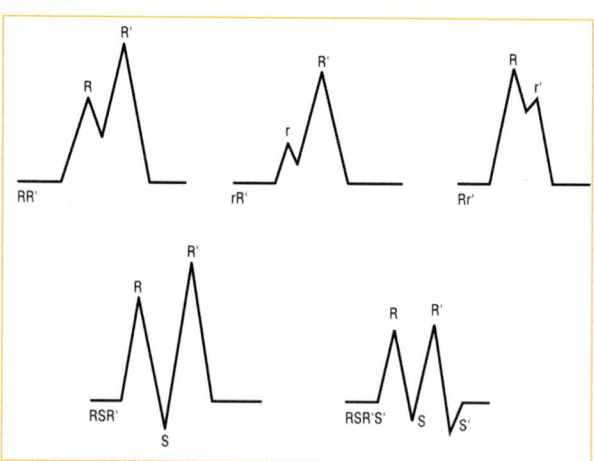

Figure 20-40 R' and S' complexes. (NOTE: The top row does not technically contain S waves. The term S wave applies only to negative components, or components that fall below the baseline. However, it is common for people to refer to any dip in a notched R wave as an S wave, regardless of whether it falls below the baseline. By following this logic further, most authors and clinicians refer to the second peak as the R' wave. Although this nomenclature is technically incorrect, it is so common that people accept this as the norm.)

R' and S' Waves

Just to make matters more interesting, let's look at some problems with the QRS waves. Changes occurring in the QRS complex can lead to bizarre complexes, and their waves are named differently if they change directions and cross the baseline. Such a wave is called an X' (X prime) wave, in which X is not an actual wave, but rather a term that can stand for either an R or S wave. R' and S' (R prime and S prime) refer to extra waves within the QRS complex. By definition, the first negative wave that we reach after the P wave is called the Q wave. The first positive deflection after the P is the R wave. Here is where it gets tricky: an S wave is the first negative component after an R wave. If we now get another upward component, we start with R'. The next negative component is S'.

A positive wave occurring after the S' would then be an R" wave (read as R double prime), and so on. Figure 20-40 ▶ shows some examples.

Individual Components of the ECG Complex

The P Wave

The P wave is usually the first wave encountered on an ECG complex (Figure 20-41 ▶). It represents the electrical depolarization of both atria. The wave starts when the SA node (also referred to as the sinus node) fires. It also includes transmission of the impulse through the three internodal pathways, the Bachman bundle, and the atrial myocytes themselves.

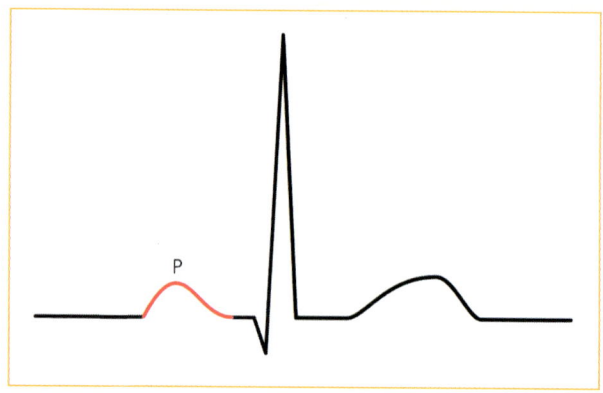

Figure 20-41 The P wave. Cardiac event represented by the P wave: Atrial depolarization. Normal duration: 0.08 to 0.11 seconds.

The duration of the wave itself can vary between 0.08 and 0.11 seconds in healthy adults. The axis of the P wave is usually directed downward and to the left, the direction the electrical impulse travels on its journey to the atrioventricular node and the atrial appendages.

The Tp Wave

The Tp wave, which represents repolarization of the atria, deflects in the opposite direction of the P wave (Figure 20-42 ▶). It is usually not seen because it occurs at the same time as the QRS wave and is obscured

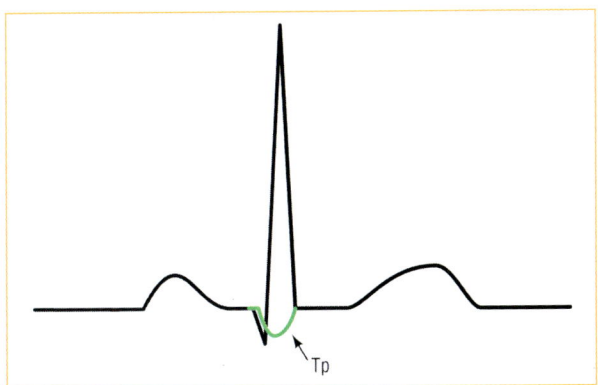

Figure 20-42 The Tp wave. Cardiac event represented by the Tp wave: Atrial repolarization. Normal duration: Usually not seen. Wave orientation: Opposite to the P wave.

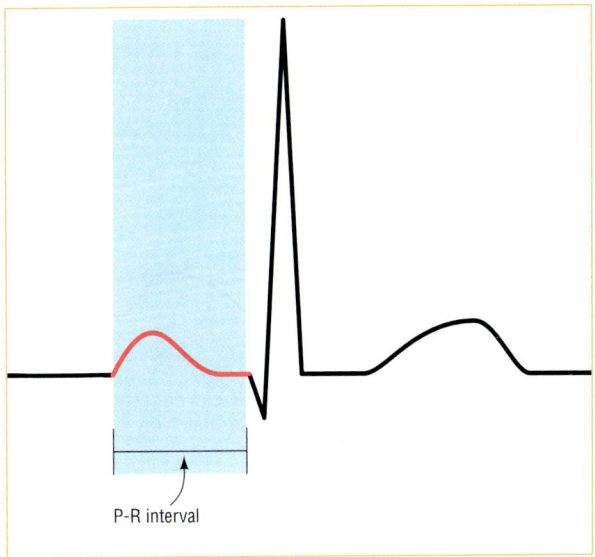

Figure 20-44 The P-R interval. Cardiac events represented by the P-R interval: Impulse initiation, atrial depolarization, and the normal delay at the AV node. Normal duration: 0.12 to 0.20 seconds.

(buried) by that more powerful complex. However, you can sometimes see it when there is no QRS after the P wave. This occurs in AV dissociation or nonconducted beats (discussed later in this chapter). You may also see it in P-R depression, or in the ST segment depression present in very fast sinus tachycardias. It appears as ST depression because the QRS comes sooner in the cycle, and the Tp wave—if it is negative—draws the ST segment downward.

The P-R Segment

The P-R segment occupies the time between the end of the P wave and the beginning of the QRS complex (Figure 20-43 ▼). It is usually found along the baseline. It can, however, be depressed by less than 0.8 mm under normal circumstances; anything greater than that indicates a pathologic condition (for example, pericarditis).

The P-R Interval

The P-R interval represents the time from the beginning of the P wave to the beginning of the QRS complex (Figure 20-44 ▲). It includes the P wave and the P-R segment, both discussed previously. The P-R interval covers all of the events from the initiation of the electrical impulse in the SA node up to the moment of ventricular depolarization. The normal duration is from 0.12 seconds to 0.20 seconds. If the P-R interval is shorter than 0.11 seconds, it is considered shortened. A P-R interval longer than 0.20 seconds is a first-degree AV block, which we will talk about in a later section. The P-R interval can be quite long, sometimes 0.40 seconds or greater. The term P-Q interval is sometimes used interchangeably if there is a Q wave as the initial component of the QRS complex.

The QRS Complex

The QRS complex represents ventricular depolarization. It is composed of two or more waves (Figure 20-45 ▶). Each wave has its own name or label. These can become quite complex. The main components are the Q, R, and S waves. By convention, the Q wave is the first negative deflection after the P wave. The Q wave can be present or absent. The R wave is the first positive deflection after the P wave. This will be the initial wave of the QRS complex if there is no Q wave present. The first

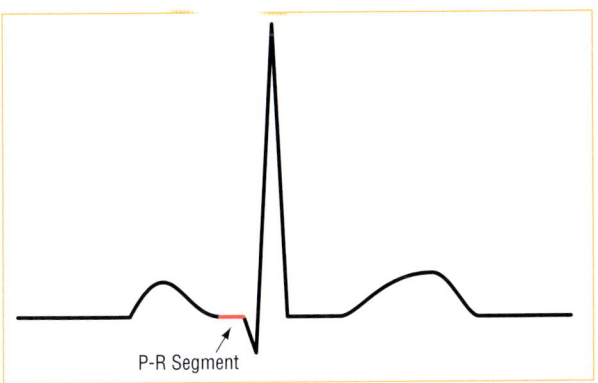

Figure 20-43 The P-R segment. Cardiac event represented by the P-R segment: Transmission of the electrical depolarization wave through the AV node, bundle of His, bundle branches, and Purkinje system.

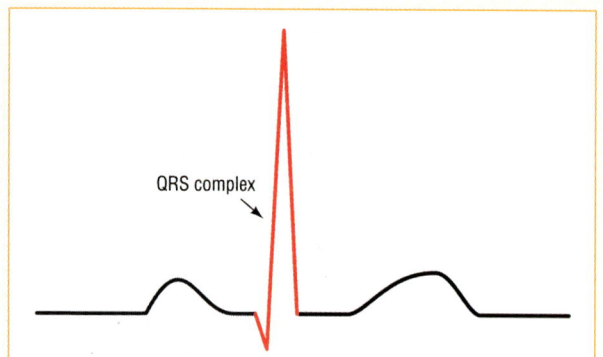

Figure 20-45 The QRS complex. Cardiac event represented by the QRS complex: Ventricular depolarization. Normal duration: 0.06 to 0.11 seconds.

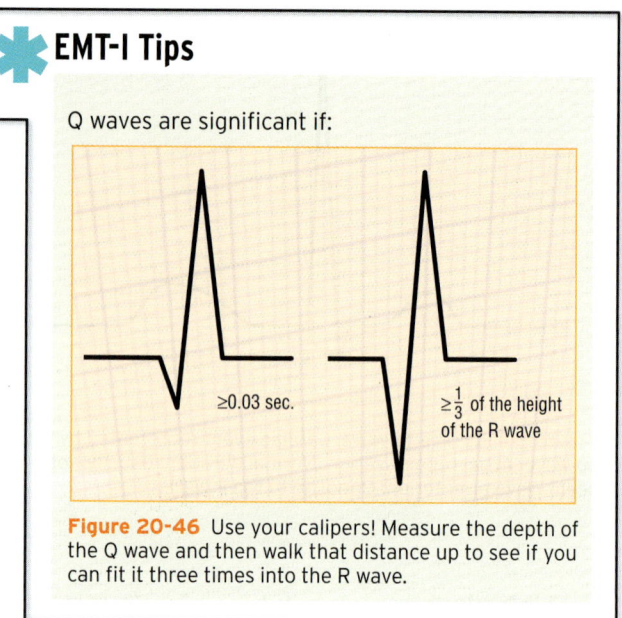

Figure 20-46 Use your calipers! Measure the depth of the Q wave and then walk that distance up to see if you can fit it three times into the R wave.

negative deflection after the R wave is the S wave. If there are additional components in the QRS complex, they will be named as prime waves (see Figure 20-40).

Q Wave Significance

The Q wave can be benign, or it can be a sign of dead myocardial tissue. A Q wave is considered significant if it is 0.03 seconds or wider or its height is equal to or greater than one third the height of the R wave. If it meets either of these criteria, it could indicate a myocardial infarction. If it doesn't, it is not a significant Q wave (Figure 20-47). Remember, only a 12-lead ECG can quantify these findings.

The Intrinsicoid Deflection

The intrinsicoid deflection is measured from the beginning of the QRS complex to the beginning of the negative downslope of the R wave in leads that begin with an R wave and do not contain a Q wave (Figure 20-48). It represents the amount of time it takes the electrical impulse to travel from the Purkinje system in the endocardium to the surface of the epicardium immediately under an electrode.

The ST Segment

The ST segment is the section of the ECG cycle from the end of the QRS complex to the beginning of the T wave. The point where the QRS complex ends and the ST segment begins is called the J point (Figure 20-49). Many times, a clear J point cannot be identified because of ST segment elevation. The ST segment is usually found along the baseline. However, it can vary slightly in healthy patients. It is important to note that in some patients, you may note ST segment depression or elevation while viewing lead II. This is not a

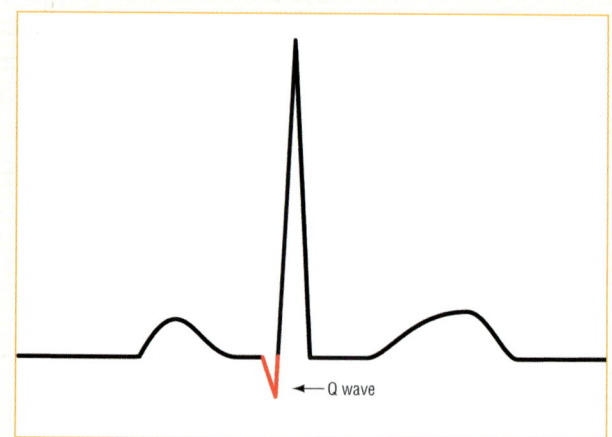

Figure 20-47 Insignificant Q wave.

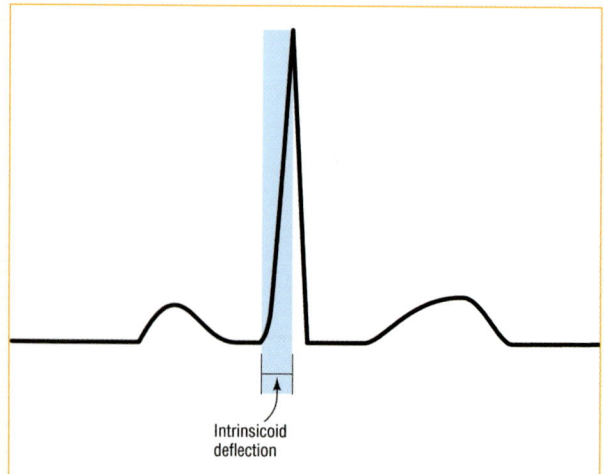

Figure 20-48 The intrinsicoid deflection.

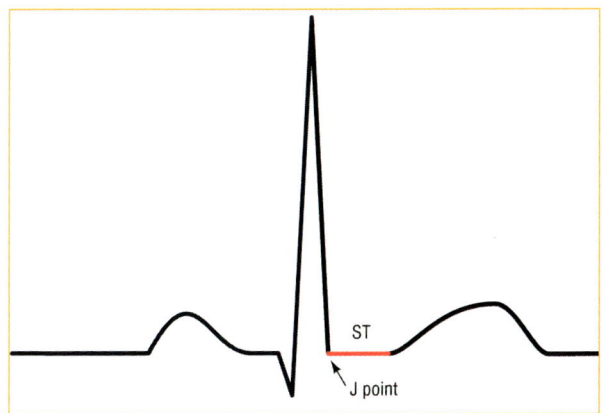

Figure 20-49 The J point. Cardiac event represented by the ST segment: Electrically neutral period between ventricular depolarization and repolarization. Normal location: At the level of the baseline.

conclusive finding of myocardial ischemia or injury. A 12-lead ECG, in conjunction with other tests performed in the hospital, must be performed to quantify these findings.

The ST segment represents an electrically neutral time for the heart. The ventricles are between depolarization (QRS complex) and repolarization (T wave). Mechanically, this represents the time that the myocardium is maintaining contraction to push the blood out of the ventricles. As you can imagine, very little blood would be expelled if the ventricles only contracted for 0.12 seconds.

The T Wave

The T wave represents ventricular repolarization Figure 20-50 ▼ . It is the next deflection—either positive or negative—that occurs after the ST segment

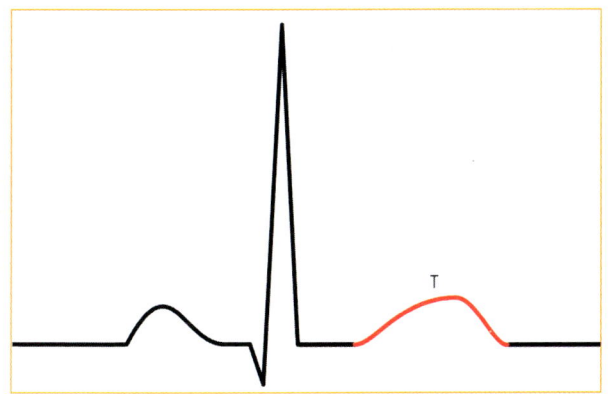

Figure 20-50 The T wave. Cardiac event represented by the T wave: Ventricular repolarization.

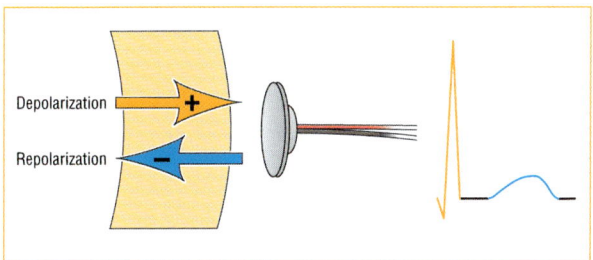

Figure 20-51 Depolarization and repolarization.

and should begin in the same direction as the QRS complex.

Why should the T wave be in the same direction as the QRS? If it represents repolarization, shouldn't it be opposite the QRS? For the answer, we need to go back to the concept of ventricular excitation. The Purkinje system is near the endocardium; therefore, electrical depolarization should begin in the endocardium and move out toward the epicardium Figure 20-51 ▲ .

You would expect repolarization to occur in the same direction because the cell that was first depolarized should be the first to repolarize, but this is not the case. Because of increased pressure on the endocardium during contraction, the repolarization wave travels in the opposite direction, from the epicardium back to the endocardium (see Figure 20-51). Remember, a negative wave—and repolarization is a negative wave—traveling away from the electrode is perceived the same as a positive wave moving toward it. Hence, the normal T wave should be in the same direction as the QRS. There are exceptions in some pathologic states.

The T wave should be asymmetrical, with the first part rising or dropping slowly and the latter part moving much faster Figure 20-52 ▶ . The way to check for symmetry of the T wave, if the ST segment is elevated, is to draw a perpendicular line from the peak of that wave to the baseline and then compare the symmetry of the two sides, ignoring the ST segment Figure 20-53 ▶ . Symmetric T waves can be normal but are usually a sign of disease.

The Q-T Interval

The Q-T interval is the section of the ECG complex encompassing the QRS complex, the ST segment, and the T wave—from the beginning of the Q to the end of the T Figure 20-54 ▶ . It represents all of the events of ventricular systole, from the beginning of ventricular depolarization to the end of the repolarization cycle. The interval varies with heart rate, electrolyte abnormalities, age, and sex. A prolonged Q-T is a harbinger of possible dysrhythmias. The Q-T interval should be no longer than one half of the preceding R-R interval (the interval between the peaks of the two preceding R waves).

The U Wave

The U wave is a small, flat wave sometimes seen after the T wave and before the next P wave (Figure 20-55 ▼). Various theories have arisen about what it represents, including ventricular depolarization and endocardial repolarization. Nobody knows for sure. It can be seen in healthy patients, especially in the presence of bradycardia. It can also be seen in hypokalemia (low potassium level). One valuable point is that there can be no possibility of hyperkalemia in the presence of a U wave (more about this later). The only other clinical significance of the U is that it can sometimes cause inaccuracy in measuring the Q-T interval.

Additional Intervals

There are a few additional intervals that we will cover as the text continues. However, let's talk about two of the most common ones now. First, there is the R-R interval, the distance between identical points (usually the peaks) of two consecutive QRS complexes

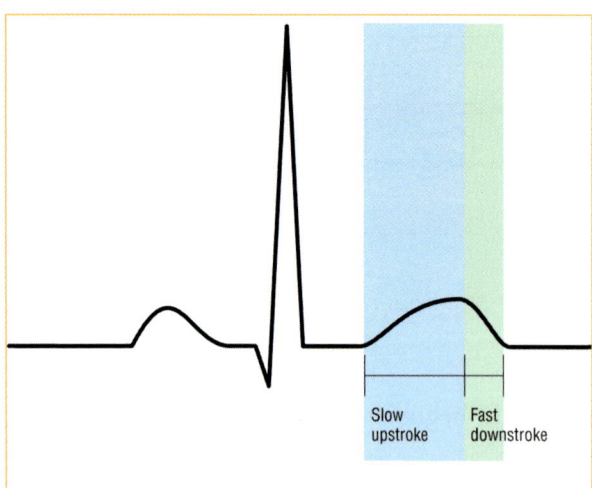

Figure 20-52 Slow upstroke and fast downstroke of the T wave.

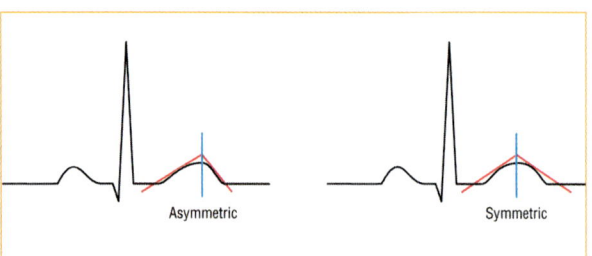

Figure 20-53 Assessing the symmetry of a T wave.

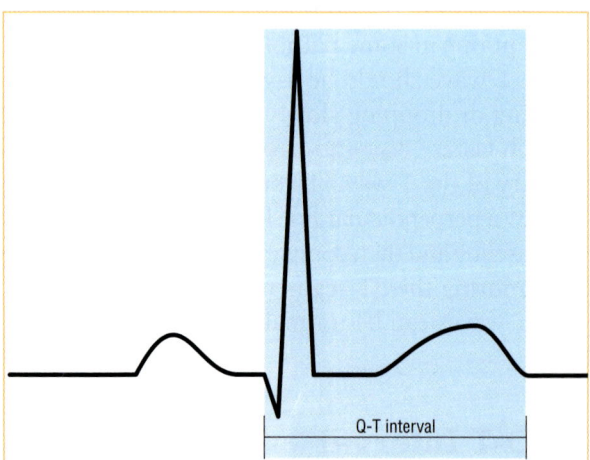

Figure 20-54 The Q-T interval. Cardiac events represented by the Q-T interval: All the events of ventricular systole and diastole. Normal duration: Variable, especially with heart rate. Usually less than half of the R-R interval.

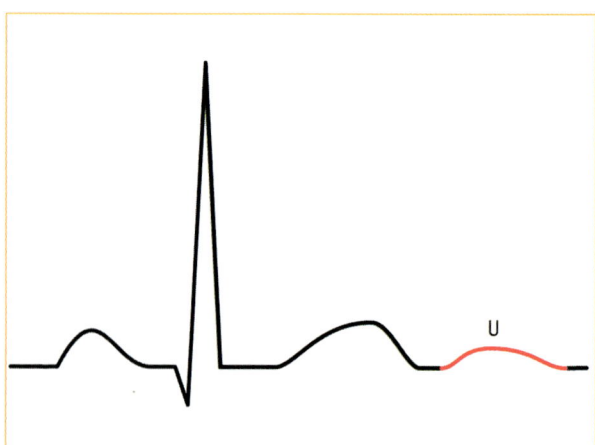

Figure 20-55 The U wave. Cardiac event represented by the U wave: Unknown. Important points: Low voltage; deflects in the same direction as the T wave. Clinical importance: Usually benign. The most important clinical significance of a U wave is that it could be a sign of hypokalemia.

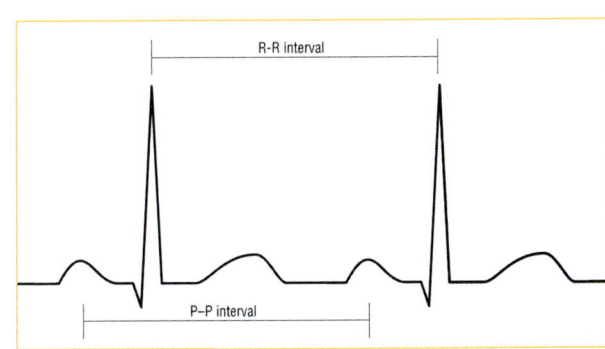

Figure 20-56 The P-P interval and the R-R interval.

Boxes and Sizes

The pen will record the ECG waves and segments onto the paper. To keep things simple, we have drawn straight horizontal lines to represent the complexes in Figure 20-57 ▼.

The ECG paper passes under the pen at a rate of 25 mm/sec. Each little box is, therefore, 1/25th of a second, or 0.04 seconds. Because a big box is made up of five little boxes, it represents 5 × 0.04 seconds = 0.20 seconds, so five big boxes make 1 second.

There are usually some small marks along the top or bottom of the strip every 3 seconds so that you can keep tabs on the time more easily. The lead should be appropriately labeled by the machine or the person obtaining the strip for easy identification. In addition, the patient's name should be labeled at the beginning or end of the strip.

When we talk about the vertical height of a wave or segment, we use millimeters; for instance, a wave that is five little boxes high would, in reality, be five millimeters high. Likewise, a darker big box is five millimeters high.

It will be very useful to keep these measurements in mind, especially when we discuss rates and widths

Figure 20-56 ▲). You will be measuring this often to evaluate the rhythm. Regular rhythms are those that have consistent R-R intervals.

Another is the P-P interval; the distance between two identical points on one P wave and the next (see Figure 20-56). This interval will be very useful in evaluating the patient for rhythm abnormalities. Examples include Wenckebach second-degree heart block, atrial flutter, and third-degree heart block.

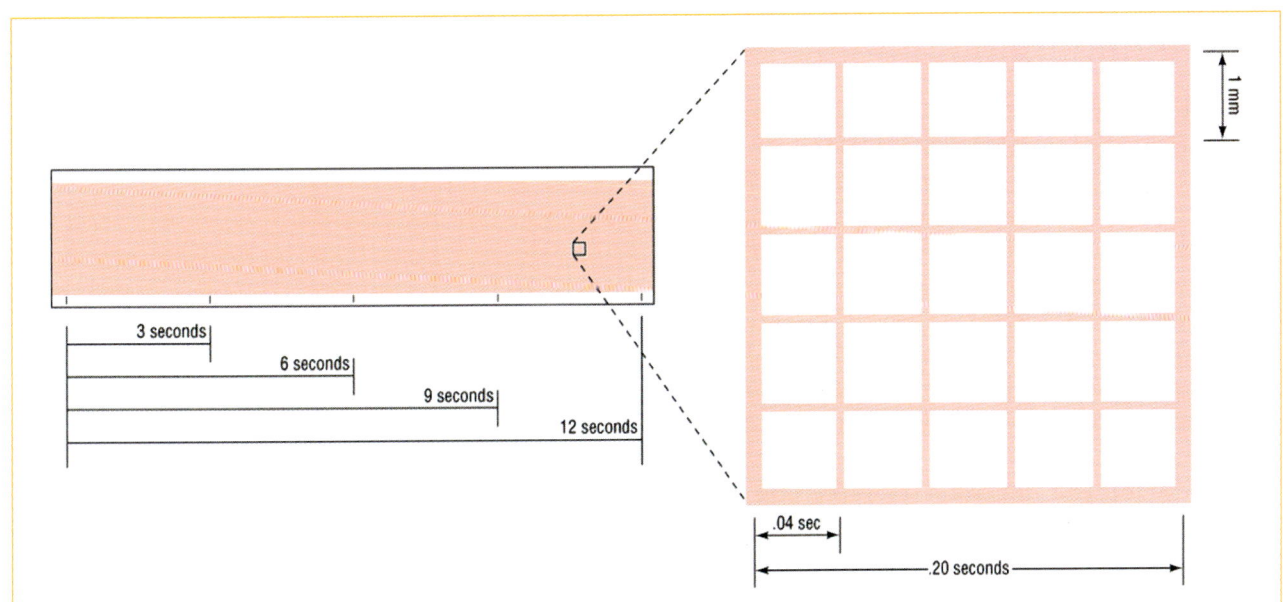

Figure 20-57 ECG paper. Height is measured in millimeters (mm) and width in milliseconds (ms).

of waves and segments. Everything on the rhythm strip is measured in millimeters or milliseconds, and you will use these measurements to describe your findings when examining the strip.

As an example, a wave can be described as being 15 mm high and 0.06 seconds wide. This would tell us that the height of the wave is 15 little boxes or three big boxes, and the width is 1.5 little boxes. With a bit of practice, you'll have this mastered.

ECG Tools

There are various tools that make reading and interpreting the ECG much easier (Figure 20-58). These include:

1. Calipers
2. ECG ruler
3. Straight edge

We'll talk about each of these in detail in this chapter. One quick comment about tools: although tools make your job easier, it is important not to completely depend on them. If you do, you will feel helpless when they are not available.

Calipers: The Clinician's Best Friend

In our opinion, it is almost impossible to interpret arrhythmias with any degree of accuracy if you do not use calipers (Figure 20-59). This is a strong statement, but it is true. It is possible to measure intervals and waves without calipers. It is even possible to evaluate consistency when you are evaluating the rhythm. We have seen people do all kinds of creative markings on pieces of paper to transfer the heights and widths of complexes. However, for accuracy and dependability, nothing beats the ECG calipers. If you don't own a set, go to your nearest medical bookstore or drafting supply house to get one. Always have them with you when you work clinically. It will simplify your life.

How do you use the calipers? Place one of the pins at the beginning of the object you are measuring, and move the other pin to the end. Then you can transfer that distance to an uncluttered part of the ECG paper to evaluate the height or the time of the measured object. The following are some simple ways to use calipers.

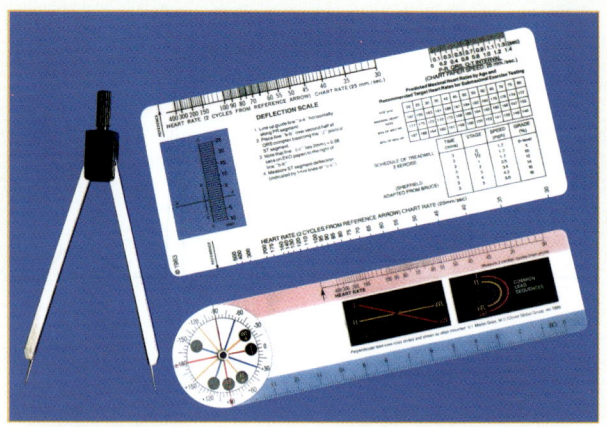

Figure 20-58 Calipers and an ECG ruler with an axis wheel and straight edge.

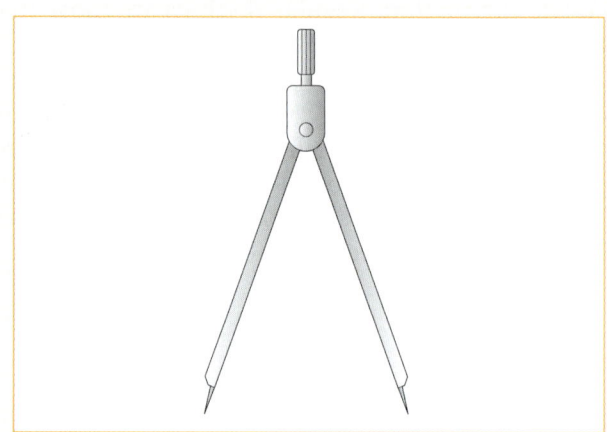

Figure 20-59 Measure distances on the ECG with calipers.

How to Use Your Calipers

Once you have measured the distance, it is easier to calculate the actual time frame on a cleaner, less cluttered area of the ECG paper (Figure 20-60). Remember, the big boxes are 0.20 seconds; there are two and a half of these in Figure 20-60, for a total of 0.50 seconds.

Now, suppose you want to see if the distance between three complexes is the same. First, measure the distance between complex A and complex B. Then, without lifting the right pin, swing the left pin to see if the distance from B to C is equal (Figure 20-61). By not moving the right pin, you are ensuring that the distances are the same. Swinging one pin over the other like this is called "walking."

You can walk the calipers back and forth across a strip to check the regularity of the complexes. You can also

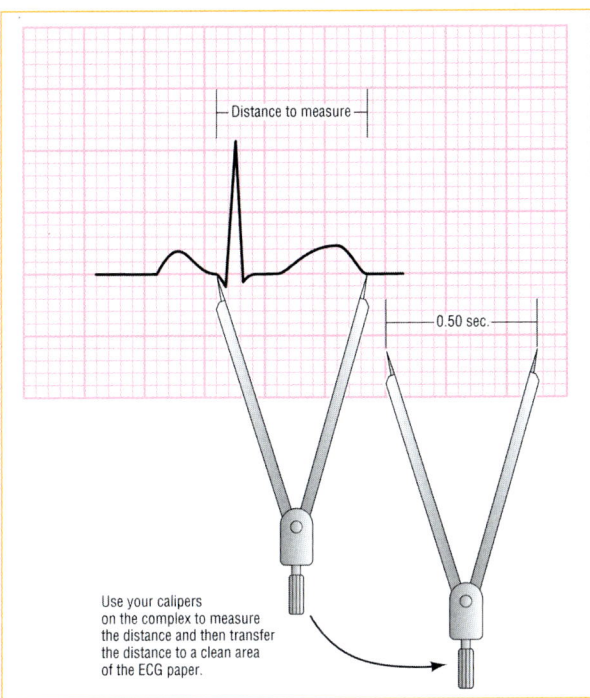

Figure 20-60 Total width of the complex is 0.50 seconds.

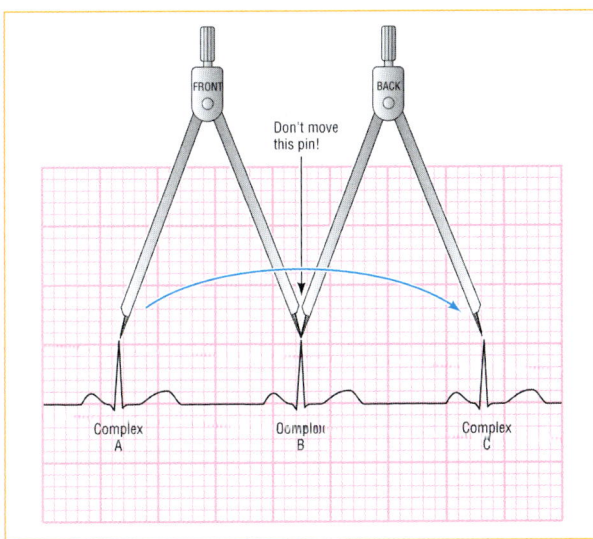

Figure 20-61 Walking the calipers. The distances are equal.

take that distance and move it anywhere you want on the paper. This technique is useful in determining third-degree heart blocks and many other ECG or rhythm abnormalities. Take your calipers and practice on some of the rhythm strips later in this chapter. Make sure you do some measurements as well.

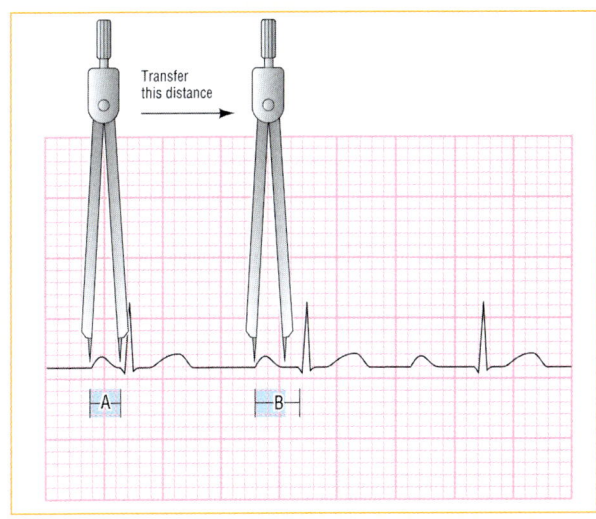

Figure 20-62 Distances A and B are not the same.

Comparing Widths

Explaining this one is a bit of overkill, but we really want you to understand the usefulness of the calipers. Suppose you wanted to see if distance A is the same as or longer than distance B (Figure 20-62▲). Position the calipers to measure distance A, then move them—transferring the distance accurately—to see if B is the same.

You will be using this technique for a great many comparisons in looking for atrioventricular blocks, aberrant beats, premature atrial contractions (PACs), PVCs, and so on.

ECG Rulers

ECG rulers (Figure 20-63▶) are not needed if you have a pair of calipers. Most rulers have one side that measures the rate and a metric ruler on the other. If you have a set of calipers and the ECG paper, you already have the same thing. ECG rulers also have some ECG criteria that are standard knowledge.

Straight Edge

Straight edges are useful in evaluating the baseline and determining whether there is any elevation or depression present. You can use a piece of paper, even the ECG paper folded in on itself (without creasing the paper—messy ECGs are tough to read). The best straight edges are clear with a line in the middle so you can see the

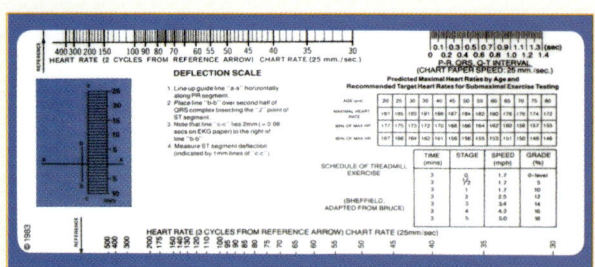

Figure 20-63 Straight-edge ruler.

whole area in question without obstructing any of the complex. You can then use the straight line to evaluate the baseline. If you wish to create additional rulers, make a copy of the one in Figure 20-64 ▼ on overhead transparency film. Your neighborhood copy store should be able to do this, preferably in color.

The Rate

When evaluating the rate of the complexes, first keep in mind that the P wave rate may be different from the QRS rate. For the purposes of this discussion, we consider QRS rates only. The same principles can be applied to obtain the P wave rate, if needed.

The rate can be obtained in various ways. If there is a computerized rate at the top of the ECG, you can usually use the rate that is given. Keep in mind, however, that this rate may be wrong. If it appears to be the wrong rate, calculate it yourself. One way of calculating the rate is to use a ruler, such as the one mentioned earlier in this chapter. There are also ways of calculating rate using the rhythm strip itself and your basic knowledge of the time intervals involved. Using your calipers with these techniques will be very helpful. Let's look at some of those ways now.

Establishing the Rate

Normal and Fast Rates

The easiest way to calculate the rate is to use the method illustrated in Figure 20-65 ▼. Find a QRS complex that starts on a thick line; this will be your starting point. Next, go to the exact spot on the next QRS complex—your end point. By tradition, we try to use the tip of the tallest wave on the QRS complex. However, you can use any spot as long as it is consistent.

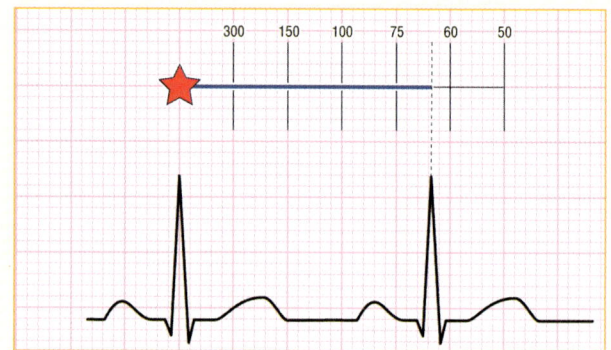

Figure 20-65 The rate is approximately 65 to 70 beats/min.

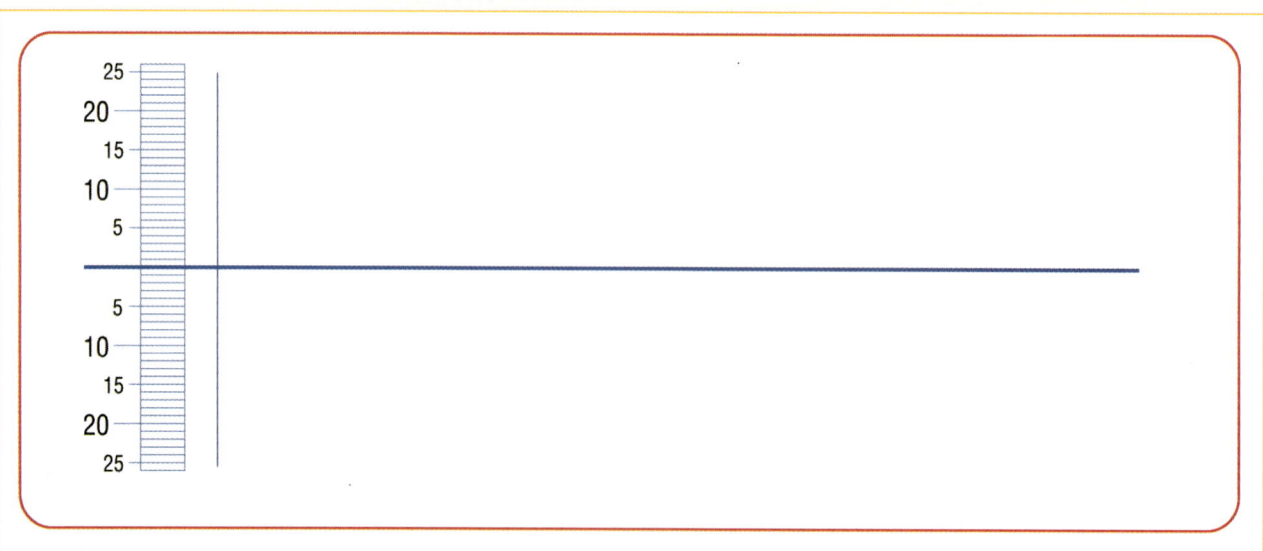

Figure 20-64 ECG straight edge.

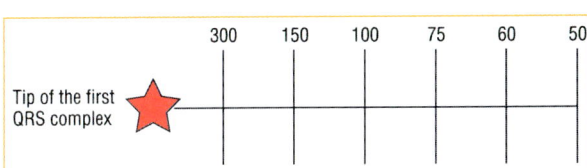

Figure 20-66 These are the rates corresponding to thick lines following the tip of the QRS complex that lands on (or is adjusted to, using calipers) an initial thick line.

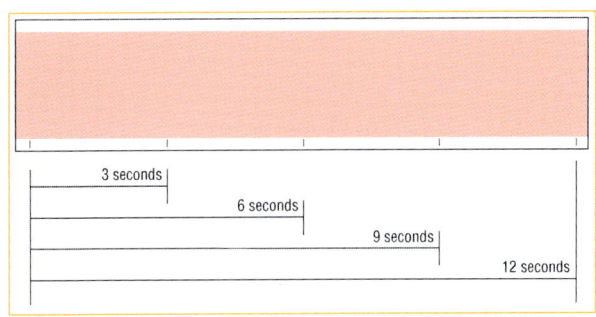

Figure 20-67 ECG paper.

Then just count the thick lines in between the two spots, using the numbers shown in **Figure 20-66**. You will have to memorize this sequence, but it is more than worth your trouble.

Another way to calculate the rate is to use your calipers to measure from the top of one complex to the top of the next. Then move the calipers—maintaining the measured distance—so that the left tip rests on a thick line, and calculate the rate as above for the distance between the two tips. The advantage here is that you don't have to hunt down a QRS that lands on a thick line to use as a starting point.

Bradycardic Rates

Do you remember the concept in **Figure 20-67**? Knowing these time intervals will be very useful when you are calculating bradycardic rhythms. Can you think of how to use these intervals to calculate the rate generally, but especially in regular and slow rhythms?

It's simple. Just count the number of cycles present in a 6-second strip, and multiply that number by 10. This will give you the number of beats in 60 seconds. You could also count the number of cycles in a 12-second strip and multiply by 5. Remember to use the fractional parts of cycles in your calculations, for example, 3.5 cycles in 6 seconds gives a rate of 35 beats per minute (3.5 cycles × 10 = 35 beats/min).

> **EMT-I Tips**
>
> (cycles in 6 seconds) × 10 = beats/min

Artifact

Artifacts are false abnormalities of the baseline present on an ECG or rhythm strip that are due to sources other than the patient's bioelectrical impulses **Figure 20-68**. The sources of these abnormalities can be anything from movement on the part of the

---

You are the Provider — Part 8

Following the appropriate interventions, your patient's rhythm has converted to a perfusing rhythm. You notice that the rhythm on the monitor is slow and the complexes are narrow.

Reassessment	Recording Time: 10 Minutes After Patient Contact
Respirations	Apneic; ventilated at 15 breaths/min
Pulse	46 beats/min, regular
Skin	Pale
Blood pressure	80/52 mm Hg
Sao_2	95% when ventilated via bag-valve-mask with 100% O_2

12. What steps can you take to determine the rhythm of this patient?

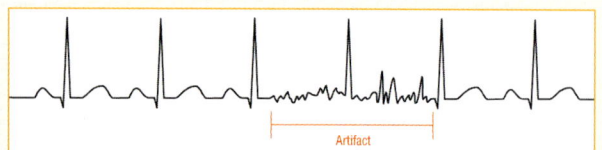

Figure 20-68 Artifact caused by a moving lead wire can result in a misinterpretation of the rhythm.

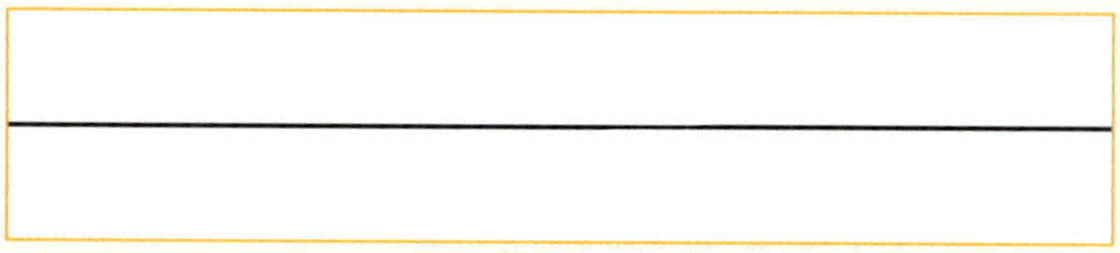

Figure 20-71 No, this patient was not in an asystolic cardiac arrest! The lead fell off his chest. When in doubt, take a look at your patient. A person cannot be sitting up eating dinner and be in asystole (lack of any electrical and mechanical activity in the heart) at the same time. Remember to always look at "the company that the arrhythmia keeps."

patient to movement of the electrical leads (wires), muscle tremors, and interference from external electrical equipment.

Many times the artifact can be easily identified and discounted. Other times, the artifact can be mistaken for the patient's rhythm or an arrhythmic event. In those cases, the artifact may lead to a misinterpretation of the rhythm and result in inappropriate, sometimes dangerous, or unnecessary treatment.

In some circumstances, as in Figure 20-69, the entire rhythm strip can be altered by the artifact. In this example, the clinicians could easily have misinterpreted the rhythm as a very dangerous rhythm known as ventricular tachycardia. Sometimes the artifact presents for only a short time, as in Figure 20-70. A quick way to verify your rhythm abnormality is to change the lead that your monitor is viewing because many times the artifact will present in only one lead. If any questions remain, remember to view the "company that the arrhythmia keeps" Figure 20-71. What we mean by this statement is that an arrhythmia does not occur in a void. Take a look at your patient and the clinical scenario before deciding on a course of action.

There is no easy way to tell what is artifact and what is the normal morphologic appearance of a rhythm. Unfortunately, it takes a lot of time and experience in ECG interpretation before you get the hang of it. A word of wisdom is to always look at what is abnormal and concentrate on that spot. Usually, that is where the answer lies, even if it is just artifact.

Major Concepts: Interpreting a Cardiac Rhythm

There are 10 points you should think about in an organized manner when approaching an ECG rhythm strip:

General:
1. Is the rhythm fast or slow?
2. Is the rhythm regular or irregular? If irregular, is it regularly irregular or irregularly irregular?

P waves:
3. Do you see any P waves?
4. Are all of the P waves the same?
5. Does each QRS complex have a P wave?
6. Is the P-R interval constant?

QRS complexes:
7. Are the P waves and QRS complexes associated with one another?
8. Are the QRS complexes narrow or wide?
9. Are the QRS complexes grouped or not grouped?
10. Are there any dropped beats?

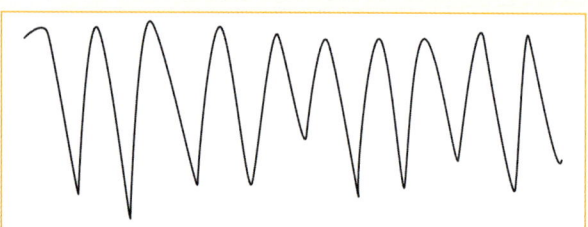

Figure 20-69 This patient was wrestling with her child. The movement of the leads caused the clinician to believe that the patient was in ventricular tachycardia. The rhythm returned to normal when the patient stopped moving.

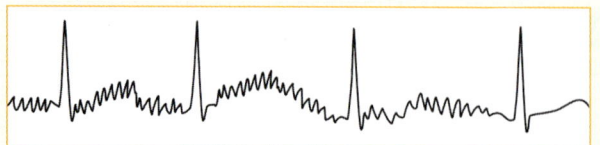

Figure 20-70 Interference by an electrical appliance in the room was the cause of this artifact. Turning off the machine caused the baseline to return to normal.

General

Is the Rhythm Fast or Slow?

Many rhythm abnormalities are associated with specific rate ranges. Therefore, it is very important to determine the rate of the rhythm in question. Decide whether you are dealing with tachycardia (>100 beats/min), bradycardia (<60 beats/min), or a normal rate.

Is the Rhythm Regular or Irregular?

Do the P waves and QRS complexes follow a regular pattern with the same intervals separating them, or are the intervals different between some or all of the beats? This is a great tool to help you narrow down the rhythm, as you will see in the upcoming pages.

There is an additional question you must answer if the rhythm is irregular: Is it regularly irregular or irregularly irregular? At first glance, this statement can be confusing. A rhythm is regularly irregular if it has some form or regularity to the pattern of the irregular complex. An example would be a rhythm in which every third complex comes sooner than the preceding two. Therefore, the intervals would be long-long-short, long-long-short, in a repeating pattern that is predictable and recurring in its irregularity.

An irregularly irregular rhythm has no pattern at all. All of the intervals are haphazard and do not repeat, with an occasional, accidental exception. Luckily, there are only three irregularly irregular rhythms: atrial fibrillation, wandering atrial pacemaker, and multifocal atrial tachycardia (discussed later). This is a differential diagnosis that you should commit to memory because it will get you out of some tight spots.

P Waves

Do you see any P waves?

The presence of P waves tells you that the rhythm in question has some atrial or supraventricular component. This is another major branch of the differential diagnosis of arrhythmias. The P waves, generated by the SA node or another atrial pacemaker, will usually reset any pacemaker down the chain.

Are all of the P waves the same?

The presence of P waves that are identical means that they are being generated by the same pacemaker site. Identical P waves should have identical P-R intervals unless an AV block is present (more later). If the P waves are not identical, consider two possibilities: there is an additional pacemaker cell firing, or there is some other component of the complex superimposed on the P wave, such as a T wave occurring at the same moment as the P wave. The presence of three or more different P wave forms with different P-R intervals defines wandering atrial pacemaker or multifocal atrial tachycardia, both described later in this chapter.

Does each QRS complex have a P wave?

An abnormal number of P waves in comparison with QRS complexes is an important point in determining whether you are dealing with some sort of AV block.

Is the P-R interval constant?

Once again, this is extremely useful in identifying a wandering atrial pacemaker or multifocal atrial tachycardia. It is also helpful in evaluating PACs with and without aberrant conduction (abnormal ventricular conduction from cell to cell that produces abnormally wide QRS complexes).

QRS Complexes

Are the P waves and QRS complexes associated with one another?

Is the P wave before a QRS complex responsible for the firing of that QRS (associated with it)? A positive answer to this question will help determine whether the entire complex is a normal beat, a premature beat, or a low-grade AV nodal block. In the discussion of ventricular tachycardia, you may note that the presence of capture and fusion beats is critical to the diagnosis. In these cases, the P wave preceding the capture or fusion beat is responsible for the complex, in contrast with the other P waves that are dissociated from their respective QRSs.

Are the QRS complexes narrow or wide?

Narrow complexes represent impulses that have traveled down the normal AV node and Purkinje network. These complexes are usually found in supraventricular rhythms, including junctional rhythms. Wide complexes indicate that the impulses did not follow the normal electrical conduction system, but instead were transmitted by direct cell-to-cell contact at some point in their travels through the heart. These wide complexes are found in PVCs, aberrantly conducted beats, ventricular tachycardia, and bundle branch blocks.

Are the QRS complexes grouped or not grouped?

This is very useful in determining the presence of an AV nodal block or recurrent premature complexes, such as bigeminy (a repeating pattern of a normal complex followed by a premature complex) and trigeminy (a repeating pattern of two normal complexes followed by a premature complex).

Are there any dropped beats?

Dropped beats occur in AV blocks and sinus arrest.

Individual Rhythms

This section shows examples of various cardiac rhythms and their respective criteria.

Supraventricular Rhythms

The term supraventricular refers to a location above the ventricles (supra = above); therefore, a supraventricular rhythm refers to a rhythm that originates above the level of the ventricles. Supraventricular rhythms typically have narrow (≤0.11 seconds) QRS complexes. Bear in mind that a supraventricular rhythm is not always a sinus rhythm; a sinus rhythm is characterized by P waves that are all upright and have the same morphologic features (form and structure), indicating that the rhythm originated in the SA node.

Normal Sinus Rhythm (NSR)

Normal sinus rhythm is shown in (Figure 20-72 ▼). Its characteristics are:
- Rate: 60–100 beats/min
- Regularity: Regular
- P wave: Present
- P/QRS ratio: 1:1
- P-R interval: Normal
- QRS width: Normal
- Grouping: None
- Dropped beats: None
- Putting it all together: This rhythm represents the normal state with the SA node functioning as the lead pacer. The intervals should all be consistent and within normal ranges. Note that this refers to the atrial rate; NSR can occur with a ventricular escape rhythm or other ventricular abnormality if AV dissociation exists.

Sinus Arrhythmia

Sinus arrhythmia is shown in (Figure 20-73 ▼). Its characteristics are:
- Rate: 60–100 beats/min
- Regularity: Varies with respiration
- P wave: Normal
- P/QRS ratio: 1:1
- P-R interval: Normal
- QRS width: Normal
- Grouping: None
- Dropped beats: None
- Putting it all together: This rhythm represents the normal respiratory variation, becoming slower during exhalation and faster on inhalation. This occurs because inhalation increases venous return by lowering intrathoracic pressure. Note that the P-R intervals are the same; only the T-P intervals (the interval from the end of the T wave of one complex to the beginning of the P wave of the next complex) vary with the respirations.

Sinus Bradycardia

Sinus bradycardia is shown in (Figure 20-74 ▶). Its characteristics are:
- Rate: Less than 60 beats/min
- Regularity: Regular
- P wave: Present
- P/QRS ratio: 1:1
- P-R interval: Normal to slightly prolonged
- QRS width: Normal to slightly prolonged
- Grouping: None
- Dropped beats: None

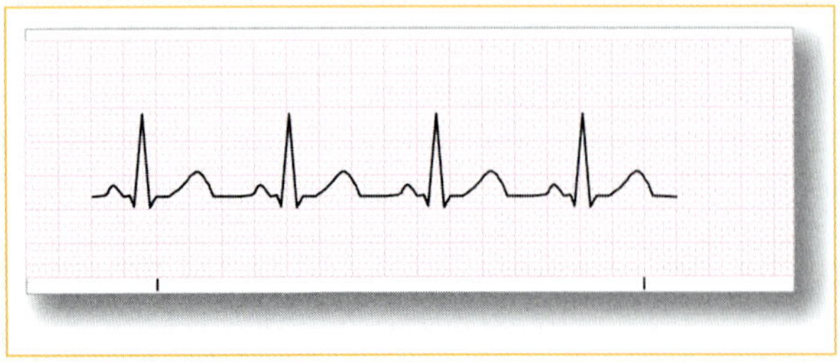

Figure 20-72 Normal sinus rhythm (NSR).

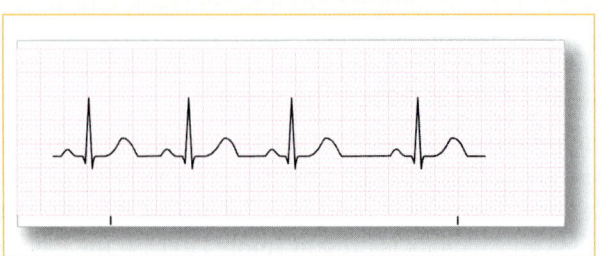

Figure 20-73 Sinus arrhythmia.

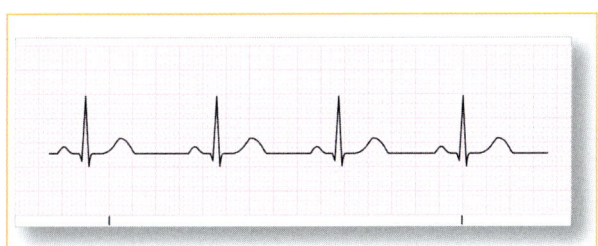

Figure 20-74 Sinus bradycardia.

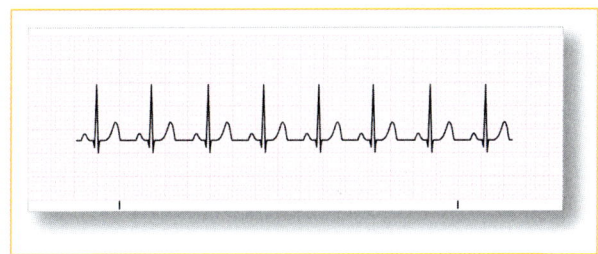

Figure 20-75 Sinus tachycardia.

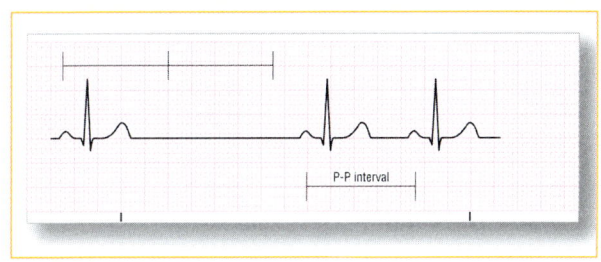

Figure 20-76 Sinus pause or arrest.

- Putting it all together: The sinus beats are slower than 60 beats/min. The origin may be in the SA node or in an atrial pacemaker. This rhythm can be caused by vagal stimulation leading to nodal slowing or by medicines such as beta blockers and is normally found in some well-conditioned athletes. The QRS complex and the P-R and Q-T intervals, may slightly widen as the rhythm slows below 60 beats/min. However, they will not widen past the upper threshold of the normal range for that interval. For example, the P-R interval may widen, but it should not widen beyond the upper range of 0.20 seconds.

Sinus Tachycardia

Sinus tachycardia is shown in Figure 20-75. Its characteristics are:
- Rate: Greater than 100 beats/min
- Regularity: Regular
- P wave: Present
- P/QRS ratio: 1:1
- P-R interval: Normal to slightly shortened
- QRS width: Normal to slightly shortened
- Grouping: None
- Dropped beats: None
- Putting it all together: This can be caused by medications or by conditions that require increased cardiac output, such as exercise, hypoxemia, hypovolemia, hemorrhage, and acidosis.

Sinus Pause or Arrest

Sinus pause or arrest is shown in Figure 20-76. Its characteristics are:
- Rate: Varies
- Regularity: Irregular
- P wave: Present except in areas of pause and arrest
- P/QRS ratio: 1:1
- P-R interval: Normal
- QRS width: Normal
- Grouping: None
- Dropped beats: Yes
- Putting it all together: A sinus pause is a variable period during which there is no sinus pacemaker working. The interval is not a multiple of the normal P-P interval. (A dropped complex that is a multiple of the P-P interval is known as an SA block, discussed next.) A sinus arrest is a longer pause, although there is no clear-cut criterion for how long a pause has to last before it is called an arrest.

Sinoatrial Block

Sinoatrial block is shown in Figure 20-77. Its characteristics are:
- Rate: Varies
- Regularity: Irregular
- P wave: Present except in areas of dropped beats
- P/QRS ratio: 1:1
- P-R interval: Normal
- QRS width: Normal
- Grouping: None
- Dropped beats: Yes
- Putting it all together: The block occurs in some multiple of the P-P interval. After the dropped

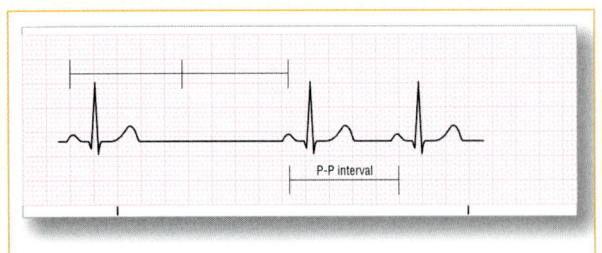

Figure 20-77 Sinoatrial block.

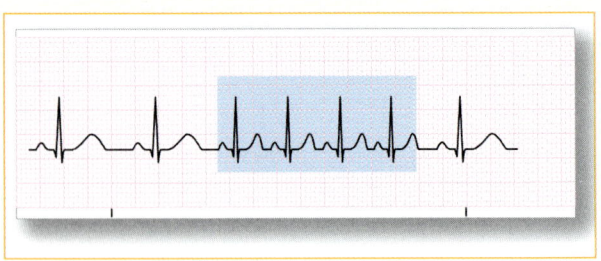

Figure 20-79 Ectopic atrial tachycardia.

beat, the cycles continue on time and as scheduled. The pathologic factor involved is a nonconducted beat from the normal pacemaker.

Premature Atrial Contraction

Premature atrial contraction is shown in Figure 20-78. Its characteristics are:

- Rate: Depends on the underlying rate
- Regularity: Irregular
- P wave: Present; in the PAC, may be a different shape
- P/QRS ratio: 1:1
- P-R interval: Varies in the PAC, otherwise normal
- QRS width: Normal
- Grouping: Sometimes
- Dropped beats: No
- Putting it all together: A PAC occurs when some other pacemaker cell in the atria fires at a rate faster than that of the SA node. The result is a complex that comes sooner than expected. Notice that the premature beat "resets" the SA node, and the pause after the PAC is not compensated; the underlying rhythm is disturbed and does not proceed at the same pace. This noncompensatory pause is less than twice the underlying normal P-P interval. With most PACs, the P wave of the premature complex will have different morphologic features than the other, normally conducted complexes.

Ectopic Atrial Tachycardia

Ectopic atrial tachycardia is shown in Figure 20-79. Its characteristics are:

- Rate: 100–180 beats/min
- Regularity: Regular
- P wave: Morphologic features of ectopic P waves are different
- P/QRS ratio: 1:1
- P-R interval: A different interval than the normal complexes
- QRS width: Normal, but can be aberrant at times
- Grouping: None
- Dropped beats: None
- Putting it all together: Ectopic atrial tachycardia occurs when an ectopic atrial focus fires more quickly than the underlying sinus rate. The P waves and P-R intervals are different because the rhythm is caused by an ectopic atrial pacemaker (a pacemaker outside the normal SA node). The episodes are usually not sustained for an extended period. Because of the accelerated rate, some ST- and T-wave abnormalities may be present transiently.

Wandering Atrial Pacemaker (WAP)

Wandering atrial pacemaker is shown in Figure 20-80. Its characteristics are:

- Rate: Variable
- Regularity: Irregularly irregular
- P wave: At least three different forms
- P/QRS ratio: 1:1
- P-R interval: Variable depending on the focus
- QRS width: Normal
- Grouping: None

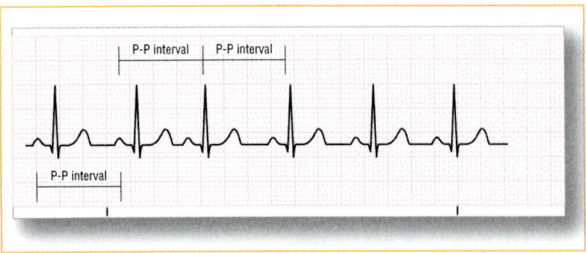

Figure 20-78 Premature atrial contraction (PAC).

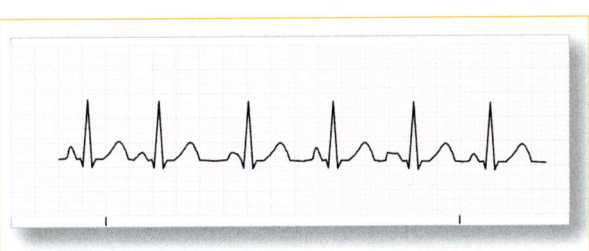

Figure 20-80 Wandering atrial pacemaker (WAP).

- Dropped beats: None
- Putting it all together: The WAP is an irregularly irregular rhythm created by multiple atrial pacemakers each firing at its own pace. The result is an ECG tracing with at least three different P wave forms with their own intrinsic P-R intervals. Think of each pacer firing from a different distance and with a different P-wave axis. The longer the distance, the longer the P-R interval. The varying P-wave axis causes differences in the morphologic features of the P waves.

Multifocal Atrial Tachycardia (MAT)

Multifocal atrial tachycardia is shown in Figure 20-81. Its characteristics are:
- Rate: More than 100 beats/min
- Regularity: Irregularly irregular
- P wave: At least 3 different forms
- P/QRS ratio: 1:1
- P-R interval: Variable
- QRS width: Normal
- Grouping: None
- Dropped beats: None
- Putting it all together: The MAT is merely a tachycardic WAP. Both MAT and WAP are commonly found in patients with severe lung disease. The tachycardia can cause cardiovascular instability at times, so it should be treated. Treatment is difficult and should be aimed at correcting the underlying problem.

Atrial Flutter

Atrial flutter is shown in Figure 20-82. Its characteristics are:
- Rate: Atrial rate commonly 250–350 beats/min; Ventricular rate commonly 125–175 beats/min
- Regularity: Usually regular, but may be variable
- P wave: Saw-toothed appearance, "F waves"
- P/QRS ratio: Variable, most commonly 2:1
- P-R interval: Variable
- QRS width: Normal
- Grouping: None
- Dropped beats: None
- Putting it all together: The F waves appear in a saw-toothed pattern such as those in this ECG tracing. (QRSs have been removed from strip B to reveal F wave shape.) The QRS rate is usually regular, and the complexes appear at some multiple of the P-P interval. The usual QRS response is 2:1 (this means that there are two F waves for each QRS complex). The ventricular response can also occur slower at rates of 3:1, 4:1, or higher. Sometimes the ventricular response will be irregular.

Rarely, you will have a truly variable ventricular response that does not fall on any multiple of the F-F interval. We call this an atrial flutter with a variable ventricular response.

Keep in mind that the saw-toothed appearance may not be obvious in all ECG tracings. Whenever you see a ventricular rate of 150 beats/min, look for the buried F waves of an atrial flutter with 2:1 block!

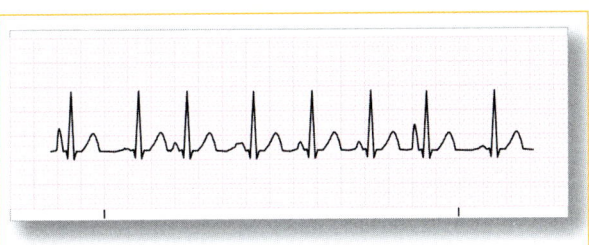

Figure 20-81 Multifocal atrial tachycardia (MAT).

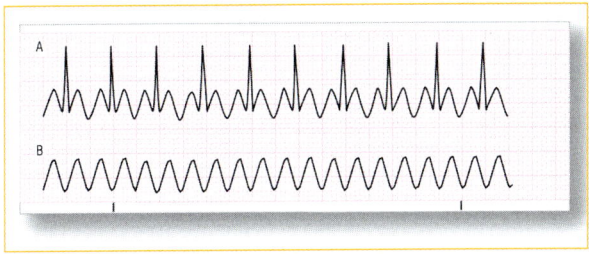

Figure 20-82 Atrial flutter.

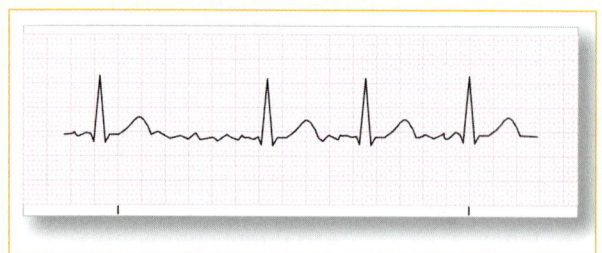

Figure 20-83 Atrial fibrillation.

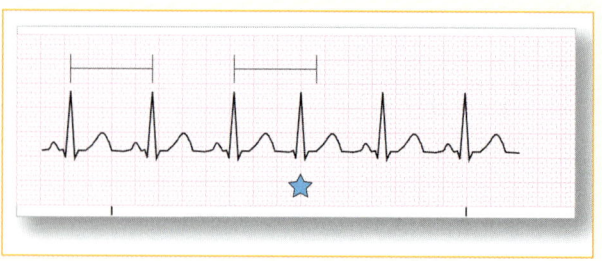

Figure 20-84 Premature junctional contraction (PJC).

Atrial Fibrillation

Atrial fibrillation is shown in Figure 20-83. Its characteristics are:
- Rate: Variable; ventricular response can be normal, fast, or slow
- Regularity: Irregularly irregular
- P wave: None; chaotic atrial activity
- P/QRS ratio: None
- P-R interval: None
- QRS width: Normal
- Grouping: None
- Dropped beats: None
- Putting it all together: Atrial fibrillation is the chaotic firing of numerous atrial pacemaker cells in a totally haphazard manner. The result is that there are no discernible P waves, and the QRS complexes are innervated haphazardly in an irregularly irregular pattern. The ventricular rate is guided by occasional activation from one of the pacemaking sources. Because the ventricles are not paced by any one site, the R-R intervals are completely random.

Junctional Rhythms

A junctional rhythm refers to any rhythm that originates in and around the AV node, in the region of the AV junction. Although junctional in nature, these rhythms are still considered supraventricular rhythms (the AV junction is above the ventricles). Junctional rhythms are not sinus in origin because the primary pacemaker is not the SA (sinus) node.

Premature Junctional Contraction (PJC)

Premature junctional contraction is shown in Figure 20-84. Its characteristics are:
- Rate: Depends on underlying rhythm
- Regularity: Irregular
- P wave: Variable (none, antegrade, or retrograde)
- P/QRS ratio: None; or 1:1 if antegrade or retrograde
- P-R interval: None, short, or retrograde; if present, does not represent atrial stimulation of the ventricles
- QRS width: Normal
- Grouping: Usually none, but can occur
- Dropped beats: None
- Putting it all together: A PJC is a beat that originates prematurely in the AV node. Because it travels down the normal electrical conduction system of the ventricles, the QRS complex is identical to the underlying QRSs. The PJCs usually appear sporadically but can occur in a regular, grouped pattern such as supraventricular bigeminy or trigeminy. There may be an antegrade or retrograde P wave associated with the complex. An antegrade P wave is one that appears before the QRS complex. The P-R interval is very short in these cases, and the P-wave axis will be abnormal (inverted in leads II and III). A retrograde P wave is one that appears after the QRS complex.

Junctional Escape Beat

Junctional escape beat is shown in Figure 20-85. Its characteristics are:
- Rate: Depends on underlying rhythm
- Regularity: Irregular

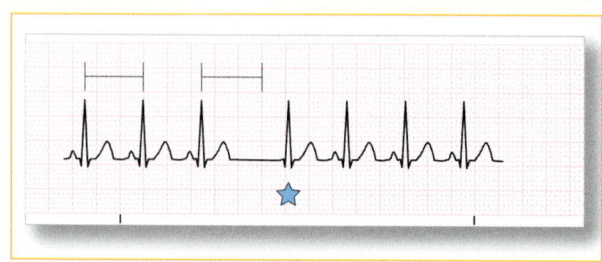

Figure 20-85 Junctional escape beat.

- P wave: Variable (none, antegrade, or retrograde)
- P/QRS ratio: None or 1:1 if antegrade or retrograde
- P-R interval: None, short, or retrograde; if present, does not represent atrial stimulation of the ventricles
- QRS width: Normal
- Grouping: None
- Dropped beats: Yes
- Putting it all together: An escape beat occurs when the normal pacemaker fails to fire and the next available pacemaker in the conduction system fires in its place. The AV nodal pacer senses that the normal pacer did not fire. So, when its turn comes up and it reaches threshold potential, it fires. The distance of the escape beat from the preceding complex is always longer than the normal P-P interval.

Junctional Escape Rhythm

Junctional escape rhythm is shown in Figure 20-86. Its characteristics are:
- Rate: 40–60 beats/min
- Regularity: Regular
- P wave: Variable (none, antegrade, retrograde)
- P/QRS ratio: None or 1:1 if antegrade or retrograde
- P-R interval: None, short, or retrograde; if present, does not represent atrial stimulation of the ventricles
- QRS width: Normal
- Grouping: None
- Dropped beats: None
- Putting it all together: A junctional escape rhythm arises as an escape rhythm when the normal pacemaking function of the atria and SA node is absent. It can also occur in the case of AV dissociation or third-degree AV block.

Accelerated Junctional Rhythm

Accelerated junctional rhythm is shown in Figure 20-87. Its characteristics are:
- Rate: 60–100 beats/min
- Regularity: Regular
- P wave: Variable (none, antegrade, retrograde)
- P/QRS ratio: None or 1:1 if antegrade or retrograde
- P-R interval: None, short, or retrograde; if present, does not represent atrial stimulation of the ventricles
- QRS width: Normal
- Grouping: None
- Dropped beats: None
- Putting it all together: This rhythm originates in a junctional pacemaker that, because it is firing faster than the normal pacemaker, takes over the pacing function. It is faster than expected for a normal junctional rhythm, pacing in the range of 60 to 100 beats/min. Pacing that exceeds 100 beats/min is known as junctional tachycardia. As with other junctional pacers, the P waves can be absent or conducted in an antegrade or retrograde manner.

Ventricular Rhythms

Ventricular rhythms are those that originate in the ventricular conduction system of the myocardium. As a general rule, these rhythms are potentially more lethal than supraventricular rhythms because of their propensity to deteriorate to life-threatening dysrhythmias (that is, V tach, V-fib). Any rhythm or complex that originates in the ventricles will have a wide (0.12 seconds) and bizarre-appearing QRS complex.

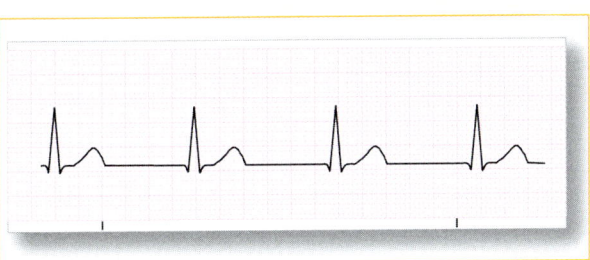

Figure 20-86 Junctional escape rhythm.

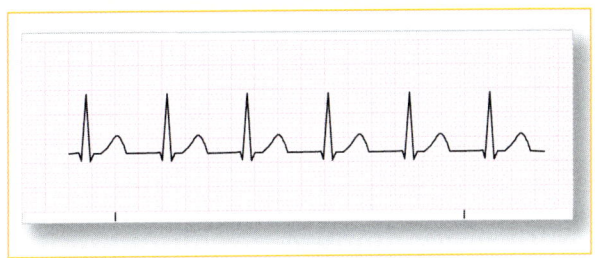

Figure 20-87 Accelerated junctional rhythm.

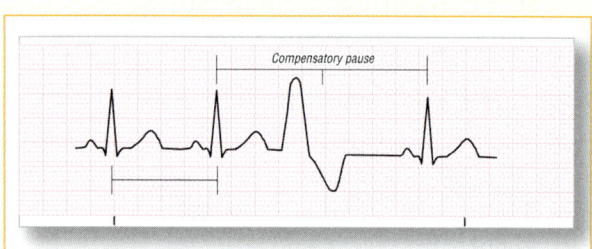

Figure 20-88 Premature ventricular contraction (PVC).

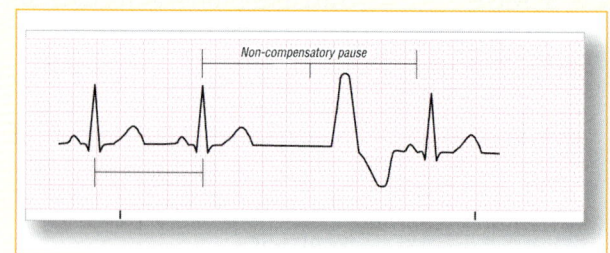

Figure 20-89 Ventricular escape beat.

Premature Ventricular Contraction

Premature ventricular contraction is shown in Figure 20-88 ▲. Its characteristics are:

- Rate: Depends on the underlying rhythm
- Regularity: Irregular
- P wave: Not present on the PVC
- P/QRS ratio: No P waves on the PVC
- P-R interval: None
- QRS width: Wide (≥0.12 seconds); bizarre appearance
- Grouping: Usually not present
- Dropped beats: None
- Putting it all together: A PVC is caused by the premature firing of a ventricular cell. The ventricular pacer fires before the normal SA node or supraventricular pacer, which causes the ventricles to be in a refractory state (not yet repolarized and unavailable to fire again) when the normal pacer fires. Hence, the ventricles do not contract at their normal time. However, the underlying pacing schedule is not altered, so the beat following the PVC will arrive on time. This is a **compensatory pause**.

Ventricular Escape Beat

Ventricular escape beat is shown in Figure 20-89 ▶. Its characteristics are:

- Rate: Depends on the underlying rhythm
- Regularity: Irregular
- P wave: None in the PVC
- P/QRS ratio: None in the PVC
- P-R interval: None
- QRS width: Wide (≥0.12 seconds); bizarre appearance
- Grouping: None
- Dropped beats: None
- Putting it all together: A ventricular escape beat is similar to a junctional escape beat, but the focus is in the ventricles. The pause is noncompensatory in this case because the normal pacer did not fire. (This is what led to the ventricular escape beat.) The pacer then resets itself on a new timing cycle and may even have a different rate.

Idioventricular Rhythm

Idioventricular rhythm is shown in Figure 20-90 ▼. Its characteristics are:

- Rate: 20–40 beats/min
- Regularity: Regular
- P wave: None
- P/QRS ratio: None
- P-R interval: None
- QRS width: Wide (≥0.12 seconds); bizarre appearance
- Grouping: None
- Dropped beats: None
- Putting it all together: An idioventricular rhythm occurs when a ventricular focus acts as the primary pacemaker for the heart. The QRS complexes are wide and bizarre, reflecting their ventricular origin. This rhythm can be found by itself or as a component of AV dissociation or

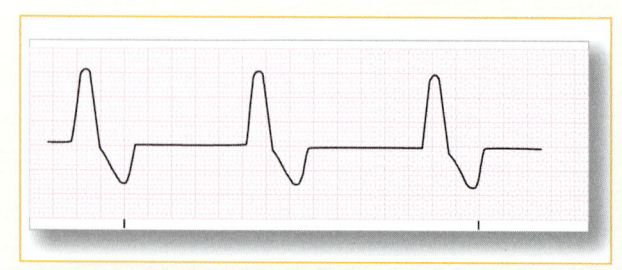

Figure 20-90 Idioventricular rhythm.

third-degree heart block. (In these latter cases, there may be an underlying sinus rhythm with P waves present.)

EMT-I Tips

Do not treat an idioventricular rhythm with antiarrhythmics! If you are successful in eliminating your last pacemaker, what do you have? Asystole!

Accelerated Idioventricular Rhythm

Accelerated idioventricular rhythm is shown in Figure 20-91 ▼. Its characteristics are:
- Rate: 40–100 beats/min
- Regularity: Regular
- P wave: None
- P/QRS ratio: None
- P-R interval: None
- QRS width: Wide (≥0.12 seconds); bizarre appearance
- Grouping: None
- Dropped beats: None
- Putting it all together: This is, basically, a faster version of an idioventricular rhythm. There are usually no P waves associated with it, in keeping with the ventricular source of the pacing. However, they can be present in AV dissociation or third-degree heart block.

Ventricular Tachycardia

Ventricular tachycardia is shown in Figure 20-92 ▶. Its characteristics are:
- Rate: 100–250 beats/min
- Regularity: Regular
- P wave: Dissociated atrial rate
- P/QRS ratio: Variable
- P-R interval: None

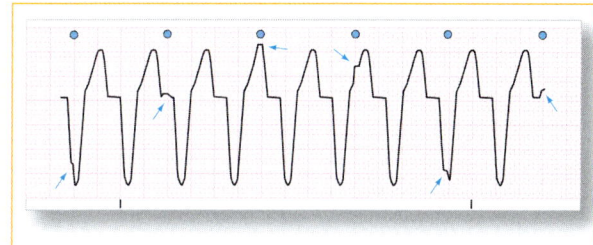

Figure 20-92 Ventricular tachycardia (V-tach).

- QRS width: Wide (≥0.12 seconds); bizarre
- Grouping: None
- Dropped beats: None
- Putting it all together: Ventricular tachycardia (V-tach) is a very fast ventricular rate that is usually dissociated from an underlying atrial rate. The rhythm depicted above is **monomorphic** V-tach, which means that all of the complexes are of the same size, shape, and direction. In this ECG tracing, you will notice irregular forms of the QRS complexes at regular intervals. These irregularities are the underlying sinus beats. (Blue dots indicate sinus beats, and arrows pinpoint the irregularities.) There are many criteria related to V-tach, which we'll take a look at now.

Capture and Fusion Beats. Occasionally, a sinus beat will fall on a spot that allows some innervation of the ventricle to occur through the normal ventricular conduction system. This forms a fusion beat Figure 20-93 ▼, which has morphologic features somewhere between the abnormal ventricular beat and the normal QRS complex. This type of complex is literally caused by two pacemakers, the SA node and the ventricular pacer. Because two areas of the ventricle are being stimulated simultaneously, the result is a hybrid—or fusion—complex with some features of both. It may help to think of this in terms of the following analogy. If you mix a

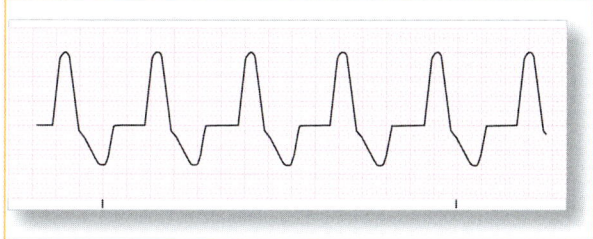

Figure 20-91 Accelerated idioventricular rhythm.

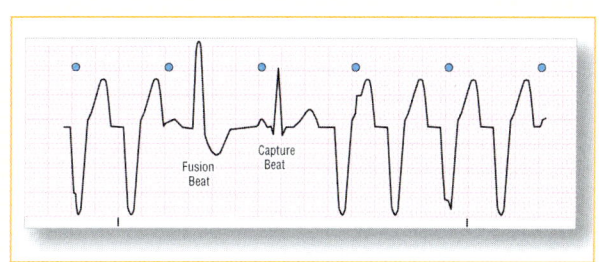

Figure 20-93 Fusion and capture beats in V-tach.

blue liquid with a yellow liquid, the result is a green liquid. A fusion beat is like the green liquid; it is the fusion of the two complexes.

A capture beat, on the other hand, is completely innervated by the sinus beat and is indistinguishable from the patient's normal complex. This is called a capture beat instead of a normal beat because it occurs in the middle of the chaos that is V-tach and is caused by chance timing of a sinus beat at just the right millisecond to "capture" or transmit through the AV node and depolarize the ventricles through the normal conduction system of the heart.

Fusion and capture beats are hallmarks of ventricular tachycardia; you will usually see them if the strip is long enough. If you see these types of complexes with a wide-complex, tachycardic rhythm, you have found V-tach.

More V-tach Indicators. There are some additional signs we should look at. You don't need to remember the names, but you should know about the Brugada and Josephson signs (Figure 20-94 ▼). The Brugada sign occurs during V-tach. The interval from the R wave to the bottom of the S wave is 0.10 seconds or more. The Josephson sign, which is just a small notching near the low point of the S wave, is another indicator of V-tach.

Torsade de Pointes (TdP)

Torsade de pointes (TdP) is shown in (Figure 20-95 ▶). Its characteristics are:
- Rate: 200–250 beats/min
- Regularity: Irregular
- P wave: None
- P/QRS ratio: None
- P-R interval: None
- QRS width: Variable
- Grouping: Variable sinusoidal pattern
- Dropped beats: None

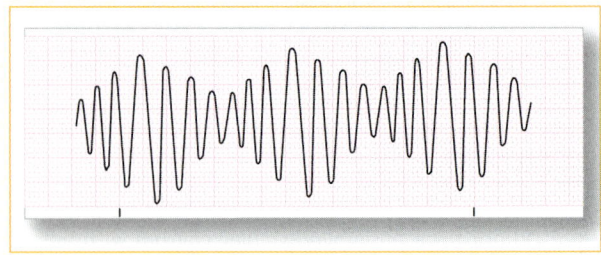

Figure 20-95 Torsade de pointes.

- Putting it all together: The dysrhythmia TdP occurs with an underlying prolonged Q-T interval. It has an undulating, sinusoidal appearance in which the axis of the QRS complexes changes from positive to negative and back in a haphazard manner. (The name, torsade de pointes, means twisting of points.) The TdP rhythm is a variant of <u>polymorphic</u> V-tach. Unlike monomorphic V-tach, the size, shape, and direction of the complexes in polymorphic V-tach are variable; it has a changing appearance. It can convert into a normal rhythm or ventricular fibrillation. Be very careful with this rhythm because it is a harbinger of death!

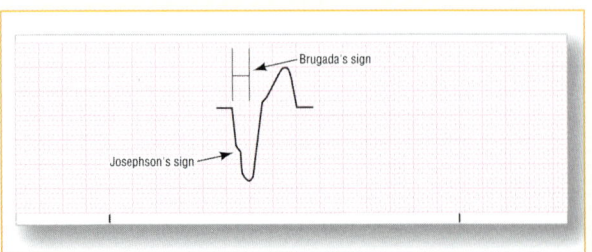

Figure 20-94 Brugada's and Josephson's signs in V-tach.

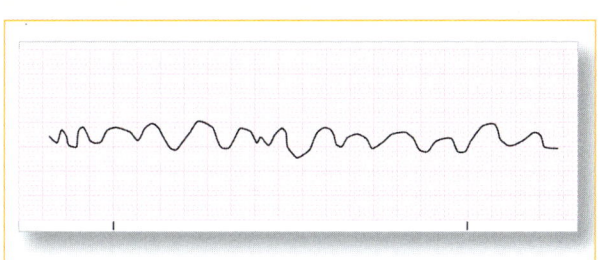

Figure 20-96 Ventricular fibrillation (V-fib).

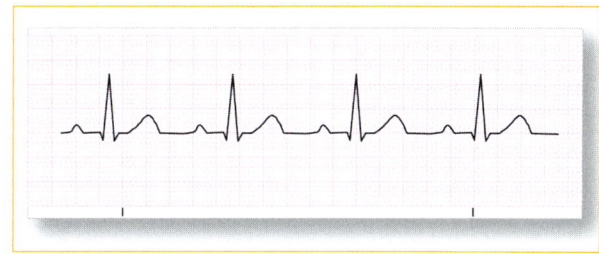

Figure 20-97 First-degree heart block.

Ventricular Fibrillation

Ventricular fibrillation is shown in Figure 20-96. Its characteristics are:
- Rate: Indeterminate
- Regularity: Chaotic rhythm
- P wave: None
- P/QRS ratio: None
- P-R interval: None
- QRS width: None
- Grouping: None
- Dropped beats: No beats at all!
- Putting it all together: If you were going to draw a picture of cardiac chaos, this would be it. The ventricular pacers are all going haywire and firing at their own pace. The result is many small areas of the heart firing at once with no organized activity.

EMT-I Tips

If your patient looks fine and is wide awake and looking at you, a lead has fallen off and this is an artifact, not V-fib.

Heart Blocks

Heart blocks (also called AV nodal blocks) refer to rhythms in which there is a partial or complete block at the AV node. A heart block can range from an abnormal delay at the AV node (first-degree heart block) to a complete blockage (third-degree heart block). A hallmark finding in a heart block is when there are more P waves than QRS complexes. As you will see, the only exception to this rule is with a first-degree heart block.

First-degree Heart Block

First-degree heart block is shown in Figure 20-97. Its characteristics are:
- Rate: Depends on underlying rhythm
- Regularity: Regular
- P wave: Normal
- P/QRS ratio: 1:1
- P-R interval: Prolonged, >0.20 seconds
- QRS width: Normal
- Grouping: None
- Dropped beats: None
- Putting it all together: First-degree heart block results from a prolonged physiologic block in the AV node. This can occur because of medication, vagal stimulation, and disease, among other causes. The P-R interval will be greater than 0.20 seconds.

Mobitz I Second-degree Heart Block (Wenckebach Block)

Mobitz I second-degree heart block (Wenckebach block) is shown in Figure 20-98. Its characteristics are:
- Rate: Depends on underlying rhythm
- Regularity: Regularly irregular
- P wave: Present
- P/QRS ratio: Variable: 2:1, 3:2, 4:3, 5:4, and so on
- P-R interval: Variable
- QRS width: Normal
- Grouping: Present and variable (see blue shading in Figure 20-98)
- Dropped beats: Yes
- Putting it all together: A Mobitz I block is also known as a Wenckebach (pronounced WENN-key-bock) block. It is caused by a diseased AV node with a long refractory period. The result is that the P-R interval lengthens between successive beats until a beat is dropped. At that point,

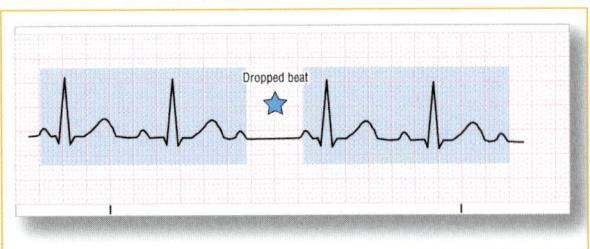

Figure 20-98 Mobitz I second-degree heart block (Wenckebach block).

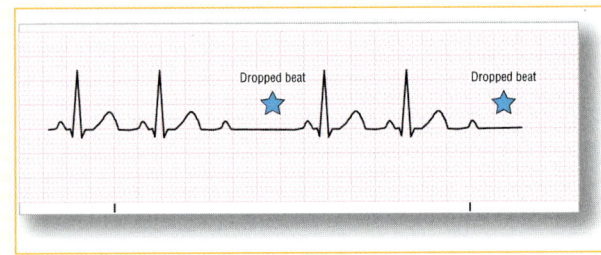

Figure 20-99 Mobitz II second-degree heart block.

> ### ✳ EMT-I Tips
>
> A word of caution about the nomenclature of blocks: The rhythm disturbances we are looking at here are AV nodal blocks. There are also bundle branch blocks, a very different phenomenon. These will be discussed later.

the cycle starts again. The R-R interval, on the other hand, shortens with each beat.

Mobitz II Second-degree Heart Block

Mobitz II second-degree heart block is shown in Figure 20-99 ▶. Its characteristics are:

- Rate: Depends on underlying rhythm
- Regularity: Regularly irregular
- P wave: Normal
- P/QRS ratio: X:X–1; for example, 3:2, 4:3, 5:4, and so on. The ratio can also be variable on rare occasions.
- P-R interval: Normal
- QRS width: Normal
- Grouping: Present and variable
- Dropped beats: Yes
- Putting it all together: In Mobitz II blocks, there are grouped beats with one beat dropped between each group. The key point to remember is that the P-R interval is the same in all of the conducted beats. This rhythm is caused by a diseased AV node, and it is a harbinger of bad things to come—namely, complete heart block.

Third-degree Heart Block

Third-degree heart block is shown in Figure 20-100 ▶. Its characteristics are:

- Rate: Separate rates for the underlying (sinus) rhythm and the escape rhythm. They are dissociated from one another.
- Regularity: Regular, but the P rate and QRS rate are different
- P wave: Present
- P/QRS ratio: Variable
- P-R interval: Variable; no pattern
- QRS width: Normal or wide
- Grouping: None
- Dropped beats: None
- Putting it all together: This is a complete block of the AV node; the atria and ventricles are firing separately. The sinus rhythm can be bradycardic, normal, or tachycardic. The escape beat can be junctional or ventricular, so the morphologic features of the QRS complexes will vary. Third-degree heart block is also referred to as complete heart block.

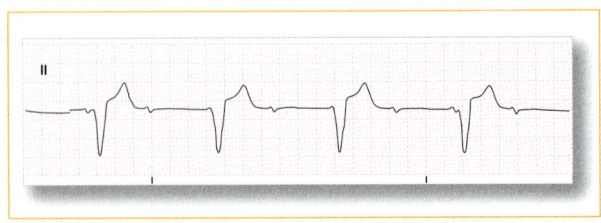

Figure 20-100 Third-degree heart block.

EMT-I Tips

What if there is a 2:1 ratio of Ps to QRSs? Is this Mobitz I or Mobitz II? In reality, you can't tell. This example is named a 2:1 second-degree block (no type is specified). Because you can't tell, assume the worst—Mobitz II. You cannot go wrong by being overly cautious with a patient's life.

EMT-I Tips

Semantics alert: If there are just as many P waves as there are QRSs, but they are dissociated, it is known as AV dissociation rather than third-degree heart block.

Premature Complexes

A premature complex is basically one that arrives ahead of schedule. The complex occurs early or prematurely compared with where it should have occurred along the strip. In musical terms, the premature complex breaks the cadence of the rhythm. Take a look at Figure 20-101 ▼. Can you find the premature complex? Of course—it is represented by the sixth gold rectangle on the strip.

Premature complexes can be sinus, atrial, junctional, or ventricular in origin. The morphologic features of the QRS complex will reflect their site of origin.

While we are on the topic of prematurity, there are some terms that you will frequently see related to premature complexes that recur at regular intervals. A premature complex that arrives every second beat is called bigeminy Figure 20-102 ▶. A premature complex that arrives every third beat is trigeminy. As you can well imagine, every fourth beat is quadrigeminy, and so forth. The common thread among all these rhythms is the sequential, repetitive occurrence of the premature complex.

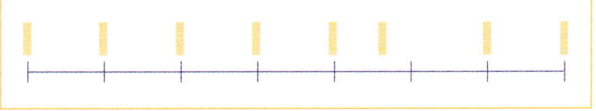

Figure 20-101 Can you spot the premature complex in the strip?

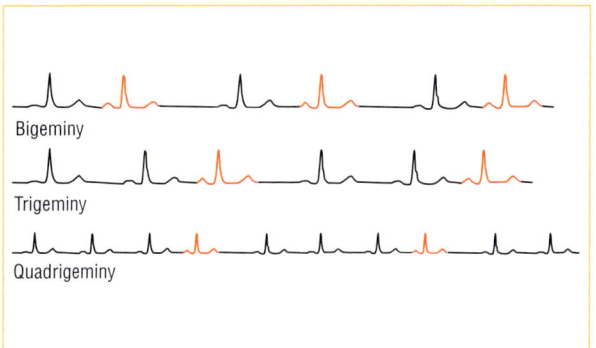

Figure 20-102 Examples of supraventricular bigeminy, trigeminy, and quadrigeminy.

An Arrhythmia vs an Event

At this point, we need to review some terminology. *A cardiac rhythm refers to the cadence or sequence of how the cardiac complexes occur.* Cardiac rhythms can be normal or abnormal and do not necessarily refer to a pathologic process. Normally, the sinus node acts as the pacemaker, and the impulse proceeds down the normal electrical conduction system to innervate the atria and the ventricles sequentially.

An arrhythmia refers to a cardiac rhythm that is pathologic in nature and is one that is created or transmitted differently than the normal process. It can begin somewhere outside the sinus node. It can travel through different pathways other than the normal electrical conduction system. It can occur at rates outside of the normal range. It can be hemodynamically stable, or it can cause hemodynamic instability. It can be fast or slow, wide or narrow.

We also should understand the difference between a rhythm and a rhythm with an overlying cardiac event that momentarily alters the cadence of the underlying rhythm. Suppose you had a strip with a clearly visible, regular cadence on it. Suddenly another pacemaker in the heart became irritable and fired early. The cadence of the rhythm is altered by the event Figure 20-103 ▼, but this is not a new arrhythmia. It is a normal rhythm with a premature complex. Always remember, *an event is not a rhythm.*

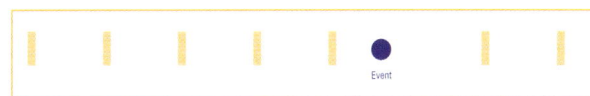

Figure 20-103 A cardiac event can alter the cadence of a rhythm.

Why the distinction? Usually novice clinicians will focus on the event and not the rhythm itself. It is usually the underlying arrhythmia that will cause the hemodynamic compromise, not the single event. Let's use an analogy to think about this another way. In emergency care, we are involved in the care of trauma patients. For a trauma patient, one of the most impressive wounds, *visually*, is a scalp laceration. They normally cause small rivers of blood to drip down the face and can be quite dramatic. However, how many people actually die of a laceration to the scalp? Very, very few. On the other hand, a blunt liver laceration does not have an impressive visual presentation, but it is often a killer. The clinician needs to look past the dramatic presentation of the scalp laceration and concentrate on the blunt injury that can kill the patient. That same mentality is how you need to approach an arrhythmia; concentrate on the rhythm and just be aware of the single event.

Escape Complexes and Rhythms

An escape complex is almost the opposite of a premature complex. Instead of occurring early in the cadence of the rhythm, it occurs late in the cadence (Figure 20-104). To understand how an escape complex occurs, remember that all cardiac tissue has the ability to function as a potential pacemaker for the heart. The sinus node has the fastest pacing cycle; the ventricular muscle has the slowest (Figure 20-105). When the primary pacemaker fails for whatever reason, the next one in succession will take over the main role.

The reason this fail-safe pacemaking system exists is so that if one pacemaker fails, there are other pacemakers to keep the heart going so the person does not die. In an escape complex, the pacemaker that is setting the main rhythm fails, and the next one takes over. This can occur for one complex or for as long as needed.

An escape rhythm occurs when the primary pacemaker fails for a prolonged period. Once again, the next pacemaker in succession will usually take over the pacemaking function for the heart.

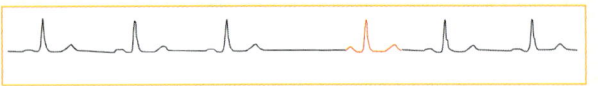

Figure 20-104 An escape complex.

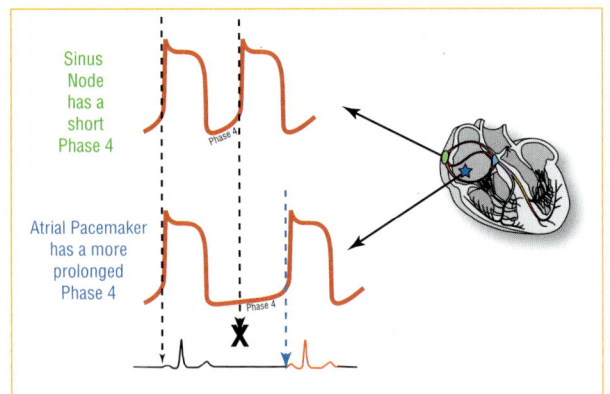

Figure 20-105 When the atrial pacemaker fails to pace at the expected time, the next pacemaker will fire according to its schedule. This creates an escape complex (blue arrow).

Ectopic Foci and Their Morphologic Features

This section deals with variations in the morphologic features of the complex based on where the complex originated in the heart. The exact location or focus that acts as the main pacemaker for a complex dictates the appearance of the complex. This is related to many factors, and we will address them individually in the pages to come. For now, take a look at (Figure 20-106) to get an overall impression of the location of a particular focus and its associated morphologic characteristics.

There are many factors that affect the morphologic features of the complexes on an ECG tracing. The main ones include the actual pacemaker site and the route

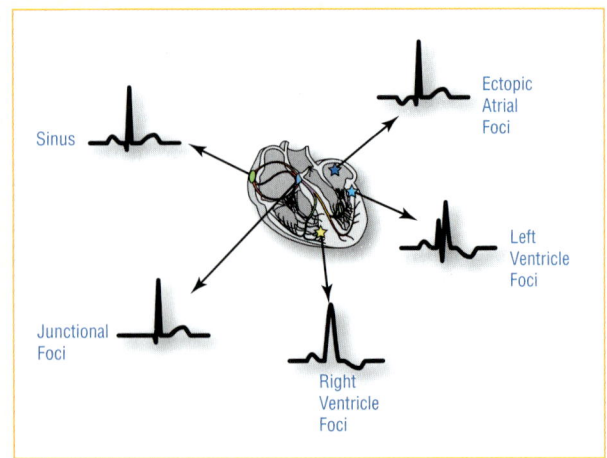

Figure 20-106 Ectopic foci and the respective morphologic characteristics of the complexes.

that the impulse has to take to cause depolarization of the entire heart.

Let's start off by looking at the ectopic atrial sites. Because we are talking about atrial sites, the changes will be seen in the P waves, and that is where we will begin. Recall that a positive vector heading toward an electrode will be interpreted on the ECG as a positive wave (Figure 20-107 ▼). A positive vector headed away from an electrode will be interpreted as a negative wave on the ECG (Figure 20-108 ▼). Vectors dictate morphologic characteristics; directions of the depolarization waves on the heart dictate vector direction and vector size.

When you have an ectopic focus acting as the pacemaker for a complex, the angle and direction of the main atrial vector (also known as the P-wave axis) will be different from one that originated in the sinus node. For simplicity, Figure 20-108 shows a vector that originated in the inferior aspect of the left atrium and travels superiorly, backward, and to the right. This vector is seen by the electrode for lead II as heading away from it and so will give rise to a completely negative or inverted P wave. As you can imagine, there are quite a large number of possible ectopic pacemakers and, therefore, quite a large number of possible P-wave forms. *The important thing clinically, is that ectopic P waves are all different morphologically from sinus P waves.* Picking up on these differences is key to making the correct interpretation.

Now, let's turn our attention to the AV node. When the AV node functions as the primary pacemaker for a complex, one of two things will happen: (1) There will be no P waves, or (2) the P wave will always be inverted in lead II.

The AV node is the only connection between the atria and the ventricles under normal circumstances. If it were not for the AV node, the atria and ventricles would function completely obliviously to one another. The AV node is, essentially, the gatekeeper for the heart, allowing communication to proceed back and forth. We saw that the gate can be opened, allowing impulses to travel back and forth between the atria and the ventricles, or it can be closed, blocking impulse transmission between the two.

Now, suppose you had a large empty container meant to hold water with two sides, compartments A and V (Figure 20-109 ▼). There is a wall in the middle acting as a dam to prevent water from traveling back and forth between the two sides. The dam has a lock in the middle with two gates that could be opened to allow movement of water back and forth between the compartments. Suppose you filled the lock, right between two gates, with water (Figure 20-110 ▶). What would happen if you opened the gate on the right? The water would flow into compartment V. Compartment A would

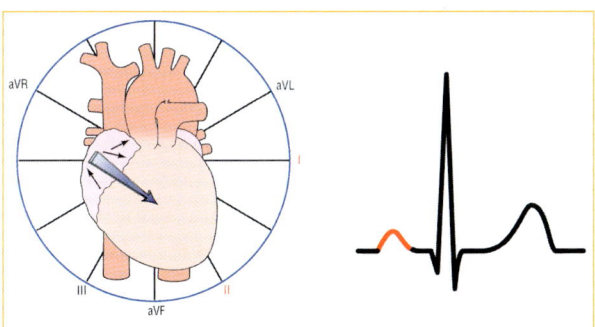

Figure 20-107 In this example, the P wave vector is headed inferiorly, backward, and to the left. Lead II sees a positive vector headed toward it, and this is represented electrocardiographically as a positive P wave in that lead. Note: Leads aVR, aVL, and aVF can only be viewed with a 12-lead ECG. You may see these terms but they are beyond the scope of basic cardiology for the EMT-I.

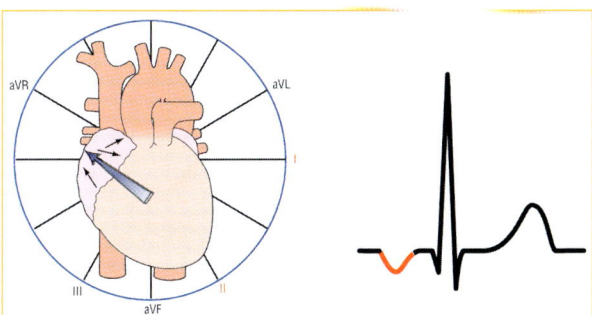

Figure 20-108 In this example, the P wave vector is headed superiorly, backward, and to the right. Lead II sees a positive vector headed away from it, and this is represented electrocardiographically as a negative P wave in that lead.

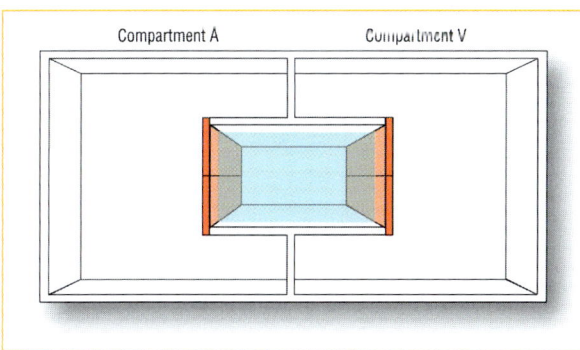

Figure 20-109 A large container with a central lock and two gates in the middle. The gates and the lock allow controlled communication between the two sides of the containers.

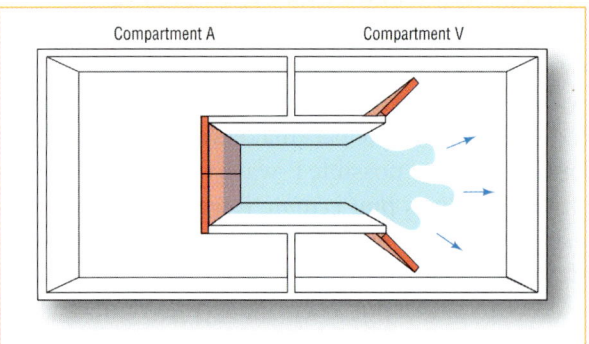

Figure 20-110 If the lock in the middle of the container were filled with water and the right gate opened, the water would flow into compartment V and spread evenly throughout that side of the container.

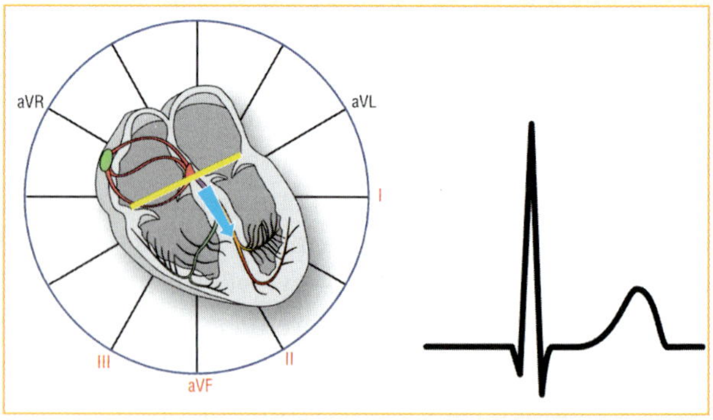

be dry and unaware of the flooding occurring in compartment V.

The same thing can happen when the AV node acts as the primary pacemaker. The junctional focus fires, causing an impulse to start to develop. This is equivalent to filling the lock with water. In our analogy, the next step would be to open the right side of the gate and allow the water to fill compartment V (Figure 20-111 ▼). In the heart, the impulse that originated in the junctional focus travels down the electrical conduction pathway, causing normal depolarization of the ventricles (Figure 20-112 ▶). This is represented on the ECG as a normal-looking QRS complex with no P waves. There are no P waves because the AV node did not allow the impulse to travel back into the atria. To put it another way, the left side of the gate was not opened.

This is what occurs if the AV node does not allow the impulse generated in a junctional focus to travel ret-

Figure 20-112 The impulse that originated in a junctional focus caused normal conduction down the electrical conduction system. The ventricles depolarized normally, forming a QRS complex with normal morphologic features.

rogradely or backward into the atria. This is one possibility. Now let's turn our attention to the other possibility.

Suppose that both gates on the lock were opened simultaneously. What would happen to the water in the lock? It would flow into both compartments at the same time (Figure 20-113 ▼). This is exactly what happens when a junctional focus fires as the pacemaker of the complex. In this case, the P wave and the QRS complex would both be formed at exactly the same time, leading to a buried P wave (Figure 20-114 ▶). The morphologic characteristics of the QRS complex may be slightly altered or may appear normal.

If the junctional focus were closer to the atrial side of the AV node, the retrograde conduction to the atria would occur faster than ventricular depolarization, and

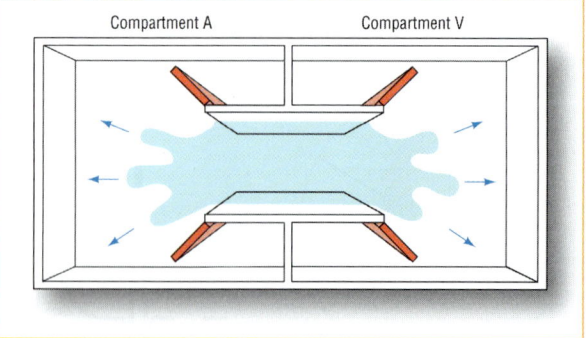

Figure 20-113 Suppose both gates on the lock opened up at the same time. The water would flow into both compartments simultaneously. In the AV node, this leads to the P wave occurring early (causing a short P-R interval) or at the same time as the QRS complex (causing the P wave to be buried in the QRS complex).

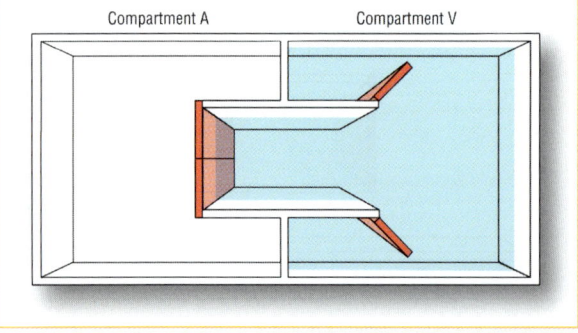

Figure 20-111 The right side of the gate was opened, releasing the contents and filling compartment V.

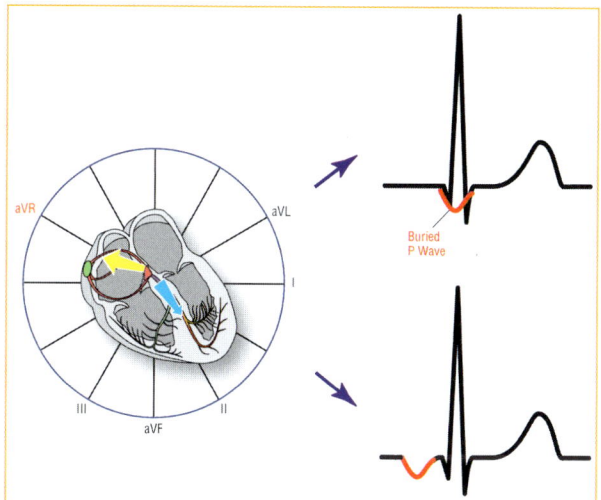

Figure 20-114 If a junctional focus acts as a primary pacemaker for a complex, the P-R interval is shorter than expected or the P wave is buried in the QRS complex. The P wave would always be inverted in leads II and III because of the direction of the vector (see yellow vector) caused by the retrograde atrial conduction of the junctional complex.

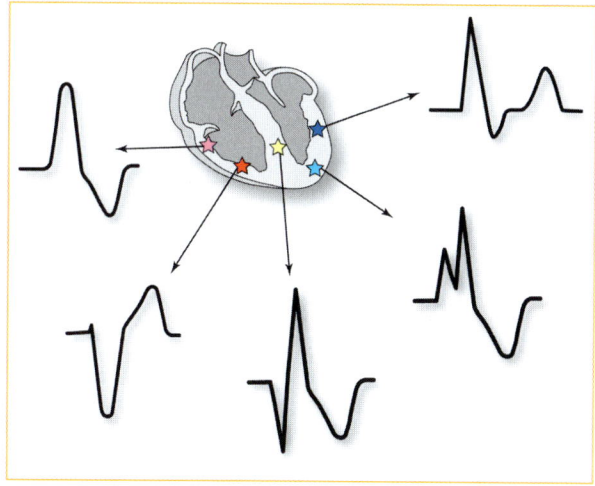

Figure 20-115 The firing of a ventricular ectopic focus leads to the formation of wide, bizarre-looking QRS complexes. The figure shows various types of possible QRS morphologic changes, but the actual appearance of a QRS complex cannot be predicted completely based on the location of the ectopic focus. In addition, the morphologic characteristics will change based on the lead used to view the complexes.

the P wave would come sooner in the cycle. This causes a shortened P-R interval.

Ectopic Foci in the Ventricles

We have seen how the morphologic changes of the complexes are caused when ectopic foci in the atria and AV node act as the primary pacemaker. Now, we turn our attention to what happens when the ventricles act as the ectopic focus.

The first thing to notice about any ventricular ectopic focus is that it will lead to very broad, bizarre-looking QRS complexes (Figure 20-115 ▶). In addition, the site of the ventricular focus will alter the morphologic features in its own way. Both of these changes can be understood more easily if you keep in mind that ECG morphologic features are dictated by vectors. So, you already have the knowledge base to figure out why this occurs. Let's see how it happens.

Use your imagination and the information you have learned so far in this chapter to try to figure out the process. How do the ventricles normally depolarize? The impulse comes down the electrical conduction pathway and spreads through the bundle of His and the left and right bundle branches and finally reaches the Purkinje system. The Purkinje system, in turn, stimulates the nearest myofibrils. From that point on, one myofib-

ril stimulates an adjoining myofibril, and the rest of the process of ventricular depolarization occurs via direct cell-to-cell stimulation. The organized sequential stimulation of the first set of myofibrils at the same time throughout the left and right ventricles greatly shortens the process of ventricular depolarization, leading to a nice, normal-looking QRS complex.

Now, what happens when an ectopic focus acts as a primary pacemaker? Is the electrical conduction system stimulated simultaneously, providing a synchronized depolarization wave to occur in both ventricles? The answer is no. When an ectopic ventricular focus fires, the only cells that become stimulated by the depolarization are the ones in direct contact with the ectopic focus. When they, in turn, fire, they stimulate only their surrounding myofibrils, and so forth. This is a process of direct cell-to-cell stimulation that is very time-consuming and does not lead to synchronized mechanical contraction. In (Figure 20-116 ▶), the cell-to-cell depolarization wave is represented by the concentric waves moving outward from the ectopic focus.

How would this direct cell-to-cell transmission of the ventricular depolarization wave look morphologically on an ECG? It depends on the vector that it forms, but it would definitely be wide because of the slow nature of the conduction. Remember, what leads to a nice, tight QRS complex is the synchronized conduction of the

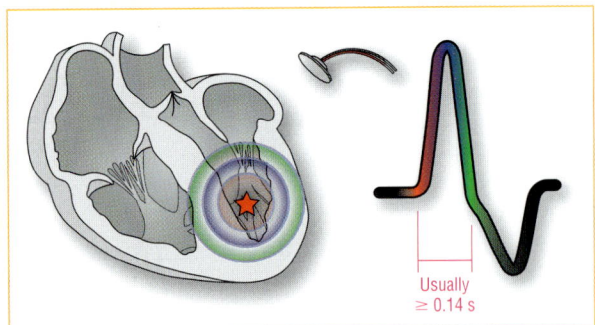

Figure 20-116 An irritable focus, represented by the red star, acts as a pacemaker and causes an impulse to occur. This gives rise to a depolarization wave that radiates outward by direct cell-to-cell transmission throughout both of the ventricles. Note the color-coded sections of the depolarization wave and the complex.

depolarization wave. An ectopic focus leads to asynchronous depolarization, which is very slow. Time on an ECG is demonstrated in the horizontal direction, hence the wide presentation on the complexes.

Now on to why the complexes have a bizarre appearance. Under normal circumstances, the synchronous depolarization of both ventricles leads to the formation of three almost simultaneous vectors Figure 20-117 ▼. These vectors give rise to distinct morphologic ECG representations that form the QRS complex: the Q wave, the R wave, and the S wave. With the firing of a ventricular pacemaker, do you have the formation of the same three distinct vectors, or do you have the formation of a haphazard series of vectors? The answer is a haphazard series of vectors. How these vectors align temporally will decide the final morphologic characteristics of the QRS complex.

Aberrancy

In electrocardiography, aberrancy relates to electrical impulses that travel along nonestablished pathways to depolarize the heart. For example, the atrial and ventricular ectopic foci that we previously discussed are aberrantly conducted. Another aspect of the term that you will very frequently hear, and the main reason for this section, is when a complex is partially transmitted along the normal electrical pathway and then becomes aberrantly conducted because of some obstruction. Let's start off this discussion by going into this process in more detail.

Suppose you had a dry riverbed. Suddenly there was a big storm leading to a buildup of water that caused a flash flood. The rising waters would take the path of least resistance that, in this case, would be the dry riverbed Figure 20-118 ▼. Now, suppose a beaver had built a dam across the riverbed. What would happen to the water flow when it hit the beaver dam? The water flow would smash into it and have to flow around the obstruction, taking any route it could. Would the flow around the obstruction be smooth as it would have been in the normal riverbed? No, because the water would

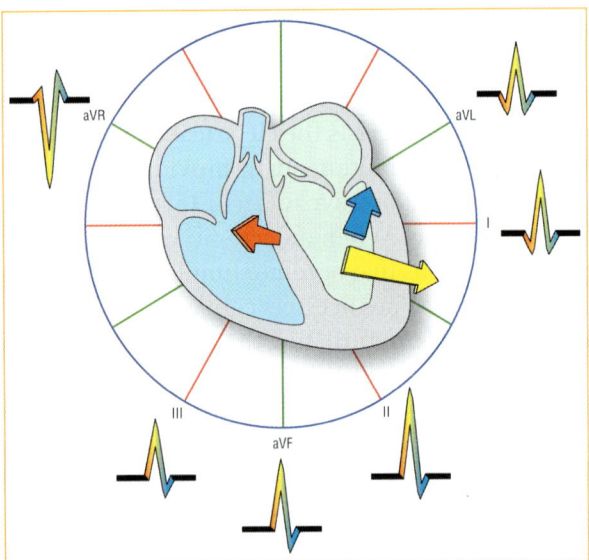

Figure 20-117 The synchronous depolarization of the ventricles by the electrical conduction system gives rise to three main vectors. The first one, represented by the red vector, will give rise to the Q wave. The second vector, represented by the yellow vector, will give rise to the R wave. The third vector, the blue vector, gives rise to the S wave. The three vectors are represented on the QRS complexes (as they appear in their particular leads) by their respective colors.

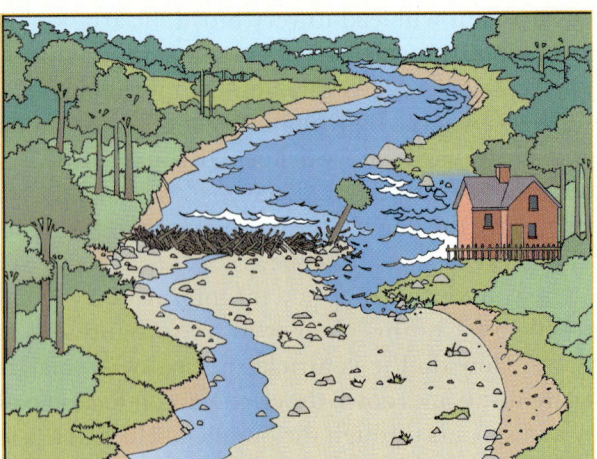

Figure 20-118 A flash flood on a river hits an obstruction. The water must find a way around the obstruction, causing turbulence and slower, abnormal flow.

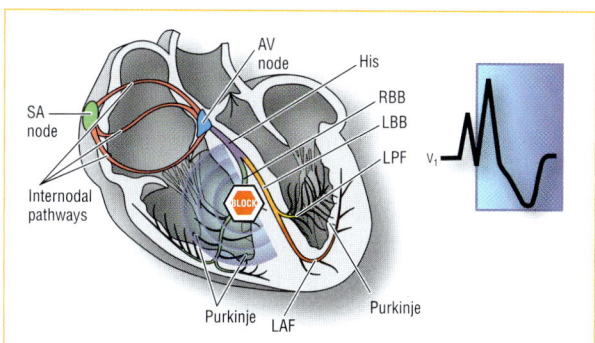

Figure 20-119 When the impulse hits an area of refractoriness in the right bundle branch, for example, the impulse is forced to continue by direct cell-to-cell transmission throughout the rest of the right ventricle. This leads to a complex that starts out normal and then ends up with a very bizarre appearance.

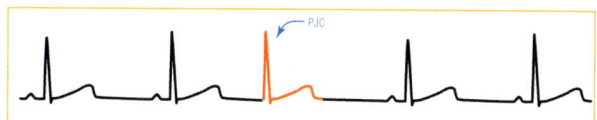

Figure 20-120 A premature junctional contraction.

have to go over millions of tiny obstacles, constantly change directions depending on elevation, and so forth. That flow creates turbulence. Turbulent flow, even though it is full of energy, is actually much slower moving than smooth, laminar flow. Let's recap: The water flows smoothly and faster before the obstruction. Once it meets the obstruction, it needs to find a way around it, which causes slow, turbulent flow of the water.

The same process can sometimes occur in the heart (Figure 20-119 ▲). The most common scenario is as follows: A normal electrical impulse is traveling down the electrical conduction system. Suddenly it hits an area that is refractory (temporarily unable to transmit the impulse), and it continues on from that spot by direct cell-to-cell transmission. As we saw before when we discussed ectopic foci, direct cell-to-cell transmission of the electrical impulse is slow and leads to aberrant vectors. Slow transmission of the impulse leads to wide complexes. Aberrant vectors lead to morphologic differences in the complexes. So, what we end up with many times is a complex that starts out looking normal and like its neighboring complexes, but suddenly there is a shift, and it looks totally different at the end.

Premature Junctional Contraction

As you can imagine, premature junctional contractions (PJCs) are junctional complexes that occur earlier than expected and are interspersed in the underlying rhythm for one or more cycles (Figure 20-120 ▶). The PJCs have the morphologic characteristics expected from any junctional complex (absent or buried P wave, inverted P waves in lead II, and narrow supraventricular QRS complexes). Usually, PJCs are associated with a non-compensatory pause because the retrogradely conducted atrial impulse typically depolarizes and resets the SA node. However, the pause may be fully compensatory when there is no retrograde conduction toward the atria.

The PJCs are fairly common electrocardiographic phenomena and can be found in people with and without structural and ischemic heart disease. They are typically caused by increased automaticity of the AV junction. They can occur singly or can be recurrent.

The coupling interval—the distance from the PJC to the previous QRS complex—can be fixed or variable. A fixed coupling interval (Figure 20-121 ▼) is commonly found in PACs and PVCs and represents an identical distance between the normal complex and the premature beat. Typically, PJCs do not have a fixed coupling interval, and the R-R interval between complexes is usually variable (Figure 20-122 ▼).

The supraventricular complexes of the PJCs typically have narrow QRS complexes associated with them. If the QRS complex is wider than 0.12 seconds, the usual causes include a preexisting bundle branch block, aberrantly conducted beats, electrolyte abnormalities, and

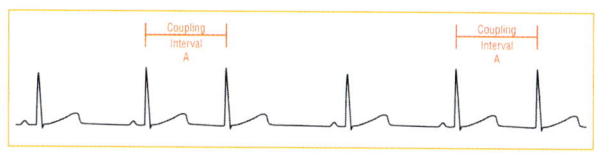

Figure 20-121 The coupling interval refers to the distance between the premature complex and the preceding normal beat found in the underlying rhythm. A fixed coupling interval is the same whenever an individual ectopic focus fires.

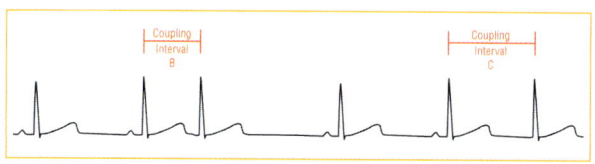

Figure 20-122 A variable coupling interval refers to variability in the coupling distance every time that the same ectopic focus fires.

fusion complexes with the T waves of the previous complexes.

PAC With Aberrancy vs PJC With Aberrancy

How can you tell if a complex is actually an aberrantly conducted PAC or an aberrantly conducted PJC? The answer is to look at the company it keeps. The events and appearance of the waves around it will be your best clues.

1. *Always look for morphologic variation in the preceding T wave.*

   We have studied buried P waves before, but this topic deserves reinforcement. Start by looking at the T waves of the preceding complexes that are normally transmitted for that patient. The morphologic characteristics of the T wave will most likely be identical from complex to complex. Mild variations may exist, but there should never be any gross differences. A gross difference in morphologic appearance, especially when associated with a premature complex, almost always signifies the presence of a buried P wave.

   The morphologic features of a T wave will usually be altered by a buried P wave (Figure 20-123). This is because the ventricular repolarization process is slow and the forces that they generate are smaller than those that occur during an actual coordinated depolarization wave. Even the relatively low forces of atrial depolarization are enough to cause an electrocardiographic fusion to occur on the strip. (Notice that this refers to a fusion on the ECG tracing because of the timing of the waves and not an actual fusion of the waves themselves within the heart as discussed in the last section.)

2. *Look for a compensatory pause.*

   The other thing that will help you to differentiate between a PAC with a buried P wave and a PJC is the type of pause involved. Usually, PACs are associated with noncompensatory pauses because the sinus node is usually reset by an ectopic atrial impulse. The pauses in PJCs can be either compensatory or noncompensatory. When there is no retrograde conduction of the depolarization wave toward the atria, PJCs are associated with compensatory pauses. When the sinus node is reset by a retrograde P wave, PJCs are associated with noncompensatory pauses. Therefore, *the presence of a compensatory pause favors the diagnosis of PJC.*

3. *Look for inverted P waves in leads II and III with short P-R intervals.*

   The P wave becomes inverted when the ectopic pacemaker is inferior and near the AV junction. By definition, therefore, a PJC will always have inverted P waves in lead II. In addition, the PJC's P wave can be before, after, or buried within the QRS complex. If the P wave occurs before the QRS complex in a PJC, the P-R interval is almost always shorter than normal since it does not have to undergo the full physiologic block in the AV node.

4. *Identify aberrantly conducted PJCs.*

   One of the toughest things in arrhythmia recognition is to correctly identify an aberrantly conducted PJC. To accomplish this feat, you need to keep a very close eye on the company it keeps and to look very closely at the area right at the start of the QRS complex.

   An aberrantly conducted complex or beat occurs when a normally transmitted depolarization wave traveling down the electrical conduction system hits an area that is refractory to impulse transmission (Figure 20-124). From that point on, the impulse has to be transmitted down to the rest of the ventricles via direct cell-to-cell transmission. Because the very early portion of the QRS complex is always transmitted down the normal electrical conduction system, that portion will always be identical to the normally conducted complexes.

   Always look at the first few milliseconds of the normally conducted QRS complex and compare it with the aberrantly conducted beat in question (Figure 20-125). As mentioned, this area is always identical to that of the normally conducted complexes. The number of milliseconds in the identical trans-

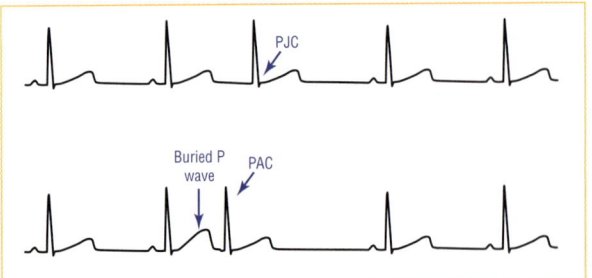

Figure 20-123 A strip showing a PJC and a strip showing a PAC with a buried P wave. Note the difference in the appearance of the T wave of the complex immediately before the PAC. The morphologic difference is due to the additive effects of the ectopic P wave and the T wave.

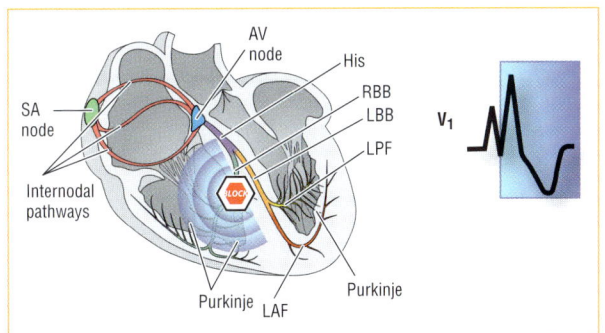

Figure 20-124 An aberrancy develops when an impulse traveling down the normal electrical conduction system hits an area of refractoriness. The cell-to-cell transmission that has to develop after that point causes electrocardiographic aberrancy.

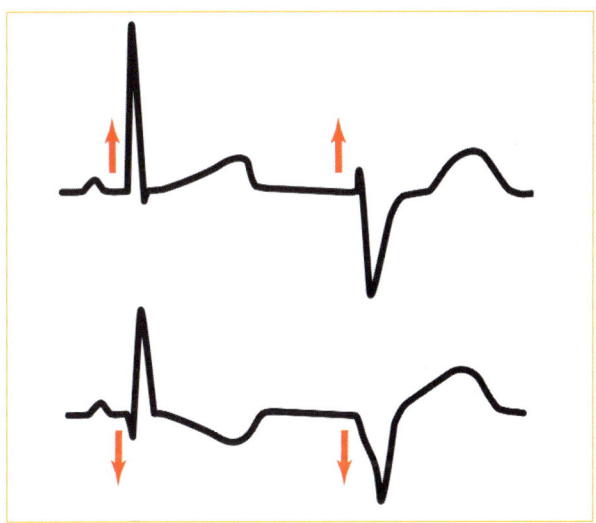

Figure 20-126 Always take a look at the direction of the start of the QRS. If the complexes are headed in the same direction, it is probably an aberrancy.

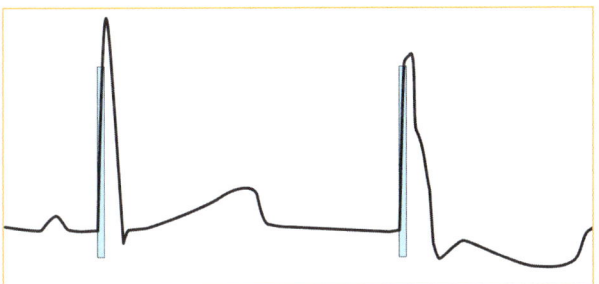

Figure 20-125 A normal sinus complex is shown in the first example, followed by an aberrantly conducted beat. Note how the initial few milliseconds of the two complexes are identical. The number of milliseconds in the identical transmission depends on the site of refractoriness that causes the aberration. If the refractory site is very close to the AV node, the amount of time will be very, very short. If the refractory site is further down the electrical conduction system, the duration of aberrancy will be longer.

mission depends on the site of refractoriness that causes the aberration. If the refractory site is very close to the AV node, the amount of time will be very, very short. If the refractory site is further down the electrical conduction system, the duration of aberrancy will be longer.

A good clinical tip to keep in mind is that if the complexes start in the same direction, especially if they occur in multiple leads, the wide complex is probably an aberrantly conducted complex **Figure 20-126**. If they start in opposite directions in multiple leads, it is most assuredly a ventricular ectopic complex.

You are the Provider   Part 9

You have determined that your patient's rhythm is sinus bradycardia. She is now breathing on her own and responds to verbal stimuli.

Reassessment	Recording Time: 12 Minutes After Patient Contact
Respirations	16 breaths/min; adequate depth
Pulse	46 beats/min, regular
Skin	Pale
Blood pressure	102/60 mm Hg
Sao$_2$	97% with 100% O_2 via nonrebreathing mask

13. What are the criteria for sinus bradycardia?

Premature Ventricular Contraction

Coupling Interval

Just like in PJCs, PVCs can have fixed or nonfixed coupling intervals. To review, the coupling interval is the distance from the previous QRS complex to the PVC. A fixed coupling interval (Figure 20-127 ▼) is a fairly common occurrence when the PVCs originate in the same ectopic focus and the depolarization wave takes the same route. Fixed coupling intervals should not be off by more than 0.08 seconds. Variable coupling distances (Figure 20-128 ▼), on the other hand, are more common in PVCs that originate from multiple ectopic pacemakers, and these PVCs will each have a different morphologic appearance.

R-on-T Phenomenon

While we are on the topic of coupling intervals, there are a couple of special types of PVCs that we should look at more closely. These include R-on-T phenomenon and end-diastolic PVCs.

Typically, PVCs occur after the previous complex has finished repolarization, in other words, after the previous T wave is finished. In certain cases, however,

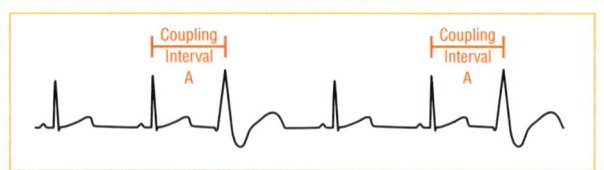

Figure 20-127 The coupling interval refers to the distance between the premature complex and the preceding normal beat found in the underlying rhythm. A fixed coupling interval is the same whenever an individual ectopic focus fires.

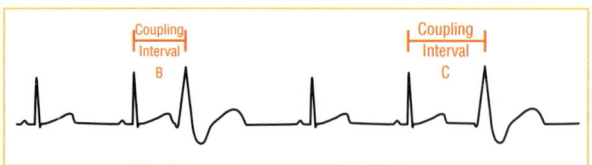

Figure 20-128 A variable coupling interval refers to a variability in the coupling distance. This can occur when the route taken by a depolarization wave is different or if the complex originated in a different ectopic focus.

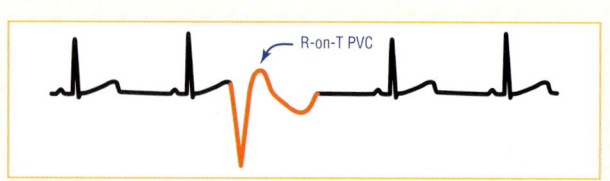

Figure 20-129 A PVC with an R-on-T phenomenon.

the PVC starts during the relative refractory period of the previous complex's T wave. This is known as the R-on-T phenomenon (Figure 20-129 ▲). This can create the potential for some very serious reentry loops and circus movements within the ventricles. These loops can lead to serious life-threatening rhythms, including ventricular tachycardia.

There has been a lot of controversy in the literature as to the true clinical importance of the R-on-T phenomenon. For a while, the thought was that the R-on-T phenomenon was very dangerous and that these PVCs had to be treated as emergencies. Then the pendulum swung in the direction of completely ignoring the R-on-T phenomenon, and the thought was that these PVCs were completely benign. Recently, the pendulum has begun to swing back in the direction of potential danger.

If there is a potential for serious clinical consequences, you should monitor the patient closely for these serious arrhythmias. In the meantime, a clinical decision based on a sound evaluation of the risk-benefit ratio of the various pharmacologic agents and your patient can be made.

End-diastolic PVC

Sometimes, when there is an underlying slow sinus bradycardia, a PVC can occur in such a way that it falls after the next normally occurring sinus P wave (Figure 20-130 ▶). These PVCs are known as end-diastolic PVCs because they occur during the late diastolic phase of the previous complex.

> **Terminology Tips**
>
> Ventricular tachycardia = 3 or more PVCs in a row at a rate of 100 beats/min or more.

Chapter 20 Cardiovascular Emergencies

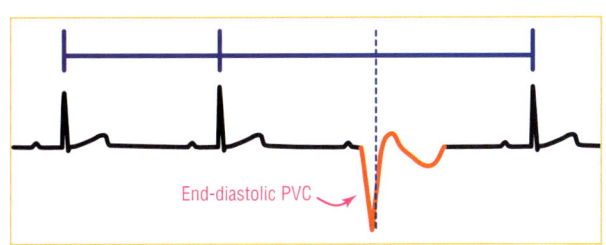

Figure 20-130 An end-diastolic PVC. Note that the PVC can easily be mistaken for an aberrantly conducted PAC or PJC.

End-diastolic PVCs have no additional clinical significance. They can, however, cause frequent misinterpretation and are often mistaken for aberrantly conducted PACs and PJCs. Luckily, this type of PVC is not frequently found.

Compensatory vs Noncompensatory Pauses

Premature ventricular contractions can be associated with compensatory (Figure 20-131 ▼) or noncompensatory (Figure 20-132 ▼) pauses. If the ectopic ventricular depolarization wave of the PVC spreads retrogradely to the atria and resets the sinus node, the pause will be noncompensatory. If the ectopic ventricular depolarization wave is blocked from retrogradely spreading to the atria, then the pause will be fully compensatory. In general, most of the pauses associated with PVCs will be fully compensatory.

Unifocal vs Multifocal PVCs

The morphologic appearance of a PVC depends on the location of the ectopic ventricular pacer that triggered the complex and the route of depolarization. If either of those two variables is different, the appearance of the PVC will be changed.

A PVC that originates in the same ectopic pacer and depolarizes via the same route through the ventricular myocardium is known as a **unifocal** PVC (Figure 20-133 ▼). These PVCs have the same coupling interval throughout the rhythm strip. They do not have to appear with a regular timing or at a specific recurring interval during the strip but can occur in a random pattern. Unifocal PVCs can appear singly or in combinations.

Multifocal PVCs (Figure 20-134 ▼) originate from different ectopic pacers or in the same ectopic

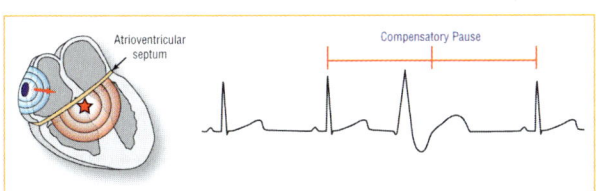

Figure 20-131 Compensatory pause. The ectopic ventricular depolarization wave does not spread retrograde to the atria. Because the sinus node is not reset, the underlying rhythm is not disturbed.

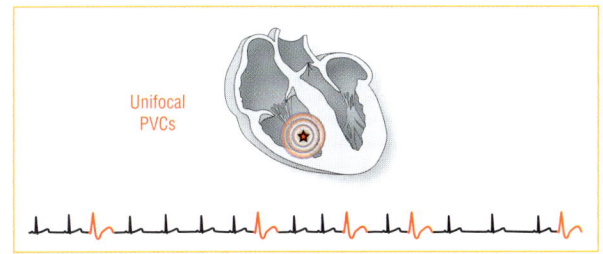

Figure 20-133 Unifocal PVCs originate in the same ectopic focus and depolarize the ventricles via the same route. The coupling interval is the same.

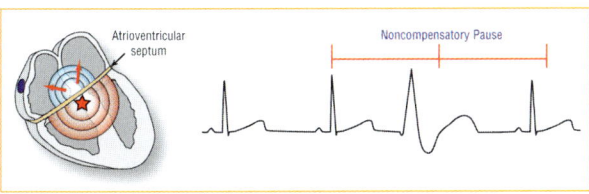

Figure 20-132 Noncompensatory pause. The ectopic ventricular depolarization wave spreads retrograde to the atria. The sinus node is reset, and the underlying rhythm or rate is changed.

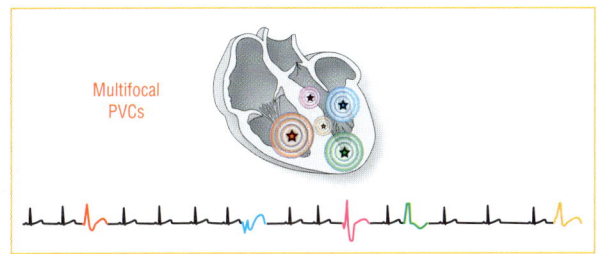

Figure 20-134 Multifocal PVCs originate in different ectopic foci or depolarize the ventricles via different routes. The coupling intervals are different.

pacemaker but take different routes to depolarize the ventricles. These PVCs occur randomly throughout the rhythm strip, and their coupling intervals will be completely different. Multifocal PVCs can appear singly or in combinations.

As mentioned earlier, the number of PVCs occurring in a minute can vary in any one patient for many reasons. The numbers of PVCs can vary because of electrolyte abnormalities, ischemia, diurnal (hormonal) changes, medications, and so on. If the number exceeds five or more per minute during an ECG strip or 20 to 30 per hour during ambulatory or Holter monitoring, they are considered frequent.

Bigeminy, Trigeminy, and More

When a PVC occurs every second complex, it is known as ventricular bigeminy (Figure 20-135 ▼). When a PVC occurs every third complex, it is known as ventricular trigeminy (Figure 20-136 ▼). Likewise, a PVC occurring every fourth complex is considered ventricular quadrigeminy (Figure 20-137 ▼). The word "ventricular" is present to designate the ectopic complexes as ventricular in origin (remember, there is also supraventricular bigeminy, and so on).

Usually, the most commonly found PVCs are unifocal and have the same coupling intervals and morphologic appearances. Multifocal PVCs are less commonly found, have different morphologic appearances, and typically do not appear with any recurring coupling interval.

Clinically, these rhythm abnormalities are stable and are not cause for alarm. The exception to this rule, however, occurs when the PVCs do not cause an adequate mechanical contraction. In these cases, the cardiac output can be dramatically altered owing to the presence of the PVCs, and clinical management and eradication of the premature complexes are indicated on an emergency basis. A good clinical habit to develop is to take the patient's pulse whenever you see a patient with bigeminy. If the palpable pulse is half of the pulse that you see on the monitor or the rhythm strip, you need to take action to eradicate the cause of the PVCs or to directly treat them. Don't forget to check the other vital signs as well!

> **EMT-I Tips**
>
> When there are three PVCs in a row, it starts to become difficult to tell whether they are a run of PVCs or ventricular tachycardia. The term salvo is typically used when the clinical impression is leaning toward the presence of ventricular tachycardia.

Couplets, Triplets, and Salvos

Bigeminy, trigeminy, and the others in that group have normal complexes interspersed between single PVCs. In this section, we are going to look at what happens when PVCs occur in sequence. When two PVCs occur sequentially, they are known as a couplet (Figure 20-138 ▼). When three PVCs occur sequentially, they are known as a triplet (Figure 20-139 ▼). The term salvo refers to a

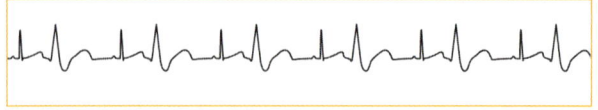

Figure 20-135 Ventricular bigeminy.

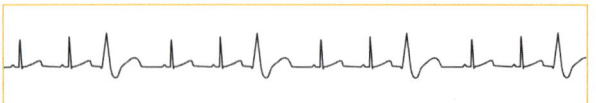

Figure 20-136 Ventricular trigeminy.

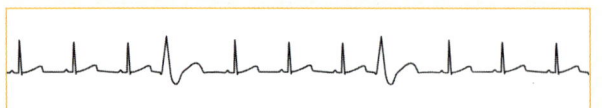

Figure 20-137 Ventricular quadrigeminy.

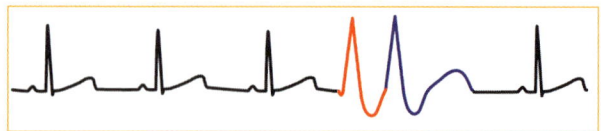

Figure 20-138 Unifocal couplet.

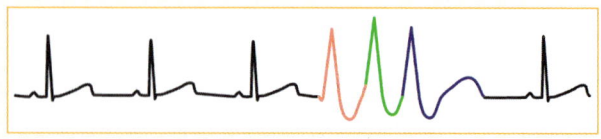

Figure 20-139 Unifocal triplet.

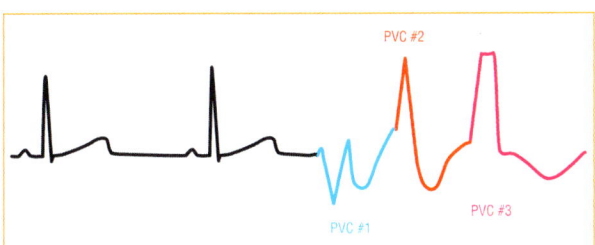

Figure 20-140 A multifocal triplet. Note the different appearance of the three ventricular beats and the varying degree of fusion between the waves.

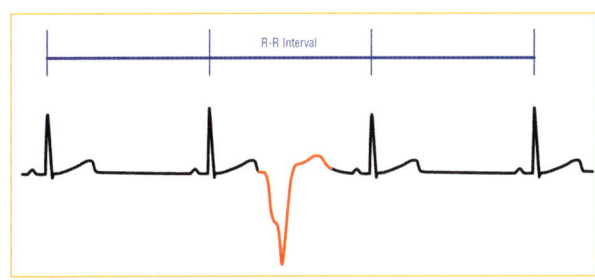

Figure 20-141 Interpolated PVC. Note that the underlying sinus rate and complexes are completely undisturbed. This can only occur if there is no ventriculoatrial activation from the PVC.

group of three or more ectopic ventricular complexes occurring sequentially.

Fusion of the various ventricular complexes and their associated waves is a very common occurrence when you are dealing with two or more sequential PVCs. The fusion can occur anywhere along the complexes and will affect the morphologic appearance of the various complexes.

Couplets and triplets can have PVCs that are unifocal or multifocal. The morphologic appearance of unifocal couplets and triplets may be slightly altered because of fusion, but the general appearance of the complexes will be the same. Multifocal couplets and triplets will show a wide variation in morphologic appearance and timing (Figure 20-140 ▲).

Clinically, unifocal couplets and triplets can be considered normal variants, but clinical correlation with your patient's condition is definitely a good idea. Multifocal couplets and triplets are a bit more troubling and may be harbingers of further, more life-threatening ventricular arrhythmias to come. Observation and treatment may be clinically indicated for these patients.

Interpolated PVC

Occasionally, a PVC occurs at such a time as to be completely sandwiched between two consecutive sinus complexes. As long as the PVC does not retrogradely depolarize the atria, the normal sinus rhythm and its associated ventricular response will continue completely undisturbed. The result is a PVC placed directly between two sinus complexes. This type of PVC is known as an interpolated PVC (Figure 20-141 ▶). These PVCs are not associated with any additional clinical significance and are just a diagnostic oddity.

Bundle Branch Blocks

In this section, we will discuss the concept of the bundle branch block (BBB) to help you formulate a practical understanding of the electrocardiographic principles involved. Bear in mind that without a 12-lead ECG, you cannot definitively interpret a BBB; however, this information will be useful for understanding other factors that may alter the appearance of the QRS complex in lead II.

We need to start off our general discussion by revisiting the electrical conduction system (Figure 20-142 ▼). Notice that the bundle of His splits off into the left and right bundle branches (LBB and RBB). The LBB, in turn, divides into the LAF and LPF. Both the RBB and the two fascicles then split into

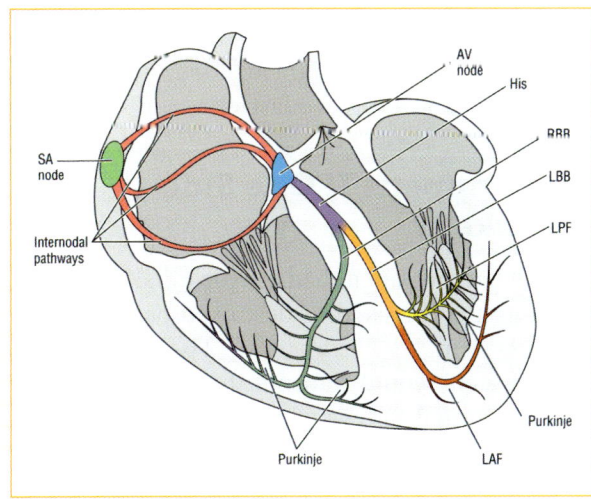

Figure 20-142 The heart and the electrical conduction system.

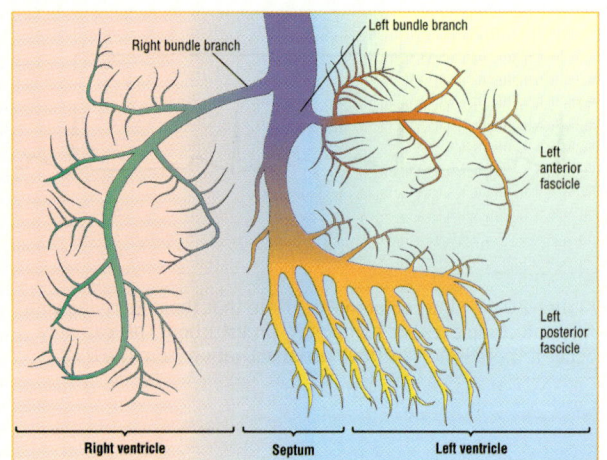

Figure 20-143 A closer look at the electrical conduction system.

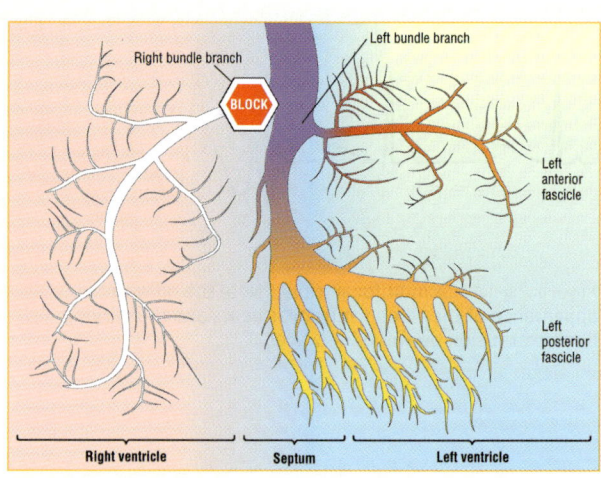

Figure 20-144 Bundle branch block.

smaller and smaller branches to form a network of terminal branches, which are collectively known as the Purkinje system (Figure 20-143). The Purkinje system allows the almost instantaneous firing of all of the ventricular cells at once.

Look at Figure 20-143. We want you to use your imagination to think about the ventricles of the heart as a flat sheet rather than a three-dimensional structure. Thinking about the system in this way will facilitate your understanding of the concepts.

Notice how the conduction system divides and innervates different areas of the heart. The LAF innervates the superior and anterior aspects of the left ventricle. The left posterior fascicle innervates the inferior and posterior aspects of the left ventricle. The RBB innervates part of the septum and the right ventricle.

Note that there is overlap of the different systems. This overlap is more prominent along the septum and along the border of the two fascicles.

What Happens If One Side Is Blocked?

Suppose that the patient had a myocardial infarction or something that blocked or destroyed part of the conduction system (Figure 20-144). The normally functioning system would transmit the impulse down the section of normal pathway the same way it always does. The sections of the heart that are innervated by those fibers would then fire instantaneously and in a coordinated manner. However, the section that is innervated by the blocked section would not receive a coordinated impulse. It would, instead, have to be depolarized by slow transmission of the impulse that is spread directly from cell to cell (Figure 20-145), starting from somewhere along the septum and spreading like a wave across the affected area of the heart.

Let's look at Figure 20-145 more closely. The impulse would travel down the LBB normally. Hence, the left ventricle and that section of the septum that is innervated by the LBB would fire normally. On the other hand,

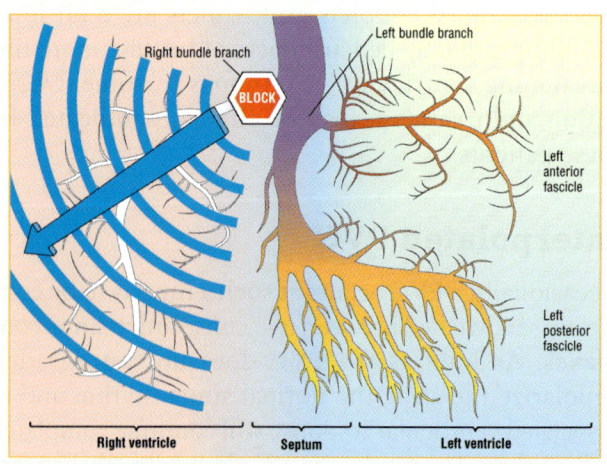

Figure 20-145 Slow depolarization caused by the bundle branch block.

the rest of the septum, and the right ventricle, would depolarize by the slower cell-to-cell route.

As you can imagine, this method of depolarizing the ventricles will give rise to abnormal-looking complexes on the ECG. Would the width of the QRS complex be increased? Yes. Why? *Because the slow cell-to-cell transmission requires a longer period to depolarize that section of the heart.* The net result is that the complexes are wider—0.12 seconds or more, to be exact.

Would the morphologic characteristics be different? Yes, they would. Once again, the morphologic features of the complex are an electrocardiographic representation of the vectors occurring in the heart during depolarization and repolarization. By adding the block, we have now created a slow-moving vector that was not there originally. In addition, because it occurs after the LBB has fired, the slow vector would be *unopposed*. This extra and unopposed vector will dramatically alter the appearance of the QRS complex.

Electrical Interventions

Defibrillation

The definition of defibrillation is to shock a fibrillating (chaotically beating) heart with specialized electrical current in an attempt to restore a normal rhythmic beat. A person in V-fib or pulseless V-tach needs immediate defibrillation to stop the chaotic activity and, hopefully, restore a normal beat. Ventricular fibrillation and pulseless V-tach are the indications for defibrillation. In contrast, asystole is not an indication for defibrillation because there is an absence of electrical activity.

To perform defibrillation, follow the steps in Skill Drill 20-6 ▶ :

1. **Determine that the cardiac rhythm is ventricular fibrillation or pulseless ventricular tachycardia** (**Step 1**).
2. If you are using paddles, apply electrode gel to the paddles before placing them on the patient's chest. **If using defibrillation pads, apply them according to the manufacturer's recommendation** (**Step 2**).
3. **Select the appropriate joules (J), and press the charge button**. For an adult, you should use 360 J monophasic (or biphasic equivalent) (**Step 3**).
4. **Reconfirm the rhythm,** and clear anyone around the patient. Make sure no one is touching the patient, stretcher, or anything else that is in contact with the patient.
5. **Clear the patient**. State, "I'm clear, you're clear, everybody's clear!" Deliver the shock (**Step 4**).
6. **Immediately perform five cycles of CPR (2 minutes)** (**Step 5**). After 2 minutes of CPR, reassess pulse and rhythm. Repeat defibrillation if needed and immediately resume CPR.

You are the Provider — Part 10

Your patient's condition improves following additional treatment en route to the hospital. You arrive and transfer care to the emergency department nurse.

Reassessment	Recording Time: 14 Minutes After Patient Contact
Respirations	18 breaths/min; adequate depth
Pulse	68 beats/min; regular
Skin	Pale
Blood pressure	116/70 mm Hg
SaO_2	98% with 100% O_2 via nonrebreathing mask

14. What causes sinus bradycardia?

Defibrillation

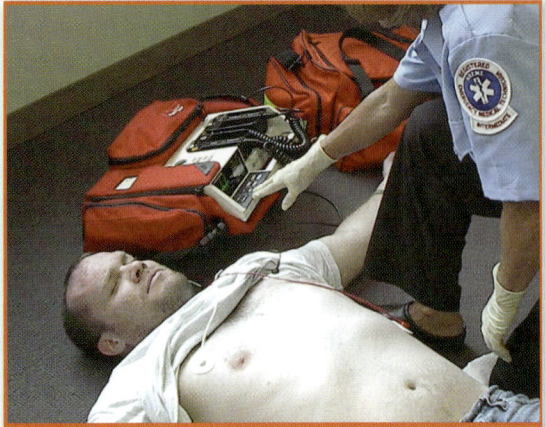

1 Determine the cardiac rhythm.

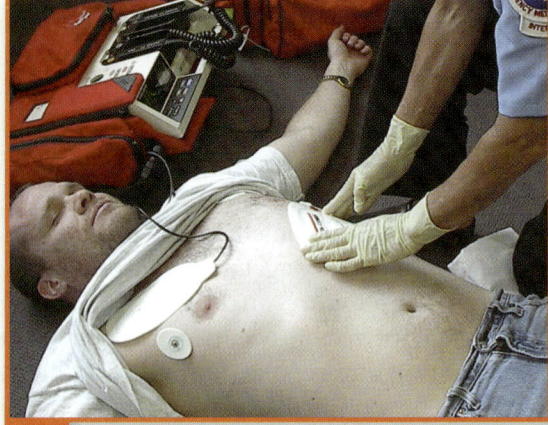

2 Apply defibrillation pads according to the manufacturer's recommendation.

(If using paddles, apply electrode gel to the paddles before placing them on the patient's chest.)

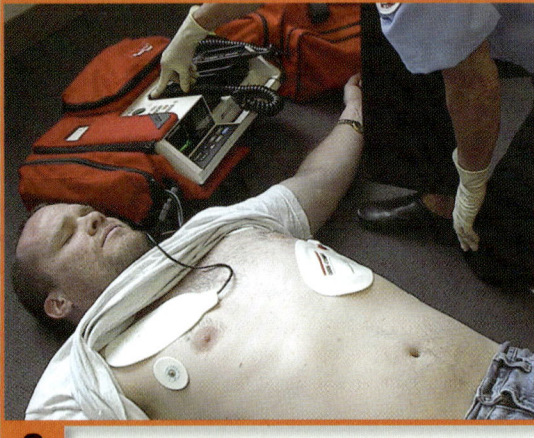

3 Continue CPR while charging.

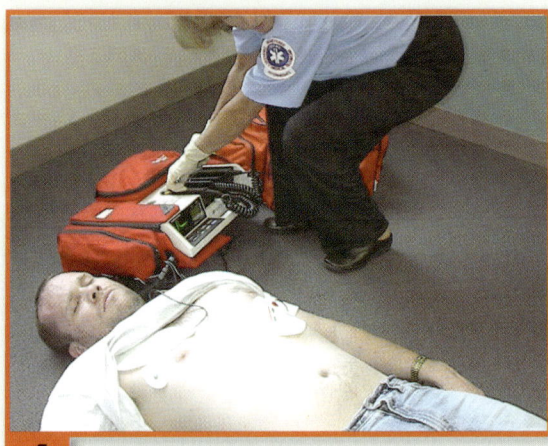

4 Reassess the rhythm, and clear anyone around the patient.

Deliver the shock.

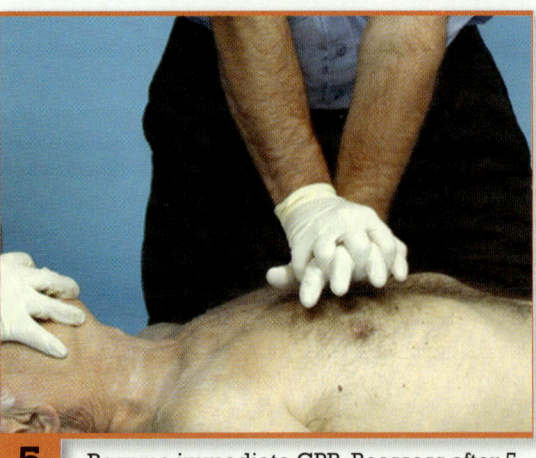

5 Resume immediate CPR. Reassess after 5 cycles (2 minutes).

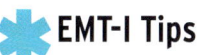

EMT-I Tips

Synchronized Cardioversion

Synchronized cardioversion is the timed delivery of energy into the myocardium to correct rapid, regular cardiac rhythms in patients who are unstable as a result of the cardiac rhythm. An internal "synchronizer" times the shock to deliver when it senses an R wave. This avoids delivering the shock during the relative refractory period (down slope of the T wave), which may precipitate V-fib.

Synchronized cardioversion involves the same steps as defibrillation; however, prior to delivering the shock, you must push the "sync" button on the monitor/defibrillator. You will know that the defibrillator has synchronized with the cardiac rhythm when the top of the R waves illuminate; on other defibrillator models, a blinking light appears above each R wave.

Unless authorized by medical control, synchronized cardioversion must be performed by a paramedic. The indications, contraindications, and adult energy settings for various cardiac dysrhythmias are as follows:

Indications
- Perfusing narrow and wide QRS complex tachycardias (rate >150 beats/min) with serious signs and symptoms linked to the tachycardia.
  - V-tach (monomorphic and polymorphic), SVT, atrial fibrillation, atrial flutter

Contraindications
- V-fib or pulseless V-tach (requires defibrillation)
- Poison- or drug-induced tachycardia
  - Treat the underlying problem with an antidote, if available.
  - The serious signs and symptoms are related to the poison or drug, not the tachycardia.
- Other health care providers being in physical contact with the patient.
  - You must ensure that **no one** is in physical contact with the patient before you perform synchronized cardioversion.

Adult Energy Settings
- Monomorphic V-tach and atrial fibrillation
  - Start with 100 J. Repeat at 200, 300, and 360 J respectively if the rhythm is not corrected.
- Polymorphic V-tach (ie, torsade de pointes)
  - Start with 200 J. Repeat at 200-300, and 360 J respectively if the rhythm is not corrected.
- Atrial Flutter or SVT
  - Start with 50 J. Repeat at 100, 200, 300, and 360 J respectively if the rhythm is not corrected.

Transcutaneous Pacing

A transcutaneous pacing system delivers pacing impulses to the heart through the skin via adhesive cutaneous electrodes, causing electrical depolarization and subsequent cardiac contraction. Immediate <u>transcutaneous pacing (TCP)</u> is indicated for patients who are hemodynamically symptomatic owing to compromising bradycardia that is too slow and unresponsive to atropine. Symptoms can include a systolic blood pressure of less than 90 mm Hg, a change in mental status, chest pain, or pulmonary edema.

To perform transcutaneous pacing, follow the steps in (Skill Drill 20-7 ▶):

1. **Determine the need for pacing** based on the presenting cardiac rhythm and the patient's clinical status, and contact medical control for authorization.
2. **Attach the three-lead cables** to continue monitoring the rhythm (**Step 1**).
3. **Apply the pacing electrodes** according to the manufacturer's recommendations. It may be necessary to carefully shave the chest of an individual with excessive chest hair (**Step 2**).
4. **Connect the electrodes to the cardiac monitor**, and select the desired heart rate. It is usually set at 80 beats/min.
5. **Slowly adjust the current setting until electrical capture is obtained.** Use the least amount of current that will provide capture (**Step 3**).
6. **Assess the patient's pulse** to ensure that the paced rate corresponds with the patient's pulse rate (**Step 4**).

You may need to administer an analgesic to make the pain of the chest wall muscle contractions tolerable.

Management

Management should follow the algorithms provided in the following sections. See Chapter 39 for a review of BLS for adults, children, and infants.

Chest Pain and Stroke

Chest pain and stroke can be very frightening to the patient and to family members. These are conditions that may prove fatal with little or no warning. It is imperative to consider psychological management along with conventional treatment when dealing with such patients. This support should also extend to the family.

Skill Drill 20-7: Transcutaneous Pacing

1. Determine the need for pacing. Attach the three-lead cables.

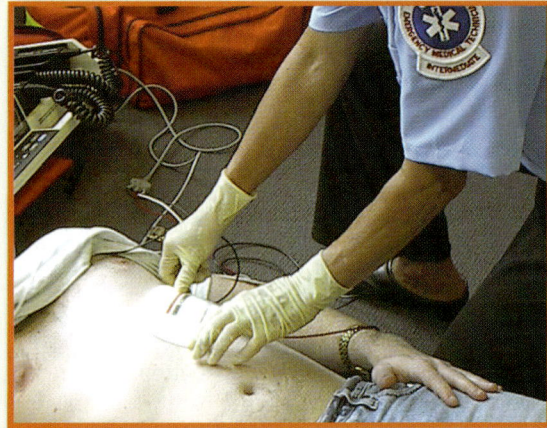

2. Apply the pacing electrodes.

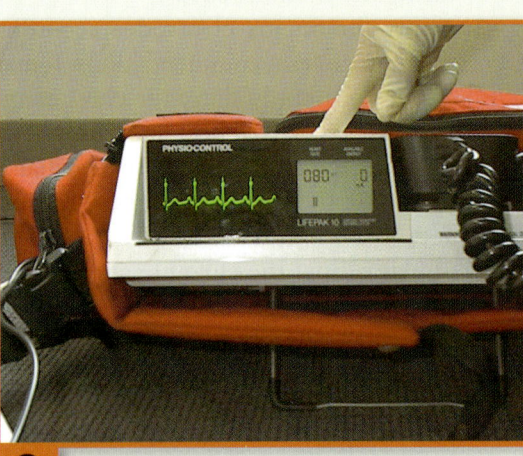

3. Connect the electrodes to the cardiac monitor, and select desired heart rate. Slowly adjust the electrical current setting until electrical capture is obtained.

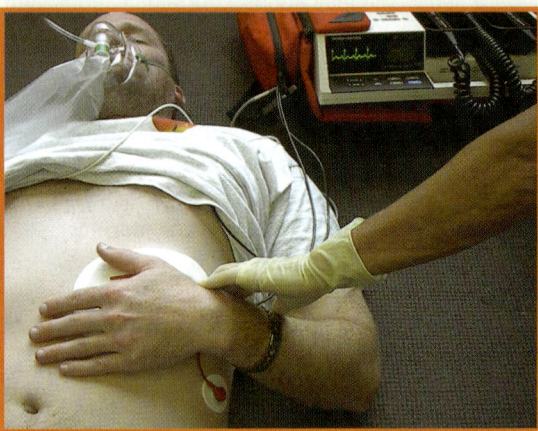

4. Assess the patient's pulse to ensure mechanical capture.

Common management modalities for any patient experiencing chest pain or signs and symptoms of a possible stroke begin with an assessment of level of consciousness, airway, breathing, and circulation. Apply high-flow oxygen, and obtain a thorough medical history. Intravenous access should be gained early, and nitroglycerin and morphine may be indicated for pain relief. Rapid transport to the closest, most appropriate facility is essential. Management of chest pain is summarized in Table 20-6 . Management of suspected stroke is summarized in Table 20-7 .

TABLE 20-6 Caring for Patients Experiencing Chest Pain

Scene safety
Initial assessment
- Responsiveness, airway, breathing, circulation

Supplemental oxygen
IV
Cardiac monitor
Vital signs

If chest pain is suggestive of cardiac origin, follow these steps:
- Medications:
  - Aspirin, 160–325 mg
  - Nitroglycerin, 0.4-mg spray or tablet (per local protocol regarding blood pressure)
  - Morphine, 2–4 mg (if pain is not relieved with nitroglycerin)

If condition persists after interventions, follow local protocols for additional care.

Tachycardias

Tachycardias fall into two categories: stable and unstable. In either case, the rapid heart rate does not allow for adequate ventricular filling and causes a decrease in cardiac output. This decrease is directly proportional to the rate.

Unstable tachycardia exists when the heart beats too fast for the patient's cardiovascular condition. This leads to serious signs and symptoms, including chest pain, dyspnea, altered mental status, pulmonary edema, hypotension, jugular venous distention, and/or orthostasis. The tachycardia is the immediate cause of the signs

TABLE 20-7 Management of Suspected Stroke

Scene safety
Initial assessment
- Responsiveness, airway, breathing, circulation

Supplemental oxygen
IV
Cardiac monitor
Vital signs

If condition is suggestive of stroke, follow these steps:
- Stroke assessment (Cincinnati Stroke Scale or Los Angeles Stroke Screen)
- Check blood glucose level
- Hospital notification and rapid transport

If condition persists after interventions, follow local protocols for any additional care.

EMT-I Tips

The first step in treating asystole is to identify that the rhythm truly is asystole. This is accomplished by verifying the rhythm in two leads. If you see asystole in lead II, switch to lead I or lead III for confirmation.

In the Field

When pacing a patient with hemodynamically unstable bradycardia, slowly increase output from the *minimum* setting until capture is achieved.

and symptoms. Unstable tachycardia requires immediate synchronized cardioversion to prevent further hemodynamic deterioration.

Stable tachycardia refers to a condition in which the patient has a heart rate of more than 100 beats/min with no significant signs or symptoms caused by the increased rate. An underlying cardiac abnormality is the cause of the patient's presentation. Treatment for stable tachycardias is aimed at slowing the rate and treating the underlying cause. Electrical cardioversion is only used if the patient's condition becomes unstable.

Management of atrial fibrillation and flutter is summarized in Table 20-8. Management of a patient with narrow-complex tachycardia is summarized in Table 20-9. Lastly, management of ventricular tachycardia—monomorphic and polymorphic—is summarized in Table 20-10.

Bradycardias

Bradycardias are simply slow rhythms of less than 60 beats/min. In symptomatic bradycardia, perfusion is poor owing to the rate. You will be concerned with treating only bradycardias that are symptomatic. Significant signs and symptoms include chest pain, dyspnea, decreased mental status, diaphoresis, hypotension, orthostasis, pulmonary edema, and CHF. Treatment is based on the degree of signs and symptoms, and consists of medications and/or transcutaneous pacing.

Asystole and *PEA* also fall in the category of bradycardias. Asystole is the absence of all electrical activity and is rarely associated with a positive outcome. Only if the cause of asystole is identified and treated in a timely manner will there be any reasonable possibility

TABLE 20-8 | Management of Tachycardia: Atrial Fibrillation or Atrial Flutter

Scene safety
Initial assessment
- Responsiveness, airway, breathing, circulation

Supplemental oxygen
IV
Cardiac monitor
Vital signs

Determine if the patient's condition is stable or unstable (serious signs/symptoms). If unstable, follow these steps:
- Pre-medicate whenever possible (sedative or narcotic analgesic)
- Synchronized cardioversion (100-200-300-360 J monophasic or biphasic equivalent) as needed to resolve rhythm (Note: Start at 50 J for atrial flutter.)
- If condition persists after interventions, follow local protocols for any additional care.

If stable, follow these steps:
- Consider need for medications:
  - Calcium channel blockers to control rapid ventricular rate (eg, diltiazem, 0.25 mg/kg)
  - Antiarrhythmics to convert rhythm (eg, amiodarone, 150 mg)
- If condition persists after interventions, follow local protocols for any additional care.

TABLE 20-9 | Management of Narrow-Complex Supraventricular Tachycardia

Scene safety
Initial assessment
- Responsiveness, airway, breathing, circulation

Supplemental oxygen
IV
Cardiac monitor
Vital signs

Determine if the patient's condition is stable or unstable. If stable, follow these steps:
- Vagal maneuvers
- Medication:
  - Adenosine, 6 mg, then 12 mg if needed (repeat 12-mg dose once if needed; total dose = 30 mg)
- If condition persists after interventions, follow local protocols for any additional care. (This could include calcium channel blockers or antiarrhythmics such as those used to treat atrial fibrillation or atrial flutter.)

If unstable and the cardiac rhythm is SVT, follow these steps:
- Pre-medicate whenever possible (sedative or narcotic analgesic)
- Synchronized cardioversion (50-100-200-300-360 J monophasic or biphasic equivalent) as needed to resolve rhythm
- If condition persists after interventions, follow local protocols for any additional care.

of survival. The term PEA refers to any semiorganized electrical activity that can be seen on the cardiac monitor despite the patient lacking a palpable pulse. As with asystole, identifying and treating the underlying cause is the key to patient survival.

Management of a patient with bradycardia is summarized in Table 20-11. Management of a patient with PEA is summarized in Table 20-12. Management of a patient with asystole is summarized in Table 20-13.

TABLE 20-10	Management of Ventricular Tachycardia

Scene safety
Initial assessment
- Responsiveness, airway, breathing, circulation

Supplemental oxygen
IV
Cardiac monitor
Vital signs

If rhythm indicates stable monomorphic ventricular tachycardia, follow these steps:
- Consider these medications (**one** of the following):
  - Amiodarone, 150 mg over 10 minutes
  - Lidocaine, 1-1.5 mg/kg
- If condition persists after interventions, follow local protocols for any additional care.

If rhythm indicates stable polymorphic ventricular tachycardia (ie, torsade de pointes), follow these steps:
- Consider this medication:
  - Magnesium sulfate, 1-2 g

If rhythm indicates unstable ventricular tachycardia, follow these steps:
- Pre-medicate whenever possible (sedative or narcotic analgesic)
- Synchronized cardioversion (100-200-300-360 J monophasic or biphasic equivalent) as needed to resolve rhythm
- If condition persists after interventions, follow local protocols for any additional care.

V-fib and Pulseless V-tach

Management of ventricular fibrillation and pulseless ventricular tachycardia is the most important management process to know for adult resuscitation. Most people who collapse in cardiac arrest are in V-fib. Management of ventricular fibrillation and pulseless ventricular tachycardia is summarized in Table 20-14. Rapid treatment according to this table provides the best scientific approach to restore spontaneous circulation. Defibrillation is the vital component for patients in ventricular fibrillation or pulseless ventricular tachycardia. A precordial thump is indicated for a witnessed arrest and, when performed immediately, may prevent the need for defibrillation.

TABLE 20-11	Management of Bradycardia

Scene safety
Initial assessment
- Responsiveness, airway, breathing, circulation

Supplemental oxygen
IV
Cardiac monitor
Vital signs

If bradycardia is causing serious signs/symptoms, follow these steps:
- Atropine, 0.5 mg (not recommended for high-degree AV block)
- Transcutaneous pacing
- Epinephrine, 2-10 µg/min
- Dopamine, 5-10 µg/kg/min

If bradycardia persists after interventions, follow local protocols for any additional care.

TABLE 20-12 Management of Pulseless Electrical Activity (PEA)

Scene safety

Initial assessment
- Responsiveness, airway, breathing, circulation

If patient is unresponsive, apneic, and has no signs of circulation, begin CPR until a monitor/defibrillator is available.

If PEA exists, follow these steps:
- Perform endotracheal intubation (or dual lumen airway device), IV therapy, continuous ECG monitoring, and CPR
- Attempt to identify and correct reversible causes:
  - **P**ulmonary embolus
  - **A**cidosis
  - **T**ension pneumothorax, tablets (drug overdose)
  - **C**ardiac tamponade
  - **H**ypovolemia, hypoxia, hypothermia, hypokalemia/hyperkalemia
- Medications:
  - Epinephrine, 1 mg (repeated every 3-5 min as needed); may administer 40 U vasopressin (*one-time dose*) in place of first or second dose of epinephrine
  - Atropine, 1 mg, if bradycardia present (repeated every 3-5 min to maximum of 3 mg)

If condition persists after interventions, follow local protocols for any additional care.

TABLE 20-13 Management of Asystole

Scene safety

Initial assessment
- Responsiveness, airway, breathing, circulation

If patient is unresponsive, apneic, and has no signs of circulation, begin CPR until a monitor/defibrillator is available.

If cardiac rhythm indicates asystole, follow these steps:
- Confirm in a second lead.
- Perform endotracheal intubation (or dual lumen airway device), IV therapy, continuous ECG monitoring, and CPR
- Attempt to identify and correct reversible causes (same as PEA)
- Medications:
  - Epinephrine 1 mg (repeated every 3-5 min as needed); may administer 40 U vasopressin (*one-time dose*) in place of first or second dose of epinephrine
  - Atropine 1 mg (repeated every 3-5 min to maximum of 3 mg)

If condition persists after interventions, follow local protocols for any additional care or for terminating efforts.

TABLE 20-14 Management of V-fib and Pulseless V-tach

Scene safety

Initial assessment
- Responsiveness, airway, breathing, circulation

If patient is unresponsive, apneic, and has no signs of circulation, begin CPR until a monitor/defibrillator is available.

If cardiac rhythm indicates V-fib or V-tach, follow these steps:
- Defibrillate one time (360 J monophasic or biphasic equivalent), followed immediately by CPR (reassess pulse and rhythm every 2 minutes); follow all shocks with immediate CPR.
- Perform endotracheal intubation (or dual lumen airway device), IV therapy, and continuous ECG monitoring.
- Attempt to identify and correct reversible causes
- Medications:
  - Epinephrine, 1 mg IV (repeated every 3-5 min)
  OR
  - Vasopressin in place of first or second dose of epinephrine, 40 U (single dose only; wait 10-20 min before initiating epinephrine therapy)
- Defibrillate at 360 J monophasic or biphasic equivalent
- If rhythm persists, use an antiarrhythmic medication (**one** of the following):
  - Amiodarone, 300 mg (repeat one time in 3-5 min at 150 mg)
  - Lidocaine, 1-1.5 mg/kg (repeat every 3-5 min; maximum 3 mg/kg)
- Defibrillate at 360 J monophasic or biphasic equivalent

If condition persists after interventions, follow local protocols for additional care.

Pediatric Needs

For pediatric patients, the energy level is set at 2 J/kg for the first shock and 4 J/kg for subsequent shocks. Follow American Heart Association pediatric guidelines and local protocols for pharmacologic management of the presenting rhythm.

EMT-I Tips

Never forget the patient!! Treat the patient, not the cardiac monitor.

You are the Provider

Summary

1. What are the risk factors for cardiovascular disease?

Age, family history, hypertension, hyperlipidemia, male sex, smoking, and carbohydrate intolerance. Possible contributing risks include diet, female sex, obesity, oral contraceptives, sedentary living, personality type, and psychosocial tensions.

2. What causes a myocardial infarction?

Complete blockage of an artery that supplies oxygen to the heart results in death to a portion of the myocardium, or a myocardial infarction.

3. What is the pacemaker function of the heart, and why do we need it?

The pacemaker dictates the rate at which the heart will cycle through its pumping action to circulate the blood. The pacemaker creates an organized beating of all of the cardiac cells, in a specialized sequence, to produce effective pumping action. It sets the pace that all of the other cells will follow.

4. What is the main pacemaker, and at what rate does it pace?

The heart's pacemaker is the SA node, found in the muscle of the right atrium. This area responds to the needs of the body, controlling the beat based on information it receives from the nervous, circulatory, and endocrine systems. The main pacemaker paces at a rate of 60 to 100 beats/min, with an average of 70 beats/min.

5. What are the causes of chest pain that you should consider in caring for this patient?

Possible causes of chest pain include angina pectoris, cholecystitis, aneurysm, hiatal hernia, pleurisy, esophageal and gastrointestinal diseases, pulmonary embolism, pancreatitis, respiratory infections, aortic dissection, pneumothorax, herpes zoster (shingles), chest wall tumors, and blunt trauma.

6. The pain of an AMI differs from the pain of angina in three ways. What are they?

The pain of AMI:
- May or may not be caused by exertion but can occur at any time, sometimes when a person is sitting quietly or even sleeping.
- Does not resolve in a few minutes; rather, it can last between 30 minutes and several hours.
- May or may not be relieved by rest or nitroglycerin.

7. What are three serious consequences of an AMI?

An AMI can have three serious consequences: sudden death, cardiogenic shock, and CHF.

8. What rhythm is this patient in?

This patient is in ventricular tachycardia (VT or V-tach). Ventricular tachycardia is a rapid heart rhythm, usually at a rate of 150 to 200 beats/min. The electrical activity starts in the ventricle instead of the atrium; therefore, the QRS complexes will be wide and bizarre. This rhythm usually does not allow adequate time between beats for the left ventricle to fill with blood. Therefore, the patient's blood pressure may fall. He or she may also feel weak or lightheaded or may even become unresponsive. In some cases, the patient may develop worsening chest pain or chest pain that was not there before onset of the dysrhythmia.

9. What should concern you about this rhythm?

Most cases of VT will be more sustained and may deteriorate into ventricular fibrillation.

10. What steps should you take when treating a conscious patient complaining of chest discomfort?

- Reassure the patient, and perform the initial assessment.
- Apply oxygen. If available, use pulse oximetry. Apply a nonrebreathing mask at 12 to 15 L/min.
- Apply the cardiac monitor, and note the presence of any dysrhythmias. Treat symptomatic patients according to local and ACLS protocols.
- Position the patient.
- Measure and record the patient's vital signs.
- If cardiac arrest occurs, follow local protocols and ACLS guidelines.
- Obtain a focused history and physical exam.
- Ask specific questions about the patient's chest discomfort. Use the OPQRST mnemonic to determine the type of pain.

Continued

You are the Provider continued

- Prepare to assist with prescribed nitroglycerin. Help the patient administer prescribed nitroglycerin.
- The mnemonic "MONA" is often used for pharmacologic interventions associated with chest pain: morphine, oxygen, nitroglycerin, and aspirin.
- The OPQRST mnemonic is used for assessing pain: onset, provocation/palliation, quality, radiation/referred, severity, and time.

11. What is your next step in the management of this patient?

If you are traveling to the hospital with an unresponsive patient, check the pulse at least every 30 seconds. If a pulse is not present, take the following steps:

- Stop the vehicle.
- If the AED is not immediately ready, perform CPR until it is available.
- Analyze the rhythm.
- Deliver a shock, if indicated, and immediately begin CPR.
- Continue resuscitation according to your local protocol.

If you are en route with a conscious adult patient who is having chest pain and becomes unresponsive, take the following steps:

- Check for a pulse.
- Stop the vehicle.
- If the AED is not immediately ready, perform CPR until it is ready.
- Analyze the rhythm.
- Deliver a shock, if indicated, and immediately begin CPR.
- Continue resuscitation according to your local protocol. If a "no shock" message is given and no pulse is present, you should start CPR, then transport.

12. What steps can the EMT-I take to determine the rhythm of this patient?

There are 10 points you should think about in an organized manner when approaching arrhythmias:

Summary

General:
- Is the rhythm fast or slow?
- Is the rhythm regular or irregular? If irregular, is it regularly irregular or irregularly irregular?

P waves:
- Do you see any P waves?
- Are all of the P waves the same?
- Does each QRS complex have a P wave?
- Is the P-R interval constant?

QRS complexes:
- Are the P waves and QRS complexes associated with one another?
- Are the QRS complexes narrow or wide?
- Are the QRS complexes grouped or not grouped?
- Are there any dropped beats?

13. What are the criteria for sinus bradycardia?

- Rate: Less than 60 beats/min
- Regularity: Regular
- P wave: Present
- P/QRS ratio: 1:1
- P-R interval: Normal to slightly prolonged
- QRS width: Normal to slightly prolonged
- Grouping: None
- Dropped beats: None
- Putting it all together: The sinus beats are slower than 60 beats/min.

14. What causes sinus bradycardia?

This rhythm can be caused by vagal stimulation leading to nodal slowing, or by medicines such as beta blockers and is normally found in some well-conditioned athletes. The QRS complex, and the P-R and Q-T intervals, may slightly widen as the rhythm slows to less than 60 beats/min. However, they will not widen past the upper threshold of the normal range for that interval. For example, the P-R interval may widen, but it should not widen beyond the upper range of 0.20 seconds.

Prep Kit

Ready for Review

- Cardiovascular diseases are the number one killer of men and women. Although older people are at a higher risk, such a sweeping generalization overlooks a staggering number of young victims. For these reasons, early recognition and early treatment are the keys to survival.

- The heart is divided down the middle into two sides, right and left, each with upper chambers called atria and lower chambers called ventricles.

- The largest of the four heart valves that keep blood moving through the circulatory system in the proper direction is the aortic valve, which lies between the left ventricle and the aorta, the body's main artery.

- The heart's electrical conduction system controls heart rate and helps to keep the atria and ventricles working together.

- The heart has a backup pacemaker system. Every cell in the conduction system is capable of setting the pace, but the intrinsic rate is slower than the cells that precede it. The further away from the SA node, the slower the pacemaker.

- Regulation of heart function is provided by the brain via the autonomic nervous system, the hormones of the endocrine system, and the heart tissue. Baroreceptors and chemoreceptors sense abnormalities in pressure and chemical composition.

- Electrolytes are responsible for initiating and conducting electrical signals in the heart. The action potential of the cardiac cell has three phases: stimulation, depolarization, and recovery.

- The two phases of the cardiac cycle are systole, the pumping phase, and diastole, the resting phase.

- Pulmonary circulation carries blood from the right side of the heart to the lungs, and back to the left side of the heart. Systemic circulation is responsible for blood flow to the rest of the body.

- During periods of exertion or stress, the myocardium requires more oxygen. This is supplied by dilation of the coronary arteries, which increases blood flow.

- Common places to feel for a pulse include the carotid, femoral, brachial, radial, ulnar, posterior tibial, and dorsalis pedis arteries.

- Low blood flow to the heart is usually caused by coronary artery atherosclerosis, a disease in which cholesterol plaques build up inside blood vessels, eventually occluding them. Occasionally, a brittle plaque will crack, causing a blood clot to form. Heart tissue downstream suffers from a lack of oxygen and, within 30 minutes, will begin to die. This is called an acute myocardial infarction (AMI), or heart attack.

- Myocardial tissues that are ischemic but are not yet dying can cause pain called angina. The pain of AMI, although the same in terms of how it is described (ie, crushing, pressure), is different from that of angina in that it can come at any time, not just with exertion; it lasts up to several hours, rather than just a few moments; and it is not relieved by rest or nitroglycerin.

- In addition to chest pain or pressure, signs of AMI include sudden onset of weakness, nausea, and sweating; sudden arrhythmia; pulmonary edema; and even sudden death.

- Heart attacks can have three serious consequences. One is sudden death, usually the result of cardiac arrest caused by abnormal heart rhythms called dysrhythmias. These include tachycardia, bradycardia, ventricular tachycardia, and, most commonly, ventricular fibrillation.

- The second consequence is cardiogenic shock. Symptoms include restlessness; anxiety; pale, clammy skin; pulse rate higher than normal; and blood pressure lower than normal. Patients with these symptoms should receive oxygen, assisted ventilation as needed, and immediate transport.

Technology

- Interactivities
- Vocabulary Explorer
- Anatomy Review
- Web Links
- Online Review Manual

Prep Kit Continued...

- The third consequence of AMI is congestive heart failure (CHF); in which the damaged myocardium can no longer contract effectively enough to pump blood through the system. The lungs become congested with fluid, breathing becomes difficult, the heart rate increases, and the left ventricle enlarges. Signs include swollen ankles from pedal edema, high blood pressure, rapid heart rate and respirations, rales, and sometimes the pink sputum and dyspnea of pulmonary edema.

- Treat a patient with CHF as you would a patient with chest pain. Monitor the patient's cardiac rhythm, give the patient oxygen via nonrebreathing face mask, and allow the patient to remain in a position of comfort.

- In treating patients with chest pain, obtain a SAMPLE history, following the OPQRST mnemonic to assess the pain; measure and record vital signs; put the patient in a comfortable position, usually sitting up; administer prescribed nitroglycerin and oxygen; and transport the patient, reporting to medical control as you do.

- If a patient is apneic and pulseless and is 8 years or older and weighs at least 55 lb, you must decide whether to use the automated external defibrillator (AED). If the patient weighs less than 55 lb or is younger than 8 years, you may use an AED if it is equipped with special pediatric pads and can deliver the reduced energy levels necessary for this patient. Otherwise, begin CPR. Note: Adult pads may be used on patients between the ages of 1 and 8 years if pediatric pads are not available. Pads must be placed on the front and back to prevent touching of the pads on the chest.

- Follow local protocols and ACLS algorithms to treat a patient in cardiac arrest. Ensure a patent airway, and obtain an advanced airway as soon as possible. Monitor cardiac rhythms and establish IV access. Pharmacologic treatment should be based on ECG monitoring and ACLS protocols.

- Termination of efforts should be based on local protocol and direct communication with online medical direction.

- The AED requires the operator to apply the pads, power on the unit, analyze the rhythm, and press the shock button. The computer inside the AED recognizes rhythms that require shocking and will not mislead you. If available, use pediatric pads for patients younger than 8 years and those who weigh less than 55 lb. Otherwise, use adult pads on pediatric patients between 1 year and 8 years of age. You may have to apply pads to the front and back.

- The three most common errors in using certain AEDs are failure to keep a charged battery in the machine, applying the AED to a patient who is moving, and applying the AED to a responsive patient with a rapid heart rate. Do not touch the patient while the AED is analyzing the heart rhythm or delivering shocks.

- In integrating use of the AED and CPR, you should perform CPR only after giving up to three shocks, if indicated. If you still cannot feel a pulse, perform CPR for 1 minute.

- If paramedics are responding to the scene, stay where you are and continue the sequence of shocks and CPR. Do not wait for the paramedics to arrive to begin defibrillation. If paramedics are not responding, begin transport after six shocks or after the machine gives three consecutive messages that no shock is advised. If an unresponsive patient has a pulse but loses it during transport, you must stop the vehicle, start CPR if the defibrillator is not ready, then apply the AED.

- The chain of survival, which is the sequence of events that must happen for a patient with cardiac arrest to have the best chance of survival, includes recognition of early warning signs and immediate activation of EMS, immediate CPR by bystanders, early defibrillation, and early advanced care. Seconds count at every stage.

- When interpreting a patient's cardiac rhythm in lead II, it is important to understand that you cannot diagnose AMI; a 12-lead ECG, among other tests performed in the hospital, is required to definitively diagnose such a condition.

- Lead II is the most common lead used by the EMT-I to view a patient's cardiac rhythm. In this lead, you can identify and, if necessary, treat life-threatening cardiac arrhythmias.

- Indications for defibrillation are ventricular fibrillation and pulseless ventricular tachycardia. Defibrillation does not work for asystole because there is no electrical activity present.

- When pacing, use the least amount of current necessary to provide capture.

Vital Vocabulary

aberrancy The abnormal conduction of an electrical impulse through the heart. This aberrant conduction gives rise to wide complexes that are morphologically different from those that have gone through the normal pathways.

absolute refractory period The period in the cell firing cycle at which it is impossible to restimulate a cell to fire off another impulse.

acute myocardial infarction (AMI) Heart attack; death of heart muscle following obstruction of blood flow to it. Acute in this context means, "new" or "happening right now."

afterload The resistance the heart must pump against, or the systemic vascular resistance.

alpha effects Stimulation of alpha receptors that results in vasoconstriction.

angina pectoris Transient (short-lived) chest discomfort caused by partial or temporary blockage of blood flow to the heart muscle.

aorta The main artery, which receives blood from the left ventricle and delivers it to all the other arteries that carry blood to the tissues of the body.

aortic arch One of three described portions of the aorta; the section of the aorta between the ascending and descending portions that gives rise to the right brachiocephalic (innominate), left common carotid, and left subclavian arteries.

aortic valve The one-way valve that lies between the left ventricle and the aorta. It keeps blood from flowing back into the left ventricle after the left ventricle ejects its blood into the aorta and is one of four heart valves.

arrhythmia An irregular or abnormal heart rhythm; also, absence of heart rhythm.

arteriosclerosis The thickening of the arterial walls that results in a loss of elasticity and concomitant reduction in blood flow.

arteries Vessels of the circulatory system that carry oxygenated blood away from the heart.

ascending aorta The first of three portions of the aorta; originates from the left ventricle and gives rise to two branches, the right and left main coronary arteries.

asynchronous Not occurring at the same time.

asystole Complete absence of heart electrical activity.

atherosclerosis A disorder in which cholesterol and possibly calcium build up inside the walls of blood vessels, eventually leading to partial or complete blockage of blood flow.

atrioventricular (AV) node The site located in the right atrium adjacent to the septum that is responsible for transiently slowing electrical conduction.

atrioventricular valves The two valves through which blood flows from the atria to the ventricles.

atrium One of two (right and left) upper chambers of the heart. The right atrium receives blood from the vena cava and delivers it to the right ventricle. The left atrium receives blood from pulmonary veins and delivers it to the left ventricle.

automaticity The ability of cardiac cells to generate an impulse to contract even when there is no external nervous stimulus.

baroreceptors Receptors in the blood vessels, kidneys, brain, and heart that respond to changes in pressure in the heart or main arteries to help maintain homeostasis.

beta effects Stimulation of beta receptors that results in increased inotropic, dromotropic, and chronotropic states.

bigeminy A premature complex that occurs at every second beat. The complexes can be supraventricular or ventricular.

blood The fluid tissue that is pumped by the heart through the arteries, veins, and capillaries and consists of plasma and formed elements or cells, such as red blood cells, white blood cells, and platelets.

bradycardia Slow heart rate, less than 60 beats/min.

bruit An abnormal "whooshing" sound indicating turbulent blood flow within a blood vessel.

Prep Kit continued...

bundle of His Part of the conduction system of the heart; a continuation of the atrioventricular node.

capillaries Microscopic, thin-walled blood vessels through which oxygen and nutrients and carbon dioxide and waste products are exchanged.

cardiac arrest A state in which the heart fails to generate an effective and detectable blood flow; pulses are not palpable in cardiac arrest, even if muscular and electrical activity continues in the heart.

cardiac cycle The repetitive pumping process that begins with the onset of cardiac muscle contraction and ends just before the beginning of the next contraction.

cardiac output The amount of blood pumped through the circulatory system in 1 minute.

cardiogenic shock A state in which not enough oxygen is delivered to the tissues of the body, caused by low output of blood from the heart. It can be a severe complication of a large acute myocardial infarction, as well as other conditions.

chemoreceptors Receptors in the blood vessels, kidneys, brain, and heart that respond to changes in chemical composition of the blood to help maintain homeostasis.

chordae tendineae cordis Small muscular strands that attach the ventricles and the valves, preventing regurgitation of blood through the valves from the ventricles to the atria.

chronotropic state Related to the control of the heart's rate of contraction.

circumflex coronary artery One of the two branches of the left main coronary artery.

compensatory pause A pause immediately following a premature complex that is longer than the interval between two normally conducted beats, allowing the rhythm to proceed, without any alteration of cycle length, around the premature complex. In essence, the pause compensates for the short interval preceding the premature complex and allows the rate to proceed on schedule.

conduction system A group of complex electrical tissues within the heart that initiate and transmit stimuli that result in contractions of myocardial tissue.

conductivity The ability of the cardiac cells to conduct electrical impulses.

congestive heart failure (CHF) A disorder in which the heart loses part of its ability to effectively pump blood, usually as a result of damage to the heart muscle and usually resulting in a backup of fluid into the lungs.

contractility The strength of heart muscle contraction.

coronary arteries Blood vessels that carry blood and nutrients to the heart muscle.

coronary artery disease (CAD) The condition that results when atherosclerosis or arteriosclerosis is present in the arterial walls.

coronary sinus The end of the great cardiac vein that collects blood returning from the walls of the heart.

cusps The flaps the comprise the heart valves.

defibrillate To shock a fibrillating (chaotically beating) heart with specialized electrical current in an attempt to restore a normal rhythmic beat.

depolarization A state in which the cell becomes more positive, moving toward equilibrium with the extracellular fluid. Depolarization takes place during the latter part of the resting state and is completed during activation by the action potential.

descending aorta One of the three portions of the aorta, it is the longest portion and extends through the thorax and abdomen into the pelvis.

diastole The relaxation phase of the heart, when the ventricles are filling with blood.

dromotropic state Related to the control of the heart's electrical conduction.

dysrhythmia An irregular or abnormal heart rhythm.

ejection fraction The portion of the blood ejected from the ventricle during systole.

electrical potential An electrical charge difference that is created by the difference in sodium and potassium concentrations across the cell membrane at any given instant.

electrocardiogram (ECG) A 12-lead electrocardiographic recording used to evaluate the heart and its rhythm.

epicardium The layer of the serous pericardium that lies closely against the heart; also called the visceral pericardium.

epinephrine A naturally occurring hormone with a greater stimulatory effect on beta receptors that also may be given as a cardiac drug.

escape complex A beat that occurs after a normal pacemaker fails to fire.

escape rhythm A rhythm that occurs after a normal pacemaker fails to fire.

excitability A property of cardiac cells that provides the cells with the ability to respond to electrical impulses.

foramen ovale An opening between the two atria that is present in the fetus but closes shortly after birth.

fossa ovalis A depression between the right and left atria that indicates where the foramen ovale had been located in the fetus.

heart A muscular, cone-shaped organ whose function is to pump blood throughout the body.

inferior vena cava The principal vein draining blood from the lower portion of the body.

inotropic state Related to the strength of the heart's contraction.

interatrial septum A membrane that separates the right and left atria.

interventricular septum A thick wall that separates the right and left ventricles.

ischemia A lack of oxygen that deprives tissues of necessary nutrients, resulting from partial or complete blockage of blood flow; potentially reversible because permanent injury has not yet occurred.

isoelectric line Baseline of a tracing on an electrocardiogram (ECG).

junctional rhythm Any rhythm that originates in and around the atrioventricular (AV) node, in the region of the AV junction; junctional rhythms are not sinus in origin because the primary pacemaker site is not in the sinoatrial (SA) node.

left anterior descending (LAD) artery One of the two branches of the left main coronary artery, which is the largest and shortest of the myocardial blood vessels. The LAD and the circumflex coronary arteries supply blood to the left ventricle and other areas.

lumen The inside diameter of an artery or other hollow structure.

mediastinum The area in the chest that lies between the lungs and contains the heart and great vessels and other structures.

mitral valve The valve in the heart that separates the left atrium from the left ventricle.

monomorphic A term used to describe a rhythm that has complexes of the same size, shape, and direction (for example, monomorphic ventricular tachycardia).

murmur An abnormal heart sound, heard as a "whooshing" sound and indicating turbulent blood flow within the heart.

myocardium Heart muscle.

necrosis Tissue death resulting from a prolonged lack of oxygen.

noncompensatory pause A pause immediately following a premature complex that alters the rhythm, causing a resetting of the pacemaker and an alteration of cycle length after the premature complex. In essence, this pause does not compensate for the short interval preceding the premature complex, and the rate is completely reset after the event.

norepinephrine A naturally occurring hormone with a greater stimulatory effect on alpha receptors that also may be given as a cardiac drug.

Prep Kit continued...

occlusion Blockage, usually of a tubular structure such as a blood vessel.

P wave The first positive wave in the normal cardiac conduction pattern, it represents movement of the electrical impulse through the atria, resulting in atrial contraction.

P-P interval The interval represented by the space between the P waves of two consecutive complexes.

P-R interval The interval that occupies the space between the beginning of the P wave and the beginning of the QRS complex.

P-R segment The segment of the complex that occupies the space between the end of the P wave and the beginning of the QRS complex.

P-wave axis The calculated electrical axis for the P waves.

papillary muscles Specialized muscles that attach the ventricles to the cusps of the valves by muscular strands called chordae tendineae cordis.

parietal layer One of two layers of the serous pericardium. It is separated from the visceral pericardium by a small amount of pericardial fluid.

pedal edema Swelling of the feet and ankles caused by collection of fluid in the tissues; a possible sign of congestive heart failure (CHF).

perfusion The flow of blood through body tissues and vessels.

pericardial fluid A serous fluid that fills the space between the visceral pericardium and the parietal pericardium and helps to reduce friction.

pericardial sac A thick fibrous membrane that surrounds the heart. Also called the pericardium.

pericardium A thick fibrous membrane that surrounds the heart. Also called the pericardial sac.

polarized state The state of the resting cell, which normally has a net negative charge with respect to the outside of the cell.

polymorphic A term used to describe a rhythm that has complexes of varying size, shape, and direction (for example, polymorphic ventricular tachycardia).

preload The pressure on the ventricles at the end of the resting phase of the heart. It is influenced by blood returned to the heart from the body, the total volume of blood in the body, the distribution of the blood throughout the body, and the action of the atria.

premature complex A complex that arrives earlier than expected for the cadence of the rhythm.

pulmonary circulation The circulatory system in the body that carries blood from the right side of the heart to the lungs and back to the left side of the heart.

pulmonic valve The semilunar valve that regulates blood flow between the right ventricle and the pulmonary artery.

Q-T interval The interval represented by the space from the beginning of the QRS complex to the end of the T wave; may vary with heart rate.

QRS complex The second positive waveform that follows the P-R segment in the normal electrical conduction pattern and represents the depolarization of the ventricles. This complex corresponds to ventricular contraction, or systole.

quadrigeminy A premature complex every fourth beat. The complexes can be supraventricular or ventricular.

R-on-T phenomenon When a premature ventricular contraction falls on the T wave of the previous complex.

R-R interval The interval represented by the space between the R waves of two consecutive complexes.

relative refractory period The latter phase of repolarization in which the cells are able to respond to a stronger-than-normal stimulus.

repolarization The process of returning to the cardiac cells' resting or polarized state that occurs once the cardiac cells depolarize.

salvo When three or more premature ventricular contractions (PVCs) occur sequentially. Commonly used when the presence of ventricular tachycardia is suspected.

semilunar valves The two valves, the aortic and pulmonic valves, that divide the heart from the aorta and pulmonary arteries.

serous pericardium The inner membrane of the pericardium, which contains two layers called the visceral pericardium and the parietal pericardium.

sinoatrial (SA) node The normal site of the origin of electrical impulses; located high in the right atrium, it is the heart's natural pacemaker.

sodium-potassium pump A molecular (ion-transporting) mechanism whereby sodium is actively moved out of a cell and potassium moved in.

ST segment The second pause that occurs in the normal electrical conduction pattern and represents the beginning of repolarization of the heart.

Starling's law A principle that states that if a muscle is stretched slightly before stimulation to contract, the muscle will contract harder; describes how increased venous return to the heart stretches the ventricles and allows for increased cardiac contractility.

stroke volume The amount of blood that the left ventricle ejects into the aorta in each contraction.

superior vena cava The principal vein draining blood from the upper portion of the body.

supraventricular A cardiac rhythm that originates above the ventricles.

synchronized Occurring at the same time.

syncope Fainting spell or transient loss of consciousness.

systemic circulation The circulatory system in the body that is responsible for blood flow in all areas of the body, except for areas covered by the pulmonary circulation (blood flow from the right side of the heart to the lungs and back to the left side of the heart).

systole Contraction of the ventricular mass with its concomitant pumping of blood into the systemic circulation.

T wave The third positive waveform in the normal electrical conduction pattern, it represents the completion of repolarization.

tachycardia Rapid heart rhythm, more than 100 beats/min.

transcutaneous pacing (TCP) A system that delivers pacing impulses to the heart through the skin via adhesive cutaneous electrodes, causing electrical depolarization and subsequent cardiac contraction.

tricuspid valve The heart valve that separates the right atrium from the right ventricle.

trigeminy A premature complex every third beat. The complexes can be supraventricular or ventricular.

tunica adventitia The outer layer of tissue of a blood vessel wall, composed of elastic and fibrous connective tissue.

tunica intima The smooth, thin, inner lining of a blood vessel.

tunica media The middle and thickest layer of tissue of a blood vessel wall, composed of elastic tissue and smooth muscle cells that allow the vessel to expand or contract in response to changes in blood pressure and tissue demand.

U wave A small, flat wave sometimes seen after the T wave and before the next P wave. It could represent ventricular depolarization and endocardial repolarization.

unifocal A term used to describe a singly occurring premature ventricular contraction (PVC) or PVCs that share a common morphologic appearance because they originate in the same ectopic focus.

veins The blood vessels that transport unoxygenated blood back to the heart.

ventricle One of two (right and left) lower chambers of the heart. The left ventricle receives blood from the left atrium (upper chamber) and delivers blood to the aorta. The right ventricle receives blood from the right atrium and pumps it into the pulmonary artery.

ventricular fibrillation Disorganized, ineffective twitching of the ventricles, resulting in no blood flow and a state of cardiac arrest.

ventricular tachycardia Rapid heart rhythm in which the electrical impulse begins in the ventricle (instead of the atrium), which may result in inadequate blood flow and eventually deteriorate into cardiac arrest.

visceral layer The layer of the serous pericardium that lies closely against the heart. Also called the epicardium.

Assessment in Action

You are called to respond to a 58-year-old man with a complaint of chest pain. When you arrive, you find Mr Sneed sitting at the dinner table. He is sweaty and pale and is clutching his chest. He states he is nauseated and short of breath. He tells you the pain is in the left side of his chest and that it moves down his arm. He began having pain about 2 or 3 hours ago but thought it was indigestion. He has taken two antacid tablets without relief. His wife finally convinced him to call an ambulance.

While you are interviewing Mr Sneed, your partner gives him oxygen and assesses his vital signs. He finds a blood pressure of 162/106 mm Hg and a bounding pulse at 110 beats/min. His respiratory rate is 20 breaths/min. Pulse oximetry reveals a saturation of 95%. The cardiac monitor shows sinus tachycardia at 110 beats/min.

Mr Sneed is moved to the ambulance where IV access is established. He is given an aspirin and two doses of nitroglycerin sublingually before the pain subsides. He has no other complications en route to the hospital and is handed over to the emergency department staff in stable condition.

1. Your interview with Mr Sneed includes the OPQRST of chest pain. What does the "R" stand for?
   - A. Revolving
   - B. Resolution
   - C. Relief
   - D. Radiation/Referred

2. Which structure of the heart is the outermost layer that contains serous fluid?
   - A. The endocardium
   - B. The myocardium
   - C. The pericardium
   - D. The echocardium

3. The MOST common cardiac dysrhythmia associated with sudden cardiac death is:
   - A. ventricular tachycardia.
   - B. ventricular fibrillation.
   - C. pulseless electrical activity.
   - D. asystole.

4. Before administering nitroglycerin to a patient with chest pain, you must ensure the patient has a systolic blood pressure of at least:
   - A. 90 mm Hg.
   - B. 100 mm Hg.
   - C. 110 mm Hg.
   - D. 120 mm Hg.

5. Basic risk factors of cardiovascular disease include all EXCEPT:
   - A. hypotension.
   - B. male sex.
   - C. smoking.
   - D. family history.

6. The deposits on the arterial walls, usually of cholesterol and other fatty substances, that cause loss of elasticity with a concomitant reduction in blood flow is known as:
   - A. a murmur.
   - B. arteriosclerosis.
   - C. atherosclerosis.
   - D. peripheral vascular disease.

Points to Ponder

Mrs White is 65 years old. She had a heart attack 3 years ago and occasionally has mild chest pain. She has noticed more difficulty breathing in the evening and has had to sleep on an extra pillow at night. She has also felt palpitations and irregularities in her heart rate. Her doctor has diagnosed congestive heart failure.

You respond to Mrs White's address in the middle of the night. She can speak to you only in broken sentences and is coughing up pink, frothy sputum. When you assess her vital signs, you find a blood pressure of 174/110 mm Hg. Her heart rate is 126 beats/min and irregular. You apply the cardiac monitor and find an irregularly irregular rhythm with no obvious P waves. Her respirations are labored at 24 breaths/min.

After giving Mrs White oxygen at 15 L/min and inserting an IV line, you contact medical control for permission to administer nitroglycerin, furosemide (Lasix), and morphine. With these drugs given, Mrs White's condition improves. Her breathing is much less labored. She is transported to the hospital, and care is handed off to the emergency department staff.

Issues: Understanding the Urgency in Care With CHF and Respiratory Distress, Understanding the Need for High-Concentration Oxygen Therapy, Using Medications in the Treatment of CHF

Diabetic Emergencies

1999 Objectives

Cognitive

5-3.1 Describe the pathophysiology of diabetes mellitus. (p 986)
5-3.2 Describe the effects of decreased levels of insulin on the body. (p 988)
5-3.3 Correlate abnormal findings in assessment with clinical significance in the patient with a diabetic emergency. (p 992)
5-3.4 Discuss the management of diabetic emergencies. (p 993)
5-3.5 Describe the mechanism of ketone body formation and its relationship to ketoacidosis. (p 988)
5-3.6 Describe the effects of decreased levels of insulin on the body. (p 988)
5-3.7 Discuss the pathophysiology of hypoglycemia. (p 991)
5-3.8 Recognize the signs and symptoms of the patient with hypoglycemia. (p 991)
5.3-9 Describe the management of a hypoglycemic patient. (p 993)
5-3.10 Integrate the pathophysiological principles and the assessment findings to formulate a field impression and implement a treatment plan for the patient with hypoglycemia. (p 992)
5-3.11 Discuss the pathophysiology of hyperglycemia. (p 988)
5-3.12 Recognize the signs and symptoms of the patient with hyperglycemia. (p 991)
5-3.13 Describe the management of the hyperglycemic patient. (p 993)
5-3.14 Differentiate between diabetic emergencies based on assessment and history. (p 990)
5-3.15 Correlate abnormal findings in the assessment with clinical significance in the patient with a diabetic emergency. (p 992)
5-3.16 Develop a patient management plan based on field impression in the patient with a diabetic emergency. (p 994)

Affective

None

Psychomotor

None

1985 Objectives

There are no 1985 objectives for this chapter.

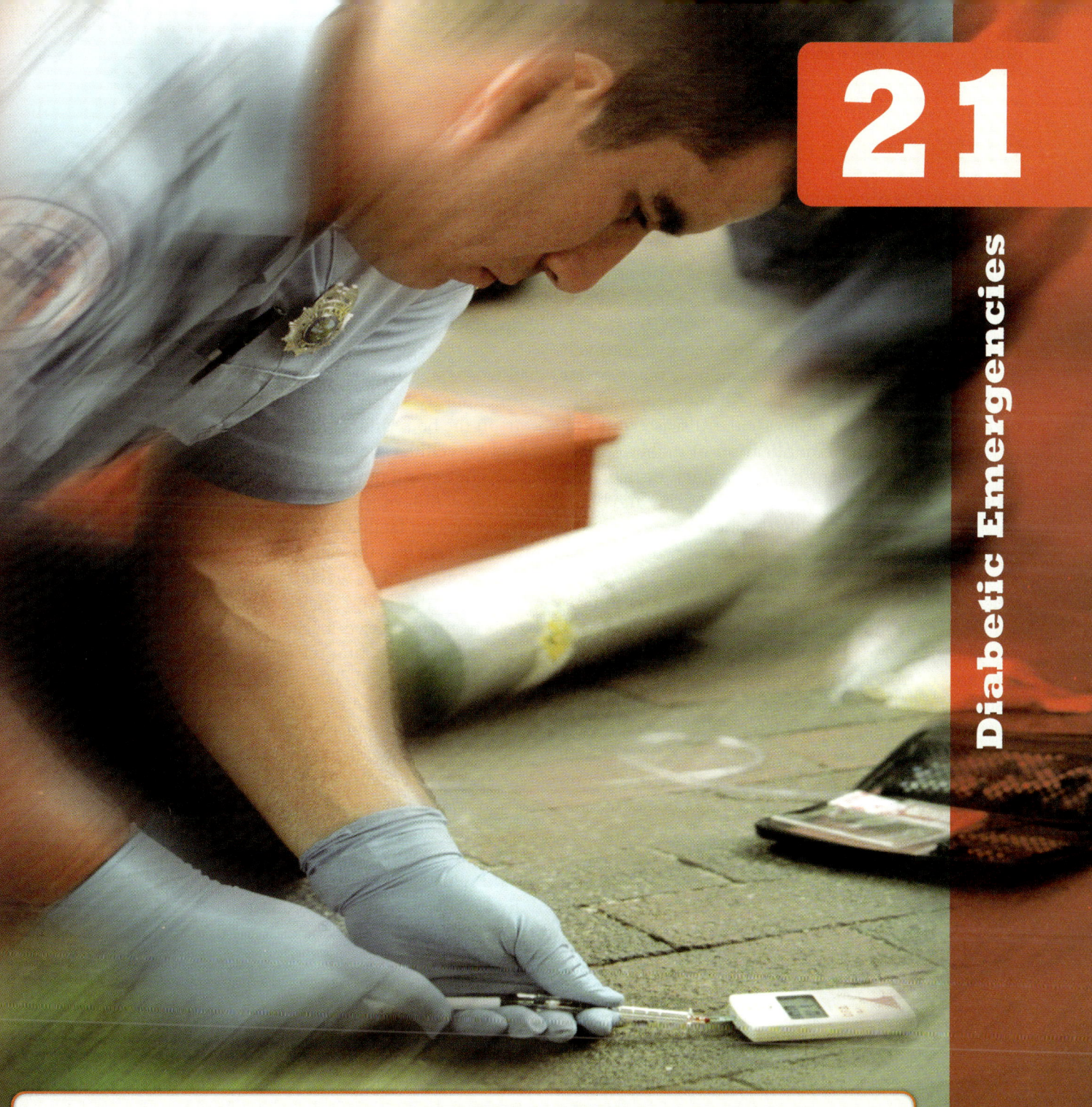

21

Diabetic Emergencies

You are the Provider

You and your partner are just preparing to sit down for dinner when a call comes in that EMS is needed for an unknown diabetic emergency. While en route, you both review what problems you might encounter on scene. This chapter will help you to manage those challenging calls involving patients with diabetes-related problems.

1. What are the two types of diabetes?
2. What are the two most common types of diabetic emergencies seen in the prehospital setting?

Diabetic Emergencies

Diabetes is a very common disease, affecting about 6% of the population. It is a metabolic disorder in which the hormone insulin, which is needed to regulate blood glucose levels, is absent or ineffective. Without treatment, blood glucose levels become too high (hyperglycemia) and can cause coma and death. If properly treated, most people with diabetes can live relatively normal lives. However, diabetes can have many severe complications that affect the length and quality of life, including blindness, cardiovascular disease, and kidney failure. Another complication of diabetes often occurs when the patient takes too much of their prescribed insulin, which, by rapidly lowering the blood glucose level, can cause a life-threatening state of hypoglycemia (low blood glucose). Therefore, as an EMT-I, you need to know the signs and symptoms of a blood glucose level that is too high or too low so that you can administer the most appropriate treatment.

This chapter explains two types of diabetes and how they are controlled, including the roles of glucose and insulin. You will learn how to distinguish between hyperglycemia and hypoglycemia, which often resemble each other. The chapter discusses how to identify and treat diabetic emergencies in the prehospital setting. Complications such as seizures, altered mental status, and myocardial infarction are also briefly discussed.

Diabetes

Defining Diabetes

Literally, the word "diabetes" means "a passer through; a siphon." Medically, the term refers to a metabolic disorder in which the body's ability to metabolize simple carbohydrates (glucose) is impaired. It is characterized by the passage of large quantities of urine containing glucose, significant thirst, and deterioration of body functions. Glucose, or dextrose, is one of the basic sugars in the body and, along with oxygen, is the primary fuel for cellular metabolism.

The central problem in diabetes is the lack or ineffective action of insulin, a hormone produced by the pancreas that facilitates the uptake of glucose from the bloodstream into the cell. A hormone is a chemical substance produced by a gland that has special regulatory effects on other body organs and tissues. Without insulin, cells begin to "starve" because insulin is needed, like a key, to let glucose into the cells.

The full name of diabetes is diabetes mellitus, which means "sweet diabetes." This refers to the presence of glucose (sugar) in the urine. Diabetes mellitus is a metabolic disorder in which the body cannot metabolize glucose, usually because of the lack of insulin; the result is a wasting of glucose in the urine. *Diabetes insipidus*, a rare condition, also involves excessive urination; however, the missing hormone is one that regulates urinary fluid reabsorption. In this book, the term "diabetes" always refers to diabetes mellitus.

If left untreated, diabetes leads to a wasting of body tissues and death. Even with appropriate medical care, some patients with particularly aggressive forms of diabetes will die at a relatively young age from one or more complications of the disease. Most patients with diabetes, however, can live a normal life span; however, they must be willing to adjust their lives, especially their dietary habits and activities, to the demands of the disease.

Types of Diabetes

Diabetes is a disease with two distinct onset patterns. It may become evident when the person is a child, or it may develop later in life, usually when the person is middle-aged. Heredity also may play a role in the development of diabetes.

In type I diabetes, most patients do not produce insulin at all. They need daily injections of supplemental, synthetic insulin throughout their lives to control blood glucose levels. Since this type of diabetes most commonly strikes children, it was formerly called "juve-

---

www.EMSzone.com/EMTI

Technology

- Interactivities
- Vocabulary Explorer
- Anatomy Review
- Web Links
- Online Review Manual

nile diabetes." It also is known as insulin-dependent diabetes mellitus (or IDDM). However, in some cases, it can develop later in life. Patients with type I diabetes are more likely to have metabolic problems and organ damage such as blindness, heart disease, kidney failure, and nerve disorders.

In type II diabetes, which usually appears later in life, patients produce inadequate amounts of insulin. In other cases, they may produce a fairly normal amount but the insulin does not function effectively. Although some patients with type II diabetes may require supplemental insulin, most can be treated with diet and non-insulin-type oral medications (hypoglycemic agents) such as chlorpropamide (Diabinase), tolbutamide (Orinase), glyburide (Micronase), glipizide (Glucotrol), metformin (Glucophage), and rosiglitazone (Avandia). These medications stimulate the pancreas to produce more insulin and, thus, lower the blood glucose level. In some cases, these medications can lead to hypoglycemia, particularly when patient activity and exercise levels are too vigorous or excessive. Patients with hypoglycemia have an abnormally low level of blood glucose. Type II diabetes was formerly referred to as adult (maturity)-onset diabetes and as non–insulin-dependent diabetes mellitus (or NIDDM). Some patients with non–insulin-dependent diabetes may, in fact, be dependent on insulin.

The two types of diabetes are equally serious, although type II diabetes is easier to regulate. Both can affect many tissues and functions other than the glucose-regulating mechanism. Both require lifelong medical management. Diabetes is a chronic systemic syndrome characterized by hyperglycemia that is secondary to a decrease in the secretion or activity of insulin. Diabetes may be an autoimmune problem, in which the body develops antibodies to its own tissues and literally destroys them. The severity of diabetes relates to the amount of insulin-producing tissue that is damaged or destroyed, as well as the age of the person at the time of onset.

The Role of Glucose and Insulin

Glucose is the major source of energy for the body, and all cells need it to function properly. Some cells will not function at all without glucose. The brain needs a constant supply of glucose, just as it does oxygen. Without glucose, or with a very low glucose level, brain cells rapidly suffer permanent damage. With the exception of the brain, insulin is needed to allow glucose to enter individual body cells to fuel their functioning. For this reason, insulin is said to be a "cellular key" Figure 21-1 ▼.

Regulation of glucose levels in the body is a complex and dynamic process that begins when absorbed carbohydrates stimulate the release of insulin from the beta cells of the islets of Langerhans in the pancreas. When released, insulin mediates the transport of glucose across the cell membrane, where it is used to produce energy. The cells then convert the glucose and 6 oxygen molecules into 38 total adenosine triphosphate (ATP) molecules through processes that include glycolysis, the conversion of glucose into energy via metabolic pathways, and the Krebs cycle. When oxygen is present during this process, aerobic metabolism occurs, the by-products of which are carbon dioxide and water. The excess glucose is stored in the liver and skeletal muscles as glycogen. When the blood glucose level drops, the alpha cells of the islets of Langerhans release the hormone glucagon to convert the stored glycogen back into glucose through a process called glycogenolysis. If

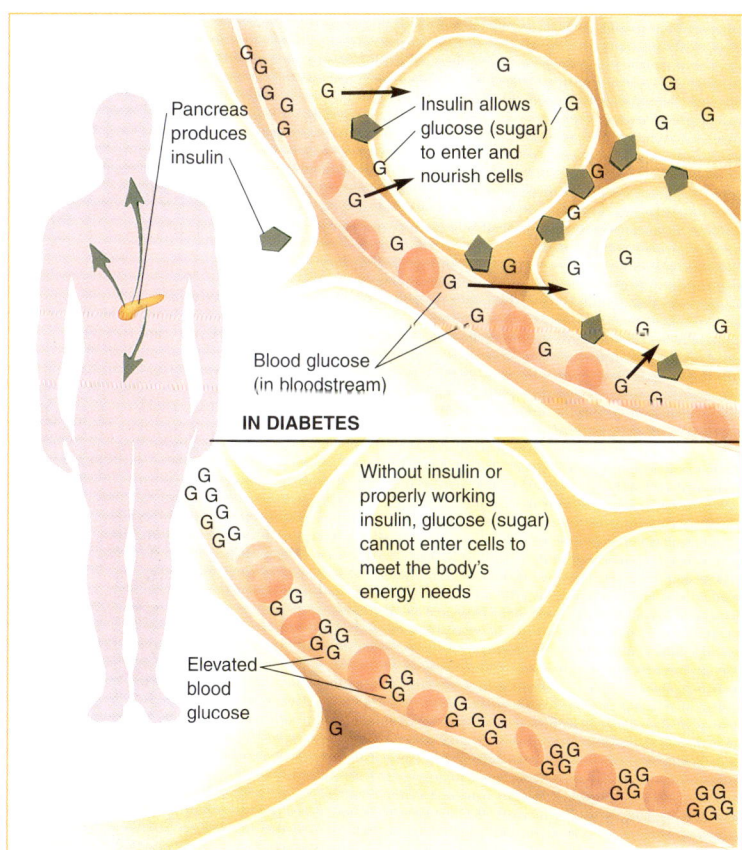

Figure 21-1 Diabetes is defined as a lack of or ineffective action of insulin. Without insulin, cells begin to "starve" because insulin is needed to allow glucose to enter and nourish the cells.

stored glycogen levels are depleted, the cells begin to metabolize fats, proteins, and other non-carbonate sources, thus producing new glucose—a process called gluconeogenesis. In healthy endocrine systems, these shifts in metabolism are tolerated and never allowed to proceed to extremes.

Without insulin, glucose from food remains in the blood and gradually rises to extremely high levels. Normally, high carbohydrate levels are tolerated and returned to normal through metabolic pathways. Problems arise when the blood glucose level remains elevated and the mechanisms that normally correct this have failed. This condition is called hyperglycemia. Once the blood glucose levels reach 200 mg/dL or more, or twice the usual amount (normally 80 to 120 mg/dL), excess glucose is excreted by the kidney. This process requires a large amount of water. The loss of water in such large amounts causes the classic symptoms of uncontrolled diabetes, the "3 Ps":

- Polyuria: frequent and plentiful urination, regardless of intake
- Polydipsia: frequent drinking of liquid to satisfy continuous thirst (secondary to the loss of excessive body water)
- Polyphagia: excessive eating as a result of cellular "hunger or starvation," seen only occasionally

Without glucose to supply energy for cells, the body must turn to other fuel sources, the most abundant of which is fat. Unfortunately, when fat is used as an immediate energy source, chemicals called "ketones" and "fatty acids" are formed as waste products and are difficult for the body to excrete. As they accumulate in blood and tissue, certain ketones can upset the pH balance and produce a dangerous condition called acidosis. The form of acidosis seen in uncontrolled diabetes is called diabetic ketoacidosis (DKA), in which an accumulation of certain acids occurs when insulin is not available in the body. Signs and symptoms of DKA include vomiting, abdominal pain, and a type of deep, rapid breathing called Kussmaul respirations. The ketones are also responsible for the sweet, fruity breath odor associated with DKA. When the acid levels in the body become too high, individual cells will cease to function. If the patient is not given proper fluid rehydration and insulin to reverse fat metabolism and restore the use of glucose as a source of energy, ketoacidosis will progress to unresponsiveness, diabetic coma, and, eventually, death.

Diabetes mellitus is treatable; however, treatment must be tailored for the individual patient. The key is to constantly balance the patient's need for glucose with the available supply of insulin by testing the blood or the urine. In the past, most patients tested their urine daily for the presence of glucose and acetone. "Acetone" is a type of ketone that indicates the presence of ketones in the blood; however, its absence does not rule out the presence of ketones in the blood. Many patients now measure the level of glucose in the blood instead, using a "blood glucose self-monitoring unit." This is a much simpler and more accurate procedure. A drop of blood from the fingertip is placed on a thin strip of chemically treated paper. The paper turns a particular color, which is compared with a color chart that matches colors with approximate blood glucose readings (Figure 21-2A ▶). Blood glucose is measured in milligrams per deciliter (100 mL) of blood and should normally range from 80 to 120 mg/dL.

Patients can also buy devices for pricking the fingertip with a fine needle (lancet), standard tables for reading the strips, or a more elaborate unit that automatically analyzes the test strip and provides a digital readout of the blood glucose level, otherwise known as a glucometer. EMT-Is are allowed to use test strips or glucometers in some systems in North America (Figure 21-2B ▶).

> **EMT-I Tips**
>
> In DKA, the body does not have sufficient insulin to transport glucose into the cells. Therefore, it uses stored fat as an energy source, producing ketones and acids as waste products. This increase in acids causes a decrease in the body's pH, resulting in "metabolic acidosis." The body must then rely on its buffer systems to attempt to return the pH balance to normal.
>
> $$\uparrow H^+ + HCO_3^- = \uparrow H_2CO_3 = H_2O + \uparrow CO_2$$
>
> ($\uparrow$Hydrogen + Sodium Bicarbonate = $\uparrow$Carbonic Acid = Water + $\uparrow$Carbon Dioxide)
>
> The chemical buffer system initially breaks down the acid into a form that can be readily expelled from the body. Remember that with metabolic acidosis, the compensatory mechanism is the respiratory system. Because carbon dioxide is an acid, an increase in the rate and depth of respirations (Kussmaul respirations) will attempt to decrease the amount of acid in the body.

Hyperglycemia

Hyperglycemia occurs in patients with diabetes who are able to produce enough insulin to prevent DKA but not enough to prevent severe hyperglycemia. It is usually accompanied by an inadequate fluid intake. Hyperglycemia can lead to another condition known as hyperglycemic hyperosmolar nonketotic coma.

Hyperglycemic hyperosmolar nonketotic coma (HHNC) is a severe form of hyperglycemia. It is characterized by severe hyperglycemia, hyperosmolality, and dehydration, but no ketoacidosis. There is an insulin deficiency present, but the exact etiology is not known. High levels of glucose in the cerebrospinal fluid lead to dehydration of the brain and altered levels of consciousness, especially in geriatric patients.

During a period of several days, HHNC causes a gradual deterioration in mental status. It is typically precipitated by infection, dehydration, or extreme cold and tends to affect geriatric patients with a history of poor health. Signs and symptoms are similar to those of DKA. The patient typically presents with an altered mental status and dehydration; however, since ketoacids are not present in the blood, Kussmaul respirations and the sweet, fruity breath odor that accompanies them, are absent. Assessment may also reveal coma, seizures, hemiparesis, aphasia, increasing mental depression, and an abnormal increase in urination. Treatment for HHNC is the same as that for DKA and consists of maintenance of airway, breathing, and circulation, as well as fluid rehydration.

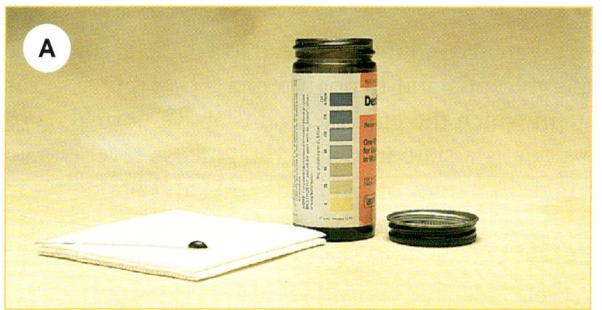

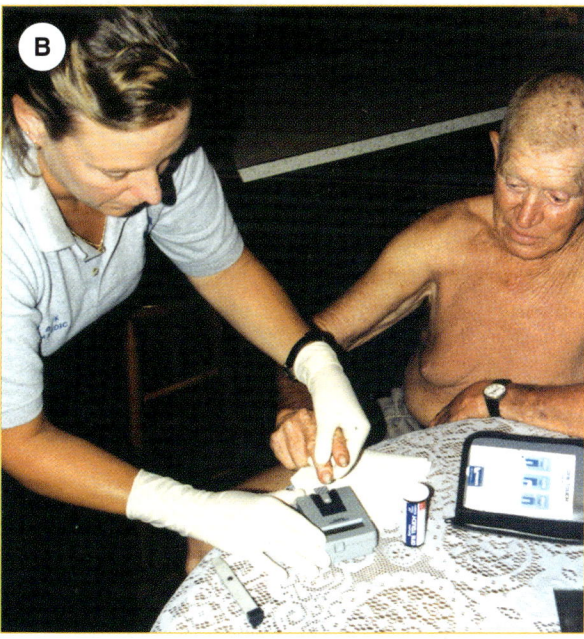

Figure 21-2 **A.** Glucose test strips for blood analysis. **B.** A blood glucose self-monitoring kit with a digital meter is a device used by patients at home or by EMT-Is.

You are the Provider — Part 2

Upon arrival, you discover that your patient is 38 years old with type I diabetes. Your initial assessment reveals:

Initial Assessment	Recording Time: Zero Minutes
Appearance	Diaphoretic, anxious
Level of Consciousness	Confused and disoriented
Airway	Open and clear
Breathing	Respiratory rate, somewhat increased and shallow
Circulation	Radial pulse, rapid and weak

3. What is the first step in caring for this patient?
4. What questions would be appropriate to ask any ill patient who has a history of diabetes?

Hyperglycemia and Hypoglycemia

Two different conditions can lead to a diabetic emergency: hyperglycemia and hypoglycemia. Hyperglycemia is a state in which the glucose level is above normal. Hypoglycemia is a state in which the glucose level is below normal. Extremes of hyperglycemia and hypoglycemia can lead to diabetic emergencies (Figure 21-3 ▼). Ketoacidosis results from prolonged and exceptionally high hyperglycemia. Diabetic coma then results when ketoacidosis is not treated adequately. Hypoglycemia, on the other hand, will progress into unresponsiveness and eventually insulin shock. The signs and symptoms of hypoglycemia and hyperglycemia can be quite similar (Table 21-1 ▶). For example, staggering and an intoxicated appearance or complete unresponsiveness can be present with both conditions. Note that your assessment of these potential emergencies should not prevent you from providing prompt care and transport as detailed in this chapter. In such emergencies, the earlier clues are gathered, the

TABLE 21-1	Characteristics of Diabetic Emergencies	
	Hyperglycemia	**Hypoglycemia**
History		
Food intake	Excessive	Insufficient
Insulin dose	Insufficient	Excessive
Onset	Gradual	Rapid, within minutes
Skin	Warm and dry	Pale and moist
Infection	Common	Uncommon
Gastrointestinal Tract		
Thirst	Intense	Absent
Hunger	Absent	Intense
Vomiting	Common	Uncommon
Respiratory System		
Breathing	Rapid, deep (Kussmaul respirations)	Normal or rapid
Odor of breath	Sweet, fruity	Normal
Cardiovascular System		
Blood pressure	Normal to low	Low
Pulse	Tachycardia	Rapid, weak
Nervous System		
Consciousness	Ranging from restlessness to coma	Irritability, confusion, seizures, or coma
Urine		
Sugar	Present	Absent
Acetone	Present	Absent
Treatment		
Response	Gradual, within 6 to 12 hours following medication and fluid	Immediately after administration of glucose

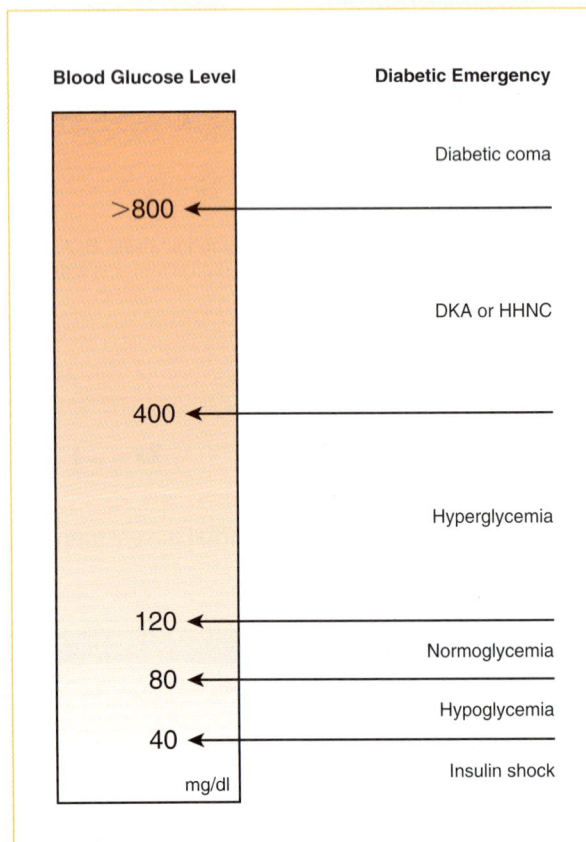

Figure 21-3 The two most common diabetic emergencies, diabetic coma and insulin shock, develop when the patient has too much or too little glucose in the blood, respectively. This scale shows blood glucose levels as they relate to various diabetic emergencies.

better the patient outcome. With specific information about the type of emergency, you can help the hospital prepare prompt, definitive care for the patient.

Diabetic Coma

Diabetic coma is a state of unresponsiveness resulting from several problems, including ketoacidosis, dehydration because of excessive urination, and hyperglycemia. Too much blood glucose by itself does not always cause diabetic coma, but on some occasions, it can lead to it.

Diabetic coma may occur in the patient who is not under medical treatment, who takes insufficient insulin, who markedly overeats, or who is undergoing a stressful event, such as an infection, illness, overexertion, fatigue, or drinking alcohol. Usually, ketoacidosis develops during a period of hours to days. The patient may ultimately be found comatose with the following physical signs:

- Kussmaul respirations
- Dehydration, as indicated by dry, warm skin and sunken eyes
- A sweet or fruity (acetone) odor on the breath, caused by the respiratory system's attempt to rid the body of blood ketones
- Tachycardia
- A normal or slightly low blood pressure
- Altered mental status
- Weight loss
- Abnormal increase in urination

Insulin Shock

Insulin shock is the result of hypoglycemia, or insufficient glucose in the blood. When insulin levels remain high, glucose is rapidly taken out of the blood to fuel the cells. If the glucose level gets too low, there may be an insufficient amount to supply the brain. If the blood glucose level remains low, unresponsiveness and permanent brain damage can quickly follow.

The brain gets its glucose without the aid of insulin because insulin cannot cross the blood-brain barrier, which regulates the substances allowed to cross into the cerebral circulation. Glucose can cross the blood-brain barrier. Proper neurologic functions and the cellular metabolism of the brain rely on a certain amount of glucose being present in the cerebral circulation. If the circulating blood glucose level of the brain drops, neural cells begin to shut down, altering the patient's level of consciousness. Because glucose is the fuel source for cellular metabolism, diminished cerebral glucose levels lead to the inability of the cells to use oxygen for aerobic cellular respiration. Cellular hypoxia develops, and the patient enters insulin shock.

Insulin shock typically occurs when the patient:

- Took too much insulin;
- Took a regular dose of insulin but did not eat enough food; or
- Had an unusual amount of activity or vigorous exercise and depleted all available glucose.

Insulin shock may also occur after the patient vomits a meal after having taken a regular dose of insulin. At times, insulin shock may occur with no identifiable predisposing factor (idiopathic).

Pediatric Needs

Diabetes in children may pose a particular management problem. First, the high levels of activity of children mean that they can use up circulating glucose more quickly than adults do, even after a normal insulin injection. Second, they do not always eat correctly and on schedule. Third, they have limited stores of liver glycogen that can be rapidly depleted. As a result, insulin shock can develop more rapidly and more severely in children than in adults.

Insulin shock develops much more quickly than diabetic coma. In some instances, it can occur in a matter of minutes. Hypoglycemia can be associated with the following signs and symptoms:

- Normal or rapid respirations
- Pale, moist (clammy) skin
- Diaphoresis (sweating)
- Dizziness, headache
- Rapid, weak pulse
- Normal to low blood pressure
- Altered mental status; aggressive, confused, lethargic, or unusual behavior
- Anxious or combative behavior
- Hunger
- Seizure, fainting, or coma
- Weakness on one side of the body (may mimic stroke)

Both extremes of diabetic coma and insulin shock produce unresponsiveness and, in some cases, death; however, the treatment modalities are different. Diabetic coma is a complex metabolic condition that usually develops over time and involves all the tissues of the body. Correcting this condition may take many hours in a well-controlled hospital setting. Insulin shock, however, is an acute condition that can develop rapidly. A patient with diabetes who has taken his or her standard insulin dose but missed lunch may develop insulin shock before eating the next meal. Giving the patient glucose will rapidly reverse the condition. Without glucose, however, the patient may have permanent brain damage. Minutes count.

Most people with diabetes understand and manage their disease well; however, emergencies occur. In addition to diabetic coma and insulin shock, patients with diabetes may have "silent" or painless heart attacks, a possibility that you should always consider. Their only symptom may be "not feeling so well." This is especially true of geriatric patients. It is imperative to maintain a high index of suspicion and treat patients aggressively. In general, patients with diabetes may experience a decreased sensitivity to pain. This is the result of a condition called diabetic neuropathy, or permanent damage of the nerve fibers.

Emergency Medical Care

You should ask the following questions of any ill patient who has a history of diabetes:

- Do you take insulin or any pills that lower your blood sugar?
- Has your medication dosage changed recently?
- Are you taking any new medications?
- Have you had any recent infections?
- Have you taken your usual dose of insulin (or pills) today?
- Have you eaten normally today?
- Have you had any illnesses, unusual amount of activity, or stress today?
- When was your last doctor's visit?

If the patient has eaten but has not taken insulin, it is more likely that DKA is developing. If the patient has taken insulin but has not eaten, the problem is more likely to be insulin shock. A patient with diabetes will often know what is wrong. If the patient is incoherent or unresponsive, attempt to obtain a medical history from family members or bystanders.

The first step is to perform an initial assessment of the patient's ABCs. Verify that the airway is open. Suction any secretions present in the airway. Assess breathing and give high-flow oxygen via nonrebreathing mask at 12 to 15 L/min. If the patient is not breathing or is breathing inadequately, assist ventilation with 100% oxygen. If the patient is unable to maintain his or her own airway, consider inserting a Combitube to secure the airway. Continue to monitor the airway as you provide care. Perform the focused history and physical examination while your partner obtains the baseline vital signs and SAMPLE history.

Consider endotracheal intubation for patients with an altered mental status and those who are unable to maintain their own airway.

> ### In the Field
>
> A patient with Kussmaul respirations may have an Sao_2 of close to 100% because of their increased rate and depth of respirations. These patients still need high-flow oxygen via nonrebreathing mask. The respirations are in response to the increased acidosis in the body. By supplying additional oxygen, you help to offset the problem.

When you are assessing a patient whom you suspect might have diabetes, check for an emergency medical identification symbol—a wallet card, necklace, or bracelet—or ask the family or patient about a history of diabetes. Remember, however, that just because a person has diabetes does not mean that the diabetes is causing the current problem. He or she might be having a myocardial infarction, stroke, or other medical emergency. For this reason, you must always perform a full, careful assessment, paying attention to the ABCs. Inform medical control that you are at the scene of a diabetic emergency. Ask the patient or family about the patient's last meal and insulin dose.

In the past, EMTs were often advised to place oral glucose gel or glucose tablets under the tongue or in the mouth of an unresponsive patient. Very little sugar is actually absorbed in this manner. The risk of choking or aspirating liquid into the lungs probably outweighs the benefits of providing such small amounts of glucose. Therefore, although glucose is very important to give to patients with diabetes with altered mental status, *you should not attempt to give anything by mouth to an unresponsive patient*, even if you suspect insulin shock. These patients need intravenous glucose. Your responsibility is to provide proper treatment and prompt transport to the hospital.

What if no one else is present, but you know that the unresponsive patient has diabetes? Then you must use your knowledge of the signs and symptoms to decide whether the problem is diabetic coma or insulin shock. Remember, however, this assessment should not prevent you from providing prompt treatment and transport. The primary visible difference will be the patient's breathing: deep, rapid respirations in diabetic coma and normal or rapid respirations in insulin shock. However, the patient with diabetes who is unresponsive and having convulsions is more likely to be in insulin shock. Any time you are unsure and unable to obtain a glucose reading, you should err on the side of caution and give glucose. The risk of increasing the glucose level of a patient who is already hyperglycemic is minimal compared with the benefit of increasing the glucose level of one who is hypoglycemic. Hypoglycemia is very detrimental to the patient's overall health and can quickly lead to other systemic problems.

Place the patient in a position of comfort. Obtain intravenous (IV) access for all patients experiencing a diabetic emergency and obtain a blood glucose analysis. For patients presenting with signs of dehydration, administer a 20-mL/kg bolus of an isotonic crystalloid solution such as normal saline or lactated Ringer's. Treatment is aimed at rehydrating the patient and providing prompt transport to an appropriate facility. Reassess after the initial bolus and repeat if needed. Reassure the patient en route, and provide general comfort measures.

Monitor the cardiac rhythm and treat arrhythmias according to standard ACLS protocols.

> **In the Field**
>
> When you are unable to measure a patient's glucose level and are unsure whether the patient is hypoglycemic or hyperglycemic, always err on the side of caution and give glucose. More glucose in a hyperglycemic patient will not cause harm, but it may save the life of a hypoglycemic patient, especially if the patient is in insulin shock.

Keep in mind that any unresponsive patient may have undiagnosed diabetes. In patients with altered mental status, you may be able to determine this in the field, if you have the proper equipment to test the patient's blood glucose. Without this critical knowledge, treat this patient as you would any other unresponsive per-

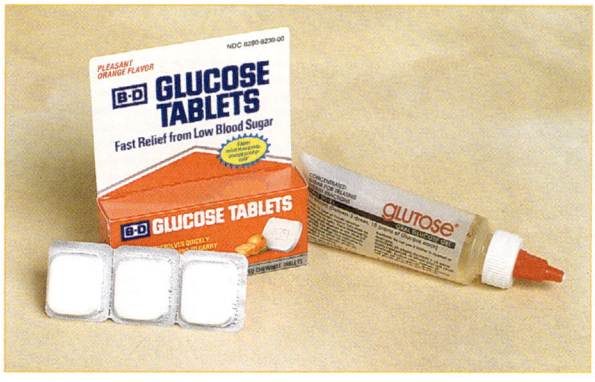

Figure 21-4 Oral glucose is commercially available in gel and tablet form. One tube of gel equals one dose.

son. Provide emergency medical care, particularly airway management, and prompt transport. At the emergency department, the diabetes and its associated complications can quickly be diagnosed.

Giving Oral Glucose

Oral glucose is available commercially in tablet form and as a gel that dissolves when placed in the mouth (Figure 21-4 ▲). One toothpaste-type tube of gel equals one dose. Trade names for the gel include Glutose and Insta-Glucose. Glucose gel, which increases blood glucose levels, should be given to any patient with a decreased level of consciousness who has a history of diabetes. The only contraindications to glucose are an inability to swallow or unresponsiveness, since aspiration (inhalation of the substance) can occur. Oral glucose itself has no side effects if it is administered properly; however, aspiration in a patient who does not have a gag reflex can have lethal results. A conscious patient (even if confused) who does not really need glucose will not be harmed by it. Therefore, do not hesitate to give it under these circumstances.

As with any patient contact, be sure to wear gloves before placing anything into a patient's mouth. After you have confirmed that the patient is conscious and able to swallow and have obtained an online or off-line order from medical control, follow these steps to administer oral glucose (Skill Drill 21-1 ▶):

1. **Examine the tube** to ensure that it is not open or broken. Check the expiration date (**Step 1**).
2. **Squeeze a generous amount** onto the bottom third of a bite stick or tongue depressor (**Step 2**).
3. **Open the patient's mouth.**

Skill Drill 21-1: Administering Glucose

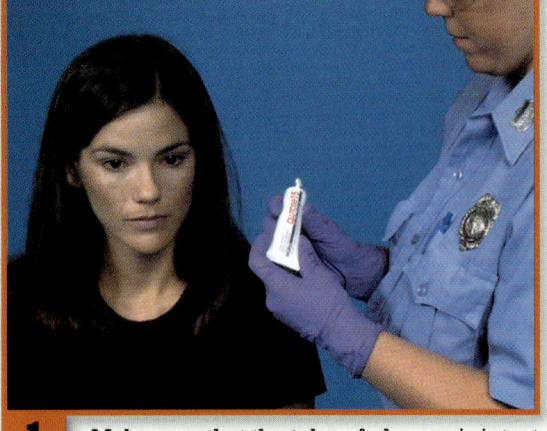

1. Make sure that the tube of glucose is intact and has not expired.

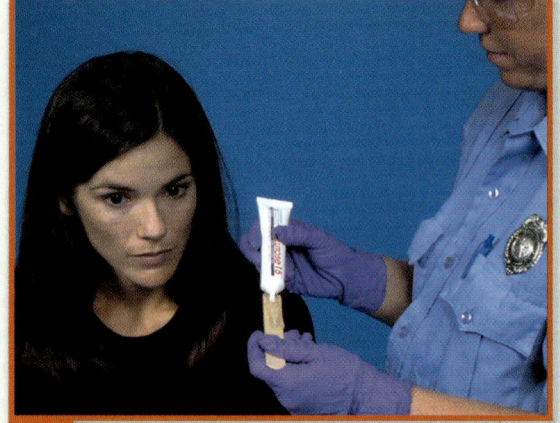

2. Squeeze the entire tube of oral glucose onto the bottom third of a bite stick or tongue depressor.

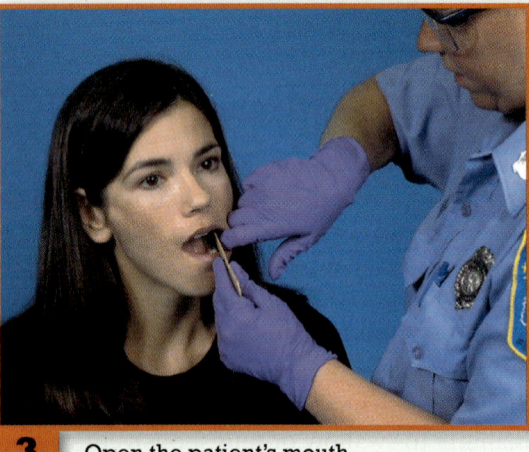

3. Open the patient's mouth. Place the tongue depressor on the mucous membranes between the cheek and the gum with the gel side next to the cheek.

4. Place the tongue depressor on the mucous membranes between the cheek and gum, with the gel side next to the cheek. Once the gel is dissolved, or if the patient becomes unresponsive or has a seizure, remove the tongue depressor (**Step 3**).

Reassess the patient regularly after giving glucose, even if you see rapid improvement in the patient's condition. Remain alert for airway problems, sudden loss of consciousness, or seizures. Provide prompt transport to the hospital; do not delay transport just to give additional oral glucose.

A patient in insulin shock (rapid onset of altered mental status, hypoglycemia) needs sugar immediately, and a patient in diabetic coma (acidosis, dehydration,

In the Field

A tube of commercially prepared cake icing is an excellent substitute for oral glucose. You may be able to find some in the patient's kitchen.

hyperglycemia) needs insulin and IV fluid therapy. These patients need prompt transport to the hospital for appropriate medical care.

For the conscious patient in insulin shock, protocols usually recommend oral glucose, which will usually reverse the reaction within several minutes. Do not be afraid to give too much sugar. The problem often will not be solved with just a sip of juice. An entire candy bar or a full glass of sweetened juice is often needed. Do not give sugar-free drinks that are sweetened with saccharin or other synthetic sweetening compounds, as they will have little or no effect. Remember that even if the patient responds after receiving glucose, he or she may still need additional treatment. Therefore, you must transport the patient to the hospital as soon as possible. Reassess the patient's blood glucose level and give additional glucose if needed.

When there is any doubt as to whether a conscious patient with diabetes is experiencing insulin shock or diabetic coma, most protocols will err on the side of giving glucose, even though the patient may have signs and symptoms of DKA. Untreated insulin shock will result in unresponsiveness and can quickly cause significant brain damage or death. Compared with the patient in DKA, the patient in insulin shock is in a far more critical condition and far more likely to experience permanent problems. Furthermore, the amount of

Geriatric Needs

You might encounter an older patient who has undiagnosed diabetes. These patients report that they have not been feeling well for a while but have not seen a physician. A patient with undiagnosed diabetes or one who is in denial or ignores the advice of his or her physician may call 9-1-1 when the signs and symptoms get worse. Nonhealing wounds, blindness, renal failure, and other complications are associated with poorly controlled or uncontrolled diabetes. As an EMT-I, you might be the first health care provider to recognize and suggest medical treatment to an elderly patient who might otherwise ignore his or her condition. It is important that you recognize the signs and symptoms of diabetes. As you obtain a SAMPLE history, ask the patient whether he or she has noticed ants in the bathroom, especially around the toilet. Ants like sugar, and excess sugar is excreted in the urine. An infestation of ants around the toilet could indicate sugar excreted in the urine and, hence, elevated blood glucose and the possibility of diabetes.

EMT-I Safety

Managing problems related to diabetes and altered mental status poses very little risk to you, because exposure to body fluids is generally very limited. However, some patients can become confused and even aggressive at times. Follow body substance isolation precautions, as you would with any other patient. Always use gloves, and wash your hands carefully after obtaining and checking a blood sample or if you perform airway techniques.

You are the Provider — Part 3

Your patient's wife reveals that he takes 32 units of 70/30 insulin every morning and 14 units of regular insulin before going to bed.

Vital Signs	Recording Time: 2 Minutes After Patient Contact
Respirations	22 breaths/min, shallow
Pulse	124 beats/min, regular and slightly weak
Skin	Pale and diaphoretic
Blood Pressure	90/52 mm Hg

5. What is the most appropriate treatment for this patient?

sugar that is typically given to such a patient is not likely to exacerbate (worsen) the condition of a patient with DKA. When in doubt, consult medical control.

Administering 50% Dextrose

The treatment available for patients experiencing insulin-related problems is the administration of 50% dextrose (D_{50}) via IV line when it is not possible to give oral glucose (for example, with an unresponsive patient). Remember to perform a blood glucose level check before administering D_{50}. It may be necessary to administer more than one dose if the patient's blood glucose level is extremely low or if the patient fails to respond fully to a single dose. Readminister the appropriate dose of D_{50} according to local protocol if the patient's condition does not improve.

D_{50} is an IV medication used with patients who have hypoglycemia. It is usually supplied in a prefilled container called a "bristojet" containing 25 g of dextrose dissolved in 50 mL of water.

Indications for the use of D_{50} include the following:
- Symptomatic hypoglycemia
  - A blood glucose reading of less than 70 mg/dL with signs and symptoms
- Altered level of consciousness for unknown reasons
- Unresponsiveness with no obtainable patient history
- Cardiac arrest with a rhythm of pulseless electrical activity (PEA) or asystole or with a history of diabetes
- Coma of unknown etiology
- Generalized hypothermia

Exercise caution when using D_{50}; contraindications include the presence of increased intracranial pressure or possible intracranial bleeding. D_{50} may also result in tissue necrosis and phlebitis caused by extravasation of dextrose outside the vein. Use caution with patients suspected of having low potassium levels, such as patients who are taking diuretics. Administering glucose in the presence of hypokalemia worsens the effects of low potassium. However, the potential for worsening the patient's hypokalemia should not be a factor when dealing with a severely hypoglycemic patient.

Doses of D_{50} are as follows:
- Adults: 25 g (50 mL) of D_{50} (or follow local protocol)
- Children 3 months to 7 years old: D_{25} (empty half of the bristojet of D_{50} and draw up normal saline to fill the tube; this will give a concentration of 25% if your service does not carry the prefilled syringes of D_{25}.)
- Newborns to 3 months old: D_{10} solution (put 2 mL of D_{50} into a syringe and add 8 mL of normal saline)

D_{50} is extremely necrotic and will cause serious damage to tissue. You must give it by IV push while carefully monitoring for infiltration into local tissue. Follow the steps shown in (Skill Drill 21-2 ▶) to administer D_{50}.

Complications of Diabetes

Diabetes is a systemic disease affecting all tissues of the body, especially the kidneys, eyes, small arteries, and peripheral nerves (Figure 21-5 ▼). Therefore, you are likely to be called to treat patients with a variety of complications of diabetes, such as heart disease, visual disturbances, renal failure, stroke, and ulcers or infections of the feet or toes. With the exception of myocardial infarction and stroke, most of these will not be acute emergencies. Considering that diabetes is a major risk factor for cardiovascular disease, people with diabetes should always be suspected of having a potential for myocardial infarction, particularly if they are older, even when they do not present with classic symptoms such as chest pain or pressure.

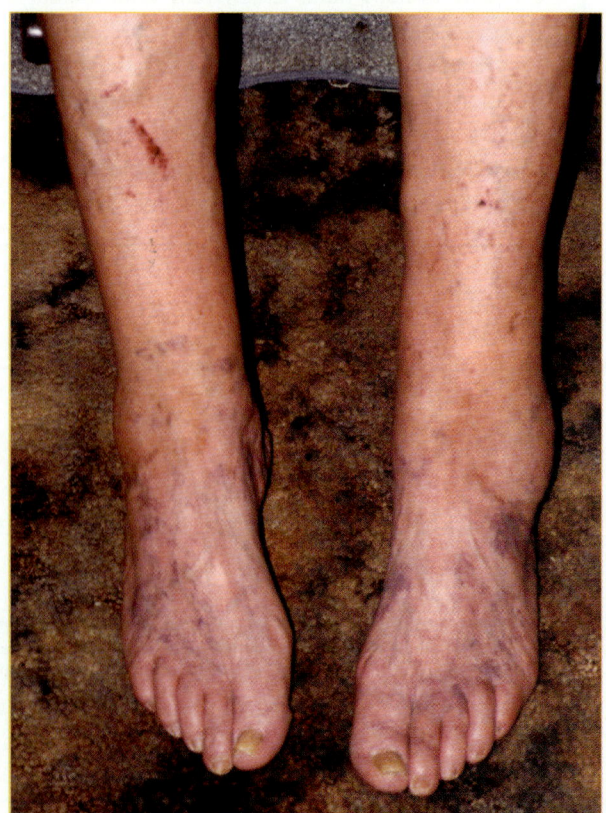

Figure 21-5 Peripheral edema and poor circulation are complications associated with long-term diabetes.

Skill Drill 21-2: Administration of D_{50}

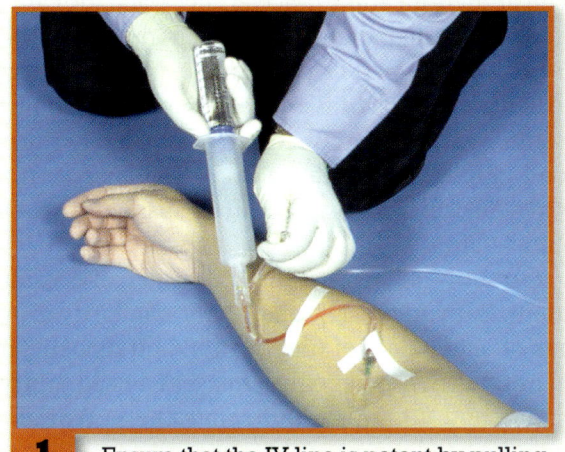

1. Ensure that the IV line is patent by pulling back on the plunger to see if blood returns through the IV tubing.

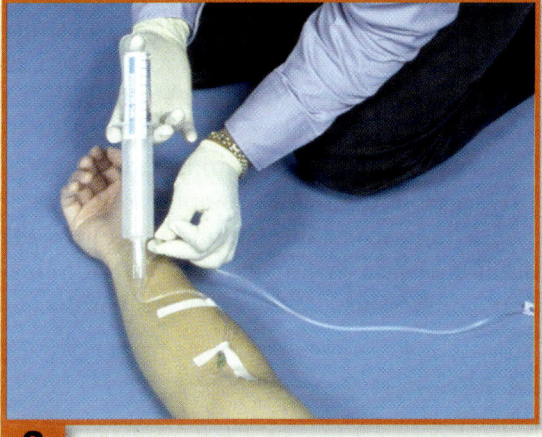

2. Crimp the IV tubing proximal to the injection port. Depress the plunger slowly to avoid rupturing the vein.

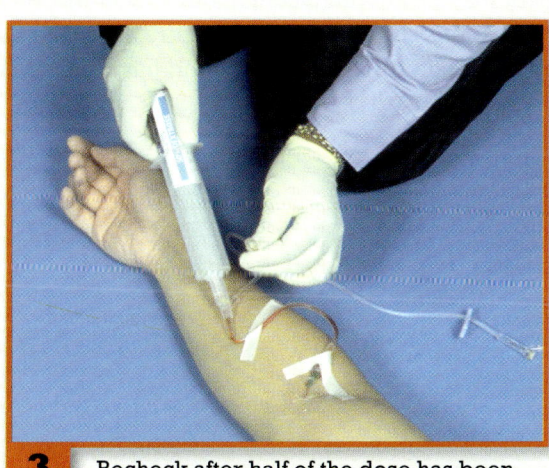

3. Recheck after half of the dose has been given by pulling back on the plunger again to check for blood return.

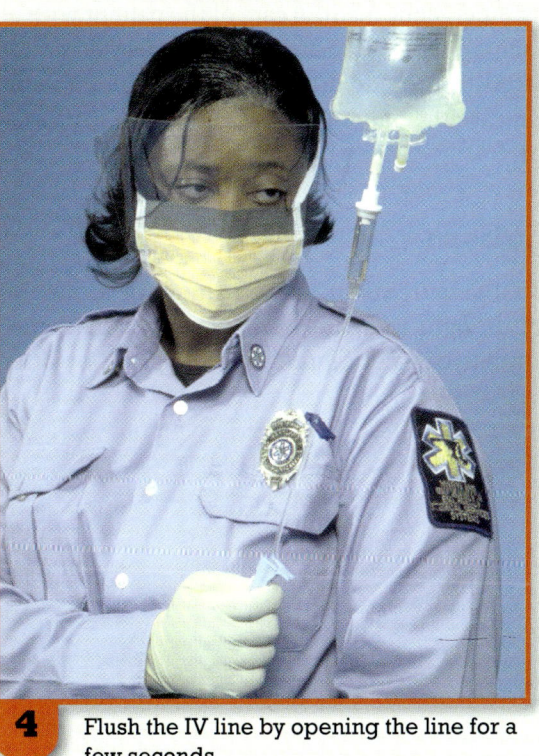

4. Flush the IV line by opening the line for a few seconds.

Seizures

Although seizures are rarely life threatening, you should consider them very serious, even in patients with a history of chronic seizures. Seizures, which may be brief or prolonged, are caused by fever, infections, poisoning, hypoglycemia, trauma, and hypoxia. They can also be idiopathic (of unknown cause). Although brief seizures are not harmful, they may indicate a more dangerous and potentially life-threatening underlying condition. Because seizures can be caused by head injury, consider trauma as a cause. In a patient with diabetes, you should consider hyperglycemia or hypoglycemia.

Emergency medical care of seizures includes ensuring that the airway is clear and placing the patient on his or her side if there is no possibility of cervical spine trauma. Do not attempt to place anything in the patient's mouth (such as a bite stick or oral airway). Be sure to have suctioning equipment readily available in case the patient vomits. Provide artificial ventilation if the patient is cyanotic or appears to be breathing inadequately. Establish IV access and provide prompt transport.

Consider endotracheal intubation to maintain the airway. Monitor cardiac rhythm and consider administration of anticonvulsants as allowed by local protocols.

Altered Mental Status

Although altered mental status is often caused by complications of diabetes, it may also be caused by a variety of conditions, including poisoning, part of the postseizure state (postictal phase), infection, head injury, and hypoxia.

Begin emergency medical care of the patient with an altered mental status by ensuring that the airway is clear. Be prepared to provide artificial ventilation and suctioning in case the patient vomits, and provide prompt transport.

Alcoholism

Occasionally, patients in insulin shock or a diabetic coma are thought to be intoxicated, especially if their condition has caused a motor vehicle crash or other incident. Confined by police in a "drunk tank," a patient with diabetes is at risk. In such situations, an emergency medical identification bracelet, necklace, or card may help to save the patient's life. Often, only a blood glucose test performed at the scene or in the emergency department will identify the real problem. In some EMS systems, you will be trained and allowed to perform the blood glucose test at the scene. Otherwise, you must always suspect hypoglycemia in any patient with altered mental status.

Certainly, diabetes and alcoholism can coexist in a patient. But you must be alert to the similarity in symptoms of acute alcohol intoxication and diabetic emergencies. Likewise, hypoglycemia and a head injury can coexist, and you must appreciate the potential even when the head injury is obvious.

Relationship to Airway Management

Patients with altered mental status, particularly those who are difficult to awaken, are at risk for losing their gag reflex. When the gag reflex is absent, patients cannot reject foreign materials in their mouth (including vomit), and their tongue will often relax and obstruct the airway. Therefore, you must carefully monitor the airway in patients with hypoglycemia, diabetic coma, or other complications such as stroke or seizure. Place the patient in a lateral recumbent position, and have suction readily available.

You are the Provider

Summary

1. What are the two types of diabetes?

Type I (IDDM) and type II diabetes (NIDDM)

2. What are the two most common types of diabetic emergencies seen in the prehospital setting?

Hypoglycemic reaction and diabetic ketoacidosis are the two most common types of diabetic-related emergencies encountered in the prehospital setting.

3. What is the first step in caring for this patient?

The first step is to perform an initial assessment of the patient's ABCs. Verify that the airway is open. Suction any secretions present in the airway. Assess the patient's breathing and give high-flow oxygen via nonrebreathing mask at 12 to 15 L/min or assist ventilations if the patient is breathing inadequately.

4. What questions would be appropriate to ask any ill patient who has a history of diabetes?

- Do you take insulin or any pills that lower your blood sugar?
- Has your medication dosage changed recently?
- Are you taking any new medications?
- Have you had any recent infections?
- Have you taken your usual dose of insulin (or pills) today?
- Have you eaten normally today?
- Have you had any illnesses, unusual amount of activity, or stress today?
- When was your last doctor's visit?

5. What is the most appropriate treatment for this patient?

The most effective treatment available for patients experiencing insulin-related problems is the administration of 50% dextrose (D_{50}) via IV when you are unable to give oral glucose (eg, patients with an altered mental status).

Prep Kit

Ready for Review

- Diabetes is a metabolic disorder caused by the lack of insulin, a hormone that enables glucose to enter the cells, where it can be used for energy. Diabetes is typically characterized by excessive urination and resulting thirst, along with deterioration of body tissues.

- There are two types of diabetes. Type I diabetes, or insulin-dependent diabetes, usually starts in childhood and requires daily insulin to control the blood glucose level. Type II diabetes, or non-insulin-dependent diabetes, usually develops in middle-age patients and can often be controlled with diet and oral medications. Both are serious systemic diseases that affect the kidneys, eyes, small arteries, and peripheral nerves, especially if the disease is uncontrolled or poorly controlled.

- Patients with diabetes have chronic complications that place them at risk for other diseases such as myocardial infarction, stroke, and infections. Most often, however, you will be summoned to treat the acute complications of blood glucose imbalance. These include hyperglycemia (excess blood glucose) and hypoglycemia (low blood glucose).

- Symptoms of hypoglycemia classically include confusion; rapid respirations; pale, moist skin; diaphoresis; dizziness; fainting; and even coma and seizures. This condition, called insulin shock, is rapidly reversible with the administration of glucose, in oral or IV form. Without treatment, permanent brain damage and death can occur.

- Hyperglycemia is usually associated with dehydration and ketoacidosis. It can result in diabetic coma, marked by rapid (often deep) respirations; warm, dry skin; a weak pulse; and a fruity breath odor. Hyperglycemia must be treated in the hospital with insulin and IV fluid rehydration.

- Since either too much or too little blood glucose can result in altered mental status, you must perform a thorough history and patient assessment. When you cannot determine the nature of the problem, it is best to treat the patient for hypoglycemia. Be prepared to give oral glucose to a conscious patient who is confused or has a slightly decreased level of consciousness and D_{50} to an unresponsive patient. Do not give oral glucose to a patient who is unresponsive or otherwise unable to swallow properly or protect his or her own airway.

- Remember, in all cases, providing emergency medical care and prompt transport is your primary responsibility.

Vital Vocabulary

acidosis A pathologic condition resulting from the accumulation of acids in the body.

diabetes mellitus A metabolic disorder in which the ability to metabolize carbohydrates (sugars) is impaired due to a lack of insulin.

diabetic coma Unresponsiveness caused by dehydration, a very high blood glucose level, and ketoacidosis.

diabetic ketoacidosis (DKA) A form of acidosis in uncontrolled diabetes in which certain acids accumulate when insulin is not available.

glucagon The hormone released from the alpha cells in the islets of Langerhans that converts glycogen to glucose when the body's blood glucose level drops.

gluconeogenesis The production of new glucose through the metabolization of non-carbohydrate sources.

glucose One of the basic sugars; it is the primary fuel, along with oxygen, for cellular metabolism.

glycogenolysis The process by which glycogen is converted to glucose; facilitated by glucagon.

glycolysis The conversion of glucose into energy via metabolic pathways.

Technology

Interactivities

Vocabulary Explorer

Anatomy Review

Web Links

Online Review Manual

hormone A chemical substance, produced by a gland, that regulates the activity of body organs and tissues.

hyperglycemia Abnormally high glucose level in the blood.

hyperglycemic hyperosmolar nonketotic coma (HHNC) Condition characterized by severe hyperglycemia, hyperosmolality, and dehydration but no ketoacidosis.

hypoglycemia Abnormally low glucose level in the blood.

insulin A hormone produced by the islet of Langerhans (an exocrine gland in the pancreas) that enables sugar in the blood to enter the cells of the body; used in synthetic form to treat and control diabetes mellitus.

insulin shock Unresponsiveness or altered mental status in a patient with diabetes caused by significant hypoglycemia; usually the result of excessive exercise or activity, failure to eat after a routine dose of insulin, or an inadvertent overdose of insulin.

islets of Langerhans Structures found in the pancreas that are composed of four types of cells; one type, the beta cell, is responsible for the production of insulin.

Kussmaul respirations Deep, rapid breathing; the result of an accumulation of certain acids when insulin is not available in the body.

polydipsia Excessive thirst persisting for long periods despite reasonable fluid intake; often the result of excessive urination.

polyphagia Excessive eating; in diabetes, the inability to use glucose properly can cause a sense of hunger.

polyuria The passage of an unusually large volume of urine in a given period; in diabetes, this can result from wasting of glucose in the urine.

type I diabetes The type of diabetic disease that usually starts in childhood and requires insulin for proper treatment and control.

type II diabetes The type of diabetic disease that usually starts later in life and often can be controlled through diet and oral medications.

Assessment in Action

You are dispatched for a possible unconscious person at the local community college during exam week. You arrive to find a 19-year-old woman, who is responsive only to painful stimuli.

Her friends say that they were on their way to have some lunch when she started acting strange and seemed to be confused. One of her friends says that she thinks she may be a diabetic. Another friend quickly responds by saying that she does not think so because the patient never talked about needing insulin shots. Your initial assessment includes a blood glucose reading of 50 mg/dL.

1. A hormone produced by the pancreas that facilitates the uptake of glucose from the bloodstream into the cell is called:
   A. glucose.
   B. insulin.
   C. glucagon.
   D. glycogen.

2. A metabolic disorder in which the body cannot metabolize glucose, usually because of the lack of insulin resulting in glucose in the urine, is called:
   A. insulin shock.
   B. diabetes insipidus.
   C. diabetes mellitus.
   D. diabetic ketoacidosis.

3. The type of diabetes in which the body does not produce any insulin is called:
   A. type I diabetes.
   B. type II diabetes.
   C. type III diabetes.
   D. type IV diabetes.

4. The condition in which the blood glucose level remains elevated and the mechanisms that normally correct this have failed is called:
   A. hypoglycemia.
   B. hyperglycemia.
   C. gluconeogenesis.
   D. glycolysis.

5. When the body is not able to use glucose for energy, it turns to other sources of energy, such as fat. This results in the formation of:
   A. ketones.
   B. glucagon.
   C. insulin.
   D. glycogen.

6. A type of deep, rapid breathing that is seen in patients with diabetic ketoacidosis (DKA) is known as:
   A. Cheyne-Stokes breathing.
   B. agonal respirations.
   C. Kussmaul respirations.
   D. neurogenic hyperventilation.

7. Normal or rapid respirations, moist skin, diaphoresis, tachycardia, and combative behavior are seen in patients experiencing:
   A. diabetic coma.
   B. hypoglycemia.
   C. diabetic ketoacidosis.
   D. hyperglycemia.

8. If not carefully assessed, patients in insulin shock or diabetic coma may be mistaken for a(n):
   A. intoxicated patient.
   B. stroke patient.
   C. psychiatric patient.
   D. any of the above.

9. The medication of choice to treat an adult patient with insulin shock is:
   A. 25 g of D_{50}.
   B. 25 g of D_{25}.
   C. 500 mL of D_5W.
   D. 1 g of glucagon.

10. A systemic disease affecting all tissues of the body, especially the kidneys, eyes, small arteries, and peripheral nerves is called:
    A. encephalopathy.
    B. diabetes mellitus.
    C. Grave's disease.
    D. vascular disease.

Points to Ponder

You are dispatched for an unconscious person at the local grocery store. Upon your arrival, you find a 35-year-old man with an altered level of consciousness. You perform a rapid assessment that includes assessment of the blood glucose. The glucometer gives a reading of only 40 mg/dL. You realize that the patient is experiencing insulin shock. You start an IV and administer 25 g of D_{50}. After about 5 minutes, the patient regains complete consciousness. He is alert and oriented to person, place, and time. You explain to him what happened and that you gave him a medication to improve his condition. You tell him that he should get checked out at the hospital. The patient does not want to go to the hospital and asks you to please remove the IV. What do you do?

Issues: Recognizing Insulin Shock, Determining the Most Effective Treatment

Allergic Reactions and Envenomations

1999 Objectives

Cognitive

5-4.1 Define allergic reaction. (p 1006)
5-4.2 Define anaphylaxis. (p 1006)
5-4.3 Define allergens. (p 1007)
5-4.4 Describe the common methods of entry of substances into the body. (p 1007)
5-4.5 List common antigens most frequently associated with anaphylaxis. (p 1007)
5-4.6 Describe physical manifestations in anaphylaxis. (p 1006)
5-4.7 Recognize the signs and symptoms related to anaphylaxis. (p 1010)
5-4.8 Differentiate among the various treatment and pharmacological interventions used in the management of anaphylaxis. (p 1012)
5-4.9 Integrate the pathophysiological principles of the patient with anaphylaxis. (p 1011)
5-4.10 Correlate abnormal findings in assessment with the clinical significance in the patient with anaphylaxis. (p 1012)
5-4.11 Develop a treatment plan based on field impression in the patient with allergic reaction and anaphylaxis. (p 1012)

Affective

None

Psychomotor

None

1985 Objectives

There are no 1985 objectives for this chapter.

22

Allergic Reactions and Envenomations

You are the Provider

You are dispatched to treat a 14-year-old girl with a possible bee sting. On arrival you find your patient seated against a rock in a park. She was on a nature hike with her middle school class. The teacher tells you the girl is allergic to bee stings and carries medicine for it. Your patient has six obvious stings, two of them on her face. The sting areas are red and swollen, and the girl says that they itch "a lot."

1. Why does the time between exposure and reaction often indicate the severity of an allergic reaction?
2. What is the primary mechanism of an allergic reaction, and how can it have an impact on airway patency?

Allergic Reactions and Envenomations

Every year, at least 1,000 Americans die of acute allergic reactions. In dealing with allergy-related emergencies, you must be aware of the possibility of acute airway obstruction and cardiovascular collapse and be prepared to treat these life-threatening complications. You must also be able to distinguish between the body's usual response to a sting or bite and an allergic reaction, which may require epinephrine. Your ability to recognize and manage the many signs and symptoms of allergic reactions may be the only thing standing between life and imminent death for a patient.

This chapter begins by describing the five categories of stimuli that may provoke allergic reactions. It then goes into considerable detail about insect stings and the typical reactions to them that occur among people who are, and those who are not, allergic to bees, wasps, yellow jackets, and hornets. You will learn what to look for in assessing patients who may be having an allergic reaction and how to care for them, including the administration of epinephrine. The chapter then describes specific bites from poisonous spiders and snakes, ticks, dogs, humans, and marine animals.

Allergic Reactions

Contrary to what many people think, an allergic reaction, an exaggerated immune response to any substance, is not caused directly by an outside stimulus, such as a bite or sting. Rather, it is a reaction by the body's immune system, which releases chemicals to combat the stimulus. Among these chemicals are histamines, which are released by the mast cells, and leukotrienes. An allergic reaction may be mild and localized, involving only hives, itching, or tenderness, or it may be severe and systemic, resulting in shock and respiratory failure. An allergic reaction occurs following contact with a specific allergen to which the patient has been previously exposed and sensitized. The patient may also experience hypersensitivity, an abnormal sensitivity in which there is an exaggerated response by the body to the stimulus or antigen.

Anaphylaxis is an extreme allergic reaction that is not always life threatening, but it typically involves multiple organ systems. In severe cases, anaphylaxis can rapidly result in death. Two of the most common signs of anaphylaxis are wheezing, a high-pitched, whistling breath sound resulting from bronchospasm and typically heard on expiration, and widespread urticaria, or hives. Urticaria consists of small areas of generalized itching or burning that appear as multiple, small, raised areas on the skin Figure 22-1.

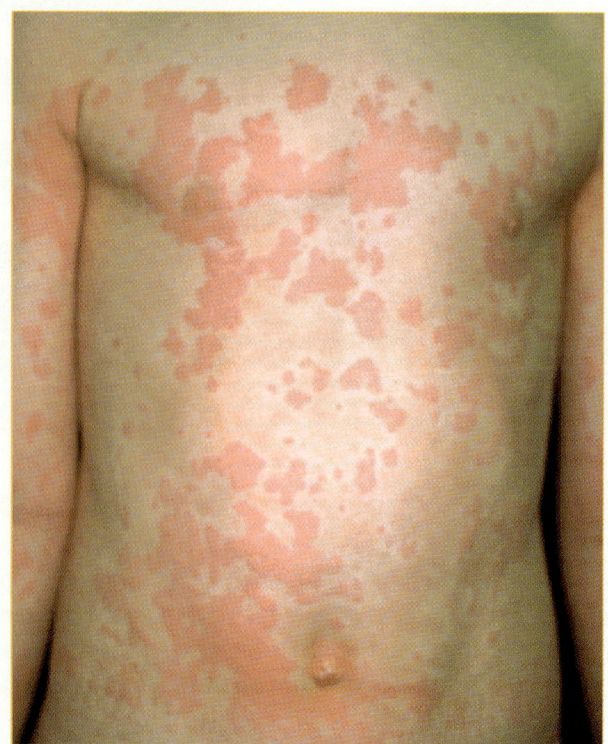

Figure 22-1 Urticaria, or hives, may appear following a sting and is characterized by multiple, small, raised areas on the skin. Urticaria may be one of the warning signs of impending anaphylactic shock.

Technology

- Interactivities
- Vocabulary Explorer
- Anatomy Review
- Web Links
- Online Review Manual

www.EMSzone.com/EMTI

EMT-I Tips

Anaphylaxis is a severe allergic reaction that may be life threatening and typically involves multiple organ systems.

Given the right person and the right circumstances, almost any substance can trigger the body's immune system and cause an allergic reaction: animal bites, food, latex gloves, or even semen can be an <u>allergen</u>, the antigen or substance causing the allergic response. The most common allergens, however, fall into the following five general categories:

- **Insect bites and stings.** When an insect bites you and injects the bite with its venom, the act is called <u>envenomation</u> or, more commonly, a sting. The sting of a honeybee, wasp, ant, yellow jacket, or hornet may cause a severe reaction with the swiftness of its injected venom. The reaction may be local, causing swelling and itchiness in the surrounding tissue, or it may be systemic, involving the entire body. Such a total body reaction would be considered an anaphylactic reaction.
- **Medications.** Injection of medications such as penicillin may cause a rapid (within 30 minutes) and severe allergic reaction. However, reactions to oral medications, such as oral penicillin, may be slower in onset (more than 30 minutes) but equally severe. The fact that a person has taken a medication once without experiencing an allergic reaction is no guarantee that he or she will not have an allergic reaction to the same medication with subsequent exposure.
- **Plants.** People who inhale dusts, pollens, or other plant materials to which they are sensitive may experience a rapid and severe allergic reaction.
- **Food.** Eating certain foods, such as shellfish or nuts, may result in a relatively slow (more than 30 minutes) reaction that still can be quite severe. The person may be unaware of the exposure or inciting agent.
- **Chemicals.** Certain chemicals, makeup, soap, latex, and various other substances can cause severe allergic reactions.

Allergens enter the body through oral ingestion, injection or envenomation, inhalation, or topical absorption (Table 22-1 ▼). Typically, the allergens that do not travel through the digestive tract cause the most severe reaction. Those that are injected or inhaled tend to cause the most severe reaction.

TABLE 22-1	Allergen Routes of Entry into the Body
■ Ingestion	
■ Injection	
■ Inhalation	
■ Absorption	

You are the Provider Part 2

As you kneel in front of the patient, you note the following:

Initial Assessment	Recording Time: Zero Minutes
Appearance	Flushed, very anxious
Level of consciousness	Alert and oriented, follows commands
Airway	Open, breathing loudly
Breathing	Respirations, rapid at 40 breaths/min
Circulation	Radial pulses, present; skin, warm and moist

3. What is the first treatment priority?
4. How should the patient be positioned?

Insect Stings

There are more than 100,000 species of bees, wasps, and hornets. Deaths from anaphylactic reactions to stinging insects far outnumber deaths from snake bites. The stinging organ of most bees, wasps, yellow jackets, and hornets is a small hollow spine projecting from the abdomen. Venom can be injected through this spine directly into the skin. The stinger of the honeybee is barbed, so the bee cannot withdraw it (Figure 22-2A ◀). Therefore, the bee leaves a part of its abdomen embedded with the stinger and dies shortly after stinging its victim. Wasps and hornets have no such handicap; they can sting repeatedly (Figure 22-2B ▼). Since these insects

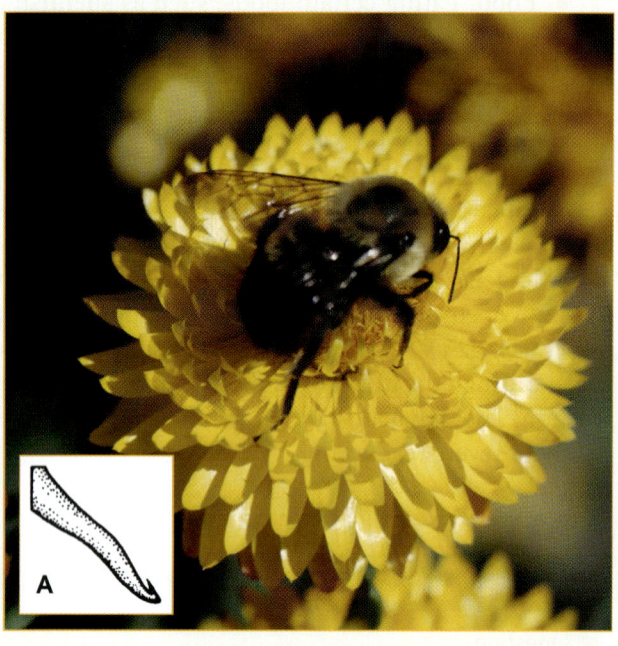
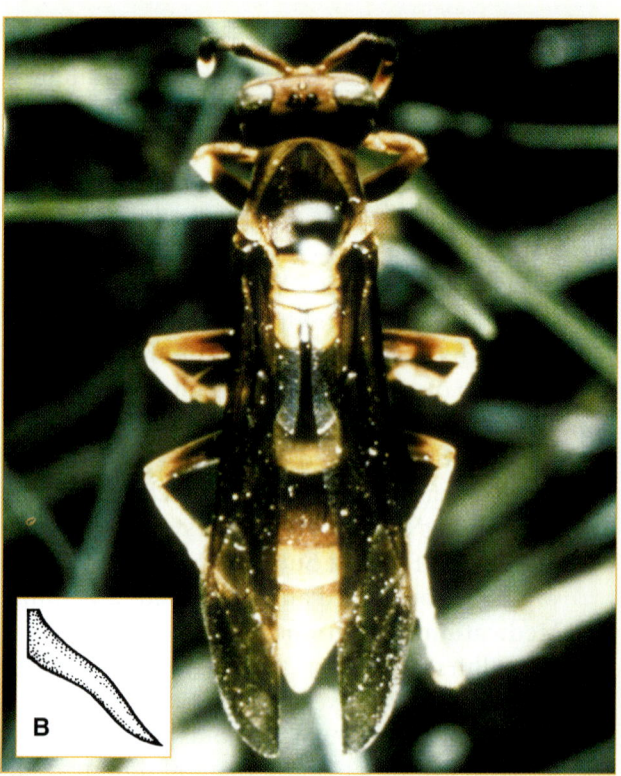

Figure 22-2 Most stinging insects inject venom through a small, hollow spine that projects from the abdomen. **A.** The stinger of the honeybee is barbed and cannot be withdrawn once the bee has stung someone. **B.** The wasp's stinger is unbarbed, meaning that it can inflict multiple stings.

You are the Provider — Part 3

The patient is allowed to remain sitting next to the teacher where she feels most comfortable. The teacher tells you that she is sure the "bees" were actually wasps.

Vital Signs	Recording Time: 2 Minutes After Patient Contact
Skin signs	Red, swollen patches on both legs, left arm, and face
Pulse rate and quality	142 beats/min, regular
Blood pressure	104/66 mm Hg
Respiratory rate and depth	40 breaths/min, labored
Sao_2	95%
Pupils	Equal and reactive to light

5. What is the term for the red, swollen areas that itch?
6. What can you do to alleviate some of the patient's anxiety?

usually fly away after stinging, it is often impossible to identify which species was responsible for the reaction.

Some ants, especially the fire ant (*Solenopsis*) Figure 22-3A ▼, also strike repeatedly, often injecting a particularly irritating toxin, or poison, at the bite sites. It is not uncommon for a patient to sustain multiple ant bites, usually on the feet and legs, within a very short period of time Figure 22-3B ▼.

Signs and symptoms of insect stings or bites are usually at the site of injury and include sudden pain, swelling, localized heat, and, in light-skinned people, redness. There may be itching and sometimes a wheal (or welt), which is a raised, swollen, well-defined area on the skin Figure 22-4 ▶. There is no specific treatment for these injuries, although applying ice sometimes makes them less irritating. The swelling associated with an insect bite may be dramatic and sometimes frightening to patients. However, these local manifestations are usually not serious.

Because the stinger of the honeybee remains in the wound, it can continue to inject venom for up to 20 minutes following the actual sting. In caring for a patient who has been stung by a honeybee, you should gently attempt to remove the stinger and attached muscle by scraping the skin with the edge of a sharp, stiff object such as a credit card Figure 22-5 ▼. Generally, *you should not use tweezers or forceps, as squeezing may cause*

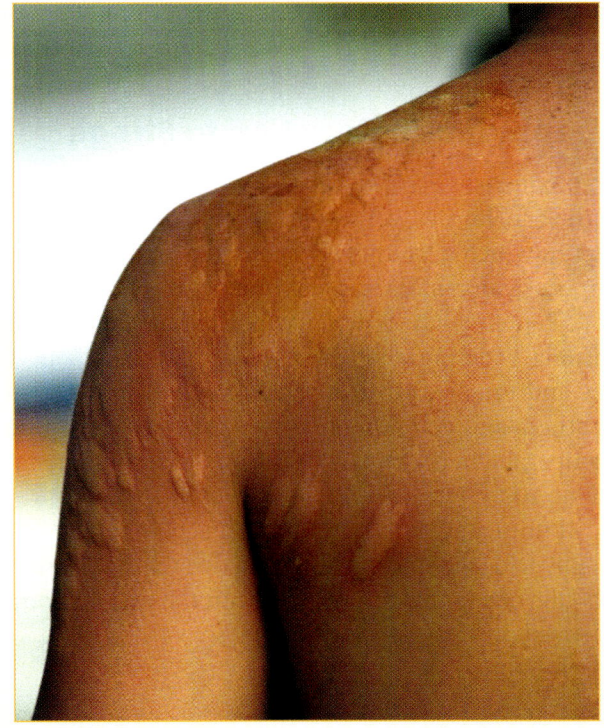

Figure 22-4 A wheal is a whitish, firm elevation of the skin that occurs after an insect sting or bite.

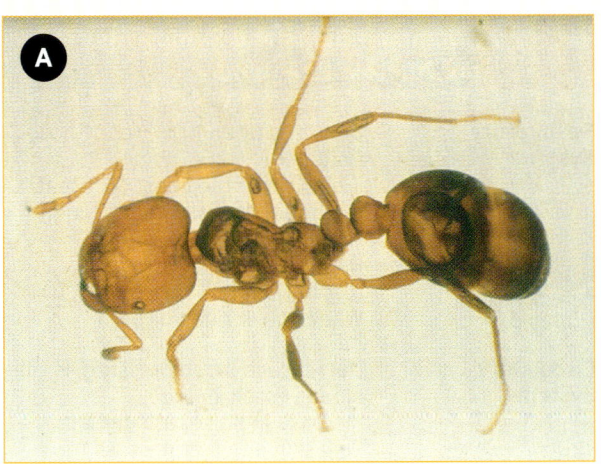

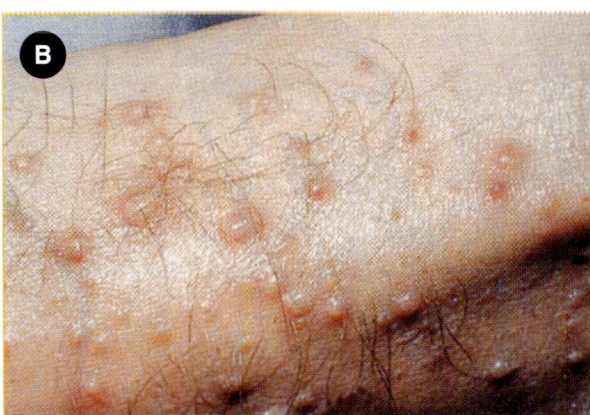

Figure 22-3 A. The fire ant. **B.** Fire ants inject an irritating toxin at multiple sites. Bites are generally found on the feet and the legs and appear as multiple raised pustules.

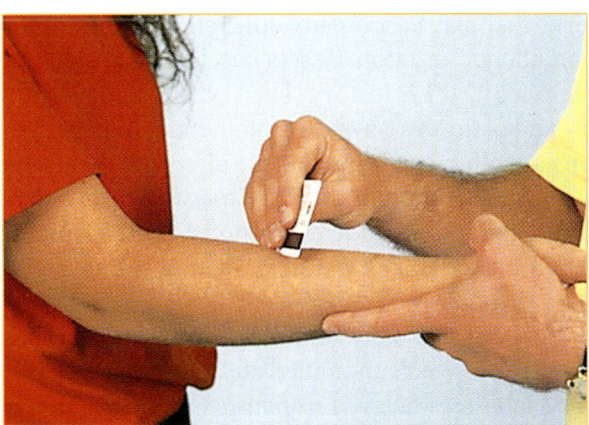

Figure 22-5 To remove the stinger of a honeybee, gently scrape the skin with the edge of a sharp, stiff object such as a credit card.

the stinger to inject more venom into the wound. Gently wash the area with soap and water or a mild antiseptic. Try to remove any jewelry from the area before swelling begins. Position the injection site slightly below the level of the heart and apply ice or cold packs to the area, but not directly on the skin, to help relieve pain and slow the absorption of the toxin. Be alert for vomiting or any signs of shock or allergic reaction, and do not give the patient anything by mouth. Place the patient in the shock position and give oxygen if needed. Monitor the patient's vital signs and be prepared to provide further support as needed.

Anaphylactic Reaction to Stings

Approximately 5% of all people are allergic to the venom of the bee, hornet, yellow jacket, or wasp. This type of allergy, which accounts for about 200 deaths per year, can cause anaphylaxis, a life-threatening allergic reaction. Patients may experience generalized itching and burning, widespread urticaria, wheals, swelling about the lips and tongue, bronchospasm and wheezing, chest tightness and coughing, dyspnea, anxiety, abdominal cramps, and hypotension. Occasionally, respiratory failure occurs.

If untreated, an anaphylactic reaction can proceed rapidly to death. In fact, more than two thirds of patients who die of anaphylaxis do so within the first half hour, so speed on your part is essential.

Patient Assessment

Begin by performing a scene size-up, which in some cases can lead you to possible answers. Next, perform your initial assessment. A patient may have bite or sting marks that may accompany other signs and symptoms of an allergic reaction. Assess baseline vital signs, and obtain a SAMPLE history. Then obtain a focused history, and perform a physical examination. Allergic symptoms are almost as varied as the allergens themselves. Your assessment of the patient experiencing an allergic reaction should include evaluations of the respiratory system, the circulatory system, mental status, and the skin (Table 22-2 ▶).

Responses to antigens may occur as a biphasic response, in which an immediate acute response is followed later by a delayed response. Or, the reaction can either be acute or delayed. Acute reactions occur immediately and as a rule produce the most life-threatening situations. Delayed reactions may take minutes to hours or longer, and the response is not usually as exaggerated.

To help minimize the effects of a delayed reaction that occurs alone or as part of a biphasic response, all patients who experience an allergic reaction should be encouraged to seek medical attention.

> **Terminology Tips**
>
> Remember, the prefix *bi-* means two. Therefore, biphasic means in two phases or stages.

Natural immunity to specific antigens is present at birth, whereas acquired immunity results from exposure to a specific antigen or pathogen through contact or via immunization with a weakened form of the substance. Allergy shots for desensitization work by injecting small amounts of the allergen that the patient is allergic to and allowing the body to produce natural antibodies to fight off that allergen the next time it is introduced into the body. Over time, the dose is grad-

TABLE 22-2	Common Signs and Symptoms of Allergic Reactions
Respiratory System	■ Sneezing or an itchy, runny nose (initially) ■ Tightness in the chest or throat ■ Irritating, persistent, dry cough ■ Hoarseness ■ Rapid, labored, or noisy respirations ■ Wheezing, stridor, or both
Circulatory System	■ Decrease in blood pressure as the blood vessels dilate ■ Increase in pulse rate (initially) ■ Pale skin and dizziness, as the vascular system fails ■ Loss of consciousness and coma
Skin	■ Flushing, itching, or burning skin; especially common over the face and upper chest ■ Urticaria over large areas of the body, both internally and externally ■ Swelling, especially of the face, neck, hands, feet, and tongue ■ Swelling and cyanosis or pallor around the lips ■ Warm, tingling feeling in the face, mouth, chest, feet, and hands
Other Findings	■ Anxiety, a sense of impending doom ■ Abdominal cramps ■ Headache ■ Itchy, watery eyes ■ Decreasing mental status

ually increased as the patient's own immune system is able to compensate and defend itself.

Wheezing may be present during an allergic reaction. It occurs because excessive fluid and mucus are secreted into the bronchial passages, and muscles around these passages tighten in response to the release of histamines and leukotrienes that the allergen induces. Exhalation, normally the passive, relaxed phase of breathing, becomes increasingly difficult as the patient tries to cough up the secretions or move air past the constricted airways. The combination of fluid in the air passages and the constricted bronchi produce the wheezing sound. Breathing rapidly becomes more difficult, and the patient may even stop breathing. Prolonged respiratory difficulty can cause a rapid heartbeat (tachycardia), shock, respiratory failure, and death. <u>Stridor</u>, a harsh, high-pitched inspiratory sound, occurs when swelling in the upper airway (near the vocal cords and throat) closes off the airway and can eventually lead to total obstruction.

Histamines also cause an increase in vascular permeability by dilating capillaries and venules and allowing plasma to seep out of the capillaries and into surrounding tissues. This results in <u>angioedema</u>, which can cause rapid swelling of the airway, and a subsequent decrease in circulating blood volume. With less volume to pump, cardiac preload is decreased, thus reducing both stroke volume and cardiac output. Unless corrected, this will lead to hypotension and inadequate tissue perfusion (shock).

Remember, the presence of hypoperfusion (shock) or respiratory distress indicates that the patient is having a severe allergic reaction that could lead to death.

> ### EMT-I Tips
>
> While one EMT-I is getting oxygen ready, the other should be assisting the patient into a supine position with the head and shoulders elevated. This will improve perfusion to the brain while easing respiratory effort.

Emergency Medical Care

Not all signs and symptoms are present in every allergic reaction. Maintain a high index of suspicion if a reaction has occurred previously and the patient has been exposed to that same substance. If the patient appears to be having an allergic reaction, perform an initial assessment and give 100% oxygen by nonrebreathing mask or assist ventilation with a bag-valve-mask device if the patient is breathing inadequately. When performing a focused history and physical examination, you should ask whether the patient has a history of allergies, what the patient was exposed to, when the exposure occurred, and how the patient was exposed. Determine the onset of symptoms, what the effects of the exposure have been, and how they have progressed. Find out what interventions have been completed before your arrival. Determine whether the patient has any prescribed, preloaded medications for allergic reactions (such as an epinephrine auto-injector), and then inform medical control of the patient's condition.

You are the Provider — Part 4

You have applied 100% oxygen via a nonrebreathing mask and have performed a focused assessment. Despite your attempts to calm the patient, she appears to be even more agitated.

Reassessment	Recording Time: 5 Minutes After Patient Contact
Skin signs	Skin is pale, diaphoretic
Pulse	156 beats/min, weak radial pulses
Blood pressure	88 mm Hg by palpation
Respirations	42 breaths/min, labored
Sao$_2$	95% (on 100% oxygen)

As you listen to her breath sounds, you hear wheezing.

7. What is causing the wheezing?

If necessary, be prepared to use standard airway procedures and positive-pressure ventilation according to the principles identified in Chapter 9.

Your assessment of the patient with an allergic reaction should include determining the patient's level of consciousness, the status of the airway and breathing effort, and baseline vital signs. The focused history and physical examination will identify problems specific to the allergic reaction. If the patient is identified as having life-threatening problems, a detailed physical examination should be performed; however, this should be accomplished en route to the hospital. When assessing the patient with an allergic reaction, determine the following:

- Is the patient able to speak?
- Is the patient restless or agitated?
- What is the level of consciousness using the **AVPU** scale (**A**lert; responsive to **V**erbal stimuli; responsive to **P**ain; **U**nresponsive)?
- Any hoarseness, stridor, or wheezing?
- What is the rate and quality of the patient's breathing and degree of respiratory distress?
- Does the patient have adequate tidal volume?
- Any accessory muscle use or decrease in breath sounds?
- What is the patient's skin color, condition, and temperature?
- Any redness, rashes, itching, or edema noted?
- Are the baseline vital signs abnormal (for example, hypotension or tachycardia)?

If the patient appears to be having a severe allergic (or anaphylactic) reaction, you should administer BLS at once and provide prompt transport to the hospital. In addition to providing oxygen, you should be prepared to maintain the patient's airway or initiate CPR. If necessary, treat for shock by placing the patient in a Trendelenburg position, maintain body heat with a blanket, and initiate intravenous therapy as discussed in Chapter 7. Placing ice over the injury site has been thought to slow absorption of the toxin and diminish swelling, but ice packs placed directly on the skin may freeze it and cause tissue and cellular damage. Like any other attempt to reduce swelling with ice, you should be careful not to overdo the icing.

In some areas, you may be allowed to assist the patient with epinephrine. Whether naturally occurring in the body (endogenous) or made by a drug manufacturer, epinephrine works rapidly to raise the blood pressure by constricting the blood vessels and increasing the strength of the cardiac contractions. Epinephrine also dilates the bronchioles, thus improving the patient's breathing. All bee sting kits should contain a prepared syringe of epinephrine, ready for intramuscular injection, along with instructions for its use. Your EMS service may or may not allow you to help patients self-administer epinephrine to combat allergic reactions or anaphylaxis. In some places, the medical director may authorize you to carry an epinephrine auto-injector (such as an EpiPen) or to assist patients who have their own EpiPen. The adult system delivers 0.3 mg of epinephrine via an automatic needle and syringe system; the infant-child system delivers 0.15 mg (Figure 22-6A ▼). (Table 22-3 ▶) summarizes the management of anaphylaxis.

If the patient is able to use the auto-injector on his or her own, your role is limited to helping. To use, or help the patient use, the auto-injector, you should first **receive a direct order from medical control** or follow local protocols or standing orders. **Follow body substance isolation precautions, and make sure the medication has been prescribed** specifically for that patient. If it has not, do not give the medication: inform medical control, and provide immediate transport. **Finally,**

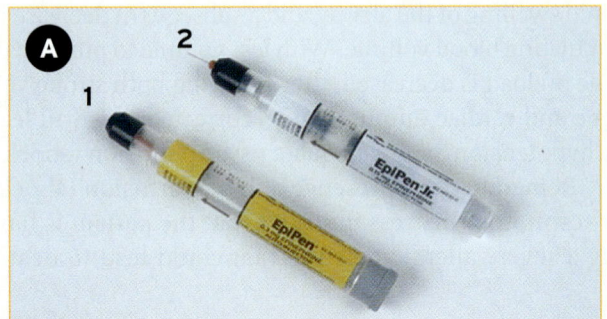

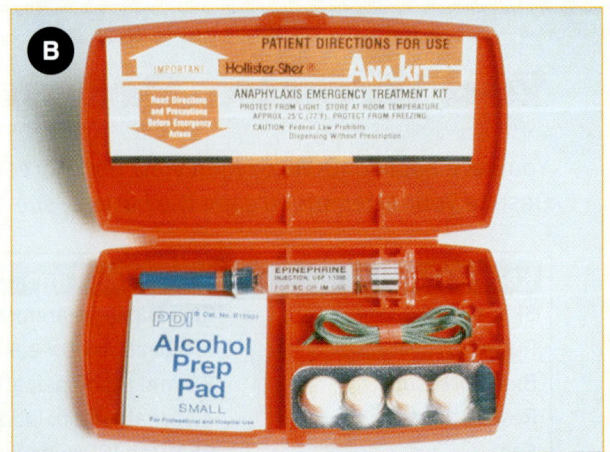

Figure 22-6 Patients who experience severe allergic reactions often carry their own epinephrine, which comes predosed in an auto-injector or a standard syringe. **A.** EpiPen auto-injectors (1-unfired adult model, 2-fired junior model). **B.** AnaKit with epinephrine syringe.

Skill Drill 22-1: Using an Auto-Injector

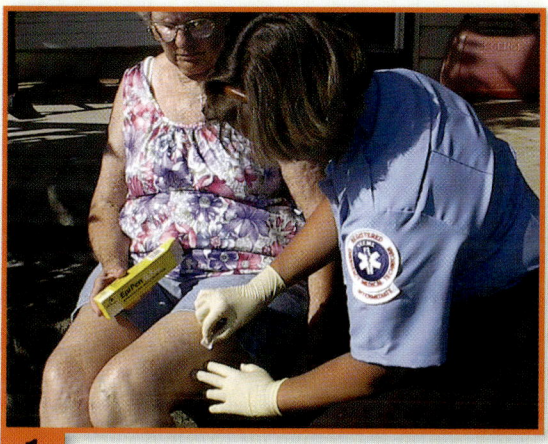

1. Remove the auto-injector's safety cap and quickly wipe the thigh with antiseptic.

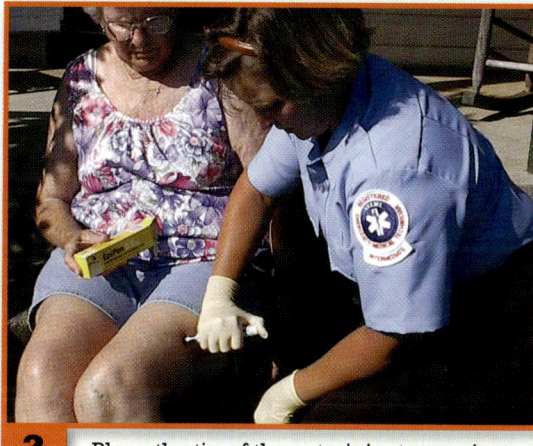

2. Place the tip of the auto-injector against the lateral thigh.

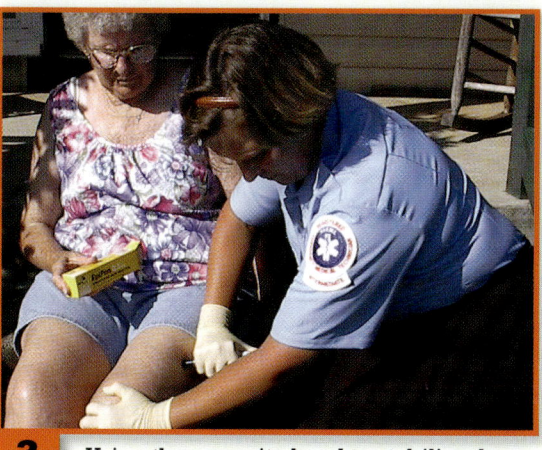

3. Using the opposite hand to stabilize the leg, push the auto-injector firmly against the thigh and hold it in place until all of the medication is injected.

TABLE 22-3 Management of Anaphylaxis

- Remove the offending agent (for example, the stinger).
- Position the patient as appropriate.
- Apply high-flow oxygen or assist ventilation as needed.
- Obtain venous access.
- Give fluid resuscitation as needed.
- Administer epinephrine via an EpiPen or AnaKit.
- Transport promptly.
- Frequently reassess the patient and provide psychological support.

make sure the medication is not discolored and that the expiration date has not passed.

Once you have completed these steps, follow the steps in **Skill Drill 22-1** to use an epinephrine auto-injector.

1. **Remove the safety cap** from the auto-injector, and, if possible, wipe the patient's thigh with alcohol or some other antiseptic. However, do not delay administration of the drug (**Step 1**).
2. **Place the tip of the auto-injector** against the lateral part of the patient's thigh, midway between the hip and the knee (**Step 2**).

Skill Drill 22-2: Using an AnaKit

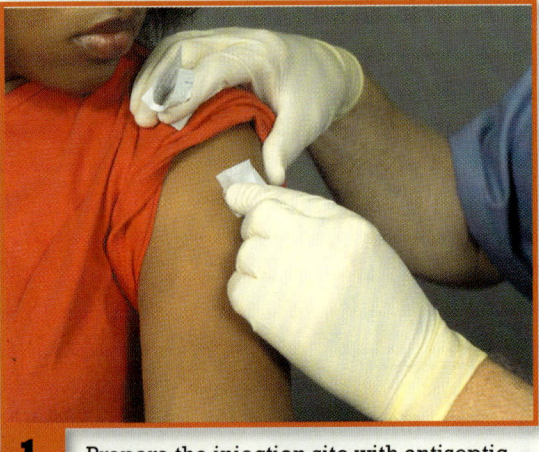

1 Prepare the injection site with antiseptic and remove the needle cover.

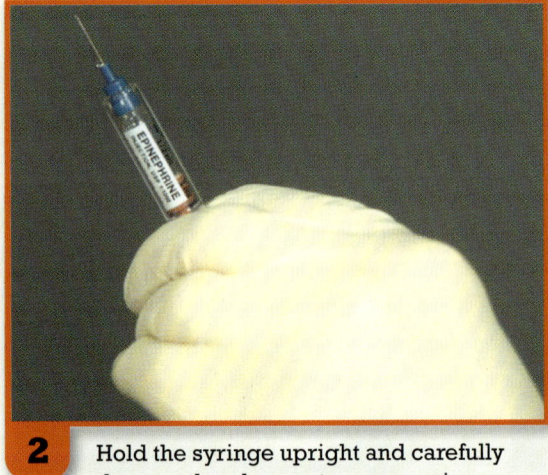

2 Hold the syringe upright and carefully depress the plunger to remove air.

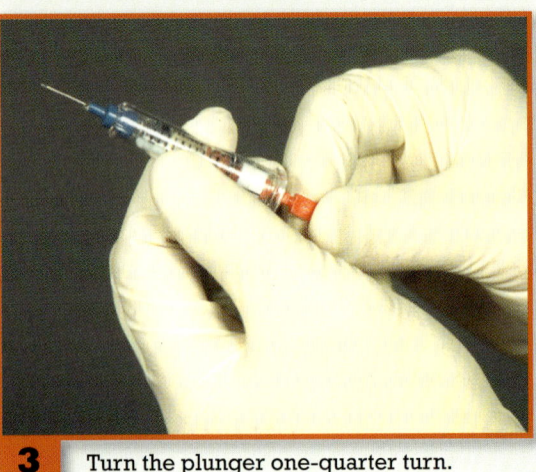

3 Turn the plunger one-quarter turn.

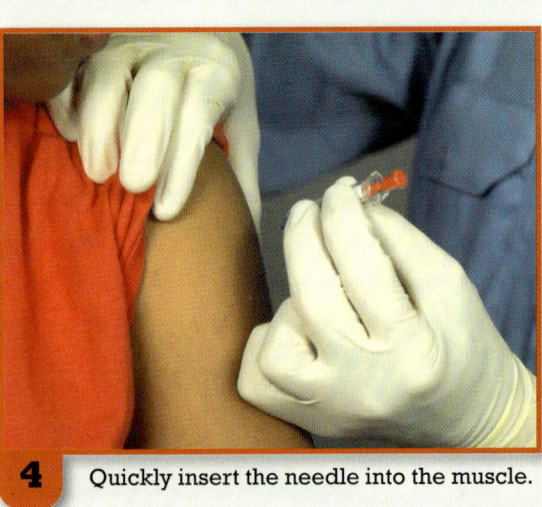

4 Quickly insert the needle into the muscle.

---

3. **Push the injector firmly** against the thigh until the injector activates. Hold steady pressure to prevent kick back from the spring in the syringe, and to prevent the needle from being pushed out of the injection site too soon. Hold the injector in place until the medication is injected (10 seconds) (**Step 3**).
4. **Remove the injector** from the patient's thigh and dispose of it in the proper biohazard container.
5. **Record the time and dose** of injection on the patient care form.
6. **Reassess and record** the patient's vital signs and clinical response after using the auto-injector.

If the patient has known allergies to insects, he or she might carry a commercial bee sting kit (AnaKit) that contains a standard syringe of epinephrine for intramuscular injection (Figure 22-6B ◀). If you will administer this epinephrine, make the same general preparations you make for an auto-injector: Obtain an order from medical control, take body substance isolation precautions, and ensure that the medicine belongs to the patient, is not discolored, and that the expiration date has not passed. Follow the steps in (Skill Drill 22-2 ▲) to administer epinephrine from an AnaKit:

1. **Prepare the injection site** with an alcohol wipe or other antiseptic, if there is time. Remove the needle cover (**Step 1**).

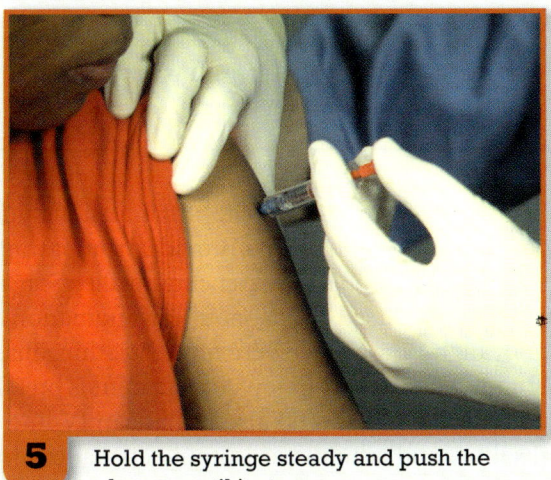

5 Hold the syringe steady and push the plunger until it stops.

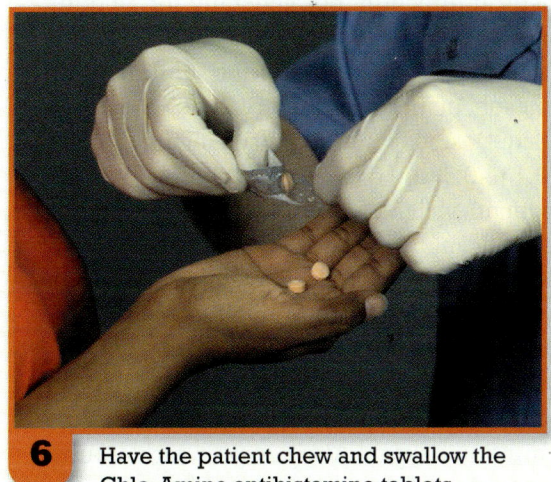

6 Have the patient chew and swallow the Chlo-Amine antihistamine tablets provided in the kit.

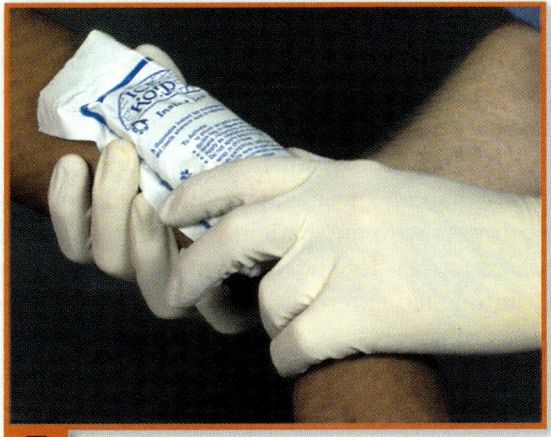

7 If available, apply a cold pack to the sting site.

2. **Hold the syringe upright** so that any air inside rises to the base of the needle. Remove the air by depressing the syringe plunger until it stops (**Step 2**).
3. **Turn the plunger** one-quarter turn (**Step 3**).
4. **Insert the needle quickly,** straight into the injection site, deep enough to place the tip into the muscle beneath the skin and subcutaneous layer (**Step 4**).
5. **Holding the syringe steady,** push the plunger until it stops, to ensure that all medication is injected (**Step 5**).
6. **Have the patient chew and swallow the Chlo-Amine antihistamine tablets** in the kit (**Step 6**).
7. If you have or can **make a cold pack,** apply it to the site of the sting to reduce swelling and minimize the amount of venom that enters the circulation (**Step 7**).

The syringe from the Anakit holds a second injection if needed.

Other bee sting kits contain some oral or injectable antihistamines, agents that block the effect of histamines. These work relatively slowly, within several minutes to 1 hour. Because epinephrine can have an effect within 1 minute, it is the primary drug to treat the life-threatening effects of the allergic reaction (for example hypotension and bronchoconstriction).

In some areas of the country, EMT-I squads can administer epinephrine for anaphylaxis. Follow your local protocols or medical direction, but generally for an adult weighing more than 50 kg, you will inject 0.3 to 0.5 mL (0.3 to 0.5 mg) of a 1:1,000 epinephrine solution intramuscularly or subcutaneously at intervals of 5 to 15 minutes, as needed. Doses for children vary, ranging from 0.1 to 0.3 mL (0.1 to 0.3 mg) of a 1:1,000 solution, depending on the patient's weight. Be aware that the medication may cause significant tachycardia and increased anxiety or nervousness. Complete the emergency care as outlined above for the patient, and provide prompt transport, closely monitoring the patient's condition, including cardiac monitoring, frequently. Remember that all patients with suspected anaphylaxis should be given high-flow, high-concentration oxygen. Also consider early intubation if the patient's status warrants it.

Because epinephrine constricts blood vessels, it may cause the patient's blood pressure to rise significantly. Monitor intravenous fluid administration carefully to prevent inadvertent fluid overloading of the patient. Other side effects of epinephrine include pallor, dizziness, chest pain, headache, nausea, and vomiting. All of these effects may cause the patient to feel anxious or excited. These side effects are worth the tradeoff when epinephrine is used in a life-threatening situation. However, if the patient has no signs of respiratory distress or shock after contact with a substance that causes an allergic reaction, continue with the focused history and physical exam. Note that patients who are not wheezing or who have no signs of respiratory compromise or hypotension should not be given epinephrine.

> **EMT-I Tips**
>
> It is much easier to obtain intravenous (IV) access before the patient's blood pressure starts to drop. Obtain IV access early.

Whether or not your emergency treatment includes epinephrine, you should always provide prompt transport for any patient who is experiencing an allergic reaction or has experienced a poisonous envenomation or bite. Apply high-flow oxygen via a nonrebreathing mask at 15 L/min or assist ventilation if the patient is breathing inadequately. You should also initiate an IV line of normal saline, and administer isotonic crystalloid fluids as needed to maintain adequate perfusion. Continue to reassess the patient's vital signs en route; remember that signs and symptoms may change rapidly. You may need to give more than one injection of epinephrine if you note that the patient has decreasing mental status, increased breathing difficulty, or a decreasing blood pressure. Be sure to consult medical control first. Current auto-injectors give only one dose, and a patient who needs more than one dose will need to have more than one injector. As with any patient you are transporting, be prepared to treat for shock, begin BLS measures, or use the automated external defibrillator if the patient develops cardiac arrest.

If the patient's condition improves, provide supportive care, including continuing oxygen therapy during transport.

You are the Provider — Part 5

Before your partner returns with the stretcher, the patient hands you an EpiPen auto-injector with her name on it. You check for clarity of the fluid and the expiration date and find it to be in order. You contact medical control and obtain an order to administer the medication.

Reassessment	Recording Time: 6 Minutes After Patient Contact
Level of consciousness	Patient is becoming progressively lethargic
Respirations	38 breaths/min, more labored, audible wheezing
Pulse	160 beats/min, weak, thready
Blood pressure	84 mm Hg by palpation
Skin	Pale, cool, diaphoretic

8. Where will you administer the EpiPen?
9. What effects do you expect from the administration of the epinephrine?

EMT-I Tips

If your medical director and protocols allow it, and your patient has an inhaled bronchodilator as well as an epinephrine auto-injector, one EMT-I can help administer the inhaler while the other administers the epinephrine.

Documentation Tips

Allergic reactions and responses to bites and stings can become rapidly life threatening. With prompt care, severe signs and symptoms may subside just as quickly. Thus, performing a multisystem exam and documenting your findings is important before and after treatment. Pay particular attention to the patient's skin condition and to the status of respiratory, circulatory, and mental functions.

Specific Bites and Envenomations

Spider Bites

Spiders are numerous and widespread in the United States. Many species of spiders bite. However, only two, the female black widow spider and the brown recluse spider, are able to deliver serious, even life-threatening venom. When you care for a patient who has sustained a spider bite, be alert to the possibility that the spider may still be in the area. Remember that your safety is of paramount importance.

Black Widow Spider

The female black widow spider (*Latrodectus mactans*) is fairly large as far as spiders go, measuring approximately 2″ long with its legs extended. It is usually black and has a distinctive, bright red-orange marking in the shape of an hourglass on its abdomen (Figure 22-7 ▶). The female is larger and more toxic than the male. Black widow spiders are found in every state except Alaska. They prefer dry, dim places around buildings, in woodpiles, and among debris.

The bite of the black widow spider is sometimes overlooked. If the site becomes numb right away, the patient may not even recall being bit. However, most black widow spider bites cause immediate localized pain and symptoms, including agonizing muscle spasms. In some cases, a bite on the abdomen causes muscle spasms so severe that the patient may be thought to have an acute abdomen, such as peritonitis. The main danger with this type of bite, however, comes from the fact that the black widow's venom is poisonous to nerve tissues (neurotoxic). Other systemic symptoms include dizziness, sweating, nausea, vomiting, and rashes. Tightness in the chest and difficulty breathing typically develop within 24 hours, as well as severe cramps, with board-like rigidity of the abdominal muscles. Generally, these signs and symptoms subside over 48 hours.

If necessary, a physician can administer a specific antivenin, a serum containing antibodies that counteract the venom, but because of a high incidence of side effects, its use is reserved for very severe bites, for aged or very feeble people, and for children younger than 5 years. The severe muscle spasms are usually treated in the hospital with IV benzodiazepines such as diazepam (Valium) or lorazepam (Ativan). In general, emergency treatment for a black widow spider bite consists of BLS for the patient in respiratory distress. Much more often, the patient will merely require relief from pain. Transport the patient to the emergency department as soon as possible for treatment of both pain and muscle rigidity. If it is possible and can be done safely, take the spider with you for positive identification.

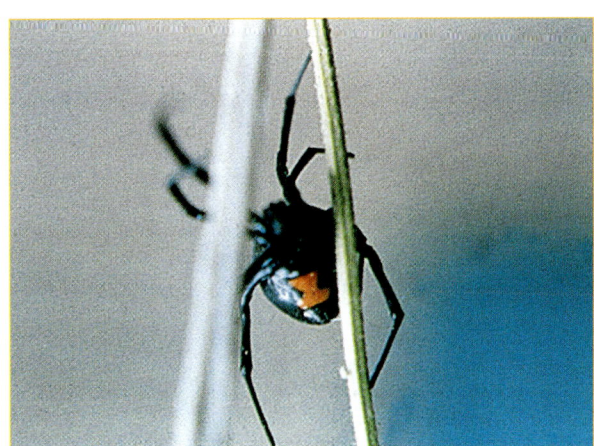

Figure 22-7 Black widow spiders are distinguished by their glossy black color and bright orange hourglass marking on the abdomen.

Brown Recluse Spider

The brown recluse spider (*Loxosceles reclusa*) is dull brown and, at 1″, somewhat smaller than the black widow Figure 22-8 ▼. The short-haired body has a violin-shaped mark that is brown to yellow on its back, which is why it is commonly referred to as the "fiddle back" spider. Although it lives mostly in the southern and central parts of the country, the brown recluse may be found throughout the continental United States. The spider is named for its tendency to live in dark areas: in corners of old, unused buildings; under rocks; and in woodpiles. In cooler areas, it moves indoors to closets, drawers, cellars, and old piles of clothing.

In contrast with the venom of the black widow spider, the venom of the brown recluse spider is not neurotoxic but cytotoxic; that is, it causes severe local tissue damage. Typically, the bite is not painful at first but becomes so within hours. The area becomes swollen and tender and develops a pale, mottled, cyanotic center and possibly a small blister Figure 22-9 ▼. During the next several days, a scab of dead skin, fat, and debris will form and dig into the skin, producing a large ulcer that may not heal unless treated promptly. Transport patients with such symptoms as soon as possible.

Brown recluse spider bites rarely cause systemic symptoms and signs. When they do, the initial treatment is BLS and transportation to the emergency department. Again, it is helpful if you can identify the spider and take it to the hospital along with the patient.

A to Z Terminology Tips

Toxic means poisonous. By adding the prefixes *cyt-* meaning *cell*, and *neuro-* meaning *nerves* or *nervous system*, the meanings of the terms *neurotoxic* and *cytotoxic* can easily be deduced.

Neurotoxin: A poison that affects the nervous tissue or system.

Cytotoxin: A poison that affects the cells locally.

In the Field

When treating a snakebite victim, take the snake along to the hospital for identification if it has been killed; however, if you are scratched or punctured by the fangs when handling it, you may also be envenomated. Use extreme caution.

Snake Bites

Snake bites are a worldwide problem of some significance. More than 300,000 injuries from snake bites occur annually, including 30,000 to 40,000 deaths. The greatest number of deaths occur in Southeast Asia and India (25,000 to 30,000 per year) and in South Amer-

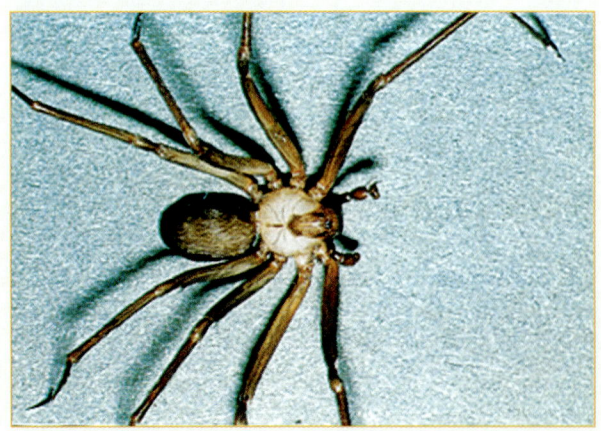

Figure 22-8 Brown recluse spiders are dull brown and have a dark, violin-shaped mark on the back.

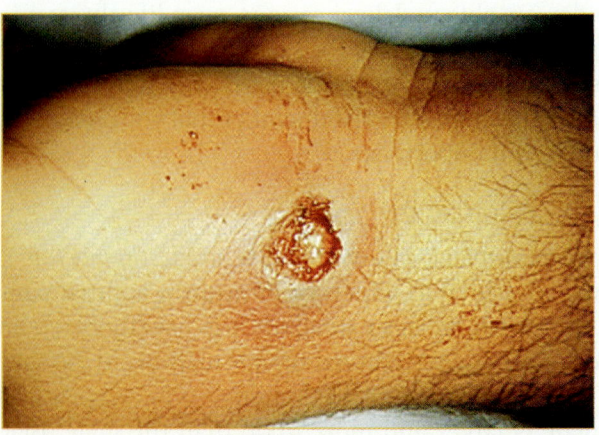

Figure 22-9 The bite of a brown recluse spider is characterized by swelling, tenderness, and a pale, mottled cyanotic center. There may also be a small blister on the bite.

ica (3,000 to 4,000 per year). In the United States, 40,000 to 50,000 snake bites are reported annually, about 7,000 of them caused by poisonous snakes. However, deaths due to snake bites in the United States are extremely rare, about 15 a year for the entire country.

Of the approximately 115 different species of snakes in the United States, only 19 are venomous. These include the rattlesnake (*Crotalus* and *Sistrurus*), the copperhead (*Agkistrodon contortrix*), the cottonmouth, or water moccasin (*Agkistrodon piscivorus*), and the coral snake (*Micrurus* and *Micruroides*) Figure 22-10 ▼. At least one of these poisonous species is found in every state except Alaska, Hawaii, and Maine. As a general rule, these creatures are timid. They usually do not bite unless provoked, angered, or accidentally injured, as when they are stepped on. There are a few exceptions to these rules. Cottonmouths are often rather aggressive, and very little provocation is needed to annoy a rattlesnake. Coral snakes, by contrast, are very shy and usually bite only when they are being handled.

Most snake bites occur between April and October, when the animals are active, and tend to involve young men who have been drinking alcohol. Texas reports the largest number of bites. Other states with a major concentration of snake bites are Louisiana, Georgia, Oklahoma, North Carolina, Arkansas, West Virginia, and Mississippi. If you work in one of these areas, you should be thoroughly familiar with the emergency care of snake bites. Remember, almost any time you are caring for a patient with a snake bite, another snake, or perhaps the same one, could come along and create a second victim: you. Therefore, use extreme caution on these calls, and be sure to wear the proper protective equipment for the area.

In general, only a third of snake bites result in significant local or systemic injuries. Often, envenomation does not occur because the snake has recently struck another animal and exhausted its supply of venom producing what is known as a "dry bite."

With the exception of the coral snake, poisonous snakes native to the United States all have hollow fangs

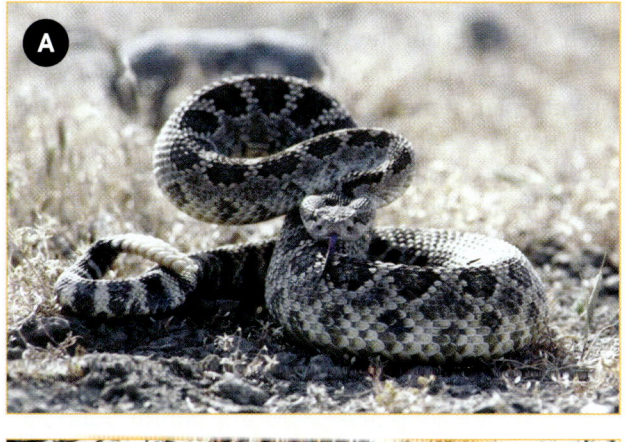

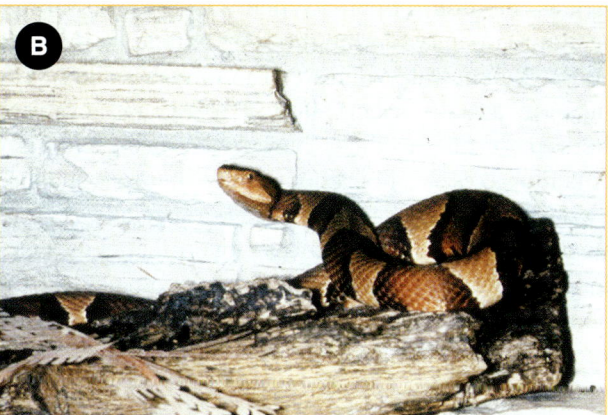

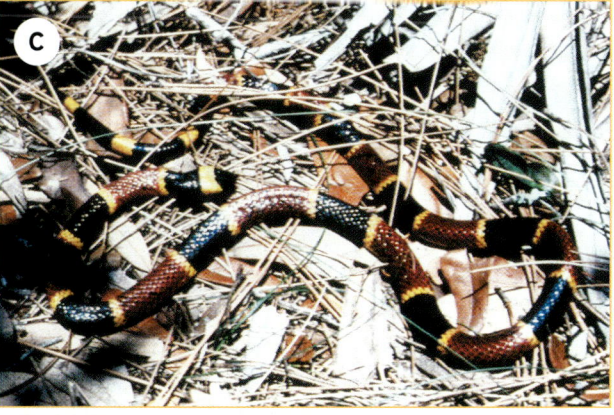

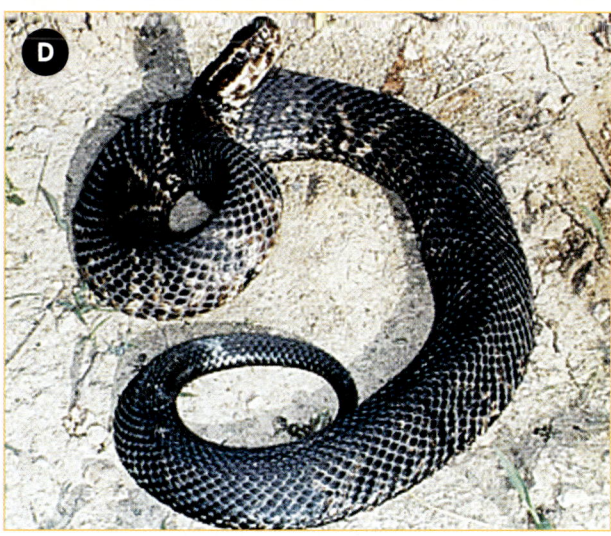

Figure 22-10 **A.** Rattlesnake. **B.** Copperhead. **C.** Coral snake. **D.** Cottonmouth.

in the roof of the mouth that inject the poison from two sacs at the back of the head. The classic appearance of the poisonous snake bite, therefore, is two small puncture wounds, usually about $\frac{1}{2}''$ apart, with discoloration, swelling, and pain surrounding them (Figure 22-11 ▼). Nonpoisonous snakes can also bite, usually leaving horseshoe-shaped teeth marks. However, some poisonous snakes have teeth as well as fangs, making it impossible to determine the type of snake responsible for a given set of teeth marks. On the other hand, fang marks are a clear indication of a poisonous snake bite.

Pit Vipers

Rattlesnakes, copperheads, and cottonmouths are all pit vipers, with triangular-shaped, flat heads (Figure 22-12 ▶). They take their name from the small pits located just behind each nostril and in front of each eye. The pit is a heat-sensing organ that allows the snake to strike accurately at any warm target, especially in the dark when it cannot see through its vertical, slitlike pupils.

The fangs of the pit viper normally lie flat against the roof of the mouth and are hinged to swing back and forth as the mouth opens. When the snake is striking, the mouth opens wide and the fangs extend; in this way, the fangs penetrate whatever the mouth strikes. The fangs are actually special hollow teeth that act much like hypodermic needles. They are connected to a sac containing a reservoir of venom, which in turn is attached to a poison gland. The gland itself is a specially adapted salivary gland, which produces powerful enzymes that digest and destroy tissue. The primary purpose of the venom is to kill small animals and to start the digestive process before they are eaten.

The most common form of pit viper is the rattlesnake. Several different species of rattlesnake can be identified by the rattle on the tail. The rattle is actually numerous layers of dried skin that were shed but failed to fall off, coming to rest against a small knob on the end of the tail. When agitated or endangered, rattlesnakes shake their tails, or rattles, to warn the invader away. Rattlesnakes have many patterns of color, often with a diamond pattern. They can grow to 6′ or more in length.

Copperheads are smaller than rattlesnakes, usually 2′ to 3′ long, with a reddish coppery color crossed with brown or red bands. These snakes typically inhabit woodpiles and abandoned dwellings, often close to areas of habitation. Although they account for most of the venomous snake bites in the eastern United States, copperhead bites are typically not fatal; however, note that the venom can destroy extremities.

Cottonmouths grow to about 4′ in length. Also called water moccasins, these snakes are olive or brown, with black cross-bands and a yellow undersurface. They are water snakes, with a particularly aggressive pattern of behavior. Although deaths from the bites of these snakes are rare, tissue destruction from the venom may be severe. Cottonmouths have been known to strike at their victims from the water.

The signs of envenomation by a pit viper are severe burning pain at the site of the injury, followed by swelling and, in light-skinned people, a bluish discoloration (ecchymosis) that signals bleeding under the skin. These signs are evident within 5 to 10 minutes after the bite has occurred, and they spread during the next 36 hours. In addition to destroying tissues locally, the venom of the pit viper can also interfere with the body's blood-clotting mechanisms and cause bleeding at various distant sites. Other systemic signs, which may or may not occur, include weakness, sweating, fainting, and shock.

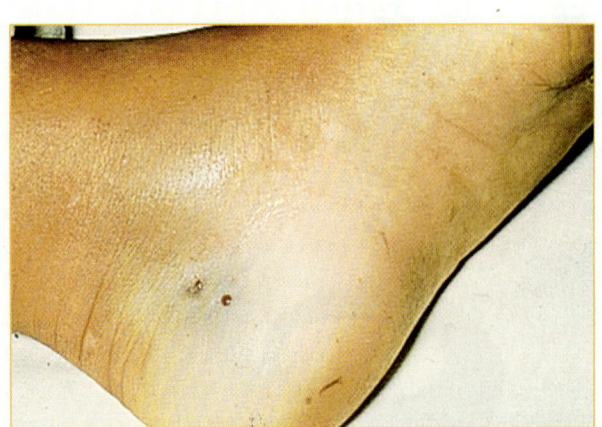

Figure 22-11 A snake bite wound from a poisonous snake has characteristic markings: two small puncture wounds about $\frac{1}{2}''$ apart, discoloration, and swelling.

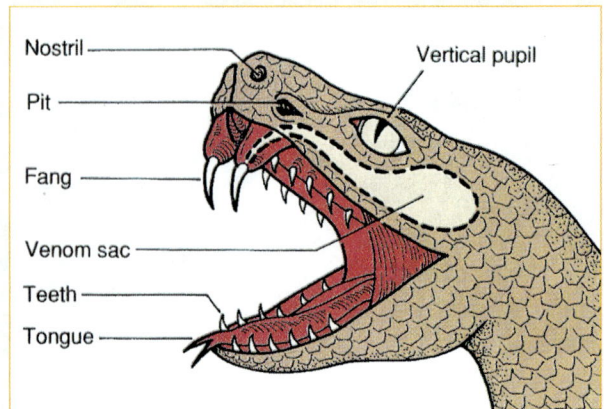

Figure 22-12 Pit vipers have small, heat-sensing organs (pits) located in front of their eyes that allow them to strike at warm targets, even in the dark.

If the patient has no local signs an hour after being bitten, envenomation more than likely did not occur. If swelling has occurred, you should mark its edges on the skin. This will allow physicians to assess what has happened and when it happened with greater accuracy. Frequently measuring the circumference of the affected extremity will allow you to determine the speed at which swelling is occurring.

In treating a snake bite from a pit viper, follow these steps:

1. Calm the patient. Have the patient lie supine, and explain that remaining still and calm will slow the spread of any venom through the system.
2. Locate the bite area; clean it gently with soap and water or a mild antiseptic. **Do not apply ice to the area as this will cause local vasoconstriction and push the venom further into the bloodstream.**
3. If the bite occurred on an arm or leg, splint the extremity to decrease movement and then place the affected extremity below the level of the heart.
4. Be alert for vomiting, which may be a sign of anxiety rather than the toxin itself.
5. Do not give anything by mouth.
6. If, as rarely happens, the patient was bitten on the trunk, keep him or her supine and calm and transport as quickly as possible.
7. Monitor the patient's vital signs, and mark the skin with a pen over the area that is swollen, proximal to the swelling, to note whether swelling is spreading. Circumferential measurement of the affected extremity will also determine the degree of swelling.
8. If signs of shock are present, place the patient in the shock position and administer 100% oxygen. Be prepared to assist ventilations if needed. Initiate IV therapy according to local protocols.
9. If the snake has been killed, as is often the case, take it with you so that physicians can identify it and administer the proper antivenin. **Be careful in handling any snake.** The fangs of a pit viper are sharp and may scratch your skin, allowing the remaining venom to penetrate.
10. Notify the hospital that you are bringing in a snake bite patient; if possible, describe the snake.
11. Transport the patient promptly to the hospital.
12. Monitor the patient's cardiac rhythm and treat any arrhythmias according to standard ACLS protocols.

If the patient shows no sign of envenomation, provide BLS as needed, place a sterile dressing over the suspected bite area, and immobilize the injury site. All patients with a suspected snake bite should be taken to the emergency department, whether they show signs of envenomation or not. Treat the wound as you would any deep puncture wound to prevent infection.

You are the Provider — Part 6

Your partner returns with the stretcher, and you assist the patient onto it. You note that her color is much better and she appears to be breathing without difficulty.

Reassessment	Recording Time: 11 Minutes After Patient Contact
Level of consciousness	Alert, oriented, jittery
Respirations	20 breaths/min, nonlabored, no wheezing
Pulse	144 beats/min, strong radial pulses
Blood pressure	98/44 mm Hg
Skin	Warm, pink, dry

You continue to give oxygen via nonrebreathing mask and start an IV en route to the hospital. On arrival at the emergency room, you give your report to the nurse and find a spare corner to complete your patient care report.

10. What IV fluid would you start for this patient, and at what rate would you run it?

If you work in an area where poisonous snakes are known to live, you should know the local protocol for handling snake bites. You should also know the address of the nearest facility where antivenin is available. This may be a nearby zoo, the local or state public health department, or a local community hospital.

> **EMT-I Tips**
>
> Evidence of the exact source of an allergic reaction or envenomation may be scarce when you arrive, or bystanders may give you incorrect information. The cause is more likely to pose a risk to responders, and added risk to the patient, if you draw incorrect conclusions about its nature. Keep your eyes and ears open, avoid making unsupported assumptions, and be curious about things that don't quite make sense.

Coral Snakes

The coral snake is a small reptile with a series of bright red, yellow, and black bands completely encircling the body. Many harmless snakes have similar coloring (such as the king snake), but only the coral snake has red and yellow bands next to one another, as this helpful rhyme suggests: "Red on yellow will kill a fellow; red on black, venom will lack."

A rare creature that lives primarily in Florida and in the desert southwest, the coral snake is a relative of the cobra. It has tiny fangs and injects the venom with its teeth by a chewing motion, leaving behind one or more puncture or scratchlike wounds. Because of its small mouth and teeth and limited jaw expansion, the coral snake usually bites its victims on a small part of the body, such as between fingers or toes.

Coral snake venom is a powerful toxin that causes paralysis of the nervous system (neurotoxic). Within a few hours of being bitten, a patient will exhibit bizarre behavior, followed by progressive paralysis of eye movements and respiration. Often, there are limited or no local symptoms.

Successful treatment, either emergency or long-term, depends on positive identification of the snake and support of vital central nervous system functions, such as breathing. Antivenin is available, but most hospitals do not stock it. Therefore, you should notify the hospital of the need for it as soon as possible. The steps for emergency care of a coral snake bite are as follows:

1. Immediately quiet and reassure the patient.
2. Flush the area of the bite with 1 to 2 quarts of warm, soapy water to wash away any poison left on the surface of the skin. **Do not apply ice to the region.**
3. Splint the extremity to minimize movement and the spread of venom at the site. Position the affected extremity below the level of the heart.
4. Check the patient's vital signs, and continue to monitor them.
5. Keep the patient warm, and elevate the lower extremities to help prevent shock. Initiate IV therapy according to local protocols.
6. Give supplemental oxygen if needed, and be prepared to assist ventilation.
7. Transport the patient promptly to the emergency department, giving advance notice that the patient has been bitten by a coral snake.
8. Give the patient nothing by mouth.
9. Monitor the patient's cardiac rhythm and treat any arrhythmias according to standard ACLS protocols.

Scorpion Stings

Scorpions are eight-legged arachnids from the biologic group Arachnida with a venom gland and a stinger at the end of their tail **Figure 22-13**. Scorpions are rare; they live primarily in the southwestern United States and in deserts. With one exception, a scorpion's sting is usually very painful but not dangerous, causing localized swelling and discoloration. The exception is the *Centruroides sculpturatus*. Although it is found naturally in Arizona and New Mexico, as well as parts of Texas, California, and Nevada, it may be kept as a pet by any-

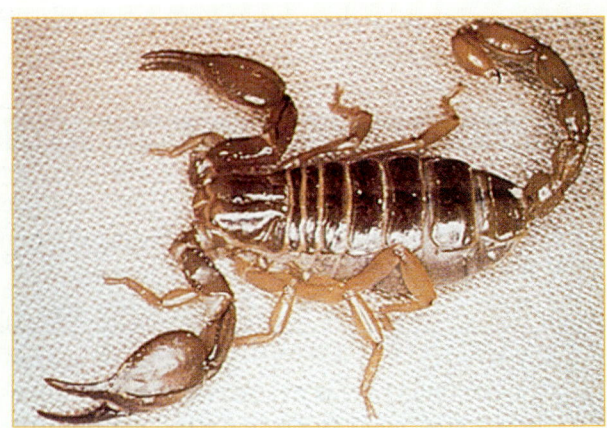

Figure 22-13 The sting of a scorpion is usually more painful than it is dangerous, causing localized swelling and discoloration.

one. The venom of this particular species may produce a severe systemic reaction that brings about circulatory collapse, severe muscle contractions, excessive salivation, hypertension, seizures, and cardiac failure. Antivenin is available but must be administered by a physician. If you are called to care for a patient with a suspected sting from a *sculpturatus*, you should notify medical control as soon as possible. Administer all the elements of BLS, and transport the patient to the emergency department as rapidly as possible. If the patient is allergic to the scorpion, regardless of the species, anaphylactic shock could occur.

Tick Bites

Found most often on brush, shrubs, trees, sand dunes, or other animals, ticks usually attach themselves directly to the skin (Figure 22-14 ▼). Only a fraction of an inch long, they can easily be mistaken for a freckle, especially since their bite is not painful. Indeed, the danger with a tick bite is not from the bite itself, but from the infecting organisms that the tick carries. Ticks commonly carry two infectious diseases: Rocky Mountain spotted fever and Lyme disease. Both are spread through the tick's saliva, which is injected into the skin when the tick attaches itself.

Rocky Mountain spotted fever, which is not limited to the Rocky Mountains, occurs within 7 to 10 days after a bite by an infected tick. Its symptoms include nausea, vomiting, headache, weakness, paralysis, and possibly cardiorespiratory collapse.

Lyme disease has received extensive publicity. It is, after acquired immunodeficiency syndrome (or AIDS), the second most rapidly growing infectious disease in the United States. Originally seen primarily in Connecticut, Lyme disease has been reported in 35 states. It occurs most commonly in the Northeast, the Great Lakes states, and the Pacific Northwest; New York State reports the largest number of cases. The first symptom, a rash that may spread to several parts of the body, begins about 3 days after the bite of an infected tick. The rash may eventually resemble a target or bull's-eye pattern in one third of patients (Figure 22-15 ▼). After a few more days or weeks, painful swelling of the joints, particularly the knees, occurs. Lyme disease may be confused with rheumatoid arthritis and, like that disease, may result in permanent disability. However, if it is recognized and treated promptly with antibiotics, the patient may recover completely.

Tick bites occur most commonly during the summer months, when people are out in the woods wearing little protective clothing. Transmission of the infection from tick to person takes at least 12 hours, so if you are called to remove a tick, you should proceed carefully and slowly. Do not attempt to suffocate the tick with gasoline or Vaseline or burn it with a lighted match; you will only burn the patient. Instead, using fine tweezers, grasp the tick by the head and pull it straight out of the skin. This method will usually remove the whole tick. Even if part of the tick is left embedded in the skin, the part containing the infecting organisms has been removed. Cleanse the area with disinfectant, and save the tick in a glass jar or other container so that it can be identified. Do not handle the tick with your fingers. Provide any necessary supportive emergency care, and transport the patient to the hospital.

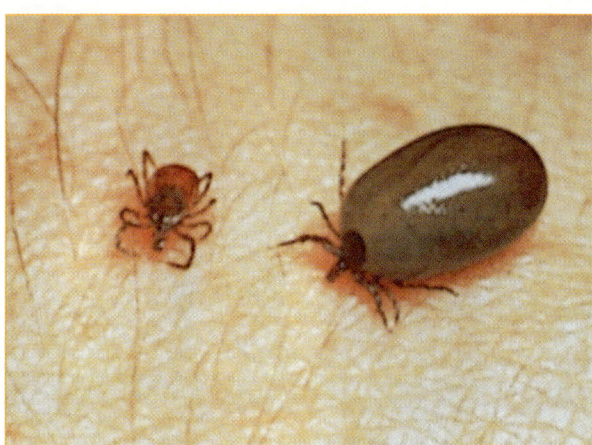

Figure 22-14 Ticks typically attach themselves directly to the skin.

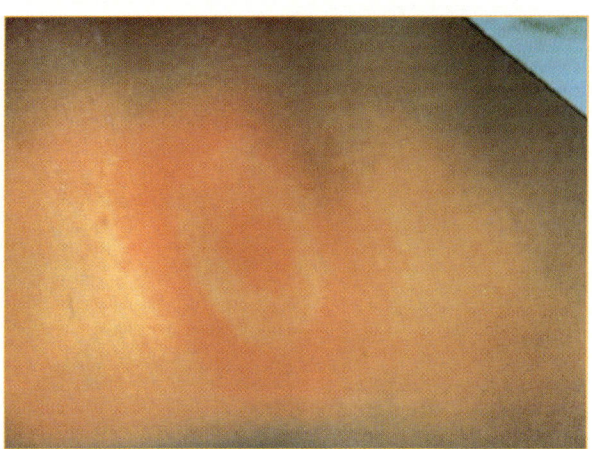

Figure 22-15 The rash associated with Lyme disease has a characteristic "bull's-eye" pattern.

Dog Bites and Rabies

Most people who are bitten by dogs do not report the incident to a physician, believing that dog bites are not serious. They can be very serious, however. A dog's mouth is heavily contaminated with virulent bacteria. You should consider all dog bites as contaminated and potentially infected wounds that may require antibiotics, tetanus prophylaxis, and suturing Figure 22-16. Occasionally, dog bites result in mangled, complex wounds that require surgical repair. For these reasons, all dog bites should be treated by a physician. Place a dry, sterile dressing over the wound, and promptly transport the patient to the emergency department. If an arm or leg was injured, splint that extremity. Often, the patient will be extremely upset and frightened, a situation that calls for calm reassurance on your part.

A major concern with dog bites is the spread of *rabies*, an acute, fatal viral infection of the central nervous system that can affect all warm-blooded animals. Although rabies is extremely rare today, particularly with widespread inoculation of pets, it still exists. Stray dogs that have not been inoculated can be carriers of the disease, as can squirrels, bats, foxes, skunks, and raccoons. The virus is in the saliva of a rabid or infected animal and is transmitted through biting or through licking an open wound. Infection can be prevented in a person who has been bitten by such an animal only by a series of special vaccine injections that must be initiated soon after the bite. Since animals that have rabies do not always show it immediately in their behavior, a person's only chance to avoid the vaccine is to find the animal and turn it over to the health department for observation, testing, or both. Refer to your local animal control procedures.

Children, particularly young ones, may be seriously injured or even killed by dogs. These dogs are not always vicious or rabid; sometimes, the child had unknowingly provoked the animal. However, you must assume that it may turn and attack you as well. Therefore, you should not enter the scene until the animal has been secured by the police or an animal control officer. Then you may carry out the necessary emergency care and transport the child to the emergency department. The EMT-I is required by law to report all animal bites to the appropriate authority, which is typically the emergency department physician.

Human Bites

The human mouth, more so than even the dog's, contains an exceptionally wide range of virulent bacteria and viruses. For this reason, you should regard any human bite that has penetrated the skin as a very serious injury. Similarly, any laceration caused by a human tooth can result in a serious, spreading infection Figure 22-17 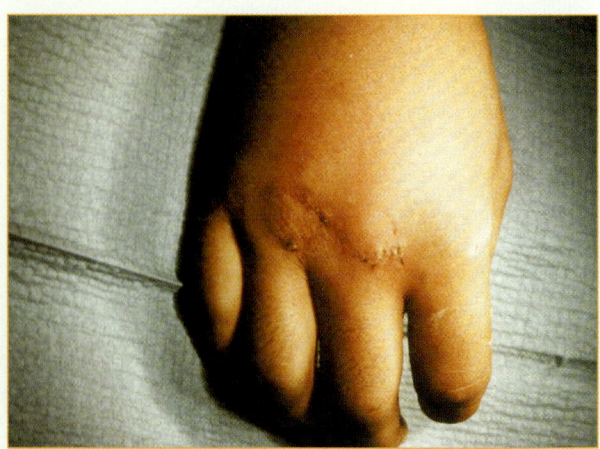. Remember this if you have occasion to treat someone who has been punched in the mouth: The person who delivered the punch may also need treatment.

Figure 22-16 Dog bite wounds should be examined at the hospital, as these wounds are heavily contaminated with virulent bacteria.

Figure 22-17 Human bites can result in serious, spreading infection. Thus, patients must be evaluated at the hospital.

The emergency treatment for human bites consists of the following steps:
1. Promptly immobilize the area with a splint or bandage.
2. Control all bleeding, and apply a dry, sterile dressing.
3. Provide transport to the emergency department for surgical cleansing of the wound and antibiotic therapy.

Injuries From Marine Animals

Coelenterates, including the fire coral, Portuguese man-of-war, sea wasp, sea nettles, true jellyfish, sea anemones, true coral, and soft coral, are responsible for more envenomations than any other marine animals **Figure 22-18 ▼**. The stinging cells of the coelenterate are called nematocysts, and large animals may discharge hundreds of thousands of them. In light-skinned people, envenomation causes very painful, reddish lesions extending in a line from the site of the sting. Systemic symptoms include headache, dizziness, muscle cramps, and fainting.

To treat a sting from the tentacles of a jellyfish, a Portuguese man-of-war, various anemones, corals, or hydras, remove the patient from the water and pour any type of alcohol on the affected area. Unlike fresh water, alcohol will inactivate the nematocysts. Do not try to manipulate the remaining tentacles; this will only cause further discharge of the nematocysts. Remove the tentacles by scraping them off with the edge of a sharp, stiff object such as a credit card. Persistent pain may respond to immersion of the area in hot water (110°F to 115°F, 43°C to 46°C) for 30 minutes. On very rare occasions, a patient may have a systemic allergic reaction to the sting of one of these animals. Treat such a patient for anaphylactic shock. Give BLS, and provide immediate transport to the hospital.

Toxins from the spines of urchins, stingrays, and certain spiny fish such as the lionfish, scorpion fish, and

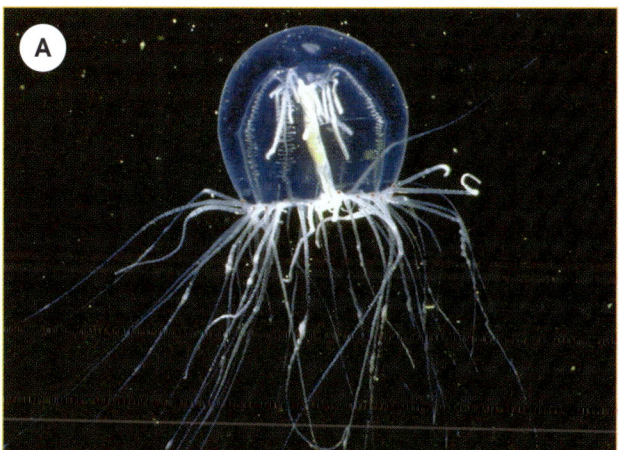

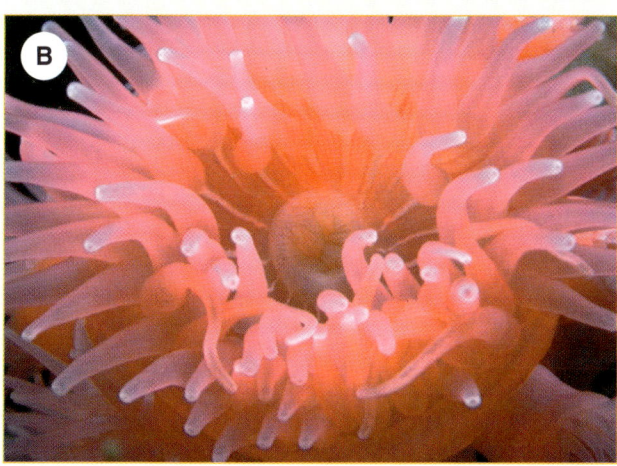

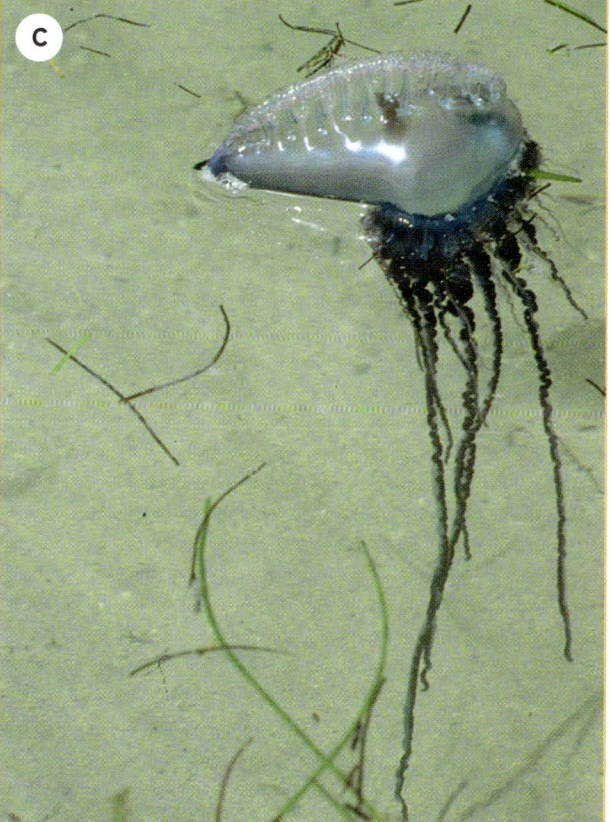

Figure 22-18 Coelenterates are responsible for many marine envenomations. **A.** Jellyfish. **B.** Sea anemone. **C.** Portuguese man-of-war.

stonefish are heat-sensitive (Table 22-4 ▼). Therefore, the best treatment for such injuries is to immobilize the affected area and soak it in hot water for 30 minutes. This will often provide dramatic relief from local pain. However, the patient still needs to be transported to the emergency department, since he or she could develop an allergic reaction or infection, including tetanus.

TABLE 22-4	Common Marine Animals With Toxins
Dogfish	Scorpion fish
Dragon fish	Sea anemone
Fire coral	Sea urchins
Hydroids	Starfish
Jellyfish	Stingray
Lionfish	Stonefish
Marine snail	Tiger fish
Portuguese man-of-war	Toadfish
Ratfish	Weever fish

If you work near the ocean, you should be familiar with the marine life in your area. The emergency treatment of common coelenterate envenomations consists of the following steps:

1. **Limit further discharge** of nematocysts by avoiding fresh water, wet sand, showers, or careless manipulation of the tentacles. Keep the patient calm, and reduce motion of the affected extremity.
2. **Inactivate the nematocysts** by applying alcohol. (Although isopropyl or rubbing alcohol is recommended, virtually any type of alcohol, including high-proof liquor or cologne, is effective.)
3. **Remove the remaining tentacles** by scraping them off with the edge of a sharp, stiff object such as a credit card. Do not use your ungloved hand to remove the tentacles, because self-envenomation may occur. Persistent pain may respond to immersion in hot water (110°F to 115°F, 43°C to 46°C) for 30 minutes.
4. **Provide transport** to the emergency department.

You are the Provider — Summary

1. Why does the time between exposure and reaction often indicate the severity of an allergic reaction?

The quicker the reaction, the more severe it tends to be.

2. What is the primary mechanism of an allergic reaction, and how can it have an impact on airway patency?

Histamine release causes bronchoconstriction, resulting in decreased airflow.

3. What is the first treatment priority?

Oxygenation—In this case a nonrebreathing mask at 15 L/min

4. How should the patient be positioned?

She should be placed in a position of comfort to facilitate breathing and minimize anxiety.

5. What is the term for the red, swollen areas that itch?

Urticaria

6. What can you do to alleviate some of her anxiety?

Talk to her soothingly and reassuringly, allow the teacher to remain with her, and encourage the teacher to assist in calming the patient.

7. What is causing the wheezing?

Constriction of the bronchioles, or lower airway passages

8. Where will you administer the EpiPen?

Lateral thigh, midway between the hip and knee

9. What effects do you expect from the administration of the epinephrine?

Increased heart rate, increased blood pressure, dilated bronchioles

10. What IV fluid would you start for this patient, and at what rate would you run it?

An isotonic crystalloid solution, such as normal saline, is appropriate. The patient is not in need of fluid resuscitation, so an IV lifeline to keep the vein open (or KVO) is all that is needed.

Prep Kit

Ready for Review

- An allergic reaction is a response to chemicals the body releases to combat certain stimuli, called allergens. Allergic reactions occur most often in response to five categories of stimuli: insect bites and stings, medications, food, plants, and chemicals. The reaction may be mild and local, involving itching, redness, and tenderness, or severe and systemic, including shock and respiratory failure.

- Anaphylaxis is a life-threatening allergic reaction mounted by multiple organ systems, which must be treated with epinephrine. Wheezing and skin wheals can be signs of anaphylaxis.

- People who know that they are allergic to bee, hornet, yellow jacket, or wasp venom often carry a bee sting kit that contains epinephrine in an auto-injector. You may help to administer this medication in this form with authorization from medical control. All patients with suspected anaphylaxis require oxygen. In assessing a person who may be having an allergic reaction, check for flushing, itching, and swelling skin; hives; wheezing and stridor; a persistent cough; a decrease in blood pressure; a weak pulse; dizziness; abdominal cramps; and headache.

- Poisonous spiders include the black widow spider and the brown recluse spider. Poisonous snakes include pit vipers, cottonmouths, copperheads, and coral snakes.

- A person who has been bitten by a pit viper needs prompt transport; clean the bite area and keep the patient quiet to slow the spread of venom. Notify the hospital as soon as possible if a patient has been bitten by a coral snake, as its venom can cause paralysis of the nervous system, and most hospitals do not have appropriate antivenin on hand.

- Patients who have been bitten by ticks may be infected with Rocky Mountain spotted fever or Lyme disease and should see a doctor as soon as possible. Remove the tick using tweezers, and save it for identification.

- Dog bites and human bites can both lead to serious infection and must be treated by a physician. Dogs can carry rabies, a fatal viral infection present in their saliva. Vaccination of the patient is necessary to prevent rabies in a person who has been bitten by a dog that cannot be captured or identified. Do not try to rescue a child who is being attacked by a dog without the help of police or animal control officers. By law, all animal bites must be reported to the appropriate authority.

- Remember that a hundred times more people die every year of allergic reactions to food, bee stings, or medications than of bites from venomous snakes or marine animals. Many venomous snake bites may be treated with antivenin. Many marine envenomations may benefit from submersion in hot water to deactivate the heat-sensitive toxins. Such treatment may be started in the field at the request of medical control.

- Always provide prompt transport to the hospital for any patient who is having an allergic reaction or has been bitten by a poisonous insect or animal. Remember that the patient's condition can deteriorate rapidly. Carefully monitor the patient's vital signs en route, especially for airway compromise.

Technology

- Interactivities
- Vocabulary Explorer
- Anatomy Review
- Web Links
- Online Review Manual

Vital Vocabulary

allergen A substance that causes an allergic reaction; also referred to as an antigen.

allergic reaction The body's exaggerated immune response to an internal or surface antigen.

anaphylaxis An extreme, possibly life-threatening systemic allergic reaction that may include shock and respiratory failure.

angioedema Plasma seepage out of the capillaries and into the surrounding tissues; may cause airway swelling and closure in patients with anaphylaxis.

antivenin A serum that counteracts the effect of venom from an animal or insect.

envenomation The act of injecting venom.

epinephrine A substance produced by the body (commonly called adrenaline), and a drug produced by pharmaceutical companies that increases blood pressure and causes bronchodilation; the drug of choice for an anaphylactic reaction.

histamines Substances released by the immune system in allergic reactions that are responsible for many of the symptoms of anaphylaxis.

hypersensitivity Abnormal sensitivity; a condition in which there is an exaggerated response by the body to the stimulus of a foreign agent.

leukotrienes Chemical substances that contribute to anaphylaxis; released by the immune system in allergic reactions.

rabid Describes an animal that is infected with rabies.

stridor A harsh, high-pitched respiratory sound, generally heard during inspiration, that is caused by partial blockage or narrowing of the upper airway.

toxin A poisonous or harmful substance.

urticaria Small spots of generalized itching and/or burning that appear as multiple raised areas on the skin; hives.

wheal A raised, swollen, well-defined area on the skin resulting from an insect bite or allergic reaction.

wheezing A high-pitched, whistling breath sound, caused by bronchoconstriction and typically heard on expiration.

Assessment in Action

You and your partner are dispatched to a local park for a patient with trouble breathing. You arrive at the scene to find a 9-year-old boy in obvious respiratory distress.

His face is swollen and he has hives around his neck. The patient tells you that he is allergic to bees and hornets and he believes that a hornet stung him. He further tells you that he has a prescribed EpiPen but he does not have it with him. You place the patient on oxygen and begin to provide care.

1. An exaggerated immune response to any substance is called:
   - A. an allergic reaction.
   - B. hypersensitivity.
   - C. anaphylaxis.
   - D. envenomation.

2. Chemicals that the body uses to combat a stimulus are called histamines. They are released by:
   - A. mast cells.
   - B. the renal system.
   - C. thrombocytes.
   - D. red blood cells.

3. Anaphylaxis is typically characterized by facial edema, difficulty breathing, and:
   - A. hypertension.
   - B. tachycardia.
   - C. bradycardia.
   - D. severe vomiting.

4. A foreign substance that causes an allergic reaction is called a(n):
   - A. antibiotic.
   - B. antihistamine.
   - C. allergen.
   - D. antibody.

5. Epinephrine works by _____ blood pressure and _____ bronchioles.
   - A. lowering, constricting
   - B. raising, constricting
   - C. raising, dilating
   - D. lowering, dilating

6. When administering epinephrine for anaphylaxis, the EMT-I must be aware of:
   - A. significant bradycardia and respiratory depression.
   - B. significant tachycardia and increased nervousness.
   - C. decreased breathing and decreased blood pressure.
   - D. significant tachycardia and decreased neurologic function.

7. Common signs and symptoms of an allergic reaction include all of the following, EXCEPT:
   - A. tightness in the chest or throat.
   - B. hypertension and bradycardia.
   - C. rapid, labored, or noisy respirations.
   - D. cool, pale skin and dizziness.

8. Approximately ____ of all people are allergic to the venom of the bee, hornet, yellow jacket, or wasp.
   - A. 5%
   - B. 10%
   - C. 15%
   - D. 20%

Points to Ponder

You are dispatched to a private residence for a possible allergic reaction. You arrive at the scene, enter the residence, and find a 20-year-old woman sitting in the living room. She has a rash on her face and neck. Her eyes are swollen and you can hear audible wheezing. The patient tells you that she is allergic to peanuts; however, she hasn't eaten any peanuts. She only had a garden salad for lunch. The patient has a blood pressure of 100/60 mm Hg, a pulse of 128 beats/min, and respirations are 24 breaths/min and labored.

What do you think is wrong with this patient?

What is the appropriate treatment for this patient?

What could have caused the patient to experience this?

Issues: Best Patient Care

Poisonings and Overdose Emergencies

1999 Objectives

Cognitive

5-5.1 Identify appropriate personal protective equipment and scene safety awareness concerns in dealing with toxicologic emergencies. (p 1035)

5-5.2 Identify the appropriate situations in which additional non-EMS resources need to be contacted. (p 1035)

5-5.3 Review the routes of entry of toxic substances into the body. (p 1037)

5-5.4 Discuss the role of the Poison Control Center in the United States. (p 1036)

5-5.5 List the toxic substances that are specific to your region. (p 1041)

5-5.6 Identify the need for rapid intervention and transport of the patient with a toxic substance emergency. (p 1035)

5-5.7 Review the management of toxic substances. (p 1040)

5-5.8 Differentiate among the various treatments and pharmacological interventions in the management of the most common poisonings by inhalation, ingestion, absorption, and injection. (p 1040)

5-5.9 Utilize assessment findings to formulate a field impression and implement a treatment plan for patients with the most common poisonings by inhalation, ingestion, absorption, and injection. (p 1037-1039, 1044)

5-5.10 Review poisoning by overdose. (p 1039)

5-5.11 Review the signs and symptoms related to the most common poisonings by overdose. (p 1035)

5-5.12 Correlate the abnormal findings in assessment with the clinical significance in patients with the most common poisonings by overdose. (p 1039)

5-5.13 Differentiate among the various treatments and pharmacological interventions in the management of the most common poisonings by overdose. (p 1039)

5-5.14 Utilize assessment findings to formulate a field impression and implement a treatment plan for patients with the most common poisonings by overdose. (p 1039)

Affective

5-5.15 Appreciate the psychological needs of victims of drug abuse or overdose. (p 1041)

Psychomotor

None

1985 Objectives

There are no 1985 objectives for this chapter.

23

Poisonings and Overdose Emergencies

You are the Provider

You are dispatched for a possible overdose. Upon arrival you find a 16-year-old girl lying on her bed. Her mother tells you that she has been depressed lately. The mother tells you that her sleeping pills are gone and that it is possible that her daughter may have taken them. This chapter will help you manage those difficult and challenging situations involving poisons and answer the following question.

1. What is your primary responsibility as an EMS provider in this situation?

Substance Abuse and Poisoning

Every day, each of us comes into contact with things that are potentially poisonous. This is not surprising when you consider that almost any substance may be a poison in certain circumstances. Different doses can turn even a remedy into a poison. Consider aspirin, which, when taken in recommended doses, is a safe and effective analgesic. Too much aspirin, however, can result in death.

Acute poisoning affects some 5 million children and adults each year. Chronic poisoning, often caused by abuse of medications and other substances, including tobacco, is much more common. Fortunately, deaths from poisoning are fairly rare. Rates of death from poisoning for children have decreased steadily since the 1960s, when safety caps were introduced for drug bottles and containers. Deaths from poisoning in adults, though, have been rising; the majority are the result of drug abuse.

Unintentional poisonings include the following:

- **Dosage errors**—These may be the result of an error on the part of the physician prescribing the medication, the person administering the medication in a health care setting (such as a nurse or an EMT-I), or simply an error on the part of the patient or family member. Elderly patients may have a problem reading the prescription label or may forget they have already taken their medication, resulting in an inadvertent overdose.
- **Idiosyncratic reactions**—These are peculiar or individual reactions to a drug or some other substance; one person reacts differently from another.
- **Childhood poisoning**—Children are naturally curious. Flavored medications, designed to improve the taste, and those shaped like cartoon characters are appealing. Unsupervised children may help themselves to their medications, resulting in an overdose. In large doses, preparations such as iron tablets may be fatal to a young child.
- **Environmental exposure**—Patients may unwittingly be exposed to toxins in their everyday environment. Carbon monoxide poisoning may occur from an old furnace or heater in an enclosed area, sprayed pesticides may expose the person to organophosphates, and large fires may lead to smoke inhalation.
- **Occupational exposures**—People working near chemicals should take the necessary precautions to protect themselves from exposure. The employer should provide personal protective equipment. Failure to take protective measures could result in an accidental exposure.
- **Neglect and abuse**—This category includes actions such as exposing a child to a toxic substance, without regard to the fact that it has been proven to be detrimental to health.

Drug and alcohol abuse generally fall under the category of "unintentional poisoning," even though the patient understands it is a possibility. What starts out as recreational use may progress to the point of accidental overdose because of impaired judgment from use of these substances.

Intentional poisoning and overdoses include the following:

- **Chemical warfare**—Our biggest concern used to be the development of nuclear arms. These weapons have now taken a backseat with the introduction of poisonous chemicals that may be introduced via venting systems, spraying, or even the postal service.
- **Assault and homicide**—Chemicals used for assault may render the victim helpless, as in the case of pepper spray, allowing the perpetrator to escape. Other chemicals, such as arsenic, may be added to food or drink in an attempted murder.
- **Suicide attempts**—People who want to kill themselves in a less violent manner may take an overdose of prescription or over-the-counter medications. Alcohol and sleeping pills are a popular combination. The person hopes he or she will simply go to sleep and not wake up. With any

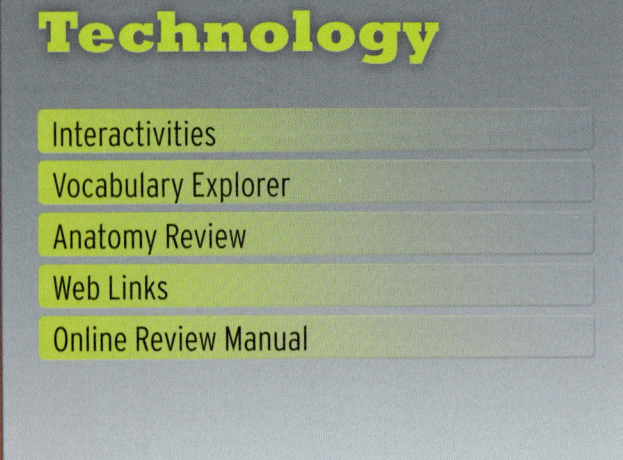

deliberate exposure to an excessive amount of any drug, consider that it may be a suicide attempt.

In this chapter, the term "poisoned" includes acute and chronic poisonings. As an EMT-I, you must recognize that patients with either type of problem may have a variety of injuries. Although you cannot stop a long-term substance abuse problem, you may be able to prevent death from the acute effects of the poison.

This chapter discusses how to identify the patient who has been poisoned and how to gather clues about the poison. It describes the different ways in which poison is introduced into the body. It then discusses the signs, symptoms, and treatment of specific poisons, including sedatives and opioids (narcotic medicines with actions similar to morphine). Food poisoning and plant poisoning are also discussed.

Identifying the Patient and the Poison

A poison is any substance with a chemical action that can damage body structures or impair body function. A poison can be introduced into the body through a variety of means. Poisons act by changing the normal metabolism of cells or by destroying them outright. Poisons may act acutely, as in an overdose of heroin, or chronically, as in years of alcohol or other substance abuse. Substance abuse is the misuse, usually knowingly, of any substance to produce a desired effect (for example, cocaine intoxication).

Your primary responsibility is to yourself and your partner by ensuring scene safety. It is imperative to recognize the potential for any personal exposure and to take necessary precautions to prevent it. This includes airway protection, body substance isolation precautions, and the use of any other specialized equipment needed. If you are not trained in these areas, you should recognize the need for additional resources and alert your dispatcher. Hazardous materials teams are specially trained to deal with all types of potentially dangerous exposures. Law enforcement may be required for assistance with maintaining control of a scene, and fire services may be used for fire suppression or decontamination. In the event of entrapment, rescue units may also be needed.

Your primary responsibility to the patient who has been poisoned is to recognize that a poisoning has occurred. Keep in mind that very small amounts of some poisons can cause considerable damage or death. If you have even the slightest suspicion that a patient has taken a poisonous substance, you should notify medical control and begin emergency treatment at once.

Symptoms and signs of poisoning vary according to the specific agent, as shown in Table 23-1. Some poisons cause tachycardia, while others cause bradycardia; some cause the pupils to dilate, while others cause the pupils to constrict. If respiration is depressed or difficult, cyanosis may occur. Some chemical compounds will irritate or burn the skin or mucous membranes, resulting in burning or blistering. The presence of such injuries at the mouth strongly suggests the ingestion (swallowing) of a poison, such as lye. If possible, ask the patient the following questions:

- What substance did you take (or were you exposed to)?
- When did you take it (or become exposed to it)?

TABLE 23-1	Toxidromes: Typical Signs and Symptoms of Specific Drug Overdoses
Opioids and Opiates	Hypoventilation and respiratory arrest Constricted pupils (miosis) Sedation and coma Hypotension Bradycardia
Sympathomimetics	Hypertension Tachycardia Dilated pupils (mydriasis) Agitation and seizures Hyperthermia
Sedatives and Hypnotics	Slurred speech Sedation and coma Hypoventilation and respiratory arrest Hypotension Bradycardia
Anticholinergics	Tachycardia Hyperthermia Hypertension Dilated pupils (mydriasis) Dry skin and mucous membranes Sedation, agitation, seizures, coma, and delirium Decreased bowel sounds
Cholinergics	Excess defecation and urination Muscle fasciculations Constricted pupils (miosis) Excess lacrimation and salivation Airway compromise Nausea and vomiting

- How much did you ingest?
- What actions have been taken before EMS arrival?
- How much do you weigh?

Try to determine the nature of the poison. Objects at the scene may provide clues: an empty bottle, a needle or syringe, scattered pills, chemicals, even an overturned or damaged plant. The remains of any nearby food or drink may also be important. Place any "suspicious" material in a plastic bag, and take it to the hospital, along with any containers you find.

Containers can provide critical information. In addition to the name and concentration of the drug, a pill bottle label may list specific ingredients, the number of pills that were originally in the bottle, the name of the manufacturer, and the dose that was prescribed. This information can help emergency department physicians determine how much has been ingested and what specific treatment may be required. For certain food poisonings, a food container that lists the name and location of the maker or the vendor may be of equal importance

EMT-I Tips

Poison Centers

There are several hundred poison centers in the United States. The phone number of your local poison center is typically found on the inside cover of your local phone book. The telephone number for the National Poison Control Center is 1-800-222-1222. Staff members at every center have access to information about virtually all of the commonly used medications, chemicals, and substances that could possibly be poisonous. They know the appropriate emergency treatment for each, including the antidote, if there is one. An <u>antidote</u> is a substance that will counteract the effects of a particular poison.

If you believe that a patient has been poisoned, you should immediately provide medical control with all relevant information: when the poisoning occurred; a description of the suspected poison, including the amount involved; and the patient's size, weight, and age. If necessary, medical control can contact the regional poison center and relay specific instructions back to you.

A medical toxicologist is a physician who specializes in caring for patients who have been poisoned. About 100 of these specialists work in specialty hospitals called medical toxicology treatment centers, located throughout the United States. At times, your medical control may divert a patient who meets certain poisoning criteria to one of these centers instead of to the closest hospital.

You and your medical control center should know the telephone number of your regional poison center and have it available in case you respond to a call for a poisoning.

You are the Provider — Part 2

As you begin your initial assessment of the patient, you note the following:

Initial Assessment	Recording Time: Zero Minutes
Appearance	Pale
Level of consciousness	Responds appropriately to painful stimuli
Airway	Open; breathing loudly
Breathing	Respirations, slow and deep
Circulation	Radial pulses, slow; skin, warm and dry to touch

2. What is the first treatment priority for this patient?
3. What are some of the ways that poisons can enter the body?

in saving the life of the patient and possibly other people who may potentially ingest the same food.

If the patient vomits, collect the material, called vomitus, in a separate plastic bag so that it can be analyzed at the hospital. After providing emergency care, collecting and bagging suspicious materials and vomitus may be the most important thing you can do for the patient. Positive identification of the substance can prevent unnecessary delays in further treatment of the patient.

How Poisons Get Into the Body

Emergency care for the patient who has been poisoned may include a range of actions from reassuring an anxious parent to instituting CPR. Most often, it will not include administering a specific antidote, because most poisons do not have one. Therefore, in general, the most important treatment for poisoning is diluting and/or physically removing the poisonous agent. How you do this depends on how the poison gets into the patient's body in the first place. The four routes of absorption of poisons into the body are as follows:

- Ingestion Figure 23-1A ▼
- Inhalation Figure 23-1B ▼
- Injection Figure 23-1C ▼
- Absorption (surface contact) Figure 23-1D ▼

Injection often can be the most worrisome route of poisoning. You can administer oxygen to a patient who has inhaled a poison, and you can give activated charcoal to one who has ingested a poison. You can flood the skin with water and wash out the eyes of one who has contacted a poison. However, you cannot remove or dilute injected poisons, a fact that makes these cases especially urgent. On the other hand, all routes of poisoning can be deadly, and each should be thought of as being equally serious.

Always consult medical control before you proceed with the treatment of any poisoning victim.

Ingested Poisons

Approximately 80% of all poisonings are by mouth (ingestion). Ingested poisons include liquids, household cleaners, contaminated food, plants, and, in the majority of cases, drugs. Poisoning by ingestion is usually accidental in children and, except for contaminated

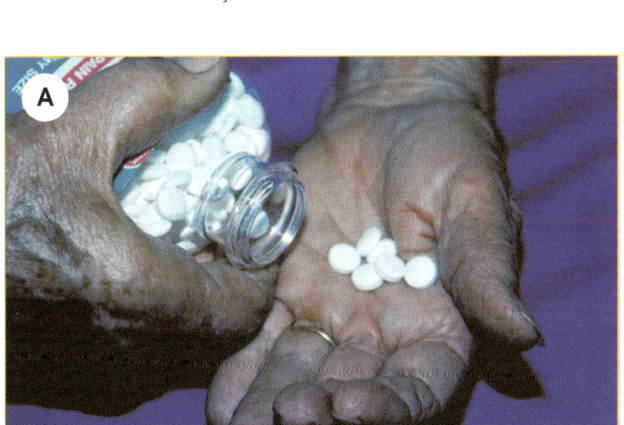
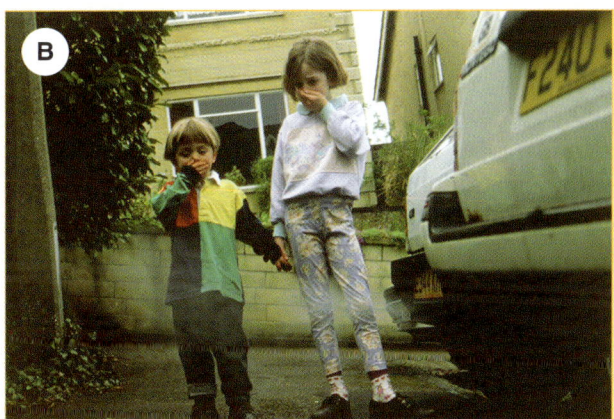
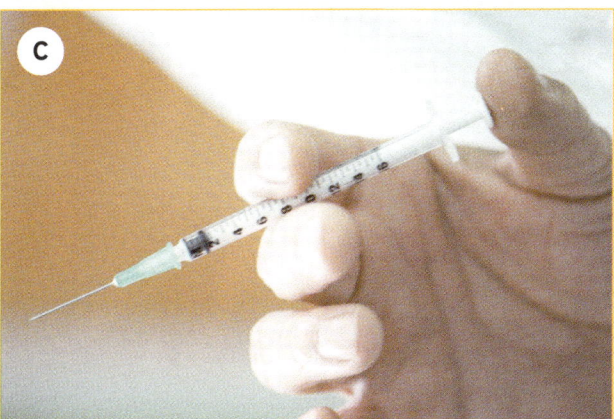
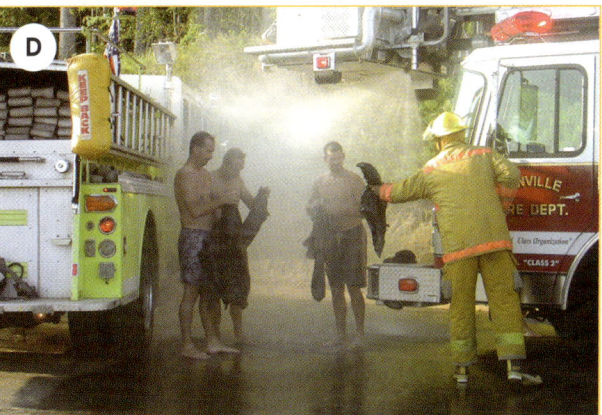

Figure 23-1 There are four routes by which a poison can enter the body. **A.** Ingestion. **B.** Inhalation. **C.** Injection. **D.** Absorption (surface contact).

food, deliberate in adults. Plant poisonings are common among children, who like to explore and often bite the leaves of various bushes or shrubs.

Your goal as an EMT-I is to rapidly remove as much of the poison as possible from the gastrointestinal tract. For most poisoning victims, this emergency treatment is sufficient.

In the past, syrup of ipecac was used to induce vomiting, but it is no longer recommended. Syrup of ipecac is usually not carried on ambulances. Today, many EMS systems allow you to carry activated charcoal on your unit. Activated charcoal is supplied as a suspension that binds to the poison in the stomach and delays digestion. Delayed digestion of the poison will buy some time until it can be removed at the hospital by gastric lavage. Therefore, it is more effective and safer than syrup of ipecac. Because activated charcoal is an inky, messy fluid, you may have to do some coaxing to get the patient to drink it; try to give it in a covered cup with a straw Figure 23-2 . Remember, you should never force this (or any other) liquid into a patient's mouth, nor should you administer any solution by mouth if the patient is not awake and alert enough to swallow it.

Although every poison will result in a specific set of symptoms and signs, you should always assess the airway, breathing, and circulation of every patient who has been poisoned. Many patients have died as a result of problems with ABC that might have been managed easily. Be prepared to provide aggressive ventilatory support and CPR to a patient who has ingested an opiate, sedative, or barbiturate, each of which can cause depression of the central nervous system (CNS), resulting in respiratory and cardiovascular depression. Whenever poisoning is involved, you should provide prompt transport to the emergency department. The patient may need other treatments that can be given only in the hospital. Paramedic backup also may be a good idea, as these providers often carry and can administer additional medications and therapies.

EMT-I Tips

While one EMT-I explains the use of activated charcoal, the other can prepare a large plastic garbage bag to hang on the patient as a bib. This will help contain the charcoal solution if the patient vomits.

Inhaled Poisons

Patients who have inhaled poison, including natural gas, certain pesticides, carbon monoxide, chlorine, or other gases, should be moved to a safe environment immediately Figure 23-3 . After the patient has been removed, assess ABCs and provide 100% supplemental oxygen or ventilatory support as needed. If you are performing the rescue, use a self-contained breathing apparatus to protect yourself from poisonous fumes. Remember that once patients are removed from the toxic environment, they are not toxic to you. However, make certain that only trained rescuers remove the patient from the poisonous environment.

Some inhaled poisons, such as carbon monoxide, are odorless and produce severe hypoxia without damaging or even irritating the lungs. Others, such as chlorine, are

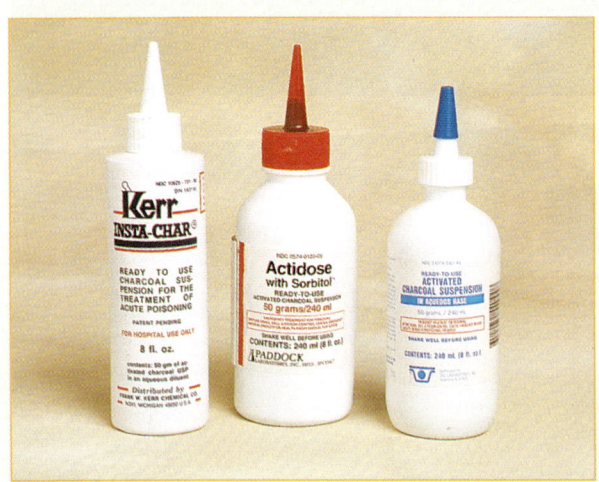

Figure 23-2 Activated charcoal comes as a premixed suspension that you should give, if local protocol allows, in a covered cup with a straw.

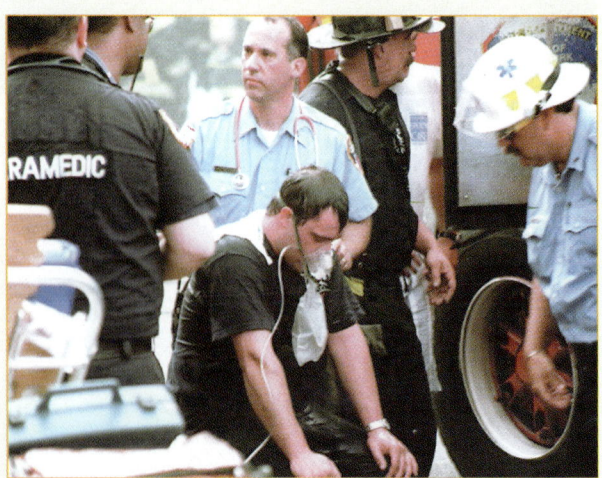

Figure 23-3 Patients who have inhaled poisons need 100% supplemental oxygen and prompt transport to the emergency department.

very irritating and cause swelling-induced airway obstruction and pulmonary edema. The patient may report the following signs and symptoms: burning eyes, sore throat, cough, chest pain, hoarseness, wheezing, respiratory distress, dizziness, confusion, and headache; in severe cases, you might note stridor. The patient may also have seizures or altered mental status. Some inhaled agents cause progressive lung damage, even after the patient is removed from direct exposure; the damage may not be evident for a few hours. Meanwhile, it may take 2 or 3 days or more of intensive care to reestablish normal lung function. For this reason, all patients who have inhaled poison require immediate transport to an emergency department. Provide 100% supplemental oxygen via nonrebreathing mask and, if necessary, ventilatory support with a bag-valve-mask device. Make sure a suctioning unit is available in case the patient vomits. As with other poisonings, it is helpful to take containers, bottles, and labels when you transport the patient to the hospital.

Injected Poisons

Poisoning by injection is almost always the result of a deliberate drug overdose, such as heroin or cocaine **Figure 23-4**. Contrary to the situations portrayed by television detectives, the only other parties who are likely to have injected a patient with poison are insects and animals.

Signs and symptoms of poisoning by injection can have a multitude of presentations, including weakness, dizziness, fever, chills, easy excitability, or unresponsiveness.

In general, injected poisons are impossible to dilute or remove, as they are usually absorbed quickly into the body or cause intense local tissue destruction. If you suspect that rapid absorption has occurred, monitor the patient's airway, provide 100% supplemental oxygen, and be alert for nausea and vomiting. Remove rings, watches, and bracelets from areas around the injection site if swelling occurs. Prompt transport to the emergency department is essential. Take all containers, bottles, and labels with the patient to the hospital.

Absorbed (Surface Contact) Poisons

Many corrosive substances will damage the skin, mucous membranes, or eyes, causing chemical burns, telltale rashes, or lesions. Acids, alkalis, and some petroleum (hydrocarbon) products are very destructive, and relatively small amounts can cause significant skin damage. Signs and symptoms of absorbed poisoning include a history of exposure, liquid or powder on the patient's skin, burns, itching, irritation, redness of the skin in light-skinned individuals, and typical odors of the substance.

Emergency treatment for a typical contact poisoning includes the following two steps:

1. Avoid contaminating yourself or others.
2. Remove the irritating or corrosive substance from the patient as rapidly as possible.

Remove all clothing that has been contaminated with poisons or irritating substances, thoroughly brush off any dry chemicals, flush the skin with running water, and then wash the skin with soap and water. When a large amount of material has been spilled on a patient, flooding the affected part for at least 20 minutes may be the fastest and most effective treatment. *If the patient has a chemical agent in the eyes, you should irrigate them quickly and thoroughly, at least 5 to 10 minutes for acid substances and 15 to 20 minutes for alkalis.* As you irrigate the eyes,

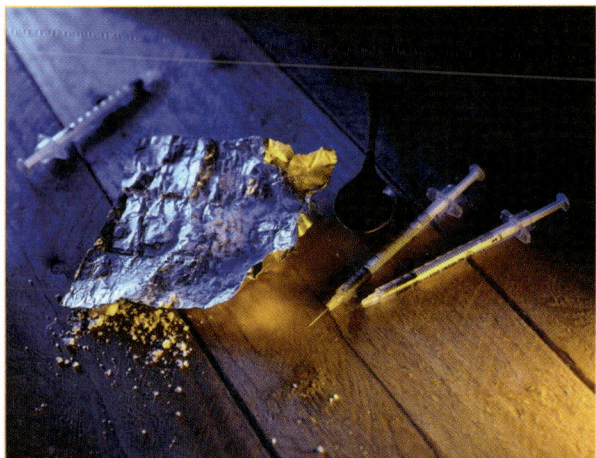

Figure 23-4 Injected poisons are impossible to dilute or remove from the body; therefore, prompt transport to the emergency department is critical.

EMT-I Safety

To minimize contamination from a patient who has had contact with a hazardous substance, one EMT-I should stay fully protected and assist the patient. This EMT-I is considered "contaminated." The other EMT-I should stay clear and have as little contact as possible, to be able to provide what is needed and drive without contaminating equipment and the front of the vehicle.

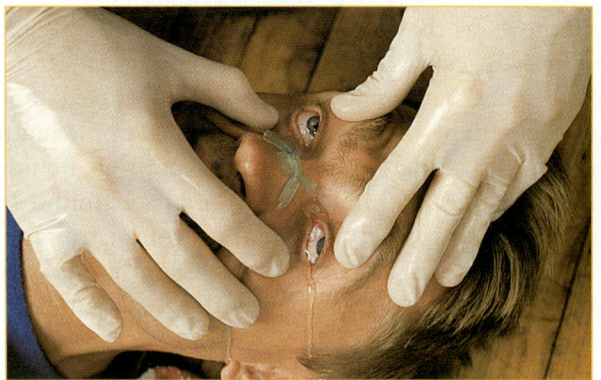

Figure 23-5 If a chemical agent is in the patient's eyes, irrigate the eyes quickly and thoroughly, ensuring that the irrigation fluid runs outward from the bridge of the nose. (Use of a nasal cannula is pictured.)

> **Documentation Tips**
>
> Take time at the scene to make thorough and legible notes about the nature of the poisoning. You can then quickly state the type and amount of substance and the time and route of exposure in your radio, verbal, and written reports. Busy hospital staff will also appreciate clear notes that can be handed over on arrival.

make sure that the fluid flows outward from the bridge of the nose to avoid inadvertent contamination of the other eye Figure 23-5 . Be sure to place a towel around the head to absorb the water and prevent it from draining into the ears.

Many chemical burns occur in industrial settings, where showers and specific protocols for handling surface burns are available. If you are called to such a scene, trained personnel will usually be there to assist you. Do not spend time trying to neutralize substances on the skin with additional chemicals. This may actually be more harmful. Instead, wash the substance off immediately with copious amounts of water.

The only time you should not irrigate the contact area with water is when a poison reacts violently with water, such as phosphorus or elemental sodium. These substances ignite when they come into contact with water. Instead, brush the chemical off the patient, remove contaminated clothing, and apply a dry dressing to any burned area. Be sure to wear gloves and the proper protective clothing.

Provide prompt transport to the emergency department for definitive care. En route, continue irrigation and provide oxygen if possible.

> **In the Field**
>
> Flush with copious amounts of water immediately if the chemical is "wet." If the chemical is "dry," be sure to brush it off the skin before flushing with water. Do not use water if the chemical is phosphorous or sodium.

Emergency Medical Care

External decontamination is important. Remove tablets or fragments from the patient's mouth, wash or brush poison from the patient's skin, and monitor the patient's breathing. Treatment focuses on support: assessing and maintaining the patient's ABCs. Gain intravenous (IV) access on any patient suspected of being exposed to poisons.

In some cases, you will give activated charcoal to patients who have ingested poison, if approved by medical control or local protocol. *Charcoal is not indicated for patients who have ingested an acid, alkali, or petroleum product; who have a decreased level of consciousness; or who are unable to swallow.*

Remember that activated charcoal adsorbs, or sticks to, many commonly ingested poisons, preventing the toxin (poison) from being absorbed into the body by the stomach or intestines. If local protocol permits, you will likely carry plastic bottles of premixed suspension, each containing up to 50 g of activated charcoal. Common trade names for the suspension are InstaChar, Actidose, and LiquiChar. The usual dose for an adult or child is 1 g of activated charcoal per kilogram of body weight. The usual adult dose is 25 to 50 g, and the usual pediatric dose is 12.5 to 25 g.

Before you give a patient charcoal, obtain approval from medical control. Next, shake the bottle vigorously to mix the suspension. The medication looks like mud, so it is best to cover the outside of the container so that the fluid is not visible and ask the patient to drink with a straw. You might need to persuade the patient to drink it, particularly if the patient is a child, but never force it. If the patient takes a long time to drink the mixture, you will have to shake the container frequently to keep the suspension from separating. Be sure to record the time when you administered the activated charcoal.

The major side effect of ingesting activated charcoal is black stools. A patient who has ingested a poison that causes nausea may vomit after taking activated charcoal, and the dose may have to be repeated. As you reassess the patient, be prepared for vomiting, nausea, and possible airway problems.

Geography-specific Toxic Emergencies

While some toxins are found in all areas of the country, others are specific only to certain geographic locations. These include environment-specific examples such as venomous snakes, spiders, and various sea creatures. These are covered in more detail in Chapter 22: Allergic Reactions and Envenomations. Other geographic-specific toxins include those associated with chemical manufacturing plants and transportation routes such as rail and highway.

Specific Poisons

Over time, a person who routinely misuses a substance needs increasing amounts of it to achieve the same result. This is called developing a tolerance to the substance. Increasing tolerance can lead to addiction. A person with an addiction has an overwhelming desire or need to continue using the agent, at whatever cost, with a tendency to increase the dosage. Addiction is not exclusive to the classic drugs of abuse, such as cocaine. Almost any substance can be abused, including laxatives, nasal decongestants, vitamins, and food.

The importance of body substance isolation precautions in caring for victims of drug abuse cannot be stressed enough. Known drug abusers have a fairly high incidence of serious and undiagnosed infections, including human immunodeficiency virus and hepatitis. These patients may bite, spit, hit, or otherwise injure you, causing you to come into contact with their blood and other body fluids. Always be sure to wear appropriate protective equipment. Use extreme caution when handling these patients and their belongings. Uncapped used needles, razor blades, and other sharp items may be found in pockets or belongings and pose a threat to the rescuer. A calm, professional approach can defuse frightening situations, but keep your safety and that of your team in the forefront of your mind. Expect the unexpected and remember: The drug user, not the drug, can pose the greatest threat.

Grouping Toxicologically Similar Agents

By grouping the agents together that are toxicologically similar, it is easier to remember the assessment and management of toxicologic emergencies. Regardless of the incident, personal safety and the ABCs are always the first considerations. Specific antidotes apply in some situations, but the basics are clearly the most important. Even though several drugs produce similar clinical patterns, grouping of these agents does not take into consideration how or why the toxin has been introduced into the body. Be sure to include the general management based on route of entry in addition to specific treatments.

Alcohol

The most commonly abused drug in the United States is ethyl alcohol (sometimes called ETOH). It affects people from all walks of life and results in more than 200,000 deaths each year. More than 50% of all traffic deaths and injuries, 67% of murders, and 33% of suicides are related to alcohol, which impairs a person's ability to think and function rationally. Alcoholism is one of the greatest national health problems, along with heart disease, cancer, and stroke.

Initially, alcohol is a CNS stimulant; however, in higher doses, it is a powerful CNS depressant. It is a sedative, a substance that decreases activity and excitement, and a hypnotic, a substance that induces sleep. In general, alcohol dulls the sense of awareness, slows reflexes, and reduces reaction time. It may also cause aggressive and inappropriate behavior and lack of coordination. However, a person who appears intoxicated may have other medical problems as well. Look for signs of head trauma, toxic reactions, or uncontrolled diabetes. Severe acute alcohol intoxication may cause hypoglycemia, which may contribute to the symptoms. At the very least, you should assume that all intoxicated patients are experiencing a drug overdose and will require thorough examination by a physician. In most states, such patients cannot legally refuse treatment or transport.

If a patient exhibits signs of serious CNS depression, you must provide respiratory support. This may be difficult, however, because depression of the respiratory system can also cause emesis, or vomiting. The vomiting may be very forceful or even bloody (hematemesis), since large amounts of alcohol irritate the stomach. Internal bleeding should also be considered if the patient appears to be in shock (hypoperfusion), as blood might not clot effectively in a patient who has a prolonged history of alcohol abuse.

A patient in alcohol withdrawal may experience frightening hallucinations or delirium tremens (DTs), a syndrome characterized by restlessness, fever, sweating, disorientation, agitation, and even seizures. These conditions may develop if patients no longer ingest the usual daily quantity of alcohol. Alcoholic hallucinations come and go. A patient with an otherwise fairly clear mental state may see fantastic shapes or figures or hear odd voices. Such auditory and visual hallucinations often precede DTs, which are a much more severe complication.

Delirium tremens may develop 1 to 7 days after a person stops drinking or when consumption levels are decreased suddenly. Again, patients may experience one or more of the following signs and symptoms:

- Agitation and restlessness
- Fever
- Sweating
- Confusion, disorientation, or both
- Delusions, hallucinations, or both
- Seizures

Provide prompt transport for these patients after you have completed your assessment and provided necessary care. A person who is experiencing hallucinations or DTs is extremely ill. Should seizures develop, treat them as you would any other seizure. The patient should not be restrained, although you must protect the patient from self-injury. Give the patient oxygen and watch carefully for vomiting. Hypovolemia may develop from sweating, fluid loss, insufficient fluid intake, or vomiting associated with DTs. If you see signs of hypovolemic shock, elevate the patient's legs 6″ to 12″, clear the airway, and turn the head to one side to minimize the chance of aspiration during transport. Establish an IV, and give a 20-mL/kg bolus of an isotonic crystalloid solution, such as normal saline. Patients experiencing DTs may not respond appropriately to suggestions or conversation, as they are often confused and frightened. Therefore, your approach should be calm and relaxed. Reassure the patient and provide emotional support.

Narcotics and Opiates

The pain relievers called opioid analgesics are named for the opium in poppy seeds, the origin of heroin, codeine, and morphine. On the list of frequently abused drugs, they have been joined by a number of synthetic opioids (opiates), with origins in the laboratory. These include meperidine (Demerol), hydromorphone (Dilaudid), propoxyphene (Darvon), oxycodone (Percocet), hydrocodone (Vicodin), fentanyl, and methadone Table 23-2. Most of these drugs have legitimate medical uses. With the exception of heroin, which is illegal in the United States, many addicts may have started using any of the opioids with an appropriate medical prescription.

Opioids, also referred to as narcotics, are CNS depressants and can cause severe respiratory depression. When administered intravenously, and in therapeutic doses, they produce a characteristic euphoric "high" or "kick." Tolerance develops rapidly, so some users may require increasing doses to experience the same effect. In general, emergency medical problems related to opioids are caused by respiratory depression, including a decreased volume of inspired air and decreased respirations, or respiratory arrest. Patients typically appear sedated and cyanotic and have constricted (pinpoint) pupils. They may also have hypotension, bradycardia, nausea, seizures, or may be in a coma.

Treatment includes supporting the ABCs. You may try to arouse patients by talking loudly to them or shaking them gently. Always give 100% supplemental oxygen, or assist ventilation as needed, and be prepared for vomiting. Many home remedies are believed to reverse the respiratory depression associated with heroin overdose, including applying ice to the groin or forcing milk into the mouth. *These are not effective therapies and frequently complicate the clinical picture.* Nevertheless, you should be aware that a patient's family or friends might have attempted inappropriate methods of resuscitation. The only effective antidotes to reverse the symptoms and signs of opioid overdose are certain narcotic antagonists such as naloxone (Narcan).

Patients will respond to naloxone within 2 minutes when it is given intravenously. Establish an IV of an isotonic crystalloid solution and give 1 to 2 mg of naloxone via IV push after contacting medical control for permis-

TABLE 23-2	Common Opioid Drugs
Butorphanol (Stadol)	Meperidine (Demerol)
Codeine	Methadone (Dolophine)
Fentanyl derivatives ("China White")	Morphine
Heroin	Oxycodone (Percodan)
Hydrocodone (Hycodan)	Pentazocine (Talwin)
Hydromorphone (Dilaudid)	Propoxyphene (Darvon)

sion. Place the patient on a cardiac monitor and be alert for dysrhythmias that may develop. Be alert for possible adverse side effects such as combativeness, increased blood pressure, tremors, nausea and vomiting, ventricular fibrillation, sweating, and tachycardia. Notify medical control of any side effects, and initiate appropriate actions. Transport promptly to the closest, most appropriate facility, providing psychological support en route.

Sedative-Hypnotic Drugs

Barbiturates and benzodiazepines have been used therapeutically for a long time. They are easy to obtain and relatively inexpensive. People sometimes solicit prescriptions from several physicians for the same hypnotics or a variety of sedative-hypnotic drugs. These drugs are CNS depressants and alter the level of consciousness, with effects similar to those of alcohol, so that the patient may appear drowsy, peaceful, or intoxicated (Table 23-3). By themselves, these drugs do not relieve pain, nor do they produce a specific high, although users often take alcohol or an opioid at the same time to boost their effects.

In general, these agents are taken by mouth. Occasionally, however, contents of capsules are suspended or dissolved in water and injected to produce a rather sudden state of ease and contentment. Unfortunately, use of IV sedative-hypnotic drugs quickly induces tolerance, so an individual requires increasingly larger doses. As a result, you are less likely to be called on to treat an acute overdose in someone who chronically abuses these drugs. However, you may be called to a scene of an attempted suicide in which the patient has taken large quantities of these drugs. In these situations, patients will have marked respiratory depression, hypotension, and bradycardia; in severe cases, the patient will be in a coma.

Sedative-hypnotic drugs may also be given to unsuspecting people as a "knock-out" drink, or "Mickey Finn." More recently, drugs such as flunitrazepam (Rohypnol), which produces an amnesiac effect, have been abused as a "date rape drug," causing the unwary individual to become sedated and even unresponsive. The individual later begins to awaken, confused and unable to remember what happened.

In general, your treatment of patients who have overdosed with sedative-hypnotic drugs and have respiratory depression is to maintain a patent airway, provide ventilatory assistance with 100% oxygen, and prompt transport. You may attempt to stimulate the person by speaking loudly or gently shaking him or her.

As with any patient who is under the influence of a CNS depressant drug, be alert for vomiting.

A specific antidote is available for acute benzodiazepine overdose. It is called flumazenil (Romazicon) and is given intravenously. Although it will reverse the sedation and respiratory depression of the benzodiazepine sedative-hypnotic drugs, it will have no effect on the signs and symptoms of overdose from ethyl alcohol, barbiturates, or narcotics. Flumazenil is typically administered in the hospital after a physician's assessment. As multidrug use becomes more common, you may find it increasingly difficult to determine what agents the patients have taken. Your best approach is to treat any obvious injuries or illnesses, keeping in mind that drug use may complicate the clinical picture and make full life support necessary. Focus on the ABCs, especially the possibility of airway problems (relaxation of the tongue, causing obstruction), vomiting, respiratory depression, and, in severe cases, cardiac arrest. Gain IV access, and promptly transport the patient to the closest appropriate facility.

Monitor the cardiac rhythm of any patient who has overdosed on a CNS depressant drug and treat arrhythmias following standard ACLS protocols. Be prepared to intubate the patient to protect their airway.

TABLE 23-3 Examples of Sedative-Hypnotic Drugs

Barbiturates	Benzodiazepines	Others
Amobarbital	Alprazolam (Xanax)	Carisoprodol (Soma)
Butabarbital	Chlordiazepoxide (Librium)	Chloral hydrate ("Mickey Finn")
Pentobarbital	Diazepam (Valium)	Cyclobenzaprine (Flexeril)
Phenobarbital	Flunitrazepam (Rohypnol)	Ethchlorvynol (Placidyl)
Secobarbital	Lorazepam (Ativan)	Ethyl alcohol (drinking alcohol)
	Oxazepam (Serax)	Glutethimide (Doriden)
	Temazepam (Restoril)	Hydrocarbon inhalants
		Isopropyl alcohol (rubbing alcohol)
		Meprobamate (Equagesic)

Psychiatric Medications

Tricyclic antidepressants are yet another form of therapeutic medications that are frequently abused. They are commonly prescribed for such conditions as depression, ADHD (attention-deficit/hyperactivity disorder), migraine headaches, Tourette syndrome, bed-wetting, obsessive-compulsive disorder (also called OCD), and panic disorders. Common tricyclic antidepressants include amitriptyline (Elavil), amoxapine (Asendin), clomipramine (Anafranil), doxepin (Sinequan), imipramine (Tofranil), and nortriptyline (Aventyl).

Tricyclic antidepressant actions are associated with increasing the available levels of the neurotransmitters serotonin and norepinephrine in the brain. They are effective for most people with serious depression, but produce a number of troublesome and potentially serious side effects. Tricyclic antidepressants often cause dry mouth, dizziness, urinary retention, delirium, constipation, orthostatic hypotension, and tachyarrhythmias; heart block can occur in patients with cardiac disease. The degree of side effects varies with each drug taken. Side effects may be additive with opioids or alcohol. Findings vary, depending on the drug taken, the dose, and the time since ingestion (Table 23-4 ▶).

Management of the toxic effects of tricyclic antidepressants starts with personal safety and assessment of the ABCs. Provide 100% supplemental oxygen and ventilatory support as needed. Establish IV access, and give a 20-mL/kg bolus of an isotonic crystalloid solution for patients who present with hypotension. Place the patient in a position of comfort, and provide psychological support. Transport immediately to the closest appropriate facility. Monitor vital signs en route, and advise medical control of any changes.

Abused Inhalants

Many abused inhalants produce several of the same CNS effects as other sedative-hypnotic drugs, but these agents are inhaled instead of ingested or injected. Some of the more common agents include acetone, toluene, xylene, and hexane, which are found in glues, cleaning compounds, paint thinners, and lacquers. Similarly, gasoline and various halogenated hydrocarbons, such as Freon, used as propellants in aerosol sprays, are also abused as inhalants. None of these inhalants are used for therapeutic purposes. Since these are products that can be bought in hardware stores, teenagers seeking a high like that obtained from alcohol commonly abuse them.

Always use special care in dealing with a patient who may have used inhalants. Their effects range from mild drowsiness to coma, but unlike most other sedative-hypnotic drugs, these agents may often cause seizures. In addition, halogenated hydrocarbon solvents can make the heart highly sensitive to the patient's own adrenaline, putting the patient at high risk for sudden cardiac death from

TABLE 23-4	Assessment Findings After Ingestion of Tricyclic Antidepressants
Early findings: ■ Dry mouth ■ Confusion ■ Hallucinations	Late findings: ■ Delirium ■ Respiratory depression ■ Hypotension ■ Hyperthermia ■ Seizures ■ Coma ■ Dysrhythmias

You are the Provider — Part 3

As you continue your assessment of this patient, you obtain the following:

Vital Signs	Recording Time: 2 Minutes After Patient Contact
Skin	Pale and cool to touch
Pulse rate/quality	42 beats/min, weak
Blood pressure	90/56 mm Hg
Respiratory rate/depth	8 breaths/min, shallow

4. What is your next step?

ventricular fibrillation (V-fib); even the action of walking may release enough adrenaline to cause a fatal ventricular arrhythmia. You must try to keep such patients from struggling with you or exerting themselves. Administer 100% supplemental oxygen, and use a stretcher to move the patient. Never allow such patients to walk to the ambulance. Prompt transport to the hospital is essential; establish IV access, and monitor vital signs en route.

Place the patient on a cardiac monitor and treat any arrhythmias according to standard ACLS protocols.

Carbon Monoxide

Carbon monoxide (CO) poisoning is common after exposure to fire or smoke in an enclosed space, improperly functioning space heaters, and inhalation of exhaust fumes in an automobile that is not well ventilated. Because carbon monoxide is colorless, odorless, and tasteless, patients may not realize they are exposed. Factors that influence the effects of carbon monoxide on a patient include the patient's inherent rate and depth of breathing, length of exposure, concentration of the gas, and differences in susceptibility. Because of impaired alveolar gas exchange, patients with preexisting respiratory illnesses are more susceptible to the effects of any toxic gas. When assessing the scene, note the presence of multiple patients experiencing the same signs and symptoms, including family pets. This is an indication of the likelihood of some type of exposure.

Carbon monoxide has an affinity for hemoglobin that is 200 times greater than that of oxygen. Oxygen-carrying capacity is decreased significantly as carbon monoxide binds to the hemoglobin molecule, resulting in severe tissue hypoxia.

It is important to note that the pulse oximeter is "blind" to carbon monoxide and may give you a falsely high reading. In other words, the patient can have an oxygen saturation of 90% or greater, yet have a significant level of carbon monoxide (carboxyhemoglobin) in the blood. Remember, the pulse oximeter is designed to detect gross abnormalities, not subtle changes. Use the device with caution in patients who might have carbon monoxide poisoning.

Assess the scene for personal hazards, and immediately move the patient to a well-ventilated area. Apply 100% supplemental oxygen, and assist ventilation as needed. Assess vital signs and gain IV access en route to the closest appropriate facility. The closest hospital with a hyperbaric chamber should be a consideration. In severe cases, the patient is placed inside the chamber, and atmospheric pressures are exerted against the body to force the carbon monoxide molecules away from the hemoglobin, thus allowing oxygenation to resume.

Reassure the patient, and provide psychological support en route to the hospital. The patient's clinical status should dictate the transport mode.

Monitor the cardiac rhythm of any patient who has inhaled a toxic substance and treat arrhythmias following standard ACLS protocols. Be prepared to intubate the patient to protect their airway.

> **In the Field**
>
> *Always* treat the patient and not the diagnostic tool. Pulse oximeters may give false readings when patients have been exposed to carbon monoxide. The same is true of cardiac monitors when the leads have detached.

Sympathomimetics

Sympathomimetics are CNS stimulants that frequently cause hypertension, tachycardia, and dilated pupils. A stimulant is an agent that produces an excited state. Amphetamines and methamphetamines ("ice") are commonly taken by mouth. In many cases, people who abuse these drugs also inject them. The drugs typically are taken to make the user "feel good," improve task performance, suppress appetite, or prevent sleepiness. They may just as easily produce irritability, anxiety, lack of concentration, and seizures. Other common examples of sympathomimetics include phentermine (Adipex) and benzedrine (racemic amphetamine sulfate). Caffeine, theophylline (Aminophylline), and phenylpropanolamine (PPA), a nasal decongestant, are all mild sympathomimetics. So-called "designer drugs," such as Ecstasy and Eve, are also frequently abused in certain areas of the country.

Sympathomimetic drugs are frequently called "uppers" (Table 23-5). Someone using one of these agents may display disorganized behavior, restlessness, and sometimes anxiety or great fear. Paranoia and delusions are also common with sympathomimetic abuse.

Cocaine, also called coke, crack, crystal, snow, freebase, rock, gold dust, blow, and lady, may be taken in a number of different ways. Classically, it is inhaled into the nose and absorbed through the nasal mucosa, damaging tissue, causing nosebleeds, and, ultimately, destroying the nasal septum. It can also be injected intravenously or subcutaneously (skin-popping). Cocaine can be absorbed through all mucous membranes and even

TABLE 23-5	Street Names for Amphetamines	
Adam	Eve	Meth
Bennies	Fen-phen	Psychodrine
Crank	Golden eagle	Speed
DOM	Ice	STP
Ecstasy	MDA	Uppers

across the skin. In any form, the immediate effects of a given dose last less than an hour.

Another method of abusing cocaine is by smoking it. Crack is pure cocaine. It melts at 93°F (34°C) and vaporizes at a slightly higher temperature. Therefore, crack is easily smoked. In this form, it reaches the capillary network of the lungs and can be absorbed into the body in seconds. The immediate outflow of blood from the heart speeds the drug to the brain, so its effect is felt at once. Smoked crack produces the most rapid means of absorption and, therefore, the most potent effect.

Cocaine is one of the most addicting substances known, more so than heroin or nicotine. Its immediate effects include excitement and euphoria. Acute cocaine overdose is a genuine emergency, as patients are at high risk for seizures and cardiac arrhythmias. Long-term cocaine abuse may cause hallucinations; patients with "cocaine bugs" think that bugs are crawling out of their skin.

In caring for patients who have been poisoned with any of the sympathomimetics, be aware that their severe agitation can lead to tachycardia and hypertension. Patients may also display paranoid behavior, putting you and other health care providers in danger. Law enforcement officers should be at the scene to restrain the patient, if necessary. Do not leave the patient unattended and unmonitored during transport.

All of these patients need to be transported to the emergency department promptly because of their risk of seizures, cardiac dysrhythmias, and stroke. You may see blood pressures as high as 250/150 mm Hg. Administer 100% supplemental oxygen, or, if needed, provide ventilatory assistance, and be prepared to provide suctioning. Assess vital signs, and gain IV access. Provide psychological support as well. If the patient is already having a seizure, you must protect them from injury.

Monitor the cardiac rhythm of any patient with a cocaine ingestion and treat arrhythmias following standard ACLS protocols. If the patient becomes unresponsive, consider intubation to protect their airway.

Transport patient to the closest appropriate facility. The patient's clinical presentation should dictate the transport mode.

Marijuana

The flowering hemp plant *Cannabis sativa*, called marijuana, is abused throughout the world. It has been estimated that as many as 20 million people use marijuana daily in the United States. Inhaling marijuana smoke from a cigarette or pipe produces euphoria, relaxation, and drowsiness. It also impairs short-term memory and the capacity to perform complex thinking and work. In some people, the euphoria progresses to depression and confusion. An altered perception of time is common, and anxiety and panic can occur. With very high doses, patients experience hallucinations.

A person who has been using marijuana rarely needs transport to the hospital. Exceptions may include someone who is hallucinating, very anxious, or paranoid. However, you should be aware that marijuana is often used as a vehicle to get other drugs into the body. For example, it may be covered with crack or PCP (phencyclidine, also known as "angel dust").

Hallucinogens

Hallucinogens alter an individual's sensory perceptions (Table 23-6). The classic hallucinogen is lysergic acid diethylamide (known as LSD). Abuse of another hallucinogen, PCP, is relatively uncommon among young adults. PCP is a dissociative anesthetic that is easily synthesized and highly potent. Its effectiveness by oral, nasal, pulmonary, and IV routes makes it easy to add to other street drugs. PCP is dangerous, as it causes severe behavioral changes in which individuals often inflict injury to themselves.

All these agents cause visual hallucinations, intensify vision and hearing, and generally separate the user from reality. The user, of course, expects that the altered sen-

TABLE 23-6	Commonly Abused Hallucinogens
Bufotenine (toad skin)	Mescaline
Dimethyltryptamine (DMT)	Morning glory
Jimson weed	Nutmeg
Lysergic acid diethylamide (LSD)	Phencyclidine (PCP)
Marijuana	Psilocybin (mushroom)

sory state will be pleasurable. Often, however, it can be terrifying. At some point, you are bound to encounter patients who are having a "bad trip." They will usually be hypertensive, tachycardic, anxious, and probably paranoid.

Many of the hallucinogens have sympathomimetic properties. Indeed, your care for a patient who is having a bad reaction to a hallucinogenic agent is the same as that for a patient who has taken a sympathomimetic. Project a calm, professional manner, and provide emotional support. Do not use restraints unless you or the patient is in danger of injury and then always within the guidelines specified by local authorities. These patients may suddenly experience hallucinations or odd perceptions, so careful monitoring throughout transport is essential. Never leave a patient who has taken a hallucinogen unattended and unmonitored.

Anticholinergic Agents

The classic description of a person who has taken too much of an anticholinergic medication is "hot as a hare, blind as a bat, dry as a bone, red as a beet, and mad as a hatter." These are medications possessing properties that, among other effects, block the parasympathetic nervous system. Common drugs with a significant anticholinergic effect include atropine, diphenhydramine (Benadryl), Jimson weed, and certain tricyclic antidepressants. With the exception of Jimson weed, these medications usually are not abused drugs but may be taken as an intentional overdose. You will find that it is often difficult to distinguish between an anticholinergic overdose and a sympathomimetic overdose. Both groups of patients may have agitation, tachycardia, and dilated pupils. Once pure anticholinergic poisoning has been diagnosed, the patient may be treated with physostigmine intravenously by staff in the emergency department, depending on the severity of the situation.

As newer, safer antidepressants such as fluoxetine (Prozac) and sertraline (Zoloft) crowd the market, you can expect to see fewer overdoses of tricyclic antidepressants such as amitriptyline (Elavil) and imipramine (Tofranil). In addition to its anticholinergic effects, a cyclic antidepressant overdose may cause more serious, indeed life-threatening, problems. This is because the medication may block the electrical conduction system in the heart, leading to lethal cardiac arrhythmias. Patients with acute cyclic antidepressant overdose must be transported immediately to the emergency department; they may appear "normal," but then seizures occur, and death can result within 30 minutes. The seizures and cardiac arrhythmias caused by a severe cyclic antidepressant overdose are best treated with IV sodium bicarbonate. If you work in a tiered system, you should consider calling for paramedic backup when you are en route to the scene.

Immediate transport to the closest appropriate facility is essential. Apply 100% supplemental oxygen, and assist ventilations as needed. Gain IV access en route to the hospital.

Weapons of Mass Destruction

Although the use of weapons of mass destruction (WMD) still remains more prevalent in wartime and is more closely associated with the military, it has become a threat during peacetime and could involve EMT-Is practicing in civilian life (see Chapter 37). We have seen WMD used to produce tragedies such as the Oklahoma bombing of a federal building. We have also seen widespread use of sarin gas, ricin, and anthrax. We now protect ourselves against terrorist attacks at events such as the Olympic Games. Protection involves military presence, and, in the event of an attack, we have military medical teams and civilian teams, which include the disaster medical assistance teams (DMATs). These DMATs are made up of experts that include physicians, nurses, respiratory therapists, EMT-Is, paramedics, and clergy. During these events, DMATs are federalized and operate under the Department of Health and Human Services.

Biological, chemical, and nuclear agents are used for mass destruction. Many different agents are used. Treatment after an attack is typically divided into three zones. The first zone is the red or hot zone, which is usually managed by the military or other highly trained individuals. In the hot zone, patients are triaged and go through early decontamination (called decon). In the next zone, the yellow or warm zone, extensive decontamination takes place by trained individuals. The last zone, the green zone or cold zone, is where EMS will treat and transport the patient. Although EMT-Is do not manage patients who are in a hot zone, they will have to manage patients after the decontamination team has completed and cleared the patients for transport. EMS providers do not enter the red or yellow area unless they are trained and are wearing the proper clothing. It is important to understand that you should never enter a situation that is potentially dangerous without proper training.

Monitor the patient's cardiac rhythm. One to two doses of sodium bicarbonate may be given as ordered by medical control.

Cholinergic Agents

Cholinergic agents are the "nerve gases" designed for chemical warfare. These agents overstimulate normal body functions that are controlled by parasympathetic nerves, resulting in salivation, mucus secretion, urination, excessive tearing, and bradycardia. Obviously, you are unlikely to run across these. However, you may be called on to care for patients who have been exposed to one of the organophosphate insecticides or certain wild mushrooms, which are also cholinergic agents. The signs and symptoms of cholinergic drug poisoning are easy to remember because of the mnemonic DUMBELS:

- Defecation
- Urination
- Miosis (constriction of the pupils)
- Bronchorrhea (discharge of mucus from the lungs)
- Emesis
- Lacrimation (tearing)
- Salivation

Another mnemonic is SLUDGE:

- Salivation
- Lacrimation
- Urination
- Defecation
- Gastrointestinal irritation
- Eye constriction and Emesis

In poisonings, these normal functions and body secretions are excessive. In addition, patients may have bradycardia or tachycardia, wheezing, bronchoconstriction, seizures, diaphoresis, headache, dizziness, nausea, or weakness, or a combination of these signs and symptoms; patients also may be comatose.

The most important consideration in caring for a patient who has been exposed to an organophosphate insecticide or other cholinergic agent is to avoid exposure yourself. Because such agents may cling to the patient's clothing and skin, decontamination may take priority over immediate transport to the emergency department. Depending on your local EMS protocol, this can be treated as a hazardous materials (or Haz-Mat) situation.

Management focuses on decontamination as the first priority. Aggressive management of the airway involves suctioning of secretions to prevent aspiration and applying 100% supplemental oxygen or assisted ventilations as needed. Establish an IV of an isotonic crystalloid solution.

Transport to the closest appropriate facility, allowing patient status to dictate the transport mode. Provide psychological support, and be alert for sudden changes in the patient's condition. Reassess the airway frequently, and consider the use of a Combitube or other dual-lumen airway device if no gag reflex is present.

Perform endotracheal intubation if definitive airway protection is needed.

Consider giving atropine to dry up secretions as ordered by medical control. Unfortunately, most EMS services do no carry enough atropine to be truly effective. Diazepam (Valium) may also be ordered to control seizure activity. Monitor the patient's cardiac rhythm and treat arrhythmias according to local and ACLS protocol. Consider intubation if the patient is unable to maintain his or her airway.

Miscellaneous Drugs

While not as common as it was 30 years ago, aspirin (acetylsalicylic acid or ASA) poisoning remains a potentially lethal condition. Ingesting too many aspirin tablets, at one time or on a long-term basis, may result in nausea, vomiting, hyperventilation, and ringing in the ears (tinnitus). Patients with this problem are frequently anxious, confused, tachypneic, and in danger of having seizures. Acute aspirin overdose may be associated with life-threatening metabolic acidosis. These patients should be transported quickly to the hospital.

Overdosing with acetaminophen is also very common, probably because it is available in so many different preparations, such as Tylenol. The good news is that acetaminophen is generally not very toxic. A healthy patient could ingest 140 mg of acetaminophen for every kilogram of body weight without serious adverse effects. The bad news is that the symptoms of an overdose generally do not appear until it is too late. For example, massive liver failure may not be apparent for a full week. And patients may not provide the information necessary for a correct diagnosis. For this reason, obtaining information at the scene is very important. By finding an empty acetaminophen bottle, you may save a patient's life. If given early enough (before liver failure occurs), a specific antidote may prevent liver damage and death.

Be extremely careful in dealing with a child who has unintentionally ingested a poisonous substance. Although such incidents usually do not lead to death, family members may be distraught, and your professional attitude will help to ease the tension. Remember, however, that a single swallow of some substances can kill a child (Table 23-7 ▶).

TABLE 23-7	Substances That Can Be Fatal if Ingested by Children

Benzocaine
Calcium channel blockers (verapamil, nifedipine, diltiazem)
Camphor
Chloroquine
Diphenoxylate (for example, Lomotil)
Hydrocarbon solvents
Methanol and ethylene glycol
Methylsalicylate (oil of wintergreen)
Phenothiazines (for example, chlorpromazine [Thorazine])
Quinine
Theophylline
Tricyclic antidepressants (for example, amitriptyline [Elavil], imipramine [Tofranil], nortriptyline [Pamelor])
Visine

Some alcohols, including methyl alcohol and ethylene glycol, are even more toxic than ethyl alcohol (drinking alcohol). Although a person with alcoholism who is unable to obtain ethyl alcohol may use them as a substitute, they are more often taken by someone attempting suicide. In either case, immediate transport to the emergency department is essential. Methyl alcohol is found in dry gas products and Sterno; ethylene glycol is found in some antifreeze products. Both cause a "drunken" feeling. If ingestion is untreated, both will also cause severe tachypnea, blindness (methyl alcohol), renal failure (ethylene glycol), and, eventually, death. Even ethyl alcohol (typical drinking alcohol) can cause respiratory arrest if ingested in too high a dose or too fast, particularly in children.

Food Poisoning

The term "ptomaine poisoning" was coined in 1870 to indicate poisoning by a class of chemicals found in rotting food. It is still used today in many news accounts of food poisoning. This is unfortunate, because the term is misleading. Food poisoning is almost always caused by eating food that is contaminated by bacteria. The food may appear perfectly good, with little or no decay or odor to suggest danger.

There are two main types of food poisoning. In one, the organism itself causes disease; in the other, the organism produces toxins that cause disease Table 23-8 . A toxin is a poison or harmful substance produced by bacteria, animals, or plants.

One organism that produces direct effects of food poisoning is the *Salmonella* bacterium. The condition called salmonellosis is characterized by severe gastroin-

Geriatric Needs

In an accidental overdose or poisoning, an older patient may have become confused about his or her drug regimen. He or she may have forgotten that the medication had been taken, repeating the dose a number of times. Or the patient could have forgotten the doctor's instructions to discard leftover medication and might have taken both the current and the older drug, resulting in an increase in effects or an untoward drug interaction.

An older patient may also intentionally overdose in an attempt to commit suicide. Geriatric patients have been known to ingest common household chemicals such as insecticides, acetaminophen, aspirin, or caustic substances in an attempt to end their lives. Be alert for any indication of an intentional overdose or poisoning, even though the patient might deny an attempted suicide.

In considering any poisoning, remember the basics. Because of the aging process, the routes of administration and decreased metabolism in older patients pose significant changes in the way the poison is absorbed into the body. In senior citizens, damage to the stomach could be more severe, because increased gastric acids can alter absorption of the poison. In addition, decreased gastric motility slows absorption by delaying emptying of the stomach and, in caustic substance ingestion, increases injury to the stomach.

If a senior citizen inhales a poison, even in tiny quantities, lung damage can be severe. Consider the decreased lung capacity and ability to exchange oxygen and carbon dioxide in the older patient's lungs. Pulmonary function can be significantly impaired with the inhalation of minute amounts of poison.

For poisons that are absorbed by or injected into the skin, reduced circulation to the skin can decrease or delay absorption into the body. Watch for an increased reaction or irritation at the skin site.

In geriatric patients, the liver may not be able to metabolize the poison as effectively and the kidneys may not be able to excrete the poison as quickly. Therefore, the drug or poison remains in the body for a longer period of time, causing additional tissue damage. When a medication is not metabolized or excreted as quickly as in younger people, the drug could accumulate to toxic levels and, ultimately, become fatal.

TABLE 23-8	Common Sources of Food Poisoning
Bacillus cereus	Giardia lamblia
Campylobacter	Rotavirus
Clostridium botulinum toxin	Salmonella
Clostridium perfringens	Shigella
Cryptosporidium	Staphylococcus toxin
Enterococcus	Vibrio parahaemolyticus
Escherichia coli	Yersinia enterocolitica

TABLE 23-9	Common Toxic Plants
Scientific Name	**Common Name**
Abrus precatorius	Jequirity bean, rosary pea
Cicuta species	Water hemlock, wild carrot
Colchicum autumnale	Autumn crocus
Conium maculatum	Poison hemlock
Convallaria majalis	Lily of the valley
Datura species	Jimson weed, stinkweed
Dieffenbachia	Dieffenbachia, dumbcane
Digitalis purpurea	Purple foxglove
Nerium oleander	Oleander, rose laurel
Nicotiana glauca	Tree tobacco
Phoradendron	Mistletoe
Phytolacca americana	Pokeweed
Rhododendron	Rhododendron, azalea
Ricinus communis	Castor bean
Solanum nigrum	Nightshade
Zigadenus species	Death camas

testinal symptoms within 72 hours of ingestion, including nausea, vomiting, abdominal pain, and diarrhea. In addition, patients with salmonellosis may be systemically ill with fever and generalized weakness. Some people are carriers of certain bacteria; although they may not become ill themselves, they may transmit diseases, particularly if they work in the food services industry. Proper cooking usually kills bacteria, and proper cleanliness in the kitchen prevents cross-contamination of uncooked foods.

The more common cause of food poisoning is the ingestion of powerful toxins produced by bacteria, often in leftovers. The bacterium *Staphylococcus*, a common culprit, is quick to grow and produce toxins in foods that have been prepared in advance and kept too long, even in the refrigerator. Foods prepared with mayonnaise, when left unrefrigerated, are a common vehicle for the development of staphylococcal toxins. Staphylococcal food poisoning usually results in sudden gastrointestinal symptoms, including nausea, vomiting, and diarrhea. Although time frames may vary from individual to individual, symptoms usually start within 2 to 3 hours after ingestion but may start as long as 12 hours after ingestion.

The most severe form of food poisoning is botulism. This often fatal disease usually results from eating improperly canned food, in which the spores of *Clostridium* bacteria have grown and produced a toxin. The symptoms of botulism are neurologic: blurring of vision, weakness, and difficulty in speaking and breathing. Symptoms may develop as long as 4 days after ingestion or as early as the first 24 hours.

In general, you should not try to determine the specific cause of acute gastrointestinal problems. After all, severe vomiting may be a sign of a self-limiting food poisoning, a bowel obstruction requiring surgery, or another poison, such as copper, arsenic, zinc, cadmium, scombrotoxin (fish poison), or mushrooms of the *Clitocybe* or *Inocybe* genus. Instead, you should obtain as much history as possible from the patient and transport promptly to the hospital. When two or more individuals in one group have the same illness, you should take some of the suspected food to the hospital. In advanced cases of botulism, you may have to assist ventilations and provide aggressive life support.

Plant Poisoning

Several thousand cases of poisoning from plants occur each year, some of them severe. Many household plants are poisonous if ingested, as they may be by children who like to nibble the leaves (Table 23-9). Some poisonous plants cause local irritation of the skin; others can affect the circulatory system, the gastrointestinal tract, or the central nervous system. It is impossible for you to memorize every plant and poison, let alone their effects (Figure 23-6). You can and should do the following:

1. Assess the patient's airway and vital signs.
2. Notify the regional poison center for assistance in identifying the plant.
3. Provide prompt transport.

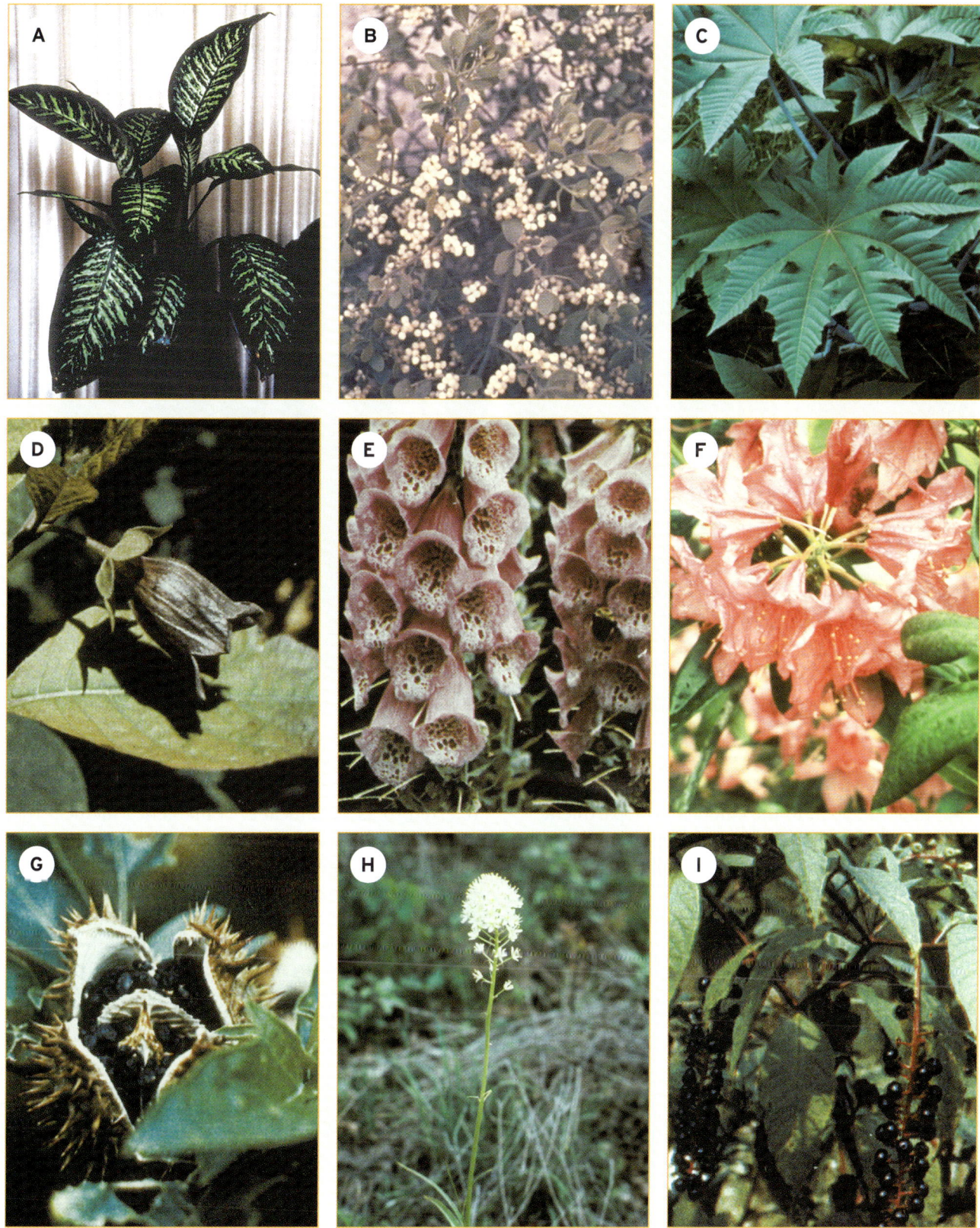

Figure 23-6 The toxins in these common poisonous plants are often ingested or absorbed through the skin. **A.** Dieffenbachia. **B.** Mistletoe. **C.** Castor bean. **D.** Nightshade. **E.** Foxglove. **F.** Rhododendron. **G.** Jimson weed. **H.** Death camas. **I.** Pokeweed.

Continued

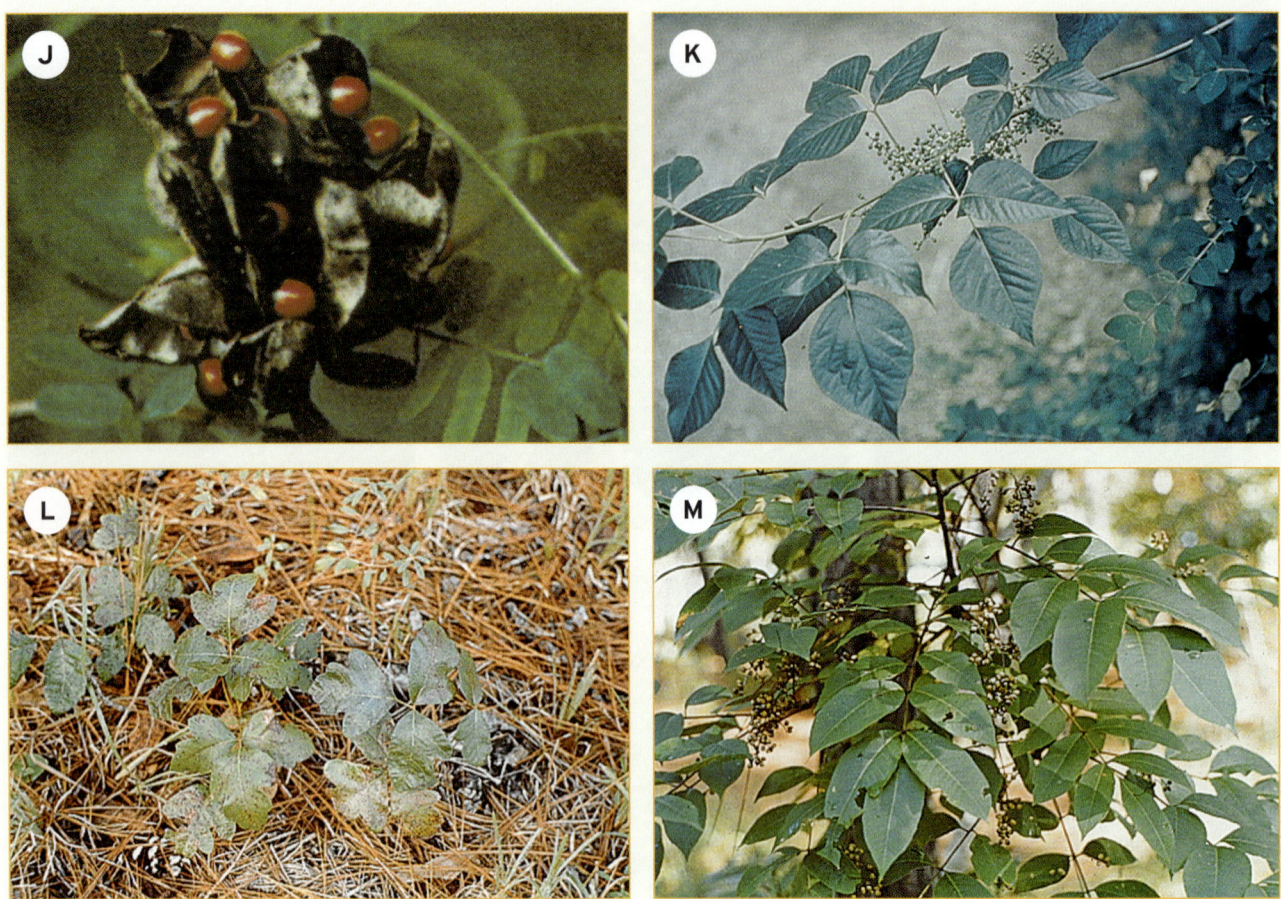

Figure 23-6—cont'd The toxins in these common poisonous plants are often ingested or absorbed through the skin. **J.** Rosary pea. **K.** Poison ivy. **L.** Poison oak. **M.** Poison sumac.

4. Take the plant to the emergency department.

Irritation of the skin and/or mucous membranes is a problem with the common houseplant called dieffenbachia, which resembles "elephant ears." When chewed, a single leaf may irritate the lining of the upper airway enough to cause difficulty in swallowing, breathing, and speaking. In rare circumstances, the airway may be completely obstructed by swelling. Dieffenbachia is also referred to as "dumbcane." Emergency medical treatment of dieffenbachia poisoning includes maintaining an open airway, giving 100% supplemental oxygen, and transporting the patient promptly to the hospital. You should continue to assess the patient for airway difficulties throughout transport, and provide positive-pressure ventilations if needed.

You are the Provider | Summary

1. What is your primary responsibility as an EMS provider in this situation?

Your primary responsibility to the patient who has been poisoned is to recognize that a poisoning has occurred.

2. What is the first treatment priority for this patient?

Treatment focuses on support: assessing and maintaining the patient's ABCs.

3. What are some of the ways that poisons can enter the body?

There are four routes by which a poison can enter the body.
A. Ingestion.
B. Inhalation.
C. Injection.
D. Absorption (surface contact).

4. What is your next step?

In general, your treatment of patients who have overdosed with sedative-hypnotics and have respiratory depression is to maintain a patent airway, provide ventilatory assistance with 100% oxygen, and provide prompt transport. You may attempt to stimulate the person by speaking loudly or gently shaking him or her. As with any patient who is under the influence of a CNS depressant drug, be alert for vomiting.

According to your level of certification, and if local protocol permits, start an IV of normal saline and administer Narcan to rule out narcotic ingestion.

Monitor the patient's cardiac rhythm and treat arrhythmias following standard ACLS protocols.

Prep Kit

Ready for Review

- Poisons act acutely or chronically to destroy or impair body cells. If you believe a patient may have taken a poisonous substance, you should notify medical control and begin emergency treatment at once. This may include administration of an antidote, usually at the hospital, if an antidote exists. It also entails collecting any evidence about the type of poison that was used and taking it to the hospital; diluting and physically removing the poisonous agent; providing respiratory support; and transporting the patient promptly to the hospital.

- A poison can be introduced into the body in one of four ways: ingestion, inhalation, injection, or absorption (surface contact). Approximately 80% of all poisonings are by ingestion, including plants, contaminated food, and most drugs. In general, activated charcoal should be used to treat patients who have ingested these substances.

- In the case of surface contact poisons, be sure to avoid contaminating yourself. You should then remove all contaminated substances and clothing from the patient, and flood the affected part with copious amounts of water.

- Move patients who have inhaled poison into the fresh air; be prepared to use supplemental oxygen via nonrebreathing mask and to provide ventilatory support via a bag-valve-mask device.

- Emergency care may be needed for some patients, especially those who have injected poison, which is almost always a deliberate act.

- People who frequently abuse a substance can develop a tolerance to it, which may lead to addiction. Always use body substance isolation precautions when caring for victims of drug abuse.

- In addition to alcohol and marijuana, commonly abused drugs fall into seven categories: opioid analgesics, sedatives-hypnotics, inhalants, sympathomimetics, hallucinogens, anticholinergics, and cholinergics. Like alcohol, drugs in the first three categories depress the CNS and can cause respiratory depression. You must support the airway in such cases and be prepared for the patient to vomit.

- Take special care with patients who have used inhalants, since the drugs may cause seizures. Sympathomimetics, including cocaine, stimulate the CNS, causing hypertension, tachycardia, seizures, and dilated pupils. These patients may be paranoid, as may patients who have taken hallucinogens.

- Anticholinergic medications, often taken in suicide attempts, can cause a person to become hot, dry, blind, red-faced, and mentally unbalanced. An overdose of cyclic antidepressants can lead to cardiac arrhythmias.

- The symptoms of cholinergic medications, which include organophosphate insecticides, can be remembered by the mnemonic DUMBELS or SLUDGE, for excessive defecation, urination, miosis, bronchorrhea, emesis, lacrimation, and salivation.

- Two main types of food poisoning cause gastrointestinal symptoms. In one type, bacteria in the food directly cause disease, such as salmonellosis; in the other, bacteria such as *Staphylococcus* produce powerful toxins, often in leftover food.

- The most severe form of food poisoning is botulism, which can first produce neurologic symptoms as late as 4 days after ingestion.

- Plant poisoning can affect the circulatory, gastrointestinal, and central nervous systems. Some plants, such as dieffenbachia, irritate the skin or mucous membranes and may cause obstruction of the airway.

Technology

www.EMSzone.com/EMTI

- Interactivities
- Vocabulary Explorer
- Anatomy Review
- Web Links
- Online Review Manual

Vital Vocabulary

addiction A state of overwhelming obsession or physical need to continue the use of a drug or agent.

antidote A substance that is used to neutralize or counteract a poison.

delirium tremens (DTs) A severe withdrawal syndrome seen in people with alcoholism who are deprived of ethyl alcohol; characterized by restlessness, fever, sweating, disorientation, agitation, and seizures; can be fatal if untreated.

emesis Vomiting.

hallucinogens Agents that produce false perceptions in any one of the five senses.

hematemesis Vomiting blood.

hypnotic A sleep-inducing effect or agent.

ingestion Swallowing; taking a substance by mouth.

opioids Any drug or agent with actions similar to morphine (a narcotic).

poison A substance whose chemical action could damage structures or impair function when introduced into the body.

sedative A substance that decreases activity and excitement.

stimulant An agent that produces an excited state.

substance abuse The misuse, usually knowingly, of any substance to produce some desired effect.

tolerance The need for increasing amounts of a drug to obtain the same effect.

toxin A poison or harmful substance produced by bacteria, animals, or plants.

vomitus Vomited material.

Points to Ponder

You are dispatched to a nightclub for a report of an unconscious patient. You arrive at the scene to find a 22-year-old woman lying on the floor in the ladies' room. The patient is crying, scared, and very upset. You and your partner talk to her and try to calm her down. Her vital signs are: pulse, 130 beats/min; blood pressure, 150/100 mm Hg; and respirations, 24 breaths/min. You notice that the patient's pupils are dilated. You ask her if she has taken anything, but she denies this. She states that she was just dancing with her friends having a good time until she started to feel sick. She states that she only drank soda water all evening.

What do you think is wrong with your patient? What type of substance might she have taken? What psychological need does this patient have, if any? How would you care for this patient?

Issues: Calming the Patient, Obtaining a Thorough History

Assessment in Action

You are dispatched to assist the local police department for a possible drug overdose. When you arrive at the scene, you find a 34-year-old man who appears to be disoriented. His friends stopped at the police department and called 9-1-1 when he started to act strange on their way home from a party.

You ask the patient if he has taken any medications or other substances. He states that he only had one marijuana joint while at the party. Because the patient is disoriented and confused, you administer oxygen, start an IV, and give him Narcan. After about 2 minutes, the patient becomes more responsive and asks you what happened.

1. Which of the following is NOT considered an unintentional poisoning?
   A. Self-injected heroin
   B. Idiosyncratic reaction
   C. Dosage error
   D. Childhood poisoning

2. Any substance with a chemical action that can damage body structures or impair body function is called a(n):
   A. allergen.
   B. poison.
   C. hormone.
   D. antigen.

3. Which of the following questions is of LEAST pertinence when assessing a patient who has ingested a poison?
   A. How much did you ingest?
   B. How much do you weigh?
   C. When did you take it?
   D. Why did you take it?

4. A substance that will counteract the effects of a particular poison is called an:
   A. antidote.
   B. antigen.
   C. allergen.
   D. antibiotic.

5. All of the following are common routes of entry for poisons into the body, EXCEPT:
   A. ingestion.
   B. radiation.
   C. injection.
   D. inhalation.

6. If local protocol allows, you may give patients who have ingested a noncaustic poison the following:
   A. syrup of ipecac.
   B. instant glucose.
   C. activated charcoal.
   D. glucagon.

7. A type of substance that decreases activity and excitement is called a(n):
   A. hypnotic.
   B. stimulant.
   C. sedative.
   D. analgesic.

8. The drug of choice for an unconscious patient with a narcotic overdose is:
   A. Romazicon.
   B. Narcan.
   C. glucagon.
   D. activated charcoal.

9. Commonly abused inhaled agents include all of the following EXCEPT:
   A. acetone.
   B. hexane.
   C. toluene.
   D. propane.

10. Carbon monoxide has an affinity for hemoglobin that is _____ times greater than oxygen.
    A. 20
    B. 50
    C. 100
    D. 200

11. Sympathomimetic agents cause which of the following physiologic effects?
    A. Tachycardia
    B. Bradycardia
    C. Respiratory depression
    D. Pupillary constriction

Neurologic Emergencies

1999 Objectives

Cognitive

5-6.1 Discuss the general pathophysiology of non-traumatic neurological emergencies. (p 1061)

5-6.2 Discuss the general assessment findings associated with non-traumatic neurologic emergencies. (p 1068)

5-6.3 Identify the need for rapid intervention and transport of the patient with non-traumatic emergencies. (p 1062)

5-6.4 Discuss the epidemiology, assessment findings, and management for stroke and intracranial hemorrhage. (p 1061, 1068, 1069)

5-6.5 Discuss the epidemiology, assessment findings, and management for transient ischemic attack. (p 1063)

5-6.6 Discuss the epidemiology, assessment findings, and management of epilepsy/seizure. (p 1064)

5-6.7 Discuss the epidemiology, assessment findings, and management for non-specific coma or altered level of consciousness/syncope/weakness/headache. (p 1066, 1072, 1073)

5-6.8 Develop a patient management plan based on field impression in the patient with neurological emergencies. (p 1074)

Affective

5-6.9 Characterize the feelings of a patient who regains consciousness among strangers. (p 1076)

5-6.10 Formulate means of conveying empathy to patients whose ability to communicate is limited by their condition. (p 1070)

Psychomotor

5-6.11 Perform an appropriate assessment of a patient with a non-traumatic neurological emergency. (p 1070)

1985 Objectives

There are no 1985 objectives for this chapter.

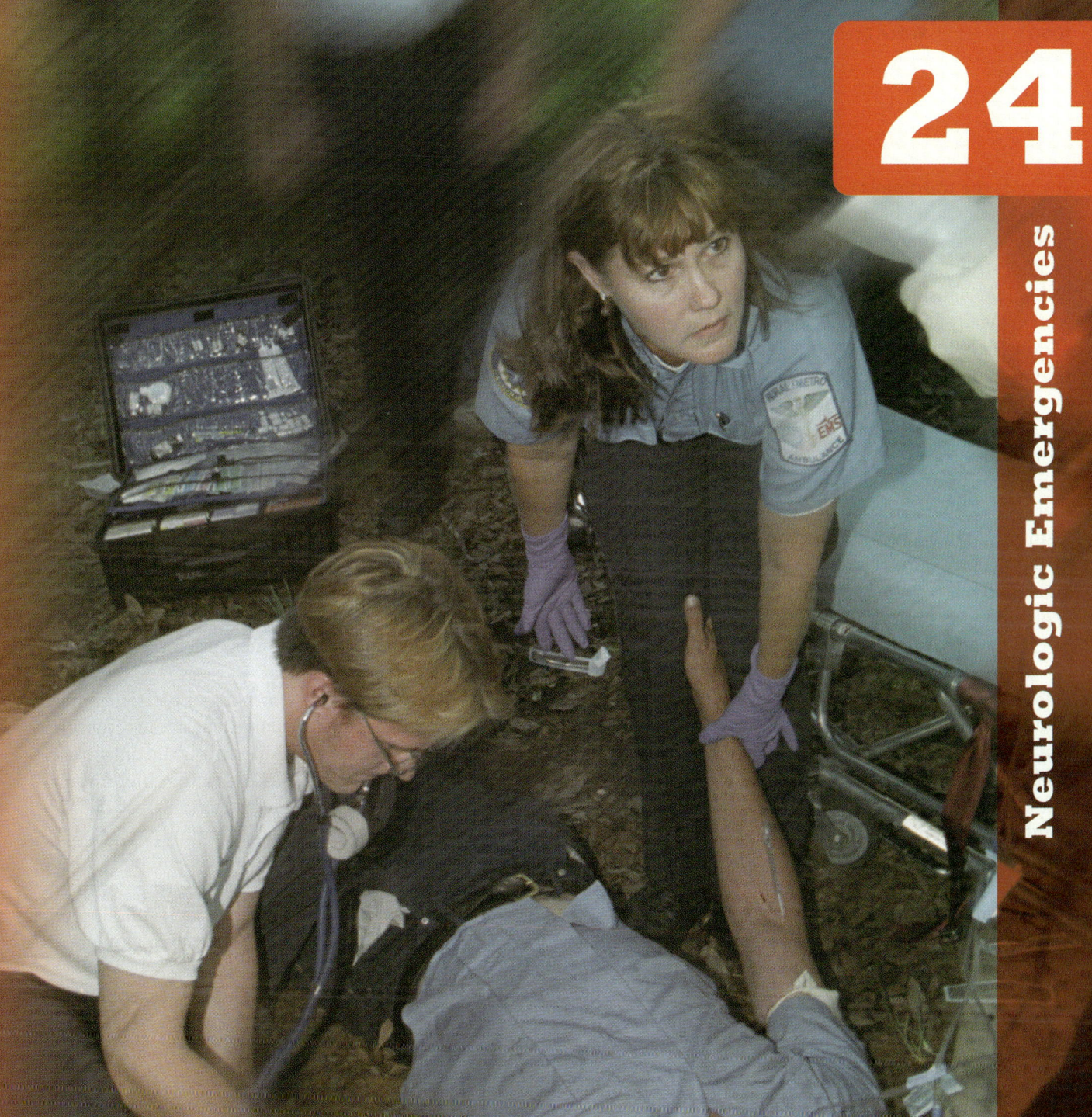

24

Neurologic Emergencies

You are the Provider

You receive a call for a male not able to speak. Upon arrival you find a 68-year-old man lying in his bed unable to get up. His wife tells you that he was fine when he went to bed last night at about 11:00 PM. When he woke up, she noted that his speech was slurred and that he was not able to move his right side.

Altered mental status can be caused by a variety of medical and traumatic conditions. It may well be one of the most challenging conditions encountered by an EMT-I.

This chapter will lay the foundation of knowledge necessary for you to provide quality care for patients with neurologic dysfunction and will also help you answer the following questions:

1. Why is the brain so dependent on a continuous supply of oxygen?
2. What is the clinical significance of a patient having a TIA (transient ischemic attack)?

Neurologic Emergencies

Stroke is the third most common cause of death in the United States, after heart disease and cancer. During the past few years, there has been a revolution in the treatment of stroke. For the most part, emergency treatment had not previously been available for patients with stroke, who typically faced years of painful rehabilitation or lifelong debilitation. Now, emergency physicians, neurologists, and neurosurgeons can help some patients with acute stroke avoid the most devastating consequences of this disease, providing that they receive prompt care.

Seizures and altered mental status also occur when there is a disorder in the brain. Seizures may occur as a result of a recent or old head injury, a brain tumor, a metabolic problem, or simply a genetic predisposition. Your ability to recognize when a seizure has occurred or is occurring is critical for the patient, because it helps direct the most appropriate treatment.

Altered mental status is a common presentation in patients with a wide variety of medical problems. You should not make assumptions about the cause of altered mental status, which can range from alcohol intoxication to stroke. Treatment varies widely, depending on the underlying cause. The care for patients with altered mental status presents a particular challenge because the patients may be difficult to handle and frustrating to treat at times. Your professionalism is paramount in these situations.

The chapter opens with a description of the structure and function of the brain and the abnormalities that occur in the most common brain disorders, including stroke, seizure, and altered mental status. It then discusses the signs and symptoms of each condition.

You will learn how to approach and assess a patient with a brain disorder and why prompt transport to an appropriate medical facility is so important. The chapter then describes key assessment and management strategies for stroke, seizure, and altered mental status.

Brain Structure and Function

The brain is the body's computer. It controls breathing, speech, and all other body functions. All your thoughts, memories, wants, needs, and desires reside in the brain. Different parts of the brain perform different functions. For example, some receive input from the senses, including sight, hearing, taste, smell, and touch; others control the muscles and movement, while others control the formation of speech.

The brain is divided into three major parts: the brain stem, the cerebellum, and the largest part, the cerebrum Figure 24-1 ▶). The brain stem controls the most basic functions of the body, such as breathing, blood pressure, swallowing, and pupil constriction. Just behind the brain stem, the cerebellum, commonly referred to as the "athlete's brain," controls muscle and body coordination. It is responsible for coordinating complex tasks that involve many muscles, such as standing on one foot without falling, walking, writing, picking up a coin, and playing the piano.

The cerebrum, which is superior to the cerebellum, is divided down the middle into the right and left cerebral hemispheres. Each hemisphere controls activities on the opposite (contralateral) side of the body and the same (ipsilateral) side of the face. The anterior (frontal) aspect of the cerebrum controls emotion and thought, the middle aspect controls touch and movement, and the posterior (occipital) aspect of the cerebrum processes sight. In most people, speech is controlled on the left side of the brain near the middle of the cerebrum.

All messages traveling to and from the brain do so along nerves. Twelve cranial nerves run directly from the brain to various parts of the head, such as the eyes, ears, nose, and face. The remaining nerves join in the spinal cord and exit the brain through a large opening in the base of the skull called the foramen magnum Figure 24-2 ▶). The 31 pairs of spinal nerves branch out from between the vertebrae in the neck and back, and they carry signals to and from the body.

Technology

www.EMSzone.com/EMT

- Interactivities
- Vocabulary Explorer
- Anatomy Review
- Web Links
- Online Review Manual

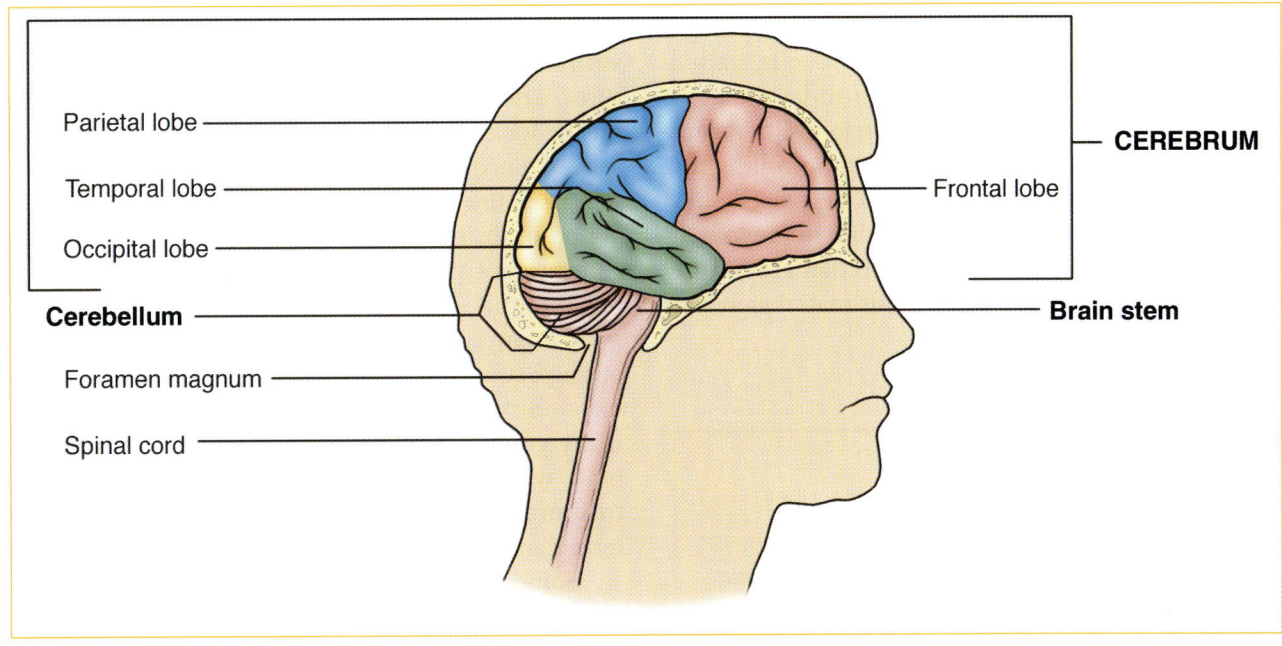

Figure 24-1 The brain lies well protected within the skull. Its major parts are the cerebrum, the cerebellum, and the brain stem.

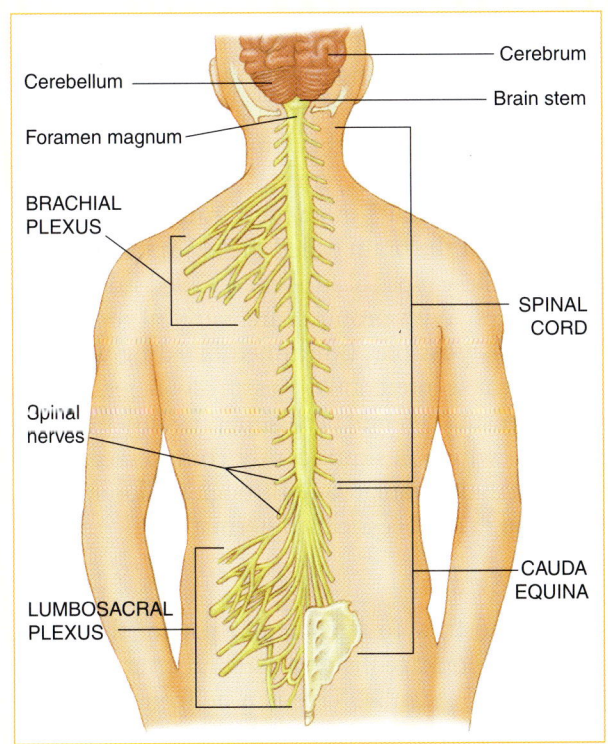

Figure 24-2 The spinal cord is the continuation of the brain stem. It exits the skull at the foramen magnum and extends down to approximately the level of the second lumbar vertebra.

Common Causes of Brain Disorders

Stroke is a common cause of brain disorder that is potentially treatable. Other brain disorders include coma, infection, and tumor. Although these specific problems are not addressed, the seizures or altered mental status that often accompanies them are discussed. The information in this section will help you better understand, communicate with, and care for patients who have experienced some type of brain disorder.

Stroke

A <u>cerebrovascular accident (CVA)</u> is an interruption of blood flow to the brain that often is sudden and results in the loss of function in the affected part of the brain. <u>Stroke</u> is the loss of brain function that results from a CVA and occurs when blood flow to a particular portion of the brain is suddenly disrupted. Without oxygen, brain cells stop working and begin to die; these dead cells are called <u>infarcted cells</u>. Once the cells are dead, medical science has little to offer. However, it may take several hours or more for cell death to occur, even when it appears that severe disability will occur. In some cases, small amounts of blood may still be getting through to the affected area of the brain. This blood may supply enough oxygen to keep a larger group of brain cells, called ischemic cells, alive, but not enough to let the cells work properly and perform their given jobs. For example, if ischemic cells are responsible for controlling the left arm, the patient will experience a decreased ability to move that arm or may not be able to move it at all. If normal blood flow is restored to that area of the brain in a timely manner, the patient may regain use of the arm.

EMT-I Tips

A stroke is also called a "brain attack." This term is used to emphasize that rapid recognition of the signs and symptoms and prompt transport to an appropriate facility can mean the difference between the patient regaining function and needing lifetime care.

New therapies, such as fibrinolytic drugs, commonly referred to as "clot busters," have been shown to reverse symptoms, thus aborting the stroke, if given within 3 hours after the onset of symptoms. These therapies may not work for all patients, and they cannot be given in certain situations, for example to patients with bleeding disorders, recent trauma, or hemorrhagic strokes (to name a few). Nevertheless, until the potential for definitive treatment is ruled out at the hospital, you should proceed under the assumption that the affected area of the brain can still be saved. The sooner the treatment is initiated, the better the chance for a positive patient outcome. Patients may not recognize the signs and symptoms of a CVA until they have progressed significantly. Rapid recognition and transport to an appropriate facility may prevent permanent damage and decrease mortality.

Interruption of cerebral blood flow may result from a thrombus, a clot that has developed locally, in this case, in a cerebral artery; arterial rupture, rupture of a cerebral artery; or a cerebral embolism, obstruction of a cerebral artery caused by a clot that was formed elsewhere, detached, and traveled to the brain.

There are two main types of stroke: *hemorrhagic* (from arterial rupture) and *ischemic* (from an embolism or thrombus).

Hemorrhagic Stroke

A hemorrhagic stroke occurs as a result of bleeding within the brain, typically when a cerebral artery ruptures. The severity of the hemorrhagic stroke depends on the location and size of the ruptured cerebral vessel. As bleeding continues within the brain, intracranial pressure increases and compresses brain tissue. When brain tissue is compressed, oxygenated blood cannot get into the area, and the surrounding cells begin to die.

Certain types of patients are at higher risk for hemorrhagic stroke. The patients at highest risk are those who have chronic, poorly controlled hypertension. After many years of high pressure, the blood vessels in the brain weaken, making them prone to rupture. Proper treatment of hypertension can help prevent this long-term damage to the blood vessels.

Some people have been born with weaknesses, called aneurysms, in the walls of the arteries. An aneurysm is a swelling or enlargement of part of an artery, resulting from weakening of the arterial wall. Many of these people have a sudden onset of a severe headache, frequently described as "the worst headache of their life," which signals the rupture of the aneurysm. Shortly after experiencing the severe headache, it is common for the patient's LOC to rapidly decrease, indicating increased intracranial pressure. When a hemorrhagic stroke occurs in an otherwise healthy young person, it is often the result of a berry aneurysm. This type of aneurysm resembles a tiny balloon (or berry) that protrudes from a cerebral artery. When the aneurysm is overstretched and ruptures, bleeding occurs in an area around the coverings (meninges) of the brain called the subarachnoid space. Therefore, these types of strokes are called subarachnoid hemorrhages. With prompt care, surgical repair of the aneurysm is possible. Continued bleeding within the brain will cause intracranial pressure to increase further, thus decreasing cerebral perfusion pressure. Eventually, the brain, which is significantly compressed, will be forced out of the cranial vault through the foramen magnum through a process called herniation.

Ischemic Stroke

When blood flow to a particular part of the brain is cut off by a blockage inside a cerebral artery, the result is an ischemic stroke. This can be from a thrombus or an embolism that obstructs blood flow. As with coronary artery disease, atherosclerosis in the blood vessels is usually the cause. Atherosclerosis is a disorder in which calcium and cholesterol build up, forming a plaque inside the walls of blood vessels. This plaque obstructs blood flow, interfering with the vessels' ability to dilate. Eventually, atherosclerosis can cause complete occlusion (blockage) of an artery Figure 24-3. In other cases, an atherosclerotic plaque in a carotid artery will rupture. A blood clot will form over the rupture in the plaque, sometimes growing big enough to completely block all blood flow through that artery. Deprived of oxygen, the parts of the brain supplied by the artery will become ischemic. Patients with ischemic strokes will have dramatic symptoms, including, among others, loss of movement on the opposite side of the body, confusion, and the inability to speak (aphasia).

If the blockage in the carotid artery is incomplete, smaller pieces of the clot may embolize (detach and travel) deep into the brain. There, a piece of clot will lodge in a branch of a cerebral artery. This cerebral embolism then obstructs blood flow Figure 24-4. Depending on the location of the obstruction, the patient may experience anything from few symptoms to an inability to move one side of the body or complete paralysis.

Transient Ischemic Attack

In some patients, normal processes in the body will destroy a blood clot in the brain. When that happens quickly, blood flow is restored to the affected area, and the patient will regain use of the affected region of the body. When stroke symptoms spontaneously subside within 24 hours, the event is called a transient ischemic attack (TIA), also referred to as a "small stroke."

Although most patients with TIAs do well, it is still a neurologic emergency. It may be a warning sign that a larger, permanent stroke is imminent. For this reason, all patients with a TIA should be evaluated by a physician to determine whether preventive action can be taken. Because it is often impossible to differentiate the symptoms of a TIA from a stroke, assume that the patient is having a stroke. Administer 100% supplemental oxygen, obtain intravenous (IV) access, and

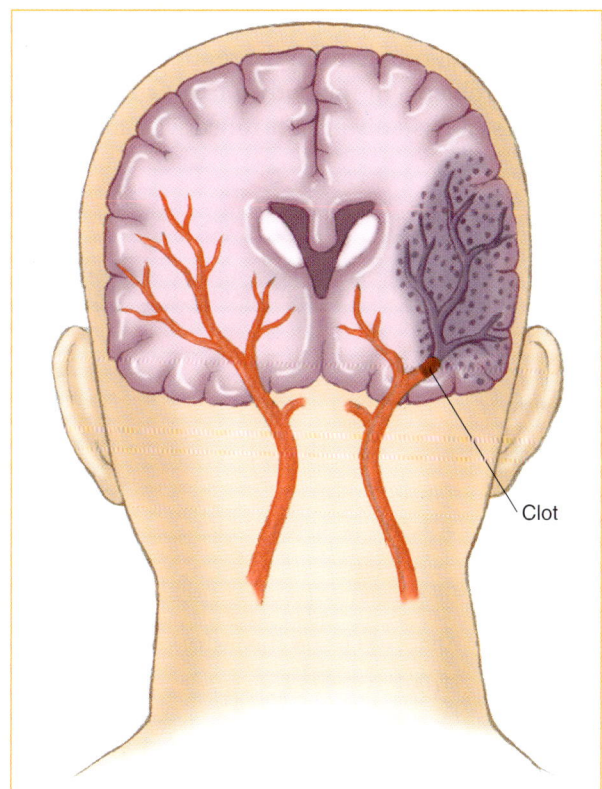

Figure 24-3 Atherosclerosis can damage the wall of a cerebral artery, producing narrowing and a clot. When the vessel is narrowed or completely blocked, blood flow to that part of the brain may be blocked, and the cells begin to die.

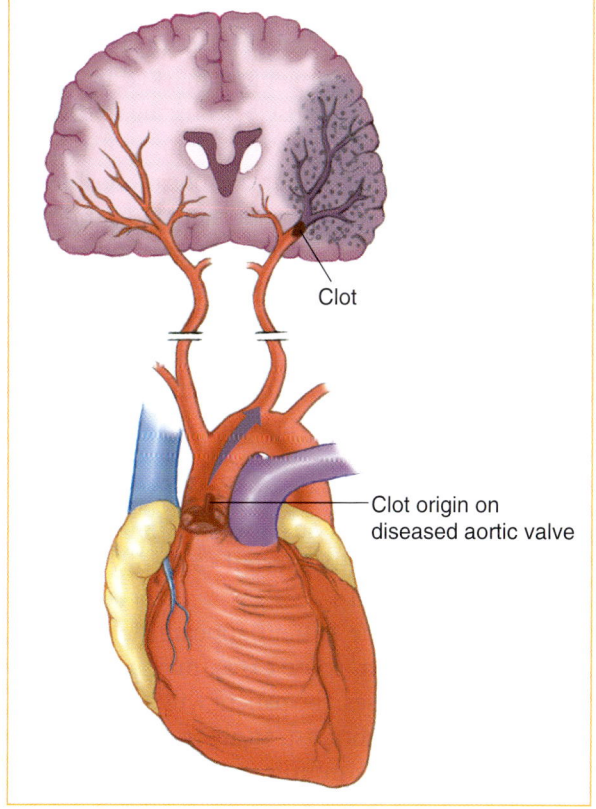

Figure 24-4 An embolus, a blood clot usually formed on a diseased heart valve, can travel through the body's vascular system, lodge in a cerebral artery, and cause a stroke.

transport the patient to the closest appropriate facility for evaluation.

Place the patient on a cardiac monitor and treat any arrhythmias according to standard ACLS protocols.

Seizures

A seizure, or convulsion, is typically characterized by unconsciousness and a generalized severe twitching of all of the body's muscles that lasts several minutes or longer. This type of seizure is often called a generalized seizure (also called a generalized tonic-clonic seizure and formerly called a grand mal seizure). In other cases, the seizure may be characterized by a brief lapse of attention in which the patient has a blank stare and does not respond to anyone. This type of seizure, called an absence seizure (formerly called petit mal seizure), typically occurs in young children.

Characteristics of Seizures

Some seizures occur on only one side of the body. Others begin on one side and gradually progress to a generalized seizure that affects the entire body. These seizures typically have a tonic phase characterized by a continuous, unremitting total muscular contraction and a clonic phase, a form of movement marked by contractions and relaxations of a muscle occurring in rapid succession. Most people with chronic seizures tolerate these events reasonably well without complications; however, in some situations, seizures may signal an underlying life-threatening condition, such as a metabolic disorder or space-occupying intracranial lesion (for example, a tumor). It is important to remember that during a generalized seizure, all muscles of the body are paralyzed, including the diaphragm and intercostal muscles. Therefore, seizure-related deaths are almost always the result of prolonged hypoxia.

Most seizures last 3 to 5 minutes and are followed by a brief period of unconsciousness and unresponsiveness. Then, a lengthy period (5 to 30 minutes or more) of what is called a postictal state occurs. During the postictal state, the patient appears sleepy, is difficult to arouse, and, in some cases, may be combative. Gradually, in most cases, the patient will begin to recover and fully awaken. In contrast, an absence seizure can last for just a fraction of a minute, after which the patient fully recovers immediately with only a brief lapse of memory of the event and no postictal state.

Generalized seizures that are prolonged (more than 10 minutes) or two generalized seizures in a row without a return of consciousness are referred to as status epilepticus, also known as status seizures. Because of the resultant prolonged hypoxia, status epilepticus is clearly a life-threatening emergency that requires prompt emergency medical care.

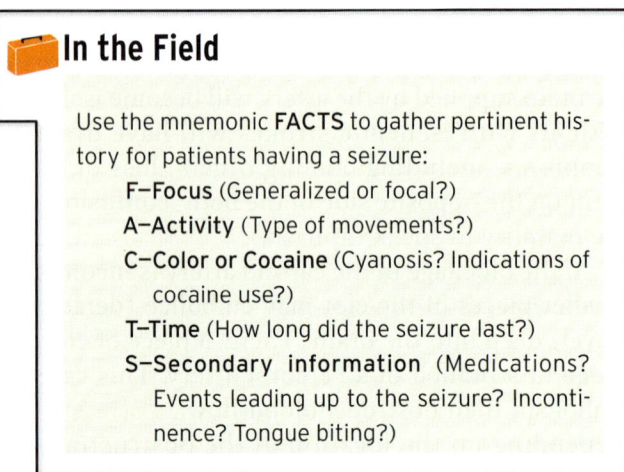

In the Field

Use the mnemonic **FACTS** to gather pertinent history for patients having a seizure:

- F—Focus (Generalized or focal?)
- A—Activity (Type of movements?)
- C—Color or Cocaine (Cyanosis? Indications of cocaine use?)
- T—Time (How long did the seizure last?)
- S—Secondary information (Medications? Events leading up to the seizure? Incontinence? Tongue biting?)

Causes of Seizures

Some seizure disorders, such as epilepsy, are congenital, which means that the patient was born with the condition. Other types of seizures may be due to a high fever, structural problems in the brain, or metabolic or chemical problems in the body (Table 24-1). Epileptic seizures can usually be controlled with medications

TABLE 24-1	Common Cause of Seizures
Type	**Cause**
Epileptic	Congenital in origin
Structural	Tumor (benign or cancerous) Infection (brain abscess) Scar from previous injury Head trauma Degenerative cerebral diseases
Metabolic	Abnormal blood chemistry Hypoglycemia Poisoning Eclampsia Drug overdose Sudden withdrawal from alcohol, medications
Febrile	Sudden high fever

such as phenytoin (Dilantin), phenobarbital (for example, Solfoton), or carbamazepine (for example, Tegretol). Patients with epilepsy will often have seizures if they stop taking their medications or if they do not take an adequate dose. In fact, most seizures are the result of medication noncompliance. In the emergency department, blood analysis will frequently show a subtherapeutic level of anticonvulsant.

Seizures may also be caused by an area of abnormality in the brain, such as a benign or cancerous tumor, an infection (brain abscess), or a scar from a previous injury. These seizures are said to have a *structural* cause; in other cases, the seizures are *metabolic*. Seizures from a metabolic cause can be caused by abnormal levels of certain blood chemicals (for example, extremely low sodium levels), hypoglycemia (low blood glucose level), poisons, drug overdoses, or sudden withdrawal from routine and heavy alcohol or sedative drug use or even from prescribed medications. Phenytoin (Dilantin), a drug that is used to control seizures, can cause seizures itself if the person takes too much. In some cases, seizures are idiopathic (of unknown cause).

Seizures can also result from sudden high fevers, particularly in children. Such seizures, known as febrile seizures, are usually unnerving for parents to observe but are generally well tolerated by the child. Nevertheless, you must transport a child who has had a febrile seizure, as this condition needs to be evaluated in the hospital. The fact that a second seizure may occur is worrisome, and if it occurs, the patient requires rapid evaluation in a hospital to identify possible causes, such as serious inflammation in the brain or tissues covering the brain (conditions known as encephalitis and meningitis, respectively; infection may also be present). Febrile seizures result from a rapid increase in body temperature. In other words, it is not necessarily how high the fever gets, but how quickly it gets there.

The Importance of Recognizing Seizures

Regardless of the type of seizure, it is extremely important for you to recognize when a seizure is occurring or whether one has already occurred. You must also determine whether this episode differs from any previous ones. For example, if the previous seizure occurred on only one side of the body and this seizure occurred over the entire body, some additional or new problem may be involved. In addition to recognizing that seizure activity has occurred and/or that something different may now be occurring, you must also recognize the postictal state and the complications of seizures.

Because most seizures involve vigorous twitching of the muscles, they use a lot of oxygen. This excessive demand consumes oxygen that was being delivered by the circulation to support the vital functions of the body. It is similar to a situation in which you exercise vigorously without giving your body a chance to rest. As a result, there is a buildup of acids in the bloodstream, and the patient may turn cyanotic (bluish lips, mucous membranes, and skin) from the lack of oxygen. Often the seizures themselves prevent the patient from breathing normally, making the problem worse.

Recognizing seizure activity also means looking at other problems associated with the seizure. For example, the patient may have fallen during the seizure episode and injured some part of the body; head injury is the most serious possibility. Patients having a generalized seizure may experience incontinence, meaning that they may lose bowel and bladder control. Therefore, one clue that unresponsive or confused patients may have had a seizure is to find that they were incontinent. Although incontinence is possible with other medical conditions, sudden incontinence is likely a sign that a seizure has occurred.

EMT-I Safety

Be on the lookout for patients who may behave violently during the postictal phase. Although most patients who have had a seizure pose no threat to EMS responders, signs of alcohol or drug abuse should heighten your awareness of the potential for dangerous behavior.

Documentation Tips

Physician evaluation of a patient who has had a seizure depends heavily on reports of the seizure pattern and changes in that pattern. Record all pertinent information about the seizure in terms of duration, areas of body movement, and possible precipitating factors (such as recent trauma, fever, medication noncompliance). This requires effective interviewing of available witnesses, family members, or caregivers.

The Postictal State

Once a seizure has stopped, the patient's muscles relax, becoming almost flaccid, or floppy, and breathing becomes labored (fast and deep) in an attempt to compensate for the buildup of acids in the bloodstream. By breathing faster and more deeply, the body can balance the pH in the bloodstream. With normal circulation and liver function, the acids clear away within minutes, and the patient will begin to breathe normally. The longer the seizure was, the longer it will take for this imbalance to correct itself. Likewise, longer and more severe seizures will result in a longer postictal phase.

In some situations, the postictal state may be characterized by hemiparesis, or weakness on one side of the body, resembling a stroke. Unlike the typical stroke, hypoxic hemiparesis spontaneously resolves within a short period of time. Most commonly, the postictal state is characterized by lethargy and confusion to the point that the patient may be combative and appear angry. You must be prepared for these circumstances, both in your approach to scene control and in your treatment of the patient's symptoms. If the patient's condition does not improve, you should consider other possible underlying problems, including hypoglycemia and infection.

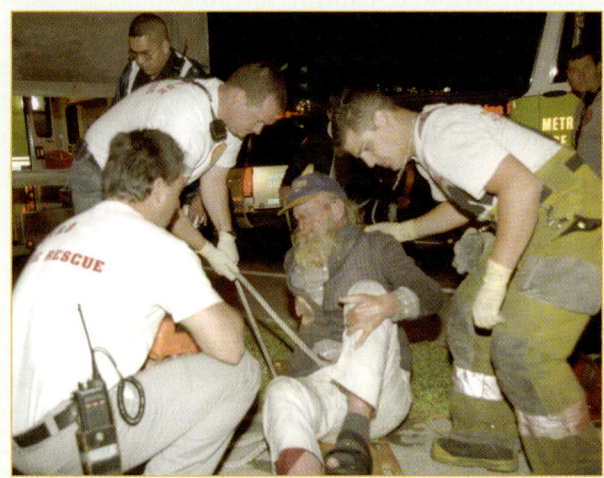

Figure 24-5 A patient with altered mental status can be unresponsive in some instances; in others, the patient may be responsive but confused.

> **EMT-I Tips**
>
> Besides recognizing that a seizure has occurred, it is important to learn whether the pattern has changed. Was this seizure different from previous ones? If so, how?

> **In the Field**
>
> When assessing a patient with altered mental status, consider the mnemonic **AEIOU-TIPS**.
>
> A—Alcohol, Acidosis
> E—Encephalitis, Epilepsy
> I—Insulin
> O—Overdose
> U—Uremia
> T—Trauma
> I—Infection
> P—Psychiatric
> S—Seizures

Altered Mental Status

Aside from stroke and seizures, the most common type of neurologic emergency that you will encounter is a patient with altered mental status. Simply put, altered mental status means that the patient is not thinking clearly or is incapable of being aroused. In some instances, patients will be unresponsive (Figure 24-5); in others, they may be responsive but confused. The range of problems is wide, and the causes are many, including common problems such as hypoglycemia (low blood glucose level), hypoxemia, intoxication, drug overdose, unrecognized head injury, brain infection, body temperature abnormalities, and uncommon conditions such as brain tumors, glandular abnormalities, and poisonings.

Hypoglycemia

The clinical picture of patients with altered mental status due to hypoglycemia is very complex. Patients can have signs and symptoms that mimic stroke and seizures. Because both oxygen and glucose are needed for brain function, hypoglycemia can mimic conditions in the brain such as those associated with stroke. In these cases, the patient may have hemiparesis, similar to what occurs as a result of a stroke. The principal difference, however, is that a patient who has had a stroke may be alert and attempting to communicate normally, whereas a patient with hypoglycemia almost always has an altered or decreased level of consciousness (Figure 24-6).

> **A to Z Terminology Tips**
>
> Hypo = low; glycemia = glucose in the blood; therefore, hypoglycemia is a low level of glucose (or sugar) in the blood.
>
> En = within; cephal = head; itis = inflammation. Encephalitis is an inflammation in the head that causes swelling of the brain.

Patients with hypoglycemia commonly, but not always, take medications that lower the blood glucose level. Thus, if the patient appears to have signs and symptoms of stroke and an altered mental status, you should report your findings to medical control and treat the patient accordingly. Check for and report medications, but remember that not all patients who have diabetes take insulin or other medications to lower the blood glucose level. Remember, also, that patients with a decreased level of consciousness should not be given anything by mouth. Again, local protocols should guide your actions.

Patients with hypoglycemia can also experience seizures, and you may arrive at the scene to find a patient in a postictal state: confused and disoriented or unresponsive. The mental status of a patient who has had a typical seizure is likely to improve; however, in a patient with hypoglycemia, the mental status is not likely to improve, even after several minutes. Therefore, you should consider the possibility of hypoglycemia in a patient who has had a seizure, especially if the blood glucose reading is low.

Likewise, you should consider hypoglycemia in a patient who has altered mental status after an injury such as a motor vehicle crash, even when there is the possibility of an accompanying head injury. As with any other patient, you should look for medical identification bracelets or medications that might confirm your suspicions.

Other Causes of Altered Mental Status

Altered mental status can occur as a result of hypoglycemia, but there are many other possibilities as well, including unrecognized head injury and severe alcohol intoxication. Your consideration of other possibilities becomes important because a patient with altered mental status may be combative and refuse treatment and transport. You should be prepared for difficult patient encounters and follow local protocols for dealing with these situations, recognizing the potential for serious underlying problems.

In most cases, a patient who appears intoxicated most likely is just that; however, you must consider other problems as well. Individuals with chronic alcoholism can have abnormalities in liver function and in their blood-clotting and immune systems, which can predispose them to intracranial bleeding, brain and bloodstream infections, and hypoglycemia.

Psychological problems and complications from medications are also possible causes of altered mental status. A person who appears to have a psychological problem may also have an underlying medical condition.

Infections are another possible cause, particularly those involving the brain or bloodstream. Infections in these areas are obviously life threatening and need immediate attention. Patients may not demonstrate typical signs of infection, such as fever, particularly if they are very young or very old or have impaired immune systems.

Altered mental status can also be caused by drug overdose or poisonings; therefore, you should monitor patients closely for accompanying cardiac and respiratory problems.

The presentation of altered mental status varies widely from simple confusion to coma. Regardless of the cause, you should consider altered mental status to be an emergency that requires immediate attention, even when it appears that the culprit may simply be alcohol intoxication or a minor car crash or fall.

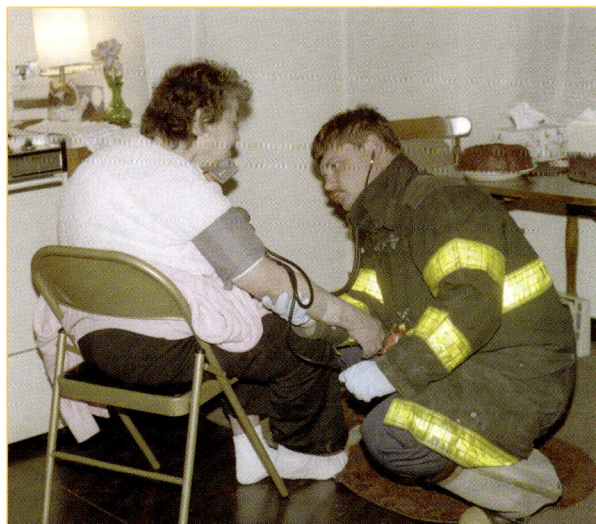

Figure 24-6 During your assessment of a patient with altered or decreased level of consciousness, consider the possibility of hypoglycemia.

Signs and Symptoms of Brain Disorders

Many different disorders can cause brain or other neurologic symptoms, which can affect level of consciousness, speech, and voluntary muscle control. As a general rule, if the brain problem is caused primarily by disorders in the heart and lungs, the entire brain will be affected. For example, without any blood flow (cardiac arrest), the patient will go into a coma and can have permanent brain damage within minutes, even if CPR is performed immediately. However, if the primary problem is in the brain, such as poor blood supply to the middle part of the left cerebral hemisphere, the patient may not be able to move some parts of the right side of the body. This might be the right arm or the right leg. Facial muscles may also be affected on one side. Low oxygen levels in the bloodstream, due to lung disease, for example, will affect the entire brain, causing anxiety, restlessness, and confusion.

Stroke

Left Hemisphere Problems

If the left cerebral hemisphere has been affected, the patient may have a speech disorder called **aphasia**, which is an inability to produce or understand speech. Speech problems vary widely. Patients may have trouble understanding speech but can speak clearly. This condition is called receptive aphasia. You can detect this problem by asking the patient a question such as "What day is today?" In response, the patient with aphasia may say, "Green." The speech is clear, but it does not make sense. Other patients will be able to understand the question but cannot produce the right sounds to answer. Only grunts or other incomprehensible sounds emerge. These patients have expressive aphasia.

Right Hemisphere Problems

If the right cerebral hemisphere of the brain is not getting enough blood, patients will have trouble moving the muscles on the left side of the body. Usually, they will understand language and be able to speak, but their words may be slurred and hard to understand. Slurred speech is referred to as **dysarthria**.

Interestingly, patients with right hemisphere strokes may be completely oblivious to their problem. If you ask these patients to lift the left arm and they cannot, they will lift the right arm instead. They seem to have forgotten that the left arm even exists. This symptom is called neglect. Patients with a problem affecting the posterior aspect of the cerebrum (occiput) may neglect certain parts of their vision. Generally, this is difficult to detect in the field, but you should be aware of the possibility. Try to sit or stand on the patient's unaffected side, because he or she may be unable to see things on the affected side.

The problem of neglect causes many patients who have had large strokes to delay seeking help. Unless caused by a ruptured cerebral artery, in which case the patient will complain of a severe headache, strokes are typically not painful. Therefore, a patient may be unaware that there is a problem until a family member or friend points out that some part of the patient's body is not functioning normally.

You are the Provider — Part 2

As you begin your assessment of this patient, you note the following:

Initial Assessment	Recording Time: Zero Minutes
Appearance	Pale and very anxious
Level of consciousness	Able to follow simple commands
Airway	Open and clear
Breathing	Respiratory rate appears normal
Circulation	Radial pulses present; skin is pale, warm, and dry

3. What is the first treatment priority?

Bleeding in the Brain

Patients who have bleeding in the brain (intracerebral hemorrhage) may present with hypertension. Sometimes, this is the cause of the bleeding, but many times it is a response to the bleeding. Hypertension may be a response of the body to shunt more oxygenated blood to the injured portion of the brain, a process called autoregulation. High blood pressure in stroke patients should not be treated in the field. Quite often, blood pressure will return to normal or drop significantly on its own.

Other Conditions

The following three conditions may simulate stroke:
- Hypoglycemia
- A postictal state
- Subdural or epidural bleeding (bleeding within the skull that compresses the brain)

Because both oxygen and glucose are needed for brain metabolism, a patient with hypoglycemia may look like a patient who is having a stroke. You should find out whether the patient has diabetes and takes insulin or a glucose-lowering medication.

A patient in the postictal state may appear to be having a stroke; however, in most cases, a patient in a postictal state will recover spontaneously, whereas a patient having a stroke will not.

Subdural and epidural bleeding usually occur as a result of trauma. The dura is a leathery covering over the brain, next to the skull. A fracture near the temporal region of the skull may cause an artery (usually the middle meningeal artery) to bleed on top of the dura, resulting in pressure on the brain (Figure 24-7A). Because the source of bleeding is from an artery, the onset of symptoms from *epidural* bleeding is usually very rapid after the injury. In other cases, the veins just below the dura may be torn and bleed, which is known as *subdural* bleeding (Figure 24-7B). Because veins tend to bleed slowly, the onset of symptoms occurs more slowly, sometimes over a period of several days.

The onset of strokelike signs and symptoms may be subtle; the original injury may not even be remembered.

Assessing the Patient

Stroke

When you are called to assist a patient with a possible stroke, you should first determine whether the patient is responsive and breathing. Friends and family members may think that the patient has had a stroke when he or she is actually in cardiac arrest.

Initial Assessment

On arrival, you should assess and care for any immediate problems with the patient's ABCs. If the patient is responsive and breathing, obtain a focused history and physical examination. Also try to speak with relatives or friends who may have seen what happened (Figure 24-8). Make a special effort to determine when the patient last appeared

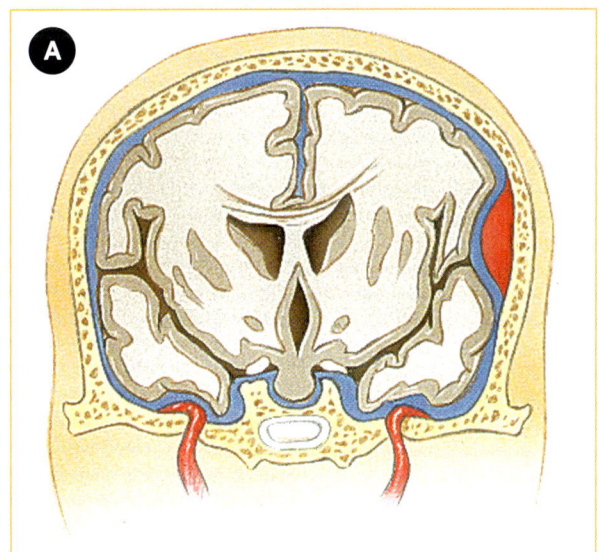

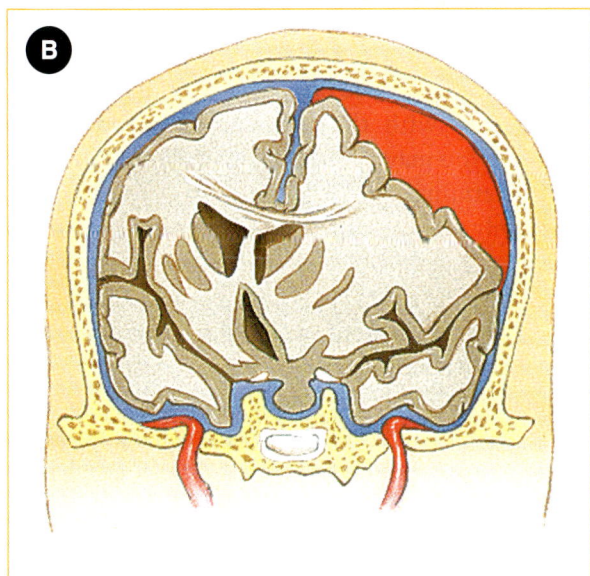

Figure 24-7 Trauma to the head can result in intracranial bleeding. **A.** Bleeding above the dura but outside the brain is epidural. **B.** Bleeding beneath the dura but outside the brain is subdural.

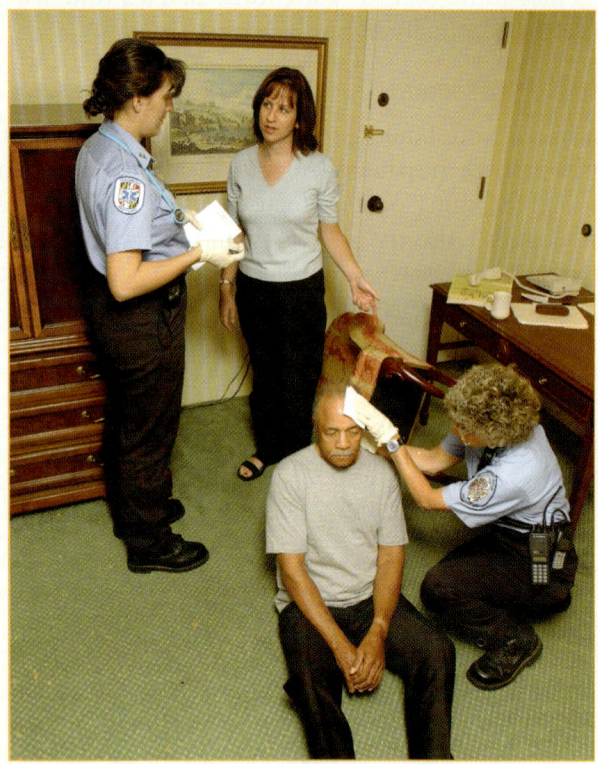

Figure 24-8 Try to speak with family members or bystanders who may have seen what happened. They may also be able to tell you when the patient last appeared "normal."

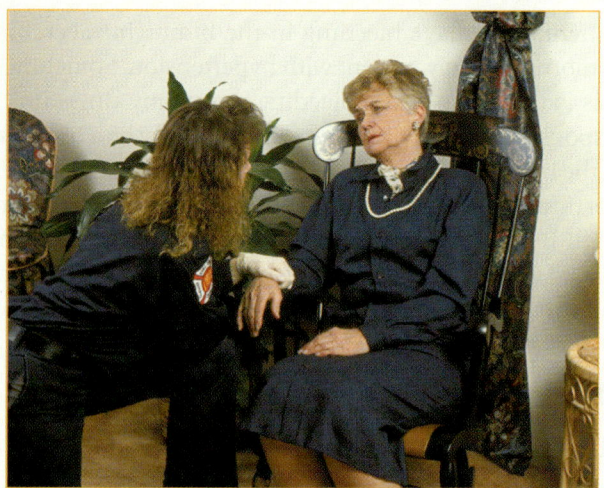

Figure 24-9 Make a special effort to establish communication with a patient who may have had a stroke. Look for indications that the patient understands you, such as a glance, gaze, squeeze of the hand, efforts to speak, or nodding of the head.

to be "normal." This will tell physicians in the emergency department whether it is safe to begin certain treatments (for example, fibrinolytic therapy) that must be given within a narrow timeframe after the onset of symptoms. Because you may be the only person on the emergency medical team with the opportunity to speak with bystanders, you may be the only one who can make this critical determination. Many times, you will be able to find out only that the patient seemed normal when he or she went to sleep the night before. Note that in such cases, the time the patient was last seen to be normal was at bedtime, not when the patient awoke with symptoms. Obtain or list all medications the patient has taken, and record the patient's general health before this episode.

Determine the patient's level of consciousness. Although a patient who has had a stroke may appear to be unconscious and unable to speak, the patient may still be able to hear and understand what is taking place. Be careful what you say, avoiding all unnecessary, negative, or inappropriate remarks. Try to communicate with the patient by looking for indications that the patient can understand you, such as a glance, gaze, motion or pressure of the hand, efforts to speak, or nodding the head.

Establishing effective communication can help calm the patient and lessen the fear that accompanies an inability to communicate 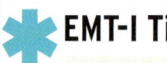.

As you perform the initial assessment, administer 100% supplemental oxygen. Then begin your focused history and physical examination, including baseline vital signs and blood glucose level. If the patient is breathing inadequately (for example, reduced tidal volume), provide assisted ventilation, protect the airway, and suction to prevent aspiration. Remember to check for any history of diabetes, seizures, or recent head injury.

> ### ✱ EMT-I Tips
>
> Assessment and initiating treatment of a patient with altered mental status can keep a team of two responders very busy, particularly because history taking often involves interviewing others. Despite the number of demands, at least one responder needs to keep a close eye on the patient for signs of airway compromise, physical danger from falling, or other risks associated with the patient's mental compromise.

Focused History and Physical Exam

As soon as possible, perform a neurologic exam as part of your focused physical exam. You should perform at least three key physical tests on patients you suspect of

TABLE 24-2	Cincinnati Stroke Scale		
Test		Normal	Abnormal
Facial Droop (Ask patient to show teeth or smile.)		Both sides of face move equally well.	One side of face does not move as well as the other.
Arm Drift (Ask patient to close eyes and hold both arms out with palms up.)		Both arms move the same, or both arms do not move.	One arm does not move, or one arm drifts down compared with the other side.
Speech (Ask patient to say, "The sky is blue in Cincinnati.")		Patient uses correct words with no slurring.	Patient slurs words, uses inappropriate words, or is unable to speak.

having had a stroke: tests of speech, facial movement, and arm movement. If any one of the three is positive (abnormal), the patient should be assumed to be having (or to have had) a stroke.

The EMT should use the Cincinnati Stroke Scale, which tests speech, facial droop, and arm drift. The entire examination is identified in Table 24-2.

To test speech, simply ask the patient to repeat a simple phrase such as "The sky is blue in Cincinnati." If the patient does this correctly, you know that he or she understands and can produce speech. If the patient cannot repeat the phrase, the problem may be with either function: understanding speech or producing it. Receptive and expressive aphasia were discussed earlier in this chapter.

To test facial movement, ask the patient to show his or her teeth (or gums, if there are no teeth). Watch to see that both sides of the face around the mouth move equally. If only one side is moving well, then you know that something is wrong with the control of the muscles on the other side. Also note any unusual breath odor, which could indicate conditions such as diabetic ketoacidosis or alcohol intoxication.

To test arm movement, ask the patient to hold both arms in front of his or her body, palms up toward the sky, with eyes closed and without moving. For the next 10 seconds, watch the patient's hands. If you see one arm drift down toward the ground, you know that side is weak. If both arms stay up and do not move, you know that both sides of the brain that control voluntary muscle movement are functioning normally.

If both arms fall to the ground, you have not really established anything. Perhaps the patient did not understand your instructions. Try the arm test again, but this time move the patient's arms into position. Another possibility to consider is that the patient is having a problem other than stroke. This is likely to be the answer if both sides of the brain are functioning abnormally.

Routine assessment of the patient with a possible stroke should include use of the Glasgow Coma Scale (GCS), which can be seen in Table 24-3.

TABLE 24-3	Glasgow Coma Scale
Eye Opening	Score
Spontaneous	4
In response to speech	3
In response to pain	2
None	1
Best Verbal Response	
Oriented conversation	5
Confused conversation	4
Inappropriate words	3
Incomprehensible sounds	2
None	1
Best Motor Response	
Obeys commands	6
Localizes pain	5
Withdraws to pain	4
Abnormal flexion	3
Abnormal extension	2
None	1
Total score: 14-15, Mild dysfunction	
Total score: 11-13, Moderate to severe dysfunction	
Total score: 10 or less, Severe dysfunction	

Transport Considerations

After you have performed the neurologic exam, prepare the patient for transport. You want to spend as little time on the scene as possible. Remember, stroke is an emergency. There may be treatment available for the patient at the hospital; however, this treatment is time-sensitive. Place the patient in a comfortable position, usually on one side, with the paralyzed side down and well protected with padding Figure 24-10. The patient's head should be elevated about 6". Continue giving 100% oxygen, or, if needed, assisted ventilations en route. Establish IV access, and obtain blood samples for analysis. Give 50% dextrose if the patient is hypoglycemic. Use an isotonic crystalloid solution at a keep-vein-open rate unless the patient is hypovolemic. If hypotensive, give a fluid bolus of 20 mL/kg to maintain adequate perfusion (for example, to maintain the radial pulses). Excessive fluids will increase bleeding and intracranial pressure in patients with hemorrhagic strokes.

Monitor the cardiac rhythm and consider intubation if the patient is unable to maintain his or her airway.

After you begin transport, you should relay the information you have obtained to the receiving hospital. Be sure to include the time that the patient was last seen to be normal, the findings of your neurologic examination, and the time you anticipate arriving at the hospital. This information will allow the emergency department to allocate the appropriate resources for the patient's arrival.

Seizures

You are typically called to care for a patient who has had a seizure because someone actually witnessed the seizure. However, you may also be called to see an unresponsive patient when the patient is found in a postictal state Figure 24-11. In other situations, you may be called to care for a patient who is having seizures and find that the patient actually has some other medical problem, such as cardiac arrest or a psychological problem. Therefore, thorough assessment is key because the information gathered at the scene may be extremely important to the hospital staff who will be caring for the patient.

In most cases, you will arrive after the seizure has ended, because they typically last only a few minutes. By the time someone recognizes the problem, calls for help, and receives a response, the patient is usually in a postictal state. Thus, you must obtain as much information from family or bystanders as possible to verify that a seizure has occurred and to obtain a description of the seizure's progression.

Initial Assessment

As with any other situation, on arrival, you should focus on the ABCs. The patient may have been eating or chewing gum at the time of the seizure, thus posing a risk for a foreign body obstruction. Bystanders may have tried to put objects in the patient's mouth "to help them breathe better," even though this practice is ill-advised. Breathing and circulation should be assessed and treated as necessary. Again, during the immediate postictal state following a major seizure, you should anticipate rapid, deep respirations and an accompanying tachycardia due to a sympathetic nervous system discharge in response to the seizure. However, respirations and heart rate should begin to slow to normal rates after several minutes. If not, you should suspect problems beyond the seizure itself.

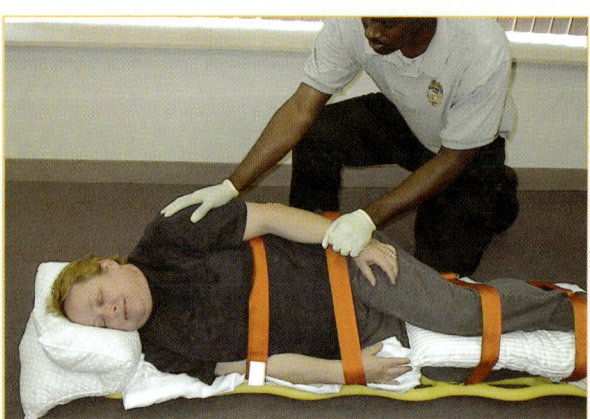

Figure 24-10 A patient who has had a stroke should be positioned with the paralyzed side down and well protected with padding. Elevate the head about 6".

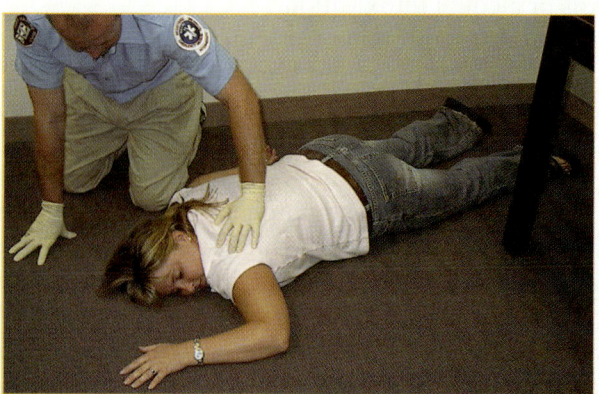

Figure 24-11 A patient who has had a seizure may be found in the postictal state when you arrive. If this is the case, be sure to ask family members or bystanders to verify that a seizure has occurred and how the seizure developed.

Focused History and Physical Exam

You should obtain a SAMPLE history, including whether the patient has a history of seizures. If so, it is important to find out how the patient's seizures typically occur and whether this episode differs in some way from previous episodes. You should also ask what medications the patient has been taking. If the patient takes phenytoin (Dilantin) and phenobarbital, he or she most likely has chronic problems. You might find that the patient ran out of medication or stopped taking medication for a while.

If the patient has no history of seizures and now has a sudden focal (not generalized) seizure, a serious condition, such as brain tumor, intracranial bleeding, or serious infection, should be suspected. You should also determine whether the patient takes medications that lower the blood glucose level, such as insulin or oral hypoglycemic agents. In other situations, you may want to inquire about drug use or potential exposure to toxins.

As you document the physical signs of the seizure, observe for recurrent seizures. If another seizure occurs, note whether it starts at a focal part of the body (for example, one arm or one leg) and then progresses to the rest of the body. Most important, evaluate the patient's mental status and monitor it frequently to verify progressive improvement. The patient should be assessed for injuries, including head lacerations, shoulder dislocation, bitten tongue, and long bone fractures. Also assess for weakness or loss of sensation on one side of the body, and reassess for improvement in such findings.

Syncopal Episodes

From time to time you will be called for a "person down" with no known cause. The patient may experience a temporary loss of consciousness, known as a syncopal episode, due to diminished cerebral blood flow. There may be an obvious explanation, such as severe dehydration or bradycardia, or there may be no signs or symptoms leading to the event.

All patients experiencing syncope should be transported to the emergency department for evaluation. Remember to protect the cervical spine if spinal trauma is suspected or cannot otherwise be ruled out. Evaluate the level of responsiveness, ABCs, and give 100% oxygen. Place the patient in a position of comfort if no trauma is suspected. Establish IV access, and determine the glucose level. Treat associated hypoglycemia or hypovolemia as previously described. Reassess frequently for any changes in mental status or vital signs.

Altered Mental Status

Although altered mental status is a relatively straightforward condition, you should attempt to categorize the severity of the problem and look for accompanying or underlying conditions as you assess the patient. Use the

 Geriatric Needs

Over time, the brain gradually deteriorates and shrinks (atrophy) as a part of the normal aging process. This can increase the risk of head injury from minor forces, because the brain can move more freely within the skull. A reduced brain mass can also reduce the patient's baseline mental status and capacity. A smaller brain can impair memory function, and with lapses in short-term memory, the geriatric patient can ask the same or similar questions repeatedly.

When you are called to care for an older patient with an altered mental status, consider the possibility of a stroke or TIA. At the scene of a motor vehicle crash involving an older driver, consider a stroke or TIA as the precipitating factor in the crash. Be alert for an altered mental state or unusual pupil response in low light (that is, constricted or unequal pupils in dim light).

Beware of headache. Although older patients have tension headaches, they are far less common in the older adult population. You should consider any headache as potentially serious.

As with the general population, older people can also have seizures. Remember that seizures are not necessarily due to epilepsy. You should consider and assess for the possibility of a drug overdose, stroke, head injury, or central nervous system infection. Status epilepticus in an older patient can have harmful effects such as hypoxia, irregular heart rhythm (dysrhythmias), hypotension, elevated body temperature, low blood glucose level, and, if the patient vomits, aspiration.

Remember that the older patient is at higher risk for central nervous system illnesses and injuries, including brain injury, TIA, stroke, and seizures. Do not be surprised to find a serious head injury with an otherwise insignificant mechanism of injury. Remember too that a syncopal episode or generalized weakness may be the only sign of a myocardial infarction in older patients.

AVPU scale (**A**lert; responsive to **V**erbal stimuli; responsive to **P**ain; **U**nresponsive) to assess the patient's level of responsiveness.

During your assessment, you should also consider other underlying medical conditions; the most important are those that are easily reversible. Therefore, you should consider hypoxemia and hypoglycemia as possible causes. Continually reassess the patient closely for depressed respirations and assist ventilation if needed. Likewise, a patient with a decreased level of consciousness may not be able to protect the airway. Therefore, you should make sure that basic airway maneuvers are followed and suctioning is available (Figure 24-12 ▶). Prompt transport is necessary, with close monitoring of vital signs en route.

Monitor the cardiac rhythm in any patient with an altered mental status and treat arrhythmias following standard ACLS protocols. Be prepared to intubate patients if they cannot protect their own airway.

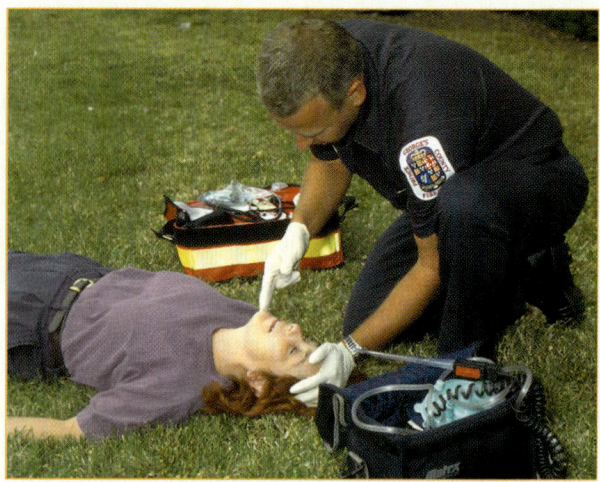

Figure 24-12 Securing and maintaining the airway in a patient who is unconscious is critical; also be sure to have suction readily available in case the patient vomits.

Emergency Medical Care

Stroke

In patients with a suspected stroke, physicians in the emergency department must determine whether there is bleeding in the brain. If there is no bleeding, the patient may be a candidate for medication to help break up the blood clot (fibrinolytic therapy) and reestablish blood flow or to help brain cells survive the reduced amount of oxygen. The only reliable way to tell whether there is bleeding is with a special type of radiographic test called a computed tomography (CT) scan. Blood is usually easy to see on the CT scan (Figure 24-13 ▶).

Most hospitals have only one CT scanner. The technician who knows how to run the machine may not be in the hospital in the middle of the night. That is why it is important that you recognize the signs and symptoms of stroke. If the emergency department staff knows that you are transporting a patient with a possible stroke, they may be able to call in the technician before you arrive, or they may decide to delay a CT scan on another

You are the Provider   Part 3

You are unable to determine the onset of the patient's symptoms. You continue your assessment of the patient and prepare to transport.

Vital Signs	Recording Time: 2 Minutes After Patient Contact
Respirations	16 breaths/min, shallow
Pulse	88 beats/min, irregular
Skin	Pale, warm, and dry
Blood pressure	208/108 mm Hg
Sao_2	95% on room air

4. What are some of the concerns that you might have regarding this patient's medical condition?
5. What are your care and transport options for this patient?

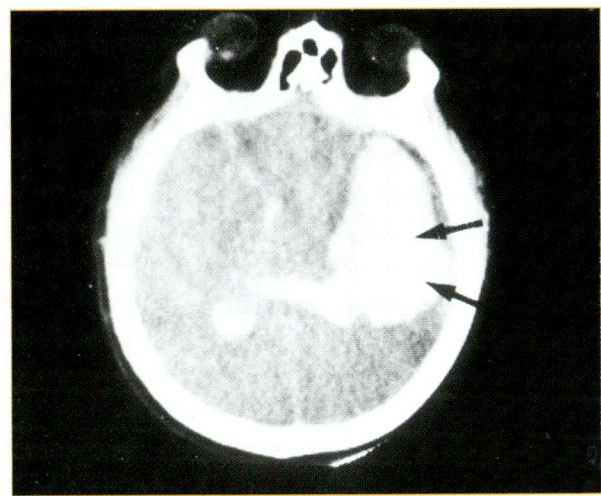

Figure 24-13 A CT scan of a ruptured cerebral aneurysm. The light area represents hemorrhage into the brain tissue (arrows).

TABLE 24-4	Tips on Patient Care

- Patients who experience a TIA typically have the same signs and symptoms as those who have a stroke. These signs and symptoms can last from minutes up to 24 hours. Therefore, the signs of stroke that you note on arrival may gradually resolve. Patients who appear to have had a TIA should be transported for further evaluation.
- Place the patient's affected or paralyzed extremity in a secure and safe position during patient movement and transport.
- Some patients who have had a stroke may be unable to communicate, but they can often understand what is being said around them. Be aware of this possibility.
- New therapies for stroke must be used shortly after the onset of symptoms. Minimize time on the scene, and notify the receiving hospital as soon as possible.

patient who has a less critical problem. Keep in mind that most treatments for stroke must be started as soon as possible after the onset of the event (Table 24-4). Few, if any, current treatments are effective if they are started more than 3 hours after the stroke begins. Even if 3 hours have passed since the onset of symptoms, prompt action on your part is essential.

Seizures

In most situations, patients who have had a seizure require definitive evaluation and treatment in the hospital. Even a patient who has a history of chronic epilepsy that is controlled with medications may have an occasional seizure, commonly referred to as a "breakthrough" seizure. These patients should also be taken to the hospital for evaluation. At the hospital, blood levels of seizure medications are checked to ensure that patients are receiving the correct dose. Clearly, patients who have just had their first seizure or those with chronic seizures who have had an episode that is "different" require immediate evaluation to rule out life-threatening conditions. Administer 100% supplemental oxygen to any patient who has experienced a seizure, whether it is the first or whether the patient has chronic seizures. This will help ameliorate any associated hypoxia. Note any medications the patient is currently taking and any previous seizures, the time of onset, the duration of the seizure activity, the number of seizures, and whether the patient regained responsiveness between seizures. Provide spinal immobilization if trauma was involved or cannot be ruled out.

Depending on local protocols, you should assess and treat the patient for possible hypoglycemia (for example, a person with diabetes who has altered mental status and takes insulin or oral agents that lower the blood glucose level). If trauma is suspected, provide spinal immobilization. Look for tongue lacerations and bleeding that may create an obstruction or lead to aspiration. Also note the presence of bladder or bowel incontinence. With recurrent seizures, protect the patient from further injury and manage the airway as needed. Establish IV access, and obtain blood samples for analysis. Give an isotonic crystalloid fluid bolus of 20 mL/kg to maintain adequate perfusion.

If you are treating a child who you suspect is having a febrile seizure, you should attempt to lower the body temperature by removing the child's clothing and cooling the child with tepid water, particularly around the head and neck, and then fanning the moistened areas. Be careful not to make the patient shiver, which will further increase temperature and precipitate another seizure.

If the patient has been exposed to a toxin or poison, you should safely remove the source if possible. Suction should be readily available in case a patient with a decreased level of consciousness begins to vomit.

In all instances, you should be patient and tolerant because many of these patients are likely to be confused and, occasionally, frightened. Many patients who experience seizures are frustrated with their condition and may refuse transport. Compassion and professional behavior are required to help convince the patient that transport is necessary for definitive care.

If the patient is actively seizing, consider the use of anticonvulsants or muscle relaxers. Monitor the cardiac rhythm and treat dysrhythmias according to ACLS or local protocols.

Pediatric Needs

Children can have altered mental status caused by strokes, seizures, and other brain emergencies. However, children who have subarachnoid hemorrhages may not have a berry aneurysm; instead, they may have a congenital problem with the blood vessels in the brain known as an arteriovenous malformation. Children who have sickle cell anemia are at particularly high risk for ischemic stroke. Treat stroke in children the same way that you do in adults.

As mentioned earlier in this chapter, seizures can result from sudden high fever, particularly in children. Remember that although febrile seizures are generally well tolerated by children, you must transport them to the hospital. The possibility of a second seizure makes transport mandatory so that if other problems develop, the child is in the hospital and can receive immediate, definitive care.

If you suspect that a patient with altered mental status has hypoglycemia and you have the ability to test for it, you should do so and treat the patient according to local protocols. Also, these patients require close monitoring, particularly of the airway, en route to the hospital.

You are the Provider — Summary

1. Why is the brain so dependent on a continuous supply of oxygen?

Without oxygen, brain cells stop working and begin to die. Medical science currently has little to offer these cells once they are dead. However, it may take several hours or more for cell death to occur, even when it appears that severe disability will occur.

2. What is the clinical significance of a patient having a TIA?

A TIA may be a warning sign that a larger, permanent stroke is imminent. Because of this, all patients with a TIA should be evaluated by a physician to determine whether preventive action can be taken.

3. What is the first treatment priority?

Upon arrival, you should assess and care for any immediate problems with the patient's ABCs. If the patient is responsive and breathing, obtain a focused history and physical exam. Also try to speak with relatives or friends who may have seen what happened. Make a special effort to determine when the patient last appeared to be normal. This will help physicians in the emergency department determine whether it is safe to begin certain treatments.

4. What are some of the concerns that you might have regarding this patient's medical condition?

The concern facing the EMT-I is that this patient may be having an ischemic or hemorrhagic stroke, and care needs to be provided expeditiously if any signs or symptoms are going to be reversed.

5. What are your care and transport options for this patient?

After you have performed a neurologic exam, you need to prepare the patient for transport. You want to spend as little time on the scene as possible. A possible stroke is an emergency. There may be treatment available for the patient at the hospital; however, this treatment is time-sensitive. Place the patient in a comfortable position, usually on one side, with the paralyzed side down and well protected with padding. The patient's head should be elevated about 6". Continue giving 100% oxygen. Establish IV access. Give 50% dextrose if the patient is hypoglycemic. Use an isotonic crystalloid solution at a keep-vein-open (KVO) rate unless the patient is hypovolemic. If the patient is hypotensive, give a fluid bolus of 20 mL/kg to maintain adequate perfusion (eg, radial pulses). Excessive fluids will increase bleeding and intracranial pressure in patients with hemorrhagic strokes.

Prep Kit

Ready for Review

- The cerebrum, the largest part of the brain, is divided into right and left hemispheres, each controlling the opposite side of the body.

- Different parts of the brain control different functions. The frontal lobe of the cerebrum controls emotion and thought; the middle controls touch and movement; the occipital lobe of the cerebrum is involved with vision. In most people, speech is controlled on the left side of the brain, near the middle of the cerebrum.

- Many different disorders can cause brain or other neurologic symptoms. As a general rule, if the problem is primarily in the brain, only part of the brain will be affected. If the problem is systemic, the whole brain will be affected.

- Stroke is a significant brain disorder because it is common and potentially treatable. Seizures and altered mental status are also common, and you must learn to recognize the signs and symptoms of each. Other causes of neurologic dysfunction include coma, infections, and tumors.

- Strokes occur when part of the blood flow to the brain is suddenly obstructed; within minutes, brain cells begin to die. Signs and symptoms of stroke include receptive or expressive aphasia, dysarthria, muscle weakness or numbness on one side, facial droop, and, sometimes, hypertension.

- You should always perform at least three neurologic tests on patients you suspect of having a stroke: test speech, facial movement, and arm movement.

- In a TIA, normal body processes break up the blood clot, restoring blood flow and ending symptoms in less than 24 hours. However, patients with TIA are at high risk for a permanent stroke. Because current treatments must be administered within 3 hours of the onset of symptoms to be most effective, you should provide prompt transport.

- Always notify the hospital as soon as possible that you are bringing in a possible stroke patient, so that staff there can prepare to test and treat the patient without delay.

- Seizures are characterized by unconsciousness and generalized twitching of all or part of the body. There are types of seizures that you should learn to recognize: generalized, absence, and febrile seizures.

- Most seizures last between 3 and 5 minutes and are followed by a postictal state in which the patient may be unresponsive, have labored breathing and hemiparesis, and may have been incontinent. It is important for you to recognize the signs and symptoms of seizures so that you can provide emergency department staff with information as you transport the patient.

- Altered mental status is also a common neurologic problem that you will encounter as an EMT-I. Signs and symptoms vary widely, as do the causes for this condition. Among the most common causes are hypoglycemia, alcohol intoxication, drug overdose, and poisoning.

- As you assess the patient with altered mental status, do not always assume intoxication; hypoglycemia is just as likely a cause. Prompt transport with close monitoring of vital signs en route is indicated.

Technology

- Interactivities
- Vocabulary Explorer
- Anatomy Review
- Web Links
- Online Review Manual

Vital Vocabulary

absence seizure Seizure that may be characterized by a brief lapse of attention in which the patient may stare and does not respond; formerly known as a petit mal seizure.

aphasia The inability to understand or produce speech.

arterial rupture Rupture of an artery. Involvement of a cerebral artery may contribute to interruption of cerebral blood flow.

atherosclerosis A disorder in which cholesterol and calcium build up inside the walls of blood vessels, forming plaque, which eventually leads to partial or complete blockage of blood flow. An atherosclerotic plaque can also become a site where blood clots can form, detach, and travel elsewhere in the circulatory system (embolize).

cerebral embolism Obstruction of a cerebral artery caused by a clot that was formed elsewhere in the body and traveled to the brain.

cerebrovascular accident (CVA) An interruption of blood flow to the brain that results in the loss of brain function; also referred to as a stroke or brain attack.

clonic phase Seizure movement marked by repetitive muscle contractions and relaxations in rapid succession.

dysarthria The inability to pronounce speech clearly, often due to loss of the nerves or brain cells that control the small muscles in the larynx.

febrile seizures Seizures that result from sudden high fever, particularly in children.

generalized seizure Seizure characterized by severe twitching of all the body's muscles that may last several minutes or more; formerly known as a grand mal seizure.

hemiparesis Weakness on one side of the body.

hemorrhagic stroke One of the two main types of stroke; occurs as a result of bleeding inside the brain.

hypoglycemia A condition characterized by a low blood glucose level.

incontinence Loss of bowel and bladder control; can be due to a generalized seizure or to other conditions.

infarcted cells Cells that die as a result of loss of blood flow.

ischemic cells Cells that receive enough blood after an event, such as a cerebrovascular accident, to stay alive but not enough to function properly.

ischemic stroke One of the two main types of stroke; occurs when blood flow to a particular part of the brain is cut off by a blockage (for example, a clot) inside a blood vessel.

postictal state Period following a seizure that lasts between 5 and 30 minutes, characterized by labored respirations and some degree of altered mental status.

seizure An episode often characterized by generalized, uncoordinated muscular activity associated with loss of consciousness; a convulsion.

status epilepticus A condition in which seizures recur every few minutes without a lucid interval or last more than 10 minutes.

stroke A loss of brain function in certain brain cells that do not get enough oxygen during a CVA. Usually caused by obstruction of the blood vessels in the brain that feed oxygen to those brain cells.

syncope Temporary loss of consciousness and postural tone caused by diminished cerebral blood flow.

thrombus Local clotting of blood in the cerebral arteries that may result in the interruption of cerebral blood flow and subsequent stroke.

tonic phase In a seizure, the steady, rigid muscle contractions with no relaxation.

transient ischemic attack (TIA) A disorder of the brain in which brain cells temporarily stop working because of insufficient oxygen, causing strokelike symptoms that resolve completely within 24 hours of onset.

Assessment in Action

You are dispatched to a private residence for a patient complaining of a severe headache. You arrive at the scene to find a 55-year-old man sitting on the couch in the living room. He tells you that he has a very bad headache.

You notice that the patient's speech is slurred as he talks to you. As you continue your assessment, you determine that the patient has some facial drooping on the left side and his right arm appears to be limp. You notify the hospital of your findings and are instructed to transport him immediately to the ED for further evaluation.

1. The cerebrum is divided into two hemispheres. Each hemisphere controls activities on the _____ side of the body and the _____ side of the face.
   A. same, opposite
   B. opposite, same
   C. same, same
   D. opposite, opposite

2. An ischemic stroke may be caused by any of the following, EXCEPT:
   A. systemic hypoxia.
   B. cerebral thrombus.
   C. intracerebral bleeding.
   D. cerebral embolism.

3. People who have a ruptured cerebral aneurysm often complain of:
   A. mild weakness and confusion.
   B. a sudden, severe headache.
   C. a sudden loss of vision in one eye.
   D. weakness in the extremities.

4. A disorder in which calcium and cholesterol build up, forming a plaque inside the walls of blood vessels, which could lead to an ischemic stroke, is known as:
   A. arteriosclerosis.
   B. atherosclerosis.
   C. atelectasis.
   D. stenosis.

5. When a patient has stroke-like symptoms that spontaneously subside within 24 hours, a _____ has occurred.
   A. ruptured cerebral aneurysm
   B. spontaneous cerebral embolism
   C. transient ischemic attack
   D. temporary cerebral infarct

6. A type of seizure characterized by a brief lapse of attention, in which the patient has a blank stare and does not respond to anyone is known as a(n):
   A. grand mal seizure.
   B. generalized seizure.
   C. focal seizure.
   D. absence seizure.

7. A state in which the seizure patient appears sleepy, is difficult to arouse, and occasionally combative, is known as the:
   A. tonic state.
   B. postictal state.
   C. clonic state.
   D. hypertonic state.

8. A mnemonic described in this chapter that should be used to gather pertinent history for patients having a seizure is:
   A. SAMPLE.
   B. AVPU.
   C. BTLS.
   D. FACTS.

9. All of the following are medications commonly prescribed to help control seizures, EXCEPT:
   A. Labetolol.
   B. Dilantin.
   C. Solfoton.
   D. Tegretol.

10. Aphasia is a term used to describe:
    A. an inability to speak.
    B. difficulty swallowing.
    C. difficulty hearing.
    D. unilateral weakness.

Points to Ponder

You are dispatched to the local high school during a basketball game for a report of an unconscious patient. Upon your arrival at the scene, you find a 16-year-old adolescent who, according to bystanders, began to violently shake while sitting in the bleachers watching the game. His friend tells you that he seized for about 2 minutes. The patient is currently semiconscious, incontinent, and diaphoretic. What actions should you take?

Issues: Best Patient Care, Working with Bystanders, Calming Frightened Patients

Nontraumatic Abdominal Emergencies

1999 Objectives

Cognitive

5-7.1 Discuss the pathophysiology of non-traumatic abdominal emergencies. (p 1084)
5-7.2 Discuss the signs and symptoms of non-traumatic acute abdominal pain. (p 1084)
5-7.3 Describe the technique for performing a comprehensive physical examination on a patient with non-traumatic abdominal pain. (p 1087)
5-7.4 Describe the management of the patient with non-traumatic abdominal pain. (p 1091)

Affective

None

Psychomotor

None

1985 Objectives

There are no 1985 objectives for this chapter.

25

Nontraumatic Abdominal Emergencies

You are the Provider

You receive a call for an unknown problem. You arrive at a local business to find a 30-year-old woman clutching her abdomen and doubled over in pain.

An acute abdomen can be the result of something as minor as indigestion or as life threatening as a ruptured aortic aneurysm. This chapter will prepare you to properly care for the patient with an acute abdomen and help you answer the following questions:

1. What does "referred pain" mean, and does it indicate a serious problem?
2. Is it a requirement that all patients complaining of abdominal pain be transported to the hospital?

Nontraumatic Abdominal Emergencies

Abdominal pain is a common complaint, but the cause is often difficult to identify, even for a physician. As an EMT-I, you do not need to determine the exact cause of acute abdominal pain. You simply need to be able to recognize a life-threatening problem and act swiftly in response. Remember, the patient is in pain and is probably anxious, requiring all your skills of rapid assessment and emotional support.

This chapter begins by explaining the physiology of the acute abdomen. It then describes the signs and symptoms of the acute abdomen and explains how to examine the abdomen. Next, it discusses the different causes of the acute abdomen and appropriate emergency medical care.

Physiology of the Acute Abdomen

Acute abdomen is a medical term referring to the sudden onset of abdominal pain that indicates an irritation of the peritoneum, the thin membrane that lines the entire abdominal cavity. This condition, called peritonitis, can be caused by an infection, a penetrating abdominal wound, a blunt injury severe enough to damage abdominal organs, and many diseases. In all cases, the major symptom is the same: severe pain. The major clinical signs are abdominal tenderness and distention.

Anatomically, the peritoneum is not one membrane, but two. The *parietal peritoneum* lines the walls of the abdominal cavity; the *visceral peritoneum* covers the surface of each of the organs in the abdominal cavity.

Two different types of nerves supply these two areas of the peritoneum. The parietal peritoneum is supplied by the same nerves from the spinal cord that supply the skin overlying the abdomen; it can therefore perceive many of the same sensations: pain, touch, pressure, heat, and cold. These sensory nerves can easily identify and localize a point of irritation. In contrast, the visceral peritoneum is supplied by the autonomic nervous system. These nerves are far less able to localize sensation. The visceral peritoneum is stimulated when distention or contraction of the hollow abdominal organs activates the stretch receptors. This sensation is usually interpreted as colic, a severe, intermittent cramping pain. Other painful sensations that occur because of an irritated visceral peritoneum may be perceived at a distant point on the surface of the body, such as the back or shoulder. This phenomenon is called referred pain.

Referred pain is the result of connections between the body's two separate nervous systems. The spinal cord supplies sensory nerves to the skin and muscles; these nerves are a part of the somatic (voluntary) nervous system. The autonomic nervous system controls the function of the abdominal organs and the caliber of the blood vessels. The nerves connecting these two systems cause the stimulation of the autonomic nerves to be perceived as stimulation of the spinal sensory nerves. For example, *acute cholecystitis* (inflammation of the gallbladder) may cause referred pain to the right shoulder, because the autonomic nerves serving the gallbladder lie near the spinal cord at the same anatomic level as the spinal sensory nerves that supply the skin of the shoulder (Figure 25-1 ▶).

Signs and Symptoms of Acute Abdomen

Peritonitis typically causes ileus, or paralysis of the muscular contractions that normally propel material through the intestine. (This movement is known as peristalsis.) The retained gas and feces, in turn, cause abdominal distention. In the presence of such paralysis, nothing that is eaten can pass normally out of the stomach or through the bowel. The only way the stomach can empty itself, then, is by emesis, or vomiting. For this reason, peritonitis is almost always associated with nausea and

Technology

- Interactivities
- Vocabulary Explorer
- Anatomy Review
- Web Links
- Online Review Manual

www.EMSzone.com/EMTI

vomiting. These complaints do not point to a particular cause, because they can accompany almost every type of gastrointestinal disease or injury.

Similarly, anorexia, loss of hunger or appetite, is a nonspecific symptom. It too, is a common complaint in gastrointestinal and abdominal disease or injury.

Peritonitis is associated with a loss of body fluid into the abdominal cavity and usually results from abnormal shifts of fluid from the bloodstream into body tissues. This decreases the volume of circulating blood and may eventually cause *hypovolemic* shock. This problem can be compounded by massive internal or external bleeding, resulting in severe inadequate perfusion (shock). The patient may have normal vital signs or, if the peritonitis has progressed further, signs of shock (such as restlessness, tachycardia, and hypotension). When peritonitis is accompanied by hemorrhage, the signs of shock are much more apparent.

> **EMT-I Tips**
>
> An acute abdomen is characterized by abdominal pain and tenderness.

Fever may or may not be present, depending on the cause of the peritonitis. Patients with diverticulitis (an inflammation of small pockets in the colon) or cholecystitis may have a substantial elevation in temperature, which may be due to the inflammatory process itself or an underlying infection. However, patients with acute appendicitis may have a normal temperature until the appendix ruptures and an abscess starts to form.

As we have seen, an acute abdomen is characterized by abdominal pain and tenderness. The pain may be sharply localized or diffuse (widespread) and will

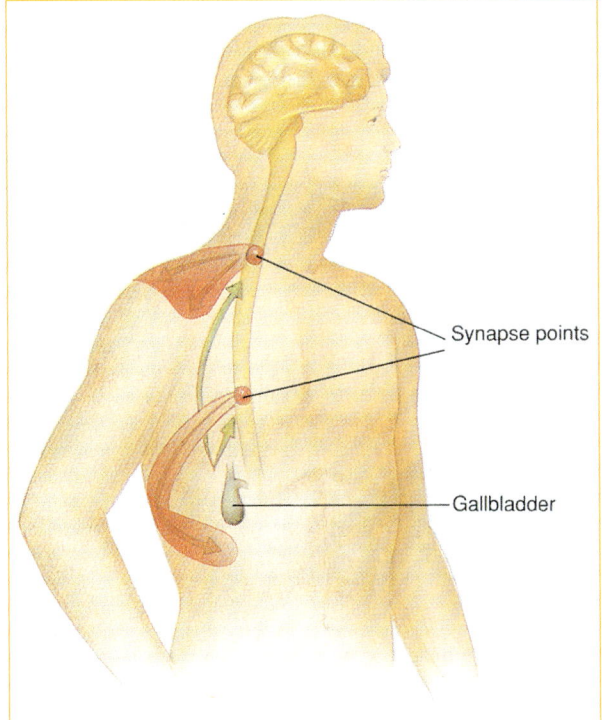

Figure 25-1 Acute cholecystitis can cause referred pain to the shoulder, as well as abdominal pain.

You are the Provider — Part 2

You approach the patient with your jump kit while your partner gets the stretcher.

Initial Assessment	Recording Time: Zero Minutes
Appearance	In severe pain; pale, diaphoretic, and moaning as she holds her stomach
Level of consciousness	Alert and oriented, but obviously in a lot of pain
Airway	Open and clear
Breathing	Respiratory rate, somewhat increased but with adequate tidal volume
Circulation	Skin, very clammy; radial pulse, rapid

3. What are some conditions that may cause abdominal pain?
4. What is your first consideration in treating this patient?

vary in severity. Localized pain gives a clue to the problem organ or area causing it. Tenderness may be minimal or so great that the patient will not allow you to touch the abdomen.

Another sign of the acute abdomen is tenseness of the abdominal muscles over the irritated area. In some instances, the muscles of the abdominal wall become rigid in an involuntary effort to protect the abdomen from further irritation. This boardlike muscle spasm, called guarding, can be seen with major problems such as a perforated peptic ulcer or pancreatitis. In some situations, patients are comfortable only when lying in one particular position, which tends to relax muscles adjacent to the inflamed organ and, thus, lessen the pain. Therefore, the position of the patient may provide an important clue. For example, a patient with appendicitis may draw up the right knee. A patient with pancreatitis may lie curled up on one side Figure 25-2 .

To gauge the degree of distention, simply look at the patient's abdomen. Distention begins shortly after muscular contractions of the bowel have ceased. Pulse and blood pressure may undergo significant change or may remain relatively normal. These findings usually reflect the severity of the process, its duration, and the amount of fluid lost into the abdomen.

Remember, the patient with peritonitis usually has abdominal pain, even when lying quietly. The patient can be quiet but have difficulty breathing and may take rapid, shallow breaths because of the pain. Usually, you will find tenderness on palpation of the abdomen or when the patient moves. The degree of pain and tenderness is usually related directly to the severity of peritoneal inflammation.

> **EMT-I Tips**
>
> When palpating the abdomen, always begin on the side opposite from the site of pain.

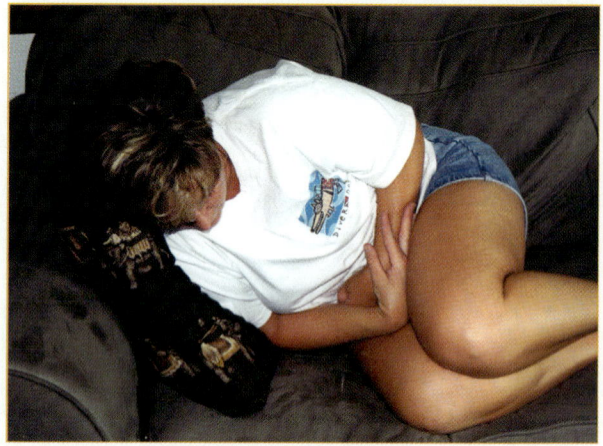

Figure 25-2 A patient experiencing abdominal pain will often curl into a fetal position to relieve the pressure on the abdomen.

You are the Provider — Part 3

Your initial questioning reveals a 30-year-old woman who ate lunch approximately an hour and a half ago. She was working at her computer when a sharp pain started in her lower abdomen.

Vital Signs	Recording Time: 2 Minutes After Patient Contact
Respirations	28 breaths/min, adequate depth
Pulse	124 beats/min, regular, radial pulses slightly weak
Skin	Pale, cool, diaphoretic
Blood pressure	112/68 mm Hg
Sao_2	97% on room air

Your partner is approaching with the stretcher.

5. What is your next step?
6. In what position will you transport this patient?

Documentation Tips

An acute abdomen usually indicates peritonitis, in which generalized signs can make it challenging to determine exactly where the problem lies, even for physicians. Knowing abdominal assessment steps well and recording your findings in detail are important early components of the process that leads to diagnosis.

The following is a checklist of common signs and symptoms of irritation or inflammation of the peritoneum that you can use to determine whether a patient has an acute abdomen:

- Local or diffuse abdominal pain and/or tenderness
- A quiet patient who is guarding the abdomen
- Rapid and shallow breathing
- Referred (distant) pain
- Anorexia, nausea, vomiting
- Vomiting blood (bright red or "coffee ground" emesis)
- Tense, often distended, abdomen
- Sudden constipation or bloody diarrhea
- Dark, tarry stool (melena)
- Painful or frequent urination
- Discolored urine accompanied by a strong odor
- Tachycardia
- Hypotension
- Fever

Use the following steps to assess the abdomen:

1. Explain to the patient what you are about to do.
2. Place the patient in a supine position with the legs drawn up and flexed at the knees to relax the abdominal muscles, unless trauma is involved, in which case the patient will remain supine and immobilized.
3. Determine whether the patient is restless or quiet; whether motion causes pain; or whether any characteristic position, distention, or obvious abnormality is present.
4. Palpate the four quadrants of the abdomen gently to determine whether it is tense (guarded) or soft Figure 25-3 ▶ . Palpate the suspect abdominal quadrant last.
5. Determine whether the patient can relax the abdominal wall on command.
6. Determine whether the abdomen is tender when palpated. Note any rigidity, guarding, or pulsating mass.

You are the Provider — Part 4

You and your partner lift the patient onto the stretcher and allow her to turn to her left side and bend her knees. This appears to ease the pain slightly. She tells you she is very nauseated. Your partner hands her an emesis bag while you apply oxygen with a nonrebreathing mask at 15 L/min.

Reassessment	Recording Time: 5 Minutes After Patient Contact
Respirations	26 breaths/min, good depth
Pulse	132 beats/min, radial pulses weak and thready
Skin	Paler, more diaphoretic
Blood pressure	94/50 mm Hg
Sao₂	98% on O₂ via nonrebreathing mask at 15 L/min

After loading the patient in the ambulance, you begin your focused history and physical exam. Upon palpation of the abdomen, you find palpable tenderness in the right lower quadrant. The abdomen is also slightly distended. You decide to transport on an emergency status based on your findings.

7. What questions should you ask in relation to the pain and medical history?
8. What condition do the vital signs and distended abdomen indicate?
9. As an EMT-I, what are your treatment options?

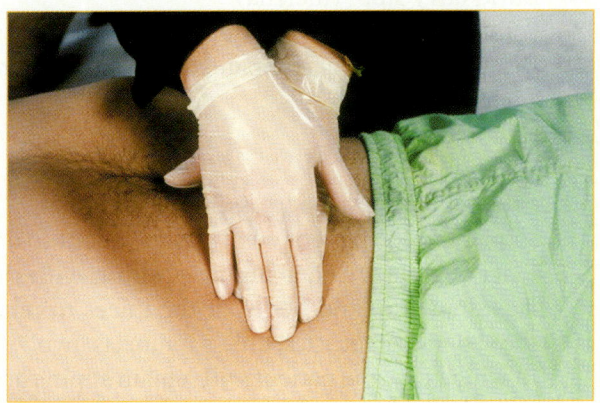

Figure 25-3 Check tenderness or rigidity by gently palpating the abdomen.

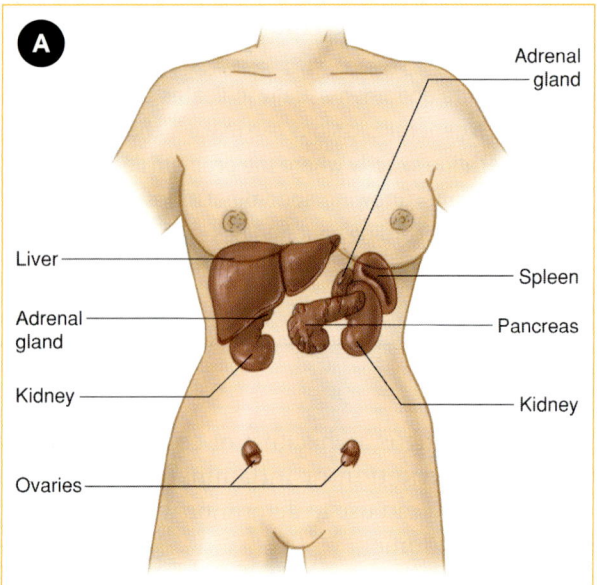

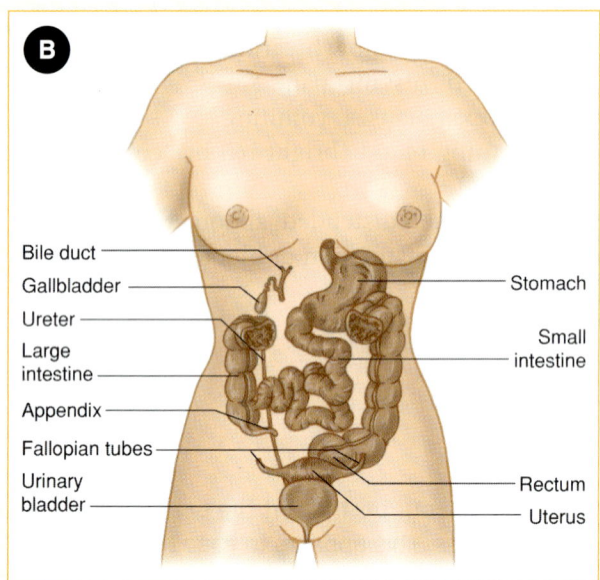

Figure 25-4 The solid and hollow organs of the abdomen. **A.** Solid organs include the liver, spleen, pancreas, kidneys, and, in women, ovaries. **B.** Hollow organs include the gallbladder, stomach, small and large intestine, and urinary bladder.

Although such an examination will yield much information, it should not be prolonged. The physician will do a much more detailed examination in the emergency department. Remember to be very gentle when palpating the abdomen. Occasionally, an organ within the abdomen will be enlarged and very fragile, and rough palpation would cause unnecessary pain and could cause further damage.

Causes of Abdominal Pain

Gastrointestinal and Urinary Tract

The abdominal cavity contains the solid and hollow organs that make up the gastrointestinal, genital, and urinary systems (Figure 25-4 ▶). Many of these organs, such as the bowel, are covered by visceral peritoneum; parietal peritoneum covers the inside aspect of the abdominal wall that forms the abdominal cavity. The entire abdominal cavity normally contains a very small amount of peritoneal fluid to bathe the organs. Any condition that allows pus, blood, feces, urine, gastric juice, intestinal contents, bile, pancreatic juice, amniotic fluid, or other foreign material to lie within or adjacent to this cavity can cause peritonitis and, thus, an acute abdomen. Technically, organs such as kidneys, ovaries, and other genitourinary structures are *retroperitoneal* (behind the peritoneum). However, because they lie next to the peritoneum, problems in these organs can lead to an acute abdomen. Therefore, nearly every kind of abdominal problem can cause an acute abdomen.

Among the common diseases that produce signs of an acute abdomen are acute appendicitis, perforated gastric ulcer, cholecystitis, and diverticulitis. The more common emergency problems, with most common locations of direct and referred pain, are listed in (Table 25-1 ▶).

Because the parietal peritoneum is richly supplied with very sensitive nerves, disease or inflammation of organs that lie behind or beneath the abdominal

TABLE 25-1	Common Abdominal Conditions
Condition	**Localization of Pain**
Appendicitis	Around navel (referred); right lower quadrant (direct)
Cholecystitis	Right shoulder (referred); right upper quadrant (direct)
Duodenal ulcer	Upper midabdomen or upper back
Diverticulitis	Left lower quadrant
Aortic aneurysm (ruptured or dissecting)	Low back and right lower quadrant
Cystitis (inflammation of the urinary bladder)	Lower midabdomen (retropubic)
Kidney infection (pyelonephritis)	Costovertebral angle
Kidney stone	Right or left flank, radiating to genitalia (referred)
Pelvic inflammation (in women)	Both lower quadrants
Pancreatitis	Upper abdomen (both quadrants); back

Geriatric Needs

An older patient is just as susceptible as a younger adult to the acute abdomen. However, the signs and symptoms might be different. Because of altered pain sensation, the geriatric patient with an acute abdomen may not feel any discomfort or may describe the discomfort as mild, even in severe conditions.

Because the older patient has decreased body temperature regulation and response, conditions such as an acute abdomen, including peritonitis, may not present with fever. However, if fever is present, it can be minimal.

Because of the older patient's response to the acute abdomen, a delay in identifying the condition and seeking medical attention may occur, putting the patient at risk for complications. You should ask about the patient's medical history, especially the history of recent illness, to identify a potential illness. Ask about abdominal discomfort, when the patient last had a bowel movement, whether she or he was constipated or had diarrhea, when the patient last ate, and whether she or he vomited. Ruling out appendicitis, bowel obstruction, and ruptured bowel can hasten proper treatment and recovery, and should therefore not be attempted in the field.

cavity can cause the signs of peritonitis. These signs and symptoms are similar to those produced by actual inflammation within the abdominal cavity. Pancreatitis, for example, can produce peritonitis that is difficult to distinguish from a perforated ulcer. Kidney stones that cause colic of the ureter are frequently associated with ileus. Infections of the urinary tract may also cause peritoneal irritation.

Uterus and Ovaries

Gynecologic problems are a common cause of acute abdominal pain. Always consider that a woman with lower abdominal pain and tenderness may have a problem related to her ovaries, fallopian tubes, or uterus.

Pain may also be related to the normal menstrual cycle. A common lower abdominal pain, often confused with appendicitis but fairly short lived, is called *mittelschmertz*. It is associated with the release of an egg from the ovary, characteristically occurring in the middle of the menstrual cycle, between menstrual periods. Mittelschmertz may also be associated with lower abdominal tenderness. Some women experience painful cramps at the time of their menstrual periods. In some, the discomfort may be crippling and the menstrual flow severe.

A common cause of an acute abdomen in women is *pelvic inflammatory disease (PID)*, an infection of the fallopian tubes and the surrounding tissues of the pelvis. With PID, acute pain and tenderness in the lower abdomen may be intense and accompanied by a high fever. If you suspect PID, promptly transport the patient to the emergency department for treatment.

Between 1% and 2% of all pregnancies are ectopic. The term *ectopic pregnancy* means that a fertilized egg has come to lie in an area outside the uterus, usually in a fallopian tube. A fallopian tube is simply not large enough to support the growth of a fetus and placenta for more than about 6 to 8 weeks. When the tube ruptures, it produces massive internal hemorrhage and acute abdominal pain, generally on one side. In this situation, the acute abdomen may be associated with the onset of hypovolemic shock. This combination mandates immediate transport to the hospital. Suspect an ectopic pregnancy in any patient of childbearing age who presents with acute abdominal distress.

Other Organ Systems

The aorta lies immediately behind the peritoneum on the spinal column. In older people, the wall of the aorta sometimes develops weak areas that swell to form an aneurysm. The development of an aneurysm, unless acutely dissecting, is rarely associated with symptoms because it occurs slowly, but if the aneurysm ruptures, massive hemorrhage may occur and, with it, the signs of acute peritoneal irritation. The patient may also experience severe back pain, because the peritoneum can, at times, be rapidly stripped away from the wall of the main abdominal cavity by the hemorrhage. Pain can also be associated with the pressure of blood on the back itself. In such instances, bleeding usually leads to profound shock. The association of acute abdominal signs and symptoms with shock requires prompt transportation. Because this is a fragile situation with a large, leaking artery, avoid unnecessary or vigorous palpation of the abdomen. Remember to handle the patient gently during transport.

Pneumonia, especially in the lower parts of the lung, may cause both ileus and abdominal pain. In this case, the problem lies in an adjacent body cavity, but the intense inflammatory response can affect the abdomen. Treat and transport this patient as you would any patient with abdominal pain.

A hernia is a protrusion of an organ or tissue through a hole in the body wall covering its normal site. Virtually any organ or tissue in the body can herniate through its covering membranes in certain circumstances. Hernias can occur as a result of the following:

- A congenital defect, as around the umbilicus
- A surgical wound that has failed to heal properly
- Some natural weakness in an area such as in the groin

You are the Provider   Part 5

En route to the hospital you interview the patient using OPQRST and SAMPLE and also ask about the possibility of pregnancy. She tells you she had a total hysterectomy 2 years ago, which rules out a possible ectopic pregnancy. Her pain was sudden in onset, and she rates it as a "10" on a 1 to 10 scale. You have placed her in the shock position and are attempting to gain intravenous (IV) access. You notice that her abdomen is even more distended.

Reassessment	Recording Time: 10 Minutes After Patient Contact
Respirations	28 breaths/min, shallow
Pulse	Absent radial pulses, 144 beats/min carotid
Skin	Extremely pale, cool, diaphoretic
Blood pressure	Unable to palpate
Mental status	Decreasing alertness

You manage to start an 18-gauge IV catheter in her left forearm.

10. What fluid will you use, and at what rate will you run it?
11. What additional treatment might you consider?

Hernias always produce a mass or lump that is usually easy to detect. Extreme obesity may interfere with the ability to detect the mass. At times, the mass will disappear back into the body cavity in which it belongs. In this case, the hernia is said to be *reducible*. If the mass cannot be pushed back within the body, it is said to be *incarcerated*.

Reducible hernias pose little risk to the patient; some people live with them for years. When a hernia is incarcerated, however, its contents may become seriously compressed by the surrounding tissue, eventually compromising the blood supply. This situation, called <u>strangulation</u>, is a serious medical emergency. Immediate surgery is required to remove any dead tissue and repair the hernia.

The following signs and symptoms indicate a serious hernia problem:

- The existence of the hernia itself
- A previously reducible mass can no longer be pushed back inside the body
- Pain at the hernia site
- Tenderness when the hernia is palpated
- Red or blue discoloration of the skin over the hernia

Any of these signs and symptoms, other than the hernia itself, is cause for prompt transport to the emergency department.

Emergency Medical Care

The signs and symptoms of an acute abdomen signal a serious medical or surgical emergency. Ensure that you provide prompt, gentle transport for the patient; do not delay transport. Carry out the following steps as quickly as possible before transport.

1. **Do not attempt to diagnose** the cause of the acute abdomen.
2. **Clear and maintain the airway.**
3. **Anticipate vomiting.** Place the patient in the recovery position or position of comfort. Most patients feel better in a lateral recumbent position with the knees pulled in toward the chest.
4. **Administer 100% supplemental oxygen** and be prepared to assist ventilation if the patient has a reduced tidal volume (shallow breathing).

You are the Provider Part 6

Upon arrival at the hospital your patient is responsive only to pain. She is receiving 100% oxygen, covered with a blanket, and in the shock position. You have two IV lines running at the appropriate rate and can barely feel her radial pulses.

Reassessment	Recording Time: 14 Minutes After Patient Contact
Respirations	24 breaths/min, good depth, Sao_2 is 98%
Pulse	Weak radial pulses, carotid pulses are strong
Blood pressure	90 mm Hg systolic by palpation
Skin	Pale, cool, diaphoretic
Mental status	Responds to painful stimuli

You turn the patient over to the charge nurse and give a detailed report of your findings. As you clean the unit in preparation for your next call, you recall the events to yourself.

12. Are you satisfied with the way you treated the patient?
13. Is there anything else you might have considered?

5. **Do not give the patient anything by mouth.** Food or fluid will only aggravate many of the symptoms, because intestinal paralysis will prevent it from passing out of the stomach. In addition, the stomach will have to be emptied before surgery if it is required.
6. **Document all pertinent information.** Onset, Provocation, Quality, Radiation, Severity, and Time (OPQRST). Note the presence of abdominal tenderness, distention, or guarding.
7. **Avoid analgesics.** Pain medications (for example, morphine, demerol) should be avoided because they may mask the patient's signs and symptoms, making the physician's examination and subsequent diagnosis more difficult.
8. **Anticipate the development of hypovolemic shock.** Monitor blood pressure. Treat the patient for shock when it is evident. Elevate the patient's legs 6 to 12 inches (shock position).
9. **Establish IV access**, and give a 20-mL/kg bolus of an isotonic crystalloid if the patient presents with signs of hypovolemia. Otherwise, maintain fluid at a keep-vein-open rate.
10. **Make the patient as comfortable as possible** for transport. Conserve body heat with blankets, as needed. Provide gentle but rapid transport and constant psychological support.
11. **Monitor vital signs**; these may change quickly.

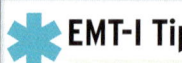

EMT-I Tips

Because abdominal pain could be the result of a cardiac event and because shock-induced hypoxia can cause cardiac arrhythmias, you should monitor the patient's cardiac rhythm and treat arrhythmias based on standard ACLS or local protocols.

You are the Provider — Summary

1. What does "referred pain" mean, and does it indicate a serious problem?

Referred pain is defined as pain in two different body locations that are related to the same problem. For example, a patient with an inflamed gallbladder commonly complains of pain to the right upper abdominal quadrant and pain to the right shoulder; however, there is no "trail" of pain in between these two points. Referred pain could indicate a potentially serious condition.

2. Is it a requirement that all patients complaining of abdominal pain be transported to the hospital?

Because there are many causes of abdominal pain, some of them potentially life-threatening, the patient who complains of abdominal pain should be evaluated in the emergency department.

3. What are some conditions that may cause abdominal pain?

There are numerous conditions that may cause abdominal pain in women. Cystitis, gallbladder problems, pancreatitis, PID, ectopic pregnancy, menstrual pain, appendicitis, and kidney infection are some of the potential causes.

4. What is your first consideration in treating this patient?

Airway is the top priority for any patient. Because this patient is alert and her breathing is of adequate depth, a nonrebreathing mask at 15 L/min is appropriate.

5. What is your next step?

Place the patient on the stretcher, and load her into the ambulance to begin your focused history and physical exam.

6. In what position will you transport this patient?

Because no trauma is suspected, this patient should be placed in a position of comfort.

7. What questions should you ask in relation to the pain and medical history?

Assess the severity of pain by using OPQRST—Onset, Provocation, Quality, Radiation, Severity, and Time—and obtain a SAMPLE history on all patients with an intact mental status. Because this patient is a woman, she should be asked discreetly about her last menstrual period and the possibility of pregnancy. Always protect the patient's privacy when asking questions.

8. What condition do the vital signs and distended abdomen point to?

This patient has classic symptoms of hypovolemic shock, possibly from a ruptured appendix.

9. As an EMT-I, what are your treatment options?

Treat for shock: 100% supplemental oxygen, keep the patient warm, position the patient appropriately, and administer IV fluids depending on patient presentation, and based on local protocol.

10. What fluid will you use, and at what rate will you run it?

Use an isotonic crystalloid solution of normal saline or lactated Ringer's. To avoid increasing internal hemorrhage, run the IV fluids (preferably using two large-bore catheters) to maintain perfusion (radial pulses), or according to local protocols, usually 20 mL/Kg followed by reassessment.

11. What additional treatment might you consider?

Keep the patient warm and place her in the shock position. Because of the patient's decreased level of consciousness and shallow breathing, you should assist ventilations with a BVM device and 100% oxygen.

12. Are you satisfied with the way you treated the patient?

You should treat the patient according to local protocols and your level of training. Not all patients have a favorable outcome, so you should not feel as if you have erred as long as you gave good, appropriate patient care.

13. Is there anything else you might have considered?

The glucose level should be checked any time a patient's mental status is altered.

Prep Kit

Ready for Review

- The acute abdomen is a medical emergency requiring prompt but gentle transport.
- The pain, tenderness, and abdominal distention associated with acute abdomen are signs of peritonitis, which may be caused by any condition that allows pus, blood, feces, urine, gastric juice, intestinal contents, bile, pancreatic juice, amniotic fluid, or other foreign material to accumulate within or adjacent to the peritoneum.
- In addition to abdominal disease or injury, problems in the gastrointestinal, genital, and urinary systems may cause peritonitis.
- Appendicitis, perforated gastric ulcer, cholecystitis, diverticulitis, and a strangulated hernia are common causes of an acute abdomen.
- Signs and symptoms of acute abdomen include pain, nausea, vomiting, and a tense, distended abdomen.
- Pain is common directly over the inflamed area of the peritoneum, or it may be referred to another part of the body. Referred pain occurs because of the connections between the two different nervous systems supplying the parietal peritoneum and the visceral peritoneum.
- Your first priorities are to assess airway, breathing, and circulation and then apply oxygen. Assist ventilation if the patient is breathing inadequately. Next, obtain a pertinent medical history: When did the symptoms begin? How have they changed over time? Where exactly is the pain? What does it feel like? How long does it last, and how intense is it? Has there been a loss of fluid volume as a result of vomiting or diarrhea?
- Take vital signs, and gently palpate the abdomen. The presence of abdominal tenderness will confirm the need to transport the patient to the emergency department in an urgent manner.
- Do not give the patient with an acute abdomen anything by mouth. Analgesics should also be avoided. In all likelihood, the bowel is paralyzed, making it impossible for food to pass out of the stomach.

Technology

- Interactivities
- Vocabulary Explorer
- Anatomy Review
- Web Links
- Online Review Manual

Vital Vocabulary

acute abdomen A condition of sudden onset of pain within the abdomen, usually indicating peritonitis; demands immediate medical or surgical treatment.

aneurysm A swelling or enlargement of a part of an artery, resulting from weakening of the arterial wall.

anorexia Lack of appetite for food.

appendicitis Inflammation of the appendix.

cholecystitis Inflammation of the gallbladder.

colic Acute, intermittent, cramping abdominal pain.

diverticulitis Inflammation of a diverticulum, usually in the colon, creating abdominal discomfort; a diverticulum is an abnormal pouch or sac.

emesis Vomiting.

guarding Involuntary muscle contractions (spasm) of the abdominal wall; an effort to protect the inflamed abdomen.

hernia The protrusion of a loop of an organ or tissue through an abnormal body opening.

ileus Paralysis of the bowel, arising from any one of several causes; stops contractions that move material through the intestine.

pancreatitis Inflammation of the pancreas.

peristalsis Waves of alternate circular contraction and relaxation of the intestines or other tubular structure to propel the contents forward.

peritoneum The membrane lining the abdominal cavity (parietal peritoneum) and covering the abdominal organs (visceral peritoneum).

peritonitis Inflammation of the peritoneum.

referred pain Pain felt in an area of the body other than the area where the cause of pain is located.

strangulation Complete obstruction of blood circulation in a given organ as a result of compression or entrapment, an emergency situation causing death of tissue.

ulcer Abrasion of the stomach or small intestine.

Prep Kit continued...

Points to Ponder

You are caring for a patient who has been experiencing periumbilical abdominal pain for several hours. He now states the pain seems to have shifted to the right lower quadrant of his abdomen. He also tells you that as long as he holds pressure on the area, the pain is diminished; but when he lets go, the pain is much worse. You perform an assessment on him, focusing on his abdomen. You repeatedly palpate the area of pain in order to determine the exact location and intensity. The patient screams out in pain and begins to vomit. You now move him to the ambulance and begin transport.

En route to the hospital, the patient becomes less responsive and his vital signs indicate hypoperfusion. You apply 100% supplemental oxygen and attempt to start an IV of crystalloid fluid, but are unsuccessful.

You arrive at the hospital 45 minutes after initial contact with the patient. A computed tomographic (CT) scan of the patient's abdomen is performed, and it is determined that his appendix has ruptured. He is quickly sent to the operating room.

Was the abdominal assessment performed appropriately? How could the patient have benefited from a short scene time and rapid transport?

Issues: Understanding Rapid assessment and Rapid Transport, Understanding Acute Abdomen as a Surgical Emergency

Assessment in Action

You are dispatched to a residence for a woman having abdominal pain. Your response time to the scene is approximately 10 minutes. Fire department first responders are en route to the scene as well.

Upon arrival at the scene, you find a 32-year-old woman lying in a fetal position in the middle of her bed. You introduce yourself and your partner to the patient and ask her what is wrong. The patient states that she was in the shower approximately 30 minutes ago when she experienced a sudden onset of severe, sharp pain in her left lower abdominal area. She feels very nauseated and is dizzy, but denies having vomited. Your partner begins to obtain her vital signs while you continue your assessment.

1. Which of the following would *not* be considered a sign or symptom of acute abdomen?

    A. Tense, distended abdomen
    B. Dark, tarry stools
    C. Intense hunger
    D. Fever

2. A serious condition that must be suspected because of the patient's age is:

    A. appendicitis.
    B. ectopic pregnancy.
    C. mittelschmertz.
    D. cholecystitis.

3. When palpating the patient's abdomen, you should begin in the:

    A. right upper quadrant.
    B. left upper quadrant.
    C. right lower quadrant.
    D. left lower quadrant.

4. Involuntary muscle contractions of the abdominal wall are considered a natural response to protect the inflamed abdomen. This is known as:

    A. guarding.
    B. colic.
    C. ilius.
    D. peristalsis.

5. Treatment for patients with an acute abdomen includes all of the following EXCEPT:

    A. diagnosing the cause of pain.
    B. maintaining the airway.
    C. avoiding analgesics.
    D. establishing IV access.

6. You find that the patient's vital signs indicate hypovolemia. Further treatment for her should include all of the following EXCEPT:

    A. 100% supplemental oxygen.
    B. 20 mL/kg of isotonic crystalloid.
    C. cardiac monitoring.
    D. IV analgesics.

Environmental Emergencies

1999 Objectives

Cognitive

5-8.1 Define "environmental emergency." (p 1102)
5-8.2 Identify risk factors most predisposing to environmental emergencies. (p 1102)
5-8.3 Identify environmental factors that may cause illness or exacerbate a pre-existing illness. (p 1102)
5-8.4 Identify environmental factors that may complicate treatment or transport decisions. (p 1102)
5-8.5 List the principal types of environmental illnesses. (p 1102)
5-8.6 Identify normal, critically high and critically low body temperatures. (p 1103, 1111)
5-8.7 Describe several methods of temperature monitoring. (p 1104)
5-8.8 Describe the body's compensatory process for over heating. (p 1111)
5-8.9 Describe the body's compensatory process for excess heat loss. (p 1102)
5-8.10 List the common forms of heat and cold disorders. (p 1103, 1108, 1111)
5-8.11 List the common predisposing factors associated with heat and cold disorders. (p 1104)
5-8.12 List the common preventative measures associated with heat and cold disorders. (p 1103, 1111)
5-8.13 Define heat illness. (p 1111)
5-8.14 Identify signs and symptoms of heat illness. (p 1111)
5-8.15 List the predisposing factors for heat illness. (p 1111)
5-8.16 List measures to prevent heat illness. (p 1111)
5-8.17 Relate symptomatic findings to the commonly used terms: heat cramps, heat exhaustion, and heat stroke. (p 1111, 1113, 1115)
5-8.18 Discuss how one may differentiate between fever and heat stroke. (p 1113)
5-8.19 Discuss the role of fluid therapy in the treatment of heat disorders. (p 1112, 1113)
5-8.20 Differentiate among the various treatments and interventions in the management of heat disorders. (p 1112, 1113, 1115)
5-8.21 Integrate the pathophysiological principles and the assessment findings to formulate a field impression and implement a treatment plan for the patient who has dehydration, heat exhaustion, or heat stroke. (p 1113, 1115)
5-8.22 Define hypothermia. (p 1103)
5-8.23 List predisposing factors for hypothermia. (p 1104)
5-8.24 List measures to prevent hypothermia. (p 1104)
5-8.25 Identify differences between mild and severe hypothermia. (p 1104)
5-8.26 Describe differences between chronic and acute hypothermia. (p 1103)
5-8.27 List signs and symptoms of hypothermia. (p 1105)
5-8.28 Correlate abnormal findings in assessment with their clinical significance in the patient with hypothermia. (p 1105)
5-8.29 Discuss the impact of severe hypothermia on standard BCLS and ACLS algorithms and transport considerations. (p 1107)
5-8.30 Integrate pathophysiological principles and the assessment findings to formulate a field impression and implement a treatment plan for the patient who has either mild or severe hypothermia. (p 1105)
5-8.31 Define near-drowning. (p 1117)
5-8.32 List signs and symptoms of near-drowning. (p 1118)
5-8.33 Discuss the complications and protective role of hypothermia in the context of near-drowning. (p 1118)
5-8.34 Correlate the abnormal findings in assessment with the clinical significance in the patient with near-drowning. (p 1118)
5-8.35 Differentiate among the various treatments and interventions in the management of near-drowning. (p 1118)
5-8.36 Integrate pathophysiological principles and the assessment findings to formulate a field impression and implement a treatment plan for the near-drowning patient. (p 1118)
5-8.37 Integrate pathophysiological principles of the patient affected by an environmental emergency. (p 1103-1105, 1111-1113, 1115)

26

5-8.38 Differentiate between environmental emergencies based on assessment findings. (p 1104-1105, 1109-1110, 1111-1114)

5-8.39 Correlate abnormal findings in the assessment with the clinical significance in the patient affected by an environmental emergency. (p 1104-1105, 1109-1110, 1111-1114)

5-8.40 Develop a patient management plan based on the field impression of the patient affected by an environmental emergency. (p 1105-1108, 1110, 1112, 1115)

Affective

None

Psychomotor

None

1985 Objectives

There are no 1985 objectives for this chapter.

Environmental Emergencies

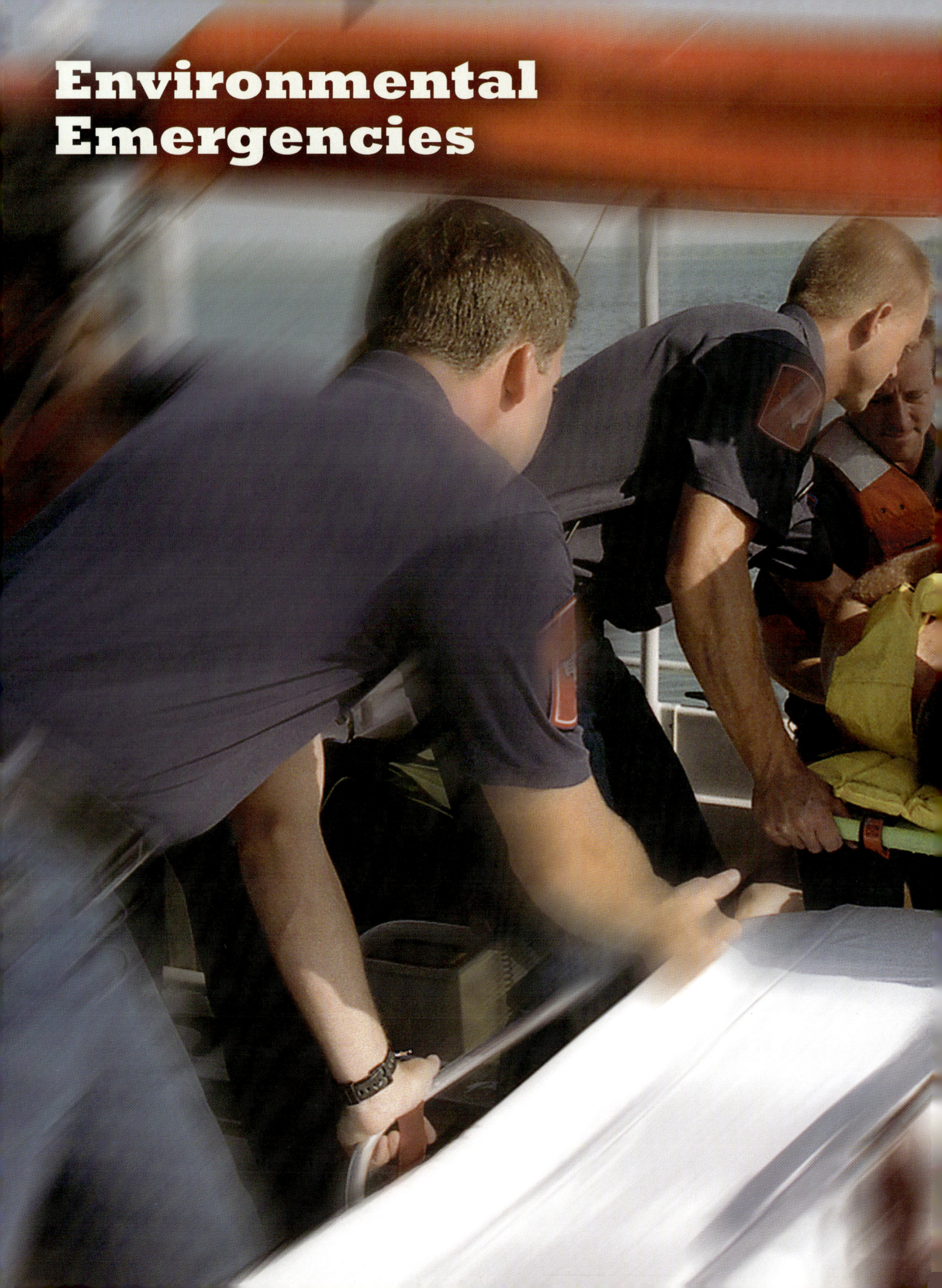

26

Environmental Emergencies

You are the Provider

You are dispatched for a "person down" on the tennis court of the local park. You arrive at the scene and find a 52-year-old man, with a history of a heart attack, making inappropriate statements. It is a hot summer day with 75% humidity.

This chapter will provide information necessary to care for patients with an environmental emergency and help you answer the following questions:

1. How does heat exhaustion differ from heatstroke?
2. How do the patient's age and medical history affect tolerance to the temperature?

Environmental Emergencies

An environmental emergency is a medical condition caused or exacerbated by the weather, terrain, atmospheric pressure, or other risk factors Table 26-1 . Heat and cold can both overwhelm the body's mechanisms for regulating temperature, including sweating and radiation of body heat into the atmosphere. A variety of medical emergencies can result from exposure to heat or cold, particularly in children, elderly people, people with chronic illnesses, and young adults who overexert themselves. The environmental impact on morbidity and mortality increases with stressors that induce or exacerbate other medical or traumatic conditions. There is also a range of medical emergencies that arise from water recreation, which can sometimes be complicated by cold temperatures. These emergencies include localized injuries and systemic illnesses. Environmental factors such as climate, season, weather, atmospheric pressure, and terrain also have a major role in the severity of environmental emergencies. As an EMT-I, you can save lives by recognizing and responding properly to these emergencies, many of which require prompt treatment in the hospital.

This chapter describes how the body regulates core temperature and the ways in which body heat is lost to the environment. It then discusses the various forms of heat-, cold-, and water-related emergencies, including how to recognize and treat hypothermia, hyperthermia, and diving injuries.

TABLE 26-1	Risk Factors for Environmental Emergencies

- Age
- General health
- Fatigue
- Predisposing medical condition
- Medications: prescription and over the counter

A to Z Terminology Tips

Hypo = low; hyper = high; thermia = temperature; therefore, hypothermia is a body temperature lower than normal, and hyperthermia is a body temperature higher than normal.

Cold Exposure

Normal body temperature must be maintained within a very narrow range for the body's chemistry to work efficiently. Homeostasis, or a constant internal balance, must be maintained. If the body, or any part of it, is exposed to a cold environment, these mechanisms may be overwhelmed. Cold exposure may cause injury to individual parts of the body, such as the feet, hands, ears, or nose, or to the body as a whole. When the entire core body temperature falls because of inadequate internal heat production (called thermogenesis), excess cold stress, or a combination of both, the condition is called hypothermia.

Because heat always travels from a warmer place to a cooler place, the body will tend to lose heat to the environment. Through thermolysis, or methods of heat loss, the body can lose heat in the following five ways:

- Conduction is the direct transfer of heat from a part of the body to a colder object, as when a warm hand touches cold metal or ice or is immersed in cold water. Heat passes directly from the body to the colder object.
- Convection occurs when heat is transferred to circulating air, as when cool air moves across the body surface. A person standing outside in windy winter weather, wearing lightweight clothing, is losing heat to the environment mostly by convection.
- Evaporation is the conversion of any liquid to a gas, a process that requires energy, or heat. Evaporation is the natural mechanism by which sweat-

ing cools the body. This is why swimmers coming out of the water feel a sensation of cold as the water evaporates from their skin. People who exercise vigorously in a cool environment may sweat and feel warm at first, but later, as their sweat evaporates, they can become exceedingly cool.

- Radiation is the loss of body heat directly to colder objects in the environment. Because heat always travels from a warm object to a cooler one, a person standing in a cold room will lose heat by radiation.
- Respiration causes body heat to be lost, as warm air in the lungs is exhaled into the atmosphere and cooler air is inhaled.

The rate and amount of heat loss by the body can be modified in three ways:

1. **Increase heat production.** One way for the body to increase its heat production is to increase the rate of cellular metabolism, as occurs in shivering.
2. **Move to an area where heat loss is decreased.** The most obvious ways to decrease heat loss from radiation and convection are to move out of a cold environment and seek shelter from wind. Simply covering the head will minimize radiation heat loss by up to 70%.
3. **Wear insulated clothing, which helps decrease heat loss in several ways.** Insulators, such as specific materials or dry, still air, do not conduct heat. Thus, layers of clothing that trap air provide good insulation, as do wool, down, and synthetic fabrics that have small pockets of trapped air. Protective clothing also traps perspiration and prevents evaporation. Sweating without evaporation will not result in cooling.

Hypothermia

Hypothermia literally means "low temperature." It occurs when the core temperature of the body falls below 95°F (35°C). The body can usually tolerate a drop in core temperature of a few degrees. However, below this critical point, the body loses its ability to regulate temperature and to generate body heat. Progressive loss of body heat then begins.

To protect itself against heat loss, the body normally constricts blood vessels in the skin; this results in the characteristic pale appearance of the hypothermic patient. As a secondary compensatory mechanism against heat loss, the body attempts to create additional heat by shivering, which is the active moving of many muscles to generate heat. Many body functions begin to slow down as cold exposure continues and these mechanisms are overwhelmed. Eventually, the functioning of key organs such as the heart and brain begins to slow. Untreated, this can lead to death.

Heat loss occurs through physiologic and environmental mechanisms. Hypothermia can develop quickly, as when someone is immersed in cold water, or more gradually, as when a lost person is exposed to the cold environment for several hours or more. The temperature does not have to be below freezing (<32°F) for hypothermia to occur. In winter, homeless people and those whose homes lack heating may develop hypothermia at higher

You are the Provider — Part 2

You and your partner approach the patient, who is in a sitting position supported by bystanders. You note that his face is flushed and he is sweating profusely.

Initial Assessment	Recording Time: Zero Minutes
Appearance	Healthy; face is flushed, and sweating profusely
Level of consciousness	Slightly confused and unsure of his surroundings
Airway and breathing	Open and clear; respirations, 24 breaths/min and deep
Circulation	Radial pulses, rapid, strong, and bounding
Skin	Warm to touch; diaphoretic

3. What is the probable cause of his increased respiratory rate and depth?
4. What is your first consideration in treating this patient?

temperatures. Even during summer, swimmers who remain in the water for extended periods are at risk of hypothermia. Like all heat- and cold-related injuries, hypothermia is more common among elderly people, children, and people who are ill, all of whom are less able to adjust to temperature extremes. Hypothermia is also common among the very young, who are unable to put on clothes to protect themselves against the cold. Infants and children are small, with a relatively large body surface area, and have less body fat than do adults. Also, because of their small muscle mass, children may not be able to shiver as effectively as adults, and infants do not shiver at all.

Patients who are in poor general health are more susceptible to cold. Patients with injuries or illness, such as burns, shock, head injury, stroke, generalized infection, injuries to the spinal cord, malnutrition, hypothyroidism, diabetes, and hypoglycemia, are more prone to hypothermia, as are patients who have taken certain drugs or poisons. Other contributing factors include fatigue, exhaustion, length and intensity of exposure, and the environmental condition itself. High humidity, wind, and low temperatures all exacerbate cold exposure. Preventive measures may decrease signs and symptoms and include appropriate dress, rest, adequate nutrition, and limiting exposure in cold environments.

Signs and Symptoms

Signs and symptoms of hypothermia increase in severity as the core temperature falls. Hypothermia generally progresses through four general stages, as shown in Table 26-2. Although there is no clear distinction among the stages, the different signs and symptoms of each will help you estimate the severity of the hypothermia. When you assess a patient in the field, you should be able to distinguish between mild and severe hypothermia.

It is important to assess the temperature of the skin close to the trunk, or core, of the body. Extremities may be cold due to exposure, yet the patient may be hemodynamically stable. To assess the patient's general temperature, pull your glove back and place the back of your hand on the patient's skin Figure 26-1. If the skin feels cool, the patient is likely experiencing a generalized cold emergency. Temperature may be measured using an oral, an axillary, a tympanic, or a rectal thermometer or through touch. If you work in a cold environment, you should carry a hypothermia thermometer, which registers lower core temperatures Figure 26-2. It must be inserted into the rectum for an accurate reading. Note that regular thermometers will not register the temperature of a patient who has significant hypothermia.

Mild hypothermia occurs when the core temperature is between 90°F and 95°F (32°C and 35°C). The patient is usually alert (may be withdrawn) and shiv-

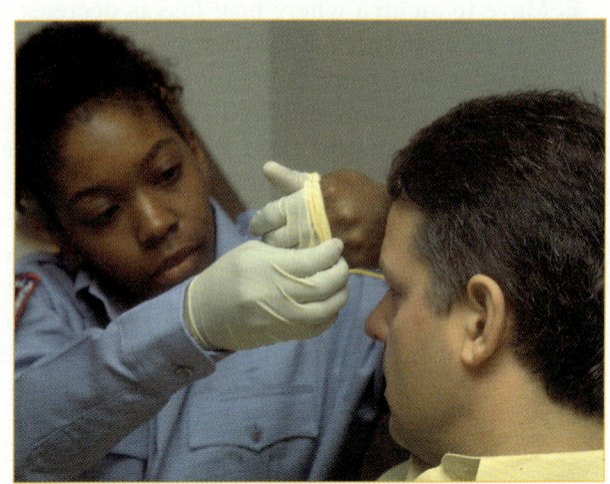

Figure 26-1 To assess a patient's temperature, pull back your glove and place the back of your hand on the patient's skin.

TABLE 26-2	Characteristics of Systemic Hypothermia			
Core Temperature	90° to 95°F (32° to 35°C)	89° to 92°F (32° to 33°C)	80° to 88°F (27° to 31°C)	<80°F (<27°C)
Signs and symptoms	Shivering, foot stamping	Loss of coordination, muscle stiffness	Coma	Apparent death
Cardiorespiratory response	Constricted blood vessels, rapid breathing	Slowing respirations, slow pulse	Weak pulse, arrhythmias, very slow respirations	Cardiac arrest
Level of consciousness	Withdrawn	Confused, lethargic, sleepy	Unresponsive	Unresponsive

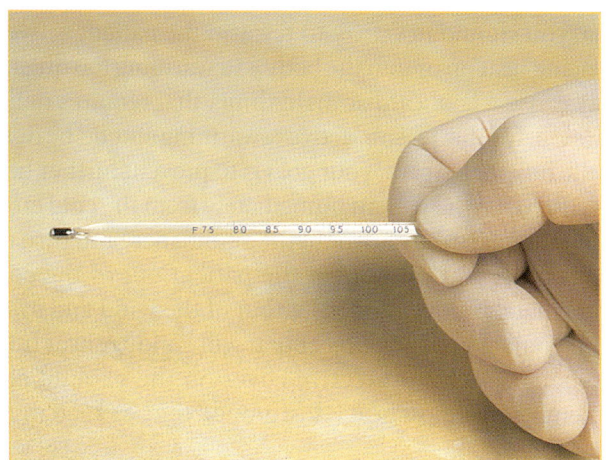

Figure 26-2 A special rectal hypothermia thermometer registers temperatures well below that of a regular thermometer.

ering in an attempt to generate more heat through muscular activity. In a further attempt to generate body heat, the patient may jump up and down and stamp his or her feet. Pulse rate and respirations are usually rapid. The skin in light-skinned people can be red but may eventually appear pale and then cyanotic.

> ### Documentation Tips
>
> Recording specific results of your early assessment is particularly valuable when the patient is hypothermic. If there is a question regarding the initiation of CPR, note the anatomic location where you checked the pulse and for how long you checked it. Also note the initial body temperature and the anatomic location where it was taken. These points will be important to hospital staff and will help protect you if medicolegal issues are ever raised.

Severe hypothermia occurs when the core temperature is less than 90°F (32°C). As the body compensates, the patient may present with signs and symptoms of a cold emergency while maintaining a normal core body temperature. The temperature is actually being maintained by thermogenesis. As energy stores of glycogen in the liver and muscles are exhausted, the core body temperature begins to drop. Shivering stops, and muscular activity decreases. At first, small, fine muscle activity such as coordinated finger motion ceases. Eventually, as the temperature falls further, all muscle activity stops.

As the core temperature drops toward 85°F (29°C), the patient becomes lethargic, usually losing interest in continuing to fight the cold. The level of consciousness decreases, and the patient may try to remove his or her own clothes. Poor coordination and memory loss follow, along with reduced or complete loss of sensation to touch, mood changes, and impaired judgment. The patient becomes less communicative, experiences joint or muscle stiffness, and has trouble speaking. The muscles eventually become rigid, and the patient begins to appear stiff or rigid.

If the temperature continues to fall to 80°F (27°C), vital signs slow; the pulse becomes weaker, and respirations decrease in rate and depth or become absent altogether. Cardiac arrhythmias may occur as the blood pressure decreases.

At a core temperature less than 80°F (27°C), all cardiorespiratory activity may cease, pupillary reaction is slow, and the patient may appear dead.

Never assume that a cold, pulseless patient is dead. Patients may survive even severe hypothermia, if proper emergency measures are carried out.

Emergency Medical Care

Even mild degrees of hypothermia can have serious consequences and complications. These include cardiac irritability and blood-clotting abnormalities. Therefore, all patients with hypothermia require immediate transport for evaluation and treatment. Management of hypothermia in the field, regardless of the severity of the exposure, consists of stabilizing the ABCs and preventing further heat loss. You should move the patient from the cold environment to prevent further heat loss. To prevent further damage to the feet, do not allow the patient to walk. Remove any wet clothing, and place dry blankets over and under the patient **Figure 26-3** ▶. Always make sure to handle the patient gently so that you will not cause pain or further injury to the skin. Do not massage the extremities. Do not allow the patient to eat or use any stimulants, such as coffee, tea, or cola, or to smoke or chew tobacco.

You can give the patient warm (102°F to 104°F), humidified oxygen if you have not already done so during the initial assessment. Next, **assess the patient's pulse for 30 to 45 seconds**, especially before considering CPR. Begin passive external rewarming, which includes wrapping the patient in blankets and turning up the heat in the patient compartment of the ambulance.

If the patient is alert and responds appropriately, the hypothermia is mild, and you can begin active exter-

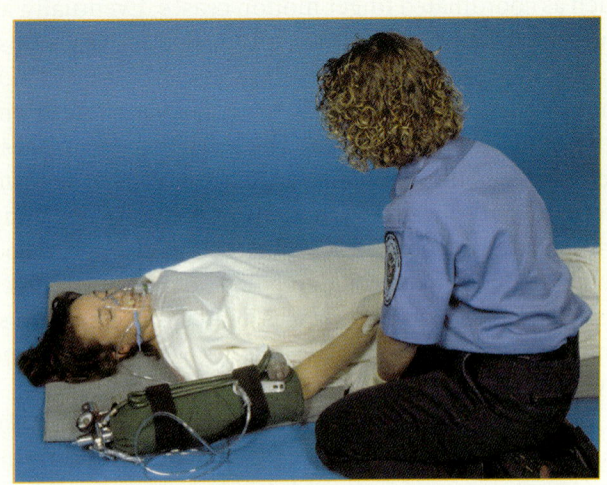

Figure 26-3 Place dry blankets over and under the hypothermic patient; give warm, humidified oxygen; assess the pulse for 30 to 45 seconds before considering CPR.

nal rewarming. Active external rewarming involves wrapping the patient in blankets and applying heat packs or hot water bottles to the groin, axillae, and base of the neck. The patient should respond favorably to this, as these are areas of high heat transfer. When giving fluid intravenously, it is crucial to warm the fluid (102°F to 104°F) before administration to prevent further heat loss. Although the rewarming effect of the intravenous (IV) fluid is minimal, it is imperative to maintain the patient's current body temperature.

Once the patient reaches the hospital, rewarming may continue by immersing the patient in warm water, 102°F to 104°F. Warm water immersion has little application in the prehospital setting because it can induce rewarming shock. It is also not practical in an out-of-hospital setting. Rewarming shock occurs as the active external rewarming causes a reflex vasodilation, subsequently lowering the blood pressure and increasing the surface area of the vessels. This may also further increase cardiac irritability due to a decreased oxygen supply to the myocardium. Rewarming shock can be easily prevented in the controlled environment of the hospital and by IV fluid administration to offset the vasodilation.

You must try to minimize further loss of body heat, especially when you cannot get to a hospital quickly. However, when the patient has moderate or severe hypothermia, you should never try to rewarm the patient actively (placing heat on or into the body). Rewarming too quickly may cause a fatal cardiac arrhythmia that requires defibrillation; for this reason, active rewarming should be done in the hospital. Again, your goal is to prevent further heat loss. Remove the patient immediately from the cold environment, place the patient in the ambulance, and turn up the heat. If you cannot get the patient out of the cold immediately, move him or her out of the wind and away from contact with any object that will conduct heat from the body. Place a protective cover on the patient, and remember that most heat is lost around the head and neck.

> **EMT-I Tips**
>
> Handle hypothermic patients *very gently*. Excessive movement increases the risk of inducing ventricular fibrillation.

If the patient is alert and shivering, you may assume that the hypothermia is relatively mild. If possible, you can give warm fluids by mouth in this case, assuming that the patient can swallow without a problem and is not nauseated. This will also help with dehydration resulting from the cold diuresis, or increased excretion of urine in a cold environment. Remove all wet clothing, and cover the patient with a blanket. Notify the hospital of the patient's condition so that staff can prepare to start rewarming as soon as you arrive.

When the patient is not shivering and is lethargic, moderate or severe hypothermia is probably present. A special low-temperature thermometer is required to take this patient's temperature, generally done through the rectum. A patient with a moderate form of hypothermia will have a core temperature between 90° and 95°F (32° to 35°C).

If you cannot feel a radial pulse, gently palpate for a carotid pulse or auscultate for an apical pulse and wait for 30 to 45 seconds before you decide that the patient is pulseless.

Physicians disagree about the wisdom of performing basic life support (BLS; that is, CPR) on a patient with hypothermia who seems to be pulseless. Such a patient actually may be in a kind of "metabolic ice box," having achieved a metabolic balance that BLS may upset. Even a pulse rate of 1 or 2 beats/min indicates cardiac activity, and cardiac activity may spontaneously recover once the body's core is warmed. However, there is evidence that when correctly performed, BLS will increase

> **EMT-I Tips**
>
> Never place hot or cold packs directly against the patient's skin. Always wrap them in a towel or cloth to prevent burning or freezing the skin, respectively.

blood flow to the critical parts of the body. For this reason, some authorities recommend starting BLS on a patient with hypothermia and no pulse. The American Heart Association recommends that CPR be started if the patient has no detectable pulse or breathing. Again, for a patient with hypothermia, this may require a prolonged pulse check. Always follow local protocols to determine whether to begin chest compressions or use an automated external defibrillator (AED). You should perform ventilation with warm, humidified oxygen. Remove wet clothing, and protect the patient from the cold and wind with blankets in a warmer environment.

If you are in an area where hypothermia is a common problem, you should have specific protocols for dealing with this situation. In all cases, consult with medical control.

Advanced Cardiac Life Support Considerations

Cardiac medications exposed to very low temperatures may be less effective, and the hypothermic patient's metabolic rate is typically too slow to effectively process them. Temperatures should always be controlled in the passenger compartment of the ambulance when not in use to maintain the efficacy and shelf life of medications. Lidocaine, for example, may paradoxically lower the fibrillatory threshold in the hypothermic heart and increase resistance to defibrillation. Follow local protocols and American Heart Association recommendations.

Advanced airway procedures should be initiated immediately for apneic patients. There is no evidence of increased risk of inducing ventricular fibrillation from orotracheal or nasotracheal intubation.

Ventricular fibrillation (or V-fib) is the cardiac rhythm seen most often in hypothermic patients. The risk of ventricular fibrillation is related to depth and duration of the hypothermia and may be induced by rough handling. It is also generally impossible to electrically defibrillate a hypothermic heart that is colder than 86°F. For this reason, medical control may order BLS treatment only with rapid transport to the closest appropriate facility.

> **In the Field**
>
> Oxygen may be warmed or cooled by taping hot packs or cold packs to the oxygen tubing. This will also work for IV fluids.

Management of Cold Exposure in a Sick or Injured Person

All patients who are severely injured are at risk for hypothermia. Keep this in mind when you are evaluating a patient with multiple injuries.

A sick or injured person who has been trapped in a cold environment may develop hypothermia or may already have problems related to cold exposure. Such patients are more susceptible than are healthy people

You are the Provider — Part 3

Your initial questioning reveals that the patient has been playing tennis since 9:00 AM without a break. It is now 11:30 AM. Bystanders tell you he has not had anything to drink and has not rested at all.

Vital Signs	Recording Time: 2 Minutes After Patient Contact
Level of consciousness	Slightly confused; knows his name but unsure of surroundings
Respirations	24 breaths/min, deep
Sao$_2$	98% on room air
Pulse	116 beats/min, strong and bounding radial pulses
Blood pressure	148/92 mm Hg
Skin	Flushed, diaphoretic

5. What is your next step in treating this patient?
6. How will you obtain consent for treatment?

to cold injury. Take the following steps promptly to prevent further cold injury:

1. **Remove wet clothing**, and keep the patient dry.
2. **Prevent conduction heat loss.** Move the patient away from any wet or cold surfaces, such as a car frame.
3. **Insulate all exposed body parts**, especially the head, by wrapping them in a blanket or any other available dry, bulky material.
4. **Prevent convection heat loss** by erecting a wind barrier around the patient.
5. **Remove the patient** from the cold environment as promptly as possible.

Gentle transportation is necessary because of myocardial irritability and the risk of inducing ventricular fibrillation. Transport the patient with the head level or slightly down. Always transport to the closest appropriate facility. The availability of cardiac bypass rewarming capabilities would be preferable in considering the destination.

Regardless of the nature or severity of the cold injury, remember that even an unresponsive patient may be able to hear you. Some patients have told of hearing themselves pronounced dead by someone who had forgotten the old saying: "No one is dead unless he is warm and dead." If you carry an AED or manual defibrillator, you should perform defibrillation if indicated. However, the AHA recommends limiting defibrillation to three shocks in patients with severe hypothermia.

Because cold muscle is a poor conductor of electricity, the cardiac monitor may show asystole, but the patient may indeed have a cardiac rhythm.

Consider endotracheal intubation to maintain the airway if needed.

Local Cold Injuries

Most injuries from cold are localized to exposed parts of the body. The extremities, particularly the feet, ears, nose, and face, are especially vulnerable to cold injury ◀ **Figure 26-4** ◀. When exposed parts of the body become very cold but not frozen, the condition is called frostnip, chilblains, or immersion foot (trench foot). When the parts become frozen, the injury is called <u>frostbite</u>.

You should determine the duration of the exposure, the temperature to which the body part was exposed, and the wind velocity during exposure. These are important factors in determining the severity of a local cold injury. You should also investigate a number of underlying factors:

- Exposure to wet conditions
- Inadequate insulation from cold or wind

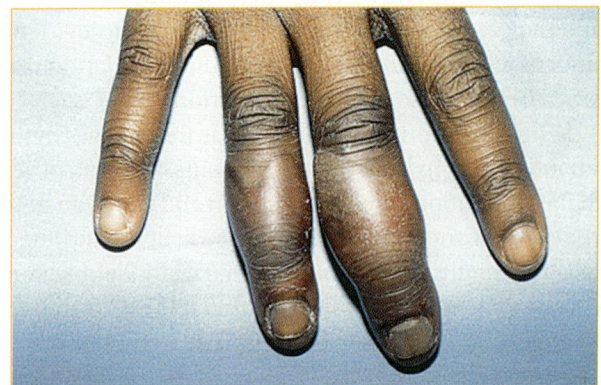
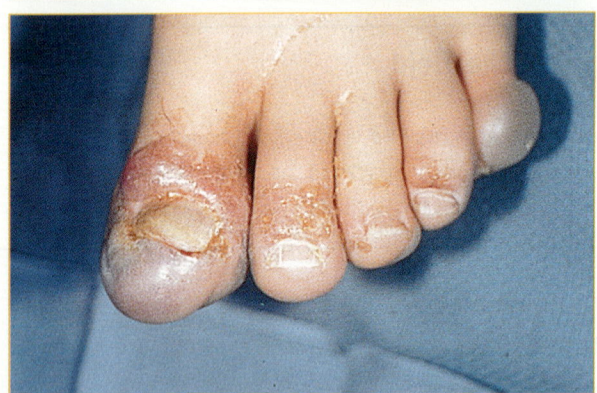
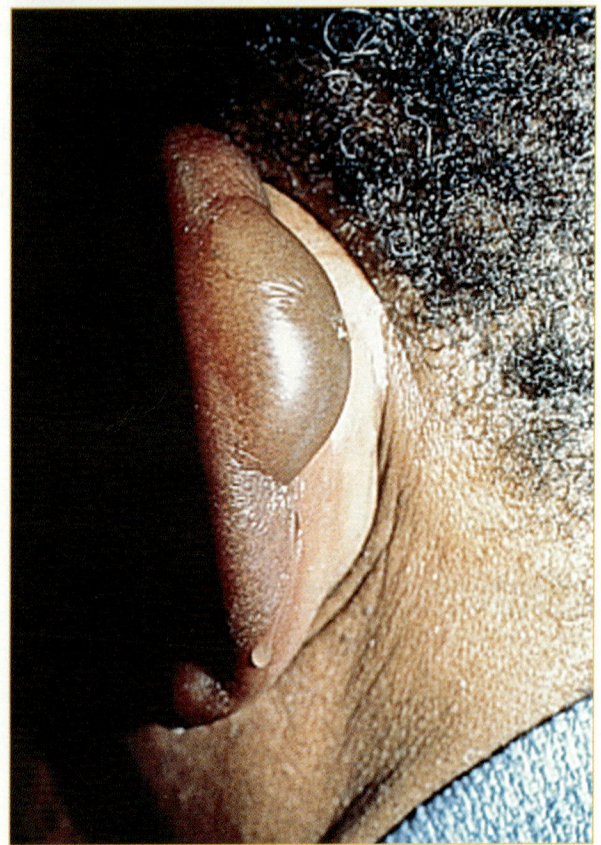

Figure 26-4 The extremities, particularly the feet, ears, nose, and face, are susceptible to frostbite.

- Restricted circulation from tight clothing or shoes or circulatory disease
- Fatigue
- Inadequate nutrition
- Alcohol or drug use or abuse
- Hypothermia
- Diabetes
- Cardiovascular disease
- Older age

In generalized hypothermia, blood is shunted away from the extremities in an attempt to maintain the core temperature. This shunting of blood increases the risk of local cold injury to the extremities, ears, nose, and face. Thus, the patient with generalized hypothermia should also be assessed for frostbite or other local cold injury. The reverse is also true. You must remember that both local and systemic cold exposure problems can occur in the same patient.

Frostnip and Immersion Foot

After prolonged exposure to the cold, the skin may be freezing while the deeper tissues are unaffected. This condition, which often affects the ears, nose, and fingers, is called frostnip. Because frostnip is usually not painful, the patient is often unaware that a cold injury has occurred. Immersion foot, also called trench foot, occurs after prolonged exposure to cold water. It is particularly common in hikers or hunters who stand for a long time in a river or lake. In both frostnip and immersion foot, the skin is pale (blanched) and cold to the touch; normal color does not return after palpation of the skin. In some cases, the skin of the foot will be wrinkled, but it can also remain soft. The patient complains of loss of feeling and sensation in the affected area.

As in all other hypothermia cases, the emergency treatment of these less severe local cold injuries consists of removing the patient from the cold, wet environment, but also rewarming the affected part. With frostnip, contact with a warm object may be all that is needed; you can use your hands, your breath, or the patient's own body. During rewarming, the affected part will often tingle and become red in light-skinned people. With immersion foot, remove wet shoes, boots, and socks, and rewarm the foot gradually, protecting it from further cold exposure.

Frostbite

Frostbite is the most serious local cold injury, because the tissues are actually frozen. Freezing permanently damages cells, although the exact mechanism by which damage occurs is not known. The presence of ice crystals within the cells may cause physical damage. The change in the water content in the cells may also cause changes in the concentration of critical electrolytes, producing permanent changes in the chemistry of the cell. When the ice thaws, further chemical changes occur in the cell, causing permanent damage or cell death, called gangrene Figure 26-5 . If gangrene occurs, the dead tissue must be surgically removed, sometimes by amputation. Following less severe damage, the exposed part will become inflamed, tender to the touch, and unable to tolerate further exposure to cold.

Frostbite can be identified by the hard, frozen feel of the affected tissues. Frostbitten parts are often hard and waxy Figure 26-6 . The injured part feels firm

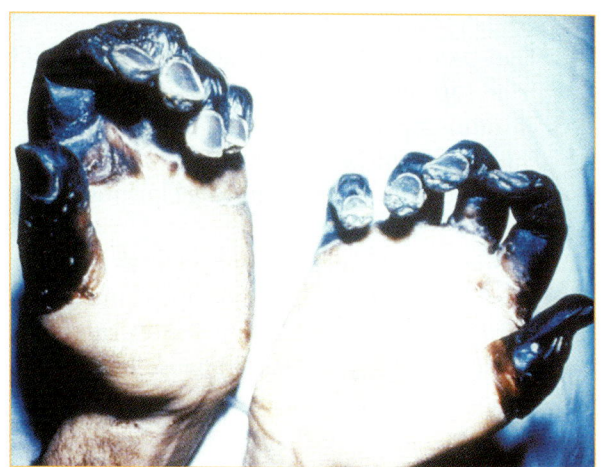

Figure 26-5 Gangrene, or permanent cell death, can occur when tissue is frozen and certain chemical changes occur in the cells.

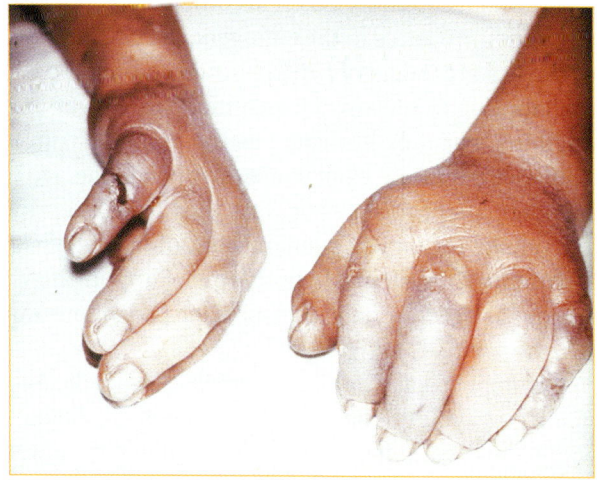

Figure 26-6 Frostbitten parts may be hard and waxy to the touch.

to frozen as you gently touch it. Blisters and swelling may be present. In light-skinned people with a deep injury that has thawed or partially thawed, the skin may appear red with purple and white areas, or it may be mottled and cyanotic.

As with a burn, the depth of skin damage will vary. With superficial frostbite, only the skin is frozen; with deep frostbite, the deeper tissues are frozen as well. You may not be able to tell superficial from deep frostbite in the field. Even an experienced surgeon in a hospital setting may not be able to tell until several days have elapsed.

Emergency Medical Care of Local Cold Injury

The emergency treatment of local cold injuries in the field should include the following steps:

1. **Remove the patient** from further exposure to the cold.
2. **Handle the injured part gently**, and protect it from further injury.
3. **Administer oxygen**, if this was not already done during the initial assessment.
4. **Remove any wet or restricting clothing** over the injured part.

With an early or superficial injury, such as frostnip or immersion foot, splint the extremity and cover it loosely with a dry, sterile dressing. Never rub injured tissues with anything, as this will cause further damage. Do not reexpose the injury to cold.

With a late or deep cold injury, such as frostbite, be sure to remove any jewelry or other potentially restrictive items from the injured part and cover the injury loosely with a dry, sterile dressing. Do not break blisters or rub or massage the area. Do not apply heat or rewarm the part. Unlike frostnip and trench foot, rewarming of the frostbitten extremity is best accomplished under controlled circumstances in the emergency department. You can cause a great deal of further injury to fragile tissues by attempting to rewarm a frostbitten part. Never apply something warm or hot, such as the exhaust from the ambulance engine or, even worse, an open flame. Do not allow the patient to stand or walk on a frostbitten foot.

Evaluate the patient's general condition for the signs or symptoms of systemic hypothermia. Support the vital functions as necessary, and transport the patient promptly to the hospital.

If prompt hospital care is not available and medical control instructs you to institute rewarming in the field, use a warm-water bath. Immerse the frostbitten part in water with a temperature between 100°F and 112°F (38°C and 44.5°C). Check the water temperature with a thermometer before immersing the limb, and recheck it frequently during the rewarming process. The water temperature should never exceed 112°F (44.5°C). Stir the water continuously. Keep the frostbitten part in the water until it feels warm and sensation has returned to the skin. Dress the area with dry, sterile dressings, placing them also between injured fingers or toes. Expect the patient to complain of severe pain.

Never attempt rewarming if there is any chance that the part may freeze again before the patient reaches the hospital. Some of the most severe consequences of frostbite, including gangrene and amputation, have occurred when parts were thawed and then refrozen.

Cover the frostbitten part with soft, padded, sterile cotton dressings. If blisters have formed, do not break them. Remember, you cannot accurately predict the outcome of a case of frostbite early in its course. Even body parts that appear gangrenous may recover following proper emergency and hospital treatment.

> **EMT-I Tips**
>
> IV fluids may be warmed by placing them over a defroster or hanging them in front of a heater vent. If fluids are warmed, be sure to test the temperature (for example, run the fluid over your inner wrist like you would a baby's bottle) before infusing them into a patient.

Cold Exposure and You

As an EMT-I, you are also at risk for hypothermia if you work in a cold environment. If cold weather search-and-rescue operations are a possibility in your assigned areas, you should receive survival training and precautionary tips. You should be thoroughly familiar with local conditions. Be aware of existing and potential weather conditions, and stay abreast of changes that are forecast for the area. Make sure proper clothing is available, and wear it whenever appropriate. Your vehicle, too, must be properly equipped and maintained for a cold environment. As with so many hazards, you cannot help others if you do not practice self-protection. Never allow yourself to become a casualty!

> **EMT-I Tips**
>
> Do not become a victim! You cannot help others if you do not practice self-protection.

Heat Exposure

Normal body temperature is 98.6°F (37°C). Complicated regulatory mechanisms keep this internal temperature constant, regardless of the ambient temperature, the temperature of the surrounding environment. In a hot environment or during vigorous physical activity, when the body itself produces excess heat, it will try to rid itself of the excess heat. The body does this by a process known as thermolysis. There are several ways that thermolysis may occur. The two most efficient are sweating (and evaporation of the sweat) and dilation of peripheral blood vessels, which brings warm blood to the skin's surface (causing flushing) to increase the rate of heat radiation. In addition, of course, the person who becomes overheated can remove clothing and try to find a cooler environment.

Ordinarily, the heat-regulating mechanisms of the body work very well and people are able to tolerate significant temperature changes. When the body is exposed to or generates more heat energy than it can lose because of inadequate thermolysis, hyperthermia results. Hyperthermia is a high core temperature, usually 101°F (38.4°C) or higher.

When the body's mechanisms to decrease body heat are overwhelmed and the body is unable to tolerate the excessive heat, illness develops. High air temperature can reduce the body's ability to lose heat by radiation; high humidity reduces the ability to lose heat through evaporation. Another contributing factor is vigorous exercise, during which the body can lose more than 1 L of sweat per hour, causing loss of fluid and electrolytes. Signs of thermolysis include diaphoresis, increased skin temperature, and flushing. Signs of thermolytic inadequacy include altered mentation and altered levels of consciousness. The patient may also present with signs of dehydration. Illness from heat exposure can cause the following problems:

- Heat cramps
- Heat exhaustion
- Heatstroke

All three forms of heat illness may be present in the same patient, because untreated heat exhaustion may progress to heatstroke. Heatstroke is a life-threatening emergency.

Persons at greatest risk for heat illnesses are children; elderly people; people with heart disease, chronic obstructive pulmonary disease, diabetes, dehydration, or obesity; and people with limited mobility. The autonomic neuropathy in diabetes interferes with vasodilation and perspiration and may interfere with thermoregulatory input, predisposing people with diabetes to heat illnesses. Elderly people, newborns, and infants exhibit poor thermoregulation. Newborns and infants are often dressed in too much clothing. Alcohol and certain drugs, including medications that dehydrate the body (such as diuretics) or decrease the ability of the body to sweat (such as antihistamines), also make a person more susceptible to heat illnesses. When you are treating someone for a heat illness, always obtain a thorough medical history that includes any medications that the patient may be taking. Obtaining a thorough patient history of the present illness should lead you to make the differentiation between a fever and a heat emergency.

Other contributing factors to heat illnesses include the length of exposure, intensity of exposure, and the environment itself. Ambient environmental conditions, such as humidity and wind, have a major role as well. This also includes indoor conditions.

Preventive measures to protect from heat emergencies include maintaining adequate fluid intake, acclimatizing to the environment, and limiting exposure. Thirst is an adequate indicator of dehydration. People working outside in high temperatures should drink water continually to replace what is lost through perspiration. In addition, adapting to the environment results in more perspiration with lower salt concentration. This increases fluid volume in the body and decreases the chances of dehydration. Spending time outdoors in the early morning or late evening when temperatures are lower, as opposed to the middle of the day, can also decrease a patient's risk.

> 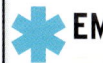 **EMT-I Tips**
>
> Keeping yourself hydrated while on duty is very important, especially during periods of heavy exertion or work in the heat. Drink at least 3 L of water per day and more when exertion or heat is involved. Urinary color and frequency correlate directly with the body's fluid level.

Heat Cramps

Heat cramps are painful muscle spasms that occur after vigorous exercise. They do not occur only when it is hot outdoors. They may be seen in factory workers and even well-conditioned athletes. The exact cause of heat cramps is not well understood. We know that sweat produced during strenuous exercise, particularly in a warm environment, causes a change in the body's balance of **electrolytes**, or salts. The result may be a loss of essential electrolytes from the cells. Dehydration may also have a role in the development of muscle cramps. Large amounts of water can be lost from the body as a result of excessive sweating. This loss of water may affect muscles that are being stressed and cause them to go into spasm.

Heat cramps usually occur in the legs or abdominal muscles. When the abdominal muscles are involved, the pain and muscle spasm may be so severe that the patient appears to have an acute abdominal problem. If a patient with a sudden onset of abdominal cramps has been exercising vigorously in a hot environment, you should suspect heat cramps.

Take the following steps to treat heat cramps in the field (Figure 26-7 ▶):

1. **Remove the patient** from the hot environment, including sunlight, a source of radiant heat gain. Loosen any tight clothing.
2. **Rest the cramping muscles.** Have the patient sit or lie down until the cramps subside.
3. **Replace fluids by mouth.** Use water or a diluted (half-strength) balanced electrolyte solution, such as Gatorade. In most cases, plain water is the most useful. Do not give salt tablets or solutions that have a high salt concentration. The patient already has an adequate amount of electrolytes circulating; they are just not distributed properly. With adequate rest and fluid replacement, the body will adjust the distribution of electrolytes, and the cramps will disappear.

If the cramps do not go away after these measures, initiate an IV line and transport the patient to the hospital. The patient may need prolonged rehydration that cannot be provided in the field.

Once the cramps are gone, the patient may resume activity. For example, an athlete can return to play once the heat cramps have disappeared. However, heavy sweating may cause the cramps to recur. Hydration by drinking a lot of water is the best preventive and treatment strategy.

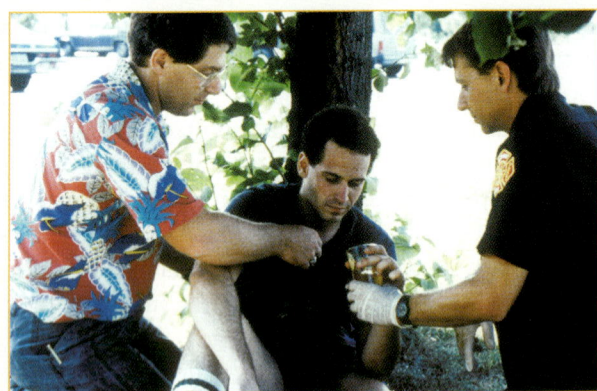

Figure 26-7 A patient with heat cramps should be moved to a cool environment as you begin your assessment and treatment.

You are the Provider Part 4

You and your partner assist the patient onto the stretcher and place him in the air-conditioned ambulance. After loosening his clothing, your partner wraps ice packs in washcloths to place around his neck and under his arms. You administer oxygen via nonrebreathing mask at 15 L/min.

Reassessment	Recording Time: 5 Minutes After Patient Contact
Respirations	20 breaths/min, deep
SaO_2	98% on oxygen
Pulse	116 beats/min, strong and bounding
Blood pressure	148/92 mm Hg
Skin	Not as flushed
Level of consciousness	Seems to be more alert and aware of his surroundings

7. What questions should you ask in relation to medical history?
8. What could be the cause of his altered mental status?
9. What are your treatment options?

> **A to Z Terminology Tips**
>
> LOC = level of consciousness, AMS = altered mental status

Heat Exhaustion

Heat exhaustion, also called *heat prostration* or *heat collapse*, is the most common illness caused by heat. It is the result of the body's losing so much water and so many electrolytes through very heavy sweating that hypovolemia (fluid depletion) occurs. For sweating to be an effective cooling mechanism, the sweat must be able to evaporate from the body. Otherwise, the body will continue to produce sweat, with further loss of body water. People standing in the hot sun, particularly those wearing several layers of clothing, such as football fans or parade watchers, may sweat profusely but experience little body cooling. High humidity will also decrease the amount of evaporation that can occur. People working or exerting themselves in poorly ventilated areas are unable to release heat through convection. Thus, people who work or exercise vigorously and those who wear heavy clothing in a warm, humid, or poorly ventilated environment are particularly prone to heat exhaustion.

In heat exhaustion, there is an increased core body temperature with some neurologic deficit. Symptoms may be due solely to dehydration combined with overexertion. The result is orthostatic hypotension. Symptoms generally resolve with rest and supine positioning. Fluids and elevation of the legs are also beneficial. Symptoms that do not resolve with rest and positioning may be due to the increased core body temperature and are predictive of impending heatstroke and must be treated aggressively.

The signs and symptoms of heat exhaustion and those of associated hypovolemia are as follows:
- Onset while working hard or exercising in a hot, humid, or poorly ventilated environment and sweating heavily
- Onset, even at rest, in an elderly person or an infant in hot, humid, and poorly ventilated environments or extended time in hot, humid environments
- Cool, clammy skin with ashen pallor
- Dry tongue and thirst
- Dizziness, weakness, or faintness, with accompanying nausea or headache
- Normal vital signs, although the pulse is often rapid and the diastolic blood pressure may be low
- Normal or slightly elevated body temperature; on rare occasions, as high as 104°F (40°C)

To treat the patient, follow the steps in **Skill Drill 26-1** ▶ :

1. **Remove excessive layers of clothing**, particularly around the head and neck (**Step 1**).
2. **Move the patient promptly** from the hot environment, preferably into the back of the air-conditioned ambulance. If outdoors, move out of the sun.
3. **Give the patient oxygen** if this was not already done during the initial assessment.
4. **Encourage the patient to lie down** and elevate the legs (supine position). Loosen any tight clothing, and fan the patient for cooling (**Step 2**).
5. **If the patient is fully alert**, encourage him or her to sit up and slowly drink up to a liter of water, as long as nausea does not develop. Never force fluids by mouth on a patient who is not fully alert or allow drinking while supine, because the patient could aspirate the fluid into the lungs.
6. **If the patient becomes nauseated**, transport positioned on the side to prevent aspiration. In most cases, these measures will reverse the symptoms, causing the patient to feel better within 30 minutes. Use more aggressive treatment, such as IV fluid therapy and close monitoring, especially in the following circumstances:
   - The symptoms do not clear up promptly.
   - The level of consciousness decreases.
   - The temperature remains elevated.
   - The person is very young, elderly, or has any underlying medical condition, such as diabetes or cardiovascular disease.
7. **Gain IV access, and give normal saline** fluid boluses of 20 mL/kg as needed if the patient is nauseated or unable to take fluid by mouth (**Step 3**).
8. **Transport the patient on his or her side** if you think the patient may be nauseated and ready to vomit, but make certain that the patient is secured (**Step 4**).
9. **Monitor the cardiac rhythm** and treat any disturbances according to local and ACLS protocols.

Skill Drill 26-1

Treating for Heat Exhaustion

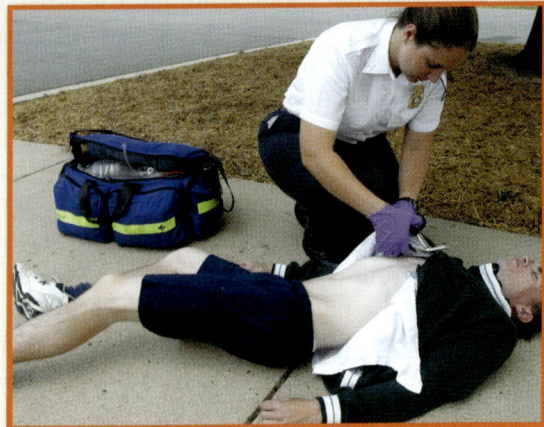

1 Remove extra clothing.

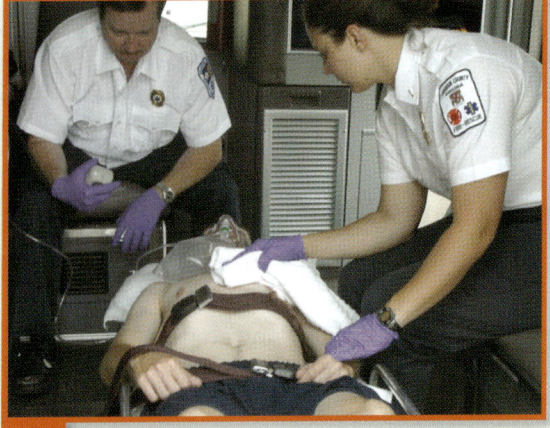

2 Move the patient to a cooler environment. Give oxygen.

Place the patient in a supine position, elevate the legs, and fan the patient.

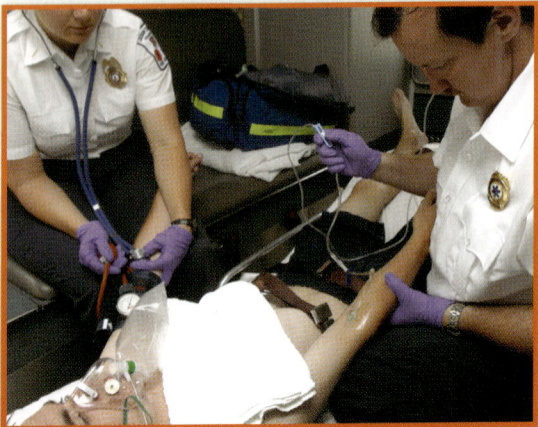

3 Establish IV access. Give normal saline fluid boluses of 20 mL/kg as needed if the patient is nauseated or unable to take fluid by mouth.

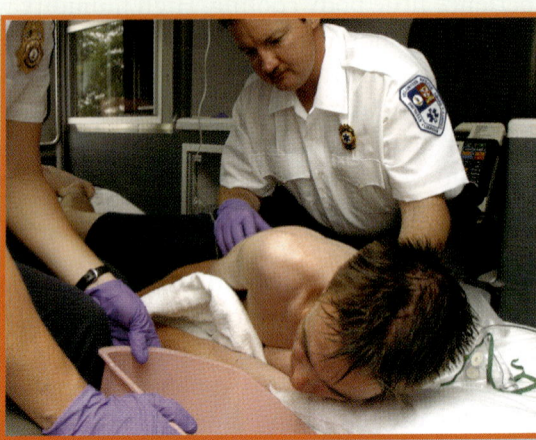

4 If the patient is nauseous or becomes nauseous, transport on the side.

Heatstroke

Heatstroke, the least common but most serious illness caused by heat exposure, occurs when the body is subjected to more heat than it can effectively remove, and normal mechanisms for getting rid of the excess heat are overwhelmed. The body temperature then rises rapidly to the level at which tissues are destroyed, with significant neurologic deficit. Organ damage occurs in the brain, liver, and kidneys. Untreated heatstroke always results in death.

Heatstroke can develop in patients during vigorous physical activity or when they are outdoors or in a closed, poorly ventilated, humid space. It also occurs during heat waves among people (particularly elderly people) who live in buildings with no air conditioning or with poor ventilation. It may also develop in children who are left unattended in a locked car on a hot day.

Many patients with heatstroke have hot, dry, flushed skin because their sweating mechanism has been overwhelmed and they are severely dehydrated. However, early in the course of heatstroke, the skin may be moist or wet because of residual sweat from earlier perspiration. For this reason, do not rule out heatstroke if the patient's skin is still moist. The body temperature rises rapidly in patients with heatstroke. It may rise to 106°F (41°C) or higher. As the body core temperature rises, the patient's level of consciousness falls.

Often, the first sign of heatstroke is a change in behavior. However, the patient then becomes unresponsive very quickly. The pulse is usually rapid and strong at first, but as the patient becomes increasingly unresponsive, the pulse becomes weaker and the blood pressure falls.

Classic heatstroke commonly presents in people with chronic illnesses. There is an increased core body temperature due to deficient thermoregulatory function. Predisposing conditions include age, diabetes, and other medical conditions. "Hot, red, dry" skin is common in these patients. Exertional heatstroke commonly presents in people who are in good general health but have an increased core body temperature due to overwhelming heat stress, which may be due to excessive ambient temperature, excessive exertion, prolonged exposure, or poor acclimatization. "Moist, pale" skin is common in these patients.

Recovery from heatstroke depends on the speed with which treatment is administered, so you must be able to identify this condition quickly. Emergency treatment has one objective: Get the body temperature down by any means available. Take the following steps when treating a patient with heatstroke:

1. **Move the patient** out of the hot environment and into the ambulance.
2. **Set the air conditioning** to maximum cooling.
3. **Remove the patient's clothing.**
4. **Give the patient oxygen** if this was not done during the initial assessment. Assist ventilations as needed.
5. **Apply cool packs** to the patient's neck, groin, and armpits Figure 26-8 .
6. **Cover the patient** with wet towels or sheets, or spray the patient with cool water and fan him or her to quickly evaporate the dampness on the skin.
7. **Aggressively and repeatedly fan** the patient with or without dampening the skin.
8. **Provide immediate transport to the hospital.**
9. **Gain IV access, and give normal saline** fluid boluses of 20 mL/kg. Repeat as needed to maintain adequate perfusion and alleviate symptoms of dehydration.
10. **Notify the hospital** as soon as possible so that the staff can prepare to treat the patient immediately on arrival.
11. **Monitor the cardiac rhythm** and treat any disturbances according to local and ACLS protocols.

EMT-I Tips

Do not cool a patient to the point of shivering, or you will increase rather than decrease the body temperature. Ice packs and cold water immersion may produce reflex vasoconstriction and shivering because of the effect on peripheral thermoreceptors. Reflex hypothermia results from overcooling.

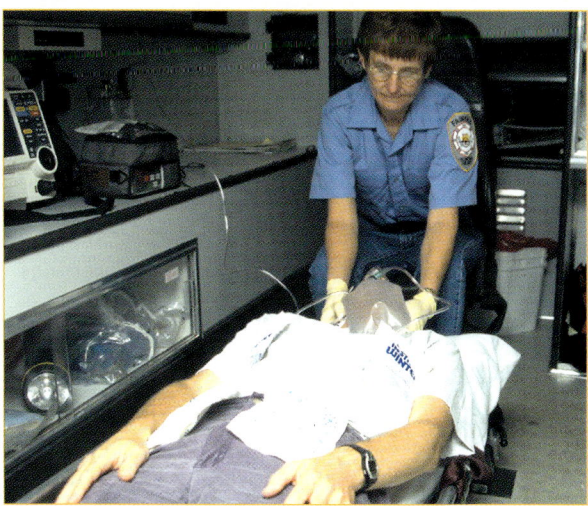

Figure 26-8 As part of treatment of heatstroke, give oxygen and place cool packs around the patient's neck, groin, and armpits.

Geriatric Needs

As we age, our bodies can lose their ability to respond to the environment. Older adults undergo changes in their ability to compensate for low or high ambient temperatures. For example, if the ambient temperature rises from 85°F to 94°F (29.5°C to 34.5°C), the older adult may not recognize the change or be able to compensate for it. Therefore, unless the person is accustomed to the heat, heatstroke can develop relatively quickly.

Shivering, a common effect of hypothermia, is the body's attempt to generate heat. However, because of a decrease in muscle mass or tone, the hypothermic older patient may not shiver. Furthermore, a decrease in muscle mass and body fat means that there is less insulation and protection from the cold. Because of the body's altered response to heat loss and its ability to gain heat, the health care provider might not suspect or report hypothermia. In caring for the geriatric patient in cold climates, be sure to protect the patient against unwanted heat loss. Cover all exposed areas with loose-fitting blankets. Give particular attention to protecting the patient's head, because heat loss from the head is substantial.

Because of reduced circulation to the skin, heat loss via conduction, convection, and radiation is significantly lower. In addition, the aging process alters the patient's ability to perspire; therefore, heat loss through evaporation is reduced. Because the older patient cannot disperse heat effectively, classic heatstroke can develop rapidly. Typically, the older adult will not go through an initial stage of heat exhaustion. During the summer, you should be acutely aware of the potential for heatstroke and factors that can predispose a patient to heat illness. Factors that increase the possibility of heatstroke include medications, diabetes, alcohol abuse, malnutrition, parkinsonism, hyperthyroidism, and obesity.

Both hypothermia and hyperthermia can occur in older patients in environmental settings that are subtle unless you are looking for them. These problems appear commonly, for example, when budget concerns prompt older people to keep heat turned down in the winter or to not use air conditioning in hot weather. Thermal emergencies can develop over time in indoor, urban environments that may not seem uncomfortable to you.

 EMT-I Tips

Even though some salt additive is beneficial, salt tablets may cause gastrointestinal irritation and ulceration and hypernatremia and should be avoided. Fluid therapy with normal saline is preferred.

Lightning Injuries

According to the National Weather Service, there are an estimated 25 million cloud-to-ground lightning flashes in the United States each year. On average, lightning kills between 60 and 70 people per year in the United States based on documented cases. While documented lightning injuries in the United States average about 300 per year, undocumented lightning injuries are likely much higher. Lightning is the third most common cause of death from isolated environmental phenomena.

The energy associated with lightning is comprised of direct current (DC) of up to 200,000 amps and a potential of 100 million volts or more. Temperatures generated from lightning vary between 20,000°F and 60,000°F.

Most lightning deaths and injuries occur during the summer months when people are enjoying outdoor activities, despite an approaching thunderstorm. Those most commonly struck by lightning include boaters, swimmers, and golfers; any type of activity that exposes the person to a large open area increases the risk of being struck by lightning.

The determining factor on whether lightning could injure or kill depends on whether a person is in the path of the lightning discharge. In addition to the visible flash that travels through the air, the current associated with the lightning discharge travels along the ground. Although some victims are injured or killed by a direct lightning strike, many victims are indirectly struck when standing near an object that has been struck by lightning, such as a tree (splash effect).

The cardiovascular and nervous systems are most commonly injured during a lightning strike; therefore, respiratory or cardiac arrest is the most common cause of lightning-related deaths. The tissue damage caused by lightning is different from that caused by other electrical-related injuries (ie, high-power-line injuries). This is because the tissue damage pathway usually occurs over the skin, rather than through it. Additionally, because the duration of a lightning strike is short, skin burns are usually superficial; full-thickness (third-degree) burns are rare. Lightning injuries are categorized as being mild, moderate, or severe:

- **Mild.** Loss of consciousness, amnesia, confusion, tingling, and other nonspecific signs and symptoms. Burns, if present, are typically superficial.
- **Moderate.** Seizures, respiratory arrest, cardiac standstill (asystole) that spontaneously resolves, and superficial burns.
- **Severe.** Cardiopulmonary arrest. Because of the delay in resuscitation, often due to remote locations, many of these patients do not survive.

Emergency Medical Care

As with any scene response, the safety of you and your partner has priority. Take measures to protect yourself from being struck, especially if the thunderstorm is still in progress. Contrary to popular belief, lightning can, and does, strike in the same place twice. Move the patient to a place of safety, preferably in a sheltered area.

If you are in an open area and adequate shelter is not available, it is important to recognize the signs of an impending lightning strike and take immediate action to protect yourself. If you suddenly feel a tingling sensation or your hair stands on end, the area around you has become charged—a sure sign of an imminent lightning strike. Curl up in a ball and lie on the ground; make yourself as small a target as possible. If you are standing near a tree or other tall object, move away as fast as possible, preferably to a low-lying area. Lightning has an affinity for objects that project from the ground (ie, trees, fences, buildings).

The process of triaging multiple victims of a lightning strike is different than the conventional triage methods used during a mass-casualty incident. When a person is struck by lightning, respiratory or cardiac arrest, if it occurs, usually occurs immediately. Those who are conscious following a lightning strike are much less likely to develop delayed respiratory or cardiac arrest; most of these victims will survive. Therefore, you should focus your efforts on those who are in respiratory or cardiac arrest. This process, called <u>reverse triage</u>, differs from conventional triage, where such patients would ordinarily be classified as deceased.

Emergency care for a lightning injury is the same as it is for other severe electrical injuries. Because the massive DC shock caused by lightning, the patient experiences massive muscle spasms (tetany), which can result in fractures of long bones and spinal vertebrae. Therefore, manually stabilize the patient's head in a neutral inline position and open the airway with the jaw-thrust maneuver. If the patient is in respiratory arrest with a pulse, begin immediate BVM ventilations with 100% oxygen. If the patient is in cardiac arrest, attach an AED as soon as possible and provide immediate defibrillation if indicated. If severe bleeding is present, control it immediately.

If you are unable to effectively ventilate the patient with a BVM, insert a Combitube or similar advanced airway device. Insert at least one large-bore IV line and provide crystalloid (ie, normal saline, lactated Ringer's) fluid boluses of 20 mL/kg to treat suspected hypovolemia and to promote the excretion of myoglobin, a chemical released by injured muscle that can result in renal damage or failure.

Due to the potential for dysrhythmias, always monitor the cardiac status of a lightning strike victim. Apply a cardiac monitor and treat cardiac dysrhythmias in accordance with standard ACLS or local protocols. Perform endotracheal intubation for patients who cannot protect their own airway or for those in respiratory or cardiac arrest. If seizures occur, administer diazepam (Valium), lorazepam (Ativan), or other medications as directed by local protocol.

Provide full spinal immobilization and transport the patient to the closest appropriate facility. If CPR or ventilations are not required, address other injuries (ie, splint fractures, dress and bandage burns) and provide continuous monitoring while en route to the hospital.

Drowning and Near Drowning

<u>Drowning</u> is death from suffocation because of submersion in water or other fluids; <u>near drowning</u> is defined as near suffocation in water or other fluids with a recovery event that lasts at least 24 hours. Patients with near drowning can, however, die of secondary complications (such as pneumonia) that occur beyond 24 hours. Drowning is often the last in a cycle of events caused by panic in the water Figure 26-9 ▶. It can happen to anyone who is submerged in water for even a short time. Struggling toward the surface or the shore, the person becomes fatigued or exhausted, which leads him or her to sink even deeper. However, drowning also occurs in mop buckets, puddles, bathtubs, and other places where the individual is not completely submerged. Small children can drown in only a few inches of water if unattended.

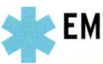

EMT-I Tips

Focus your efforts on lightning strike victims who appear "dead." Many of these patients can be successfully resuscitated.

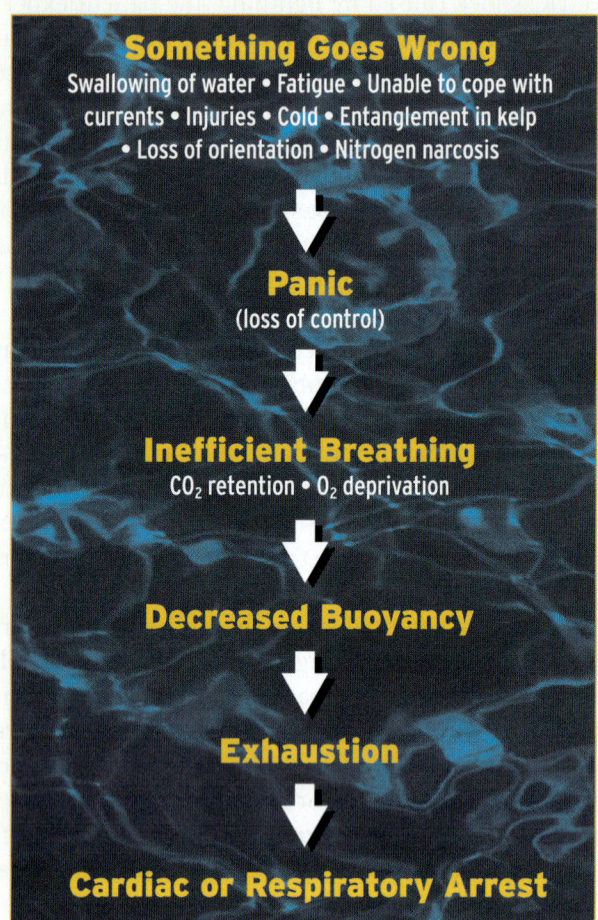

Figure 26-9 Panic in the water often precedes drowning.

diving reflex may actually slow metabolism to the point of protecting vital organs, such as the brain, heart, lungs, and kidneys. Hypoxia is always the first concern, but all near-drowning victims should be treated for hypothermia.

> **EMT-I Tips**
>
> All near-drowning patients should be transported for evaluation.

> **EMT-I Tips**
>
> The cold-water near-drowning patient may require more care than two EMT-Is can provide by themselves. Airway management and ventilation needs can make it difficult to remove wet clothing, treat hypothermia, and perform further assessment unless additional trained help is available. On this type of call, consider requesting backup before you encounter the patient.

Emergency Medical Care

Treatment begins with rescue and removal from the water. When necessary, artificial ventilation should begin as soon as possible, even before the victim is removed from the water. At the same time, you must stabilize and protect the patient's spine when a long fall or dive has occurred (or if this is a possibility when no information is provided). Associated cervical spine injuries are possible, especially in diving mishaps. If the patient does not have a possible spinal injury, you can turn the patient quickly to the left side to allow draining from the upper airway. Note that water will not drain from the lungs. If there is evidence of upper airway obstruction by foreign matter, remove the obstruction manually or by suction, if available. If necessary, use abdominal thrusts, followed by assisted ventilations. Administer oxygen if this was not done during the initial assessment, either by nonrebreathing mask for patients who are breathing adequately or via bag-valve-mask device for those requiring assisted ventilation. *Do not perform abdominal thrusts unless a foreign body airway obstruction is present. Doing so will increase the risk of regurgitation of water and aspiration.*

Check for a pulse immediately after the patient is removed from the water. It may be difficult to locate a pulse because of constriction of the peripheral blood

Inhaling very small amounts of fresh or salt water can severely irritate the larynx, sending the muscles of the larynx and the vocal cords into spasm, called laryngospasm. The average person experiences this to a mild degree when a bit of a drink is inhaled and the patient coughs and seems to be choking for a few seconds. This is the body's attempt at self-preservation, because laryngospasm prevents more water from entering the lungs. But this can be too much of a good thing in severe cases such as water submersion, because the patient's lungs cannot be ventilated when significant laryngospasm is present. Instead, progressive hypoxia occurs until the patient becomes unconscious. At this point, the spasm relaxes, making rescue breathing possible. Of course, if the patient has not already been removed from the water, the patient may now inhale deeply, and more water may enter the lungs. In 85% to 90% of cases, significant amounts of water enter the lungs of the drowning victim.

Hypothermia is also a major consideration in near drownings. Heat loss is rapid, particularly if the patient is actively flailing about, which expends a lot of energy. However, hypothermia may also be beneficial. The mammalian

EMT-I Tips

You must ensure the safety of rescue personnel before a water rescue can begin. If the patient is conscious and still in the water, you should perform a water rescue. An old saying sums up the basic rule of water rescue: "Reach, throw, and row, and only then go." First, try to reach for the patient (Figure 26-10A ▶). If that does not work, then throw the patient a rope, a life preserver, or any floatable object that is available (Figure 26-10B ▶). For example, an inflated spare tire, rim and all, will float well enough to support two people in the water. Next, use a boat if one is available (Figure 26-10C ▶). Do not attempt a swimming rescue unless you are trained and experienced in the proper techniques (Figure 26-10D ▶). Even then, you should always wear a helmet and a personal flotation device (Figure 26-11 ▶). Too many well-meaning individuals become victims while attempting a water rescue. A panicked swimmer will make every effort to remain above water, even if this means submerging the rescuer in the process. In cold climates or cold water, rapid hypothermia is a concern for rescuers as well. Be prepared for this potential event.

If you work in a recreation area near lakes, rivers, or an ocean, you must have a prearranged plan for water rescue. This plan should include access to and cooperation with local personnel who are trained and skilled in water rescue; these personnel should help develop the protocols for water rescue. Because the success of any water rescue depends on how rapidly the patient is removed from the water and ventilated, make sure you always have immediate access to personal flotation devices and other rescue equipment.

vessels and low cardiac output. Nevertheless, if the pulse is undetectable, start CPR if the patient is unresponsive.

Even if resuscitation in the field appears completely successful, you must always transport near-drowning patients to the hospital. Symptoms may not appear for 24 hours or more after resuscitation. Adult respiratory distress syndrome (ARDS) or renal failure may occur after resuscitation. Inhalation of any amount of fluid can lead to delayed complications lasting for days or weeks.

Make sure that the patient is kept warm, especially after cold-water immersion. Make sure blankets and protection from the environment are provided as needed. If ventilation equipment is not available but oxygen is, you can breathe the oxygen in yourself and give mouth-to-mask ventilation until rescue equipment arrives. In this method, your expired air will have a higher percentage of oxygen.

You are the Provider — Part 5

The patient tells you he had a massive heart attack 4 years ago but has been fine since then. He is allergic to penicillin and sulfa drugs. He was not feeling well yesterday and did not eat or drink much. He has only had coffee this morning.

Reassessment	Recording Time: 10 Minutes After Patient Contact
Level of consciousness	Improved
Respirations	20 breaths/min, adequate depth
Pulse	96 beats/min, strong
Blood pressure	136/84 mm Hg
Skin	Warm and dry

Your partner climbs into the front of the ambulance to drive to the local hospital while you attempt to gain IV access.

10. What size IV catheter would you choose?
11. What fluid will you use, and at what rate will you run it?

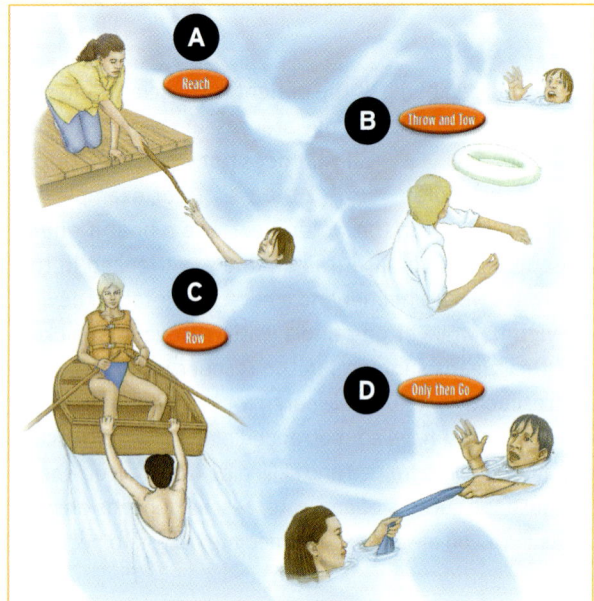

Figure 26-10 Basic rules of water rescue. **A.** Reach the person from shore. If you cannot reach the person from shore, wade closer. **B.** If an object that floats is available, throw it to the person. **C.** Use a boat if one is available. **D.** If you must swim to the person, use a towel or board for him or her to hold onto. Do not let the person grab you.

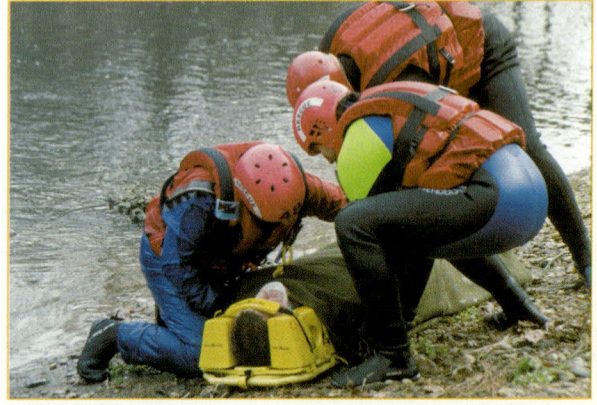

Figure 26-11 When performing water rescue, you must wear proper protective equipment, including a personal flotation device.

Spinal Injuries in Submersion Incidents

Submersion incidents may be complicated by spinal fractures and spinal cord injuries. You must assume that spinal injury exists with the following conditions:

- The submersion has resulted from a diving mishap or long fall.
- The patient is unconscious, and no information is available to rule out the possibility of a mechanism causing neck injury.
- The patient is conscious but complains of weakness, paralysis, or numbness in the arms or legs.
- You suspect the possibility of spinal injury despite what witnesses say.

Most spinal injuries in diving incidents affect the cervical spine. When spinal injury is suspected, the neck must be protected from further injury. This means that you will have to stabilize the suspected injury while the patient is still in the water. Follow the steps in (**Skill Drill 26-2** ▶):

1. **Turn the patient supine.** Two rescuers are usually required to turn the patient safely, although in some cases one rescuer will suffice. Always rotate the entire upper half of the patient's body as a single unit. Twisting only the head, for example, may aggravate any injury to the cervical spine (**Step 1**).
2. **Open the airway, and begin ventilation.** Immediate ventilation is the primary treatment of all drowning and near-drowning patients. As soon as the patient is face up in the water, use a pocket mask if it is available. Have the other rescuer support the head and trunk as a unit while you open the airway and begin artificial ventilation (**Step 2**).
3. **Float a buoyant backboard under the patient** as you continue ventilation (**Step 3**).
4. **Secure the head and trunk to the backboard** to eliminate motion of the cervical spine. Do not remove the patient from the water until this is done (**Step 4**).
5. **Remove the patient from the water, on the backboard** (**Step 5**).
6. **Remove wet clothes, and cover the patient with a blanket.** Give supplemental oxygen if the patient is breathing adequately; positive-pressure ventilation if apneic or breathing inadequately. Begin CPR if there is no pulse. Effective chest compressions are impossible to perform when the patient is still in the water (**Step 6**).
7. Consider endotracheal intubation to maintain the airway if needed. Place patient on a cardiac monitor and treat any dysrhythmias according to local and ACLS protocols.

Recovery Techniques

On occasion, you may be called to the scene of a drowning and find that the patient is not floating or visible in the water. An organized rescue effort in these circumstances

Stabilizing a Suspected Spinal Injury in the Water

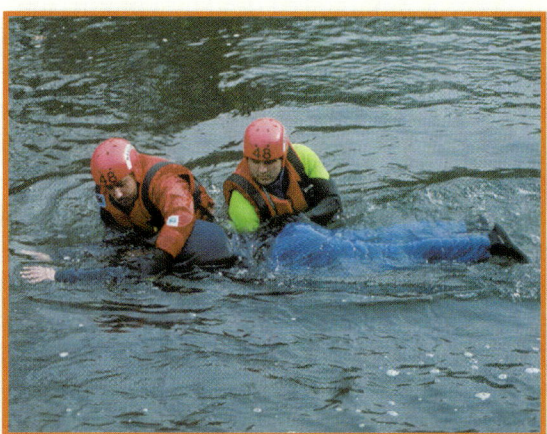

1 Turn the patient to a supine position by rotating the entire upper half of the body as a single unit.

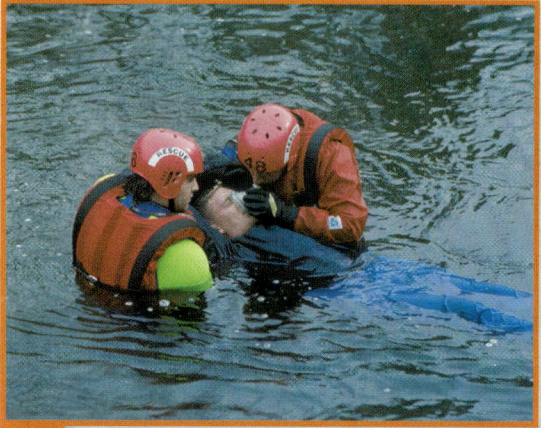

2 As soon as the patient is turned, begin artificial ventilation using the mouth-to-mouth method or a pocket mask.

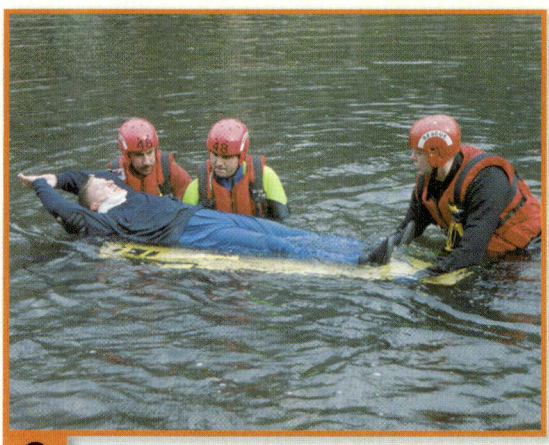

3 Float a buoyant backboard under the patient.

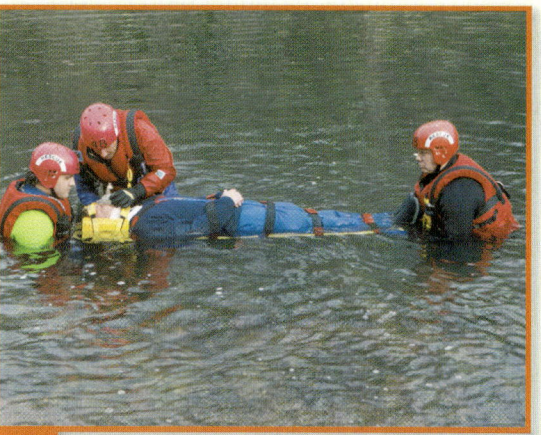

4 Secure the patient to the backboard.

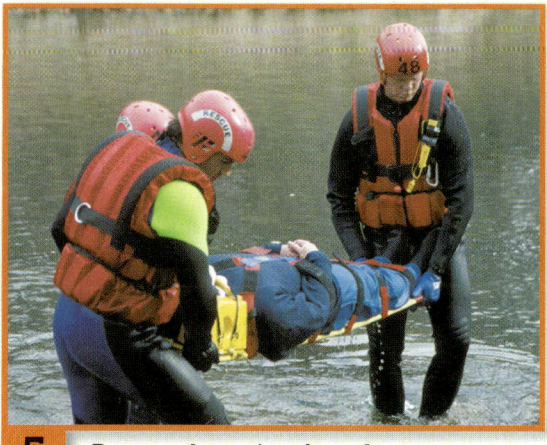

5 Remove the patient from the water.

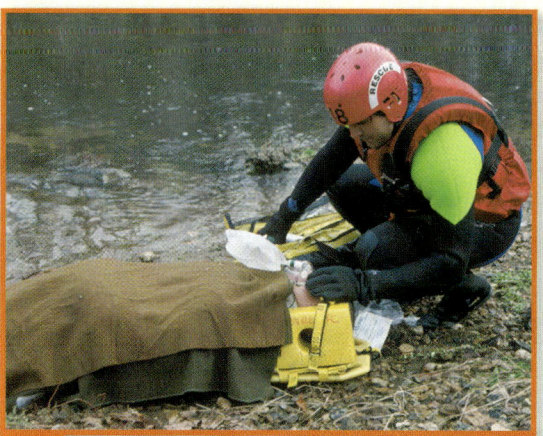

6 Cover the patient with a blanket, and apply oxygen if breathing.

Begin CPR if breathing and pulse are absent.

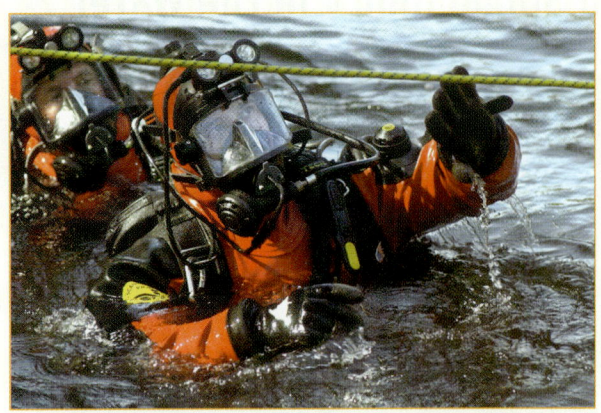

Figure 26-12 Never attempt a deep-water rescue without proper training and equipment.

calls for personnel who are experienced with recovery techniques and equipment, including snorkel, mask, and scuba gear. Scuba (self-contained underwater breathing apparatus) gear is a system that delivers air to the mouth and lungs at atmospheric pressures that increase with the depth of the dive Figure 26-12.

As a last resort, when standard procedures for recovery are unsuccessful, you may have to use a grappling iron or large hook to drag the bottom for the victim. Although the hook could seriously wound the patient, it may be the only effective way to bring him or her to the surface for resuscitation efforts.

Resuscitation Efforts

You should *never* give up on resuscitating a cold-water drowning victim. When a person is submerged in water that is colder than body temperature, heat will be conducted from the body to the water. The resulting hypothermia can protect vital organs from the lack of oxygen. In addition, exposure to cold water will occasionally activate certain primitive reflexes, which may preserve basic body functions for prolonged periods. In one case, a 2½-year-old girl recovered after being submerged in cold water for at least 66 minutes. Continue to provide full resuscitative efforts until the patient recovers or is pronounced dead by a physician.

Also, whenever a person dives or jumps into very cold water, the diving reflex (also known as the mammalian diving reflex), slowing of the heart rate caused by submersion in cold water, may cause immediate bradycardia, a slow heart rhythm. Loss of consciousness and drowning may follow. However, the person may be able to survive for an extended time under water because of a lowering of the metabolic rate and decreased oxygen demand and consumption associated with hypothermia. For this reason, you should continue full resuscitation efforts no matter how long the patient has been submerged.

Diving Emergencies

Most serious water-related injuries are associated with dives, with or without scuba gear. Some of these problems are related to the nature of the dive; others result from panic. Panic is not restricted to the person who is frightened by water. It can even happen to an experienced diver or swimmer.

There are more than 3 million scuba sport divers in the United States, and approximately 200,000 new divers are trained annually. Medical problems relating to scuba diving techniques and equipment are becoming increasingly common. These problems are separated into three phases of the dive: descent, bottom, and ascent.

Descent Emergencies

Descent problems are usually due to the sudden increase in pressure on the body as the person dives deeper into the water. Some body cavities cannot adjust to the increased external pressure of the water; the result is severe pain. The usual areas affected are the lungs, the sinus cavities, the middle ear, the teeth, and the area of the face surrounded by the diving mask. Usually, the pain caused by these "squeeze problems" forces the diver to return to the surface to equalize the pressures, and the problem clears up by itself. A diver who continues to complain of pain, particularly in the ear, after returning to the surface should be transported to the hospital.

A person with a perforated tympanic membrane (ruptured eardrum) may develop a special problem while diving. If cold water enters the middle ear through a ruptured eardrum, the diver may lose his or her balance

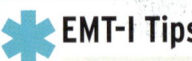**EMT-I Tips**

Never give up on resuscitating a cold-water drowning victim.

and orientation. As a result, the diver may ascend too quickly, causing further problems.

Emergencies at the Bottom

Problems related to the bottom of the dive are rarely seen. They include inadequate mixing of oxygen and carbon dioxide in the air the diver breathes and accidental feeding of poisonous carbon monoxide into the breathing apparatus. Both are the result of faulty connections in the diving gear. These situations can cause drowning or rapid ascent; they require emergency resuscitation and transport of the patient.

Another problem encountered in deep diving is nitrogen narcosis, or narcosis of the deep. It is normally associated with diving in excess of 100 feet. Because of the increase of nitrogen in the body, divers notice lightheadedness similar to a drunken state. The danger is that the diver may not recognize the problem and may not deal with the situation rationally. The diver may dive deeper, thereby compounding the problem. The effect is similar to the effects of nitrous oxide (laughing gas), giving the diver a feeling of euphoria. Should narcosis be encountered, the diver should ascend until the feeling is corrected.

Ascent Emergencies

Most of the serious injuries associated with diving are related to ascending from the bottom and are referred to as ascent problems. These emergencies usually require aggressive resuscitation. Two particularly dangerous medical emergencies are air embolism and decompression sickness (also called "the bends").

> **EMT-I Tips**
>
> As a diver descends, the gases in the body take up less space, allowing for more gas within the body. As the diver ascends, the gas bubbles get larger, and, unless the diver continually breathes out to rid the body of the excess gas, rupture of gas-filled organs may occur.
>
> Boyle's law states that if the temperature stays the same, the volume of gas gets smaller at the same rate that the surrounding pressure increases and density increases.

Air Embolism

The most dangerous and most common emergency in scuba diving is air embolism, a condition involving bubbles of air in the blood vessels. Air embolism may occur on a dive as shallow as 6′. The problem starts when the diver holds his or her breath during a rapid ascent. The air pressure in the lungs remains at a high level, while the external pressure on the chest decreases. As a result, the air inside the lungs expands rapidly, causing the alveoli in the lungs to rupture and forcing air into the bloodstream. The air released from this rupture can cause the following injuries:

- Air may enter the pleural space and compress the lungs (pneumothorax).
- Air may enter the mediastinum (the space within the thorax that contains the heart and great vessels), causing a condition called pneumomediastinum.
- Air may enter the bloodstream and create bubbles of air in the vessels called air emboli.

Pneumothorax and pneumomediastinum both result in pain and severe dyspnea. An air embolus will act as a plug and prevent the normal flow of blood and oxygen to a specific part of the body. The brain and spinal cord are the organs most severely affected by air embolism because they require a constant supply of oxygen.

The following are potential signs and symptoms of air embolism:

- Blotching (mottling of the skin)
- Froth (often pink or bloody) at the nose and mouth
- Severe pain in muscles, joints, or abdomen
- Dyspnea
- Localized pleuritic (sharp) chest pain
- Dizziness, nausea, and vomiting
- Dysphasia (difficulty speaking)
- Difficulty with vision
- Paralysis, coma, or both
- Irregular pulse and even cardiac arrest

> **Terminology Tips**
>
> Pneumo = air; thorax = thoracic cavity; therefore, a pneumothorax is air within the thoracic cavity, but outside the lungs.

Decompression Sickness

Decompression sickness, commonly called the bends, occurs when bubbles of gas, especially nitrogen, obstruct the blood vessels. This condition results from too rapid an ascent from a dive. During the dive, nitrogen that is being breathed dissolves in the blood and tissues because it is under pressure. When the diver ascends, the external pressure is decreased, and the dissolved nitrogen forms small bubbles within the tissues. These bubbles can lead to problems similar to those that occur in air embolism (blockage of tiny blood vessels, depriving parts of the body of their normal blood supply), but severe pain in certain tissues or spaces in the body is the most common problem.

The most striking symptom is abdominal and/or joint pain so severe that the patient literally doubles over or "bends." Dive tables and computers are available to show the proper rate of ascent from a dive, including the number and length of pauses that a diver should make (staged ascent). However, even divers who stay within these limits can experience the bends.

Even after a "safe dive," decompression sickness can occur from driving a car up a mountain or flying in an unpressurized airplane that climbs too rapidly to a great height. However, the risk of this diminishes after 24 to 48 hours. The problem is exactly the same as ascent from a deep dive: a sudden decrease of external pressure on the body and release of dissolved nitrogen from the blood that forms bubbles of nitrogen gas within the blood vessels.

You may find it difficult to distinguish between air embolism and decompression sickness. As a general rule, air embolism occurs immediately on return to the surface, whereas the symptoms of decompression sickness may not occur for several hours. The emergency treatment is the same for both. It consists of BLS followed by recompression in a hyperbaric chamber, a chamber or a small room that is pressurized to more than atmospheric pressure (Figure 26-13 ▶). Recompression treatment allows the bubbles of gas to dissolve into the blood and equalizes the pressures inside and outside the lungs. Once these pressures are equalized, gradual decompression can be accomplished under controlled conditions to prevent the bubbles from re-forming.

In treating patients who are suspected of having air embolism or decompression sickness, you should follow these accepted treatment steps:

1. Remove the patient from the water. Try to keep the patient calm.
2. Begin BLS, and administer oxygen or positive-pressure ventilation as needed.
3. Place the patient in a left lateral recumbent position with the head down.

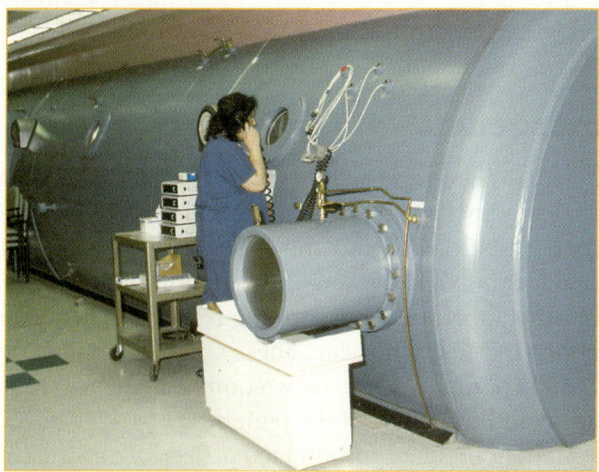

Figure 26-13 A hyperbaric chamber, usually a small room, is pressurized to more than atmospheric pressure and used in the treatment of decompression sickness and air embolism.

4. Provide prompt transport to the nearest recompression facility for treatment.
5. Consider endotracheal intubation to maintain the airway if needed. Place patient on a cardiac monitor and treat any dysrhythmias according to local and ACLS protocols.

Injury from decompression sickness is usually reversible with proper treatment. However, if the bubbles block critical blood vessels that supply the brain or spinal cord, permanent central nervous system injury may result. Therefore, the key in emergency management of these serious ascent problems is to recognize that an emergency exists and treat as soon as possible. Administer oxygen and provide rapid transport.

Any patient with suspected hypoxia following a water-related incident should be placed on a cardiac monitor and observed for arrhythmias.

Other Water Hazards

You must give close attention to the body temperature of a person who is rescued from cold water. Treat hypothermia caused by immersion in cold water the same way you treat hypothermia caused by cold exposure. Prevent further heat loss from contact with the ground, stretcher, or air, and transport the patient promptly.

A person swimming in shallow water may experience breath-holding syncope, a loss of consciousness caused by a decreased stimulus for breathing. This happens to swimmers who breathe in and out rapidly and deeply before entering the water in an effort to expand their capacity to stay underwater. While increasing the oxygen level, this hyperventilation lowers the carbon dioxide level. Because an elevated level of carbon dioxide in the blood is the strongest stimulus for breathing, the swimmer may not feel the need to breathe even after using up all the oxygen in his or her lungs. The emergency treatment for breath-holding syncope is the same as that for drowning or near drowning (Figure 26-14 ▶).

Injuries caused by boat propellers, sharp rocks, water skis, or dangerous marine life may be complicated by immersion in cold water. In these cases, remove the patient from the water, taking care to protect the spine, and administer oxygen. Apply dressings and splints if indicated, and monitor the patient closely for any signs of immersion or cold injury.

You should be aware that a child who is involved in a drowning or near drowning may be the victim of child abuse. Although it may be difficult to prove, such incidents should be handled according to laws regarding suspected child abuse.

Prevention

Appropriate precautions can prevent most immersion incidents. Each year, many small children drown in residential pools. All pools should be surrounded by a fence that is at least 6′ high, with slats no farther apart than 3″ and self-closing, self-locking gates. The most common problem is lack of adult supervision, even when attention is not given for a few seconds. Half of all teenage and adult drownings are associated with the use of alcohol. As a health care professional, you should be involved in public education efforts to make people aware of the hazards of swimming pools and water recreation.

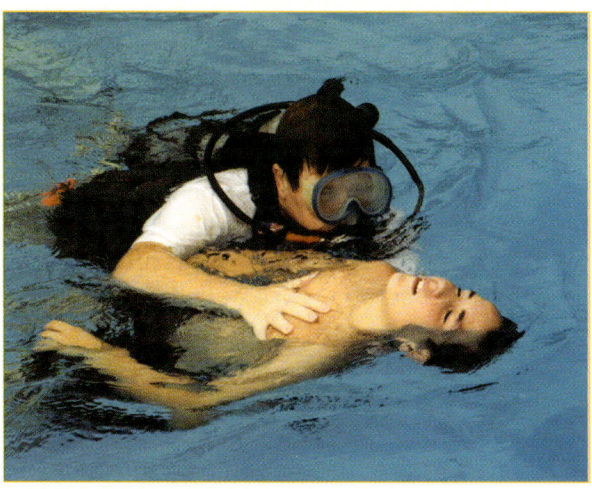

Figure 26-14 Even the best swimmer can panic and become a victim. Only properly trained personnel should attempt a rescue.

You are the Provider   Part 6

You initiate an IV line with a 16-gauge catheter and normal saline at a keep-vein-open rate and check his blood glucose level. He asks if he can sit up a little more, and you raise the head of the stretcher. He tells you that he feels slightly nauseated, so you grab an emesis bag and hand it to the patient as your partner pulls into the ambulance dock at the hospital.

Reassessment	Recording Time: 18 Minutes After Patient Contact
Level of consciousness	Alert and oriented to person, place, and time
Respirations	20 breaths/min, good air exchange
Pulse	88 beats/min, regular
Blood pressure	136/70 mm Hg
Glucose level	101 mg/dL

You turn your patient over to the nurse and give her a report including history, treatment, and response to treatment.

12. Is there anything else you could have done?

You are the Provider | Summary

1. How does heat exhaustion differ from heatstroke?

The patient with heat exhaustion, although dehydrated, maintains the ability to remove heat from the body (ie, sweating), thus preventing dangerous elevations in core body temperature. The patient with heatstroke, however, has lost the mechanisms to remove heat from the body; therefore, his or her core body temperature increases significantly, resulting in permanent brain damage or death if not promptly treated.

2. How do the patient's age and medical history affect tolerance to the temperature?

As we age, our ability to effectively regulate body temperature decreases, resulting in a lower tolerance to extremes of heat or cold. Additionally, medical problems (past or present), such as acute MI or diabetes, weaken the body to a certain degree, and may also have a negative impact on thermoregulatory function.

3. What is the probable cause of his increased respiratory rate and depth?

His core body temperature is elevated, and one of the methods of removing excess heat is through respiration.

4. What is your first consideration in treating this patient?

Remove him from the hot environment, and assess ABCs.

5. What is your next step in treating this patient?

Apply high-flow oxygen, and attempt to cool the patient while continuing to assess for any life-threatening injuries.

6. How will you obtain consent for treatment?

The patient is treated under implied consent because of his altered mental status.

7. What questions should you ask in relation to medical history?

Try to obtain a SAMPLE history if the patient is coherent enough or if bystanders are familiar. Determine if he currently has any medical problems, such as cardiac or respiratory problems or diabetes, which may be exacerbated by overheating.

8. What could be the cause of his altered mental status?

Heat exhaustion may be the most obvious, but never assume that is the only problem. Hypoglycemia, hypoxia, stroke, and seizure, are but a few conditions that may cause altered mental status.

9. What are your treatment options?

Consider the possible causes of altered mental status. Apply high-flow oxygen, and check pulse oximetry to help rule out hypoxia. Check the blood glucose level to rule out hypoglycemia. Ask the patient and bystanders who know the patient about a history of seizures or stroke. Assess the patient for hemiparesis and unequal pupils. Remember that all of this is done after assessing and treating ABCs.

10. What size IV catheter would you choose?

In case rapid fluid boluses are needed, a 14- or 16-gauge catheter should be used.

11. Which fluid will you use, and at what rate will you run it?

An isotonic crystalloid, such as normal saline, is the fluid of choice. You only want to hydrate the patient, not overload him with fluid. Because his blood pressure is adequate, it is better to run the fluid slowly and continue to oxygenate and cool the patient en route to the hospital.

12. Is there anything else you could have done?

Continually reassess your patient, and pay particular attention to any slight change in mental status. Ice packs may be placed on the oxygen or IV tubing to help with cooling. If available, humidified oxygen is another option.

Prep Kit

Ready for Review

- Cold illness can be either a local or a systemic problem. Local cold injuries include frostbite, frostnip, and immersion foot.
- Frostbite is the most serious because tissues actually freeze with this injury, causing cellular damage. All patients with a local cold injury should be removed from the cold environment and protected from further exposure.
- You can rewarm frostnipped parts, including immersion foot, with your warm hands or breath. On the other hand, you can cause further damage to a frost-bitten part by attempting to rewarm it in the field. If this is necessary because you cannot transport the patient to the hospital, immerse the part in water at a temperature between 100°F and 112°F (38°C and 44.5°C).
- Patients who are exposed to the cold can also become hypothermic. The key to treating such patients is to stabilize vital functions and prevent further heat loss. Do not attempt to rewarm patients who have moderate to severe hypothermia, because they are prone to developing arrhythmias unless handled very carefully.
- Even if you cannot find a pulse, do not consider a patient dead until he or she is "warm and dead." Local protocol will dictate whether or not such patients receive CPR or defibrillation in the field.
- The body's regulatory mechanisms normally maintain body temperature within a very narrow range around 98.6°F (37°C). The body can increase its core temperature by increasing its metabolism, for example, by shivering. In general, however, body temperature is regulated by losing heat to the atmosphere.
- Regulation of body temperature can occur via five mechanisms: conduction, convection, evaporation, radiation, and respiration. Of these, evaporation, convection, and radiation are the most important.
- The very young and the very old, as well as patients with certain diseases and medication regimens, are at increased risk of heat or cold injuries because their thermoregulatory mechanisms are not as efficient as those of other patients.
- Heat illness can take three forms: heat cramps, heat exhaustion, and heatstroke.
- Heat cramps are painful muscle spasms that occur with vigorous exercise. They usually go away if you remove the patient from the hot environment, rest the affected muscles, and replace lost fluids (by drinking a lot of water).
- Heat exhaustion, a more systemic illness, occurs when the body loses so much water and so many electrolytes that it becomes dehydrated.
- Patients with heat exhaustion may be cool and clammy, weak or faint, confused, and have a headache. The pulse is often rapid. Body temperature can be high, and the patient may or may not still be sweating. Treatment includes removing the patient, if feasible, from the heat. IV fluids are usually necessary as the patient will typically complain of nausea.
- Heat exhaustion can progress to heatstroke. This is a life-threatening emergency, usually fatal if untreated. Patients with heatstroke may or may not still be sweating, but they will usually be dry and will have high body temperatures. Changes in mental status can include coma. Rapid lowering of the body temperature in the field can save the life of a patient with heatstroke. Fanning dampened skin and placement of cold packs around the neck, armpits, and groin are key.
- Drowning and near-drowning incidents can occur even in areas that are not associated with water recreation. The first rule in caring for victims of such incidents is to be sure not to become a victim yourself. Take care to protect the spine when removing patients from the water, since spinal cord injuries, especially cervical spine injuries, are often involved in drownings. Be aware of the possibility of hypothermia, especially in cold water immersions.

Technology

- Interactivities
- Vocabulary Explorer
- Anatomy Review
- Web Links
- Online Review Manual

- While some injuries associated with scuba diving are immediately apparent, others may show up hours later. Most significant injuries occur during ascent. Patients with air embolism or decompression sickness may have pain, paralysis, or altered mental status. Be prepared to transport such patients to a recompression facility with a hyperbaric chamber.

Vital Vocabulary

air embolism Air bubbles in the blood vessels.

ambient temperature The temperature of the surrounding environment.

bends Common name for decompression sickness.

bradycardia Slow heart rate, less than 60 beats/min.

breath-holding syncope Loss of consciousness caused by a decreased breathing stimulus.

conduction The loss of heat by direct contact (for example, when a body part comes into contact with a colder object).

convection The loss of body heat caused by air movement (for example, breeze blowing across the body).

core temperature The temperature of the central part of the body (that is, the heart, lungs, and vital organs).

decompression sickness A painful condition seen in divers who ascend too quickly, in which gas, especially nitrogen, forms bubbles in blood vessels and other tissues; also called "the bends."

diving reflex Slowing of the heart rate caused by submersion in cold water; also called the mammalian diving reflex.

drowning Death from suffocation by submersion in water.

electrolytes Certain salts and other chemicals that are dissolved in body fluids and cells.

environmental emergency A medical condition caused or exacerbated by the weather, terrain, atmospheric pressure, or other local factors.

evaporation Conversion of water or another fluid from a liquid to a gas.

frostbite Damage to tissues as the result of exposure to cold; frozen body parts.

heat cramps Painful muscle spasms usually associated with vigorous activity in a hot environment.

heat exhaustion A form of heat injury in which the body loses significant amounts of fluid and electrolytes because of heavy sweating; also called heat prostration or heat collapse.

heatstroke A life-threatening condition of severe hyperthermia caused by exposure to excessive natural or artificial heat, marked by warm, dry skin; severely altered mental status; and death if untreated.

hyperbaric chamber A chamber, usually a small room, pressurized to more than atmospheric pressure.

hyperthermia A condition in which core temperature rises to 101°F (38.4°C) or more.

hypothermia A condition in which core temperature falls below 95°F (35°C) after exposure to a cold environment.

laryngospasm A severe constriction of the larynx and vocal cords.

near drowning Survival, at least temporarily, after suffocation in water.

radiation The direct loss of body heat to colder objects in the environment, or heat gain from warmer objects such as the sun.

respiration The loss of body heat as warm air in the lungs is exhaled into the atmosphere and cooler air is inhaled.

reverse triage A triage process in which efforts are focused on those who are in respiratory and cardiac arrest, and different from conventional triage where such patients would be classified as deceased. Used in triaging multiple victims of a lightning strike.

scuba A system that delivers air to the mouth and lungs at various atmospheric pressures, increasing with the depth of the dive; stands for self-contained underwater breathing apparatus.

thermogenesis The physiologic process of heat production in the body.

thermolysis The process of heat loss; methods include conduction, convection, radiation, evaporation, and respiration.

Assessment in Action

You are dispatched for a "player down" at a local basketball tournament. The temperature is near 100°F and there is little breeze. Upon arriving at the scene, the event coordinator advises you that a player "went down" after his second game. He directs you to the patient who is lying on the sidewalk in the shade.

You note that his skin is warm and very moist. He is breathing 24 breaths/min, with a pulse rate of 100 beats/min and bounding. He complains of a headache and muscle cramps, especially in his legs and abdomen. He also states he is very nauseated but has not vomited.

After moving the patient to the ambulance, you turn the air conditioner on. You place ice packs under his arms and around his neck. You then determine that IV fluids should be administered and the patient should be transported. The patient receives 100% oxygen and you gain IV access. The patient is placed on his left side and transported to the ED.

1. The two most efficient means of thermolysis are:
   A. sweating and constriction of peripheral blood vessels.
   B. sweating and dilation of peripheral blood vessels.
   C. increased heart rate and respiratory rate.
   D. decreased heart rate and respiratory rate.

2. Hyperthermia is defined as a core temperature of:
   A. 101°F or higher.
   B. 98.7°F or higher.
   C. 37°C or higher.
   D. 32°C or higher.

3. Persons at greatest risk for heat illness include:
   A. people with heart disease.
   B. people with diabetes.
   C. the elderly and young.
   D. all of the above.

4. When exertion or heat is involved, you should drink:
   A. 1 L of water per day.
   B. 2 L of water per day.
   C. 3 L of water per day.
   D. 4 L or more of water per day.

5. A patient complains of heat cramps, but denies having nausea. You should administer:
   A. Gatorade.
   B. plain water.
   C. salt tablets.
   D. electrolyte solutions.

6. If it is necessary to replace fluids by the IV route, the correct bolus amount for the adult patient is:
   A. 10 mL/kg.
   B. 20 mL/kg.
   C. 30 mL/kg.
   D. 40 mL/kg.

Points to Ponder

You are responding to a motor vehicle accident when dispatch informs you that the car left the roadway and entered a lake. First responders and a volunteer dive team are en route to the scene as well. Your response time to the scene is 30 minutes.

As you arrive at the scene, rescue divers are bringing a small child onto the bank. She is limp and lifeless in their arms. One of the first responders takes the young girl from the diver and rushes toward you, frantically screaming that she is not breathing. When you assess her, you determine that she is pulseless and apneic. Her face is cyanotic and her skin is cold to the touch.

A law enforcement officer advises that they are unable to locate the driver of the car. Your partner tells him that the child has died. You remind your partner that cold water drowning patients may be able to be resuscitated, even after prolonged submersions. BLS is started with no initial response. The patient's wet clothing is removed and she is covered with dry blankets. Medical control orders BLS care and rapid transport only until the patient is rewarmed in the ED.

On arrival at the hospital, the patient is actively rewarmed. Her pulse returns; however, she remains apneic and is placed on a ventilator. Two weeks later, she was discharged from the hospital with full neurologic function.

Why did medical control order BLS care only? Why would this small child be more likely to respond to resuscitation after a prolonged submersion than would an adult?

Issues: Understanding the Mammalian Dive Reflex, Longer Resuscitation in Hypothermic Patients

Behavioral Emergencies

1999 Objectives

Cognitive

5-9.1 Distinguish between normal and abnormal behavior. (p 1132)
5-9.2 Discuss the pathophysiology of behavioral emergencies. (p 1134)
5-9.3 Discuss appropriate measures to ensure the safety of the patient, EMT-Intermediate, and others. (p 1135)
5-9.4 Identify techniques for a physical assessment in a patient with behavioral problems. (p 1134)
5-9.5 Describe therapeutic interviewing techniques for gathering information from a patient with a behavioral emergency. (p 1136)
5-9.6 List factors that may indicate a patient is at increased risk for suicide. (p 1138)
5-9.7 Describe circumstances in which relatives, bystanders, and others should be removed from the scene. (p 1137)
5-9.8 Describe medical/legal considerations for managing a patient with a behavioral emergency. (p 1140)
5-9.9 List situations in which the EMT-Intermediate is expected to transport a patient against his will. (p 1141)
5-9.10 Describe methods of restraint that may be necessary in managing a patient with a behavioral emergency. (p 1142)
5-9.11 Formulate a field impression based on the assessment findings for patients with behavioral emergencies. (p 1138)
5-9.12 Develop a patient management plan based on the field impression for patients with behavioral emergencies. (p 1139)

Affective

5-9.13 Advocate for empathetic and respectful treatment for individuals experiencing behavioral emergencies. (p 1138)

Psychomotor

5-9.14 Demonstrate safe techniques for managing and restraining a violent patient. (p 1142)

1985 Objectives

There are no 1985 objectives for this chapter.

27

Behavioral Emergencies

You are the Provider

You are called to a scene where an 81-year-old man has assaulted his 79-year-old wife. Family members are present. The man is in the kitchen and is still displaying violent behavior. His wife is in the bedroom and presents with some discoloration to the left side of her face.

Behavioral emergencies can be very challenging calls for a variety of reasons. This chapter will give you insights into how you can safely and effectively manage these calls and will help you answer the following questions:

1. Is law enforcement always necessary at scenes for patients with a behavioral emergency?
2. What type of information obtained during the patient history might suggest to you that there is a high risk for suicide?

Behavioral Emergencies

As an EMT-I, you can expect to deal often with patients undergoing a psychological or behavioral crisis. The crisis may be due to a medical condition, mental illness, mind-altering substances, stress, and many other causes. This chapter discusses various kinds of behavioral emergencies, including those involving overdoses, violent behavior, and mental illness. You will learn how to assess a person who exhibits signs and symptoms of a behavioral emergency and what kind of emergency care may be required in these situations. The chapter also covers legal concerns in dealing with disturbed patients. Finally, it describes how to identify and manage the potentially violent patient, including the use of restraints.

Myth and Reality

Everyone experiences an emotional crisis at some point in life, some more severe than others. Perfectly healthy people may have some of the symptoms and signs of mental illness from time to time. Therefore, you should not assume that you have a mental illness when you behave in certain ways that are discussed in this chapter. For that matter, you also avoid that same assumption about a patient in any given situation.

The most common misconception about mental illness is that if you are feeling "bad" or "depressed," you must be "sick." That is simply untrue. There are many perfectly justifiable reasons for feeling depressed, including divorce, loss of a job, and the death of a relative or friend. For the teenager who just broke up with his girlfriend of 12 months, it is altogether normal to withdraw from ordinary activities and to feel "blue." This is a normal reaction to a crisis situation. However, when a person finds that Monday morning blues last until Friday, week after week, he or she may indeed have a behavioral problem.

Many people believe that all individuals with mental health disorders are dangerous, violent, or otherwise unmanageable. This is untrue. Only a small percentage of people with mental health problems fall into these categories. As an EMT-I, however, you may be exposed to a higher proportion of violent patients. After all, you are seeing people who are, by definition, considered to be having an emergency; otherwise, your assistance would not have been requested. You are there because family members or friends felt unable to manage the patient by themselves. This may be a result of the use or abuse of drugs or alcohol. It may be that the patient has a long history of mental illness and is reacting to a particularly stressful event.

While you cannot determine what has caused a person's behavioral problem, you may be able to predict that the person will become violent. The ability to predict violence is an important assessment tool for the EMT-I.

Defining Behavioral Emergencies

Behavior is what you can see of a person's response to the environment: his or her actions. Sometimes, it is obvious what a person is responding to: A person is punched, and he or she runs away or bursts into tears or hits back. Sometimes, it is less clear, as when someone is depressed for complex reasons.

Most of the time, people respond to the environment in reasonable ways. Over the years, they have learned to adapt to a variety of situations in daily life, including various stressors. This is called adjustment. There are times, however, when the stress is so great that the normal methods of adjusting do not work. When this happens, a person's behavior is likely to change, even if only temporarily. This new behavior may not be appropriate, or normal.

For a concept of normal behavior, there exists some disagreement over what is "normal." There is no clear idea or ideal model. The idea of what is normal tends to vary by cultural or ethnical groups. It is basically classified as what society accepts.

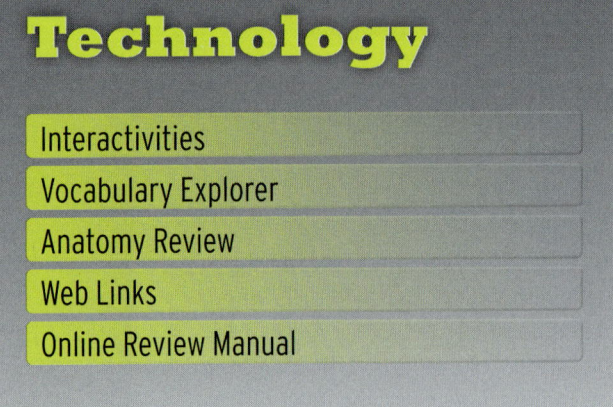

www.EMSzone.com/EMTI

- Interactivities
- Vocabulary Explorer
- Anatomy Review
- Web Links
- Online Review Manual

Abnormal or maladaptive behavior is anything that deviates from society's norms and expectations. It tends to interfere with the person's well-being and ability to function. It may also be harmful to an individual or group.

The definition of a **behavioral crisis** or emergency is any reaction to events that interferes with the **activities of daily living (ADL)** or has become unacceptable to the patient, family, or community. For example, when someone experiences an interruption of the daily routine, such as washing, dressing, and eating, chances are his or her behavior has become a problem. For that person, at that time, a behavioral emergency may exist. If the interruption of daily routine tends to recur on a regular basis, the behavior is also considered a *mental health* problem. It is then a pattern, rather than an isolated incident.

For example, a person who experiences a panic attack after having a heart attack is not necessarily mentally ill. Likewise, you would expect a person who is fired from a job to have some sort of reaction, often sadness and depression. These behavioral problems are short-term and isolated events. However, the person who reacts with a fit of rage, attacking people and property or going on a "bender" for a week, has gone beyond what society considers appropriate or normal behavior. That person is clearly undergoing a behavioral emergency. Usually, if an abnormal or disturbing pattern of behavior lasts for at least a month, it is regarded as a matter of concern from a mental health standpoint. For example, chronic **depression**, a persistent feeling of sadness and despair, may be a symptom of a mental or physical disorder. This type of long-term problem would be considered a mental health disorder.

A person who is no longer able to respond appropriately to the environment may be having what is called a psychological or psychiatric emergency. When a psychiatric emergency arises, the patient may show agitation or violence or become a threat to self or others. This is more serious than a more typical behavioral emergency that causes inappropriate behavior such as interference with ADL or intolerable actions. An immediate threat to the person involved or to others in the immediate area, including family, friends, bystanders, and EMT-Is, should be considered a psychiatric emergency. For example, a person might respond to the death of a spouse by attempting suicide. On the other hand, although this is a major life disruption, it does not have to involve violence or harm to an individual. Disruption can take many forms; not all involve violence, nor are they all psychiatric emergencies.

> **Documentation Tips**
>
> The medicolegal issues associated with responses to behavioral emergencies put added emphasis on thorough and specific documentation. Record detailed, objective findings that support the conclusion of abnormal behavior (for example, withdrawn, will not talk, crying uncontrollably), and quote the patient's own words when appropriate. ("Life isn't worth living any more." or "The voices are telling me to kill people.") Avoid subjective, judgmental statements, because these create the impression that you based your care on personal bias rather than the patient's needs.

The Magnitude of Mental Health Problems

According to the National Institutes of Mental Health, at one time or another, one in five Americans have some type of **mental disorder**, an illness with psychological

---

You are the Provider — Part 2

You and your partner discuss the options; then you approach the woman while your partner radios the dispatcher to check the arrival of law enforcement. The woman tells you that she is fine and only wants help for her husband. This has never happened before. Her vital signs are within normal limits, and she is refusing treatment.

3. Is she allowed to refuse treatment?
4. How will you determine whether she is competent to make that decision?

or behavioral symptoms that may result in impaired functioning. The mental disorder can be caused by a social, psychological, genetic, physical, chemical, or biologic disturbance.

Pathology: Causes of Behavioral Emergencies

Although sudden grief, emotional conflicts, and other psychological problems can cause behavioral emergencies, sudden illness, recent trauma, drug or alcohol intoxication, and diseases of the brain, such as Alzheimer's disease, can produce abnormal behavior as well. Likewise, altered mental status can arise from hypoglycemia, hypoxia, and exposure to excessive heat or cold. Behavioral emergencies constitute serious mental health problems and incapacitate more people than all other health problems combined. As an EMT-I, you are not responsible for diagnosing the underlying cause of a behavioral or psychiatric emergency. However, you should know the two basic categories of diagnosis a physician will use: organic (physical) and functional (psychological).

> **EMT-I Tips**
>
> You should know the two basic types of underlying causes of behavioral emergencies: organic (physical) and functional (psychological).

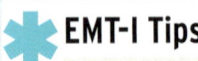 Organic brain syndrome (OBS) is a temporary or permanent dysfunction of the brain caused by a disturbance in the physical or physiologic functioning of brain tissue, such as the disturbances listed in the preceding paragraph. For example, hypoglycemia could cause organic brain syndrome. A functional disorder is one in which the etiology cannot be traced to an obvious change in the actual structure or physiology of the brain itself. Causes of organic brain syndrome may also be psychosocial, such as childhood trauma, parental deprivation, or dysfunctional family structure. They may also be sociocultural, such as environmental violence, death of a loved one, economic or employment problems, or prejudice and discrimination. Something has gone wrong, but the etiology cannot be identified definitively as brain dysfunction. Schizophrenia is a good example of a functional disorder.

These two types of disorders can look very much alike. Altered mental status, or a change in the way a person thinks or behaves, is one indicator of central nervous system disease. A patient displaying bizarre behavior may actually have an acute medical illness that is the cause, or a partial cause, of the behavior. Recognizing this possibility may allow you to save a life.

There are many misconceptions relating to mental disorders. The public tends to have the mistaken belief that abnormal behavior is always bizarre and that all patients with mental disorders and diseases are unstable and dangerous. This fallacy causes people with mental disorders to be shunned and mistrusted when many are capable of holding regular jobs and leading normal lives. There is also the misconception that mental disorders are incurable. Even though the patient may not be "cured," most disorders can be controlled with medication. Finally, many people believe that having a mental disorder is a cause for embarrassment and shame. People with a mental disorder or disease, when properly treated, are no different from those who have high blood pressure or a seizure disorder. Most are indistinguishable from any other person. Education of the public is the key to removing these doubts and fears and assisting people with mental problems to lead the most productive lives possible.

> **A to Z Terminology Tips**
>
> HTN = hypertension; Dx = diagnosis; Hx = history

Safe Approach to a Behavioral Emergency

All the regular EMT-I skills—assessment, providing care, patient approach, history-taking, and patient communication—are used in behavioral emergencies. However, other management techniques may also be necessary. It is beyond the scope of this chapter to discuss all of these techniques, but you should follow general guidelines to ensure your safety at the scene of a behavioral emergency (Table 27-1).

Assessing a Behavioral Emergency

When evaluating a situation that is considered a behavioral emergency, the first things to consider are your safety and how the patient is responding to the environment (Table 27-2). Is the situation unduly dan-

TABLE 27-1 Safety Guidelines for Behavioral Emergencies

- **Assess the scene.** If the patient is armed or has potentially harmful objects in his or her possession, have these removed by law enforcement personnel before you provide care.
- **Be prepared to spend extra time.** It may take longer to assess, listen to, and prepare the patient for transport.
- **Have a definitive plan of action.** Decide who will do what. If restraint is needed, how will it be accomplished?
- **Identify yourself calmly.** Try to gain the patient's confidence. If you begin shouting, the patient is likely to shout louder or become more excited. A low, calm voice is often a quieting influence.
- **Be direct.** State your intentions and what you expect of the patient.
- **Stay with the patient.** *Do not let the patient leave the area, and do not leave the area yourself unless law enforcement personnel can and will stay with the patient.* Otherwise, the patient may go to another room and obtain weapons, lock himself or herself in the bathroom, or take pills.
- **Encourage purposeful movement.** Help the patient get dressed and gather appropriate belongings to take to the hospital.
- **Express interest in the patient's story.** Let the patient tell you what happened or what is going on now in his or her own words. However, do not play along with auditory or visual disturbances.
- **Keep a safe distance from the patient.** Everyone needs personal space. Furthermore, you want to be sure you can move quickly if the patient becomes violent or tries to run away. Do not physically talk down to or directly confront the patient. A squatting, 45° angle approach is usually not confrontational; however, it may hinder your movements. Do not allow the patient to get between you and the exit.
- **Avoid fighting with the patient.** You do not want to get into a power struggle. Remember, the patient is not responding to you in a normal manner; he or she may be wrestling with internal forces over which neither of you has control. You and others may be stimulating these inner forces without knowing it. If you can respond with understanding to the feeling that the patient is expressing, whether this is anger, fear, or desperation, you may be able to gain his or her cooperation. If it is necessary to use force, ensure that you have adequate help and move toward the patient quietly and with assured firmness.
- **Be honest and reassuring.** If the patient asks whether he or she has to go to the hospital, the answer should be, "Yes, that is where you can receive medical help."
- **Do not judge.** You may see behavior that you dislike. Set those feelings aside, and concentrate on providing emergency medical care.

gerous to you and your partner? Do you need immediate law enforcement backup? Does the patient's behavior seem typical or normal given the circumstances? For example, a patient who has just been assaulted has good reason to be fearful of other people, including you. On the other hand, if you ask a person, "Do you know where you are?" and he or she replies, "The planet Venus" (and does not seem to be joking), you may conclude that the person is disoriented, regardless of the cause.

A behavioral crisis puts tremendous stress on a person's coping mechanisms, including natural abilities and training. The person is actually incapable of responding

You are the Provider — Part 3

Police arrive on the scene and stand by as the couple's son attempts to talk with his father. The patient agrees to talk with you and your partner. He is very agitated and will not allow you to take his vital signs.

Findings	Recording Time: 5 Minutes After Arrival on Scene
Level of consciousness	Alert, confused, very agitated
Respirations	26 breaths/min, adequate depth
Posture	Pacing, tense, clenching and unclenching fists, shouting
Medical history	Hypertension, angina, recently diagnosed with Alzheimer's disease

5. Is the patient a threat to himself? To others?
6. How will you convince him to allow you to transport him to the hospital?

TABLE 27-2	Questions to Ask When Evaluating a Behavioral Crisis
<ul><li>How does the patient respond to you?</li><li>Does the patient answer your questions appropriately?</li><li>Is the patient withdrawn or detached?</li><li>Is the patient hostile or friendly? Too friendly?</li><li>Does the patient understand why you are there?</li><li>How is the patient dressed? Is the dress appropriate for the time of year and occasion? Are the clothes clean or dirty?</li><li>Are the patient's movements coordinated or jerky and awkward? Does he or she appear to be agitated?</li><li>Are the patient's movements purposeful? Are the movements helping to accomplish a task, such as sitting down and putting on a pair of shoes, or do they appear to be aimless, such as rocking back and forth in the chair?</li><li>Has the patient harmed himself or herself? Is there damage to the surroundings?</li><li>What are the patient's facial expressions? Are they bland and flat or expressive? Does the patient show joy, fear, or anger as appropriate? To what degree?</li></ul>	<ul><li>Does the patient appear relaxed or stiff and guarded?</li><li>Are the patient's vocabulary and expressions what you would expect under the circumstances? Are they in line with the patient's social and educational background?</li><li>Is the patient easily distracted?</li><li>Are the patient's responses to what is going on around him or her appropriate?</li><li>Is the patient's memory intact? Check orientation to time, place, and person: Do you know what day/month/year it is? Do you know where you are? Do you know who I am?</li><li>Is the patient alert and able to speak logically and coherently?</li><li>What is the patient's mood? Does he or she seem agitated, elated, or abnormally depressed?</li><li>Does the patient appear fearful or worried?</li><li>Does the patient express disordered thoughts, delusions, or hallucinations? That is, does he or she appear to be seeing, hearing, or responding to people or situations that are not evident to you?</li></ul>

reasonably to the demands of the environment. This state may be temporary, as in an acute illness, or longer-lived, as in a complex, chronic mental illness. In either case, the patient's perception of reality may be compromised or distorted.

"Reflective listening" is a technique frequently used by mental health professionals to gain insight into a patient's thinking. It involves repeating back to your patient what they have said, encouraging them to expand on their thoughts. Although it often requires more time to be effective than is available in an EMS setting, it may be a helpful tool for you to use when other techniques are unsuccessful.

Sometimes a patient experiencing a behavioral or psychiatric emergency will not respond at all to your questions. In those cases, you may be able to determine a lot about the patient's emotional state from facial expressions, pulse, and respirations. Tears, sweating, and blushing may be significant indicators of state of mind. Also, make sure that you look at the patient's eyes; a patient who has a blank gaze or rapidly moving eyes may be experiencing central nervous system depression or some type of extra stress Figure 27-1 ▶.

When trying to determine the etiology of the patient's condition, you should consider four major areas as possible contributors:

- Is the patient's central nervous system functioning properly? For example, the patient may be experiencing diabetic problems, particularly hypoglycemia. He or she may have been poisoned or may be responding to physical trauma. Any of these situations could cause the patient to behave in an unusual or irrational manner.
- What is the general condition of the patient's environment? Is the patient dressed appropriately? Clean?

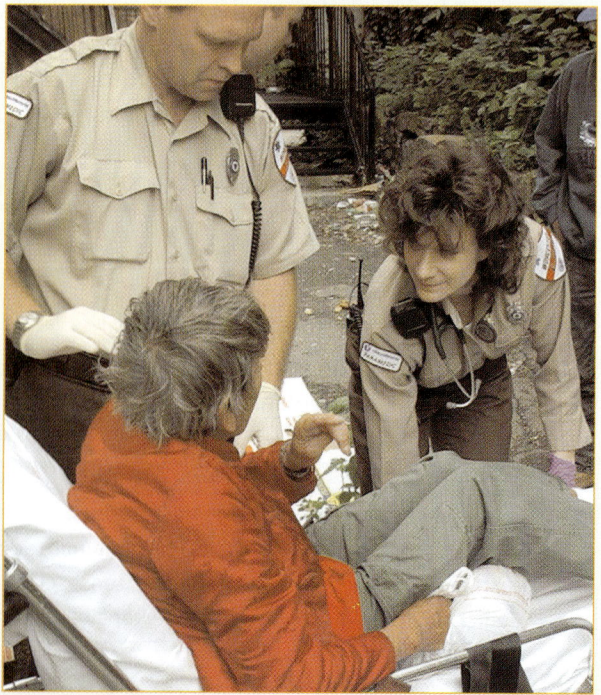

Figure 27-1 Making eye contact with a patient can provide useful clues about their emotional state.

- Is there any evidence of substance abuse? Are hallucinogens or other drugs or alcohol a factor? Does the patient see strange things? Is everything distorted? Do you smell alcohol on the patient's breath?
- Are **psychogenic** circumstances, symptoms, or illness (caused by mental rather than physical factors) involved? These might include the death of a loved one, severe depression, a history of mental illness, threats of suicide, or some other major interruption of ADL.

Family, friends, and observers may be of great help in answering these questions. Together, with your observations and interaction with the patient, they should provide enough data for you to assess the situation. This assessment has two primary goals: recognizing major threats to life and reducing the stress of the situation as much as possible.

Geriatric Needs

In an older patient, consider Alzheimer's disease and dementia as possible causes of abnormal behavior. In these cases it is essential to obtain information from relatives, friends, or extended care facility staff. Determining the patient's baseline mental status will be essential in guiding your treatment and transport decisions.

Terminology Tips

Tx = treatment

EMT-I Tips

When assessing a patient in a behavioral emergency, it can be useful to obtain information separately from a relative or caregiver. Splitting up the history-taking process in this way often yields valuable information and can help reduce the potential for violence when there is tension between the people involved.

Initial Assessment

When performing your initial assessment, it is important to limit the number of people around the patient. Remember to stay alert to potential danger. A patient in unstable condition may become violent at any time. Watch for signs of agitation or aggression.

As with any patient, the first step is to determine the presence of any life-threatening medical conditions. Perform a rapid assessment of the ABCs, and provide any

You are the Provider — Part 4

By talking quietly to the patient, you convince him to sit down and allow your partner to take his vital signs. He cannot explain his actions and denies striking his wife. He does not know his son and feels like they are all "ganging up on him."

Vital Signs	Recording Time: 12 Minutes After Patient Contact
Level of consciousness	Alert, confused, still agitated
Respirations	24 breaths/min, is 98% on room air SaO_2
Pulse	118 beats/min, strong
Blood pressure	180/110 mm Hg
Skin	Warm and dry

7. What type of treatment does this patient need?
8. What other questions might you ask the family members?

required intervention. Observe for any signs of overt behavior and give close attention to body language, such as abnormal posture or threatening gestures. While assessing mental status, note any evidence of rage, elation, hostility, depression, fear, anger, anxiety, confusion, or any other abnormal behavior. Talk to the patient as you continue your assessment, and explain all procedures that you intend to perform.

Focused History and Physical Exam

Once any life-threatening emergencies have been addressed, remove the patient from the crisis or disturbing situation. Center questions on the immediate problem to avoid confusion. Establishing a good rapport with the patient will enable you to provide better care. Use therapeutic interviewing techniques by engaging in active listening, being supportive and empathetic, limiting interruptions, and respecting the patient's personal space. Limit physical contact to minimize patient apprehension. Avoid using any threatening actions, statements, or questions, and approach slowly and purposefully.

When talking with the patient, it is important to evaluate the potential for suicide or harm to others. Factors that increase the risk include recent depression, recent loss of a family member or friend, financial setback, drug use, or evidence of a detailed plan. If the patient has gone so far as to actually establish a plan, there is a great risk of carrying it out.

Be sure to note any physical assessment findings or somatic complaints. Document the intellectual function: Is the patient oriented? Memory intact? Able to concentrate? Appropriate judgment? Does the patient have disordered thoughts, delusions, hallucinations, or unusual worries or fears or express suicidal or homicidal threats? Also note the speech pattern and content. Is the speech garbled or unintelligible? What is the patient's mood like? What about appearance and hygiene? And finally, is the patient's motor activity normal? Be sure to accurately document all findings.

Suicide

The single most significant factor that contributes to suicide is depression. Any time you encounter an emotionally depressed patient, you must consider the possibility of suicide. Risk factors for suicide are listed in Table 27-3.

TABLE 27-3 Risk Factors for Suicide

- Depression, any age
- Previous suicide attempt (Of successful suicides, 80% were preceded by at least one attempt.)
- Current expression of wanting to commit suicide or sense of hopelessness
- Family history of suicide
- Older than 40 years, particularly for single, widowed, or divorced people and people with alcoholism or depression (Men in this category who are older than 55 years have an especially high risk.)
- Recent loss of spouse, significant other, family member, or support system
- Chronic debilitating illness or recent diagnosis of serious illness
- Holidays (especially Christmas)
- Financial setback, loss of job, police arrest, imprisonment, or some sort of social embarrassment
- Substance abuse, particularly with increasing use
- Parent had alcoholism
- Severe mental illness
- Anniversary of death of loved one, job loss, divorce, or other important event
- Unusual gathering or new acquisition of things that can cause death, such as purchase of a gun, a large volume of pills, or increased use of alcohol

It is a common misconception that people who threaten suicide never commit it. This is not correct. Suicide is a cry for help. Threatening suicide is an indication that someone is in a crisis he or she cannot handle. Immediate intervention is necessary.

Whether or not the patient has any of these risk factors, you must be alert to the following warning signs:

- Does the patient have an air of tearfulness, sadness, deep despair, or hopelessness that suggests depression?
- Does the patient avoid eye contact, speak slowly or haltingly, and project a sense of vacancy, as if he or she really isn't there?
- Does the patient seem unable to talk about the future? Ask the patient whether he or she has any vacation plans. Suicidal people consider the future so uninteresting that they do not think about it; people who are seriously depressed consider the future so distant that they may not be able to think about it at all.
- Is there any suggestion of suicide? Even vague suggestions should not be taken lightly, even if presented as a joke. If you think that suicide is a possibility, do not hesitate to bring the subject

up. You will not "give the patient ideas" if you ask directly, "Are you considering suicide?"

- Does the patient have any specific plans relating to death? Has the patient recently prepared a will? Given away significant possessions or advised close friends what he or she would like done with them? Arranged for a funeral service? These are critical warning signs.

Consider also the following additional risk factors for suicide:

- Are there any unsafe objects in the patient's hands or nearby (for example, a sharp knife, glass, poisons, or a gun)?
- Is the environment unsafe (for example, an open window in a high-rise building, a patient standing on a bridge or precipice)?
- Is there evidence of self-destructive behavior (for example, partially cut wrists, large alcohol or drug intake)?
- Is there an imminent threat to the patient or others?
- Is there an underlying medical problem?

Remember, the suicidal patient may be homicidal as well. Do not jeopardize your life or the lives of your fellow EMT-Is. If you have reason to believe that you are in danger, you must obtain police intervention. In the meantime, try not to frighten the patient or make him or her suspicious.

Management Considerations

First and foremost, treat existing medical problems. Always start with the ABCs. Maintain safety for the patient and for yourself. By placing the patient on the stretcher with the straps in place, you are more in control of the situation if it turns violent. Control violent situations by restraining the patient if needed.

> **In the Field**
>
> Altered mental status may be a sign of hypoxia or hypoglycemia. Never withhold oxygen from any patient or discount its use because the patient has a history of mental problems. Check the patient's blood glucose level to rule out hypoglycemia.

Remain with the patient at all times. Avoid challenging the patient's personal space. Always ask permission before touching the patient, and explain procedures before you perform them. Remember to document only objective findings and avoid being judgmental. The patient did not ask for this problem, and it must be viewed as any other type of illness.

You are the Provider Part 5

Your partner is able to convince the patient that his blood pressure is elevated and that he needs to go to the hospital for treatment. You bring in the stretcher and allow the patient to walk over and sit without assistance, taking care to properly fasten the stretcher straps. Once the patient is loaded into the ambulance, your partner talks with him and administers oxygen while you check on his wife once more.

Reassessment	Recording Time: 17 Minutes After Patient Contact
Level of consciousness	Confused, not quite as agitated
Respirations	22 breaths/min, adequate depth
Pulse	98 beats/min, regular
Blood pressure	180/110 mm Hg
Blood glucose level	112 mg/dL

9. Who should ride in the back with the patient? Why?
10. Should you start an IV? Why or why not?
11. Should the patient be restrained?

Medicolegal Considerations

The medical and legal aspects of emergency medical care become more complicated when the patient is undergoing a behavioral or psychiatric emergency. Nevertheless, legal problems are greatly reduced when an emotionally disturbed patient consents to care. Therefore, gaining that patient's confidence is a critical task for the EMT-I.

Mental incapacity can take many forms, including unresponsiveness (as a result of hypoxia, drugs, or hypoglycemia), temporary but severe stress, or depression. Once you have determined that a patient has impaired mental capacity, you must decide whether he or she requires immediate emergency medical care. A patient in a mentally unstable condition may resist your attempts to provide care. Nevertheless, you must not leave the patient alone. Doing so may expose you to civil action for abandonment or negligence. In such situations, you should request that law enforcement personnel handle the patient. Another reason for seeking law enforcement support is that a patient who resists treatment often threatens EMT-Is and others. Violent or dangerous individuals who do not require medical care must be taken into custody by the police.

Geriatric Needs

As the population ages, you will begin to see more patients in the older-than-65 age group. In responding to an increasing number of geriatric patients, you will probably notice some behavioral or mental health problems, including depression, dementia, and delirium. These mental status changes can affect your ability to thoroughly assess and treat the ill or injured geriatric patient. Understanding the causes of altered behavior in an older patient will help you provide better patient care.

Depression is one of the more common mental status problems that you will see in the older population. While a lot of attention has been given to depression in younger adults, the media have not given much coverage to the older adult's mental health challenges. As an EMT-I, you can recognize a problem and perhaps prevent suicide in the depressed older person.

Depression has a number of causes, some organic, some psychological, and some cultural. Organic causes of depression include an emotional response to a major illness such as cancer or dementia. Furthermore, some medications can induce a feeling of depression, especially when interacting with other prescription or over-the-counter drugs. Finally, changes in the endocrine system, such as menopause, can elicit depression.

With all the possible causes of depression, an older adult can feel helpless and hopeless. A depressed person can be argumentative or placid. He or she might trivialize complaints, not wanting to be a bother to anyone. Someone who sees no way out of his or her situation may turn to suicide. Be alert for suicidal gestures and ideation, even though they may not be obvious.

While depression can create behavioral problems in older patients, dementia is another cause of abnormal behavior. The most common cause of dementia is primary progressive dementia, also known as Alzheimer's dementia. It is estimated that 10% of the population older than 65 years and 50% of the population older than 85 years have Alzheimer's dementia. Currently, there is no cure for Alzheimer's disease, and the patient's life expectancy can range from 7 to 20 years following diagnosis.

During the progression of the disease, the patient can develop openly hostile behavior and might kick, yell at, pinch, and hit you, your partner, or the caregiver. You might need to restrain the violent patient, but do so gently and only to the point at which the violent behavior stops.

Other causes of altered behavior include diabetic emergencies, heat- and cold-related illnesses, poisoning, overdose, strokes and transient ischemic attacks, and infection. It is interesting that although the mechanism is not understood, urinary tract infection or constipation can alter an older person's behavior.

As the EMT-I responding to a call for help, you should accept the possibility of depression in the older patient. Do not discount the patient's feelings or devalue his or her emotions. Be alert for suicide gestures, and pay attention to any statements about death. To obtain the patient's cooperation, you can elicit his or her help in providing care for the acute illness or injury. A smile and a touch can go a long way in alleviating fear in all of your patients, especially older patients.

Consent

When a patient is not mentally competent to grant consent for emergency medical care, the law assumes that there is implied consent. For example, the consent of an unresponsive patient is implied. The law refers to this as the emergency doctrine: consent is implied because of the necessity for immediate emergency treatment, and if the patient were conscious, he or she would consent to emergency care. In a situation that is not immediately life threatening, emergency medical care or transportation may be delayed until the proper consent is obtained. Contact medical control or follow local protocols when in doubt.

In cases involving psychiatric emergencies, however, the matter is not always clear-cut. Does a life-threatening emergency exist or not? If you are not sure, you should request the assistance of law enforcement personnel.

Limited Legal Authority

As an EMT-I, you have limited legal authority to require or force a patient to undergo emergency medical care when no life-threatening emergency exists. Patients have the right to refuse care. However, most states have legal statutes regarding the emergency care of mentally ill and drug-impaired people. These statutory provisions permit law enforcement personnel to place such a person in protective custody so that emergency care can be given. Medical direction may also order transport of a patient against his or her will. You should be familiar with your local and state laws regarding these situations.

The typical provision states that "any police officer who has reasonable cause to believe that a person is mentally ill and dangerous to himself, herself, or others or gravely disabled, may take such person into custody and take or cause such person to be taken to a general hospital for emergency examination…" Again, because these provisions vary, you should become familiar with those in your state.

The general rule of law is that a competent adult has the right to refuse treatment, even if lifesaving care is involved. In psychiatric cases, however, a court of law would probably consider your actions in providing lifesaving care to be appropriate, particularly if you have a reasonable belief that the patient would harm himself, herself, or others without your intervention. Additionally, a patient who is in any way impaired, whether by mental illness, medical condition, or intoxication, may not be considered competent to refuse treatment or transportation. These situations are among the most perilous you will encounter from a legal standpoint. When in doubt, consult your supervisor, police, or medical control. Always maintain a pessimistic attitude toward your patients' condition—assume the worst and hope for the best. Err on the side of treatment and transport. It is far easier to defend yourself against charges of battery than it is to justify abandonment.

> **EMT-I Tips**
>
> When a patient is not mentally competent to grant consent for emergency medical care, the law assumes that there is implied consent.

Restraint

Ordinarily, restraint of a person must be ordered by a physician, a court order, or a law enforcement officer. If you restrain a person without authority in a nonemergency situation, you expose yourself to a possible lawsuit, as well as to personal danger. Legal actions against the EMT-I can involve charges of assault, battery, false imprisonment, and violation of civil rights. You may use restraints only to protect yourself or others from bodily harm or to prevent the patient from causing injury to himself or herself . In either case, you may use only reasonable force as necessary to control the patient, something that different courts may define differently. For this reason, you should always

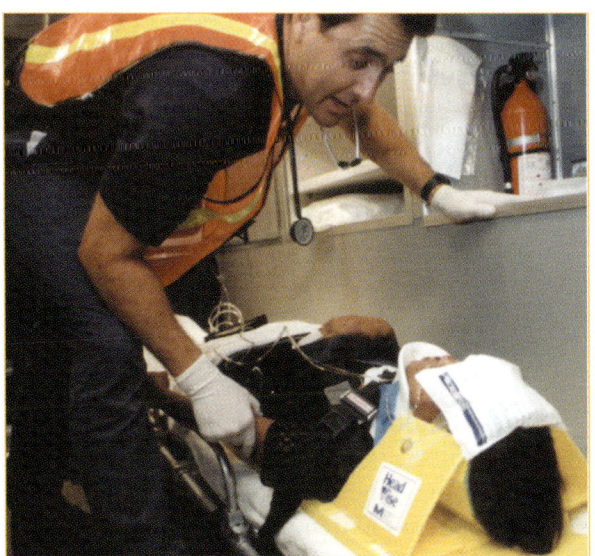

Figure 27-2 You may use restraints only to protect yourself or others or to prevent a patient from causing injury to himself or herself.

consult medical control and contact law enforcement for help before restraining a patient.

In fact, you should routinely involve law enforcement personnel if you are called to assist a patient in a severe behavioral or psychiatric crisis. They will provide physical backup in managing the patient, can serve as the necessary witness, and will provide legal authority should physical restraint become necessary. A patient who is restrained by law enforcement personnel is in their custody.

Always try to transport a disturbed patient without restraints if possible. Once the decision has been made to restrain a patient, however, you should carry it out quickly. Be aware of body substance isolation precautions. If the patient is spitting, place a surgical mask over his or her mouth and over your own and your partner's.

Make sure you have adequate help to restrain a patient safely. **At least four people should be present to carry out the restraint**, each being responsible for one extremity. Before you begin, discuss the plan of action. As you prepare to restrain the patient, stay outside the patient's range of motion.

> **In the Field**
>
> If you do not have four people to restrain a violent patient, you should call the dispatcher and request additional assistance.

When subduing a violent patient, use the minimum force necessary. You should avoid acts or physical force that may cause injury to the patient. The level of force will vary depending on the following factors:

- The degree of force that is necessary to keep the patient from injuring himself or herself, or others
- A patient's gender, size, strength, and mental status
- The type of abnormal behavior the patient is exhibiting. You should use only restraint devices that have been approved by your state's health department for this purpose; soft, wide leather or cloth restraints are preferred over police-type handcuffs.

Acting at the same time, the police officers should secure the patient's extremities with approved equipment. Somebody, preferably you or your partner, should continue to talk to the patient throughout the process. Remember to treat the patient with dignity and respect at all times. Also, monitor the patient for vomiting, airway obstruction, and cardiovascular stability, because the patient cannot fend for himself or herself. Drug or alcohol intoxication may cause violent behavior but then lead to physical problems such as vomiting or aspiration as well. Never place your patient face down because it is impossible to adequately monitor the patient and may inhibit the breathing of an impaired or exhausted patient. Be careful not to place restraints in such a way that that respiration is compromised. Reassess airway and breathing continuously. You should make frequent checks of circulation on all restrained extremities, regardless of patient position (Figure 27-3). Document the reason for the restraint and the technique that was used. Be especially careful if a combative patient suddenly becomes calm and cooperative. This is not the time to relax but to secure the situation. The patient may suddenly become combative again and injure someone. Keep in mind that you may use reasonable force to defend yourself against an attack by an emotionally disturbed patient. It is extremely helpful to have (and document) witnesses in attendance, even during transport, to protect against false accusations. EMT-Is have been accused of sexual misconduct and other physical abuse in such circumstances.

> **Documentation Tips**
>
> After restraining a patient, document the reason for doing so and the method you used. Check pulse and motor and sensory function in all extremities, make any adjustments needed to ensure adequate function, and record your actions and findings in detail.

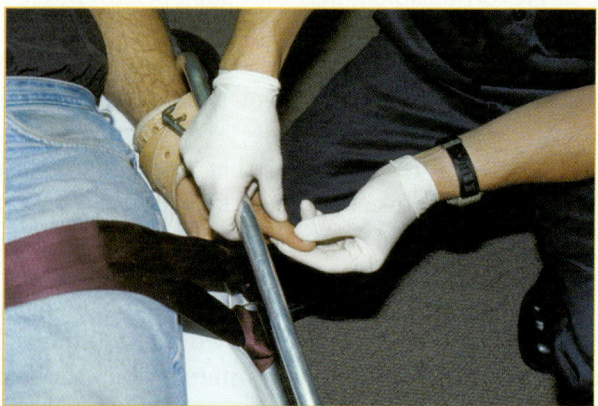

Figure 27-3 Assess airway and circulation frequently while the patient is restrained.

The Potentially Violent Patient

Violent patients make up only a small percentage of those undergoing a behavioral or psychiatric crisis. However, the potential for violence by such a patient is always an important consideration for the EMT-I. Although a large body size may be intimidating, there is no correlation between the size of the patient and the potential for violence.

Use the following list of risk factors to assess the level of danger:

- **History.** Has the patient previously exhibited hostile, overly aggressive, or violent behavior? Ask people at the scene, or request this information from law enforcement personnel or family.
- **Posture.** How is the patient sitting or standing? Is the patient tense, rigid, or sitting on the edge of his or her seat? Such physical tension is often a warning signal of impending hostility.
- **The scene.** Is the patient holding or near potentially lethal objects such as a knife, gun, glass, poker, or bat (or near a window or glass door)?
- **Vocal activity.** What kind of speech is the patient using? Loud, obscene, erratic, and bizarre speech patterns usually indicate emotional distress. Someone using quiet, ordered speech is not as likely to strike out as someone who is yelling and screaming. However, do not discount the possibility of violent behavior in the quiet patient.
- **Physical activity.** The motor activity of a person undergoing a psychiatric crisis may be the most telling factor of all. The patient who has tense muscles, clenched fists, or glaring eyes; is pacing; cannot sit still; or is fiercely protecting personal space requires careful watching. Agitation may predict a quick escalation to violence.

Other factors to consider in assessing a patient's potential for violence include the following:

- Poor impulse control
- A history of truancy, fighting, and uncontrollable temper
- Low socioeconomic status, unstable family structure, or inability to keep a steady job
- Tattoos, especially those with gang identification or statements such as "Born to Kill" or "Born to Lose"
- Substance abuse
- Depression, which accounts for 20% of violent attacks
- Functional disorder (If the patient says that voices are telling him or her to kill, believe it.)

You are the Provider — Part 6

Your partner is able to maintain a pleasant conversation with the patient en route to the hospital. The patient is calm when you transfer him to the emergency department staff.

Reassessment	Recording Time: 24 Minutes After Patient Contact
Level of consciousness	Confused but calm
Respirations	20 breaths/min, adequate depth
Pulse	84 beats/min, regular
Blood pressure	180/102 mm Hg
Skin	Warm and dry

12. What could you and your partner do to help prevent the patient from becoming agitated again when transferring his care to the emergency department staff?

You are the Provider

1. Is law enforcement always necessary at scenes for patients with altered mental status?

You must ensure that any scene is safe prior to entering—not just scenes involving patients with an altered mental status. Although there are numerous causes of an altered mental status besides a behavioral emergency, it would be prudent to have law enforcement present, if possible. Follow local protocols regarding related issues.

2. What type of information obtained during the patient history might suggest to you that there is a high risk for suicide?

It should be noted that many people commit suicide without exhibiting any warning signs. However, when you are obtaining a history from the patient or family member of the patient, signs that suggest a high risk for suicide include, among others, severe depression, loss of a job, marital discord, death of a loved one, financial difficulties, recent acquisition of a weapon, recent diagnosis of a serious illness, or the giving away of personal possessions.

3. Is she allowed to refuse treatment?

Yes. As long as she is mentally competent she may refuse care.

4. How will you determine whether she is competent to make that decision?

Thoroughly questioning the patient can determine her mental status. She should be alert to person, place, time, and event.

5. Is the patient a threat to himself? Others?

He is a potential threat to himself and others because of his agitation and altered mental status. A patient who is confused is not easy to reason with and may react with violence.

6. How will you convince him to allow you to transport him to the hospital?

He cannot legally refuse transport, but it would be much easier to talk him into it and have him go willingly. He might go more willingly if you convince him he needs to be transported for a reason other than a mental disorder.

7. What type of treatment does this patient need?

If he is taking medication, it might not be serving its purpose and the dosage may need to be evaluated or he may need another type of medication. His blood pressure is high and needs to be treated. He also needs a current mental evaluation.

8. What other questions might you ask of family members?

You may ask the following questions to evaluate a behavioral crisis:

- How does the patient respond to you?
- Does the patient answer your questions appropriately?
- Is the patient withdrawn or detached?
- Is the patient hostile or friendly? Too friendly?
- Does the patient understand why you are there?
- How is the patient dressed? Is the dress appropriate for the time of year and occasion? Are the clothes clean or dirty?
- Are the patient's movements coordinated or jerky and awkward? Does he or she appear to be agitated?
- Are the patient's movements purposeful? Are the movements helping to accomplish a task, such as sitting down

Summary

and putting on a pair of shoes, or do they appear to be aimless, such as rocking back and forth in the chair?
- Has the patient harmed himself or herself? Is there damage to the surroundings?
- What are the patient's facial expressions? Are they bland and flat or expressive?
- Does the patient show joy, fear, or anger as appropriate? To what degree?
- Does the patient appear relaxed or stiff and guarded?
- Are the patient's vocabulary and expressions what you would expect under the circumstances? Are they in line with the patient's social and educational background?
- Is the patient easily distracted?
- Are the patient's responses to what is going on around him or her appropriate?
- Is the patient's memory intact? Check orientation to time, place, and person: Do you know what day/month/year it is? Do you know where you are? Do you know who I am?
- Is the patient alert and able to speak logically and coherently?
- What is the patient's mood? Does he or she seem agitated, elated, or abnormally depressed?
- Does the patient appear fearful or worried?
- Does the patient express disordered thoughts, delusions, or hallucinations? That is, does he or she appear to be seeing, hearing, or responding to people or situations that are not evident to you?

9. Who should ride in the back with the patient? Why?

Your partner, because he has already established a good rapport with the patient.

10. Should you start an IV? Why or why not?

The patient is not in need of fluid, and you cannot give drugs; therefore, starting an IV would probably only further agitate him. The patient's stable hemodynamic status does not warrant an IV.

11. Should the patient be restrained?

As long as he is cooperative and calm, there is no need to restrain him at this point. However, you should make sure that all of the stretcher straps are firmly in place and be alert to any slight change of behavior or attitude.

12. What could you and your partner do to help prevent the patient from becoming agitated again when transferring his care to the emergency department staff?

Continue to communicate with the patient and constantly reassure him. It would also help to keep him in a secluded area. Introducing the patient and giving a thorough report to the staff will eliminate the need for the patient to answer the same questions repeatedly, which would further increase his agitation.

Prep Kit

Ready for Review

- Behavioral emergencies can present the EMT-I with great difficulties in patient management. Your major responsibility in these situations is to defuse potentially life-threatening incidents and reduce the impact of the stressful condition without exposing yourself to unnecessary risks.

- While only a small percentage of people with mental health disorders are dangerous to themselves or others, you may be exposed to a higher proportion of violent situations in your daily activities. There are a number of warning signs of violence, including a history of hostile behavior, rigidity, loud and erratic speech patterns, agitation, and depression.

- A behavioral emergency is any reaction to events that interferes with the ADL. A person who is no longer able to respond appropriately to the environment may be having a more serious psychiatric emergency. Not all behavioral emergencies involve a mental health problem, however. Some emergencies are a temporary response to a traumatic event.

- Underlying causes of behavioral emergencies fall into two categories: organic and functional disorders.

- Assessing a person who may be having a behavioral crisis involves observing the person, talking with the person, and talking with friends, family members, and witnesses to the person's behavior. You are looking for indications that the person's thoughts, feelings, and reactions are inappropriate for the circumstances. Remember to always assess ABCs.

- Consider contributing factors in four areas: central nervous system dysfunction, environmental factors or clues, drug or alcohol use, and psychogenic circumstances such as the death of a loved one or other major interruption of normal life.

- The threat of suicide requires immediate intervention. Depression is the most significant risk factor for suicide. Others include personal or family history of suicide attempts, chronic debilitating illness, financial setback, and severe mental illness.

- As an EMT-I, you have limited legal authority to require a patient to undergo emergency medical care in the absence of a life-threatening emergency. Most states have provisions allowing law enforcement personnel to place mentally impaired persons in custody so that such care can be provided. You should always involve law enforcement personnel any time you are called to assist a patient with a severe behavioral or psychiatric crisis.

- Always consult medical control and contact law enforcement for help before restraining a patient. If there is an immediate threat, leave the area until law enforcement secures the scene. If restraints are required, use the minimum force necessary. Assess the airway and circulation frequently while the patient is restrained, and maintain a constant dialogue with the patient throughout the restraining process.

- In providing emergency medical care for a patient having a behavioral emergency, be direct, honest, and calm; have a definitive plan of action; stay with the patient at all times, but do not get too close; express interest in the patient's story, but do not judge his or her behavior. Always treat patients with respect.

Technology

- Interactivities
- Vocabulary Explorer
- Anatomy Review
- Web Links
- Online Review Manual

Vital Vocabulary

activities of daily living (ADL) The basic activities a person usually accomplishes during a normal day, such as eating, dressing, and washing.

altered mental status A change in the way a person thinks and behaves that may signal disease in the central nervous system or other contributing factors.

behavior How a person functions or acts in response to his or her environment.

behavioral crisis The point at which a person's reactions to events interfere with activities of daily living; a behavioral crisis becomes a psychiatric emergency when it causes a major life interruption, such as attempted suicide.

depression A persistent mood of sadness, despair, and discouragement; depression may be a symptom of many different mental and physical disorders, or it may be a disorder in and of itself.

functional disorder A disorder in which there is no known physiologic reason for the abnormal functioning of an organ or organ system.

mental disorder An illness with psychological or behavioral symptoms and/or impairment in functioning, caused by a social, psychological, genetic, physical, chemical, or biologic disturbance.

organic brain syndrome (OBS) Temporary or permanent dysfunction of the brain, caused by a disturbance in the physical or physiologic functioning of brain tissue.

psychogenic A symptom or illness that is caused by mental factors as opposed to physical ones.

Assessment in Action

You are dispatched to the home of a 57-year-old man who is threatening suicide. The police are at the scene and advise you that it is safe to enter. When you arrive, you find the patient pacing in the living room. He is agitated and shouting about losing his job. He repeatedly yells, "I am a loser." As you introduce yourself, the patient does not acknowledge you. He continues to pace while clenching his fists and grinding his teeth.

Your partner talks with his wife in the kitchen. She tells you that her husband has been like this all morning. She says he has recently lost his job and he is concerned about the bills that are due. She also tells you that he purchased a gun last week and that it is in the bedroom.

You continue to talk to the patient, who seems to have calmed down slightly. He tells you he has a pounding headache and allows you to take his vital signs. You explain to him the need for EMS transport and evaluation at the hospital. He agrees to transport but tells you he wants to get his jacket from the bedroom. You do not allow him to go to the bedroom but instead ask his wife to retrieve the jacket.

The patient is placed on the stretcher and the straps are secure. He remains calm and cooperative. You transport him without further incident to the ED where he receives counseling and treatment for depression and suicidal ideation.

1. When the patient does not acknowledge your introduction, you should:
   A. shout your name loudly to be sure he knows who you are.
   B. step closer to him and repeat your name.
   C. calmly continue to talk to him.
   D. place your hand on his shoulder.

2. Risk factors for suicide include all of the following EXCEPT:
   A. financial gain.
   B. depression.
   C. debilitating illness.
   D. marital discord.

3. The two basic types of underlying causes of behavioral emergencies are:
   A. social and economic.
   B. organic and functional.
   C. functional and social.
   D. economic and functional.

4. Organic brain syndrome (OBS) may be a permanent or temporary dysfunction of the brain. Causes of OBS include:
   A. childhood trauma.
   B. parental deprivation.
   C. hypoglycemia.
   D. all of the above.

5. If you determine that it is necessary to restrain a patient, you should:
   A. move slowly to avoid upsetting the patient.
   B. place the patient in handcuffs.
   C. ensure the presence of at least 2 people.
   D. ensure the presence of at least 4 people.

6. Once you have restrained a violent patient, you must:
   A. document the reason for doing so and the method used.
   B. assess sensory and motor function in all extremities.
   C. monitor the patient's airway and breathing status.
   D. all of the above.

Points to Ponder

You are called to a local nursing home for a resident who is "out of control." You find an older man sitting in a chair. The staff reports that while trying to get him to go to the dining room, he became verbally abusive. They continued to insist on moving him and he struck an aide with his cane. He is now swinging the cane in the air and shouting for everyone to leave him alone.

As you approach the patient, you speak slowly and calmly. You stay far enough away so that he cannot strike you with the cane. The patient responds to you in a normal tone, but still insists that he wants to be left alone. He tells you he is not hungry and does not want to go to the dining room. Slowly, you move closer to him and ask him to give you his cane. As soon as he hands the cane to you, a staff member shouts at him and moves closer to him. Your partner stops the aide and takes him aside to calm him down. The patient begins to cry and states that he doesn't want to hurt anyone.

You assess the patient's vital signs and find them to be within normal limits. You explain to the patient that he should go to the hospital for evaluation. He agrees to transport and is placed on the stretcher and secured with straps. You determine that additional restraints are not necessary. During transport, the patient remains calm and carries on pleasant conversation.

Issues: Organic Causes of Behavioral Emergencies in Older Persons, Approaching a Patient Experiencing a Behavioral Emergency, Using Restraints When Dealing With a Behavioral Emergency

Gynecologic Emergencies

1999 Objectives

Cognitive

5-10.1 Review the anatomic structures and physiology of the female reproductive system. (p 1152)

5-10.2 Describe how to assess a patient with a gynecological complaint. (p 1154)

5-10.3 Explain how to recognize a gynecological emergency. (p 1154)

5-10.4 Describe the general care for any patient experiencing a gynecological emergency. (p 1156)

5-10.5 Describe the pathophysiology, assessment, and management of specific gynecological emergencies, including:
   a. Pelvic inflammatory disease
   b. Ruptured ovarian cyst
   c. Ectopic pregnancy
   d. Vaginal bleeding (p 1157, 1158)

5-10.6 Describe the general findings and management of the sexually assaulted patient. (p 1159)

Affective

5-10.7 Value the importance of maintaining a patient's modesty and privacy while still obtaining necessary information. (p 1155)

5-10.8 Defend the need to provide care for a patient of sexual assault, while still preventing destruction of crime scene information. (p 1159)

5-10.9 Serve as a role model for other EMS providers when discussing or caring for patients with gynecological emergencies. (p 1156)

Psychomotor

5-10.10 Demonstrate how to assess a patient with a gynecological complaint. (p 1156)

5-10.11 Demonstrate how to provide care for a patient with:
   a. Excessive vaginal bleeding
   b. Abdominal pain
   c. Sexual assault (p 1156, 1157, 1159, 1160)

1985 Objectives

There are no 1985 objectives for this chapter.

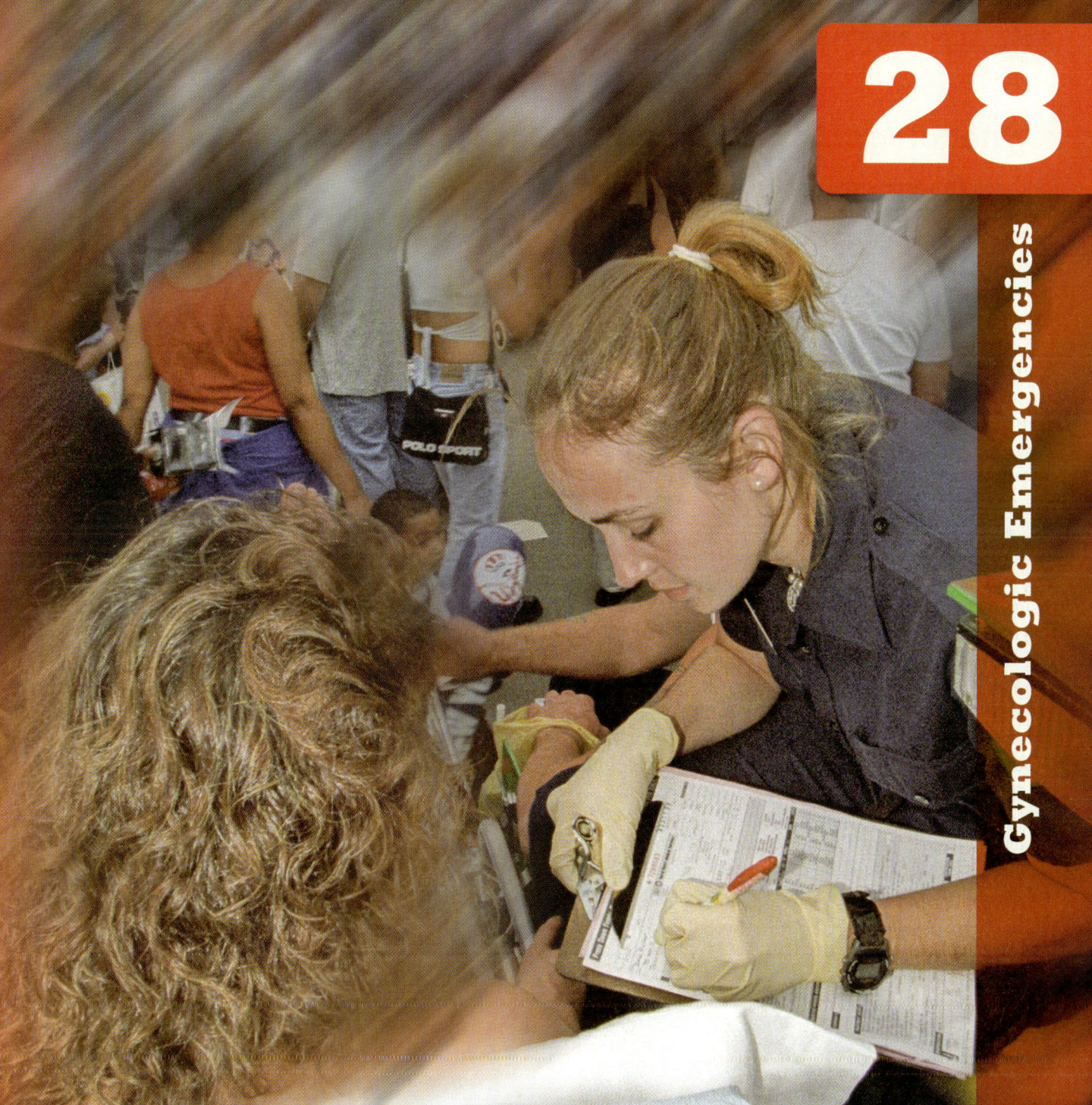

28

Gynecologic Emergencies

You are the Provider

You are dispatched for an unknown medical emergency. Upon arrival you find a 24-year-old woman complaining of the sudden onset of severe abdominal pain. She denies being pregnant and is not able to stand up straight. This chapter will help the EMT-I handle those sensitive calls involving gynecologic emergencies and answer the following questions:

1. What types of gynecologic emergencies may be encountered by the EMT-I?
2. What is the importance of acquiring a detailed history of this patient?

Gynecologic Emergencies

Occasionally, women who are in their childbearing years will have major gynecologic problems requiring urgent medical care. These include excessive bleeding and soft-tissue injuries to the external genitalia. These genital parts have a rich nerve supply, making such injuries very painful.

Disorders in the female reproductive system can also lead to gynecologic emergencies. These disorders include acute or chronic infection, hemorrhage, rupture of a cyst, and rupture of an ectopic pregnancy. Some conditions can be life-threatening without prompt intervention. The reproductive system is very vascular, and the potential for bleeding is great.

Treat lacerations, abrasions, and tears with moist, sterile compresses, using local pressure to control bleeding and a diaper-type bandage to hold the dressings in place. Leave any foreign bodies in place after stabilizing them with bandages. Because the origin of the bleeding is in an area that you cannot directly control, never pack or place dressings in the vagina, as they will only have to be removed in the emergency department. Continue to assess the patient while transporting her to the emergency department. Contusions and other blunt trauma will require careful in-hospital evaluation.

Although you might not know the exact cause of a gynecologic emergency, you should treat the patient as you would any other victim of blood loss: Observe body substance isolation (BSI) precautions, ensure maintenance of the airway, give oxygen, take and document vital signs, and treat for shock while arranging for prompt transport.

This chapter will help you learn how to make the decision of whether a life-threatening emergency exists and how to determine the need for proper prehospital intervention and transport. Finally, the chapter discusses gynecologic emergencies unrelated to childbirth.

Anatomy of the Female Reproductive System

The visible external female genitalia is known as the vulva. It is composed of the mons pubis (the pad of fatty tissue and coarse skin that lies over the pubic symphysis), the labia majora (the outer lip-shaped structure) and labia minora (the inner lip-shaped structure), the clitoris (the small erectile body partially hidden by the labia minora) that is covered by the prepuce or foreskin, the vestibule (small space at the beginning) of the vagina and its glands, the opening of the urethra (canal for the discharge of urine extending from the bladder to the outside of the body), and of the vaginal orifice (opening of the vagina). The hymen is a fold of mucous membrane that partially covers the entrance to the vagina. Contrary to popular belief, presence or absence of the hymen does not denote virginity. Pregnancy has occurred with the hymen intact. The perineum, or pelvic floor, lies between the vulva and the anus (the outlet of the rectum) Figure 28-1 ▶.

The vagina is the outermost cavity of a woman's reproductive system and forms the lower part of the birth canal. It is about 8 to 12 cm long, begins at the cervix (the neck of the uterus) and ends as an external opening of the body. Essentially, the vagina completes the passageway from the uterus to the outside world for the delivering infant. The cervical canal is the passageway from the uterus to the opening into the vagina. The uterus, or womb, is the muscular organ where the fetus grows. It is responsible for contractions during labor and ultimately helps push the infant through the birth canal. The uterus is made up of the fundus (the uppermost part of the uterus; farthest from the cervical opening), body (the principal mass of the uterus), uterine cavity (the space within the uterus), the endometrium (the inner layer of the uterine wall), and the myometrium (the muscular wall of the uterus).

The fallopian tubes, or uterine tubes, are tubes or ducts that extend from the uterus and terminate near the ovary on each side. Their purpose is to carry a mature egg, or ovum, from the ovary to the uterus and spermatozoa from the uterus toward the ovary. The female sex cell is known as an oocyte and is released by the ovaries. The ovaries are almond-shaped bodies that lie

Technology

- Interactivities
- Vocabulary Explorer
- Anatomy Review
- Web Links
- Online Review Manual

www.EMSzone.com/EMTI

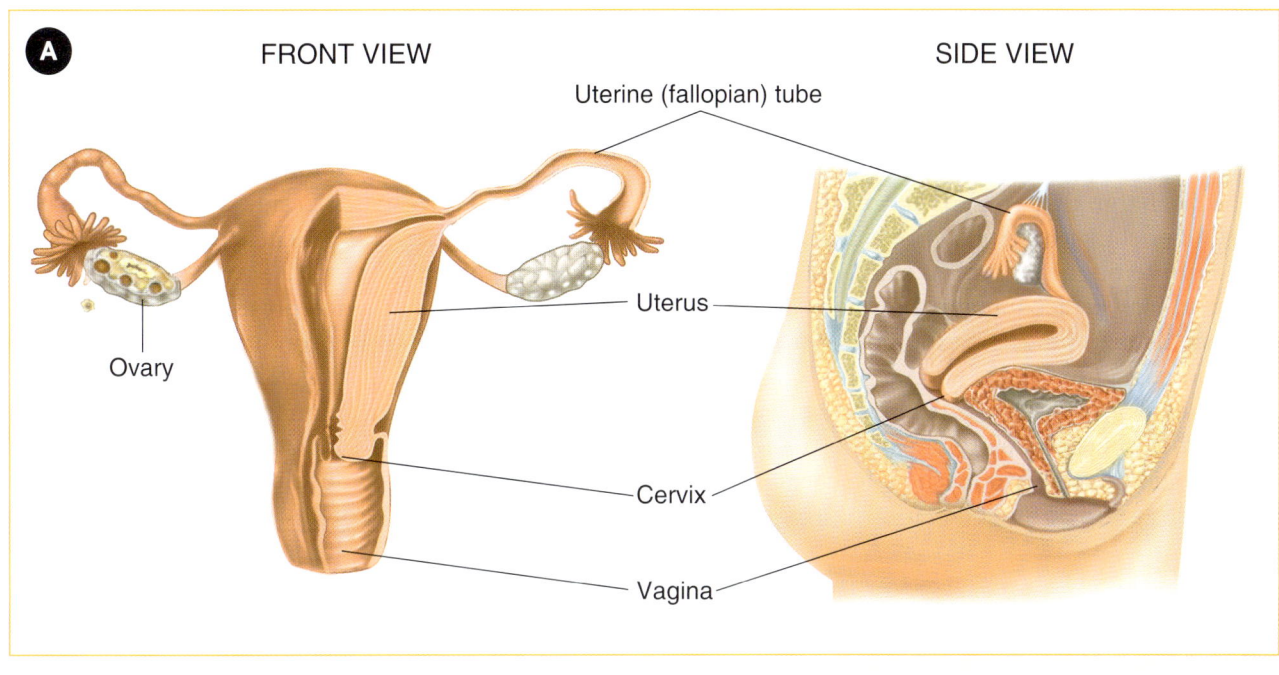
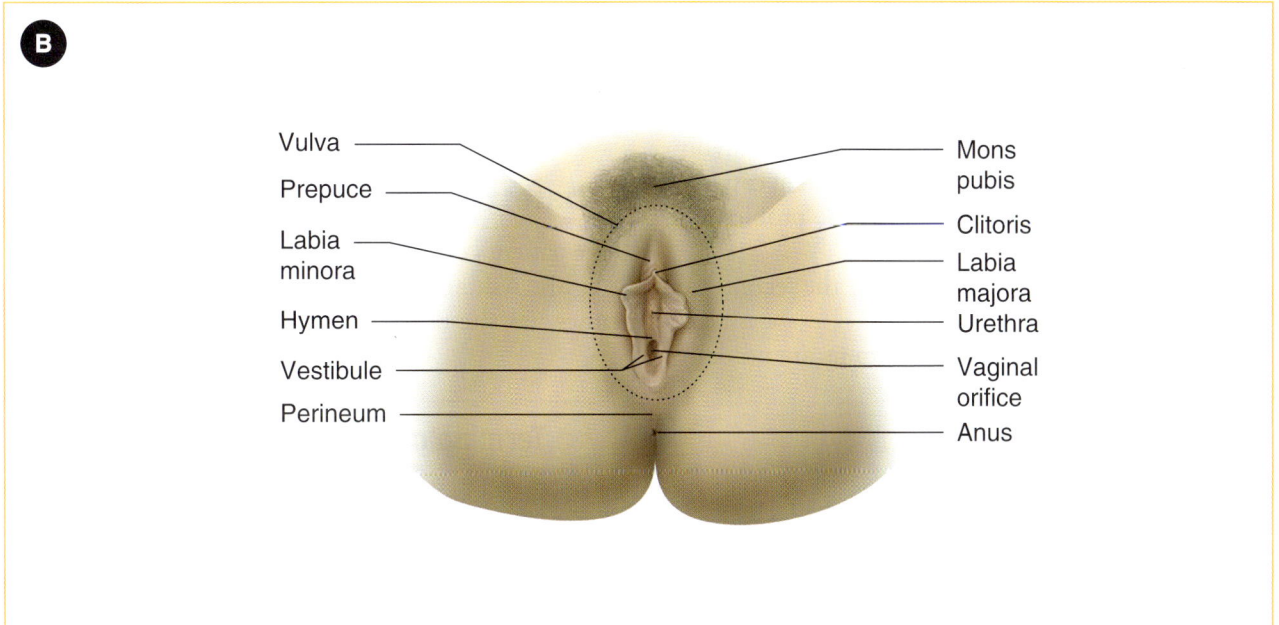

Figure 28-1 The anatomy of the female reproductive system. **A.** Front and side views. **B.** External genitalia.

on either side of the pelvic cavity. The two functions of the ovaries are to produce ova (mature oocytes) and the hormones estrogen and progesterone. These hormones are secreted by the corpus luteum, a small yellow endocrine structure that develops within a ruptured ovarian follicle (sac), and are responsible for development and maintenance of secondary sexual characteristics, preparation of the uterus for pregnancy, and development of the mammary glands.

Normal Physiology

Each month as the level of hormones rise in the female, certain characteristic changes take place. The hormones stimulate the development of the eggs in the ovaries, and cause the endometrium of the uterus to thicken in anticipation of implantation of a fertilized egg. The egg (ovum) is released from the ovary following the breaking of a follicle. This occurs around

14 days after the beginning of the menstrual cycle. If an egg is fertilized and implants in the uterus, menses is usually suspended until such time as the pregnancy ends. If no fertilized egg implants, menstruation begins. Menstruation is the cyclic shedding of the uterine lining that occurs approximately every 28 days. It is a normal discharge that is made up of blood, mucus, and cellular debris from the uterine mucosa. The flow averages 25 to 60 mL. A typical cycle lasts from 4 to 6 days and may be accompanied by signs and symptoms such as cramping, bloating, breast tenderness, and mood changes.

The initial onset of menstruation, known as menarche, occurs during puberty. Menopause is the cessation of menstruation and ovarian function. It generally occurs between the ages of 35 and 60 years. The average age is the late 40s.

General Assessment

When assessing a patient with a possible gynecologic emergency, it is essential to obtain a detailed history of the present illness. Gynecologic emergencies often have the same signs and symptoms as emergencies involving other abdominal organs. Assess the patient carefully to determine the nature and extent of the problem. Be sure to include the following:

- SAMPLE—Remember to include the second part of the "L," last menstrual cycle
- What, if any, associated symptoms are noted:
  - Fever?
  - Diaphoresis?
  - Syncope?
  - Diarrhea?
  - Constipation?
  - Urinary cramping?

The nature and location of pain may also give clues to the origin of the problem. Is the pain localized or diffuse? Is it constant, or does it come and go? Is there any radiation or referred pain? Rebound tenderness? Remember to ask specifically:

- Describe any pain or discomfort.
  - OPQRST?
  - Abdominal pain?
  - Dysmenorrhea (painful menstruation)?
- Are there any aggravating factors?
  - Ambulation?
  - Dyspareunia (pain during sexual intercourse)?
  - Defecation?
- Alleviating factors?
  - Positioning?
  - Ceasing activity?

Other medical problems may present as an abdominal problem. Cardiac pain may be misinterpreted as epigastric pain. Other conditions may also exacerbate gynecologic emergencies. Besides obtaining a SAMPLE history, be sure to ask the patient about previous episodes of this type of problem.

- What is the patient's present health?
  - Any preexisting conditions?
  - Any previous surgeries?

Once the determination is made that the problem is gynecologic, questions should be aimed at signs and symptoms and gynecologic history. Focus your questioning on the patient's normal menstrual cycle, any changes, any discharge, irritation, or trauma. Note any changes in the menstrual cycle, and consider the possibility of pregnancy in any female of childbearing age. If there is any discharge, does it have an odor? What is the consistency? Address any trauma. Consider the mechanism of injury and the need for law enforcement, especially if sexual assault has occurred.

Obstetric History

The patient's obstetric history should be addressed thoroughly. Ask about previous pregnancies. How many times has she been pregnant? How many pregnancies

> **A to Z Terminology Tips**
>
> Gravida = number of pregnancies; para = number of pregnancies carried to term; abortus = fetus that weighs less than 500 g or is younger than 20 weeks' gestation; abortion = termination of pregnancy before the fetus is able to survive (a spontaneous abortion is called a miscarriage)

> **Documentation Tips**
>
> Suppose your patient is pregnant and has had two previous children with no miscarriages. It can be documented on the patient care report as G3, P2, A0.

have been carried to full term resulting in live birth? How many miscarriages or clinical abortions?

Ask whether the patient has ever had an ectopic pregnancy. If so, how far along was the pregnancy? Has she ever has a cesarean section? A patient with a history of an obstetric problem tends to be more susceptible to repetitive problems.

When was the patient's last menstrual cycle? How long did it last? Was it normal in duration and amount of flow? Ask the patient about any bleeding between periods (breakthrough bleeding). A patient who has a regular menstrual cycle is more likely to recognize a problem than one who has an irregular cycle. Determine regularity and how this occurrence differs from usual.

Consider the possibility of pregnancy in any woman of childbearing age even if contraception has been used. Remember that some women will continue to have menstrual cycles even though they are pregnant. The flow tends to be lighter and may only be "spotting." Therefore, the presence of bleeding does not rule out pregnancy. Ask the patient about a missed or late period. Is there any breast tenderness? Has the patient noticed a need to urinate frequently without an increased fluid intake? Is there any nausea and/or vomiting that may be morning sickness? And finally, discreetly question the patient to determine whether she is sexually active and whether she has had unprotected sex.

History of Gynecologic Problems

Determine whether the patient has a history of gynecologic problems and whether she has had any infections. If so, did she seek medical treatment? What was the diagnosis? If she thinks she may be having a repeated episode, has she taken any medication or used any over-the-counter treatment? Is there any history of miscarriages, abortions, or ectopic pregnancies?

If the patient is currently bleeding, try to estimate the amount of blood that has been lost. What color is the blood? Is it dark like the normal menstrual flow, or is it bright red? How many pads are soaked per hour? Take any clots or soaked pads along with the patient to the hospital in a plastic bag. How long has the bleeding been going on?

If the patient is complaining of vaginal discharge, note the color, amount, and any odor. Is there any irritation or pain associated with the discharge? Is there any burning or irritation with urination?

Inquire about the use of contraceptives. What type is used? Is the patient consistent with use? And finally, determine whether there has been any history of trauma to the reproductive system.

When asking patients about sensitive subjects, be sure to do so in a quiet manner away from bystanders. If the patient seems to be emotionally distressed, assess the cause and degree of distress. This may require moving the patient to the ambulance to remove her from the

You are the Provider — Part 2

As you begin your assessment of this patient, you note the following:

Initial Assessment	Recording Time: Zero Minutes
Appearance	Pale and very anxious
Level of consciousness	Oriented to time, place, and person
Airway	Open and clear
Breathing	Respirations, rapid and shallow
Circulation	Radial pulses, weak and thready

3. What is the first treatment priority?

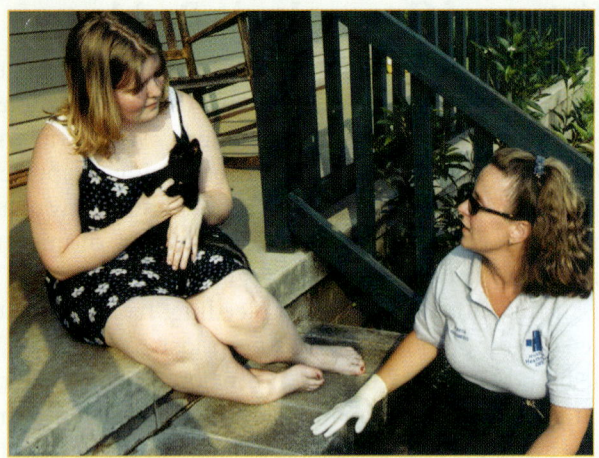

Figure 28-2 Respect the privacy of teenagers by questioning them away from parents or other bystanders.

source of the problem. This is especially true in cases of suspected abuse. Be considerate of the patient's emotional needs and ask only the questions pertinent to your evaluation of her physical status. Your sensitive and caring manner can help you serve as a role model to others.

> ### In the Field
>
> Most teenage girls feel uncomfortable discussing gynecologic problems in front of their parents. They may even refuse to seek help to avoid the embarrassment of the situation. Allow them the opportunity to talk privately, and assure them of your discretion (Figure 28-2). In most cases, a parent will be required to authorize treatment of a minor, but in the case of pregnancy the minor becomes "emancipated" and is legally able to give or refuse consent. Sexually transmitted diseases are also confidential issues in some areas and do not require parental consent for treatment. Regardless, stress the need for the patient to seek treatment for any gynecologic problem.

Physical Exam

The physical exam is performed in the same manner as the examination for other medical emergencies, with special consideration for the female reproductive system. Approach the patient with a comforting attitude. Protect the patient's modesty by placing a sheet over her and removing only the items of clothing necessary to perform your assessment. Maintain privacy during the examination and while interviewing the patient. It is also important to be considerate of the patient's needs and the reason for her discomfort. If the patient has a history of a sexually transmitted disease (for example, acquired immunodeficiency syndrome [AIDS], genital herpes, gonorrhea), it is imperative to treat the patient appropriately and without moral judgment.

Begin with an assessment of the level of consciousness. Any alteration in mental status could indicate a serious problem. Assess the patient's general appearance. What is the color of the skin and mucous membranes? Is there any cyanosis, pallor, or flushing? Cyanosis is a sign of respiratory insufficiency. Pallor can indicate shock, and flushing may be seen with fever from infection. Note any signs of shock, and recognize the need for immediate treatment and transport.

Take baseline vital signs. Include any orthostatic changes. Hypotension in a patient with abdominal pain may be a sign of internal bleeding in the absence of external hemorrhage. Tachycardia and changes in respiration might also signal shock. Note the color and amount of any bleeding or discharge. If there is any evidence of clots and/or tissue, be sure to take it with the patient to the hospital.

Expose and examine the abdomen to look for any discoloration or swelling. Palpate for any masses, tenderness, guarding, distention, or rebound tenderness. If the patient is complaining of discomfort in a particular area, always begin your assessment in the quadrant farthest away from the area of complaint, and palpate the painful area last.

General Management

Be sure to take BSI precautions. As with every patient, ABCs come first. Assess the airway and breathing. Apply 100% supplemental oxygen, and assist ventilation as needed for the inadequately breathing patient. Assess circulatory status, noting the presence of peripheral pulses and any signs of shock. Intravenous (IV) access may be obtained but typically is not necessary. If, however, the patient is demonstrating signs of shock or has excessive vaginal bleeding, establish at least one IV line using a large-bore (14- or 16-gauge) IV catheter in a large vein. Use an isotonic crystalloid solution such as normal saline or lactated Ringer's. Adjust the flow rate based on the patient's presentation. If the patient is showing any signs of hypovolemia, give a 20-mL/kg bolus and reassess the patient. Consider establishing a second IV line.

Monitor and evaluate for serious bleeding. Place absorbent dressings against the vagina; however, **never** pack dressings in the vagina. Discourage the use of tampons, and keep count of all pads used to help the physician estimate blood loss. With shock, place the patient in the shock position and keep warm.

Place the patient on a cardiac monitor and be alert for any rhythm disturbances. Pharmacologic interventions are generally not recommended. Analgesics may mask signs and symptoms, making a diagnosis difficult. They may also mask a deteriorating condition such as shock. Contact medical control for further instructions.

Place the patient in a position of comfort based on the presentation. Some patients with abdominal pain find it more comfortable to lie in a lateral recumbent position. Place the patient on the left side so that she will be facing you instead of the wall of the ambulance. Some patients prefer a knee-chest position, whereas others prefer the hips raised and the knees bent. In the event of shock, place the patient in the shock position.

Consider the possibility of pregnancy, and be prepared for a possible delivery. Anticipate the presence of an ectopic pregnancy based on signs and symptoms. If an ectopic pregnancy is suspected, be alert for possible hypovolemic shock in the event of rupture.

Evaluation by a physician is necessary. Transport the patient to the closest appropriate facility. This may include one with a labor and delivery department or a trauma center with surgical intervention capabilities. Consider emergency transport based on the patient's presentation.

Provide psychological support en route to the hospital. Keep the lines of communication open, and answer questions as honestly as possible. Remain calm, and provide reassuring, gentle care. Remember to protect the patient's privacy and modesty as much as possible.

Specific Gynecologic Emergencies

Pelvic Inflammatory Disease

Pelvic inflammatory disease (PID) is caused by an acute or chronic infection in the organs of the female pelvic cavity. Its onset is typically acute, within approximately 1 week of the menstrual period. Initial access by the infecting organism is through the vagina, where it ascends to other organs including the cervix, uterus, fallopian tubes, ovaries, uterine and ovarian support structures, and the liver. The chief symptoms of PID are pelvic pain and fever.

Complications that may accompany PID include sepsis, abscess formation, generalized peritonitis, and infertility. Scarring may cause tubal infertility and increase the risk of ectopic pregnancy.

Specific assessment findings include lower abdominal pain, possible fever, vaginal discharge, and dyspareunia (pain during sexual intercourse). The patient

---

You are the Provider — Part 3

You reassure your patient that her privacy will be respected. She is receiving 100% oxygen via nonrebreathing mask and has been placed on a cardiac monitor. Your additional assessment findings are as follows:

Vital Signs	Recording Time: 2 Minutes After Patient Contact
Respirations	28 breaths/min, shallow
Pulse	132 beats/min, regular
Skin	Pale, cool, and clammy
Blood pressure	90/60 mm Hg
SaO_2	97% on 100% oxygen

4. What additional treatment modalities are indicated for this patient?

will generally walk doubled-over and guard the abdomen. Their gait tends to be shuffling to avoid excessive movement of the abdominal muscles. Patients also appear ill. Care includes a position of comfort and transport to an appropriate facility.

Ruptured Ovarian Cyst

An ovarian cyst is a fluid-filled sac attached to the inside or outside of the ovary. As the cyst enlarges, it can contain an enormous amount of fluid. The cyst may need to be removed surgically to relieve pressure or to treat infection. Complications include possible significant internal bleeding; however, this is rare.

A sudden onset of severe lower abdominal pain may be present. Most patients have unilateral pain that may radiate from the abdomen to the back. Rupture of the cyst may result in some vaginal bleeding.

Ectopic Pregnancy

Ectopic pregnancy occurs about once in every 200 pregnancies. Vaginal bleeding may be the only sign of an ectopic pregnancy, a pregnancy that develops outside the uterus, most often in a fallopian tube. The leading cause of maternal death during the first trimester is internal hemorrhage into the abdomen following rupture of an ectopic pregnancy. For this reason, you should consider the possibility of an ectopic pregnancy in women who have missed a menstrual cycle and complain of sudden stabbing and usually unilateral pain in the lower abdomen. A history of PID, tubal ligation, or previous ectopic pregnancy should heighten your suspicions for a possible ectopic pregnancy. Consider the possibility of an ectopic pregnancy in any female of reproductive age who has abdominal pain.

An ectopic pregnancy occurs when the ovum develops outside the uterus. Numerous causes may affect the normal pathway of the ovum, preventing it from implanting in the uterus. Previous surgical adhesions, PID, a tubal ligation (having the fallopian tubes surgically tied to prevent pregnancy), or an intrauterine device, or IUD, may interfere with the movement of a fertilized egg. Generally it is the fallopian tubes that are affected, but on rare occasions, implantation may occur elsewhere in the pelvic cavity. Because the fallopian tubes are extremely narrow, even the slightest growth of the egg will cause symptoms; therefore, ectopic pregnancy is an early first trimester emergency, typically occurring within the first 6 to 8 weeks of pregnancy.

The cells begin to divide and the zygote grows, even though this process occurs without the aid of oxygen or nutrients. Therefore, there is no viable fetus that can be removed and implanted in the uterus. Eventually the fallopian tube will rupture if the ectopic pregnancy is not caught in time. This can lead to a life-threatening emergency. The patient usually presents with signs of hypovolemic shock.

The patient might complain of severe abdominal pain that radiates to the back. Vaginal bleeding may be absent or minimal. She will generally report amenorrhea, or absence of the menstrual period, even if she does not know she is pregnant. If rupture occurs, bleeding may be excessive. Expect signs and symptoms of shock. Ask the patient about additional relevant history. If the patient has had abdominal surgery, surgical adhesions may be present. Ask whether she has had PID or a tubal ligation, uses an IUD, or has had a previous ectopic pregnancy.

Monitor the patient for impending shock, including orthostatic vital signs. Note the presence and volume of vaginal blood. A ruptured ectopic pregnancy is a true medical emergency. In addition to the general management, establish a second IV line with a large-bore catheter and place the patient in the shock position if signs and symptoms of shock are present. Transport the patient rapidly to the closest appropriate facility.

Vaginal Bleeding

Vaginal bleeding can be as simple as a normal menstrual cycle or as extreme as a ruptured uterus. Never assume that your emergency call for vaginal hemorrhage is due to normal menstruation. The patient may experience menorrhagia, or heavy vaginal bleeding. Carefully ask the patient about the amount of bleeding, and treat her appropriately based on presenting signs and symptoms.

Always assume that any bleeding during the first or second trimester of a known or possible pregnancy might indicate a spontaneous abortion or miscarriage; especially if the last menstrual cycle was more than 60 days ago. Ask the patient about any previous similar events. Are there any large clots or pieces of tissue? If so, take these to the emergency department for further evaluation. This can be a very tragic time for the patient, so emotional support is extremely important.

Any vaginal bleeding during the third trimester of pregnancy is a serious emergency. Placenta previa presents with bright red bleeding, and placenta abruptio presents with dark bleeding. We will address these further in Chapter 33: Obstetric Emergencies.

Other causes of vaginal bleeding include the following:
- Onset of labor
- PID and other infections
- Trauma
- Lesions from previous surgeries or disease processes.

A physician should evaluate any vaginal bleeding differing in amount and duration from the normal menstrual cycle. The reproductive organs are very vascular, and any bleeding may be life threatening. Hemorrhage can quickly lead to hypovolemic shock and death.

When assessing a patient complaining of vaginal bleeding, be sure to inquire about the onset of symptoms. Does the onset coincide with the normal menstrual cycle? Was there any trauma involved? Is there any chance of pregnancy? Is there a history of bleeding? Check for signs of impending shock, including orthostatic vital signs. Note the presence and volume of bleeding, and remember to take any tissue or clots to the hospital for evaluation.

Traumatic Abdominal Pain

The incidence of vaginal bleeding due to traumatic causes is on the increase. Causes include the following:
- Straddle injury: This type of injury occurs when a female falls onto an object, such as the bar of a boy's bicycle, causing trauma to the external genitalia and perineum.
- Blows to the perineum: A blow to the perineum may be associated with falls or assault.
- Blunt force to the lower abdomen from assault or seat belt injuries: Any blunt force to the lower abdomen has the potential to rupture organs or cause serious injury. This usually occurs from a lap belt during an automobile accident but may be attributed to assault.
- Foreign bodies inserted into the vagina: This injury may be self-inflicted or the result of a sexual assault.
- Abortion attempt: Trauma occurs when the female uses an object such as a clothes hanger in an attempt to abort her pregnancy. This can cause massive trauma and extensive bleeding.
- Soft tissue injury: Sexual assault and vigorous sexual activity can cause soft-tissue injury.

Any or all of the pelvic organs may be affected. Patients generally present with a variety of signs and symptoms that can include severe bleeding, pain, and hypovolemic shock. Specific assessment findings are consistent with severe internal injuries. Management should be based on patient presentation.

Sexual Assault

Sexual assault and rape are all too common. Although most victims are women, men and children are also victims. Often, you can do little beyond providing compassion and transportation to the emergency department. In some cases, the patients will have suffered multiple-system trauma and will also need treatment for shock.

Do not examine the genitalia of a victim of sexual assault unless obvious bleeding requires you to apply a dressing. Discourage the patient from washing, douching, urinating, or defecating until after a physician has completed an examination; this will help to preserve any evidence of a crime. If oral penetration has occurred, discourage the patient from eating, drinking, brushing the teeth, or using mouthwash until he or she has been examined.

Treat all other injuries according to appropriate procedures and protocols for your EMS system. Observe BSI precautions. Obtain the patient's history, perform a physical exam that is limited to the affected part(s) of the body, and provide treatment as quickly, quietly, and calmly as possible. Examine the genitalia only if necessary, such as in the case of severe injury to the area. Do not use invasive procedures unless the situation is critical. Check for any other physical injury. Make efforts to shield the patient from curious onlookers. Explain all procedures before performing an examination. Avoid touching the patient without permission. Do not ask about the patient's sexual history or practices, and do not ask questions that may cause the patient to have guilt feelings.

The patient may refuse assistance or transport, often because he or she wants to maintain privacy and avoid public exposure. For adults who are mentally competent, this is the patient's right. In such cases, you should follow your system's refusal of treatment policy or procedure for sexual assault victims without judging or being condescending to the patient. Your compassion is the best tool to gain the patient's confidence to get further help. Common reactions may range from anxiety to withdrawal and silence. Denial, anger, and fear are normal behavior patterns. Maintain a professional attitude, and be aware of your own feelings and prejudices.

Psychological support is very important. Provide a safe environment and respond to the victim's wishes to talk or not to talk. Offer to call the local rape crisis center for the patient. The center will have an advocate meet the patient at the hospital and provide support throughout the physical examination. Provide reassurance to the patient, and remember that confidentiality is critical.

In addition to the usual treatment principles that apply to all victims of trauma, you should follow these special steps with patients who have been sexually assaulted:

1. Because you may have to appear in court as much as 2 or 3 years later, you must document the patient's history, assessment, treatment, and response to treatment in *detail*. Do not speculate or interject opinion. Record only the facts.
2. Make airway maintenance a major priority.
3. Complete the SAMPLE history in an objective and nonjudgmental manner.
4. Follow any crime scene policy established by your system to protect the scene and preserve any potential evidence for the police to collect. Do not disturb the scene, if possible. If the patient will tolerate being wrapped in a sterile burn sheet, this may help investigators find any hair, fluid, or fiber from the alleged offender.
5. Do not examine the genitalia unless there is major bleeding. If an object has been inserted into the vagina or rectum, do not attempt to remove it.
6. To reduce the patient's anxiety, make sure the EMT-I performing the assessment is the same sex as the patient whenever possible.
7. Discourage the patient from bathing, voiding, or cleaning any wounds until hospital personnel have completed an assessment. Handle the patient's clothes as little as possible, placing articles and any other evidence in *paper* bags. Always wear gloves when handling evidence. Do not use plastic bags, because condensation buildup in the plastic bag can potentially destroy any evidence. If a female patient insists on urinating, have her do so in a sterile urine container (if available). Also, have her deposit the toilet paper in a paper bag. Seal and mark the bag for the police. This can be critical evidence.

You are the Provider   Summary

1. What types of gynecologic emergencies may be encountered by the EMT-I?

- Pelvic inflammatory disease
- Ruptured ovarian cyst
- Ectopic pregnancy
- Vaginal bleeding
- Excessive vaginal bleeding
- Abdominal pain
- Sexual assault

2. What is the importance of acquiring a detailed history of this patient?

When assessing a patient with a possible gynecologic emergency, it is essential to obtain a detailed history of the present illness. Gynecologic emergencies often have the same signs and symptoms as those emergencies involving other abdominal organs.

3. What is the first treatment priority?

As with every patient, ABCs come first. Assess the patient's airway and breathing and provide oxygen as needed.

4. What additional treatment modalities are indicated for this patient?

If the patient is demonstrating signs of shock, as this patient is, the EMT-I should establish at least one IV line with a large-bore catheter and give a 20-mL/kg bolus of an isotonic crystalloid solution and reassess the patient. Consider establishing a second IV line.

Monitor and evaluate the patient for serious bleeding.

Place the patient in a position of comfort. Some patients with abdominal pain find it more comfortable to lie in a lateral recumbent position. Place the patient on the left side so that she will be facing you instead of the wall of the ambulance.

Prep Kit

Ready for Review

- Occasionally you will be called for a patient experiencing a gynecologic emergency unrelated to pregnancy. This may include excessive bleeding, soft-tissue injuries, or infection.
- The reproductive system is very vascular, and there is a great potential for massive hemorrhage. Familiarity with a woman's anatomy and normal physiology will prepare you to deal with most common gynecologic problems.
- The majority of patients experiencing a gynecologic emergency will be treated in the same manner regardless of the cause. Bleeding should be controlled, and the patient's ABCs should be monitored closely. Watch for developing signs of shock, and treat appropriately. Transport in the proper mode to the closest appropriate facility.
- History has a major role in caring for a patient with a gynecologic emergency. Along with a detailed history of the present illness, ask the patient about any previous gynecologic problems and her obstetric history. Consider the possibility of ectopic pregnancy in any patient of childbearing age with abdominal pain.
- Always question the patient in privacy to maintain confidentiality.
- Perform a detailed physical exam, with close attention to preserving the patient's privacy. Expose only the areas that you need to examine, and cover the patient with a sheet. Monitor the patient closely for changes that may indicate that shock is developing.
- Excessive bleeding is a serious emergency. Cover the vagina with a sterile pad; change the pad as often as necessary, and take all used pads to the hospital for examination. Pharmacologic interventions are generally not indicated. Contact medical control for further instructions.
- Use local pressure and a diaper-type bandage to hold dressings in place when treating nonobstetric injuries to the external genitalia. Never place dressings in the vagina. Treat patients with these injuries as you would any other victim of blood loss.
- In the case of sexual assault or rape, treat for shock if necessary, and record all the facts in detail. Follow any crime scene policy established by your system to protect the scene and any potential evidence. Discourage the patient from washing, douching, or voiding until a physician has examined him or her.

Vital Vocabulary

abortion Delivery of the fetus and placenta before 20 weeks; a spontaneous abortion is called a miscarriage.

anus The outlet of the rectum.

cervix The lower one third, or neck, of the uterus.

clitoris The small erectile body partially hidden by the labia minora. It is covered by the prepuce or foreskin.

dysmenorrhea Painful menstruation.

ectopic pregnancy A pregnancy that develops outside the uterus, typically in a fallopian tube.

endometrium The inner layer of the uterine wall.

fallopian tubes (or uterine tubes) Tubes or ducts that extend from near the ovaries and terminate at the uterus.

fundus The uppermost part of the uterus, farthest from the cervical opening.

hymen A fold of mucous membrane that partially covers the entrance to the vagina.

labia majora The outer lip-shaped structure of the vagina.

labia minora The inner lip-shaped structure of the vagina.

menarche The initial onset of menstruation occurring during puberty.

Technology

- Interactivities
- Vocabulary Explorer
- Anatomy Review
- Web Links
- Online Review Manual

menopause The cessation of the menstrual cycle and ovarian function.

menstruation The cyclic shedding of the uterine lining that occurs approximately every 28 days.

mons pubis The pad of fatty tissue and coarse skin that lies over the pubic symphysis.

myometrium The muscular wall of the uterus.

oocyte The female sex cell.

ovaries Almond-shaped bodies that lie on either side of the pelvic cavity. Their functions are to produce ova and certain hormones.

perineum The area of skin between the vagina and the anus.

placenta abruptio Premature separation of the placenta from the wall of the uterus.

placenta previa A condition in which the placenta develops over and partially or completely covers the cervix.

prepuce The foreskin that covers the clitoris.

urethra Canal for the discharge of urine extending from the bladder to the outside of the body.

uterus The muscular organ where the fetus grows, also called the womb; responsible for contractions during labor.

vagina The outermost cavity of a woman's reproductive system; the lower part of the birth canal.

vaginal orifice Opening of the vagina.

vestibule Small space at the beginning of an opening.

vulva The visible external female genitalia.

Points to Ponder

The police department is at the scene of a reported sexual assault. They have called for your assistance to care for a woman who has apparently been raped. You arrive to find a 50-year-old woman lying on her bed. There is a female officer in the bedroom with the patient and other officers are in the living room.

The patient is covered with a comforter and is crying. She has an obvious bruise to her face and you notice a blood stain on the bed. You ask the female officer to remain in the room with you as you continue your assessment of the patient. You fully explain to the patient your need to remove the comforter and assess her for other injuries. She agrees and allows you to proceed with your assessment. You find a 3-inch laceration to the inner thigh that is still bleeding. You do not see any evidence of life-threatening bleeding to the genitalia. You tell your patient that you must stop the bleeding to her thigh and explain how you are about to proceed. You apply direct pressure to the injury and bandage it when the bleeding stops.

The patient is moved to the stretcher and placed on a sterile burn sheet to preserve evidence. Her vital signs are within normal limits. You attempt to calm and reassure her en route to the ED. After delivering the patient to the hospital, you carefully record all of her statements to you, using quotations when possible.

Issues: Need to Protect the Crime Scene in Sexual Assault, Support and Compassion to Victims of Sexual Assault, Treating Associated Injuries Without Assessing Genitalia

Assessment in Action

You are dispatched to a suburban area for a woman having abdominal pain. You arrive at the scene and are met at the door by a young man who tells you his wife is sick. He directs you to the bathroom where you find a 20-year-old woman sitting on the toilet. She tells you she has been having severe abdominal pain for the last 3 to 4 hours and is now experiencing light vaginal bleeding.

After placing a pad over the vaginal area, you assist the patient to the stretcher, secure her in place, and move her to the ambulance. You note that she is pale and diaphoretic and that her skin is cool to the touch. She is breathing at 24 breaths/min and her heart rate is 110 beats/min. Your partner takes her blood pressure and finds it to be 90/60 mm Hg. Palpation of her abdomen reveals tenderness in the right lower quadrant with radiating pain to her back.

When interviewing the patient, she tells you that she has a history of endometriosis and frequently suffers abdominal pain and cramping; however, this episode is much worse. She believes she is pregnant, but her menstrual cycles are very irregular so she is not sure. She has a 2-year-old daughter and has had one miscarriage.

You place the patient on 100% oxygen and initiate an IV of normal saline. En route to the ED, you place the patient on a cardiac monitor.

1. How would you document this patient's obstetric history?
   A. P3 G1 A1
   B. G2 P1 A1
   C. G3 P2 A1
   D. P3 G2 A1

2. Your initial bolus of IV fluid should be:
   A. 20 mL/kg.
   B. 30 mL/kg.
   C. 40 mL/kg.
   D. 50 mL/kg.

3. After you give a fluid bolus, the patient's blood pressure is 84/46 mm Hg and her heart rate is 120 beats/min. You should:
   A. run the IV at 125 mL/h.
   B. double the initial bolus.
   C. start a second IV line.
   D. monitor her only.

4. You suspect this patient may be experiencing an ectopic pregnancy, which is:
   A. the same thing as a miscarriage.
   B. a pregnancy that develops outside of the uterus.
   C. a pregnancy that develops inside of the uterus.
   D. the cessation of the menstrual cycle.

5. Ectopic pregnancies occur in 1 out of every:
   A. 200 pregnancies.
   B. 500 pregnancies.
   C. 100 pregnancies.
   D. 1,000 pregnancies.

6. The leading cause of maternal death in the first trimester of pregnancy is internal hemorrhage from:
   A. a spontaneous miscarriage.
   B. a ruptured ectopic pregnancy.
   C. pelvic inflammatory disease.
   D. a ruptured ovarian cyst.

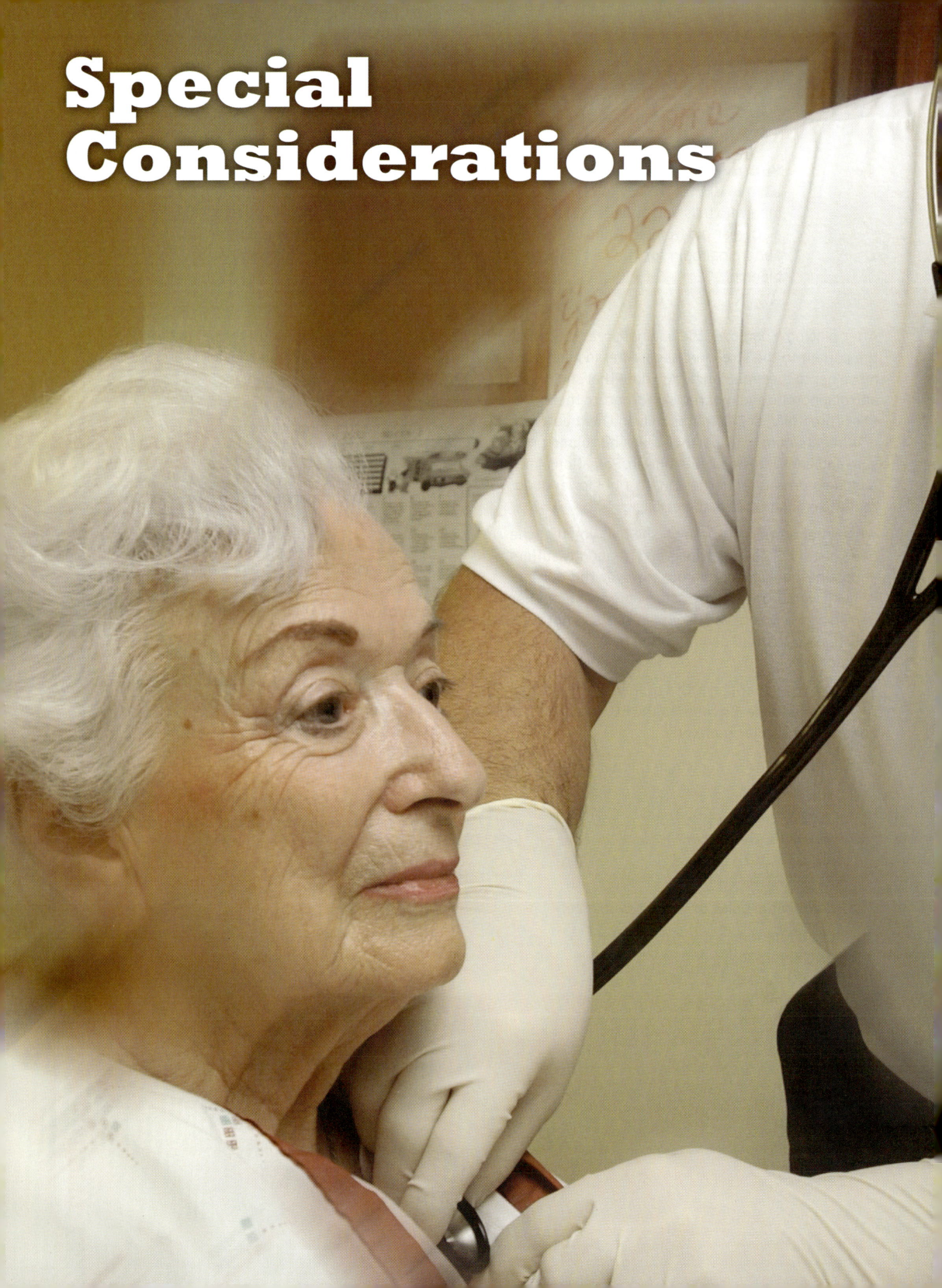

Special Considerations

Section 7

29	Obstetric Emergencies	1166
30	Neonatal Resuscitation	1200
31	Pediatric Emergencies	1228
32	Geriatric Emergencies	1336

Obstetric Emergencies

1999 Objectives

Cognitive

6-1.1 Review the anatomic structures and physiology of the reproductive system. (p 1168)
6-1.2 Identify the normal events of pregnancy. (p 1173)
6-1.3 Describe how to assess an obstetrical patient. (p 1173)
6-1.4 Identify the stages of labor and the EMT-Intermediate's role in each stage. (p 1179)
6-1.5 Differentiate between normal and abnormal delivery. (p 1189)
6-1.6 Identify and describe complications associated with pregnancy and delivery. (p 1189)
6-1.7 Identify predelivery emergencies. (p 1175)
6-1.8 State indications of an imminent delivery. (p 1180)
6-1.9 Differentiate the management of a patient with predelivery emergencies from a normal delivery. (p 1175, 1179)
6-1.10 State the steps in the predelivery preparation of the mother. (p 1180)
6-1.11 State the steps to assist in the delivery of a newborn. (p 1180)
6-1.12 Describe how to care for the newborn. (p 1186)
6-1.13 Describe how and when to cut the umbilical cord. (p 1187)
6-1.14 Discuss the steps in the delivery of the placenta. (p 1188)
6-1.15 Describe the management of the mother post-delivery. (p 1188)
6-1.16 Describe the procedures for handling abnormal deliveries. (p 1189)
6-1.17 Describe the procedures for handling complications of pregnancy. (p 1189)
6-1.18 Describe the procedures for handling maternal complications of labor. (p 1188)
6-1.19 Describe special considerations when meconium is present in amniotic fluid or during delivery. (p 1184)
6-1.20 Describe special considerations of a premature baby. (p 1180)

Affective

6-1.21 Advocate the need for treating two patients (mother and baby). (p 1187)
6-1.22 Value the importance of maintaining a patient's modesty and privacy during assessment and management. (p 1182)
6-1.23 Serve as a role model for other EMS providers when discussing or performing the steps of childbirth. (p 1168)
6-1.24 Value the importance of body substance isolation. (p 1180)

Psychomotor

6-1.25 Demonstrate how to assess an obstetric patient. (p 1173, 1175)
6-1.26 Demonstrate how to provide care for a patient with:
   1. Excessive vaginal bleeding
   2. Abdominal pain (p 1175)
6-1.27 Demonstrate how to prepare the obstetric patient for delivery. (p 1180)
6-1.28 Demonstrate how to assist in the normal cephalic delivery of the fetus. (p 1182)
6-1.29 Demonstrate how to deliver the placenta. (p 1188)
6-1.30 Demonstrate how to provide postdelivery care of the mother. (p 1188)
6-1.31 Demonstrate how to assist with abnormal deliveries. (p 1189)
6-1.32 Demonstrate how to care for the mother with delivery complications. (p 1189)

1985 Objectives

There are no 1985 objectives for this chapter.

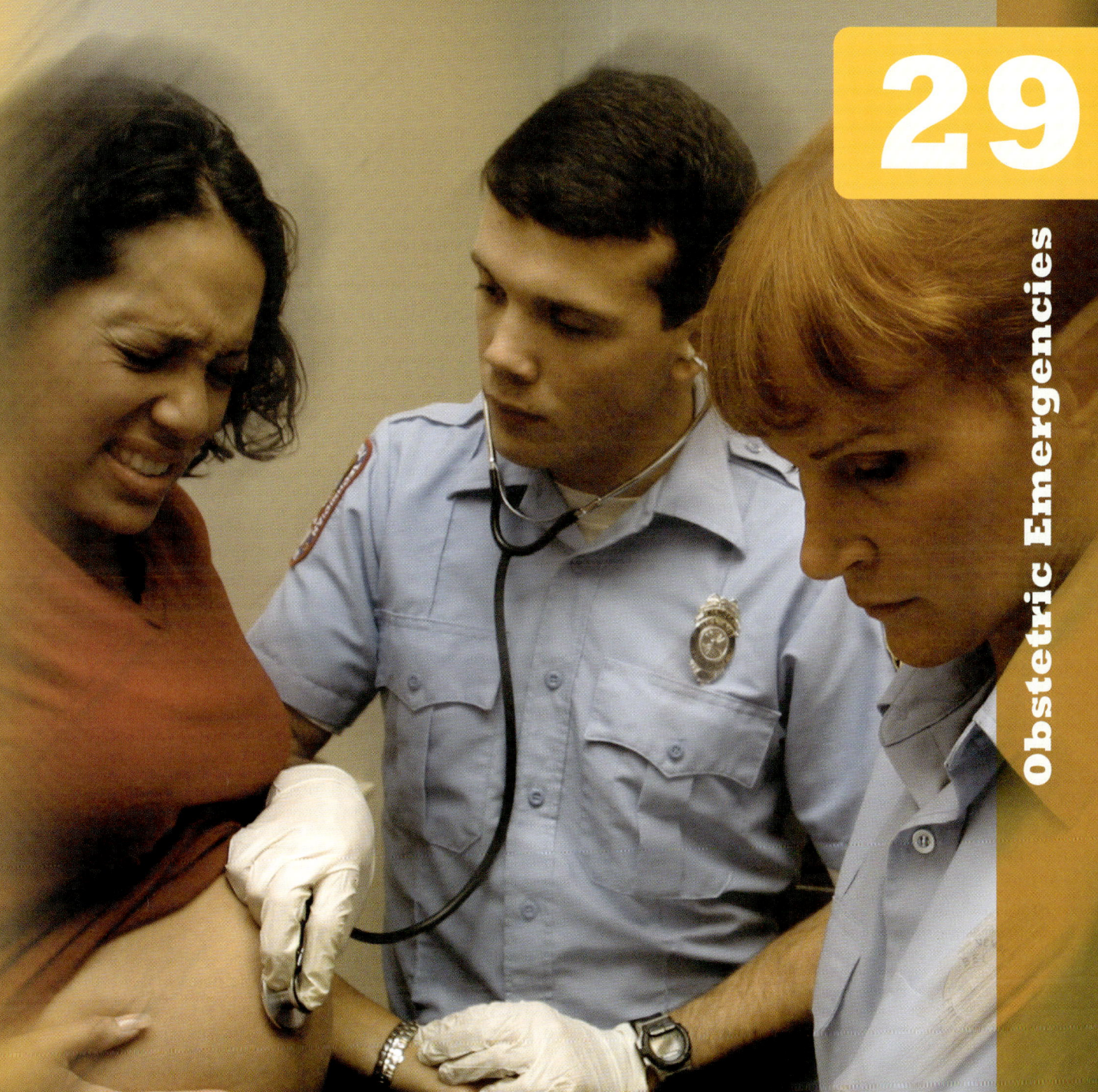

29

Obstetric Emergencies

You are the Provider

You and your partner are dispatched to 2201 Smith Way for a 35-year-old woman in labor. En route, the dispatcher informs you that the patient is alone and her contractions are 2 to 3 minutes apart.

1. What considerations should be made before your arrival?
2. What do you anticipate with her age and time between contractions?

Introduction

Most births are uneventful and require little or no medical intervention beyond basic interventions, such as suctioning, drying, and warming the baby; others, however, may be life threatening to both the woman and baby. This chapter will help prepare you to be an active, positive part of the birthing process.

Obstetric Emergencies

Arriving at the scene of a woman in labor can cause anxiety and fear on the part of both the EMT-I and the expecting parents. Parents expect to deliver their child in the controlled setting of a hospital delivery room. The prehospital provider would also prefer that delivery occur in the hospital. Unfortunately, if labor progresses quickly or other factors intervene, you may have to deliver the infant in the field. Using the knowledge acquired from this chapter, the out-of-hospital birth can be just as safe and healthy as one that occurs in the hospital. The birthing process usually requires little help from the health care provider, only supportive care of the pregnant woman and infant.

This chapter will describe and discuss the normal anatomical and physiologic changes that occur during pregnancy, the normal process of childbirth, and common antepartum, peripartum, and postpartum complications so that you will be prepared to care for both normal and abnormal deliveries. You will learn how to assess whether delivery is going to occur in the field or not and how to proceed if field delivery is necessary.

Technology

- Interactivities
- Vocabulary Explorer
- Anatomy Review
- Web Links
- Online Review Manual

www.EMSzone.com/EMTI

The Female Reproductive System

The Ovaries

The ovaries are the female reproductive organs and usually are located one on each side of the lower abdominal quadrants (Figure 29-1). The ovaries are suspended in place by a peritoneal fold, the mesovarium, and two ligaments, the suspensory ligament and the ovarian ligament.

The ovaries produce the precursors to mature eggs, the oocytes. In addition, they produce hormones that regulate female reproductive function and secondary sexual characteristics such as pubic hair and breast development. Within the ovaries, oocytes undergo a maturation process, called oogenesis, resulting in production of an ovum, a mature egg.

During the reproductive years of a woman's life, the pituitary gland releases hormones at roughly monthly intervals. These hormones, follicle-stimulating hormone (FSH) and luteinizing hormone (LH), stimulate one oocyte to undergo meiosis, the process of cell division that results in the formation of a mature ovum. A mature ovum is released into one of the fallopian tubes during ovulation and is then ready for fertilization by a sperm (Figure 29-2).

The Fallopian Tubes

The fallopian tubes are hollow tubes or ducts that extend from the uterus to the region of the ovary. These tubes serve as a passage for the movement of an ovum from the ovary and for sperm from the uterus upward.

Each fallopian tube opens directly into the peritoneal cavity in an expanded area called the infundibulum. The opening of the fallopian tube is the ostium, which is surrounded by long thin processes called fimbriae. The fimbriae help direct an ovum into the fallopian tube following ovulation. Once inside the tube, movement of cilia (hair-like projections) on the cell surfaces results in passage of the ovum toward the uterus.

The Uterus

The uterus is a pear-shaped organ located in the midline of the lower abdomen that allows implantation, growth, and nourishment of a fetus during pregnancy. The top portion is called the fundus, and the main portion of the uterus is the body. The cervix is the part of the uterus that extends into the vagina. The uterine

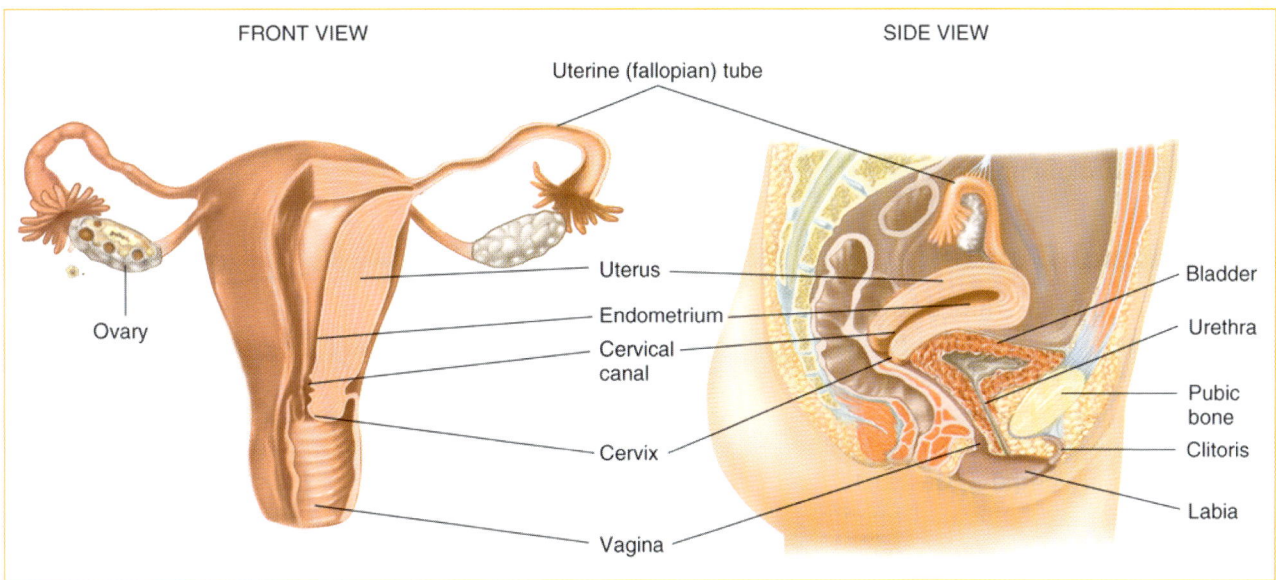

Figure 29-1 The female reproductive tract.

canal continues as the cervical canal, which opens at the tip of the cervix (the cervical os) into the vagina.

The broad ligament, round ligament, and uterosacral ligament hold the uterus in place. The uterine walls are composed of three layers. The perimetrium is the outside, serous membrane coating. The myometrium is the middle layer and contains thick smooth muscle. The innermost layer of the uterus, the endometrium, is divided into two layers. The deep basal layer is connected directly to the myometrium. The functional layer lines the cavity itself and undergoes menstrual changes and sloughing during the female menstrual cycle.

During the menstrual cycle, an ovum matures, forming a graafian follicle, or developed ovum. At ovulation, this follicle ruptures through the surface of the ovary. If fertilization occurs, the fertilized egg proceeds through the fallopian tube to implant in the uterus. If fertilization does not occur, a series of hormonal changes causes the remnants of the follicle, called the corpus luteum, to be sloughed, along with the uterine lining.

The menstrual cycle is a recurring cycle, beginning at menarche, which is the time of the first menstrual cycle, and ending at menopause. During each cycle, the lining of the uterus thickens in preparation for pregnancy. If pregnancy does not occur, this functional layer is shed during menstruation. The average menstrual cycle is 28 days, with day one being the first day of menstrual flow (Figure 29-3 ▶).

The length of menstruation varies somewhat among women. Gonadotropin-releasing hormone (GnRH) from the hypothalamus, FSH and LH from the pituitary gland, and estrogen and progesterone from the ovaries stimulate the uterine lining at different stages during the menstrual cycle.

The Vagina

The vagina is a muscular tube that forms the lower part of the female reproductive tract. It is the female organ of copulation and receives the male penis during sexual intercourse. The muscular walls of the vagina are able to expand, allowing the vagina to stretch greatly during childbirth. Mucous membranes on the surface of the vagina secrete a protective fluid and produce lubricating secretions during sexual intercourse.

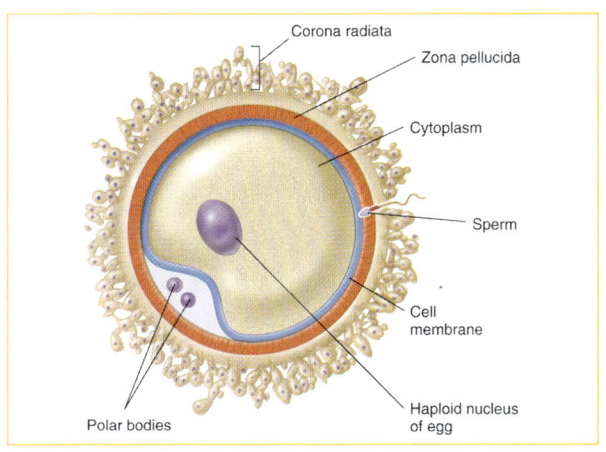

Figure 29-2 Fertilization.

The hymen is a thin mucous membrane that covers the vaginal opening. It may completely close the orifice or be completely or partially torn during intercourse or trauma. The presence or absence of a hymen is not a reliable indicator of virginity.

The External Genitalia

The area between the urethral opening and the anus is the perineum. It includes skin, the external genitalia, and underlying tissues. Two anatomic triangles make up this area. The anterior urogenital triangle contains the external genitalia; the posterior anal triangle contains the anal opening. Several deep muscles provide support to the perineal structures (Figure 29-4 ▶).

The female external genitalia are referred to as the vulva or pudendum. A pair of skin folds, the labia minora, borders the vestibule, which is a space into which the vagina and the urethra open. The clitoris is located in the anterior margin of the vestibule. It contains erectile tissue, the corpus cavernosus, which becomes engorged with blood as a result of sexual excitement. The labia minora unite over the clitoris, forming the prepuce. Lateral to the labia minora are two prominent, rounded folds of skin, the labia majora (see Figure 29-4). These structures unite anteriorly over the pubic symphysis at the mons pubis.

The Mammary Glands

Breasts contain the organs of milk production (lactation), the mammary glands. Mammary glands are actually modified sweat glands. In both male and female breasts, there is an external raised nipple that is surrounded by the pigmented areola. In the female breast, the areolar glands produce secretions that protect the nipple and areola during nursing.

The female mammary glands contain 15 to 20 glandular lobes covered by a variable amount of fatty tissue (Figure 29-5 ▶). This superficial fat gives the breast its form. The lobes produce milk, which is stored in the lactiferous sinuses and expressed from the nipple. The mammary glands are supported by a group of mammary ligaments that extend from the fascia over the pectoralis major muscles to prevent excess sagging of the breasts. With aging, however, the ligaments weaken, allowing the breasts to sag to a variable extent.

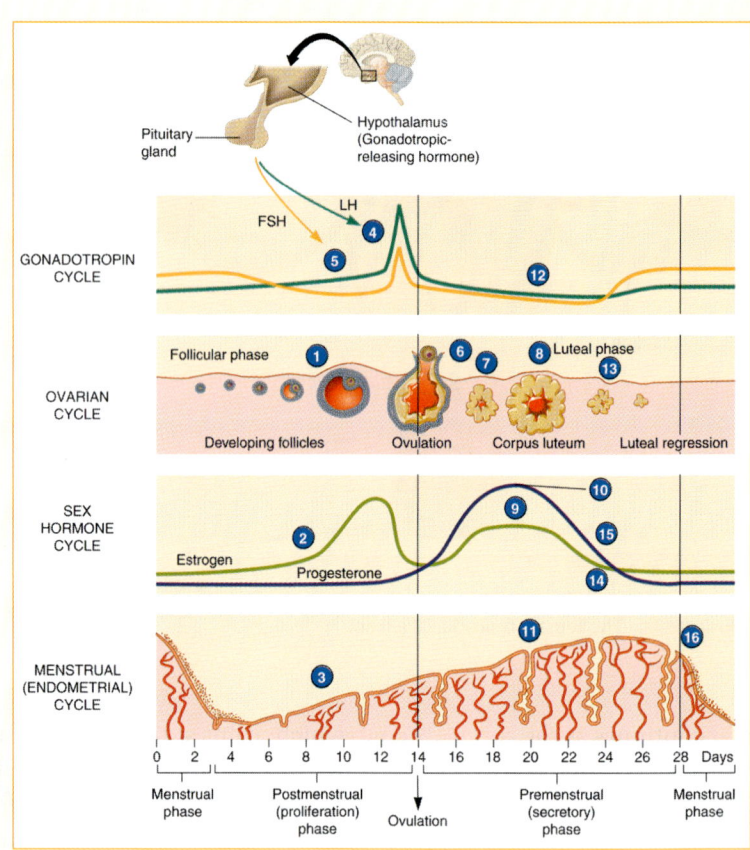

Figure 29-3 The menstrual cycle.

Gestation

Normal Gestation

Gestation refers to the process of fetal development following fertilization of an egg, and is stimulated by production of the hormone human chorionic gonadotropin (hCG). This hormone stimulates the corpus luteum to produce progesterone, which is essential for normal continuation of the pregnancy.

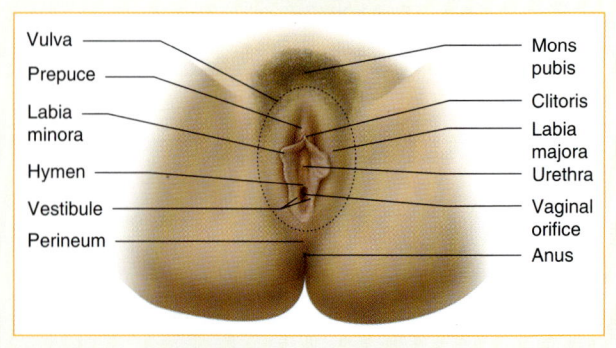

Figure 29-4 The female external genitalia.

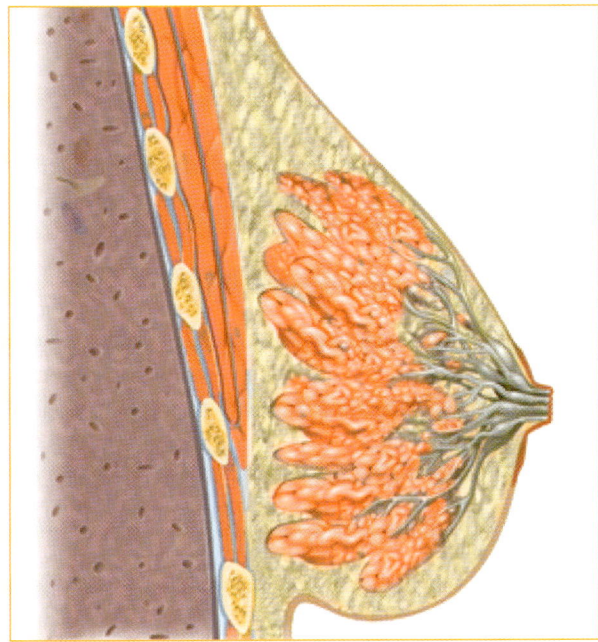

Figure 29-5 The mammary glands.

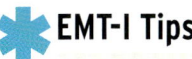

EMT-I Tips

Fallopian tubes—Normal site of fertilization.
Uterus—Normal site of implantation.

undergoes progressive cell divisions. When the zygote contains approximately 32 cells, it usually implants into the uterine wall, which has been thickened by progesterone in preparation for implantation. Implantation usually occurs approximately 7 days after fertilization. The inner group of zygote cells (the embryoblast) becomes the embryo; the outer group of cells (the trophoblast) becomes the placenta Figure 29-6 ▼. From the time of fertilization to end of the eighth week, the developing zygote is referred to as an embryo; beyond the ninth week, it is referred to as a fetus. Approximately three weeks after fertilization, the placenta is formed in the uterus and merges the fetal and maternal tissue to provide nutrients to and eliminate waste products from the developing fetus.

The placenta is attached to the endometrium on one side and surrounds the fetus on the other side. It is a highly vascular organ that provides gas exchange for the developing fetus Figure 29-7 ▶. It allows oxygen and carbon dioxide to diffuse across the placental barrier between the fetal and maternal blood. The maternal and fetal blood do not mix. The gases, nutrients, waste products, hormones, and other dissolved

When ovulation occurs and an ovum is released from the woman's ovary, it begins to travel down the fallopian tube toward the uterus. Fertilization occurs when sperm and an ovum meet, usually in the distal third of the fallopian tube. The fertilized egg, called the zygote (also called the blastocyst), moves through the fallopian tube toward the uterus. At the same time, the zygote

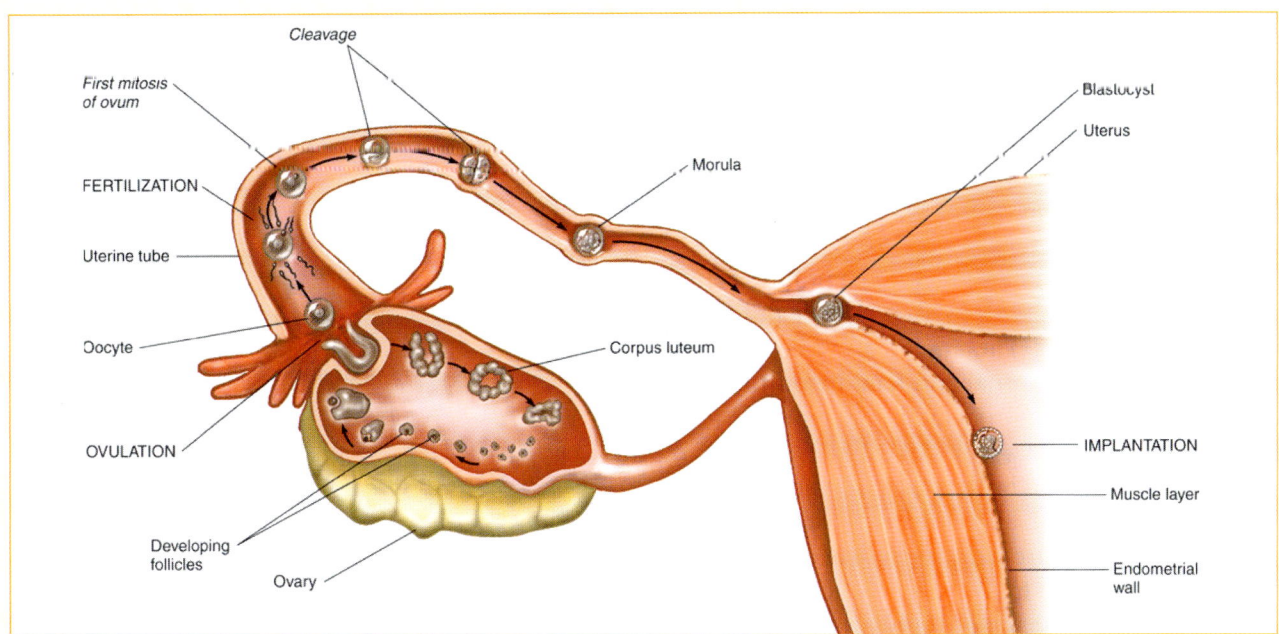

Figure 29-6 Fertilization and implantation of the embryo.

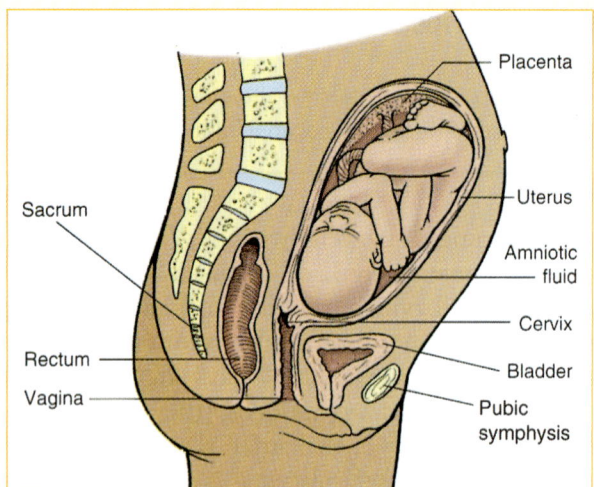

Figure 29-7 Anatomic structures of the pregnant woman.

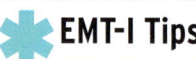

Obstetric Terminology

Understanding certain terms unique to the pregnant patient will allow you to more accurately communicate the patient's obstetric history with other health care providers. Gravida is a term used to describe the number of times a woman has been pregnant; para is a term used to describe the number of times a pregnant woman has delivered a viable baby. For example, if a woman has been pregnant twice, but had a miscarriage during her first pregnancy and one healthy child, she would be gravida 2, para 1. A woman who is pregnant for the first time would be gravida 1, para 0. Once she delivers a viable baby, however, she then becomes gravida 1, para 1.

Primigravida refers to a woman who is pregnant for the first time, while multigravida refers to a woman who has been pregnant two or more times.

Nullipara refers to a woman who has never delivered a viable baby, although she may have been pregnant before and miscarried or otherwise did not deliver a viable baby. Conversely, multipara refers to a woman who has delivered two or more viable babies. Grand multipara refers to a woman who has delivered seven or more viable babies.

particles diffuse across the semipermeable membrane in the placenta. The nutrients required for the rapid growth that occurs are carried to the fetus and its waste products from metabolism are removed. The placenta secretes hormones that promote the growth of the fetus as well as prepare the pregnant woman for labor, delivery, and milk production and release. Finally, the placenta acts as a barrier and filter to allow some substances to cross from the maternal blood supply into the fetus and preventing drugs and other harmful substances from crossing.

The fetus is connected to the placenta and therefore, to the pregnant woman by the umbilical cord. This hose-like structure contains two arteries and one vein. You can remember which direction they carry blood by considering them to be fetal blood vessels. The arteries (like all arteries) carry blood away while the vein carries blood towards the fetus. Therefore, the umbilical arteries carry deoxygenated blood and waste products away from the fetus; the umbilical vein carries oxygenated blood and nutrients to the fetus **Figure 29-8**.

The amniotic sac (also called the amniotic membranes) forms and fills with fluid to protect and cushion the developing fetus. The amniotic fluid is produced by the filtration of maternal and fetal blood through blood vessels in the placenta and by excretion of fetal urine into the amniotic sac. Amniotic fluid is swallowed by the fetus and removed by the placenta, where it passes into the mother's blood. The amount of amniotic fluid peaks at about 1 L before reducing to half a liter by the time the fetus is full term. If the amniotic sac ruptures before labor occurs, the fetus is at higher risk for complications, including trauma and infection. This is called premature rupture of membranes.

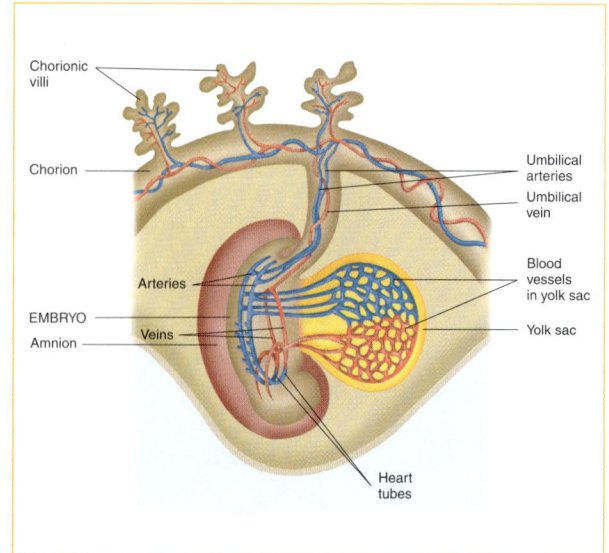

Figure 29-8 The placental-fetal circulation. During fetal development, the fetus receives all nutrients from the mother via the umbilical vein. Wastes are removed through the two umbilical arteries and are excreted by the mother.

EMT-I Tips

A missed menstrual period often is the first indication of pregnancy. The third week of the embryonic development coincides with the first missed menstrual period. Thus, by the time pregnancy is suspected, the embryo has already undergone 2 weeks of development.

It is crucial that a woman becomes aware of a pregnancy as soon as possible because the embryonic period is a time of high susceptibility to teratogens, external substances that may cause birth defects.

Trimesters of Pregnancy

Pregnancy is divided into three trimesters Figure 29-9 ▶. The first trimester extends from the last menstrual cycle through week 12 of the pregnancy. Major events in the first trimester include a positive pregnancy test result (blood or urine hCG) at 8 to 10 days, a palpable uterine fundus at the pubic symphysis at week 12, and audible fetal heart tones noted on Doppler ultrasound. All major fetal organ systems begin to develop during the embryonic period (weeks 3 through 8) Figure 29-10 ▶. From the embryonic period until delivery, organ systems undergo continuing maturation and development.

The second trimester extends from week 13 through week 27. The major events are a palpable uterine fundus between the pubic symphysis and the umbilicus at week 16, the first fetal movements (quickening) at weeks 16 through 18 in a woman who has had one or more previous pregnancies, and fetal heart tones that become audible with a fetoscope at weeks 17 through 20. In addition, female and male genitalia may be distinguished by ultrasound at week 18, first fetal movements (quickening) are noted in a woman's first pregnancy at weeks 18 through 20, and the uterine fundus is palpable at the umbilicus at week 20. At weeks 25 through 27, the lungs become capable of respiration and produce surfactant, a liquid protein substance that coats the alveoli in the lungs. Infants born at the end of the second trimester have a 70% to 80% chance of surviving an extrauterine environment.

The third trimester extends from week 28 until term, or week 40. The major events of the third trimester include the presence of papillary light reflex in the fetus, descent of the fetal head to the pelvic inlet (lightening), and rupture of the amniotic sac. Once the amniotic sac has

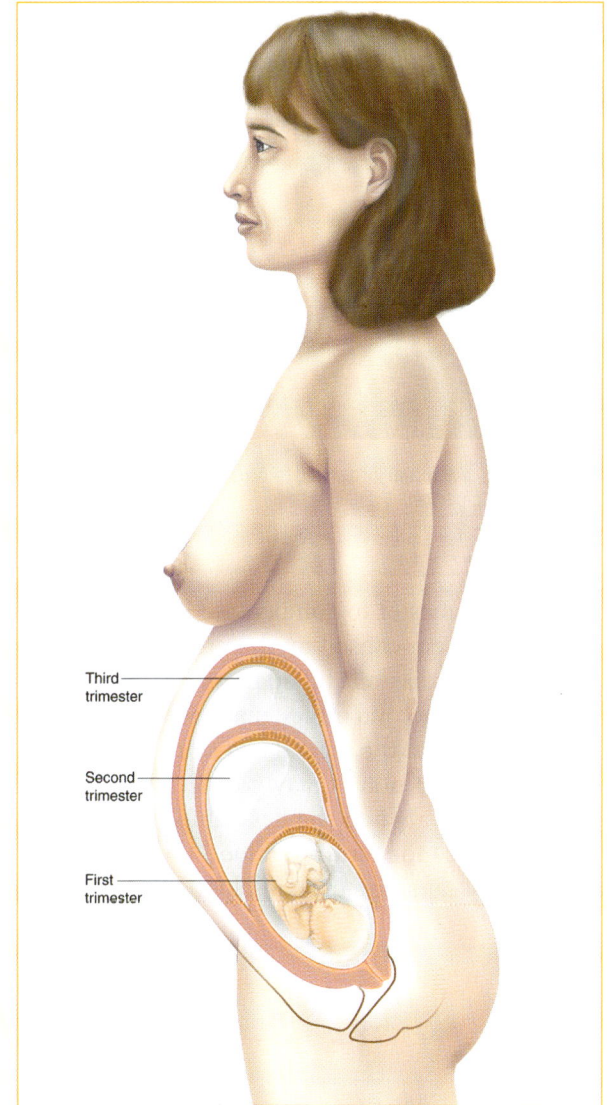

Figure 29-9 The three trimesters of pregnancy.

ruptured, the fetus must be delivered within 24 hours due to the risk of infection. At the end of the third trimester, the fetus typically weighs 7.0 to 7.5 lb (3,300 g).

Normal Maternal Changes of Pregnancy

During pregnancy, a woman's body undergoes several changes in order to support the growing fetus. The maternal cardiovascular system undergoes dramatic changes during pregnancy. The total blood volume increases by about 50% by 40 weeks and the red blood cells increase in number by about 30%. The heart rate elevates by 10 to 20 beats/min, and the cardiac output rises by 30%

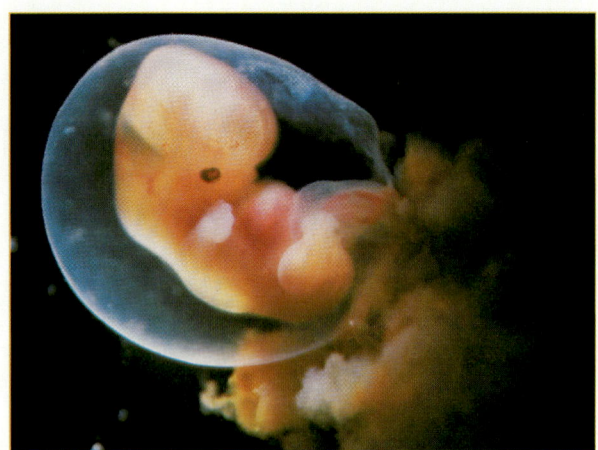

Figure 29-10 All major organ systems begin to develop during the embryonic period.

by the third trimester to compensate for the extra volume in the system caused by the growth of the fetus. The systolic and diastolic blood pressures drop by 10 to 15 mm Hg by the second trimester and return to near normal by full term. In the second and third trimesters the gravid (pregnant) uterus may compress the woman's inferior vena cava when she lies supine. This can significantly reduce the return of blood to the heart (preload), thereby causing a drop in blood pressure.

The respiratory minute volume of the patient increases by about 40% by full term to accommodate the increased blood volume and demand for oxygen from the fetus. A patient's tidal volume is the amount of air that goes in or out of the lungs with each breath. If you multiply the amount of air that goes in and out (tidal volume) by the number of breaths per minute (respiratory rate), you know the amount of air that goes in and out of the lungs per minute (minute volume). In order to increase the minute volume, a patient may increase the respiratory rate, tidal volume, or both. In pregnancy, the patient initially increases the tidal volume. Once the gravid uterus grows superiorly to lie against the diaphragm, the patient may not be able to fully inspire the tidal volume needed to maintain adequate minute volume. If so, the respiratory rate increases to compensate for the reduced tidal volume.

Because of this increase in the amount of air that goes in and out of the lungs, the amount of CO_2 that the patient exhales increases. This causes a relative respiratory alkalosis for the patient, which may cause dizziness and shortness of breath. Remember that the placenta is a semipermeable membrane like those you learned about in the fluid and electrolyte section. Dissolved particles and gasses tend to diffuse from areas of higher concentration to lower concentration. The CO_2 produced by the fetus travels to the placenta and has a higher

You are the Provider — Part 2

On arrival, you find a pregnant woman who is sitting up in her bed. She tells you her "water broke" and her contractions are very long and close together. Your partner applies high-flow oxygen and you ask her how many weeks she is into her pregnancy. She tells you she is in her 38th week; she has had prenatal care and there have been no complications during her pregnancy. You also find out that this is her fourth pregnancy and she has three children. As her next contraction begins, she tells you that she thinks the baby is close to coming.

Vital Signs	Recording Time: 3 Minutes After Patient Contact
Respirations	36 breaths/min, with adequate tidal volume
Pulse	118 beats/min, full and regular
Blood pressure	126/80 mm Hg
Level of consciousness	Alert and oriented to person, place, time, and event
SaO_2	98% (on supplemental oxygen)

3. What should you ask her about the amniotic fluid?
4. What specific questions do you have regarding this patient's medical history?
5. How do her gravida and para numbers affect your patient care decisions?

concentration of CO_2 than that of the maternal blood; therefore, diffusion occurs toward the maternal side of the placenta.

The pregnant woman often experiences gastrointestinal complaints at some time during the pregnancy. The "morning sickness" of nausea and sometimes vomiting occurs most commonly between the eighth and 14th week of pregnancy. As the uterus grows later in the pregnancy, the stomach and intestines of the woman are compressed and pushed superiorly. This may result in heartburn, a burning sensation around the epigastrium. If the patient is unconscious and has no gag reflex, the risk of regurgitation and aspiration also increases. The peristalsis of the bowels decreases from the pressure of the uterus on the gastrointestinal tract and so digestion slows, often resulting in constipation. Decreased gastrointestinal function could also affect the absorption of medications, resulting in prolonged blood levels.

The pregnant woman gains approximately 20 pounds during a full-term pregnancy. If the patient gains significantly more weight than average she may be at risk for several of the disorders of pregnancy that we will discuss later. The pregnant woman can normally have edema that will be driven by gravity to the lower extremities.

Emergencies Prior to Delivery

Most pregnant women are healthy, but some may be ill when they conceive or become ill during pregnancy. The best way to promote a healthy infant is to ensure that the pregnant woman maintains adequate oxygenation, ventilation, and perfusion.

Many complications can occur during the pregnancy that can threaten the health or life of both the woman and fetus. We will examine the most common of these conditions.

Early in the pregnancy the woman often experiences nausea, vomiting, weight gain, and stops having menstrual cycles. One of the common early pregnancy emergencies that you will care for is vaginal bleeding. This can be a sign of several conditions that range from benign to life-threatening.

Abortion

The most common cause of vaginal bleeding during the first and second trimesters is <u>abortion</u> or miscarriage. The term abortion does not imply any cause and simply means that the fetus is released from the uterus before 20 weeks of gestation. It can be spontaneous, without any known cause (idiopathic), or it could be induced by trauma, medications, or other medical causes. The rate of miscarriage in women who have a known pregnancy is about 20%, or 1 in 5 pregnancies, so this is a common occurrence. A threatened abortion occurs when the fetus may abort, but may also remain in the uterus to develop normally. The message for you to give to your patient is that you cannot be sure what the problem is in the field. She should try to remain calm and the physician will determine the best course of action.

There is no specific treatment that you must provide to the patient with a suspected abortion. The patient should receive high-flow oxygen, a large-bore IV line of an isotonic crystalloid (ie, normal saline or lactated ringers) in case fluid boluses are required for severe bleeding and shock, and transport to an appropriate hospital. You should support her emotionally and try to keep her calm. You should not give her false reassurance by telling her that everything will be all right or that her baby is fine. You cannot honestly answer her questions about the outcome of the pregnancy based on your limited prehospital evaluation. The patient needs a thorough evaluation in the hospital.

Ectopic Pregnancy

Another cause of first trimester bleeding is the implantation and growth of the embryo outside of the uterus. This <u>ectopic pregnancy</u> can implant in the fallopian tube, on the ovary, in the abdominal cavity or peritoneum, or in the cervix. The most common place to find an ectopic pregnancy is in the fallopian tube (referred to as a tubal pregnancy). During the first trimester, the embryo grows rapidly. It quickly grows into the walls of the fallopian tube, where it causes tearing and finally ruptures the tube. As this occurs, the woman usually feels lower abdominal pain and cramping. She usually, but not always, has vaginal bleeding. Depending on

Terminology Tips

Ectopic means outside of the normal area. An *ectopic pregnancy* occurs when the embryo implants in an area outside of the uterus. Implantation in a fallopian tube is most common and is referred to as a "tubal pregnancy."

where the embryo implants, the bleeding may be internal or external and may be scant or profuse. This is probably the most life-threatening emergency for the pregnant woman during the first trimester. The embryo will not survive and must be removed to save the woman. If the fallopian tube actually ruptures, she will present to you in severe shock and possibly cardiac arrest from massive hemorrhage.

The treatment of the patient with a suspected ectopic pregnancy is focused on supporting the ABCs. She should receive high-flow oxygen, at least one large-bore (14- or 16-gauge) IV line of an isotonic crystalloid, and rapid transport to a hospital that can provide immediate surgery. If she is already in shock, she should receive 20-mL/kg fluid boluses to maintain perfusion and receive airway management as indicated.

Hypertension

In the United States, one out of every 10 to 20 women will experience some degree of hypertension during pregnancy. In some women, this is a preexisting condition; the woman had hypertension before she became pregnant. In other women, hypertension is the result of a condition called preeclampsia, also referred to as pregnancy-induced hypertension (PIH). The most common of these hypertensive disorders of pregnancy is preeclampsia. Preeclampsia is an increase in blood pressure after the 20th week of gestation. It is accompanied by a protein release in the urine and often by edema, particularly in the upper body. The protein in the urine will not typically be detected by EMS and edema can be normal for the pregnant woman. The most important feature of preeclampsia for the EMT-I to recognize is hypertension. In the first trimester the blood pressure typically increases slightly; it decreases below the baseline during the second trimester, and returns to the baseline during the third trimester. It is important to obtain an accurate blood pressure in order to suspect preeclampsia and determine the patient's baseline blood pressure before becoming pregnant. You should suspect preeclampsia if the blood pressure of a woman in her second or third trimester is above 140 systolic or 90 diastolic. If she had hypertension before becoming pregnant, an increase of 30 mm Hg systolic or 15 mm Hg diastolic over that blood pressure is clinically significant.

Preeclampsia is characterized by the following signs and symptoms:
- Headache
- Swelling in the hands, face, and feet
- Anxiety
- Nausea/vomiting

In severe preeclampsia, you may also find:
- Pulmonary edema/shortness of breath
- Confusion or other altered level of consciousness
- Visual disturbances, like blurry vision or scotomata (seeing spots)
- Upper abdominal pain
- Myoclonus (hyperactive reflexes)

Preeclampsia can cause a decrease in perfusion to the fetus as a result of the vasospasm that causes the increase in blood pressure. There is also the risk of fetal cerebral hemorrhage from the hypertension. Preeclampsia is most life-threatening to the fetus and woman if seizures occur.

Eclampsia is a seizure in a pregnant woman who has preeclampsia and no other cause for the seizure. A woman who is an epileptic and has a seizure may or may not be eclamptic. Eclampsia may occur before labor, during labor, or after delivery of the infant. A woman may have only one seizure or may have continuous or multiple seizures (status epilepticus).

The treatment of a woman with preeclampsia is mostly supportive. You should ensure adequate breathing, oxygenation, and circulation and try to keep the patient calm. The patient should be kept in a position of comfort and monitored closely. At a minimum, she should receive supplemental oxygen to prevent fetal distress and an IV line at a keep-vein-open rate for medication administration if it becomes necessary.

If a seizure occurs, you must protect the patient from being injured during the seizure. Administer oxygen and maintain an open airway. You should be ready to provide suctioning or other aggressive airway maneuvers, if necessary.

Place the patient on a cardiac monitor and consider intubation if needed to control the airway. Medical control or local protocol will likely direct you to administer magnesium sulfate to the patient in eclampsia. The recommended dose is 2 to 4 g (diluted in 50 to 100 mL of normal saline) administered by slow IV bolus over 5 minutes. The mechanism of action for magnesium is unknown when administered for eclampsia, but may be because of its CNS depressant properties.

If magnesium sulfate is unsuccessful at terminating the seizure, or if it recurs, you may need to administer diazepam (Valium). The dose of Valium varies but is most commonly administered at 5 to 10 mg via slow (over 1 to 2 minutes) IV administration.

Supine Hypotensive Syndrome

Another common finding in the pregnant patient is hypotension when lying supine, called supine hypotensive syndrome or vena cava compression syndrome, which may be an issue when a woman is injured and must be immobilized. This happens mainly in the second and third trimesters of pregnancy when the woman lies supine and is a result of compression of the inferior vena cava by the weight of the gravid uterus. The condition is most easily treated by placing the woman onto her left side, which causes the uterus to shift off of the vena cava. This simple maneuver will cause an increase in cardiac output, thereby increasing maternal blood pressure and perfusion. If the patient must be immobilized on the long backboard, you should place blanket rolls or something similar under the right side of the board. The patient is placed on her left side because the inferior vena cava is found slightly right of midline on most people.

Gestational Diabetes

Another possible complication of pregnancy is gestational diabetes. During pregnancy, some women develop a problem metabolizing carbohydrates. In this condition, the pancreas will still secrete insulin; however, progesterone (the pregnancy hormone) makes the cells resistant to the uptake of the insulin. As a result, the patient's blood glucose levels rise because the glucose cannot enter the cells. To compensate for this increase, the body secretes more insulin. Gestational diabetes predisposes the patient to the same complications associated with diabetes mellitus (DM)—hyperglycemia or hypoglycemia. Usually, gestational diabetes spontaneously resolves following delivery; however, the patient may be prone to DM later in life.

A woman who has diabetes may also become pregnant. The increase in energy required for maternal health and fetal growth may cause fluctuations in her blood glucose levels. She may require a special diet or a change in medications or dosages.

The EMT-I should be aware of the possibility of diabetes complicating a pregnancy. If you encounter a woman who is pregnant with an altered or decreased mental status, you should suspect diabetes and check her blood glucose level. If hypoglycemia is present, administer 25 g of dextrose 50% IV. This should be given slowly through a large IV line. If hyperglycemia or diabetic ketoacidosis (DKA) is present, crystalloid fluid boluses may be necessary to treat the associated dehydration. Several fluid boluses may be required, as DKA is commonly associated with severe hypovolemia, possibly even shock. IV fluids will also promote the excretion of excess glucose from the body.

If a woman with preexisting or gestational diabetes does not control her blood glucose levels throughout her pregnancy, she may have problems during labor and delivery. The fetus may grow to a larger than average size. If the fetus grows too large, it may not fit through the birth canal, a shoulder may become stuck on the inside of the cervix or it may be injured during the delivery. Additionally, diabetes (gestational or DM) in a pregnant woman predisposes the newborn to hypoglycemia.

Late Pregnancy Complications

In the later stages of pregnancy, problems may occur with the placenta that may pose a risk to the health of the fetus or woman. Sometimes when the fetus implants in the uterus, the placenta starts to grow at the bottom of the uterus over the cervical os. This condition, called placenta previa, usually causes no problems until the pregnancy is near term and the fetus starts to descend into the birth canal (Figure 29-11). When the fetus

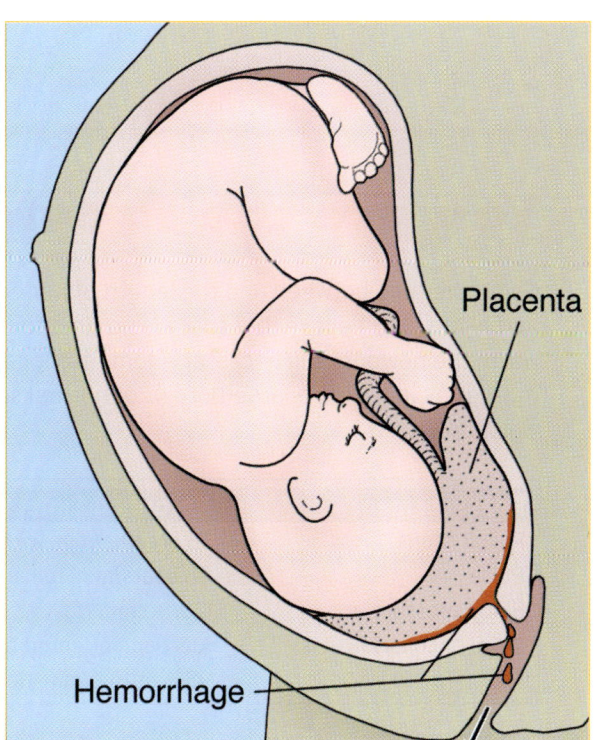

Figure 29-11 In placenta previa, the placenta develops over and covers the cervix.

descends, the uterus starts to contract and the cervical os starts to dilate. As a result, small blood vessels are torn and the patient may have some hemorrhage. This bleeding is usually external through the vagina and is typically bright red. This bleeding is usually, though not always, painless. The patient may show signs of shock depending on how much blood is lost.

Another problem that can occur with the placenta is more commonly life threatening, especially for the fetus. The placenta can separate from the endometrium before labor or delivery. Because of the many blood vessels that attach the two, this can result in severe hemorrhage. Depending on the position of the bleeding compared to the position of the placenta, hemorrhaging may be internal or external. This condition, called abruptio placentae or placental abruption, can occur spontaneously as a result of maternal hypertension, trauma, or maternal cocaine use Figure 29-12 . It most commonly occurs during the third trimester of pregnancy. A patient with an abruption typically presents with severe abdominal pain commonly described as a tearing sensation and dark venous blood from the vagina and often will appear sicker than what you would expect from the amount of external blood loss that you see.

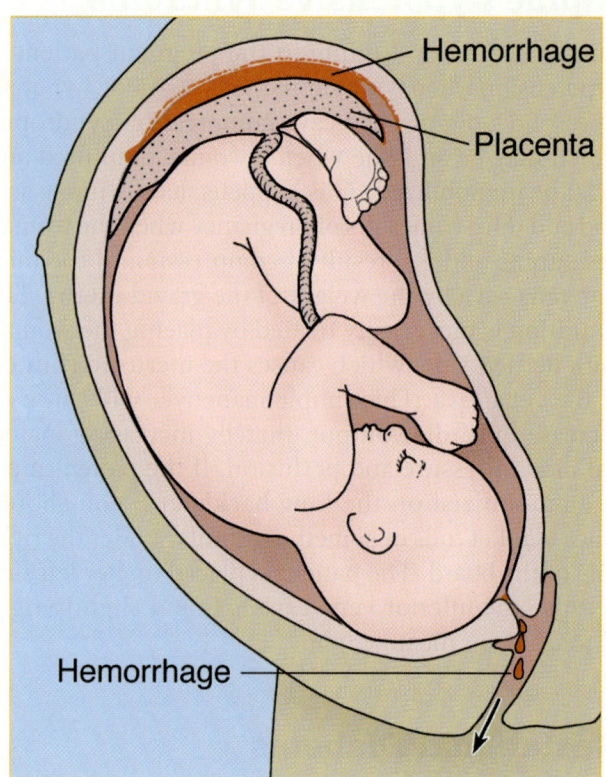

Figure 29-12 In placenta abruptio, the placenta separates prematurely from the walls of the uterus.

You are the Provider — Part 3

Given the time between and the length of her contractions along with her history of multiple pregnancies and births, you believe that there is no time to transport. You prepare your equipment to suction, dry, and warm the newborn (all necessary items are located in your sterile OB kit). Your partner takes care of the mother by initiating a large-bore IV of normal saline in her left arm and helping her disrobe from the waist down.

Reassessment	Recording Time: 10 Minutes After Patient Contact
Respirations	36 breaths/min, with adequate tidal volume
Pulse	118 beats/min, full and regular
Blood pressure	126/80 mm Hg
Level of consciousness	Alert and oriented to person, place, time, and event
Sao$_2$	98% at 15 L/min, nonrebreathing mask

6. What items will you need to assist in the birth of the baby?
7. If delivery was not imminent, how would you transport her and why?
8. What are some actions you can take before the call to prepare for deliveries in the field?

Significant amounts of blood can leak internally into the abdomen, and peritonitis (inflammation of the peritoneum) may develop. You may find that the abdomen is distended beyond normal, although this is a subjective assessment in a woman who is pregnant.

Any trauma to which the pregnant woman is exposed is dangerous to both her and the fetus. Any pregnant woman involved in a motor vehicle crash, fall, assault, or other injury must be evaluated in the emergency department. Even a minor slip and fall or car crash can result in serious trauma to the fetus. Along with a placental abruption, one of the most serious injuries that can occur from trauma is a uterine rupture, which usually results from blunt trauma to the abdomen. The uterine wall tears and the fetus and amniotic fluid are exposed to the internal abdomen of the woman. This causes significant bleeding that may be internal, external, or both. One possible sign of uterine rupture is being able to palpate fetal body parts through the abdominal wall. In a normal pregnancy, because of the muscular uterus, you cannot feel specific parts of the fetus easily. The patient usually complains of severe abdominal pain, and the abdomen may be rigid from peritonitis.

The treatment for any of the previously described complications in late pregnancy is similar. For placenta previa, abruption, and uterine rupture, you treat the woman symptomatically. Administer high-flow oxygen or assisted ventilation if needed. If the patient presents with signs and symptoms of shock, administer crystalloid fluid boluses of 20 mL/kg and provide rapid transport to the hospital. In choosing your transport destination, keep in mind that your patient may require surgical intervention. This may alter your destination depending on local protocol.

When a pregnant woman's system is stressed from shock, the body will attempt to save itself. The patient may shunt blood away from the uterus and fetus to maintain adequate blood flow to her own vital organs. The best way to save the fetus in this situation is to save the woman. If the woman dies, the chance for survival of the fetus is poor. The most important care you can provide therefore includes airway management, high-flow oxygen, adequate fluid resuscitation, and rapid transport.

Stages of Labor

There are three stages of labor. The first stage begins with the onset of contractions and ends when the cervix is fully effaced and dilated; however, because prehospital providers are not trained or authorized to assess for cervical effacement and dilation, the end of the first stage of labor is typically determined in the field by the presence of crowning, when the baby's head is visible at the vaginal opening.

Because the cervix has to be stretched thin by uterine contractions until the opening is large enough for the infant to pass through into the vagina, the first stage is usually the longest. The average length of the first stage of labor is 12.5 hours for the nulliparous patient and 7 hours in the multiparous patient. The second stage of labor is from the point of full cervical effacement and dilation (or crowning [in the field]) until the baby is delivered. The average length of time for the second stage of labor is 80 minutes for the nulliparous patient and 30 minutes for the multiparous patient. The third stage of labor begins with the delivery of the baby and ends with the delivery of the placenta. This stage takes an average of 20 to 30 minutes. Occasionally the placenta is delivered immediately after the baby is delivered. You may not know what stage the woman is in unless the baby's head is crowning or the baby has already delivered. Questioning the woman and visually inspecting the vaginal area for the presence of crowning are usually your only sources of information regarding the stage of labor the patient is in.

The onset of labor starts with contractions of the uterus. As the fetus descends into the birth canal (vagina), the pressure on the amniotic sac causes its rupture (rupture of membranes [ROM]). This is the release of the amniotic fluid that has cushioned the fetus during development.

If you were not present when the rupture of membranes occurred, you should ask if there was a foul odor to the amniotic fluid and determine its color. The fluid should be clear or nearly clear and not have a strong odor. If it is brown or black or has a strong odor, it may be an indication of meconium staining. Meconium, a thick, tarry substance, is the baby's first bowel

EMT-I Tips

Braxton-Hicks contractions, or false labor, can be felt at any time during the pregnancy. The uterus is *practicing* for the actual delivery. The differences between Braxton-Hicks contractions and contractions from actual labor include:

- No regular pattern
- No increase in intensity
- Little or no pain

movement (BM), and can pass into the amniotic fluid. Normally, the baby's first BM occurs within the first 24 hours after delivery. If the fetus is distressed while in utero, the first BM may occur prior to delivery. This causes concern because meconium can be aspirated into the baby's lungs, resulting in potentially life-threatening sepsis. If meconium is present when the baby is born, you may have to alter the sequence of initial resuscitation and perform more invasive suctioning of the trachea. This will be discussed in more detail in Chapter 30: Neonatal Resuscitation.

During the onset of labor, initial uterine contractions are often irregular. The woman may feel only a backache or abdominal cramping. As the labor progresses, the frequency and intensity of contractions increase. As the baby prepares for birth, the uterine contractions become regular and last about 30 to 60 seconds each. The length of labor varies greatly. As a general rule, it is longer in a nulliparous patient and becomes shorter in a multiparous patient. During premature labor, the contractions may not become regular or last as long as contractions in full-term pregnancies. The infant is smaller and does not require as much stretching of the birth canal to pass.

When you are assessing a pregnant woman in labor, you have to determine whether delivery will happen at the scene or if there is time to provide transport to the hospital. Consider delivering an infant at the scene under the following circumstances:

- Delivery is expected within a few minutes (ie, crowning is present)
- A natural disaster, bad weather, or some other type of catastrophe makes it impossible to reach the hospital
- No transportation is available

How do you determine whether delivery is going to occur within a few minutes? First, look for crowning. Second, ask the pregnant woman the following questions:

- How many weeks gestation are you and when are you due?
  - The more premature the infant, the more resuscitation and care it is likely to require. Knowing the gestational age can also help you select the correct-sized equipment for the infant.
- Is this your first baby?
- Are you having contractions? How far apart are the contractions? How long do the contractions last?
  - Contractions are timed from the beginning of one contraction until the beginning of the next. If they are less than 5 minutes apart and regular, delivery may be imminent.
- Do you feel the urge to move your bowels?
  - This indicates that the baby has entered the birth canal and is resting on top of the mother's rectum.
- Have you had any spotting or bleeding?
- Have you had a gushing of fluid from the vagina?
- Were any of your previous children (if she has had any) delivered by cesarean section?

Also consider asking the following questions:

- Have you had a complicated pregnancy is the past?
- Do you use illicit drugs, drink alcohol, or take any medications?
  - Many depressant drugs and alcohol pass through the placental barrier to the fetus. If they have been recently ingested, the baby may be born with respiratory depression and require aggressive resuscitation.
- Is there a possibility that this is a multiple birth?
  - Multiple births are often of lower birth weight and if they require invasive care, you may need additional assistance for each baby in addition to the mother.
- Does your physician expect any complications?
- Have you had routine prenatal care for this pregnancy?

If the patient has already had a child she may be able to tell you when she is about to deliver. If she believes that she is ready, make immediate preparations for delivery.

Preparing for Delivery

If birth is imminent, you should prepare your equipment and the patient for the delivery. Begin by placing the patient on high-flow oxygen by nonrebreathing mask, if this is not already done. Even if your patient is

EMT-I Safety

It is important that you always follow BSI precautions to protect yourself from exposure to body fluids. There is a high potential of exposure to body fluids during childbirth.

Documentation Tips

EDC—*Estimated date of confinement*—This is the due date.
Gravida—number of pregnancies including this one
Para—number of live births
Abortus—number of miscarriages, stillbirths, or surgical abortions

For a patient with a due date of December 25, 2004, who is pregnant for the fourth time, has had two live births, and has had one miscarriage, the documentation would be as follows:
EDC—12/25/04
G-4
P-2
A-1

not currently hypoxic, she will have an oxygen reserve that can protect her and the fetus if complications occur. If there is time, you should start a large-bore IV line of an isotonic crystalloid on the pregnant woman. IV access will be necessary if you have to administer medications or if fluid boluses are needed for excessive postpartum bleeding.

During contractions, inspect the vagina for crowning. Do not touch the vaginal area until you are sure that delivery is imminent. In general, do not touch the vaginal area except during delivery (under certain circumstances) and when your partner is present. Spread the pregnant woman's legs apart gently, explaining that you are doing so to decide whether the baby should be delivered immediately or if she should be transported to the hospital for delivery

Once labor has begun, there is no way it can be slowed down or stopped in the field. Never attempt to hold the pregnant woman's legs together; doing so would only complicate the delivery and cause potential injury to the infant. Do not allow the pregnant woman to get up to go to the bathroom. Instead, reassure her that the sensation of needing to move her bowels is normal and that it means she is about to deliver.

If you decide to deliver the infant at the scene, remember that you are only *assisting* the pregnant woman with the delivery. Your part is to help, guide, and support the infant as it is born. You should use BSI precautions at all times. For childbirth, this means at least gloves, a gown, and goggles or a face shield. Try to limit distractions for yourself and for the patient. You want to appear calm and reassuring while protecting the patient's modesty. If delivery is imminent with crowning, prepare to deliver the baby. If you have concerns about the delivery, you should contact medical control for further guidance. Always recognize your own limitations, and when you are unsure about what to do, transport the patient. If delivery must occur during transport, stop the vehicle and have your partner(s) assist with the delivery. Once delivery of the infant and any needed resuscitation have occurred, you may resume transport to the hospital.

Your emergency vehicle should always be equipped with a sterile emergency OB kit containing the following items **Figure 29-13** ▼:

- Surgical scissors or a scalpel
- Umbilical cord clamps
- Umbilical tape or ties
- A small rubber bulb syringe
- Towels
- 4″ × 4″ gauze sponges and/or 2″ × 10″ gauze sponges
- Sterile gloves
- Infant blanket
- Sanitary napkins
- A neonatal or infant size bag-valve-mask
- Goggles
- A plastic bag
- A gown

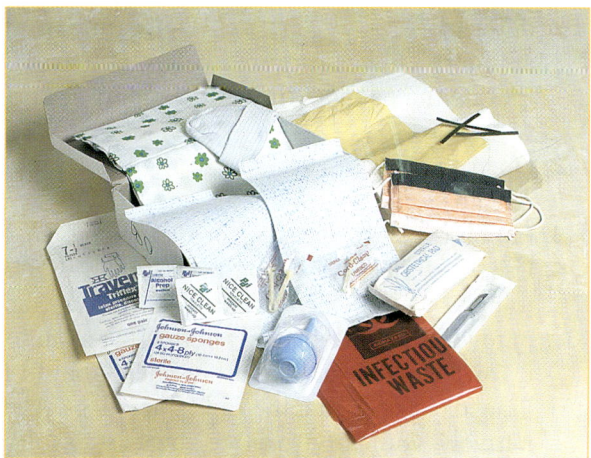

Figure 29-13 Your unit should contain a sterile OB kit. Items usually found in this kit are listed above.

Patient Position

The patient should be disrobed from the waist down. She should have her lower half covered by a sheet or blanket. Try to limit the patient's exposure and preserve her modesty as much as you can while helping her to move into a semi-Fowler's position. Place the patient on a firm surface that is padded with blankets, folded sheets, or towels. Put a pillow or blankets beneath her hips to elevate them about 2″ to 4″. Support the patient's head, neck, and upper back with pillows and blankets. If delivery is occurring in an automobile, the patient should lie on the seat, with one foot on the floor and the other on the seat, with the upper knee and hip bent.

If the emergency delivery is occurring at home, you should move the patient to the floor or other sturdy flat surface. You will find it easier to work on a firm surface than on a bed. Elevate the patient's hips and support her head with pillows. Have her keep her legs and hips flexed, with her feet flat on the surface beneath her and her knees spread apart. Track the progression of the delivery closely at all times. You do not want an abrupt delivery, when the head pops out uncontrollably, to occur. This could result in neck injuries or other injuries to the infant.

Preparing the Delivery Field

Take the following steps to prepare the area where the infant will be born:

1. If there is enough time, place towels or sheets on the floor around the delivery area to help soak up the amniotic fluid that will be released when the amniotic sac ruptures and any blood that comes from the release of the mucous plug or during delivery (Figure 29-14A). Determine if the amniotic sac has ruptured before you arrived. Elevate the patient's hips and support her head with pillows.
2. Open the OB kit carefully so that its contents remain sterile.
3. Put on the sterile gloves, goggles, and gown.
4. Use the sterile sheets and towels from the OB kit to make a sterile delivery field. Place one sheet or towel under the patient's buttocks, and unfold it toward her feet. The other sheet should be draped over her abdomen and upper legs. Alternatively, you can use three sheets: (1) folded under the buttocks, (2) placed between the legs, just below the vagina, and (3) placed across the abdomen (Figure 29-14B).

Delivering the Infant

Your partner should be at the patient's head to comfort, soothe, and reassure her during the delivery. The patient may want to grip someone's hand. She may yell or say nothing at all. During delivery some women will remain very calm while others will have an emotional reaction and cry. It is not uncommon for women to become nauseous, and some may vomit. If this occurs, have your partner turn the patient's head to the side so that her mouth and airway can be cleared with suction, as needed.

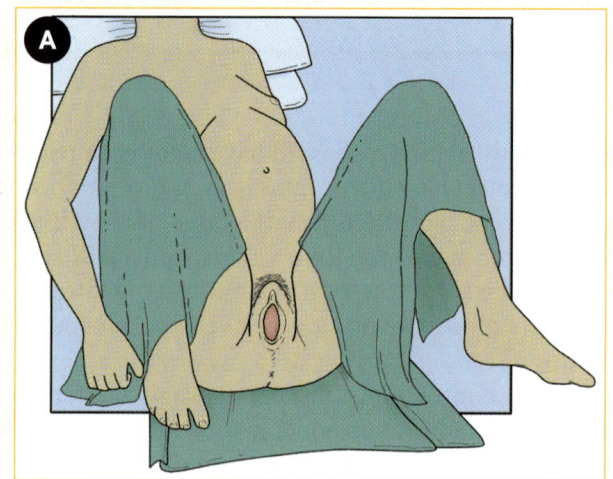

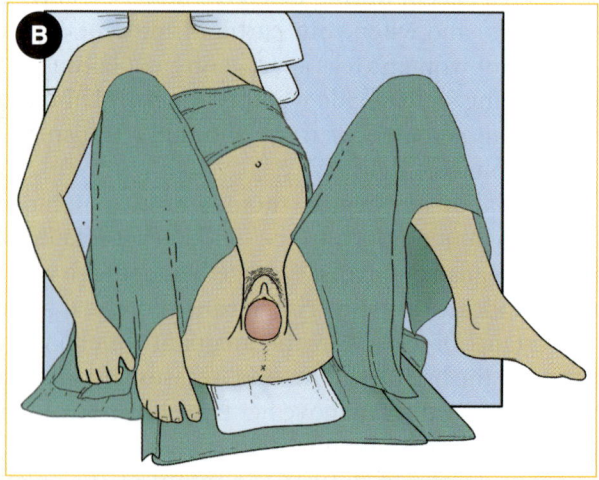

Figure 29-14 Preparing the delivery field. **A.** Place sheets or towels under the mother, elevate the woman's hips, and support her head with one or two pillows. **B.** Use sterile sheets and towels from the OB kit to make a clean delivery field. Place one sheet under her buttocks, drape the other over her abdomen, and place drapes over the thighs.

You must continually assess the patient for crowning. Do not allow an abrupt delivery to occur. Position yourself so that you can see the vagina at all times. Time the patient's contractions from the beginning of one to the beginning of the next to determine the frequency of the contractions. In addition, time the duration of each contraction. You do this by feeling the patient's abdomen from the moment the contraction begins (uterus and abdomen tightening) to the moment it ends (uterus and abdomen relaxing). The full-term delivery usually occurs when the contractions are 1 to 2 minutes apart and last from 30 to 60 seconds. Premature labor may not exhibit this pattern because the infant's smaller size may not require the full coordinated contractions that a larger infant requires. Remind the patient to take quick, short breaths during each contraction but not to strain. In between contractions, encourage the patient to rest and breathe deeply through her mouth.

Follow the steps in **Skill Drill 29-1** to deliver the infant. These steps are described in more detail here.

1. **Allow the patient to push the infant's head out. Support it as it emerges**, placing your gloved hand over the bony parts of the head and applying slight pressure to prevent an explosive delivery. Tell the patient to stop pushing while you suction fluid from the infant's mouth first, then the nostrils using the bulb syringe. Remember to squeeze the syringe before inserting it into the infant's mouth or nose (**Step 1**).
2. **Feel at the neck to see if the cord is wrapped** around it. If it is, gently lift it over the infant's head without pulling hard on the cord. Tell the patient to resume pushing at this point.
3. Once the infant's head is delivered, the upper shoulder will be visible. **Gently guide the head down slightly, if needed, to help deliver that shoulder** (**Step 2**).

You are the Provider — Part 4

While you put on the rest of your PPE, your partner moves the patient to the floor, props her hips up on thick blankets, and drapes her lower body with a sheet. The patient tells you she feels the need to push. With her next contraction, you see a head crowning from the vagina. On her next contraction she pushes, and the head is now out. You instruct her not to push, and you gently support the infant's head while suctioning the mouth then nose. You note no cord around the infant's neck. On the next contraction, you gently guide the infant's head in a downward motion and the top shoulder comes out. With the next contraction comes the other shoulder, then finally the entire infant. You hold the infant in warm, dry blankets and begin to clean him off. You then place the clamps on the umbilical cord, and gently cut it.

Reassessment	Recording Time: 15 Minutes After Patient Contact
Respirations	30 breaths/min, with adequate tidal volume
Pulse	128 beats/min, full and regular
Blood pressure	126/80 mm Hg
Level of consciousness	Alert and oriented to person, place, time, and event
SaO_2	98% at 15 L/min on nonrebreathing mask
First Apgar Score	**Recording Time: 1 Minute After Birth**
Skin color	1
Heart rate	2
Irritability	1
Muscle tone	2
Respiratory effort	2
	Total: 8

9. Because newborns are so susceptible to heat loss, what are some techniques you can utilize?
10. Why is it important to always have your hands on the newborn from the moment of crowning?

4. **Support the head and upper body as the shoulders deliver.** You may need to gently guide the head up slightly to deliver the lower shoulder (**Step 3**).
5. Once the body is delivered, handle the infant firmly but gently. It will be slippery. **Make sure the infant's neck is in a neutral position to keep the airway open** (**Step 4**).
6. **Place the first clamp approximately** 7″ from the infant's body and the second 3″ farther. Once they are firmly in place, cut between the clamps (**Step 5**).
7. **The placenta delivers itself,** usually within 20 to 30 minutes after birth of the baby. Never pull on the end of the umbilical cord in an attempt to speed delivery of the placenta (**Step 6**).

Delivering the Head

Watch the infant's head as it begins to exit the vagina; it must be supported as it emerges. It may take two, three, or more contractions for the delivery of the head to occur from the time it begins to crown. Once it is obvious that the head is coming out farther with each contraction, you should place your gloved hand over the emerging bony parts of the head and exert very gentle pressure on it, decreasing the pressure slightly between contractions. This will allow the head to come out smoothly, preventing an explosive delivery and the possibility of trauma to the baby. You should position yourself between the patient's legs during delivery. Be careful that you do not poke your fingers into the infant's eyes or into the fontanelles on the head. The anterior fontanelle is located at the front of the head, near the brow, and the posterior fontanelle is near the back of the head. The brain is covered only by skin and membranes at these spots.

Gentle pressure, exerted horizontally across the perineum with a sterile gauze pad, may reduce the risk of perineal tearing as the infant is emerging (Figure 29-15▶). Also be prepared for the possibility that the patient may have a bowel movement because of pressure on the rectum.

Unruptured Amniotic Sac

Usually, the amniotic sac will break or rupture at the beginning of labor. The sac may also rupture during contractions. If the amniotic sac has not ruptured by this point, it will appear as a fluid-filled sac (like a water balloon) emerging from the vagina. This situation is serious, as the sac will suffocate the infant if it is not removed. If it has not spontaneously ruptured, you may puncture the sac by pulling it away from the infant and tearing it with your fingers or a clamp, away from the infant's face, only as the head is crowning, not before. As the sac is punctured, amniotic fluid will gush out. Push the ruptured sac away from the infant's face as the head is delivered. Clear the infant's mouth and nose immediately, using the bulb syringe and gauze sponge.

If the amniotic fluid is green or brown instead of clear or has a foul odor, suspect meconium staining. Meconium can cause two problems: a depressed newborn and airway obstruction. If an infection has resulted from meconium aspiration prior to birth, the infant may respond only to prolonged resuscitation or may not respond at all.

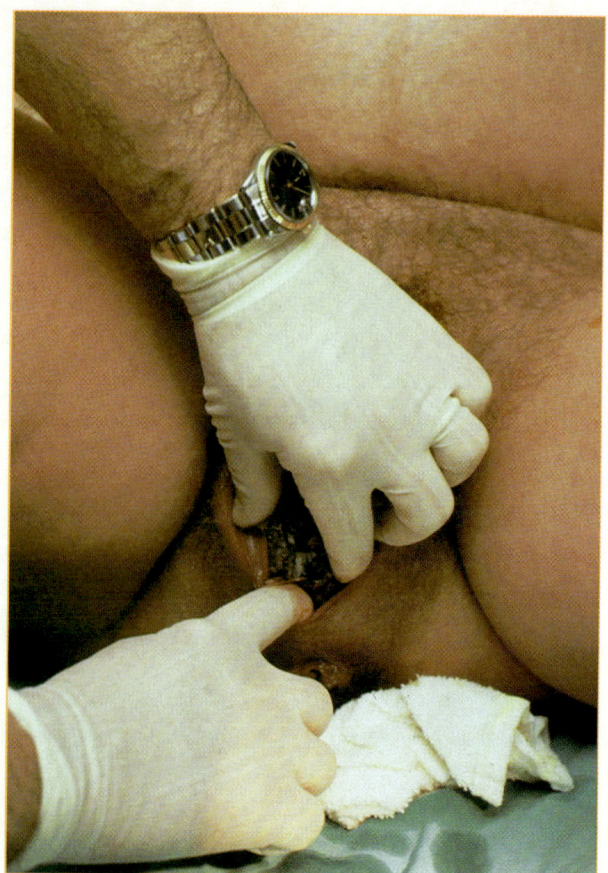

Figure 29-15 Applying gentle pressure on the perineum may reduce the risk of tearing as the infant emerges.

Delivering the Infant

Skill Drill 29-1

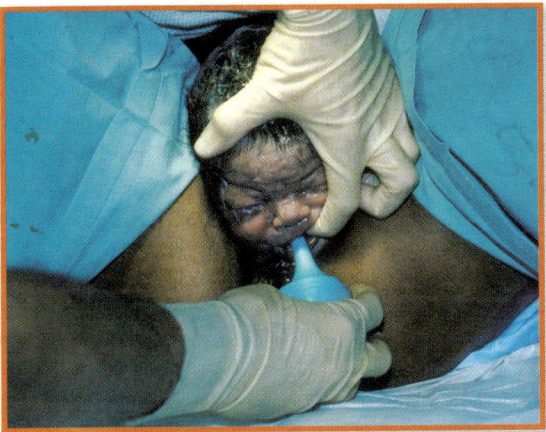

1 Support the bony parts of the head with your hands as it emerges. Suction fluid from the mouth, then the nostrils.

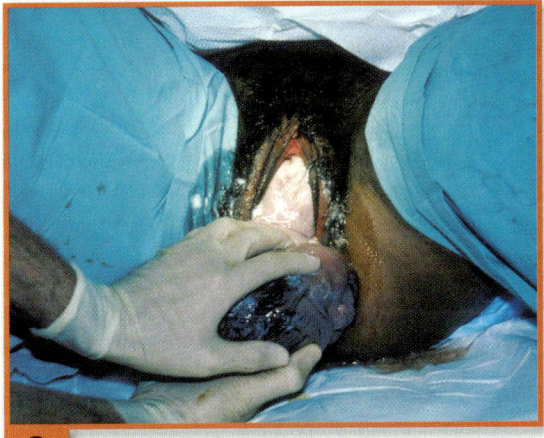

2 As the upper shoulder appears, guide the head down slightly, if needed, to help deliver the shoulder.

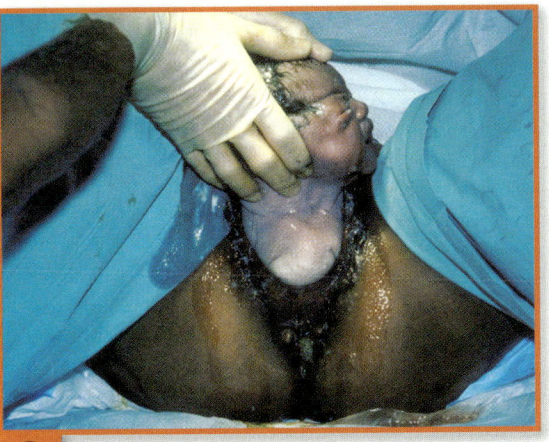

3 Support the head and upper body as the shoulders deliver. Guide the head up slightly if needed to deliver the lower shoulder.

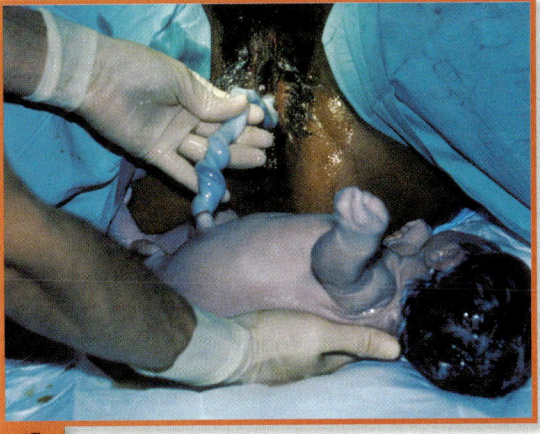

4 Handle the slippery delivered infant firmly but gently, keeping the neck in neutral position to maintain the airway.

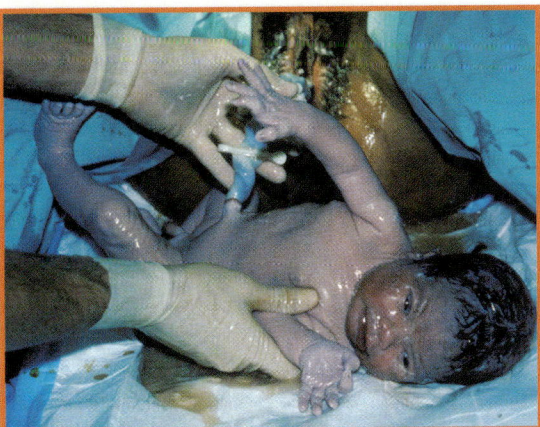

5 Place the first clamp 7" from the infant's body and the second 3" farther and cut between them.

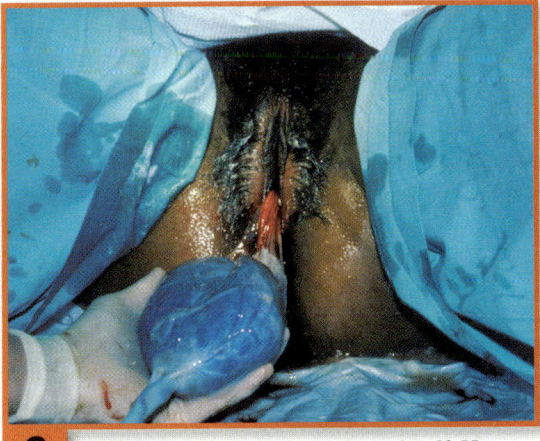

6 Allow the placenta to deliver itself. Never pull on the cord to speed up placental delivery.

Thick meconium can obstruct the airway of the newborn. Suctioning the baby's mouth and oropharynx before delivery of the body may prevent some meconium aspiration. Recent research has shown, however, that meconium aspiration usually happens days to weeks before birth. The resulting infection can develop into a serious pneumonia that usually requires advanced treatment in the neonatal intensive care unit (NICU). If thick meconium is present, you may need to perform direct tracheal suctioning using a meconium aspirator. The steps required for this will be explained in Chapter 30: Neonatal Resuscitation.

Umbilical Cord Around the Neck

Once the infant's head has been delivered, it usually rotates to one side. As soon as the head is delivered, use the index finger of one hand to feel whether the umbilical cord is wrapped around the neck while your other hand supports the head. The cord wrapped around the neck is called a nuchal cord. It is usually loose and easy to remove from around the infant's neck; simply slip the cord gently over the infant's head or shoulder. A nuchal cord that is wound tightly around the neck could cause the infant to asphyxiate. It must therefore be released from the neck immediately. If you cannot slide the cord over the infant's head, you must cut it before the delivery can continue. Start by placing two clamps 2″ apart on the cord and cutting between the clamps. If the cord is wrapped more than once around the neck, a rare event, you must clamp and cut only once. Once you have cut the cord, unwrap it from around the neck. Handle the cord very carefully; it is fragile and easily torn. If it does tear, severe hemorrhage can occur from the mother, infant, or both. Fortunately, the cord is usually not wrapped around the infant's neck and does not have to be clamped and cut until after the entire infant has been born. However, you must always check for the presence of a nuchal cord.

Now that you have delivered the infant's head (and removed the cord if needed), suction the amniotic fluid from the infant's airway before the delivery proceeds. You must ask the mother not to push while you are doing this, although her desire to do so will be very strong. While supporting the infant's head with one hand, quickly suction the fluid from the mouth and then the nose. If you suction the nose first, you may stimulate the infant to breathe, resulting in potential aspiration of the fluid in the mouth. Since infants are nose breathers, stimulation of the nose may cause a gasping response. When you suction the airway, fully compress the bulb syringe before it is inserted into the infant's mouth. Release the bulb to suction fluids and mucus into the syringe. Make sure the syringe does not touch the soft tissues of the mouth and nose. Discard the fluid into a towel, and repeat the procedure, suctioning the mouth and nose two or three times each, or until they are clear.

In the Field

Keep a towel or sheet handy to wipe your hands and to help hold the infant because it will be very slippery. Some EMT-Is will wrap 2″ tape backwards around their gloved hands to provide a better gripping surface.

Delivering the Body

By the time you are finished suctioning, the mother will probably be pushing again, and the infant's shoulder will be visible in the vagina. The infant's head is the largest part of the body. Once the head is delivered, the rest of the infant usually delivers easily. Support the head and upper body as the shoulders deliver. Do not pull the infant from the birth canal. When the abdomen and hips appear, support them with your other hand. Grasp the infant's feet as they are born. Handle the infant firmly but carefully. It will be slippery and usually covered with a harmless, white, cheesy substance called vernix caseosa.

Postdelivery Care

As soon as the entire infant is born, dry the infant off and wrap it immediately in a blanket or towel, and place it on one side, with the head slightly lower than the rest of its body. Wrap the infant so that only the face is exposed, making sure that the top of the head is covered. Make sure that the infant's neck is in a neutral position to maintain an open airway. Newborns are very sensitive to cold, so if it is at all possible, you should keep the blanket or towel warm before you use it. Use a sterile gauze pad to gently wipe the infant's mouth, and again suction the mouth and nose. Suctioning the nose is particularly important, since infants breathe through their noses. If you prefer, you can pick up and cradle the infant in your arm at the level of the mother's vagina while doing this, but always keep the head slightly downward to help prevent aspiration. After suctioning, keep the infant at the same level as the mother's vagina until the umbilical cord is cut. If the infant is higher than the vagina, blood will be transfused back through the umbilical cord to the placenta, resulting in fetal hypovolemia.

A newborn's body temperature can drop very quickly, so dry and wrap the infant as soon as possible. Only then will you clamp and cut the umbilical cord. Once the infant is born, the umbilical cord is of no further use to either mother or infant.

Postdelivery care of the umbilical cord is important, as infection is easily transmitted through the cord to the baby. Using the two clamps from the OB kit, clamp the cord between the mother and the infant, about 7" from the infant. Place the second clamp about 3" farther than the first clamp. Once the clamps are firmly in place, carefully cut the cord between them with sterile scissors or a scalpel, using great care. Remember the cord is fragile. If handled roughly, it could be torn from the infant's abdomen, resulting in fatal hemorrhage. Once the clamps are in place, there is no need to rush.

> ### 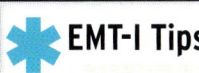 EMT-I Tips
>
> As a infant delivers, you must divide your attention between two patients. This can keep two EMT-Is busy, even when things go well. To ensure that the needs of one patient do not result in neglecting the other patient, designate one member of the crew to provide primary care to each patient. Call for help early if you suspect that both patients will need special care, or that one will require resuscitation.

> ### Documentation Tips
>
> Recording time of birth will ensure that the information is available for the birth certificate. It also provides you with a starting point from which to time the intervals for Apgar scores. This is even more important with multiple births. You will be busy; consider asking a family member to act as "timekeeper."

You are the Provider — Part 5

You now pick up the patient and place her on the gurney. You give the infant to the mother and encourage her to breast-feed. You assist with the delivery of the placenta en route to the hospital and note no significant bleeding from the mother during transport. Shortly before arrival at the hospital, you reassess the mother and the infant's Apgar score.

Reassessment	Recording Time: 20 Minutes After Patient Contact
Respirations	24 breaths/min, with adequate tidal volume
Pulse	112 beats/min, full and regular
Blood pressure	118/70 mm Hg
Level of consciousness	Alert and oriented to person, place, time, and event
SaO_2	98% at 15 L/min on nonrebreathing mask
Apgar Score	**Recording Time: 5 Minutes After Birth**
Skin color	2
Heart rate	2
Irritability	2
Muscle tone	2
Respiratory effort	2
	Total: 10

11. Why is it important to transport after delivery of the infant?
12. If the newborn is depressed, what are common methods of stimulation?

After you have cut the cord, tie the end coming from the infant. If it was a nuchal cord, now is the time to tie it. Do not use ordinary string, twine, or any type of wire; these materials may cut through the soft, fragile tissues of the cord. Place a loop of the special "umbilical tape" around the cord about 1" nearer to the infant than to the clamp. Tighten the tape slowly so that it does not cut the cord, and then tie firmly with a square knot. Cut the ends of the tape, but do not remove either clamp. The part of the cord that is protruding from the mother's vagina will be delivered when the placenta delivers.

By now, the infant should be pinkish and breathing on his or her own. You can now give the infant, wrapped in a warm blanket, to your partner; and he or she can monitor the infant and complete the infant's initial care. You should reassess the mother and prepare for delivery of the placenta. If the mother's condition is stable, you may give the infant to her. She may want to begin breast-feeding the infant.

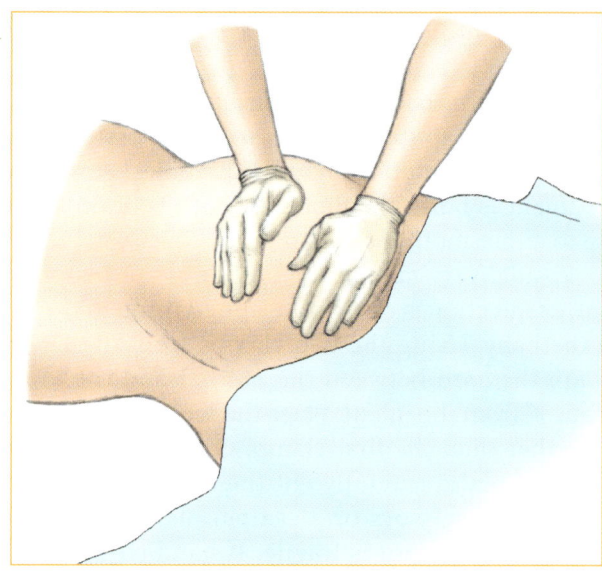

Figure 29-16 To massage the uterus, place one hand with fingers fully extended just above the mother's pubic bone and use your other hand to press down into the abdomen and gently massage the uterus in a circular motion until it becomes firm.

Delivery of the Placenta

The placenta is attached to the end of the umbilical cord that is coming out of the mother's vagina. As with the infant, you need only assist with the delivery. The uterus will deliver the placenta. This usually happens within a few minutes of the birth, although it may take as long as 30 minutes. Never pull on the end of the umbilical cord in an attempt to speed delivery of the placenta. This can cause tearing of the cord, the placenta, or both, and cause serious, perhaps life-threatening, hemorrhage.

The normal placenta is round, about 7" in diameter and about 1" thick. The side that faces toward the fetus while in utero is smooth and covered with a shiny membrane; the side that attaches to the uterine wall is rough and divided into lobes. Wrap the entire placenta and umbilical cord in a towel and place them in the plastic bag. The placenta and remaining cord must be transported to the hospital. Hospital personnel will examine them to make certain that the entire placenta has been delivered. If a piece of the placenta has been retained inside the mother, it could cause persistent bleeding or infection.

After delivery of the placenta and before transport, place a sterile pad or sanitary napkin over the vagina and straighten the mother's legs. You can help to slow postpartum bleeding by gently massaging the uterine fundus with a firm, circular motion; this will promote uterine contraction **Figure 29-16**. If the mother breast-feeds the infant, this can also help slow the postpartum vaginal bleeding. Both massaging the uterus and having the baby stimulate the mother's nipples by nursing will cause a release of <u>oxytocin</u>. This is a hormone produced in the posterior pituitary gland that will help to contract the uterus and slow bleeding.

Some bleeding, usually less than 500 mL, occurs before the placenta delivers. The following are emergency situations:

- More than 30 minutes elapse, and the placenta has not delivered.
- There is more than 500 mL of bleeding before delivery of the placenta.
- There is significant bleeding after the delivery of the placenta.

If one of these events occur, provide rapid transport of the mother and infant to the hospital. Place a sterile pad or sanitary napkin over the mother's vagina to collect any blood. Never pack the vagina with dressings in an attempt to control the hemorrhage; these will only have to be removed at the hospital. Besides, the bleeding is coming from a source that you cannot control. Place the mother in the shock position (legs elevated 6" to 12"), apply a blanket to keep her warm, and administer 100% oxygen and isotonic fluid boluses (20 mL/kg) to maintain perfusion.

EMT-I Tips

During an abnormal or complicated delivery, you should call early for paramedic assistance and contact medical control as needed.

Abnormal or Complicated Delivery Emergencies

Most infants deliver head first and without any problems. Occasionally you may be called to help a woman with an abnormal delivery. These problems are rare, but can be life-threatening for both the woman and infant. You should call early for paramedic assistance and contact medical control as needed. The definitive treatment for many of these problems is a cesarean section; therefore, rapid transport to the hospital is crucial to the survival of the infant. This section will prepare you to provide the best care possible for patients with abnormal or complicated deliveries and know when to initiate rapid transport rather than attempt delivery at the scene.

Breech Delivery

The presentation is the position in which an infant is born—the part of the body that comes out first. Most infants are born head first, or a vertex presentation. Occasionally, the buttocks or both feet come out first. This is called a breech presentation (Figure 29-17 ▶). The infant who presents breech is at greater risk for delivery trauma. Prolapsed umbilical cords (the umbilical cord comes out of the vagina before the infant) are more common in breech deliveries. Fortunately, breech deliveries are usually slow and there is time to get the patient to the hospital. If the infant's buttocks have already passed through the vagina, delivery is under way, and you must prepare to assist. You should call for paramedic backup and contact medical control if time is available. In general, if the mother does not deliver within 10 minutes of the buttocks presentation, provide rapid transport. You should have medical control guide you in this difficult situation. The infant that presents breech can deliver vaginally, but often requires advanced assistance that cannot be provided in the prehospital setting.

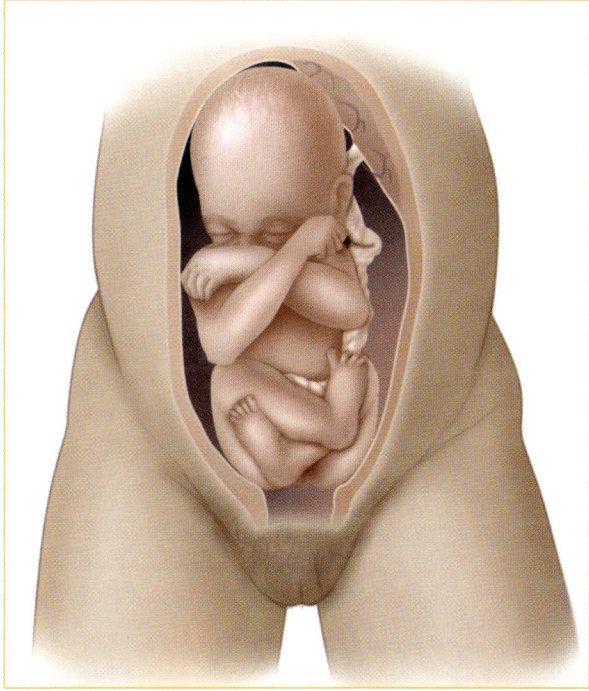

Figure 29-17 An infant in a breech presentation presents with the buttocks first. Breech deliveries are usually slow, so you will often have time to transport the patient to the hospital.

The preparations for a breech delivery are the same as those for a vertex delivery. Position the patient, unwrap the emergency delivery kit, and place yourself and your partner as you would for a normal delivery. Allow the buttocks and legs to deliver spontaneously, supporting them with your hand to prevent rapid expulsion. The buttocks will usually come out easily. Let the legs dangle on either side of your arm while you support the trunk and chest as they are delivered. The head is almost always face down and should be allowed to deliver spontaneously. If the delivery of the head stalls, you must keep the infant's airway open: Make a "V" with your gloved fingers, and place them into the vagina. You must push the walls of the vagina away from the mouth and nose of the infant. This is a true emergency and requires rapid transport. *Breech presentation is one of only two circumstances in which you should put your fingers into the vagina.*

Limb Presentations

On rare occasions, the presenting part of the infant is neither the head nor buttocks, but is a single arm, leg, or foot. This is called a limb presentation

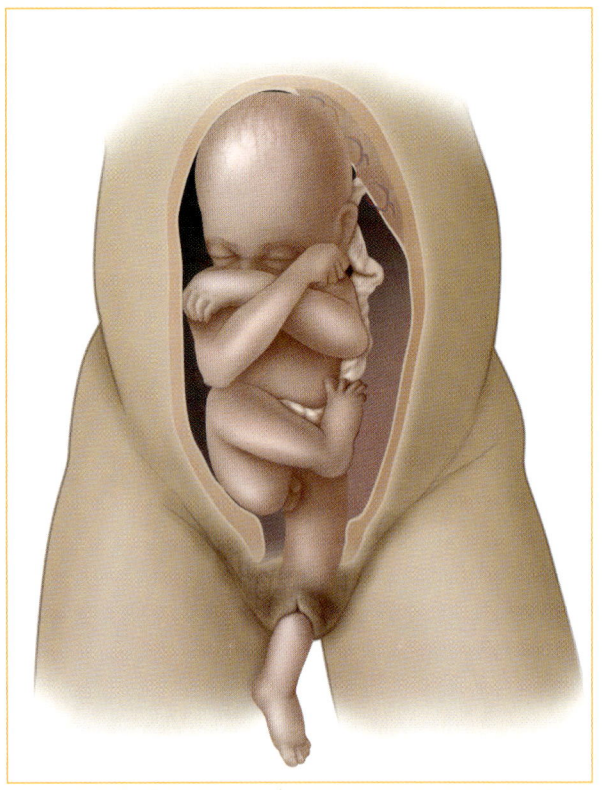

Figure 29-18 In very rare instances, an infant's limb, usually a single arm or leg, presents first. This is a very serious situation, and you must provide prompt transport for hospital delivery.

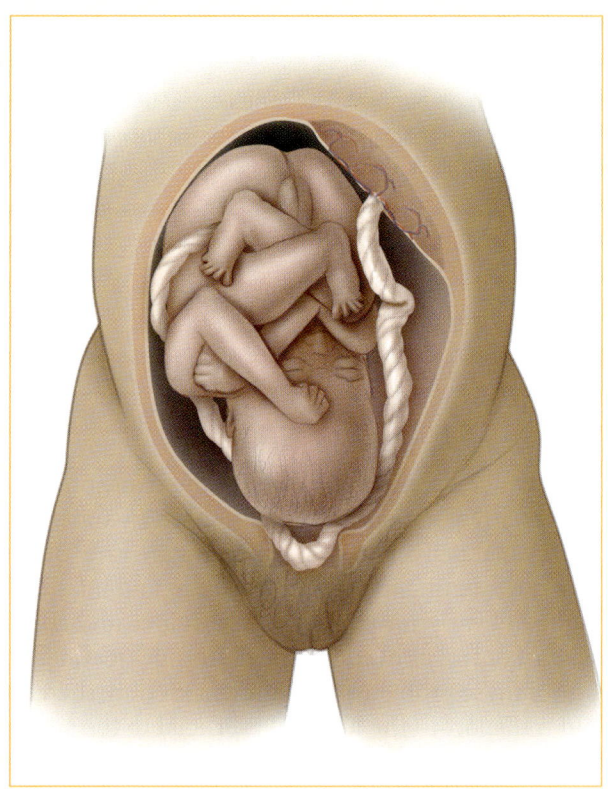

Figure 29-19 A prolapsed umbilical cord, another rare situation, is very dangerous and must be cared for at the hospital.

Figure 29-18 ▲). You cannot successfully deliver such as presentation in the field. These infants must be delivered surgically in the hospital. If you are faced with a limb presentation, you must transport the patient to the hospital immediately. If a limb is protruding, cover it with a sterile towel. Never try to push it back in, and never pull on it. Place the mother on her back with her head down and hips elevated. One of your goals is to prevent further trauma to the infant that could result from the patient's continued pushing. Your other goal is to transport the patient rapidly and safely to the hospital. Contact medical control and the receiving hospital to make certain they are prepared for your arrival. You should administer high-flow oxygen to the woman and closely monitor her condition en route.

Prolapsed Cord Presentation

Another rare presentation that may occur is the prolapse of the umbilical cord. When it occurs, the prolapsed cord usually presents when the amniotic sac ruptures. If the umbilical cord comes out of the vagina before the infant, the blood supply to the infant may be interrupted (Figure 29-19 ▲). As the infant starts to exit the cervix, the cord will be pressed against the pelvis. This can slow or stop the blood supply to and from the infant. This is another presentation that requires surgical intervention.

Your goal in the treatment of this patient is to prevent the woman from pushing and compressing the umbilical cord. If possible, place the patient in Trendelenburg's position, with her head down and lower extremities elevated. You may also use pillows or folded sheets to accomplish this position. Alternatively, the patient may be placed in a knee-chest position—kneeling and bent forward, face down. Either of these positions is meant to use gravity to help keep the weight of the infant off of the prolapsed cord.

You must now insert a gloved hand into the vagina and gently push the presenting part away from the umbilical cord. You should push with only enough pressure to keep the pulsations in the umbilical cord. You should be very careful because too much pressure could cause head or neck damage to the infant. *Note that this is the only other time you should insert your hand into the vagina.*

Do not attempt to push the cord back into the vagina. Wrap a sterile towel, moistened with saline, around the exposed cord. Administer high-flow oxygen to the patient and transport her rapidly. You may also try to have the patient take short, panting breaths, which may prevent full contractions and the urge to push.

Prolapsed Uterus

Another complication that may occur is a prolapsed or inverted uterus. While uncommon, it may be the result of a rapid delivery or pulling on the umbilical cord prior to delivery of the placenta. If the uterus prolapses, appropriate care includes **one** attempt at replacement by using the *palm* of the hand to try and push it back inside the body. If this does not work, cover it with moist dressings and transport while providing supportive care. Never use your fingers to try and replace a prolapsed uterus as this may cause it to tear and result in massive hemorrhage.

EMT-I Tips

There are only two instances when you should insert your hand inside the patient's vagina.

- Breech delivery when the head will not deliver—Use your first two fingers to make a "V" over the infant's face and nose to push the wall of the vagina away from the infant's face and allow the infant to breathe. You may also place oxygen tubing in the palm of your hand to provide blow-by oxygen to the infant.
- Cord presentation and the weight of the baby is cutting off blood flow—Insert your hand and gently lift the head off of the cord to allow blood flow to the infant. You should feel the pulse return in the cord when the pressure is removed.

You are the Provider

1. What considerations should be made before your arrival?

A discussion about how you will approach the call should occur between you and your partner. This discussion should include who will care for the woman and who will deliver the newborn (should it become necessary). A call to the hospital would also be appropriate so the hospital can notify their OB staff.

2. What do you anticipate with her age and time between contractions?

Given her age, she is more likely to have had previous pregnancies and births. This decreases the time of labor and delivery. Also, as women age, the likelihood increases for complications during pregnancy. The time between contractions leads you to believe that delivery is very close.

3. What should you ask her about the amniotic fluid?

You should ask her about the color of the amniotic fluid. If the amniotic fluid was discolored or smelled badly, this could indicate meconium in the amniotic fluid, which is a sign of fetal distress.

4. What specific questions do you have regarding this patient's medical history?

It is significant to determine if the patient has received prenatal care, if she has experienced any complications during this pregnancy, if she has any medical conditions (such as diabetes or preeclampsia), how many pregnancies and births she has had, any associated complications with each pregnancy and birth, and if each birth was a vaginal delivery.

5. How do her gravida and para numbers affect your patient care decisions?

The more pregnancies and births she has experienced, the more likely her labor and delivery time will decrease.

6. What items will you need to assist in the birth of the baby?

A sterile OB kit.

7. If delivery was not imminent, how would you transport her and why?

You would place her on her side (preferably the left side) to avoid the hypotension associated with a gravid uterus pressing down and obstructing blood flow through the vena cava.

Summary

8. What are some actions you can take before the call to prepare for deliveries in the field?

Preparation for prehospital delivery of a newborn begins with training. Because theses types of medical emergencies are infrequent, you must train at a minimum on a quarterly basis. You must also inspect your rig to ensure that all equipment necessary for delivery is available. In addition to a sterile OB kit, it is helpful to make a pediatric "first in" bag which will carry all necessary equipment to handle pediatric patients of all ages. This should be stocked with appropriate-sized bag-valve-masks and associated face pieces, length-based resuscitation tape, and other assorted items appropriate to your scope of practice.

9. Because newborns are so susceptible to heat loss, what are some techniques you can utilize?

You can ensure there are no drafts (open windows or doors), increase the ambient air temperature in your location, and use warm, clean blankets to wrap the newborn, not the same blankets you used to dry the infant. OB kits should contain a knit cap to place on the infant's head. If one isn't available, the head must still be covered to avoid significant heat loss.

10. Why is it important to always have your hands on the infant from the moment of crowning?

You must assist the infant and mother during delivery by supporting the baby's weight. This will prevent an explosive delivery, which can cause trauma to both mother and newborn.

11. Why is it important to transport after delivery of the baby?

Even a successful delivery of the infant does not guarantee there will be no complications with the mother. Delivery of the placenta can safely occur en route to the facility, which will also minimize the time to definitive care should a significant complication arise such as excessive bleeding.

12. If the newborn is depressed, what are common methods of stimulation?

Suctioning, warming, drying, and flicking the soles of the infant's feet or briskly rubbing the lateral thorax are all methods of stimulation that occur as or after the infant is born. Should the Apgar score be unacceptable, these methods can be reassessed/repeated along with ventilations via bag-valve-mask device and oxygen.

Prep Kit

Ready for Review

- When ovulation occurs and a mature egg is released, it travels down the fallopian tubes toward the uterus. If sperm are present, fertilization may occur.
- The zygote should implant into the lining of the uterus.
- The umbilical cord connects mother and fetus through the placenta. The placenta acts as a barrier and a filter.
- As the fetus grows, the different structures that are recognizable begin to form.
- The heart beats starting at the fourth week of development.
- All fetal organs have formed by the eighth week of development.
- By the 20th week, the pregnant woman can feel the fetus move.
- By the 24th week, the fetus begins to have respiratory effort.
- By the 28th week, the fetus can breathe.
- Full term is considered 40 weeks after conception.
- During pregnancy, the woman's body undergoes many changes to support and protect the developing fetus. Menstruation ceases, the total blood volume increases, the heart rate elevates, blood pressure changes, the respiratory minute volume increases, and gastrointestinal complaints such as morning sickness and heartburn can occur.
- Emergencies can occur prior to delivery. The most common cause of vaginal bleeding during the first and second trimesters is abortion (miscarriage).
- Abortion does not imply any cause and simply means that the fetus is released from the uterus before 20 weeks of gestation.
- In the field, keep the pregnant woman calm during a predelivery emergency; the hospital will determine the best course of action.
- Ectopic pregnancy occurs when the embryo implants in the fallopian tube, ovary, in the abdominal cavity, or the cervix. This is the most life-threatening emergency for the pregnant woman during the first trimester.
- One out of every 10 to 20 women experience hypertension during pregnancy. The most common disorder is preeclampsia, an increase in blood pressure after the 20th week of gestation.
- Preeclampsia can lead to cerebral hemorrhage or seizures.
- Be aware of the possibility of diabetes complicating a pregnancy.
- In the later stages of pregnancy, problems may occur with the placenta.
- Placenta previa is a condition where the placenta develops over and covers the cervix—partially or completely.
- Abruptio placentae is the premature separation of the placenta from the wall of the uterus. This is very dangerous for both the woman and the fetus.
- Uterine rupture can occur after the mother experiences trauma. Uterine rupture causes significant bleeding that may be internal, external, or both.
- There are three stages of labor. The first stage of labor begins with the onset of contractions and ends when the cervix is fully effaced and dilated. Because prehospital care providers cannot assess for cervical effacement and dilation, the end of the first stage of labor in the field occurs when the fetal head crowns from the vaginal opening.
- The second stage of labor is from the point of full dilation and effacement (crowning [in the field]) until the infant is delivered.
- The third stage of labor is from the delivery of the infant until the delivery of the placenta.
- You will assist with the delivery of the baby at the scene when delivery can be expected within a few minutes, when a natural disaster makes it impos-

Technology

- Interactivities
- Vocabulary Explorer
- Anatomy Review
- Web Links
- Online Review Manual

www.EMSzone.com/EMTI

sible to reach the hospital, or when no transportation is available.
- Remember that your job is to help, guide, and support the infant as it is born. Always contact medical control for guidance if you have concerns.
- Abnormal or complicated deliveries include breech deliveries (buttocks first), limb presentations (arm, leg, or foot first), and prolapsed umbilical cord (umbilical cord first). Quickly transport the patient with a limb presentation or prolapsed umbilical cord to the hospital.
- The only times you should place a finger or hand into the vagina are to keep the walls of the vagina from compressing the infant's airway during a face-down breech presentation or to push the infant's head away from the umbilical cord if it is prolapsed.

Vital Vocabulary

abortion Delivery of the fetus and placenta before 20 weeks of gestation; miscarriage.

abruptio placentae (placental abruption) Premature separation of the placenta from the wall of the uterus.

amniotic fluid Fluid produced by the filtration of maternal and fetal blood through blood vessels in the placenta and by excretion of fetal urine into the amniotic sac.

amniotic sac The fluid-filled, bag-like membrane in which the fetus develops.

anal triangle The posterior triangle of the perineum that contains the anal opening.

areola The pigmented ring around the nipple in the breast.

areolar glands Glands that produce secretions that protect the nipple and areola during nursing.

birth canal The vagina and cervix.

blastocyst The zygote.

breasts Structures that contain the organs of milk production.

breech presentation Delivery in which the buttocks come out first.

broad ligament One of several ligaments that support the uterus.

cervical canal A continuation of the uterine canal that opens at the tip of the cervix.

cervical os The opening of the uterus at the cervix.

cervix The lower one-third, or neck, of the uterus.

cilia Hairs on cell surfaces that aid in movement and transport.

clitoris Located in the anterior margin of the vestibule, it contains erectile tissue that becomes engorged with blood as a result of sexual excitement.

corpus cavernosus The erectile tissue found in the clitoris and penis.

corpus luteum The remnants of an unfertilized graafian follicle that hormonal changes allow to be sloughed during menstruation.

crowning The appearance of the infant's head at the vaginal opening during labor.

eclampsia Convulsions (seizures) resulting from severe hypertension in the pregnant woman.

ectopic pregnancy A pregnancy that develops outside the uterus, typically in a fallopian tube.

embryo Term used to describe the developing infant from fertilization to the end of the eighth week of gestation.

embryoblast The inner group of zygote cells; becomes the embryo.

embryonic period The period of gestation between weeks 3 and 8 in which all major organ systems begin to develop.

endometrium The innermost layer of the uterine wall.

estrogen A hormone released from the ovaries that stimulates the uterine lining during the menstrual cycle.

fallopian tube The two hollow tubes or ducts that extend from the uterus to the region of the ovary and serve as a passage for the egg and sperm.

fetoscope A device used for listening to fetal heart tones.

fetus The developing, unborn infant inside the uterus; the embryo becomes the fetus at the beginning of the ninth week.

fimbriae Long thin finger-like processes at the end of the fallopian tubes that surround the ostium.

follicle-stimulating hormone (FSH) A hormone released from the pituitary gland at roughly monthly inter-

Prep Kit continued...

vals that helps to stimulate one oocyte to undergo meiosis.

fundus The top portion of the uterus.

gestation The process of fetal development following fertilization of an egg.

gestational diabetes Condition in which progesterone (the pregnancy hormone) makes the cells resistant to insulin, resulting the potential hypoglycemia or hyperglycemia; typically resolves following delivery.

gonadotropin-releasing hormone (GnRH) The hormone produced in the hypothalamus that causes the pituitary to release the gonadotrophic substances luteinizing hormone and follicle-stimulating hormone.

graafian follicle A mature or developed ovum.

grand multipara A woman who has delivered seven or more viable infants.

gravid Pregnant.

gravida A term used to describe the number of times a woman has been pregnant.

human chorionic gonadotropin (hCG) A hormone that stimulates the corpus luteum to produce progesterone during the first eight weeks of gestation.

hymen The thin mucous membrane that covers the vaginal opening.

infundibulum The space formed in the peritoneum by the distal end of the fallopian tubes.

labia majora Two prominent, rounded folds of skin lateral to the labia minora of the female external genitalia.

labia minora A pair of skin folds in the female external genitalia that border the vestibule.

lactiferous sinuses The area in the mammary glands in which milk is stored.

limb presentation A delivery in which the presenting part is a single arm, leg, or foot.

luteinizing hormone (LH) A hormone released from the pituitary gland at roughly monthly intervals that helps to stimulate one oocyte to undergo meiosis.

mammary glands The organs of milk production in the breasts.

mammary ligaments Structures that support the mammary glands and prevent excessive sagging of the breasts.

meconium A dark green material in the amniotic fluid that can cause lung disease in the newborn; the baby's first bowel movement.

meiosis The process of cell division that occurs during the formation of a mature ovum.

menarche The first menstrual cycle; the onset of menses.

menopause The ending of the menstrual cycle (menses).

menstrual cycle A cycle lasting approximately 28 days in which physiologic changes occur in the uterus and associated reproductive organs.

menstruation The period in the menstrual cycle of sloughing and discharge of the functional layer of the endometrium.

mesovarium The peritoneal fold that helps hold the ovaries in place.

mons pubis A rounded flat pad over the female pubic symphysis.

multigravida A woman who has been pregnant more than once.

multipara A woman who has delivered two or more viable infants.

myoclonus Hyperactive reflexes; seen in women with preeclampsia.

myometrium A thick smooth muscle that forms the middle layer of the uterine wall.

nipple An external raised protuberance on the breast surrounded by the areola.

nuchal cord An umbilical cord that is wrapped around the infant's neck.

nullipara A woman who has never delivered a viable infant.

oocytes The precursors to a mature egg.

oogenesis The maturation process that results in production of an ovum, or egg.

ostium The opening in the infundibulum formed by the fallopian tubes.

ovarian ligament One of the two ligaments that help to hold the ovaries in place.

ovaries The female reproductive organs.

ovulation The release of a mature egg (ovum) into the fallopian tube from the ovary.

ovum A mature egg released by the ovary during ovulation.

oxytocin A hormone secreted in the pituitary gland that promotes uterine contractions.

para A term used to describe the number of times a woman has delivered a viable (live) infant.

perimetrium A serous membrane coating that makes up the outside layer of the uterine wall.

perineum The area of skin between the urethral opening and the anus.

peritonitis Inflammation of the peritoneum (the lining of the abdominal cavity).

placenta Tissue attached to the uterine wall that nourishes the fetus through the umbilical cord.

placenta previa A condition in which the placenta develops over and covers the cervix.

preeclampsia A condition during pregnancy characterized by hypertension, protein in the urine, and edema; a precursor to eclampsia.

premature rupture of membranes Rupture of the amniotic sac prior to the onset of labor; increases risk of fetal infection or injury.

prepuce A structure in the female external genitalia that is formed where the labia minora unite over the clitoris.

presentation The position in which an infant is born; the part of the infant that appears first.

primigravida A woman's first pregnancy.

progesterone A hormone of pregnancy; prepares the uterine lining in preparation for implantation of a fertilized egg.

prolapsed umbilical cord A situation in which the umbilical cord comes out of the vagina before the infant.

pudendum The female external genitalia; also called the vulva.

round ligament One of several ligaments that supports the uterus.

sperm Male gametes that are produced in the testicles.

supine hypotensive syndrome Low blood pressure resulting from compression of the inferior vena cava by the weight of the gravid uterus when the mother is supine.

surfactant A liquid protein substance that coats the alveoli in the lungs.

suspensory ligament One of the two ligaments that help to hold the ovaries in place.

teratogens External substances that may cause birth defects.

term A full 40-week pregnancy.

trimesters Three segments of time, each made up of approximately 3 months, that comprise the length of a pregnancy.

trophoblast The outer group of zygote cells; becomes the placenta.

ultrasound A special device that uses sound waves to determine the location and shape of internal tissues and organs.

umbilical cord The conduit connecting woman to infant via the placenta; contains two arteries and one vein.

urogenital triangle The anterior triangle of the perineum that contains the external genitalia.

uterine canal The canal portion of the uterus that extends from the uterus and continues as the cervical canal.

uterine rupture Rupture of the uterus, usually by trauma, that can result in life-threatening hemorrhage in the woman and fetus.

uterosacral ligament One of several ligaments that supports the uterus.

uterus The muscular organ where the fetus grows, also called the womb; responsible for contractions during labor.

vagina The muscular tube that forms the lower part of the female reproductive tract; the birth canal.

vernix caseosa White, cheesy substance that covers the fetus.

vestibule The space into which the vagina and the urethra open.

vulva The female external genitalia; also called the pudendum.

zygote A fertilized egg.

Assessment in Action

You are dispatched to a home for a woman in labor. You find a 24-year-old female lying on her bed. She tells you that contractions began several hours ago, but she was waiting for her husband to get home from work. She thought she would be able to wait, but when her water broke she decided to call an ambulance.

1. You will transport the patient if:
   A. crowning is present.
   B. the patient has the urge to move her bowels.
   C. contractions are greater than 3 minutes.
   D. bulging of the perineum is present.

2. You examine the patient and determine that crowning is present. The patient's stage of labor is:
   A. first stage, which involves dilation of the cervix.
   B. first stage, which involves delivery of the infant.
   C. second stage, which involves dilation of the cervix.
   D. second stage, which involves delivery of the infant.

3. Important information to obtain from the patient, along with the reason why you want to obtain that information, is:
   A. due date, because that will help you determine how long the labor will last.
   B. color of amniotic fluid, because that will help you determine what respiratory support the infant may need.
   C. number of infants she is carrying, because that will help you determine whether labor will be prolonged.
   D. use of depressants, because that will affect the patient's ability to deliver the infant.

4. The patient tells you that she is having a contraction. You should do all of the following EXCEPT:
   A. time the contraction.
   B. inspect the vagina for crowning.
   C. hold the patient's legs together.
   D. reassure the patient.

5. Proper BSI precautions for assisting with childbirth include:
   A. gloves, gown, and goggles.
   B. gloves and goggles.
   C. gloves and gown.
   D. gloves.

6. You have assessed the patient and have found that this is her third child, she has had a normal pregnancy, and her due date was 2 weeks ago. Her water broke an hour ago, contractions are 1 minute apart and last 90 seconds, and crowning occurs with contractions. You should do all of the following EXCEPT:
   A. administer oxygen and initiate an IV.
   B. have the patient move her bowels.
   C. move the patient to a firm surface.
   D. inspect the vagina with each contraction.

7. The infant's head has been delivered. You should do all of the following EXCEPT:
   A. support the head.
   B. suction the infant's mouth and nose.
   C. check around the neck for the cord.
   D. have the patient push to deliver the rest of the infant.

8. You find that the cord is wrapped very tightly around the infant's neck. You should:

   A. clamp and cut the cord.
   B. slip the cord over the head.
   C. pull on the cord to release it from the uterine wall.
   D. transport the patient immediately.

9. The infant, a girl, has been delivered. You should immediately:

   A. dry her off and keep her cool.
   B. clamp and cut the cord.
   C. suction the airway.
   D. position her above the level of the vagina.

10. The placenta is delivering and you note heavy bleeding. You should do all of the following EXCEPT:

    A. massage the fundus.
    B. pack the vagina.
    C. have the mother breast-feed the infant.
    D. transport the mother immediately.

Points to Ponder

You are on the scene of a woman in labor. She is 6 months' pregnant, this is her fourth child, and her contractions are 1 minute apart. As you are questioning her, the amniotic sac ruptures. You check the patient and discover the cord and one leg protruding from the vagina. The legs and trunk deliver very quickly because of the small size of the infant, but the head does not deliver. The cord is not pulsating. You are unsure of how to handle this situation. You position the mother on the stretcher, supporting the infant, and transport. When you arrive at the hospital, the physician delivers the infant but the resuscitation attempt fails.

What additional help should you have given this infant?

Issue: Preparing Yourself to Handle Obstetric Emergencies, Life and Death Situations

Neonatal Resuscitation

1999 Objectives

Cognitive

6-2.1 Define the term newborn. (p 1204)

6-2.2 Define the term neonate. (p 1204)

6-2.3 Identify important antepartum factors that can affect childbirth. (p 1206)

6-2.4 Identify important intrapartum factors that can term the newborn high risk. (p 1206)

6-2.5 Identify the primary signs utilized for evaluating a newborn during resuscitation. (p 1208)

6-2.6 Formulate an appropriate treatment plan for providing initial care to a newborn. (p 1208)

6-2.7 Identify the appropriate use of the Apgar score in caring for a newborn. (p 1210)

6-2.8 Calculate the Apgar score given various newborn situations. (p 1210)

6-2.9 Determine when ventilatory assistance is appropriate for a newborn. (p 1211)

6-2.10 Prepare appropriate ventilation equipment, adjuncts, and technique for a newborn. (p 1211)

6-2.11 Determine when chest compressions are appropriate for a newborn. (p 1212)

6-2.12 Discuss appropriate chest compression techniques for a newborn. (p 1212)

6-2.13 Reassess a patient following chest compressions and ventilations. (p 1212)

6-2.14 Determine when blow-by oxygen delivery is appropriate for a newborn. (p 1211)

6-2.15 Discuss appropriate blow-by oxygen delivery devices and technique for a newborn. (p 1207)

6-2.16 Assess patient improvement due to assisted ventilations. (p 1212)

6-2.17 Discuss the initial steps in resuscitation of a newborn. (p 1209)

6-2.18 Assess patient improvement due to blow-by oxygen delivery. (p 1212)

6-2.19 Discuss appropriate transport guidelines for a newborn. (p 1219)

6-2.20 Describe the epidemiology, including the incidence, morbidity/mortality and risk factors for meconium aspiration in the neonate. (p 1219)

6-2.21 Discuss the pathophysiology of meconium aspiration in the neonate. (p 1219)

6-2.22 Discuss the assessment findings associated with meconium aspiration in the neonate. (p 1219)

6-2.23 Discuss the management/treatment plan for meconium aspiration in the neonate. (p 1219)

6-2.24 Describe the epidemiology, including the incidence, morbidity/mortality and risk factors for bradycardia in the neonate. (p 1212)

6-2.25 Discuss the pathophysiology of bradycardia in the neonate. (p 1212)

6-2.26 Discuss the assessment findings associated with bradycardia in the neonate. (p 1212)

6-2.27 Discuss the management/treatment plan for bradycardia in the neonate. (p 1212)

6-2.28 Describe the epidemiology, including the incidence, morbidity/mortality, and risk factors for respiratory distress/cyanosis in the neonate. (p 1213)

6-2.29 Discuss the pathophysiology of respiratory distress/cyanosis in the neonate. (p 1213)

6-2.30 Discuss the assessment findings associated with respiratory distress/cyanosis in the neonate. (p 1213)

6-2.31 Discuss the management/treatment plan for respiratory distress/cyanosis in the neonate. (p 1213)

6-2.32 Describe the epidemiology, including the incidence, morbidity/mortality, and risk factors for hypothermia in the neonate. (p 1220)

6-2.33 Discuss the pathophysiology of hypothermia in the neonate. (p 1220)

6-2.34 Discuss the assessment findings associated with hypothermia in the neonate. (p 1220)

6-2.35 Discuss the management/treatment plan for hypothermia in the neonate. (p 1220)

6-2.36 Describe the epidemiology, including the incidence, morbidity/mortality, and risk factors for cardiac arrest in the neonate. (p 1211)

6-2.37 Discuss the pathophysiology of cardiac arrest in the neonate. (p 1211)

6-2.38 Discuss the assessment findings associated with cardiac arrest in the neonate. (p 1211)

6-2.39 Discuss the management/treatment plan for cardiac arrest in the neonate. (p 1211)

Affective

6-1.40 Demonstrate and advocate appropriate interaction with a newborn/neonate that conveys respect for their position in life. (p 1208)

6-1.41 Recognize the emotional impact of newborn/neonate injuries/illnesses on parents/guardians. (p 1222)

6-1.42 Recognize and appreciate the physical and emotional difficulties associated with separation of the parent/guardian and a newborn/neonate. (p 1222)

6-1.43 Listen to the concerns expressed by parents/guardians. (p 1222)

6-1.44 Attend to the need for reassurance, empathy, and compassion for the parent/guardian. (p 1222)

Psychomotor

6-2.45 Demonstrate preparation of a newborn resuscitation area. (p 1207)

6-2.46 Demonstrate appropriate assessment technique for examining a newborn. (p 1208)

6-2.47 Demonstrate appropriate assisted ventilations for a newborn. (p 1211)

6-2.48 Demonstrate appropriate insertion of an orogastric tube. (p 1214)

6-2.49 Demonstrate appropriate chest compression and ventilation technique for a newborn. (p 1212)

6-2.50 Demonstrate the initial steps in resuscitation of a newborn. (p 1209)

6-2.51 Demonstrate blow-by oxygen delivery for a newborn. (p 1211)

1985 Objectives

There are no 1985 objectives for this chapter.

Neonatal Resuscitation

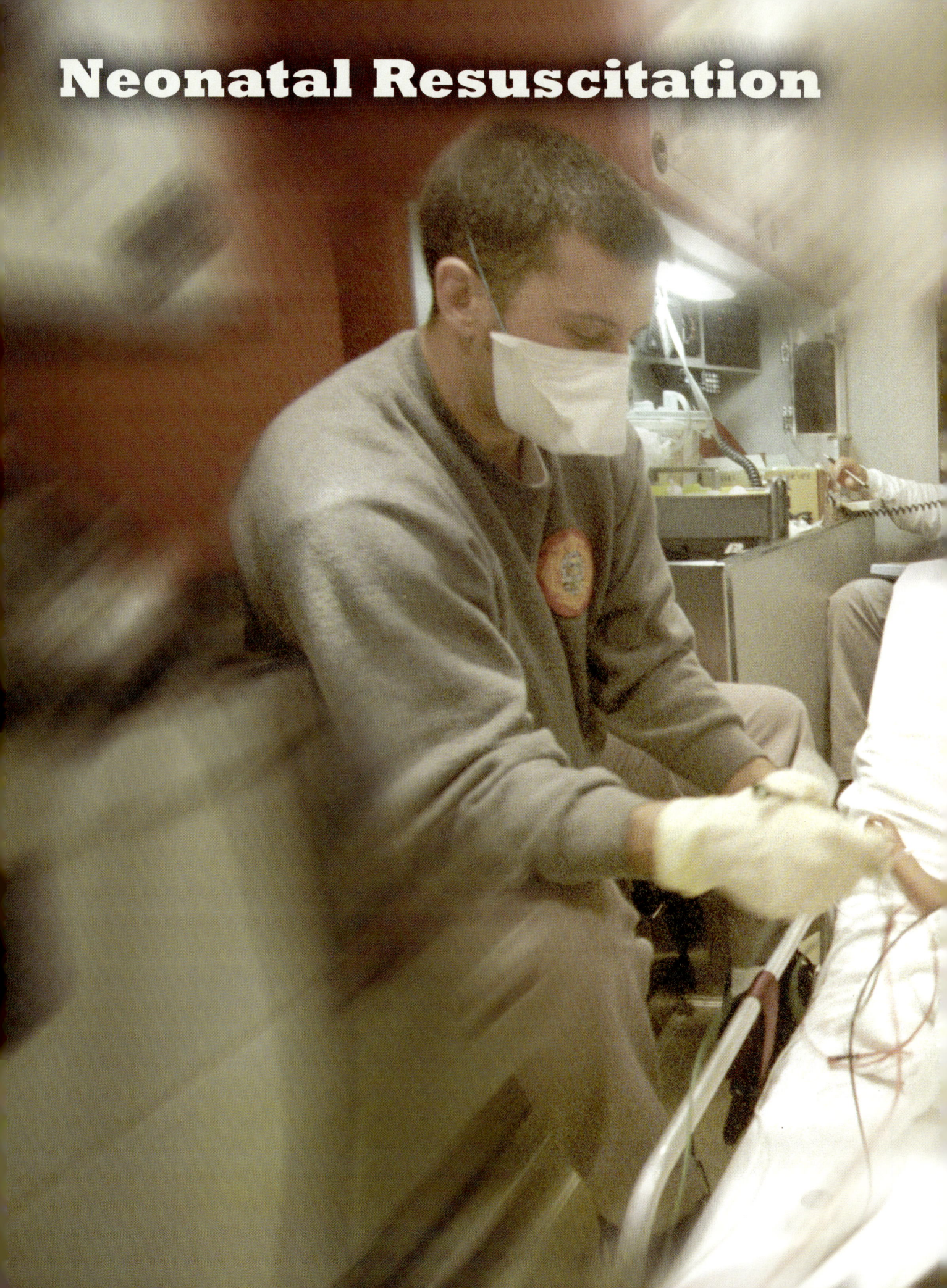

30

Neonatal Resuscitation

You are the Provider

You are called to a local shopping mall for a woman complaining of severe abdominal pain. The caller was an employee of one of the stores who stated that the patient was in one of their dressing rooms and that she was in so much pain that she couldn't get up off the floor.

1. What are the possible causes of the abdominal pain in this patient?
2. What important pieces of information would you want to obtain on initial assessment of the patient?

Neonatal Emergencies

According to the American Academy of Pediatrics (AAP), 90% of newborns are healthy at birth and require little more than basic care from the EMT-I; little, if any, assistance is needed to initiate spontaneous and regular respirations. However, 10% of newborns will require some assistance to initiate adequate breathing after birth and 1% will require extensive resuscitation in order to survive. This chapter will give you the knowledge base in order to provide the safest, most effective care to a healthy as well as a distressed newborn.

Neonatal Pathophysiology

Fetal Oxygenation In Utero

A newborn is a recently born baby and is generally considered "newborn" for the first few hours of its life. During the first 28 days of life, a baby is considered to be a neonate. Between the ages of 1 month and 1 year, a baby is referred to as an infant. The newborn phase is a period of great physiologic change, including the initiation of breathing with exchanging of oxygen (O_2) and carbon dioxide (CO_2) in the lungs, closing of blood vessels that were necessary for life in utero, and the pumping of blood into those vessels that were previously closed. These physiologic changes must, and usually do, occur within the first few seconds following birth.

Oxygen is critical for survival of the newborn, both before and after birth. In utero, the oxygen consumed by the fetus diffuses across the placental membrane from the maternal circulation to the fetal circulation.

Before birth, a small percentage of fetal blood passes through the lungs of the fetus—just enough to keep the lung tissue (parenchyma) alive. Because the fetal lungs in utero do not function as a source of gas exchange, they require less oxygen. Although the fetal lungs are expanded in utero, the alveoli are filled with fluid rather than air. Additionally, the blood vessels that deliver oxygen to, and remove carbon dioxide from, the lungs are markedly constricted.

Prior to birth, most of the blood from the right side of the fetal heart bypasses the lungs through the foramen ovale. The foramen ovale is an opening between the right and left atria, through which blood passes since it does not require oxygenation in the fetal lungs. The little blood that does not pass through the foramen ovale is diverted away from the lungs by the ductus arteriosus. The ductus arteriosus, which serves as a bridge between the left pulmonary artery and the aorta, temporarily reroutes oxygenated blood from the woman, away from the lungs of the fetus, and directly into its systemic circulation.

Fetal Transition

Following birth, the newborn will no longer be connected to the placenta; therefore, it must depend on its own lungs as the only source for oxygen intake and carbon dioxide removal. Over a matter of seconds, the lungs must therefore fill with oxygen and the pulmonary vasculature must relax (dilate) in order to perfuse the alveoli. This will allow the alveoli to absorb oxygen and become functional units of the respiratory system; they must be able to absorb oxygen and participate in pulmonary gas exchange.

Normally, there are three major physiologic changes that occur in the fetus within seconds after birth. In most cases, these changes occur spontaneously, with little support required from the EMT-I. These physiologic changes include the following:

- Fluid in the alveoli is absorbed into the lung tissue and is replaced by air. This process is facilitated when the newborn begins to breathe spontaneously. The more effective the newborn's initial breaths, the faster and more effective the fluid is removed from the alveoli. Once this occurs, oxygen in the air is able to diffuse into the pulmonary blood vessels that surround the alveoli.

Technology

- Interactivities
- Vocabulary Explorer
- Anatomy Review
- Web Links
- Online Review Manual

www.EMSzone.com/EMTI

- The umbilical cord (which contains two arteries and one vein) is clamped, thus removing the low-resistance placental circuit, resulting in an increase in the newborn's systemic blood pressure.
- The alveoli become distended and are able to hold oxygen. As a result, the blood vessels in the lungs dilate, which, together with the increased systemic blood pressure, facilitates an increase in pulmonary blood flow and decreased blood flow through the ductus arteriosus. Increased pulmonary blood flow absorbs the alveolar oxygen and the oxygen-enriched blood is returned to the left side of the heart, where it is distributed to the systemic circulation.

As pulmonary blood vessels continue to dilate and blood levels of oxygen increase, the ductus arteriosus constricts and blood flows preferentially into the lungs, picking up more oxygen to be transported throughout the body. Following this fetal transition process, the neonate is now breathing and oxygenating its own blood. As oxygen levels in the blood continue to increase, the neonate's skin turns from cyanotic to pink.

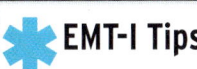

EMT-I Tips

Once the umbilical cord has been clamped, the fetus no longer receives prostaglandin-E2 from the placenta. Prostaglandin-E2 is a hormone that causes the ductus arteriosus to remain open (patent). Without this hormone, the ductus arteriosus constricts and eventually closes.

Fetal Distress

In a small percentage of newborns, problems occur during the fetal transition process previously discussed, or they may occur following delivery. If fetal distress occurs in utero, the problem is usually caused by compromised blood flow in the placenta or umbilical cord; after delivery, the cause is usually the result of an airway or breathing problem. Fetal distress can result from the following:

- The neonate's initial respiratory efforts are inadequate and not strong enough to force fluid from the alveoli.
- Foreign material, such as meconium, blocks the airway and prevents adequate breathing.
- Excessive blood loss (ie, maternal trauma) or decreased myocardial contractility.
- Sustained pulmonary arteriole constriction (pulmonary hypertension).

If the normal sequence of fetal transition is interrupted, the systemic arterial blood may not become oxygenated. In addition to constriction of the pulmonary vasculature, the arterioles of the bowels, kidneys, muscle, and skin will constrict in order to maintain

EMT-I Tips

Using a Doppler or even a regular stethoscope, you should be able to auscultate fetal heart tones to detect the presence of abnormalities.

You are the Provider   Part 2

When you arrive, you find a woman lying on the floor of the store dressing room, writhing in pain. She has apparently been incontinent of urine. She is 16 years old and her mother is with her. The mother tells you that the pain started approximately 20 minutes ago and is intermittent, coming about every 1 to 2 minutes. The patient describes it as a cramping type pain. She denies any trauma and has eaten nothing out of the ordinary today. When asked if there is a possibility of pregnancy, she initially doesn't answer. When questioned again, she states that she could be pregnant and has experienced weight gain over the last 7 to 8 months. Her mother is clearly stunned by this information.

3. What are your significant findings so far?
4. What are your next steps?

perfusion to the vital organs of the body (heart and brain). However, if oxygen deprivation continues, cardiac output will fall, resulting in decreased blood flow to all of the body's organs. Inadequate systemic perfusion can result in brain damage (anoxic brain injury), damage to other organs, or death. Clinical findings of fetal distress include the following:

- Persistent cyanosis and/or bradycardia secondary to systemic hypoxia
- Hypotension resulting from decreased coronary perfusion, decreased cardiac output, or blood loss
- Respiratory depression or apnea caused by insufficient oxygen delivery to the brain
- Poor muscle tone from hypoxia and hypercarbia in the muscles

Newborn Bradycardia

Newborn bradycardia (heart rate <100 beats/min) is almost always the result of hypoxia, usually from inadequate respiratory effort or secretions in the airway. However, the risk of fetal morbidity and mortality is minimal if hypoxia is detected quickly and corrected. Other conditions, though less common, can also cause newborn bradycardia. These include increased intracranial pressure (ICP) and acidosis.

Anticipating the Need for Resuscitation

On the basis of the presence of certain antepartum and intrapartum risk factors, you may be able to predict which newborns may require resuscitation following birth. There are a number of factors that can affect the newborn and increase the likelihood of the need for resuscitation. Gathering information through a thorough maternal history may allow you to anticipate a problematic delivery or distressed newborn Table 30-1 .

If time permits, you should also ask the pregnant woman the following additional questions to further prepare yourself for a possible neonatal resuscitation:

1. **What is your due date or how many weeks pregnant are you?**
   The more premature the newborn, the more resuscitation and care the newborn is likely to require. The lungs of the premature newborn may not have yet secreted surfactant, resulting in increased alveolar surface tension and inadequate pulmonary function. The skin of a premature baby is thin and lacks the subcutaneous fat that helps maintain body temperature. The gestational age can also help you select the correct-sized equipment for the baby if resuscitation is required.

2. **How many infants are you expecting?**
   Multiple births are often of lower birth weight and premature. If they require invasive care, you may need another ambulance to care for multiple infants as well as the mother.

3. **Has your amniotic sac ruptured? If so, what was the color and consistency of the fluid? Did it smell?**
   Thick, dark, or foul-smelling amniotic fluid can be an indication of meconium staining. If meconium has been aspirated, the newborn may have depressed respiratory function and need advanced airway management (discussed later in this chapter).

4. **Have you had any depressant drugs or alcohol within the last four hours?**
   Many depressant drugs and alcohol pass through the placental barrier to the fetus. You should be

TABLE 30-1	Risk Factors for Neonatal Resuscitation

Antepartum risk factors
- Diabetes
- Cardiac disease
- Hypertension
- Preeclampsia or eclampsia
- Multiple gestation
- Mother's age <16 years or >35 years
- Inadequate or no prenatal care
- Postterm gestation (>40 weeks)
- History of perinatal morbidity or mortality
- Use of illicit drugs, certain medications, alcohol, or cigarettes

Intrapartum risk factors
- Placental abnormalities (previa or abruptio)
- Premature labor
- Meconium-stained amniotic fluid
- Rupture of membranes greater than 24 hours prior to delivery
- Abnormal fetal presentation (ie, breech, limb presentation)
- Prolapsed umbilical cord
- Prolonged labor or precipitous delivery
- Bleeding

specifically concerned about narcotics, such as heroin and morphine; sedative-hypnotics (benzodiazepines), such as diazepam (Valium) and temazepam (Restoril); barbiturates, such as phenobarbital; and other drugs that can depress the central nervous system. If they have been recently ingested, the newborn may be born with respiratory depression and require aggressive airway support and potential medication therapy.

Resuscitation Equipment

Basic Equipment

The necessary resuscitation equipment must be present at every delivery, even if you don't anticipate problems. Although a thorough, accurate maternal history can help you identify the potential for a distressed newborn, it is not possible to identify all of the potential problems that you may encounter. Table 30-2 lists the minimum basic equipment and supplies that should be present at all deliveries. Many of these items are usually contained within the OB kit that you carry on the ambulance.

TABLE 30-2 | Basic Neonatal Resuscitation Equipment

Suction equipment
- Bulb syringe
- Mechanical suction device and tubing
- Suction catheters (5F to 12F)

Oxygen and ventilation equipment
- Neonatal-sized BVM device capable of delivering 100% oxygen
- Assortment of BVM face masks
  - Term and premature sizes
  - Cushion-rim masks are preferred
- Oxygen source with flowmeter
- Oropharyngeal airways
- Pediatric or newborn-size oxygen mask and oxygen supply tubing

Miscellaneous equipment
- Blankets and towels
- Stethoscope (neonatal head preferred)
- Umbilical cord clamps
- Sterile scalpel
- Plastic bag for the placenta

In the Field

In the absence of a warmer, blankets or towels may be warmed by wrapping them around chemical hot packs.

EMT-I Safety

During the birth and resuscitation of the newborn, you must protect yourself from the splashing of blood and other body fluids. Minimum BSI precautions include gloves, goggles or a face shield, and a gown.

Advanced Life Support Equipment

Although few newborns require aggressive resuscitation and advanced life support, the equipment and supplies necessary to perform advanced interventions must be present and fully operational. A kit prepared in advance will ensure that the equipment, if needed, is immediately accessible.

Venous Access

Venous access is usually not needed in the newborn because problems are almost always the result of respiratory insufficiency and hypoxia; airway and ventilation management are the primary treatments. However, if fluid resuscitation or medications are necessary, you must be able to access the newborn's venous circulation. Isotonic crystalloids (such as normal saline or lactated Ringer's), IV catheters (22 to 24 gauge), and pediatric intraosseous (IO) catheters should be included in your ALS kit.

If venous access is not obtainable, certain medications can be given via the endotracheal tube. These include epinephrine (Adrenaline) and naloxone (Narcan).

You may also carry umbilical vein catheters (UVCs) if your local protocols allow umbilical vein catheterization. Umbilical catheterization by prehospital care providers is a controversial procedure. While this route of vascular access in experienced hands is effective and quick, the prehospital care provider rarely needs it and complications can occur.

Endotracheal Intubation

Endotracheal intubation may be necessary if the distressed newborn's airway cannot be managed effectively with basic means (a BVM device) or if prolonged ventilatory support is needed. Additionally, certain medications can be instilled down the ET tube if venous access is not available. The following intubation equipment should be available, if needed:

- Laryngoscope with straight blades
  - Size 0 (preterm); size 1 (term)
- Extra bulbs and batteries for laryngoscope
- Endotracheal tubes
  - Sizes 2.5 mm to 4.0 mm
- Stylet (optional)
- Device to secure the ET tube
- ET_{CO_2} detector

Medications

Pharmacologic interventions may be required if the newborn fails to respond to less invasive resuscitation interventions. Although this is a rare event, the following medications, which will be discussed later in this chapter, should be available:

- Epinephrine (Adrenaline) 1:10,000—0.1 mg/mL
- Naloxone (Narcan)—0.4 mg/mL
- 10% dextrose (D_{10})—0.1 g/mL
- Sodium bicarbonate ($NaHCO_3$)—4.2% solution (0.5 mEq/mL)
- Syringes (1, 3, 5, 10, 20, and 50 mL)

and in need of further assessment and, if necessary, resuscitation.

If the answer to *all* of the questions in Table 30-3 is yes, you may proceed with routine care, which consists of drying and warming the newborn and suctioning the mouth and nose—interventions that are carried out on *every* newborn, regardless of the appearance at birth. If the answer to *any* of the questions is no, you must proceed with the initial steps of resuscitation and determine the need for further interventions.

Depressed Newborn Resuscitation

Depressed newborn resuscitation refers to the series of interventions used to stimulate spontaneous breathing. When the newborn remains depressed after drying, warming, and clearing the airway, resuscitation must proceed without delay. The inverted pyramid (Figure 30-1 ▼) shows the need for interventions in depressed newborns. BLS is usually all that is required following delivery and therefore makes up the broad top areas of the inverted pyramid. In contrast, ALS interventions such as intubation and medication administration are rarely required and make up the smaller, lower areas of the pyramid.

Interventions Immediately Following Delivery

Assessment of the Newborn

Assessment of the newborn should begin immediately following delivery. At birth, a rapid assessment focusing on certain key elements (Table 30-3 ▼) will determine if the newborn has transitioned successfully and only requires simple supportive care or is in distress

TABLE 30-3	Immediate Assessment of the Newborn

- Is the amniotic fluid clear of meconium?
- Is the infant breathing or crying?
- Does the newborn have good muscle tone?
- Is the skin color pink?
- Is this a term gestation?

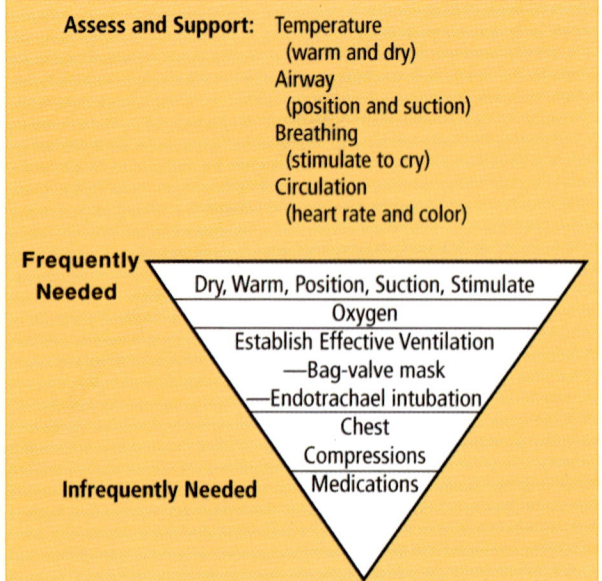

Figure 30-1 Guidelines for neonatal resuscitation as recommended by the American Heart Association.

The Initial Steps of Resuscitation

The initial steps of resuscitation, which comprise the uppermost portion of the inverted pyramid, are aimed at stimulating the infant to begin spontaneous, effective breathing. They consist of drying, warming, positioning, suctioning, and stimulating the neonate. In most newborns, these initial steps are all that are required to initiate effective breathing.

> **EMT-I Tips**
>
> To help remember the initial steps of neonatal resuscitation, remember the saying "Do What Probably Seems Simple," which stands for:
> Drying (**Do**)
> Warming (**What**)
> Positioning (**Probably**)
> Suctioning (**Seems**)
> Stimulation (**Simple**)

Drying and Warming the Newborn

When infants are born, they are covered with a slippery, wet, cheesy substance called <u>vernix caseosa</u>. This material must be quickly dried from the newborn to prevent hypothermia. Towels, preferably warmed, must therefore be present immediately following delivery. Thoroughly dry the newborn, particularly the head, which can be a source of significant body heat loss. In the controlled environment of a delivery room, a radiant warmer is present to provide thermal management; however, this is a luxury that you will not have in the prehospital setting. Therefore, when responding to a call for a possible delivery, ensure that the heater in the back of the ambulance is turned on, regardless of the time of season. The hypothermic newborn will likely not respond to even the most simple and basic resuscitation measures (such as BVM ventilations or blow-by oxygen).

Positioning the Newborn

After adequately drying and warming the newborn, position the newborn on a flat surface and ensure an open airway. The newborn's head is larger than an older child's or adult's compared to its overall body size, which leads to flexion of the neck and airway obstruction when placed in a supine position. Avoid this by extending the head *slightly* and place the airway in a neutral position. Conversely, the occiput may force the neck forward, resulting in flexion of the neck. It may be necessary to place a folded towel in between the newborn's shoulders to facilitate optimum head positioning (**Figure 30-2 ▼**). Alternatively, you can place the infant on its side (laterally recumbent), which will facilitate draining of residual fluid from the airway.

Suctioning the Airway

Initial suctioning of the newborn was performed as soon as its head delivered. However, to ensure that as much fluid as possible is cleared from the lungs, additional suctioning will be necessary. Secretions may be cleared from the mouth and nose with a bulb syringe or suction catheter (**Figure 30-3 ▶**). The mouth is suctioned before the nose to prevent aspiration if the newborn gasps when the nose is suctioned. Aspiration of secretions can cause serious respiratory problems. If there are copious secretions in the newborn's airway, turn its head to the side prior to suctioning.

If you are using a mechanical suction unit, the suction pressure should be set so that when the suction tubing is blocked, the negative pressure (vacuum) reads approximately 100 mm Hg.

When you are suctioning the newborn's airway, especially when using a catheter, avoid vigorous or deep suctioning. Stimulation of the posterior pharynx during the first few minutes after birth can produce a vagal response, resulting in severe bradycardia or apnea. Brief, gentle suction is usually adequate to remove secretions.

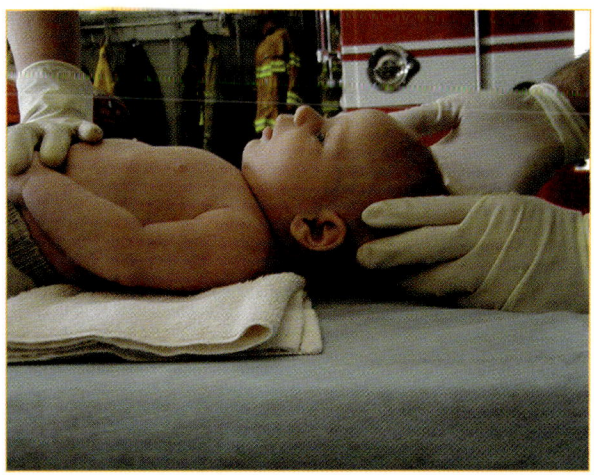

Figure 30-2 To avoid airway obstruction, it may be necessary to place a folded towel in between the newborn's shoulders.

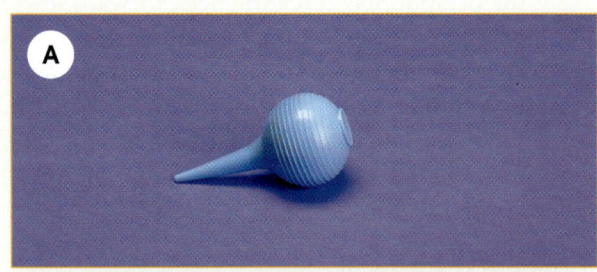
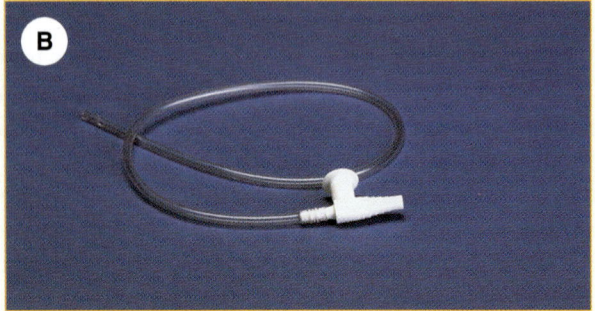

Figure 30-3 **A.** Bulb syringe. **B.** Suction catheter.

Stimulation

Both drying and suctioning provide stimulation to the newborn. In many cases, these steps are all that is needed to initiate effective respirations. If the newborn still does not have adequate respirations, additional tactile stimulation may be provided *briefly* to stimulate breathing.

There are only two acceptable and safe methods for providing tactile stimulation to the newborn: slapping or flicking the soles of the feet and gently rubbing the back, trunk, or extremities. Vigorous stimulation is not helpful and may result in injury to the newborn. *Never shake an infant!*

Continued use of tactile stimulation in an apneic newborn is wasting precious time. Begin positive pressure ventilations with a BVM device and 100% oxygen immediately if *brief* tactile stimulation fails to initiate breathing.

Essential Parameters

Following the initial steps of resuscitation, the need for and extent of further resuscitation is based on the assessment of three key parameters: respiratory effort, heart rate, and color. The Apgar score (Table 30-4 ▼) is an objective method of quantifying the newborn's condition and assessing its response to resuscitation; it is performed at 1 and 5 minutes following birth. However, resuscitation, if needed, must be initiated before the first score is assigned. *Therefore, the Apgar score is not used to determine the need for resuscitation, what interventions are necessary, or when to use them.*

Each of the five signs is assigned a value of 0, 1, or 2. The five values are then added and the sum becomes the Apgar score. Most newborns will have a score of 7 or 8 at 1 minute and a score of 8 to 10 at 5 minutes.

If the newborn required only supportive care at birth because the immediate assessment revealed that it was vigorous, a term gestation, and the amniotic fluid was clear of meconium (see Table 30-3), it would be appropriate to obtain an Apgar score at the appropriate intervals. *It should be reemphasized, however, that respiratory effort, heart rate, and color (not the Apgar score) should be immediately assessed in newborns who are depressed.*

TABLE 30-4 Apgar Score

Sign	Score 2	Score 1	Score 0
Appearance	Entire infant is pink.	Body is pink, but hands and feet remain blue.	Entire infant is blue or pale.
Pulse	>100 beats/min	<100 beats/min	Absent pulse
Grimace or irritability	Infant cries and tries to move foot away from finger snapped against its sole.	Infant gives a weak cry in response to stimulus.	Infant does not cry or react to stimulus.
Activity or muscle tone	Infant resists attempts to straighten out hips and knees.	Infant makes weak attempts to resist straightening.	Infant is completely limp, with no muscle tone.
Respiration	Rapid respirations	Slow respirations	Absent respirations

Assess Respiratory Effort

Crying is proof of breathing. Normally, a newborn's respiratory rate will be between 40 and 60 breaths/min. Breathing effort may be slightly irregular in normal newborns. Signs such as gasping, grunting, retractions, or nasal flaring, indicate increased work of breathing and respiratory distress. Respiratory distress in the newborn can be caused by the following conditions, which, if untreated, may result in cardiac arrest:

- Primary lung or heart disease
- Primary pulmonary hypertension
- Central nervous system disorders
- Mucous obstruction of nasal passages
- Spontaneous pneumothorax
- Choanal atresia (congenital blockage of the nares)
- Meconium aspiration
- Amniotic fluid aspiration
- Lung immaturity (usually secondary to surfactant deficiency)
- Pneumonia
- Shock and sepsis
- Metabolic acidosis
- Diaphragmatic hernia

Management of Apnea or Inadequate Respiratory Effort

If breathing is not visible (apnea) in the newborn, immediate positive pressure ventilations are required. Apnea in newborns presents in two forms: primary apnea or secondary apnea. **Primary apnea** will often reverse with simple stimulation by touching and by suctioning. **Secondary apnea** will not reverse without assisted ventilation. If the newborn is apneic or has gasping respirations following the initial steps of resuscitation, further stimulation is not likely to improve ventilation. Because both primary and secondary apnea can occur in utero and are difficult to differentiate, assume the infant has secondary apnea and begin positive pressure ventilations with 100% oxygen immediately.

In situations in which positive pressure ventilation is indicated, you should use a neonatal or infant-sized BVM device. The appropriately sized mask should cover the infant's mouth and nose, but not the eyes **Figure 30-4**. Make sure you have a good mask-to-face seal. Using gentle pressure, make the chest rise with each ventilation. Because additional fluids may need to be cleared from the alveoli, it may be necessary to bypass the pop-off valve on the BVM device during the first few breaths to achieve higher inspiratory pressures **Figure 30-5**. Ventilations in the neonate are provided at a rate of 40 to 60 breaths/min.

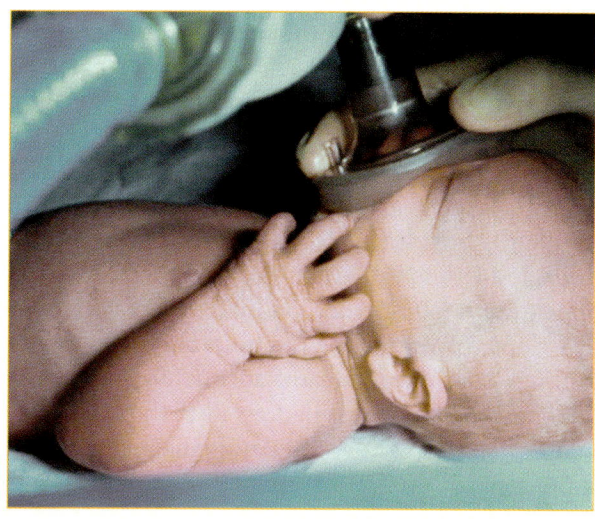

Figure 30-4 Use a neonatal or infant-sized BVM, ensuring that you cover both the infant's nose and mouth, but not the eyes. Ventilate with 100% oxygen at a rate of 40 to 60 breaths/min.

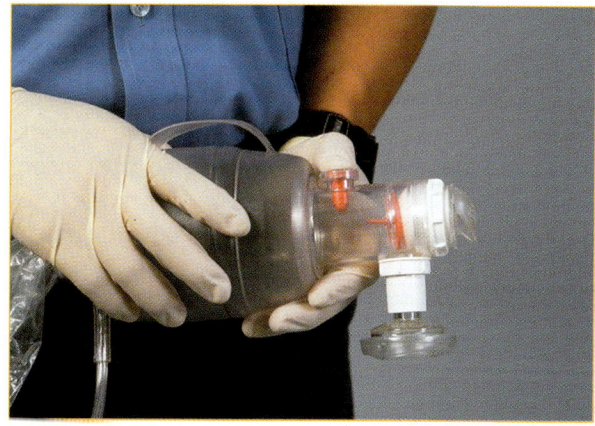

Figure 30-5 If a pop-off valve is present, occlude it to achieve higher inspiratory pressures.

In the Field

Oropharyngeal airways are rarely needed to maintain a patent airway in the newborn. The newborn's airway can usually be maintained by proper positioning. In certain situations, however, oropharyngeal airways may be needed to keep the newborn's mouth open during ventilations.

Positive pressure ventilation (PPV) is successful if you see both sides of the newborn's chest rise and hear breath sounds bilaterally. Do not ventilate the newborn with too much pressure, as this can cause damage to the lungs (barotrauma), resulting in a potential pneumothorax.

After 30 seconds of adequate ventilations, assess the heart rate. If the heart rate is at least 100 beats/min and the infant is breathing adequately, you can stop ventilations and assess the infant's color. Do not suddenly stop ventilations. Instead, gradually decrease the rate and volume of ventilations to determine whether the infant will continue to breathe adequately on his or her own. If not, continue ventilations until the infant does. You may find that gently stimulating the infant by flicking the soles of the feet or rubbing the torso will help maintain effective respirations.

Assess Heart Rate

In newborns, bradycardia (heart rate, <100 beats/min) is usually due to hypoxia, not primary cardiac disease. The crying, active newborn usually has an adequate heart rate. Assess heart rate carefully in a newborn who is not active or who requires positive pressure ventilation. This means either listening to the heart with a stethoscope (apical pulse) or palpating the base of the umbilical cord (Figure 30-6). A quick way to calculate the newborn's heart rate is to count the number of beats in 6 seconds and simply add a 0 to that number. Alternatively, you can multiply the number of beats in 6 seconds by 10.

Management of Newborn Bradycardia

Treat heart rates of fewer than 100 beats/min with positive pressure ventilation and 100% oxygen, even if respirations are normal. In most infants with bradycardia, ventilation improves the heart rate to more than 100 beats/min immediately and no further treatment is necessary.

If the heart rate is fewer than 60 beats/min, continue ventilation and begin chest compressions. Even though the infant has a pulse, the heart rate and cardiac output are not adequate for the metabolic needs of a newborn.

There are two ways to perform chest compressions in the newborn. For the preferred method, follow the steps in Skill Drill 30-1.

1. **Find the proper position:** one fingerwidth below an imaginary line drawn between the nipples on the middle third of the sternum (**Step 1**).
2. With a normal, full-term infant, **place both hands around the infant so that your thumbs are side by side**, resting on the middle third of the sternum, and the rest of your fingers encircle the thorax. In premature or very small infants, you may have to place one thumb over the other to perform chest compressions (**Step 2**).
3. **Press the two thumbs gently against the sternum.** The newborn's chest is easy to compress. Use only enough force to compress the sternum to a depth of approximately one third the anteroposterior diameter of the chest (about $\frac{1}{2}''$ to $\frac{3}{4}''$) (**Step 3**).

If your hands are too small to encircle the chest, you should use the middle and ring fingers of one hand to provide the compressions while your other hand supports the infant's back.

BVM ventilation is performed during a pause after every third compression. Avoid giving a compression and a ventilation simultaneously, since one will decrease the effectiveness of the other. You should deliver compressions and ventilations in a 3:1 ratio, for a combined total of 120 "events" per minute, 90 compressions and 30 ventilations. Keep in mind that adequate ventilation is absolutely critical to the successful resuscitation of the neonate.

Reassess the newborn after 30 seconds of positive pressure ventilation and chest compressions. If the heart rate is above 60 but below 100 beats/min, discontinue chest compressions and continue ventilations until the heart rate increases to more than 100 beats/min. If the heart rate remains below 60 beats/min, continue PPV and chest compressions and consider administering medications (discussed later in this chapter).

If prolonged ventilatory support or certain medications will be needed for the newborn, you should perform endotracheal intubation.

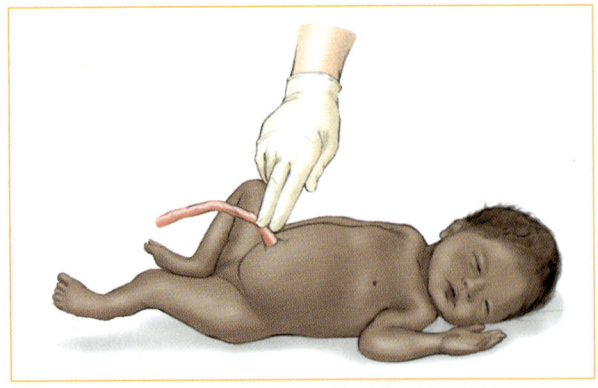

Figure 30-6 Feel for a pulse at the base of the umbilical cord.

Skill Drill 30-1: Giving Chest Compressions to a Newborn

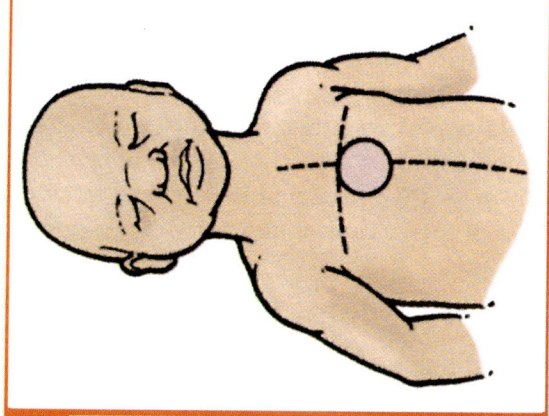

1 Find the proper position: just below the nipple line, middle of the lower third of the sternum.

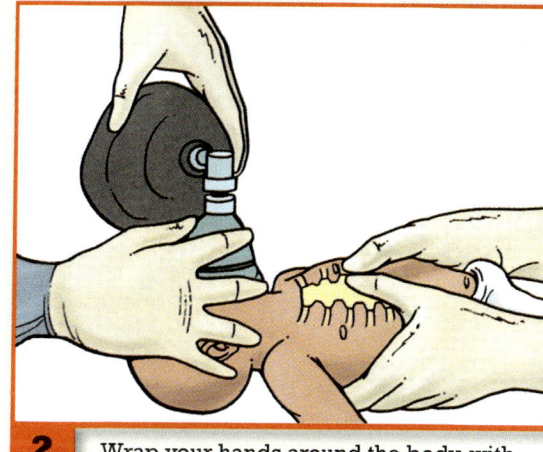

2 Wrap your hands around the body, with your thumbs resting at that position.

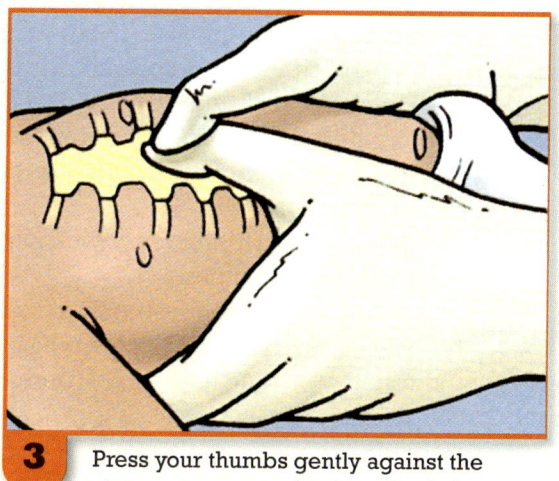

3 Press your thumbs gently against the sternum, compressing to a depth that is approximately one third the anteroposterior diameter of the chest.

Deliver compressions and ventilations in a 3:1 ratio.

Assess Color

Assessing skin color in newborns has several unique features. In utero, the infant depends on placental delivery of oxygen, and, compared to adults, the fetal oxygen concentrations are very low. The fetus has several ways to live and grow in this low-oxygen environment. When the infant is born and has not begun to breathe air, it will appear cyanotic. This is normal until effective spontaneous breathing occurs, at which time the skin usually "pinks up" rapidly.

Management of Newborn Cyanosis

If the infant has cyanosis, determine if it is central (on the trunk and face) or peripheral (limited to the hands and feet). This difference will help with decision making and treatment. If <u>central cyanosis</u> is present, administer oxygen because true hypoxia is present. Apply free-flow oxygen directly to the infant's face; avoid blowing oxygen directly into the eyes ▶ Figure 30-7 ▶. Using oxygen tubing or a pediatric face mask, set the flowmeter at 5 L/min and hold the tubing or mask

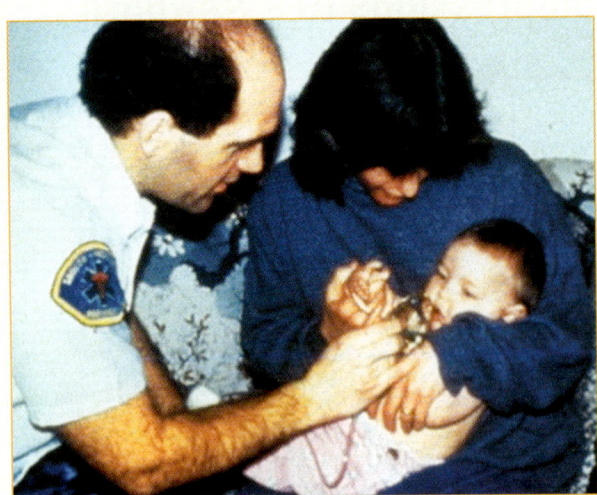

Figure 30-7 Administer free-flow oxygen to the newborn with central cyanosis.

approximately ½″ from the infant's nose and mouth. Continually assess the newborn's color while providing free-flow oxygen. If after 30 seconds of free-flow oxygen central cyanosis persists, perform positive pressure ventilation with 100% oxygen. If the cyanosis dissipates, gradually withdraw the oxygen until you are certain the newborn remains pink on room air. *Never abruptly withdraw oxygen from any newborn.*

<u>Peripheral cyanosis</u>, limited to the hands and feet, is also termed <u>acrocyanosis</u>. This is a common finding in newborns through the first 24 to 48 hours of life and requires no therapy.

Advanced Life Support Interventions

As previously discussed, most newborns require only BLS interventions to stimulate effective breathing; few will require positive pressure ventilation or chest compressions. However, approximately 1% of newborns will require aggressive resuscitation and ALS interventions because of severe cardiopulmonary depression.

Orogastric Tube Insertion

Newborns that require positive pressure ventilation for longer than 2 minutes should have an <u>orogastric (OG) tube</u> inserted and left in place. During ventilations, air is forced into the oropharynx, where it is free to enter both the trachea and the esophagus. If the airway is properly positioned, most of the air will enter the trachea and the lungs. Some air, however, may enter the esophagus and be forced into the stomach. Air that is forced into the stomach will cause gastric distention, and may result in the following complications:

- Upward pressure on the diaphragm, preventing full lung expansion.
- Regurgitation of gastric contents, which may be aspirated during ventilations.

The problems associated with gastric distention can be reduced by inserting an OG tube, suctioning gastric contents, and leaving the tube in place to act as a vent for air that enters the stomach.

You are the Provider   Part 3

Upon inspection of the patient, you determine that she is crowning. You call for another ambulance and ask your partner to get the OB kit and resuscitation equipment. You and your partner prepare for imminent delivery. Once the baby is delivered, you notice that the baby is listless with the following vital signs:

Initial Assessment	Recording Time: Zero Minutes
Respirations	20 breaths/min
Pulse	50 beats/min
Color	Central cyanosis

5. What are your priorities for treating this newborn?
6. Are medications indicated for this newborn?

Inserting an Orogastric Tube in the Newborn

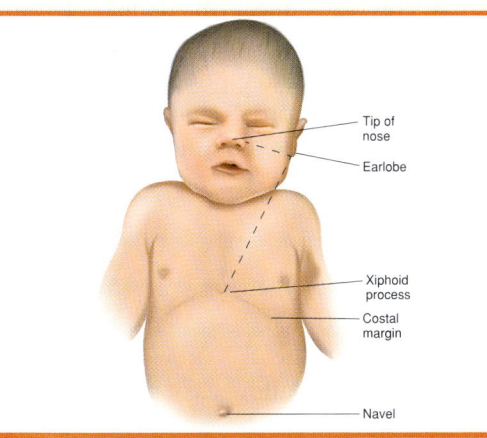

1 Measure for correct depth: from the tip of the nose to the earlobe and from the earlobe to the xiphoid process.

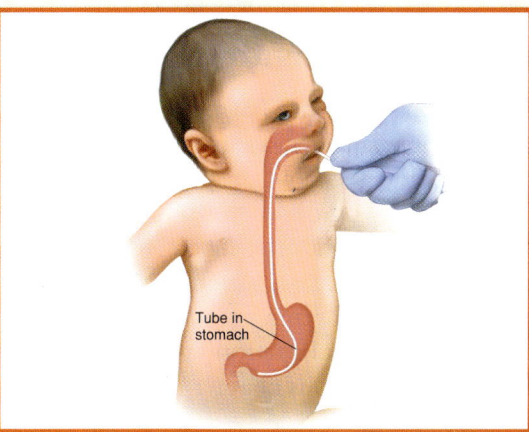

2 Insert the tube to the appropriate depth. Leave the nose open to allow for ventilations.

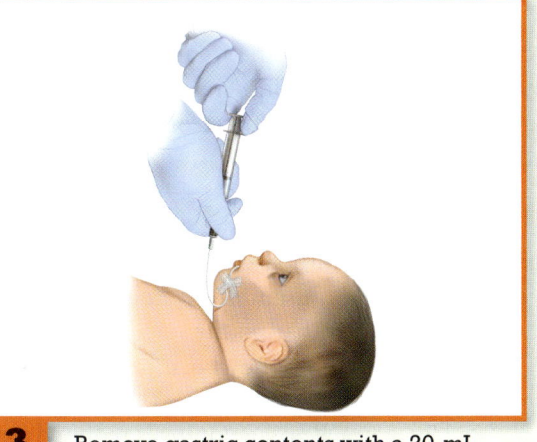

3 Remove gastric contents with a 20-mL syringe. Remove the syringe and leave the tip of the tube open to allow air to vent from the stomach. Tape the tube to the newborn's cheek.

For OG tube insertion, you will need an 8F feeding tube and a 20-mL syringe. To insert an OG tube in the newborn, follow the steps in Skill Drill 30-2.

1. **Measure for the correct depth.** The length of the inserted OG tube should be equal to the distance from the tip of the nose to the earlobe and from the earlobe to the xiphoid process. Note the centimeter marking at this place on the tube (**Step 1**).
2. **Insert the tube through the mouth to the appropriate depth.** The nose should be left open for ventilation, which can be resumed as soon as the tube has been placed (**Step 2**).
3. **Attach a 20-mL syringe and remove gastric contents.** Remove the syringe and leave the end of the tube open to vent air from the stomach.
4. **Tape the tube to the newborn's cheek** to ensure that the tube stays in the stomach (**Step 3**).

The OG tube will not interfere with the mask-to-face seal if an 8F feeding tube is used and the tube exits from the side of the mask over the newborn's cheek. A larger tube may make it difficult to obtain an adequate mask-to-face seal; a smaller tube may become obstructed by secretions.

Endotracheal Intubation

Because ventilations in the newborn, if needed, are usually of short duration and often stimulate effective breathing within a few minutes, endotracheal intubation is rarely necessary. However, under certain circumstances (Table 30-5), endotracheal intubation may be necessary.

Other indications that may require intubation in the newborn, such as extreme prematurity, diaphragmatic hernia, and tracheal suctioning for meconium, will be discussed later in this chapter.

Intubation Equipment

If endotracheal intubation becomes necessary during a neonatal resuscitation, you must quickly prepare the required equipment. Optimally, you should have a neonatal airway kit, with all the necessary equipment, within your pediatric airway kit, if you have one.

As your partner is preoxygenating the newborn with a BVM device and 100% oxygen, prepare the following equipment:

- **Laryngoscope blades**
  - Preterm—size 0 (straight)
  - Full term—size 1 (straight)
    - Straight blades are generally preferred because they facilitate easier lifting of the floppy, omega-shaped epiglottis in the newborn. Additionally, straight blades, because they are not placed in the vallecular space, are not as likely to result in vagal-induced bradycardia.
- **Endotracheal tubes**
  - Use uncuffed ET tubes.
  - Avoid tapered tubes; use a tube with a uniform diameter.
  - If possible, use an ET tube with a black line near the end of the tube
    - This black line is called the vocal cord guide. Such tubes are meant to be inserted so that the vocal cord guide is placed at the level of the vocal cords. This will position the distal end of the tube slightly above the carina.
- **Other equipment**
  - Tape or a commercial securing device
  - Suction
  - Free-flow oxygen
  - Stylet (optional)
    - Usually, the ET tube itself will be rigid enough to allow easy placement; however, if you use a stylet, make sure that it does not protrude beyond the distal tip of the tube and that it can be easily removed following placement of the tube.

There are several ways to determine the correct-sized ET tube for the newborn. You can use anatomic clues, such as the diameter of the infant's little fingernail, or you can follow the guidelines in (Table 30-6), in which the appropriate tube size is based on the newborn's weight and gestational age.

Intubation Technique

The technique for intubating the newborn is the same as it is for infants and children. Follow these general guidelines when intubating the newborn:

- Preoxygenate the newborn prior to performing intubation
  - Unless tracheal suctioning is required for meconium (discussed later)
- When possible, use a pediatric-sized laryngoscope handle
- Use the appropriate-sized ET tube (see Table 30-6)

TABLE 30-5	Indications for Endoctracheal Intubation in the Newborn

- BVM ventilations are not resulting in adequate chest rise
- Ventilatory support is needed for a prolonged period of time
- Chest compressions are necessary
  - Intubation may facilitate the coordination of chest compressions and ventilations and maximize the efficiency of each positive pressure breath
- If epinephrine is required to stimulate the heart, a common route to administer the drug is via the ET tube

TABLE 30-6	Determining the Correct ET Tube Size for the Newborn	
Tube size	Weight	Gestational age
2.5 mm	<1,000 g (1 kg)	<28 weeks
3.0 mm	1,000–2,000 g (1–2 kg)	28–34 weeks
3.5 mm	2,000–3,000 g (2–3 kg)	34–38 weeks
3.5–4.0 mm	>3,000 g (3 kg)	>38 weeks

- Lift, do not pry, when obtaining a laryngoscopic view of the vocal cords
  - This will avoid damage to the deciduous baby teeth that lie beneath the gums
- Provide free-flow oxygen during the intubation procedure
  - This will minimize the risk of bradycardia and hypoxia that can be associated with intubation
- Limit the intubation attempt to a *maximum of 20 seconds*

Following placement of the ET tube, you must assess the newborn to ensure proper placement. Auscultate over the epigastrium and both lungs as primary confirmation; use an end-tidal CO_2 ($ETCO_2$) detector as a means of secondary confirmation. For the newborn, use a pediatric $ETCO_2$ detector, also referred to as a capnographer **Figure 30-8**. Also, note the cm marking on the ET tube at the infant's gums. Secure the tube in place and frequently monitor the position of the tube (ie, auscultation, capnography).

Venous Access

As previously discussed, venous access is not usually needed in newborns; most problems can be corrected with oxygenation and ventilation. Obtain venous access only for fluid delivery or for administration of essential medications. IV access sites include the peripheral veins in the antecubital fossa and the saphenous veins just anterior to the medial malleolus at the ankle. Intraosseous (IO) access can be obtained at the proximal tibia—as with older children.

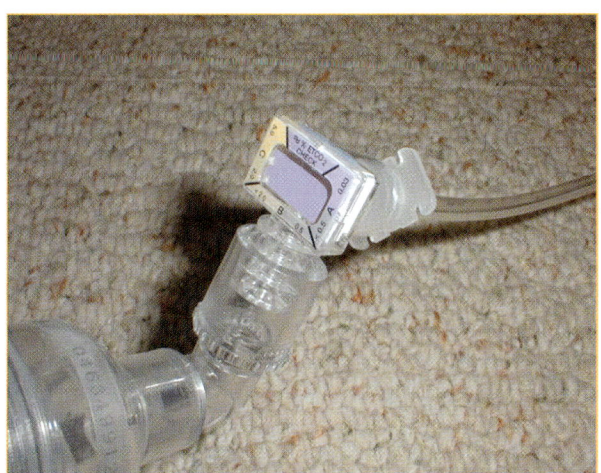

Figure 30-8 Use a pediatric $ETCO_2$ detector in newborns.

For EMS systems using umbilical vein catheterization, consider giving all medications and IV fluids this way. Do not place the umbilical catheter in too far, but place it to a depth where blood return is first seen. This will help keep the catheter out of the portal venous system and avoid complications of certain drugs entering the liver.

Signs of Newborn Hypovolemia

If there has been a placental abruption or previa or blood loss from the umbilical cord, the newborn may be in hypovolemic shock. In some cases, the newborn may have lost blood into the maternal circulation and there will be signs of shock without obvious evidence of blood loss.

Newborns in shock will appear pale and have weak pulses. They may have persistent tachycardia or bradycardia, and cardiovascular function will often not improve in response to effective ventilation, chest compressions, and cardiac medications.

Treatment of Newborn Hypovolemia

For suspected hypovolemia in the newborn, administer 10 mL/kg of an isotonic crystalloid (such as normal saline or lactated Ringer's) over 5 to 10 minutes. Although hypovolemia should be corrected fairly quickly, some clinicians are concerned that rapid fluid administration in a newborn may result in intracranial hemorrhage. Reassess the newborn and provide additional fluids as needed.

> **EMT-I Tips**
>
> Treat a hypovolemic newborn as you would an acute trauma patient with life-threatening blood loss who needs blood products. If venous access is needed due to bleeding, transport the newborn immediately and attempt IV or IO access on the way to the hospital.

Medication Therapy

Medications represent the lowermost portion of the inverted pyramid; therefore, they are the least likely interventions needed during neonatal resuscitation. This section will cover medications that may be necessary to treat refractory cardiovascular compromise, metabolic acidosis, and CNS depression caused by suspected maternal narcotic use **Table 30-7**. Other medications may be indicated; refer to your local protocols or contact medical control as needed.

Epinephrine

Epinephrine, a drug that increases heart rate (chronotropy), myocardial contractility (inotropy), and systemic vascular resistance, is indicated if the newborn's heart rate remains below 60 beats/min after 1 minute of adequate positive pressure ventilations and chest compressions. *Epinephrine is not indicated before you have established adequate ventilation; you will be wasting valuable time that should be focused on establishing effective ventilation and oxygenation.*

If indicated, epinephrine is administered in a dose of 0.1 to 0.3 mL/kg of a 1:10,000 solution via rapid administration. Repeat this dose every 3 to 5 minutes as needed, while ensuring effective ventilations and chest compressions to adequately circulate the drug.

If venous access is established, it is preferable to administer epinephrine via that route; however, epinephrine can also be administered via the endotracheal tube. To ensure that the drug reaches the lungs, consider inserting a 5F feeding tube into the ET tube and injecting the epinephrine through the feeding tube. After injecting the medication, flush the feeding tube with 0.5 mL of normal saline to clear the drug from the feeding tube. The feeding tube is then removed and positive pressure ventilation provided to effectively distribute the medication into the lungs.

Sodium Bicarbonate

Although the use of sodium bicarbonate during neonatal resuscitation is controversial, it may be helpful to correct metabolic acidosis that has resulted from a buildup of lactic acid. Lactic acid is formed during anaerobic metabolism—a condition that occurs when the tissues do not receive sufficient oxygen. Severe acidosis will result in decreased myocardial contractility and decreased pulmonary blood flow, thus preventing the lungs from adequately oxygenating the blood.

Sodium bicarbonate, however, can be harmful, especially if given too early in the resuscitation. You must ensure that ventilation and oxygenation are adequate. When sodium bicarbonate mixes with lactic acid, CO_2 is formed. Therefore, the lungs must be adequately ventilated to remove the CO_2. Sodium bicarbonate is rarely administered during neonatal resuscitation in the prehospital setting. To ensure the most appropriate dosage and avoid causing harm to the newborn, metabolic acidosis must be quantified with an arterial blood gas analysis—a capability that does not exist in the prehospital setting.

Under certain circumstances, such as a lengthy transport time to the hospital, medical control may order you to administer sodium bicarbonate to the newborn who has not responded to other therapy. The appropriate dose is 1 to 2 mEq/kg (2 to 4 mL/kg of a 4.2% solution) via IV, IO, or if available, umbilical vein administration. Sodium bicarbonate is very caustic and should never be given via the ET tube. Regardless of the route administered, give sodium bicarbonate slowly—no faster than 1 mEq/kg/min.

> **EMT-I Tips**
>
> **NEVER** give sodium bicarbonate via the ET tube and **NEVER** give it if adequate ventilation and oxygenation have not been established. Consult medical control prior to administering sodium bicarbonate to the newborn.

Naloxone

In the hospital setting, it is common for a woman in labor to be given narcotic analgesics for pain. However, in the prehospital setting, this is not the case; narcotic use is typically the result of maternal addiction (ie, heroin).

Naloxone (Narcan) is a narcotic antagonist that reverses the CNS depression caused by excessive narcotic administration. While it can be given with relative safety in the hospital to the newborn whose mother was administered a narcotic 4 hours prior to birth, *it should not be given to the newborn of a mother who is suspected of being addicted to narcotics (ie, needle tracks, known drug abuser)*. If the mother is addicted, so is her infant; giving Naloxone under these circumstances can precipitate an acute withdrawal seizure in the newborn.

Naloxone, if administered to the newborn in the prehospital setting, is given in a dose of 0.1 mg/kg (0.4 mg/mL solution) via ET, IO, or IV administration.

TABLE 30-7 Medications Used During Neonatal Resuscitation

Drug	Dose	Route*
Epinephrine	0.1–0.3 mL/kg	IV, IO, ET
Sodium bicarbonate	1–2 mEq/kg	IV or IO
Naloxone	0.1 mg/kg	IV, IO, ET
Dextrose 10%	2 mL/kg	IV or IO

*IV indicates intravenous; IO, intraosseous; and ET, endotracheal.

Although it can be given via the intramuscular (IM) or subcutaneous (SC) routes, the onset of action will be delayed. The duration of action of the narcotic often exceeds that of naloxone, necessitating repeat doses. Therefore, observe the newborn carefully, support ventilations, and be prepared to administer additional doses.

As with any medication, it is important to follow local protocols or contact medical control regarding the use of medications in the newborn. In most cases, your transport time will dictate the administration of certain medications.

Dextrose

Neonatal hypoglycemia—defined as a blood glucose level less than 40 mg/dL—can result from a variety of factors. Among the most common are infants born to diabetic mothers, prematurity (less than 37 weeks or 5.5 pounds [2.5 kg]), and fetal distress secondary to shock, hypoxemia, and hypothermia.

Signs of hypoglycemia in the newborn are often subtle and nonspecific. The newborn commonly presents with irritability, cyanosis, and poor feeding. Untreated hypoglycemia can lead to seizures, permanent neurological damage, and even death.

Check the blood glucose level of any newborn who is not responding to resuscitative efforts or otherwise has signs of hypoglycemia. If the blood glucose level is less than 40 mg/dL, administer 2 mL/kg of 10% dextrose (0.2 g/kg of a 0.1 g/mL concentration) IV push or via the umbilical vein (if it is cannulated).

Special Considerations

Meconium Staining and Aspiration

If the pregnant woman describes a foul odor or dark liquid when her amniotic sac broke, you should suspect meconium staining. Meconium is the fecal matter that is produced in utero. Normally, meconium is not expelled until after birth. Sometimes it is expelled while the fetus is still inside the mother's uterus. If this occurs, the fecal matter can pass into the fetal mouth and airway. If this happens, meconium aspiration can produce

You are the Provider — Part 4

After you provide 30 seconds of CPR and ventilations with a BVM device, the infant's breathing and heart rate stabilize. You clamp and cut the umbilical cord, wrap the infant up in a blanket, and prepare both the young woman and her infant for transport. The assessment of the infant reveals the following:

Reassessment	Recording Time: 1 Minute After Patient Contact
Respirations	30 breaths/min
Pulse	110 beats/min
Appearance	Pink body, blue extremities
Grimace-irritability	Weak cry to stimulus
Muscle tone	Weak attempts to resist straightening

Reassessment of the infant at the 5-minute mark is as follows:

Reassessment	Recording Time: 5 Minutes After Patient Contact
Respirations	50 breaths/min
Pulse	120 beats/min
Appearance	Pink
Grimace-irritability	Weak cry to stimulus
Muscle tone	Resists straightening

7. What were the 1-minute and 5-minute Apgar scores for this newborn?
8. What are your priorities during the transport to the hospital?

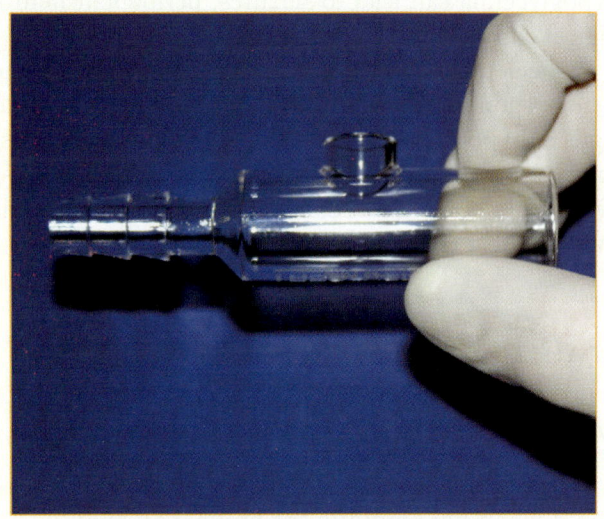

Figure 30-9 Meconium aspirator.

serious pneumonia or airway obstruction that can interfere with the newborn's ability to breathe adequately upon birth.

If meconium is present, you must alter the normal sequence of resuscitation. Once the head of the fetus is delivered, suction the mouth and nose several times if you have enough time between contractions. After birth, if the newborn is immediately crying and breathing (evidence of adequate breathing), has good muscle tone, and is rapidly becoming pink, then treat the delivery as normal.

If the newborn is not immediately vigorous, you must quickly intubate the newborn and suction the trachea. Because meconium is thick, a regular suction catheter will become easily occluded. Therefore, you should use a meconium aspirator to perform tracheal suctioning (Figure 30-9 ▲). This device attaches to the standard 15/22-mm fitting on the proximal end of the endotracheal tube; the ribbed end attaches to the suction machine. While visualizing the vocal cords, insert the ET tube in between the vocal cords. Then, while applying your thumb to the open port on the meconium aspirator, suction the hypopharynx while withdrawing the ET tube. In this manner, you are using the ET tube as the suction catheter. You should repeat this while your partner assesses and monitors the newborn. Continue tracheal suctioning until you have cleared all meconium from the airway **or** the newborn develops bradycardia. At this point, you must proceed with resuscitation.

Many times, meconium aspiration occurs in utero. If there is an infection, the damage has already been done. Your job is to remove any meconium that you can and to begin resuscitation immediately. If meconium aspiration has occurred, you should anticipate that the newborn may not respond to conventional treatment and may need prolonged resuscitation.

Hypothermia

A newborn does not have a lot of body fat. The skin of the newborn is also thinner and less able to compensate for ambient temperature changes. You should always try to keep the newborn protected from the environment. After you initially dry the newborn, discard the wet towels and immediately wrap the newborn in dry towels or blankets. The temperature in the ambulance should be turned up to an uncomfortable level for you and your crew. This will help maintain a comfortable level for the newborn.

Diaphragmatic Hernia

Sometimes the fetal diaphragm does not develop normally. If there is a hole in the diaphragm, the bowels may move into the thoracic cavity. This is a diaphragmatic hernia. Once the fetus is born, the newborn may have difficulty breathing and may require ventilatory assistance and intubation. The lung is collapsed and may have formed improperly because of the pressure from the bowels.

Twins

Twins occur about once in every 80 births. There is sometimes a familial predisposition to having twins. The mother may suspect that she is having twins because she has an unusually large abdomen. Usually twins are diagnosed early in pregnancy by ultrasound or physical examination by a physician. Because of the increased use of hormones, in vitro fertilization, and other infertility treatments, the incidence of multiple births is increasing in the United States. When you must assist in the delivery of twins or multiple births, you must call for an additional crew for each newborn.

Twins and multiple newborns are usually smaller than single newborns; they may also be premature. The delivery is typically not difficult or prolonged. If a pregnant woman has not received prenatal care, consider the possibility that you are dealing with twins any time the first newborn is small or the mother's abdomen remains fairly large after the birth. If twins are present, the second infant will usually be born within 45 minutes of the first. About 10 minutes after the first birth, contractions will begin again, and the birth process will repeat itself.

> **In the Field**
>
> Identical twins are formed from the same egg so they are generally attached to the same placenta. Fraternal twins develop from two separate eggs; therefore, they each have their own placenta.

The procedure for delivering twins is the same as that for single infants. Clamp and cut the cord of the first newborn as soon as it has been born and before the second newborn is delivered. The second newborn may deliver before or after the first placenta. There may be only one placenta, or there may be two. When the placenta has been delivered, check whether there is one umbilical cord or two. If two cords are coming out of one placenta, the twins are called identical. If only one cord is coming out of the placenta, the twins are called fraternal, and there will be two placentas.

Occasionally, the two placentas of fraternal twins are fused, so you might think that you are dealing with identical twins. Remember, if you see only one umbilical cord coming out of the first placenta, there is still another placenta to be delivered. However, if both cords are attached to one placenta, the delivery is over. Identical twins are of the same gender; fraternal twins may be of different genders, or they may be the same.

Record the time of birth of each twin separately. Twins may be so small in weight that they look premature; handle them very carefully and keep them warm.

Delivering a Newborn of an Addicted Mother

A pregnant woman's use of some legal and many illicit drugs and alcohol can cause damage to a fetus. The effects of the drugs on the newborn may include prematurity, low birth weight, and severe respiratory depression. This may be exacerbated if the mother has not received prenatal care. Fetal alcohol syndrome is the term used to describe the specific condition of newborns delivered by mothers who have abused alcohol during their pregnancy. These newborns may be developmentally delayed or have other birth defects.

The newborn of an addicted mother will need immediate hospital care. Carry out the delivery as outlined earlier, but be prepared to perform an aggressive resuscitation.

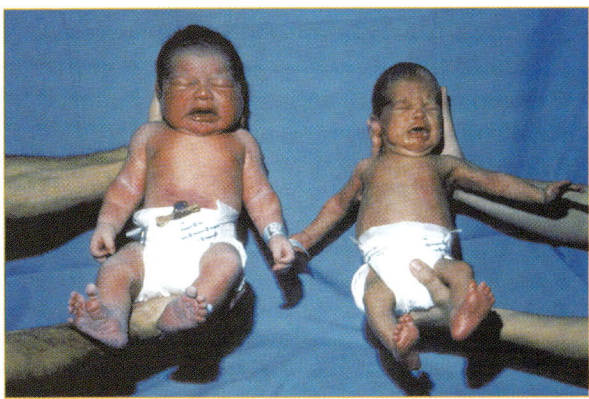

Figure 30-10 Premature newborns (at right) are smaller and thinner than full-term newborns (at left).

Premature Newborn

The usual gestational period (the period of fetal development) is 9 calendar months or 40 weeks. A normal, single newborn will weigh approximately 7 to 8 pounds at birth. Any newborn that delivers before 37 weeks of gestation or weighs less than 5.5 lbs at birth is considered to be premature. This determination is not always easy to make. Often, the exact gestational age cannot be determined. The estimate using the mother's reported last menstrual period as well as ultrasound measurements can be wrong. There are also women who deny that they are pregnant at all and receive no prenatal care. A premature newborn is smaller and thinner than a full-term newborn, and its head is proportionately larger in comparison with the rest of its body **Figure 30-10** . The vernix caseosa that is found on the full-term infant will be missing on the premature infant or will be minimally present. There will also be less body hair. Premature babies are often born with a deficiency of surfactant, resulting in increased alveolar surface tension. Therefore, positive pressure ventilations may be difficult to perform. Be careful, however, and do not become overzealous while ventilating a premature infant; doing so may result in a pneumothorax.

Premature newborns need special care to survive. Often, they require more advanced resuscitation, such as endotracheal intubation. With such care, newborns as small as 1½ lb have survived and developed normally. Follow these procedures when you are handling a premature newborn:

1. **Keep the newborn warm.** Dry the newborn as soon as he or she is born, and then remove the wet towels. Wrap the newborn in a warm blanket, exposing the face but covering the head.

Keep the newborn in a place where the temperature is between 90°F and 95°F (between 32.2°C and 35°C).

2. **Keep the mouth and nose clear of mucus.** Like all newborns, premature newborns are nose breathers, and their small nasal passages can easily be obstructed. Use the bulb syringe to suction the mouth and nostrils frequently. Handle the newborn very gently.
3. **Carefully observe the cut end of the cord** attached to the newborn, and be sure that it is not bleeding. The loss of even a few drops of blood can be very serious.
4. **Give oxygen.** Administer oxygen by mask or by the free-flow technique. Be prepared to support ventilations.
5. **Do not infect the newborn.** Premature newborns are very susceptible to infection. Protect them from contamination. Do not breathe directly into the newborn's face. Your mask will help to create a barrier. Keep everyone else as far away from the newborn as possible.
6. **Notify the hospital.** Does your system have a neonatal (newborn) transport team with specialized personnel and equipment for the care of premature and sick newborns? If so, be sure to contact the hospital before leaving the scene so that medical control can decide whether to call in the team. If not, you should still notify the hospital as soon as possible so that staff can be ready to receive the premature newborn and mother. Avoid unnecessary on-scene delays.

> **EMT-I Tips**
>
> The time surrounding the birth of an infant is a very anxious and stressful time for the parents. Even during a normal delivery, they cannot wait to count the number of fingers and toes and to make sure the baby is fine. It becomes more difficult when there is a problem with the neonate. Try to reassure the mother as you work with a distressed infant. It is best not to separate the two unless you are resuscitating the baby. Do your best to address the concerns of the parent(s) and to assuage their fears.

You may have access to a specialized premature newborn carrier (isolette), which can be used for immediate care as well as transport. Carrier supplies may include a quilted pad, newborn blanket, diaper, thermometer, suction tube and suction bulb, sterile Kelly clamp, and, most important, hot water bottles and an oxygen cylinder with the necessary attachments. Fill the hot water bottles, and pad them well so that they do not come into direct contact with the newborn's skin. Place one on the bottom of the carrier and one on each side of the space for the newborn. Once you have wrapped the newborn in a blanket and placed it inside the carrier, secure the carrier inside the vehicle.

Keep the temperature of the vehicle at 90°F to 95°F (32.2°C to 35°C) while the newborn and mother are being transported to the hospital. If a special carrier is not available, you must keep the premature newborn warm with additional blankets, thermal packets, and warmed patient compartments. Any delays will lower the newborn's body temperature.

Fetal Death

Unfortunately, you may find yourself delivering a fetus that has died in the mother's uterus before labor (stillborn). This will be a true test of your medical, emotional, and professional abilities. Grieving parents will be emotionally distraught and perhaps even hostile. All of your professionalism and support skills will be required.

The onset of labor may be premature, but labor will otherwise progress normally in most cases. If an intrauterine infection has caused the fetus's death, you may note an extremely foul odor. The delivered fetus may have skin blisters, skin sloughing, and a dark discoloration, depending on the stage of decomposition. The head will be soft and perhaps grossly deformed.

Do not attempt to resuscitate an obviously dead newborn. However, it is very difficult to determine the chances of survival for a newborn in the field. The youngest premature newborn to survive was born at 22 weeks' gestation and weighed less than $1\frac{1}{2}$ pounds at birth. To be safe, you should attempt resuscitation on any newborn that has no signs of decomposition. Some newborns have been born so early that their eyelids were fused shut at birth and survived. You will not always be able to tell in the field whether a newborn is a stillbirth from one that has a reversible cardiac arrest from a complication that has just occurred.

You are the Provider — Summary

1. What are the possible causes of the abdominal pain in this patient?

The patient could have experienced trauma, or there could be a medical cause for the pain. It is important to quickly rule out potential life-threatening injuries or illnesses such as trauma or ectopic pregnancy. Many causes of abdominal pain are not life-threatening and can only be identified by extensive testing in the hospital.

2. What important pieces of information would you want to obtain on initial assessment of the patient?

- Have you experienced any trauma?
- Is there a possibility that you may be pregnant?

3. What are your significant findings so far?

This 16-year-old appears to be in labor. Her water has broken. If she is pregnant, she has apparently kept it a secret and has not received prenatal care. You are therefore unable to determine the term of the pregnancy. All of these findings indicate a high-risk delivery, and you need to be prepared to resuscitate the newborn upon delivery.

4. What are your next steps?

Protecting the patient's privacy as much as possible, you need to question the patient more about the pregnancy while removing her pants and underpants to inspect the vaginal area for signs of amniotic fluid or crowning.

5. What are your priorities for treating this newborn?

If the infant does not respond to drying and warming, initiate CPR with a BVM and 100% oxygen.

6. Are medications indicated for this newborn?

Medications are only indicated after an initial 60 seconds of BLS resuscitation. If after 60 seconds the newborn's pulse is still below 60 beats/min, you could consider administering epinephrine.

7. What were the 1-minute and 5-minute Apgar scores for this newborn?

The 1-minute Apgar score is 6. At 5 minutes, the score is 9.

8. What are your priorities during the transport to the hospital?

- Keep the newborn warm.
- Reassess the newborn continually for changes in heart rate, respirations, or color.
- Provide supplemental oxygen to the newborn.
- Keep the newborn's mouth and nose clear of mucus.
- Watch the end of the cord for bleeding.
- Protect the newborn from infection.

Prep Kit

Ready for Review

- The newborn phase lasts from the first few minutes to the first hours after birth. The newborn phase is a period of great physiologic change.
- More than 90% of newborns breathe spontaneously without any advanced interventions. About 10% of newborns require some assistance, and 1% of newborns require advanced resuscitation techniques.
- Certain factors such as maternal diabetes, hypertension, and drug use can increase the chance that the newborn will require resuscitation.
- If you suspect that the newborn will need resuscitation, have all of the equipment open and ready for use.
- Keep all newborns warm to maintain their body heat.
- Three criteria are used to assess the need for further resuscitation in newborns—respirations, heart rate, and color.
- If the newborn's breathing is slow, absent, or inadequate or if the newborn's heart rate is below 100 beats/min, begin ventilations with a BVM device and 100% oxygen at a rate of 40 to 60 breaths/min.
- If the newborn's condition remains unchanged, consider medications that may help in resuscitation.
- The Apgar score is designed to measure the degree of fetal transition or the success of resuscitation. Most healthy newborns will have a score of 7 or 8 at 1 minute and a score of 8 to 10 at 5 minutes. The Apgar score is not used to determine the need for or extent of resuscitation.
- Special considerations in newborn resuscitation include meconium staining and aspiration, hypothermia, diaphragmatic hernia, twins, newborns with fetal alcohol syndrome, and fetal death.
- A premature newborn needs special care and resuscitation to survive.

Vital Vocabulary

acidosis A pathologic condition resulting from the accumulation of lactic acid in the blood.

acrocyanosis Cyanosis of the hands and feet; a normal finding in the newborn that may last for 24 to 48 hours following birth.

antepartum The phase before delivery of the newborn.

Apgar score A scoring system for assessing the status of a newborn that assigns a number value to each of the five areas of assessment.

apical pulse Auscultating the heart rate through the chest wall.

barotrauma Damage to a newborn's lungs resulting from excessive ventilatory pressure.

central cyanosis Cyanosis to the infant's face and trunk; indicates hypoxia.

diaphragmatic hernia A hole or defect in the diaphragm in which a portion of the bowel herniates into the thoracic cavity.

ductus arteriosus Small artery that connects the left pulmonary artery to the aorta; diverts blood away from the fetal lungs while in utero.

Technology

www.EMSzone.com/EMTI

- Interactivities
- Vocabulary Explorer
- Anatomy Review
- Web Links
- Online Review Manual

fetal alcohol syndrome A condition in infants who are born to women who are addicted to alcohol; characterized by physical and mental retardation and a variety of congenital abnormalities.

fetal transition Occurs when the fluid in the fetal lungs is replaced with air, the ductus arteriosus constricts, and the baby begins adequate oxygenation of its own blood.

foramen ovale Opening between the right and left atria, through which blood passes.

gestational period The period of fetal development from fertilization until birth.

infant A baby in the first 12 months of life.

intrapartum The phase that occurs during delivery.

inverted pyramid A diagram that demonstrates the frequency of interventions needed during newborn resuscitation.

meconium The newborn's first bowel movement; usually occurs following birth, but may occur if the fetus is distressed in utero.

meconium aspirator A device used in conjunction with an ET tube to suction meconium from the newborn's airway.

neonate The phase of life that occurs during the first 28 days after birth.

newborn The phase from the first few minutes to the first hours after birth.

orogastric (OG) tube Tube that is inserted through the mouth and into the stomach; used to decompress the stomach.

peripheral cyanosis Cyanosis of the hands and feet; also referred to as acrocyanosis.

portal venous system Special venous drainage system that takes blood from the intestines to the liver.

premature A newborn that delivers before 36 weeks' gestation or weighs less than 5 lb at birth.

primary apnea Apnea that can often be reversed with tactile stimulation and suctioning.

prostaglandin-E2 Hormone that causes the ductus arteriosus to remain open (patent).

secondary apnea Apnea that is not reversed with tactile stimulation and suctioning; requires positive pressure ventilations to reverse.

tactile stimulation Method of stimulating a newborn to breathe by flicking or slapping the soles of the feet or rubbing the lateral thorax.

umbilical vein catheter (UVC) A special catheter designed to be inserted into the umbilical vein.

umbilical vein catheterization Inserting a UVC into the umbilical vein; an alternate route for administering drugs and IV fluids to the newborn.

vernix caseosa Slippery, cheesy-like substance that covers the newborn at birth.

vocal cord guide Black line on the distal end of the ET tube; used to properly position the tube in between the vocal cords.

Assessment in Action

You are on the scene of a woman in labor. Your history and physical exam reveal a 24-year-old woman in active labor. She is at 30 weeks' gestation. Crowning is present and you expect delivery within minutes.

1. On the basis of your assessment findings, you should do all of the following EXCEPT:
   A. prepare neonatal airway equipment.
   B. protect yourself by applying appropriate PPE.
   C. administer oxygen to the patient.
   D. transport the patient immediately.

2. You have delivered a baby boy. He is cyanotic and not breathing. You should immediately:
   A. suction the airway.
   B. transport the infant immediately.
   C. wrap the infant in warm blankets.
   D. ventilate the infant with high-flow oxygen.

3. Respiratory management guidelines for your patient include:
   A. inserting a nasal airway.
   B. hyperventilating with high-flow oxygen.
   C. ventilating by completely deflating the BVM device with each ventilation.
   D. opening the airway by placing the infant in the neutral or slightly extended position.

You have provided respiratory care for 30 seconds. You reassess the infant and find a pulse of 50 beats/min, no respirations, and cyanosis. The infant is not crying but weakly resists straightening the legs.

4. What is the infant's Apgar score?
   A. 1
   B. 2
   C. 3
   D. 4

5. You should immediately:
   A. ventilate the infant for 30 seconds then reassess.
   B. begin chest compressions.
   C. hyperventilate the infant with high-flow oxygen then reassess.
   D. administer epinephrine.

6. AHA CPR guidelines for the newborn include:
   A. compressions are delivered at a rate of 140.
   B. compression to ventilation ratio is 3:1.
   C. compressions are performed using the heel of one hand.
   D. compressions are performed over the mid-sternum.

7. One minute after treatment the infant's pulse is 80 beats/min, respirations are 20 breaths/min, and the trunk is pink. You should:
   A. continue chest compressions.
   B. continue assisting ventilations.
   C. hyperventilate the patient with high-flow oxygen.
   D. administer epinephrine.

Several minutes later the infant's pulse is 120 beats/min, respirations are 40 breaths/min, and the infant has a weak cry. The infant's lips and hands are cyanotic but he strongly resists straightening of his legs.

8. What is the patient's Apgar score?
   A. 6
   B. 7
   C. 8
   D. 9

9. Your treatment will include:
   A. continuing chest compressions.
   B. continuing to assist ventilations.
   C. administering oxygen.
   D. monitoring the infant's condition only.

Points to Ponder

You arrive on the scene of a woman in labor. Your assessment reveals that contractions are 1 minute apart, the water broke an hour ago, and crowning occurs with contractions. You decide to prepare for immediate delivery.

You open your OB kit, apply the appropriate PPE, and position the mother for delivery. You ask no further questions and perform no further assessment. The infant appears to deliver normally but is not breathing. As you scramble to assemble the necessary respiratory equipment, you notice that the mother is bleeding heavily. Your partner takes over care of the infant while you massage the fundus to slow the bleeding and call for additional help. Several minutes pass. The bleeding has slowed, but only because the mother is now in cardiac arrest. The mother does not survive. After the call you learn that the mother did not have a normal pregnancy. An ultrasound recently revealed that she had an abruptio placenta. You also learn that meconium staining was present when the water broke.

What should you have done differently?

Issues: Importance of Assessment and Preparation, Problem Pregnancies, Thorough History Taking

Pediatric Emergencies

1999 Objectives

Cognitive

6-3.1 Identify methods/mechanisms that prevent injuries to infants and children. (p 1234)

6-3.2 Identify the growth and developmental characteristics of infants and children. (p 1235)

6-3.3 Identify anatomy and physiology characteristics of infants and children. (p 1238)

6-3.4 Describe techniques for successful assessment of infants and children. (p 1242)

6-3.5 Identify the common responses of families to acute illness and injury of an infant or child. (p 1242)

6-3.6 Describe techniques for successful interaction with families of acutely ill or injured infants and children. (p 1242)

6-3.7 Outline differences in adult and childhood anatomy and physiology. (p 1238)

6-3.8 Discuss pediatric patient assessment. (p 1244)

6-3.9 Identify "normal" age group related vital signs. (p 1249)

6-3.10 Discuss the appropriate equipment utilized to obtain pediatric vital signs. (p 1250)

6-3.11 Determine appropriate airway adjuncts for infants and children. (p 1259)

6-3.12 Discuss complications of improper utilization of airway adjuncts with infants and children. (p 1260, 1262)

6-3.13 Discuss appropriate ventilation devices for infants and children. (p 1264)

6-3.14 Discuss complications of improper utilization of ventilation devices with infants and children. (p 1265)

6-3.15 Discuss appropriate endotracheal intubation equipment for infants and children. (p 1267)

6-3.16 Identify complications of improper endotracheal intubation procedure in infants and children. (p 1269)

6-3.17 Define respiratory distress. (p 1285)

6-3.18 Define respiratory failure. (p 1285)

6-3.19 Define respiratory arrest. (p 1285)

6-3.20 Describe the epidemiology, including the incidence, morbidity/mortality, risk factors, and prevention strategies for respiratory distress/failure in infants and children. (p 1285)

6-3.21 Discuss the pathophysiology of respiratory distress/failure in infants and children. (p 1285)

6-3.22 Discuss the assessment findings associated with respiratory distress/failure in infants and children. (p 1285)

6-3.23 Discuss the management/treatment plan for respiratory distress/failure in infants and children. (p 1286)

6-3.24 List the indications for gastric decompression for infants and children. (p 1272)

6-3.25 Differentiate between upper and lower airway obstruction. (p 1252)

6-3.26 Describe the epidemiology, including the incidence, morbidity/mortality, risk factors, and prevention strategies for croup in infants and children. (p 1286)

6-3.27 Discuss the pathophysiology of croup in infants and children. (p 1286)

6-3.28 Discuss the assessment findings associated with croup in infants and children. (p 1287)

6-3.29 Discuss the management/treatment plan for croup in infants and children. (p 1287)

6-3.30 Describe the epidemiology, including the incidence, morbidity/mortality, risk factors, and prevention strategies for foreign body aspiration in infants and children. (p 1252)

6-3.31 Discuss the pathophysiology of foreign body aspiration in infants and children. (p 1254)

6-3.32 Discuss the assessment findings associated with foreign body aspiration in infants and children. (p 1254)

6-3.33 Discuss the management/treatment plan for foreign body aspiration in infants and children. (p 1254)

6-3.34 Describe the epidemiology, including the incidence, morbidity/mortality, risk factors, and prevention strategies for epiglottitis in infants and children. (p 1287)

6-3.35 Discuss the pathophysiology of epiglottitis in infants and children. (p 1287)

6-3.36 Discuss the assessment findings associated with epiglottitis in infants and children. (p 1288)

6-3.37 Discuss the management/treatment plan for epiglottitis in infants and children. (p 1288)

6-3.38 Describe the epidemiology, including the incidence, morbidity/mortality, risk factors, and prevention strategies for asthma/bronchiolitis in infants and children. (p 1288)

6-3.39 Discuss the pathophysiology of asthma/bronchiolitis in infants and children. (p 1289)

6-3.40 Discuss the assessment findings associated with asthma/bronchiolitis in infants and children. (p 1289)

6-3.41 Discuss the management/treatment plan for asthma/bronchiolitis in infants and children. (p 1289)

6-3.42 Describe the epidemiology, including the incidence, morbidity/mortality, risk factors, and prevention strategies for pneumonia in infants and children. (p 1290)

6-3.43 Discuss the pathophysiology of pneumonia in infants and children. (p 1291)

6-3.44 Discuss the assessment findings associated with pneumonia in infants and children. (p 1291)

6-3.45 Discuss the management/treatment plan for pneumonia in infants and children. (p 1291)

6-3.46 Describe the epidemiology, including the incidence, morbidity/mortality, risk factors, and prevention strategies for foreign body lower airway obstruction in infants and children. (p 1291)

6-3.47 Discuss the pathophysiology of foreign body lower airway obstruction in infants and children. (p 1291)

6-3.48 Discuss the assessment findings associated with foreign body lower airway obstruction in infants and children. (p 1291)

6-3.49 Discuss the management/treatment plan for foreign body lower airway obstruction in infants and children. (p 1291)

6-3.50 Discuss the common causes of shock in infants and children. (p 1292)

6-3.51 Evaluate the severity of shock in infants and children. (p 1292)

6-3.52 Describe the epidemiology, including the incidence, morbidity/mortality, risk factors, and prevention strategies for shock in infants and children. (p 1291)

6-3.53 Discuss the pathophysiology of shock in infants and children. (p 1292, 1294)

6-3.54 Discuss the assessment findings associated with shock in infants and children. (p 1292)

6-3.55 Discuss the management/treatment plan for shock in infants and children. (p 1292)

6-3.56 Identify the major classifications of pediatric cardiac rhythms. (p 1296, 1297)

6-3.57 Describe the epidemiology, including the incidence, morbidity/mortality, risk factors, and prevention strategies for cardiac dysrhythmias in infants and children. (p 1296, 1297)

6-3.58 Discuss the pathophysiology of cardiac dysrhythmias in infants and children. (p 1296)

6-3.59 Discuss the assessment findings associated with cardiac dysrhythmias in infants and children. (p 1296)

6-3.60 Discuss the management/treatment plan for cardiac dysrhythmias in infants and children. (p 1296-1299)

6-3.61 Describe the epidemiology, including the incidence, morbidity/mortality, risk factors, and prevention strategies for tachydysrhythmias in infants and children. (p 1296)

6-3.62 Discuss the pathophysiology of tachydysrhythmias in infants and children. (p 1296)

6-3.63 Discuss the assessment findings associated with tachydysrhythmias in infants and children. (p 1296)

6-3.64 Discuss the management/treatment plan for tachydysrhythmias in infants and children. (p 1296, 1297)

6-3.65 Describe the epidemiology, including the incidence, morbidity/mortality, risk factors, and prevention strategies for bradydysrhythmias in infants and children. (p 1297)

Pediatric Emergencies

6-3.66 Discuss the pathophysiology of bradydysrhythmias in infants and children. (p 1297)

6-3.67 Discuss the assessment findings associated with bradydysrhythmias in infants and children. (p 1297)

6-3.68 Discuss the management/treatment plan for bradydysrhythmias in infants and children. (p 1297)

6-3.69 Discuss the primary etiologies of cardiopulmonary arrest in infants and children. (p 1297)

6-3.70 Discuss basic cardiac life support (CPR) guidelines for infants and children. (p 1274)

6-3.71 Identify appropriate parameters for performing infant and child CPR. (p 1274)

6-3.72 Integrate advanced life support skills with basic cardiac life support for infants and children. (p 1250)

6-3.73 Describe the epidemiology, including the incidence, morbidity/mortality, risk factors, and prevention strategies for seizures in infants and children. (p 1274, 1299)

6-3.74 Discuss the pathophysiology of seizures in infants and children. (p 1299)

6-3.75 Discuss the assessment findings associated with seizures in infants and children. (p 1299)

6-3.76 Discuss the management/treatment plan for seizures in infants and children. (p 1300)

6-3.77 Describe the epidemiology, including the incidence, morbidity/mortality, risk factors, and prevention strategies for hypoglycemia in infants and children. (p 1305)

6-3.78 Discuss the pathophysiology of hypoglycemia in infants and children. (p 1305)

6-3.79 Discuss the assessment findings associated with hypoglycemia in infants and children. (p 1306)

6-3.80 Discuss the management/treatment plan for hypoglycemia in infants and children. (p 1306)

6-3.81 Describe the epidemiology, including the incidence, morbidity/mortality, risk factors, and prevention strategies for hyperglycemia in infants and children. (p 1306)

6-3.82 Discuss the pathophysiology of hyperglycemia in infants and children. (p 1306)

6-3.83 Discuss the assessment findings associated with hyperglycemia in infants and children. (p 1306)

6-3.84 Discuss the management/treatment plan for hyperglycemia in infants and children. (p 1306)

6-3.85 Discuss age appropriate vascular access sites for infants and children. (p 1277)

6-3.86 Discuss the appropriate equipment for vascular access in infants and children. (p 1276)

6-3.87 Identify complications of vascular access for infants and children. (p 1279)

6-3.88 Identify common lethal mechanisms of injury in infants and children. (p 1310)

6-3.89 Discuss anatomical features of children that predispose or protect them from certain injuries. (p 1310)

6-3.90 Describe aspects of infant and children airway management that are affected by potential cervical spine injury. (p 1313)

6-3.91 Identify infant and child trauma patients who require spinal immobilization. (p 1314)

6-3.92 Discuss fluid management and shock treatment for infant and child trauma patient. (p 1314)

6-3.93 Discuss the pathophysiology of trauma in infants and children. (p 1311)

6-3.94 Discuss the assessment findings associated with trauma in infants and children. (p 1318)

6-3.95 Discuss the management/treatment plan for trauma in infants and children. (p 1318)

6-3.96 Discuss the assessment findings and management considerations for pediatric trauma patients with the following specific injuries: head/neck injuries, chest injuries, abdominal injuries, extremities injuries, burns. (p 1315-1317)

6-3.97 Define child abuse. (p 1321)

6-3.98 Define child neglect. (p 1324)

6-3.99 Describe the epidemiology, including the incidence, morbidity/mortality, risk factors, and prevention strategies for abuse and neglect in infants and children. (p 1321)

6-3.100 Discuss the assessment findings associated with abuse and neglect in infants and children. (p 1321, 1324)

6-3.101 Discuss the management/treatment plan for abuse and neglect in infants and children. (p 1324)

6-3.102 Define sudden infant death syndrome (SIDS). (p 1307)

6-3.103 Discuss the parent/caregiver responses to the death of an infant or child. (p 1308)

6-3.104 Describe the epidemiology, including the incidence, morbidity/mortality, risk factors, and prevention strategies for SIDS infants. (p 1307)

6-3.105 Discuss the pathophysiology of SIDS in infants. (p 1307)

6-3.106 Discuss the assessment findings associated with SIDS infants. (p 1307)

6-3.107 Discuss the management/treatment plan for SIDS in infants. (p 1308)

Affective

6-3.108 Demonstrate and advocate appropriate interactions with the infant/child that conveys an understanding of their developmental stage. (p 1242)

6-3.109 Recognize the emotional dependence of the infant/child to their parent/guardian. (p 1242)

6-3.110 Recognize the emotional impact of the infant/child injuries and illnesses on the parent/guardian. (p 1242)

6-3.111 Recognize and appreciate the physical and emotional difficulties associated with separation of the parent/guardian of a special needs child. (p 1242, 1284)

6-3.112 Demonstrate the ability to provide reassurance, empathy, and compassion for the parent/guardian. (p 1242)

Psychomotor

2.1.86 Perform manual airway maneuvers for pediatric patients, including:
   a. Opening the mouth
   b. Head-tilt/chin-lift maneuver
   c. Jaw-thrust without head-tilt maneuver
   d. Modified jaw-thrust maneuver
   (p 1246, 1247, 1255)

6-3.113 Demonstrate the appropriate approach for treating infants and children. (p 1242)

6-3.114 Demonstrate appropriate intervention techniques with families of acutely ill or injured infants and children. (p 1242)

6-3.115 Demonstrate an appropriate assessment for different developmental age groups. (p 1235)

6-3.116 Demonstrate appropriate technique for measuring pediatric vital signs. (p 1248)

6-3.117 Demonstrate the use of a length-based resuscitation device for determining equipment sizes, drug doses, and other pertinent information for a pediatric patient. (p 1260)

6-3.118 Demonstrate the techniques/procedures for treating infants and children with respiratory distress. (p 1263)

6-3.119 Demonstrate proper technique for administering blow-by oxygen to infants and children. (p 1263)

6-3.120 Demonstrate the proper utilization of a pediatric non-rebreather oxygen mask. (p 1263)

6-3.121 Demonstrate appropriate use of airway adjuncts with infants and children. (p 1259)

6-3.122 Demonstrate appropriate use of ventilation devices for infants and children. (p 1265)

6-3.123 Demonstrate endotracheal intubation procedures in infants and children. (p 1268)

6-3.124 Demonstrate appropriate treatment/management of intubation complications for infants and children. (p 1269)

6-3.125 Demonstrate proper placement of a gastric tube in infants and children. (p 1273)

6-3.126 Demonstrate appropriate technique for insertion of peripheral intravenous catheters for infants and children. (p 1276)

6-3.127 Demonstrate appropriate technique for administration of intramuscular, subcutaneous, rectal, endotracheal, and oral medication for infants and children. (p 1280)

6-3.128 Demonstrate appropriate technique for insertion of an intraosseous line for infants and children. (p 1278)

6-3.129 Demonstrate age appropriate interventions for infants and children with an obstructed airway. (p 1254, 1256)

Pediatric Emergencies

6-3.130 Demonstrate appropriate airway control maneuvers for infant and child trauma patients. (p 1319)

6-3.131 Demonstrate appropriate treatment of infants and children requiring advanced airway and breathing control. (p 1259, 1266)

6-3.132 Demonstrate appropriate immobilization techniques for infant and child trauma patients. (p 1314)

6-3.133 Demonstrate treatment of infants and children with head injuries. (p 1314, 1315)

6-3.134 Demonstrate appropriate treatment of infants and children with chest injuries. (p 1316)

6-3.135 Demonstrate appropriate treatment of infants and children with abdominal injuries. (p 1316)

6-3.136 Demonstrate appropriate treatment of infants and children with extremity injuries. (p 1316)

6-3.137 Demonstrate appropriate treatment of infants and children with burns. (p 1316)

6-3.138 Demonstrate appropriate parent/caregiver interviewing techniques for infant and child death situations. (p 1309)

6-3.139 Demonstrate proper infant CPR. (p 1274)

6-3.140 Demonstrate proper child CPR. (p 1274)

6-3.141 Demonstrate proper techniques for performing infant and child defibrillation. (p 1280)

1985 Objectives

There are no 1985 objectives for this chapter.

31

Pediatric Emergencies

You are the Provider

You and your partner are called to the scene of a 9-year-old boy struck by a car. You arrive to find the boy on the ground with an obvious, angulated femur fracture. Bystanders state that he was riding on a side street and was struck by a car traveling approximately 25 miles per hour. The boy was thrown to the ground and was apparently unresponsive for a brief period. He was not wearing a helmet.

Although relatively infrequent, serious pediatric calls can be very stressful and taxing situations. The EMT-I *must* be prepared to handle the unique demands that sick or injured children present. This chapter will prepare you for the challenges of pediatric assessment and management and help you answer the following questions:

1. What are the anatomic and physiologic differences between pediatric and adult patients?
2. How must the EMT-I adjust his or her assessment and treatment to accommodate the unique challenges of a child?

Unique Needs of Children

It is not uncommon for the prehospital professional to experience anxiety when responding to a call involving a pediatric patient. Assessment and management of infants and children present a unique challenge to the EMT-I. Unlike their adult counterparts, pediatric patients, especially infants and small children, cannot provide you with the historical information that is usually easily obtained from an adult, such as events preceding the incident, what happened, medical history, and where they hurt.

In addition to caring for the sick or injured child, you must also be prepared to deal with parents or caregivers. Many times, they can provide you with the vital information that you need; other times, they panic, are demanding, or are otherwise of little assistance to you.

It is often said that children are not simply small adults—a statement that could not hold more truth. Unlike adults, children have special needs that require the EMT-I to adjust assessment and management strategies accordingly. This chapter will discuss those special needs, including the epidemiology of pediatric injury and illness, the role of the EMT-I in pediatric mortality and morbidity reduction, anatomic and physiologic differences between children and adults, and the assessment and management of pediatric medical and trauma emergencies.

Epidemiology

Approximately 10% of all EMS calls involve a sick or injured child. While pediatric emergencies account for a relatively small percentage of an EMS system's call volume, pediatric mortality has become a significant health concern in the United States, with approximately 20,000 pediatric deaths occurring each year.

Pediatric Trauma

Trauma is the leading killer of children in the United States. More children die of trauma-related injuries annually than all other causes combined. The types of injuries in children differ, depending on their age. Infants and toddlers are most commonly injured as the result of falls or abuse. Older children and adolescents are usually injured as a result of motor vehicle crashes.

Other common causes of traumatic injury and death include injuries inflicted by suicide or homicide, burns, drownings, and sports-related injuries.

Pediatric Illness

As an EMT-I, you will also respond to calls for ill children. Some diseases, such as croup, bronchiolitis, and febrile seizures, are unique to children. However, children often experience the same illnesses that affect adults.

The severity of illnesses in children can range from a simple upper respiratory infection to cardiopulmonary arrest. Thorough familiarity with common pediatric illnesses and disease processes will enable you to provide early, aggressive intervention—the key to reduced morbidity and mortality.

Injury and Illness Prevention

Children are at higher risk for injury and illness than adults. In addition, the adverse effects of injuries and illnesses tend to be more severe in children than they are in adults. As an EMT-I, you should consider it your responsibility to actively engage in programs aimed at reducing the incidence of pediatric illness and injury; preventing an injury before it occurs is far better than attempting to manage the consequences after the fact.

An effective injury or illness prevention program should focus on factors that can be changed or altered. Although many of the factors that result in pediatric illness and injury (such as weather, time of year) cannot

---

Technology

- Interactivities
- Vocabulary Explorer
- Anatomy Review
- Web Links
- Online Review Manual

www.EMSzone.com/EMTI

be changed, others can. For example, providing education to parents regarding a safe living environment may prevent many common household injuries. Ensuring that electrical outlets are covered and that cabinets containing medications or toxic substances are adequately secured requires little effort on the part of the parents or caregivers and may help to save their child's life.

Other injury prevention programs should focus on the appropriate use of car seats, the use of helmets when riding bicycles or skateboarding, and education regarding the use of drugs and alcohol. Unfortunately, many parents do not take the time to educate their children about the consequences of drug and alcohol use.

Although many pediatric illnesses cannot be prevented, parents or caregivers should be educated about the recognition of certain illnesses and when it is appropriate to seek medical attention. Many childhood illnesses that could otherwise have been treated successfully early in their course are allowed to progress to the point at which the child becomes critically ill. You must now manage the negative consequences of the illness, the outcome of which is not always positive.

Although training in infant and child CPR and treatment for airway obstructions is mandatory for licensed child care facilities, community-wide programs addressing this important training should also be offered.

Continuing Education

Because most of your work involves sick or injured adults, you must ensure a good working knowledge base and continued competency in caring for children; this does not stop after your initial training. You should attend continuing education programs that focus on the care of sick or injured children. Such programs include Pediatric Education for Prehospital Professionals (also called PEPP) and Pediatric Advanced Life Support (also called PALS), among others.

Other sources of continuing education include attendance at conferences and seminars, reading pediatric-related articles in magazines (such as *EMS Magazine*, *JEMS*), and even spending time in facilities that specialize in pediatric care, such as pediatric intensive care units and pediatric emergency departments.

As previously mentioned, prehospital care providers often experience anxiety when responding to the scene of a sick or injured child. The most effective remedy for this is to constantly strive to increase your knowledge of pediatrics and to remain current in trends in pediatric management.

Growth and Development

Adulthood begins at age 21 years. On this, the medical community has agreed. But when does childhood end? Many EMS systems use 18 years, others use 14 years, and still others use 12 or 16 years. Even though there are specific issues that are important to different age groups, there are also some general rules that apply when you are caring for children of any age (Table 31-1 ▶).

Between birth and adulthood, many physical and emotional changes occur in children. While each child is unique, the thoughts and behaviors of children as a whole are often grouped into stages: infancy, the toddler years, preschool age, school age, and adolescence. Children in each stage grapple with different developmental issues.

How you examine children and how you help them to cope with the emergency depend on several practical

You are the Provider — Part 2

As you approach the child, you note that he is lying supine on the ground and not moving. When you begin manual stabilization of his cervical spine, he responds by crying but will not answer questions or interact appropriately. His airway is open, and his respirations appear normal. His skin, however, is very pale.

3. What kind of response would you expect from a school-age child?
4. Even though you have not performed a thorough, detailed assessment, based on your initial observations would you consider this patient in critical or stable condition? What does your "gut feeling" tell you?

> **TABLE 31-1** | **Helpful Tips in Caring for Infants and Children**
>
> 1. **Try to remain calm and appear confident.** Children are used to having other people take charge. They are also easily frightened by noise, so speak with a soft voice whenever possible.
> 2. **Remember that you provide care for the whole family, not just the child.** Children are quick to pick up on caregivers' fear and anxiety. It may calm both parties if you can establish good rapport with the caregivers and allow them to help with the child's care, when practical. To avoid confusion, refrain from using technical terms.
> 3. **Honesty is the best policy.** Telling a child or caregiver that a procedure won't hurt (when you know that it will) or that it will be over quickly (when you know that it won't) can boomerang: Once you lose their trust, any additional procedures that you attempt are more likely to be met with resistance.
> 4. **Tell both the caregivers and the child what is happening as often as you can.** Lack of information is stressful for everyone; the imagination can run wild in an effort to make sense of what is going on. In children, we call this a frightening fantasy; in caregivers, we call it a worst-case scenario.
> 5. **Keep the family together as much as possible.** When children are critically ill or injured, this is not always possible, but children and their caregivers generally feel safer when they are together. Parents can sometimes be encouraged to help by holding the child's hand, talking to the child, or telling a story.
> 6. **Provide hope and reassurance to the caregivers and to the child.** Even when you are very concerned about the child's condition, be careful not to eliminate hope in the patient and family. Children especially need reassurance, rewards, and praise during painful events. Remember, however, that no one can be absolutely positive of the outcome; therefore, you must use caution and avoid providing false hope to the patient and the family.

considerations, including the child's hemodynamic stability and mental status, the anticipated transport time, the availability of other personnel, and the protocols in your area.

The Infant

Infancy is usually defined as the first year of life; the first 28 days of life is called the neonatal period. A newborn is a neonate that is a few hours old. The perinatal period is the period around birth and includes the time from 20 or 28 weeks of pregnancy through 1 or 4 weeks after birth, depending on the source.

At first, infants respond mainly to physical stimuli such as light, warmth, cold, hunger, sound, and taste. Crying is one of their main avenues of expression during this period. After the first few months, however, they learn to coo, smile, roll over, and recognize their parents and/or caregivers. Infants are usually not afraid of strangers because they become the center of attention in most families. However, by the end of their first year, they may show signs of preferring to be with their caregivers and may cry if they are separated from them **Figure 31-1**.

The Toddler

After infancy, until about 3 years of age, a child is called a toddler. During this period, children begin to walk and explore the environment. They are able to open doors, drawers, boxes, and bottles. Because they are explorers by nature and are not afraid, injuries in this age group are more frequent.

Stranger anxiety develops early in this period. Toddlers may resist separation from caregivers and be afraid to let others hold them or come near them. Because of their newly found independence, they may also be very unhappy about being restrained or held for procedures **Figure 31-2**.

Two-year-olds in particular have a well-deserved reputation for having their own ideas about almost everything, which is why these years are often called the "terrible twos." Toddlers have a hard time describing or localizing pain. Pain in the abdomen may be "My tummy hurts," and

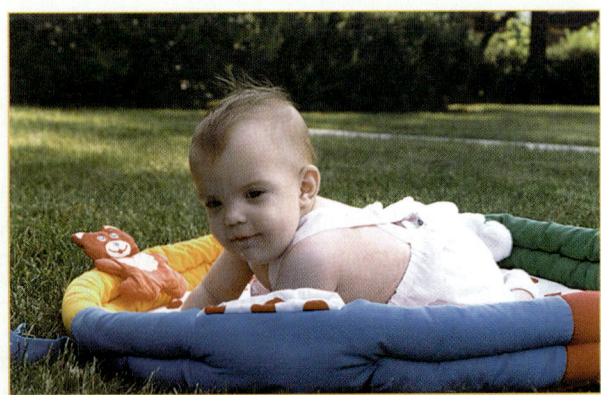

Figure 31-1 Infants are usually not afraid of strangers, but as they reach 6 months to 1 year, they may show signs that they prefer to be with their caregivers.

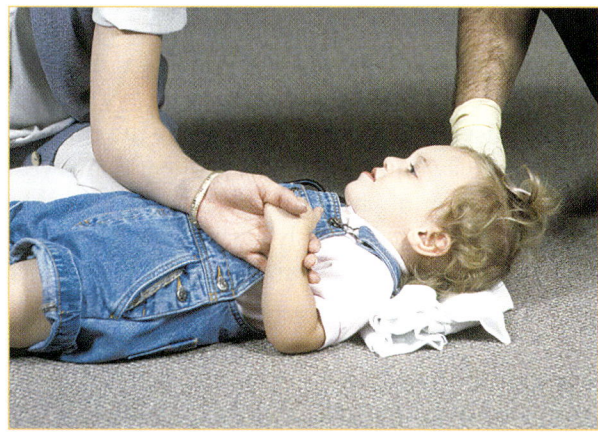

Figure 31-2 Because of their newly found independence, toddlers may be unhappy about being restrained or held for procedures.

examination may reveal tenderness throughout the body. This is not because the child is trying to be difficult but because he or she cannot tell the difference.

The Preschool-Age Child

Preschool-age children (ages 3 to 5) are able to use simple language quite effectively and have lively imaginations Figure 31-3. They can understand directions, be much more specific in describing their sensations, and identify painful areas when asked.

Preschool-age children have a rich fantasy life, which can make them particularly fearful about pain and change involving their bodies. At this age, they often believe that their thoughts or wishes can cause injury or harm to themselves or to others. They can believe that an injury was due to a bad deed they did earlier in the day.

The School-Age Child

School-age children (ages 6 to 12 years) are beginning to act more like adults. They can think in concrete terms, respond sensibly to direct questions, and help take care of themselves. Your assessment, therefore, is more like an adult assessment; talk to the child, not just the parent, when obtaining the medical history Figure 31-4.

School-age children can understand the difference between emotional and physical pain. They also have concerns about the meaning of pain. Give them simple explanations about what is causing their pain and what will be done about it. Games and conversation may distract them. Ask them to describe their favorite place, their pets, or their toys. Ask the caregiver's advice in choosing the right distraction.

Rewarding the school-age child after a procedure can be very helpful in his or her recovery, but only reward a child for completing the procedure.

The Adolescent

The adolescent (ages 12 to 18 years) is usually able to think abstractly and can participate in decision making. This is a period when the focus of their strength has moved from parents to peers. They are very concerned about body image and how they appear to their peers and to others. They may have strong feelings about

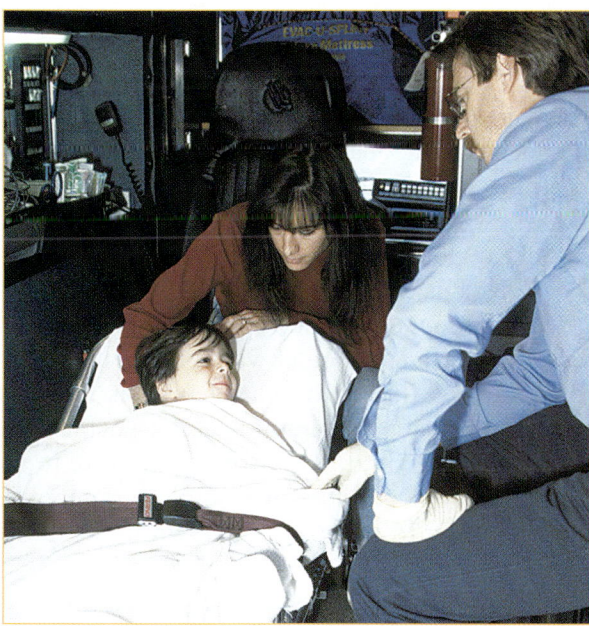

Figure 31-3 Preschool-age children have vivid imaginations, so much of the history must still be obtained from the caregiver.

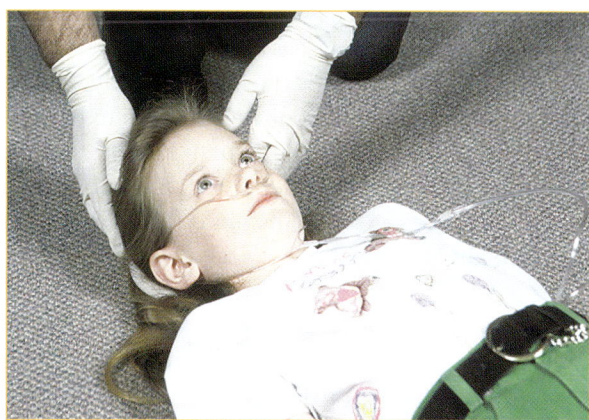

Figure 31-4 School-age children are more like adults in that they can answer your questions and help take care of themselves.

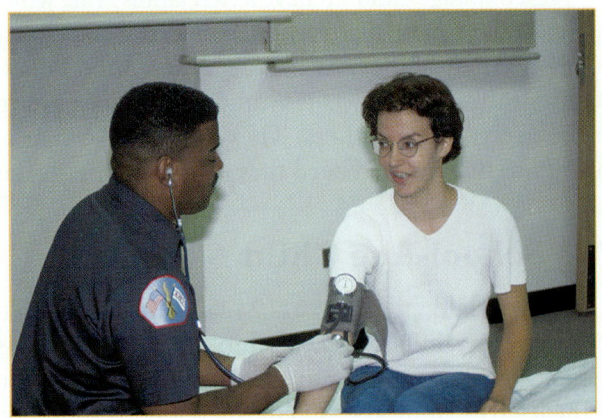

Figure 31-5 Respect the adolescent's privacy at all times; give the patient whatever information he or she requests.

being observed during procedures, even—or especially—by their caregivers.

Respect the adolescent's privacy at all times. Remember that adolescents can often understand very complex concepts and treatment options; you should provide them with information when they request it 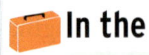. You will find them more helpful and understanding of necessary procedures.

Adolescents have a clear understanding of the purpose and meaning of pain. Whenever possible, explain any necessary procedures well in advance. Assess their pain by facial and body expression and by asking questions; adolescents can be very stoic and may not request relief from pain even when they need it. To distract them, find out what they are interested in, such as sports, books, movies, or friends, and get them talking about this.

Anatomy and Physiology

There is no other time in our lives that our bodies are growing and changing as fast as during childhood. Infants quickly change once outside the mother's body. Toddlers learn to walk and talk. School-age children explore the world without thought of consequences. The anatomic and physiologic changes and differences can create difficulties with assessment of the child if the EMT-I does not understand them.

The Head

The child's head is proportionally larger than an adult's, specifically the occipital region of the skull. The child's face, however, is smaller in comparison with the size of the head. Because of their proportionally larger heads, infants and children are especially prone to head trauma, such as during a fall, in which gravity takes them head first. Because of the proportionally larger occiput, special care must be taken when positioning the child's airway. In seriously injured children younger than 3 years, place a thin layer of padding under the back to obtain a neutral position. In seriously ill children younger than 3 years, place a folded sheet under the occiput to obtain a sniffing position.

During infancy, the anterior and posterior fontanelles are open. The fontanelles are areas where the infant's skull bones have not fused together, thus allowing compression of the head during the birthing process and for rapid growth of the brain. By the time the child reaches the age of approximately 18 months, both of the fontanelles have closed.

The fontanelles are an important anatomic landmark when assessing a sick or injured infant. Bulging of the fontanelles suggests increased intracranial pressure; sunken fontanelles suggest dehydration. These conditions will be discussed later in this chapter.

> **In the Field**
>
> Always assess the fontanelles in the infant.
> Bulging = increased intracranial pressure
> Sunken = dehydration

The Airway

To manage the pediatric airway effectively, you must first understand the anatomic differences between adults and children. To start with, the heart is higher in a child's chest, and the lungs are smaller. The opening to the trachea (glottic opening) is higher in the neck, and the neck itself is shorter.

The anatomy of a child's airway differs from that of an adult in five principal ways. These differences will influence the treatment decisions that you make about pediatric patients, including whether intervention is needed and, if so, what procedure to use. The anatomy of a child's airway and other important structures differ from those of an adult in the following ways:

- A larger, rounder occiput (posterior aspect of the skull), which, as previously discussed, requires careful positioning of the airway.

- A proportionally larger tongue relative to the size of the mouth and a more anterior location in the mouth. The child's tongue is also larger relative to the small mandible and can easily block the airway.
- A floppy, U-shaped epiglottis that is larger than an adult's, relative to the size of the airway. The epiglottis is a key anatomic landmark when providing advanced airway management (that is, endotracheal intubation).
- The larynx is higher (at the C3 to C4 level) and is more anterior. This is another important consideration when performing advanced airway management.
- A narrower airway at all levels. In relation to the adult, whose airway is narrowest at the level of the vocal cords, the narrowest portion of the child's airway is at the level of the cricoid cartilage, which is inferior to the glottis (subglottic).

Because of the smaller diameter of the trachea in infants, which is about the same diameter as a drinking straw, their airway is easily obstructed by secretions, blood, and swelling. The trachea, which is likened to a piece of corrugated tubing, is easily collapsible in children; therefore, when they experience respiratory distress, the trachea tends to draw into the neck; this is called tracheal tugging.

Because the intercostal muscles are not well developed in children, movement of the diaphragm, their major muscle in respiration, dictates the amount of air they inspire (tidal volume). This is why infants and small children are often referred to as "belly breathers." Gastric distention, a more common and significant complication in pediatric patients, can interfere with movement of the diaphragm, resulting in hypoventilation and increased risk of regurgitation with aspiration.

Until the age of approximately 4 to 6 months, infants are obligate nosebreathers. Therefore, if the nasal passages are blocked by secretions, they may not have the intuition to open their mouths to breathe.

The EMT-I must have a thorough understanding of the anatomic and physiologic difference in the child's airway to provide appropriate management. With the aforementioned anatomic differences, it is important to remember the following:

- Keep the nares clear in infants younger than 6 months
- Avoid hyperextension of the child's neck; this may result in reverse hyperflexion and kinking of the trachea
- Keep the airway clear of all secretions; even a small amount of particulate matter may result in an airway obstruction
- Use care when managing the child's airway, such as when inserting airway adjuncts; the soft tissues are very delicate and prone to swelling. In many cases, the child's airway can be maintained by correct positioning, thereby negating the use of airway adjuncts (that is, oral or nasal airways)

Special consideration must also be given to the infant or child when performing advanced airway techniques, such as endotracheal intubation (discussed later in this chapter). Figure 31-6 illustrates the major differences between pediatric and adult airways.

Chest and Lungs

The tissues of the lungs are more fragile in a child, and the ribs are softer and more pliable. As a result, significant compression injuries to the chest may injure vital intrathoracic organs (such as the heart, lungs, great vessels), often without obvious signs of external injury.

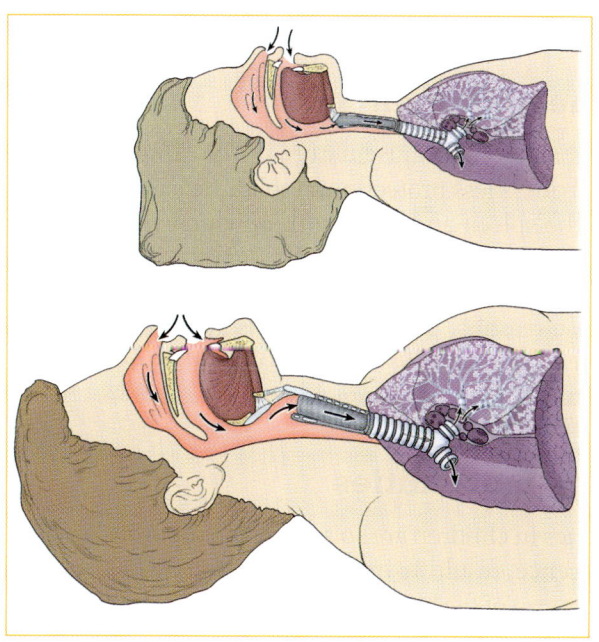

Figure 31-6 The anatomy of a child's airway differs from that of an adult's in several ways. The back of the head is proportionally larger in a child, so positioning requires more care. The tongue is proportionally larger and more anterior in the mouth. The trachea is smaller in diameter and more flexible. The airway itself is lower and narrower.

When assessing a sick or injured child, expect the ribs to be positioned horizontally. Rib fractures occur less frequently in children but are not uncommon following trauma or abuse.

The fragile parenchyma of the child's lungs makes them prone to barotrauma (pressure trauma) as the result of injury or overzealous ventilation. The respiratory muscles in a child are more immature and fatigue more quickly than an adult's; therefore, the child tends to tire more easily as a result of respiratory distress. In addition, because of the thin wall of the child's chest, breath sounds are easily transmitted to all areas of the chest, making it difficult when assessing for a chest injury (such as pneumothorax) or for correct placement of an advanced airway device.

The child's mediastinum is more mobile than an adult's. Therefore, you may see a more pronounced mediastinal shift as the result of a tension pneumothorax.

EMT-I Tips

Since the pediatric patient's ribs and sternum are much more pliable than those of an adult, expect more injuries to the underlying organs and structures.

The Abdomen

The abdominal musculature in the child is immature and offers less protection to solid, vascular organs such as the spleen and liver, both of which are proportionally larger and more vascular in children. In addition, the abdominal organs are nearer to one another. For these reasons, pediatric patients are at higher risk for splenic and hepatic injuries than adults; multiple organ injuries are more common.

The Extremities

Bones in children are softer and more porous until adolescence, resulting in incomplete fractures (greenstick fracture) of the bone. Treat any sprain or strain as though a fracture exists, and immobilize the injury accordingly.

Injury to the epiphyseal plate (growth plate) of the bone during its development, or inadvertent puncture of the growth plate during intraosseous cannulation (discussed later), may result in abnormalities in normal bone growth and development.

Skin and Body Surface Area

In comparison with adults, infants and children have thinner and more elastic skin, a larger body surface area (BSA)/weight ratio, and less subcutaneous (fatty) tissue. These factors contribute to the following:

- Increased risk of injury following exposure to temperature extremes
- Increased risk of hypothermia and dehydration
- Increased severity of burns
  - Many burns that would ordinarily be classified as minor or moderate in adults are classified as severe in children

EMT-I Tips

Because of their thinner skin and proportionally larger BSA/weight ratio, burns are more severe in a child and thus are a leading cause of death in the pediatric age group.

The Respiratory System

Proportionally, tidal volume in children is similar to that in adolescents and adults; however, their metabolic oxygen demand is doubled. In addition, their functional residual capacity is smaller, resulting in proportionally smaller oxygen reserves.

An infant needs to breathe faster than an older child. The child's lungs will grow and develop better abilities to handle the exchange of oxygen as the child ages. A respiratory rate of 40 to 60 breaths/min is normal for newborns, while teenagers are expected to have rates closer to the adult range. Breathing also requires the use of the chest muscles and the diaphragm.

Infants have very little use of their chest muscles to make their chests expand during inspiration; they use the diaphragm (belly breathers). Anything that puts pressure on the abdomen of an infant or young child can block the movement of the diaphragm and cause respiratory compromise. Young children also experience muscle fatigue much more quickly than older children, which can lead to respiratory failure if a child has had to breathe hard for long periods.

The EMT-I must be aware that infants and children, especially during respiratory distress, are highly susceptible to hypoxia because of their decreased oxygen reserves, increased oxygen demand, and easily fatigued respiratory muscles.

Cardiovascular System

Children rely mainly on their heart rate to maintain adequate cardiac output. An infant's heart rate can be 200 beats/min or more if the body needs to compensate for injury or illness. Because this is the primary method for the child's body to compensate for decreased oxygenation, the EMT-I must be aware of the normal heart rate ranges when evaluating children. Suspect shock when an infant or child presents with tachycardia. Bradycardia, however, usually indicates severe hypoxia and must be managed aggressively.

Children have limited but vigorous cardiac reserves. Proportionally, they have a larger circulating blood volume compared with adults; however, their absolute blood volume is less, approximately 70 mL/kg. Because of these factors, injured children can maintain their blood pressure for longer periods than adults, even though they are still in shock (hypoperfusion). In other words, a proportionally larger volume of blood loss must occur in the child before hypotension develops. Hypotension, when it occurs in a child, is an ominous sign and often indicates impending cardiopulmonary arrest.

The ability of a child to constrict blood vessels (vasoconstriction) provides the ability to keep vital organs well perfused. Constriction of the blood vessels can be so profound that blood flow to the periphery of the body diminishes. Signs of vasoconstriction can include weak peripheral (for example, radial) pulses, delayed capillary refill (in children younger than 6 years), and pale, cool extremities.

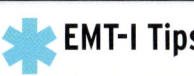

> **EMT-I Tips**
>
> When assessing a sick or injured child, be aware that bradycardia is most often the result of hypoxia; therefore, treatment is aimed at ensuring adequate oxygenation and ventilation. In addition, despite the presence of a normal blood pressure, a child, even more so than an adult, may still be in shock.

The Nervous System

The nervous system continually develops throughout childhood; however, until it is fully developed, the neural tissue is very fragile and easily damaged.

The brain and spinal cord are less well protected by the developing skull and spinal vertebrae. As a result, it takes less force to cause brain and spinal cord injuries in children than in adults. Brain injuries in young children, when they occur, are frequently more devastating. In addition, injury to the spinal cord may occur without injury to the spinal column itself.

You are the Provider — Part 3

You and your partner concur that the child's condition is critical. You administer high-flow oxygen; as your partner gathers the immobilization equipment, you perform a rapid trauma assessment and obtain a set of vital signs.

Vital Signs	Recording Time: 3 Minutes After Patient Contact
Respirations	24 breaths/min, adequate depth
Pulse	68 beats/min, regular and slightly weak
Skin	Pale and cool
Blood pressure	108/52 mm Hg
Level of consciousness	Responds only with moans and crying

5. On the basis of your initial exam, what are the most significant findings, and are they immediate life threats?
6. What are your initial priorities for treatment?

Metabolic Differences

Infants and children have limited stores of glycogen and glucose, which are rapidly depleted as a result of injury or illness. Because it takes glucose to produce energy and energy is required to maintain body temperature, infants and children are highly susceptible to hypothermia. The risk of hypothermia is further increased because of the child's larger BSA/weight ratio. When assessing and treating a newborn (neonate), you must remain aware that these young infants lack the ability to shiver—one of the body's ways of producing heat.

Significant hypovolemia and electrolyte derangements are also more common in children as a result of severe vomiting and diarrhea.

It is critical to keep the child warm during transport and take measures to prevent the loss of body heat. To conserve body heat, be sure to cover the child's head, which because of its proportionally large size, is a source of significant heat loss.

Pediatric Assessment

General Considerations

Young children will not be able to provide you with information needed to make treatment decisions (such as medical history, medications). Furthermore, children often cannot tell you where they hurt. Therefore, you must rely on a parent or caregiver to obtain as much information as you can.

It is important to remember that when children are sick or injured, you may have several patients to treat rather than just one. Family members, especially the primary caregiver, often need help or support when medical emergencies or problems develop. A calm parent usually helps to contribute to a calm child. An agitated parent usually means the child will act the same way. Make sure that you are calm, efficient, professional, and sensitive as you deal with children and their families. When possible, allow parents or caregivers to participate in the care of the child. This often helps to calm them and make them feel as though they are making a positive contribution to the situation. If the child is not critically ill or injured, allow him or her to remain on the parent or caregiver's lap.

It is common for parents or caregivers to become angry and demanding when their child is sick or injured. The EMT-I must realize that this anger is not directed toward him or her; it is a manifestation of the parents' or caregivers' fear of the situation. You must remain compassionate, calm, and professional and avoid responding negatively to the family's response; this would clearly exacerbate the situation.

Each child and situation is unique; therefore, you may have to modify your assessment of the child based on his or her age. In general, however, you should follow the same general approach to patient assessment for children as you do for adults Figure 31-7.

Scene Size-up

As with any EMS call, the scene size-up begins by ensuring that you and your partner have taken the appropriate body substance isolation (BSI) precautions. On arriving at the scene, observe for any hazards or potential hazards that may pose a threat to you or your partner. Resist the temptation to hastily access the patient because you know it is a child. Personal safety must always remain your priority.

As you enter the scene, note the position in which the child is found. Observe the area for clues to the mechanism of injury (MOI) or nature of illness (NOI); these observations will help guide your assessment and management priorities.

Note the presence of any pills, medicine bottles, or household chemicals that would suggest possible ingestion by the child. If the child has been injured—a motor vehicle crash, fall, or pedestrian incident—carefully observe the scene or vehicle (if involved) for clues to the potential severity of the child's injuries.

You must not discount the possibility of child abuse. Conflicting information from the parents or caregivers, bruises or other injuries that are not consistent with the MOI described, or injuries that are not consistent with the child's age and developmental abilities should increase your index of suspicion for abuse. Child abuse will be discussed in greater detail later in this chapter.

EMT-I Tips

Sick or injured children should not be separated from their parents unless aggressive resuscitation is needed. The stress produced by separation anxiety can worsen a sick child's condition. If you need to separate the parent and child, try to leave them within eyesight and talking distance of one another to minimize the stress of the situation.

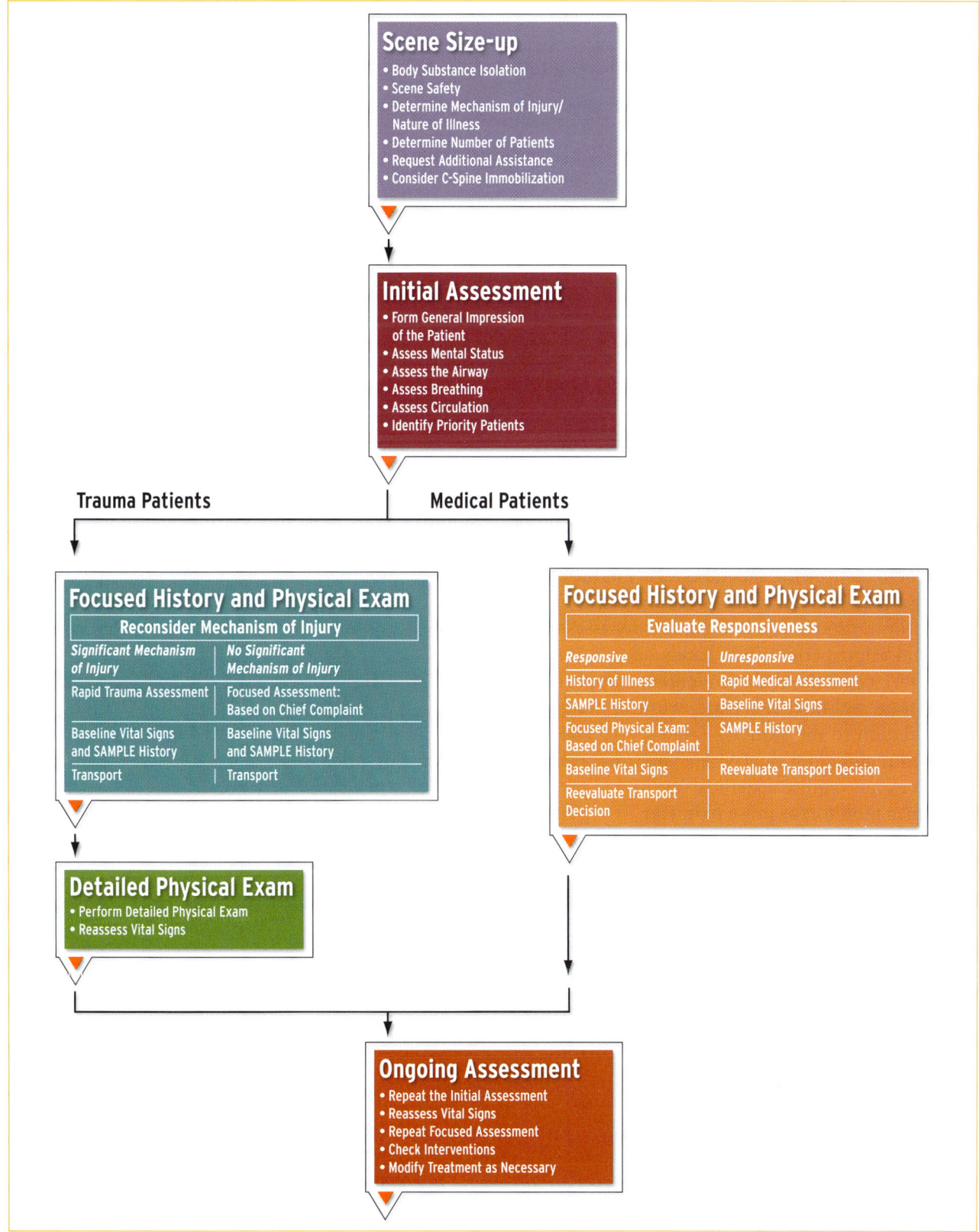

Figure 31-7 Base your assessment approach to a child on the same general steps you use for adults.

Initial Assessment

Many components of the pediatric initial assessment can be accomplished by simple observation when you first enter the scene or room. As with the adult, the objective of the initial assessment is to identify and treat immediate or potential threats to life.

The initial assessment begins by forming a general impression of the child's condition and of the environment in which he or she is found. Also note the degree of interaction between the parent or caregiver and the child; ask the parent or caregiver if the child is acting normally. Determine whether the child recognizes his or her parent or caregiver; failure to do so is an ominous sign and indicates a very sick child!

Pediatric Assessment Triangle

The pediatric assessment triangle (PAT) is a structured assessment tool that allows you to rapidly form a general impression of the infant's or child's condition without touching him or her. Its intent is to provide a "first glance" assessment to identify the general category of the child's physiologic problem and to establish urgency for treatment and/or transport. The PAT is a cursory assessment of the child before performing a hands-on assessment.

The PAT consists of three elements: appearance (muscle tone and mental status), work of breathing, and circulation to the skin Figure 31-8 . The only equipment required for the PAT are your own eyes and ears; it does not require a stethoscope, blood pressure cuff, cardiac monitor, or pulse oximeter.

Appearance

Evaluating the child's appearance involves noting the level of consciousness or interactiveness and muscle tone—signs that will provide you with information about

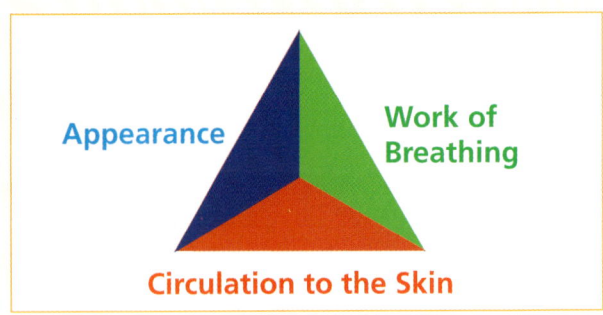

Figure 31-8 The three components of the pediatric assessment triangle (PAT) include appearance, work of breathing, and circulation to the skin.

the adequacy of the child's cerebral perfusion and overall function of the central nervous system.

Much of the information regarding the child's level of consciousness can be obtained by using the PAT. In addition, you can evaluate the child's level of consciousness by using the AVPU scale, modified as necessary for the child's age Table 31-2 .

The modified Glasgow Coma Scale (GCS) can be used to determine the degree of disability in children

TABLE 31-2	The AVPU Scale

Alert: Normal interactiveness for age

Verbal
- Appropriate: Responds to name
- Inappropriate: Nonspecific or confused

Painful
- Appropriate: Withdraws from pain
- Inappropriate: Sound or movement without purpose or localization of pain

Unresponsive: No response to any stimulus

You are the Provider Part 4

You and the firefighters on scene begin to rapidly immobilize the patient on a long board, and your partner continues the assessment. She informs you that the boy has an obvious right femur fracture and one pupil that is significantly larger than the other. He is still not responding appropriately. While relaying this information, the child has a seizure.

7. What is the etiology of the seizure, and how might it be different from the most common pediatric seizures?
8. How must you adjust your immediate treatment priorities?

EMT-I Tips

Identifying an abnormal appearance by using the PAT is a more effective way to detect subtle changes in a child's level of consciousness than the AVPU scale. Many children with mild to moderate illness or injury are "alert" on the AVPU scale, although they may have an abnormal appearance.

In the Field

Carrying an EMS field guide or placing a copy of the modified GCS on the wall of the ambulance or in the trauma kit will help you remember how to calculate this difficult formula.

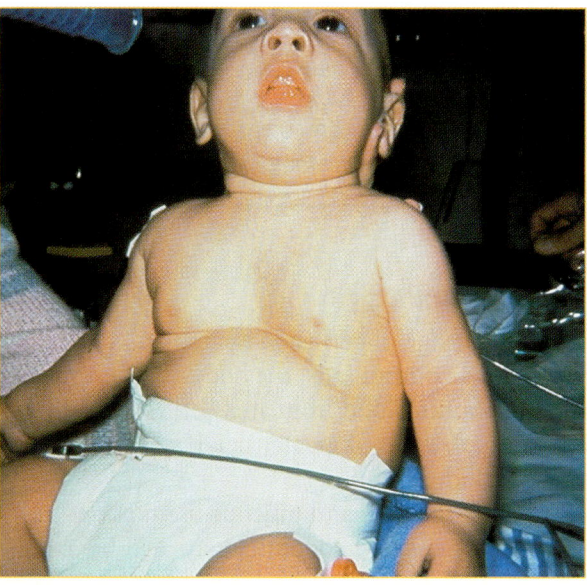

Figure 31-10 A limp child who is unable to maintain eye contact may be critically ill or injured.

with neurologic injuries (such as head trauma). However, it is a complicated scale that requires memorization and numeric scoring—tasks that may be impractical or difficult to accomplish in critical situations.

An infant or child with a normal level of consciousness will act appropriately for his or her age; he or she will have good muscle tone and will maintain good eye contact **Figure 31-9 ▼**. An abnormal level of consciousness is characterized by age-inappropriate behavior or interactiveness, poor muscle tone, or poor eye contact with the caregiver or EMT-I **Figure 31-10 ▶**.

Work of Breathing

A child's work of breathing increases as the body attempts to compensate for abnormalities in oxygenation and ventilation. Increased work of breathing often manifests as <u>tachypnea</u>, <u>retractions</u> of the intercostal muscles or sternum **Figure 31-11 ▼**, or the way the child positions himself or herself.

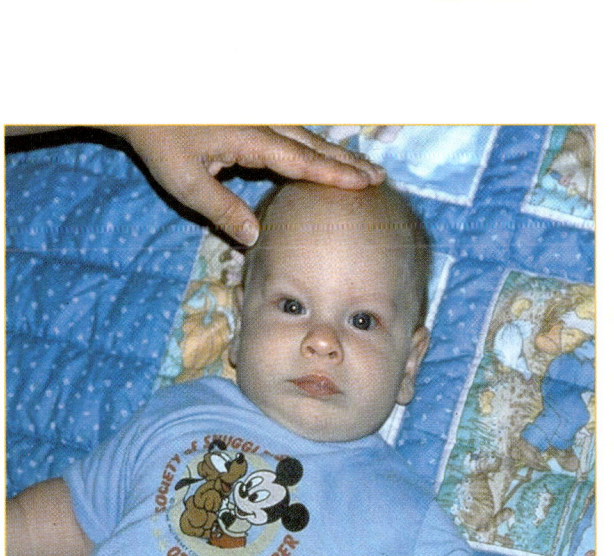

Figure 31-9 An infant or child with a normal level of consciousness will maintain good eye contact.

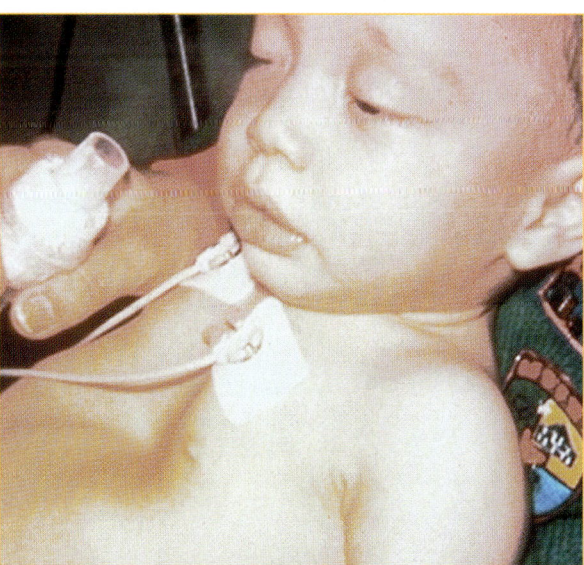

Figure 31-11 Retractions of the intercostal muscles or sternum indicate increased work of breathing.

Terminology Tips

Tachy = rapid
Pnea = related to breathing
Tachypnea = rapid breathing

Circulation to the Skin

An important sign of perfusion is circulation to the skin. When cardiac output falls, the body, through vasoconstriction, shunts blood from areas of lesser need, such as the skin, to areas of greater need, such as the brain, heart, and kidneys.

Pallor of the skin and mucous membranes may be seen in compensated shock; it may also be a sign of anemia (a deficiency of red blood cells or hemoglobin) or hypoxia. Mottling is caused by constriction of peripheral blood vessels and is another sign of poor perfusion Figure 31-12.

Cyanosis is a blue discoloration of the skin and mucous membranes that reflects a decreased level of oxygen in the blood. Cyanosis is a late sign of respiratory failure or shock; its absence should not be used to rule out such conditions. *Never wait for the development of cyanosis before administering oxygen!*

Acrocyanosis, cyanosis of the hands and feet, is a normal finding in newborns and infants younger than 2 months and occurs when they are cold.

Vital Functions

After forming your general impression of the child's condition using the PAT, perform a hands-on assessment of the child's vital functions—airway, breathing, and circulation—and treat any immediate or potential threats to life. As previously discussed, your assessment of the child may require modification based on his or her age, but the overall assessment flow is essentially the same as it is for adults.

Airway Assessment

If the infant or child is conscious and the airway is open, you can proceed with assessment of respiratory adequacy. However, if the child is unresponsive, you must ensure that the airway is properly positioned and that it is clear of mucus, vomitus, blood, and foreign bodies.

If trauma has been ruled out, open the child's airway with the head tilt–chin lift maneuver Figure 31-13. If the child has been involved in trauma or trauma is suspected, use the jaw-thrust maneuver to open the airway Figure 31-14. The modified jaw-thrust, which accomplishes the same goal as the jaw-thrust maneuver—to avoid manipulating the spine—is performed by placing your thumbs on both zygomas and your index or middle fingers (depending on the size of your hand) at the angle of the jaw. The jaw is then thrust forward with your index or middle fingers using the zygomas as a point of leverage.

In the Field

Use caution when opening the airway of a pediatric patient via the head tilt–chin lift. You can overextend the neck and actually close off the trachea.

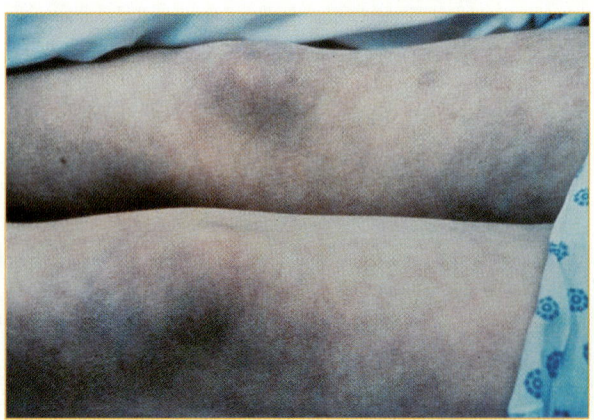

Figure 31-12 Mottling of the skin is a sign of poor perfusion and is the result of constriction of peripheral blood vessels.

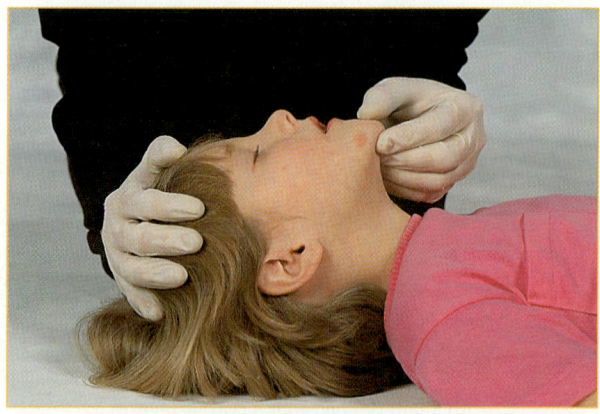

Figure 31-13 Use the head tilt–chin lift maneuver to open the airway of a child without trauma.

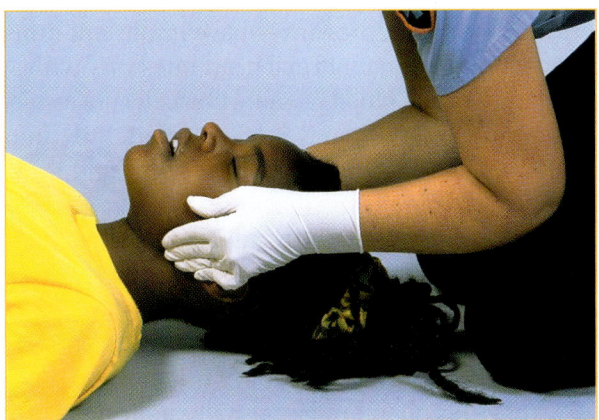

Figure 31-14 Use the jaw-thrust maneuver in a child with possible spinal injury.

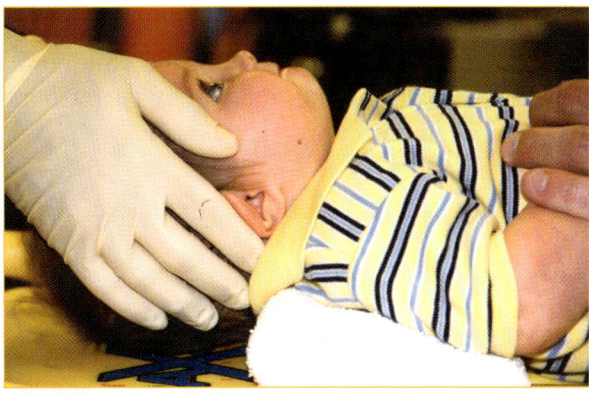

Figure 31-15 The airway should be placed in a neutral position to keep the trachea from kinking when the head is flexed or hyperextended.

Positioning the airway correctly is critical in pediatric emergency care. Position the airway in a sniffing position (unless trauma is suspected), which may require the placement of a folded sheet or towel behind the head or shoulders (Figure 31-15 ▶). When the head is bent back (hyperextended) or forward (flexed), the airway may become obstructed because of kinking of the trachea.

After the child's airway has been opened, ensure that it is clear of potential obstructions (such as mucus, blood, foreign bodies). Next, establish whether the child can maintain his or her own airway spontaneously (without the use of airway adjuncts) or whether adjuncts will be necessary to maintain airway patency. Techniques of airway management will be discussed later in this chapter.

Breathing Assessment

Assess the child's breathing by using the look, listen, and feel technique, noting the degree of air movement at the nose and mouth and determining whether the chest is rising adequately.

If the child is conscious and not in need of immediate intervention (such as suctioning or assisted ventilation), assessing respirations is usually easier with the child sitting on the caregiver's lap. Listen for abnormal respiratory sounds (Table 31-3 ▶) and note any signs of increased respiratory effort.

When observing the child's respiratory effort, note the presence of any signs of increased work of breathing, including the following:

- **Accessory muscle use**: Contractions of the muscles above the clavicles (supraclavicular)
- **Retractions**: Drawing in of the muscles between the ribs (intercostal retractions) or of the sternum during inspiration
- **Head bobbing**: The head lifts and tilts back during inspiration, then moves forward during expiration
- **Nasal flaring**: The nares widen; usually seen during inspiration
- **Tachypnea**: Increased respiratory rate

As the child begins to tire, retractions often become weak and ineffective and the accessory muscles become less prominent during breathing. Bradypnea, a decrease in the respiratory rate, is an ominous sign and indicates impending respiratory arrest. Do not mistake bradypnea for a sign of improvement; it usually indicates that the child's condition has deteriorated. Therefore, you must be prepared to begin ventilatory assistance.

TABLE 31-3 | Abnormal Respiratory Sounds

- **Stridor**: High-pitched inspiratory sound; indicates a partial upper airway obstruction (such as in croup or from a foreign body)
- **Wheezing**: High- or low-pitched sound heard usually during expiration; indicates a partial lower airway obstruction (such as in asthma, bronchiolitis)
- **Grunting**: An "uh" sound heard during exhalation; reflects the child's attempt to keep the alveoli open; indicates inadequate oxygenation
- **Absent breath sounds (despite increased work of breathing)**: Indicates a complete upper or lower airway obstruction (such as foreign body, severe asthma, pneumothorax)

Circulatory Assessment

When assessing circulation, you must first control any active bleeding. Remember, infants and children can tolerate only small amounts of blood loss before circulatory compromise occurs.

Guidelines used to assess adult circulatory status—heart rate and blood pressure—have important limitations in children. First, normal heart rates vary with age in children. Second, blood pressure is usually not assessed in children younger than 3 years; it offers little information about the child's circulatory status and is usually difficult to obtain.

Pulses may be difficult to palpate if they are weak, very fast, or very slow. In infants, palpate the brachial pulse or femoral pulse. In children older than 1 year, palpate the carotid pulse (Figure 31-16). Note the rate and quality of the pulse: Is it weak or strong? Is it normal, slow, or fast? Strong peripheral pulses usually indicate that the child is not hypotensive; however, this does not rule out the possibility of compensated shock. Weak or absent peripheral pulses indicate decreased perfusion. Weak <u>central pulses</u> indicate significant hypotension and decompensated shock. The absence of a central pulse (that is, brachial or femoral in infants, carotid in older children) indicates the need for CPR.

Tachycardia may be an early sign of hypoxia or shock, but it may also reflect less serious conditions such as fever, anxiety, pain, and excitement. Like respiratory rate and effort, heart rate should be interpreted within the context of the overall history, PAT, and entire initial assessment.

A trend of increasing or decreasing heart rate may be quite useful and may suggest worsening hypoxia or shock or improvement after treatment. When hypoxia or shock becomes critical, <u>bradycardia</u> occurs. As with slowing respirations, bradycardia in a child is an ominous sign and often indicates impending cardiopulmonary arrest.

Feel the skin for temperature and moisture at the same time you assess the child's pulse. Is the skin warm and dry or cold and clammy? Estimate the <u>capillary refill time (CRT)</u> by squeezing the end of a finger or toe for several seconds and then observing the return of blood to the area (Figure 31-17). Color should return in less than 2 seconds after you let go. The CRT is used to assess <u>end-organ perfusion</u>. It is most reliable in children younger than 6 years; however, factors such as cold temperatures may affect the CRT.

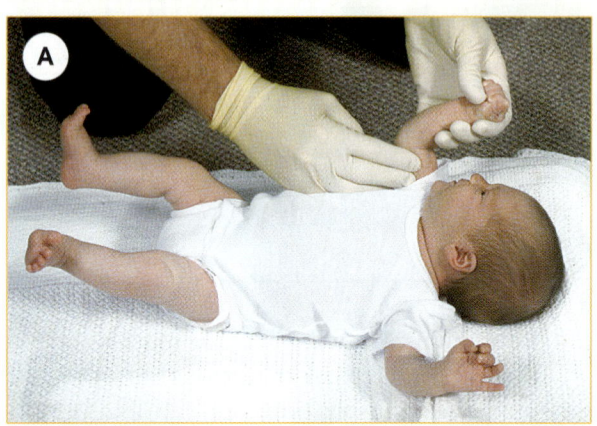
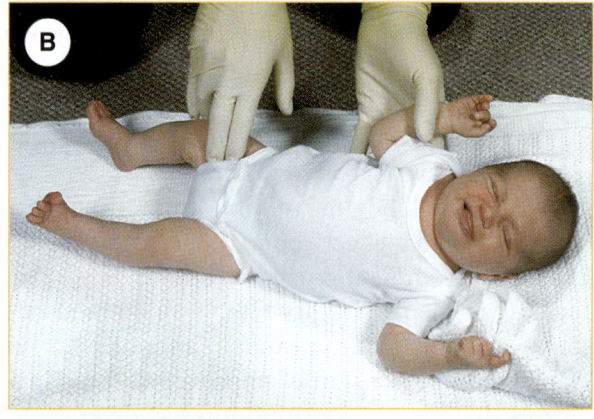
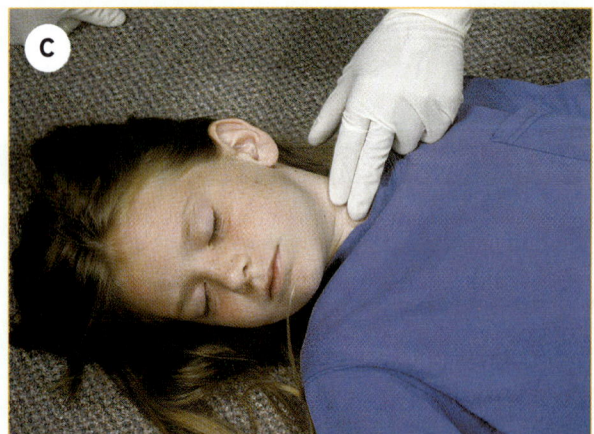

Figure 31-16 **A.** Palpate the brachial pulse in infants. **B.** Palpate the femoral pulse as a second choice. **C.** In children older than 1 year, palpate the carotid pulse.

Pediatric Vital Signs

You should take a child's vital signs in the field because you are the eyes, ears, and hands of medical control. During your assessment, you should obtain a complete set of baseline vital signs, including respirations, pulse, and blood pressure (when possible).

Respiratory rates may be difficult to interpret. Rapid respiratory rates may simply reflect high fever, anxiety, pain, or excitement. Normal rates, on the other hand, may occur in a child who has been breathing rapidly with increased work of breathing for some time and is now becoming tired. Count the respirations for at least 30 seconds and then double that number (if counted for 30 seconds). In infants and children younger than 3 years, evaluate respirations by assessing the rise and fall of the abdomen.

Assess the pulse rate by counting for at least 1 minute, noting its quality and regularity. Consider taking an **apical pulse** in infants and small children. An apical pulse is obtained by auscultating heart tones over the chest with a stethoscope.

Note that normal vital signs in pediatric patients vary with the age of the child (Table 31-4 ▼). Remem-

> **Documentation Tips**
>
> Assessment and reassessment of vital signs should be recorded on the patient care form. This important information will allow you to trend the child's vital signs, noting whether his or her condition is improving or deteriorating. It will also provide the physician at the hospital with the same valuable information.

ber that your approach to taking vital signs also varies with the age of the child. Be gentle, talk to the child, assess respirations and pulse next, and assess blood pressure last (Figure 31-18 ▼). Warm your stethoscope on your hands or a cloth before placing it on the skin. You may also want to let the child hold the equipment or

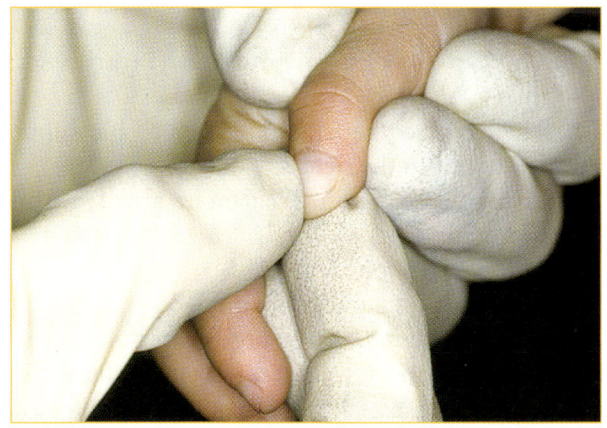

Figure 31-17 Estimate the CRT by squeezing the end of a finger or toe for several seconds until the nailbed blanches. Normal color should return within 2 seconds after you let go.

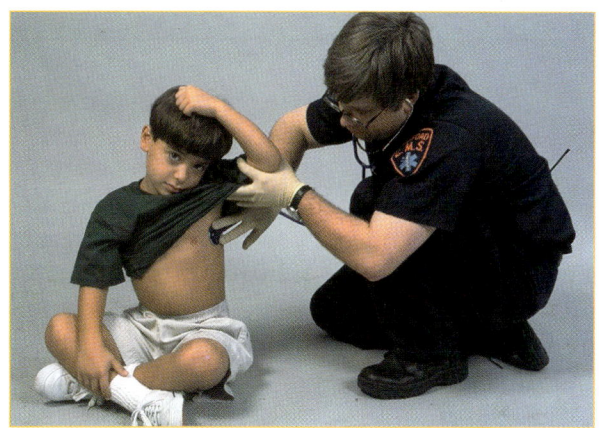

Figure 31-18 Always take vital signs in the field. Begin by talking to the child, then assess respirations and pulse, followed by blood pressure.

TABLE 31-4	Vital Signs by Age		
Age	Respirations (breaths/min)	Pulse (beats/min)	Systolic Blood Pressure (mm Hg)
Newborn: 0 to 1 month	40-60	120-160	50-70
Infant: 1 month to 1 year	30-60	100-160	70-95
Toddler: 1-3 years	24-40	90-150	80-100
Preschool age: 3-5 years	22-34	80-140	80-100
School age: 6-12 years	18-30	70-120	80-110
Adolescent: 12-18 years	12-16	60-100	90-110
Older than 18 years	12-20	60-100	90-140

stethoscope before placing it on him or her; this may help to reduce the child's anxiety.

It is important to use appropriately sized equipment when assessing a child's vital signs. To obtain an accurate reading of the child's blood pressure, you must use a cuff with a bladder length equal to approximately two thirds of the child's upper arm measured from the acromion to the tip of the olecranon 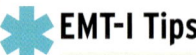. A blood pressure cuff that is too small may give you a falsely high reading, whereas a cuff that is too large may give you a falsely low reading.

> **EMT-I Tips**
>
> To estimate the *lower limit of normal* for the systolic blood pressure in a child older than 1 year, use the following formula:
>
> (Age [in years] × 2) + 70 = Systolic Blood Pressure

Transport Decision

After you have completed the initial assessment and initiated any treatment, you must make a crucial decision: Is immediate transport to the hospital indicated, or is additional assessment and treatment required at the scene? If the child is in hemodynamically stable condition, you may elect to perform a focused history and physical examination at the scene.

However, immediate transport is indicated if the scene is unsafe for the child or if any of the following conditions exist:

- A significant MOI
  - Same MOIs for the adult (see Chapter 10), in addition to the following:
    - Fall from more than 10′ or three times the child's height
    - Bicycle crash
- A history compatible with a serious illness
- A physiologic abnormality noted during the initial assessment
- A potentially serious anatomic abnormality
- Significant pain

In addition to the preceding factors, the EMT-I should also consider the following when making a transport decision:

- The type of clinical problem (injury versus illness)
- The expected benefits of advanced life support treatment in the field
- Local EMS system treatment and transport protocols
- The EMT-I's comfort level
- Transport time to the hospital

If the child's condition is urgent, perform a rapid assessment, if applicable, and initiate immediate transport. Additional assessment and treatment should occur en route to the hospital.

If the child's condition is nonurgent, perform a focused history and physical examination at the scene, provide additional treatment as needed, and then transport.

Transition Phase

If the child's condition does not require immediate transport, the <u>transition phase</u> can be used to allow the infant or child to become familiar with you and your equipment. This will help to alleviate the child's anxiety, allowing you to perform a more thorough and accurate assessment.

It is important to remember that sick or injured children are afraid and do not understand why you are there and what you are doing. As a result, they are less likely than an adult to trust you. The transition phase will facilitate the trust-building process between you and the child.

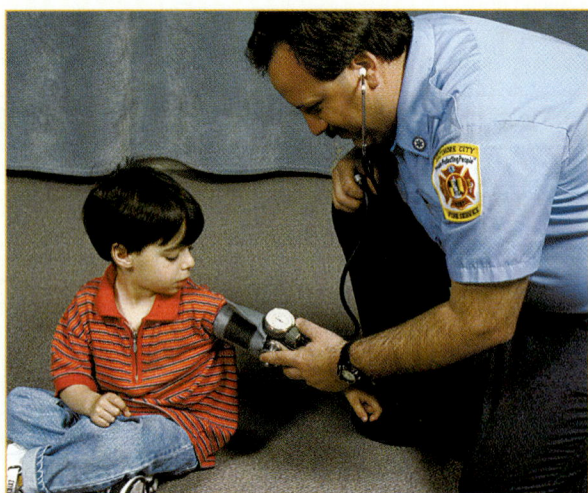

Figure 31-19 When measuring a child's blood pressure, use the proper cuff size. The bladder length should be approximately equal to two thirds of the child's upper arm length.

Focused History and Physical Exam

As with the adult, a focused history and physical exam of the child should be performed at the scene, unless his or her condition dictates immediate transport. The purpose of the focused history and physical exam is to obtain additional, specific information about the child's illness or injury.

Focused History

Your approach to the focused history will depend on the age of the patient. Historical information for an infant, toddler, or preschool-age child will need to be obtained from the parent or caregiver. When dealing with a school-age child or young adolescent, you will usually be able to obtain most of the information from the patient.

Information about sexual activity, the possibility of pregnancy, or the use of illicit drugs or alcohol should be obtained from an older adolescent patient in private. Most of these patients will be reluctant to provide this information in the presence of their parents. When asking such questions, assure the adolescent that this information is important and is needed to provide the most appropriate care.

The focused history is performed to obtain further information about the child's chief complaint. This, together with an evaluation of the child's medical history, may provide clues to the underlying illness or injury and other conditions that may exist.

When interviewing the parent or older child about the chief complaint, obtain the following pertinent information:

- Nature of the illness or injury
- How long the patient has been sick or injured
- Presence of fever
- Effects of the illness or injury on the child's behavior
- Change in bowel or bladder habits
- Presence of vomiting or diarrhea
- Frequency of urination

When obtaining information about the child's medical history, inquire whether the child is currently under the care of a physician, has any chronic illnesses, takes any medications on a regular basis, or has any known drug allergies.

Physical Exam

The focused physical exam should be performed on all children without life-threatening illnesses or injuries and who do not require a rapid assessment. Focus your assessment on the area(s) of the body affected by the illness or injury.

Young children should be assessed starting at the feet and ending at the head; older children can be assessed using the head-to-toe approach, as with adults. The extent of the physical exam will depend on the situation and may include the following:

- Pupils
  - Note the size, equality, and reactivity of the pupils to light
- Capillary refill (in children younger than 6 years)
  - Normal CRT should be less than 2 seconds
  - As discussed earlier, assess CRT by blanching the finger or toenail beds; the soles of the feet may also be used
  - Cold temperatures will increase CRT, making it a less reliable sign
- Level of hydration
  - Assess skin turgor, noting the presence of tenting
  - In infants, note whether the fontanelles are sunken or flat
  - Ask the parent or caregiver how many diapers the infant has soiled over the last 24 hours
  - Determine whether the child is producing tears when crying; note the condition of the mouth. Is the oral mucosa moist or dry?
- Pulse oximetry Figure 31-20
  - Oxygen saturation (SaO_2) should be monitored on any moderately ill or injured child
  - Monitoring SaO_2 is an excellent means of assessing the effectiveness of arterial oxygen saturation
  - Shock or hypothermia can alter the reading on the pulse oximeter

> **EMT-I Tips**
>
> If the child has experienced a traumatic injury, perform a physical exam before obtaining a focused history. The extent of your physical exam will depend on the severity of the child's injuries: a rapid assessment if the child has sustained a significant mechanism of injury or a focused exam for isolated, non-life-threatening injuries.

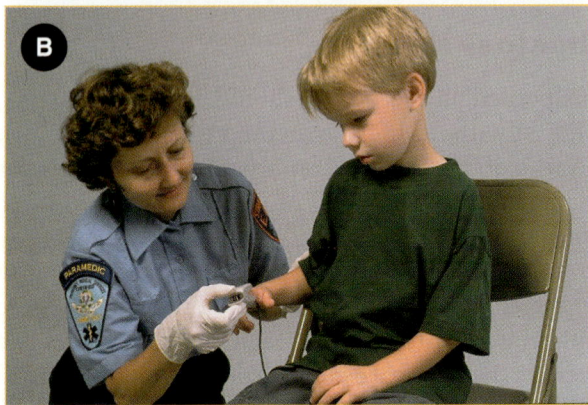

Figure 31-20 **A.** Various pulse oximeter probes wrap around or clip onto a digit or earlobe. **B.** Pulse oximetry is an excellent tool for assessing the effectiveness of breathing.

If the child's condition suggests a cardiac etiology, apply a cardiac monitor and assess his or her cardiac rhythm. The cardiac monitor is also a useful tool for monitoring fluctuations in the child's heart rate. Treat any dysrhythmias according to PALS guidelines or local protocol.

Ongoing Assessment

Reassess the child's condition as the situation dictates; every 15 minutes for a child in stable condition and at least every 5 minutes for a child in unstable condition.

The physiologic safeguards in infants and children can decompensate with alarming unpredictability; therefore, continually monitor respiratory effort, skin color and condition, and level of consciousness or interactiveness. Frequently reassess oxygen saturation, vital signs, and temperature. If the child's condition deteriorates, immediately repeat the initial assessment and adjust your treatment accordingly.

Pediatric Airway Management

Because respiratory failure is the most common cause of cardiopulmonary arrest in the pediatric population, the airway must remain patent and breathing must remain adequate at all times. You must be prepared to intervene immediately for any child with an airway problem.

This section will review the principles of basic airway management in infants and children, including correct airway positioning, airway obstruction removal techniques, and methods to ensure a patent airway and provide adequate oxygenation and ventilation.

Manual Airway Positioning

In conscious infants and children, you should allow them to assume a position of comfort; this will help alleviate anxiety and avoid potential exacerbation of their condition.

As previously discussed, positioning the airway is critical in pediatric emergency care. Recall that incorrect positioning (that is, hyperextension, flexion) may result in tracheal kinking and obstruction of the airway. Remember to open the infant or child's airway with a jaw-thrust maneuver if trauma is suspected or cannot be ruled out; use the head tilt–chin lift maneuver if trauma has been ruled out.

Follow the steps in (Skill Drill 31-1 ▶) to position the airway in a child or infant.

1. **Place the patient on a firm surface** such as a short backboard or pediatric immobilization device (**Step 1**).
2. **Fold a small towel to a thickness of approximately 1″**, and place it under the patient's shoulders or back (**Step 2**).
3. **Place tape across the child's forehead** to limit rolling of the head during transport (**Step 3**).

Foreign Body Upper Airway Obstruction

Mild or severe foreign body obstruction of the upper airway most commonly occurs in toddlers and preschool-age children (1 to 4 years); however, it can occur at any age. Children can (and do) obstruct the airway with any object that they can fit into the mouth, such as hot dogs, balloons, grapes, and coins (Figure 31-21 ▶).

Skill Drill 31-1: Positioning the Airway in a Child

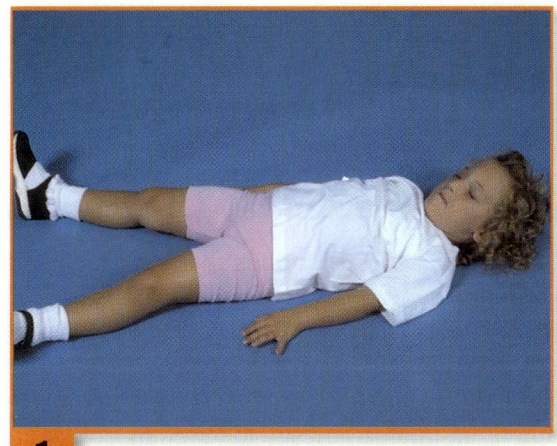

1 Position the child on a firm surface.

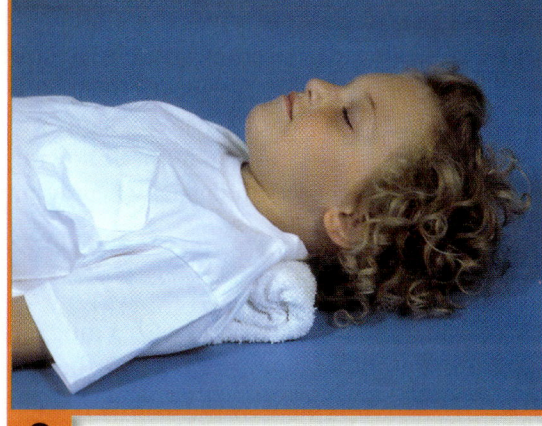

2 Place a folded towel about 1″ thick under the shoulders and back.

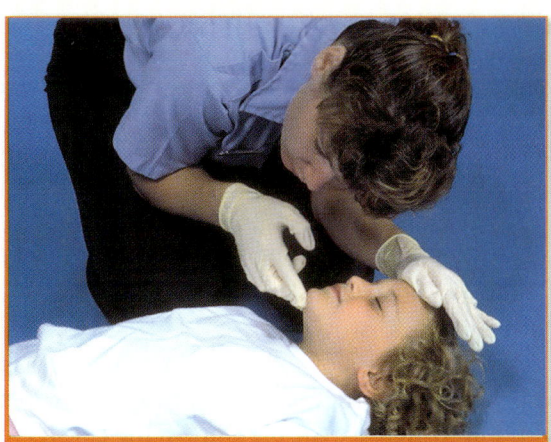

3 Immobilize the forehead to limit movement.

In cases of trauma, a child's teeth may have been dislodged into the airway. Blood, vomitus, or other thick secretions can also a cause mild or severe airway obstruction.

If interventions to relieve the obstruction are not initiated immediately, or if interventions are unsuccessful, respiratory arrest—followed by cardiac arrest—will quickly occur. Foreign body airway obstructions are classified as follows:

- Mild airway obstruction
- Severe airway obstruction

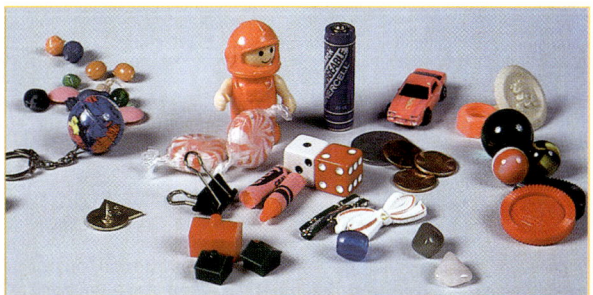

Figure 31-21 Any number of objects can obstruct a child's airway. Some of the more common ones include batteries, coins, toys, buttons, and candy.

Mild Upper Airway Obstruction

Most children with a mild foreign body airway obstruction will show signs of mild respiratory distress. Although they appear irritable or anxious, they are able to move enough air to support adequate oxygenation and ventilation. In addition to respiratory distress, signs of a mild upper airway obstruction include the following:

- Stridor, a high-pitched sound usually heard during inspiration
- Muffled or hoarse voice
- Drooling or pain in the throat

When assessing the infant or child with a mild airway obstruction, you will often discover that the parent or caregiver witnessed the child placing an object into his or her mouth.

If air exchange is adequate, as evidenced by a strong, effective cough, good skin color, and a normal level of consciousness, you should encourage the child with a mild airway obstruction to continue coughing (if he or she is old enough to understand you), provide supplemental oxygen (if tolerated), and transport the child to the hospital, allowing him or her to assume a position of comfort (Figure 31-22). Interventions other than oxygen and transport may precipitate a severe airway obstruction. Monitor the child closely for signs of inadequate air exchange, and be prepared to treat him or her for a severe airway obstruction.

EMT-I Tips

Infants or children presenting with acute respiratory distress in the absence of fever should be suspected of having a foreign body airway obstruction.

Severe Upper Airway Obstruction

A severe airway obstruction is characterized by little or no air movement, inability to speak or cry, a decreased level of consciousness, and cyanosis. Rapid identification and treatment of a severe airway obstruction is crucial to the infant or child's survival; if not treated promptly, respiratory arrest—followed by cardiac arrest—will quickly occur.

Management of Airway Obstruction in a Child

If there is reason to believe that an unresponsive child has a foreign body obstruction, check the upper airway to see whether the obstructing object is visible. The best way to do this is to grasp the tongue and jaw between your finger and thumb and lift to open the mouth; this is called the tongue-jaw lift (Figure 31-23A). If the object is visible, try to remove it using a finger sweep motion (Figure 31-23B). *Never perform blind finger sweeps in infants or children; doing so may push the object further into the airway.*

Chest compressions are recommended to relieve a severe airway obstruction in an unresponsive infant or child. These increase the pressure in the chest, creating an artificial cough that may force a foreign body from the airway.

(Skill Drill 31-2) shows the steps for performing chest compressions to an *unresponsive* child you suspect has a severe foreign body airway obstruction.

1. **Place the child in a supine position** on a firm, flat surface (**Step 1**).
2. **Inspect the upper airway** using the tongue-jaw lift. If you can see the foreign object, try to remove it (**Step 2**).
3. **Attempt rescue breathing.** If the first try is unsuccessful, reposition the child's head and try again (**Step 3**).
4. **If ventilation is still unsuccessful,** perform chest compressions (**Step 4**).
5. **Open the airway** using the tongue-jaw lift and visualize the airway (**Step 5**).

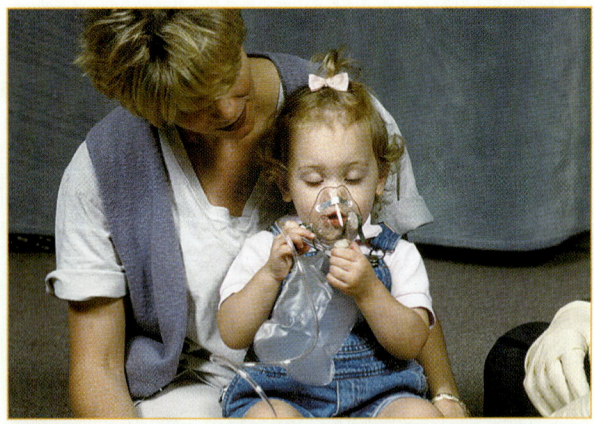

Figure 31-22 If a child has a mild airway obstruction, do not intervene except to give supplemental oxygen and allow the child to remain in whatever position is most comfortable.

6. **If you see the foreign body**, remove it. *Only attempt to remove objects you can actually see. Blind sweeps may push the object back into the airway.*
7. **Attempt rescue breathing.** If the foreign body is not expelled on the first attempt, reposition the child's head and try again.
8. **If the airway remains obstructed**, repeat the chest compressions (**Step 6**).

The following steps are used to remove a foreign body obstruction from a *conscious* child who is in a standing position **Figure 31-24**:

1. **Kneel on one knee behind the child**, and circle his or her body with both arms around the patient's chest. Prepare to give abdominal thrusts by placing your fist just above the patient's umbilicus and well below the xiphoid process. Place your other hand over that fist.
2. **Give the child rapid, distinct abdominal thrusts** in an upward direction. Be careful to avoid applying force to the lower rib cage or sternum.
3. **Repeat this standing technique** until the child expels the foreign body or becomes unresponsive.
4. **If the child becomes unresponsive**, place him or her supine on a firm, flat surface and inspect the airway using the tongue-jaw lift. If you can see the foreign body, try to remove it.
5. **Attempt rescue breathing.** If the first attempt fails, reposition the head and try again.
6. **If the airway remains obstructed**, repeat the abdominal thrusts.

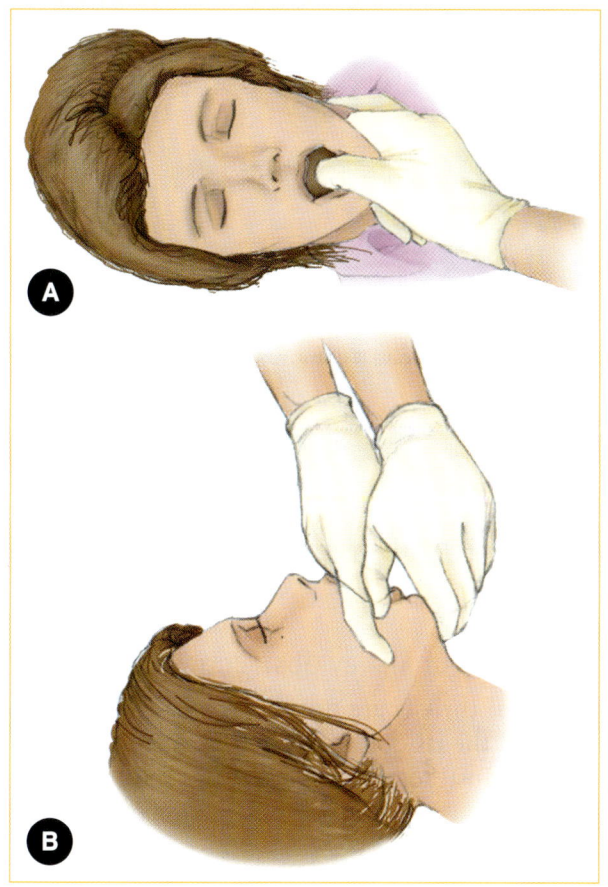

Figure 31-23 **A.** Use the tongue-jaw lift to open the mouth in an unresponsive child. **B.** If the object is visible, remove it by using a finger sweep.

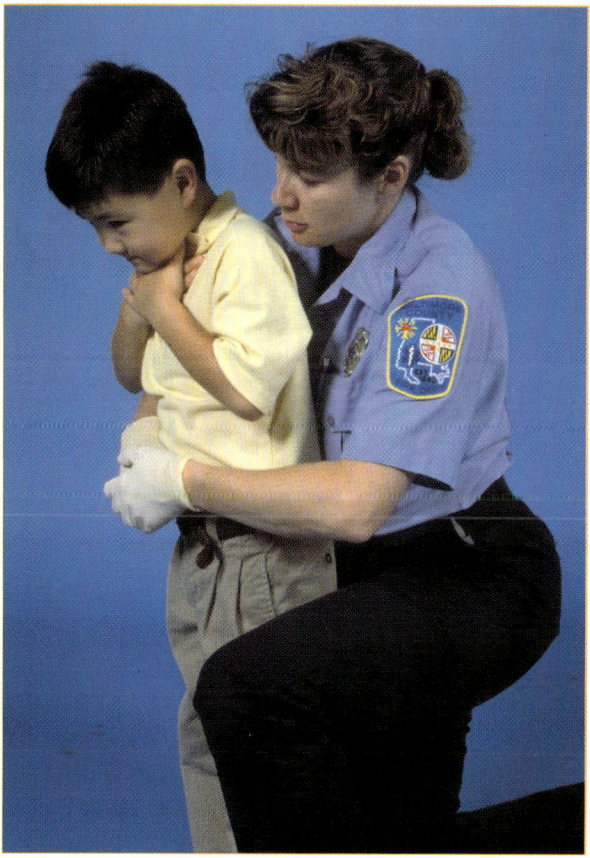

Figure 31-24 To relieve a foreign body airway obstruction in a child who is standing, kneel behind the child, wrap your arms around his or her body, and place your fist just above the umbilicus and well below the xiphoid process.

Skill Drill 31-2

Removing a Foreign Body Airway Obstruction in an Unresponsive Child

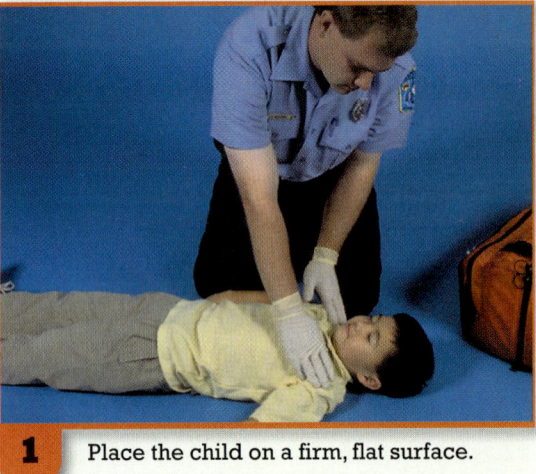

1. Place the child on a firm, flat surface.

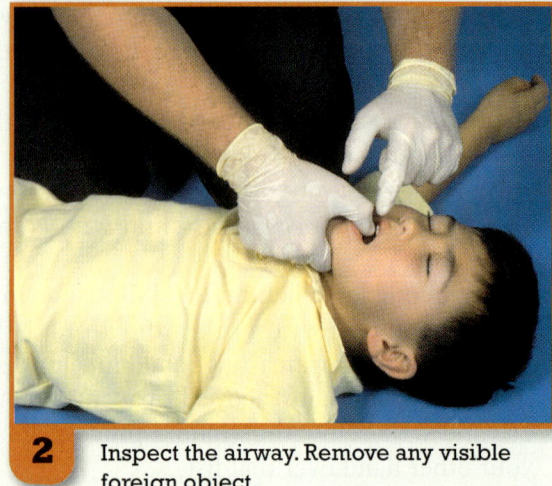

2. Inspect the airway. Remove any visible foreign object.

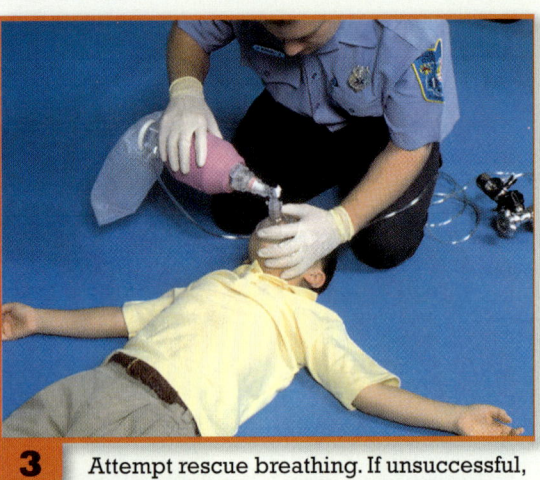

3. Attempt rescue breathing. If unsuccessful, reposition the head and try again.

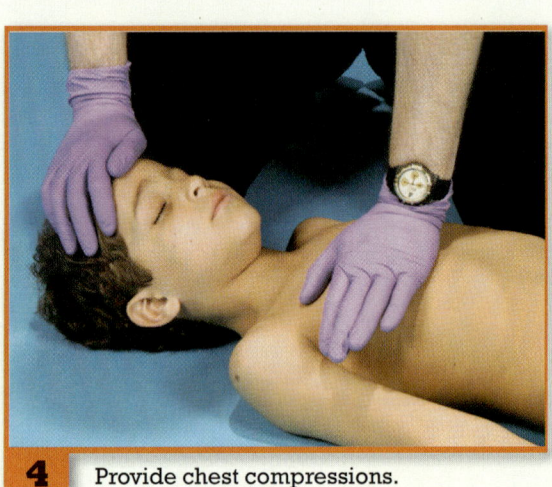

4. Provide chest compressions.

If you manage to clear the airway obstruction in an unresponsive child (older than 1 year), but he or she remains apneic and pulseless, begin CPR and attach the automatic external defibrillator (AED) as soon as possible. Use the appropriately sized AED pads for children. If, after several attempts, you are unable to relieve the obstruction, transport immediately and coordinate a rendezvous with a paramedic unit, if possible.

Management of Airway Obstruction in an Infant

Abdominal thrusts are not recommended for infants because of the risk of injury to the immature abdominal organs. Instead, perform back slaps and chest thrusts to try to clear a severe airway obstruction in a conscious infant as follows (Figure 31-25 ▶):

1. **Hold the infant face down**, with the body resting on your forearm. Support the infant's head

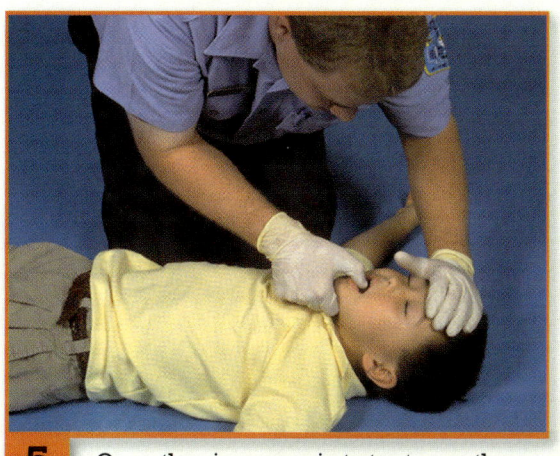

5 Open the airway again to try to see the object. Try to remove the obstruction only if you can see it.

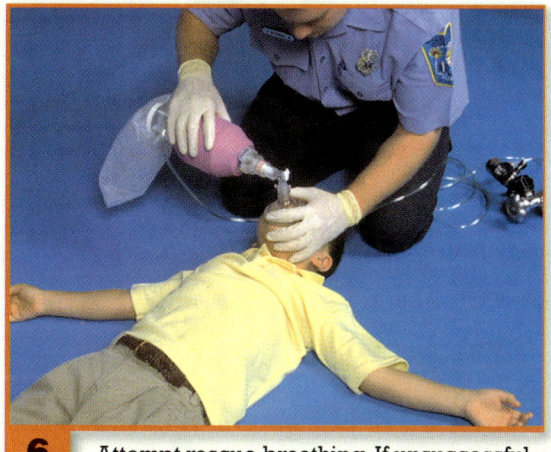

6 Attempt rescue breathing. If unsuccessful, reposition the head and try again.

Repeat chest compressions if obstruction persists.

and face with your hand, and keep the head lower than rest of the body.

2. **Deliver five back slaps** between the shoulder blades, using the heel of your hand.
3. **Place your free hand behind the infant's head and back**, and bring the infant upright on your thigh, sandwiching the infant's body between your two hands and arms. The infant's head should remain below the level of the body.
4. **Give five quick chest thrusts** in the same location and manner as for chest compressions, using two fingers placed on the lower half of the sternum. For larger infants, or if you have small hands, you can perform this step by placing the infant in your lap and turning the infant's whole body as a unit between back blows and chest thrusts.
5. **Check the airway.** If you can see the foreign body now, remove it. If not, repeat the cycle as often as necessary or until the infant becomes unresponsive.
6. **If the infant becomes unresponsive**, perform CPR.

If the infant regains consciousness, place him or her in the recovery position, administer 100% oxygen, and transport immediately. If you are unable to relieve the obstruction after several attempts, begin immediate transport and coordinate a rendezvous with a paramedic unit, if possible.

Removal of an Airway Obstruction With Magill Forceps

In the setting of complete airway obstruction, the EMT-I can make the difference between life and death. Immediate removal of an airway foreign body can often be achieved using BLS procedures.

Sometimes, however, the foreign body is deeper in the airway or embedded in tissue, so that basic maneuvers are unsuccessful. In such cases, using Magill forceps (Figure 31-26 ▶) and direct laryngoscopy may be the only option for removal.

Follow these steps to remove a foreign body airway obstruction using Magill forceps and direct laryngoscopy (Figure 31-27 ▶):

1. **Hold the laryngoscope handle with your left hand.**
2. **Open the mouth** by using thumb pressure on the chin.
3. **Insert a pediatric straight blade into the mouth**, and lift the tongue with the blade.
4. **Exert gentle traction upward along the axis of the laryngoscope handle** at a 45° angle, and

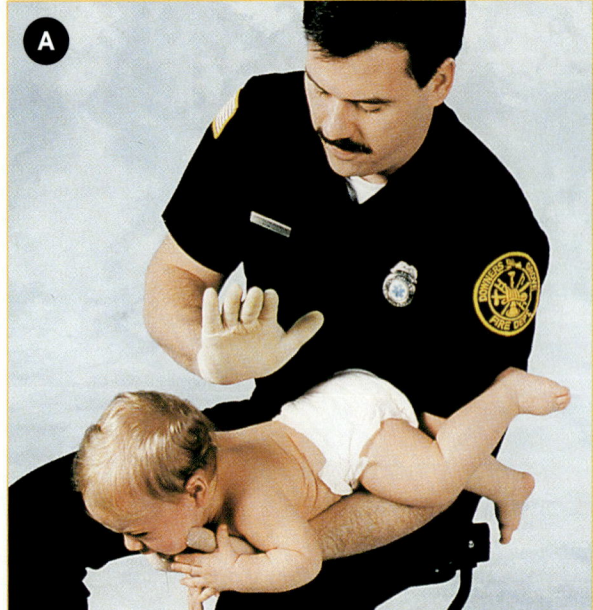

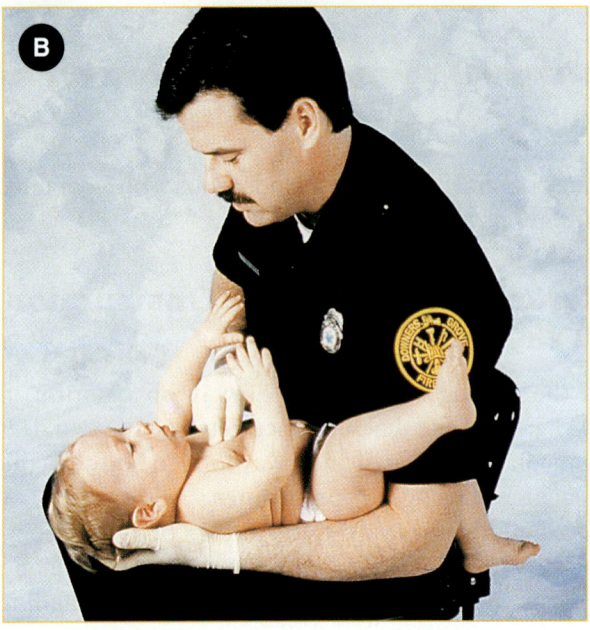

Figure 31-25 Perform back slaps and chest thrusts to clear a foreign body airway obstruction in a conscious infant. **A.** Hold the infant face down with the body resting on your forearm. Support the jaw and face with your hand, and keep the head lower than the rest of the body. Give the infant five back slaps between the shoulder blades, using the heel of your hand. **B.** Give the infant five quick chest thrusts, using two fingers placed on the lower half of the sternum.

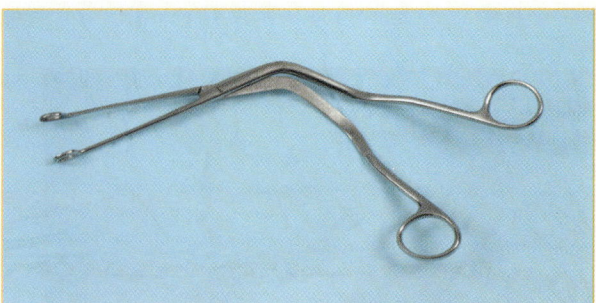

Figure 31-26 Magill forceps.

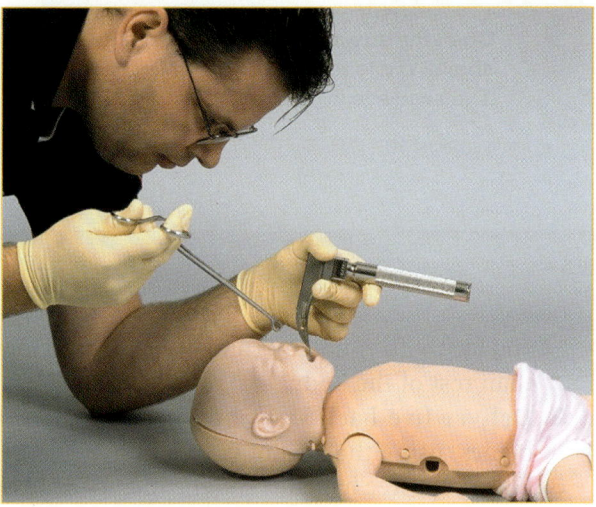

Figure 31-27 Using Magill forceps and direct laryngoscopy to remove a foreign body airway obstruction.

7. **Insert the Magill forceps** into the mouth with the tips closed.
8. **Grasp the foreign object and remove** while looking directly at it (Figure 31-28 ▶).
9. **Look at the airway** to ensure that it is clear of debris. Remove the laryngoscope blade.

Suctioning

Suctioning is a critical part of pediatric airway management. Thick secretions can occlude the airway; thin secretions can be aspirated into the lungs. If aspiration occurs, mortality increases significantly.

To suction an infant or child's airway, you can use a bulb syringe, flexible suction catheter, or rigid (tonsil-tip) suction catheter (Figure 31-29 ▶). For newborns and

advance the blade. *Do not use the teeth or gums for leverage.*
5. **Watch the tip until the foreign body is visible.** Do not go past the vocal cords.
6. **Use suction to improve visibility** if secretions are present.

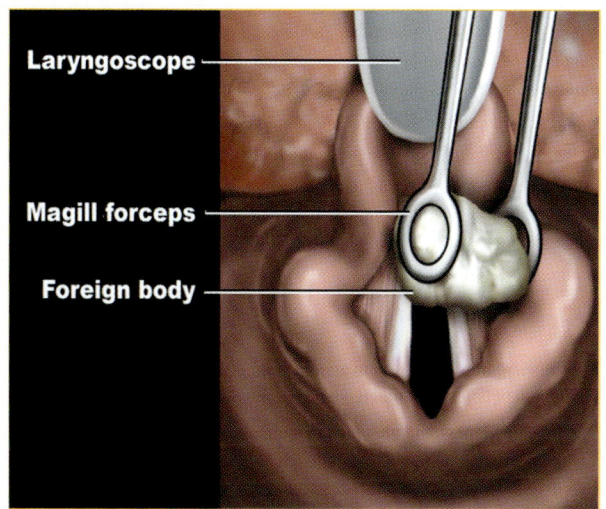

Figure 31-28 Grasping a foreign object with the Magill forceps.

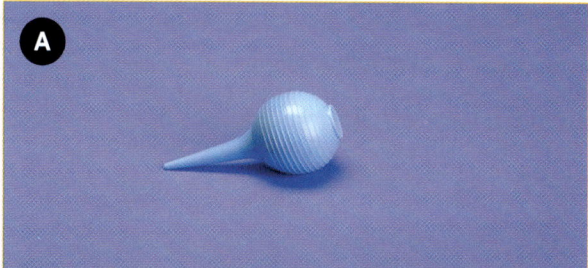

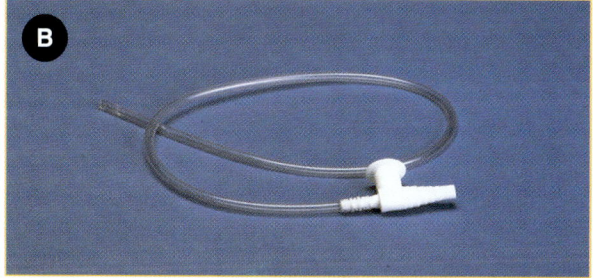

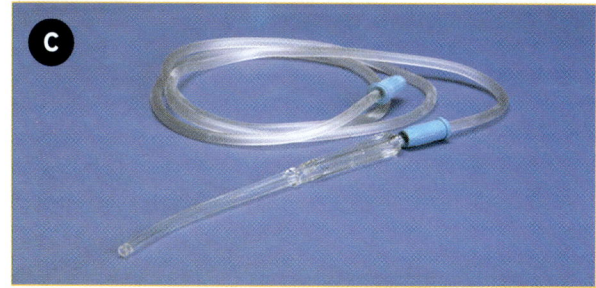

Figure 31-29 **A.** Bulb syringe. **B.** Flexible suction catheter. **C.** Rigid suction catheter.

infants, use the bulb syringe; the flexible or rigid catheter can be used in infants and children.

Because suction removes oxygen directly from the child's body, you should avoid vigorous suctioning and follow these guidelines:

- Avoid upper airway stimulation, which can cause bradycardia and hypoxia
- Decrease suction negative pressure to 100 mm Hg or less
- Suction *only* when withdrawing the catheter
- Limit suction time to 10 seconds in children and 5 seconds in infants

When suctioning the airway of an infant or child, apply a cardiac monitor and observe for bradycardia. If bradycardia occurs, stop suctioning immediately and oxygenate the child.

Airway Adjuncts

In children with inadequate ventilation, regardless of the cause, you should use an airway adjunct to maintain a patent airway. Airway adjuncts are devices that help to maintain the airway and include oropharyngeal airways and nasopharyngeal airways.

Placing the adjuncts correctly starts with choosing the appropriately sized equipment Table 31-5 ▶. If an airway adjunct is not the correct size for the child's size and age, it may cause more harm than good.

Oropharyngeal Airway

An oropharyngeal (oral) airway is designed to keep the tongue from blocking the airway, and it makes suctioning the airway, if necessary, easier. An oropharyngeal airway should be used for pediatric patients who are unresponsive and cannot maintain their own airway spontaneously. However, this adjunct should not be used in conscious patients or those who have a gag reflex. Use of an oropharyngeal airway in a patient with a gag reflex may stimulate vomiting, increasing the risk of aspiration. In addition, this adjunct should not be used in children who have ingested a caustic (corrosive) or petroleum-based product because it may induce vomiting as well.

Skill Drill 31-3 ▶ shows the preferred technique for inserting an oropharyngeal airway in a child.

1. **Determine the appropriately sized airway** by measuring from the corner of the mouth to the

TABLE 31-5	Pediatric Equipment: Getting the Size Right
The best way to identify the appropriately sized equipment for a pediatric patient is to use the length-based resuscitation tape, which can determine weight and height in patients weighing up to 34 kg Figure 31-30 ▼).	The proper sequence for using the length-based resuscitation tape is as follows: 1. Place the patient supine on a flat surface. 2. Lay the tape next to the patient with the multicolored side up. 3. Place the red end of the tape at the top of the patient's head. 4. Place one hand, side down, on top of the patient's head, covering the red box at the end of the tape. 5. Starting from the patient's head, run the side of your free hand down the tape. 6. Stretch the tape out the full length of the child, stopping at the heel. If the child is longer than the tape, stop here and use the appropriate adult technique. 7. Place your free hand, side down, at the bottom of the child's heel. 8. Note the color or letter block and weight range on the edge of the tape where your hand is. Say the color or letter out loud. 9. Select the appropriately sized equipment by matching the color or letter on the tape to the color or letter on the equipment.

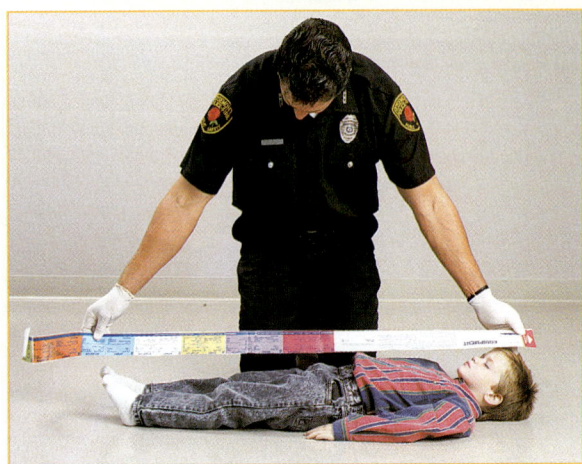

Figure 31-30 Use of a length-based resuscitation tape is one way to identify the correct size for pediatric equipment, including basic and advanced airway devices and medication doses.

earlobe or by using the length-based resuscitation tape to measure the patient.

2. **Place the airway next to the face** with the flange at the level of the central incisors and the bite block segment parallel to the hard palate. The tip of the airway should reach the angle of the jaw (**Step 1**).
3. **Position the patient's airway.** In medical patients, use the head tilt–chin lift maneuver, avoiding hyperextension; you may place a towel under the patient's shoulders. If the patient has a traumatic injury, use the jaw-thrust maneuver and provide in-line spinal stabilization (**Step 2**).
4. **Open the mouth** by applying pressure on the chin with your thumb.
5. **Insert the airway** by depressing the tongue with a tongue blade to the base of the tongue and inserting the airway directly over the tongue blade. If a tongue blade is not available, point the airway tip toward the roof of the mouth to depress the tongue. Gently rotate the airway into position as it passes through the mouth toward the curve of the tongue. Insert the airway until the flange rests against the lips.
6. **Reassess the airway** after insertion (**Step 3**). Take care to avoid injuring the hard palate as you insert the airway. Rough insertion can cause bleeding, which may aggravate airway problems and may even cause vomiting. Note also that if the patient's airway is too small, the tongue may be pushed back into the pharynx, obstructing the airway. If the oropharyngeal airway is too large, it may obstruct the larynx.

Nasopharyngeal Airway

A nasopharyngeal (nasal) airway is also an airway adjunct. It is usually well tolerated and is not as likely as the oropharyngeal airway to cause vomiting. Unlike the oropharyngeal airway, the nasopharyngeal airway is used for conscious patients or patients with altered levels of consciousness. In pediatric patients, the nasopharyngeal airway is typically used in association with respiratory failure. It is rarely used in infants younger than 1 year.

Skill Drill 31-3: Inserting an Oropharyngeal Airway in a Child

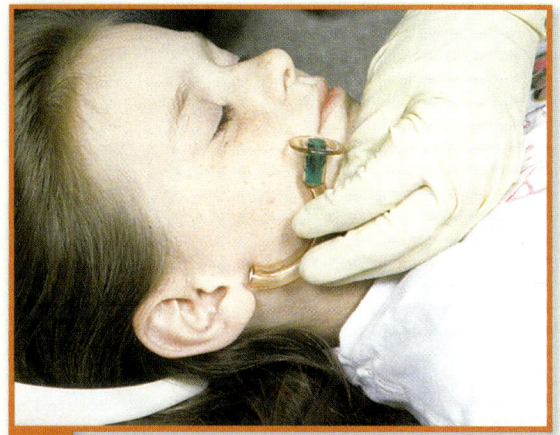

1. Determine the appropriately sized airway by visualizing the device next to the patient's face.

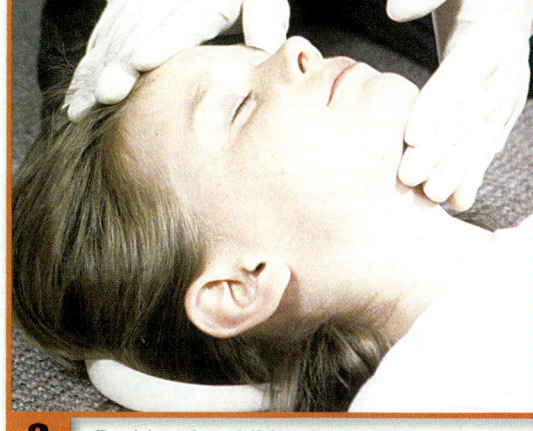

2. Position the child's airway with the appropriate method.

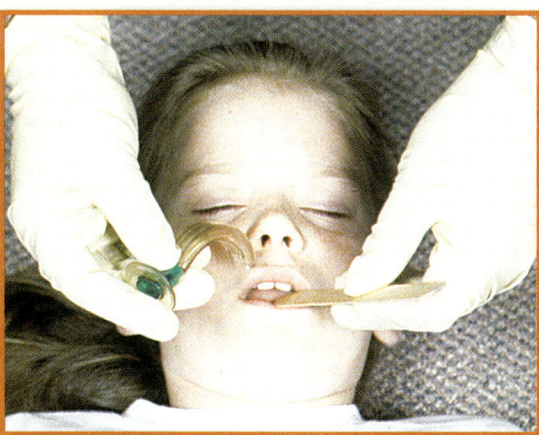

3. Open the mouth.
Insert the airway until the flange rests against the lips.
Reassess the airway.

A nasopharyngeal airway should not be used in patients with nasal obstruction or head trauma (possible skull fracture) or in patients with moderate to severe head trauma because this adjunct could increase intracranial pressure in these patients.

Follow the steps in **Skill Drill 31-4** to insert a nasopharyngeal airway in a child.

1. **Determine the appropriately sized airway.** The external diameter of the airway should not be larger than the diameter of one of the external openings of the nose, called <u>nares</u>, and there should be no <u>blanching</u> (turning white) of the naris after insertion.
2. **Place the airway next to the patient's face** to make sure the length is correct. The airway should extend from the tip of the nose to the tragus of the ear. The <u>tragus</u> is the small cartilaginous projection in front of the opening of the ear.
3. **Position the patient's airway**, using the techniques described for the oropharyngeal airway (**Step 1**).
4. **Lubricate the airway** with a water-soluble lubricant.

Inserting a Nasopharyngeal Airway in a Child

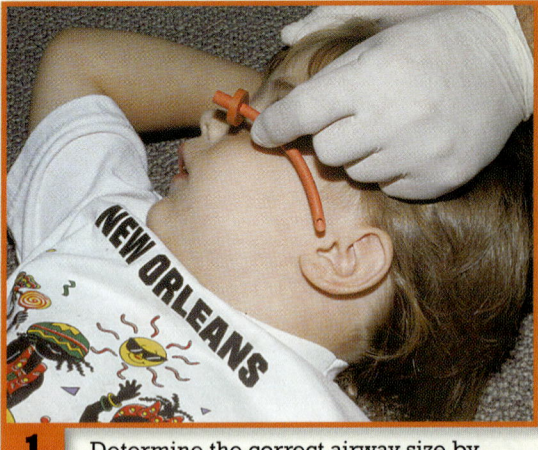

1 Determine the correct airway size by comparing its diameter with the opening of the nostril (nare).

Place the airway next to the patient's face to confirm correct length.

Position the airway appropriately.

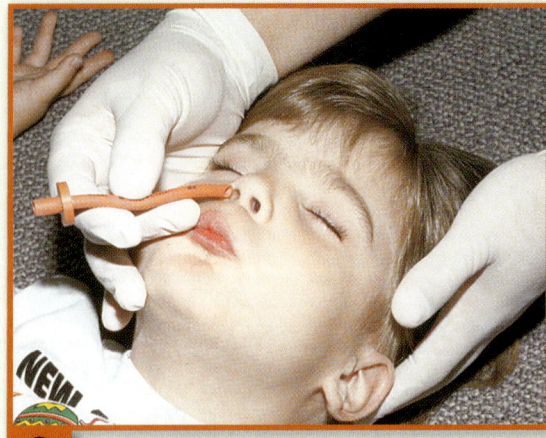

2 Lubricate the airway.

Insert the tip into the right nare with the bevel pointing toward the septum.

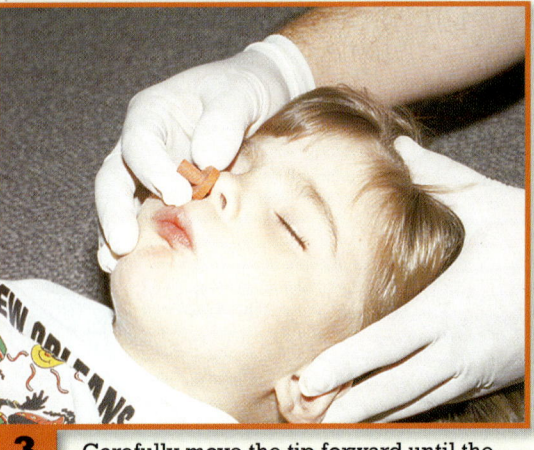

3 Carefully move the tip forward until the flange rests against the outside of the nostril.

Reassess the airway.

---

5. **Insert the tip into the right nare** (nostril opening) with the bevel pointing toward the <u>septum</u>, or central divider in the nose (**Step 2**).
6. **Carefully move the tip forward following the curvature of the nose** until the flange rests against the outside of the nostril. If you are inserting the airway on the left side, insert the tip into the left nare upside down, with the bevel pointing toward the septum. Move the airway forward slowly about 1″ until you feel a slight resistance, and then rotate the airway 180°.
7. **Reassess the airway** after insertion (**Step 3**).

As with the oropharyngeal airway, there can be problems with the nasopharyngeal airway. An airway with a small diameter may easily become obstructed by mucus, blood, vomitus, or the soft tissues of the pharynx. If the airway is too long, it may stimulate the vagus nerve and slow the heart rate or enter the esophagus, causing gastric distention. Inserting the airway in responsive patients may cause spasm of the larynx and result in vomiting.

Nasopharyngeal airways should not be used when patients have facial trauma because the airway may tear soft tissues and cause bleeding into the airway.

Oxygenation

After opening the airway, you should assess the patient's ventilation status. Look, listen, and feel for breathing. Remember to observe chest rise in older children and abdominal rise in younger children and infants. Skin condition indicates the amount of oxygen getting to the tissues of the body. Pallor, mottling, or cyanosis indicates inadequate levels of oxygen in the blood.

All ill or injured infants and children should receive supplemental oxygen. The method of oxygen delivery will be determined by the adequacy of the patient's breathing, or tidal volume.

Oxygen Delivery Devices

In treating infants and children who require supplemental oxygen, the following devices and techniques can be used:

- Nonrebreathing mask at 15 L/min provides up to 90% oxygen concentration.
- Blow-by technique at 6 L/min provides more than 21% oxygen.

Children need enough air to be delivered for adequate gas exchange in the lungs. Therefore, use of a nonrebreathing mask or the blow-by technique is indicated only for patients who have adequate respiratory rates and tidal volumes. Tidal volume is the amount of air that is delivered to the lungs in one inhalation. Because the nonrebreathing mask and blow-by technique deliver oxygen passively, positive-pressure ventilations with a bag-valve-mask (BVM) device are needed in children with inadequate breathing.

Nonrebreathing Mask

A nonrebreathing mask delivers up to 90% oxygen to the patient and allows the patient to exhale all carbon dioxide without rebreathing it Figure 31-31 ▼. To apply a nonrebreathing mask to a child do the following:

1. **Select the appropriately sized** pediatric nonrebreathing mask. The mask should extend from the bridge of the nose to the cleft of the chin.
2. **Connect the tubing** to an oxygen source set at 12 to 15 L/min.
3. **Adjust the oxygen flow** as needed to match the patient's respiratory rate and depth. The reservoir bag should neither deflate completely nor fill completely during the respiratory cycle.

Blow-by Technique

The blow-by technique does not deliver a high concentration of oxygen; however, if the child will not tolerate a nonrebreathing mask, the blow-by technique is better than no oxygen at all.

After ensuring a patent airway and maintaining proper head position, administration of oxygen via the

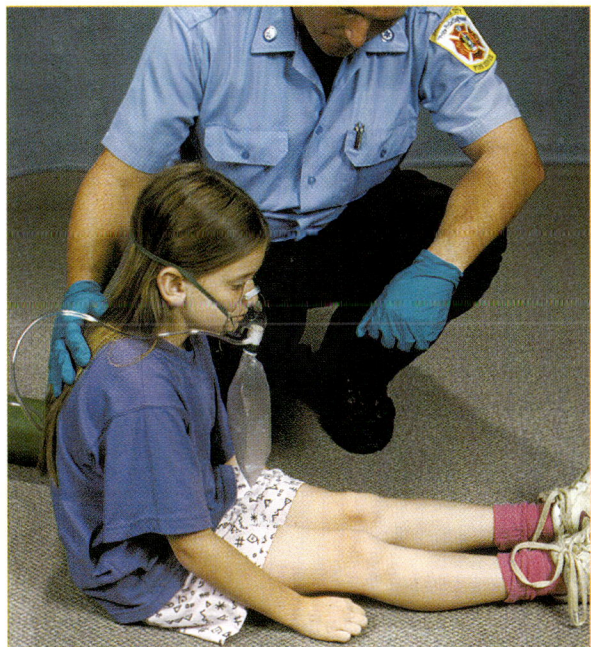

Figure 31-31 A pediatric nonrebreathing mask delivers up to 90% oxygen and allows the patient to exhale carbon dioxide without rebreathing it.

> **In the Field**
>
> Nasal cannulas are rarely used to administer oxygen in pediatric patients. Infants and children are usually not tolerant of the device, which causes anxiety and increased oxygen demand. Agitating an already hypoxic infant or child may exacerbate the condition.

blow-by technique may require assistance from the parent or caregiver. Allowing a parent or caregiver to hold the device near the child's face may facilitate his or her tolerance. To administer blow-by oxygen do the following:

1. **Place oxygen tubing through a small hole in the bottom of a 6- to 8-oz paper or Styrofoam cup** Figure 31-32 ▼). A cup is a familiar object that is less likely than an oxygen mask to frighten young children. You may be able to use an oxygen mask with an older child if you make it a game. For example, pretend that the mask belongs to a popular action hero.
2. **Connect the oxygen tubing to an oxygen source** set at 6 L/min.
3. **Hold the cup (or mask) approximately 1″ to 2″ away from the child's nose and mouth.** Remember, the child may be more tolerant of the device if it is held by a parent or caregiver.

> **In the Field**
>
> If using an oxygen mask to deliver oxygen via the blow-by technique, you must use a simple face mask. A nonrebreathing mask, because of the one-way valve, will not deliver oxygen unless it is applied firmly to the child's face.

Ventilation

If an infant or child is not breathing adequately (that is, inadequate tidal volume, fast or slow rate), positive-pressure ventilatory support will be necessary. Recall that devices such as the nonrebreathing mask cannot deliver oxygen via positive pressure; therefore, they would be inappropriate to use for an infant or child with inadequate breathing. Adequate tidal volume is necessary for passive oxygen (for example, when using a nonrebreathing mask) to be drawn into the lungs.

An infant or child with inadequate breathing is in imminent danger of respiratory arrest, which, if not treated promptly, will lead to cardiopulmonary arrest.

This section will discuss the methods of providing positive-pressure ventilation to an infant and a child, including the use of a BVM device, cricoid pressure, endotracheal intubation, and gastric decompression.

BVM Device

Assisting ventilation with a BVM device is indicated for patients who have respirations that are too fast or too slow to provide adequate tidal volume, who are unresponsive, or who do not respond in a purposeful way to painful stimuli. For obvious reasons, BVM ventilations would be indicated if the child is apneic.

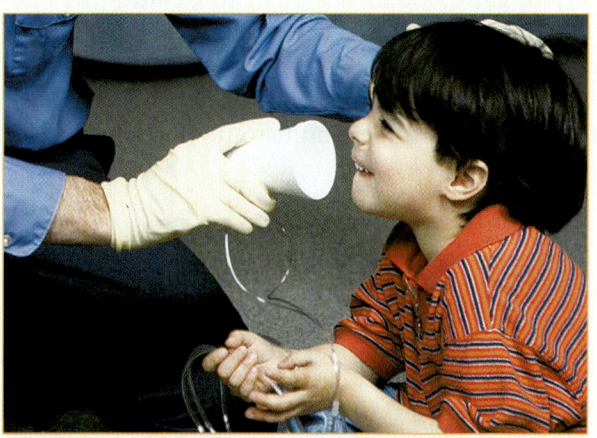

Figure 31-32 Blow-by techniques may be used because oxygen masks often frighten children. Make a small hole in a 6- to 8-oz paper or Styrofoam cup. Connect the oxygen tubing to an oxygen source, and hold the cup about 1″ to 2″ from the child's face.

You are the Provider   Part 5

The seizure stops after 2 minutes; however, the child's respirations become slow and irregular.

9. Is this child in immediate need of ventilatory management?
10. What are the signs of impending respiratory arrest?

Assist ventilation of an infant or child using a BVM device in the following way:

1. **Ensure that you have the appropriate equipment in the right size.** The mask should be the proper size so that it extends from the bridge of the nose to the cleft of the chin, avoiding compression of the eyes (Figure 31-33 ▼). The mask is transparent, so you can observe for cyanosis and vomiting. In addition, mask volume should be small to decrease dead space and avoid rebreathing; however, the bag should contain at least 450 mL of air. Use an infant bag rather than a neonatal bag for children older than 1 year. Older children and adolescents may need an adult bag. Make sure that there is no pop-off valve on the bag, or, if there is one, make sure that you can hold it shut as necessary to achieve adequate chest rise.
2. **Maintain a good seal** with the mask on the face. An inadequate mask-to-face seal will result in inadequate tidal volume delivery and a decreased concentration of delivered oxygen.
3. **Ventilate at the appropriate rate and volume** by delivering each breath over 1 second—just enough to produce visible chest rise. Allow adequate time for exhalation.

Errors in technique, including providing too much volume with each breath, squeezing the bag too forcefully, and ventilating at too fast a rate, can result in gastric distention or a pneumothorax. An inadequate mask-to-face seal or improper head position can lead to inadequately delivered tidal volume and hypoxia.

Even with the best technique, the patient may regurgitate and aspirate the contents of his or her stomach.

Perform one-rescuer BVM ventilation in an infant or child according to the steps in (Skill Drill 31-5 ▶).

1. **Open the airway**, and insert the appropriate airway adjunct (**Step 1**).
2. **Hold the mask on the patient's face** by using the E-C clamp method. Form a C with the thumb and index finger along the mask while the other three fingers form an E along the mandible. With infants and toddlers, support the jaw with only your third finger. Be careful not to compress the area under the chin because you may push the tongue into the back of the mouth and block the airway. Keep fingers on the mandible.
3. **Make sure the mask forms an airtight seal** on the face. Maintain the seal while checking that the airway is open (**Step 2**).
4. **Squeeze the bag**, using the correct ventilation rate; 12 to 20 breaths/min for infants and children.
5. **Allow 1 second per ventilation**, providing adequate time for exhalation (**Step 3**).
6. **Assess effectiveness of ventilation** by watching for adequate bilateral rise and fall of the chest (**Step 4**).

Two-Rescuer BVM Ventilation

This procedure is similar to one-rescuer ventilation except that it requires two rescuers, one to maintain an adequate mask-to-face seal and maintain the patient's head position and the other to ventilate the patient. Although this technique is more effective in delivering adequate tidal volume, you may not always be able to dedicate two EMT-Is to the patient's airway.

Cricoid Pressure

Cricoid pressure (the Sellick maneuver) can and should also be used with pediatric patients to minimize the risks of gastric distention, regurgitation, and aspiration during positive pressure ventilation.

Locating the cricoid ring may be more challenging because the laryngeal prominence is less obvious in

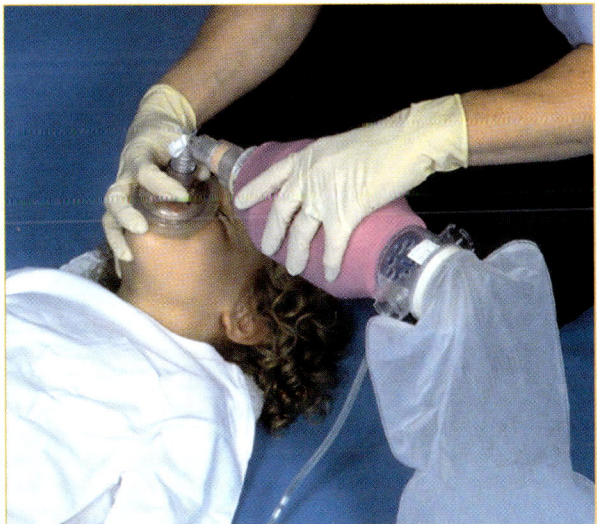

Figure 31-33 Proper mask size for BVM ventilation is critical. The mask should extend from the bridge of the nose to the cleft of the chin, avoiding compression of the eyes.

Skill Drill 31-5

One-Person BVM Ventilation on a Child

1. Open the airway, and insert the appropriate airway adjunct.

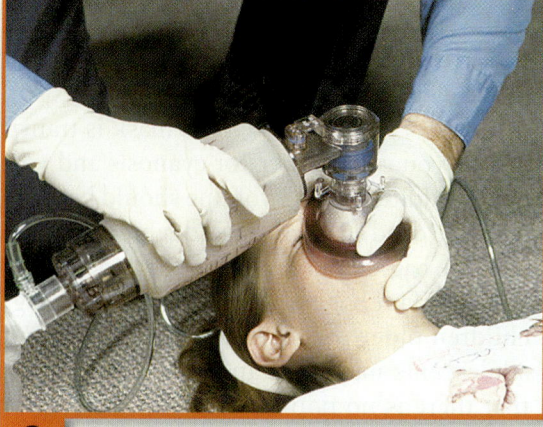

2. Hold the mask on the patient's face with a one-handed head tilt–chin lift technique ("E-C grip").

Ensure a good mask-to-face seal while maintaining the airway.

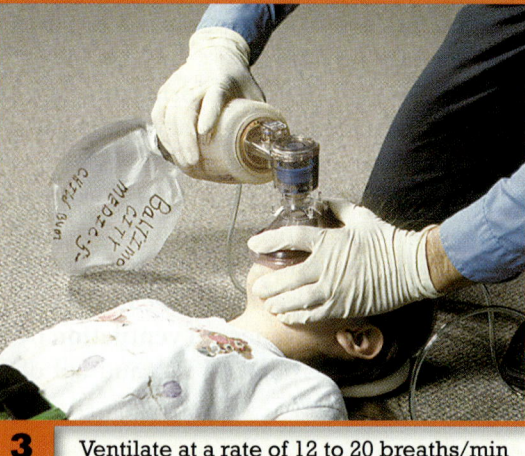

3. Ventilate at a rate of 12 to 20 breaths/min for the infant and child.

Allow adequate time for exhalation.

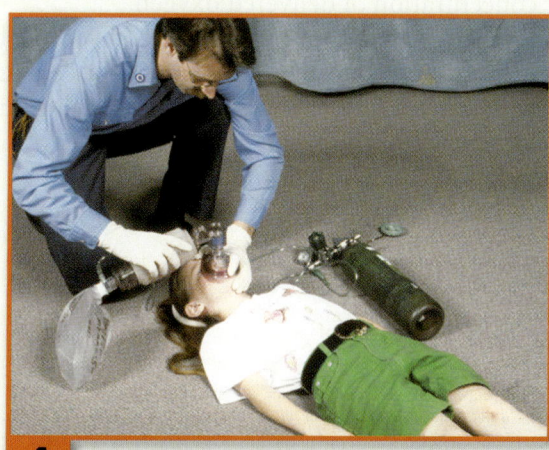

4. Assess effectiveness of ventilation by watching bilateral rise and fall of the chest.

---

children. Only minimal pressure is needed, and excessive pressure can actually cause tracheal compression and airway obstruction **Figure 31-34**.

Endotracheal Intubation

Although endotracheal intubation has been considered the "gold standard" for prehospital airway management, recent studies have suggested that effective BVM ventilations can be as effective in the EMS setting when transport times are short. Indications for endotracheal intubation for pediatric patients are as follows:

- Cardiopulmonary arrest
- Respiratory arrest
- Respiratory failure
- Traumatic brain injury
- Unresponsiveness
- Inability to maintain a patent airway
- Need for prolonged ventilatory support
- Need for endotracheal administration of certain resuscitative medications

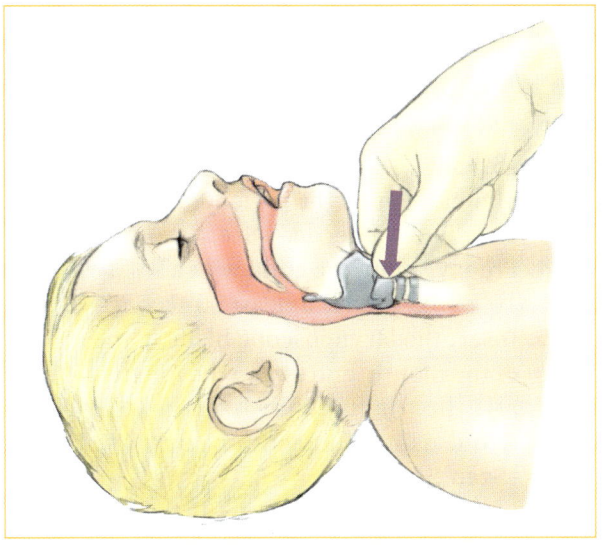

Figure 31-34 Applying posterior cricoid pressure on an infant or child. Excessive pressure can cause airway obstruction.

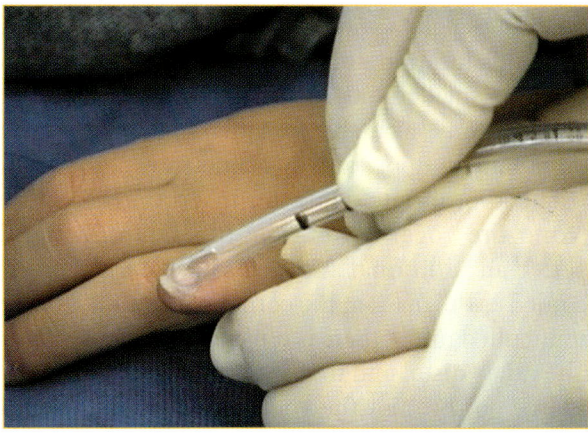

Figure 31-35 The width of the child's small fingernail can be used to estimate the inside diameter of the ET tube.

While some of these indications are similar to those for BVM ventilation, endotracheal intubation is indicated when BVM ventilation is ineffective. As with the adult patient, the most important part of pediatric endotracheal intubation is preparation and equipment selection. Some of the anatomic differences listed earlier in this chapter have a role in successful intubation because proper airway position is critical.

Equipment for Endotracheal Intubation

Any size laryngoscope handle can be used, although many prefer the thinner pediatric handles. Straight (Miller, or Wis-Hipple) blades are preferred because they make it easy to lift the floppy epiglottis. If a curved (Macintosh) blade is used, the tip of the blade is positioned in the vallecula to lift the jaw and epiglottis to visualize the vocal cords.

The appropriately sized blade extends from the patient's mouth to the tragus of the ear. Acceptable means of measuring include using the length-based resuscitation tape and following these general guidelines:
- Premature newborn: Size 0 straight blade
- Full-term newborn to 1 year: Size 1 straight blade
- 2 years to adolescent: Size 2 straight blade
- Adolescent or older: Size 3 straight or curved blade

Endotracheal (ET) tube size can be selected by using a variety of methods: length-based resuscitation tape; anatomic clues, such as the size of the child's nostril or width of the small fingernail (Figure 31-35); and general guidelines (Table 31-6). For children older than 1 year, you can use either of the following formulas:
- (Age [in years] ÷ 4) + 4
  - For example, a 4-year-old child would need a 5.0-mm tube (4 ÷ 4 + 4 = 5.0)
- (Age [in years] + 16) ÷ 4
  - For example, a 6-year-old child would need a 5.5-mm tube (16 + 6 ÷ 4 = 5.5)

One key point is to use uncuffed ET tubes until 8 to 10 years of age. A cuff at the cricoid ring is unnecessary

TABLE 31-6 General Guidelines for Selecting Pediatric ET Tubes

Age	Endotracheal tube, mm	Insertion depth, cm
Premature newborn	2.0-2.5 uncuffed	5.0-8.0
Term newborn	3.0-3.5 uncuffed	8.0-9.5
Infant	3.5-4.0 uncuffed	9.5-11.0
Toddler (1-3 years)	4.0-5.0 uncuffed	11.0-14.0
Preschool (3-5 years)	5.0-5.5 uncuffed	14.0-15.5
School age (6-10 years)	5.5-6.5 uncuffed	15.5-18.5
School age (10-12 years)	6.5 cuffed	18.5
Adolescent	7.0-8.0 cuffed	20.0-23.0

to obtain a seal in young children. Furthermore, a cuff can cause ischemia and damage the mucosa of the trachea at this location. It is important to have a tube that is one size smaller and one that is one size larger than expected always available for situations in which there is variability in upper airway diameter.

The appropriate depth for insertion is 2 to 3 cm beyond the vocal cords. The tube should then be inserted an additional 2 to 3 cm. The depth should be recorded as the mark at the corner of the child's mouth. For uncuffed tubes, there is often a black glottic marker at the tube's distal end to use as a guide. When you see this line go through the vocal cord, stop. For cuffed tubes, when the cuff is just below the vocal cords, stop. Another guideline is to insert the tube to a depth that is equal to three times the inside diameter of the ET tube minus 1. (For example, a 3.5-mm tube should be inserted to a depth of 9.5 cm [$3.5 \times 3 = 10.5$] $- 1 = 9.5$).

The use of a stylet is based on personal preference. If you use a stylet, insert it into the ET tube stopping at least 1 cm from the end of the tube; a stylet that protrudes beyond the end of the ET tube can cause damage to the oral mucosa and vocal cords. Pediatric stylets will fit into tubes sized 3.0 to 6.0 mm, whereas adult stylets are used for tubes sized 6.0 mm or larger. With the stylet in place, bend the ET tube into a gentle upward curve. In some cases, bending the tube into the shape of a hockey stick is beneficial.

Preparation for Endotracheal Intubation

The child should be preoxygenated with a BVM device and 100% oxygen for at least 30 seconds before attempting intubation using the "squeeze, release, release" technique previously described. Adequate preoxygenation cannot be overemphasized because respiratory failure or arrest is the most common cause of cardiopulmonary arrest in the pediatric population. During this time, you must also ensure that the child's head is in the proper position—the <u>neutral position</u> for those with suspected spinal trauma or the sniffing position for those without trauma. An airway adjunct can be inserted if needed to ensure adequate ventilation.

Stimulation of the parasympathetic nervous system and bradycardia can occur during intubation; therefore a cardiac monitor should be applied if available. A pulse oximeter should be used before, during, and after the intubation attempt to monitor the patient's pulse rate and oxygen saturation.

To perform endotracheal intubation in the infant or child, follow the steps listed in (Skill Drill 31-6 ▶):

1. **Take BSI precautions** (gloves and face shield) (**Step 1**).
2. **Check, prepare, and assemble your equipment** (**Step 2**).
3. **Manually open the patient's airway,** and insert an adjunct if needed (**Step 3**).
4. **Preoxygenate the child** with a BVM device and 100% oxygen for at least 30 seconds (**Step 4**).
5. **Insert the laryngoscope blade** in the right side of the mouth, and sweep the tongue to the left. Lift the tongue with firm, gentle pressure. Avoid using the teeth or gums as a fulcrum (**Step 5**).
6. **Identify the vocal cords**. If the cords are not visible, instruct your partner to apply cricoid pressure (**Step 6**).
7. **Introduce the ET tube** in the right corner of the patient's mouth (**Step 7**).
8. **Pass the ET tube through the vocal cords** to approximately 2 to 3 cm below the vocal cords. Inflate the cuff if a cuffed tube is used (**Step 8**).
9. **Attach an end-tidal carbon dioxide** ($ETCO_2$) detector (**Step 9**).
10. **Attach the BVM device,** ventilate, and auscultate for equal breath sounds over each lateral chest wall high in the axillae. Ensure absence of breath sounds over the abdomen (**Step 10**).
11. **Secure the ET tube,** noting the placement of the distance marker at the patient's teeth or gums, and reconfirm tube placement (**Step 11**).

EMT-I Tips

Do not exceed *20 seconds* during any single intubation attempt in an infant or child.

Securing the ET Tube

While there are several methods of using tape to secure ET tubes, no single method is failsafe. One person should always hold the tube in place while another secures the device. The American Heart Association recommends the use of a commercially manufactured tube-securing device for adults and children, when possible 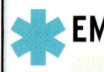 .

Confirmation of ET Tube Position

Three methods to confirm ET tube position include clinical assessment (that is, auscultating breath sounds, monitoring oxygen saturation), use of end-tidal carbon dioxide ($ETCO_2$) detectors, and use of esophageal detector bulbs or syringes. Most of the process of confirmation of ET tube placement is identical to that used in adults. However, there are several important factors that must be considered when using some of these devices in children.

- The adult colorimetric $ETCO_2$ detector cannot be used for children weighing less than 15 kg. The pediatric one can be used for any infant or child Figure 31-37.
- The esophageal bulb or syringe cannot be used with children younger than 5 years weighing less than 20 kg.
  - Because the tracheal walls in children are more collapsible and there is a reduced volume of exhaled air, the bulb or syringe may not fill quickly, giving you the false impression that the ET tube is in the esophagus, when it is actually in the trachea.

Indications for Immediate ET Tube Removal

As with adults, undetected esophageal placement of the ET tube can have disastrous results in children. Frequent monitoring of proper tube placement, especially during any move of the patient (such as from the ground to the stretcher) is essential. The following clinical findings indicate immediate removal of the ET tube:

- No chest rise with ventilation
- Absence of breath sounds during auscultation
- Presence of epigastric gurgling sounds or vomitus in the ET tube
- Failure to confirm proper tube position with detection devices

If inadvertent esophageal intubation has occurred, immediately remove the ET tube and preoxygenate the child for at least 30 seconds before any further intubation attempts.

Complications of Endotracheal Intubation

Although the ET tube is an excellent means of securing a patent airway, the procedure is not without risk. First and foremost, you must assume that the child's stomach is full; emergency patients rarely present on an empty stomach. Have suction readily available in case stimulation of the airway with the laryngoscope causes vomiting.

As previously noted, *a single intubation attempt in the infant or child should not exceed 20 seconds*. Prolonged intubation attempts will likely result in bradycardia and hypoxia. Closely monitor the child's cardiac rhythm and oxygen saturation during any intubation attempt.

Be very careful when manipulating infants' and children's airways with the laryngoscope. The soft tissues of their upper airway are very fragile and easily damaged. Do not use the gums or teeth for leverage because this may result in dislodgement and potential aspiration of broken teeth.

The need to frequently monitor the position of the ET tube cannot be overemphasized. Inadvertent extubation or unrecognized esophageal intubation can be lethal.

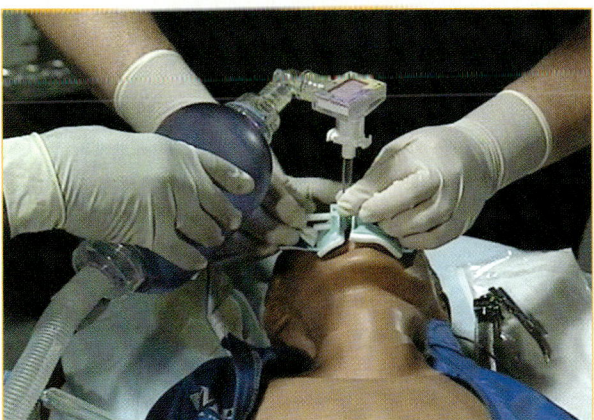

Figure 31-36 Commercially manufactured ET tube holders should be used to secure the tube in place.

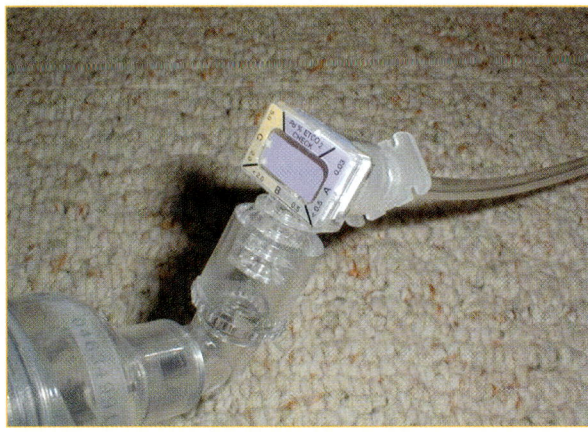

Figure 31-37 Use the pediatric $ETCO_2$ detector for infants and children weighing less than 15 kg.

Performing Pediatric Endotracheal Intubation

Skill Drill 31-6

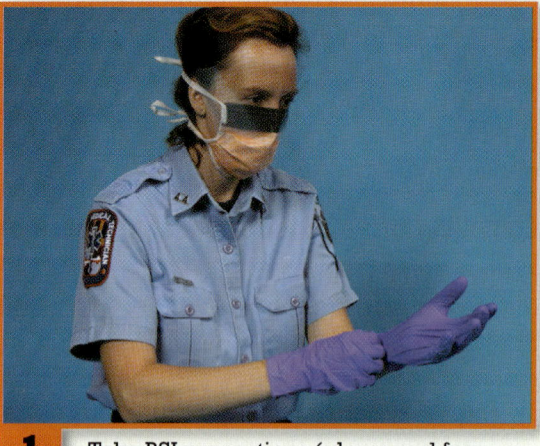

1 Take BSI precautions (gloves and face shield).

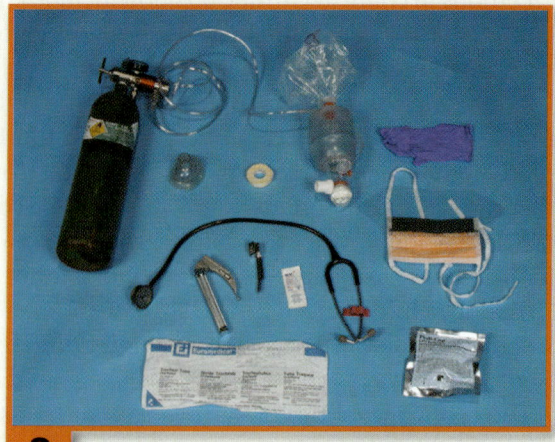

2 Check, prepare, and assemble your equipment.

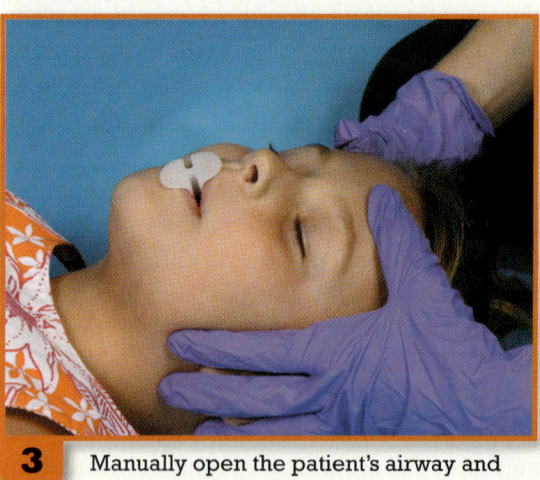

3 Manually open the patient's airway and insert an adjunct if needed.

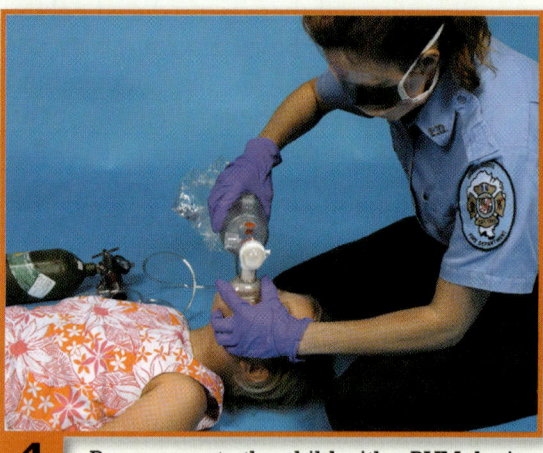

4 Preoxygenate the child with a BVM device and 100% oxygen for at least 30 seconds.

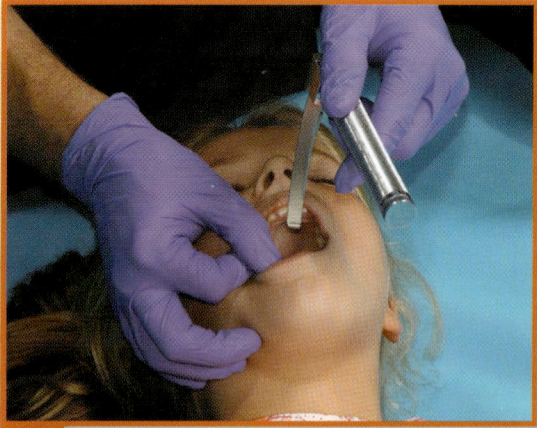

5 Insert the laryngoscope blade in the right side of the mouth, and sweep the tongue to the left. Lift the tongue with firm, gentle pressure. Avoid using the teeth or gums as a fulcrum.

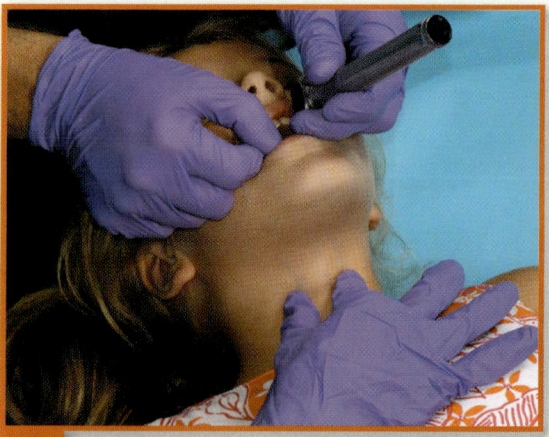

6 Identify the vocal cords. If the cords are not visible, instruct your partner to apply cricoid pressure.

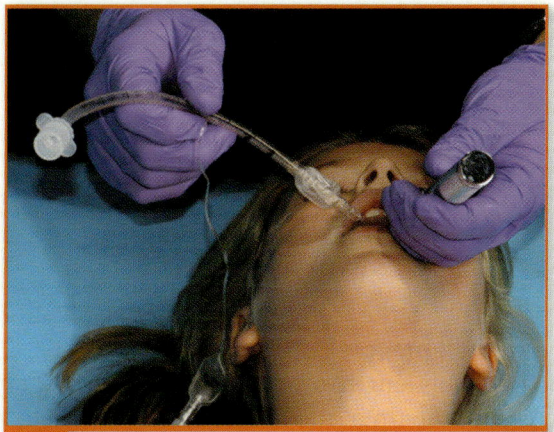

7 Introduce the ET tube in the right corner of the patient's mouth.

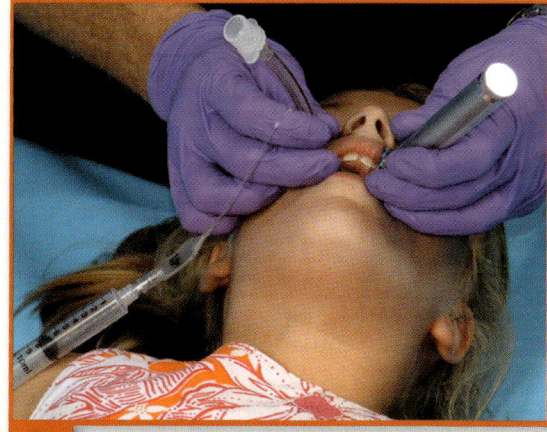

8 Pass the ET tube through the vocal cords to approximately 2 to 3 cm below the vocal cords. Inflate the cuff if a cuffed tube is used.

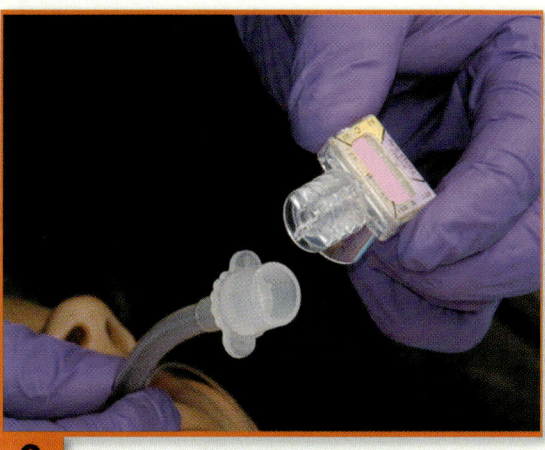

9 Attach an ETCO$_2$ detector.

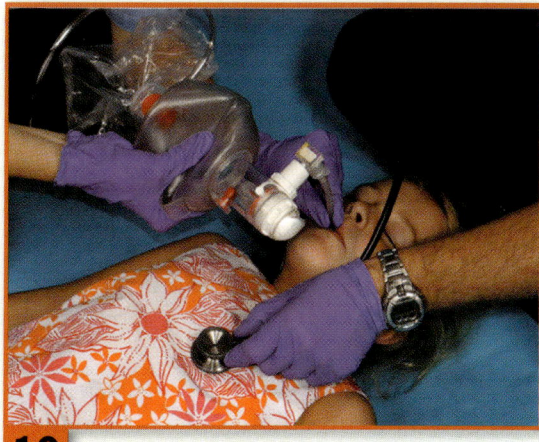

10 Attach the BVM device, ventilate, and auscultate for equal breath sounds over each lateral chest wall high in the axillae. Ensure absence of breath sounds over the abdomen.

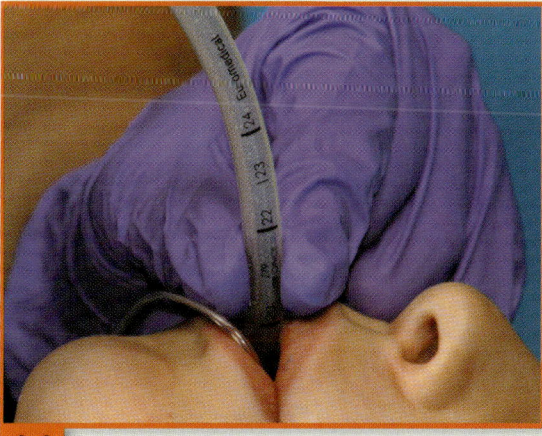

11 Secure the ET tube, noting the placement of the distance marker at the patient's teeth or gums, and reconfirm tube placement.

Documentation Tips

Pulse rate and oxygen saturation should be documented before, during, and after an intubation attempt. Once the tube has been positioned, document the depth of the tube as measured at the right-hand corner of the patient's mouth.

TABLE 31-7	Methods of Determining NG and OG Tube Sizes

- Use a length-based resuscitation tape (see Table 31-5).
- Select a tube size that is the same as the size of the patient's nostril, through which it should pass with minimal resistance.
- Use a tube size twice the ET tube size that the child would need (a child who needs a 5.0-mm ET tube needs a 10 French OG or NG tube).

Gastric Decompression*

During positive-pressure ventilation, it is common to inflate the stomach, as well as the lungs, with air. Gastric distention slows downward movement of the diaphragm and decreases tidal volume, making ventilation more difficult and necessitating higher inspiratory pressures. In addition, gastric distention increases the risk that the patient will vomit and aspirate stomach contents into the lungs. Placement of a nasogastric (NG) tube or an orogastric (OG) tube decompresses the stomach and makes assisted ventilation easier.

Gastric decompression with an NG or OG tube is contraindicated in unresponsive children with a poor or absent gag reflex and an unsecured airway. In such cases, you should perform endotracheal intubation first to decrease the risk of vomiting and aspiration.

Preparation of Equipment

To perform NG or OG tube insertion, you will need the following equipment and supplies:

- The appropriate size NG or OG tube
- A 30- to 60-mL syringe with a funnel-tipped adaptor for manual removal of stomach contents through the tube
- Mechanical suction
- Adhesive tape
- Water-soluble lubricant

Follow these steps to prepare the patient and the equipment for NG or OG tube placement:

1. Select the proper size tube. Sizing techniques are outlined in Table 31-7.
2. Measure the tube on the patient. The length of the tube should be the same as the distance from the lips or tip of the nose (depending on whether the NG or OG route is used) to the earlobe PLUS the distance from the earlobe to the xiphoid process Figure 31-38.
3. Mark this length on the tube with a piece of tape. When the tip of the tube is in the stomach, the tape should be at the lips or nostril.
4. Place the patient in a supine position.
5. Assess the gag reflex. If the patient is unresponsive and has a poor or absent gag reflex, perform endotracheal intubation before gastric tube placement.
6. In a trauma patient:
   a. Maintain in-line stabilization of the cervical spine if a neck injury is possible.
   b. Choose the OG route of insertion if the patient has a severe head or midfacial injury
7. Lubricate the end of the tube.

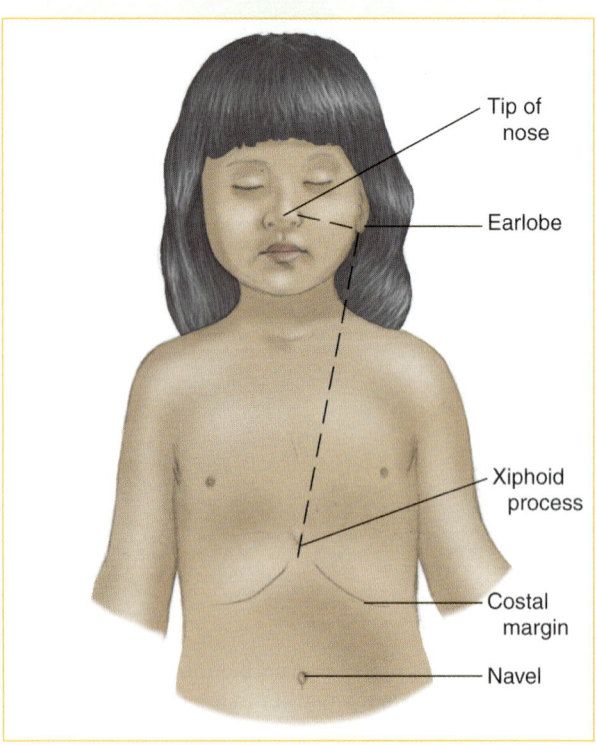

Figure 31-38 Technique for measuring the distance to insert an NG or OG tube.

---

*Used with permission of the American Academy of Pediatrics, *Pediatric Education for Prehospital Professionals*, Elk Grove Village, IL, American Academy of Pediatrics.

NG Tube Insertion

Follow these steps to insert an NG tube in an infant or child:

1. Insert the tube gently through the nostril, directing the tube straight back. *Do not angle the tube superiorly*.
2. If the tube does not pass easily, try the opposite nostril or a smaller tube. *Never force the tube*.
3. If NG passage is unsuccessful, use the OG approach.

OG Tube Insertion

Follow these steps to insert an OG tube in an infant or child:

1. Insert the tube over the tongue, using a tongue blade if necessary to facilitate insertion.
2. Advance the tube into the hypopharynx, then insert rapidly into the stomach.
3. If coughing, choking, or change in voice occurs, immediately remove the tube; it may be in the trachea.

Assessing Placement of the NG and OG Tubes

Follow these steps to confirm successful placement of the NG or OG tube:

1. Check tube placement by aspirating stomach contents. Use a syringe with an appropriate adaptor to quickly instill 10 to 20 mL of air through the tube while auscultating over the left upper quadrant. If there is a rush of air (or gurgling) heard over the stomach, the placement is correct.
2. If correct placement cannot be confirmed, remove the tube.
3. Secure the tube to the bridge of the nose or to the cheek, using adhesive tape **Figure 31-39**.
4. Aspirate air from the stomach, using a 30- to 60-mL catheter-tipped syringe, or connect the tube to mechanical suction at a low, continuous, or intermittent setting.

Complications of NG or OG Tube Insertion

As with endotracheal intubation, you must be aware of the potential complications associated with the placement of an NG or OG tube. These include the following:

- Placement of the tube into the trachea, resulting in hypoxia
- Vomiting and aspiration of stomach contents
- Airway bleeding or obstruction

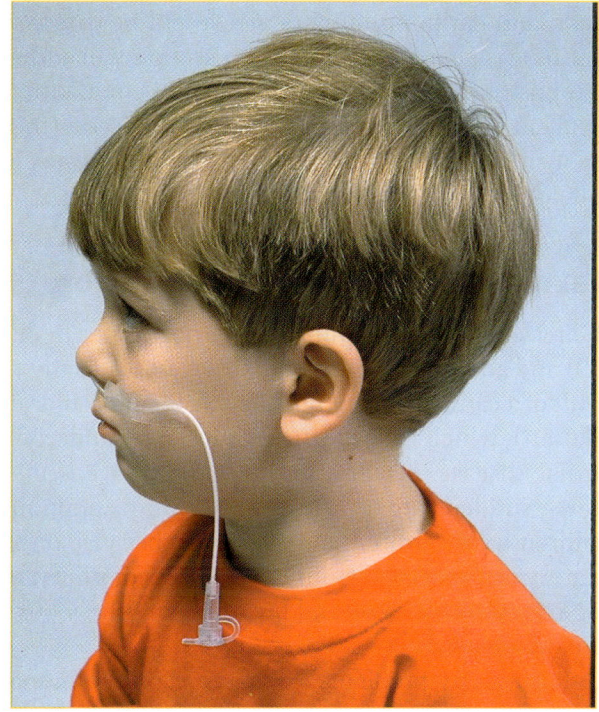

Figure 31-39 Proper method for securing an NG or OG tube.

- Passage of the tube into the cranium
  - This can occur if you insert an NG tube into a patient with severe head or midfacial trauma. The tube may be inadvertently passed through the fracture and into the brain. Signs of severe head trauma include nasal bleeding or clear nasal secretions, which may contain cerebrospinal fluid (cerebrospinal fluid rhinorrhea).

Circulation

As previously discussed, assessment of circulation in the infant or child is best performed by assessing signs of end-organ perfusion, such as level of consciousness, capillary refill time (children younger than 6 years), and condition of the skin. Use of the PAT can often identify problems with circulation, allowing you to immediately intervene and prevent a potentially catastrophic event.

In addition to respiratory failure, shock is a common cause of cardiopulmonary arrest in children as well. Failure to recognize the signs and symptoms of shock and begin prompt treatment may result in permanent brain damage or possibly death.

Although the signs, symptoms, and treatment of shock and cardiopulmonary arrest will be discussed later in this chapter, the following section will address methods of maintaining and improving circulation in the infant or child, including CPR, vascular access (intravenous [IV] and intraosseous [IO]), IV fluid resuscitation, and resuscitative medications.

Cardiopulmonary Resuscitation

The reasons for cardiopulmonary arrest differ in children and adults. In adults, cardiac arrest is usually the result of a cardiac dysrhythmia (such as ventricular fibrillation), which is itself usually caused by underlying cardiac disease. Because most children have healthy hearts, sudden cardiac arrest is rare. More commonly, children have cardiopulmonary arrest because of respiratory or circulatory failure from illness or injury. For this reason, the airway and breathing are the focus of pediatric BLS.

Respiratory problems leading to cardiopulmonary arrest in children can have a number of different causes, including the following:

- Injury, both blunt and penetrating
- Infection of the respiratory tract or another organ system
- A foreign body in the airway
- Near drowning
- Electrocution
- Poisoning or drug overdose
- Sudden infant death syndrome (SIDS)

The techniques for assessing responsiveness and opening and maintaining a patent airway (basic and advanced) were discussed earlier in this chapter. Therefore, in this section, the techniques for chest compressions in the infant and child will be discussed and demonstrated.

For chest compressions to be effective, the patient should be placed on a firm, flat surface with the head at the same level as the body. If you need to carry an infant while providing CPR, your forearm and hand can serve as the flat surface. Follow the steps in (Skill Drill 31-7 ▶) to perform infant chest compressions:

1. **Place the infant on a firm surface**, using one hand to keep the head in an open airway position. You can also use a pad or wedge under the shoulders and upper body to keep the head from tilting forward.
2. Imagine a line drawn between the nipples. **Place two fingers in the middle of the sternum**, about ½″ below the level of the imaginary line (one fingerbreadth) (**Step 1**).
3. **Using two fingers, compress the sternum** about one third to one half the depth of the chest. Compress the chest at a rate of 100 compressions/min. The ratio of compressions to breaths should be 30:2 with one rescuer and 15:2 with two rescuers.
4. **After each compression, allow the sternum to return briefly to its normal position.** Allow equal time for compression and relaxation of the chest. Do not remove your fingers from the sternum, and avoid jerky movements (**Step 2**).
5. **Coordinate rapid compressions and ventilations** in a ratio of 30:2 with one rescuer and 15:2 with two rescuers, making sure the infant's chest rises with each ventilation. You will find this easier to do if you use your free hand to keep the head in the open airway position. If the chest does not rise or rises only a little, use a chin lift to open the airway.
6. **Reassess the infant for signs of spontaneous breathing or pulses** after every five cycles of CPR or 2 minutes (**Step 3**).

(Skill Drill 31-8 ▶) shows the steps for performing chest compressions in children between ages 1 year and the onset of puberty (12 to 14 years of age).

1. **Place the child on a firm surface**, and use one hand to maintain the head in a tilted-back position (**Step 1**).
2. **Using two fingers of the other hand, locate the bottom of the sternum** by tracing the lower margin of the rib cage to the notch where the ribs and sternum meet. Place the heel of one or two hands between the nipple line. Avoid compression over the lower tip of the sternum, which is called the <u>xiphoid process</u> (**Step 2**).
3. **Compress the chest** about one third to one half its total depth. Compress the chest at a rate of 100 compressions/min. Compression and relaxation should be about the same duration. Use smooth movements. Hold your fingers off the child's ribs, and keep the heel of your hand (or hands) on the sternum.
4. **Coordinate rapid compressions and ventilations** in a ratio of 30:2 with one rescuer and 15:2 with two rescuers, making sure the chest rises with each ventilation. At the end of each cycle of chest compressions, pause for 2 ventilations (**Step 3**).

Performing Infant Chest Compressions

Skill Drill 31-7

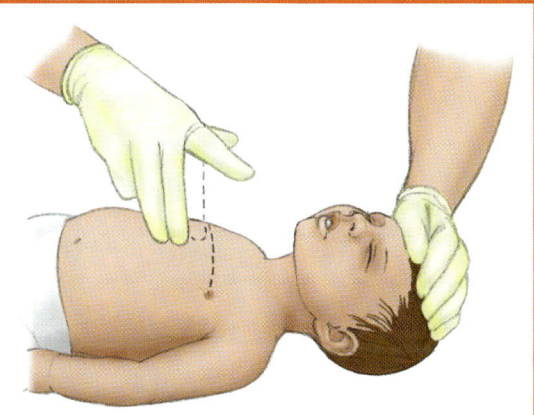

1 Position the infant on a firm surface while maintaining the airway.

Place two fingers in the middle of the sternum just below a line between the nipples.

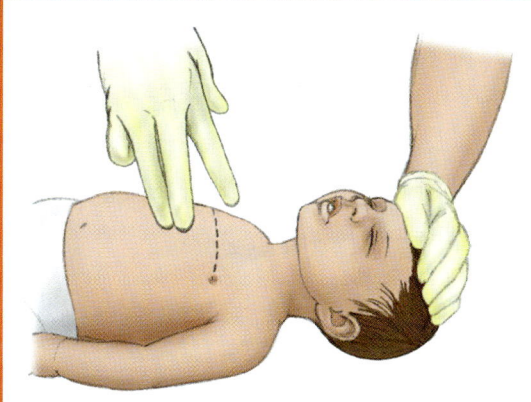

2 Use two fingers to compress the chest $1/3$ to $1/2$ its depth at a rate of 100 times/min.

Allow the sternum to return briefly to its normal position between compressions.

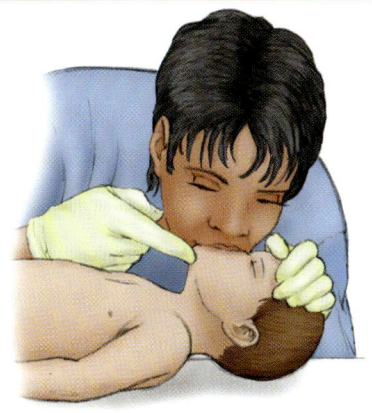

3 Coordinate rapid compressions and ventilations in a ratio of 30:2 with one rescuer and 15:2 with two rescuers.

Check for return of breathing and pulse after five cycles of CPR or 2 minutes.

5. **Reassess the child for signs of spontaneous breathing and pulses** after five cycles of CPR or 2 minutes.
6. **If the child resumes effective breathing**, place him or her in the recovery position (**Step 4**).

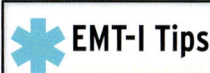 **EMT-I Tips**

For children older than 1 year, incorporate the AED into the sequence of CPR.

Skill Drill 31-8: Performing Chest Compressions on a Child

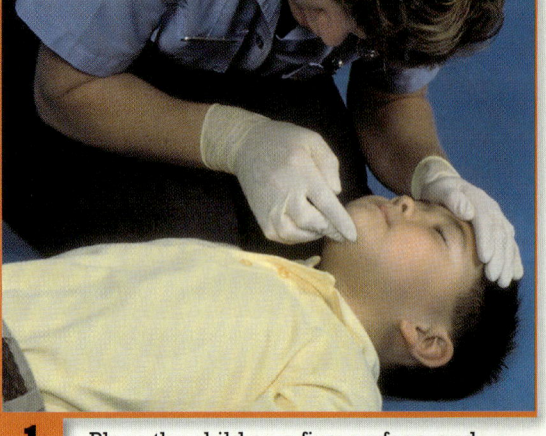

1. Place the child on a firm surface, and maintain the airway with one hand.

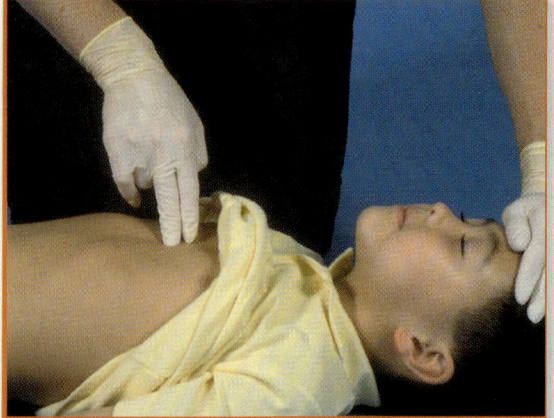

2. Place the heel of your other hand over the lower half of the sternum, avoiding the xiphoid.

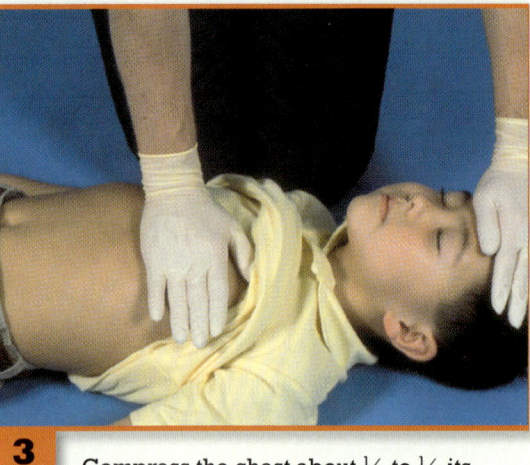

3. Compress the chest about ⅓ to ½ its depth at a rate of 100/min.

Coordinate compressions with ventilations in a ratio of 30:2 with one rescuer and 15:2 with two rescuers, pausing for ventilations.

4. Reassess for breathing and pulse after five cycles of CPR.

If the child resumes effective breathing, place him or her in the recovery position.

Intravenous Access

Although IV therapy is not performed as frequently in children as it is in adults, the technique, indications, and contraindications in the infant and child are the same as they are for adults. In addition, the same IV solutions and equipment used for adults can be used for pediatric patients (see Chapter 7), with a few exceptions.

Catheters

If you are using an over-the-needle catheter ("angiocath") to start a pediatric IV, the 20-, 22-, 24-, and 26-gauge catheters are best for insertion **Figure 31-40**. Butterfly catheters are useful for pediatric patients and can be placed in the same locations as over-the-needle catheters and in visible scalp veins. However, butterfly catheters are associated with a higher rate of infiltra-

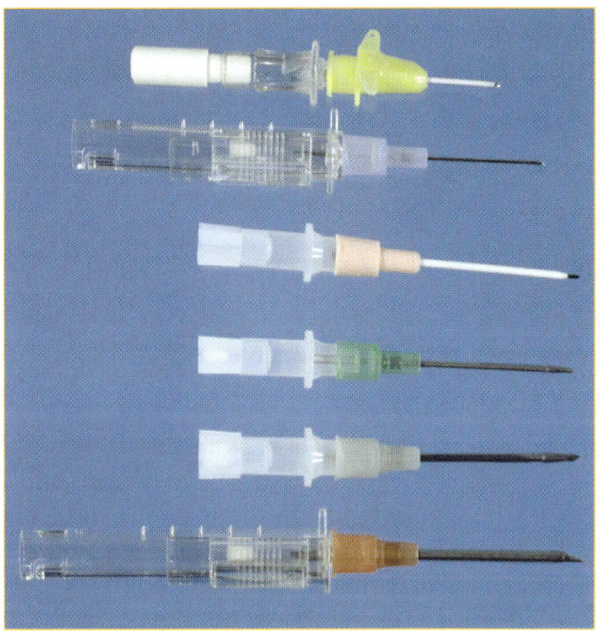

Figure 31-40 Note the difference in sizes of IV catheters.

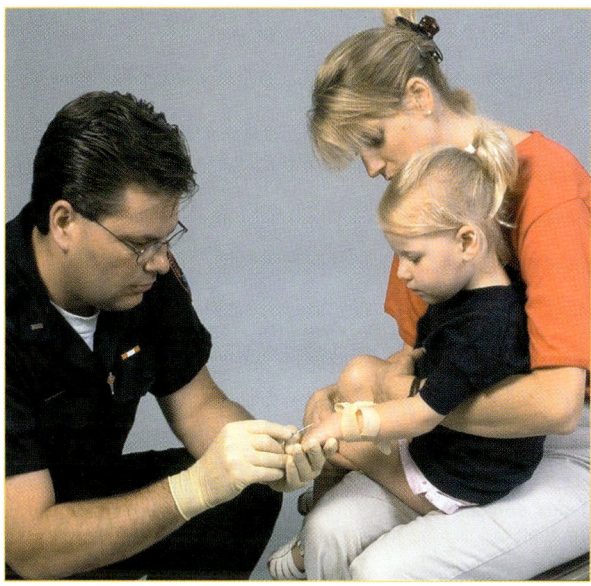

Figure 31-41 If possible, allow the child to sit on the parent or caregiver's lap when starting an IV. Secure the child's legs to avoid kicking.

tion because a stainless steel needle lies in the vein, instead of the Teflon catheter or an over-the-needle catheter.

Administration Sets

Fluid control for pediatric patients is important. Using a special type of microdrip set called a <u>Volutrol</u> allows you to fill the large drip chamber with a specific amount of fluid and administer only this amount to avoid fluid overload. The 100-mL calibrated drip chamber on the Volutrol can be shut off from the IV bag.

If your EMS system does not use the Volutrol, a regular microdrip administration set can be used; however, use caution when administering fluid through these administration sets.

IV Locations

When starting the IV, take both the child and the parent or caregiver into consideration. The parent can become as stressed as the child. If the condition of the child permits, take time to thoroughly explain the procedure to both the child and the parent or caregiver. When possible, allow the infant or child to sit on the parent or caregiver's lap when starting the IV **Figure 31-41**.

The younger the child, the fewer choices you have for IV sites. Hand veins are painful and difficult to manage in younger children; however, they remain the location of choice for starting peripheral IVs.

Protecting the IV site after it has been established is critical and is sometimes best accomplished by immobilizing the site with an arm board before cannulation. One of the better techniques for starting pediatric IVs is to use a penlight to illuminate the veins on the back of the hand. Shine the light through the palm side of the hand to illuminate the veins on the dorsal aspect of the hand. Once a suitable site is located, mark the vein with a pen so you can find the location after you turn off the penlight. Proceed with starting the IV, using the mark you created as a guide. Sometimes the best choice is an antecubital vein, especially if the child is critically ill or injured and needs fluid resuscitation or medication therapy. illustrates the different sites for starting IVs in infants and children.

> ### ✳ EMT-I Tips
>
> Most pediatric patients do not require prehospital IV therapy. Do not start an IV in an infant or child unless it is absolutely necessary (for example, if cardiac arrest or shock occur). Remember that unnecessarily agitating a child can exacerbate the child's condition, especially if already hypoxic.

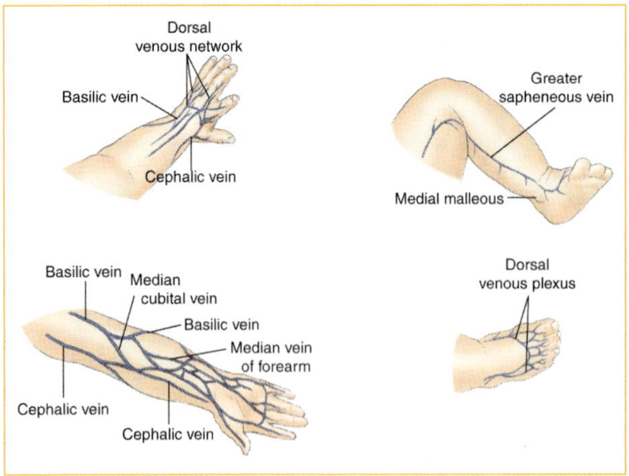

Figure 31-42 Sites for IVs in infants and children are the hands, antecubital fossa, the saphenous veins at the ankle, and the feet.

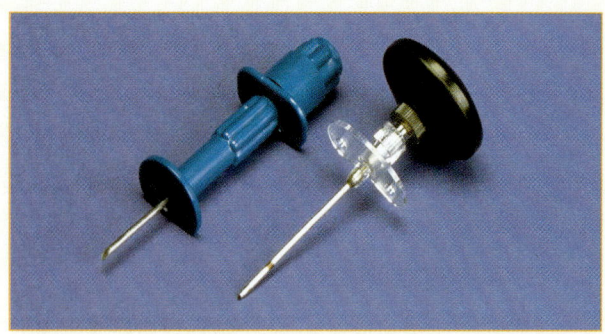

Figure 31-43 IO needles.

IO Infusion

Intraosseous (IO) infusion is used for emergency vascular access in pediatric patients as defined by protocol when immediate IV access is difficult or impossible. When placed correctly, the IO needle will rest in the medullary canal, the space within the bone that contains bone marrow. An IO should be attempted if you are unable to obtain IV access within three attempts *or* 90 seconds in a critically ill or injured pediatric patient. Often these children are experiencing a life-threatening situation such as cardiac arrest, status epilepticus, or progressive shock. An IO infusion is contraindicated if a secure IV line is available or if a fracture (or possible fracture) exists in the same bone in which you plan to insert the IO needle.

The IO needle is usually inserted in the proximal tibia with a special IO needle Figure 31-43 ▶. A commonly used IO catheter is the Jamshedi needle. This double needle, consisting of a solid-bore needle inside a sharpened hollow needle, is pushed into the bone with a screwing, twisting action. Once the needle pops through the bone, the solid needle is removed, leaving the hollow steel needle in place. Standard IV tubing is then attached to this catheter.

Anything that can be administered intravenously can be administered through an IO line (such as isotonic fluids, medications). The IO lines require full and careful immobilization because they rest at a 90° angle to the bone and are easily dislodged. Stabilization is critical for these lines to maintain adequate flow. Stabilize the IO needle in the same manner that you would any impaled object. Follow the steps in Skill Drill 31-9 ▶ to establish an IO infusion in the pediatric patient:

1. **Check selected IV fluid for proper fluid**, clarity, and expiration date. Look for any discoloration or particles floating in the fluid. If found, discard and choose another bag of fluid.
2. **Select the appropriate equipment**, including an IO needle, syringe, saline, and extension set (**Step 1**). A three-way stopcock may also be used to facilitate easier fluid administration.
3. **Select the proper administration set.** Connect the administration set to the bag. Prepare the administration set. Fill the drip chamber and flush the tubing. Make sure all air bubbles are removed from the tubing.
4. **Prepare the syringe and extension tubing (Step 2).**
5. **Cut or tear the tape.** This can be done at any time before IO puncture.
6. **Take BSI isolation precautions.** This must be done before IO puncture.
7. **Identify the proper anatomic site** for IO puncture (**Step 3**). To miss the epiphyseal (growth) plate, you should measure two fingerbreadths below the knee on the medial side of the leg.
8. **Cleanse the site appropriately.** Follow aseptic technique by cleansing in a circular manner from the inside out.
9. **Perform the IO puncture**, involving the following steps:
   Stabilize the tibia. Place a folded towel underneath the knee and hold in such a manner as to keep your fingers away from the site of puncture. Insert the needle at the proper angle.
10. **Insert the needle at a 90° angle** to the leg. Advance the needle with a twisting motion until a "pop" is felt (**Step 4**). Unscrew the cap, and remove the stylet from the needle (**Step 5**).

11. **Attach the syringe and extension set** to the IO needle. Pull back on the syringe to aspirate blood and particles of bone marrow to ensure placement.
12. **Slowly inject saline** to ensure proper placement of the needle. Watch for infiltration, and stop the infusion immediately if noted. It is possible to fracture the bone during insertion of the IO. If this happens, you should remove the IO needle and switch to the other leg.
13. **Connect the administration set**, and adjust the flow rate as appropriate. Fluid does not flow well through an IO needle, and boluses are given by administering the fluid using the syringe (**Step 6**).
14. **Secure the needle with tape**, and support it with a bulky dressing. Stabilize in place in the same manner that an impaled object is stabilized. Use bulky dressings around the catheter, and tape securely in place. Be careful not to tape around the entire circumference of the leg, which could impair circulation and create compartment syndrome.
15. **Dispose of the needle in the proper container** (**Step 7**).

Complications of IO Infusions

As with any invasive procedure, there are potential complications with IO infusion that you must be aware of. With proper technique, the following potential complications may be avoided:

- Compartment syndrome
- Failed infusion
- Growth plate injury
- Bone and muscle inflammation caused by infection (osteomyelitis)
- Skin infection
- Bony fracture

Fluid Resuscitation

As previously mentioned, appropriate fluid administration in the pediatric patient is crucial; IV fluids must be administered based on the child's clinical condition. If too much fluid is administered, overload can result and cause acute left-sided heart failure and pulmonary edema. Conversely, administering insufficient fluid volumes will not be effective in treating the child's condition. Use of a microdrip administration set, Volutrol, or IV infusion pump is highly recommended to prevent a "runaway IV."

Fluid resuscitation for the infant or child in hypovolemic shock begins with an initial bolus of 20 mL/kg of an isotonic crystalloid solution (for example, normal saline, lactated Ringer's), followed by a careful reassessment. Administer further boluses of 20 mL/kg as needed to maintain adequate perfusion.

In children who require multiple IV fluid boluses, you should carefully and frequently assess their breath sounds, noting signs of pulmonary edema (for example, rales, rhonchi).

In the Field

Remember to ask the parent or caregiver how much the child weighs and then convert the weight in pounds to kilograms. If the weight of the child is unknown, use the following formula to estimate the weight in kilograms:

(Age [in years] × 2) + 8 = Weight in kilograms

When administering IV fluids or medications, it is crucial to obtain as accurate an estimate of the child's weight as possible.

You are the Provider   Part 6

Transport is begun to a trauma center located 25 miles away. You ask a fire fighter to drive the ambulance because your partner's assistance is needed in the back with the patient. Your BVM ventilations have been adequate thus far, but you are concerned about the long transport time and the development of gastric distention. Therefore, you decide to perform endotracheal intubation.

11. What are the most significant challenges of intubation in the pediatric patient?

Skill Drill 31-9

Pediatric IO Infusion

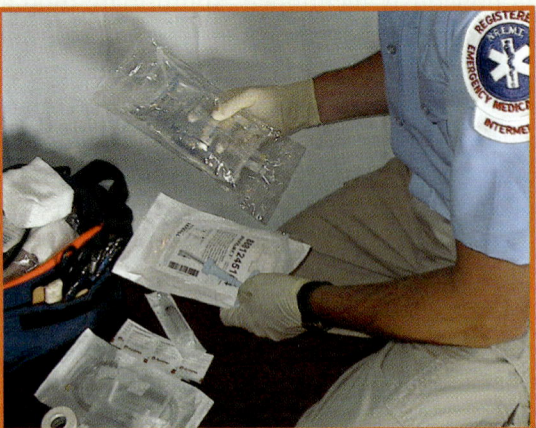

1. Check selected IV fluid for proper fluid, clarity, and expiration date.

Select the appropriate equipment, including an IO needle, syringe, saline, and extension.

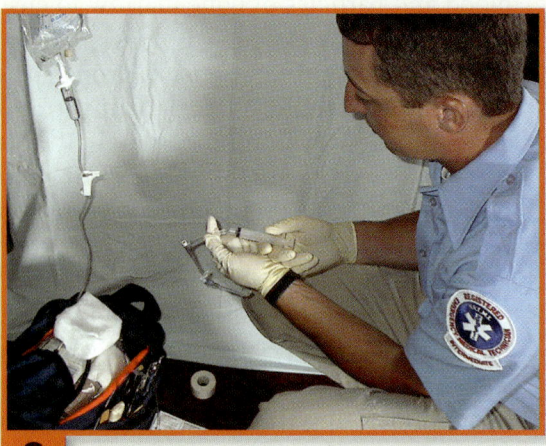

2. Select the proper administration set. Connect the administration set to the bag. Prepare the administration set. Prepare the syringe and extension tubing.

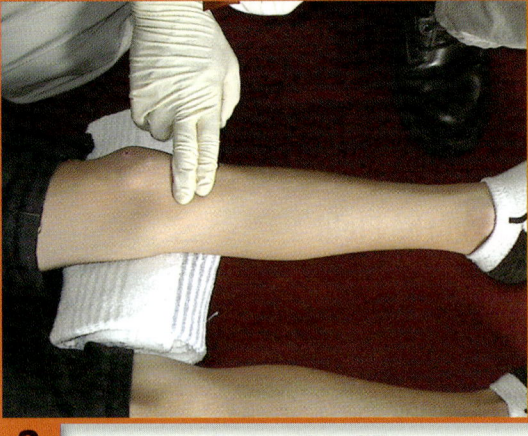

3. Cut or tear the tape. Take BSI precautions. Identify the proper anatomic site for IO puncture.

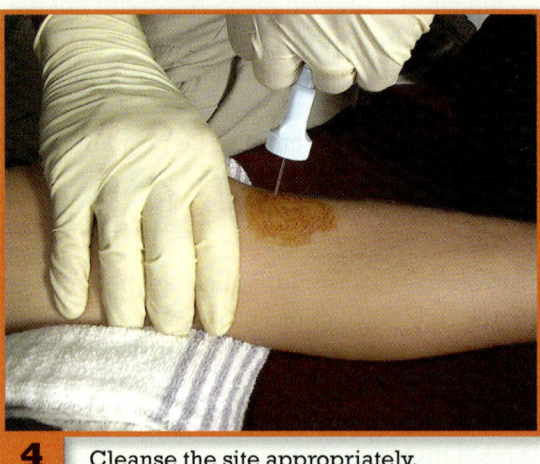

4. Cleanse the site appropriately. Stabilize the tibia. Insert the needle at the proper angle. Advance the needle with a twisting motion until a "pop" is felt.

Medication Therapy

Because most cases of cardiopulmonary arrest in infants and children are related to respiratory failure, oxygen is the most common medication that you will administer to them in the prehospital setting. Most pediatric emergencies can be managed by maintaining a patent airway, administering 100% oxygen, and transporting to the hospital.

In some cases, however, the EMT-I will encounter a child who requires a medication in addition to oxygen. Table 31-8 lists the common medications used during pediatric resuscitation. Additional medications will be addressed throughout the remainder of this chapter, as applicable.

Manual Defibrillation

Ventricular fibrillation (V-fib) and pulseless ventricular tachycardia (V-tach) are less commonly seen in children than in adults; therefore, defibrillation is usually

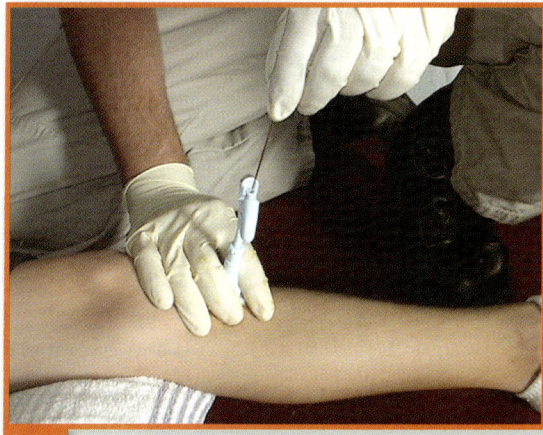

5 Unscrew the cap, and remove the stylet from the needle.

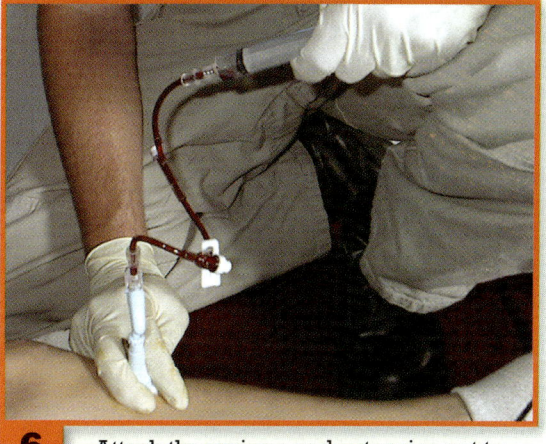

6 Attach the syringe and extension set to the IO needle.

Pull back on the syringe to aspirate blood and particles of bone marrow to ensure placement.

Slowly inject saline to assure proper placement of the needle.

Watch for infiltration, and stop the infusion immediately if noted.

Connect the administration set, and adjust the flow rate as appropriate.

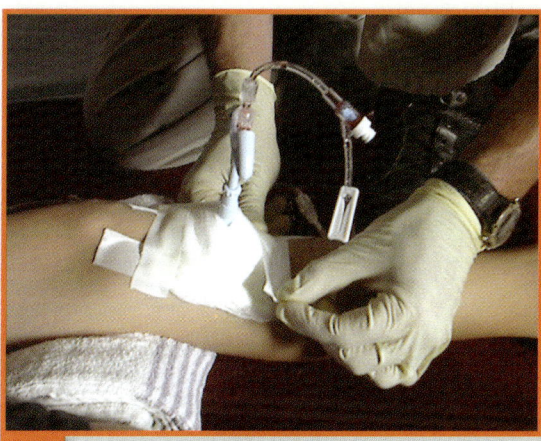

7 Secure the needle with tape, and support it with a bulky dressing.

Dispose of the needle in the proper container.

---

not required during resuscitation of infants and children. Bradydysrhythmias are more common in the pediatric population during cardiac arrest; however, conditions such as electrocution, congenital heart defects, and myocarditis can result in V-fib or pulseless V-tach.

As with adults, immediate defibrillation is just as crucial in infants and children with V-fib or pulseless V-tach. Therefore, on determining that the infant or child is pulseless and apneic, a rapid assessment of the cardiac rhythm is required to assess the need for defibrillation.

Follow these steps to perform manual defibrillation in the infant or child:

1. Confirm unresponsiveness, pulselessness, and apnea.
2. Begin CPR if a defibrillator is not immediately available.
3. Select the proper paddle size (Table 31-9 ▶).
4. Apply conductive gel to the paddles. Place one paddle on the anterior chest wall to the right of the sternum, inferior to the clavicle; place the

TABLE 31-8 Medications Used in Pediatric Resuscitation*

Adenosine
- 0.1 mg/kg (up to 6.0 mg) via rapid IV or IO administration; follow with ≥ 5 mL normal saline flush
  - Second dose: 0.2 mg/kg
  - Maximum single dose: 12 mg

Amiodarone
- 5 mg/kg via rapid IV or IO administration
  - Maximum single dose: 300 mg
  - Maximum cumulative dose: 15 mg/kg per day

Atropine Sulfate†
- 0.02 mg/kg via rapid IV, IO, or ET administration
  - Minimum single dose: 0.1 mg
  - Maximum single dose: 0.5 mg for a child; 1.0 mg for an adolescent
  - Maximum total dose: 1.0 mg for a child; 2.0 mg for an adolescent
- 0.03 mg/kg ET (absorption may be unreliable)

Dopamine
- 2-20 µg/kg/min titrated to desired effect
  - Usual initial dose is 5-10 µg/kg/min
  - If infusion dose is >20 µg/kg/min, consider using an epinephrine infusion

Epinephrine†
- *Bradycardia (repeat every 3-5 minutes)*
  - IV or IO: 0.01 mg/kg (0.1 mL/kg of 1:10,000 solution)
  - Through the ET tube: 0.1 mg/kg (0.1 mL/kg of 1:1,000 solution)
- *Cardiac arrest (repeat every 3-5 minutes)*
  - IV or IO: 0.01 mg/kg (0.1 mL/kg of 1:10,000 solution)
  - ET route: 0.1 mg/kg (0.1 mL/kg of 1:1,000 solution)
- *Maintenance infusion*
  - Start at 0.1 µg/kg/min
  - Titrate to desired effect (0.1-1.0 µg/kg/min)

Glucose‡
- 0.5-1.0 g/kg via IV or IO administration
  - Maximum doses
    - 5% Dextrose (D_5W): 10-20 mL/kg
    - 10% Dextrose ($D_{10}W$): 5-10 mL/kg
    - 25% Dextrose ($D_{25}W$): 2-4 mL/kg

Lidocaine†
- 1 mg/kg via rapid IV, IO, ET tube administration
  - Maximum dose of 100 mg
    - Maintenance infusion: 20-50 µg/kg/min
- ET dose: 2-3 mg/kg

Naloxone†
- 0.1 mg/kg up to 2 mg IV/IO for total reversal of narcotic effects
- If total reversal not required, smaller doses (1-5 µg/kg) may be used. Titrate to effect. May be given via the ET route, but other routes are preferred.

*Additional medications not listed may be administered according to local protocol or at the discretion of medical control.
†For ET tube administration, dilute medication with normal saline to a volume of 3-5 mL and follow with several positive pressure ventilations.
‡Administer into a large vein; ensure the IV is patent; dextrose may cause local tissue necrosis if it extravasates.

TABLE 31-9 Pediatric Defibrillation Paddle Size

- Older than 12 months *or* >10 kg: 8-cm (adult) paddles
- Up to 12 months *or* <10 kg: 4.5-cm (pediatric) paddles
- Paddles selected should be the largest size that allows good chest contact over the entire paddle surface area and distinct separation between the two paddles.

other paddle on the left midclavicular line at the level of the xiphoid process Figure 31-44 ▼ . Apply firm pressure to the paddles.

a. For children older than 12 months *or* who weigh more than 10 kg, you may use anterior-posterior paddle placement Figure 31-45 ▶ .

5. Assess the cardiac rhythm to confirm the presence of V-fib or pulseless V-tach.
6. Select the appropriate energy setting, and charge the defibrillator.
7. Verbally **and** visually ensure that nobody is in contact with the patient; stop CPR if it is in progress.

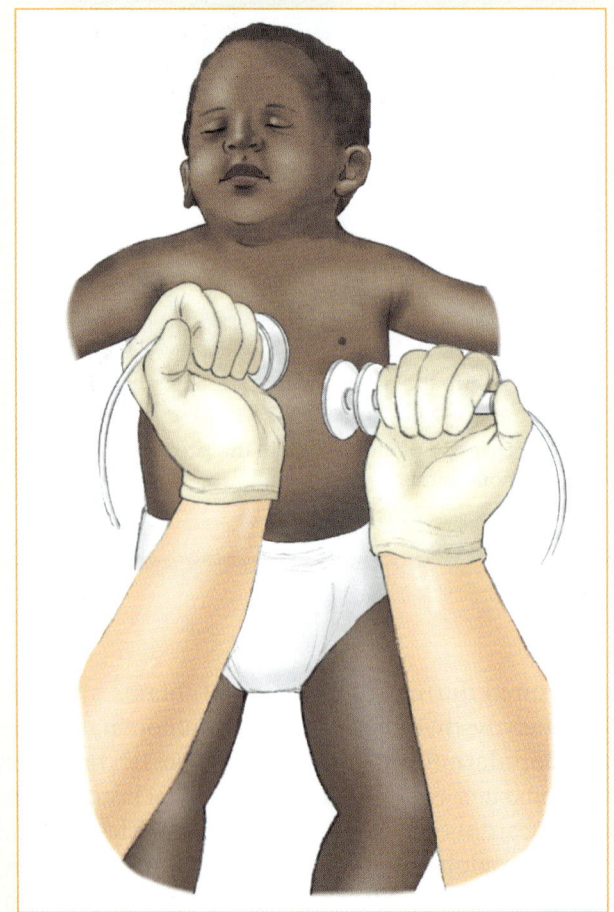

Figure 31-44 Site for paddles on the anterior chest wall.

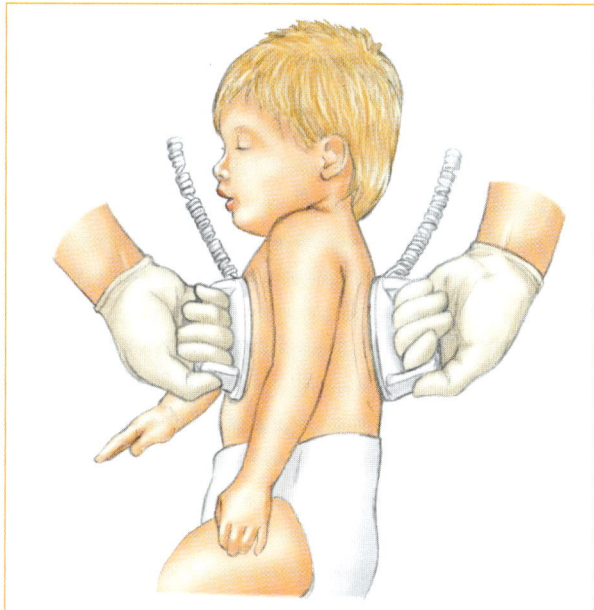

Figure 31-45 Site for paddles with child on side and paddles placed in anterior-posterior position.

8. Deliver the shock at the appropriate energy setting.
9. Resume immediate CPR.
10. Reassess the patient's cardiac rhythm and pulse every 2 minutes.
11. Insert an advanced airway, establish an IV line, and begin medication therapy if indicated; repeat defibrillation after every 2 minutes of CPR for refractory V-fib or pulseless V-tach.

The initial energy setting for defibrillation for pediatric patients is 2 joules (J) per kg. Further defibrillation should occur at 4 J/kg for subsequent shocks.

Many EMS systems use pregelled defibrillator pads instead of paddles. If your system uses defibrillator pads, place them in the same location as you would when using an AED. When applying the pads, ensure that there are no air pockets in the pad-skin interface; this may result in skin burns and decreased defibrillation effectiveness.

EMT-I Safety

Before performing defibrillation, visually **and** verbally ensure that nobody is in contact with the patient. Use the phrase "I'm clear, you're clear, we're all clear."

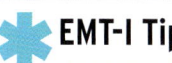 EMT-I Tips

Synchronized cardioversion is the timed delivery of energy into the myocardium to correct rapid, regular cardiac rhythms in patients who are in unstable condition as a result of the cardiac rhythm. An internal synchronizer times the shock to deliver when it senses an R wave. This avoids delivering the shock during the relative refractory period (down slope of the T wave), which may precipitate V-fib.

Synchronized cardioversion involves the same steps as defibrillation; however, before delivering the shock, you must push the "sync" button on the monitor/defibrillator. You will know that the defibrillator has synchronized with the cardiac rhythm when the tops of the R waves illuminate; on other defibrillator models, a blinking light appears above each R wave.

Unless an EMT-I is authorized by medical control, synchronized cardioversion must be performed by a paramedic. The indications, contraindications, and pediatric energy settings for synchronized cardioversion are as follows:

Indications
- Perfusing narrow QRS complex tachycardias with serious signs and symptoms linked to the tachycardia
  - Supraventricular tachycardia (SVT)
    - Heart rate greater than 180 beats/min in the child
    - Heart rate greater than 220 beats/min in the infant
- Perfusing wide QRS complex tachycardia with serious signs and symptoms linked to the tachycardia
  - V-tach

Contraindications
- V-fib or pulseless V-tach (requires defibrillation)
- Poison- or drug-induced tachycardia
  - Treat the underlying problem with an antidote, if available.
  - The serious signs and symptoms are related to the poison or drug, not the tachycardia.
- Other health care providers in physical contact with the patient
  - You must ensure that **no one** is in physical contact with the patient before you perform synchronized cardioversion.

Pediatric Energy Settings
- 0.5–1.0 J/kg
  - If unsuccessful, repeat at 2 J/kg as needed

Transport Considerations

The mode of transport (that is, code I versus code III) is dependent on the infant or child's clinical condition. Although you should follow local protocols and guidelines regarding the appropriate transport mode, unnecessary use of lights and siren may only increase the anxiety level of the child, parent, or caregiver. In addition, the use of lights and siren increases your risk of being involved in an accident; many drivers may not hear or see you until you are right behind them. Regardless of the transport mode, always drive with due regard for other drivers around you.

When managing a critically ill or injured child, you should never delay transport to perform procedures that can just as easily be performed en route to the hospital. Although you will possess new skills as an EMT-I, never forsake simple BLS interventions (that is, opening the airway) for the purpose of performing advanced life support interventions (such as intubation).

The appropriate transport destination is also dependent on the child's clinical condition. In general, critically ill or injured patients should be transported to the closest appropriate facility, usually a trauma center. However, when making your transport decision, consider the length of transport and the availability of specialized pediatric facilities. For example, it may be more beneficial to the patient to travel an additional 5 to 10 miles, bypassing hospitals of lesser capability, to a facility that specializes in pediatric trauma or medical emergencies. Early access to specialty care can improve the child's outcome. Exercise sound judgment, and always follow local protocols about transport issues.

Psychological Support and Communication Strategies

At the scene and during transport, you should continue to provide emotional support to the child and his or her family. Many times, using the parent or caregiver to assist in making the child more comfortable, especially during painful procedures (such as IV therapy), is beneficial to all (Figure 31-46 ▶). It facilitates your ability to assess and treat the child, it calms the child, and it helps to alleviate anxiety in the parent or caregiver.

Remember that infants, toddlers, preschoolers, and school-age patients do not favor separation from their parent or caregiver (separation anxiety); infants and children have a natural fear of strangers. Therefore, if the child's condition is stable, allow him or her to remain with the parent or caregiver. Also, before performing any procedure, provide time for the child to become

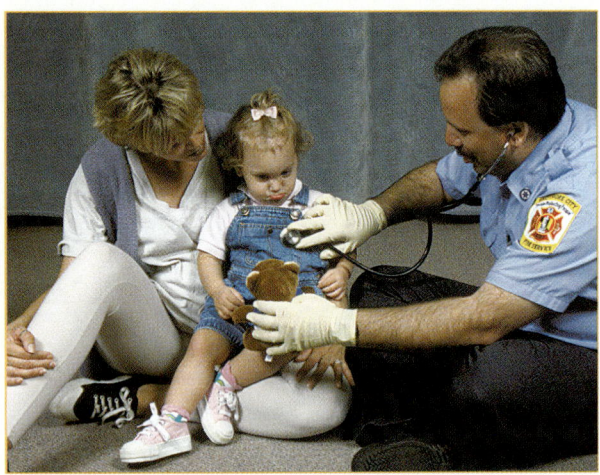

Figure 31-46 Use the parent or caregiver to assist you in calming the child.

familiar with the equipment that you will be using, such as letting the child listen to your own heartbeat with a stethoscope.

Children will become naturally fearful of you if you tower over them; therefore, when possible and practical, position yourself at the same level as the child; this will facilitate communication and minimize fear and anxiety. Allowing the child to hold onto a favorite toy or blanket may help further minimize fear.

When speaking to the child, use terminology that is appropriate for his or her age; use simple, nonmedical terms when communicating with the parent or caregiver as well. Information exchange will be more accurate and effective if the parent or caregiver understands what you are asking and saying.

Crying and fear are inherent responses of sick or injured children; therefore, you should allow them to express these feelings. However, you should let children know that certain physical actions, such as hitting, biting, and spitting, are not permitted.

Pediatric Medical Emergencies

As with adults, you will encounter a variety of pediatric medical emergencies as an EMT-I, some of which are unique to pediatric patients. Typically, these emergencies will be airway or respiratory-related; however, problems that affect other body organs or systems may be encountered as well. This section will discuss medical emergencies that are generally unique to the pediatric patient.

Respiratory Compromise

There are many causes of respiratory compromise in children. Although you might not be able to identify the exact cause, you must be able to recognize the signs and symptoms and provide appropriate treatment in order to prevent respiratory or cardiopulmonary arrest.

You will face some special challenges in caring for sick and injured children. Infants and children are not simply small adults. They come in a variety of sizes, and their anatomy and physiology differ from those of adults. Despite the differences between children and adults, like adults, providing adequate oxygenation and ventilation is the first step to achieving the best possible outcome for the patient, regardless of the underlying problem.

Respiratory compromise causes varying levels of pulmonary gas exchange impairment; it is categorized in three phases of severity: respiratory distress, respiratory failure, and respiratory arrest.

Phases of Respiratory Compromise

Respiratory distress represents the earliest phase of respiratory compromise and is most prominently noted by an increase in the child's work of breathing. In the early stages of respiratory distress, respirations are often too fast for the patient's age. If, like most people, you find it hard to memorize normal vital sign ranges for infants and children, keep reference charts handy for this purpose. Respirations of greater than 60 breaths/min are a sign of a problem. But remember, you are treating the child, not the numbers. A child breathing at a rate of 60 breaths/min who is playing happily does not need assisted ventilation; a child breathing at a rate of 60 breaths/min who is lying unresponsive on the floor does.

Initially, as the child with respiratory distress is compensating, arterial CO_2 tension in the blood decreases. However, as respiratory distress increases, and the child's condition deteriorates, arterial CO_2 tension begins to increase. Respiratory distress in children is characterized by the following clinical signs:

- Normal mental status (initially), progressing to irritability or anxiety
- Tachypnea
- Nasal flaring, as the body tries to increase the size of the airway
- Grunting respirations, as the body attempts to keep the alveoli expanded at the end of expiration
- Tachycardia
- Head bobbing
- Accessory (intercostal) muscle use; remember that in young children, the diaphragm is the major muscle of ventilation
- Retractions, or movements of the child's flexible rib cage
- The tripod position; in older children this position will maximize their ability to breathe
- Improvement of cyanosis (if present) with supplemental oxygen

If promptly treated, most children with respiratory distress will have a positive outcome; however, if treatment is delayed, the child will quickly deteriorate to respiratory failure.

Respiratory failure indicates that the body has used up its available energy stores and cannot continue to support the extra work of breathing. At this point, the child's respiratory efforts are ineffective to support adequate minute volume. Resultantly, respiratory acidosis develops secondary to excessive CO_2 retention. Respiratory failure in children is characterized by the following clinical signs:

- Decreased level of consciousness
- Marked tachypnea followed by bradypnea
- Marked retractions followed by agonal breathing
- Poor muscle tone
- Marked tachycardia followed by bradycardia
  - Bradycardia is defined as a heart rate less than 80 beats/min in the child; less than 100 beats/min in the infant
  - Bradycardia in children is almost always related to a lack of oxygen and is an ominous sign
- Central cyanosis

If any of the above signs are noted during your assessment of the child with a respiratory problem, you must act immediately. Failure to aggressively manage the child with respiratory failure will quickly result in respiratory arrest, followed by cardiopulmonary arrest.

Respiratory arrest, the last phase of respiratory compromise before cardiopulmonary arrest, must be treated aggressively in order to prevent death. Respiratory arrest in children is characterized by the following clinical signs:

- Unresponsive
- Bradypnea followed by apnea
- Absent chest wall motion
- Limp muscle tone
- Bradycardia followed by asystole
- Profound cyanosis

Emergency Medical Care

Emergency medical care for the infant or child with respiratory compromise depends on the severity of his or her condition. In all cases, you must ensure a patent airway and adequate breathing.

When assessing airway patency, you must determine if the airway can be maintained by simple positioning, or if airway adjuncts (ie, oral or nasal airway) or advanced airway management are required.

An infant or child in respiratory distress or early respiratory failure needs supplemental oxygen. Remember, anxiety, agitation, or crying may increase the effort or work of breathing, so use whichever method that seems least upsetting to the child: nonrebreathing mask or blow-by oxygen (Figure 31-47 ▼). You may need to get creative by distracting the child with games, a toy, or talking.

If the child has progressed to respiratory failure or respiratory arrest, it will be necessary to separate him or her from the parent or caregiver. Begin assisted ventilation with 100% oxygen immediately, using the BVM device that is appropriate for the child's age. If the child is unresponsive, use cricoid pressure to minimize the incidence of gastric distention and to decrease the risk of vomiting with aspiration.

If BVM ventilations do not improve the child's condition, it will be necessary to perform endotracheal intubation. Consider inserting a nasogastric or orogastric tube if gastric distention is impairing your ability to effectively ventilate the child.

Obtain vascular access in the event that pharmacological interventions are necessary. However, because these procedures can be time-consuming, consider performing them en route to the hospital. Transport mode is dictated by the child's condition, as is the destination facility. It is important to be aware of facilities in your area that are equipped to care for critically ill infants and children.

During transport, it is important to provide emotional support to the parent or caregiver by keeping them apprised of the situation.

Perform frequent ongoing assessments of the child during transport. Signs of clinical improvement include improvement of skin color and condition, increasing oxygen saturation, increasing heart rate, and improvement in mental status.

Upper Airway Diseases

Assessment and management of the infant and child with a foreign body upper airway obstruction was discussed earlier in this chapter. Therefore, this section will focus on the assessment and management of respiratory emergencies involving the upper and lower airway that result from infectious processes and inflammation.

Croup

Croup, also known as *laryngotracheobronchitis*, is a viral infection of the upper airway that most commonly affects children between 6 months and 4 years of age; it rarely occurs in older children.

Croup involves an inflammatory process of the upper respiratory tract involving the subglottic (below the vocal cords) region. Most children with croup do well with treatment; however, if left untreated, the infection can lead to airway obstruction secondary to inflammation and progressive narrowing of the airway (Figure 31-48 ▶). Spasmodic croup, another form of croup, is not the result of an infection, and occurs most commonly in the middle of the night; there is usually no previous history of an upper respiratory infection (URI).

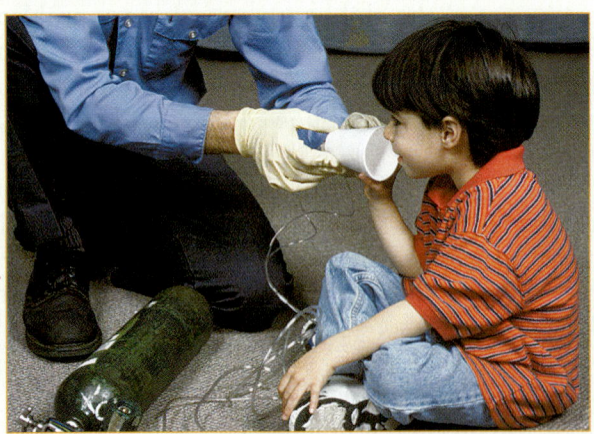

Figure 31-47 A child in respiratory distress needs supplemental oxygen; you should select whichever method that seems least upsetting to the child.

> **In the Field**
>
> **DO NOT** do anything to agitate a child with suspected croup or epiglottitis. Doing so could create a laryngospasm and closure of the airway.

Assessment Findings

The signs and symptoms of croup usually appear following a recent (within the past 1 to 2 days) cold or other upper respiratory infection. Typically, the child appears relatively well during the day; however, at night, a harsh or brassy cough develops—often likened to a barking seal or dog. Mild to moderate croup may spontaneously resolve within a few hours; however, it can recur for two or three consecutive nights.

A child with severe croup appears sick. He or she begins to experience inspiratory stridor—a sign of progressive upper airway narrowing. Fever, if present, is typically low-grade, ranging from 100°F and 101°F. Additionally, the following signs and symptoms may be observed during your assessment:

- Increased work of breathing
  - Intercostal and supraclavicular retractions
  - Tracheal tugging
  - Nasal flaring
- Signs of hypoxia
  - Tachycardia
  - Restlessness or anxiety
  - Decreased oxygen saturation
  - Cyanosis (a late sign)

Emergency Medical Care

Emergency care for a child with suspected croup begins by ensuring a patent airway and adequate oxygenation and ventilation. The administration of humidified or nebulized oxygen via mist at 4 to 6 L/min often provides symptomatic relief. Oxygen can be delivered via nonrebreathing mask or the blow-by technique.

Avoid agitating the child and allow him or her to remain with the parent or caregiver when possible. IV therapy is usually not needed for the child with croup and should therefore be avoided. Additionally, simple measures such as taking a blood pressure may also cause agitation. Most children with croup respond well to treatment. Rarely does the disease progress to respiratory failure.

Depending on local protocol, you may administer beta-2 agonists (ie, albuterol) or steroidal anti-inflammatory medications (ie, Solu-Medrol), to treat severe croup. Contact medical control as needed regarding the pharmacological management of croup.

Epiglottitis

Epiglottitis, also known as *acute supraglottic laryngitis*, is an acute bacterial infection that results in rapidly forming cellulitis (tissue swelling) of the epiglottis and its surrounding structures Figure 31-49 . The epiglottis becomes cherry red and swollen.

Although epiglottitis can occur at any age, it typically affects children between 3 and 7 years of age. Epiglottitis is most commonly caused by the *Haemophilus influenzae* type B bacteria. Unlike croup, which is usually self-limiting and rarely life-threatening, epiglottitis can cause a true life-threatening emergency secondary to complete upper airway obstruction.

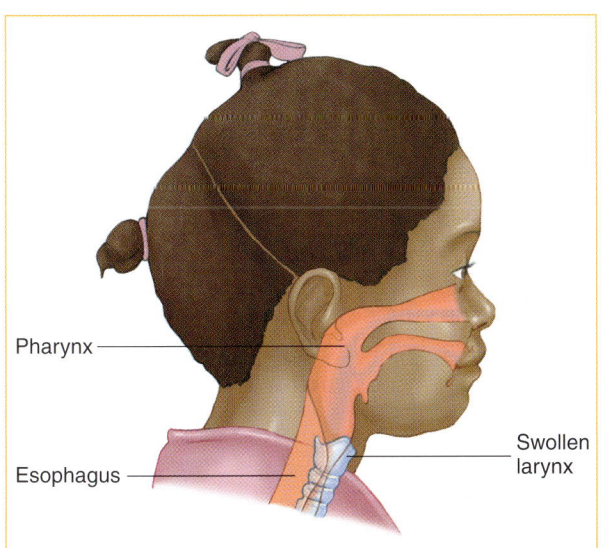

Figure 31-48 Croup can result in progressive narrowing of the upper airway secondary to inflammation, resulting in an upper airway obstruction.

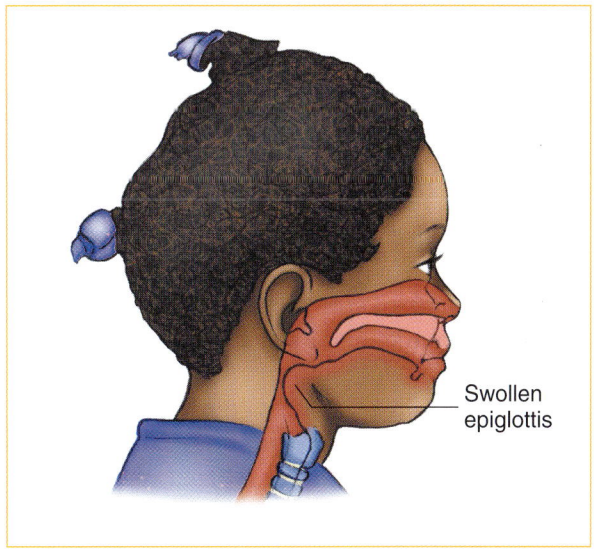

Figure 31-49 Epiglottitis is an acute bacterial infection that can cause airway obstruction in children.

Fortunately, the incidence of epiglottitis has decreased over past years and is now an uncommon occurrence in children. This is the result of the *Haemophilus* flu vaccine, which children are now receiving as a part of their regular childhood immunizations.

Assessment Findings

Initially, the clinical presentation of epiglottitis is similar to that of croup; the child often appears to have a mild upper respiratory infection. As with croup, the child later awakens in the middle of the night; however, he or she typically presents with a high fever (as high as 104°F), a brassy cough, and respiratory distress of varying severity.

Epiglottitis, unlike croup, progresses rapidly and results in narrowing of the upper airway. In addition to increased work of breathing (ie, retractions, accessory muscle use) and varying degrees of hypoxia, epiglottitis is characterized by the following clinical signs:

- Stridor
- Muffled voice
- Drooling
  - The result of the child not being able to swallow his or her saliva
- Difficulty swallowing (dysphagia)
- Sore throat
- Sitting fully upright

Children with epiglottitis usually have no history of the disease. However, the signs and symptoms, when they progress, typically occur over a short span of time (6 to 8 hours). Epiglottitis can rapidly progress to respiratory failure and arrest.

Emergency Medical Care

Begin management of a child with epiglottitis by ensuring a patent airway and adequate ventilation. Administer supplemental oxygen, preferably humidified, via nonrebreathing mask or the blow-by technique. Be sure to use the technique that is least intimidating to the child, and allow the parent or caregiver to assist, if possible.

If the airway becomes completely obstructed, two-rescuer BVM ventilations are usually effective in achieving adequate tidal volume.

Unless the upper airway is completely obstructed, endotracheal intubation is contraindicated. Inserting a laryngoscope into the child's mouth may result in laryngospasm and rapid obstruction of the airway. Intubation is also contraindicated if your transport time to the hospital is short.

If the child's condition necessitates intubation, use a stylet and an ET tube that is 1 or 2 times smaller than you would normally use. This will facilitate placement of the tube through the narrowed glottic opening. Performing chest compressions during visualization of the airway may facilitate location of the vocal cords, as bubbles may be seen at the glottic opening as the chest is compressed.

Rapidly transport the child with epiglottitis to the closest appropriate facility. Notify the receiving hospital early regarding the child's status. Avoid any activities that will increase the child's fear and anxiety. Unless your transport time is lengthy and the child is in need of medication therapy, IVs should not be attempted. Additionally, avoid other potentially agitating procedures, such as taking a blood pressure. Allow the child to assume a position of comfort; if appropriate, allow the child to remain with the parent or caregiver.

Unless it is necessary to perform advanced airway management, *never visualize the airway or place anything into the mouth of a conscious child with epiglottitis*. Doing so may cause laryngospasm and complete obstruction of the airway.

> **EMT-I Tips**
>
> **Never** examine the oropharynx in a conscious child with respiratory distress. If epiglottitis is present, doing so may result in severe laryngospasm and complete upper airway obstruction. Remember, croup is a viral infection with a slow onset and epiglottitis is a bacterial infection with a rapid onset.

Lower Airway Diseases

A lower airway disease affects the bronchioles or the lungs themselves. In contrast to upper airway diseases, which commonly present with stridor, diseases of the lower airway often present with wheezing, rales, or rhonchi, in addition to increased work of breathing and hypoxia of varying severity. Lower airway diseases include asthma, bronchiolitis, pneumonia, and foreign body lower airway obstruction.

Asthma

Asthma is an acute spasm and inflammation of the bronchioles in the lungs (bronchospasm) and is associated with excessive mucus production Figure 31-50 ▶). In approximately 50% of cases, asthma occurs before the age of 10 years; it rarely occurs in infants younger than

1 year. Because of the hyperreactive airways, asthma is commonly referred to as a reactive airway disease (RAD).

Asthma is typically encountered in children with a preexisting history of the disease. In between attacks, the child is usually asymptomatic. However, an acute attack can be caused by various triggers, including upper respiratory infections, allergies, changes in environmental temperature, physical exertion, and emotional stress.

An acute asthma attack occurs when the hyperreactive bronchioles become narrowed, causing a reduction of expiratory airflow through them. The initial response during an acute asthma attack is the result of the immune system's response to the trigger, which releases chemicals called histamines. As the attack progresses, mucous membrane swelling of the bronchiolar walls swell and mucus plugging of the bronchiolar lumen further restricts expiratory airflow. Pulmonary gas exchange is impaired, and the child becomes hypoxemic.

Assessment Findings

The signs and symptoms of an acute asthma attack vary, depending on the severity of the attack. During your assessment, you should determine if the child has been prescribed a metered-dose inhaler (MDI) containing a beta$_2$ agonist (ie, Albuterol) or other medication. If so, determine how many puffs, if any, he or she took prior to your arrival.

You will typically find the child sitting up, in a preferential position, and in obvious respiratory distress. When you are evaluating breathing, you will often note a prolonged expiratory phase, indicating the child's difficulty in expelling air from his or her lungs.

Wheezing is commonly heard during auscultation of the chest, usually during expiration. During a more severe asthma attack, however, wheezing may become so loud that it is audible without a stethoscope. Other signs include tachycardia, tachypnea, and agitation.

Ask the child (if old enough) or parent/caregiver if the child has ever been intubated or admitted to the ICU for his or her asthma. If the answer to either of these questions is yes, you must prepare to aggressively treat the child, if necessary.

Emergency Medical Care

As with any respiratory emergency, you must first ensure airway patency and breathing adequacy. Then, direct your treatment toward the following goals:

- Improvement of ventilation
- Correction of hypoxia
- Relief of bronchospasm and inflammation

Administer oxygen by the method most tolerated by the child: a nonrebreathing mask or the blow-by technique. Depending on how many, if any, puffs the child has taken from his or her MDI prior to your arrival, you may assist him or her with the medication as directed by medical control.

Other than oxygen, the primary pharmacologic agent used for an acute asthma attack is a beta-$_2$ agonist. Albuterol (Ventolin, Proventil) seems to be the most commonly administered bronchodilator. Other medications, however, such as metaproterenol (Alupent), or isoetharine (Bronkosol), may be administered depending on local protocols. Albuterol (or other beta-$_2$ agonists) are administered through a nebulizer. To facilitate the child's breathing of the medication through the mouthpiece of the nebulizer, tape two tongue blades together to make a nose clip Figure 31-51.

The pediatric dose of Albuterol depends on the child's weight, and may need to be repeated based on the child's clinical response. Correct dosing is as follows:

- **Less than 15 kg:** Albuterol (5 mg/mL) at 2.5 to 5.0 mg (0.5 to 1.0 mL), diluted in 3 mL of normal saline.
- **Greater than 15 kg:** Albuterol (5 mg/mL) at 5 to 10 mg (1 to 2 mL), diluted in 3 mL of normal saline.

Depending on your transport time, medical control may also order the administration of corticosteroids (ie, Solu-Medrol) to help reduce bronchiole inflammation.

Children experiencing a prolonged asthma attack tend to tire quickly. If the child is showing signs of respiratory

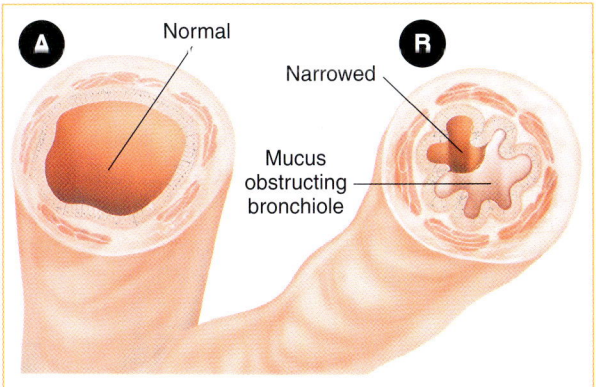

Figure 31-50 Asthma is an acute spasm of the bronchioles. **A.** Cross-section of a normal bronchiole. **B.** The bronchiole in spasm; a mucus plug has formed and partially obstructed the bronchiole.

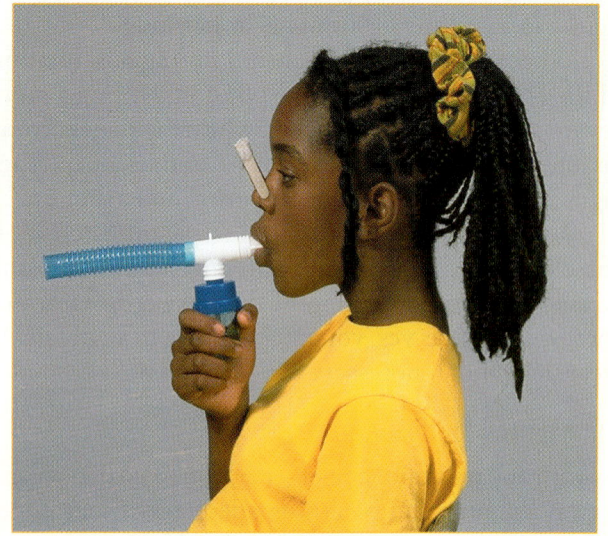

Figure 31-51 A nose clip can help the child breathe through the mouthpiece of the nebulizer.

failure (ie, shallow breathing, progressive lethargy, poor muscle tone), begin assisted ventilations with a BVM device and 100% oxygen. If needed, bronchodilator therapy can be administered during positive pressure ventilations with a small volume in-line nebulizer.

Endotracheal intubation may be necessary if prolonged ventilatory support is needed or if BVM ventilations are ineffective. Additionally, any critically ill child should be placed on a cardiac monitor.

Additional treatment consists of monitoring the child's oxygen saturation and transporting promptly to the hospital. If the child's condition will allow, do not separate him or her from the parent or caregiver.

Status asthmaticus, a severe and prolonged asthma attack, is characterized by a "quiet chest," indicating profound bronchospasm and minimal air movement. Status asthmaticus is usually unresponsive to conventional asthma therapy and is a dire emergency. Although the treatment for status asthmaticus is essentially the same as it is for a mild or moderate asthma attack, it is more aggressive and must be performed en route to the hospital. Many children with status asthmaticus will experience respiratory failure secondary to severe hypoxia, acidosis, and physical exhaustion, and will require assisted ventilations, or, if necessary, advanced airway management.

Medical control or local protocol may dictate the administration of epinephrine 1:1000 subcutaneously in children with severe respiratory distress or failure resulting from a reactive airway disease. Follow local protocols regarding the appropriate pediatric dosage.

Bronchiolitis

Bronchiolitis, another form of reactive airway disease, is a viral infection that results in inflammation and constriction of the bronchioles. It most commonly occurs during the winter months in children younger than 2 years. Although there are a number of viruses that can cause bronchiolitis, respiratory syncytial virus (RSV) appears to be the most common. Most children, once being exposed to RSV, will develop lifelong immunity; however, this is usually not the case in infants, who have inherently immature immune systems.

Assessment Findings

Bronchiolitis can be difficult to distinguish from asthma; both disease processes present with respiratory distress and expiratory wheezing. However, the following historical and assessment findings generally support a field impression of bronchiolitis:

- Children with bronchiolitis tend to have a family history of asthma
- Because bronchiolitis is caused by a viral infection, a low-grade fever is usually present; fever is usually not associated with asthma
- Asthma rarely occurs in infants younger than 1 year; whereas bronchiolitis is common in this age group

Emergency Medical Care

Emergency care for an infant or child with bronchiolitis is the same as it is for asthma. Administer supplemental oxygen, preferably humidified, as tolerated by the child. As with asthma, infants and small children often tire quickly following prolonged periods of respiratory distress; therefore, you must be prepared to assist ventilations as needed.

In addition, continuous monitoring of the child's oxygen saturation is essential. Transport the child to the hospital for evaluation. If his or her condition permits, do not separate the child from the parent or caregiver.

Consider administering a beta$_2$ agonist (ie, albuterol), in the same dose for asthma, via nebulizer if the child presents with respiratory distress. If BVM ventilations are required but ineffective, or if the child requires prolonged ventilatory support, perform endotracheal intubation. Continuously monitor the child's cardiac rhythm.

Pneumonia

Pneumonia is a common disease process that infects the lower airway and the lung. Although it can occur at any age, in pediatric patients it is most commonly seen in infants, toddlers, and preschoolers (ages 1 to 5 years).

Pneumonia can be caused by a virus or bacteria; less commonly is it the result of a fungus. In children, pneumonia is usually caused by a virus. As children get older, however, the incidence of bacterial pneumonia increases.

Assessment Findings

The signs and symptoms of pneumonia depend on the severity of the disease. Varying levels of respiratory distress are commonly observed and the child often appears anxious. In addition, the following clinical signs are often seen with pneumonia:

- Unilaterally diminished breath sounds
- Rales
- Rhonchi (localized or diffuse)
- Chest pain
- Fever

Children with pneumonia typically have a recent history of a cough or cold, or a lower airway infection (ie, bronchitis).

Emergency Medical Care

Emergency care for the child with pneumonia begins by ensuring a patent airway and adequate breathing. Administer supplemental oxygen therapy using the most tolerated method (ie, nonrebreathing mask, blow-by), and transport the patient to the hospital. Allow the child to assume a position of comfort. Allow the parent or caregiver to remain with the child, unless the child's condition will not allow it.

Vascular access is generally not indicated for children with pneumonia; however, if the child's condition warrants medication therapy, establish IV or IO access en route to the hospital.

Assist ventilations with a BVM device and 100% oxygen if the child shows signs of respiratory failure (ie, shallow respirations, progressive lethargy, poor muscle tone). Continuously monitor the child's oxygen saturation.

If BVM ventilations are ineffective or if prolonged ventilatory support will be required, perform endotracheal intubation. Apply a cardiac monitor and assess the child's cardiac rhythm.

Foreign Body Lower Airway Obstruction

Occasionally, a child will aspirate a small object, such as a nut, seed, or small toy, into the lower airway. Depending on the size and position of the object, it may partially or completely obstruct airflow into the affected lung. Because the child still has one functional lung, rapid progression to respiratory failure or arrest is rare. If respiratory failure or arrest does occur, it is usually the result of prolonged respiratory distress and physical exhaustion.

Assessment Findings

The infant or child with a foreign body lower airway obstruction appears anxious. If the object is large, he or she will present with respiratory distress. Because the object is irritating to the tissues of lower airway, a severe cough is common. Other clinical findings include the following:

- Unilaterally diminished breath sounds
- Unilateral rales or rhonchi
- Chest pain

The parent or caregiver typically reports seeing the infant or child placing something into his or her mouth before the symptoms began.

Emergency Medical Care

Emergency care for the infant or child with a foreign body lower airway obstruction begins by ensuring airway patency and adequate ventilation. Administer supplemental oxygen by the method most tolerated by the child (ie, nonrebreathing mask, blow-by).

Avoid agitating the child because this may cause a partial foreign body lower airway obstruction to become a complete obstruction. Allow the child to assume a position of comfort and avoid separation of him or her from the parent or caregiver, if possible.

Vascular access is generally not necessary unless the child's condition becomes critical and he or she needs medication therapy. Definitive therapy involves visualizing and removing the foreign body with a bronchoscope. This procedure must be performed at the hospital.

Shock

Shock (hypoperfusion) is an abnormal condition characterized by inadequate delivery of oxygen and nutrients to the tissues and inadequate removal of metabolic substrates from the body. Shock is the second most common cause of cardiopulmonary arrest in the pediatric age group; respiratory failure is the most common. As with the adult, however, early recognition and prompt intervention can prevent permanent disability or death.

Compared to adults, children can compensate for shock for longer periods of time, maintaining adequate perfusion due to vasoconstriction. Unfortunately, however, when hypotension occurs, it does so quickly and unpredictably, and may result in rapid deterioration to cardiopulmonary arrest.

Common causes of shock in the pediatric population include hypovolemia (from trauma or illness) and sepsis. Although less common, allergic reactions and poisonings can result in shock. Shock from a primary cardiac event is rare in infants and children.

Classifications of Shock

In children as well as adults, shock is classified as being compensated (early) or decompensated (late or irreversible). The signs and symptoms vary, depending on the degree of shock the child is in. Although infants and children have little ability to increase myocardial contractility to meet increased metabolic demands, they do compensate vigorously by increasing heart rate and peripheral vascular resistance. All children in shock should receive 100% supplemental oxygen or assisted ventilation as needed, thermal management, and rapid transport to an appropriate facility. Unless it is absolutely critical, time-consuming procedures (ie, IV, IO access) should be performed en route. Treatment for the specific types of shock will be addressed later in this section.

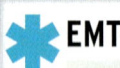

EMT-I Tips

Carefully assess any infant or child with suspected shock. At first, the signs and symptoms may be subtle and hard to detect. A thorough assessment and history and a keen eye will enable you to recognize shock in its earliest stages.

Compensated Shock

Compensated (early) shock occurs when the body is actively compensating through the mechanisms previously described (tachycardia, vasoconstriction). During this early stage of shock, the child's blood pressure remains normal; however, because of vasoconstriction, signs of decreased peripheral perfusion are present. Compensated shock in infants and children is characterized by the following clinical signs:
- Irritability or anxiety
- Tachycardia
- Tachypnea
- Weak peripheral pulses, strong central pulses
- Delayed capillary refill (>2 seconds)
  - Most reliable in children less than 6 years of age
  - May be affected by cold temperatures
- Cool, pale extremities
- Normal systolic blood pressure
- Decreased urinary output

Provided that the early signs and symptoms of shock are promptly recognized and treatment and transport are initiated early, most children with compensated shock will have a positive outcome.

Decompensated Shock

Decompensated (late) shock occurs when the body is no longer able to effectively compensate for decreased perfusion. It is typically characterized by a drop in blood pressure, which signifies failure of the body's compensatory mechanisms.

Decompensated shock in infants and children is characterized by the following clinical signs:
- Lethargy or coma
- Marked tachycardia or bradycardia
- Marked tachypnea or bradypnea
  - Bradycardia and bradypnea in an infant or child with shock are ominous signs and indicate impending cardiopulmonary arrest.
- Markedly delayed capillary refill
- Cool, pale, dusky, mottled extremities
- Markedly decreased urinary output
- Hypotension

With aggressive treatment, decompensated shock *may* be reversible. Unfortunately, because of the prolonged insult to the cardiovascular system, vital organs such as the brain, heart, and kidneys are often permanently damaged; therefore, the child usually dies of multiple organ failure.

General Shock Management

Upon recognition of the signs of shock, begin immediate and aggressive management and rapid transport to an appropriate facility. Time-consuming interventions (ie, IV or IO access) should be attempted en route. General shock management, which focuses on maintaining a patent airway, administering oxygen, and providing warmth, is listed in (Skill Drill 31-10 ▶).

1. **Ensure that the airway is open.** Provide spinal immobilization if indicated.
2. **Assess breathing adequacy.** Be prepared to assist ventilations if necessary.
3. **Control bleeding** if present (**Step 1**).
4. **Administer 100% supplemental oxygen** via nonrebreathing mask. Continue to monitor airway and breathing (**Step 2**).

General Shock Management

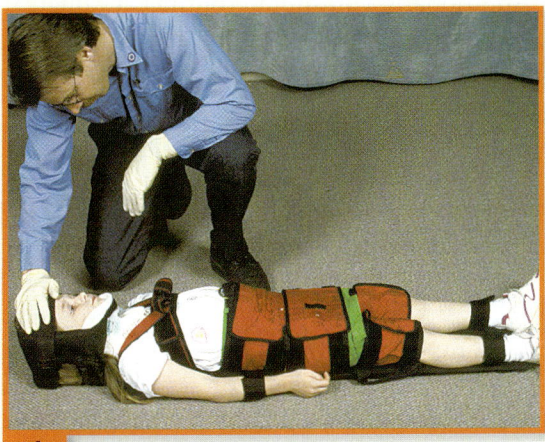

1 Open the airway.
Provide spinal immobilization if indicated.
Assess breathing and be prepared to ventilate.
Control any bleeding.

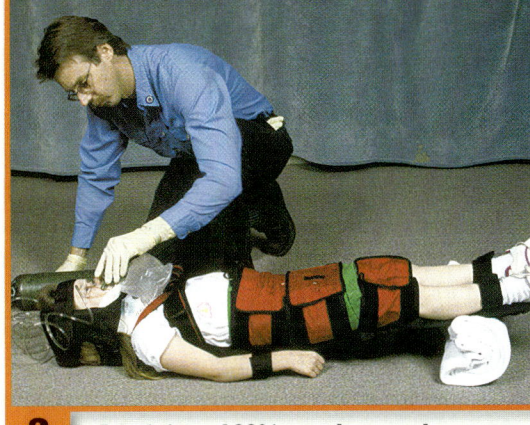

2 Administer 100% supplemental oxygen.

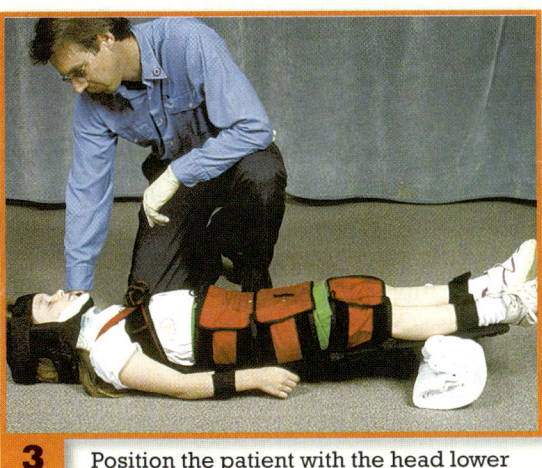

3 Position the patient with the head lower than the feet.

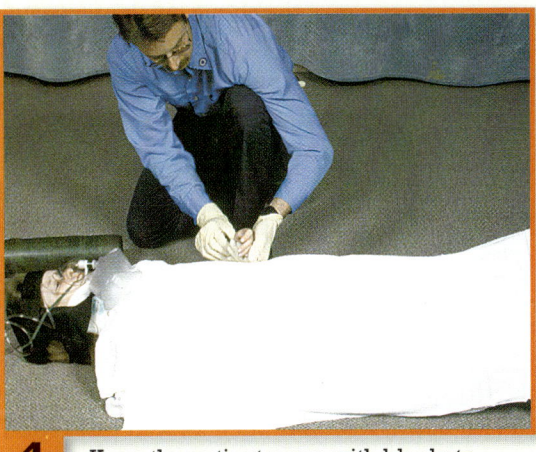

4 Keep the patient warm with blankets.
Transport immediately.
Gain IV access and give a 20-mL/kg bolus of an isotonic crystalloid solution.
Continue to monitor vital signs.
Allow a caregiver to accompany the child if possible.

5. **Position the patient** with the head lower than the feet by elevating the legs with blankets (**Step 3**).
6. **Keep the patient warm** with blankets and by turning up the heat in the patient compartment.
7. **Provide immediate transport** to the closest appropriate facility.
8. **Initiate an IV** of an isotonic crystalloid solution and give a **20-mL/kg bolus** to maintain radial (or brachial in the infant) pulses.
9. **Continue monitoring vital signs** en route to the hospital.
10. **Allow a caregiver** to accompany the child whenever possible (**Step 4**).

Place any child in shock on a cardiac monitor and be alert for cardiac dysrhythmias. If the child becomes unresponsive, perform endotracheal intubation to definitively secure the airway.

Etiologies of Shock

Regardless of the etiology of shock, the end result is the same—inadequate tissue perfusion. However, to most appropriately treat the infant or child with shock, you must understand its underlying cause.

As we progress into the section on assessment and management of the different etiologies of shock, bear in mind that the following four mechanisms must remain intact at all times in order for adequate perfusion to continue:

1. A functional heart
2. A functional respiratory system
3. Intact vasculature
4. Adequate volume

Failure of *one or more* of the above mechanisms will result in shock. For example, if the heart fails to perform adequately, cardiogenic shock develops; respiratory shock develops if the respiratory system fails; neurogenic shock develops if the vasculature dilates; and hypovolemic shock develops if too much blood or water is lost from the body.

Hypovolemic Shock

Hypovolemic shock, the most common type of shock encountered in infants and children, is the result of decreased circulating volume, such as water or blood. In infants and children, hypovolemic shock is often the result of dehydration or blood loss (internal or external). Dehydration in children is usually the result of viral gastroenteritis, which causes excessive vomiting and diarrhea. Excessive perspiration or respiratory excursion can also cause significant dehydration. Hypovolemia from blood loss may be the result of blunt or penetrating trauma, as seen with falls, motor vehicle crashes, and child abuse.

Assessment Findings

The signs and symptoms of hypovolemic shock depend on whether the child is compensating or decompensating. Early signs of shock include irritability and anxiety, tachypnea, tachycardia, delayed capillary refill time, and a normal systolic blood pressure, among others. Late signs of shock include lethargy, absent peripheral pulses, and hypotension.

Additionally, you should routinely evaluate infants and children with suspected hypovolemia for signs of dehydration, including the following:

- Poor skin turgor
- Decreased saliva
- Absence of tears when crying
- Sunken fontanelle (in infants)
- Dry mucosa (ie, eyes, mouth)

Emergency Medical Care

Treat infants and children in hypovolemic shock with 100% supplemental oxygen or assisted ventilation as needed. If trauma is suspected or cannot be ruled out, immobilize the spine.

Establish vascular access and administer normal saline or lactated Ringer's fluid boluses of 20 mL/kg as needed to maintain adequate perfusion. After each fluid bolus, reassess the child; several fluid boluses are often needed in children with severe hypovolemia.

Transport the child to the closest appropriate facility. If trauma is the cause of the hypovolemia, the closest trauma center should be your destination. Unless he or she is immobilized, allow the child to assume a comfortable position. Provide emotional support as needed to the child and parent or caregiver.

If the child becomes unresponsive, or if BVM ventilations (if needed) are ineffective, perform endotracheal intubation.

Distributive Shock

Distributive shock, a relatively uncommon cause of shock in children, occurs when vascular tone is decreased, resulting in massive vasodilation and systemic venous pooling of blood. Because there is no actual loss of blood, patients with distributive shock are said to be experiencing relative hypovolemia. In other words, relative to the larger vascular container, the normal blood volume is inadequate to meet the metabolic needs of the body. Distributive shock can be caused by the following conditions:

- Sepsis (infection)
- Spinal cord injury
- Anaphylaxis

Septic shock occurs when an invading organism, usually a bacterium, attacks the blood vessels, preventing them from constricting. Resultantly, the blood vessels dilate, blood pressure falls, and tissue perfusion decreases. Although a number of infections can result in septic shock (ie, ear infections, pneumonia), meningitis (inflammation of the meninges covering the brain and spinal cord) is commonly associated with septic shock in children.

Compared to adults, infants and children are especially prone to sepsis because of their immature immune systems. The signs and symptoms of sepsis, which vary depending on the severity of the infection, include poor feeding, irritability, fever, and vomiting and diarrhea.

If the infection is not treated promptly with antibiotics, septic shock may occur and result in death. The signs of septic shock include those of sepsis with additional signs such as an altered mental status, tachycardia and tachypnea, delayed capillary refill, and eventual hypotension.

Emergency medical care for septic shock includes ensuring airway patency and adequate breathing, administering 100% supplemental oxygen or assisted ventilation if the child is in respiratory failure, vascular access, and 20-mL/kg boluses of an isotonic crystalloid solution to maintain perfusion. Immediate transport to an appropriate facility is essential.

Consider a vasopressor, such as dopamine, if IV fluids fail to increase tissue perfusion.

Neurogenic shock occurs when sympathetic nervous system control over the cardiovascular system is lost. Recall that the sympathetic nervous system, through the release of epinephrine and norepinephrine, is responsible for constriction of the blood vessels, increased myocardial contractility, and increased heart rate. When communication between the sympathetic nervous system and the heart and blood vessels is blocked (ie, spinal cord injury), epinephrine and norepinephrine can no longer exert their normal effects.

Unlike other types of shock (ie, hypovolemia), neurogenic shock presents with a different clinical picture. Instead of the usual tachycardia, the patient presents with bradycardia—a result of unopposed parasympathetic nervous system stimulation. Because the effects of epinephrine and norepinephrine on the vasculature are lost, the patient presents with dry skin (warm or cool) instead of the classic moist or clammy skin. Blood pressure falls as a result of widespread vasodilation (relative hypovolemia).

Emergency medical care for neurogenic shock includes ensuring airway patency and adequate breathing, administering 100% supplemental oxygen or assisted ventilation if the child is in respiratory failure, vascular access, and 20-mL/kg boluses of an isotonic crystalloid solution to maintain perfusion. Because spinal cord injury is the common cause of neurogenic shock (hence the term, "spinal shock"), full spinal immobilization is critical. Provide prompt transport to the closest appropriate facility.

Consider a vasopressor, such as dopamine, if IV fluids fail to increase tissue perfusion.

Anaphylactic shock is caused by an exaggerated immune response resulting from exposure to an allergen to which the patient was previously sensitized. This exaggerated immune response causes the release of histamines, among other chemicals, that cause constriction of the bronchioles, dilation of the blood vessels, and leakage of fluid into the interstitial space. As a result, the patient experiences respiratory compromise, relative hypovolemia (from vasodilation), and angioedema (caused when fluid enters the interstitial space). In addition to signs of shock, the patient with anaphylaxis usually presents with the following:

- Rash or hives (urticaria)
- Facial and airway swelling (the result of angioedema)

There is a difference between an allergic reaction and anaphylaxis. An allergic reaction does not result in hemodynamic compromise; anaphylaxis does. The treatment, therefore, will depend on the severity of the patient's condition. If anaphylactic shock is not treated immediately, death will result from respiratory failure and decreased tissue perfusion.

Any patient with an allergic reaction should receive 100% oxygen; be prepared to assist ventilations if necessary. If the child has a history of severe allergic reactions, he or she may have a prescribed epinephrine autoinjector (EpiPen junior), which contains 0.15 mg of epinephrine, or an AnaKit, which contains a prefilled syringe of epinephrine and an antihistamine (ie, Chlo-Amine, Benadryl). If the child is demonstrating signs of an allergic reaction, obtain authorization from medical control and assist the child with, or administer, the epinephrine. The steps for administering epinephrine via autoinjector and prefilled syringe were discussed in Chapter 22.

For an allergic reaction without signs of shock, administer epinephrine 1:1,000 subcutaneously, followed by diphenhydramine (Benadryl) via IM injection. If anaphylactic shock is present, obtain IV or IO access and administer epinephrine 1:10,000, followed by diphenhydramine (both via the IV or IO route). Be prepared to perform endotracheal intubation if signs of airway swelling and severe respiratory compromise are present.

Cardiogenic Shock

Cardiogenic shock is caused by failure of the heart (pump failure) to meet the metabolic needs of the body. Unless a congenital heart defect is present, children, unlike adults, rarely experience cardiogenic shock secondary to primary cardiac damage (ie, myocardial infarction). Instead, cardiogenic shock in children is usually the result of secondary cardiac damage (ie, toxic ingestion, near-drowning, etc).

The signs and symptoms of cardiogenic shock vary depending on whether the child is compensating or decompensating. Additionally, the following clinical signs, which indicate backing up of blood into the lungs and systemic circulation, are often observed:

- Rales
- Jugular venous distention
- Enlarged liver (hepatomegaly)
- Peripheral edema

Emergency medical care for the infant or child with cardiogenic shock begins by ensuring airway patency and adequate breathing. Administer 100% supplemental oxygen and be prepared to assist ventilations if needed. Establish vascular access and administer 20 mL/kg of normal saline or lactated Ringer's solution as needed to maintain adequate perfusion. Transport the child to the closest appropriate facility, allowing him or her to maintain a position of comfort.

Attach a cardiac monitor. If a tachydysrhythmia is the suspected cause of cardiogenic shock, consider the administration of 0.1 mg/kg of adenosine via rapid IV or IO push. Be prepared to perform endotracheal intubation if the child cannot protect his or her own airway.

Cardiac Dysrhythmias

Cardiac dysrhythmias such as ventricular fibrillation, ventricular tachycardia, and supraventricular tachycardia, are uncommon in infants and children. Most dysrhythmias—when they occur in children—are slow and indicate inadequate oxygenation. Nonetheless, you may be called to treat an infant or child with a variety of dysrhythmias, some of which may result in serious cardiovascular compromise or death if not promptly treated. For an in-depth analysis of cardiac dysrhythmias, refer to Chapter 20.

Tachydysrhythmias

Tachydysrhythmias, which are uncommon in infants and children, are defined as cardiac rhythms that exceed the maximum normal heart rate estimated for the child or infant's age. Tachydysrhythmias can have narrow or wide QRS complexes. When they occur in infants and children, tachydysrhythmias are rarely the result of a primary cardiac event; they often indicate a secondary cause.

Supraventricular Tachycardia

Supraventricular tachycardia (SVT) is a narrow QRS complex tachycardia characterized by a heart rate greater than 220 beats/min in the infant or greater than 180 beats/min in the child. Although the exact cause of SVT in children is unknown, it may cause inadequate perfusion secondary to decreased ventricular filling time and decreased cardiac output. Most children, however, can tolerate fast heart rates relatively well.

Emergency medical care for an infant or child with SVT will depend on his or her hemodynamic status—are they stable or unstable?

The stable child with SVT should be treated with 100% supplemental oxygen and prompt transport to the hospital. If IV or IO access is available, administer the following medications:

- **Adenosine, 0.1 mg/kg**
  - May be repeated at 0.2 mg/kg if needed.

If the infant or child is unstable, as evidenced by hypotension, an altered mental status, or poor skin color, synchronized cardioversion will be required; however, this procedure must be performed by a paramedic. Therefore, you should immediately transport the child with continuous cardiac monitoring and arrange a rendezvous with a paramedic unit, if possible.

In the Field

If permitted by local protocol or medical control, the EMT-I may perform synchronized cardioversion. Start with 0.5 to 1.0 J/kg. If unsuccessful, repeat the procedure with 2 J/kg.

Ventricular Tachycardia with a Pulse

Ventricular tachycardia (V-tach) and other ventricular dysrhythmias are uncommon in children. They are almost always the result of a secondary cause (ie, drug ingestion) rather than a primary cardiac event. On rare occasions, you may encounter an infant or child with a ventricular dysrhythmia caused by a congenital heart defect.

V-tach is characterized by wide QRS complexes and an exceedingly high heart rate. As with SVT, treatment for V-tach with a pulse depends on whether the child's condition is stable or unstable.

The stable child with V-tach with a pulse should be treated with 100% supplemental oxygen and promptly transported to the hospital. If IV or IO access is available, administer one of the following medications:

- Amiodarone, 5 mg/kg
- Lidocaine, 1 mg/kg

If the infant or child is unstable, as evidenced by hypotension, an altered mental status, or poor skin color, synchronized cardioversion will be required; however, this procedure must be performed by a paramedic. You should immediately transport the child and arrange a rendezvous with a paramedic unit, if possible. V-tach may rapidly deteriorate to V-fib. Therefore, continuous cardiac monitoring is essential. Be prepared to defibrillate the child if he or she becomes pulseless and apneic.

Bradydysrhythmias

Bradydysrhythmias, characterized by narrow QRS complexes and slow heart rates, are the most common cardiac dysrhythmias that you will encounter in the pediatric patient. The most common cause of bradycardia in the infant or child is hypoxia. In some children, bradycardia may be the result of increased parasympathetic tone; however, this is rare. Bradycardia is defined as a heart rate of less than 100 beats/min in the infant and less than 80 beats/min in the child.

If the condition of the child with a bradydysrhythmia is stable, provide 100% supplemental oxygen and transport the child to the hospital with continuous monitoring en route. An abnormally slow heart rate in a child deserves evaluation at the hospital.

Because hypoxia is the most common cause of bradycardia in children, those children whose conditions are unstable (ie, hypotension, altered mental status, poor skin color) should receive ventilatory assistance with a BVM and 100% oxygen. If BVM ventilations are ineffective and/or the child's heart rate does not improve, perform endotracheal intubation.

If, despite adequate oxygenation and ventilation, the infant or child's heart rate is less than 60 beats/min, begin chest compressions at the appropriate rate and depth. Obtain IV or IO access and perform the following interventions, as needed:

- Epinephrine
  - IV or IO: 0.01 mg/kg (0.1 mL/kg of a 1:10,000 solution)
  - ET: 0.1 mg/kg (0.1 mL/kg of a 1:1,000 solution)
    - Repeat epinephrine (IV, IO, or ET) every 3 to 5 minutes as needed

- Atropine*
  - 0.02 mg/kg via IV, IO, or ET administration (minimum dose of 0.1 mg)
    - May repeat once
- Consider transcutaneous cardiac pacing (TCP)

EMT-I Tips

Remember, bradycardia in infants and children is almost always the result of severe hypoxia. Provide ventilatory assistance with 100% oxygen before considering pharmacologic therapy.

Absent Rhythms

An absent rhythm is one that does not produce a pulse; therefore, the child will be in cardiopulmonary arrest. In children, asystole is the most commonly encountered absent rhythm. Less commonly, you will encounter a child with V-fib, pulseless V-tach, or pulseless electrical activity (PEA). Unfortunately, because these rhythms indicate prolonged hypoxia, the mortality rate is high.

Asystole

Asystole represents a total absence of electrical and mechanical activity. On the cardiac monitor, it will appear as a flatline; there are no electrical complexes. The conditions of many children deteriorate from a bradydysrhythmia to asystole if immediate treatment is not initiated; the prognosis is usually poor.

Upon detecting asystole on the cardiac monitor, you should check another lead configuration or turn up the gain sensitivity to rule out the possibility of fine V-fib.

Emergency medical care for asystole includes CPR, endotracheal intubation, IV or IO access and the following pharmacologic interventions:

- Epinephrine
  - IV or IO: 0.01 mg/kg (0.1 mL/kg of a 1:10,000 solution)
  - ET: 0.1 mg/kg (0.1 mL/kg of a 1:1,000 solution)
    - Repeat epinephrine (IV, IO, or ET) every 3 to 5 minutes as needed

---

*Give atropine before epinephrine for bradycardia that you suspect is caused by increased parasympathetic tone or primary AV block.

Pulseless Electrical Activity (PEA)

Pulseless electrical activity (PEA) is characterized by an organized cardiac rhythm on the cardiac monitor; however, the child does not have a palpable pulse.

Emergency medical care for PEA includes CPR, intubation, IV or IO access, and the following medications:

- Epinephrine
  - IV or IO: 0.01 mg/kg (0.1 mL/kg of a 1:10,000 solution)
  - ET: 0.1 mg/kg (0.1 mL/kg of a 1:1,000 solution)

EMT-I Tips

In addition to the aforementioned treatment for all arrhythmias–cardiac arrest or otherwise–treatment should focus on identifying and treating any potential underlying causes. Use the mnemonic "6H and 6T" when considering the potential underlying causes. This mnemonic stands for:

- Hypoxemia
  - Check ET tube placement
  - Ensure 100% oxygen delivery
- Hypovolemia
  - Administer a 20-mL/kg bolus of an isotonic crystalloid
  - Assess for signs of hypovolemia (ie, dehydration, trauma)
- Hypothermia
  - Assess core body temperature
  - Provide thermal management
- Hyperkalemia or hypokalemia
  - Continue resuscitative efforts
  - Provide immediate transport
- Hypoglycemia
  - Assess the blood blucose level of *any* sick or injured child
  - Administer the appropriate dose and concentration of dextrose if needed
- Hydrogen ion (acidosis)
  - Ensure adequate oxygenation and ventilation *first*
  - Consult medical control regarding sodium bicarbonate administration
- Tamponade (cardiac)
  - Administer 20-mL/kg boluses of an isotonic crystalloid
  - Immediate transport; definitive treatment is a pericardiocentesis
- Tension pneumothorax
  - Assess breath sounds
  - Perform needle decompression as needed
- Toxins (poisons and drugs)
  - Look for evidence of drug or poison ingestion
  - Consider administering naloxone (Narcan)
    - Up to 5 years of age (up to 20 kg): 0.1 mg/kg
    - ≥5 years of age (or >20 kg): 2.0 mg
- Thromboembolism (coronary) or Thromboembolism (pulmonary)
  - Continue resuscitative efforts
  - Provide immediate transport
- Trauma

Some causes of lethal cardiac arrhythmias (cardiac arrest or non-cardiac arrest), if identified early, can potentially be corrected. If no underlying cause is detected, or the suspected cause cannot be treated in the field, continue resuscitative efforts, transport immediately, and contact medical control en route.

- Repeat epinephrine (IV, IO, or ET) every 3 to 5 minutes as needed

V-fib and Pulseless V-tach

V-fib and pulseless V-tach are treated as the same rhythm in infants and children, although they appear different as two different dysrhythmias on the cardiac monitor. As a primary event, V-fib and pulseless V-tach are rare in children; however, they can be the result of secondary causes, such as electrocution or a toxic ingestion.

Emergency medical care for V-fib or pulseless V-tach includes the following:

- **Defibrillation**
  - 2 J/kg initially, then 4 J/kg for subsequent shocks
- **CPR**
- **Endotracheal intubation**
- **IV or IO access**
- **Epinephrine**
  - IV or IO: 0.01 mg/kg (0.1 mL/kg of a 1:10,000 solution)
  - ET: 0.1 mg/kg (0.1 mL/kg of a 1:1,000 solution)
    - Repeat epinephrine (IV, IO, or ET) every 3 to 5 minutes as needed
- **Repeat defibrillation at 4 J/kg as needed**
  - Repeat defibrillation as needed after 2 minutes of CPR following each medication
- **Antiarrhythmic** (*one* of the following)
  - Amiodarone, 5 mg/kg via IV or IO administration
  - Lidocaine, 1 mg/kg via IV, IO, or ET administration
- **Repeat defibrillation at 4 J/kg every 2 minutes as needed, followed by immediate CPR.**

Other Medical Emergencies

Seizures

A seizure is the result of disorganized electrical activity in the brain. It can be very frightening to people around the patient. Therefore, it is important to reassure the family and to approach assessment and management in a calm, step-by-step manner.

Assessment Findings

Seizures in children may appear in several different ways including shaking of the whole body or movement in a single arm or leg. Seizures can also appear as lip smacking, eyes blinking, or staring off into space. In a true seizure, movements cannot be stopped on command or by holding an extremity. The duration of movement varies from patient to patient.

There are several general categories of seizures. In the course of an epileptic episode, a patient may experience one or more of these types of seizures:

- **Generalized (grand mal) seizures** appear as back-and-forth motions of both upper and lower extremities. The patient is unresponsive to verbal commands or painful stimulation.
- **Partial seizures** may appear as movement in one limb, lip smacking, or eye deviation only (eyes turned to either side or up or down).
- **Absence (petit mal) seizures** appear as an unresponsiveness period without any movement and may last seconds to minutes.

Altered mental status and the inability of others to stop a movement or range of movements in the affected limb are common to grand mal and partial seizures. Many patients feel pins and needles, hear sounds, have a metallic taste in their mouth, or see hallucinations before the seizure (aura). In all but absence seizures, there is a <u>postictal period</u> of extreme fatigue or unresponsiveness after the seizure for anywhere from a few minutes to several hours. During this time, the patient may appear sleepy and/or confused and is not able to interact appropriately. A short period of seizure activity is generally not harmful to the patient. After 30 minutes or more, however, the brain may become hypoxic, and continued seizure activity can be harmful. <u>Status epilepticus</u> is a continuous seizure, or multiple seizures without a return to consciousness, for 30 minutes or more.

If you can identify the cause of the seizure, you will be better able to monitor the patient for any potential complications associated with the underlying problem (Table 31-10 ▼). In particular, be alert for the presence of medications, possible poisons, and indications of abuse or neglect.

TABLE 31-10	Common Causes of Seizures
■ Child abuse	
■ Electrolyte imbalance	
■ Fever	
■ Hypoglycemia (low blood glucose level)	
■ Idiopathic (no cause can be found)	
■ Infection	
■ Ingestion	
■ Hypoxia	
■ Medications	
■ Poisoning	
■ Previous seizure disorder	
■ Recreational drug use	
■ Head trauma	

Febrile Seizures

Febrile seizures are common in children between the ages of 6 months and 6 years and are caused by an abrupt rise in body temperature. Most pediatric seizures are due to fever alone, which is why they are called febrile seizures. These seizures typically occur on the first day of a febrile illness, are characterized by generalized tonic-clonic seizure activity, and last less than 15 minutes with a short postictal phase or none at all. They may be a sign of a more serious problem, such as meningitis. Obtain a history from the caregivers, as these children may have had a prior febrile seizure.

> **EMT-I Tips**
>
> A febrile seizure is caused by an abrupt rise in body temperature. It is not necessarily how high the fever gets, but how quickly it gets there.

If you are called to care for a child who has had a febrile seizure, you often will find that the patient is awake, alert, and fully interactive when you arrive. Keep in mind that a persistent fever can lead to another seizure. Carefully assess the ABCs, begin cooling measures with tepid water (not cold), and provide prompt transport; all children with febrile seizures need to be seen in the hospital setting Figure 31-52 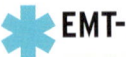.

Emergency Medical Care

Although medical management of seizures in the hospital setting may vary according to cause, your assessment and management of these patients remain essentially the same from patient to patient. First, ensure that the scene is safe for you and your partner and for the patient. Next, perform an initial assessment, focusing on the ABCs. If possible, obtain a brief history from the caregivers about previous serious illnesses or seizures and current medication or trauma.

Securing and protecting the airway are your priority. To avoid obstruction from the tongue falling back into the airway, place a child who is having a seizure or who is postictal in the recovery position if you can do so Figure 31-53.

In the case of trauma, place the head in a neutral inline position and ensure that the cervical spine is protected with spinal precautions. Be ready to use suction to prevent aspiration of stomach contents, blood, or vomitus. Do not place your fingers or any other object in the mouth of a patient who is having a seizure.

A patient who is actively seizing or who is postictal may not be breathing adequately. Assessing the rate and depth of respirations in this situation can be difficult but is essential. Patients may have shallow, rapid breathing or may have occasional deep respirations. Signs that a patient is not breathing adequately include the following:

- Very slow respirations
- Very shallow breaths (reduced tidal volume)
- Cyanotic or pale lips
- Snoring respirations caused by the tongue blocking the airway

Ensure a patent airway and deliver oxygen by nonrebreathing mask or the blow-by technique. If there are no signs of improvement, begin BVM ventilations with appropriately sized equipment.

If the child remains unresponsive after the seizure or requires prolonged ventilatory support, consider performing endotracheal intubation. *Do not attempt intubation during an active seizure.*

Figure 31-52 Following a febrile seizure, carefully assess the child's ABCs. Then begin cooling measures and prepare the child for transport.

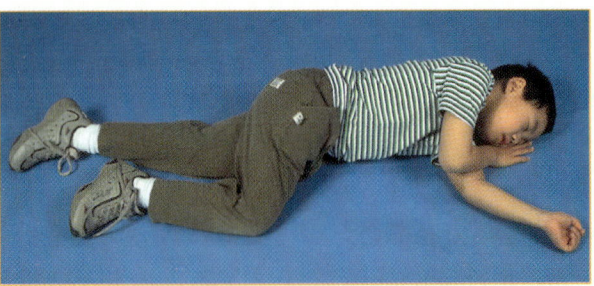

Figure 31-53 A child in the postictal (confused) state following a seizure should be placed in the recovery position.

Patients who are experiencing a seizure usually maintain adequate blood pressure and pulse rate unless the seizure is caused by an underlying circulatory or neurologic problem or trauma, including bleeding, heart problems, or brain injury. Nevertheless, you must evaluate the pulse and blood pressure and re-evaluate them. Once the ABCs have been addressed, assessment and management should proceed as follows. If the patient is actively seizing, note the type of movement and position of the eyes, as this information may be very helpful for hospital staff in making a diagnosis. If there is a fever, begin cooling measures such as removing clothing and placing towels moistened with tepid water on the child. A child with febrile seizures can seize again if the temperature remains high. Do not use alcohol or cold water to cool a patient. Make sure the patient is protected from hitting the sides of the stretcher or nearby equipment. Bring any medications or possible poisons at the scene to the hospital with the patient. If the patient is in status epilepticus, call for paramedic backup, as medication is required to stop the seizures.

Establish IV or IO access and obtain a blood glucose reading and administer glucose if the child is hypoglycemic.

To terminate the seizure, administer the following medication:

- **Diazepam (Valium)***
  - 1 month to 5 years of age: 0.2 to 0.5 mg via slow IV or IO administration
    - Repeat every 2 to 5 minutes as needed
    - Maximum dose of 2.5 mg
  - 5 years of age and older: 1 mg via slow IV or IO administration
    - Repeat every 2 to 5 minutes as needed
    - Maximum dose of 5.0 mg

Documentation Tips

The physician who evaluates your patient after a seizure will need information on the seizure pattern and changes in that pattern. Record all pertinent information about factors that may have triggered the seizure, including its duration, areas of body movement, and the patient's return to consciousness afterward. Witnesses, family members, or caregivers will be important sources of information.

*Diazepam may be administered rectally. Contact medical control as needed.

Altered Level of Consciousness

People who are aware of themselves and their surroundings are said to be conscious. Nonverbal infants may demonstrate consciousness by following a person's face or an object (tracking), by babbling and cooing, or by crying. Infants and children may exhibit an altered level of consciousness (also called altered mental status) in many ways, including lack of response to vocal commands and pain, combative behavior, confusion, thrashing about, drifting into and out of an alert state, or a change in the pitch and nature of their cry.

Common causes of altered level of consciousness in a pediatric patient can be found in the mnemonic AEIOU-TIPS:

- Alcohol
- Epilepsy, endocrine, or electrolyte abnormalities
- Insulin or low blood glucose levels
- Opiates or other CNS depressant drugs
- Uremia
- Trauma or temperature
- Infection
- Psychogenic or poison
- Shock, stroke, or shunt obstruction

Your first step in caring for a patient with an altered level of consciousness is to assess the ABCs and provide appropriate care as necessary. As you determine responsiveness, remember to use the AVPU scale. Then obtain a brief history from the patient's caregivers, focusing on the following points:

- Does the patient have any illnesses?
- Does the patient take any medications? When was the last dose?
- Did the patient ingest any substances (eg, poisons, drugs, or plant material)?
- Has the patient been ill?
- Has the patient had any behavior problems?

Next, observe the patient's pupils: Are they dilated or pinpoint? Do they react to a light by constricting (Figure 31-54)? Are the eyes turned to the right, left, up, or down? Is the patient staring without moving his or her eyes? Is the patient posturing (Figure 31-55)?

Once you have completed your initial assessment, immediately secure the airway. Provide supplemental oxygen with a nonrebreathing mask. If respirations are inadequate, provide assisted ventilation with a BVM device.

Consider endotracheal intubation for definitive airway protection. Also, attach a cardiac monitor and assess the child's cardiac rhythm.

If you suspect trauma, log roll the child onto a backboard, apply a cervical collar, and fully immobilize the

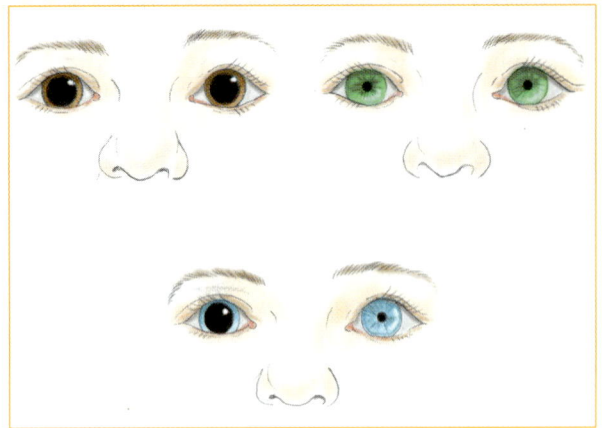

Figure 31-54 Observe a child's eyes for changes in pupillary size.

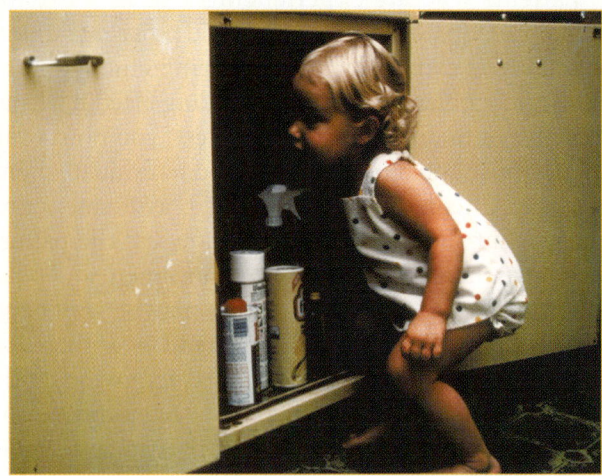

Figure 31-56 A curious child will try to taste or swallow almost any substance. A common victim of accidental ingestion of dangerous compounds is the unwatched toddler.

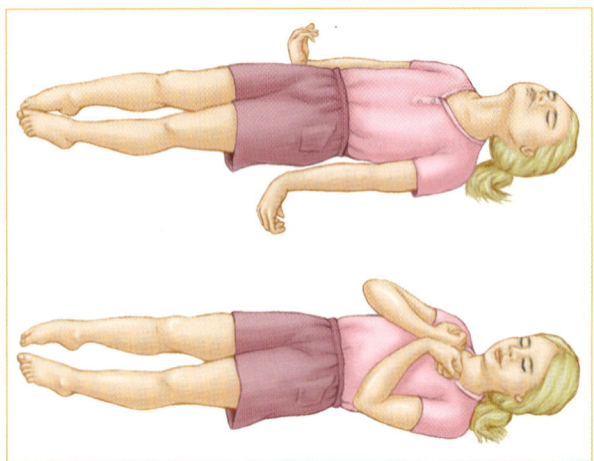

Figure 31-55 Observe a child for posturing.

spine. If the child is actively seizing, follow the care described earlier in this chapter on seizures. Remember to call for paramedic backup as necessary. Regardless of the cause, you should support the patient's vital functions and provide prompt transport.

Poisoning

Poisoning is common among children. It can occur by ingesting, inhaling, injecting, or absorbing a toxic substance (Figure 31-56). The signs and symptoms of poisoning vary widely, depending on the substance and the age and weight of the child (Table 31-11). The child may appear normal at first, even in serious cases, or he or she may be confused, sleepy, or unresponsive.

Infants may be poisoned as a result of being fed a harmful substance by a sibling or a caregiver or as a result of child abuse. Infants can be exposed to drugs and poisons left on floors and carpeting. They can also be exposed in a room or automobile in which harmful and illicit drugs, such as crack, cocaine, or PCP, are being smoked. Toddlers are curious and often ingest poisons when they find them in the home or garage. For example, some people store petroleum products in soda bottles. Toddlers may believe the substance to be soda. Adolescents are more likely to have ingested alcohol and street drugs while at parties or in a suicide attempt.

After you have completed your initial assessment and addressed any immediate life-threats, you should ask the caregiver the following questions:

- What is the substance(s) involved?
- Approximately how much of the substance was ingested or involved in the exposure (eg, number of pills, amount of liquid)?

TABLE 31-11	Common Sources of Poisoning in Children

- Alcohol
- Aspirin and acetaminophen
- Household cleaning products such as bleach and furniture polish
- Houseplants
- Iron
- Prescription medications of family members
- Street drugs
- Vitamins

- What time did the incident occur?
- How much does the child weigh?
- Are there any changes in behavior or level of consciousness?
- Was there any choking or coughing after the exposure? (These can be signs of airway involvement.)

Because a child's level of consciousness may be affected by the poison, your care will be guided by how awake and alert the child appears. For a child who is responsive, your protocols may dictate that you contact medical control and your local poison control center to report the situation. Focus on the ABCs, keeping in mind that the child's condition may change over time. Assess the patient's level of consciousness and support the vital functions as necessary, including giving supplemental oxygen. If the patient is combative and/or agitated, protect yourself from injury. Do not administer syrup of ipecac (if this is still used in your EMS system) unless directed to do so by medical control. Call for paramedic backup if the patient's condition becomes unstable. As you prepare the patient for transport, try to find the container that held the suspected poison, collect any vomitus from the child and place it in a plastic bag, and take both to the emergency department.

If the child is unresponsive, make sure that you focus immediately on the ABCs, and be prepared to provide artificial ventilation if necessary. Give supplemental oxygen, and then call medical control to report the situation. Provide transport to the emergency department, keeping in mind that the child's condition could change at any time.

Fever

Fever is a common reason parents call 9-1-1. Simply defined, fever is an increase in body temperature, usually in response to an infection. Body temperatures of 100.4°F (38°C) or higher are considered to be abnormal. Fevers have many causes and are rarely life-threatening events. However, you should not underestimate the potential seriousness of fevers, such as those that occur in conjunction with a rash. You should try to determine whether the fever is a sign of serious illness, such as meningitis. Common causes of a high temperature in a child include the following:

- Infection, such as pneumonia, meningitis, or urinary tract infection
- Neoplasm (cancer)
- Drug ingestion
- Collagen vascular disease, including arthritis and systemic lupus erythematosus
- High environmental temperature

Note that there are other conditions in which the body temperature increases that are not a fever. Hyperthermia differs from fever in that it is an increase in body temperature caused by an inability of the body to cool itself. Hyperthermia is typically seen in warm environments, such as a closed car on a hot day.

Emergency medical care of a child with a fever begins with an initial assessment of the ABCs, caring for immediate life threats as needed. Be sure to wear personal protective equipment, especially if meningitis is a possibility. Look carefully at the child to obtain a general impression: Does the child look sick? Then report your findings to medical control. Assess the patient's level of consciousness, and obtain vital signs. Evaluate the child for signs and symptoms of shock. If the child feels very warm, remove any covering so that the skin is exposed. Begin cooling measures en route, preferably by placing wet, cool (not cold) towels over the child's body and head. Unless associated with shock or severe dehydration, IV therapy is generally not necessary in a child with fever.

Meningitis

Meningitis is an inflammation of the tissue, called the meninges, that covers the spinal cord and brain. It is caused by an infection by bacteria, viruses, fungi, or parasites. If left untreated, meningitis can lead to permanent brain damage or death. Being able to recognize a patient who may have meningitis is an important skill for the EMT-I.

Meningitis can occur in both children and adults, but some individuals are at greater risk than others, as follows:

- Males
- Newborn infants
- Children whose immune systems have been weakened by AIDS or cancer
- Children who have any history of brain, spinal cord, or back surgery
- Children who have had head trauma
- Children with shunts, pins, or other foreign bodies within their brain or spinal cord

At especially high risk are children with a ventriculoperitoneal (VP) shunt. These special needs children have tubing that can usually be seen and felt just under the scalp.

The signs and symptoms of meningitis vary, depending on the age of the patient. Fever and altered level of consciousness are common symptoms of meningitis in patients of all ages. Changes in level of consciousness can range from a mild or severe headache to confusion, lethargy, and/or an inability to understand commands or interact appropriately. The child may also experience a seizure, which as described earlier may be a first sign of meningitis. Assess the level of consciousness using the AVPU scale. Infants younger than 2 to 3 months can have apnea, cyanosis, fever, or hypothermia.

In describing children with meningitis, physicians often use the term "meningeal irritation" or "meningeal signs" to describe pain that accompanies movement. Bending the neck forward or back increases the tension within the spinal canal and stretches the meninges, causing a great deal of pain (nuchal rigidity). This results in the characteristic stiff neck of children with meningitis, who will often refuse to move their neck, lift their legs, or curl into a "C" position, even if coached to do so. One sign of meningitis in an infant is increasing irritability, especially when being handled. Another sign is a bulging fontanel.

One form of meningitis deserves special attention. Neisseria meningitidis is a bacterium that causes a rapid onset of meningitis symptoms, often leading to shock and death. Children with N meningitidis typically have small, pinpoint, cherry-red spots or a larger purple/black rash. This rash may be on part of the face or body. These children are at serious risk of sepsis, shock, and death.

All patients with possible meningitis should be considered highly contagious and infectious. Therefore, you should use BSI precautions whenever you suspect meningitis and follow up with the hospital to learn the patient's final diagnosis. If you have been exposed to saliva and respiratory secretions from a child with N meningitidis, you should receive antibiotics to protect yourself and others from the bacteria. This is particularly true if you managed the patient's airway. If you were not in close contact with the patient or his or her respiratory secretions, you do not need treatment.

In taking the history of a child with meningitis, pay particular attention to the following details:

- Onset of illness, including any upper respiratory symptoms such as runny nose, cough, or other cold symptoms
- Presence and duration of fever
- Level of activity
- Change in behavior in older children, irritability in younger children

Emergency medical care of a patient who is believed to have meningitis should begin with an initial assessment of the ABCs and immediate care of life threats. Some patients may experience episodes of cyanosis and/or apnea. If the patient is old enough to follow commands and respond, either verbally or nonverbally, determine responsiveness by asking, "What is your name?" "How old are you?" and "Hold up two fingers." Remember that you should be wearing appropriate protective equipment before you start caring for the child.

After you have secured the airway, give supplemental oxygen by mask or the blow-by technique, as tolerated. You should be prepared to assist ventilations with a BVM device if necessary. Assess the patient's vital signs, keep him or her warm, and watch for signs and symptoms of shock. If the patient's vital signs are unstable, obtain vascular access and administer IV fluids as needed to maintain adequate perfusion.

Perform endotracheal intubation if BVM ventilations are ineffective or if the child will require prolonged ventilatory support. Monitor the cardiac rhythm.

> **EMT-I Safety**
>
> Some forms of meningitis are highly contagious. Use BSI precautions whenever you suspect meningitis, including mask and eye protection when there is coughing, sneezing, or any other possibility of contact with the patient's respiratory secretions. Local protocols may also call for putting a mask on the patient.

Dehydration

Dehydration occurs when fluid losses are greater than fluid intake. The most common cause of dehydration in children is vomiting and diarrhea. If left untreated, dehydration can lead to shock and eventually death. Infants and children are at greater risk than adults for dehydration because their fluid reserves are smaller than those in adults. Life-threatening dehydration can overcome an infant in a matter of hours. Again, your ability to recognize a child with this condition is a critical part of your job.

Dehydration can be described as mild, moderate, or severe. The severity of the dehydration can be gauged by looking at several clues (Table 31-12). For example, an infant with mild dehydration may have dry lips and gums, decreased saliva, and fewer wet diapers throughout the day (Figure 31-57). As the dehydration grows more severe, the lips and gums may become very dry, the eyes may look sunken, and the infant may be sleepy and/or irritable, refusing bottles. The skin may be loose and have no elasticity (tenting); this is called poor skin turgor. Also, infants may have sunken fontanelles.

TABLE 31-12	Vital Signs and Symptoms of Dehydration		
	Mild Dehydration	**Moderate Dehydration**	**Severe Dehydration**
Pulse	Normal	Increased	Increased; 160 or greater is a sign of impending shock
Level of activity	Normal or slowed	Slowed	Variable, weak to unresponsive
Urine output	Decreased	Decreased	No output
Skin	Normal	Cool, mottled; poor turgor	Cool, clammy; poor turgor; delayed capillary refill time
Mouth	Saliva may have drooling, bubbles	Dry mucous membranes	Dry mucous membranes
Eyes	Normal	Tears	Sunken eyes; lack of tears when crying
Anterior fontanelle	Normal to sunken	Sunken	Very sunken
Level of consciousness	Normal	Altered	Altered; lethargic
Blood pressure	Normal	Normal	Normal to low when shock sets in

Young children can compensate for fluid losses by decreasing blood flow to the extremities and directing it to vital organs such as the brain and heart. Children who are moderately to severely dehydrated may have mottled, cool, clammy skin and delayed capillary refill. Respirations will usually be increased. Be aware that blood pressure may remain normal until the child is in shock.

Emergency medical care should include careful attention assessing the ABCs and obtaining baseline vital signs. However, if the dehydration is severe, IV or IO access should be obtained and crystalloid fluid boluses of 20 mL/kg should be given as needed. All children with signs and symptoms of moderate to severe dehydration should be transported to the emergency department.

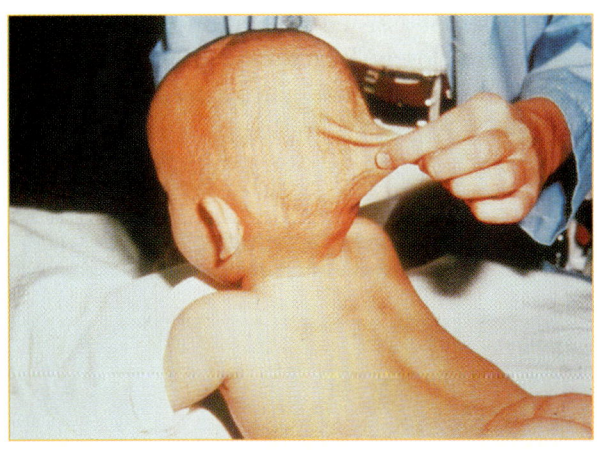

Figure 31-57 An infant with mild dehydration may exhibit "tenting" or poor skin turgor.

Hypoglycemia

Hypoglycemia is defined as an abnormally low blood glucose level. Infants and children have limited stores of glucose, which can be quickly depleted in times of illness, injury, or stress. You must recognize that hypoglycemia is a life-threatening emergency that requires immediate treatment. If hypoglycemia is unrecognized or treatment is delayed, permanent brain damage or death can result.

> **EMT-I Tips**
>
> Although hypoglycemia is more common in patients with diabetes, physical exertion, illness, or injury can result in hypoglycemia in the nondiabetic child. Remember to assess blood glucose levels in all ill or injured children with an altered mental status or bizarre behavior.

Assessment Findings

General signs and symptoms of hypoglycemia include hunger, malaise, tachycardia, tachypnea, diaphoresis, and tremors. The severity of the patient's clinical presentation depends on how low the blood glucose level has dropped. Hypoglycemia can be classified as being mild, moderate, and severe (Table 31-13). You should obtain a blood glucose reading in any infant or child that you suspect is hypoglycemic. Normal blood glucose levels range from 80 to 120 mg/dL.

In children with a known history of diabetes, ask the parent or caregiver the following questions. Allow the child to answer the questions if he or she is old enough and understands what you are asking:

1. Have you taken your insulin today? If so, what was the dosage?
2. Has your medication recently changed?
3. When was the last time that you ate? What did you eat?
4. Have you been playing outside or otherwise exerting yourself?

Emergency Medical Care

Management of hypoglycemia begins by administering 100% oxygen or assisted ventilation if needed. Monitor vital signs closely. Treat the symptomatic child with glucose if his or her blood glucose reading is less than 80 mg/dL.

If the child is conscious and alert enough to swallow, administer oral glucose as allowed by local protocol. If, however, the child has an altered mental status or is otherwise incapable of swallowing, administer IV glucose in the following dosages:

- Younger than 2 years: 25% dextrose (D_{25}), 2 to 4 mL/kg
  - Dilute 50% dextrose (D_{50}) 1:1 with normal saline to make D_{25}
- Older than 2 years: 50% dextrose (D_{50}), 1 to 2 mL/kg

If an IV cannot be established, insert an intraosseous needle. If vascular access (IV or IO) is not available, medical control may order the administration of 1 mg of glucagon via IM injection.

Repeat a blood glucose reading 10 to 15 minutes following the administration of glucose. If the patient is still symptomatic and his or her blood glucose reading remains below 80 mg/dL, repeat the glucose as needed.

Hyperglycemia

Hyperglycemia is an abnormally high blood glucose level. It can either be the presenting problem in a child with new-onset diabetes mellitus or it may occur as a complication in a child with a known history of diabetes. If not recognized or promptly treated, hyperglycemia can result in severe dehydration and diabetic ketoacidosis (DKA), both of which are potentially life-threatening.

Assessment Findings

During your assessment of the child with suspected hyperglycemia, you will typically find that a dose of insulin was missed, a greater proportion of food was eaten compared to the dose of insulin, or the insulin pump malfunctioned.

Like hypoglycemia, the signs and symptoms of hyperglycemia depend on how high the level of blood glucose is (Table 31-14). During your assessment, ask the same questions of the child or parent as you did for suspected hypoglycemia.

Emergency Medical Care

Management of hyperglycemia begins by administering 100% oxygen or assisted ventilation if needed. Monitor vital signs closely. Obtain IV access and administer 20-mL/kg boluses of normal saline or lactated Ringer's solution as needed to maintain adequate perfusion. Children with hyperglycemia and DKA are often severely dehydrated.

TABLE 31-13 Signs and Symptoms of Hypoglycemia

Mild
- Hunger
- Weakness (malaise)
- Tachypnea
- Tachycardia

Moderate
- Diaphoresis (sweating)
- Tremors
- Irritability
- Vomiting
- Mood swings
- Blurred vision
- Stomach ache
- Headache
- Dizziness

Severe
- Decreased level of consciousness
- Seizures

TABLE 31-14	Signs and Symptoms of Hyperglycemia

Early
- Polydipsia (excessive thirst)
- Polyuria (excessive urination)
- Weight loss

Acute (dehydration and early ketoacidosis)
- Weakness
- Abdominal pain
- Generalized body aches
- Anorexia (loss of appetite)
- Nausea and vomiting
- Signs of dehydration (except for decreased urinary output)
  - Warm, dry skin
  - Poor turgor
- Fruity breath odor
- Tachypnea
- Hyperventilation
- Tachycardia

Late (ketoacidosis)
- Coma
- Deep and slow or fast respirations (Kussmaul's respirations)
- Signs of shock from severe dehydration

Closely monitor the patient's ABCs and be prepared to adjust your treatment accordingly. The patient in DKA desperately needs insulin; however, this is not a drug that is administered in the prehospital setting. Therefore, immediate transport to the closest appropriate facility is critical.

If you are unable to obtain IV access, insert an intraosseous needle. If the patient's respiratory status deteriorates, be prepared to perform endotracheal intubation. Monitor the cardiac rhythm.

In the Field

If you are unable to determine whether a child with an altered mental status has hypoglycemia or hyperglycemia (ie, glucometer failure), administer glucose. If the child is in DKA, the extra sugar will likely not cause further harm. However, if he or she is hypoglycemic, sugar could save his or her life. Remember the adage, "When in doubt, give sugar."

Sudden Infant Death Syndrome

The unexpected death of an infant is called sudden infant death syndrome (SIDS) when, after a complete autopsy, the cause of death remains unexplained. SIDS is the leading cause of death in infants younger than 1 year; most cases occur in infants between 2 and 4 months of age.

Although it is impossible to predict SIDS, there are several known risk factors:
- Mother younger than 20 years
- Mother smoked during pregnancy
- Low birth weight
- The baby is placed on his or her stomach in a crib

Deaths due to SIDS can occur at any time of the day; however, these children are often discovered in the morning when the parents go in to check on the infant. If you are the first provider at the scene of suspected SIDS, you will face three tasks: assessment and management of the patient, communication and support of the family, and assessment of the scene.

Assessment and Management

SIDS is a diagnosis of exclusion. All other potential causes must first be ruled out, a process that may take physicians quite a while. An infant who has been a victim of SIDS will be pale or blue, not breathing, pulseless, and unresponsive. Other causes for such a condition include the following:
- Overwhelming infection
- Child abuse
- Airway obstruction from a foreign object or as a result of infection
- Meningitis
- Accidental or intentional poisoning
- Hypoglycemia (low blood glucose level)
- Congenital metabolic defects

Regardless of the cause, assessment and management of the infant remain the same. Remember that what you find in assessing the infant and the scene may provide important diagnostic information.

Begin with an assessment of the ABCs and provide interventions as necessary. Depending on how much time has passed since the child was discovered, he or she may show signs of postmortem changes. These include stiffening of the body, called rigor mortis, and dependent lividity, which is the pooling of blood in the lower parts of body or those that are in contact with the floor or bed.

If the child shows such signs, call medical control. In some EMS systems, a victim of SIDS may be declared dead on the scene. Deciding whether to start CPR on a child who shows clear signs of rigor mortis or dependent lividity can be very difficult. Family members may consider anything less as withholding critical care. In this situation, the best course of action may be to initiate CPR and transport the patient and the family to the nearest emergency department, where the family can receive more extensive support (follow local protocols). If there is no evidence of postmortem changes, begin CPR immediately.

As you assess the infant, pay special attention to any marks or bruises on the child before performing any procedures, including CPR. Also note any intervention such as CPR that was done by the parents before you arrived.

Communication and Support of the Family

The death of a child is a very stressful event for a family. It also tends to evoke strong emotional responses among health care providers, including EMS personnel. Part of your job at this point is to allow the family to express their grief in ways that may differ from your own cultural, religious, and personal practices. Provide support in whatever ways you can.

Many times family members will ask specific questions about the event: Why did this happen? How did this happen? Let them know that their concerns will be addressed but that answers are not immediately available. Always use the infant's name in speaking to family members. If possible, allow the family to spend time with the infant and to ride in the ambulance to the hospital.

Scene Assessment

Carefully inspect the environment, following local protocols, noting the condition of the scene where the caregivers found the infant. Your assessment of the scene should concentrate on the following:

- Signs of illness, including medications, humidifiers, thermometers, etc
- The general condition of the house (Note any signs of poor hygiene.)
- Family interaction. Do not allow yourself to be judgmental about family interactions at this time. Note and report any behavior that is clearly not within the acceptable range, such as physical and verbal abuse.
- The site where the infant was discovered. Note all items in the infant's crib or bed, including pillows, stuffed animals, toys, and small objects.

The death of a child is difficult for everyone involved: parents, relatives, friends, and health care professionals. You should arrange for a proper debriefing after your involvement with the case comes to a close. This can be a session with a trained counselor or a group discussion with your colleagues or the entire health care team.

Apparent Life-Threatening Event

Infants who are not breathing and are cyanotic and unresponsive when found by their families sometimes resume breathing and color with stimulation. These children have had what is called an <u>apparent life-threatening event (ALTE)</u>, sometimes called "near-miss SIDS." In addition to cyanosis and apnea, a classic ALTE is characterized by a distinct change in muscle tone (limpness) and choking or gagging. After the event, a child may appear healthy and show no signs of illness or distress. Nevertheless, you must complete a careful assessment and provide immediate transport to the emergency department.

Pay strict attention to management of the airway. Assess the infant's history and, if possible, the environment. Allow caregivers to ride in the ambulance. If asked, explain that you cannot say what caused the event and

 EMT-I Tips

Most parents of children who die suddenly will experience extremely strong emotional responses for a long time after the death. Counseling and support services begin with your care, including immediate referral to longer term services. You can usually make this referral through social services personnel in a hospital you work with, something you should know about in advance. Many communities also support groups for families who lose children, including SIDS deaths. Make sure the parents are aware of available services, offer to put them in touch while you are there, and leave the contact information in written form for their later reference even if you have helped them make the contact.

that this is something that the physician will have to determine at the hospital.

Death of a Child

As with SIDS, the death of a child from any cause poses special challenges for EMS personnel. In addition to any medical treatment the child may require, you must be prepared to offer the family a high level of support and understanding as they begin the grieving process (Table 31-15). First, the family may want you to initiate resuscitation efforts, which may or may not conflict with your EMS protocols. If the child is clearly deceased and, under protocol, can be declared dead in the field, but the family is so distraught that they insist that resuscitation efforts be made, initiate CPR and transport the child.

The extent of your interaction with the family will depend, to some degree, on the number of providers available at the scene. Always introduce yourself to the child's caregivers and ask about the child's date of birth and medical history. If and when the decision is made to start or stop resuscitation efforts, inform the family immediately. Find a place for family members where they can watch resuscitation without being in the way. Do not, in any case, speculate on the cause of the child's death. The family will want to see the child and should be asked whether they want to hold the child and say good-bye. Parents may be experiencing strong feelings of denial.

The following interventions are helpful in caring for the family at this time:

- Learn and use the child's name rather than the impersonal "your child."
- Speak to family members at eye level, maintaining good eye contact with them.
- Use the word "dead" or "died" when informing the family of the child's death; euphemisms such as "passed away" or "gone" are not effective.
- Acknowledge the family's feelings ("I know this is devastating for you"), but never say "I know how you feel," even if you have experienced a similar event; the statement will anger many people.
- Offer to call other family members or clergy if the family wishes.
- Keep any instructions short, simple, and basic. Emotional distress may limit their ability to process information.
- Ask each adult family member individually whether he or she wants to hold the child.
- Wrap the dead child in a blanket, as you would if he or she were alive, and stay with the family while they hold the child. Ask them not to remove tubes or other equipment that was used in an attempted resuscitation.

Remember that each individual and each culture expresses grief in a different way, some more visibly than others. Some will require intervention; others will not. Most caregivers feel directly or indirectly responsible for the death of a child and may express this immediately; this does not mean that they actually are respon-

TABLE 31-15 How You Can Help the Family of a Deceased Child

When arriving on site:
- Introduce yourself quickly.
- Obtain a brief history.
- When possible, one provider should stay with the family.

If resuscitation is attempted:
- Give brief, frequent updates and explanations.
- Allow family members to stay within viewing distance if they wish.
- Allow family members to accompany the child to the hospital when possible.

If no resuscitation is performed:
- Sit down with the family.
- Inform the family immediately.
- Explain why no resuscitation will be attempted.
- Offer to arrange for religious support, including baptism or last rites.

Beginning the grieving process:
- Learn and use the child's name.
- Allow family to express emotions; be nonjudgmental.
- Give brief explanations and answers.
- Explain to the family that the cause of death is still unknown.
- Allow time for questions.

Do:
- Tell the family how sorry you are.
- Tell the family whom they can call if they have questions later.
- Give written instructions and referrals.

Don't:
- Say, "I know how you feel."
- Say, "You have other children" or "You can have other children."
- Attempt to answer the question "Why did this happen?"
- Try to tell family that they will be feeling better in time.

sible. Sometimes, it is helpful to address the issue of guilt by saying, "Many caregivers feel responsible for their child's death. Are you feeling that?" Parents often have questions that you should be prepared to answer (Table 31-16). Although you should keep the possibility of abuse or neglect in mind, your role is not that of investigator. Any further inquiry is the responsibility of law enforcement.

Some EMS systems arrange for home visits after the death of a child so that EMS providers and family members can come to some sort of closure together. This also gives the family an opportunity to ask any remaining questions about the event. However, you need special training for such visits.

Again, coping with the death of a child can be very stressful for health care professionals. You may find yourself with unexpected feelings of pain and loss. It is helpful to take some time before going back on the job to work through your feelings and to talk about the event with your EMS colleagues. Be alert for signs of posttraumatic stress in yourself and others: nightmares, restlessness, difficulty sleeping, lack of appetite, or a constant need for food. Consider the need for professional help if these signs or symptoms continue. All EMS programs should have critical incident stress management protocols and debriefing teams available for traumatic incidents.

Although you may experience the death of a child as a failure, your skill at coping with this kind of emotional event can be a great comfort to the family, helping them to accept their loss and begin the long process of grieving.

Pediatric Trauma Emergencies

Trauma is the number one killer of children in the United States. More children die of trauma-related injuries in 1 year than of all other causes combined. As an EMT-I, you will frequently treat injured children; therefore, you must have a thorough understanding of how trauma affects them. The quality of care in the first few minutes after a child has been injured can have an enormous impact on that child's chances for complete recovery.

Treatment of traumatic injuries in children starts with understanding these injuries as completely as possible. The types of injuries differ, depending on the age of the child. Infants and toddlers are most commonly hurt as a result of falls or abuse. Older children and adolescents are usually injured as a result of mishaps involving automobiles. According to information collected by the National Pediatric Trauma Registry (NPTR) during the last 10 years, the automobile is the most significant threat to the well-being of the child. Approximately 41% of all injuries that the NPTR recorded in this time period were related to vehicular mishaps, including those involving bicycles and pedestrians. Other common causes of traumatic injury and death include falls, gunshot wounds, blunt injuries, and sports activities. Another extremely serious and troublesome cause of injury is child abuse.

Anatomic Differences

By now, you know that children are not simply small adults. They differ in many ways other than size. Children have less circulating blood than adults do. Children also lose body heat more easily than adults do because children have a larger body surface area in relation to body mass. A child's bones have not finished growing; they are more flexible and elastic than those in an adult. Fat is distributed in a child in a somewhat different way than in an adult, so vital organs in the abdomen and the chest of a child are less well insulated. Therefore, a child may experience significant injuries to internal organs

TABLE 31-16 Common Questions Following Death of a Child

Q Was there pain?
A This often can be answered by a simple "No." If you are uncertain, you may give an indirect answer such as "We really don't know what patients feel in these circumstances."

Q What did he (or she) die of?
A Do not answer this question; you would probably be guessing at this point. Instead, say, "Hopefully an autopsy will provide that answer."

Q Why did this happen?
A Do not attempt to answer this question either, as the answer depends on one's own individual philosophy or religion. "I wish I had an answer for you" is usually the most appropriate response.

Q What happens now?
A This question usually concerns the next few minutes or the next hour. If you know, you should give the family a general idea of what will happen. For example, if there is no history of illness, you can say that "the coroner (or medical examiner) will be examining [the child's name], and then he (or she) will be taken to the mortuary."

but have little or no evidence of external trauma. This is especially true of chest injuries. Because a child's ribs are softer and more flexible than those of an adult, they may compress the underlying lungs and heart, causing life-threatening conditions without obvious external damage Figure 31-58 .

Given these anatomic differences, you must be able to recognize severe injuries in children and to identify potentially life-threatening injuries so that you can provide prompt emergency medical care. This begins with your scene size-up. Look for the child's level of activity, work of breathing, and skin color. This information is quickly gained and is the beginning of your ABCs. Complete the initial assessment by:

- Evaluating the child's responsiveness
- Ensuring that the child has an open airway and is breathing
- Assisting ventilation and giving supplemental oxygen to the child, if necessary
- Assessing the child's circulation by obtaining a pulse (brachial, carotid, femoral) and blood pressure, evaluating for external bleeding, and assessing skin color, temperature, and capillary refill

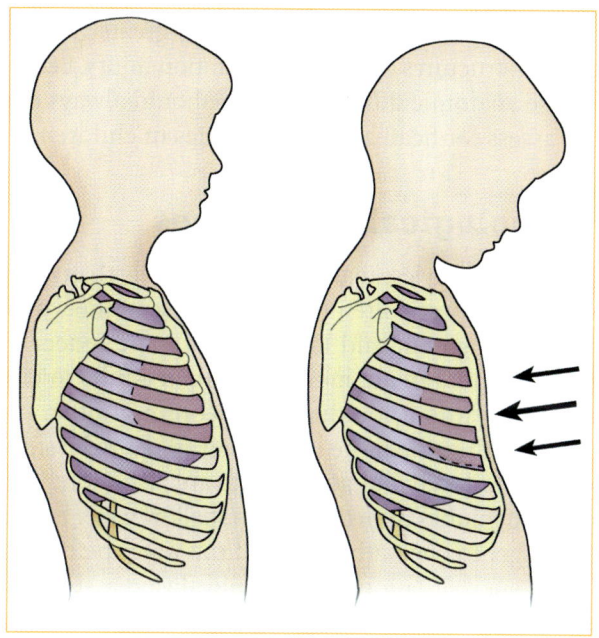

Figure 31-58 A child's ribs are softer and more flexible than an adult's. As a result, compression of the lungs and heart, causing serious injury, can occur with no obvious external injury.

Injury Patterns

Although you are not responsible for diagnosing injuries in children, your ability to recognize and report serious injuries will provide critical information to hospital staff. For this reason, it is important for you to understand the special physical and psychological characteristics of children and what makes them more likely to have certain kinds of injuries. Situations that are unique to children also make them more susceptible to injury, such as their need to ride in child safety seats, their involvement in specific mishaps with motor vehicles, and their participation in organized sports.

Physical Differences

Children are smaller than adults; therefore, when they are hurt in the same type of accident as an adult, the location of their injuries may differ from those in an adult. For example, the bumper of a car will strike an adult in the lower leg, whereas that same bumper will strike a child in the pelvis. In a crash involving sudden deceleration, an adult might injure a ligament in the knee; in that same accident, a child might injure the bones in the leg.

Children's bones and soft tissues are less well developed than those of adults; therefore, the force of an injury affects these structures somewhat differently than

You are the Provider   Part 7

You successfully intubate the child and confirm correct tube placement. As your partner ventilates the child, you perform a detailed physical examination.

12. On the basis of the mechanism of injury (25 mph frontal motor vehicle impact, no helmet, loss of consciousness), what injury patterns should you suspect and where should you examine further for injuries?

it does in an adult. Because a child's head is proportionately larger than an adult's, it exerts greater stress on the neck structures during a deceleration injury. Because of these anatomic differences, you should always carefully assess for head and neck injuries in children.

Psychological Differences

Children are also less mature psychologically than adults; therefore, they are often injured because of their undeveloped judgment and their lack of experience. For example, children are more likely than adults to cross the street without looking for oncoming traffic. As a result, children are more likely than adults to be struck by cars. Children and adolescents are also more likely to sustain injuries from diving into shallow water because they forget to check the depth of the water before they dive. In such situations, you should always assume that the child has serious head and neck injuries. Other common injuries include wrist injuries from in-line roller skating and ankle fractures from bicycle crashes. Note that these examples do not apply to all children or all adults. In fact, some children have more common sense than some adults. However, you should be aware of these injury patterns when you are called to respond to pediatric emergencies.

Child Safety Seats

Children are often injured or killed in motor vehicle crashes. Those who are not restrained in child safety seats are at greater risk for head, neck, and spinal injuries. Although child safety seats are effective in decreasing the severity of injuries, children may still sustain abdominal and lower spinal injuries as the result of trauma caused by improperly used passenger restraints. Infants are especially prone to injuries of the head and neck due to weaker neck muscles and their larger head and should be in a rear-facing seat until 1 year of age. Although head, neck, and spinal injuries are less common in restrained passengers, they are certainly possible. Therefore, you should always immobilize the patient's cervical spine Figure 31-59 .

Young children, especially those who have been restrained in a child safety seat, may be critically injured or killed by airbags if they are riding in the front passenger seat of a car Figure 31-60 . This occurs because the child safety seat is positioned too close to the airbag. When the airbag deploys, the child may sustain a devastating spinal or head injury. For this reason, child safety seats should never be placed in the front seat of a vehicle that is equipped with passenger airbags.

Automobile Collisions

Children playing or riding a bicycle can dart out in front of motor vehicles without looking. In such a situation, the driver may have very little time to slow down or stop to prevent hitting the child. The area of greatest injury varies, depending on the size of the child and the height of the bumper at the time of impact Figure 31-61 . When vehicles slow down at the moment of impact, the bumper dips slightly, causing the point of impact with the child to be lowered. The exact area that is struck depends on the child's height and the final position of the bumper at the time of impact.

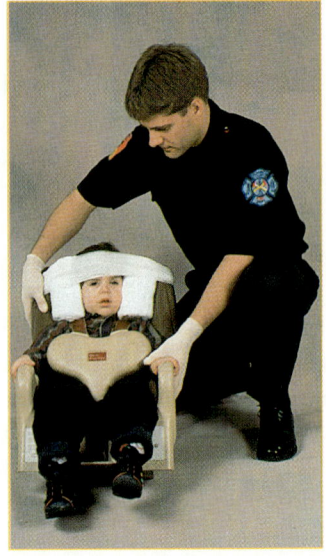

Figure 31-59 Even though head, neck, and spinal injuries are less common in children who are restrained, they are still possible. Therefore, you should always immobilize the patient's cervical spine.

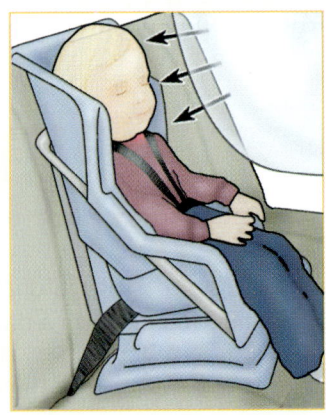

Figure 31-60 Children riding in a child safety seat in the front passenger seat of a car may be injured or killed by the force of a deploying airbag.

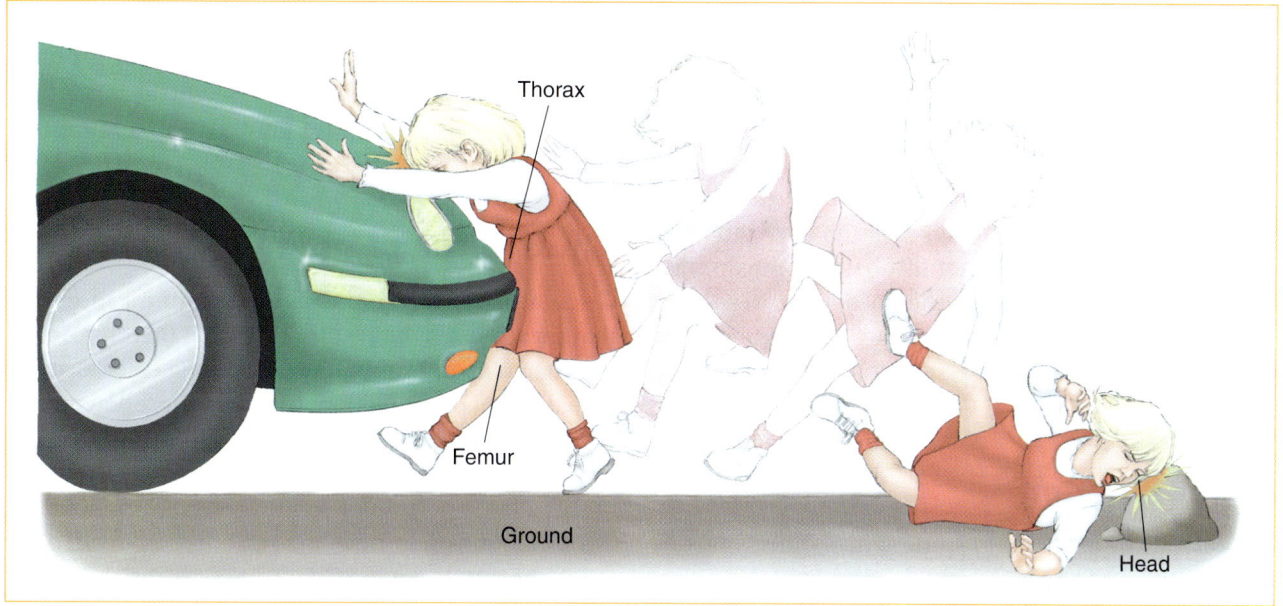

Figure 31-61 The exact area that is struck depends on the child's height relative to the position of the bumper at the time of impact.

Children who are injured in these situations often sustain high-energy injuries to the head, spine, abdomen, pelvis, or legs.

Sports Activities

Children, especially those who are older or adolescents, are often injured in organized sports activities. Head and neck injuries can occur after high-speed collisions in contact sports such as football, wrestling, ice hockey, field hockey, soccer, or lacrosse. Remember to immobilize the cervical spine when caring for children with sports-related injuries. You should also be familiar with your local protocols related to helmet removal, and/or follow the guidelines presented in Chapter 17.

Special Considerations

Special considerations should be taken into account when managing the pediatric trauma patient. Management strategies for the injured infant or child will often require modifications from those in adults to accommodate the special needs of pediatric patients.

Airway Control

Because of the unique characteristics of the child's airway, the following factors should be taken into consideration when managing an injured child's airway:

- Maintain manual stabilization of the child's cervical spine with the head in a neutral position. The sniffing position, used to position the airway in an uninjured child, may compromise a spinal injury and should therefore be avoided
- All trauma patients must receive 100% supplemental oxygen. Additionally, because children often experience respiratory failure or arrest following trauma, you must be prepared to assist ventilations with a BVM device and 100% oxygen.
  - Remember that shallow or grossly irregular respirations will not provide adequate tidal volume; closely monitor the child's respiratory effort and be prepared to intervene immediately.
- Airway patency must be maintained with a jaw-thrust maneuver; if any secretions (ie, blood, mucus, vomitus) are in the mouth, they must be removed with suction.
  - You cannot manage a child's breathing if his or her airway is not patent; obtain and

maintain a patent airway first, then provide any required treatment

If BVM ventilations are not providing adequate tidal volume, are otherwise ineffective, or if prolonged ventilatory support is required, perform endotracheal intubation. Remember to maintain the child's head in a neutral in-line position during intubation. Two personnel will be required to achieve this most effectively.

Even if the child has been intubated, you should consider placing a gastric tube to decompress the stomach. If the child's injury or injuries will require surgical intervention, his or her stomach will have to be emptied.

Immobilization

Immobilization of a child's spine will require special modifications and appropriately sized equipment. Take the following into consideration when performing spinal immobilization in the injured child:

- As with the adult, use a rigid cervical collar. If you do not have the appropriately sized cervical collar (common with infants), use rolled towels and place them around the child's head to maintain stabilization of his or her head.
  - Remember that a cervical collar that is too large or too small may cause more harm than good to the child.
- If an injured child is found in his or her safety seat following a motor vehicle crash, immobilize him or her in the safety seat, unless the child's condition is critical and he or she requires aggressive management.
  - Children get used to riding in their car seats; it becomes their "personal space." Removing a child from his or her environment may cause agitation and anxiety, making assessment and management more difficult.
- If available, use a pediatric immobilization device for the injured child. If such a device is not available, you can improvise by using a vest-style extrication device (turned upside down) to provide full-body immobilization.
- A short immobilization device (ie, short wooden backboard) is optimum for immobilizing infants and small children. If using a long backboard, use padding to encircle the child; secure the child in place with tape, straps or triangular bandages (cravats).

Remember to immobilize infants, toddlers, and preschoolers in a supine position with in-line stabilization of the cervical spine. This may be accomplished by placing padding from the shoulders to the hips. This will help to prevent them from sliding around on the backboard. Techniques of pediatric immobilization will be discussed and demonstrated later in this chapter.

Fluid Management

Circulatory compromise is less common in children than in adults as the result of trauma; therefore, airway management and ventilatory support takes priority over management of circulation. Consider the following when you are establishing vascular access in the injured child:

- Large-bore IV catheters should be inserted into a large peripheral vein whenever possible.
- Because definitive care can only be provided at the hospital, never delay transport for the purpose of starting an IV; this procedure should be performed en route to the hospital.
- To maintain perfusion in a child, administer an initial bolus of 20 mL/kg using an isotonic crystalloid solution (ie, normal saline, lactated Ringer's).
  - Frequently reassess the child's vital signs and provide additional IV fluid boluses of 20 mL/kg if no improvement is noted following the initial bolus.
  - If the child's condition does not improve following two boluses of an isotonic crystalloid, blood loss is likely severe and will probably need surgical intervention. Provide rapid transport with continuous monitoring of the child en route.

If IV access cannot be obtained within three attempts or 90 seconds, insert an intraosseous needle to gain access to the vascular system. Also monitor the cardiac rhythm.

Traumatic Brain Injury

Assessment and management of the brain-injured patient are based on recommendations from the Brain Trauma Foundation. Head trauma is a leading cause of traumatic death in children. Children, because of their proportionately large head, are at higher risk for head trauma especially following a motor vehicle crash or a fall.

Early recognition and aggressive management can reduce mortality and morbidity from traumatic brain injury. Without prompt care, traumatic brain injuries can, and often do, result in permanent damage or death.

Using the modified Glasgow Coma Scale (GCS), head injuries in children are categorized as being mild, moderate, and severe:

- *Mild:* GCS is 13 to 15
- *Moderate:* GCS is 9 to 12
- *Severe:* GCS is less than 9

The GCS can be a difficult scale to memorize. For this reason, you should keep a copy of it on your ambulance wall or within an EMS field guide.

Complications of severe head trauma include intracranial bleeding and cerebral edema, which result in increased intracranial pressure (ICP). Signs of ICP include hypertension, bradycardia, and abnormal breathing patterns—a trio of clinical findings referred to as Cushing's triad. A common respiratory pattern seen following severe brain trauma is rapid, deep breathing, which progresses to slow, deep breathing and alternating periods of apnea (Cheyne-Stokes respirations). Abnormal breathing following a severe head injury suggests pressure on the brainstem. In infants, bulging fontanelles are an indicator of increased ICP.

Without prompt treatment, ICP will result in herniation of the brain, which occurs when the pressure within the cranium forces the brain through the foramen magnum, the large opening at the base of the skull through which the spinal cord passes. Herniation often results in permanent brain damage (even with prompt treatment) or death. Signs of herniation include the following:

- Asymmetrical (unequal) pupils
- Posturing
  - Decorticate (flexor) posturing is characterized by flexion of the arms and extension of the legs.
  - Decerebrate (extensor) posturing is characterized by extension of the arms and legs.

Management for the brain-injured patient focuses on maintaining cerebral perfusion—accomplished by ensuring airway patency and adequate breathing—and providing rapid transport, preferably to a facility that specializes in pediatric trauma care.

The method of providing oxygenation must be based on the adequacy of the child's breathing. In general, 100% oxygen should be administered to a child with a traumatic brain injury. Assist ventilations at a normal rate for the child if he or she has a GCS that is less than 9 or is breathing inadequately. *Do not hyperventilate a brain-injured patient unless signs of herniation are present.* Signs of brain herniation, which would indicate the need for hyperventilation, include the following:

- Unresponsive
- Asymmetrical pupils *or* bilaterally unreactive (fixed) and dilated pupils
- Decerebrate (extensor) posturing *or* flaccid paralysis
- Active seizures

It cannot be overemphasized that aggressive treatment and rapid transport to a trauma center are crucial to the survival of the infant or child with a traumatic brain injury.

Injuries to Specific Body Systems

Head Injuries

Head injuries are common in children. This is due, in part, to the fact that the size of a child's head, in relation to the body, is larger than that of an adult. The signs and symptoms of head injury in a child are similar to those in an adult, but there are some important differences. Nausea and vomiting are common signs and symptoms of head injury in children; however, it is easy to mistake these for an abdominal injury or illness. You should suspect a serious head injury in any child who experiences nausea and vomiting after a traumatic event.

Your single most important step in caring for a child with a head injury is to maintain adequate oxygenation and ventilation. Whenever you suspect trauma, you should immobilize the cervical spine and use the jaw-thrust maneuver to open the airway, as the child's tongue may have relaxed back into the throat, blocking the airway. As you immobilize the child onto a backboard, avoid using sandbags to immobilize the head (Figure 31-62). If the child begins to vomit and the board has to be turned to the side, the weight of the bags on the head could cause additional injury.

Do not hyperventilate the child with severe head injury unless signs of brain herniation (ie, unequal

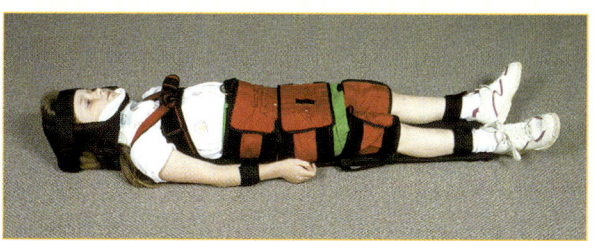

Figure 31-62 Use a proper pediatric immobilization device rather than sandbags to immobilize the head of a child. If you need to turn the board to the side if the child vomits, sandbags could shift and cause further injury.

pupils, decerebrate posturing, unresponsiveness) are present.

Respiratory failure or arrest can occur as a result of head injuries in children. You should be prepared to assist ventilations or provide rescue breaths in any child who has evidence of severe head injury.

Obtain vascular access and administer IV fluids as needed to maintain a systolic blood pressure of at least 80 to 90 mm Hg in the child with a head injury. Hypotension in the patient with a traumatic brain injury can cause a decrease in cerebral perfusion, resulting in permanent brain damage or even death. However, if the child is hypertensive, avoid fluid boluses because they may further increase intracranial pressure. Guidelines for the assessment and management of brain trauma were discussed earlier in this chapter.

Chest Injuries

Chest injuries in children are usually the result of blunt trauma rather than penetrating objects. Remember that children have very soft, flexible ribs that can be compressed a great deal without breaking. Keep this in mind as you assess a child who has sustained high-energy blunt trauma to the chest. Even though there may be no external sign of injury, such as broken ribs, contusions, or bleeding, there may be significant injuries within the chest.

Abdominal Injuries

Abdominal injuries are very common in children. Remember, though, that children can compensate for significant blood loss better than adults without signs or symptoms of shock developing. They can also have a serious injury without early external evidence of a problem. All children with abdominal injuries should be monitored for signs and symptoms of shock, including a weak, rapid pulse; cold, clammy skin; decreased capillary refill (an early sign); confusion; and decreased systolic blood pressure (a late sign). Even in the absence of signs and symptoms of shock, or with only very few signs and symptoms, you should remain cautious about the possibility of internal injuries.

Children can lose a large portion of their blood volume before hypotension develops Figure 31-63 ▶. This is potentially dangerous for two reasons. First, infants and children have less blood circulating in their bodies than adults do, so the loss of even a small volume of fluid can lead to shock. Second, children can tolerate a lower proportional blood loss than adults before developing signs and symptoms of shock. Stated differently, when children develop hypotension as a result of hemorrhage, more profound shock is already present than in adults who first develop hypotension from blood loss. Whereas 30 to 40% blood loss is what is required to predictably produce systolic hypotension in healthy adults, greater than 25% blood volume loss in children significantly increases the risk of shock. Thus children are less tolerant of blood loss overall than are adults.

You should always suspect hidden internal injuries in children after a high-energy trauma. One of the problems associated with abdominal injuries in children is the presence of air in the stomach. Children, especially those who have had a traumatic injury, tend to swallow air. Air in the stomach can cause distention and interfere with your assessment. Air can also accumulate in the stomach with artificial ventilation, making it less effective. This is one of the reasons to use the jaw-thrust maneuver to position the airway, as it decreases the amount of air accumulating in the stomach.

Injuries of the Extremities

Children have immature bones with active growth centers. Growth of long bones occurs from the ends at specialized growth plates. These growth plates, or epiphyseal plates, are potential weak spots in the bone and are often injured as a result of trauma. In general, children's bones bend more easily than those of an adult. As a result, incomplete or greenstick fractures can occur.

Extremity injuries in children are generally managed in the same manner as those in adults. Painful deformed limbs with evidence of broken bones should be splinted. Specialized splinting equipment, such as a traction splint for fractures of the femur, should be used only if it fits the child. You should not attempt to use adult immobilization devices on a child unless the child is large enough to properly fit in the device.

Burns

Children can be burned in a variety of ways. The most common involve exposure to hot substances such as scalding water in a bathtub, hot items on a stove, or exposure to caustic substances such as cleaning solvents or paint thinners Figure 31-64 ▶. You should suspect possible internal injuries from chemical ingestion when

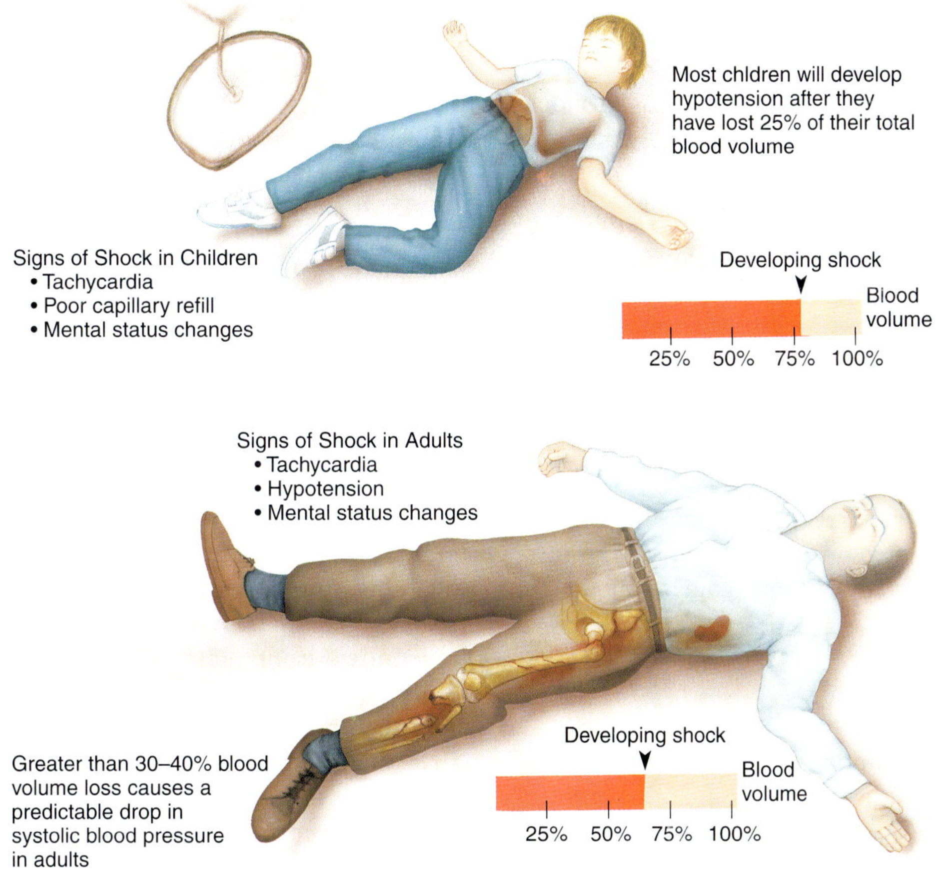

Figure 31-63 Children tolerate a lower total blood volume loss and a lower proportional loss of blood volume than adults do before developing severe shock.

you see a child who has burns, particularly around the face and mouth.

One common problem following burn injuries in children is infection. Burned skin cannot resist infection as effectively as normal skin can. For this reason, aseptic technique should be used in handling the skin of children with burn wounds.

As when you are caring for adults, when caring for children you should first remove all clothing from the burned skin as part of a complete exposure of the patient. Leaving charred clothing in place prevents you from clearly assessing the patient. In addition, the clothing may still be hot and continue to burn the underlying skin if it is not removed. After chemical burns, it is particularly important to remove the clothing rapidly because chemical materials that are retained within the clothing may also cause damage to the underlying skin.

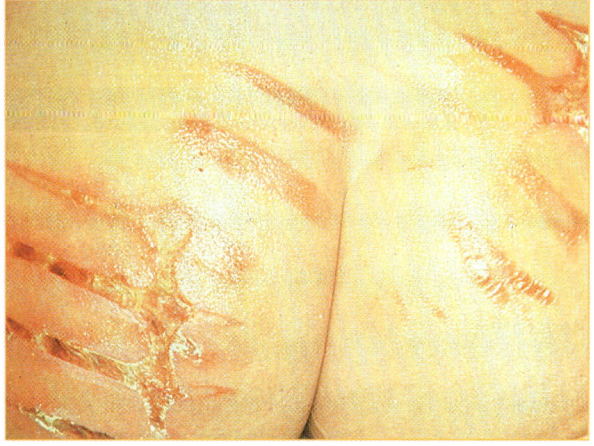

Figure 31-64 The most common burns in children involve exposure to hot surfaces. This child's buttocks were placed against a hot heating grate.

After the skin has been exposed, you should place dry, sterile dressings on the skin as soon as possible to decrease the risk of infection.

Obtain vascular access, preferably in a nonburned area, and administer 20-mL/kg boluses of normal saline or lactated Ringer's fluid if the child is in shock. Reassess the child's condition and administer additional IV fluids as needed.

Insert an intraosseous catheter if you are unable to obtain IV access.

You must learn your local protocols regarding the immediate referral of children to burn centers. Table 31-17 provides some general guidelines to follow in assessing a child who has been burned. These guidelines may help you to determine which children should be treated primarily at specialized burn centers. Also note that you should consider the possibility of child abuse in any burn situation. Make sure you report any information about your suspicions to hospital staff.

Submersion Injury

Submersion injuries include near drowning and drowning. In submersion situations, you must always take steps to ensure your own safety when retrieving the patient from the water.

Drowning is the second most common cause of unintentional death among children in the United States; children younger than 5 years are at particular risk. At this age, children often fall into swimming pools and lakes, but many drown in bathtubs and even buckets. Older adolescents, who account for the most drownings after toddlers, drown when swimming or boating; alcohol is frequently a factor.

The principal injury from submersion is lack of oxygen. Even a few minutes (or less) without oxygen affect the heart, lungs, and brain, causing life-threatening problems such as cardiac arrest, respiratory difficulty, and coma. Submersion in icy water can rob the body of heat, causing hypothermia. While a very few, very cold victims of submersion hypothermia have survived long periods in cardiac arrest in icy water, most people in this situation die. Diving into the water, of course, increases the risk of neck and spinal cord injuries.

Assessment and reassessment of the ABCs are critical in submersion injuries. First assess breathing and pulse because the patient may be in cardiac or respiratory arrest. Immediately check breathing effort, skin color, and capillary refill in addition to vital signs. Always immobilize the cervical spine of patients who were diving. Lung injuries may progress, causing breathing difficulty over time, so be sure to reassess the patient frequently during transport.

If you cannot effectively ventilate the patient, consider the possibility of a foreign body airway obstruction; water alone does not obstruct the airway. If you can see the object, be sure to use removal techniques that are appropriate to the patient's age.

If it is within your scope of practice, consider using a nasogastric tube to protect the airway in unresponsive patients, as they will usually vomit. Always have a suction device ready in case of vomiting or water in the airway.

Perform endotracheal intubation if BVM ventilations are required, but ineffective. The child should also be intubated if prolonged ventilatory support will be required and the cardiac rhythm should be monitored.

Remove wet clothing so that the patient does not get colder. Keep the patient warm and monitor vital functions during transport.

A child may appear completely normal after being submersed and then have problems minutes or hours later. This is called secondary drowning and happens when the lungs are filled with fluid from within the lung (pulmonary edema).

Emergency Medical Care

Emergency medical care of a child who has experienced a traumatic injury immediately focuses on the ABCs, as with all patients.

TABLE 31-17	Severity of Burns in Children
Severity of Burn	**Body Area Involved**
Minor	Partial-thickness burns involving less than 10% of the body surface
Moderate	Partial-thickness burns involving 10% to 20% of the body surface
Critical	Any full-thickness burn
	Any partial-thickness burn involving more than 20% of the body surface
	Any burn involving the hands, feet, face, airway, or genitalia

Airway

You should be alert for airway problems in all children who have sustained traumatic injuries. Children who are awake, alert, and talking generally have open airways; however, unresponsive children, even those who are initially breathing on their own with signs of an open airway, are at risk for airway obstruction. Look and listen for signs indicating abnormal airflow through the upper airway. If stridor—an abnormal airway sound made by turbulent airflow—is present, use the jaw-thrust maneuver to keep the airway open. One advantage of this maneuver is that it minimizes the risk of damage to the cervical spine because it keeps the head in a neutral position.

Because nausea and vomiting are common in children with traumatic head injuries, you must be prepared for it. Keep suctioning equipment readily available so that you can suction the mouth and oropharynx as necessary to keep the airway open. Be prepared to turn a backboard to one side if the child vomits Figure 31-65 ▶. Remember that you should not use sandbags to stabilize the cervical spine in children. If you must turn the backboard to allow for vomiting, the weight of the sandbags may cause additional head injury when the backboard and patient are turned.

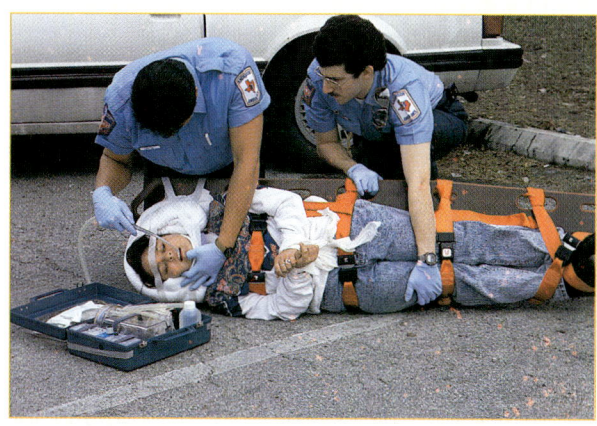

Figure 31-65 Turn the backboard to the side and suction the mouth when an immobilized child vomits.

Breathing

You should give supplemental oxygen to all children with possible head, chest, or abdominal injuries or any evidence of shock to correct hypoxia. Children who are breathing on their own should be given high-concentration oxygen via a nonrebreathing mask. Care should be taken to ensure that the mask fits the child properly; adult masks used on children

---

You are the Provider   Part 8

With an estimated time of arrival at the trauma center of 5 minutes, you perform a reassessment of the child, which reveals the following:

Reassessment	Recording Time: 15 Minutes After Patient Contact
Respirations	Ventilated at a rate of 20 breaths/min
Pulse	54 beats/min, regular and bounding
Skin	Pale
Blood pressure	140/92 mm Hg
Level of consciousness	Unresponsive, moans occasionally
Pupils	Asymmetrical, left pupil dilated and nonreactive

On the basis of altered mental status, asymmetrical pupils, and the bradycardia, you assume this patient has a severe brain injury.

13. On the way to the trauma center, what are some treatment options to help deal with the potentially rising intracranial pressure?

typically leak, making oxygen administration less effective (**Figure 31-66**).

You should be prepared to assist with ventilation in children with inadequate breathing. For children who have had traumatic injuries, use a child-sized BVM device and ventilate at a rate of 12 to 20 breaths/min, or one breath every 3 to 5 seconds.

Hyperventilation is indicated in children with severe head trauma *only* when signs of brain herniation are present. Signs of brain herniation include unresponsiveness, a unilaterally dilated and nonreactive pupil, bilaterally fixed and dilated pupils, decerebrate (extensor) posturing, or flaccid paralysis. Follow your local protocols regarding hyperventilation of the brain-injured patient.

Perform endotracheal intubation to protect the airway of an unresponsive child with a severe traumatic injury.

EMT-I Tips

An injured child with serious airway or breathing problems is likely to need full-time attention from two EMT-Is. The need for a driver, and often for added help with patient care, makes it important to start arranging early for backup from another unit—possibly even before you arrive at the scene.

Immobilization

Immobilization is necessary for all children who have possible head or spinal injuries after a traumatic event. Follow the steps in **Skill Drill 31-11**:

1. **Maintain the child's head in a neutral position** by placing a towel under the child's shoulders (**Step 1**).
2. **Place an appropriately sized cervical collar** on the patient (**Step 2**).
3. **Carefully log roll the child** onto the immobilization device (**Step 3**).
4. **Secure the patient's torso** to the immobilization device first (**Step 4**).
5. **Secure the child's head** to the immobilization device (**Step 5**).
6. **Complete immobilization** by ensuring that the child is strapped in properly (**Step 6**).

Immobilization can be difficult to perform due to the child's body proportions. Young children require padding under the torso to maintain a neutral position. At around 8 to 10 years of age, children no longer require padding underneath the torso in order to form a neutral position. Instead, they can simply lie supine on the board. However, another complication may occur if a child is put onto an adult-sized backboard. Because a child's body is narrower than an adult's, it will require padding along the sides in order to be properly secured on an adult-sized backboard

Follow the steps in **Skill Drill 31-12** to immobilize an infant:

1. **Carefully stabilize the infant's head in a neutral position** and lay the seat down into a reclined position on a hard surface (**Step 1**).

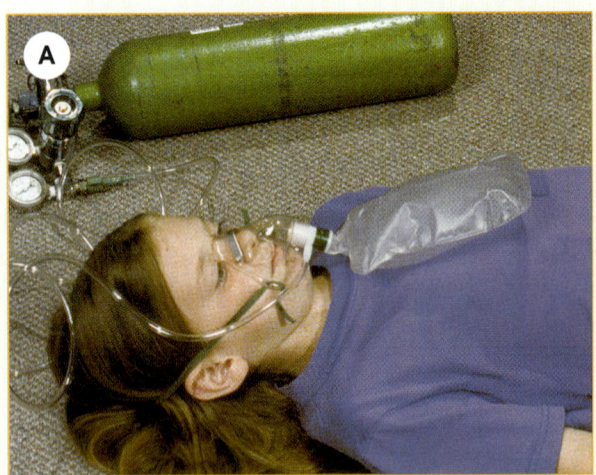
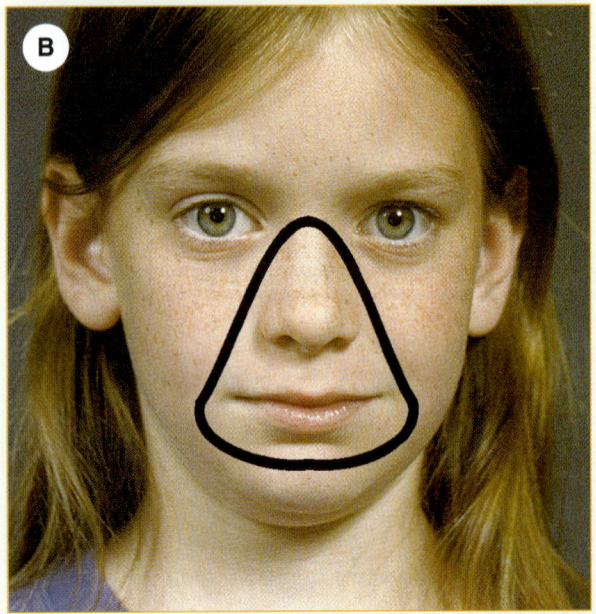

Figure 31-66 **A.** Use a properly fitting nonrebreathing mask to deliver supplemental oxygen. **B.** Area covered on a child's face with a properly fitting mask.

2. **Position a pediatric board or other similar device** between the patient and the surface on which the infant is resting (**Step 2**).
3. **Carefully slide the infant into position** on the board (**Step 3**).
4. **Make sure the infant's head is in a neutral position** by placing a towel under the infant's shoulders (**Step 4**).
5. **Secure the torso first** and place any padding to fill any voids (**Step 5**).
6. **Secure the infant's head** to the board (**Step 6**).

As with all patients who have unstable or potentially unstable injuries, immediate transport is indicated. The identification of the nearest appropriate facility depends on local protocols and the capabilities of local hospitals. In some areas of the country, you may be directed to take the patient directly to a pediatric trauma center or to arrange for air transport to a pediatric trauma center. In other areas of the country, children are evaluated primarily at local hospitals and are then transferred to a pediatric trauma center. You should be familiar with the local guidelines and protocols regarding transport issues.

Child Abuse

The term <u>child abuse</u> means any improper or excessive action that injures or otherwise harms a child or infant; it includes physical abuse, sexual abuse, neglect, and emotional abuse. The intentional injury of a child, whether physical or emotional, is not rare in our society. More than 2 million cases of child abuse are reported to child protection agencies annually. Many of these children suffer life-threatening injuries, and some die. If suspected child abuse is not reported, the child is likely to be abused again and again, perhaps suffering permanent injuries or even death. Therefore, you must be aware of the signs of child abuse and neglect, and of your responsibility to report suspected abuse to law enforcement or child protection agencies.

Signs of Abuse

As an EMT-I, you will be called to homes because of a reported injury to a child. If you suspect that physical or sexual abuse is involved, you should ask yourself the following questions:

- Is the injury typical for the developmental level of the child?
- Is the method of injury reported by the parent or caregiver consistent with the child's injuries?
- Is the caregiver behaving appropriately (concerned about the child's well-being)?
- Is there evidence of drinking or drug use at the scene?
- Was there a delay in seeking care for the child?
- Is there a good relationship between the child and the caregiver?
- Does the child have multiple injuries at different stages of healing?
- Does the child have any unusual marks or bruises that may have been caused by cigarettes, grids, or branding injuries?
- Does the child have several types of injuries, such as burns, fractures, and bruises?
- Does the child have any burns on the hands or feet that involve a glove distribution (marks that encircle a hand or foot in a pattern that looks like a glove)?
- Is there an unexplained decreased level of consciousness?
- Is the child clean and an appropriate weight for his or her age?
- Is there any rectal or vaginal bleeding?
- What does the home look like? Clean or dirty? Is it warm or cold? Is there food?

Your assessment in the field will allow a better assessment by the medical staff later. An easy way to remember these is the mnemonic CHILD ABUSE shown in **Table 31-18**.

As you assess the child, look for and pay particular attention to the following signs **Figure 31-67**.

TABLE 31-18	CHILD ABUSE Mnemonic for Assessing Possible Child Abuse

Consistency of the injury with the child's developmental age
History inconsistent with injury
Inappropriate parental concerns
Lack of supervision
Delay in seeking care
Affect
Bruises of varying ages
Unusual injury patterns
Suspicious circumstances
Environmental clues

Skill Drill 31-11: Immobilizing a Child

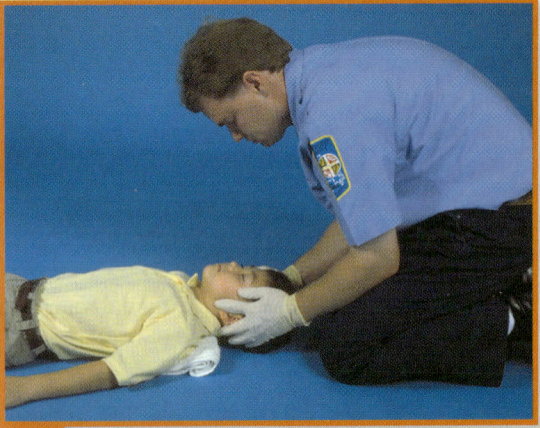

1 Use a towel under the shoulders to maintain the head in neutral position.

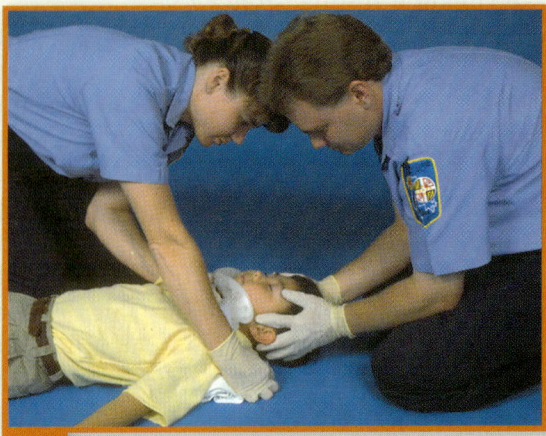

2 Apply an appropriately sized cervical collar.

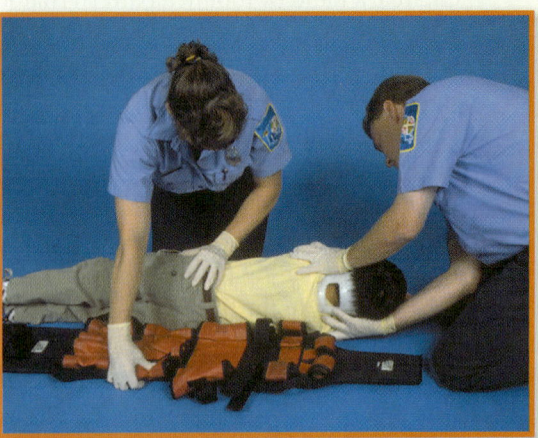

3 Log roll the child onto the immobilization device.

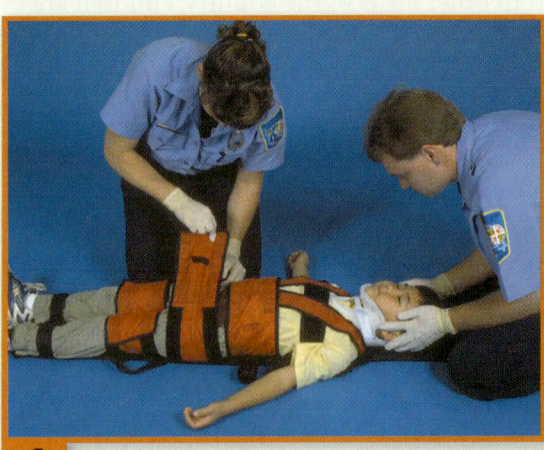

4 Secure the torso first.

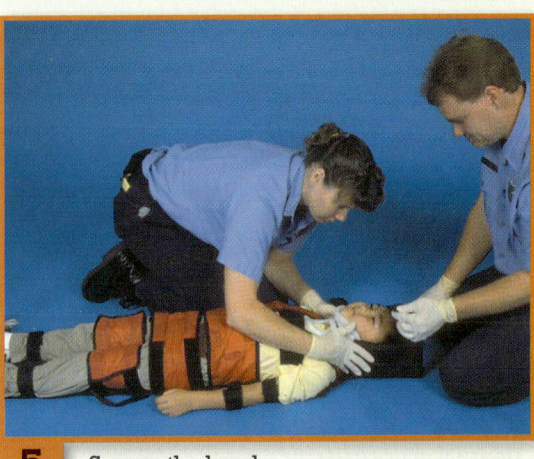

5 Secure the head.

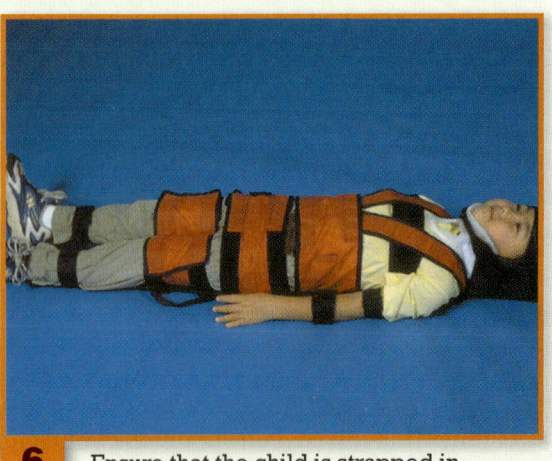

6 Ensure that the child is strapped in properly.

Immobilizing an Infant

Skill Drill 31-12

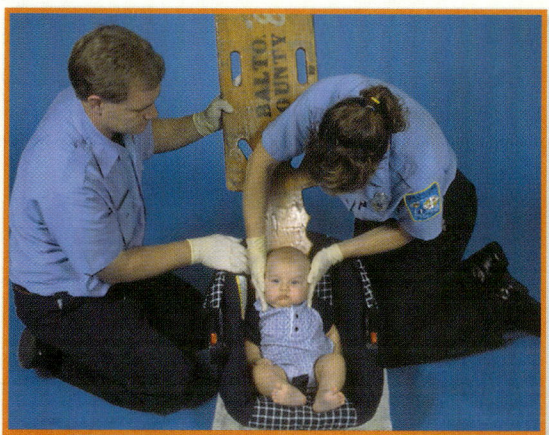
1 Stabilize the head in neutral position.

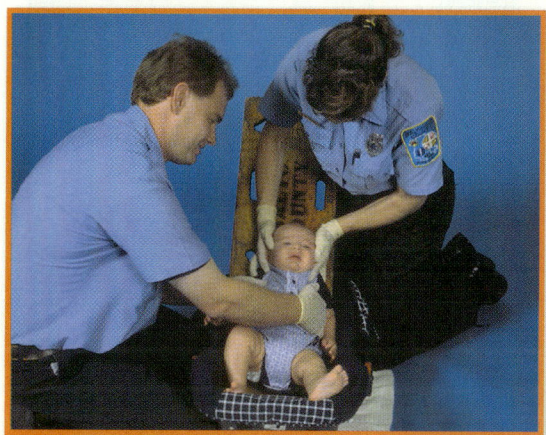
2 Place an immobilization device between the infant and the surface on which he or she is resting.

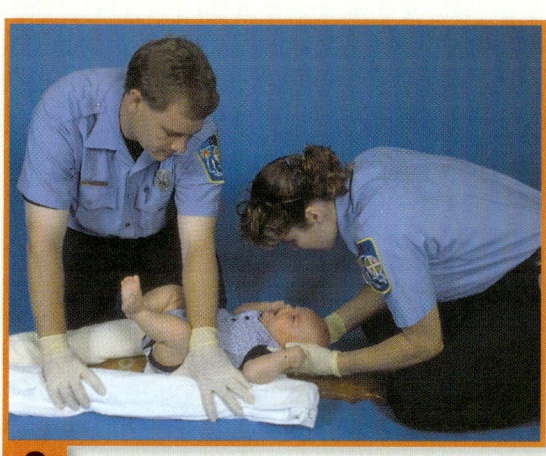
3 Slide the infant onto the board.

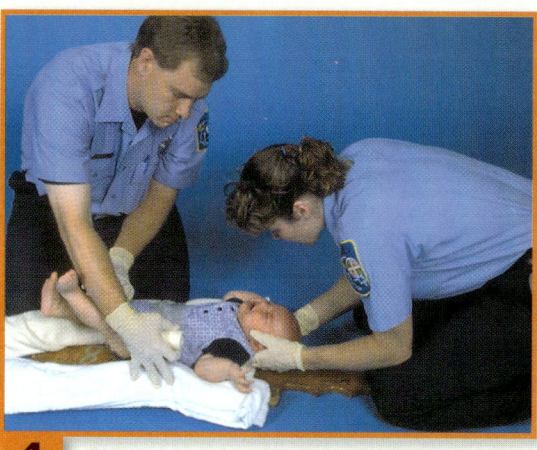
4 Place a towel under the shoulders to ensure neutral head position.

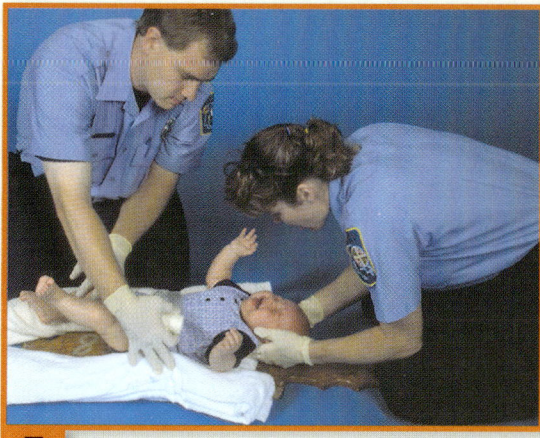
5 Secure the torso first; pad any voids.

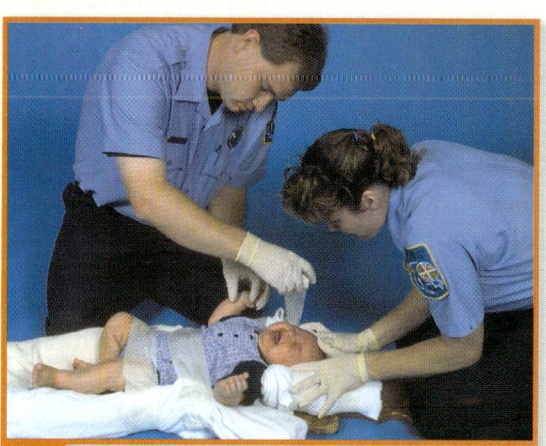
6 Secure the head.

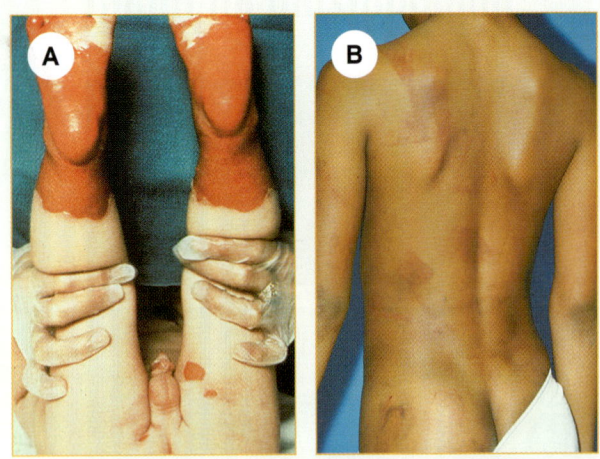

Figure 31-67 Signs of child abuse. **A.** Scald. **B.** Multiple injuries at different stages of healing.

Bruises

Observe the color and location of any bruises. New bruises are pink or red. Over time, bruises turn blue, then green, then yellow-brown and faded. Note the location. Bruises to the back, buttocks, or face are suspicious and are usually inflicted by someone else.

Burns

Burns to the penis, testicles, vagina, or buttocks are usually inflicted by someone else, as are burns that encircle a hand or foot to look like a glove. You should suspect abuse if the child has cigarette burns or grid pattern burns.

Fractures

Fractures of the humerus or femur do not normally occur without major trauma, such as a fall from a high place or a motor vehicle crash. Falls from bed are not usually associated with fractures.

Shaken Baby Syndrome

Infants may sustain life-threatening head trauma by being shaken or struck on the head, a life-threatening condition called shaken baby syndrome. With this condition, there is bleeding within the head and damage to the cervical spine as a result of intentional, forceful shaking. The infant will be found unresponsive, often without evidence of external trauma. The call for help may be for an infant who has stopped breathing or is unresponsive. The infant may appear to be in cardiopulmonary arrest, but what has likely occurred is that the shaking tore blood vessels in the brain, resulting in bleeding around the brain. The pressure from the blood results in a coma.

Neglect

Children who are neglected are often dirty or too thin or appear developmentally delayed because of lack of stimulation. You may observe such children when you are making calls for unrelated problems. Report all cases of suspicious neglect.

Symptoms and Other Indicators of Abuse

An abused child may appear withdrawn, fearful, or hostile. You should be particularly concerned if the child refuses to discuss how an injury occurred. Occasionally, the parent or caregiver will reveal a history of several "accidents." Be alert for conflicting stories or a marked lack of concern from the parents or caregiver. Remember, the abuser may be a parent, caregiver, relative, or friend of the family. Sometimes the abuser is an acquaintance of a single parent.

Emergency Medical Care

Your priority is to care for ABCs, as in all other instances. Care for all wounds, splint fractures, and keep the infant or child warm and comfortable. Provide transport in all instances in which you suspect abuse has occurred. You are not there to solve the problem or to accuse a parent or caregiver. In fact, you need their cooperation, as you cannot transport a child without consent from the parent or guardian. Sometimes, you can persuade a parent to allow transport if you say that the child may need special x-rays or tests. If the parent still refuses and you are concerned about the child's well-being, consult law enforcement.

EMT-Is in all states must report all cases of suspected abuse, even if the emergency department fails to do so. Most states have special forms for reporting. Supervisors are generally forbidden to interfere with the reporting of suspected abuse, even if they disagree with the assessment. You do not have to prove that there has been abuse. Law enforcement and child protection agencies are mandated to investigate all reported cases.

Sexual Abuse

Children of any age and either gender can be victims of sexual abuse. Most victims of rape are older than age 10 years, although younger children may be victims as well. This type of sexual abuse is often the result of long-standing abuse by relatives.

Your assessment of a child who has been sexually abused should be limited to determining the type of dressing any injuries require. Sometimes, a sexually abused child is also beaten. Therefore, you should treat any bruises or fractures as well. Do not examine the genitalia of a young child unless there is evidence of bleeding, or there is an injury that must be treated.

In addition, if you suspect that a child is a victim of sexual abuse, do not allow the child to wash, urinate, or defecate before a physician completes an exam. Although this step is difficult, it is important to preserve evidence. If the abused child is a girl, ensure that a female EMT-I or police officer remains with the child unless locating one will delay transport.

You must maintain professional composure the entire time you are assessing and caring for a sexually abused child. Assume a concerned, caring demeanor, and shield the child from onlookers and curious bystanders. Obtain as much information as possible from the child and any witnesses. The child may be hysterical or unwilling to say anything at all, especially if the abuser is a relative or family friend. You are in the best position to obtain the most accurate firsthand information about the incident. Therefore, you should record any information carefully and completely on the patient care report.

Transport all children who are victims of sexual assault. Sexual abuse of a child is a crime. Cooperate with law enforcement officials in their investigations.

EMS Response to Pediatric Emergencies

After care and transport of a sick or injured child, you may experience a wide range of powerful emotions. These emotions result from the call itself or from your previous experience (or inexperience) in caring for infants and children. You may feel anxious if you have not had much experience in dealing with infants and children. You may also think of your own children or the children of a loved one.

As a result, you must be prepared to care for children. Practice with children and pediatric equipment is necessary. As you know, children are not simply small adults. However, many of the skills and principles you use to care for adults can be applied to children. You must simply remember there are differences in anatomy and emotions.

After difficult incidents involving children, debriefing is helpful in working through the stress and trauma. It is also a means to help you in the future if you are faced with similar situations. The ability to seek help after difficult episodes is a sign of maturity and confidence.

You are the Provider — Summary

1. What are the most important anatomic and physiological differences between pediatric and adult patients?

Proportionately larger head size, pliable bones, responsive cardiovascular systems, and relatively exposed abdominal organs all are tremendously important when considering the pediatric patient.

2. How must we adjust our assessment and treatment to account for these challenges?

We must have a higher index of suspicion for injuries, particularly to the head, chest, and abdomen, and we must aggressively treat all life threats to prevent cardiopulmonary arrest.

3. What kind of response would you expect from a school-age child?

Developmentally speaking, the school-age child should interact and answer questions. Anxiety would be expected, but no response is abnormal.

4. Even though you have not performed a detailed assessment, based on your initial observations would you consider this patient in critical or stable condition? What does your "gut feeling" tell you?

Your "gut feeling" or "view from the door" should tell you immediately that something is wrong. An unresponsive child with a major mechanism of injury is clearly a critical situation.

5. On the basis of your initial exam, what are the most significant findings and are they immediate life threats?

The child's color is pale, and he is not moving or responding appropriately. Any one of these findings could be potentially life-threatening; his condition is clearly critical.

6. What are you initial priorities for treatment?

Perform an initial assessment, with simultaneous cervical spine stabilization. Address all life threats as they are discovered.

7. What is the etiology of the seizure and how might it be different than the most common pediatric seizures?

You should suspect that this child is experiencing a seizure secondary to brain trauma. Most seizures in children are relatively benign (ie, febrile seizures) and require very little treatment. This child's seizure suggests increased intracranial pressure.

8. How must you adjust your immediate treatment priorities?

With a seizing child (or any seizure patient for that matter) your priorities must be to protect the airway and breathing and terminate the seizure. If possible, obtain vascular access and administer an anticonvulsant medication (ie, Valium).

9. Is this child in immediate need of ventilatory management?

Absolutely! Slow, irregular respirations will not produce adequate tidal volume. As a result, minute volume will fall and the child will become more hypoxic.

10. What are the signs of impending respiratory arrest?

Very fast or very slow respirations, gasping or grunting respirations, decreased chest movement or lung sounds, altered mental status and/or poor muscle tone, and cyanosis (a late sign).

11. What are the most significant challenges of intubation in the pediatric patient?

Smaller airway structures and a proportionately larger tongue. These challenges can be overcome by adjusting your technique and using the appropriately sized intubation equipment.

12. On the basis of the mechanism of injury (25-mph frontal motor vehicle impact, no helmet, loss of consciousness), what injury patterns should you suspect and where should you examine further for injuries?

You should be suspicious for head, abdominal, thoracic, and lower extremity injuries.

13. On the way to the trauma center, what are some treatment options to help deal with the potentially rising intracranial pressure?

Maintain adequate oxygenation and ventilation. In addition, administer IV fluid boluses of 20 mL/kg if hypotension occurs. Hypotension (<80 mm hg in the child) in the brain-injured patient can compromise cerebral perfusion.

Prep Kit

Ready for Review

- The airway in a child has a smaller diameter than the airway in an adult and is therefore more easily obstructed.
- Because the diaphragm is the principal muscle of respiration in children and infants, gastric distention can create breathing difficulties.
- You will need to carry special sizes of airway equipment for pediatric patients.
- Use a length-based resuscitation tape to determine the appropriately sized equipment for children.
- Use the pediatric assessment triangle (PAT) to obtain a general impression of the infant or child.
- In treating possible respiratory failure in a child, always position the airway in a neutral position.
- Use an airway adjunct to maintain an open airway: an oropharyngeal airway in an unresponsive patient, and a nasopharyngeal airway in a conscious patient (unless he or she has sustained head trauma).
- Appropriate oxygen delivery devices include the blow-by technique at 6 L/min, a nonrebreathing mask at 12 to 15 L/min, and a BVM device at 12 to 15 L/min.
- Use a BVM device with a child whose breathing and tidal volume are inadequate and who has an altered level of consciousness. If BVM ventilations are ineffective or if the child will require prolonged ventilatory support, perform endotracheal intubation.
- There are three keys to successful use of the BVM device in a child: (1) Have the appropriate equipment in the right size, (2) maintain a good face to mask seal, and (3) ventilate at the appropriate rate and volume: 12 to 20 breaths/min for an infant or child, or one breath every 3 to 5 seconds. Squeeze gently, and stop squeezing as the chest wall begins to rise.
- Children younger than 5 years often obstruct their upper and lower airway with a variety of foreign objects.
- If the child is conscious, encourage him or her to cough to clear the airway.
- If the child is unresponsive, you should first use the tongue-jaw lift and finger sweeps to try to remove an object that you can see. Never perform blind finger sweeps in infants or children with an airway obstruction.
- In treating an unresponsive infant or child with severe airway obstruction, perform chest compressions, alternating with attempts at artificial breathing.
- In a conscious child who is sitting or standing, apply abdominal thrusts from behind. Continue to perform abdominal thrusts until the obstruction is relieved or the child loses consciousness. In a conscious choking infant, give back slaps and chest thrusts.
- A child who is in early respiratory distress may be breathing too slowly or too fast. Rates greater than 60 breaths/min are a sign of a problem and may require assisted ventilation, especially if tidal volume is reduced (ie, shallow breathing). Look for signs of extra effort to breathe, including nasal flaring and grunting respirations; these may give way to cyanosis—a late sign.
- You must intervene immediately if bradycardia develops in a child in respiratory distress. Use the least upsetting method to administer supplemental oxygen, adding assisted ventilations if it becomes necessary. Consider intubation to definitively secure the airway.
- Cardiac dysrhythmias, such as V-fib and V-tach, are uncommon in children. When dysrhythmias occur, they usually present as bradydysrhythmias.

Technology

- Interactivities
- Vocabulary Explorer
- Anatomy Review
- Web Links
- Online Review Manual

Prep Kit Continued...

- Many bradydysrhythmias in children can be successfully treated with ventilatory assistance and 100% oxygen, thereby negating the use of pharmacologic agents.

- V-fib and pulseless V-tach are treated with immediate defibrillation and pharmacologic interventions.

- Seizures in children may appear as a shaking of the whole body (generalized), a movement in a single arm or leg or eye (partial), or momentary unresponsiveness (absence seizure).

- Complications of seizures are due to injury from seizure motion, airway obstruction, or poor breathing effort.

- Do not put anything into the mouth of a seizing child. Do position the child so that the tongue is not an obstruction, and be prepared to suction secretions or vomitus.

- Febrile seizures, occurring on the first day of a fever, may be a sign of a more serious problem such as meningitis. Begin cooling measures and transport the patient to the hospital.

- Other childhood conditions that require immediate transport include altered level of consciousness, which you may assess using the AVPU scale; severe dehydration; and poisoning.

- The best way to cool a child with a fever is with wet towels that are at room temperature, not cold.

- Children with meningitis will have a fever, altered level of consciousness, and irritability, along with neck pain.

- All patients with possible meningitis should be considered highly contagious and infectious. *Neisseria meningitidis* infection, characterized by tiny red spots or a large purple rash, is a fast-moving, dangerous form of meningitis.

- If you have been exposed to respiratory secretions from a child with this form of the disease, you should take antibiotics.

- Infants and children can go into shock after the loss of even a small volume of fluid or blood, which may be caused by an injury, dehydration, severe infection or allergic reaction, heart disease, or a collapsed lung.

- Children who are in shock often have increased respirations but normal blood pressure until the condition is severe. Changes in skin color and capillary refill are important signs of shock.

- Establish vascular access in any infant or child in shock; administer 20-mL/kg boluses of normal saline or lactated Ringer's solution as needed to maintain adequate perfusion.

- The most common cause of dehydration in children is vomiting and diarrhea. Life-threatening dehydration can develop in an infant in hours. You can determine whether a child's dehydration is mild, moderate, or severe by assessing the child's urine output, level of activity, mental status, skin tone, and pulse.

- BLS for infants and children consists of determining responsiveness and assessing airway, breathing, and circulation.

- If the child is unresponsive but breathing adequately, place him or her in the recovery position unless you suspect a spinal injury. Use the head tilt–chin lift or jaw-thrust maneuver to open the airway in a child who is unresponsive and not breathing.

- If a child is not breathing, provide rescue breathing while keeping the airway open. Breathe for an infant or child between ages 1 year and the onset of puberty (12 to 14 years of age) at a rate of one breath every 3 to 5 second or 12 to 20 breaths/min.

- To provide CPR in an infant, compress the chest at a ratio of 30:2 compressions to ventilations with one rescuer and 15:2 with two rescuers; use two or three fingers, and compress the lower half of the sternum to a depth that is one half to one third the diameter of the chest.

- In children, use the same depth and rate of compressions as you did for the infant; however, use the heel of one or both hands (depending on the child's size) to compress the chest; avoid compressing the xiphoid process.

- A victim of sudden infant death syndrome (SIDS) will be pale or blue, not breathing, pulseless, and unresponsive. He or she may show signs of postmortem changes, including rigor mortis and dependent lividity; if so, call medical control to report the situation.

- If family members insist or protocols mandate, you should initiate CPR and transport infant and family to the emergency department, where the family can receive more extensive support. If the child does not have any evidence of postmortem changes, begin CPR immediately.
- Carefully inspect the environment where a SIDS victim was found, looking for signs of illness, abusive family interactions, and objects in the child's crib.
- Provide support for the family in whatever way you can, but do not make judgmental statements. Allow them to spend time with the child and ride in the ambulance to the hospital.
- Any death of a child is stressful for family members and for health care providers.
- In dealing with the family, acknowledge their feelings, keep any instructions short and simple, use the child's name, and maintain eye contact.
- Be prepared to respond to philosophical as well as medical questions, in most cases by indicating concern and understanding; do not be specific about the cause of death.
- Be alert for signs of posttraumatic stress in yourself and others after dealing with the death of a child.
- It can help to talk about the event and your feelings with your EMS colleagues.

Vital Vocabulary

accessory muscle use A sign of increased work of breathing characterized by chest wall muscle contractions during breathing.

acrocyanosis cyanosis of the hands and feet in newborns and infants younger than 2 months; occurs when the infant is cold; this is a normal finding.

adolescent Person between 12 and 18 years of age.

agonal breathing Slow, shallow, irregular breathing pattern.

altered level of consciousness A mental state in which infants and children may be unresponsive, combative, or confused, may thrash about, or may drift into and out of an alert state; also called altered mental status.

anaphylactic shock Caused by a severe allergic reaction; histamines and other chemicals from the immune system result in severe bronchospasm and vasodilation.

anemia A deficiency of red blood cells.

angioedema Swelling of the soft tissues when fluid enters the interstitial space; may be severe enough to compromise breathing if the airway is involved.

antihistamine Medications, such as diphenhydramine (Benadryl), that are used to block the release of histamines from the immune system; stops an allergic reaction.

apical pulse Obtained by auscultating heart tones over the chest with a stethoscope.

apneic Characterized by absence of breathing.

apparent life-threatening event (ALTE) An event that causes unresponsiveness, cyanosis, and apnea in an infant, who then resumes breathing with stimulation.

asthma Acute spasm and inflammation of the bronchioles in the lungs.

asystole Total absence of electrical and mechanical activity in the heart; appears as a "flatline" on the cardiac monitor.

AVPU scale Used to assess level of consciousness; recorded as being alert, verbally responsive, responsive to pain, or unresponsive.

barotrauma Trauma caused by increased pressure.

blanching Turning white.

blow-by technique Method of delivering oxygen by holding a face mask or similar device near the infant or child's face; used when a nonrebreathing mask is not tolerated.

bradycardia A slow heart rate; less than 80 beats/min in children; less than 100 beats/min in infants.

bradydysrhythmias Narrow QRS complex cardiac rhythms with a slow heart rate; the most common cardiac dysrhythmia seen in children; usually the result of severe hypoxia.

bradypnea Slow respiratory rate; ominous sign in a child; indicates impending respiratory arrest.

bronchiolitis A viral infection that results in inflammation and constriction of the bronchioles; seen most commonly in children younger than 2 years.

Prep Kit continued...

bronchoscope An instrument used to visualize and inspect the large bronchi.

bronchospasm Narrowing or constriction of the bronchioles; caused by an acute inflammatory response, such as asthma.

capillary refill time (CRT) The amount of time that it takes for blood to return to the capillary bed after applying pressure to the skin or nailbed; indicates the status of end-organ perfusion; reliable in children younger than 6 years.

cardiogenic shock Caused by failure of the heart to meet the metabolic needs of the body; an uncommon cause of shock in children.

central cyanosis Cyanosis to the central (core) part of the body; indicates significant hypoxemia.

central pulses Pulses that are closest to core (central) part of the body where the vital organs are located.

cerebrospinal fluid rhinorrhea Drainage of cerebrospinal fluid from the nose.

child abuse Any improper or excessive action that injures or otherwise harms a child or infant; includes physical abuse, sexual abuse, neglect, and emotional abuse.

compensated (early) shock The maintenance of perfusion to the vital organs by decreasing peripheral perfusion; systolic blood pressure is maintained at or near normal.

cricoid pressure The application of posterior pressure to the cricoid cartilage; minimizes gastric distention and the risk of vomiting and aspiration during ventilations; also referred to as Sellick's maneuver.

croup Infection of the airway below the level of the vocal cords, usually caused by a virus; also referred to as laryngotracheobronchitis.

cyanosis A blue discoloration of the skin and mucous membranes; indicates decreased levels of oxygen in the blood.

decompensated (late) shock Occurs when the body is no longer able to effectively compensate for decreased perfusion; characterized by a drop in blood pressure.

dehydration A state in which fluid losses are greater than fluid intake into the body, leading to shock if untreated.

dependent lividity Pooling of the blood in the lower parts of the body after death.

diabetic ketoacidosis (DKA) A potentially life-threatening complication of diabetes mellitus; caused by severe hyperglycemia; results in cellular production of ketones (acids) and severe dehydration.

distributive shock Massive vasodilation and systemic venous pooling of blood caused by a loss of vascular tone; uncommon type of shock seen in children.

dysphagia Difficulty swallowing.

end-organ perfusion The status of perfusion to the vital organs of the body; determined by assessing capillary refill time (CRT).

end-tidal carbon dioxide ($ETco_2$) detectors Determine the presence of carbon dioxide in exhaled air; used as a secondary device for confirmation of correct ET tube placement.

epiglottitis An acute bacterial infection that results in rapid swelling of the epiglottis and surrounding tissues; also referred to as acute supraglottic laryngitis.

epiphyseal plate The growth plate of the bone; responsible for normal bone growth and development.

febrile seizure Seizure relating to fever.

fontanelles Areas where the infant's skull has not fused together; usually disappear at approximately 18 months of age.

functional residual capacity The volume of air remaining in the lungs following exhalation; also referred to as oxygen reserve.

gastric decompression Removal or air or other contents from the stomach.

gastric distention Inflation of the stomach with air; a complication of positive pressure ventilation or when an infant or child breathes too fast and too deep.

greenstick fracture An incomplete fracture of a bone; seen in children, whose bones are pliable and may not completely fracture.

grunting An "uh" sound heard during exhalation; reflects the child's attempt to keep the alveoli open; a sign of increased work of breathing.

head bobbing The head lifts and tilts back during inspiration, then moves forward during expiration; a sign of increased work of breathing.

hepatomegaly Enlargement of the liver.

histamines Chemicals released by the immune system that cause an inflammatory response, such as that seen with asthma or an allergic reaction.

hyperglycemia An abnormally high blood glucose level.

hypoglycemia An abnormally low blood glucose level.

hypovolemic shock Caused by a loss of blood or water from the body; the most common type of shock seen in infants and children.

infancy The first year of life.

intraosseous (IO) infusion Method of delivering fluids or medications into the medullary canal of the bone; used when IV access cannot be quickly obtained.

Jamshedi needle A double needle, consisting of a solid-bore needle inside a sharpened hollow needle; used to access the medullary canal for intraosseous infusion.

length-based resuscitation tape A tape that estimates an infant or child's weight on the basis of length and lists appropriate drug doses and equipment sizes on the tape.

mediastinum The space in between the lungs that contains the trachea, heart, great vessels, and a portion of the esophagus.

medullary canal The space within the bone that contains bone marrow.

meningitis Inflammation of the meninges that cover the spinal cord and the brain.

minute volume The volume of air breathed into and out of the respiratory system each minute.

nares The external openings of the nostrils.

nasal flaring Widening of the nares during inspiration; commonly seen in infants; indicates increased work of breathing.

nasogastric (NG) tube A tube that is inserted into the stomach via the nose; used for gastric decompression.

nasopharyngeal (nasal) airway A basic airway adjunct inserted into a nostril; prevents the tongue from blocking the airway; better tolerated in semiconscious patients with a gag reflex; rarely used in infants.

nebulizer A device that aerosolizes medications for inhalation into the lungs.

Neisseria meningitidis A form of bacterial meningitis characterized by rapid onset of symptoms, often leading to shock and death.

neonatal Referring to the first 28 days of life.

neurogenic shock Occurs when sympathetic nervous system control over the cardiovascular system is lost; results in massive vasodilation, bradycardia, and decreased perfusion.

neutral position An in-line position of the head with the rest of the body; used to maintain the airway in patient's with suspected spinal trauma.

newborn Another term for neonate.

nonrebreathing mask Supplemental oxygen delivery device that contains a reservoir to prevent rebreathing of carbon dioxide; used for patients with adequate breathing; delivers up to 90% oxygen.

nuchal rigidity A stiff or painful neck; commonly associated with meningitis.

occiput The posterior (back) aspect of the head.

orogastric (OG) tube A tube that is inserted into the stomach via the mouth; used for gastric decompression.

oropharyngeal (oral) airway A basic airway adjunct inserted into the mouth; designed to keep the tongue from blocking the airway; used only in unresponsive patients without a gag reflex.

osteomyelitis Infection of the bone and muscle; a potential complication of intraosseous infusion.

parenchyma The tissue of an organ itself.

pediatric assessment triangle (PAT) A structured assessment tool that allows you to rapidly form a general impression of the infant or child without touching him or her; consists of assessing appearance, work of breathing, and circulation to the skin.

pericardiocentesis Insertion of a needle through the chest wall and into the pericardium to remove fluid; definitive treatment for a pericardial tamponade.

perinatal period The period around birth and includes the time from 20 or 28 weeks of pregnancy through 1 or 4 weeks after birth.

pneumonia A common disease that infects the lower airway and the lung; most commonly seen in infants, toddlers and preschoolers; characterized by fever and respiratory distress.

Prep Kit continued...

postictal period The period immediately following a seizure, characterized by extreme tiredness or listlessness.

preschool-age Between 3 and 5 years of age.

pulseless electrical activity (PEA) An organized cardiac rhythm on the cardiac monitor in the absence of a palpable pulse.

rales A crackling breath sound caused by the flow of air through liquid in the lungs; a sign of lower airway obstruction.

reactive airway disease (RAD) A term used to describe any condition that causes hyperreactive bronchioles and bronchospasm.

relative hypovolemia Caused when the vascular space enlarges and cannot accommodate the body's normal blood volume; no actual blood loss occurs.

respiratory arrest Absence of breathing; the most common precursor to cardiopulmonary arrest in children.

respiratory distress The earliest phase of respiratory compromise; most prominently noted by an increased work of breathing.

respiratory failure Occurs when the body has used up its available energy stores and cannot continue to support the extra work of breathing.

respiratory syncytial virus (RSV) A virus that commonly causes bronchiolitis; usually results in life-long immunity following exposure.

retractions Drawing in of the intercostal muscles and sternum during inspiration; a sign of increased work of breathing.

rigor mortis Stiffening of the body after death.

school-age Between 6 and 12 years of age.

separation anxiety Fear of being separated from a dependent, such as a parent or caregiver; common in young children.

sepsis A state of infection.

septic shock Caused by massive sepsis (infection); bacteria attack the blood vessels and prevent them from constricting.

septum A central divider, such as the nasal septum.

shaken baby syndrome Bleeding within the head and damage to the cervical spine as a result of intentional, forceful shaking of an infant or small child.

shock An abnormal condition characterized by inadequate delivery of oxygen and nutrients to the tissues and inadequate removal of metabolic substrates from the body; also called hypoperfusion.

sniffing position Optimum head position for the uninjured child who requires airway management.

spasmodic croup Noninfectious form of croup; presents in the same fashion as viral croup, but in the absence of infection.

status asthmaticus A severe and prolonged asthma attack; characterized by minimal or absent wheezing and minimal to no air movement; cannot be treated successfully with conventional asthma therapy.

status epilepticus The term used to describe a continuous seizure, or multiple seizures without a return to consciousness, for 30 minutes or more.

stridor High-pitched inspiratory breathing sound; indicates a partial upper airway obstruction.

subglottic Below the glottis and vocal cords.

sudden infant death syndrome (SIDS) Unexpected death of an infant or young child that remains unexplained after a complete autopsy.

supraventricular tachycardia (SVT) A narrow QRS complex tachycardia characterized by a heart rate greater than 220 beats/min in the infant or greater than 180 beats/min in the child.

synchronized cardioversion The timed delivery of energy into the myocardium to correct rapid, regular cardiac rhythms in patients who are unstable.

tachydysrhythmias Cardiac rhythms that exceed the maximum normal heart rate estimated for the child or infant's age.

tachypnea Increased respiratory rate.

tenting A condition where the skin remains depressed after you remove your finger; indicates overhydration.

tidal volume The amount of air that is delivered to the lungs in one inhalation.

toddler A child between 1 and 3 years of age.

tongue-jaw lift Grasping the tongue and jaw between your finger and thumb and lifting to open the mouth; used to visualize the airway for foreign bodies.

tonic-clonic seizure A seizure that features rhythmic back-and-forth motion of an extremity and body stiffness.

tracheal tugging Pulling of the trachea into the neck during inspiration; a sign of increased work of breathing.

tragus The small cartilaginous projection in front of the opening of the ear.

transition phase Utilized to allow the infant or child to become familiar with you and your equipment; only appropriate if the child's condition is stable.

tripod position An abnormal position to keep the airway open; it involves leaning forward onto two arms stretched forward.

ventricular tachycardia (V-tach) A wide QRS complex tachycardia with an exceedingly high rate; uncommon in children.

Volutrol A special type of microdrip set; allows you to fill a large drip chamber with a specific amount of fluid to avoid fluid overload.

wheezing High- or low-pitched sound heard usually during expiration; indicates a partial lower airway obstruction.

xiphoid process The lower cartilaginous tip of the sternum.

Assessment in Action

You are dispatched to a motor vehicle crash scene involving a car and a pedestrian. On arrival you find a 5-year-old boy lying in the roadway. He was struck by a vehicle and thrown approximately 10'.

1. As you approach the patient you can visually evaluate all of the following EXCEPT:
   A. interactiveness and movement.
   B. breathing sounds and effort.
   C. skin condition and temperature.
   D. mechanism of injury and bleeding.

2. As you assess the patient you should consider all of the following to be abnormal findings EXCEPT:
   A. diaphragmatic breathing.
   B. emotions of a younger age.
   C. cyanosis of the extremities.
   D. quiet behavior.

3. During the initial assessment you should:
   A. intubate immediately if the child is not breathing.
   B. recognize that respiratory compromise is a critical finding.
   C. apply a cervical collar and then assess ABCs.
   D. assess ABCs immediately then immobilize cervical spine.

4. The most common injuries seen when a child is struck by a vehicle include all of the following EXCEPT:
   A. chest injury.
   B. femur fracture.
   C. abdominal injury.
   D. head injury.

Your assessment reveals an unresponsive 5-year-old child. He is pale, his extremities are cyanotic, and he is cool to the touch. His respirations are rapid, his pulse is rapid and regular, and his capillary refill is delayed. You note a large hematoma to the left side of his head and his abdomen is slightly distended.

5. Your patient's status is:
   A. load and go because he is in ventilatory failure.
   B. load and go because he has a cardiac dysrhythmia.
   C. load and go because he is hypothermic.
   D. load and go because he is in shock.

6. Your immediate treatment will consist of:
   A. initiating an IV and administering a 20-mg/kg bolus.
   B. synchronized cardioversion.
   C. elevating the foot of the backboard.
   D. immobilization and oxygen.

7. You will manage your patient's airway and breathing by:
   A. inserting an oropharyngeal airway along the natural curve of the airway and squeezing the bag-valve-mask device only until the chest rises.
   B. opening the airway using a jaw-thrust technique and ventilating using a demand valve device.
   C. inserting an oropharyngeal airway using the rotation technique and ventilating every 3 seconds.
   D. opening the airway using the head tilt-chin lift technique and fully deflating the bag-valve-mask device with each ventilation.

As you are moving the patient to the ambulance you note that the patient has stopped breathing. Assessment also reveals the patient has no pulse. The monitor shows asystole.

8. You should immediately:
   A. initiate an IV and administer a 20 mg/kg-bolus.
   B. initiate CPR.
   C. hyperventilate the patient.
   D. defibrillate the patient.

9. When performing CPR on your patient you will:
   A. compress the chest 1½" to 2".
   B. compress the chest with two fingers.
   C. compress the chest at a rate of 100 times a minute.
   D. assess the pulse at the brachial artery.

10. Intubation guidelines for your patient include:
    A. use a curved blade size 2.
    B. prepare size 6, 6.5, and 7 tubes.
    C. confirm placement prior to securing the tube in place.
    D. limiting your intubation attempt to a maximum of 30 seconds.

Points to Ponder

You arrive on the scene of a respiratory distress call to find a 4-year-old girl sitting on her mother's lap. The mother tells you that the child was playing quietly when she suddenly started coughing and wheezing. You notice that she has a very weak cough and is cyanotic. You treat the child for an airway obstruction, but her condition worsens. In an effort to remove the object by visualizing the airway, you insert a laryngoscope into the mouth. As you do so, the child stops breathing. You are unable to intubate or ventilate the child because the airway is swollen shut. Your further attempts at resuscitation fail.

What went wrong?

Issues: Understanding Respiratory Distress and Cardiopulmonary Arrest in a Child; Providing an Adequate Assessment Before Initiating Treatment

Geriatric Emergencies

1999 Objectives

Cognitive

6-4.1 Describe dependent and independent living environments. (p 1341)

6-4.2 Identify local resources available to assist the elderly and discuss strategies to refer at-risk patients to appropriate community services. (p 1340)

6-4.3 Discuss expected physiological changes associated with aging. (p 1342)

6-4.4 Describe common psychological reactions associated with aging. (p 1342)

6-4.5 Discuss problems with mobility in the elderly. (p 1348, 1351)

6-4.6 Discuss problems with continence and elimination. (p 1345)

6-4.7 Describe communication strategies used to provide psychological support. (p 1353)

6-4.8 Discuss factors that may complicate the assessment of the elderly patient. (p 1348)

6-4.9 Discuss common complaints, injuries, and illnesses of elderly patients. (p 1349)

6-4.10 Discuss pathophysiology changes associated with the elderly in regards to drug distribution, metabolism, and elimination. (p 1345)

6-4.11 Discuss the impact of polypharmacy, dosing errors, medication non-compliance, and drug sensitivity on patient assessment and management. (p 1354)

6-4.12 Discuss various body system changes associated with age. (p 1344)

6-4.13 Discuss the assessment and management of the elderly patient with complaints related to the following body systems:
- Respiratory
- Cardiovascular
- Nervous
- Endocrine
- Gastrointestinal (p 1344-1346)

6-4.14 Describe the assessment of nervous system diseases in the elderly, including cerebral vascular disease, delirium, dementia, Alzheimer's disease, and Parkinson's disease. (p 1346, 1360)

6-4.15 Discuss the assessment of an elderly patient with gastrointestinal problems, including GI hemorrhage and bowel obstruction. (p 1358)

6-4.16 Discuss the normal and abnormal changes with age related to toxicology. (p 1345)

6-4.17 Discuss the assessment of the elderly patient with complaints related to toxicology. (p 1354)

6-4.18 Describe the assessment and management of the elderly patient with toxicological problems. (p 1354)

6-4.19 Discuss the assessment and management of the patient with environmental considerations. (p 1339)

6-4.20 Discuss the normal and abnormal changes of the musculoskeletal system with age. (p 1346)

6-4.21 Discuss the assessment and management of the elderly patient with complaints associated with trauma. (p 1356)

Affective

6-4.22 Demonstrate and advocate appropriate interactions with the elderly that convey respect for their position in life. (p 1353)

6-4.23 Recognize and appreciate the many impediments to physical and emotional well being in the elderly. (p 1353)

Psychomotor

6-4.24 Demonstrate the ability to assess a geriatric patient. (p 1348)

6-4.25 Demonstrate the ability to apply assessment findings to the management plan for a geriatric patient. (p 1348)

1985 Objectives

There are no 1985 objectives for this chapter.

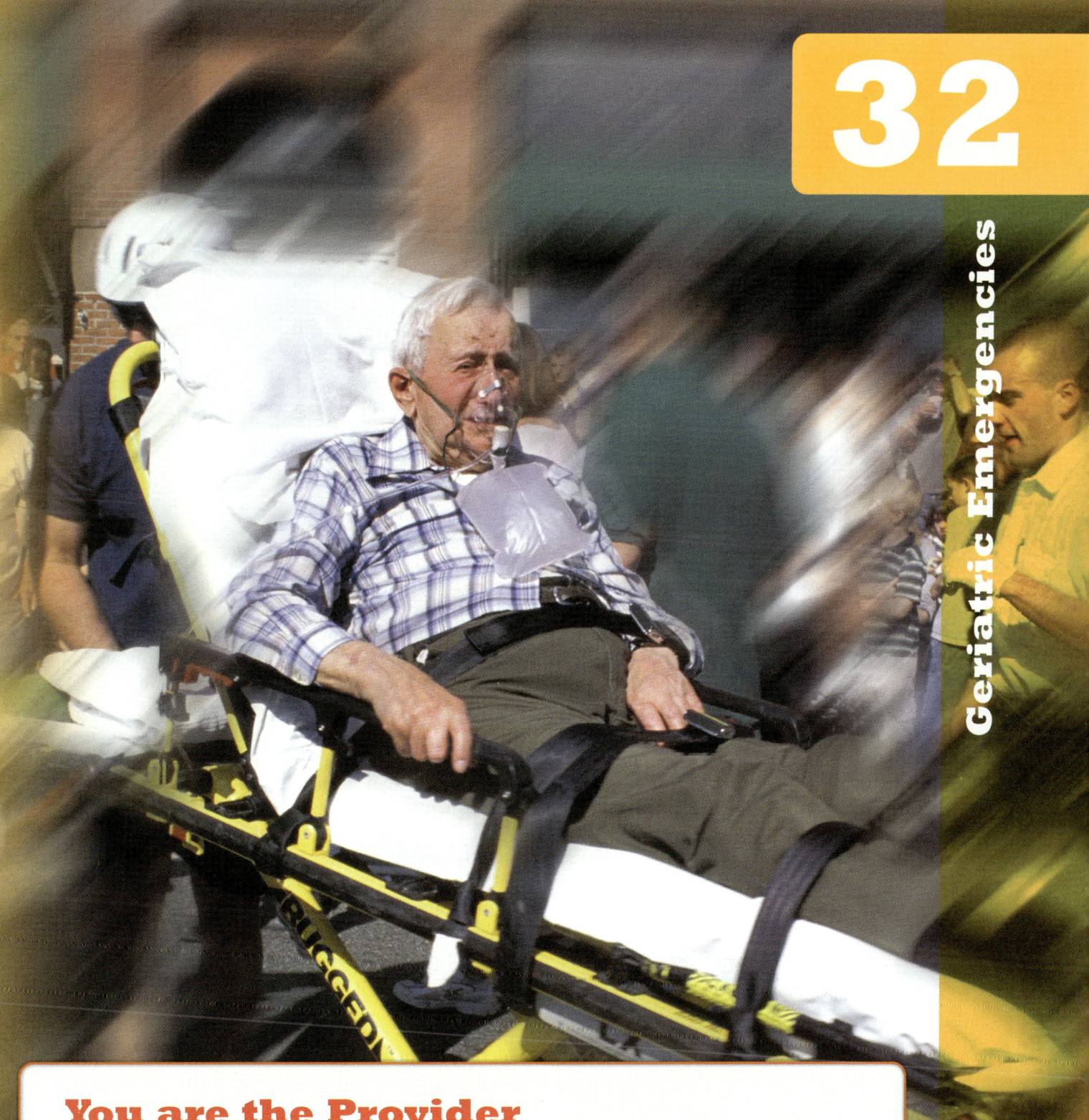

32

Geriatric Emergencies

You are the Provider

You are dispatched to a neighborhood outside your normal response district for a medical alert alarm. The dispatch center was alerted by the alarm company and is advised that there is an elderly couple at the residence. The alarm company attempted to call the residence but there was no answer. The alarm company also advises you that noises can be heard from inside the residence via the monitoring device. Your local police have also been notified and are responding as well.

1. On the basis of the limited information that you have been given, what type of call for assistance do you start to think of?
2. Do the words "elderly" and "medical alarm" automatically bring to mind a biased view of geriatric patients?
3. How do these stereotypes affect patient care? Can providers be guilty of practicing ageism without even realizing it?

Geriatric Emergencies

The term "geriatric" is becoming an integral part of medicine today. Treatment, prevention, and management of disease and disability in later life are becoming more important than ever due to an aging society (Figure 32-1). For some time, EMS education approached the treatment of geriatric patients with the same considerations as those for younger adults. Now, this is beginning to change.

Geriatric patients, or older patients, are generally considered to be persons who are older than 65 years. A decline in our body systems starts in our late 20s and progresses slowly throughout our lifespan. Think of yourself and subtle changes you have seen as a result of aging. Perhaps you have noticed a slight deficit in eyesight or hearing, or difficulty in doing activities you had no problem doing ten years ago. The reality is that we all age, and older persons will become a larger percentage of the population in the new century.

According to the most recent US Census Data, almost 35 million individuals are older than 65 years, which is equal to one in every eight persons, or approximately 12% of the population. Why is the number so large? Remember that people today are living longer than they did 15 to 20 years ago. Advances in medical care and preventive measures have been instrumental in this increased longevity. A child born in 2001 can expect to live 77 years, which is a 30-year increase from a child born in the year 1900. It is projected that by the year 2030, the population of older people will be greater than

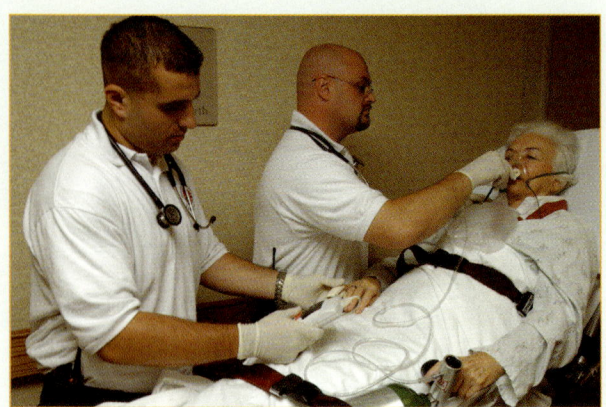

Figure 32-1 Working with geriatric patients is a large part of being an EMS provider.

70 million. This number represents a very significant evolutionary trend for the EMT-I because older people are the major users of the EMS system and health care systems in general. Approximately 34% of EMS calls involve older people. These calls may be confusing to the EMT-I because the classic presentation of medical conditions common in younger patients may not be present in older patients. An acute MI may present in an atypical fashion; nonspecific symptoms such as weakness, dizziness, or nausea are not uncommon. Some older patients may not experience chest pain or pressure (ie, silent MI). An aging body can mask serious medical conditions. Older patients frequently have chronic medical problems and may be taking numerous medications for their illnesses. Providing effective treatment for this growing number of patients will require you to understand the issues related to aging and how you may have to modify some of your assessment and treatment approaches.

We should respect the wealth of knowledge that elderly patients have to offer. In many countries, the elderly are treated with reverence. In many other cultures the elderly are seen as a valuable resource of history. In Japan, there is a "Respect for the Aged Day." Many people in the United States, however, look upon elderly people as burdens to society. As an EMT-I, you must remember to treat every patient the way you would want your loved ones to be treated.

The GEMS Diamond

There are many acronyms in the prehospital setting to help you remember steps in your assessment and treatment. The American Geriatrics Society, in association

Technology

- Interactivities
- Vocabulary Explorer
- Anatomy Review
- Web Links
- Online Review Manual

www.EMSzone.com/EMTI

with the National Council of State EMS Training Coordinators, has developed a mnemonic to help providers recall key themes when dealing with geriatric patients. The GEMS diamond was designed to assist the prehospital professional in the assessment and treatment of elderly patients (Table 32-1). You will be reminded of each theme within this chapter.

"G" of the GEMS diamond is to recognize that the patient is a geriatric patient. The EMT-I's thought process needs to be geared to the possible problems of an aging patient.

"E" of the GEMS diamond stands for an environmental assessment. Assessment begins with scene safety and BSI. If a scene is not safe, attempt to make it safe. If you walk into a room and trip over a rug, should you mention it or act as if nothing happened? Assessment of the environment can help give clues regarding the patient's condition. Contributing factors to the patient's condition may be directly related to something within their environment. The EMT-I can have a profound effect on the patient by suggesting changes in potentially hazardous items found during a home safety check. Preventive interventions for geriatric patients include reviewing the home environment to ensure that safe and livable conditions exist, providing information on preventing falls, and making referrals to appropriate social services agencies when needed. Preventive care is very important for an elderly patient, who may not carefully study the environment or may not realize where risks exist. EMT-Is who respond to the homes of elderly patients are in an ideal position not only to provide immediate help, but also to provide key information to others in the health care and social services systems. Often, simple preventive measures can help the elderly to avoid further injury, costly medical treatment, and death.

"M" of the GEMS diamond stands for medical assessment. Older patients tend to have a variety of medical problems and may be on numerous prescription, over-

TABLE 32-1 The GEMS Diamond

G Geriatric Patients
- Present atypically
- Deserve respect
- Experience normal changes with age

E Environmental Assessment
- Check the physical condition of the patient's home: Is the exterior of the home in need of repair? Is the home secure?
- Check for hazardous conditions that may be present (eg, poor wiring, rotted floors, unventilated gas heaters, broken window glass, clutter that prevents adequate egress).
- Are smoke detectors present and working?
- Is the home too hot or too cold?
- Is there a fecal or urine odor in the home? Is bedding soiled or urine soaked?
- Is food present in the home? Is it adequate and unspoiled?
- Are liquor bottles present? If so, are they lying empty?
- If the patient has a disability, are appropriate assistive devices (eg, a wheelchair or walker) present?
- Does the patient have access to a telephone?
- Are medications out of date, unmarked, or from many physicians?
- If living with others, is the patient confined to one part of the home?
- If the patient is residing in a nursing facility, does the care appear to be adequate to meet the patient's needs?

M Medical Assessment
- Older patients tend to have a variety of medical problems, making assessment more complex. Keep this in mind in all cases—both trauma and medical. A trauma patient may have an underlying medical condition that could have caused, or may be exacerbated by, the injury.
- Obtaining a medical history is important in older patients, regardless of the chief complaint.
- Initial assessment
- Ongoing assessment

S Social Assessment
- Assess activities of daily living (eating, dressing, bathing, toileting)
- Are these activities being provided for the patient? If so, by whom?
- Are there delays in obtaining food, medication, or other necessary items? The patient may complain of this, or the environment may suggest this.
- If in an institutional setting, is the patient able to feed himself or herself? If not, is food still sitting on the food tray? Has the patient been lying in his or her own urine or feces for prolonged periods of time?
- Does the patient have a social network? Does the patient have a mechanism to interact socially with others on a daily basis?

the-counter, and herbal medications. Obtaining a thorough medical history is very important in older patients.

"S" stands for social assessment. There are numerous social agencies that are readily available to help the older patient. Many agencies can provide assistance to our older population, but they must be made aware of the need. Older patients may believe that these social agencies are for "other people" or for the indigent. Many older people also are too proud to ask for help, or don't want anyone else to know they need assistance. Some older people are wary of finances and believe that nothing is ever "free" or that there may be a "catch" involved. Consider obtaining information pamphlets about some of the agencies for older people in your area. If you have these brochures with you and encounter a person in need, you can provide them with this valuable information. Social agencies that deal with the older population will be more than happy to share a listing of the services they provide. If they don't provide direct assistance, they can refer you to someone who can.

Some agencies can provide home meal delivery on a daily or weekly basis. The intent is to provide a meal that is nutritious, but this service also allows the older person contact with someone from the outside. Another benefit that the older population may take advantage of is that health clubs (in association with health insurance companies and aging agencies) may have certain times of the day set aside for a structured exercise program specific for them. This type of program not only provides physical stimulation but provides a social gathering as well. Another social and physical event for seniors may be "mall walking." A local mall may offer early morning access for exercise or walking. Check for the availability of these services in your area. In many areas of the country, home safety checks are being performed. The goal behind these checks is to prevent an injury or fall to the older population. EMS personnel will visit the homes and suggest preventive safety measures such as nonslip rugs, grab handles, and other safety devices. There are also church and/or social agencies that may have social programs for older persons Figure 32-2 .

> **In the Field**
>
> Unless you have a true emergency situation, take care when removing an older patient's clothing for assessment. Use scissors wisely—this may be the only sweater, coat, or undergarment belonging to that person.

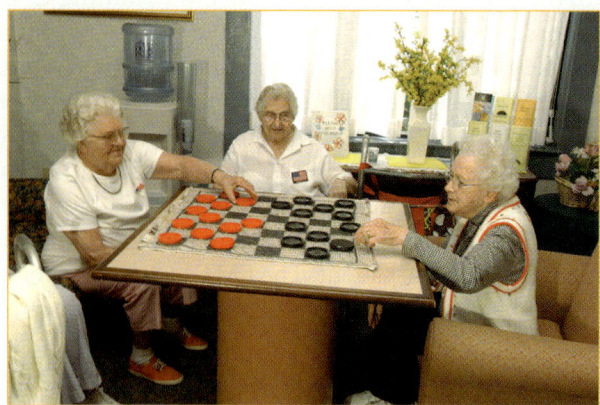

Figure 32-2 Some social agencies have programs for older people.

The Economic Impact of Aging

As an EMT-I, you need to be aware of the economic impact of aging. Many older people today did not have the benefit of retirement planning. Money may be tight. The Social Security Administration reports that the four major sources of income for older people are social security, income from assets, pensions, and earnings. Of these four sources, 91% of older people report Social Security as their major source of income. For many older people, this is their only source of income, causing them to balance their needs on a monthly basis. Older people may not seek medical assistance because of the concern over cost.

The cost of prescriptions for older persons may cause some patients to either skip days of their medication or cut their dosage in half. According to Families USA Foundation, the average annual prescription spending

> **EMT-I Tips**
>
> Of the 40 million Medicare beneficiaries, approximately:
> - 34% (14 million) have no prescription medication coverage
> - 30% (12 million) have inadequate prescription medication coverage (unreliable, costly, or both)
> - 12% (5 million) have Medicaid coverage
> - 24% (10 million) have retirement coverage from prior employment
>
> Nearly two-thirds (64%) of Medicare beneficiaries have no coverage or inadequate coverage (unreliable, costly, or both).

per older person is more than $1,200 and is projected to be $2,800 in 2010. Therefore, many older people who have reached retirement age continue to be a part of the workforce to supplement their limited income.

Independent and Dependent Living

Not all geriatric patients that you are called to assist will be living in a nursing home; in fact, only a small percentage of older people live in nursing homes. Many older patients are able to live independently. You may also encounter a senior citizen who is the primary caregiver for his or her parent or parents. Many times these patients will be in the same home in which they grew up. Be aware that many of these same patients have a fear that if you take them to the hospital, they will never see their home again.

Most healthy older adults strive to live independently. They may believe that they are able to care for themselves and handle activities of daily living (ADLs). When one of the adults becomes ill and can no longer take care of himself or herself, that person becomes dependent upon others in the home. Depending on the age and health of the others in the home, someone else may become a caregiver. Many older couples or friends and family who live together can provide basic assistance for each other; however, some older patients do not have family or friends to assist them. They are totally dependent on themselves, may attempt to do everything on their own, and may not seek available assistance. Patients who become isolated from outside social events are susceptible to self-abuse or alcohol or medication abuse.

> ### In the Field
>
> Oftentimes you will encounter a couple who has been together for many years with no immediate family. In times of crisis, the patient is cared for and the spouse is forgotten due to the situation. If the spouse cannot drive, there may be no way for him or her to get to the hospital, and he or she may not be able to contact the hospital to follow up on the loved one's progress. You can help by simply asking a bystander, fire fighter, police officer, or anyone who is not directly caring for the patient to help the spouse into the passenger seat of the ambulance and to fasten the seat belt so that when you are ready to go, the spouse is ready also. This request only takes a few minutes for you but is so important to the spouse.

What happens when an individual is unable to care for himself or herself? For financial reasons or previous experience, the family may decide to provide care to the older patient in the home. They may seek the help of a visiting nurse agency. Outsiders, as well as the EMT-I, may believe the patient can receive better care in a dependent care facility. You need to remember that families have their reasons for wanting an older patient to stay in a familiar home environment. Sometimes older patients refuse to accept that they need assistance, and may not be aware of the danger in insisting on caring for themselves. The care of an older patient may fall upon a spouse or family members who may have

You are the Provider — Part 2

A neighbor arrives to let you into the home. As the door opens you notice an older woman lying on the living room floor. She is conscious, alert, and complaining of pain to her hip. You look around and notice that the home is not well kept. It appears the patient may have tripped over a loose rug on the floor. The patient states she was heading toward the bedroom for a distress call from her husband. The police officer returns from the bedroom and states that no one is in the room, much to your surprise. Your partner returns from the bedroom and tells you that a hospital bed in the room appears to have been used recently.

4. Do you now have enough resources on scene to deal with two potential patients? Are there other methods to determine if there is actually another patient?
5. What types of questions do you feel would be appropriate for this patient?
6. Do you feel that it is an appropriate time to question your patient about the status of her husband?

additional medical problems themselves. You may respond to a home or facility for a patient only to find out that the caregiver is actually more in need of care than the patient. The stress of caring for a chronically ill person can become overwhelming. Caregivers may be so focused on caring for the patient that they neglect their own health care and/or social needs. For example, a caregiver may be afraid to leave the house, may limit social interactions, and may need help for his or her own stress.

Dependent living (sometimes known as residential care) has many different levels of assistance. The level is based on two factors. One is based upon the needs of the person, while the other is based upon restrictions that are placed upon the individual. Dependent care can range from the least restrictive retirement community to the structured skilled nursing facility and dementia/Alzheimer's specialty care facilities.

Leading Causes of Death

The leading causes of death in older people include heart disease, cancer, stroke, COPD, pneumonia, diabetes, and trauma. Contrary to popular belief, people do not die of "old age." The oldest documented person lived for 122 years. The aging physiology of older people makes them more vulnerable than younger people to the effects of disease and injury. In addition, acute illness and trauma are more likely to involve organ systems beyond those initially involved. For example, an older person who has fallen and fractured a hip may have pneumonia during recovery because of a weakened immune system. Table 32-2 lists the risk factors that affect mortality in older patients.

TABLE 32-2	Risk Factors Affecting Mortality in Older Patients

- Age older than 75 years
- Living alone
- Recent death of a spouse or significant other
- Recent hospitalization
- Incontinence (inability to hold urine or feces)
- Immobility
- Unsound mind

Physiologic Changes That Accompany Age

As we get older, our anatomy and physiology changes. In general, a 65-year-old person cannot expect to have the same degree of physical performance as when he or she was 30 years old. By the time a person reaches age 65 years, the amount of total body water and the numbers of total body cells have decreased by as much as 30%. Generally, after 30 years of age, organ systems begin to deteriorate at a rate of approximately 1% per year. The heart muscle thickens, the arteries becomes less elastic, maximum vital capacity of the lungs may decline as much as 40% between the ages of 20 and 65. However, the aging process does not necessarily mean that a person will experience disease.

Common stereotypes about older persons include the presence of mental confusion, illness, a sedentary lifestyle, and immobility. Although these perceptions are common, they are usually very far from the truth. Older persons can continue to stay fit and active even though they will not be able to perform at the same level as they did in their youth Figure 32-3 . Most older individuals lead very active lives, participating in sports and in the community, and they are generally healthy despite the aging process. What happens to our body system when we age?

- Motor nerves begin to deteriorate, reaction time decreases
- Steady increase in blood pressure
- Decreased ability to maintain normal body temperature
- Muscles become less flexible and strength declines

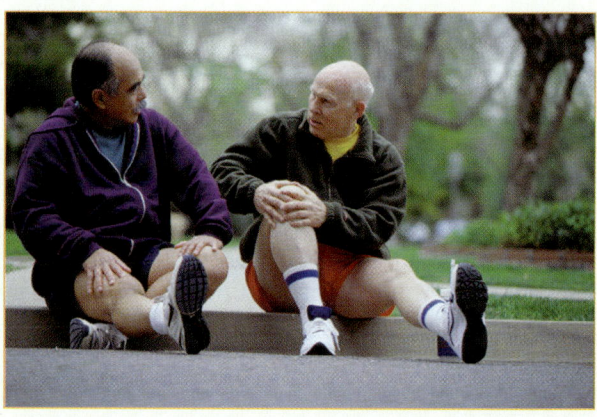

Figure 32-3 Older people can continue to stay fit and active.

- O_2/CO_2 exchange in the lungs and at the cellular level declines, body fatigues at faster rate than when younger
- Metabolism rate decreases, weight gain may result

Skin

Collagen, a protein that is the chief component of connective tissue and bones, decreases as we age, making the skin wrinkled, thinner, and more susceptible to injury. Because the elasticity of the skin has declined, bruising becomes more common because the peripheral blood vessels cannot constrict and stop the bleeding as quickly. This causes a greater number of bruises as well as large hematomas from minimal trauma. The healing process takes longer as we age because of a decrease in the blood flow to the capillaries. There are also fewer sweat glands, and older skin feels dry. The body's ability to regulate heat is also affected by the decrease in the sweat glands. Remember these changes when you respond to a home and the patient may be wearing multiple layers of clothing. Less fat rests under the skin, making pressure sores more common in the older, bed-bound patient 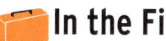. These sores (also called decubitus ulcers) form when the patient lies in the same position for a long period of time, allowing the body to cut off the blood flow to an area of already thin skin, which in turn results in tissue death and development of a pressure sore. It is for this reason that those confined to a bed or stationary position need special care and a regular regimen of documented position changes every one to two hours.

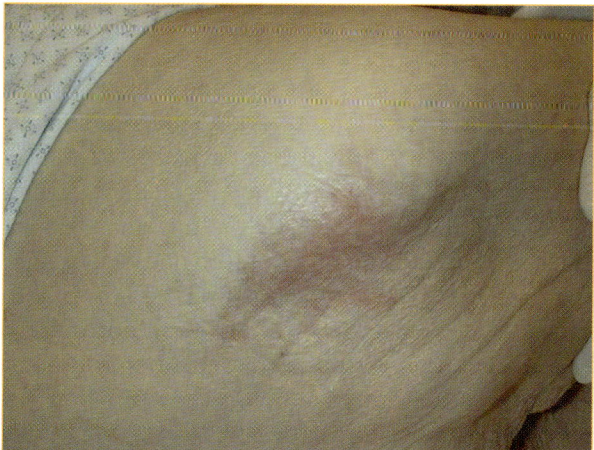

Figure 32-4 A pressure sore. This sore is in stage 1, meaning it is in the early stages of development.

Senses

Studies show that changes to the senses increase as we age. In our 40s, hearing begins to decline. As we age into our 50s, vision and tactile senses decrease. Taste senses begin to change in our 60s, although the ability to smell does not begin to diminish until our 70s.

Vision

As people age, the pupils of the eyes begin to lose the ability to handle changes in light and require more time to adjust, which can make driving and walking more hazardous. Light changes and the increase of glare can cause problems of visual acuity and depth perception. Cataracts, clouding of the lenses or their surrounding membranes, interfere with vision and make it difficult to distinguish colors and see clearly, increasing the likelihood of falls, and account for some mistakes when an older person is taking medication.

Glaucoma, which affects peripheral vision, is a group of diseases that affect the optic nerve and the clogging of the drainage canals, resulting in increased intraocular pressure. This disease is a gradual process and affects nearly 3 million people. Vision loss from cataracts can be repaired with surgery; however, vision loss from glaucoma is not able to be restored. Many older patients depend on their prescription glasses. Misplaced glasses can make the easiest task become impossible. Changes in the vision of older people may include limited depth perception or an inability to see things clearly (even with prescription lenses).

Macular degeneration is a disease that reduces the center of vision. The macula in the retina of the eye is responsible for detailed vision such as reading. This disease may cause small or large items to seem different than they really are. Color perception can also vary within both eyes. Patients with macular degeneration have the ability to see outlines of subjects but the center portion of the object may appear as a dark spot.

> ### In the Field
> When treating a patient with a visual impairment, always stay in direct contact with the patient. If you are not touching the patient, allow him or her to rest a hand on your arm or leg for their comfort. Also explain any procedures in advance so that your patient is not taken by surprise.

Hearing

Changes in the inner ear make hearing high-frequency sounds difficult—muffled sounds are sometimes not even heard. For this reason, increasing the volume of your voice may not make it any easier for the patient to hear your words. These changes can also cause problems with balance, increasing the risk of falls. To compensate for the hearing deficits, many older patients are prescribed hearing-assistance devices (eg, hearing aids). Approximately 75% of older patients have some type of hearing deficit. These devices, however, do not always return hearing to normal levels. Simple actions such as helping patients to insert their hearing device will increase your ability to communicate. Many audiologists have brochures to help patients with these devices. It would be beneficial for you to read this same information and obtain additional training about inserting a hearing aid and how to make minor repairs. A buildup of <u>cerumen</u> (earwax) may also contribute to hearing problems.

EMT-I Tips

Always position yourself so that you are on the "good" side of the patient with a hearing deficit. Because hearing deficits usually involve the loss of high-frequency sounds, yelling in the patient's ear will only serve to further distort the patient's hearing.

Taste

Changes in appetite may occur because of a decrease in the number of taste buds. By the time we are in our 70s, we have approximately one-third fewer taste buds. Although these changes are gradual over our lifetime, the salty and sweet sensation appears to be among the first to diminish. It is important to note that a patient with diminished taste may not be able to discern fresh food from spoiled food. Older people commonly add large amounts of salt to their food in an attempt to improve its taste. Patients with a history of hypertension and limited sodium intake restrictions may need to consider alternate seasonings.

Touch

The sense of touch decreases from loss of the end nerve fibers. This loss, in conjunction with the slowing of the peripheral nervous system, can create situations where an older person can have a delayed reflex reaction when touching something hot, resulting in a burn. The touch of a provider's hand is very comforting and reassuring and should be considered in your assessment. Many older patients may grasp your hand as a means for comfort or during severe pain episodes.

Smell

The sense of smell is among the last to diminish. However, factors such as upper respiratory infections (ie, the common cold), which older persons are more prone to, can affect the sense of smell.

Respiratory System

Although the alveoli become enlarged, their elasticity decreases, making it harder to expel the used air in an older person's lung tissue. This lack of elasticity, caused by a decrease in pulmonary surfactant, results in a decreased ability to exchange oxygen and carbon dioxide, which causes an increase in residual volume. The body's receptors that monitor the changes in oxygen and carbon dioxide slow with age, which causes lower pulse oximetry readings even in healthy individuals. A decrease in the number of cilia that line the bronchial tree lessens the ability to cough and therefore increases the chances of infections such as pneumonia. A patient who is having trouble breathing may have decreased use of the accessory muscles because of the decrease in muscle mass that accompanies aging Figure 32-5▶. This decrease in muscle mass and strength associated with the respiratory system may also increase the likelihood of an airway obstruction from either secretions or food particles.

Cardiovascular System

Cardiac output, which is the amount of blood pumped from the heart in one minute, is a measure of the workload of the heart. Normally, an increased demand on the cardiovascular system is compensated for by increasing the heart rate, increasing the contraction of the heart, and constricting the blood vessels to nonvital organs in order to shunt blood to vital organs. It is estimated that the heart will beat approximately 3 billion times in a lifetime. Over this period of time it is normal that the electrical conduction system will show signs of wear. The cells of the sinoatrial node (the heart's primary pacemaker) will decrease in number and in function; therefore, dysrhythmias may begin to develop. Aging decreases a person's ability to increase heart rate, increase cardiac contraction strength, and constrict, or narrow, blood

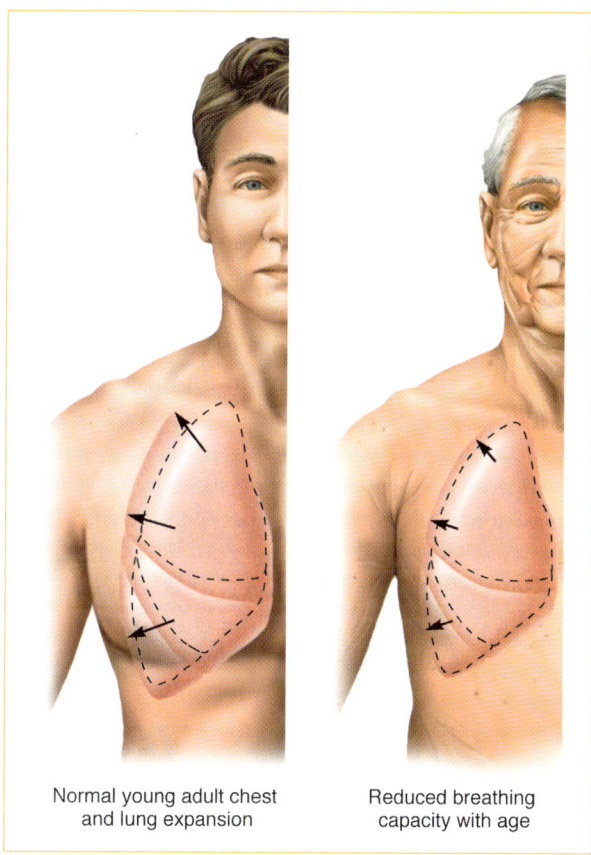

Figure 32-5 Breathing capacity can decrease by up to 50% during the aging process.

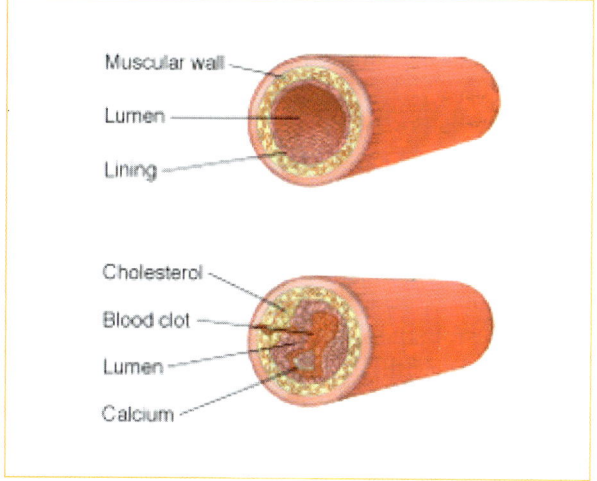

Figure 32-6 Atherosclerosis, the buildup of fatty plaque on arterial walls, may progress to the point that the plaque occludes the artery.

vessels (called <u>vasoconstriction</u>) because of stiffer vessels. Many older patients are at risk for <u>atherosclerosis</u>, an accumulation of fatty material in the arteries 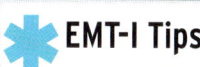. Major complications of atherosclerosis include myocardial infarction and stroke. The presence of <u>arteriosclerosis</u>, a disease that causes the arteries to thicken, harden, and calcify, increases the risk of stroke, heart disease, hypertension, and bowel infarction. Older people are also at an increased risk for an <u>aneurysm</u>, a weakening in the wall of a blood vessel (usually an artery), resulting in an area of dilation or "ballooning" of the vessel. Severe blood loss occurs when an aneurysm ruptures.

Renal System

In older people, kidney function declines because of a 30% to 40% decrease in the number of and function of nephrons. Nephrons are the cells that make up the kidney. In addition to removing waste products from the body in general, the kidneys are also important in eliminating certain medications from a person's system. With a decrease in renal function, levels of medications may rise—perhaps to toxic levels. For this reason, the prescribing theory for older patients is to start low and go slow. Many patients will need to have therapeutic blood levels drawn when placed on a new medication or when there is a change in dosing. Electrolyte disturbances are also more likely to occur as a result of decreased filtration of the blood.

> **EMT-I Tips**
>
> Due to the amount of time that drugs remain in the system of an older person, it is often recommended that half doses are given to any person older than 70 years or to those persons with known renal or liver dysfunction. Follow your local protocols and medical direction in these cases.

Nervous System

The number of neurons (nervous system cells) in some areas of the body may decrease by as much as 45%. By age 85 years, a 10% reduction in brain weight and size can result in increased risk of head trauma, due to a larger area in the skull in which the brain can move during injury. Short-term memory impairment, a decrease in the ability to perform psychomotor skills, and slower reflex times are all normal in the aging process. This decline may make assessment of the older patient challenging. It is important to know an older patient's normal abilities to determine the patient's current status.

Specific Neurologic Conditions and Problems

Parkinson's Disease. Parkinson's disease involves the nerve cells in the motor area of the brain. A patient with Parkinson's disease may present with uncontrollable shaking beginning unilaterally and progressing to other areas (including the face); the shaking appears to increase during times of stress. It normally can be seen when a patient is sitting still. Parkinson's is due to a breakdown of the cells causing a deficiency of dopamine, which causes the messages to be improperly sent. Dopamine is a neurotransmitter that carries messages to the body.

Alzheimer's Disease. Scientists are not sure what causes Alzheimer's disease; however, they believe it is caused by a problem surrounding the death of neurons in the brain. The disease begins gradually, with difficulty performing routine tasks and/or forgetting recent events. As it advances, personality changes, impaired judgment, and impaired ability to communicate thoughts or ideas become more prominent. Alzheimer's disease is the most common form of dementia, affecting 10% of persons older than 65 years and almost 50% of persons older than 85 years. Approximately 56% of patients with dementia have some stage of Alzheimer's disease.

Musculoskeletal System

As the disks between the vertebrae begin to narrow, and a decrease in height of between 2″ and 3″ may occur through a lifespan. A decrease in the amount of muscle mass often results in less strength, and fractures are more likely to occur because of a decrease in bone density (osteoporosis). Posture also changes as flexion at the neck and an anterior curling of the shoulders produce a condition called **kyphosis** (also called humpback, hunchback, or Pott's curvature), making immobilization of older persons more challenging.

Gastrointestinal System

A decrease in the volume of saliva and gastric juices causes older people to experience a dry mouth, making it harder to masticate (chew) and begin to digest foods. A slowing of the intestinal tract may cause constipation or fecal impaction. Decreased liver function makes it harder to detoxify the blood and eliminate substances such as medications and alcohol.

This can make it difficult for patients and their physician to find the appropriate dosage when taking new medications.

Immune System

Sepsis occurs as the result of an infection. Infection is usually caused by germs (ie, bacteria, viruses, fungi) and may affect a part of (local) or the entire (systemic) body. The degree of sepsis can vary, from such a common occurrence as a dental abscess to the more severe sepsis, which affects more than one of the body's organs or systems. Septic shock occurs when hypoperfusion occurs following severe systemic infection. The signs and symptoms of septic shock may be fever, respiratory distress, increased pulse rate, generalized weakness, and hypotension. Site-specific infections may allow other signs and symptoms to be present. A patient with a urinary tract infection may have a foul odor associated with the urine and sometimes pain upon urinating or cloudy urine. Patients may develop infections through their lungs, through a urinary catheter, or even through intravenous access.

Advance Directives

Many individuals today are making use of **advance directives**, which are specific legal documents that direct relatives and caregivers about what kind of medical treatment the patient wishes to receive if he or she cannot speak for himself or herself. An advance directive is also commonly called a living will. Mentally competent adults and emancipated minors have the right to consent to or decline treatment, provided that they are competent to do so. The definition of competence is often hotly debated, but a person who is older than 18 years, alert to person, place, and time, not intoxicated, and who understands the consequences of his or her decision, is generally deemed competent. Unfortunately, patients who are unresponsive or in a medical crisis are not able to inform medical personnel about their wishes to consent to or decline treatment. It is dangerous to take someone else's word for what the patient's wishes are; this is the reason that written advance directives have been developed.

Advance directives may also take the form of "Do Not Resuscitate" (DNR) orders, sometimes called "Do Not Attempt Resuscitation" (DNAR) orders. DNR orders give you permission not to attempt resuscitation for a patient in cardiac arrest. However, for a DNR order to be valid, in general, the patient's medical problems must be clearly stated, and the form must be signed by the patient or legal guardian and by one or more physicians. In most states, the form must be dated within the preceding 12 months. Even in the presence of a DNR order, you are still obligated to provide supportive measures that may include oxygen delivery, pain relief, and comfort when you can. DNR does not mean do not treat. Learn and become familiar with your state laws regarding this issue.

A durable power of attorney for health care is an advance directive that is exercised by an individual who has been authorized by the patient to make medical decisions for the patient. Be sure to follow your service's protocol when faced with any advance directive.

Dealing with advance directives has become more common for EMS providers as more individuals are electing to use hospice services and spend their final days at home (Figure 32-7 ▶). Although advance directives may be in place, family members or caregivers who are faced with the final moments of their loved one's life or when the patient's condition worsens often panic and call 9-1-1. Family members and caregivers may then become upset if you take resuscitative action and begin transportation to the hospital. It is important to understand that many family members or caregivers call 9-1-1 because they do not want to be alone during such a stressful time.

Another common situation is the transportation of patients from nursing facilities. Specific guidelines vary from state to state; however, you should consider the following general guidelines:

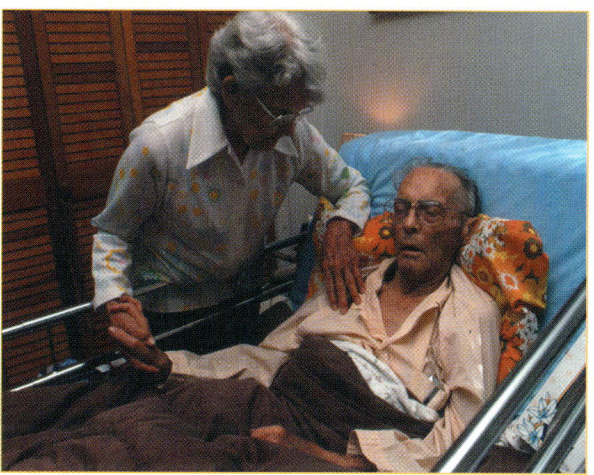

Figure 32-7 More individuals are electing to use hospice services and to receive care in their own home.

- Patients have the right to refuse treatment, including resuscitative efforts, provided that they are competent and able to communicate their wishes.
- A DNR order is valid in a health care facility only if it is in the form of a written order by a physician.
- You should periodically review state and local protocols and legislation regarding advance directives.
- When you are in doubt or when there are no written orders, you should begin resuscitative measures.

It is essential that every EMT-I become familiar with his or her state regulations and local protocols regarding advance directives. Every service should also

You are the Provider   Part 3

Your assessment shows a 67-year-old woman who is lying in a left lateral recumbent position. She is complaining of severe pain to the left side. She states that last night she got up to respond to a call for assistance from her husband. The patient denies having any medical history or taking medications, although medication bottles are visible from where you are standing. The patient is unsure of her last oral intake or whether she has any allergies.

7. What methods can you use to find out a patient's medical or prescribed medication history?
8. Are there other methods to determine a patient's history or medications if the patient is unsure or unresponsive?

provide additional training on the actions you should take when presented with advance directives. When in doubt, your best course of action is to take resuscitative action that is appropriate to the situation and to practice sound medical treatment. In a court of law, it is easier to defend why you attempted resuscitation as opposed to not attempting resuscitation.

Patient Assessment

Any time you assess a patient, start with the same basic approach: scene size-up, initial assessment, and a focused history and physical exam. Assessing an older patient is no different; however, there are some issues that may require you to modify your approach to the initial assessment or become more aware of some conditions that may affect older patients.

Scene Size-up

As you approach any scene, you must be keenly aware of the environment and the reason you were called. Recall the "E" of the GEMS diamond. Activities of daily living such as the ability to move around, talk on the telephone, prepare and eat meals, perform basic cleaning skills, and attend to personal hygiene are essential for continued health in all individuals. For older people, normal aging or a disease process may make activities of daily living difficult and cause a cascade of problems. For example, suppose that a 70-year-old woman, who trips on a loose carpet, falls and breaks her hip. She lives alone and has no one to help her with cooking and other daily activities. Her hip is treated, but in the following months of therapy, she fears the thought of falling again and does as little as she can. She becomes weaker and begins to have some difficulty walking, lifting even small objects, shopping, and making meals. She loses some weight and becomes weaker and is eventually forced to move to an adult care facility because of her need for constant help. All of this was the result of a simple fall.

When you first arrive at a patient's residence, you should look for important clues to determine not only your safety, but also that of the patient. The environment will provide a great deal of important information if you know where to look and what to look for.

The general condition of the home will give you some important clues. Are there hazards, such as steep stairs, missing or loose handrails, or other things that could cause a fall Figure 32-8 ? Is it evident that the person may be having difficulty keeping the house clean?

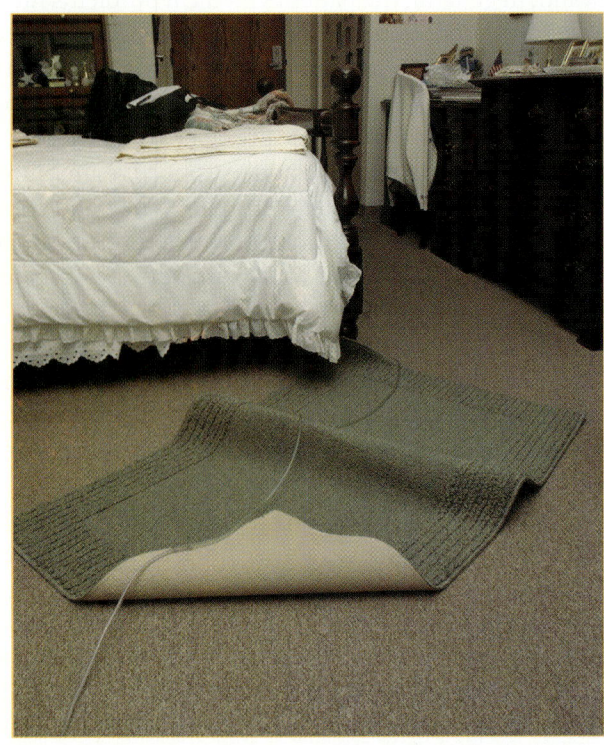

Figure 32-8 Loose rugs may increase the chance of the patient falling.

Is there evidence of adequate food, water, heat, lighting, and ventilation? Are there many pill bottles around, indicating treatment for multiple disease processes? Does someone else live there who can help to answer your questions? These are very important scene clues that can provide a wealth of information before you even make contact with the patient.

Initial Assessment

The sequence of the initial assessment is the same for pediatric, adult, and geriatric patients. However, you should not make any assumptions about an older patient's level of consciousness. Never assume that an altered mental status is normal. Altered mental status indicates some level of brain dysfunction and is a serious problem. The best rule of thumb is to always compare the patient's current level of consciousness or ability to function with the level or ability before the problem began. Do not assume that confusion or unresponsiveness is normal behavior for anyone. In many cases, you will have to rely on a family member or caregiver to determine the patient's baseline level of consciousness and how it has changed as a result of the event Figure 32-9 .

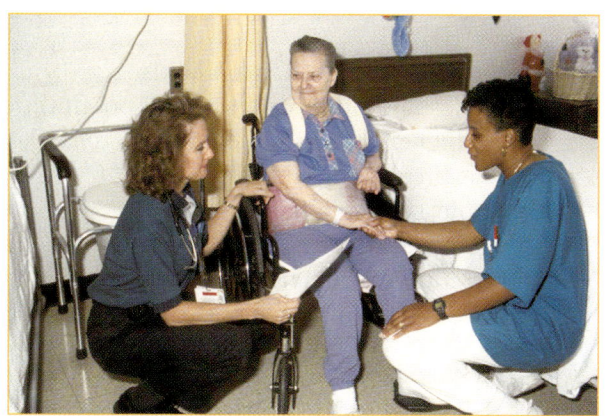

Figure 32-9 Interview family members, friends, and caregivers as part of your assessment of an older patient.

During the initial assessment, you will assess the patient's chief complaint and ABCs. If a life-threatening condition exists, you will have to perform emergency treatment before continuing your assessment. The initial assessment sets the tone and helps you to decide whether the patient requires a rapid resuscitative approach or a slower, contemplative one. In many cases, the slower, contemplative approach is all that is needed.

> **EMT-I Tips**
>
> To minimize distraction and confusion, have only one responder speak to the patient at a time. Another responder can gather the medical history from relatives or a caregiver or examine the scene for helpful information.

Most Common Geriatric Complaints

An older patient can have multiple complaints or the primary complaint can be caused by a secondary complaint. Many patients will only reveal a lesser complaint during questions asked in your assessment. Additionally, they may not consider the secondary complaint to be important. Determining the chief complaint can be extremely difficult at times. As an EMT-I, you will have to play the role of detective many times to determine the actual complaint. The more facts and information that you can obtain from the patient and bystanders or caregivers, the more informed your treatment decision will be. The patient who is in respiratory distress may not be complaining about the shortness of breath, but may be complaining of feeling dizzy. Are the two complaints related? A patient who is hypoxic will complain of being dizzy. Older patients can develop a tolerance to their diseases. Many have been able to modify their lifestyles around their diseases. In addition, some older patients don't want to bother anyone. This mindset causes a delay in seeking help and may exacerbate the patient's condition. Many older patients attribute their medical condition merely to the process of aging.

Shortness of Breath

Many of your older patient contacts involve a patient who is complaining of respiratory distress, either acutely or chronically. Remember that, in addition to the shortness of breath, another condition may be an underlying cause. Obtaining an accurate pertinent medical and prescribed medication history may help you determine the etiology of the problem (ie, respiratory versus cardiac). If the patient has a history of pedal edema, discomfort of the chest and hypertension, the cause may be cardiac related. A productive cough and signs of emphysema point toward a respiratory condition. Patients in respiratory distress should not be overwhelmed with questions. Many times a bystander or family member may be able to answer your questions. Consider asking your patient to nod yes or no in response to questions. It is important to find out whether the patient has a history of respiratory problems and what, if any, medications they are taking. Determining the onset of symptoms is a crucial part of your initial patient contact (using the OPQRST-I mnemonic). Patients experiencing respiratory distress should receive supplemental oxygen as soon as possible and be observed for signs of inadequate breathing, which would necessitate assisted ventilations. Nonrebreathing masks can be intimidating to an older patient; they may want to remove the mask to answer your questions. If you remove the patient's glasses, replace them once you have applied the mask. If the patient cannot tolerate the nonrebreathing mask, use a nasal cannula. Some older patients with COPD may be on home oxygen. Many of these patients will medicate themselves. Medications taken prior to your arrival may affect your treatment, so gather this important information, if possible.

Chest Pain

Older patients may experience and present with chest pain differently than the general population. Patients may delay calling for assistance and believe the pain will go away just as in previous episodes. The OPQRST-I mnemonic of pain in the older patient is important. Remember that the pain threshold of older patients may be different. If the patient has a history of angina, determine if this episode is different from previous events. Is the patient taking the medication that is prescribed for the condition? Many times the patient will not use the term pain, but may use the word "discomfort" or "fluttering."

> **In the Field**
>
> It is important to remember that an older person experiencing a myocardial infarction may only complain of dyspnea, weakness, or a syncopal episode. There may be no associated pain. Instead of asking about pain directly say, "Describe to me exactly how you feel."

Altered Mental Status

An altered mental status is not normal. You need to rapidly determine if this is a patient who requires immediate transport. When you are assessing a patient who is exhibiting signs of altered mental status, it is important to determine the onset of symptoms. Ascertain what is normal for this patient and if the patient has a pertinent history that may be attributed to the complaint. If the patient is a diabetic, have the appropriate medications been taken? Is it possible the patient may have taken the wrong medication or taken alcohol with medications? Because of cost concerns, many older patients will try medications that are not prescribed for them. They may be taking a medication that is prescribed for a spouse who has a similar problem, or worse, a completely different problem.

Potential causes of altered mental status can be remembered using the VITAMINS C & D mnemonic:

- **V**ascular: stroke, brain, embolism
- **I**nflammation: inflammation of the blood vessels in the brain
- **T**oxins: carbon monoxide poisoning
  Trauma: concussion, intracerebral hemorrhage
  Tumors: primary brain tumor, or metastasis (developed elsewhere and spread to the brain)
- **A**utoimmune: production of immune system components against a normal structure in the body
- **M**etabolic: liver or renal failure, hypoglycemia, hyperglycemia, hypothyroidism or hyperthyroidism, hyperosmolar hyperglycemic nonketotic coma (HHNC)
- **I**nfection: meningitis, encephalitis
- **N**arcotics and other drugs: many possibilities, with a higher chance of mental status changes if there is preexisting CNS disease
- **S**ystemic: sepsis, hypoxia
- **C**ongenital: seizures
- **D**egenerative: Alzheimer's disease and other dementias, Parkinson's disease

Abdominal Pain

The geriatric patient who complains of abdominal pain will be among the most frustrating for the EMT-I. The reason for frustration is trying to determine what may be causing the pain. One half of older patients presenting with abdominal pain will require hospital admission and one third will need surgical interventions. Acute versus chronic pain may help in your assessment, and the mnemonic OPQRST-I of pain may help you determine what is happening to your patient. There are numerous causes of acute abdominal pain in the geriatric population, including inflammation, infection, and ischemic disorders. The patient may have a difficult time localizing the pain and describing whether or not the pain is radiating or referred. The cause of the pain may be something as life threatening as an aneurysm or simple epigastric pain following eating a spicy meal. Nonetheless, it is more important for you to provide supportive care and transport the patient for a definitive diagnosis, rather than attempting to determine the exact etiology of the pain.

Dizziness or Weakness

Obtaining an accurate history of a patient complaining of dizziness or weakness is often difficult with an older patient. This complaint can be caused by a cardiac problem, infections with the inner ear, hypotension, or hypertension. During your assessment, it is important to check the patient's pulse, motor, and sensation in all extremities as the patient may be experiencing a stroke. Ask the patient if the weakness, dizziness, or both are always present or if it only occurs during certain activity.

Fever

Many times you may be called for a patient who has a fever. This is the body's immune response to combat an infection. Consider the circumstances surrounding the fever. Is the patient unresponsive or does the patient have an altered mental status? Is the patient septic? When was the fever first noticed?

Trauma

Trauma to an older person can be more debilitating than trauma to a younger person. Consider what may happen to the patient following trauma: bone fractures, recovery, and a possible nursing home stay. Was there an underlying medical cause that lead to the traumatic event? Did the patient have a syncope episode before the fall or the motor vehicle crash?

Pain

The OPQRST-I mnemonic will help you understand more about the patient's pain. Remember that as the body ages, pain sensation changes. Many older patients live with pain on a daily basis. Activities of daily living are often modified because of the pain. Consider the current weather when assessing a patient's pain; many patients experience an exacerbation of pain when the weather changes. Is the pain of an acute onset, or has it been developing over a period of days or weeks? Were over-the-counter medications used? If so, did they help to alleviate the pain?

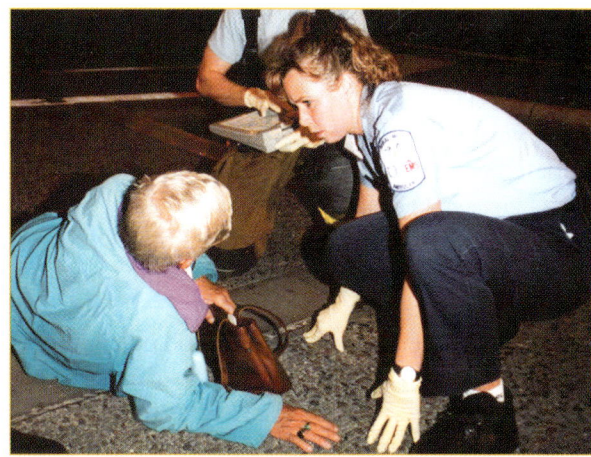

Figure 32-10 When you are assessing a patient for a fall, look for clues about what may have caused or contributed to the event.

> **EMT-I Tips**
>
> If the patient tells you that their pain is chronic, determine if its onset was slow and progressive or acute. The patient may have experienced an acute onset of pain a week ago; however, because the pain worsened, EMS was called. Many patients will interpret an acute onset of gradually worsening pain as being "chronic."

Falls

When you are assessing a patient who experienced a fall, always consider what factors may have contributed to the event Figure 32-10 ▶). Did the patient wake up in the middle of night to go to the bathroom and trip? Did the patient miss a step because of visual impairment? Many older patients will be able to tell you how many steps they have in their home. Counting the stairs as they ascend or descend may help them be more aware and in control of their body mechanics. Did the patient trip over a loose item such as a rug? Patients with walking assist devices also are prone to falls. When patients are found after a fall, it is important to try to find out how long they have been on the ground. Use your keen sense of awareness to investigate the surroundings and the potential mechanism of injury, especially if the patient is unable to recall the events that may have caused the fall. If you are called early in the morning and the previous night's dinner is still on the table, the patient may have fallen 12 to 16 hours earlier. Look for other clues such as mail and newspapers building up outside. Also consider the neighbors. Although they can be a valuable source of information, you must be careful to maintain the patient's privacy. Clues are also important when you may be called for a medical alert activation. Find out if it is an inactivity alarm or a distress alarm. Consider who has a key to gain entry to check on the patient. Many times this may be the person who calls for assistance. Consider these factors if you have to force entry to check on the welfare of a patient. Responsibilities vary according to jurisdiction as to who is allowed to force entry. Find out what laws and policies exist within your EMS system.

Nausea, Vomiting, and Diarrhea

The complaint of nausea, vomiting, and diarrhea needs to be investigated to determine the underlying cause. The foundation of these complaints may be attributed to conditions inside or outside the gastrointestinal tract. If an older patient is complaining only of nausea, this does not mean that vomiting and/or diarrhea will not soon follow. Remember that nausea may be the older patient's complaint during a cardiac episode. There are many possible causes of gastrointestinal complaints. During the assessment of the patient, determining the onset may provide a clue to possible causes. Viral gastroenteritis, which your patient may self-diagnose as the "stomach flu," is a common finding.

It is estimated that there are more than 90 million yearly episodes of diarrhea with the adult population. Geriatric patients are at risk for dehydration as a result of diarrhea. Drug-related diarrhea and associated nausea and vomiting usually occur after a new medication is initiated or after a change in dosage. Infectious agents such as viruses and bacteria can cause acute diarrhea, which, if it lasts less than 4 weeks, is considered an illness. Chronic diarrhea is defined as lasting longer than the 4-week period.

Geriatric patients are at risk for food poisoning, also known as bacterial gastroenteritis, due to existing medical conditions such as dementia. Patients may ingest contaminated food without even being aware of it because of sensory decline due to the aging process and improper hygiene. Symptoms of *Salmonella* usually begin within 12 to 72 hours of eating and may be of only 2- to 3-days' duration. *Staphylococcus aureus* will have a more rapid onset, usually within 2 to 8 hours, and the symptoms are typically more severe.

During your assessment of the patient who reports having nausea, vomiting, or diarrhea, remember to ask if there is any unusual color associated with the vomiting and/or diarrhea. Take note in your environmental assessment if there are basins or waste baskets near the patient, and look inside to see any abnormal emesis or if it appears to be blood tinged. Bright red bleeding is not normal and must be noted in your report. Bloody emesis or diarrhea is a clinically significant finding and may indicate serious gastrointestinal bleeding.

There are many causes of nausea, vomiting, and diarrhea. In addition to those mentioned above, patients with lactose intolerance, constipation, reaction to certain cancer medications and treatments, and bowel obstructions may present with nausea, vomiting, or diarrhea. Prepare for episodes of vomiting while assessing your patient and also during transport; have your suction ready. Many patients are unable to provide much if any warning prior to vomiting.

Focused History and Physical Exam

It is often said that 80% of a medical diagnosis is based on the patient's history. The history is a key component in helping to assess a patient's problem. In addition to clearing the airway and managing the ABCs, obtaining a thorough history is one of the most important things you can do. An inaccurate or inadequate history can lead to an incorrect field impression, which may result in an inappropriate treatment plan.

You are the Provider — Part 4

Initial vital signs are as follows:

Vital Signs	Recording Time: 5 Minutes After Patient Contact
Respirations	20 breaths/min, nonlabored
Pulse	50 beats/min, weak but regular
Blood pressure	142/92 mm Hg
Level of consciousness	Alert and oriented
Breath sounds, Sao_2	Lungs are clear bilaterally; Sao_2, 96% on room air

Pulse, motor, and sensation are present in all extremities. Your partner relays that medications prescribed to the patient are Dilantin, Diabinase, Lasix, Digoxin, and Zoloft. In addition, over-the-counter medications of aspirin and an antacid are found. The prescriptions appear to have been used in compliance with fill dates on the bottle. Dosage requirements seem to have been followed. The prescription for Zoloft, a medication for depression and social anxiety disorder, appears to be less than 1 week old.

9. Is it possible that a medication error may be the cause of the patient's fall?
10. Is it important that a list of all the medications be provided to the receiving facility?

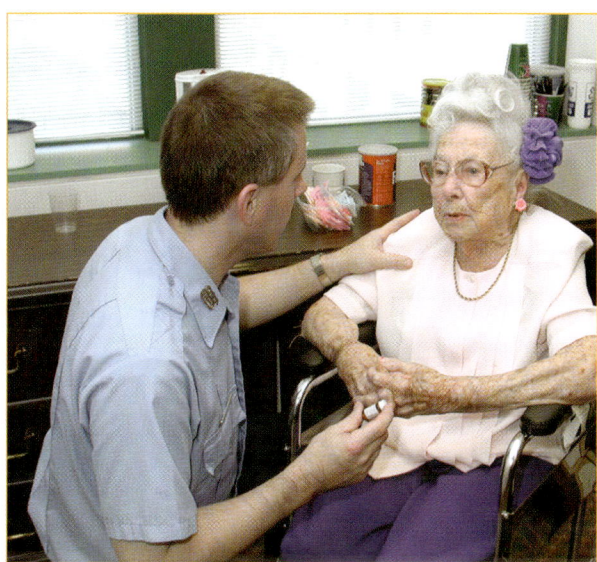

Figure 32-11 As you assess an older patient, make eye contact and grasp the patient's hand to feel for temperature, grip, and skin condition.

To obtain an accurate history, patience and good communication skills are essential. An older patient's diminished sight, hearing, and speaking ability may hamper communications Figure 32-11 ▲ . If possible, take a few moments to have the patient put in his or her dentures or hearing aid or, if necessary, assist the patient in doing any of these things. All of these items can help the patient to communicate with you more effectively.

Communicating With Older Patients

Communication is the key to a productive encounter with a patient. Consider your own personal communication skills. Does the patient understand what you are saying, asking, or doing? Maintaining eye contact and speaking in a steady tone will assist you in communicating with the patient. You may be required to repeat a question or statement when it appears that the patient does not comprehend what you are asking or saying. Verbal and nonverbal communications are important tools of the EMT-I. Verbal communication is the actual spoken word as well as the tone of your voice. Nonverbal communication includes body position, eye contact, and gestures. Remember that just because a patient is older, you should not assume that they are unable to communicate. Patients who have had a stroke may become very frustrated because they are unable to communicate their thoughts. It is important to remain patient and not pressure the patient into answering a question; this will merely add to their frustration.

Create an engaging and friendly environment for good communication by reducing the volume on your own portable radios and making sure that the television or radio volume in the home is turned low or off. Remember to look at the patient during your initial contact. When the patient is sitting in a chair, bend down or position yourself at the patient's level to speak directly to the patient and allow the patient to see your face. Avoid asking questions of the patient while you are looking elsewhere. When asking your patient questions or when making statements, you should avoid the perception of being judgmental, especially as it relates to the patient's reason for calling EMS or for the patient's noncompliance with prescribed medications.

While you are communicating with the patient, it is important that you know that the patient understands what is being said. This can be accomplished by repeating the answer to the patient. This eliminates any confusion as to what was actually said. It also allows for corrections to be made. If a patient is complaining of chest pain and you ask when it first started, the patient may respond that they have had chest pain for weeks. Your response back to the patient should include a statement such as, "This pain has been bothering you for weeks?" The patient then may adjust their comment to tell you that the current pain has only been present for the last 2 hours. This method of communicating allows for both parties to understand what is being said and to make any corrections if needed.

A poor history-gathering technique can hamper communications. You must be able to gain your patient's confidence, which is best accomplished by treating the patient with respect, taking a slow deliberate approach, and explaining what you are doing. First, ask the patient what his or her name is, and then address the patient using courtesy titles, such as "Mr.," "Mrs.," or "Ms.," and his or her last name. Avoid being overly familiar with the patient, and do not use first names or nicknames unless the patient asks you to. Older adults of a different ethnic background than yours may have different styles of communication and interaction. Become familiar with the different ethnic groups in your community and observe their style of interaction. Some patients may require a more personable approach, whereas other patients may prefer a more formal approach. Also be aware that some older adults from different ethnic groups may have different beliefs about health care and aging.

When there are multiple responders, everyone asks questions, sometimes several at a time. This is a poor technique that results in a haphazard history regardless

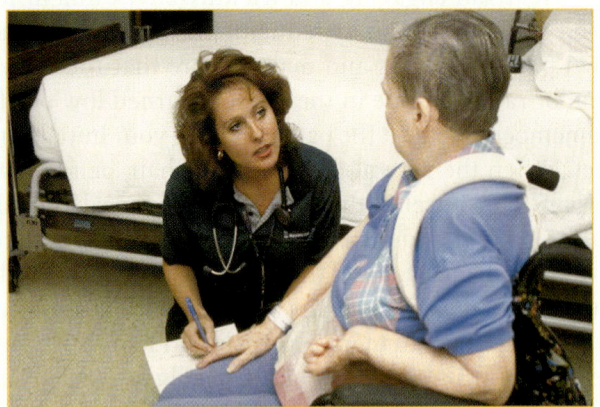

Figure 32-12 A slow, deliberate approach to the patient history, with one EMT-I asking the questions, is generally the best strategy in assessing an older patient.

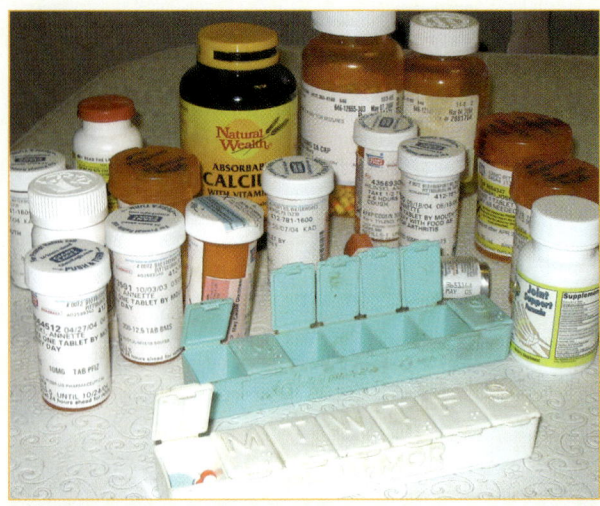

Figure 32-13 Older patients are often prescribed multiple medications.

of the patient's age. For older patients who may have communication or perceptual problems, it makes obtaining a thorough or SAMPLE history almost impossible. In addition, many individuals are reluctant to discuss their problems in front of a crowd. Be sure to have one EMT-I obtain the patient's history, one question at a time, providing as much privacy as possible Figure 32-12.

When speaking to an older patient, ask as many open-ended questions as possible, and use closed-ended questions to clarify points. It is better to ask, "Please tell me about the pain you are feeling" rather than, "Is the pain sharp or dull?" While taking the history, write down any key points on a notepad to avoid asking the same question repeatedly. After interviewing the patient, ask family members or caregivers to clarify what you just learned from the patient. Be careful not to offend the patient. Taking a few minutes to obtain an accurate history saves time in the long run by providing information on which appropriate treatment decisions can be based.

Past medical conditions can provide information about the patient's current problem. Older patients often have more than one disease process at a time, and the symptoms of one disease may make the assessment of another more difficult.

Use of Multiple Medications

Older patients are often prescribed multiple medications Figure 32-13. **Polypharmacy** is a common finding in geriatric patients. Polypharmacy, or the simultaneous use of many medications, is also noted when a patient is prescribed more than five medications per day. People older than 75 years use about 11 prescriptions per year compared to 2 to 3 for people in their 20s and 30s. Older patients often seek medical care from multiple physicians and may feel embarrassed to tell one physician what another physician has prescribed, which can lead to the patient taking the same medication twice. Prescription use can be even more difficult when the bottles are marked with different names for the same medication.

Obtain a list of medications and dosages. Information regarding the medications a patient is currently taking is vital. In addition, find out whether the patient has recently started or stopped taking any of the medications, is taking any over-the-counter (OTC) medications, or has taken any "home remedies." Herbal medication use has increased, and many patients will take OTC medications and are not aware of the potential interactions with any other medications they may be taking. Older patients should consult with their physician or pharmacist when adding OTC medications or herbal supplements to their daily regimen of prescribed medications.

Medication interactions and noncompliance with instructions for taking prescribed drugs are common and may contribute to the patient's symptoms or problem. Any information the patient tells you about recent modifications in medication dosages or medication changes should be included in your patient care report. Some older patients believe that the side effects of medication interaction are just signs of getting old. Older patients who have difficulty opening the prescription bottle may not take that prescribed medication; even those with easy-open lids are difficult for someone with arthritis. Some older patients are being treated by multiple physicians; it is important that all health care providers involved in the care of the patient are aware of other medications that are being prescribed.

> **In the Field**
>
> Many people do not believe herbal remedies to be "medications" because they are not prescribed by a physician. Be sure to question the patient about any herbal remedies and take them along with you to the hospital.

Many older patients will have a written list of their medication names and dosages. Some agencies have provided medication lists for older patients to use. Some of these are known as the "Envelope of Life" or "Vial of Life" and are placed in the refrigerator (Figure 32-14 ▼). A sticker or magnet that is affixed to the refrigerator or front door will alert EMS providers that there is important patient information available.

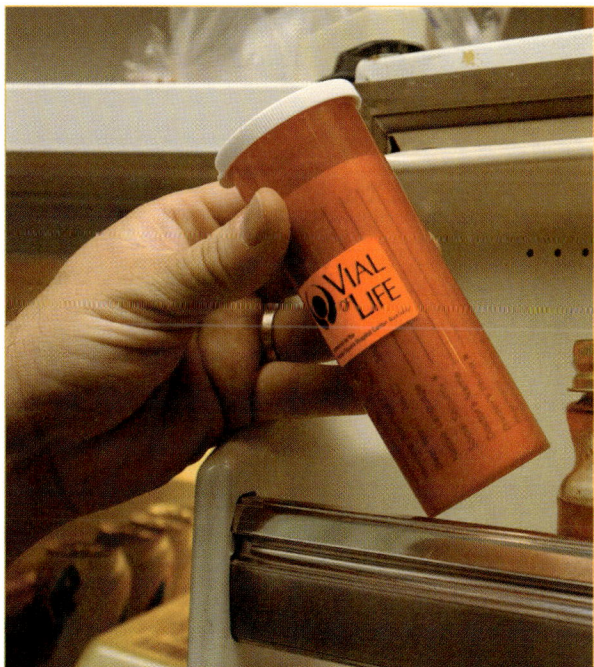

Figure 32-14 Medication containers such as the Vial of Life can be provided to older patients to keep track of medical information.

Like any other item, these aids are beneficial if they are kept up to date. This document contains the patient's medical history, current medications, and any allergies.

Some patients may not recall the actual name of the medication and may refer to them by color or what they are prescribed for. "I take the little blue one for my heart at night and the pink one for my blood pressure twice a day." This information may also be helpful in determining pertinent past history. The opposite end of the spectrum is possible when a patient hands you a shopping bag full of medications. Many of the bottles may be empty or outdated and there may be numerous medications from different doctors or hospitals. Look at compliance and the fill dates on the bottles. This tool may help you to determine if the patient has been taking his or her medications regularly.

There are many commercially available medication reminders and containers. The most common is the weekly pill box. This box is divided into days of the week. The patient (or another responsible party) fills the box with the medication for the week, separated into the 7 days. Many older patients rely upon this pill box to recall if they have taken their medication for the day. As an EMT-I, you can be aware of the patient's medication compliance by looking to see if the daily box is open. Many patients will leave open those days in which they have taken their medication. It is important to find out who fills the box and on what day it is normally filled. There are also electronic versions of the same device that will emit a beeping sound when it is time to take the medication.

Additional Considerations

Be aware that the sensation of pain may be diminished in an older patient, leading you to underestimate the severity of his or her condition. This diminished sensation is associated with the aging nervous system. For example, 20% to 30% of older patients have "silent" myocardial infarctions (heart attacks), without the typical symptom of chest pain. In addition, fear of hospitalization often causes the patient to either understate or minimize their symptoms.

During the focused physical examination, be aware that older people are more prone to hypothermia than are younger people. Be sure to keep the patient warm and maintain body temperature. Inspection and palpation can be hampered by multiple layers of clothing. Remove only the clothing that is necessary for an accurate assessment, and cover the patient back up when you are finished. Preserve the patient's dignity at all times.

Response to Nursing and Skilled Care Facilities

Nursing homes or skilled care facilities are common locations in which the EMT-I will encounter an older patient. Before you provide transport for the patient, you should find out the following critical information from the nursing staff:

- What is the patient's chief complaint today?
- What is the patient's admitting diagnosis? In other words, what is the initial problem that lead to admission to the facility?

To determine the nature of the problem, you will usually have to compare the patient's present condition with his or her condition before the onset of the symptoms. Ask the staff about the patient's mobility, activities of daily living (ADL), and ability to speak. This will help to establish the patient's baseline condition and determine whether today's behavior differs from it.

Many facilities that are transferring patients will include a transfer record that contains the patient's medical history, medication lists and dosages, previous diagnoses, vital signs, allergies, and additional information Figure 32-15 ▼. These records provide you, as well as other health care providers that will be involved in the care of the patient, with essential information and will save time, especially when the patient cannot speak for himself or herself. Be sure to obtain this essential record before leaving for the hospital and relay it to the hospital staff when giving your report.

Trauma

Mechanism of Injury

Falls are the leading cause of trauma, death, and disability in older patients. Most patients survive; however, a significant number require hospitalization. Motor vehicle trauma is the second leading cause of trauma death in the geriatric population. An older patient is five times more likely than a younger patient to be fatally injured in a car crash, even though excessive speed is rarely a causative factor in the older age group. Pedestrian accidents and burns are also common mechanisms

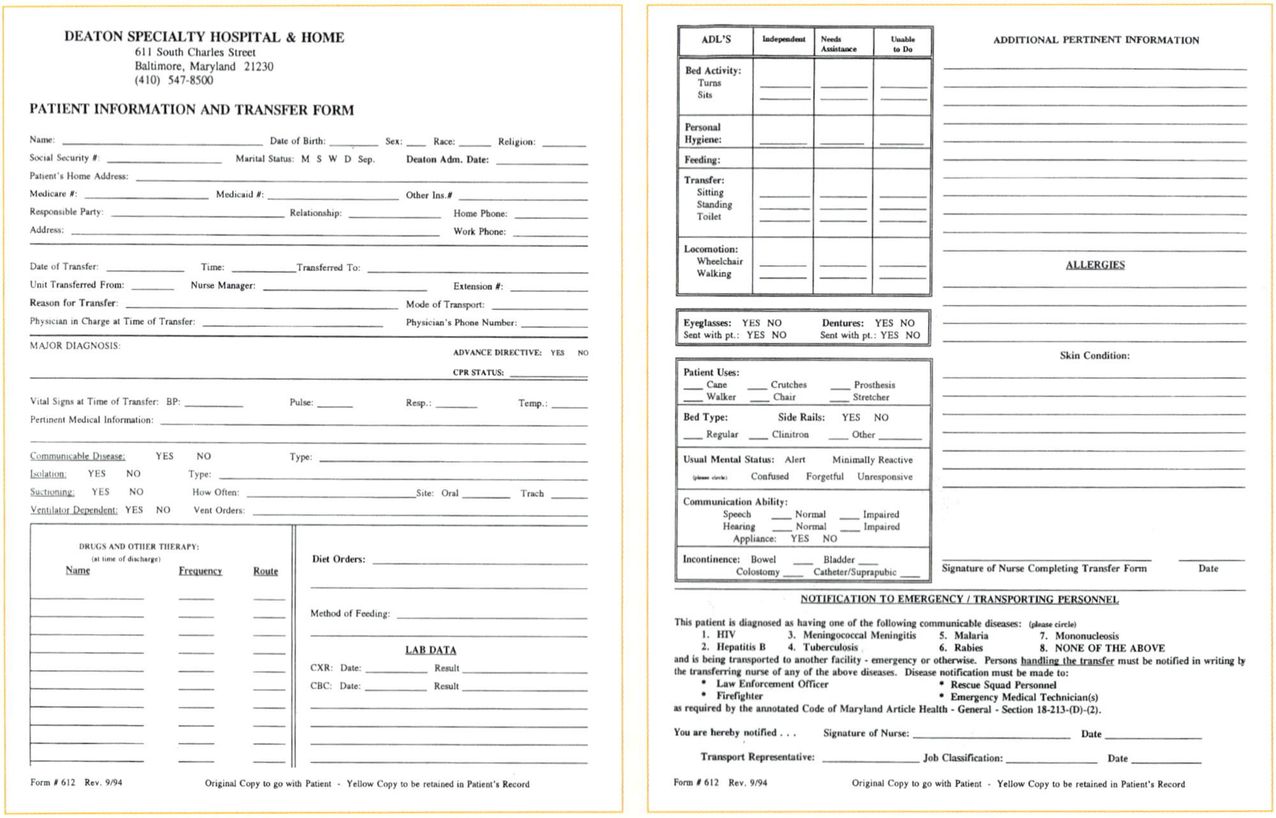

DEATON SPECIALTY HOSPITAL & HOME
611 South Charles Street
Baltimore, Maryland 21230
(410) 547-8500

PATIENT INFORMATION AND TRANSFER FORM

Name: ______ Date of Birth: ______ Sex: ___ Race: ______ Religion: ______
Social Security #: ______ Marital Status: M S W D Sep. Deaton Adm. Date: ______
Patient's Home Address: ______
Medicare #: ______ Medicaid #: ______ Other Ins.# ______
Responsible Party: ______ Relationship: ______ Home Phone: ______
Address: ______ Work Phone: ______

Date of Transfer: ______ Time: ______ Transferred To: ______
Unit Transferred From: ______ Nurse Manager: ______ Extension #: ______
Reason for Transfer: ______ Mode of Transport: ______
Physician in Charge at Time of Transfer: ______ Physician's Phone Number: ______

MAJOR DIAGNOSIS: ADVANCE DIRECTIVE: YES NO
CPR STATUS: ______

Vital Signs at Time of Transfer: BP: ______ Pulse: ______ Resp.: ______ Temp.: ______
Pertinent Medical Information: ______

Communicable Disease: YES NO Type: ______
Isolation: YES NO Type: ______
Suctioning: YES NO How Often: ______ Site: Oral ______ Trach ______
Ventilator Dependent: YES NO Vent Orders: ______

DRUGS AND OTHER THERAPY:
(at time of discharge)
Name Frequency Route

Diet Orders: ______
Method of Feeding: ______

LAB DATA
CXR: Date: ______ Result ______
CBC: Date: ______ Result ______

Form # 612 Rev. 9/94 Original Copy to go with Patient - Yellow Copy to be retained in Patient's Record

ADL'S	Independent	Needs Assistance	Unable to Do
Bed Activity: Turns, Sits			
Personal Hygiene:			
Feeding:			
Transfer: Sitting, Standing, Toilet			
Locomotion: Wheelchair, Walking			

Eyeglasses: YES NO Dentures: YES NO
Sent with pt.: YES NO Sent with pt.: YES NO

Patient Uses:
___ Cane ___ Crutches ___ Prosthesis
___ Walker ___ Chair ___ Stretcher

Bed Type: Side Rails: YES NO
___ Regular ___ Clinitron ___ Other ______

Usual Mental Status: Alert Minimally Reactive
(please circle) Confused Forgetful Unresponsive

Communication Ability:
Speech ___ Normal ___ Impaired
Hearing ___ Normal ___ Impaired
Appliance: YES NO

Incontinence: Bowel ___ Bladder ___
Colostomy ___ Catheter/Suprapubic ___

ADDITIONAL PERTINENT INFORMATION

ALLERGIES

Skin Condition:

Signature of Nurse Completing Transfer Form Date

NOTIFICATION TO EMERGENCY / TRANSPORTING PERSONNEL

This patient is diagnosed as having one of the following communicable diseases: (please circle)
1. HIV 3. Meningococcal Meningitis 5. Malaria 7. Mononucleosis
2. Hepatitis B 4. Tuberculosis 6. Rabies 8. NONE OF THE ABOVE
and is being transported to another facility - emergency or otherwise. Persons handling the transfer must be notified in writing by the transferring nurse of any of the above diseases. Disease notification must be made to:
• Law Enforcement Officer • Rescue Squad Personnel
• Firefighter • Emergency Medical Technician(s)
as required by the annotated Code of Maryland Article Health - General - Section 18-213-(D)-(2).

You are hereby notified . . . Signature of Nurse: ______ Date ______
Transport Representative: ______ Job Classification: ______ Date ______

Form # 612 Rev. 9/94 Original Copy to go with Patient - Yellow Copy to be retained in Patient's Record

Figure 32-15 A transfer record from a long-term care facility contains vital information for members of the medical team.

of injury in older patients, resulting in death, serious injury, or disability.

Systemic Impact of Aging and Trauma

You must consider the aging body's decreasing ability to isolate simple trauma when you are assessing and caring for an older patient. An isolated hip fracture in a healthy 25-year-old is rarely associated with systemic decline. However, the same injury in an 85-year-old patient can produce a systemic impact that results in deterioration, shock, and life-threatening hypoxia or multiple end-organ system failure, a dangerous condition in which the body tissues and cells do not have enough oxygen. Although an injury may be considered isolated and not alarming in most adults, an older patient's overall physical condition may lessen the body's ability to compensate for the effects of even simple injuries. Younger patients have the ability to increase their heart rate, constrict their blood vessels, and breathe faster and deeper to compensate for injuries. The aging body has a heart that can no longer beat as fast, vessels that cannot constrict as well due to atherosclerosis, and lungs that do not exchange oxygen as well.

Your assessment of the patient's condition and stability must include past medical conditions, even if they do not appear to be related to the current problem. For example, suppose you respond to a call for a patient with a history of unstable angina who sustains a simple isolated fracture of the ankle. You must consider this patient to be potentially unstable and provide prompt transport; the stress associated with the simple injury could result in an exacerbation of the patient's angina.

Falls and Trauma

A medical condition such as syncope (fainting), a cardiac rhythm disturbance, or a medication interaction may lead to a fall that causes injury to the patient. Whenever you assess an older patient who has fallen, it is important to determine why the fall occurred. Sometimes, a recent history of starting or stopping blood pressure medication is enough to cause a patient to become dizzy and fall. Consider that the fall may have been caused by a medical condition, and look carefully for clues from the patient, bystanders, and the environment. Although the trauma that the patient sustains from the fall can be serious, you should also consider that if a medical condition caused the fall, it could exacerbate, or be exacerbated by, the injury.

When you respond to a motor vehicle crash, be alert to the possibility that a medical emergency may have caused the accident, especially in single-vehicle collisions with no apparent cause.

Because brain tissue atrophies with age, older persons are more likely to sustain closed head injuries, such as subdural hematomas. These hematomas can go

You are the Provider — Part 5

The patient appears to be in moderate to severe discomfort. On a pain scale of 0 to 10, she describes her pain as an 8. As you continue to assess the patient, she appears to be more aware of her surroundings. She is placed on a backboard with a vacuum padding to ease the discomfort. You notice outward rotation of her left hip as she is placed on the board. The patient expresses concern about her husband in the other room and says she can't leave the house and leave him all alone. As you are moving the patient to the ambulance you overhear a neighbor talking about how this patient "hasn't been the same since her husband died 3 weeks ago." They explain that the patient has become isolated and depressed. She was the sole caregiver of her husband who died due to complications from a stroke. Her home, which was always clean and tidy, has become unkempt since her husband died. She had no family and refused help from any of her neighbors. She did, however, recently agree to seek help for her depression.

11. How important is additional padding of the voids for this patient?
12. Would an orthopaedic "scoop" stretcher be of any use in moving this patient onto the backboard?
13. How can you relay to the patient that her husband is not in the house?
14. Is this information important to provide to social services personnel at the receiving facility?

unnoticed because the blood has a void to fill before it can produce pressure in the skull, showing the familiar signs of head trauma.

As a result of decreased bone mass and strength from <u>osteoporosis</u>, a generalized bone disease that is commonly associated with postmenopausal women, older patients are prone to fractures, especially in areas such as the hip. With age, the spine stiffens as a result of atrophy of intervertebral discs, and the vertebrae become brittle. Compression fractures of the spine are also more likely to occur in older patients.

Because of the amount of flexion that occurs in the spinal column, hip, or knee of older patients, use of conventional splints and backboards to immobilize the patient may be difficult or impossible unless a lot of padding is used. What is considered a normal anatomic position for children and adults is often very abnormal for some older trauma patients. You should try to determine the patient's baseline condition and what was normal for the patient before the accident. Trying to force a patient with pronounced joint flexion into "normal" anatomic position can be very painful for the patient and may cause further harm. Some devices, such as traction splints, simply do not work on patients with flexed hips and knees. Splinting devices, such as vacuum mattresses that conform to body contours, may be a better choice for immobilization than a conventional backboard (Figure 32-16).

Remember that when you treat an older trauma patient, you must assess the injuries and carefully look for the potential underlying cause of the incident.

Cardiovascular Emergencies

Syncope

You should always assume that <u>syncope</u>, or fainting, in an older person is a life-threatening problem until proven otherwise. Syncope is the result of a temporary interruption of blood flow to the brain. Syncope has many causes, some more serious than others. Regardless, an older person who has experienced a loss of consciousness should be transported to the hospital and examined to determine the cause. (Table 32-3) shows some of the causes of syncope in an older patient.

Myocardial Infarction

The classic symptoms of a myocardial infarction (MI, or heart attack) are often not present in older people. As stated previously, as many as one third of older patients have "silent" myocardial infarctions in which the usual chest pain is not present. (Table 32-4) shows signs and symptoms that are commonly noted in older patients who are experiencing a myocardial infarction.

The Acute Abdomen

Because of an aging nervous system, abdominal complaints in older patients are extremely difficult to assess. A number of life-threatening abdominal problems are common in older patients. Internal bleeding may be a cause of the patient's abdominal complaint, which can lead to shock and death. Abdominal aortic aneurysm (AAA) is one of the most rapidly fatal conditions. It is the 13th leading cause of death in the United States. Major risk factors for AAA include being older than 60 years, smoking, hypertension, and a family history of AAA.

With an AAA, the walls of the aorta weaken and blood begins to leak into the layers of the vessel, causing the aorta to bulge like a bubble on a tire. If enough blood is lost into the vessel wall itself, shock occurs. If the wall bursts, it rapidly leads to fatal blood loss. If the aneurysm is detected early, there is a chance to repair the vessel before rupture and fatal blood loss occur.

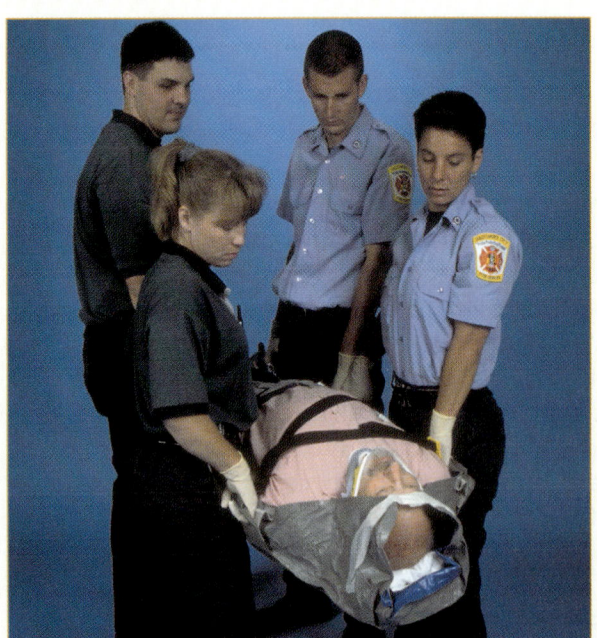

Figure 32-16 Vacuum mattresses that conform to body contours are a good choice for immobilizing older patients.

TABLE 32-3	Possible Causes of Syncope in an Older Patient
Cardiac dysrhythmias/myocardial infarction	The heart is beating too fast or too slow, the cardiac output drops, and blood flow to the brain is interrupted. An MI can also cause syncope.
Vascular and volume	Medication interactions can cause venous pooling and vasodilation, widening of a blood vessel, resulting in a drop in blood pressure and inadequate blood flow to the brain. Another cause of syncope can be a decrease in blood volume because of hidden bleeding from a condition such as a leaking aortic aneurysm.
Neurologic	A transient ischemic attack (TIA) or a "small stroke" can sometimes cause syncope.

TABLE 32-4	Common Signs and Symptoms of Myocardial Infarction in an Older Patient
Dyspnea	Dyspnea, the feeling of shortness of breath or difficulty in breathing, is a common complaint in older people and is commonly associated with an MI. It is often combined with other symptoms, such as nausea, weakness, and sweating. Chest pain associated with angina typically has an onset during periods of stress or exertion. In older persons, chest pain is often not present, but exertional dyspnea is noted. As the disease progresses, dyspnea may occur without exertion. Dyspnea in older people may be the equivalent of chest pain in younger people who are having angina or an MI. In addition, congestive heart failure and acute pulmonary edema may result from the "silent" MI.
Generalized weakness	Generalized weakness (malaise) can be caused by many things. However, you should suspect an MI in a patient with a sudden onset of weakness. Weakness is often associated with sweating.
Syncope/confusion/altered mental status	Syncope can have many causes, and in older people, none of these causes should be presumed to be minor. Syncope often has a cardiac etiology. Altered mental status is usually a signal of poor blood supply to the brain, often from cardiac dysrhythmia and MI.

A patient with an abdominal aortic aneurysm most commonly reports abdominal pain radiating through to the back with occasional flank pain. If the AAA becomes large enough, it can be felt as a pulsating mass just above and slightly to the left of the umbilicus during your physical examination. Occasionally, the AAA causes a decrease in blood flow to one of the legs, and the patient complains of some discomfort in the affected extremity. Assessment may also reveal diminished or absent pulses in the extremity. Compensated shock (early shock) and decompensated shock (late shock) as a result of blood loss are common occurrences. Because of a decrease in blood volume and decreased blood flow to the brain, the patient may experience syncope. You should treat the patient for shock and provide prompt transport to the hospital.

Another cause of abdominal pain and shock is gastrointestinal bleeding, which can occur for a variety of reasons and is usually heralded by vomiting of blood or material that looks like coffee grounds, called hematemesis. Bleeding that travels through the lower digestive tract usually manifests as black or tarry stools, called melena, while frank red blood in the stool (hematochezia) usually means a local source of bleeding such as hemorrhoids. A patient with gastrointestinal bleeding may experience weakness, dizziness, or syncope. Bleeding into the gastrointestinal system can be life threatening because of the potential for blood loss and shock.

Bowel obstructions occur frequently in the geriatric population. The gastrointestinal tract slows with aging and the patient can experience problems having bowel movements. Straining in an attempt to have a bowel movement can stimulate the vagus nerve, resulting in vasovagal syncope, where the heart rate drops to the point where the patient becomes dizzy or passes out. This patient will usually be stable upon your arrival, but requires transport to rule out other causes of the syncopal episode. Another reason for bowel obstruction in older patients is the use of narcotic analgesics, which also decrease GI function.

Altered Mental Status

Because there are stereotypical perceptions about older people, we may expect them to forget names or not be able to remember events or learn new things. However, these types of changes in mental status are not part of the normal aging process. They may be part of a slow deterioration of a condition or a disease of rapid onset, neither of which is normal. To determine the onset of this change in mental status, you must compare the patient's ability to function with that of the recent past. This will help to establish a baseline and give some perspective regarding the onset of the change. The two terms that are often used to describe a change in mental status are "delirium" and "dementia."

Delirium is a change in mental status that is marked by the inability to focus, think logically, and maintain attention. Acute anxiety may be present in addition to the other symptoms. Usually, memory remains mostly intact. Delirium is commonly marked by an acute or recent onset and is a "red flag"—a serious, potentially life-threatening problem—for some type of new health problem. Delirium may be caused by tumors, fever, or drug or alcohol intoxication or withdrawal. Delirium can be present from metabolic causes as well. Any time a patient has an acute onset of delirious behavior, you should rapidly assess the patient for the following three conditions:

- Hypoxia
- Hypovolemia
- Hypoglycemia

Any of these three conditions, if left unrecognized or untreated, may be rapidly fatal. Delirium is short in its onset and usually correctable if identified early.

Dementia is the slow onset of progressive disorientation, shortened attention span, and loss of cognitive function. Dementia develops slowly over a period of years rather than a few days. Alzheimer's disease or genetic factors may cause dementia. Dementia is usually considered irreversible and is an expected course of the pathophysiologic neurologic disease process. The patient's history and determination of function in the recent past are key factors in determining the difference between delirium and dementia. A demented patient may be experiencing a delirious event. Delirium is caused by emergent problems; dementia is not.

EMT-I Tips

Dementia and delirium are two completely different entities, yet they both present with alterations in mental status. Dementia is a chronic problem (ie, Alzheimer's disease), while delirium is an acute problem (ie, hypoglycemia). Because both delirium and dementia can present in a similar manner, it is important to determine the patient's baseline mental status.

Elder Abuse

Reports and complaints of abuse, neglect, and other related problems among the nation's geriatric population are on the rise. Elder abuse is defined as any action or inaction on the part of an older person's family member, caregiver, or other associated person who takes advantage of the older person's person, property, or emotional state; it is sometimes called parent battering.

The prevalence of elder abuse is not fully known for several reasons, including the following:

- Elder abuse is a problem that has been largely hidden from society.
- The definitions of abuse and neglect among older people vary.
- Victims of elder abuse are often hesitant to report the problem to law enforcement agencies or human and social welfare personnel.
- Most commonly seen as financial abuse, which may not be as visibly obvious.

You are the Provider — Part 6

The patient was admitted to the hospital following diagnosis of a hip fracture. Surgery and rehabilitation were performed and the patient was referred to social services. It is believed that her fall may have been caused by the addition of new medications in addition to the trip hazard of the loose rug. She now has become an advocate for injury and illness prevention in older people in the neighborhood.

An older adult who is being abused by his or her relative or caregiver may feel ashamed or guilty. The abused individual may feel shame, anger, or guilt (or all three) for being in an abusive situation. If the caregiver/abuser is a family member, the abused person may fear retribution or anger from other family members for reporting the abuse to an outside agency. Many families do not want an outside agency in "their business," and the abused older person may feel like a traitor for reporting abuse.

If the abuser is not a family member, the abused older person may feel frightened to report the abuse for fear of alienating the agency that is providing the supposed "care." The older person may then feel as if he or she will have nowhere to turn for care. In some areas of the country, there is a lack of formal reporting mechanisms, and some states lack clear statutory provisions that require that elder abuse be reported.

The physical and emotional signs of abuse, such as rape, spouse beating, or nutritional deprivation, are often overlooked or inaccurately identified. Older women in particular are not likely to report incidents of sexual assault to law enforcement agencies. Patients with sensory deficits, senility, and other forms of altered mental status, such as drug-induced depression, may not be able to report abuse.

Elder abuse occurs most often in women older than 75 years. The abused person is often frail with multiple chronic medical conditions, has dementia, and may suffer from an impaired sleep cycle, sleepwalking, and periods of shouting at others. The individual may be incontinent and is generally dependent on others for activities of daily living.

Abusers of older people are often sufferers of child abuse themselves, and the abuse that is inflicted upon the person may be done in retaliation. Most abusers are not trained in the particular care that the older person requires and have little relief time from the constant care demands of their own family. The stress associated with this situation may lead to abusive behavior.

The abuser may also suffer from marked fatigue, be unemployed with financial difficulties, or be a substance abuser. With a careful eye, you can recognize the clues to these stressful situations and help guide the family toward programs in the community that are geared to helping the whole family. Programs such as adult day care, meals on wheels, or many local individualized programs help to decrease the stress put on the family, thus decreasing the risk of abuse.

Abuse is not restricted to the home; environments such as nursing homes, convalescent homes, and continuing care centers (assisted-living facilities) are also sites where older people sustain physical, psychological, or pharmacologic abuse. Often, care providers in these environments consider older people to represent management problems or categorize them as obstinate and undesirable patients.

Assessment of Elder Abuse

While you are assessing the patient, you should try to obtain an explanation of what happened. You should suspect abuse when answers to questions about what caused the injury are concealed or avoided.

You must also suspect abuse when you are given unbelievable answers from anyone other than the patient, the possible abuser, or significant witnesses. You should be suspicious if you think, "Does this make sense?" or "Do I really believe this story?" while reviewing the patient's history. If you see burns, especially cigarette burns or physical marks that indicate that certain parts of the patient's body have been scalded systematically, you must also suspect abuse. As an EMT-I, you may be the first health care provider to observe the signs of possible abuse. Information that may be important in assessing possible abuse includes the following:

- Repeated visits to the emergency department or clinic
- A history of being "accident prone"
- Soft-tissue injuries
- Unbelievable or vague explanations of injuries
- Psychosomatic complaints
- Chronic pain
- Self-destructive behavior
- Eating and sleep disorders
- Depression or a lack of energy
- Substance and/or sexual abuse

You should remember that many patients who are being abused are so afraid of retribution that they make false statements. An older patient who is being abused by family members may lie about the origin of abuse for fear of further abuse or being thrown out of the home. In other cases of elder abuse, sensory deprivation or dementia may hinder adequate explanation.

In addition to the lifesaving care that you can provide the patient, your examination of the patient can help to reduce further trauma from abuse through its very identification. Repeated abuse can lead to a high risk of death. A preventive measure in reducing additional maltreatment of the patient is identification of the abuse by emergency medical providers. This may allow for

TABLE 32-5	Categories of Elder Abuse

Physical
- Assault
- Neglect
- Dietary
- Poor maintenance of home
- Poor personal care

Psychological
- Benign neglect
- Verbal
- Being treated as an infant
- Deprivation of sensory stimulation

Financial
- Theft of valuables
- Embezzlement

referral and protective services of human, social, and public safety agencies (Table 32-5).

Signs of Physical Abuse

Signs of abuse may be quite obvious or subtle. Inflicted bruises are usually found on the buttocks and lower back, genitals and inner thighs, cheeks or earlobes, upper lip and inside the mouth, and neck. Pressure bruises caused by the human hand may be identified by oval grab marks, pinch marks, or hand prints. Human bites are typically inflicted on the upper extremities and can cause lacerations and infection. You should inspect the patient's ears for indications of twisting, pulling, or pinching or evidence of frequent trauma to the external ears.

You should also investigate multiple bruises in various states of healing by questioning the patient and reviewing the patient's activities of daily living.

Burns are a common form of abuse. Typical abuse from burns are caused by contact with cigarettes, matches, heated metal, forced immersion in hot liquids, chemicals, and electrical power sources.

It may be difficult to see a failure to thrive in an older patient who has been abused. You should observe the patient's weight and try to determine whether the patient appears undernourished or has been unable to gain weight in the current environment. Does the patient have a ravenous appetite? Has medication been withheld? Is money being withheld, so the patient cannot buy food or medicine? You should also check for signs of neglect, such as evidence of a lack of hygiene, poor dental hygiene, poor temperature regulation, or lack of reasonable amenities in the home.

You must regard injuries to the genitals or rectum with no reported trauma as evidence of sexual abuse in any patient. Older patients with an altered mental status may never be able to report sexual abuse. In addition, many women do not report cases of sexual abuse because of fear, shame, and a desire to forget the incident.

Documentation Tips

As with other legally complex and emotionally charged issues, the possibility of elder abuse demands particularly careful documentation. Be thorough, objective, and factual, avoiding unsupported opinions and personal judgments. You may be called on to explain your report in a legal proceeding.

You are the Provider

Summary

1. On the basis of the limited information that you have been given, what type of call for assistance do you start to think of?

The dispatch for a medical alarm should alert you to the possibility that an older patient may have fallen on the floor and needs assistance. Many times, EMS responds to an alarm only to find out that a patient is not even home. The more information you can obtain, the better—such as, is it inactivity alarm, or was the alert button activated? You need to make sure that there really is no patient inside. Your agency would be the best authority on this subject.

2. Do the words of "elderly" and "medical alarm" automatically bring to mind a biased view of geriatric patients?

The preconceived notion that it is another "lift assist" call makes us prejudiced. Do we raise the tone of our voice because the patient is older? If so, that is a subtle form of ageism. Making up our minds about the cause of the call before we even arrive dictates our response.

3. How do these stereotypes affect patient care? Can providers be guilty of practicing ageism without even realizing it?

It can be frustrating to be dispatched to the same patient on a frequent basis. If this patient has just fallen down, do we assess the patient or do we just help them back into the chair and return to service? We can prevent these calls by evaluating the patient and the environment and, if necessary, referring the patient for social assistance.

4. Do you now have enough resources on scene to deal with two potential patients? Are there other methods to determine if there is actually another patient?

The older patient is found on the floor and there is talk of another patient. Should you call for additional resources before a second patient is found? The answer is that it is a judgment call that you will be able to make as you gain additional field experience. Assessing an older patient who is found on the floor requires you to ask the same questions that you would ask any other patient. Is it a medical or trauma patient? This patient may be both.

During your scene size-up and initial assessment, you should determine the number of patients and whether you need additional resources. In this scenario, it is a little different because you are unable to find your second patient. In many communities police officers will respond on calls if there is a possibility that forced entry will be needed. This police officer would be a great resource to survey the home to see whether there is another patient. It is possible that even an older patient can harm you.

5. What types of questions would be appropriate for this patient?

Asking your patient questions regarding the incident, including a SAMPLE history, is the most appropriate at this time. Additional questions will be based upon the patient's response to your questions. Remember that a patient who is lying on the floor with a possible hip injury may not understand the relevance of "last oral intake." You may have to rephrase your question, asking the patient when the last time he or she had anything to eat or drink. The answer to this simple question may help you determine how long the patient may have been on the floor.

6. Do you feel that it is an appropriate time to question your patient about the status of her husband?

Questioning your patient as to the whereabouts of the second patient is appropriate. The patient may have had a memory lapse, or she may believe that the patient is still in the home.

7. What methods can you use to find out a patient's medical or prescribed medication history?

Surveying the home for a medical history must be done with caution, especially if you or your partner needs to survey the home alone. If possible, a witness should accompany you or your partner to avoid accusations that items of value were removed. Also, ask the patient whether it is alright to look for medications in a specific area, such as the kitchen or bathroom.

Continued

You are the Provider continued

8. Are there other methods to determine a patient's history or medication use if the patient is unsure or unresponsive?

Most older people will store their medications in the kitchen area or dining area. Bathrooms and bedrooms are also where you can find prescription bottles. Don't forget the refrigerator; the patient may have the "Vial of Life."

9. Is it possible that a medication error may be the cause of the patient's fall?

Yes. Medication errors account for many emergency department visits for the geriatric population.

10. Is it important that a list of all the medications be provided to the receiving facility?

Yes. The patient's medications may be a contributing factor to the current condition and additional medical history and information about multiple physician visits can be obtained from previously prescribed medications.

11. How important is additional padding of the voids for this patient?

Additional padding completes the splinting and immobilization process. Be aware of the need to fill the void on kyphotic patients even if there is no suspected cervical spine injury. In addition to these items, filling the voids increases the patient's comfort and provides a more secure feeling.

12. Would an orthopaedic "scoop" stretcher be beneficial in moving this patient onto the backboard from the floor?

Moving a patient with a possible hip injury can be accomplished by log rolling the patient onto the uninjured side and placing the backboard underneath. This method allows you to assess the patient's back but may cause additional discomfort for the patient when returned to the supine position. The orthopaedic scoop stretcher will assist you in moving the patient from the floor onto the backboard and minimize the amount of movement; however, it does not allow you to fully assess the patient's back for any additional injuries. The main goal in moving the patient from the floor is to limit the amount of movement. You may at times have to become very creative in how you will move patients from the position in which they are found.

13. How can you relay to the patient that her husband is not in the house?

There are numerous methods to deal with a patient's question; your approach should always include telling the truth.

14. Is this information important to provide to the social services at the receiving facility?

You need to document all of your findings, including the environment in your patient care report. The more information that you provide to the receiving facility, the better able they are to find the appropriate services for this patient. As an EMT-I, you need to be an advocate for the geriatric population. There are numerous resources available out there not only for your benefit, but also the patient's. Recall the GEMS diamond on all your calls that involve older patients.

Summary

Prep Kit

Ready for Review

- Management of older patients can present you with many challenges that are not encountered with younger patients and confront you with a host of different problems that may be quite difficult and frustrating to solve.
- The health problems of older people are multifaceted, and frequent barriers to communication can be expected.
- Although assessment of the older patient involves the same basic approach as with any other patient, you may have to take a slower approach to the older patient. To obtain an adequate history and physical exam will require patience, but it is time well spent.
- The injury or medical condition may be worse than is indicated by the existing signs and symptoms, and the injuries and conditions that are found will have a more profound effect than they would in a younger patient.
- In addition to the critical needs that an underlying medical problem may cause, the older patient's condition is more unstable than a younger patient's and has an increased possibility for sudden, rapid deterioration.
- The prevalence of elder abuse is not fully known because many patients do not report it. Abusers are often family members who must care for the older person in addition to caring for their own spouses and children.
- Elder abuse also occurs in nursing, convalescent, and continuing care centers. Elder abuse can be gruesome, vulgar, and barbaric; however, your responsibility is to provide potentially lifesaving care to the patient and try to reduce additional abuse through identification of the problem.
- You must be careful to obtain an accurate history of the patient, be compassionate, and communicate your findings effectively. Be an advocate for your geriatric patients.
- The duty that we owe to our elders should be no less than we would expect in our own golden years.

Vital Vocabulary

activities of daily living (ADLs) Activities of daily living include cooking and caring for oneself, bathing, housework, and personal hygiene as well as toilet activities.

advance directives Written documentation that specifies medical treatment for a competent patient should he or she become unable to make decisions.

aneurysm A weakening in the wall of a blood vessel, usually an artery.

arteriosclerosis A disease that is characterized by hardening, thickening, and calcification of the arterial walls.

atherosclerosis The most common form of arteriosclerosis in which fatty material is deposited and accumulates in the innermost layer of medium- and large-sized arteries.

cataract Clouding of the lens of the eye or its surrounding transparent membrane.

cerumen Earwax.

collagen A protein that is the chief component of connective tissue and bones.

compensated shock The early stage of shock, in which the body can still compensate for hypoperfusion.

decompensated shock The late stage of shock, when blood pressure is falling.

delirium An acute change in mental status marked by the inability to focus, think logically, and maintain attention.

dementia The slow onset of progressive disorientation, shortened attention span, and loss of cognitive function.

Technology

- Interactivities
- Vocabulary Explorer
- Anatomy Review
- Web Links
- Online Review Manual

Prep Kit continued...

dependent living A type of care in which a person receives assistance based upon his or her needs or restrictions; can range from the least restrictive retirement community to the structured skilled nursing facility and dementia/Alzheimer's specialty care facilities. Sometimes known as residential.

dyspnea Shortness of breath or difficulty breathing.

elder abuse Any action or inaction on the part of an elderly individual's family member, caregiver, or other associated person that takes advantage of the elderly individual's person, property, or emotional state; also called granny beating or parent battering.

hematemesis Vomited blood, which may be bright red or dark, or if the blood has been partially digested, may look like coffee grounds.

hypoxia A dangerous condition in which the body does not have enough oxygen.

kyphosis A condition in which the back becomes hunched over due to an abnormal curvature of the spine.

macular degeneration Deterioration of the central portion of the retina.

melena Black, tarry stools caused by digested blood that has traveled through the digestive tract.

osteoporosis A generalized bone disease, commonly associated with postmenopausal women, in which there is a reduction in the amount of bone mass leading to fractures after minimal trauma in either sex.

polypharmacy Simultaneous use of many medications.

syncope Fainting, often caused by an interruption of blood flow to the brain.

vasoconstriction Narrowing of a blood vessel.

vasodilation Widening of a blood vessel.

Assessment in Action

You are dispatched to a local shopping center for a patient who is not acting right. You find an 83-year-old man sitting on a bench, looking dazed. An employee from a nearby store tells you the patient has been sitting here for hours, and the employee finally decided to call 9-1-1.

1. Evaluation of the scene should include all of the following EXCEPT:
   A. looking for potential environmental causes.
   B. looking at the general condition of the patient.
   C. looking in the patient's pockets for medical information.
   D. determining the need for spinal immobilization.

2. When conducting your initial assessment, you should expect to find:
   A. altered mental status.
   B. altered respiratory status.
   C. altered circulatory status.
   D. no abnormalities.

3. Evaluating the chief complaint in an older patient can be difficult because geriatric patients often:
   A. have numerous complaints.
   B. have serious medical conditions that present with only vague symptoms.
   C. have only complaints related to the aging process.
   D. amplify the severity of their complaints.

4. When assessing your patient you should not:
   A. explain what you are doing to your patient.
   B. question the patient regarding pain.
   C. assume abnormalities are normal.
   D. question the patient regarding his medications.

5. When communicating with your patient you should:
   A. repeat the patient's answers.
   B. avoid eye contact when possible.
   C. address the patient as honey or sweetie.
   D. ask the same question more than once.

6. You begin to speak with the patient and he responds to some questions. You ask which medications he is on. He states that he takes numerous medications, but does not respond when you ask what they are for. You should:
   A. call the patient's physician.
   B. ask the patient if he has a list of medications with him.
   C. call the patient's pharmacist to obtain his medication list.
   D. consider the information unobtainable.

7. You engage the patient in further conversation. You find out that he went to a new doctor three days ago and was put on a new medication. This may be important information for all of the following reasons EXCEPT:
   A. the patient may have inadvertently taken the same medication twice.
   B. the new medication may be masking other symptoms.
   C. the new medication may counteract another medication.
   D. the new medication has not had time to take effect.

www.EMSzone.com/EMT

Assessment in Action

8. When you are conducting a focused history and physical exam, you should:
   A. monitor the patient's level of consciousness.
   B. not assess severity because older persons have a decreased sensation to pain.
   C. remove excess clothing to prevent the patient from becoming overheated.
   D. perform a focused rapid head-to-toe assessment.

Your assessment reveals the following information: the patient was dizzy and is unaware how long he has been at the shopping center. There are no obvious injuries; his BP is 104/60 mm Hg and his pulse is 50 beats/min and irregular.

9. This patient's condition should be considered:
   A. significant because it is clear that he has been abused.
   B. significant because of his altered mental status.
   C. nonsignificant because this is probably normal for his age.
   D. nonsignificant because no injuries were noted on exam.

10. Your treatment should include:
    A. oxygen, IV, atropine.
    B. pacing, oxygen, transport.
    C. IV, atropine, pacing.
    D. oxygen, IV, transport.

Points to Ponder

You respond to a nursing home for a patient who fell. On arrival you find an 84-year-old woman lying in bed with several staff members with her. The patient has an obvious deformity to her left thigh. Staff members tell you that the patient fell out of her wheelchair and that she suffers from numerous medical problems, including senility. Once in the ambulance the patient tells you that one of the aides was mad at her and twisted her leg on purpose as she lay in bed. You attribute these comments to her senility and do not relay the information to the ER or proper authorities. Several weeks later you return to the nursing home for the same patient. This time she is in cardiopulmonary arrest and does not survive. An autopsy reveals that the patient was suffocated.

Could this death have been prevented? What should you have done differently?

Issues: Understanding Subtle Signs of Elder Abuse, Reporting Elder Abuse to Authorities

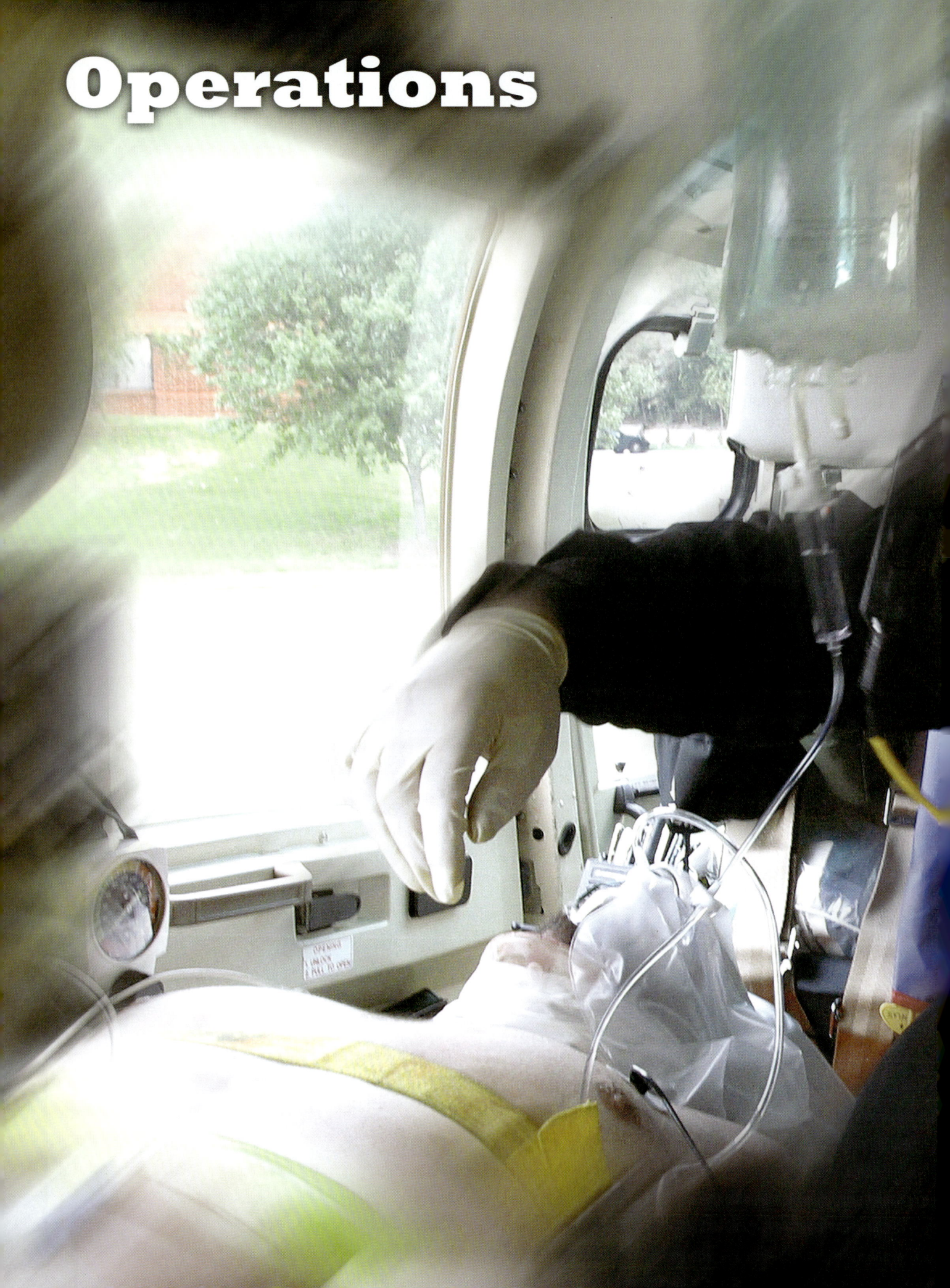
Operations

Section 8

33	Ambulance Operations	1372
34	Lifting and Moving	1402
35	Gaining Access	1444
36	Special Operations	1460
37	Response to Terrorism and Weapons of Mass Destruction	1490

Ambulance Operations

1999 Objectives

There are no 1999 objectives for this chapter.

1985 Objectives

1.2.8 Describe GSA/KKK Ambulance standards. (p 1374)

1.2.9 Define the American College of Surgeons Essential Equipment List and how it relates to local state laws. (p 1377)

1.2.17 Discuss replacement of equipment and supplies. (p 1394)

1.6.54 Describe the benefits and complications of lights and sirens and when they should be used. (p 1389)

Additional Objectives*

Cognitive

1. Discuss the medical and nonmedical equipment needed to respond to a call. (p 1377)
2. List the phases of an ambulance call. (p 1375)
3. Describe the general provisions of state laws relating to the operation of the ambulance and privileges in any or all of the following categories:
   - speed
   - warning lights
   - siren
   - right-of-way
   - parking
   - turning (p 1389)
4. List contributing factors to unsafe driving conditions. (p 1386)
5. Describe the considerations that should be given to:
   - request for escorts
   - following an escort vehicle
   - intersections (p 1390)
6. Discuss "Due Regard for Safety of All Others" while operating an emergency vehicle. (p 1390, 1397)
7. State what information is essential in order to respond to a call. (p 1384)
8. Discuss various situations that may affect response to a call. (p 1385)
9. Differentiate between the various methods of moving a patient to the unit based upon injury or illness. (p 1392)
10. Apply the components of the essential patient information in a written report. (p 1393)
11. Discuss the elements that dictate the use of lights and siren to the scene and to the hospital. (p 1390)
12. Summarize the importance of preparing the unit for the next response. (p 1394)
13. Identify what is essential for completion of a call. (p 1393)
14. Distinguish among the terms cleaning, disinfection, high-level disinfection, and sterilization. (p 1395)
15. Describe how to clean or disinfect items following patient care. (p 1394)

Affective

16. Explain the rationale for appropriate reporting of patient information. (p 1393)
17. Explain the rationale for having the unit prepared to respond. (p 1394)

Psychomotor

None

*These are noncurriculum objectives.

33

Ambulance Operations

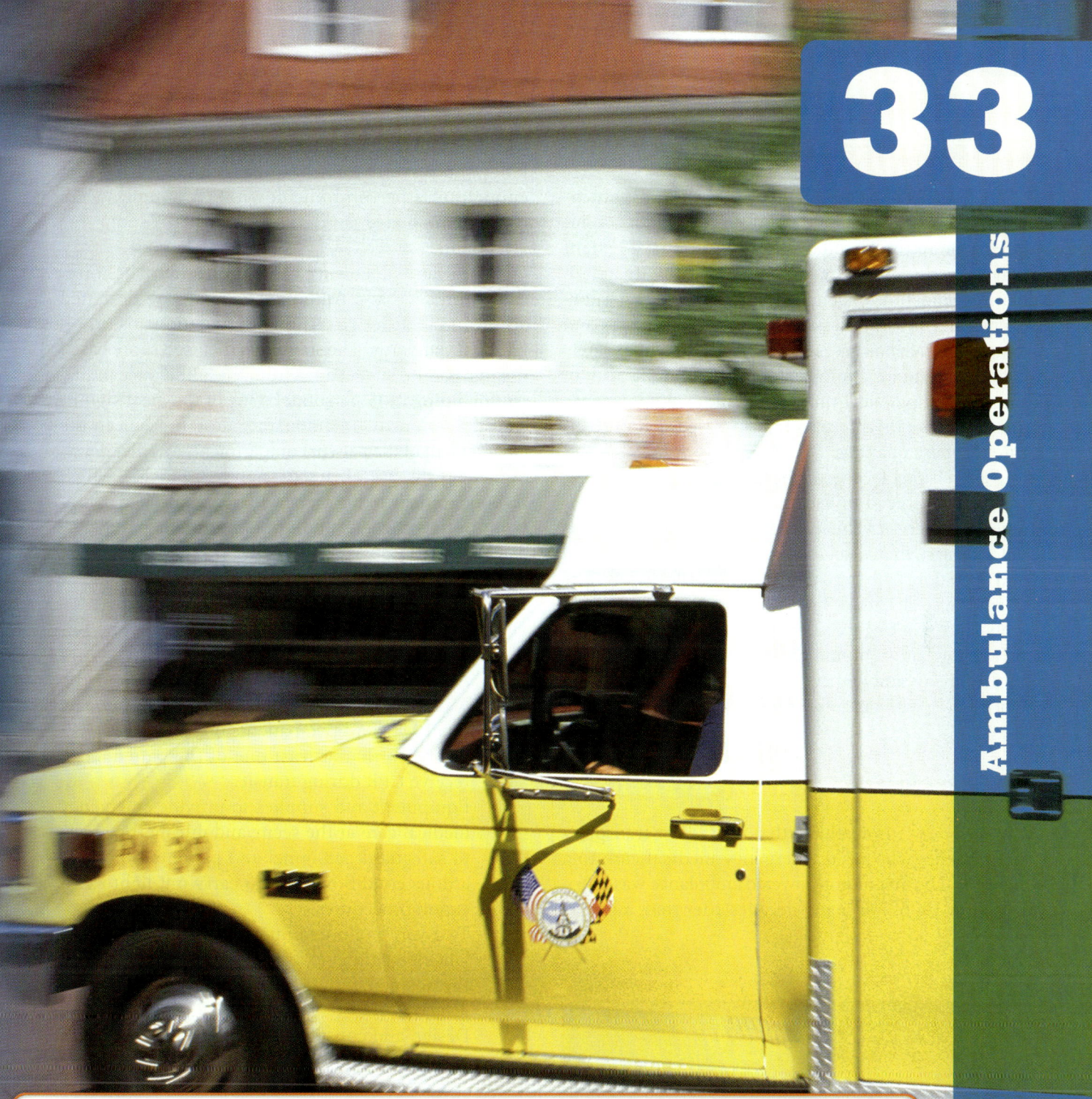

You are the Provider

You and your partner are on duty one Friday evening when you receive a call for an injury accident. Dispatch tells you that the police officer on scene is telling you "to step it up."

Every day, thousands of Americans will dial 9-1-1 for some emergency. Within minutes, an ambulance is en route to the scene bringing specially trained and equipped prehospital providers to their side.

This chapter will begin to acquaint you with the emergency response vehicle along with its contents that are your "tools of the trade." It will also help you answer the following questions:

1. What are the nine phases of an ambulance call?
2. Why is having "due regard for the safety of others" essential when responding to a call?

Ambulance Operations

Many patients have said that one of the most frightening parts of being suddenly ill or injured is the ambulance ride to the hospital. Already anxious, a patient may be made more so by a fast, bumpy ride with a siren blaring. Sometimes, such a ride is truly lifesaving. However, in most cases, excessive speed is unnecessary and dangerous. What is necessary is that the patient is safely transported to an appropriate medical care facility in the shortest practical time. This takes common sense and defensive driving techniques. Speed is no substitute for these qualities.

This chapter focuses on the techniques and judgment that you will need to learn to drive an ambulance or ambulance service vehicle. It begins with a look at ambulance design, then discusses emergency vehicle control and operation, both important factors in safe driving. The chapter also discusses how to equip and maintain an ambulance, parking considerations, the effects of weather on driving, and common hazards that are encountered in driving an ambulance. Finally, it describes how to work safely with air ambulances.

Emergency Vehicle Design

An **ambulance** is a vehicle that is used for transporting patients who need emergency medical care to a hospital. The first motor-powered ambulance was introduced in 1906. For many decades after that, a hearse was the vehicle that was most often used as an ambulance, because it was the only vehicle with room enough for a person to lie down. Few supplies were carried on board, and there was little space for attendants.

The hearse-ambulance has gone the way of its horse-drawn predecessor. Ambulances today are designed according to strict government regulations based on national standards. The standards themselves are based in large part on suggestions from the ambulance industry, including EMS personnel. One of the most significant developments in ambulance design has been the enlargement of the patient compartment. Another development is the use of **first-responder vehicles**, which respond initially to the scene with personnel and equipment to treat the sick and injured until an ambulance can arrive.

As defined by the National Academy of Sciences-National Research Council, the modern ambulance is a vehicle for emergency medical care that has the following features:

- A driver's compartment
- A patient compartment that can accommodate two EMTs and two patients on stretchers, positioned so that at least one of the patients can receive CPR during transit
- Equipment and supplies to provide emergency medical care at the scene and during transport, to safeguard personnel and patients from hazardous conditions, and to carry out light extrication procedures
- Two-way radio communication so that ambulance personnel can speak with the dispatcher, the hospital, public safety authorities, and medical control
- Design and construction that ensure maximum safety and comfort

Each state establishes its own standards for licensing or certifying ambulances; however, most use the federal specifications (KKK-A-1822C, 1990) that cover the following three types of basic ambulance designs (Figure 33-1 ▶) and (Table 33-1 ▶).

The six-pointed **Star of Life®** emblem (Figure 33-2 ▶) identifies vehicles that meet federal specifications as licensed or certified ambulances. It should be affixed to the sides, rear, and roof of the ambulance. Local regulatory authorities determine what emblems may be displayed on the side of an ambulance. (Figure 33-3 ▶) illustrates some of the required features of a licensed or certified ambulance.

Technology

- Interactivities
- Vocabulary Explorer
- Anatomy Review
- Web Links
- Online Review Manual

www.EMSzone.com/EMT

Chapter 33 Ambulance Operations 1375

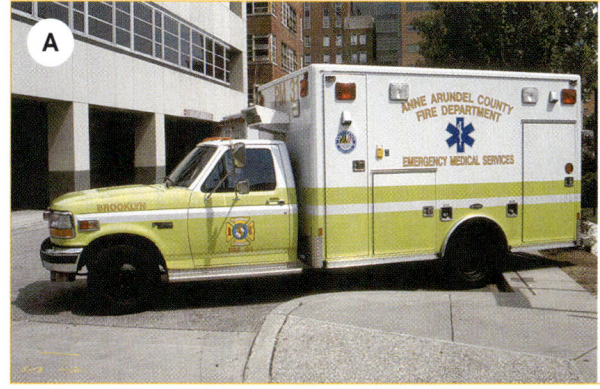
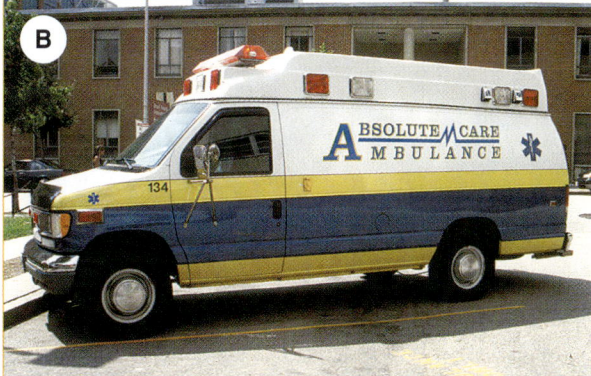
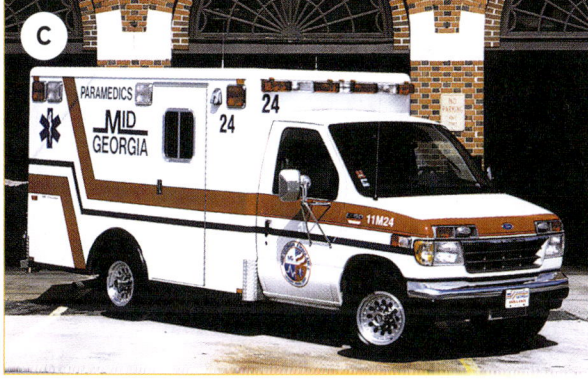

Figure 33-1 **A.** The conventional, truck cab-chassis has a modular ambulance body that can be transferred to a new chassis (Type I). **B.** The standard van ambulance has a forward-control integral cab body (Type II). **C.** The specialty van ambulance has a forward-control integral cab body (Type III).

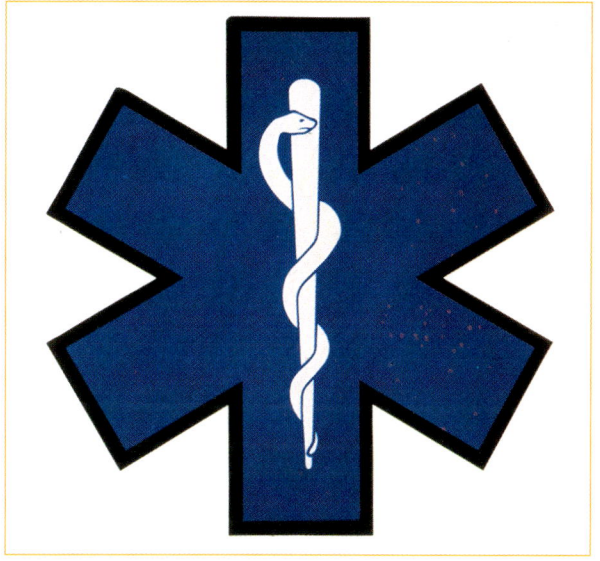

Figure 33-2 The Star of Life®.

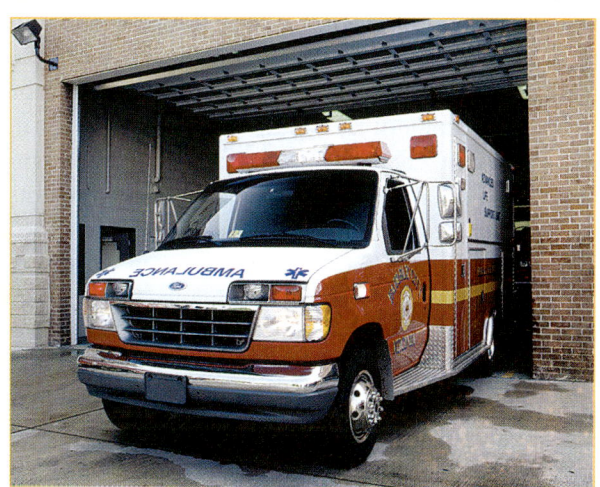

Figure 33-3 Warning lights and public address systems are required on licensed or certified ambulances.

TABLE 33-1	Basic Ambulance Designs
Type I	Conventional, truck cab-chassis with a modular ambulance body that can be transferred to a newer chassis as needed
Type II	Standard van, forward-control integral cab-body ambulance
Type III	Specialty van, forward-control integral cab-body ambulance

Phases of an Ambulance Call

An ambulance call has nine phases: preparation, dispatch, en route, arrival at scene, transfer of patient to ambulance, en route to receiving facility (transport), at receiving facility (delivery), en route to station, and postrun, as shown in Table 33-2 ▶. These nine phases address the vehicle and its crew, and their roles in a response to a medical emergency. The details of patient care are not included in these nine phases.

TABLE 33-2	Phases of an Ambulance Call

- Preparation for the call
- Dispatch
- En route
- Arrival at scene
- Transfer of the patient to the ambulance
- En route to the receiving facility (transport)
- At the receiving facility (delivery)
- En route to the station
- Postrun

The Preparation Phase

Making sure that equipment and supplies are in their proper place and ready for use, and that the vehicle is in good working order with appropriate fluid levels, fuel, tire pressure, etc, is an important part of preparing for the call. Some services have special personnel to stock and clean the ambulances. Items that are missing or that do not work are of no use to you or the patient. As a general rule of thumb, the more complex a piece of equipment is, and the harder it is to learn to use, the more likely it is to malfunction during an emergency. Many EMS items have never been rigorously tested under field conditions and could turn out to be expensive mistakes. For this reason, new equipment should only be placed on an ambulance after consulting with the medical director.

Equipment and supplies should be durable and, to the extent possible, standardized. This makes it easy to quickly exchange equipment with other ambulances or with the emergency department, thus saving time during patient transfer.

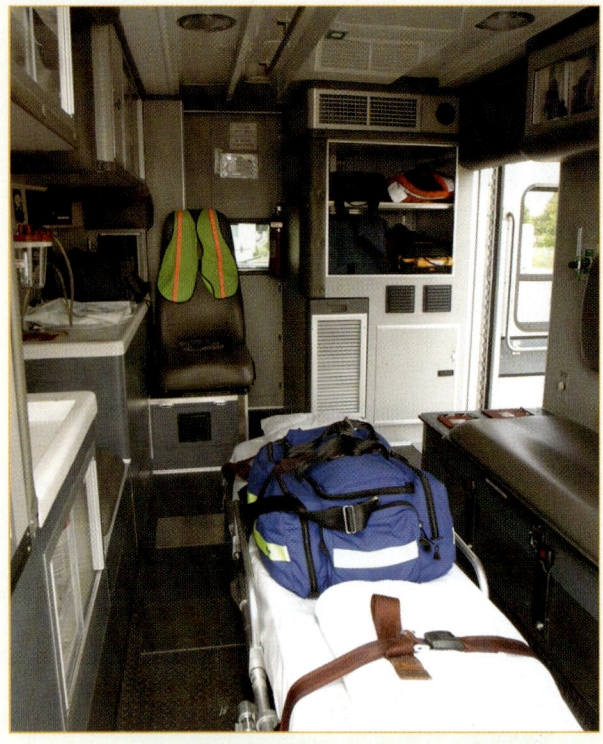

Figure 33-4 Store equipment and supplies in the ambulance according to how urgently and how often they are used.

Store equipment and supplies in the ambulance according to how urgently and how often they are used **Figure 33-4**. Give priority to items that are needed to care for life-threatening conditions. These include equipment for airway management, artificial ventilation, and oxygen delivery. Place these items within easy reach, at the head of the stretcher. Place items for cardiac care, control of external bleeding, and monitoring blood pressure at the side of the stretcher.

You are the Provider — Part 2

You arrive on scene to find that a car has hit a bridge abutment. The scene is safe and there are two victims trapped in the front seat of the car. You recognize that you will need to extricate both victims before you will be able to treat and transport.

3. What is included in the preparation phase of an ambulance call?
4. What items on your squad are needed to care for life-threatening conditions and where should they be stored?

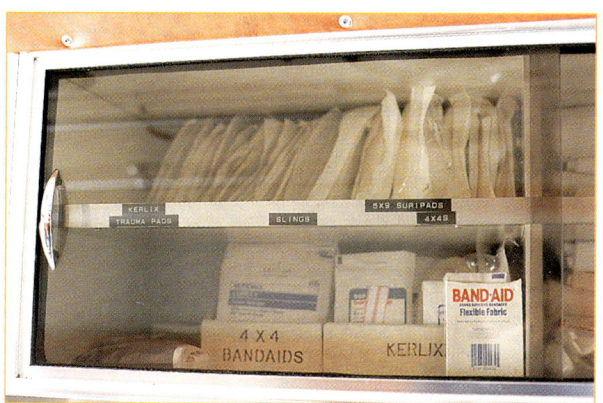

Figure 33-5 Containers should be placed in cabinets and drawers with transparent fronts for quick identification.

Storage cabinets and kits should open easily. They should also close securely so that they do not fly open while the ambulance is in motion. Cabinet and drawer fronts should be transparent so that you can quickly identify their contents; if they are not, be sure to label each container Figure 33-5 ▲.

Medical Equipment

As an EMT-I, you have access to a large variety of medical equipment and supplies, far more than can be described here. The American College of Surgeons Essential Equipment List was used in the past but is no longer relevant. Certain items must be available on the ambulance at all times.

Basic Supplies. Table 33-3 ▶ lists the common supplies carried on ambulances.

Airway Management. Airway management equipment that should be carried on ambulances includes the following:
- Oropharyngeal airways for adults, children, and infants
- Nasopharyngeal airways for adults and children
- Two sets of equipment for advanced airway procedures if your service is authorized by state regulation and the medical director to perform these: one in the ambulance and one in the jump kit that you carry to the patient

Ventilation Devices. It is important that two portable artificial ventilation devices that operate independently of an oxygen supply are carried on the ambulance: one for use in the ambulance and one for use outside the ambulance or as a spare. These devices include pocket masks and bag-valve-mask (BVM) devices. In addition, BVM devices capable of oxygen enrichment that, when attached to an oxygen supply with the oxygen reservoir in place, are able to supply almost 100% oxygen, should also be carried on the ambulance. Devices should be either disposable or easy to clean and <u>decontaminate</u>, which means to remove radiation, chemical, or other hazardous materials.

Masks for these devices come in a variety of sizes, from infant to adult, and are necessary materials to carry on the ambulance. The masks should be transparent so that you can monitor the patient's respirations, notice any color changes in the patient, and detect vomiting. Adult- and pediatric-size BVMs should be used with the appropriately sized mask to deliver the proper volume of oxygen-enriched air to the patient. In some regions, barrier devices for ventilation may be carried on the ambulance, depending on the preference of the medical director. Oxygen-powered devices are also available to provide ventilation to a patient. The

TABLE 33-3	Common Supplies

- Pillows and pillowcases
- Sterile sheets
- Blankets
- Towels
- Disposable emesis bags or basins
- Boxes of disposable tissue
- Bedpan (optional)
- Urinals (one male, one female; optional)
- Thermometers (one oral, one rectal, one hypothermia)
- Blood pressure cuffs (pediatric, adult, large adult)
- Stethoscope
- Pair of trauma shears
- Package of disposable drinking cups
- Unbreakable container of water
- Package of wet wipes
- Chemical cold and heat packs
- Sterile irrigation fluid
- Restraining devices
- Package of plastic bags for waste or severed parts
- Latex, vinyl, or other disposable gloves (various sizes)
- Sharps container (minimum)
- Set of hearing protectors
- Infection control kits (goggles, masks, waterproof gowns)

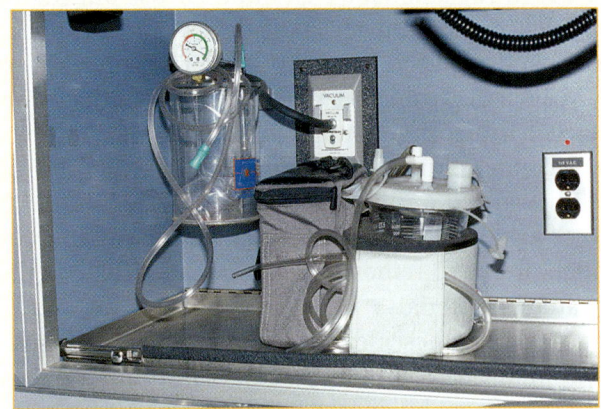

Figure 33-6 The ambulance should carry both a mounted suctioning unit and a portable unit.

EMT-I should follow local guidelines in identifying the specific ventilation equipment carried on the ambulance.

Suctioning Unit. The ambulance should carry both portable and mounted suctioning units (Figure 33-6 ▲). These units must be powerful enough to provide an airflow of 30 L/min at the end of the tube and a vacuum of 300 mm Hg when the tube is clamped. The suctioning force must be adjustable for use on infants and children. The units should include large-bore, nonkinking suction tubing with rigid and flexible suction catheters.

The installed unit should include a suction yoke, an unbreakable collection bottle, water for rinsing the suction catheters, and suction tubing, all easily accessible when you are sitting at the head of the stretcher. The tubing must reach the patient's airway, regardless of the patient's position. All components of the suctioning unit must be disposable or made of material that is easily cleaned and decontaminated.

Oxygen Delivery. The ambulance should carry at least two oxygen supply units: one portable and one installed. The portable unit should be located near a door or in the jump kit, for easy use outside the ambulance. It should have a minimum capacity of 300 L of oxygen and be equipped with a yoke, pressure gauge, flowmeter, oxygen supply tubing, nonrebreathing mask, and nasal cannula. This unit must be able to deliver oxygen at a variable rate between 2 to 15 or 2 to 25 L/min, depending on the regulator. At least one extra portable 300-L cylinder should be kept on the ambulance. Many services equip the backup cylinder with its own yoke, gauge, regulator, and tubing so that it can be used for a second patient.

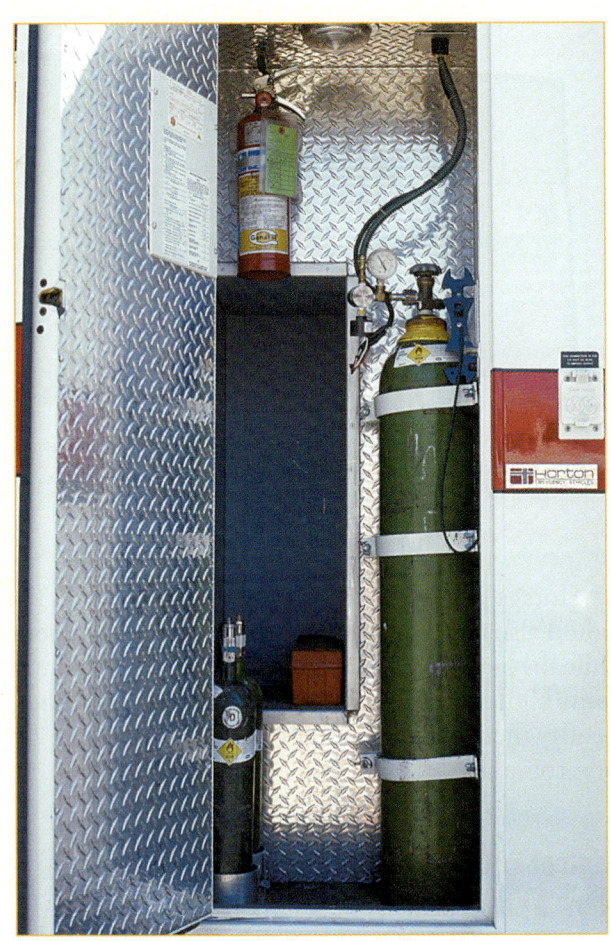

Figure 33-7 An oxygen unit with a capacity of 3,000 L of oxygen should be mounted on the ambulance.

The mounted oxygen unit should have a capacity of 3,000 L of oxygen (Figure 33-7 ▲). It should also be equipped with visible flowmeters that are capable of delivering 2 to 25 L/min that are accessible when you are at the head of the stretcher. Oxygen masks, with and without nonbreathing bags, should be transparent, and disposable, in sizes for adults, children, and infants.

Ambulance services that often transport patients on runs lasting longer than 1 hour should consider using a disposable, single-use humidifier for the mounted oxygen system. On runs of less than 1 hour, humidification may increase a patient's risk of infection unless the equipment is rigorously maintained.

CPR Equipment. A CPR board provides a firm surface under the patient's torso so that you can give effective chest compressions (Figure 33-8A). It also establishes an appropriate degree of head tilt (Figure 33-8B). If you do not have a special CPR board, you can place a long or short backboard under the patient on the stretcher. Use a tightly rolled sheet or towel to raise the patient's shoulders 3″ to 4″; this will also keep the patient's head in a position of maximum backward tilt and keep the shoulders and chest in a straight position. Caution: Do not use this roll to hyperextend the neck if you suspect a spinal injury.

Mechanical devices that operate on compressed gas and deliver chest compressions and ventilations are also available.

Basic Wound Care Supplies. Table 33-4 lists the basic supplies for dressing and bandaging open wounds that should be included on the ambulance.

Splinting Supplies. Examples of supplies for splinting fractures and dislocations that may be carried on ambulances (Figure 33-9) are listed in Table 33-5.

TABLE 33-4	Basic Wound Care Supplies

- Sterile sheets
- Large safety pins
- Adhesive tape in several widths
- Self-adhering, soft roller bandages, 4″ x 5 yd
- Self-adhering, soft roller bandages, 2″ x 5 yd
- Sterile dressings, gauze, 4″ x 4″
- Sterile dressings, ABD or laparotomy pads, usually 6″ x 9″ or 8″ x 10″
- Sterile universal trauma dressings, usually 10″ x 36″, folded into 9″ x 10″ packages
- Sterile, occlusive, nonadherent dressings (aluminum foil sterilized in original package)
- An assortment of band-aids

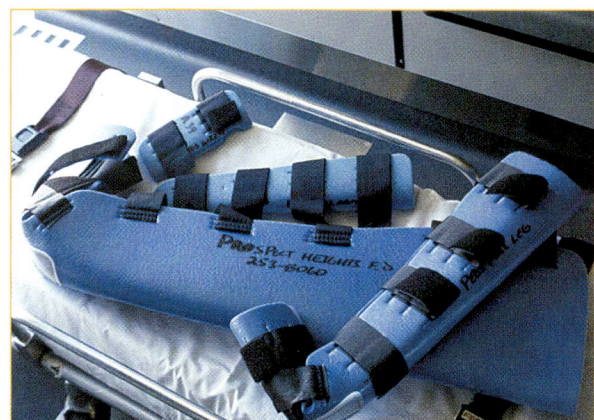

Figure 33-9 Supplies for splinting fractures and dislocations should be carried on the ambulance.

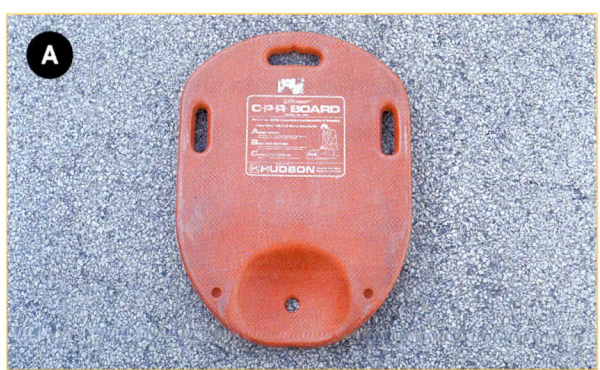

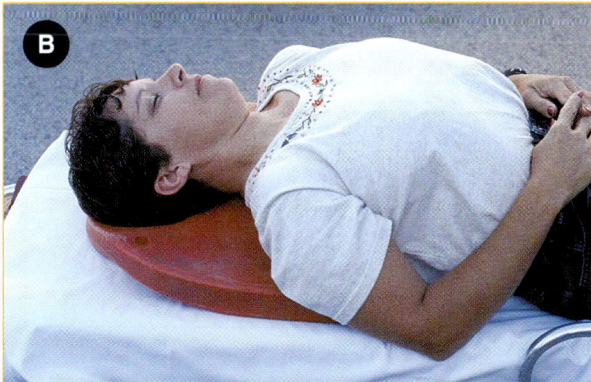

Figure 33-8 **A.** A CPR board should be carried on the ambulance. **B.** A patient on a CPR board has the appropriate degree of head tilt for effective artificial ventilation.

TABLE 33-5	Splinting Supplies

- Adult-size traction splint
- Child-size traction splint
- A variety of arm and leg splints, such as inflatable, vacuum, cardboard, plastic, foam, wire-ladder, or padded board. The number and type of splints should be determined by state regulations and your medical director.
- A variety of triangular bandages and roller bandages
- A short backboard device
- A long backboard
- Cervical collars in an adjustable size or a variety of sizes
- Adult-size pneumatic antishock garment (PASG), previously called MAST trousers

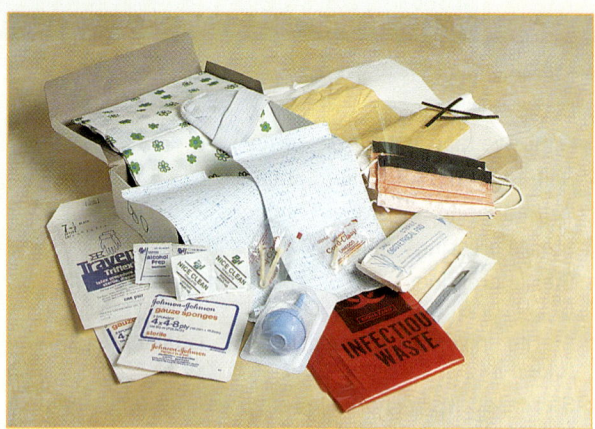

Figure 33-10 A sterile emergency obstetric kit must be carried on the ambulance.

TABLE 33-6	Emergency OB Kit

- Pair of surgical scissors
- Hemostats or special cord clamps
- Umbilical tape or sterilized cord
- Small rubber bulb syringe
- Towels
- Gauze sponges
- Pairs of sterile gloves
- Sanitary napkins
- A plastic bag
- Baby blanket

Childbirth Supplies. You must carry a sterile emergency obstetric (OB) kit (Figure 33-10 ▲) that includes the supplies listed in (Table 33-6 ▶).

Medications. It is important that the ambulance carry the items listed in (Table 33-7 ▶). Be certain that you have the telephone number and radio frequency of medical control or the local poison control center with you on the ambulance. The back of your clipboard is a good place to keep this information.

TABLE 33-7	Medications and Other Supplies

- Activated charcoal
- Drinkable water and cups
- Oral glucose
- Oxygen
- Supplies for irrigating the skin and eyes
- Other regional equipment, depending on the area and local protocol

Automated External Defibrillator. Semiautomated defibrillation equipment, as permitted by regulation and the local medical director, should always be carried on the ambulance (Figure 33-11 ▶).

You are the Provider Part 3

Your first patient has been extricated. As you approach her, you notice the following:

Initial Assessment	Recording Time: Zero Minutes
Appearance	In pain, pale, and diaphoretic
Level of consciousness	Responsive verbally
Airway	Open
Breathing	Respiratory rate increased with increased work of breathing
Circulation	Skin appears pale and clammy; radial pulse, weak and rapid

5. To adequately care for this patient's airway needs, what airway equipment should be carried on every ambulance?
6. To ensure that you have an adequate supply of oxygen, what are the two types of oxygen containers that should be carried on every ambulance?

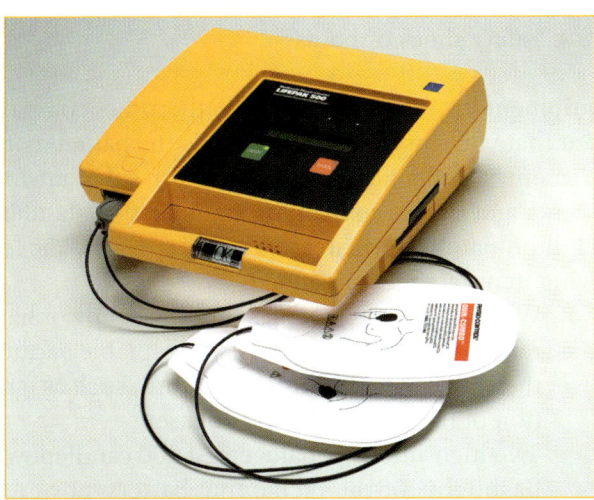

Figure 33-11 Every BLS unit should carry an automated external defibrillator.

TABLE 33-8	Items Carried in a Jump Kit

- Latex, vinyl, or other gloves
- Triangular bandages
- Trauma shears
- Adhesive tape in various widths
- Universal trauma dressings
- Self-adhering soft roller bandages, 4″ x 5 yd and 2″ x 5 yd
- Oropharyngeal airways in adult, child, and infant sizes*
- BVM device with masks for adults, children, and infants*
- Blood pressure cuff
- Stethoscope
- Penlight
- Sterile gauze dressings, 4″ x 4″
- Sterile dressings (ABD or laparotomy pads), 6″ x 9″ or 8″ x 10″
- Thermometer
- Adhesive strips
- Oral glucose
- Activated charcoal

*These might be carried in a separate airway kit, along with the portable oxygen cylinder.

The Jump Kit. The ambulance must be equipped with a portable, durable, and waterproof jump kit that you can carry to the patient Figure 33-12 . Think of the jump kit as the "5-minute kit," containing anything you might need in the first 5 minutes with the patient except for the semiautomated external defibrillator, possibly the oxygen cylinder, and portable suctioning unit. The jump kit must be easy to open and secure. Table 33-8 lists the items that are typically contained in a jump kit.

Patient Transfer Equipment. Each ambulance should carry the following patient transfer equipment:
- A primary wheeled ambulance stretcher
- A folding stretcher
- A collapsible chair device or stair chair for use in narrow spaces
- A roll up backboard (Reeve's stretcher)

The collapsible and folding stretchers may be combined into one unit. Stretchers must be easy to move, store, clean, and disinfect. The folding stretcher should keep the patient elevated above the floor when in the flat, extended position. The wheeled stretcher should be adjustable in height Figure 33-13 . When it is secured

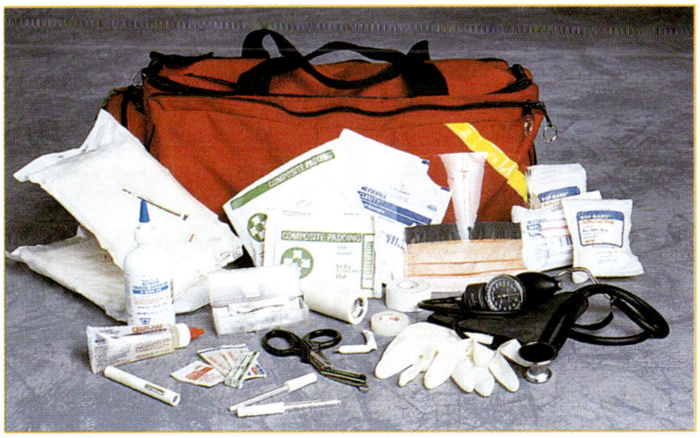

Figure 33-12 A portable jump kit contains anything you may need during the first 5 minutes with the patient except for the automated external defibrillator and possibly the oxygen cylinder and portable suctioning unit.

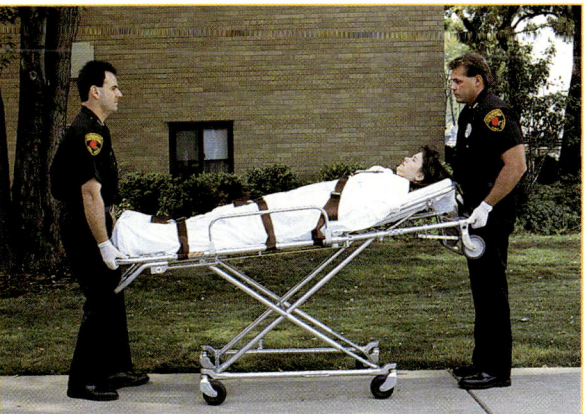

Figure 33-13 The wheeled ambulance stretcher is adjustable in height.

in the lowest position, the top should be 11″ to 15″ above the floor of the ambulance. You should be able to tilt the head of the stretcher upward to at least a 60° semisitting position and tilt the entire stretcher into 10° to 15° of Trendelenburg's position (head down) for airway care and treatment of shock. Stretchers must be at least 76″ long and 23″ wide and must be provided with fasteners to secure them firmly to the floor or side of the ambulance during transport. Stretcher restraints should be capable of holding the stretcher in place in case the vehicle rolls over. Make sure there are at least two restraining devices for the patient, such as deceleration or stopping straps over the shoulders, to prevent the patient from continuing to move forward in case the ambulance suddenly slows or stops.

Moving the patient to the ambulance can be done in different ways, depending on the injury or illness. Some patients can walk easily to the ambulance, which is sometimes easier and safer than trying to use a stretcher. For patients with spinal injuries, using a backboard or other immobilizing device, such as a Kendrick Extrication Device (KED), is usually best. For some patients with medical problems, especially patients with respiratory problems, transport with the patient sitting upright may allow the patient the most comfort and safety.

Safety and Operations Equipment. In addition to medical equipment, a properly stocked ambulance carries several kinds of equipment for responder safety, rescue operations, and locating emergency scenes. To do the job effectively, EMS personnel will need the following equipment:

- Personal protective equipment
- Equipment for work areas
- Preplanning/navigation guides
- Extrication equipment

Personal Safety Equipment. You should always carry personal protective equipment that allows you to work safely in a limited variety of hazardous or contaminated situations. These situations include the edges of a structural fire or explosion, vehicle extrication, and in crowds. The equipment should protect you from exposure to blood and other potentially infectious body fluids. Note that you will not be equipped to face all HazMat and other exposure situations that you may encounter; this is the job of specially trained HazMat technicians and response teams. Your equipment might include the following:

- Face shields
- Gowns, shoe covers, caps
- Turnout gear
- Helmets with face shields or safety goggles
- Safety shoes or boots

Equipment for Work Areas. A weatherproof compartment that you can reach from outside the patient compartment should hold equipment for safeguarding patients and EMTs, controlling traffic and bystanders, and illuminating work areas **Figure 33-14**. The following items are recommended:

- Warning devices that flash intermittently or have reflectors (road flares are not acceptable because they can pose an additional hazard, such as ignition of flammable liquids or gases)
- Two high-intensity halogen 20,000 candlepower flashlights of the recharging battery-powered, stand-up type
- Fire extinguisher, type BC, dry powder, size 5 lb minimum
- Hard hats or helmets with face shields or safety goggles
- Portable floodlights

Preplanning and Navigation. Make sure you have detailed street and area maps in the driver's compartment of the ambulance, along with directions to key locations, such as local hospitals. Become familiar with the roads and traffic patterns in your town or city so that you can plan alternative routes to common destinations. Pay particular attention to ways around fre-

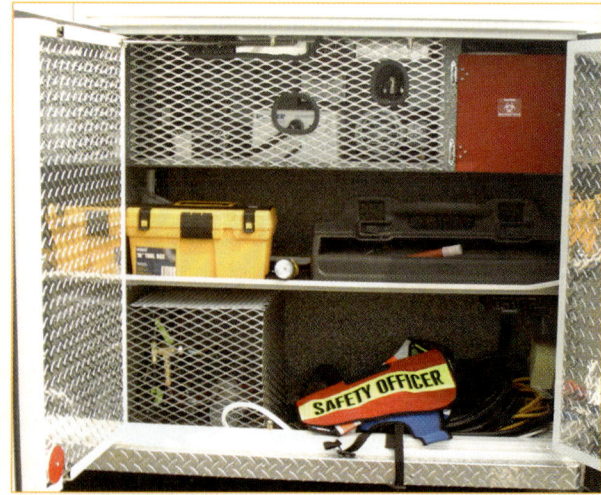

Figure 33-14 The ambulance should have a weatherproof compartment that can be reached from outside the patient compartment. It should hold equipment for safeguarding patients and EMTs, controlling traffic, and illuminating work areas.

quently opened bridges, congested traffic, or blocked railroad crossings. Often, switching to an alternative route will save more time than driving faster. Also become familiar with special facilities and locations within your regional operating area, such as other medical facilities, airports, arenas and stadiums, and chemical or research facilities that might pose unusual problems (staging areas may be pre-defined for emergency operations).

Extrication Equipment. A weatherproof compartment outside the patient compartment should contain equipment that is needed for simple, light extrication, even if an extrication and rescue unit is readily available. Table 33-9 lists the items that should be included in the compartment.

If rescue and extrication services are not readily available, additional equipment may be needed.

Personnel

Every ambulance must be staffed with at least one EMT-I in the patient compartment whenever a patient is being transported; two EMTs are strongly recommended. Some services may operate with a non-EMT driver and a single EMT-I in the patient compartment.

TABLE 33-9 Extrication Equipment

- 12″ wrench, adjustable, open-end
- 12″ screwdriver, standard square bar
- 8″ screwdriver, Phillips head #2
- Hacksaw with 12″ carbide wire blades
- Vise-grip pliers, 10″
- 5-lb hammer with 15″ handle
- Fire ax, butt, 24″ handle
- Wrecking bar with 24″ handle. This may be in a combination tool with a hammer and ax.
- 51″ crowbar, pinch point
- Bolt cutter with 1″ to 1¼″ jaw opening
- Folding shovel, pointed blade
- Tin snips, double action, 8″ minimum
- Gauntlets, reinforced, leather covering past midforearm; one pair per crew member
- Rescue blanket
- Ropes, 5,400-lb tensile strength in 50′ lengths in protective bags
- Mastic knife (able to cut seat belt webbing)
- Spring-load center punch
- Pruning saw
- Heavy duty 2″ x 4″ and 4″ x 4″ shoring (cribbing) blocks, various lengths

Daily Inspections

Being fully prepared means that you and your team must inspect both the ambulance and equipment daily to ensure that everything is in proper working order. The ambulance inspection should include the following:

- Fuel levels
- Oil levels
- Transmission fluid levels
- Engine cooling system and fluid levels
- Batteries
- Brake fluid
- Engine belts
- Wheels and tires, including the spare, if there is one. Check inflation pressure and look for signs of unusual or uneven wear.
- All interior and exterior lights
- Windshield wipers and fluid
- Horn
- Siren
- Air conditioners and heaters
- Ventilating system
- Doors. Make sure they open, close, latch, and lock properly.
- Communication systems, vehicle and portable
- All windows and mirrors. Check for cleanliness and position.

Check all medical equipment and supplies at least daily, including all the oxygen supplies, the jump kit, splints, dressings and bandages, backboards and other immobilization equipment, and emergency OB kit. Is the equipment functioning properly? Are the supplies clean? Are there enough of them? All battery-operated equipment, including the defibrillator, should be operated and checked each day. Rotate the batteries according to an established schedule and manufacturer's guidelines.

Documentation Tips

Because mechanical aspects of emergency work such as driving and moving patients strongly impact your safety and that of others, your service should have specific procedures for daily inspections. Following them protects you physically, and documenting your compliance is an important legal protection. Procedures should call for dating and either signing or initialing the checksheets, and for storing them where they can be found later if needed.

Safety Precautions

A final part of the preparation phase is reviewing safety precautions. These precautions, which include standard traffic safety rules and regulations, should be followed on every call. Check to make sure that safety devices, such as seat belts, are in proper working order.

The Dispatch Phase

Dispatch must be easy to access and in service 24 hours a day (Figure 33-15 ▶). It may be operated by the local EMS or by a shared service that also covers law enforcement and the fire department. The dispatch center might serve only one jurisdiction, such as a single city or town, or it might be an area or regional center serving several communities or an entire county. In either case, it should be staffed by trained personnel who are familiar with the agencies they are dispatching and the geography of the service area. For every emergency request, the dispatcher should gather and record the following minimum information:

- The nature of the call
- The name, present location, and call-back telephone number of the caller
- The location of the patient(s)
- The number of patients and some idea of the severity of their conditions
- Any other special problems or pertinent information about hazards or weather conditions

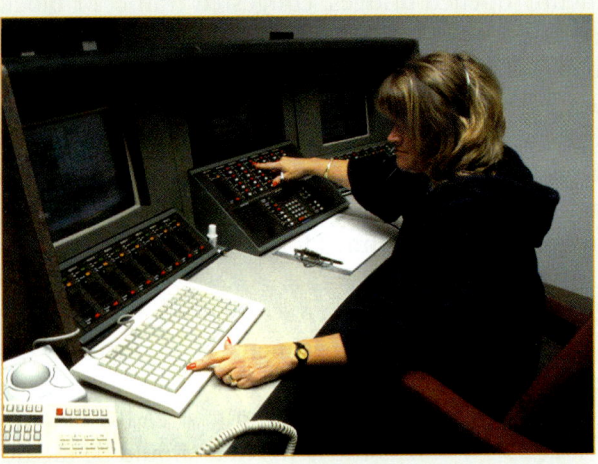

Figure 33-15 The dispatcher is the key communications link throughout all phases of the ambulance run.

Many areas implement emergency medical dispatching, which provides the caller with instructions for patient care before the ambulance arrives.

En Route to the Scene

As you and your partner prepare to respond to the scene, make sure you fasten your seat belts and shoulder harnesses before you move the ambulance. At this point, you should inform dispatch that your unit is responding and confirm the nature and location of the call. This

---

You are the Provider Part 4

Your second victim is still pinned in the vehicle. He has obvious trauma to his head. He was the unrestrained driver of the vehicle. As you approach him, you note the following:

Initial Assessment	Recording Time: Zero Minutes
Appearance	Pale, diaphoretic
Level of consciousness	Unresponsive
Airway	Open
Breathing	Respiratory rate, slow
Circulation	Skin, clammy and pale; radial pulse, slow and bounding

7. Your squad was able to successfully extricate the first patient and is working to extricate this patient. What extrication equipment should be carried on every ambulance?

is also an excellent time to ask for any other available information about the location. For example, you might learn that the patient is on the third floor or that the best door to use is around the side of the house.

While en route, the team should prepare to assess and care for the patient. Review dispatch information about the nature of the call and the location of the patient. Assign specific initial duties and scene management tasks to each team member, and decide what type of equipment to take initially. Depending on your operation procedures, you may also decide which stretcher to bring to the patient.

Driver Characteristics

In many ways, the en route or response phase of the call is the most dangerous for you. Collisions between automobiles and emergency vehicles cause many serious injuries among EMS personnel (Figure 33-16). Therefore, drivers should be screened carefully. Not everyone who drives an automobile is qualified to drive an emergency vehicle. In some states, you must successfully complete an approved emergency vehicle operations course before you are allowed to drive the ambulance on emergency calls. In any state, diligence and caution are important characteristics, as are a positive attitude about your ability and tolerance of other drivers.

One basic requirement is physical fitness. Many crashes occur as a result of physical impairment of the driver. You should not be driving if you are taking medications that may cause drowsiness or slow your reaction times. These include cold remedies, analgesics, or tranquilizers. And, of course, you should never drive or provide medical care after drinking alcohol.

Another requirement is emotional fitness. Emotions should not be taken lightly. Personality often changes once an individual gets behind a steering wheel. Emotional stability is closely related to the ability to operate under stress. In addition to knowing exactly what to do, you must be able to do it under trying conditions.

The proper attitude is very important for the driver of an ambulance. Being able to drive to your destination without interruption and to move into the opposite lane are valuable, time-saving skills that must be practiced consistently. Do not ever get behind the wheel thinking that you can do whatever you like.

In addition to training and experience, the good judgment and knowledge that you need to drive an ambulance requires practice. Remember, even the best drivers can benefit from practice.

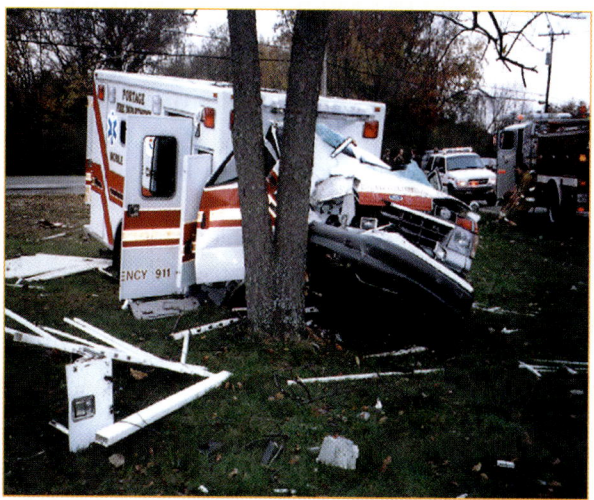

Figure 33-16 The en route or response phase may be the most dangerous part of the call.

Safe Driving Practices

Safe driving is a very important part of the emergency care of sick and injured patients.

The first rule of safe driving in an emergency vehicle is that speed does not save lives; good care does. The second rule is that the driver and all passengers must wear seat belts and shoulder restraints at all times. These are the most important items of safety equipment on every ambulance. Other EMTs should wear restraints en route to the scene and whenever they are not performing direct patient care. Patients should also be properly restrained.

Learn how your vehicle accelerates, corners, sways, and stops. For example, disc booster brakes make braking more efficient but increase sway. You must know exactly how your particular vehicle will respond to steering, braking, and accelerating under various conditions.

Getting a feel for the proper brake pressure comes with experience and practice. Each vehicle has a different braking action. For example, the brakes on types I and III vehicles have a heavier feel than the brakes on a type II vehicle. Braking on a diesel-powered unit will be different from braking on an identically equipped gasoline-powered unit. Certain heavy vehicles use air

 EMT-I Tips

> The proper attitude is very important for the driver of an ambulance. The good judgment needed to drive an ambulance requires practice—even for the best drivers.

brakes, which have yet another feel. Get to know each vehicle you drive, and be sure you understand its braking characteristics and the best downshifting techniques.

The EMT driver often assumes that motorists and pedestrians will do the right thing when an emergency vehicle is in the vicinity. This is a mistake. Motorists may indeed pull over to the nearest curb and stop or drive as close to the curb as possible, but you cannot take this behavior for granted. At any time, a motorist might stop suddenly in front of the ambulance or pull to the left. Both of these motorist responses may result in a crash. Always assume the driver has not heard your siren or seen you until proven otherwise by his or her actions.

When you are driving an ambulance on a multi-lane highway, you should usually stay in the extreme left-hand (fast) lane. This allows other motorists to move over to the right when they see or hear you approach.

Most important, you must always drive defensively. Never rely on what another motorist will do unless you get a clear visual signal. Even then, you must be prepared to take defensive action in the case of a misunderstanding, panic, or careless driving on the part of the other driver.

> ### EMT-I Safety
>
> Ambulance crashes that kill EMTs, patients, or occupants of other vehicles are disturbingly common. Many of them could be prevented by the driver of the ambulance. Attending thoroughly to your own driving skills, driving according to established standards, and dealing with any obvious deficiencies in your partner's driving skills are all crucial to your safety on the job.

The Problem of Excessive Speed. Only in extreme life-and-death emergencies is speed an important factor. In most instances, if you properly assess and stabilize the patient at the scene, speed during transport is unnecessary and undesirable. Regardless of the situation, you should never travel at a speed that is unsafe for the given road conditions.

Studies have shown conclusively that excessive speeds are unnecessary and, in most cases, do not add to patient survivability. More often, using excessive speed while driving to and from the scene has resulted in crashes in which the EMT, patient, and occupants of other vehicles are killed.

Consider these factors:
1. **Expertise** on the part of the dispatcher, resulting in calls being given a high priority only when this is truly indicated. Dispatching requires a trained, experienced EMT or emergency medical dispatcher. Only someone with training and a working knowledge of emergency calls can determine the urgency of a call, especially when the caller is excited and distraught.
2. **Adequate equipment in the ambulance.** If you have the equipment and supplies that are necessary to stabilize the patient, you will be able to properly care for the patient en route without the need for speeding to the hospital.
3. **Adequate training of the EMT-I.** With adequate training and confidence in your ability to care for the patient, your role extends beyond simply acting as a chauffeur.
4. **Adequate driving ability.** This is the most important factor. If you understand the added risks that go with high-speed driving and the principles of safe ambulance operation, you will tend to choose safety over speed.
5. **Recognition of siren syndrome.** The siren may have a psychological effect on drivers. Recognizing this will help you become aware of your or other drivers' tendencies to drive faster and faster in the presence of sirens. Although a siren signifies a request for drivers to yield right of way, drivers do not always yield right-of-way.

Emergency Vehicle Control. As the driver of an ambulance, you have only two ways to control the vehicle: by changing its direction or changing its speed. Either maneuver requires a continuous rolling contact between the surface of the tires and the surface of the road. Two factors are involved in this contact. The first is the <u>coefficient of friction</u>, which is a measure of the tire's grip on the road; <u>friction</u> is resistance to the motion of one body against another. The second factor is the <u>footprint</u> of the tire, which is the area of contact between the tire and surface of the road. On the typical ambulance, the footprint is about 8" long and as wide as the tire.

The coefficient of friction may vary widely on different parts of the same road, depending on the condition of the surface, the age of the road, and the weather. It also varies according to the tire's tread design and wear. As a driver, you must constantly evaluate the road surface: At a given speed, how much frictional force can the tires apply before the ambulance becomes unstable?

This is especially important in cornering, in which additional centrifugal force is acting on the vehicle.

Steering Techniques. Steering technique includes the way you hold the steering wheel, the way it moves, and the timing of the movements. Hold the wheel with your hands at the ten-o'clock and two-o'clock positions. This allows you to turn the wheel without removing either hand; one hand pulls while the other slides so that they remain parallel. Your hands should not pass the twelve-o'clock or six-o'clock positions, because they will cross and become tangled; instead, let the hand that was pulling start to slide, and use the opposite hand to pull.

Timing of steering wheel movements relates to the speed of the vehicle. All vehicles lag somewhat when responding to steering input. The faster the speed, the greater the lag.

Chassis Set. The chassis is the vehicle frame of the ambulance. Chassis set is the transfer of weight (center of mass) to different points on the chassis. Basically, the weight of a vehicle is concentrated over one of three points on the chassis: the front wheels, the rear wheels, or the center between the front and rear wheels. The transfer of weight from one point to another is caused by acceleration, or increasing speed, or deceleration, or slowing down. When a vehicle accelerates, the weight is transferred to the rear; the front wheels lose some traction, which means that you lose some ability to steer. The ambulance will have a tendency to travel in a straight line. With braking, the opposite weight shift occurs; this is why the rear end of the vehicle tends to slide to the outside of a curve when cornering.

Vehicle Size and Distance Judgment. Vehicle length and width are critical factors in maneuvering, driving, and parking an emergency vehicle. They are especially important with types I and III vehicles, which are wider than they look from behind the steering wheel. To brake and pass effectively, you must know the width and length of your vehicle. Crashes often occur when the vehicle is backing up. Always use someone outside the ambulance as a ground guide when you are backing up, to avoid any surprises. Vehicle size and weight will greatly influence braking and stopping distances. Good peripheral vision and depth perception will help you to judge distances, but they are no substitute for intensive training, experience, and frequent evaluation of the vehicle.

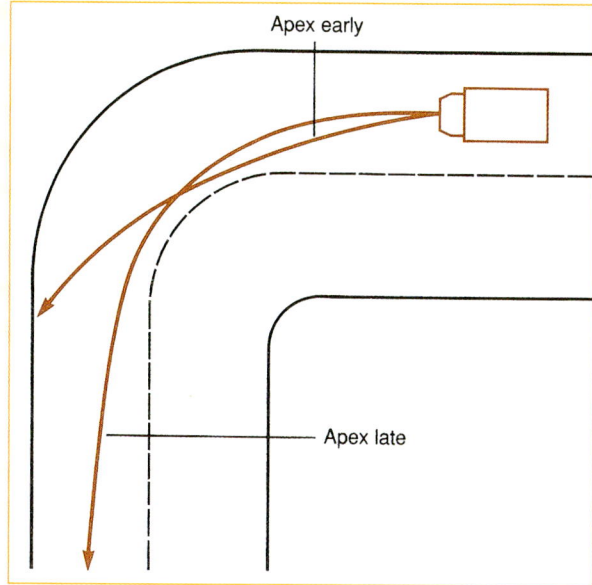

Figure 33-17 To keep the ambulance in the proper lane on a curve, you must know the vehicle's present position and projected path and take the corner at the correct speed.

Road Positioning and Cornering. Road position means the position of the vehicle on the roadway relative to the inside or outside edge of the paved surface. To corner efficiently, you must know the vehicle's present position and its projected path. The aim is to take the corner at the speed that will put you in the proper road position as you exit the curve (Figure 33-17). The process works in the following way: The apex of the turn through a curve is the point at which the vehicle is closest to the inside edge of the curve. If you reach the apex early in the curve, the vehicle will be forced toward the outside of the roadway as it exits the curve. If you reach the apex late in the curve, the vehicle will tend to stay on the inside of the roadway; this helps you to keep the vehicle in the proper lane.

Controlled Acceleration. Controlled acceleration is the use of acceleration to control the vehicle; it is done by applying foot pressure on the accelerator pedal. Acceleration is most efficient when the vehicle is traveling in a straight line, because the force of linear acceleration is equally distributed to the rear wheels. If you accelerate in a curve or during a turn, however, you force the vehicle to the outside of the curve. If acceleration in this direction becomes excessive, the vehicle may drift out of control and become unstable. Accelerate as you come out of the curve to provide stability to the vehicle.

Controlled Braking. Controlled braking is the use of the brakes to control the vehicle. Brakes not only control the movement of the vehicle, causing it to slow or stop; they also help to control its direction. Braking while the vehicle is traveling in a straight line is the safest, most efficient method. Braking in a turn causes a loss of efficiency. You might not notice this at low speed, but it becomes more apparent at higher speeds. Applying the brakes while cornering is not an effective way to slow the vehicle and may actually cause a skid or spin. Instead, maintain your speed by simultaneously easing off brake pressure and increasing accelerator pressure. Getting the feel for the proper brake pressure comes with experience and practice driving your assigned vehicle.

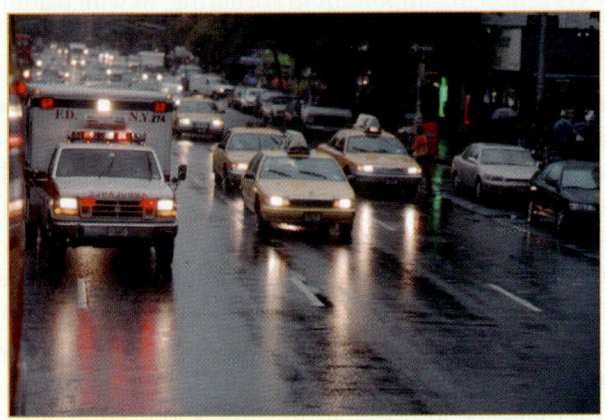

Figure 33-18 Modify your speed according to changing weather, road, and driving conditions.

> **In the Field**
>
> ALWAYS BRAKE IN A STRAIGHT LINE!

Weather and Road Conditions

You should be constantly alert to changing weather, road, and driving conditions 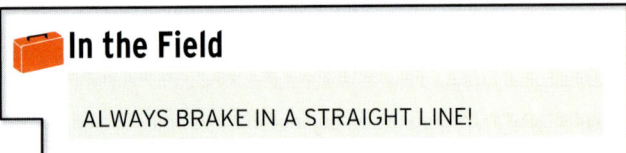. Whether going to or coming from an emergency, you must modify your speed according to road conditions. Take warnings of ice or hazardous conditions seriously, and be prepared to take an alternative route, if necessary. During a major disaster, all public safety and emergency services should be coordinated. If you run into unexpected traffic congestion, notify the dispatcher so that other emergency vehicles can select alternative routes.

Even the most careful drivers will occasionally run into unexpected situations that may require special driving skills. However, if you drive at a speed that is appropriate for the weather and road conditions, you will minimize these situations. For example, it is safer if you decrease speed in weather situations involving fog, rain, snow, or ice.

Hydroplaning. On a wet road, a tire usually displaces the water on the road surface and stays in direct contact with the road. However, at speeds greater than 30 mph, the tire may be lifted off the road as water "piles up" under it; the vehicle feels as if it were floating. This is known as <u>hydroplaning</u>. At higher speeds on wet roadways, the front wheels may actually be riding on a sheet of water, robbing the driver of control of the vehicle. If hydroplaning occurs, you should gradually slow down without jamming on the brakes. Shimmying the steering wheel may also help to cut through the water and allow the tires to regain road surface, but this technique requires a great deal of practice.

Water On the Roadway. Wet brakes will slow the vehicle and pull it to one side or the other. If at all possible, avoid driving through large pools of standing water; often, you cannot tell how deep they are. If you must drive through standing water, make sure to slow down and turn on the windshield wipers. After driving out of the pool, lightly tap the brakes several times until they are dry. If the vehicle is equipped with anti-lock brakes, apply a steady, light pressure to dry the brakes. Driving through moving water should be avoided at all times.

Decreased Visibility. In areas where there is fog, smog, snow, or heavy rain, common sense tells you to slow down after warning cars behind you. At night, use only low headlight beams for maximum visibility without reflection. You should always use headlights during the day to increase your visibility to other drivers. Also, watch carefully for stopped or slow-moving cars.

Ice and Slippery Surfaces. A light mist on an oily, dusty road can be just as slippery as a patch of ice. Good all-weather tires and an appropriate speed will reduce traction problems significantly. If you are in an area that often has snowy or icy conditions, consider using studded snow tires, if they are permitted by law. You should be especially careful on bridges and overpasses when

> **EMT-I Tips**
>
> Although preventing skids and sliding is ideal, you are likely to skid or slide at least occasionally, especially if you live in climates with ice and snow. Your training should include the technique for correcting slides during turns. If you are likely to drive on ice and snow, you should practice until it becomes automatic—at low speeds in an area where there is no danger of collisions. Remember that four-wheel-drive and front-wheel-drive vehicles behave differently in slides than their rear-wheel-drive counterparts.

temperatures are close to freezing. These road surfaces will freeze much faster than surrounding road surfaces because they lack the warming effect of the ground underneath.

Laws and Regulations

Regulations regarding vehicle operations vary from state to state and from city to city, but some things are the same everywhere. Drivers of emergency vehicles have certain limited privileges in every state. However, these privileges do not lessen their liability in a crash. In fact, in most cases, the driver is presumed to be guilty if a collision occurs while the ambulance is operating with warning lights and siren. Motor vehicle crashes are the single largest source of lawsuits against EMS personnel and services.

While on an emergency call, emergency vehicles typically are exempt from usual vehicle operations. If you are on an emergency call and are using your warning lights and siren, you may be allowed to do the following:

- Park or stand in an otherwise illegal location
- Proceed through a red traffic light or stop sign after stopping
- Drive faster than the posted speed limit
- Make a turn that is normally illegal
- Travel left of center to make an otherwise illegal pass

Remember that these exemptions vary by state and local jurisdiction. Therefore, you should check your local statutes for regulations in your area.

An emergency vehicle is never allowed to pass a school bus that has stopped to load or unload children and is displaying its flashing red lights or extended "stop arm." If you approach a school bus that has its lights flashing, you should stop before reaching the bus and wait for the driver to make sure the children are safe, close the bus door, and turn off the warning lights. Only then may you carefully proceed past the stopped school bus.

You are the Provider Part 5

You are transporting the female patient and your reassessment shows that your patient's condition is deteriorating.

Vital Signs	Recording Time: 8 Minutes After Patient Contact
Respirations	24 breaths/min
Pulse	154 beats/min
Skin	Pale and diaphoretic
Blood pressure	88/52 mm Hg
Sao_2	88% on 15 L/min oxygen via nonrebreathing mask

8. Your partner, who is driving, is using lights and siren. What are the three basic principles that govern the use of warning lights and siren on an ambulance?
9. While on an emergency call such as this, using your warning lights and sirens, what might you be able to do?

Use of Warning Lights and Siren. Three basic principles govern the use of warning lights and siren on an ambulance:

1. The unit must be on a true emergency call to the best of your knowledge.
2. Both audible and visual warning devices must be used simultaneously.
3. The unit must be operated with due regard for the safety of all others, on and off the roadway.

The siren is probably the most overused piece of equipment on an ambulance. In general, the siren does not help you as you drive, nor does it really help other motorists. Motorists who are driving at the speed limit with the windows up, the radio on, and the air conditioner or heater set on high may not hear the siren until the ambulance is very close. If the radio is particularly loud, they may not hear the siren at all.

If you do have to use the siren, be sure to warn the patient before you turn it on. Be especially mindful not to increase the speed of the ambulance just because the siren is in use. Always travel at a speed that will allow you to stop safely at all times, especially so that you are prepared for drivers who do not give you the right-of-way. Never assume that warning lights and sirens will allow you to drive through a congested area without stopping or slowing down. Slow down to ensure that all drivers are stopping as you approach an intersection, then proceed with due caution.

Some ambulance headlights are equipped with a high-beam flasher unit. These are the most visible, effective warning devices for clearing traffic in front of the vehicle.

Right-of-way Privileges. A right-of-way privilege is just that: a privilege. State motor vehicle statutes or codes often grant an emergency vehicle, such as an ambulance, the right to disregard the rules of the road when responding to an emergency. However, in doing so, the operator of an emergency vehicle must not endanger people or property under any circumstances.

Consider this case: An ambulance is approaching an intersection that is controlled by a four-way stop sign. The ambulance, with lights and audible warning device functioning, proceeds through the intersection without slowing or stopping and crashes into a car coming from its right. Did the operator of the ambulance act appropriately by going through the intersection in this manner?

Right-of-way privileges for ambulances vary from state to state. Some states allow you to proceed through a red light or stop sign after you stop and make sure it is safe to go on. Other states allow you to proceed through a controlled intersection "with due regard," using flashing lights and siren. This means that you may proceed only if you consider the safety of all people who are using the highway. If you fail to use due regard, your service might be sued if a crash occurs. If you are found to be at fault, you may personally have to pay punitive damages or face both civil and criminal sanctions.

Get to know your local right-of-way privileges. Exercise them only when it is absolutely necessary for the patient's well-being. The use of lights and audible warning devices is a matter of state and local practice and protocol.

Use of Escorts. Using a police escort is an extremely dangerous practice. When other motorists hear a siren and see a police car passing, they might assume that the police car is the only emergency vehicle and not see the ambulance. The only time an escort is justified is when you are in unfamiliar territory and truly need a guide more than an escort. In such cases, neither vehicle should use any warning lights or sirens. If you are being guided by a police car, make sure that you follow at a safe distance.

Intersection Hazards. Intersection crashes are the most common and usually the most serious type of collision in which ambulances are involved. Always be alert and careful when approaching an intersection. If you are on an urgent call and cannot wait for traffic lights to change, you should still come to a momentary stop at the light; look around for other motorists and pedestrians before proceeding into the intersection.

Motorists who "time the traffic lights" present a serious hazard. You may arrive at an intersection while the light is green. At the same time, a motorist who is timing the lights on the cross street arrives at the intersection. The motorist has a red light but knows that it is about to turn green and is expecting to go through. The stage is now set for a serious crash.

Another common intersection hazard occurs when the driver of one emergency vehicle follows another emergency vehicle through an intersection without assessing the situation carefully. A motorist who has yielded the right-of-way to the first vehicle may proceed into the intersection without expecting a second vehicle. You should exercise extreme caution in these situations. To signal motorists that a second unit is approaching, use a siren tone that is different from that of the first vehicle.

TABLE 33-10	Guidelines for Safe Ambulance Driving

Keep in mind the following guidelines whenever you are en route to a call:

1. Select the shortest and least congested route to the scene at the time of the dispatch.
2. Avoid routes with heavy traffic congestion; know alternative routes to each hospital during rush hours.
3. Avoid one-way streets; they may become clogged. Do not go against the flow of traffic on a one-way street, unless absolutely necessary.
4. Watch carefully for bystanders as you approach the scene. Curiosity seekers rarely move out of the way.
5. Park the ambulance in a safe place once you arrive at the scene. If you park facing into traffic, turn off your headlights so that they do not blind oncoming cars unless they are needed to illuminate the scene. If the vehicle is blocking part of the road, keep your warning lights on to alert oncoming motorists; otherwise, turn them off.
6. Drive within the speed limit while transporting patients, except in the rare extreme emergency.
7. Go with the flow of the traffic.
8. Use the siren as little as possible en route.
9. Always drive defensively.
10. Always maintain a safe following distance. Use the "4-second rule": Stay at least 4 seconds behind another vehicle in the same lane.
11. Try to maintain an open space or cushion in the lane next to you as an escape route in case the vehicle in front of you stops suddenly.
12. Use your siren if you turn on the emergency lights, except when you are on a freeway.
13. Always assume that other drivers will not hear the siren or see your emergency lights.

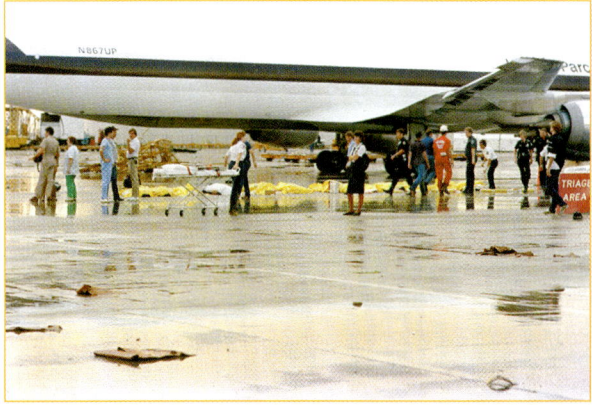

Figure 33-19 Once you arrive at the scene, you should report to dispatch and ask for backup, rescue, or HazMat units as needed.

Guidelines for Safe Ambulance Driving

Table 33-10 ▲ lists the guidelines to follow when you are en route to a call.

Arrival at the Scene

Once you reach the scene, you should inform dispatch that you have arrived and give a brief report of what you see. Also report any unexpected situations, such as the need for backup units, a heavy rescue unit, or a HazMat team Figure 33-19 ▶. Do not enter the scene if there are any hazards to you. If there are dangerous hazards at the scene, the patient should be moved before you begin care. The patient may have to be moved by others if you are not appropriately equipped or trained.

Immediately size up the scene by using the following guidelines:
- Look for safety hazards.
- Evaluate the need for additional units or other assistance.
- Determine the mechanism of injury in trauma patients or the nature of the illness in medical patients.
- Evaluate the need to stabilize the spine.
- Make sure that you follow BSI precautions. The type of care that you expect to give will dictate what personal protective equipment you should wear.

If you are the first EMT-I at the scene of a mass casualty incident, quickly estimate the number of patients Figure 33-20 ▶. Inform dispatch that backup units are needed at the scene. Mass casualty incidents involve complex organization of personnel under the incident command system (see Chapter 36). In this system, individual EMT-Is may be assigned roles to do such things as begin the triage process, assist in treating patients, and loading patients for transportation to a hospital.

Safe Parking

In assessing the situation, you must decide where to park the ambulance. Pick a position that will allow for efficient traffic control and flow around a crash scene. Do not park alongside the scene, as you may block the movement of other emergency vehicles. Instead, park about 100′ past the scene on the same side of the road. It is best to park uphill and/or upwind of the

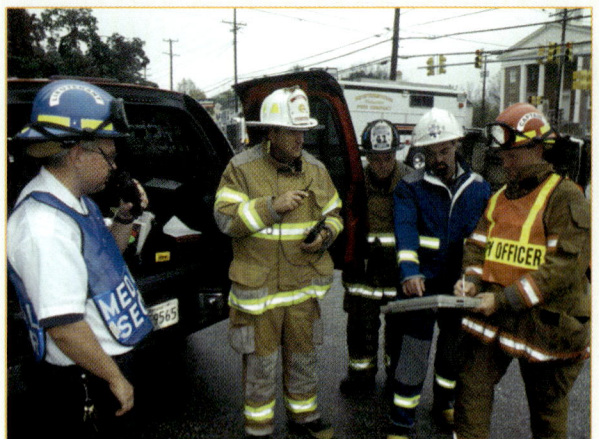

Figure 33-20 At a mass-casualty incident, follow instructions from the incident commander assigning your roles. These could include assisting with triage, treating patients, or loading patients for transportation to the hospital.

scene if smoke or hazardous materials are present Figure 33-21 ▼ . If you must park on the back side of a hill or curve, leave your warning lights or devices on. Do the same when parking at night. Always park so as to provide a cushion of space between your vehicle and operations at the scene. Assume that someone will collide with your vehicle and strike personnel on the scene.

Stay away from any fires, explosive hazards, downed wires, or structures that might collapse. Be sure to set the parking brake. If your vehicle is blocking part of the roadway, leave the emergency warning lights on. If your vehicle has them, leave only the flashing yellow lights on. Other drivers tend to drive toward emergency vehicles with flashing red or red and white lights. Within these safety guidelines, you should try to park your ambulance as close to the scene as possible to facilitate emergency medical care. If necessary, you can temporarily block traffic to unload equipment and to load patients quickly and safely. If you must do this, try to do it quickly so that traffic is not blocked any longer than is absolutely necessary. Also, park in a location that will not hamper you leaving the scene.

Traffic Control

After ensuring your own safety, your first responsibility at a crash scene is to care for the patients. Only when all the patients have been treated and the emergency situation is under control should you be concerned with restoring the flow of traffic. If the police are slow to arrive at the scene, you might then need to take action.

The purpose of traffic control is to ensure an orderly traffic flow and to prevent another crash. Under ordinary circumstances, traffic control is difficult. A crash or disaster scene presents serious additional problems. Passing motorists often "rubberneck," paying little attention to the roadway in front of them. Some curiosity seekers may park down the road and return on foot, creating still other hazards. As soon as possible, place appropriate warning devices, such as reflectors, on both sides of the crash. Remember, the main objectives in directing traffic are to warn other drivers, to prevent additional crashes, and to keep vehicles moving in an orderly fashion so that care of the injured is not interrupted.

The Transfer Phase

In almost every case, you will provide lifesaving care right where you find the patient, before moving the patient to the ambulance. You may then begin less critical measures, such as bandaging and splinting. Next, you must package the patient for transport, securing him or her to a device such as a backboard, a scoop stretcher, or the wheeled ambulance stretcher. Then move to the ambulance, and properly lift the patient into the patient compartment.

No matter how careful the driver may be, riding to the hospital while lying on one's back on a stretcher can be uncomfortable and even dangerous. So be sure to secure the patient with at least three straps across the body Figure 33-22 ▶ . Use deceleration or stopping straps over the shoulders to prevent the patient from

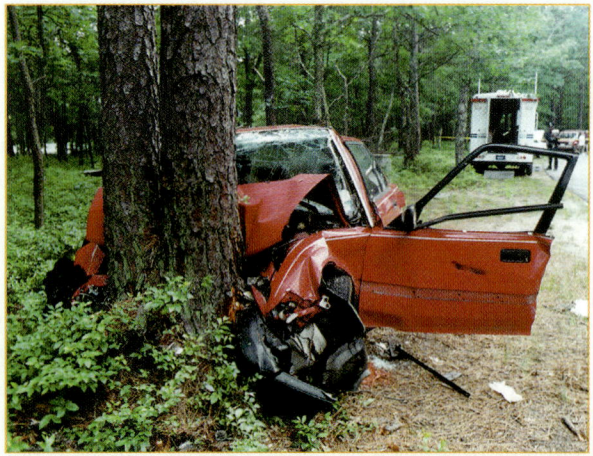

Figure 33-21 Park the ambulance about 100′ past the scene on the same side of the road. Park uphill or upwind of the scene if hazardous materials are present.

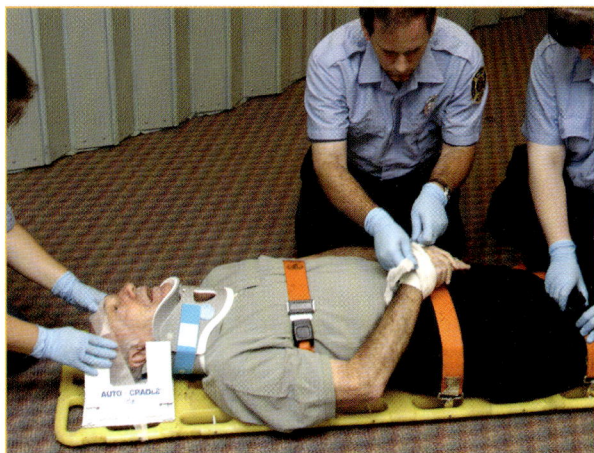

Figure 33-22 Be sure to secure the patient appropriately for protection during transport.

continuing to move forward in case the ambulance suddenly slows or stops.

The Transport Phase

Inform dispatch when you are ready to leave with the patient. Report the number of patients you have and the name of the receiving hospital. Even though you have already assessed and treated the patient, you should continue to monitor him or her en route. These ongoing assessments may uncover changes in the patient's vital signs and overall condition. Be sure to recheck the patient's vital signs en route. The frequency of checking vital signs depends on the situation, but checking them every 15 minutes for a stable patient and every 5 minutes for an unstable patient is a practice that many services use. In addition, it is important that you continually reassess the patient's clinical situation, and record and address new problems and the patient's responses to earlier treatment.

At this time, you should also contact the receiving hospital. Inform medical control about your patient(s) and the nature of the problem(s). Depending on the number of EMT-Is on your team and how much care the patient needs, you might also want to begin working on your written report while en route.

Finally, and most importantly, do not abandon the patient emotionally. Do not become so involved in paperwork and ongoing assessments that you ignore the patient's fears. You are there to help the patient as a person, so use this time to reassure him or her. Some patients, such as the very young or elderly, may benefit from added attention during transport. Be aware of the differing levels of need of different patients.

The Delivery Phase

Inform dispatch as soon as you arrive at the hospital. Then follow these steps to transfer the patient to the receiving hospital:

1. Report your arrival to the triage nurse or other arrival personnel.
2. Physically transfer the patient from the stretcher to the bed directed for your patient.
3. Present a complete verbal report at the bedside to the nurse or physician who is taking over the patient's care.
4. Complete a detailed written report, and leave a copy with an appropriate staff member.

The written report should include a summary of the history of the patient's current illness or injury with pertinent positives and negatives, mechanism of injury, and findings on your arrival. In addition, you should list vital signs and briefly mention relevant past medical or surgical history, as well as information regarding medication and allergies. Also, be sure to include any treatment and its effect that occurred in the prehospital setting.

While at the hospital, you may be able to restock any items that were used during the run, such as oxygen masks or dressings and bandages **Figure 33-23**. Remember, though, that your priority is transfer of the patient and patient information to the hospital staff. Restocking the ambulance comes second.

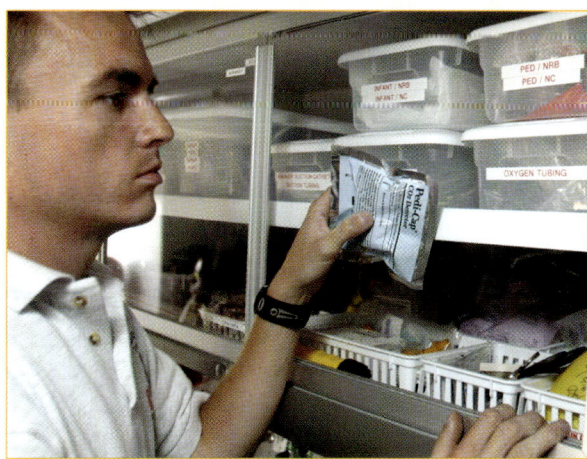

Figure 33-23 After transferring the patient and relating patient information to the hospital staff, you should restock any items that were used during the run.

The Postrun Phase

During the postrun phase, you should complete and file any additional written reports and again inform dispatch of your status, location, and availability.

You are also responsible for maintaining the ambulance so that it is safe and available on a moment's notice. This means routine inspections. Use a written checklist to document needed repairs or replacement of equipment and supplies. In addition, you must ensure that the following steps are taken after each trip:

- Scrub blood, vomitus, and other substances from the floors, walls, and ceilings with soap and water.
- Clean and decontaminate the inside of the ambulance, according to state and local regulations. (You can use a 10% solution of bleach in water to clean the ambulance after any contamination.)
- Dispose of any contaminated waste in the manner prescribed by your agency.
- Clean the outside of the ambulance as needed.
- Replace or repair broken or damaged equipment without delay.
- Replace any other equipment or supplies that were used.
- Refuel the vehicle if the fuel tank is below required reserves. The oil level should be checked each time the vehicle is refueled.

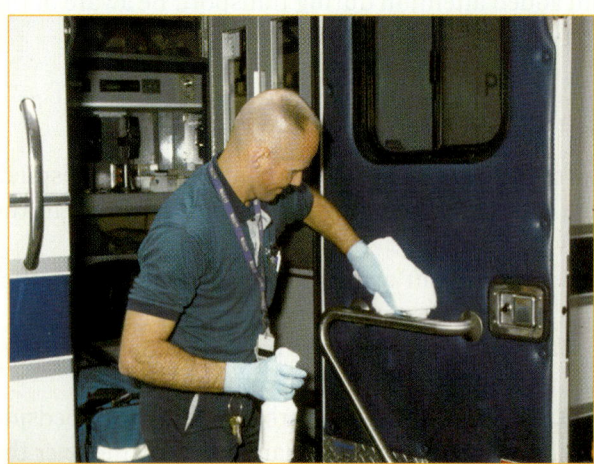

Figure 33-24 Be sure to clean and disinfect the ambulance and equipment at the station if you did not do so at the hospital.

En Route to the Station

Once you leave the hospital, inform dispatch whether or not you are in service and where you are going. As soon as you are back at the station, you should do the following:

- Clean and disinfect the ambulance and any equipment that was used, if you did not do so before leaving the hospital **Figure 33-24**.
- Restock any supplies you did not get at the hospital.

You are the Provider   Part 6

Your second patient has severe head trauma. Due to the prolonged extrication, you have determined that aeromedical transport would be the best means of transport for this patient. Further assessment of this patient reveals the following:

Vital Signs	Recording Time: 2 Minutes After Patient Contact
Respirations	8 breaths/min, shallow
Pulse	48 beats/min, bounding
Skin	Pale and diaphoretic
Blood pressure	160/90 mm Hg
Sao_2	96% on 100% oxygen by nonrebreathing mask

10. What is the survival of this patient dependent upon?

It is important that you know the meanings of the terms "cleaning," "disinfection," "high-level disinfection," and "sterilization," as follows:

- Cleaning. The process of removing dirt, dust, blood, or other visible contaminants from a surface.
- Disinfection. The killing of pathogenic agents by directly applying a chemical made for that purpose to a surface.
- High-level disinfection. The killing of pathogenic agents by the use of potent means of disinfection.
- Sterilization. A process, such as the use of heat, that removes all microbial contamination.

Dispose of any contaminated materials that are not disinfected by placing them in the appropriate containers used for biohazard disposal.

Prescheduled Preventative Maintenance Checks

The ambulance chassis and engine components are subjected to significantly greater stresses than the typical automobile or truck. For this reason, the manufacturer's recommendations for periodic maintenance must be strictly followed, especially regarding lubrication, oil and filter changes, transmission and differential service, brakes, wheel alignment, wheel bearings, and steering components. Many services now use a Hobbs or engineer hour meter, which assesses hours of engine use, in addition to the odometer to help determine periodic maintenance requirements.

As is the case with emergency medical care report forms, local and individual differences will affect inspection routines. Your ambulance service should develop its own inspection forms for all three kinds of inspections so that nothing is overlooked. These forms should be filed for inspection and legal documentation and should be kept for at least 3 years.

Air Medical Operations

Air ambulances are used to evacuate medical or trauma patients. They land at or near the scene, and transport patients to trauma facilities every day in many areas.

There are two basic types of air medical units: fixed-wing and rotary-wing, otherwise known as helicopters (Figure 33-25 ▶). Fixed-wing aircraft generally are used for interhospital patient transfers over distances greater than 100 to 150 miles. For shorter distances, ground transport or rotary-wing aircraft are more efficient.

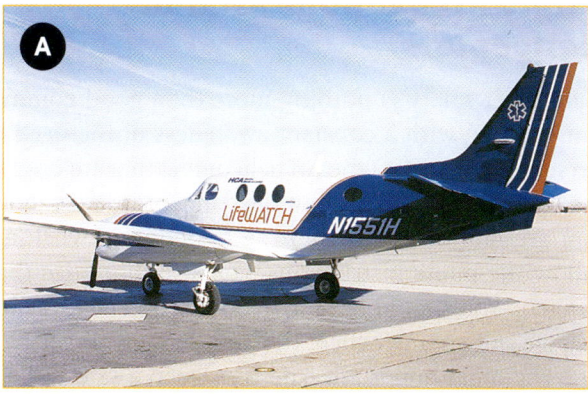

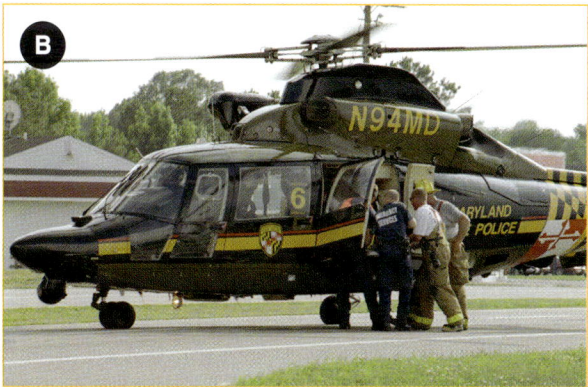

Figure 33-25 A. Fixed-wing aircraft are generally used to transfer patients from one hospital to another over distances greater than 100 to 150 miles. **B.** A rotary-wing aircraft, or helicopter, is used to help provide emergency medical care to patients who need to be transported quickly over shorter distances.

Specially trained medical flight crews accompany all air ambulance flights. Your role in fixed-wing aircraft transfers probably will be limited to providing ground transport for the patient and medical flight crew between the hospital and the airport.

Rotary-wing aircraft have become an important tool in providing emergency medical care. Trauma patient survival is directly related to the time that elapses between injury and definitive treatment. Most helicopters that are used for emergency medical operations fly well in excess of 100 mph in a straight line, without road or traffic hazards. The crew may include EMTs, paramedics, flight nurses, or physicians.

You should be familiar with the capabilities, protocols, and methods for accessing helicopters in your area. Helicopter services provide training for EMT-Is in ground operations and safety. The following discussion is an introduction to safe operations, and is not intended to be substituted for the more extensive courses available locally.

Safety Precautions Around Helicopters

Helicopter safety is nothing more than good common sense, along with a constant awareness of the need for personal safety. The types of helicopters that are used for medical operations vary, but the dangers are the same. If you are familiar with the way helicopters work and follow the pilot's instructions, you will minimize these dangers. You should be sure to do nothing near the helicopter and go only where the pilot or crew directs you.

The most important rule is to keep a safe distance from the aircraft whenever it is on the ground and "hot," which means when the tail rotor is spinning. This means that every EMT-I should stay outside the landing zone perimeter unless directed by the pilot or a member of the flight crew that they are to come to the aircraft. Usually, the flight crew will come to the EMT-Is carrying their own equipment and not require any assistance inside the landing zone. If you are asked to enter the landing zone, stay away from the tail rotor; the tips of its blades move so rapidly that they are invisible. In fact, never approach the helicopter from the rear, even if it is not hot. If you must move from one side of the helicopter to another, go around the front. Never duck under the body, the tail boom, or the rear section of the helicopter; the pilot cannot see in these areas. The proper approach area is between the nine-o'clock and three-o'clock positions as the pilot faces forward (Figure 33-26).

Another area of concern is the height of the main rotor blade. On many aircraft, it is flexible and may dip as low as 4' off the ground (Figure 33-27). When you approach the aircraft, walk in a crouched position. Wind gusts can alter the blade height without warning, so be sure to protect equipment as you carry it under the blades. Air turbulence created by the rotor blades can blow off hats and loose equipment. These, in turn, can become a danger to the aircraft and personnel in the area.

When accompanying a flight crew member, you must follow directions exactly. Never try to open any aircraft door or move equipment unless a crew member tells you to. When told to approach the aircraft, use extreme caution and pay constant attention to hazards.

Landing Sites

Although a helicopter can fly straight up and down, this is the most dangerous mode of operation. The safest and most effective way to land and take off is similar to that used by fixed-wing aircraft. Landing at a slight angle allows for safer operations. Takeoff combines a gradual

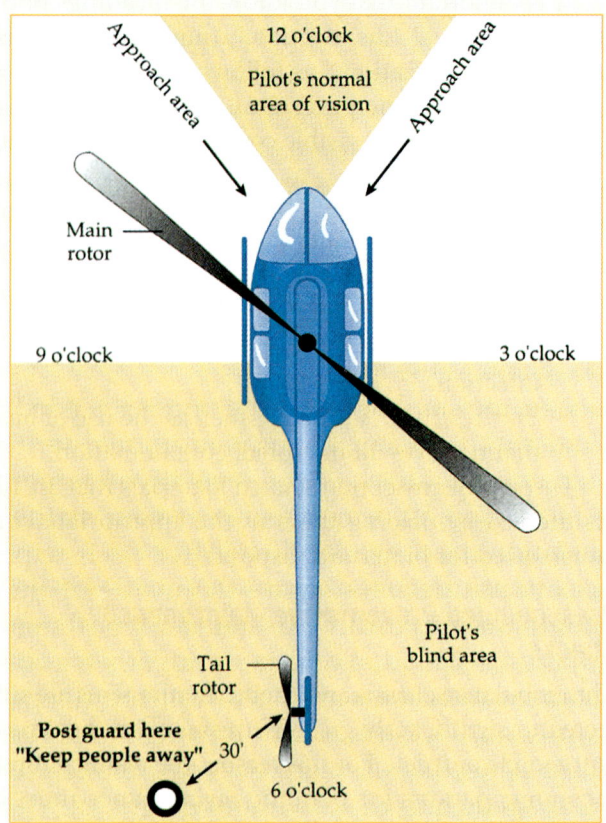

Figure 33-26 Approach a helicopter between the nine-o'clock and three-o'clock positions as the pilot faces forward.

lift and forward motion to travel up and out on a slight angle.

Clearing a landing site is another important role you can play. Look for loose debris, electric or telephone wires, poles, or any other hazards that might interfere with the safe landing of the helicopter. If you note any hazards, inform the pilot by radio or other signal. The

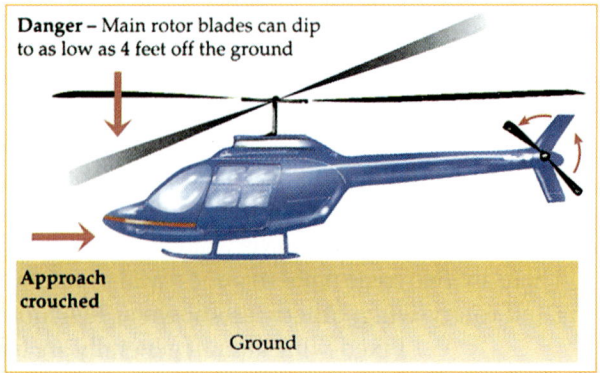

Figure 33-27 The main rotor blade of the helicopter is flexible and may dip as low as 4' off the ground.

pilot will usually "overfly," or survey the site, before final approach and landing to ensure that all potential dangers are identified. Depending on the time, temperature, winds, and the aircraft's weight, you might need to mark the proposed site with flags, lights, or other signaling devices. A clear landing zone that is at least 100′ by 100′ is recommended.

If the helicopter must land on a grade, extra caution is advised. The main rotor blade will be closer to the ground on the uphill side. In this situation, approach the aircraft from the downhill side only (Figure 33-28 ▶). Do not move the patient to the helicopter until the crew has signaled that they are ready to receive you. A flight crew member will direct and assist you in loading the patient.

Nighttime operations are considerably more hazardous than daytime operations because of the darkness. The pilot may fly over the area with the helicopter's lights on to spot obstacles and the shadows of overhead wires, which can be hard to see. Do not shine spotlights, flashlights, or any other lights in the air to help the pilot; they may temporarily blind the pilot. Instead, direct light beams toward the ground at the landing site. Even after the helicopter has landed, you should not aim lights

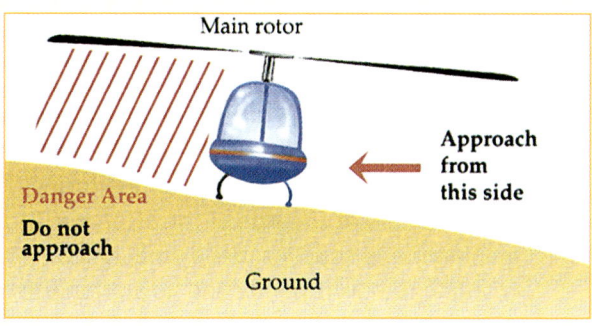

Figure 33-28 Approach a helicopter on a grade from the downhill side only.

anywhere near it. Of course, smoking, open lights or flames, and flares are prohibited within 50′ of the aircraft at all times.

For further information on air ambulances, see the following publications:

- DOT publication HS805-703, Air Ambulance Guidelines, February 1981
- DOT publication HS806-841, Proceedings: National MEDEVAC Helicopter Conference

You are the Provider

1. What are the nine phases of an ambulance call?

1. Preparation for the call
2. Dispatch
3. En route
4. Arrival at scene
5. Transfer of the patient to the ambulance
6. En route to the receiving facility (transport)
7. At the receiving facility (delivery)
8. En route to the station
9. Postrun

2. Why is having "due regard for the safety of others" essential when responding to a call?

Because it is necessary that the patient be safely transported to an appropriate medical care facility in the shortest practical time. This takes common sense and defensive driving techniques. Speed is no substitute for these qualities. EMT-Is must always travel at a speed that will allow them to stop safely at all times,

Summary

especially so that they are prepared for drivers who do not give them the right-of-way. Never assume that warning lights and sirens will allow you to drive through a congested area without stopping or slowing down. Slow down as you approach an intersection to ensure that all drivers are stopping, then proceed with due caution.

3. What is included in the preparation phase of an ambulance call?

Making sure that equipment and supplies are in their proper place and ready for use and that the vehicle is in good working order with appropriate fluid levels, fuel, tire pressure, etc, is an important part of preparing for the call.

4. What items on your squad are needed to care for life-threatening conditions and where should they be stored?

Equipment for airway management, artificial ventilation, and oxygen delivery are necessary.

Continued

You are the Provider continued   Summary

Place these items within easy reach, at the head of the stretcher. Place items for cardiac care, control of external bleeding, and monitoring blood pressure at the side of the stretcher. Store equipment and supplies in the ambulance according to how urgently and how often they are used.

5. To adequately care for this patient's airway needs, what airway equipment should be carried on every ambulance?

Airway management equipment that should be carried on ambulances includes the following:

- Oropharyngeal airways for adults, children, and infants
- Nasopharyngeal airways for adults and children
- Two sets of equipment for advanced airway procedures if your service is authorized by state regulation and the medical director to perform these: one in the ambulance and one in the jump kit that you carry to the patient

6. To ensure that you have an adequate supply of oxygen, what are the two types of oxygen containers that should be carried on every ambulance?

The ambulance should carry at least two oxygen supply units: one portable and one installed.

7. Your squad was able to successfully extricate the first patient and is working to extricate this patient. What extrication equipment should be carried on every ambulance?

- 12" wrench, adjustable, open-end
- 12" screwdriver, standard square bar
- 8" screwdriver, Phillips head #2
- Hacksaw with 12" carbide wire blades
- Vise-grip pliers, 10"
- 5-lb hammer with 15" handle
- Fire ax, butt, 24" handle
- Wrecking bar with 24" handle. This may be in a combination tool with a hammer and ax.
- 51" crowbar, pinch point
- Bolt cutter with 1" to $1\frac{1}{4}$" jaw opening
- Folding shovel, pointed blade
- Tin snips, double action, 8" minimum
- Gauntlets, reinforced, leather covering past mid-forearm; one pair per crew member
- Rescue blanket
- Ropes, 5,400-lb tensile strength in 50" lengths in protective bags
- Mastic knife (able to cut seat belt webbing)
- Spring-load center punch
- Pruning saw
- Heavy duty 2" x 4" and 4" x 4" shoring (cribbing) blocks, various lengths

8. Your partner, who is driving, is using lights and siren. What are the three basic principles that govern the use of warning lights and siren on an ambulance?

1. The unit must be on a true emergency call to the best of your knowledge.
2. Both audible and visual warning devices must be used simultaneously.
3. The unit must be operated with due regard for the safety of all others, on and off the roadway.

9. While on an emergency call such as this, using your warning lights and sirens, what might you be able to do?

If you are on an emergency call and are using your warning lights and siren, you may be allowed to do the following:

- Park or stand in an otherwise illegal location
- Proceed through a red traffic light or stop sign after stopping
- Drive faster than the posted speed limit
- Make a turn that is normally illegal
- Travel left of center to make an otherwise illegal pass

Remember that these exemptions vary by state and local jurisdiction. Therefore, you should check your local statutes for regulations in your area.

10. What is the survival of this patient dependent upon?

Trauma patient survival is directly related to the time that elapses between injury and definitive treatment. Most helicopters that are used for emergency medical operations fly well in excess of 100 mph in a straight line, without road or traffic hazards.

Prep Kit

Ready For Review

- An ambulance is an emergency medical vehicle that contains a driver's compartment, a patient compartment, equipment and supplies to provide care at the scene and during transport, and two-way radio communication. It must be designed and constructed to ensure maximum safety and comfort.

- Ambulances should be white on the outside with an orange stripe, and should have blue lettering and reflective emblems. The Star of Life®, a six-pointed emblem that identifies ambulances that meet federal specifications, may be displayed on the sides, rear, and roof of the ambulance.

- The ambulance should be climate-controlled, insulated, and easy to clean. The patient compartment should be large enough to accommodate two stretcher patients, two EMTs, and all the necessary equipment and supplies to take care of patients.

- The nine phases of an ambulance call are preparation for the call, dispatch, en route to the scene, arrival at the scene, transferring the patient to the ambulance, en route to the receiving facility, at the receiving facility, en route to the station, and postrun.

- Specific patient care supplies should be carried on the ambulance, including basic medical equipment, airway management equipment and ventilation devices, suctioning equipment, oxygen delivery equipment, CPR equipment, and basic wound care supplies.

- In addition, you must ensure that splinting supplies, childbirth supplies, and appropriate medications are on board.

- An automated external defibrillator, as permitted by medical control, should always be carried on the ambulance. A jump kit, patient transfer equipment, nonmedical supplies, and initial extrication and rescue equipment are also needed.

- The driver must be qualified to drive the ambulance; he or she must be physically and emotionally fit, and have the proper attitude. The driver must know and follow safe driving practices.

- In addition to ground ambulances, air ambulances in the form of fixed-wing aircraft or helicopters are used to evacuate patients, land at a crash scene, and transport patients to trauma facilities.

Vital Vocabulary

acceleration The process of increasing speed.

air ambulances Fixed-wing aircraft and helicopters that have been modified for medical care; used to evacuate and transport patients with life-threatening injuries to treatment facilities.

ambulance A specialized vehicle for treating and transporting sick and injured patients.

chassis The vehicle frame.

chassis set Transfer of the weight (center of mass) of the ambulance to different points on the chassis.

cleaning The process of removing dirt, dust, blood, or other visible contaminants from a surface.

coefficient of friction A measure of the grip of the tire on the road surface.

CPR board A device that provides a firm surface under the patient's torso.

deceleration The process of slowing down.

decontaminate To remove or neutralize radiation, chemical, or other hazardous material from clothing, equipment, vehicles, and personnel.

disinfection The killing of pathogenic agents by direct application of chemicals.

first-responder vehicle A specialized vehicle used to transport EMS equipment and personnel to the scenes of medical emergencies.

footprint The area of contact between the ambulance tire and the road surface.

friction Resistance to the motion of one body against another.

Technology

- Interactivities
- Vocabulary Explorer
- Anatomy Review
- Web Links
- Online Review Manual

www.EMSzone.com/EMT

Prep Kit continued...

high-level disinfection The killing of pathogenic agents by using potent means of disinfection.

hydroplaning A condition in which the tires of a vehicle may be lifted off the road surface as water "piles up" under them, making the vehicle feel as though it is floating.

jump kit A portable kit containing items that are used in the initial care of the patient.

Star of Life® The six-pointed star that identifies vehicles that meet federal specifications as licensed or certified ambulances.

sterilization A process, such as heating, that removes microbial contamination.

Points to Ponder

You are transporting a patient to the hospital and the family is following you in a private vehicle. You notice that the family goes through a stop sign with you, and then goes through a red light with you. You go through the next red light without slowing. A vehicle entering the intersection from your left swerves, narrowly avoiding the ambulance, but broadsides the family's vehicle.

What problems do you identify with this scenario? How could this tragedy have been avoided?

Issues: Understanding the Procedures Required for Emergency Driving and the Dangers Involved; Due Regard for the Safety of Others

Assessment in Action

You and your EMT-B partner have just started your shift. You are working out of a busy downtown station in a major city. You are conducting your vehicle inspection when you are dispatched to an emergency.

1. While completing your vehicle inspection, you should ensure that:
   A. the airway equipment is conveniently located at the foot of the stretcher.
   B. the regulator is detached from the oxygen tank.
   C. you have an adequate supply of PPE.
   D. the medications have expired.

2. Your dispatch information typically includes all of the following EXCEPT:
   A. call location is Buck's Diner at 1234 Main Street.
   B. patient's name is Gladys Peabody.
   C. nature of the problem is chest pain.
   D. number of patients is one.

3. While responding to this call, you should keep in mind all of the following rules of safe driving EXCEPT:
   A. you should clear your own intersections.
   B. you and your partner should be properly restrained.
   C. you should know your ambulance characteristics.
   D. you should assume motorists see you.

4. You should also remember that the most common location for collisions is:
   A. on hills.
   B. on curves.
   C. at intersections.
   D. on straight roadways.

5. As you arrive on the scene, you observe a crowd standing around a person lying on the sidewalk. You should quickly:
   A. determine whether additional units are needed.
   B. immediately move the patient to the ambulance.
   C. park the ambulance so that the roadway is blocked.
   D. ask a bystander what happened, then assess the patient's ABCs.

6. You are transporting your patient to the hospital. Factors that may inhibit your partner's ability to control the ambulance include all of the following EXCEPT:
   A. weather.
   B. excessive speed.
   C. poor judgment.
   D. wearing restraints.

7. Your partner should keep in mind the principles governing the use of lights and siren, which include all of the following EXCEPT:
   A. the siren is used only at intersections.
   B. a true emergency situation is involved or suspected.
   C. lights and siren are used together.
   D. the ambulance is operated with due regard for the safety of others.

8. You have treated and transported your patient. Your activities at the hospital will include all of the following EXCEPT:
   A. completing a written report.
   B. helping the patient walk from the ambulance into the hospital.
   C. restocking supplies that were used on the call.
   D. providing hospital staff with a complete verbal report.

9. The killing of pathogenic agents by the use of potent means of disinfection is called:
   A. cleaning.
   B. disinfecting.
   C. high-level disinfection.
   D. sterilization.

www.EMSzone.com/EMT

Lifting and Moving

1999 Objectives

There are no 1999 objectives for this chapter.

1985 Objectives

1.6.50 Describe how the patient is immobilized to the stretcher, and to the ambulance. (p 1427-1430, 1433-1435)

Additional Objectives*

Cognitive

1. Define body mechanics. (p 1404)
2. Discuss the guidelines and safety precautions that need to be followed when lifting a patient. (p 1406, 1415)
3. Describe the safe lifting of cots and stretchers. (p 1414)
4. Discuss the guidelines and safety precautions for carrying patients and/or equipment. (p 1406, 1415)
5. Discuss one-handed carrying techniques. (p 1410)
6. Describe correct and safe carrying procedures on stairs. (p 1412, 1416)
7. State the guidelines for reaching and their application. (p 1417)
8. Describe correct reaching for log rolls. (p 1418)
9. State the guidelines for pushing and pulling. (p 1418)
10. Discuss the general considerations of moving patients. (p 1419)
11. State three situations that may require the use of an emergency move. (p 1419)
12. Identify the following patient-carrying devices.
    - Wheeled ambulance stretcher
    - Portable ambulance stretcher
    - Stair chair
    - Scoop stretcher
    - Long spine board
    - Basket stretcher
    - Flexible stretcher (p 1413, 1416, 1430, 1435-1438)
13. List the steps in performing rapid extrication. (p 1423)

Affective

14. Explain the rationale for properly lifting and moving patients. (p 1464)

Psychomotor

15. Working with a partner, prepare each of the following devices for use, transfer a patient to the device, properly position the patient on the device, move the device to the ambulance, and load the patient into the ambulance: wheeled ambulance stretcher, portable ambulance stretcher, stair chair, scoop stretcher, long spine board, basket stretcher, and flexible stretcher. (p 1413, 1416, 1430, 1435-1438)

*These are noncurriculum objectives.

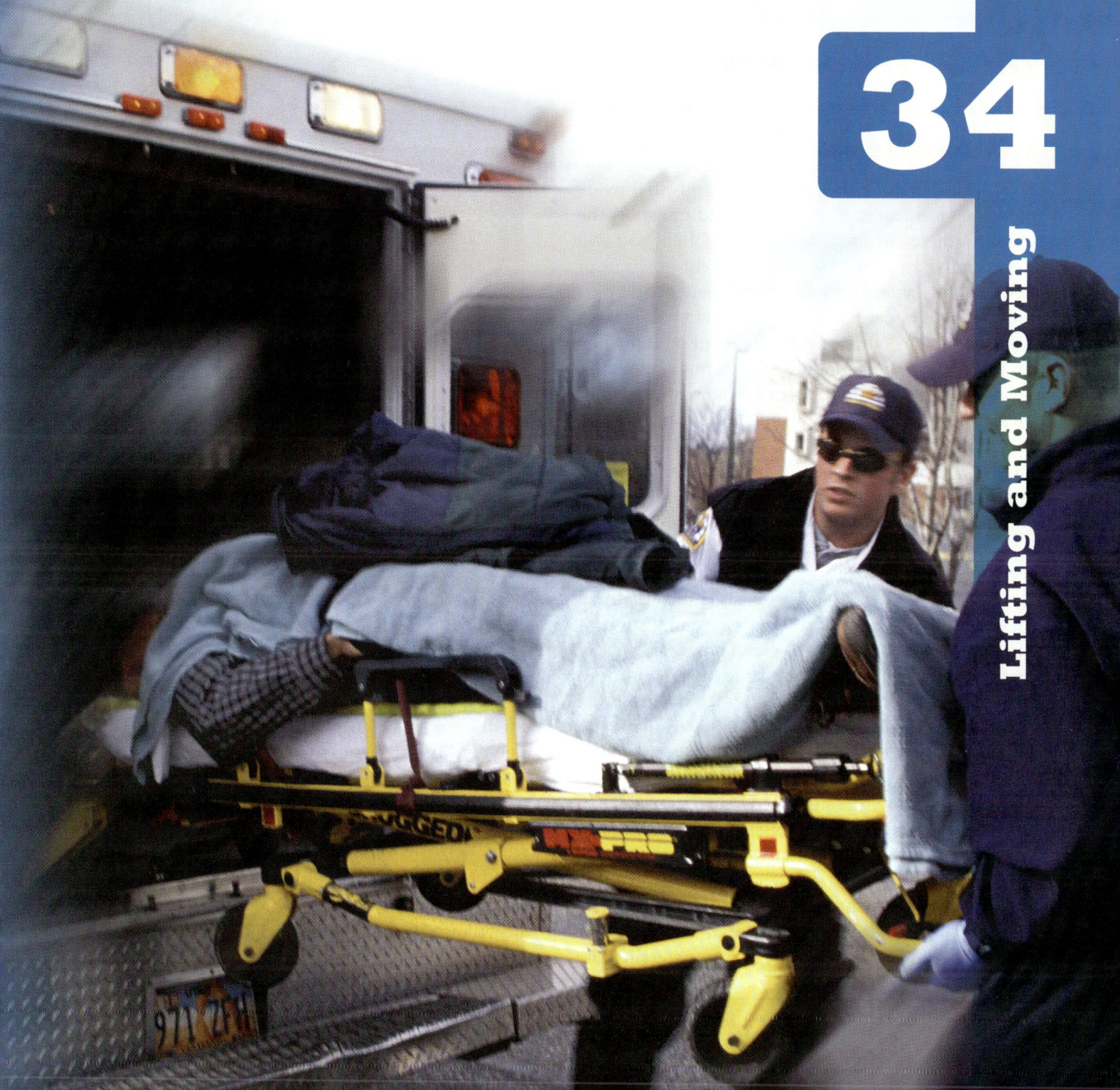

34

Lifting and Moving

You are the Provider

You and your partner are called to the scene of a man who has fallen in his bathroom. When you and your partner arrive on the scene, you find a 38-year-old man lying prone over the edge of the bathtub, with his torso in the bathtub and his legs outside of the bathtub. The patient is conscious and alert.

The vast majority of the calls that you respond to as an EMS provider involve lifting and moving patients. Understanding the basic principles of body mechanics, as well as developing the ability to weigh multiple options based upon patient need, will help you make appropriate decisions. This chapter will prepare you to do that as well as answer the following questions:

1. Does the patient need an *emergency*, *urgent*, or *nonurgent* move?
2. How can you accomplish this move in the safest way possible?

Lifting and Moving Patients

You will have to move the patient frequently to provide emergency medical care in the field and transport the patient to the emergency department. Often, you will have to move the patient into a different position or location. Once you have assessed the patient and provided emergency care, you and your team will have to move the patient onto a long backboard or cot. Then you must move the patient to the waiting ambulance and load the patient into the patient compartment. After you arrive at the hospital, you must unload the patient, move him or her to the correct examining room, and transfer the patient from the cot to the emergency department bed. To avoid injury to the patient, yourself, or your partners, you will have to learn how to lift and carry the patient properly, using proper body mechanics and a power grip. To be able to move a patient safely and properly in the various situations that you will encounter in the field, you will have to learn how to perform emergency body drags and lifts, rapidly move a patient from a car onto the cot, assist a patient from a chair or bed onto the cot, and lift a patient from the floor onto the cot. In addition, you will need to move a patient from the bed onto the cot or carry a patient up or down stairs. You and your team will have to know how to place a patient with a suspected spinal injury onto a long backboard and package patients with and without suspected spinal injury. At times, you and your team will need to move a patient who weighs more than 300 lb or carry a patient on a trail or across rugged terrain. You will need to know the special techniques for loading and unloading the cot and transferring the

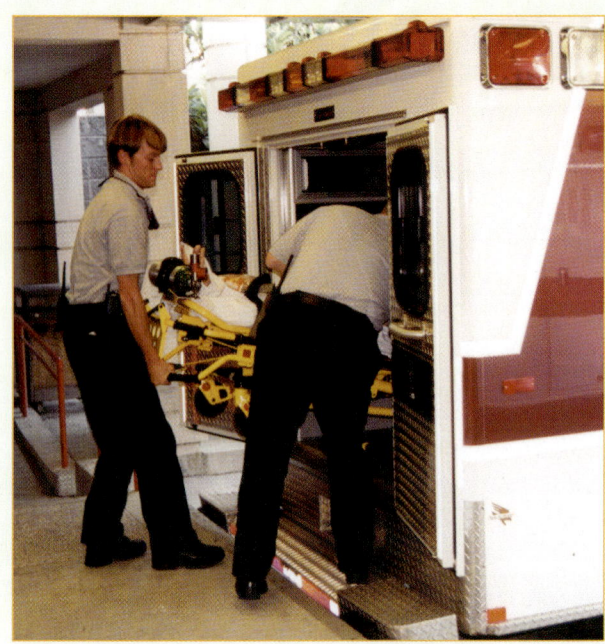

Figure 34-1 Loading and unloading patients requires good physical conditioning to reduce your risk of injury.

patient from the cot to an examining table or bed in the emergency department Figure 34-1.

Lifting and carrying are dynamic processes. To ensure that no individual suddenly bears unexpected, dangerous weight and to reduce the risk of injury to an EMT-I or the patient, you must know where rescuers should be positioned and how to give and receive lifting commands so that all parties act simultaneously. You will also need to know how to prepare patient-moving devices, such as a wheeled ambulance stretcher (also called an ambulance cot or simply "the cot"), stair chair, backboard, scoop stretcher, folding ambulance stretcher, basket stretcher, or flexible stretcher, and when and how to use them. This chapter will cover lifting, carrying, and reaching techniques as well as principles of moving patients, including emergency, urgent, and nonurgent moves. In addition, different types of equipment and patient positioning will be discussed in detail.

Body Mechanics

Anatomy Review

The shoulder girdle rests on the rib cage and is supported by the vertebrae that lie inferior to it. The arms are connected to and hang from the shoulder girdle. When the person is standing upright, the individual

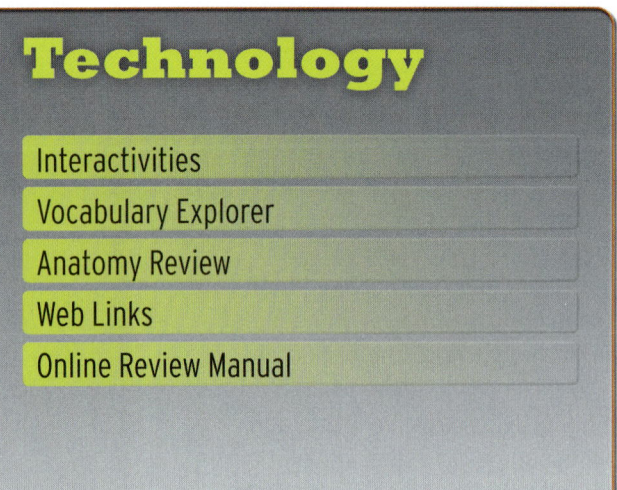

weight-bearing vertebrae are stacked on top of each other and aligned over the sacrum. The sacrum is both the mechanical weight-bearing base of the spinal column and the fused central posterior section of the pelvic girdle.

When a person is standing upright, the weight of anything being lifted and carried in the hands is reflected onto the shoulder girdle, the spinal column inferior to it, the pelvis, and then the legs Figure 34-2. In lifting, if the shoulder girdle is aligned over the pelvis and the hands are held close to the legs, the force that is exerted against the spine occurs in an essentially straight line down the strong-stacked vertebrae in the spinal column. Therefore, with the back properly maintained in an upright position, very little strain occurs against the muscles and ligaments that keep the spinal column in alignment, and significant weight can be lifted and carried without injury to the back Figure 34-3. However, you may injure your back if you lift with your back curved or, even if straight, bent significantly forward at the hips Figure 34-4. With the back in either of these positions, the shoulder girdle lies significantly anterior

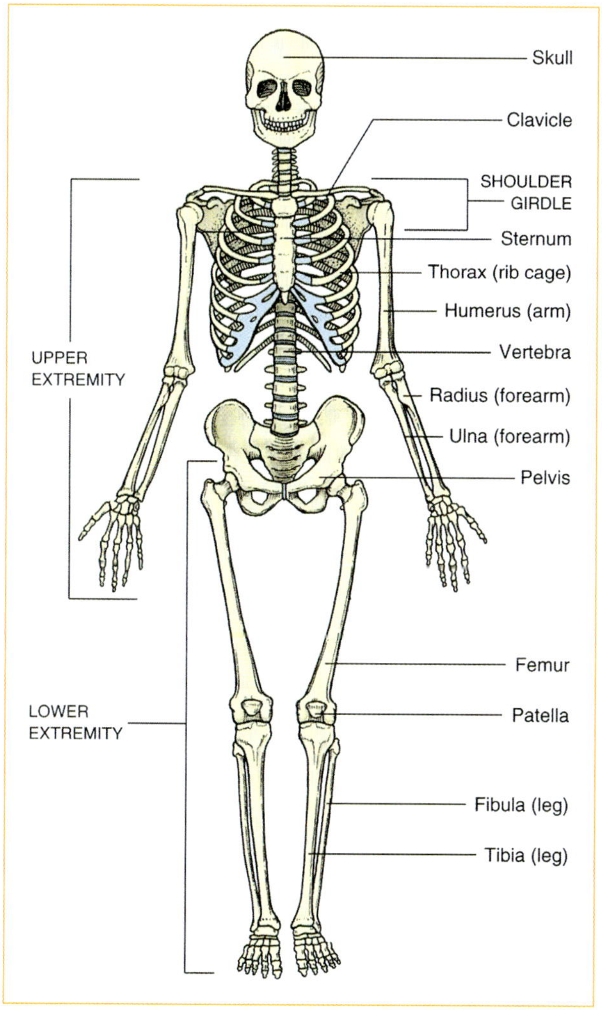

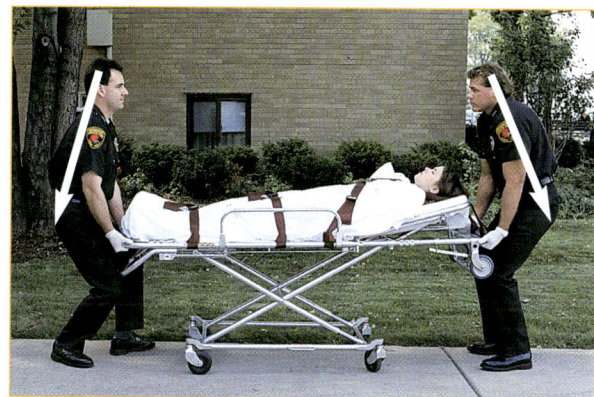

Figure 34-3 If your body is properly aligned when you lift, the line of force exerted against the spine occurs in an essentially straight line down the vertebrae. In this way, the vertebrae support the lift.

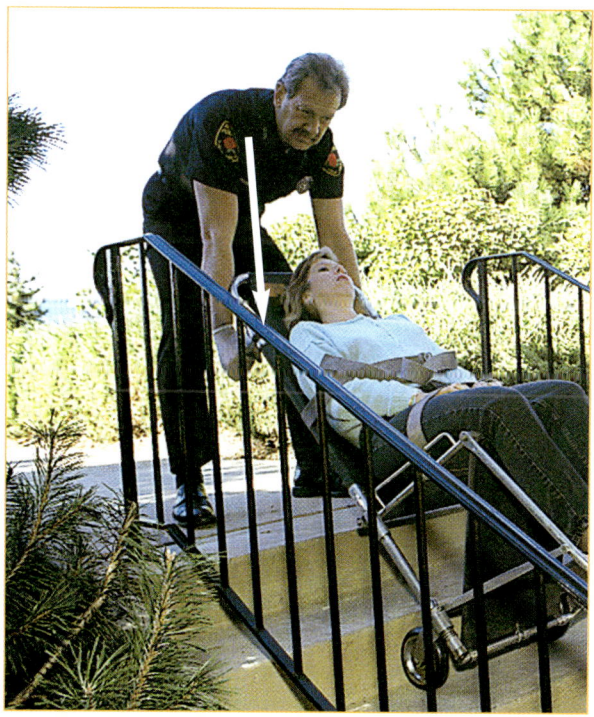

Figure 34-4 You may be injured if you lift with your back curved, as the lifting force is exerted primarily across, rather than down, the spinal column. When this occurs, the muscles of the back, not the vertebrae, are supporting the lift.

Figure 34-2 When you are standing upright, the weight of anything that you lift and carry in your hands is borne by the shoulder girdle, the spinal column, the pelvis, and the legs.

to the pelvis, and the force of lifting is exerted primarily across, rather than down, the spinal column. When this occurs, the weight is supported by the muscles of the back and ligaments that run from the base of the skull to the pelvis, keeping the spinal column in alignment, rather than by each vertebral body and disk resting on those aligned below it. In addition, the upper spine and torso serve as a lever so that the force that is exerted against the muscles and ligaments in the lumbar and sacral regions, as a result of the mechanical advantage produced, is many times that of the combined weight of your upper body and the object you are lifting. Therefore, the first key rule of lifting is to always keep the back in a straight, upright (vertical) position and to lift without twisting.

When lifting, you should spread your legs about 15" apart (shoulder width) and place your feet so that your center of gravity is properly balanced between them. Then, with the back held upright, bring your upper body down by bending the legs. Once you have properly grasped the patient or cot and made any necessary adjustments in the location of your feet, lift the patient by raising your upper body and arms and by straightening your legs until you are again standing. Because the leg muscles are exercised by walking, climbing stairs, or running, they are well developed and extremely strong. Therefore, as well as being the safest way to lift, lifting by extending the properly placed flexed legs is also the most powerful way to lift. This method is appropriately called a <u>power lift</u>. The power lift position is also useful for individuals who have weak knees or thighs.

Even if the back is held properly upright, the same adverse force across the spinal column and leverage against the lower back will occur if you lift a heavy object with your arms outstretched so that your hands are significantly anterior to the plane described by the front of the torso. Therefore, you should *never* lift a patient or other heavy object while reaching any significant distance in front of your torso or face. Whenever you are lifting or carrying a patient, be sure to hold your arms so that your hands are almost immediately adjacent to the plane described by your anterior torso (the anterior torso and imaginary lines extended vertically above and below it). Always keep the weight that you are lifting as close to your body as possible.

Lateral force across the spine and sideways leverage against the lower back must also be avoided. If you lift with only one arm or with the arms extended more to one side than the other, more force will be exerted against one side of the shoulder girdle than the other, causing lateral force to be exerted across the spinal column. To prevent this, keep your arms approximately the same distance apart as when hanging at each side of the body, with the weight distributed equally and properly centered between them. If the weight is not balanced between both arms or properly centered between the shoulders when you are preparing to lift, turn your body and/or move to the left or right until the weight is properly balanced and centered. To lift safely and produce the maximal power lift, you should take the following steps (**Skill Drill 34-1**):

1. **Tighten your back in its normal upright position** and use your abdominal muscles to lock it in a slight inward curve.
2. **Spread your legs apart about 15"**, and bend your legs to lower your torso and arms.
3. **With arms extended down each side of the body**, grasp the cot or backboard with your hands held palm up and just in front of the plane described by the anterior torso and imaginary lines extending vertically from it to the ground.
4. **Adjust your orientation and position** until the weight is balanced and centered between both arms (**Step 1**).
5. **Reposition your feet** as necessary so that they are about 15" apart with one slightly farther forward and rotated so that you and your center of gravity will be properly balanced between them. Be sure to straddle the object, keep your feet flat, and distribute your weight to the balls of the feet or just behind them (**Step 2**).
6. **With the arms extended downward**, lift by straightening your legs until you are fully standing. Make sure your back is locked in and that your upper body comes up before your hips (**Step 3**).

Reverse these steps whenever you are lowering the cot. Always remember to avoid bending at the waist.

Your safety, as well as that of the other EMT-Is and the patient, depends on the use of proper lifting techniques and having and maintaining a proper hold when lifting or carrying a patient. If you do not have proper hold of the cot, or of the patient in a body lift, you will

> ### EMT-I Safety
>
> EMT-I and patient safety depends on proper lifting techniques and maintaining a proper hold while lifting and carrying. Loss of grasp by one EMT-I may cause injury to another team member as well as the patient.

Performing the Power Lift

Skill Drill 34-1

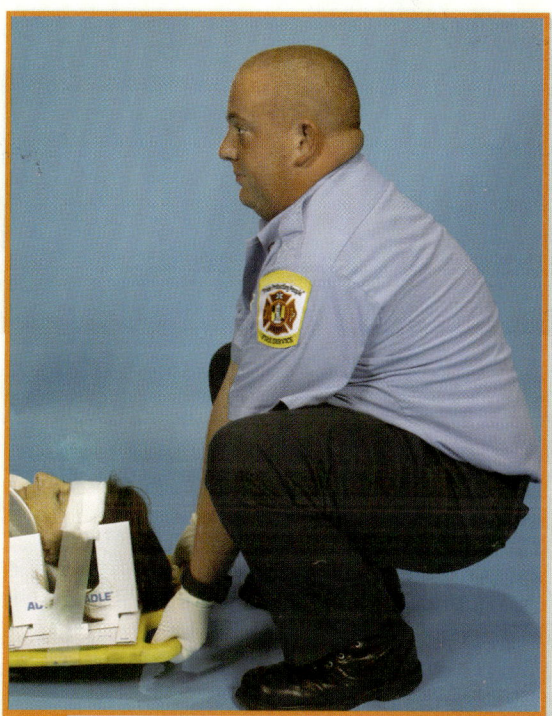

1 Lock your back into an upright, inward curve. Spread and bend your legs. Grasp the backboard, palms up and just in front of you. Balance and center the weight between your arms.

2 Position your feet, straddle the object, and distribute weight.

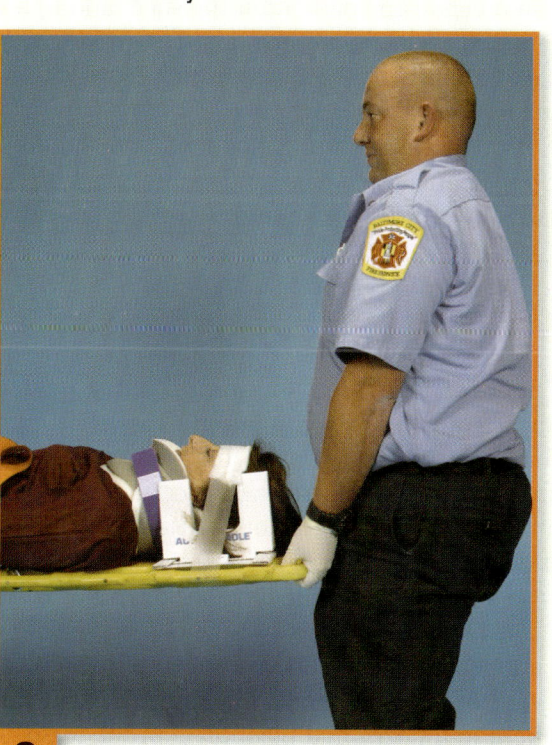

3 Straighten your legs and lift, keeping your back locked in.

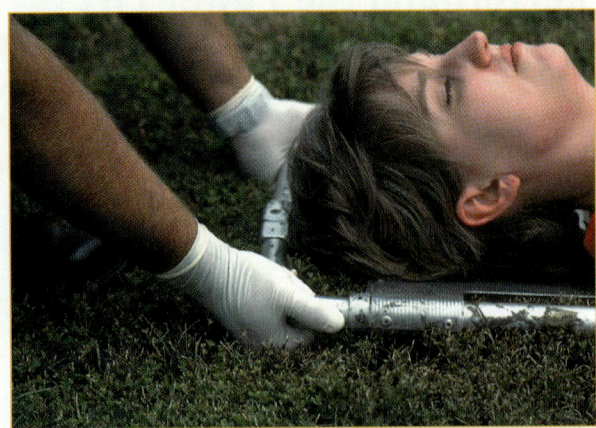

Figure 34-5 To perform the power grip, grasp the handle of the litter with your palms up and your thumb extending up. Make sure your hands are about 10" apart and that your fingers are all at the same angle. The underside of the handle should be fully supported by the palm of your hand.

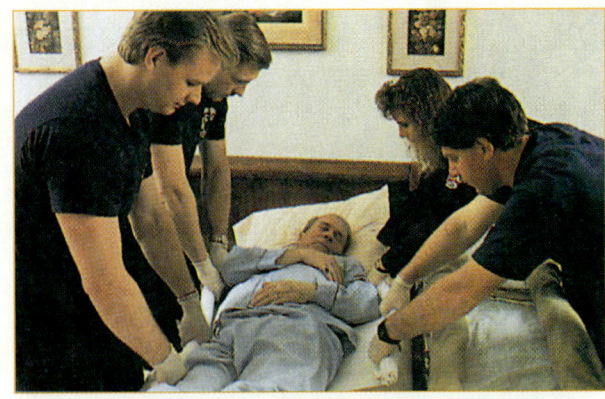

Figure 34-6 When lifting a patient by a bedsheet, you should center the patient on the sheet and tightly roll up the excess fabric on each side. This produces a cylindrical handle that provides a strong way to grasp the fabric.

not be able to bear a proper share of the weight, and there is an increased chance that you can suddenly lose your grasp with one or both hands. If you temporarily lose your grasp with one or both hands, the position and weight distribution of the cot changes suddenly, and the other members of the team must quickly reach beyond a safe distance to avoid dropping the patient. As a result, sudden excessive force may be placed across each one's spine, causing lower back injury.

You should use the <u>power grip</u> to get the maximum force from your hands whenever you are lifting a patient (Figure 34-5 ▲). The arm and hand have their greatest lifting strength when facing palm up. Whenever you grasp a cot or backboard, your hands should be at least 10" apart. Each hand should be inserted under the handle with the palm facing up and the thumb extended upward. You should then advance the hand until the thumb prevents further insertion and the cylindrical handle lies firmly in the crease of the curved palm. Curl your fingers and thumb tightly over the top of the handle. All your fingers should be at the same angle. To have the proper power grip, make sure that the underside of the handle is fully supported on your curved palm with only the fingers and thumb preventing it from being pulled sideways or upward out of the palm.

If you must lift the object higher once you have lifted by extending your legs, you will be able to "curl" the object higher by using your biceps to flex the arms while maintaining the power grip and weight supported in the palms.

You should *never* grasp a cot or backboard with the hand placed palm down over the handle. In lifting with the palm down, the weight is supported by the fingers rather than the palm. This hand orientation places the tips of the fingers and thumb under the handle. If the weight forces them apart, your grasp on the handle will be lost.

When lifting a patient by a sheet or blanket, you should center the patient on the sheet and tightly roll up the excess fabric on each side. This produces a cylindrical handle that provides a strong, secure way to grasp the fabric (Figure 34-6 ▲).

When directly lifting a patient, you should tightly grip the patient in a place and manner that will ensure that you will not lose your grasp on the patient.

Weight and Distribution

Whenever possible, you should use a device that can be rolled to move a patient. However, in case a wheeled device is not available, you must make sure that you understand and follow certain guidelines for carrying a patient on a cot. (Table 34-1 ▶) shows the guidelines.

If a patient is supine on a backboard or is lying or in a semi-sitting position on the cot, his or her weight is not equally distributed between the two ends of the device. Between 68% and 78% of the body weight of a patient in a horizontal position is in the torso. Therefore, more of the patient's weight rests on the head end of the device than on the foot end.

TABLE 34-1	Guidelines for Carrying a Patient on a Cot

- Be sure that you know or can find out the weight to be lifted and the limitations of the team's abilities.
- Coordinate your movements with those of the other team members while constantly communicating with them.
- Do not twist your body as you are carrying the patient.
- Keep the weight that you are carrying as close to your body as possible while keeping your back in a locked-in position.
- Be sure to flex at the hips, not at the waist, and bend at the knees, while making sure that you do not hyperextend your back by leaning back from your waist.

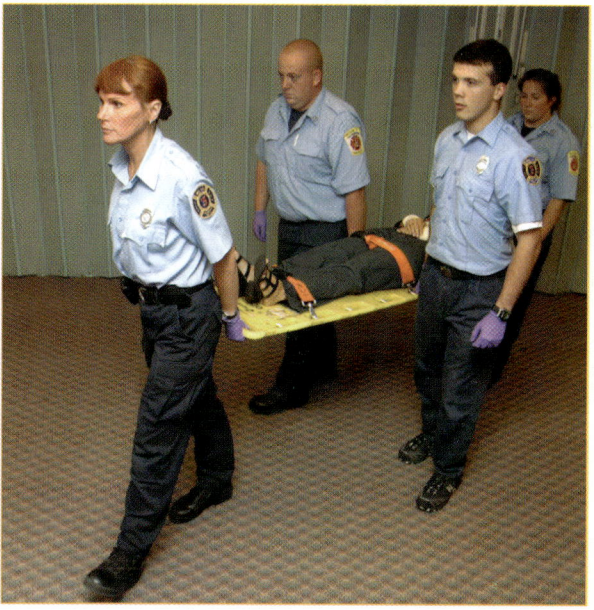

Figure 34-7 The diamond carry requires four rescuers, one each at the head of the backboard, the foot end, and each side of the patient's torso.

A patient on a backboard or cot should be lifted and carried by four rescuers in a <u>diamond carry</u>, with one EMT-I at the head end of the device, one at the foot end, and one at each side of the patient's torso (Figure 34-7 ▶ Skill Drill 34-2 ▶). Follow these steps to perform the diamond carry:

1. To best balance the weight, the EMT-Is at each side should be located so that they are able to grasp the board or stretcher with one hand adjacent to the distal edge of the patient's pelvis and the other midthorax. **All four lift the device while facing in toward the patient (Step 1)**.
2. **Once the device has been lifted**, the EMT-I at the foot end turns around to face forward **(Step 2)**.
3. **The EMT-I at each side** should turn the head-end hand palm down and then release the other hand **(Step 3)**.
4. **The EMT-Is at the sides turn toward the patient's feet.** All four should be facing the same direction and will be walking forward when carrying the patient **(Step 4)**.

You are the Provider — Part 2

Your assessment shows that the patient is stable. The patient complains of significant cervical pain and tenderness. The patient slipped on a wet floor and fell headfirst, striking his head on the wall and falling into the bathtub. The patient has no other complaints. The patient's vital signs are as follows:

Vital Signs	Recording Time: Zero Minutes
Respirations	16 breaths/min, adequate depth
Pulse	92 beats/min, regular
Blood pressure	Strong radial pulse, auscultated pressure deferred until patient removed from current location
Skin	Warm, dry, pink

3. What is the urgency of this move?
4. What are your primary considerations when planning this move?

Skill Drill 34-2

Performing the Diamond Carry

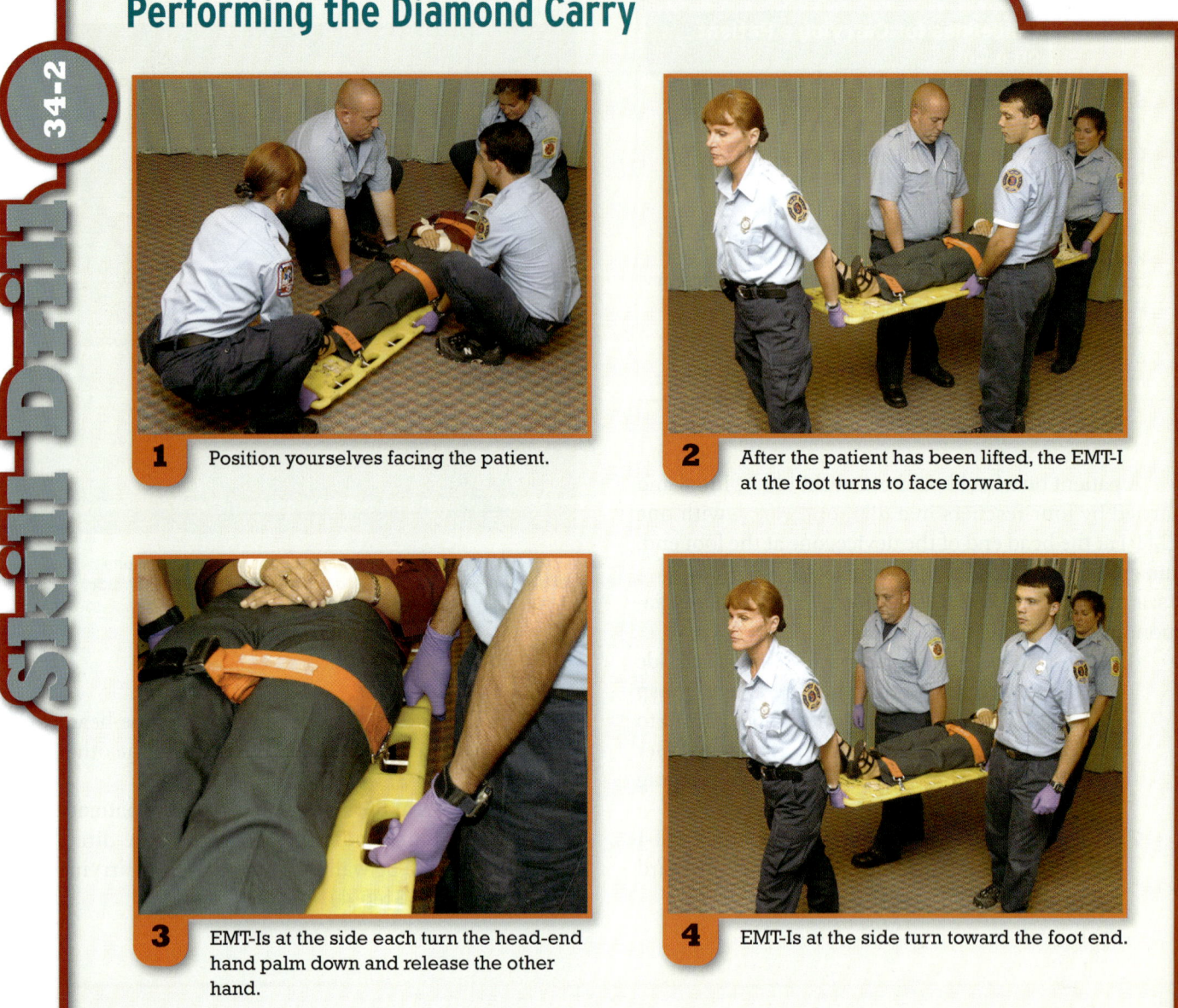

1. Position yourselves facing the patient.
2. After the patient has been lifted, the EMT-I at the foot turns to face forward.
3. EMT-Is at the side each turn the head-end hand palm down and release the other hand.
4. EMT-Is at the side turn toward the foot end.

A patient on a backboard or stretcher should be carried feet first to place the lightest load on the EMT-I at the patient's feet, who, to walk forward, must turn and grasp the handles with his or her back to the device. Carrying the patient feet first will also allow a conscious patient to see in the direction of movement.

It is important that you and your team use the correct lifting techniques to lift the cot. You must also make sure that your team members are of the same approximate height and strength, if possible.

One method of lifting and carrying a patient on a backboard is the one-handed carrying technique (Skill Drill 34-3). With this method, four or more EMT-Is each use one hand to support the backboard so that they are able to face forward as they are walking. Here are the steps:

1. **Before lifting the backboard**, be sure that at least two EMT-Is are on each side of the backboard facing each other and using both hands (**Step 1**).
2. **Lift the backboard** to carrying height using correct lifting techniques including a locked-in back (**Step 2**).
3. Once you have lifted the backboard to carrying height, you and your partners **turn in the direction you will be walking** and switch to using one hand (**Step 3**).

Performing the One-Handed Carrying Technique

Skill Drill 34-3

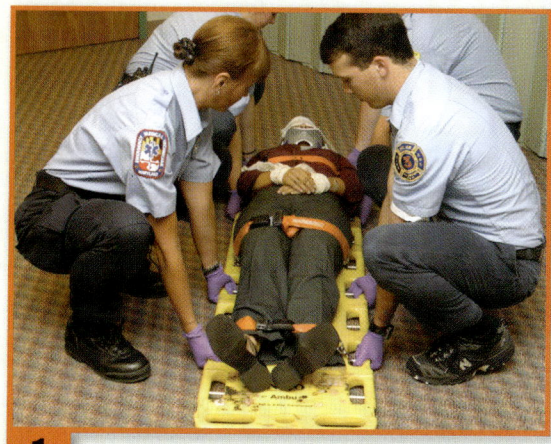

1 Face each other and use both hands.

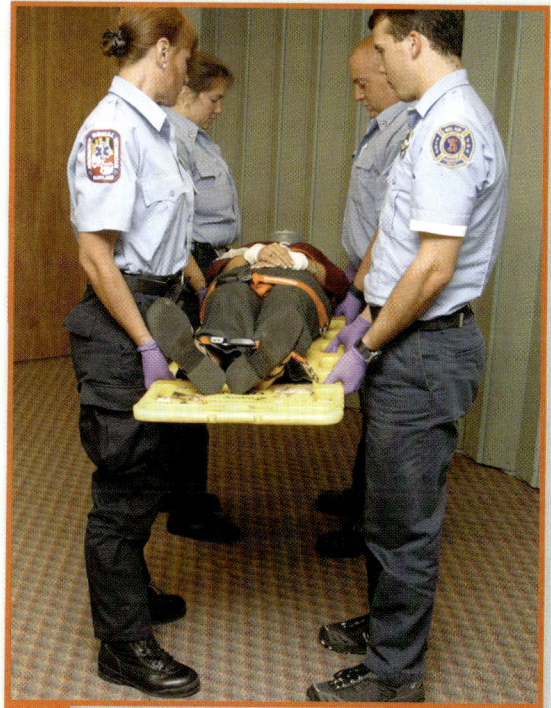

2 Lift the backboard to carrying height.

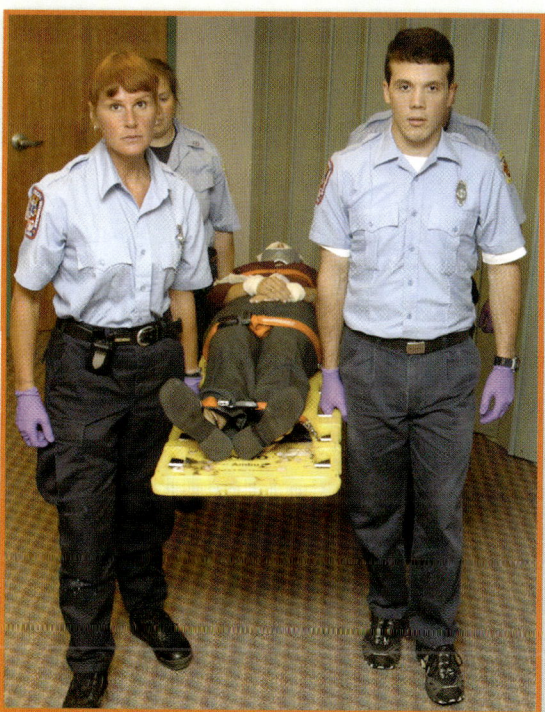

3 Turn in the direction you will walk and switch to using one hand.

Be sure to pick up and carry the backboard with your back in the locked-in position. If you need to lean to either side to compensate for a weight imbalance, you have probably exceeded your weight limitation. If this occurs, you may need to add helpers or reevaluate the carry, or you might injure yourselves or drop the patient.

A diamond carry is more stable than a carry in which there are two EMT-Is at each side of the backboard with no one at the patient's head or feet. With two EMT-Is at each side, each EMT-I can only hold the backboard or cot with one hand when turned to face in the same direction. However, both carrying methods are recommended and widely used in the field.

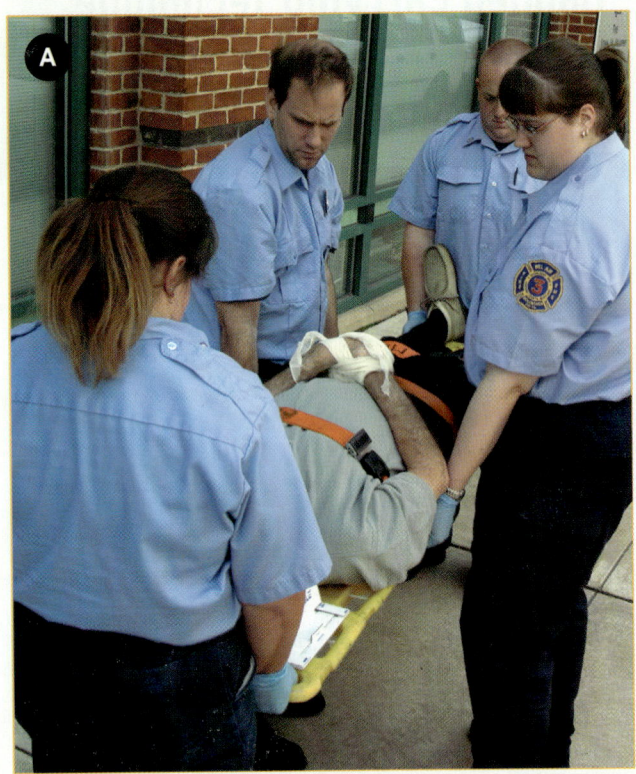
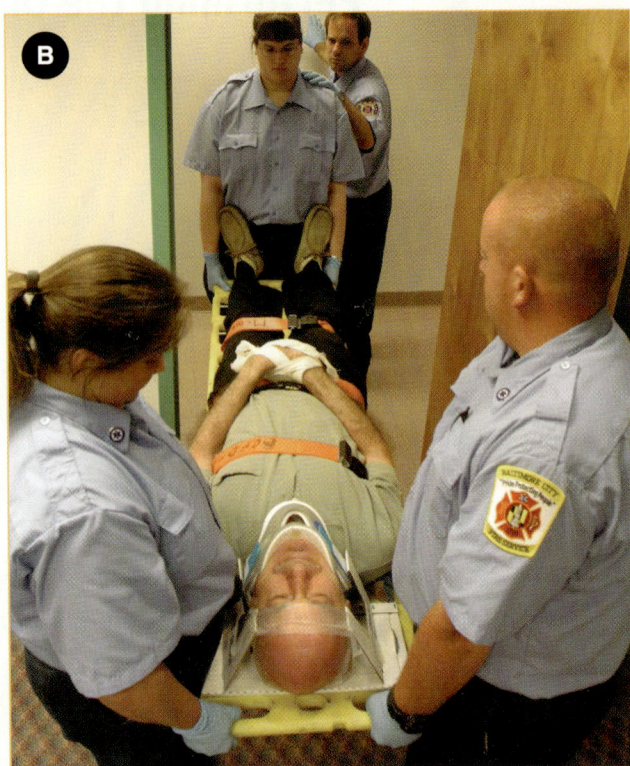

Figure 34-8 Carrying a patient through a narrow doorway or hallway. **A.** Stop and turn in to face the patient until you move through the passage. **B.** If the doorway or hallway is very narrow, the EMT-Is at the side will need to move. One should move next to the EMT-I at the head and share the load. The other should move in front of and support the back of the EMT-I carrying the foot end to steady and guide him or her through the passage.

The diamond carry is recommended when a patient must be carried in a building (Figure 34-8). If you must carry a patient through a narrow doorway or hallway, simply stop and have all the EMT-Is turn until each is again facing in toward the patient. Then, by taking small, slow steps, you can move through the doorway. If the doorway is too narrow for the EMT-Is at the sides of the backboard to fit through, have one go through the doorway before the backboard or stretcher. As the other three EMT-Is slowly move through the doorway, the EMT-I who walked through before the backboard should grasp the backboard from the other side of the doorway before the EMT-I who is still at the side of the backboard reaches the doorway and must let go.

Sometimes, if a doorway, hallway, or stairwell is very narrow, it will only be possible to carry the backboard or stretcher from the head and foot ends. When this occurs, the EMT-Is who were lifting and carrying at each side should relocate to help those at each end. One should move next to the EMT-I at the head end and share the load with him or her. The other should move in front of and grasp the belt of the EMT-I carrying the foot end, and steady and guide him or her.

When you must carry a patient up or down a flight of stairs or other significant incline, use a stair chair if possible. When you must use a backboard or stretcher, be sure that the patient is anatomically secured to the device in such a way that he or she cannot slide significantly when the stretcher is at an angle (Skill Drill 34-4):

1. **Apply a strap** that passes tightly across the upper torso and through each armpit, but not over the arms, to hold the patient in place while leaving the arms free. The strap is secured to the handles at both sides of the backboard so that it cannot slide toward the foot end of the board. Strap the patient securely to the backboard (**Step 1**).
2. **When you carry the patient down stairs** or an incline, make sure the backboard or stretcher is carried with the foot end first so that the head end is elevated higher than the foot end. The straps will prevent the patient from sliding down or off the backboard (**Step 2**).
3. **When you carry a patient up stairs** or an incline, the elevated head end of the backboard or stretcher should go first (**Step 3**).

Skill Drill 34-4: Carrying a Patient on Stairs

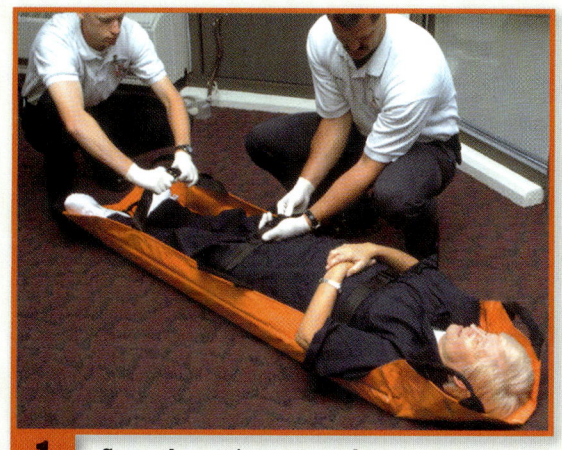

1 Strap the patient securely.

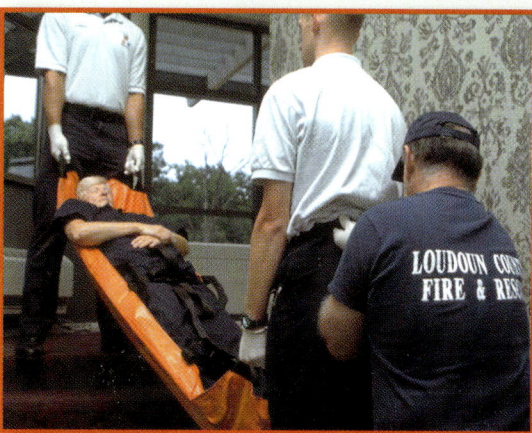

2 Carry a patient down stairs with the foot end first, head elevated.

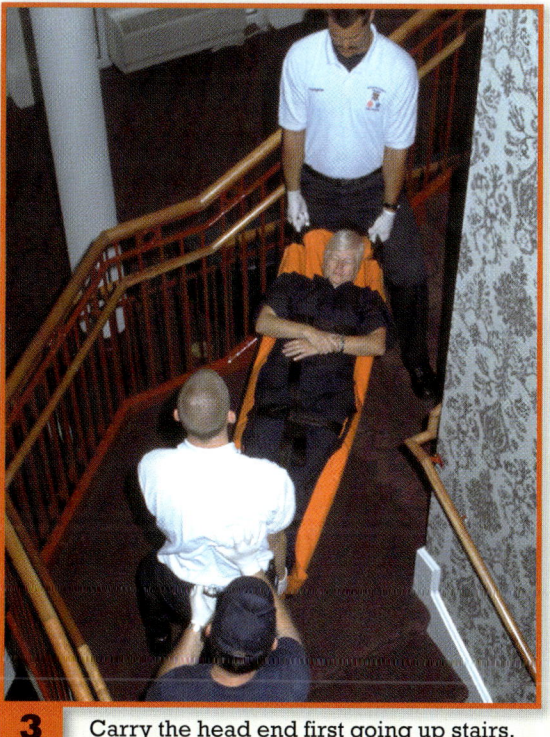

3 Carry the head end first going up stairs.

Whenever possible, you should use the patient's armpits as anatomic anchors and support points when you use a direct body lift or drag to move the patient or when assisting a patient who can stand.

The <u>wheeled ambulance stretcher</u> or cot, which is a specially designed cot that can be rolled along the ground, weighs between 40 and 70 lb, depending on its design and features **Figure 34-9 ▶**. Because its weight must be added to that of the patient, it is generally not taken up or down stairs or to other locations where the patient must be carried rather than rolled for any significant distance. When the patient is upstairs, you should bring the wheeled ambulance stretcher to the ground floor landing and prepare it for the patient. You should then take either a wheeled stair chair or a backboard upstairs. Both of these devices are considerably

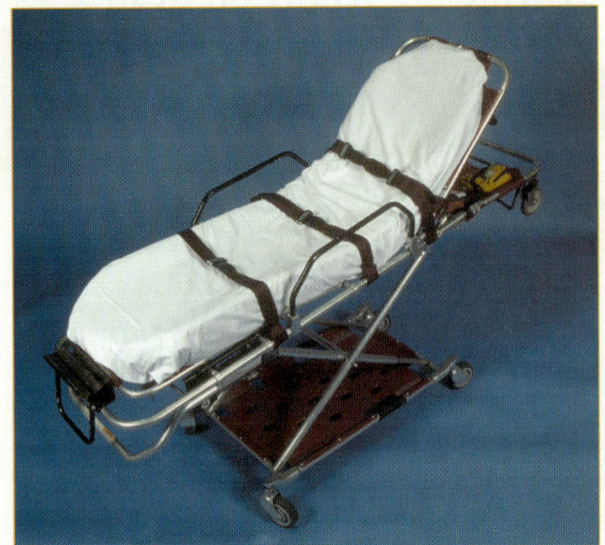

Figure 34-9 The wheeled ambulance stretcher is specially designed to roll along the ground.

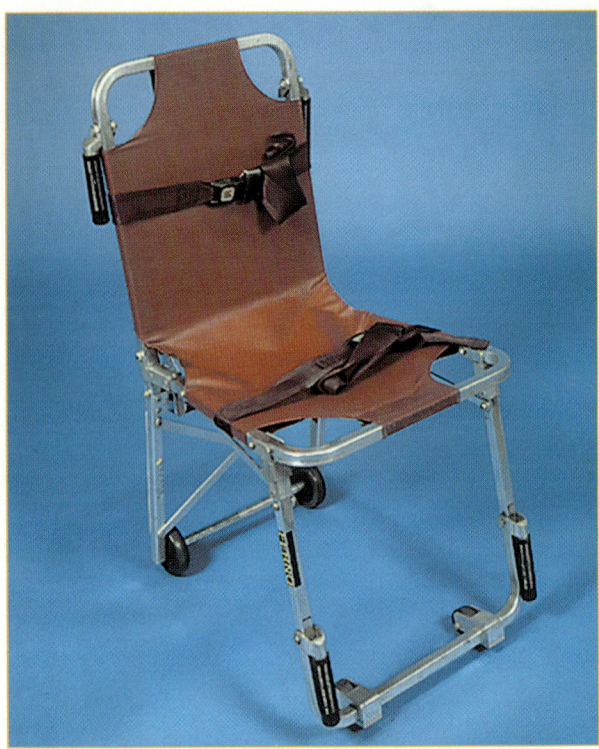

Figure 34-10 A wheeled stair chair can be used to transfer a conscious patient up or down a flight of stairs.

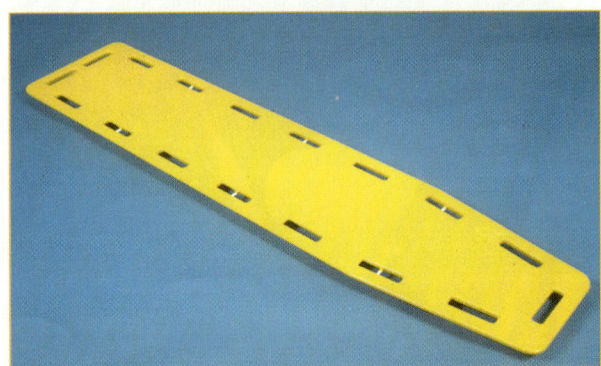

Figure 34-11 A backboard is used to transfer patients who must be moved in a supine or immobilized position.

lighter than a wheeled cot and may be used to carry the patient down to the waiting cot. Use a wheeled <u>stair chair</u> to bring a conscious patient down to the waiting cot if the patient's condition allows him or her to be placed in a sitting position (Figure 34-10 ▶). Once the cot has been reached, transfer the patient from the stair chair onto the cot. When the patient is in cardiac arrest, must be moved in a lying position, or must be immobilized, secure the patient onto a backboard. A <u>backboard</u>, which is a device that provides support to patients whom you suspect have hip, pelvic, spinal, or lower extremity injuries, is also called a spine board, trauma board, or longboard (Figure 34-11 ▶). You can then carry the patient on the backboard down the stairs to the prepared cot. Once you reach the cot, place both the board and patient on the cot and secure them with additional straps.

Directions and Commands

To safely lift and carry a patient, you and your team must anticipate and understand every move, and each move must be executed in a coordinated manner. The team leader should indicate where each team member is to be located and rapidly describe the sequence of steps that will be performed to ensure that the team knows what is expected of it before any lifting is

> **EMT-I Tips**
>
> Since lifting and moving techniques require a team leader to coordinate and direct the process, it will save time and prevent confusion to establish either informal practices or formal procedures that tell all team members—in advance—who will be in charge of these activities.

initiated. If you must lift and move the patient through a number of separate stages, the team leader should first give an abbreviated overview of the stages, followed by a more detailed explanation of each stage just before it will occur.

Orders that will initiate the actual lifting or moving or any significant changes in movement should be given in two parts: a preparatory command and a command of execution. For example, if the team leader says "All ready to stop. STOP!," the "All ready to stop" will get your attention, identify who should act, and prepare them to act; the declarative "STOP!" will indicate the exact moment for execution. Commands of execution should be delivered in a louder voice. Often, a countdown is helpful when you need to lift a patient. To avoid confusion in using a countdown, always clarify whether "three" is to be a part of the preparatory command or whether it is to serve as the order to execute. You can say "We're going to lift on three. One-two-THREE!" or "I'm going to count to three and then we're going to lift. One-two-three-LIFT!"

Additional Lifting and Carrying Guidelines

You should estimate how much the patient weighs before attempting to lift him or her. Commonly, adult patients weigh between 100 and 210 lb. If you use the correct technique, you and one other EMT-I should be able to safely lift this weight. Depending on your individual strength, you and another EMT-I may be able to safely lift an even heavier patient. However, because it is quite a bit safer to have four rescuers lift, you should try to use four rescuers whenever the available resources allow. *You should know how much you can comfortably and safely lift and should not attempt to lift a proportional weight (the share of the weight that you will bear) that exceeds this amount.* If you find that lifting the patient places strain on you, call for the lifting to be stopped and the patient to be lowered. You should then obtain additional help before again attempting to lift the patient. Be sure to communicate clearly and frequently with your partner and other rescuers whenever you are lifting a patient.

You should *not* attempt to lift a patient who weighs more than 250 lb with fewer than four rescuers, regardless of individual strength. Protocols should include a method to rapidly summon additional help to lift and carry such a patient or, as in the case of a cardiac arrest, provide and maintain the necessary care in the field and when moving and transporting the patient. In addition, you must know, or be able to find out, the weight limitations of the equipment you are using and how to handle patients who exceed the weight limitations. Special techniques, equipment, and resources generally are required to move any patient who weighs more than 300 lb to the ambulance. These resources should be summoned when you arrive.

Because more than half of a patient's weight is distributed to the head end of the backboard or cot, the strongest of the available EMT-Is should be located at the head end of the device. Even with four or more EMT-Is carrying the patient, the strain on the EMT-I carrying the head end of the device will be increased when you must negotiate a narrow area or flight of stairs. In carrying a patient up or down a flight of stairs, proportionally greater weight will also be distributed to the EMT-I who is carrying the foot end when the backboard or cot becomes angled because of the incline. You should anticipate this and, in such cases, make sure the two strongest EMT-Is are positioned at the head and foot ends of the board. Because of the incline of the stairway, if one of the two EMT-Is is considerably taller than the other, it will be easier if the shorter of the two is at the head end and the taller is at the foot end.

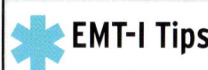

EMT-I Tips

Know your limits! Never hesitate to call for assistance when the patient's weight exceeds your lifting capabilities.

The dynamics that are involved in carrying a patient down a flight of stairs or for any significant distance will not allow you to carry as much proportional weight as you can to safely lift or support the patient during a move onto a nearby backboard or cot. Therefore, if you feel that you are approaching your maximum lifting capacity as you are moving the patient onto a backboard or cot, you should not attempt to lift and carry the patient for any significant distance or down a flight of stairs. You can again attempt to lift and carry the patient after you have decreased the amount of proportional weight you will be carrying by changing your position on the device or that of the others on the team or have obtained additional help.

You should try to use a stair chair instead of a cot, whenever possible, to carry a patient down stairs.

Skill Drill 34-5

Using a Stair Chair

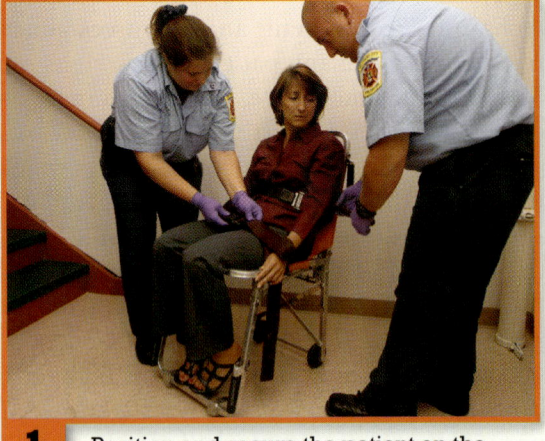

1 Position and secure the patient on the chair.

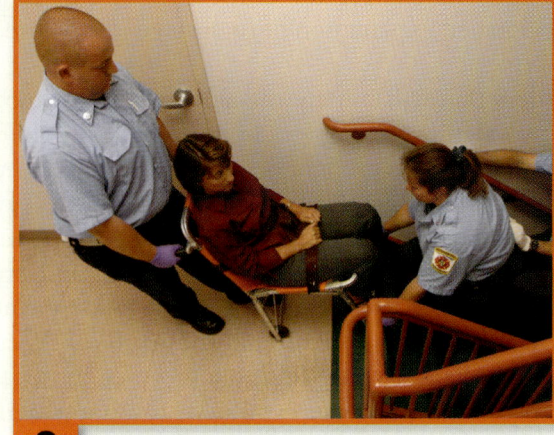

2 Take your places at the head and foot of the chair.

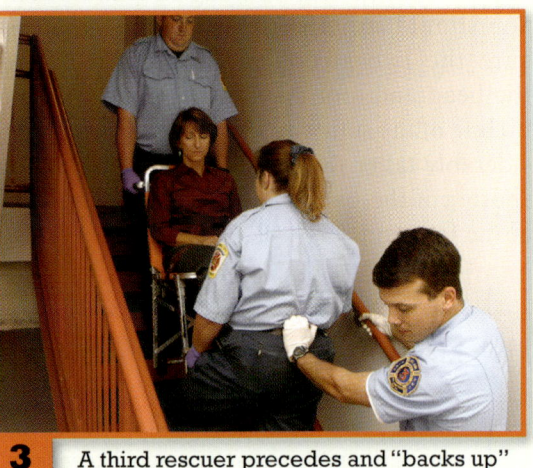

3 A third rescuer precedes and "backs up" the rescuer carrying the foot.

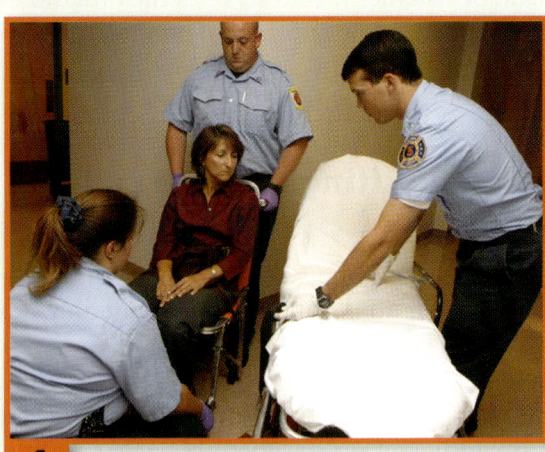

4 Lower the chair to roll on landings, or for transfer to the cot.

Follow the steps in Skill Drill 34-5:

1. **Secure the patient to the stair chair with straps.** At a minimum, use a lap belt at the hips and a strap around the chest. You should also use some method to secure the arms and hands so the patient does not reach out to grasp something and throw the carrying team off balance (**Step 1**).
2. **Rescuers take their places around the patient** seated on the chair: one at the head and one at the foot. The rescuer at the head will give directions to coordinate the lift and carry (**Step 2**).
3. **A third rescuer precedes the two carrying the chair** to open doors, spot them on stairs, and so on. For lengthy carries, the third responder can also rotate into the carrying team to provide breaks for the other two (**Step 3**).
4. **When reaching landings and other flat intervals** in the carry, lower the chair to the ground and roll it rather than carrying. When reaching the level where the cot awaits, roll the chair into position next to the cot in preparation for transferring the patient (**Step 4**).

As with other carries, always remember to keep your back in a locked-in position and to flex at the hips, not the waist. You should also bend at the knees and keep the patient's weight and your arms as close to your body as possible. Try to avoid any unnecessary lifting and carrying of the patient. If an assist, log roll, or body drag will not harm or jeopardize the patient, use one to move the patient onto the backboard or cot.

Principles of Safe Reaching and Pulling

When you use a body drag to move a patient, the same basic body mechanics and principles apply as when lifting and carrying. *Your back should always be locked and straight*, not curved or bent laterally, and you should avoid any twisting so that the vertebrae remain in normal alignment. When you are reaching overhead, avoid hyperextending your back. When you are pulling a patient who is on the ground, you should always kneel to minimize the distance that you will have to lean over (Figure 34-12A ▶). To keep your reach within the recommended distance, reach forward and grasp the patient so that your elbows are just beyond the anterior torso (Figure 34-12B ▶). When you are pulling a patient who is at a different height from you, bend your knees until your hips are just below the height of the plane across which you will be pulling the patient (Figure 34-12C ▶). During pulling, you should extend your arms no more than about 15″ to 20″ in front of your torso. Reposition your feet (or knees, if kneeling) so that the force of pull will be balanced equally between both arms and the line of pull will be centered between them (Figure 34-12D ▶). Pull the patient by slowly flexing your arms. When you can pull no

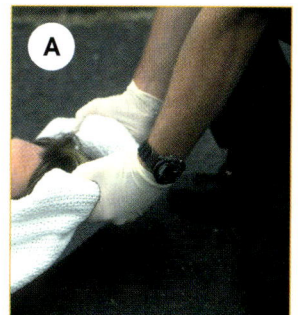
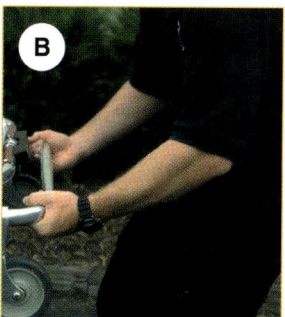
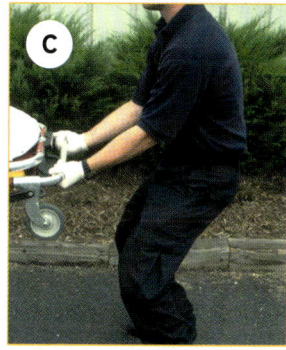
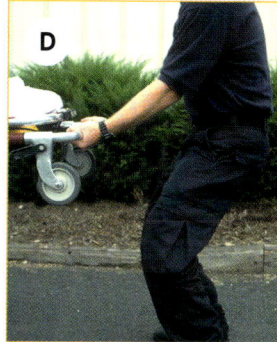

Figure 34-12 Reaching and pulling safely. **A.** Kneel to pull a patient who is on the ground. **B.** When pulling, your elbows should only extend just beyond the anterior torso. **C.** Bend your knees to pull a patient who is at a different height than you are. **D.** Position your feet or knees to balance the force of pull.

You are the Provider — Part 3

You call for assistance and the local fire department sends an engine company with four EMT-I/fire fighters. Your partner climbs into the bathtub to perform cervical spine immobilization. You and your partner agree that you cannot properly apply a cervical collar at this time because of the position of the patient. You decide that the best way to move the patient is to lift him out of the bathtub and move him to the backboard once assistance arrives on the scene. A quick recheck of the vital signs shows the following:

Vital Signs	Recording Time: 2 Minutes After Patient Contact
Respirations	14 breaths/min, adequate depth
Pulse	92 beats/min, regular
Blood pressure	Strong radial pulse
Skin	Warm, dry, pink

5. How can you and your partner safely lift this patient while maintaining appropriate spinal immobilization?
6. What do you need to think about and be prepared for once you have lifted the patient?

farther because your hands have reached the front of your torso, stop and move back another 15″ to 20″. Then, when properly positioned, repeat the steps. You should alternate between pulling the patient by flexing your arms and then repositioning yourself so that your arms are again extended with your hands about 15″ in front of your torso. By not moving yourself and the patient simultaneously, you will prevent undesirable jostling of the patient and the chance that sudden unscheduled force will occur across your spine. You should also try to prevent injury to yourself by avoiding situations that involve strenuous effort lasting more than 1 minute.

If you must drag a patient across a bed, you will have to kneel on the bed to avoid reaching beyond the recommended distance. Then follow the steps described until the patient is within 15″ to 20″ of the bed's edge. You can then complete the drag while standing at the side of the bed. Rather than dragging the patient by his or her clothing, use the sheet or blanket under the patient for this purpose.

Unless the patient is on a backboard, transfer a patient from the cot to a bed in the emergency department or the patient's hospital room with a body drag. With the cot at the same height as the bed and held firmly against its side, you and another EMT-I should kneel on the hospital bed and, in the manner previously described, drag the patient in increments until he or she is properly centered on the bed. When transferring the patient onto a narrow examining table, rather than kneeling on the table, you can usually drag the patient while standing against the opposite side.

Sometimes during a body drag, you and another EMT-I may have to pull the patient with one of you on each side of the patient. You will have to alter the usual pulling technique to prevent pulling sideways and producing adverse lateral leverage against your lower back. You should position yourself by kneeling just beyond the patient's shoulder and facing toward his or her groin (Figure 34-13A ▶). By extending one arm across and in front of your chest, you can grasp the armpit and, with the other arm extended in front and to the side of the torso, the patient's belt. Then, by raising your elbows and flexing your arms, you can pull the patient with the line of force at the minimum angle possible (Figure 34-13B ▶).

Generally, when log rolling a patient onto his or her side, you will initially have to reach farther than 18″ (Figure 34-14 ▶). To minimize this distance, kneel as close to the patient's side as possible, leaving only enough room so that your knees will not prevent the patient from being rolled. When you lean forward, keep your

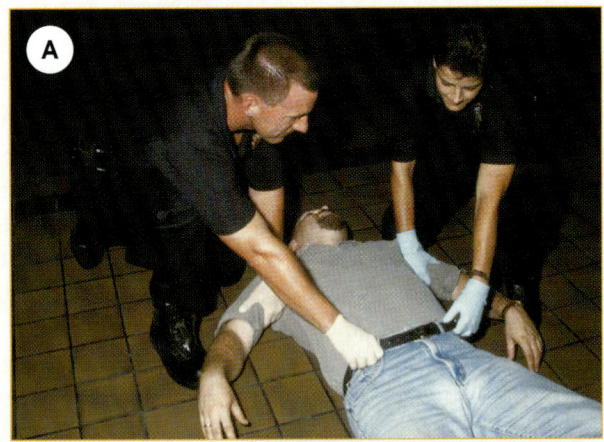
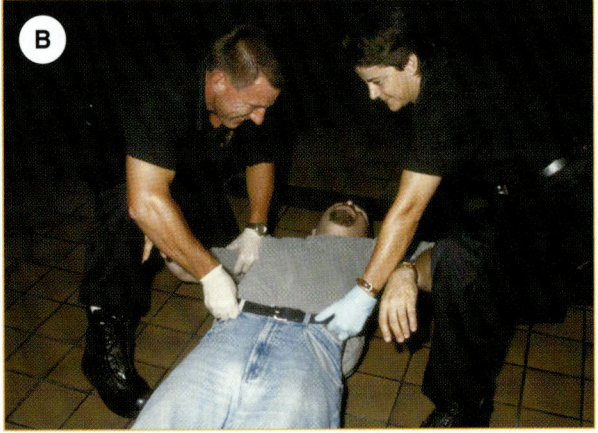

Figure 34-13 A body drag with an EMT-I on each side of the patient. **A.** Kneel just beyond the patient's shoulder facing his or her groin. Extend one arm across and in front of your chest, and grasp the armpit. Extend your other arm in front and to the side of the patient's torso, and grasp the patient's belt. **B.** Raise your elbows and flex your arms to pull the patient.

back straight, and lean solely from the hips. Be sure to use your shoulder muscles to help with the roll. To minimize the amount of time you are extended like this and to support the patient's weight, roll the patient without stopping until the patient is resting on his or her side. Some EMS experts consider that, during a log roll, you should pull rather than push the patient. Local protocols will guide your training in this area.

When you are rolling the wheeled ambulance stretcher, make sure that it is elevated (Figure 34-15 ▶). Pull the stretcher from the foot end. Make sure your arms are held close to your body, and be careful to avoid reaching significantly behind you or hyperextending your back. Your back should be locked, straight, and untwisted. While you are walking and pulling the stretcher, bend slightly forward at the hips. As you walk, your legs are pulled back with the feet on the ground, your pelvis is moved forward, and the movement of the pelvis

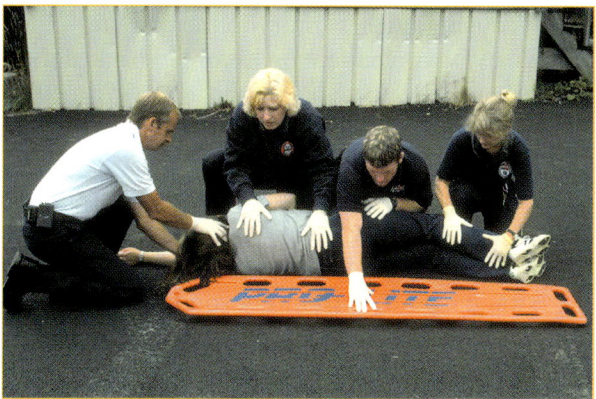

Figure 34-14 When placing a patient onto a backboard, roll the patient onto his or her side. Kneel as close to the patient's side as possible, leaving only enough room so that your knees will not prevent the patient from being rolled. Lean forward, keeping your back straight and leaning solely from the hips. Use your shoulder muscles to help with the roll.

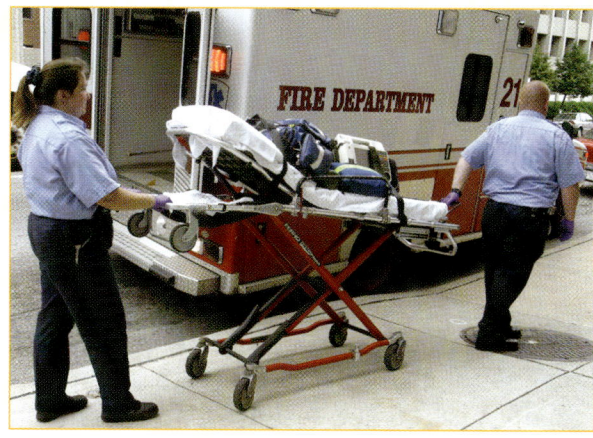

Figure 34-15 Push the stretcher from the head end. If you are guiding the cot from the foot end, make sure your arms are held close to your body, and be careful to avoid reaching significantly behind you or hyperextending your back. Your back should be locked, straight, and untwisted.

is transferred to the stretcher through your straight torso and firmly held arms. You should try to keep the line of the pull through the center of your body by bending your knees.

A second EMT-I should guide the head end and assist you by pushing with his or her arms held with the elbows bent so that the hands are about 12″ to 15″ in front of the torso. To protect your elbows from injury, you should never push an object with your arms fully extended in a straight line and the elbows locked. When you push with the elbow bent but firmly held from bending further, the strong muscles of the arm serve as a shock absorber if the wheels or foot end of the stretcher strikes an obstacle that causes its progress to be suddenly slowed or stopped. You must be sure that you push from the area of your body that is between the waist and shoulder. If the weight you are pushing is lower than your waist, you should push from a kneeling position. Be careful that you do not push or pull from an overhead position.

General Considerations

Moving a patient should normally be done in an orderly, planned, and unhurried fashion. This approach will protect both you and the patient from further injury and reduce the risk of worsening the patient's condition when he or she is moved. At a minimum, on most calls you will have to lift and carry the patient to the wheeled ambulance stretcher, move the stretcher and patient to the ambulance, and load the stretcher into the patient compartment.

You will often have to include several additional steps to place the patient onto a backboard and/or carry him or her down a flight of stairs. You will also have to add a stop at the top of the stairway so that everyone can reposition for carrying the patient down the stairs. Repositioning usually requires lowering the backboard to the ground and lifting it again when all EMT-Is are in their proper places. If you are carrying the patient in a stair chair, the additional step occurs after you have descended the stairs and reached the stretcher. At that point, you will have to assist or lift the patient from the stair chair onto the stretcher.

You should carefully plan ahead and select the methods that will involve the least lifting and carrying. Remember to always consider whether there is an option that will cause less strain to you and the other EMT-Is.

Emergency Moves

You should use an <u>emergency move</u> to move a patient before initial assessment and care are provided when there is some potential danger, and you and the patient must move to a safe place to avoid possible serious harm or death. The presence of fire, explosives, or hazardous materials and your inability to protect the patient from other hazards or gain access to others in a vehicle who need lifesaving care are all situations in which you should use an emergency move.

The only other time you should use an emergency move is if you cannot properly assess the patient or provide immediate potentially critical emergency care because of the patient's location or position.

If you are alone and danger at the scene makes it necessary for you to use an emergency move, regardless of a patient's injuries, you should use a drag to pull the patient along the long axis of the body. This will help to keep the spinal column in line as much as possible. When performing an emergency move, one of your primary concerns is the danger of aggravating an existing spinal injury. Remember that it is impossible to remove a patient quickly from a vehicle while providing as much protection to the spine as you would give by using an immobilization device. However, if you follow certain guidelines during the move, you can usually move a patient from a life-threatening situation without causing further injury to the patient.

You can move a patient on his or her back along the floor or ground by using one of the following methods.

- Pull on the patient's clothing in the neck and shoulder area Figure 34-16A.
- Place the patient onto a blanket, coat, or other item that can be pulled Figure 34-16B.
- Rotate the patient's arms so that they are extended straight on the ground beyond his or her head, grasp the wrists, and, with the arms elevated above the ground, drag the patient Figure 34-16C.
- Place your arms under the patient's shoulders and through the armpits, and, while grasping the patient's arms, drag the patient backward Figure 34-16D.

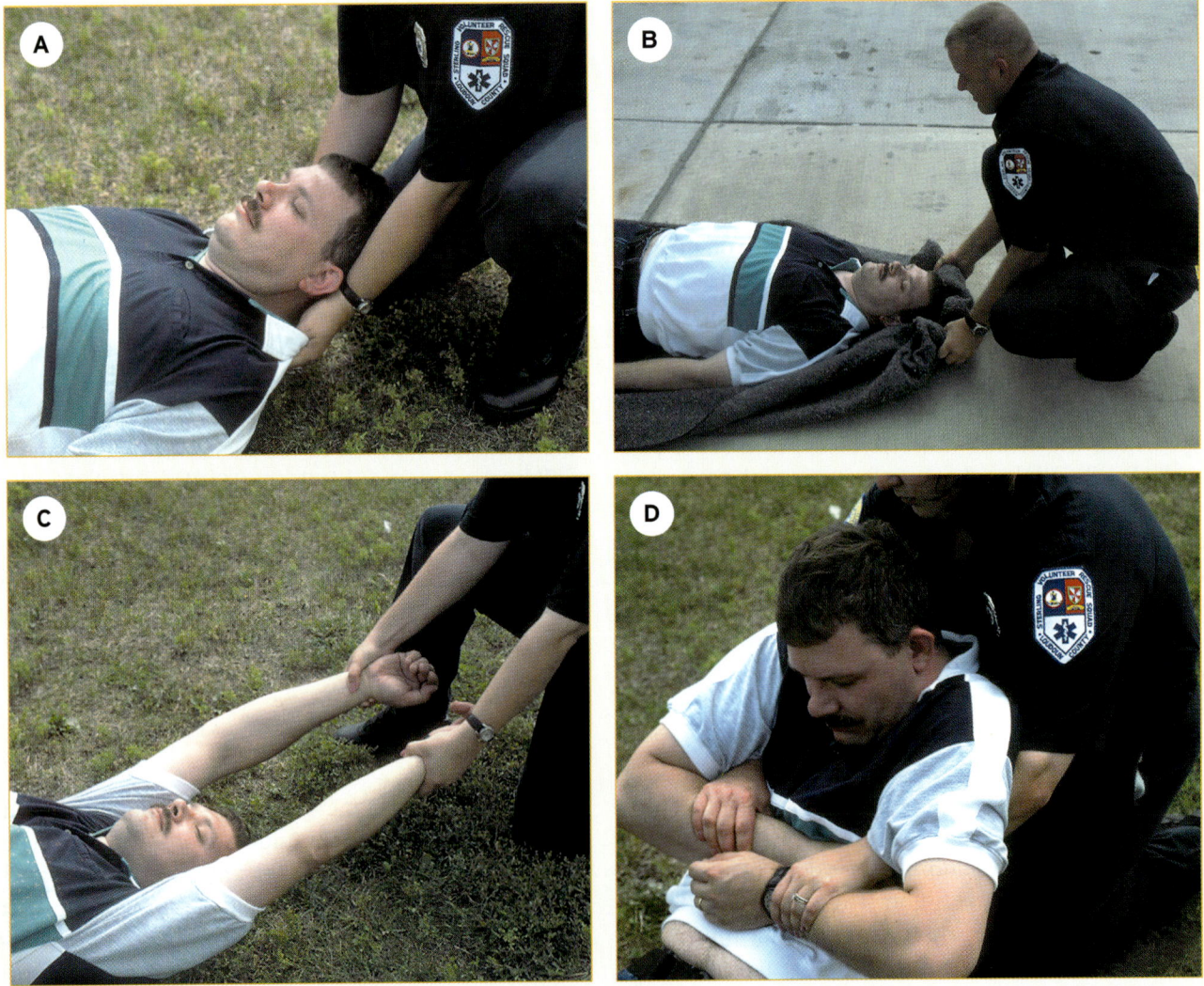

Figure 34-16 Dragging methods. **A.** Emergency clothes drag. **B.** Blanket drag. **C.** Arm drag. **D.** Arm-to-arm drag.

If you are alone and must remove an unconscious patient from a car, you should first move the patient's legs so they are clear of the pedals and are against the seat. Then rotate the patient so that his or her back is positioned facing the open car door. Next, place your arms through the armpits and support the patient's head against your body (Figure 34-17A ▶). While supporting the patient's weight, drag the patient from the seat. If the legs and feet clear the car easily, you can rapidly drag the patient to a safe location by continuing this method (Figure 34-17B ▶). If the legs and feet do not clear the car easily, you can slowly lower the patient until he or she is lying on his or her back next to the car, clear the legs from the vehicle, and, as previously described, use a long-axis body drag to move the patient a safe distance from the vehicle.

You should use one-person techniques to move a patient only if a potentially life-threatening danger exists and you are alone or, because of the pressing nature of the danger, your partner is moving a second patient simultaneously. Additional one-rescuer drags, carries, and lifts are shown in (Figure 34-18 ▶).

Urgent Moves

An urgent move may be necessary for moving a patient with an altered level of consciousness, inadequate ventilation, or shock (hypoperfusion). An extreme weather condition may also make an urgent move necessary. In some cases, patients must be urgently moved from the location or position in which they are found. When a patient who is sitting in a car or truck must be urgently moved, you should use the rapid extrication technique.

Rapid Extrication Technique

The long backboard, short backboard, and vest-type devices are known as immobilization devices. Normally, you would use an extrication-type vest or half-backboard device to immobilize a seated patient with a suspected spinal injury before removing the patient from the car. However, using either of these devices usually requires between 6 and 8 minutes, in some cases even longer. By using the rapid extrication technique instead, the patient can be moved from sitting in the car to lying supine on a backboard in 1 minute or less. (Table 34-2 ▶) describes the situations in which you should use the rapid extrication technique.

In such cases, the delay that occurs in applying an extrication-type vest or half-board is contraindicated.

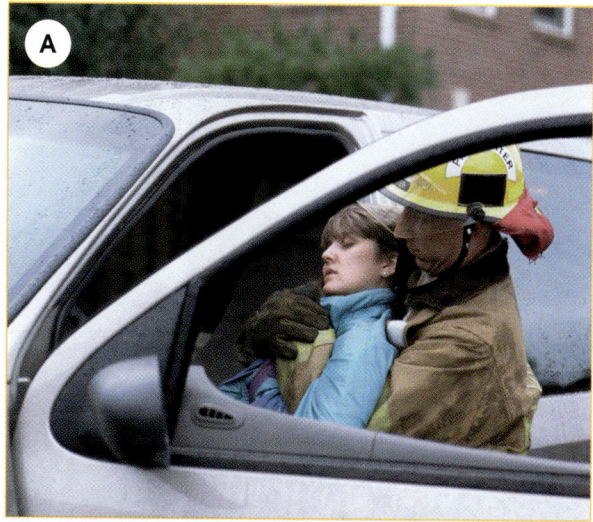

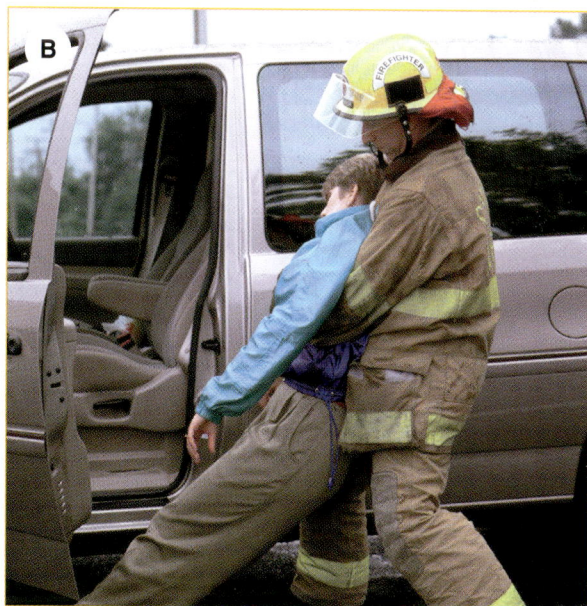

Figure 34-17 One-person technique for moving an unconscious patient from a car. **A.** Grasp the patient under the arms. **B.** Pull the patient down into a supine position.

TABLE 34-2	Situations in Which to Use the Rapid Extrication Technique

- The vehicle or scene is unsafe.
- The patient cannot be properly assessed before being removed from the car.
- The patient needs immediate intervention that requires a supine position.
- The patient's condition requires immediate transport to the hospital.
- The patient blocks the EMT-I's access to another seriously injured patient.

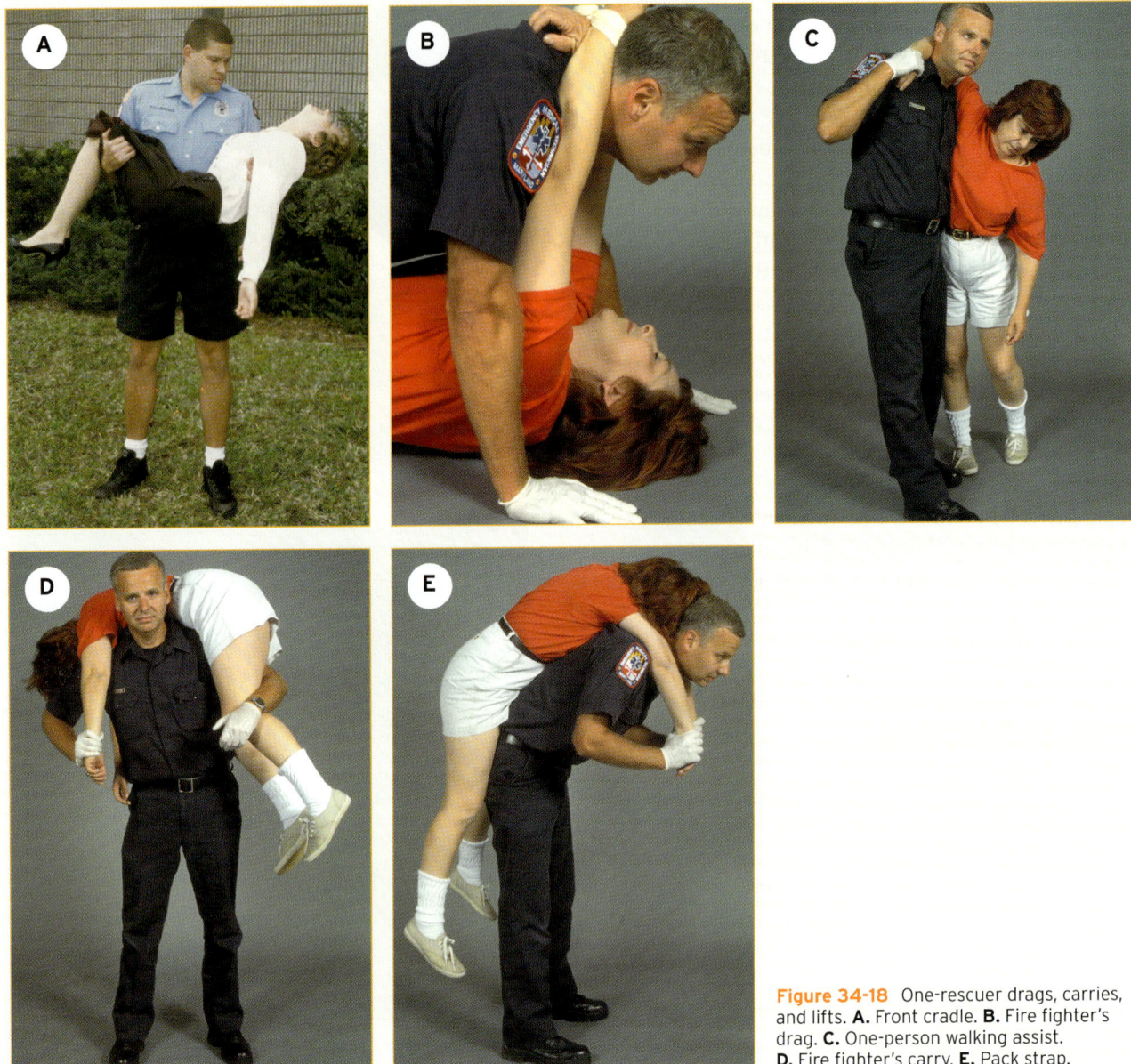

Figure 34-18 One-rescuer drags, carries, and lifts. **A.** Front cradle. **B.** Fire fighter's drag. **C.** One-person walking assist. **D.** Fire fighter's carry. **E.** Pack strap.

However, the manual support and immobilization that you provide when using the rapid extrication technique produce a greater risk of spine movement. You should not use the rapid extrication technique if no urgency exists.

The rapid extrication technique requires a team of three EMT-Is who are knowledgeable and practiced in the procedure. You should take the following steps when using the rapid extrication technique Skill Drill 34-6 :

1. **First EMT-I applies manual in-line support** of the patient's head and cervical spine from behind. Support may be applied from the side, if necessary, by reaching through the driver's side doorway (**Step 1**).

2. **Second EMT-I serves as team leader** and, as such, gives the commands, coordinating moves until the patient is supine on the backboard. Because the Second EMT-I lifts and turns the patient's torso, he or she must be physically capable of moving the patient. Second EMT-I works from the driver's side doorway. If First EMT-I is also working from that doorway, Second EMT-I should stand closer to the door hinges toward the front of the vehicle. Second EMT-I

applies a cervical immobilization device and performs the initial assessment (**Step 2**).

3. **Second EMT-I provides continuous support** of the patient's torso until the patient is supine on the backboard. Once Second EMT-I takes control of the torso, usually in the form of a body hug, he or she should not let go of the patient for any reason. Some type of cross-chest shoulder hug usually works well, but you will have to decide what method works best for you on any given patient. You must remember that you cannot simply reach into the car and grab the patient; this will only twist the patient's torso. You must rotate the patient as a unit.

4. **Third EMT-I works from the front passenger's seat** and is responsible for rotating the patient's legs and feet as the torso is turned, ensuring that they are free of the pedals and any other obstruction. With care, Third EMT-I should first move the patient's nearer leg laterally without rotating the patient's pelvis and lower spine. The pelvis and lower spine rotate only as Third EMT-I moves the second leg during the next step. Moving the nearer leg early makes it much easier to move the second leg in concert with the rest of the body. After Third EMT-I moves the legs together, they should be moved as a unit (**Step 3**).

These first steps of the rapid extrication technique direct the team to their starting positions and responsibilities. First EMT-I applies in-line support and immobilization of the head and neck and actually 'counts' the move. Second EMT-I gives orders and supports the torso. Third EMT-I moves and supports the patient's legs. The team is now ready to move the patient.

5. **The patient is rotated 90°** so that the back is facing out the driver's door and the feet are on the front passenger's seat. This coordinated movement is done in three or four short, quick "eighth turns." Second EMT-I coordinates the sequence of moves and the First EMT-I directs each quick turn by saying, "Ready, turn" or "Ready, move." Hand position changes should be made between moves.

6. **In most cases, First EMT-I will be working from the back seat.** At some point, either because the doorpost is in the way or because he or she cannot reach farther from the back seat, First EMT-I will be unable to follow the torso rotation. At that time, Third EMT-I should assume temporary in-line support of the head and neck until First EMT-I can regain control of the head from outside the vehicle. If a fourth EMT-I is present, Fourth EMT-I stands next to Second EMT-I. Fourth EMT-I takes control of the head and neck from outside the vehicle without involving Third EMT-I. As soon as the change has been made, the rotation can continue (**Step 4**).

7. **Once the patient has been fully rotated**, the backboard should be placed against the patient's buttocks on the seat. Do not try to wedge the backboard under the patient. If only three EMT-Is are present, be sure to place the backboard within arm's reach of the driver's door before the move so that the board can be pulled into place when needed. In such cases, the far end of the board can be left on the ground. When a fourth EMT-I is available, First EMT-I exits the rear seat of the car, places the backboard against the patient's buttocks, and maintains pressure in toward the vehicle from the far end of the board. (Note: When the door opening allows, some EMT-Is prefer to insert the backboard onto the car seat before the patient is rotated.)

EMT-I Tips

The person holding the c-spine always calls the move.

8. **As soon as the patient has been rotated** and the backboard is in place, Second EMT-I and Third EMT-I lower the patient onto the board while supporting the head and torso so that neutral alignment is maintained. First EMT-I holds the backboard until the patient is secured (**Step 5**).

9. **Next, Third EMT-I must move across the front seat** to be in position at the patient's hips. If Third EMT-I stays at the patient's knees or feet, he or she will be ineffective in helping to move the body's weight. The knees and feet follow the hips.

10. **Fourth EMT-I maintains manual in-line support** of the head and now takes over giving the commands. If a fourth EMT-I is not present, you can direct a volunteer to assist you. Second EMT-I maintains direction of the

Skill Drill 34-6

Performing Rapid Extrication Technique

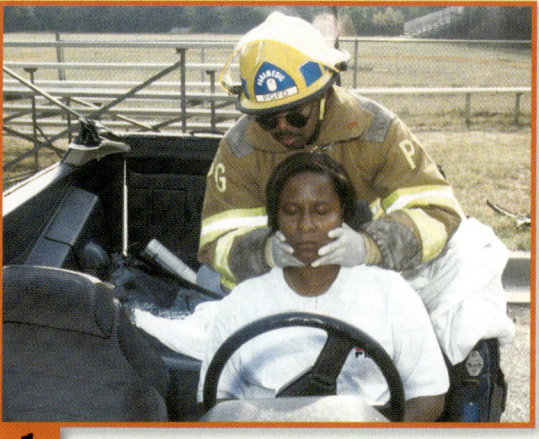

1 First EMT-I provides in-line manual support of the head and cervical spine.

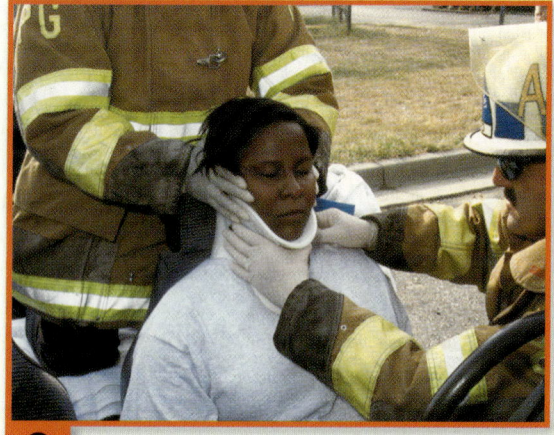

2 Second EMT-I gives commands, applies a cervical collar, and performs the initial assessment.

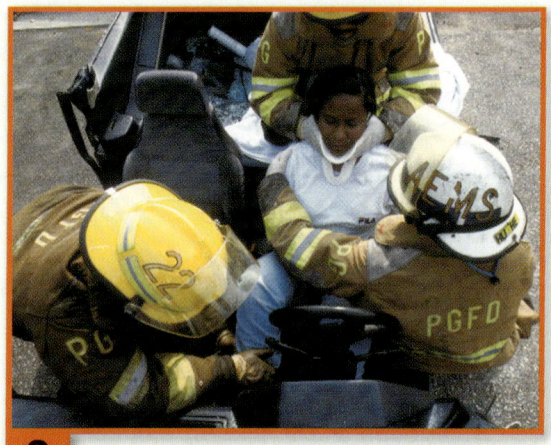

3 Second EMT-I supports the torso. Third EMT-I frees the patient's legs from the pedals and moves the legs together, without moving the pelvis or spine.

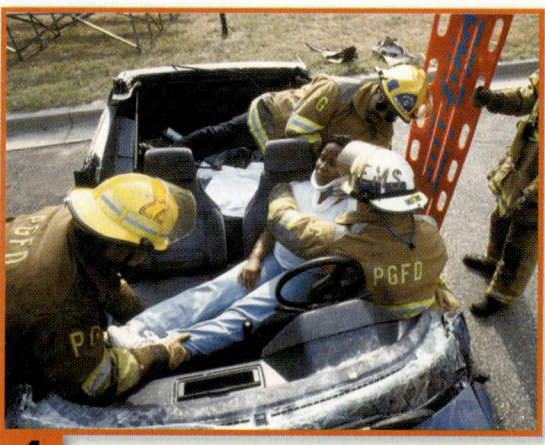

4 Second and Third EMT-Is rotate the patient as a unit in several short, coordinated moves. First EMT-I (relieved by Fourth EMT-I or bystander as needed) supports the head and neck during rotation (and later steps).

extrication. Second EMT-I stands with his or her back to the door, facing the rear of the vehicle. The backboard should be immediately in front of Third EMT-I. Second EMT-I grasps the patient's shoulders or armpits. Then, on command, Second EMT-I and Third EMT-I slide the patient 8″ to 12″ along the backboard, repeating this slide until the patient's hips are firmly on the backboard (**Step 6**).

11. At that time, **Third EMT-I gets out of the vehicle** and moves to the opposite side of the backboard, across from Second EMT-I. Third EMT-I now takes control at the shoulders, and Second EMT-I moves back to take control of the hips. On command, these two EMT-Is move the patient along the board in 8″ to 12″ slides until the patient is placed fully on the board (**Step 7**).

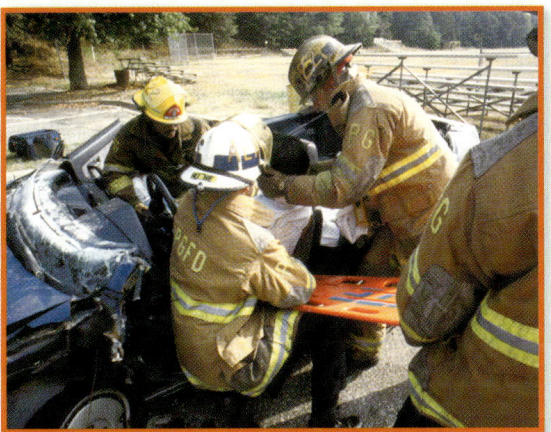

5 First (or Fourth) EMT-I places the backboard on the seat against the patient's buttocks.

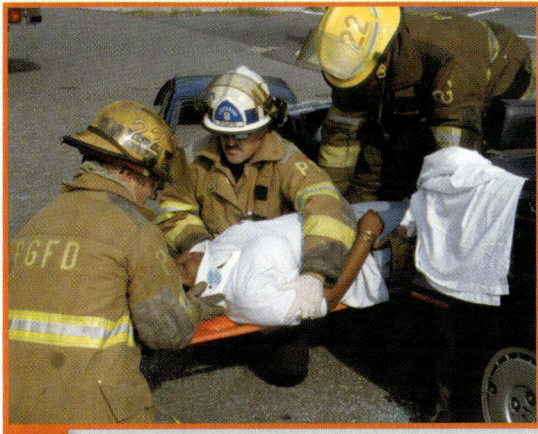

6 Third EMT-I moves to an effective position for sliding the patient.

Second and Third EMT-Is slide the patient along the backboard in coordinated, 8" to 12" moves until the hips rest on the backboard.

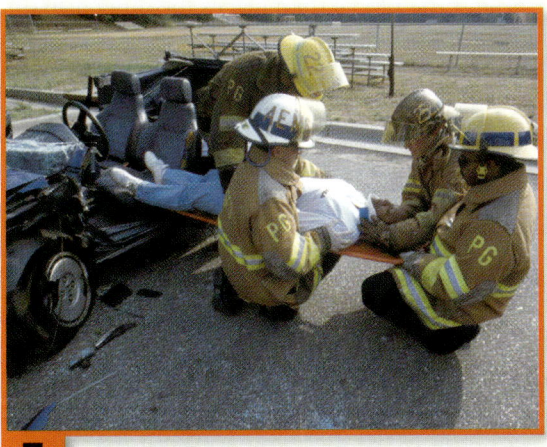

7 Third EMT-I exits the vehicle, moves to the backboard opposite Second EMT-I, and they continue to slide the patient until patient is fully on the board.

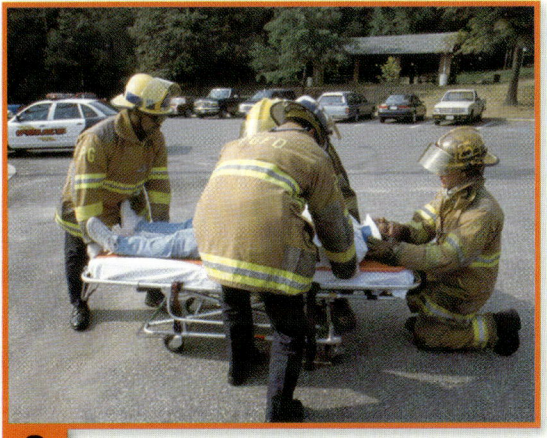

8 First (or Fourth) EMT-I continues to stabilize the head and neck while Second and Third carry the patient away from the vehicle.

12. **First (or Fourth) EMT-I continues to maintain manual in-line support** of the head. Second EMT-I and Third EMT-I now grasp their side of the board, and then carry it and the patient away from the vehicle onto the prepared cot nearby (**Step 8**).

In some cases, you will be able to rest the head end of the backboard on the cot while the patient is moved onto the backboard. In others, you will not. Once the backboard and patient have been placed on the cot, you should begin lifesaving treatment immediately. If you used the rapid extrication technique because the scene was dangerous, you and your team should immediately move the cot a safe distance away from the vehicle before you assess or treat the patient.

The steps of the rapid extrication technique must be considered a general procedure to be adapted as needed. Two-door cars differ from four-door models.

Larger cars differ from smaller compact models, pickup trucks, and full-size sedans and four-wheel-drive vehicles. You will handle a large, heavy adult differently from a small adult or child. Every situation will be different—a different car, a different patient, and a different crew. Your resourcefulness and ability to adapt are necessary elements to successfully perform the rapid extrication technique.

Nonurgent Moves

When both the scene and the patient are stable, you should carefully plan how to move the patient. If your patient move is rushed or not well planned, it may result in discomfort or injury to the patient, you, and your team. Before you attempt any move, the team leader must be sure that there are enough personnel, any obstacles have been identified or removed, the proper equipment is available, and the procedure and path to be followed have been clearly identified and discussed.

In nonurgent situations, you and your team may choose one of several methods for lifting and carrying a patient. Three general methods are presented here, which may serve as a basis for your plan. You may adapt these procedures to meet your needs on a case-by-case basis.

Direct Ground Lift

The direct ground lift is used for patients with no suspected spinal injury who are found lying supine on the ground. You should use this lift when you have to lift and carry the patient some distance to be placed on the cot. If you find the patient semiprone or lying on his or her side, you should first roll the patient onto his or her back. Ideally, the direct ground lift should be performed by three EMT-Is; however, it can be done with only two. The direct ground lift is performed as follows:

1. **Line up on one side of the patient** with First EMT-I at the patient's head, Second EMT-I at the patient's waist, and Third EMT-I at the patient's knees. All EMT-Is kneel on one knee, preferably the same knee Figure 34-19A .
2. **The patient's arms should be placed on his or her chest if possible.**
3. **First EMT-I places one arm under the patient's neck and shoulders** and cradles the patient's head. First EMT-I then places the other arm under the patient's lower back.
4. **Second EMT-I places both arms under the waist**, and the first and third EMT-Is slide their arms either up to the midback or down to the buttocks as appropriate.

You are the Provider   Part 4

The four additional EMT-I/fire fighters arrive on the scene. With their assistance, you and your partner carefully lift the patient out of the bathtub. After placing the patient supine on the backboard, you perform a complete focused history and physical exam. The exam reveals a stable patient with pain and tenderness to the distal cervical/proximal thoracic spine area with good movement, strength, and feeling in all extremities, and no other complaints. Vital signs are listed below. You apply a cervical collar and secure the patient to the backboard with straps and a head immobilizer. In order to move the patient to the ambulance, you have to take him down a set of eight steps outside the front door.

Vital Signs	Recording Time: 5 Minutes After Patient Contact
Respirations	14 breaths/min
Pulse	96 beats/min, regular
Blood pressure	132/86 mm Hg
Skin	Warm, dry, pink

7. What is the best way to accomplish this move?
8. Do you have any special strapping considerations when preparing this patient to move?

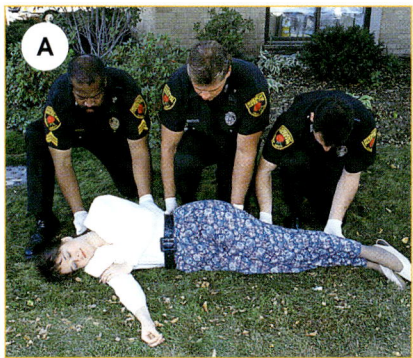 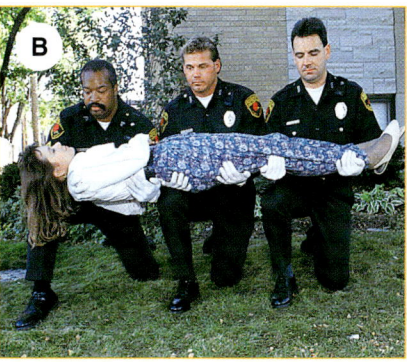 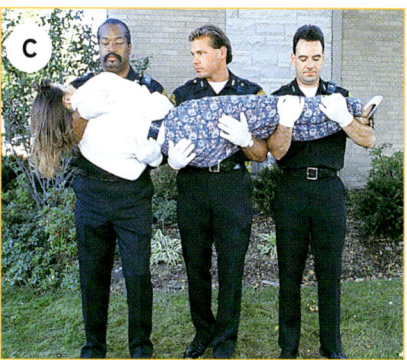

Figure 34-19 The direct ground lift. **A.** Line up on one side of the patient, with one EMT-I at the head, one at the waist, and one at the patient's knees. Place the patient's arms on his or her chest. **B.** On command, lift the patient to knee level. **C.** On command, roll the patient toward your chest, then stand and carry the patient to the cot.

5. Third EMT-I places one arm under the patient's knees and the other above the buttocks.
6. On command, the team lifts the patient up to knee level as each EMT-I rests an arm on his or her knee (Figure 34-19B).
7. As a team and on signal, each EMT-I rolls the patient in toward his or her chest. Again on signal, the team stands and carries the patient to the cot (Figure 34-19C).
8. The steps are reversed to lower the patient onto the cot.

Extremity Lift

The extremity lift may also be used for patients with no suspected extremity or spinal injuries who are supine or in a sitting position on the ground. The extremity lift may be especially helpful when the patient is in a very narrow space or there is not enough room for the patient and a team of EMT-Is to stand side by side.

Communication is the key to success with this lift. You and your partner must coordinate your movements through direct verbal commands. You should perform the extremity lift as follows (Skill Drill 34-7):

1. First EMT-I kneels behind the patient's head as Second EMT-I kneels at the patient's feet. The two EMT-Is are facing each other.
2. The patient's hands should be crossed over his or her chest.
3. First EMT-I places one hand under each of the patient's armpits. First EMT-I grasps the patient's wrists and pulls the upper torso until the patient is in a sitting position (**Step 1**).
4. First EMT-I reaches his or her arms through the patient's armpits and grasps the patient's forearms, or his or her own wrists.
5. Second EMT-I moves to a position between the patient's legs, facing in the same direction as the patient, and slips his or her hands under the patient's knees (**Step 2**).
6. Both EMT-Is move up to a standing position and make sure they are balanced with a good grip on the patient.
7. As the EMT-I at the head gives the command, both stand fully upright and move the patient to the stretcher (**Step 3**).

You will be less likely to injure yourself if you bend at the hips and knees and use your legs for lifting. However, this lift and carry method increases pressure on the patient's chest, so the patient may be uncomfortable in this position.

Transfer Moves

There are several ways to transfer the patient from a bed onto the cot.

Direct Carry

Transfer a supine patient from a bed to the cot using the direct carry method. Position the cot parallel to the bed, with the head of the cot at the foot of the bed. Be sure that you prepare the cot by unbuckling the straps and remove any other items from it (Figure 34-20A). Both you and your partner should face the patient while standing between the bed and the cot. You should slide one arm under the patient's neck and cup the patient's

Skill Drill 34-7

Extremity Lift

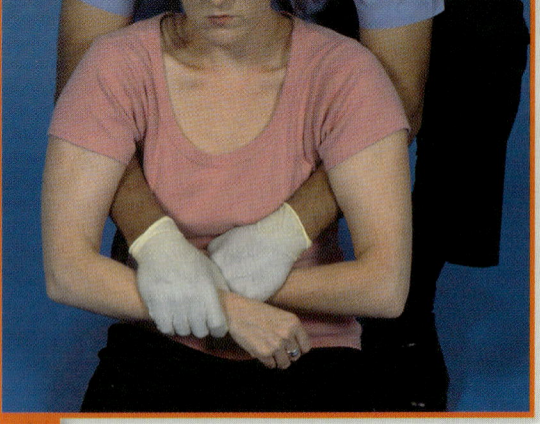

1 Patient's hands are crossed over the chest. First EMT-I grasps patient's wrists or forearms and pulls patient to a sitting position.

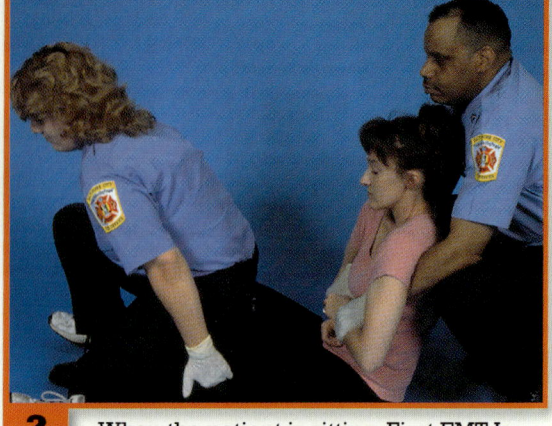

2 When the patient is sitting, First EMT-I passes his or her arms through patient's armpits and grasps the patient's opposite (or his or her own) forearms or wrists.

Second EMT-I kneels between the legs, facing the feet, and places his or her hands under the knees.

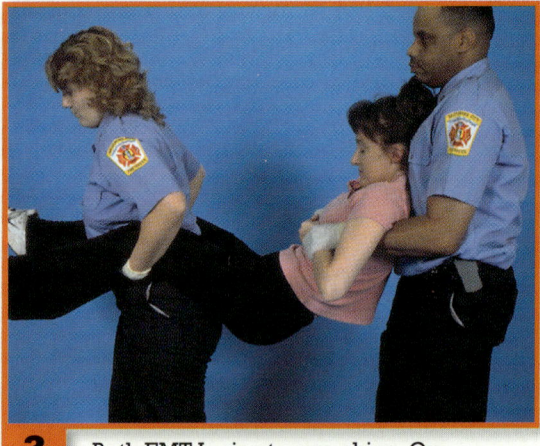

3 Both EMT-Is rise to crouching. On command, both lift and begin to move.

---

shoulder. Your partner should slide his or her hand under the patient's hip and lift slightly. You should then slide your other arm under the patient's back, and your partner should place both arms underneath the patient's hips and calves (Figure 34-20B ▶). Slide the patient to the edge of the bed, and lift and curl the patient toward your chests. You and your partner should then rotate to the cot and gently place the patient onto it (Figure 34-20C ▶).

Draw Sheet Method

To move the patient onto a cot, use the draw sheet method. Place the cot next to the bed, making sure it is at the same height as the bed and rails are lowered and straps are unbuckled. Be sure to hold the cot to keep it from moving. Loosen the bottom sheet underneath the patient, or log roll the patient onto a blanket (Figure 34-21A ▶). Reach across the cot, and grasp the sheet or blanket firmly at the patient's head, chest, hips, and knees (Figure 34-21B ▶). Gently slide the patient onto the cot (Figure 34-21C ▶).

Other Carries

Other carries are performed in the following manner:
- Place a backboard next to the patient and, after using a log roll or slide to move the patient onto the backboard, secure the patient and lift and carry the backboard to the nearby prepared cot.

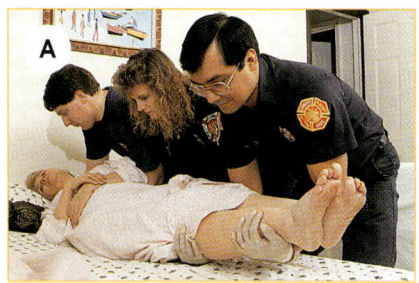 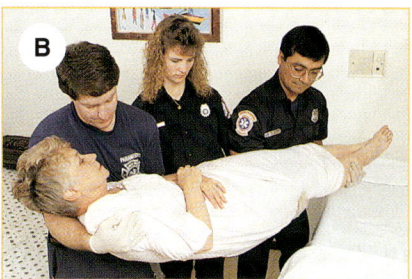 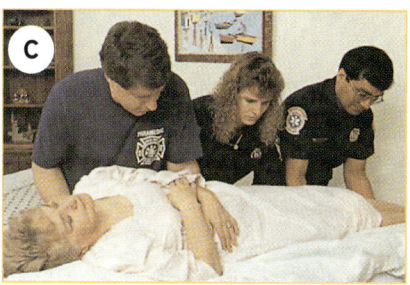

Figure 34-20 The direct carry method. **A.** Bring the cot in parallel to the bed with the patient's feet facing the head of the cot. Secure the cot to prevent it from rolling. **B.** Lift the patient in a smooth, coordinated fashion. Slowly walk the patient around, and position him or her over the cot. **C.** Slowly and gently lower the patient onto the cot.

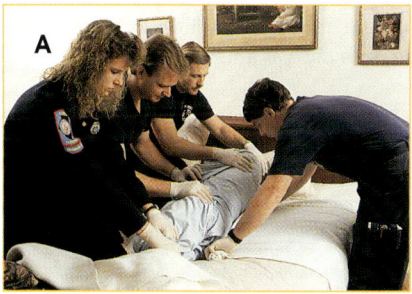 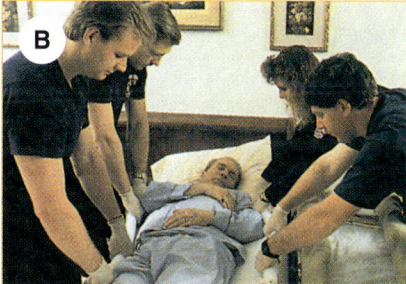 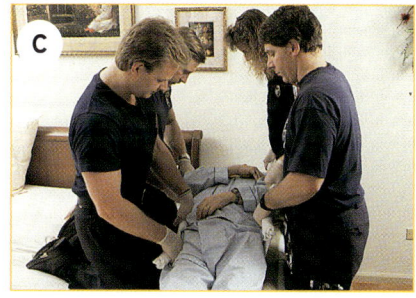

Figure 34-21 The draw sheet method. **A.** Log roll the patient onto a sheet or blanket. **B.** Bring the cot in parallel to the bed. Gently pull the patient to the edge of the bed. **C.** Transfer the patient to the cot.

- Insert the halves of a scoop stretcher under each side of the patient, and fasten the two sides together. Lift and carry the patient to the nearby prepared cot. Follow the steps below **Skill Drill 34-8**. (Note that you can also log roll a patient onto a scoop stretcher that is already locked together.)
  1. **With the scoop stretcher separated**, measure the length of the scoop and adjust to the proper length (**Step 1**).
  2. **Position the stretcher**, one side at a time. One EMT-I lifts the patient's side slightly by pulling on the far hip and upper arm, while the other EMT-I slides the stretcher into place (**Step 2**).
  3. **Lock the stretcher ends together** by engaging their locking mechanisms one at a time and continuing to lift the patient slightly as needed to avoid pinching (**Step 3**).
  4. **Apply and tighten straps** to secure the patient to the scoop stretcher before transferring to the cot (**Step 4**).
- Assist an able patient to the edge of the bed, and, placing the patient's legs over the side, help the patient to sit up. Move the cot so that its foot end touches the bed near the patient. Help the patient to stand and rotate so that he or she can sit down on the center of the cot. Lift the patient's legs, and rotate them onto the cot while your partner lowers the torso onto the cot.

To avoid the strain of unnecessary lifting and carrying, you should use the draw sheet method or assist an able patient to the cot whenever possible.

To move a patient from the ground or the floor onto the cot you should use one of the following methods:
- Lift and carry the patient to the nearby prepared cot using a direct body carry.
- Use a log roll or long-axis drag to place the patient onto a backboard, and then lift and carry the backboard to the cot. Place both the backboard and the patient onto the cot.
- Use a scoop stretcher.
- Log roll the patient onto a blanket **Figure 34-22A**, centering the patient on the blanket and rolling up the excess material on each side. Lift the patient by the blanket, and carry him or her to the nearby cot **Figure 34-22B**.

Skill Drill 34-8

Using a Scoop Stretcher

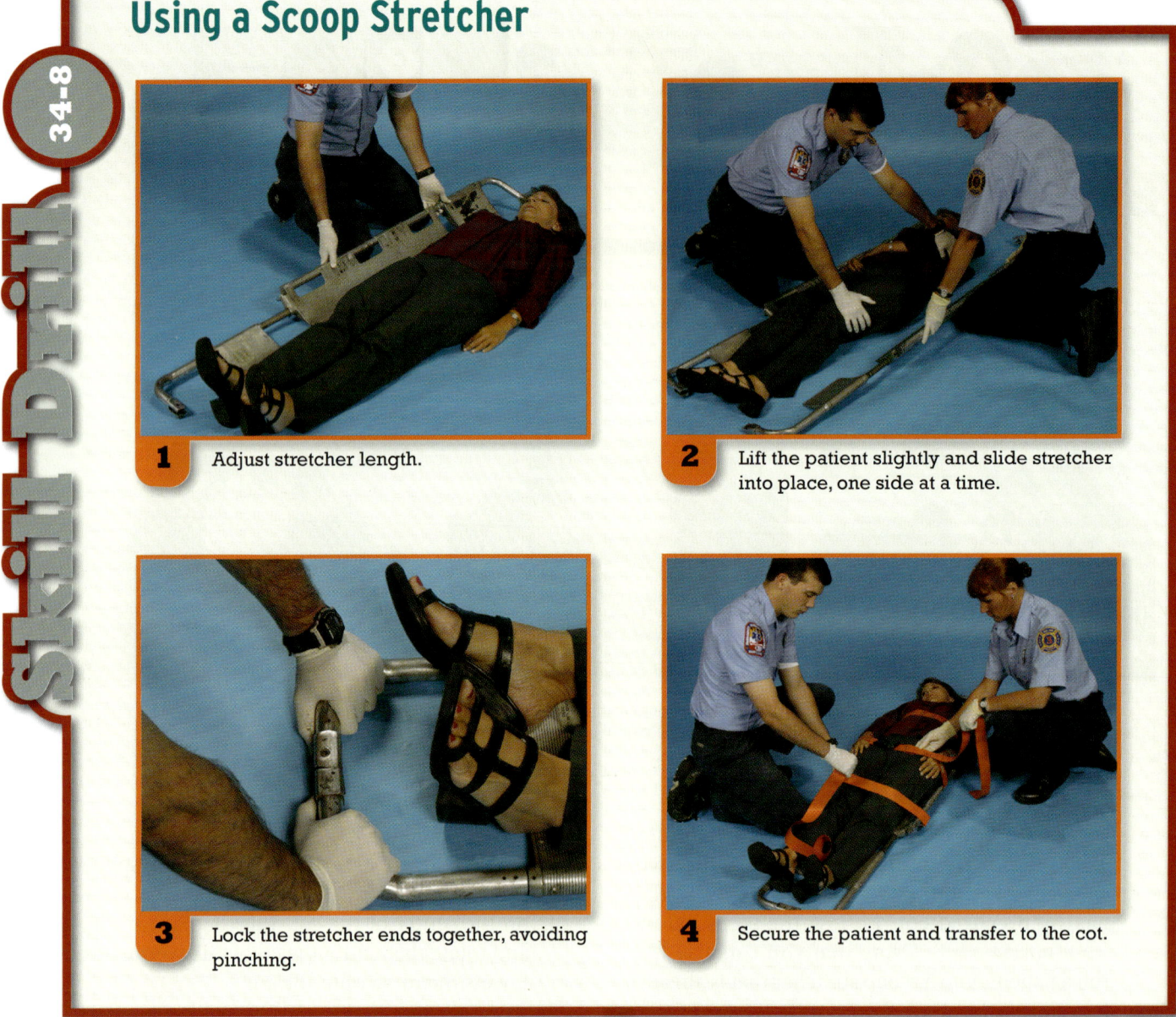

1. Adjust stretcher length.
2. Lift the patient slightly and slide stretcher into place, one side at a time.
3. Lock the stretcher ends together, avoiding pinching.
4. Secure the patient and transfer to the cot.

If a patient is sitting in a chair and cannot assist you, transfer the patient from the chair to a stair chair Figure 34-23 ▶).

Patient-Moving Equipment

The Wheeled Ambulance Stretcher

The wheeled ambulance stretcher, or cot, is the most commonly used device to move and transport patients. Only when you must transport two patients in the same ambulance should it be necessary to transport one patient on a folding stretcher or backboard placed on the long squad bench.

Most patients are placed directly on the cot. However, you will need to place and secure patients with a possible spinal injury or multiple system trauma onto a backboard. Patients who may need CPR or must be carried down (or up) a flight of stairs while supine should also be placed on a backboard. The backboard and patient are then secured onto the cot.

You can use a stair chair to carry a patient who can tolerate being in a sitting position down a flight of stairs to the prepared cot, which is waiting in the lower hallway. You should then transfer the patient from the chair to the cot.

In most instances, it is best if you pull the foot end of the cot while your partner guides it from the head end. When the cot must be carried, it is best if four

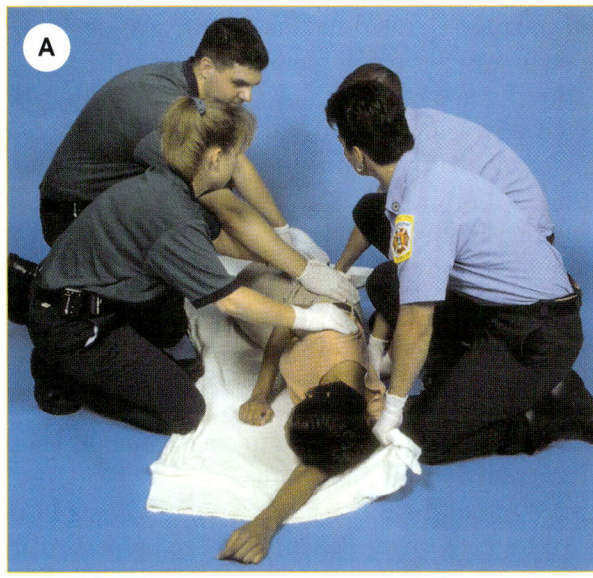

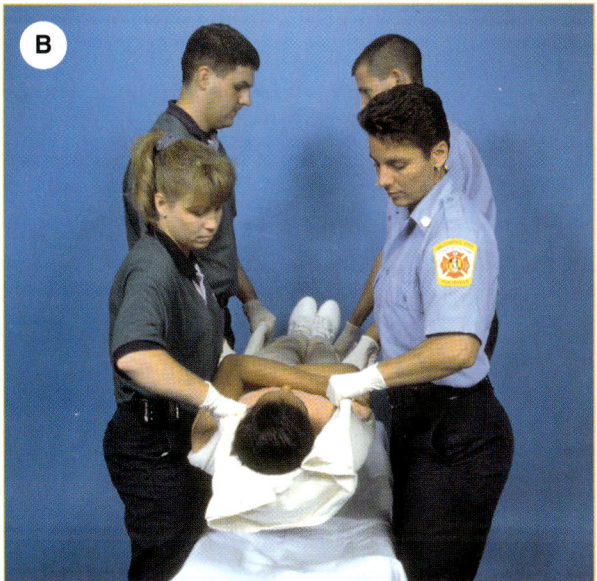

Figure 34-22 Log rolling a patient on the ground. **A.** Log roll the patient onto a blanket. **B.** Lift the blanket and transfer the patient to the cot.

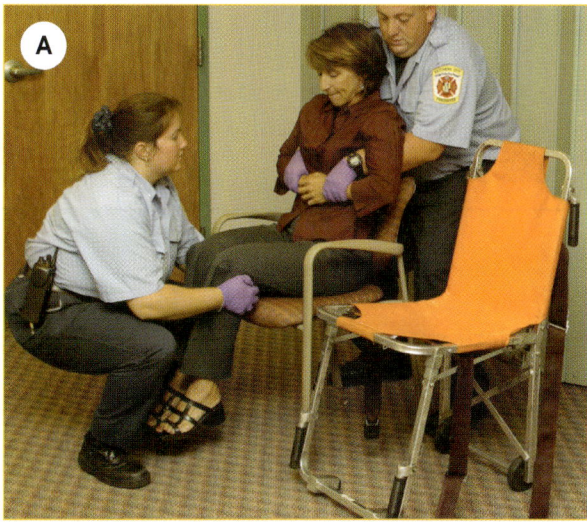

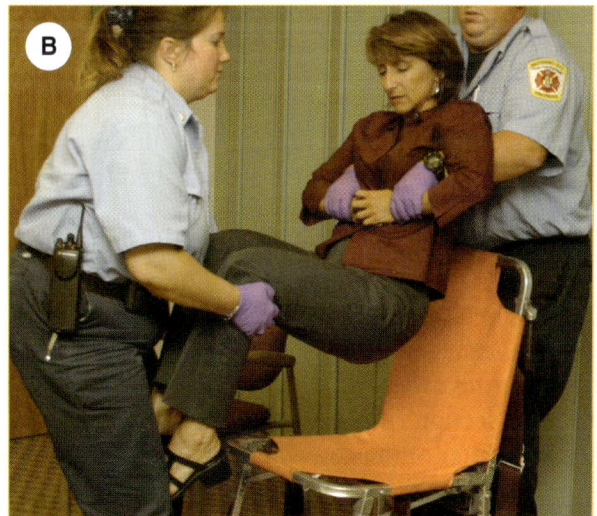

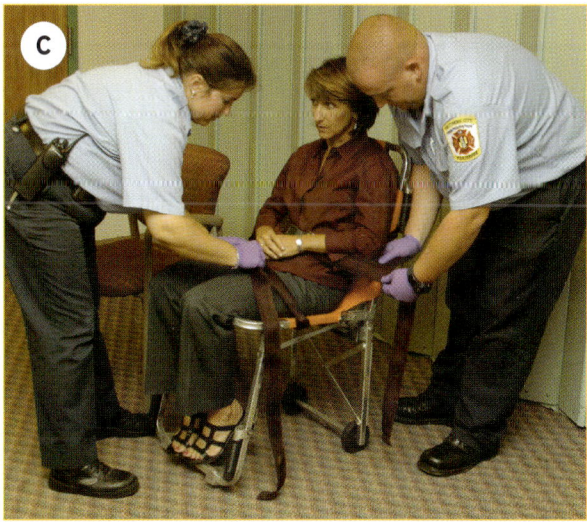

Figure 34-23 Moving a patient from a chair to a stair chair. **A.** Slide your arms through the patient's armpits, and grasp the patient's crossed forearms. Second EMT-I grasps the patient's legs at the knees. **B.** Gently lift the patient onto the locked stair chair. **C.** Position and secure the patient on the stair chair.

rescuers are available to carry it. There is more stability with a four-person carry, and the carry requires less strength. One EMT-I should be positioned at each corner of the cot to provide an even lift. A four-person carry is much safer if the cot must be moved over rough ground. If only two EMT-Is are available, or if limited space will allow room for only two EMT-Is to carry the cot, there is risk that the cot will become unbalanced. In a two-person carry, the two EMT-Is should stand facing each other, with one person at the head end of the cot and the other at the foot end. With this type of carry, one EMT-I will have to walk backward.

> **EMT-I Tips**
>
> The wheeled ambulance stretcher, or cot, is the most commonly used device to move and transport patients.

Features

The modern cot is available in a number of different models, which may include different features (Figure 34-24). Before going on a call, you should be fully familiar with the specific features of the cot that your ambulance carries. You must know where the controls to adjust and lock each feature are located and how each works.

The cot has a specific head end and foot end. The cot has a strong horizontal rectangular tubular metal main frame to which all of its other parts are attached. The cot should be pulled, pushed, and lifted only by its main frame or handles, which are attached to the main frame specifically for this purpose.

On most models, a second tubular frame made up of three sections is attached within or above the main frame. A metal plate is fastened to each of the three sections between its sides. This plate serves as the platform on which the cot mattress and patient are supported. The head section runs from the head end of the cot to near the center of the cot, where the patient's hips will be. Hinges at the area where the hips will be allow the head end to be elevated and the patient's back to be positioned at any desired angle from flat to fully upright. The head end of the cot is designed to be elevated or moved down only when a tilt control is purposely released. At all other times, the back will remain locked at the position in which it was placed. The frame and plates that lie from the hips to the foot end of the cot are divided into two hinged sections. These sections may be connected so that the foot end can be drawn in toward the knees, causing the frame and plates to hinge upward under the patient's knees to elevate them as desired. This feature is not found in all models.

A retractable guardrail is attached along the central portion of the main frame of the cot at each side and is lowered out of the way when a patient is being loaded onto the cot. Once the patient has been properly placed on the cot, the handle is drawn up and locked in an elevated position perpendicular to the surface of the cot. The patient cannot roll off either side of the cot even if a securing strap becomes released. The guardrail at each side can be lowered only if its locking handle is released.

The underside of the main frame of the cot is supported on a folding undercarriage that has a smaller horizontal rectangular frame and four large rubber casters at its bottom end. The folding undercarriage is designed so that the litter can be adjusted to any height from about 12" above the ground, which is the desired height when the stretcher is secured in the ambulance, to 32" to 36" above the ground, which is the desired height when the stretcher is being rolled. Because you are able to lock the cot at any height between its lowest height and its fully extended height, it can be locked at the same height as any bed or examining table to allow the patient to be slid from one to the other. This permits you to transfer the patient without the need for any additional lifting. The controls for folding the undercarriage are designed so that the cot remains locked at its present height when the controls are not being activated. As an additional safety feature on most cots, the main frame must be slightly lifted so that the undercarriage becomes unweighted before it will fold, even if the control is pulled. Therefore, if the handle is accidentally pulled, the elevated cot will not suddenly drop. Controls for elevating and lowering most cots are located at the foot end and at one or both sides. You and your partner must use the proper lifting mechanics to lift the wheeled ambulance stretcher.

The mattress on a cot must be fluid resistant so that it does not absorb any type of potentially infectious material, including water, blood, or other body fluid.

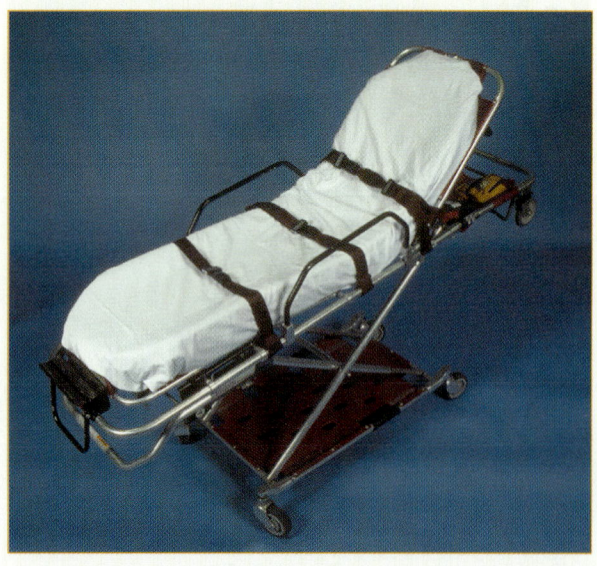

Figure 34-24 An ambulance stretcher (cot).

Documentation Tips

Ensure a thorough patient care report by including details of how you moved the patient. For instance: "Moved patient to stretcher with draw-sheet lift."

Moving the Cot

Whenever a patient has been placed onto the cot, one EMT-I must hold the main frame to make sure that it cannot roll. When the cot is elevated, the main frame and the patient extend considerably beyond the wheels at both the head end and foot end of the cot. Therefore, whenever a patient is on an elevated cot, you must ensure that it is held firmly between two hands at all times so that even if the patient moves, the cot cannot tip (Figure 34-25).

If the loaded cot must be carried down a short flight of steps, be sure to first retract the undercarriage; however, this is not necessary when the cot must be lifted over a curb, single step, or obstacle of a similar height (Figure 34-26). Remember, if the patient must be carried up or down a full flight or several flights of stairs, you should prepare the cot and leave it on the ground floor at the bottom (or top) of the stairs. Use a backboard or stair chair to carry the patient up or down the stairs to the waiting cot.

These are the steps to load the cot into an ambulance (Skill Drill 34-9):

1. **Tilt the head end of the main frame upward** and place it into the patient compartment with the wheels on the floor. The two additional wheels that extend just below the head end are attached to the main frame and will enable this movement (**Step 1**).
2. **With the patient's weight supported** by these two head-end wheels and the EMT-I at the foot end of the cot, move to the side of the main frame and release the undercarriage lock to lift the undercarriage up to its fully retracted position. The wheels of the undercarriage and the two on the head end of the main frame will now be on the same level (**Step 2**).
3. **Simply roll the cot** the rest of the way into the back of the ambulance, where it will rest on all six wheels (**Step 3**).
4. **Secure the cot** in the ambulance with the strong clamps that fasten around the undercarriage when the cot is pushed into them. The clamps are located in a rack on the floor or side of the patient compartment (**Step 4**).

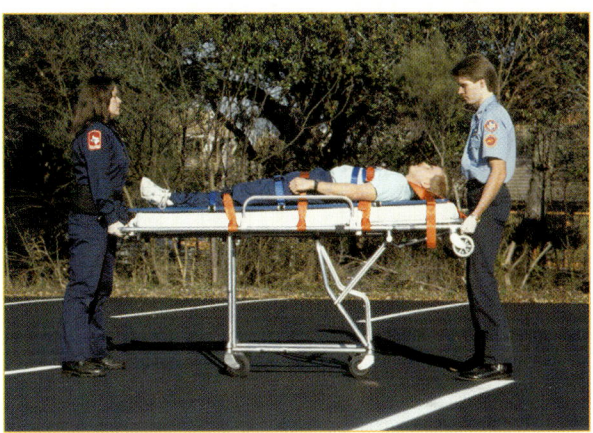

Figure 34-25 Make sure that you hold the main frame of the cot when it is elevated so that even when the patient moves, the cot does not tip.

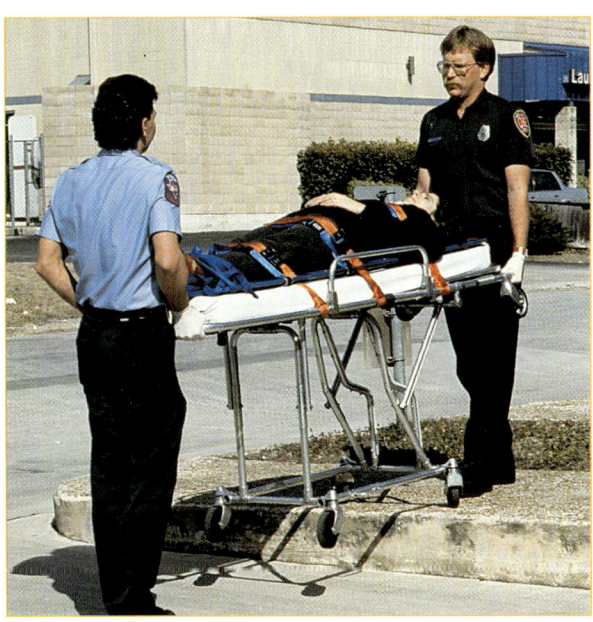

Figure 34-26 You need not retract the undercarriage of the cot when lifting it over a curb, single step, or obstacle of similar height.

The clamps will hold the cot in place until they are released at the hospital. You can control and release the clamps with a single handle that is positioned so that you can activate it when standing on the ground at the open back doors of the ambulance when the cot is to be unloaded. The cot is designed to be rolled on regular flat surfaces. If the patient must be moved over a lawn

Skill Drill 34-9

Loading a Cot into an Ambulance

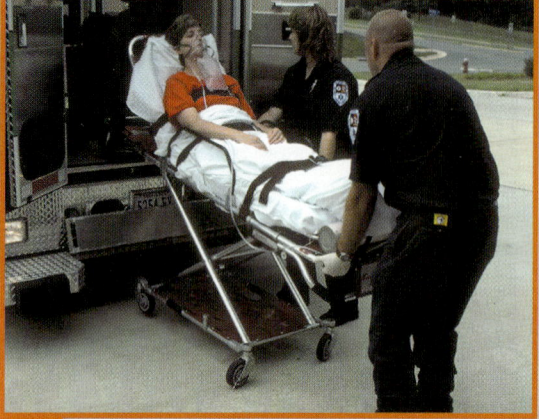

1 Tilt the head of the cot upward, and place it into the patient compartment with the wheels on the floor.

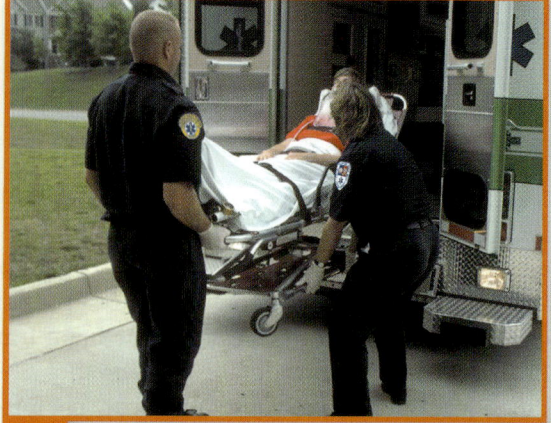

2 Second rescuer on the side of the cot releases the undercarriage lock and lifts the undercarriage.

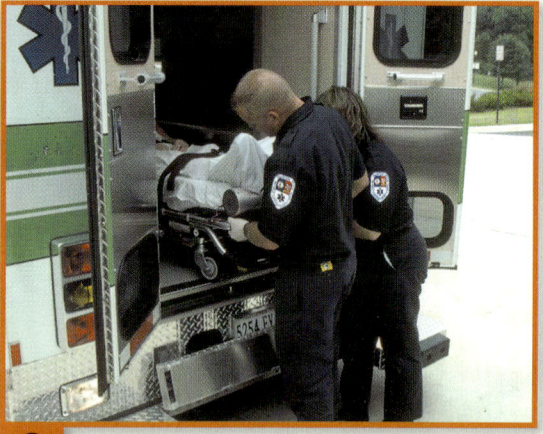

3 Roll the cot into the back of the ambulance.

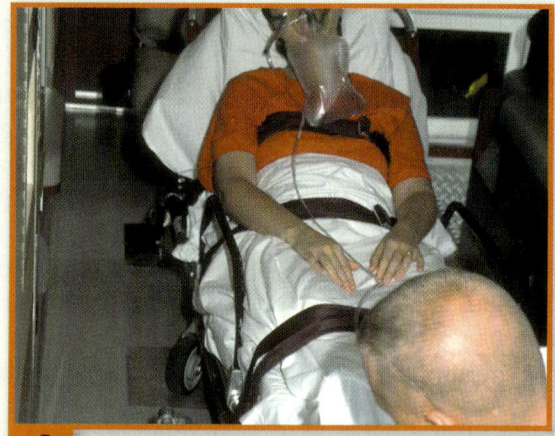

4 Secure the cot to the brackets mounted in the ambulance.

or other irregular surface, you must lift and carry the cot over the terrain.

An IV pole is attached to many cots. The IV pole can be unfolded or extended above the main frame to hold an IV bag above the patient while you move the cot to the ambulance. Some wheeled ambulance stretchers even include a carrier to hold an electrocardiogram (ECG) monitor or automated external defibrillator (AED) and portable oxygen unit. If the model you use does not include these features, you will have to secure the portable oxygen unit and ECG monitor or AED to the top surface of the cot mattress at the patient's legs.

The extra wheels below the head end of the main frame of the cot are not featured on some older or less expensive wheeled ambulance stretchers. These cots are not self-loading. When you reach the back of the ambulance with such a cot, you must lower it until the undercarriage is in its lowest retracted position and then, with you and your partner at each side of the cot, lift it to the height of the floor of the ambulance and roll it into

TABLE 34-3	Guidelines for Loading the Cot into the Ambulance

- Make sure there is sufficient lifting power.
- Follow the manufacturer's directions for safe and proper use of the cot.
- Make sure that all cots and patients are fully secured before you move the ambulance.

the track that locks it into place. Table 34-3 ▲ shows the guidelines that you must follow to load the cot into the ambulance.

Portable/Folding Stretchers

A portable stretcher is a stretcher with a strong rectangular tubular metal frame and rigid fabric stretched across it Figure 34-27 ▼. Portable stretchers do not have a second multipositioning frame or adjustable undercarriage. Some models have two wheels that fold down about 4″ underneath the foot end of the frame and legs of a similar length that fold down from the head end at each side. The wheels make it easier to move the loaded stretcher. The legs should not be used as handles.

Some portable stretchers can be folded in half across the center of each side so that the stretcher is only half its usual length during storage. Many ambulances carry a portable stretcher to use if a patient is in an area that is difficult to reach with a wheeled ambulance stretcher or a second patient must be transported on the squad bench of the ambulance.

A portable stretcher weighs much less than a wheeled stretcher and does not have a bulky undercarriage. However, because most models do not have wheels, you and your team must support all of the patient's weight and any equipment along with the weight of the stretcher.

Flexible Stretchers

Several types of flexible stretchers, such as the SKED, Reeves, or Navy stretcher, are available and can be rolled up across either the stretcher's width or, in the case of the SKED, its length, so that the stretcher becomes a smaller tubular package for storage and carrying Figure 34-28 ▼. When you must carry the equipment

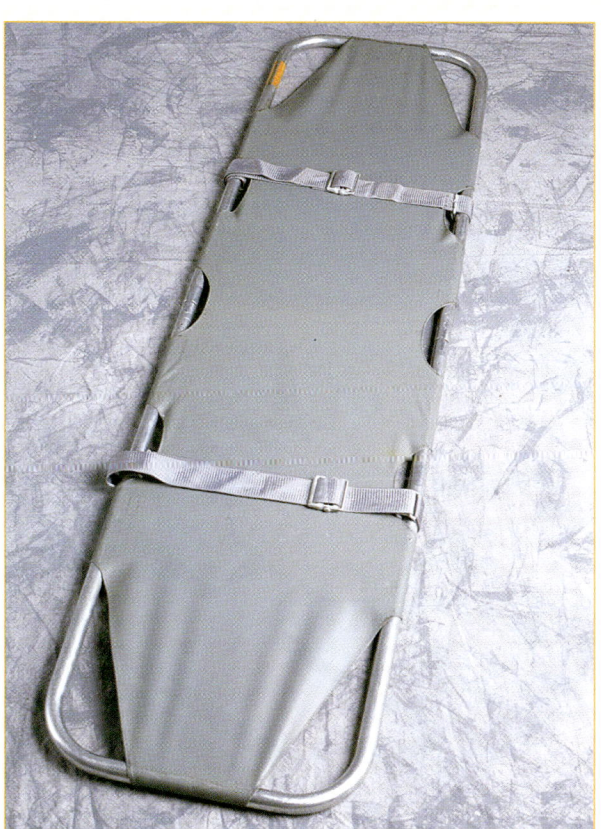

Figure 34-27 A portable stretcher.

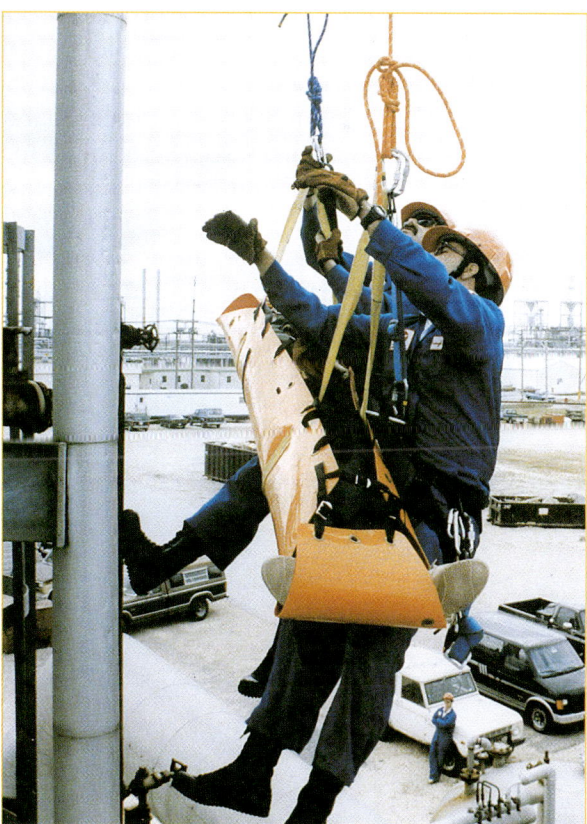

Figure 34-28 A flexible stretcher.

a considerable distance from the nearest place that the ambulance can be located, this is an important consideration. A flexible stretcher forms a rigid stretcher that conforms around the patient's sides and does not extend beyond them. When these stretchers are extended, they are particularly useful when you must remove a patient from or through a confined space. The SKED stretcher can also be used if the patient must be belayed or rappelled by ropes.

The flexible stretcher is the most uncomfortable of all the various devices; however, it provides excellent support and immobilization. When the stretcher is wrapped around the patient and the straps are secured, the patient is completely immobilized. The stretcher can then be lowered by rope or slid down a flight of stairs by resting it on the front edge of each step.

Backboards

Backboards are long, flat boards made of rigid, rectangular material (Figure 34-29 ▼). Backboards were originally made of wood but are now made of other materials as well, mostly plastic. They are used to carry patients and to immobilize supine patients with suspected spinal injury or other multiple trauma. Backboards can also be used to move patients out of awkward places. They are 6′ to 7′ long and are commonly used for patients who are found lying down. Parallel to the sides and ends of the backboard are a number of long holes that are about $\frac{1}{2}''$ to 1″ from the outer edge. These holes form handles and handholds so that the board can be easily grasped, lifted, and carried. The handles and adjacent holes also allow straps used to secure and immobilize the patient to the backboard to be secured to each side and end of the backboard at any needed location.

For many years, backboards were made of thick marine plywood whose surface was sealed with polyurethane or another marine varnish. Wooden backboards are still used in some places. If wooden backboards are used, you must follow infection control procedures before you can reuse the backboards. Where wooden backboards are no longer used, they have generally been stored so that they will be available in the event of a multiple-casualty situation. Newer backboards are made of plastic materials that will not absorb blood or other infectious substances.

You can use a short backboard, called either a short backboard or a half-board, to immobilize the torso, head, and neck of a seated patient with a suspected spinal injury until you can immobilize the patient on a backboard. Short backboards are 3′ to 4′ long. The original short wooden backboard has generally been replaced with a vest-type device that is specifically designed to immobilize the patient until he or she is moved from a sitting position to supine on a backboard (Figure 34-30 ▼). The vest-type devices are easier to use

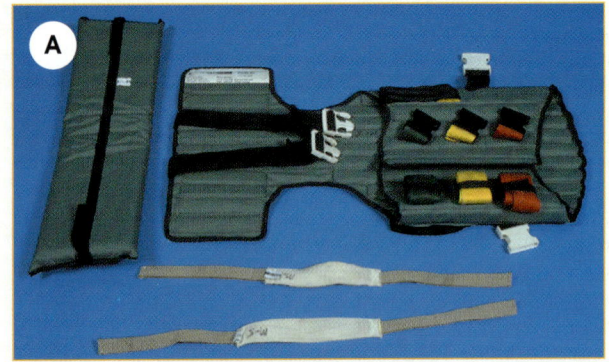

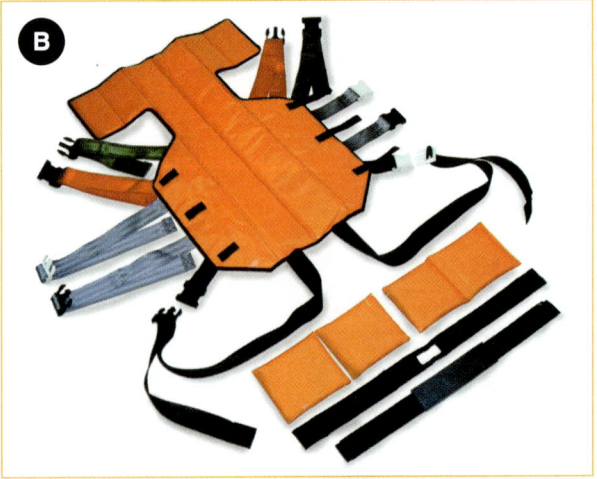

Figure 34-30 Vest-type short immobilization devices. **A.** KED. **B.** Oregon-type vest-style device.

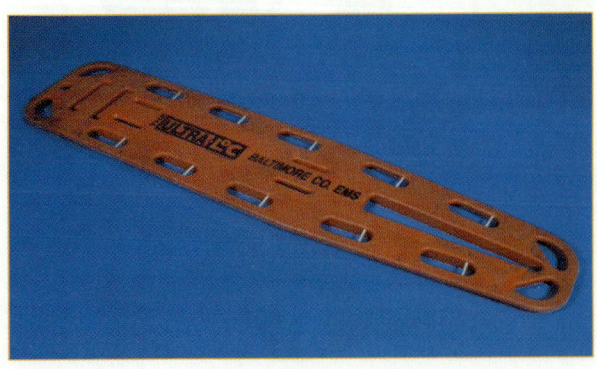

Figure 34-29 A long backboard.

than the wooden backboard. The vest-type pictured is the Kendrick Extrication Device (KED).

Basket Stretchers

You should use a rigid basket stretcher, often called a Stokes litter or Stokes basket, to carry a patient across uneven terrain from a remote location that is inaccessible by ambulance or other vehicle Figure 34-31. If you suspect that the patient has a spinal injury, you should first immobilize him or her on a backboard and then place the backboard into the basket stretcher. Once you have reached the ambulance and wheeled ambulance stretcher, you can remove the patient and backboard from the basket stretcher and place them on the cot.

Basket stretchers either are made of plastic with an aluminum frame or have a full steel frame that is connected by a woven wire mesh. The wire basket is very uncomfortable for the patient unless the wire is padded. Either type can be used to carry a patient across fields, rough terrain, or trails or on a toboggan, boat, or all-terrain vehicle.

Basket stretchers surround and support the patient, yet their design allows water to drain through holes in the bottom. Basket stretchers are also used for technical rope rescues and some water rescues. Not all basket stretchers are rated or appropriate for each of these specialized rescue uses. The types of basket stretchers that are acceptable for specialized rescue must be determined by individuals with additional special training.

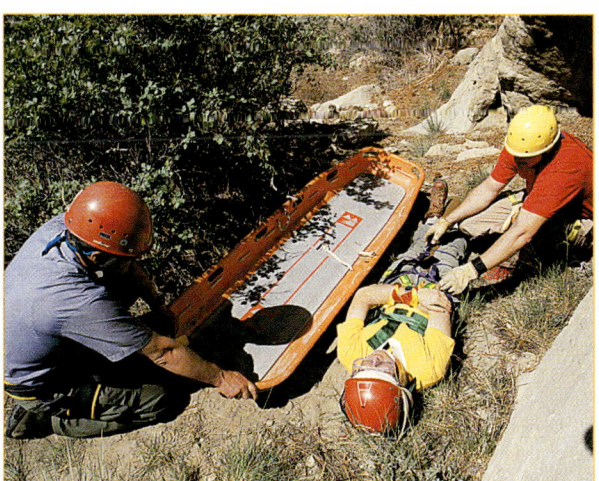

Figure 34-31 A basket stretcher.

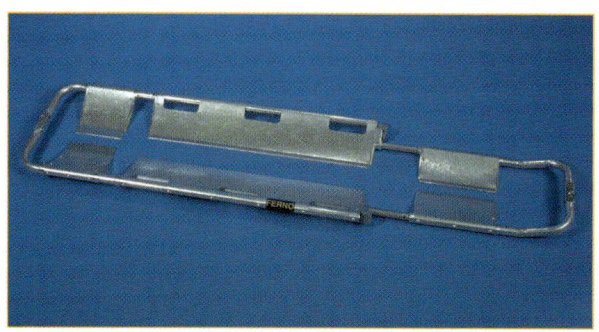

Figure 34-32 A scoop stretcher.

Scoop Stretcher

The scoop stretcher, also referred to as an orthopaedic stretcher or split litter, is designed to be split into two or four pieces Figure 34-32. These sections are fitted around a patient who is lying on the ground or another relatively flat surface. The parts are reconnected, and the patient is lifted and placed on a long backboard or stretcher. A scoop stretcher may be used for patients who have been struck by a motor vehicle.

A scoop stretcher is efficient; however, both sides of the patient must be accessible. You must also pay special attention to the closure area beneath the patient so that clothing, skin, or other objects are not trapped. As with the long backboard, you must fully stabilize and secure the patient before moving him or her; however, you cannot slip a scoop stretcher under the long axis of the patient's body. Scoop stretchers are narrow, well constructed, and compact and have excellent body support features but are not adequate when used alone for standard immobilization of a spinal injury. You and your team should practice often with a scoop stretcher to be ready for using it with a patient.

Stair Chairs

Stair chairs are folding aluminum frame chairs with fabric stretched across them to form a seat and seat back Figure 34-33. They have fold-out handles to help you carry their head and foot ends up or down a flight of stairs, and most have rubber wheels at their back with casters in front so that they can be rolled along the floor and make turns. Stair chairs serve as an adjunct for moving a patient up or down stairs to the ground floor, where the prepared wheeled ambulance stretcher is waiting. You can roll the stair chair on the floor until you reach the stairwell, then carry it (rather than roll and bump it) up or down the stairs. Once you reach the ground floor,

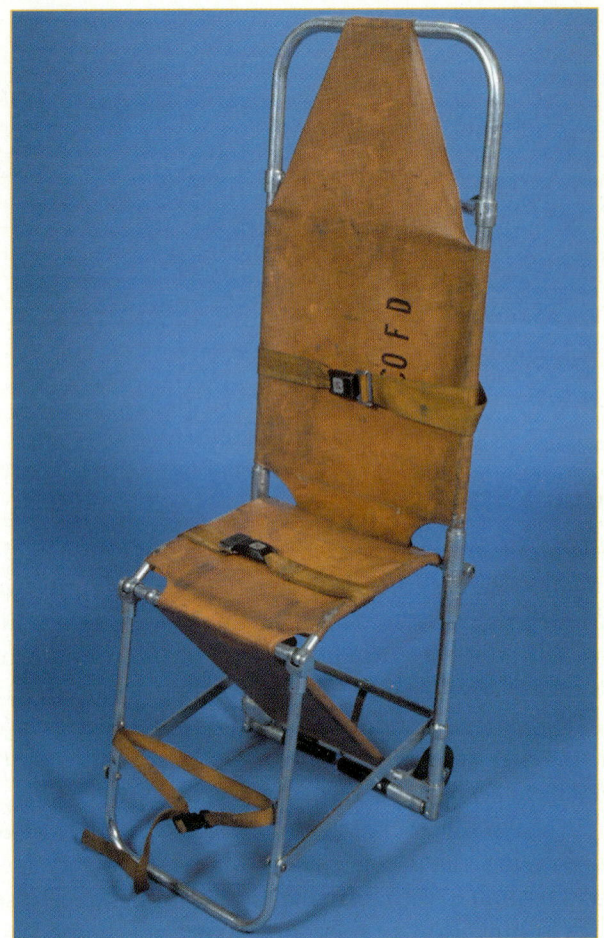

Figure 34-33 A stair chair.

you can roll it to the waiting cot and assist or lift the patient onto the cot.

Be sure to follow manufacturer's directions for maintenance, inspection, repair, and upkeep for any device that you use as patient-handling equipment.

Moving and Positioning the Patient

Every time you have to move a patient, you must take special care that neither you, your team, nor the patient is injured. Patient packaging and handling are technical skills that you will learn and perfect through practice and training.

Training and practice are required to use all the equipment that is described in this chapter. You must master the skills necessary for their use and understand the advantages and limitations of each device. Practice each technique with your team often so that when you must move a patient, you can perform the move quickly, safely, and efficiently. After each patient transfer, you and your team should evaluate the appropriateness of the technique that you used, as well as your technical skill in completing the transfer. You must also be sure to maintain your equipment according to the manufacturer's instructions. Using clean, well-maintained equipment is but one part of providing high-quality patient care.

After you deliver the patient to the emergency department, you and your team must begin preparing for your next call. Review the positive points about the transport. Discuss changes that would improve the next run. This process of review and evaluation identifies the following:

- Procedures that need more practice
- Equipment that needs to be cleaned or repaired
- Skills that you need to review or acquire

Most important, a critical review helps you and your team to become more confident and better-skilled EMT-Is.

Certain patient conditions, such as head injury, shock, spinal injury, and pregnancy, call for special lifting and moving techniques. Patients with chest pain or difficulty breathing should sit in a position of comfort, as long as they are not hypotensive. Patients with suspected spinal injuries must be immobilized on a long backboard. Patients who are in shock should be packaged and moved in a supine position or with their legs elevated 6″ to 12″. Pregnant patients who are hypotensive should be positioned and transported on their left sides. Move an unresponsive patient with no suspected spinal injury into the recovery position by rolling the patient onto his or her side without twisting the body. Transport a patient who is nauseated or vomiting in a position of comfort, but be sure that you are positioned appropriately to manage the airway.

You are the Provider — Summary

1. Does the patient need an *emergency*, *urgent*, or *nonurgent* move?

It is important to assess the patient and the situation to determine whether you need to move this patient quickly, possibly sacrificing good body mechanics and appropriate spinal immobilization, or if you can move at a slower, more determined pace. If the patient's condition allows, it is always better to take your time, plan the move, and, when necessary, call for additional assistance.

2. How can you accomplish this move in the safest way possible?

When making your decision about how to move a patient, it is important to consider your options for providing a stable lift for the patient while using good body mechanics. Too often, impatient providers make decisions that compromise patient safety or result in an injury to one of the EMS providers.

3. What is the urgency of this move?

This patient is stable and, given the unusual position, would benefit from additional assistance and a well-planned move. This would be a nonurgent move.

4. What are your primary considerations when planning this move?

Given the possibility of a spinal injury, it is important to move the patient while taking appropriate spinal precautions. Given the tight quarters of most bathrooms and the number of obstacles, you must also consider what additional equipment and resources you would need to accomplish the move safely. Primary considerations would include: clear leadership and direction, maintaining cervical spine immobilization during the move, moving the patient into a neutral, in-line position, getting the patient onto the backboard, and lifting safely.

5. How can you safely lift this patient while maintaining appropriate spinal immobilization?

You need to try to figure out a way to lift this patient while keeping your back straight. Appropriate application of a cervical collar here would be difficult if not impossible. If you have enough people, assign one rescuer to maintain the head and place four rescuers around the patient (two on either side of the patient). The rescuers at the patient's sides should slide their arms under the patient at the key lifting points and hold onto the rescuers arms directly across from them. The key lifting points are as follows: shoulders at the level of the armpits, pelvis, and just proximal to the knees. The third lifting point is just proximal to the knees in this situation because the patient is prone. If the patient is supine, the lifting point is just distal to the knee. Under the command of the rescuer at the head, lift the patient straight up into a neutral, in-line position as you lift. Move the patient out to a location where you have more room and lower the patient to the floor. You can then log roll the patient onto a backboard.

You could also accomplish this move by using straps at the key lifting points instead of the rescuers locking their arms. This would allow the rescuers to be in a better position to use their legs for lifting. Lifting straps were once very popular lifting adjuncts for EMS providers, but have become less so in recent years. Straps can give you better leverage in many lifting situations and should be considered an important option.

This is just one possible method for lifting this patient. The situation and location will dictate which method is used to move the patient.

You are the Provider continued

6. What do you need to think about and be prepared for once you have lifted the patient?

You need to consider the space limitations and obstacles that will affect moving the patient out of the bathroom once he has been lifted from the bathtub. Make sure you have this planned out ahead of time. You will need to find a location to transfer the patient to the backboard that will afford the most room to maneuver, and consider how the transfer will take place. For instance, if you opted to use straps to lift the patient, you may be able to roll the patient as you lower him to the backboard. Of course, all rescuers would have to be comfortable with this maneuver in order to accomplish it safely.

Once the patient is supine on the backboard, the cervical collar should be placed if you have not been able to apply it previously.

Summary

7. What is the best way to accomplish this move?

Once the patient is secured to the backboard, use a diamond carry to move the patient down the stairs to the stretcher.

8. Do you have any special strapping considerations when preparing this patient to move?

When carrying a patient up or down stairs, additional strapping should be used around the patient's feet and over his shoulders to prevent sliding up and down the backboard.

Prep Kit

Ready for Review

- The first key rule of lifting is to always keep your back in an upright position and lift without twisting. You can lift and carry significant weight without injury as long as your back is in the proper upright position.
- The power lift is the safest and most powerful way to lift.
- The safety of you, your team, and the patient depends on the use of proper lifting techniques and maintaining a proper hold when lifting or carrying a patient. If you do not have a proper hold, you will not be able to bear your share of the weight, or you may lose your grasp with one or both hands and possibly cause a lower back injury to one or more EMT-Is. It is always best to move a patient on a device that can be rolled. However, if a wheeled device is not available, you must understand and follow certain guidelines for carrying a patient on a cot.
- You must constantly coordinate your movements with those of the other team members and make sure that you communicate with them.
- When lifting a cot, you must make sure that you and your team use correct lifting techniques. You and your team should also be of similar height and strength.
- If you must carry a loaded backboard or cot up or down stairs or other inclines, be sure that the patient is tightly secured to the device to prevent sliding. Be sure to carry the backboard or cot foot end first so that the patient's head is elevated higher than the feet.
- Directions and commands are an important part of safe lifting and carrying. You and your team must anticipate and understand every move and execute it in a coordinated manner. The team leader is responsible for coordinating the moves.
- You should try to use four rescuers whenever resources allow. You should also know how much you can comfortably and safely lift and not attempt to lift more than this amount. Rapidly summon additional help to lift and carry a weight that is greater than you are able to lift.
- The same basic body mechanics apply for safe reaching and pulling as for lifting and carrying. Keep your back locked and straight, and avoid twisting. Do not hyperextend your back when reaching overhead.
- You should normally move a patient with nonurgent moves in an orderly, planned, and unhurried fashion, selecting methods that involve the least amount of lifting and carrying.
- At times, you may have to use an emergency move to move a patient before providing initial assessment and care. You should perform an urgent move if a patient has an altered level of consciousness, inadequate ventilation or shock, or in extreme weather conditions.
- The wheeled ambulance stretcher, or cot, is the most commonly used device to move and transport patients. Other devices that are used to lift and carry patients include portable stretchers, flexible stretchers, backboards, basket stretchers (Stokes litters), scoop stretchers, and stair chairs.
- Whenever you are moving a patient, you must take special care so that neither you, your team, nor the patient is injured. You will learn the technical skills of patient packaging and handling through practice and training.
- Training and practice are also required to use all the equipment that is available to you. You must practice each technique with your team often so that you are able to perform the move quickly, safely, and efficiently.

Technology

- Interactivities
- Vocabulary Explorer
- Anatomy Review
- Web Links
- Online Review Manual

www.EMSzone.com/EMTI

Prep Kit continued...

Vital Vocabulary

backboard A device that is used to provide support to a patient who is suspected of having a hip, pelvic, spinal, or lower extremity injury. Also called a spine board, trauma board, or longboard.

basket stretcher A rigid stretcher commonly used in technical and water rescues that surrounds and supports the patient yet allows water to drain through holes in the bottom; also called a Stokes litter.

diamond carry A carrying technique in which one EMT-I is located at the head end, one at the foot end, and one at each side of the patient; each of the two EMT-Is at the sides uses one hand to support the stretcher so that all are able to face forward as they walk.

direct ground lift A lifting technique that is used for patients who are found lying supine on the ground with no suspected spinal injury.

emergency move A move in which the patient is dragged or pulled from a dangerous scene before initial assessment and care are provided.

extremity lift A lifting technique that is used for patients who are supine or in a sitting position with no suspected extremity or spinal injuries.

flexible stretcher A stretcher that is a rigid carrying device when secured around a patient but can be folded or rolled when not in use.

portable stretcher A stretcher with a strong rectangular tubular metal frame and rigid fabric stretched across it.

power grip A technique in which the litter or backboard is gripped by inserting each hand under the handle with the palm facing up and the thumb extended, fully supporting the underside of the handle on the curved palm with the fingers and thumb.

power lift A lifting technique in which the EMT-I's back is held upright, with legs bent, and the patient is lifted when the EMT-I straightens the legs to raise the upper body and arms.

rapid extrication technique A technique to move a patient from a sitting position inside a vehicle to supine on a backboard in less than 1 minute when conditions do not allow for standard immobilization.

scoop stretcher A stretcher that is designed to be split into two or four sections that can be fitted around a patient who is lying on the ground or other relatively flat surface; also called a split litter or orthopaedic stretcher.

stair chair A lightweight folding device that is used to carry a conscious, seated patient up or down stairs.

wheeled ambulance stretcher A specially designed stretcher that can be rolled along the ground. A collapsible undercarriage allows it to be loaded into the ambulance; also called the cot or an ambulance cot.

Assessment in Action

You are on the scene treating a woman for weakness, dizziness, and headache and are ready to move her to the ambulance.

You are in a third floor apartment, which is accessible only via a narrow stairway. The patient weighs 300 pounds and cannot tolerate sitting up.

1. Proper lifting techniques to keep in mind when you lift this patient include all of the following EXCEPT:
   A. lock your back in its normal upright position.
   B. reach with the arms and lift with your arms.
   C. spread your legs about 15" and bend at the knees.
   D. balance the patient's weight between your arms.

2. When carrying the patient down the stairs you should:
   A. secure the patient to the cot and use a diamond carry.
   B. use a diamond carry and go down the stairs head first.
   C. secure the patient to the cot and use two people to carry the patient.
   D. secure the patient to a backboard and go down the stairs feet first.

3. Prior to lifting and moving the patient you should do all of the following EXCEPT:
   A. identify a team leader for the move.
   B. determine what resources you need.
   C. put the strongest EMT-I at the patient's head.
   D. evaluate the weight limitations of the equipment.

4. To protect yourself, as well as this patient, you should:
   A. have the patient walk to the ambulance.
   B. communicate with your partner as the two of you lift the patient.
   C. have the family help you carry the patient.
   D. know your limitations and refrain from exceeding them.

5. The patient could be moved using the:
   A. direct carry or draw sheet method.
   B. extremity lift or direct carry.
   C. draw sheet method or extremity lift.
   D. stair chair or direct carry.

6. When moving the patient from the bed to the cot using the draw sheet method you should:
   A. not log roll the patient.
   B. grasp the sheet at the head and the feet.
   C. use the sheet to slide the patient to the cot.
   D. position the cot at the foot of the bed.

7. When moving the patient via the cot you should do all of the following EXCEPT:
   A. keep one hand on the cot at all times.
   B. ensure the cot fastens into the ambulance.
   C. know how to operate the cot.
   D. lower the cot when moving down the stairs.

Points to Ponder

You and your partner are carrying a patient down a flight of stairs. You knew the patient's weight was on the border of requiring assistance, but decided to move the patient on your own. You and your partner decided that you could handle it if you used the stair chair. As you are about half way down the stairs, you lose your grip and drop the patient. Your efforts to stop the patient from falling are in vain, as your hand is crushed between the wall and the stair chair. The patient tips over, and slides face first down the stairs. He is seriously injured. Your partner is pulled over with the stair chair. He lands on the patient and suffers injuries to his back and legs.

What should you have done to prevent these injuries?

Issues: Injuries Caused By Improper Lifting, Knowing Your Equipment and Your Limitations in Lifting

Gaining Access

1999 Objectives
There are no 1999 objectives for this chapter.

1985 Objectives
1.6.51 Describe patient extrication. (p 1446)

Additional Objectives*

Cognitive
1. Describe the purpose of extrication. (p 1446)
2. Discuss the role of the EMT-I in extrication. (p 1446)
3. Identify what equipment for personal safety is required for the EMT-I. (p 1447)
4. Define the fundamental components of extrication. (p 1446)
5. State the steps that should be taken to protect the patient during extrication. (p 1448)
6. Evaluate various methods of gaining access to the patient. (p 1449)
7. Distinguish between simple and complex access. (p 1450)

Affective
None

Psychomotor
None

*These are noncurriculum objectives.

35

Gaining Access

You are the Provider

You are dispatched to the scene of a motor vehicle crash, in which a small passenger car has struck a utility pole. As you arrive at the scene, you note that the utility pole is down and its wires are across the hood of the car. You immediately notify the power company.

This chapter will review fundamental principles of safety and extrication as they pertain to gaining access to your patients. In addition, it will also help you answer the following questions:

1. What functions does the EMS team perform at the scene of an incident?
2. What is the connection between good communication, an accurate scene size-up, and the overall safety of the operation?

Gaining Access

As an EMT-I, you will usually not be responsible for rescue and extrication. Rescue involves many different processes and environments. It also requires training beyond the level of the EMT-I. In this chapter, you will learn basic concepts of extrication.

The chapter begins with a discussion of personal safety and patient safety. Gaining access is the next phase of extrication discussed. This includes how to gain access to patients and how to keep patients and bystanders safe in the process. Your main concern is reaching the patient so that you can begin providing care. In most instances, once you have reached the patient, extrication will occur around you and the patient. Communication between the EMT-I caring for the patient and rescue personnel performing the extrication is vital. Removal is the final phase of extrication; the patient's spine is immobilized and he or she is placed on the ambulance stretcher.

Fundamentals of Extrication

During all phases of rescue, your primary concern is safety, and your primary role is to provide emergency medical care and prevent further injury to the patient. You will provide care as extrication goes on around you unless this proves to be too dangerous for you or the patient. **Extrication** is the removal from entrapment or from a dangerous situation or position. **Entrapment** means to be caught within a closed area with no way out, or to have a limb or other body part trapped. In the context of this chapter, extrication means removal of a patient from a wrecked automobile. However, the same principles and concepts apply to other situations.

You will need to coordinate your efforts with those of the rescue team. If you respect their job, they will respect yours. You should communicate with members of the rescue team throughout the extrication process. Start talking to the rescue team leader as soon as you arrive at the scene. Under the incident command system (described in Chapter 36), the rescue operations are integrated as a separate group. The EMT-I becomes a member of this group, and will enter the vehicle and provide care for the patient(s) when approved by the extrication leader.

At any accident scene, four different basic functions must be addressed **Figure 35-1**. When possible, responders work in well-defined separate teams to ensure clear lines of responsibility and organization. Each team focuses on and is responsible for a different function:

- Fire fighters are responsible for extinguishing any fire, preventing additional ignition, ensuring that the scene is safe, and washing down any spilled fuel.
- Law enforcement is responsible for traffic control and direction, maintaining order at the scene, investigating the crash or crime scene, and establishing and maintaining lines so that bystanders are kept at a safe distance and out of the way of rescuers.
- The rescue team is responsible for properly securing and stabilizing the vehicle, providing safe entrance and **access** to patients (the ability to reach the patient), extricating any patients, ensuring that patients are properly protected during extrication or other rescue activities, and providing adequate room so that patients can be removed properly.
- EMS personnel are responsible for assessing and providing immediate medical care, triage and assigning priority to patients, packaging the patient, providing additional assessment and care as needed once the patient has been removed, and providing transport to the emergency department.

Good communication among team members and clear leadership are essential to safe, efficient provision of proper emergency care. Although your input at the scene is important, one member of your team must be

Technology

- Interactivities
- Vocabulary Explorer
- Anatomy Review
- Web Links
- Online Review Manual

www.EMSzone.com/EMTI

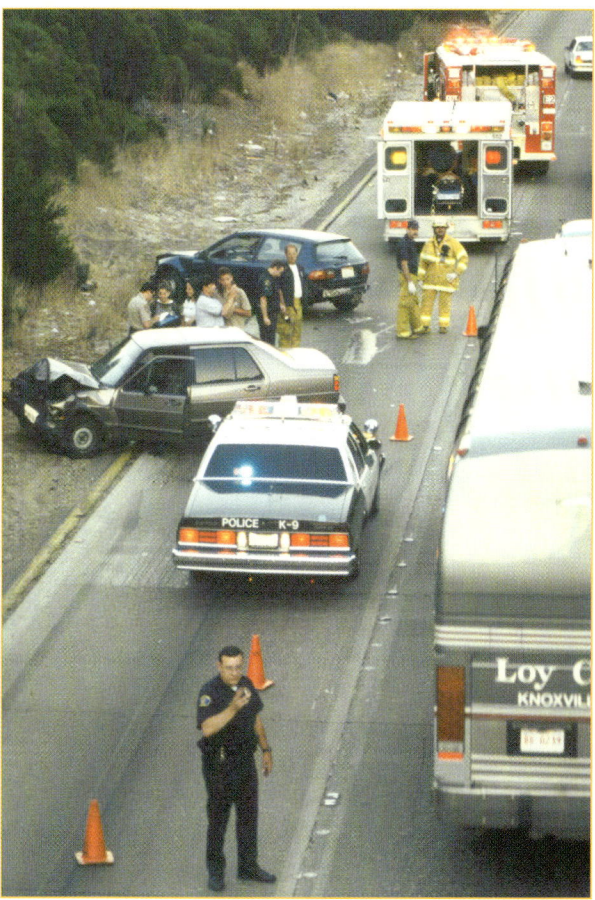

Figure 35-1 Every crash requires cooperation, as each responder has a specific role at the scene. Fire fighters, law enforcement, the rescue team, and EMS personnel all have individual roles.

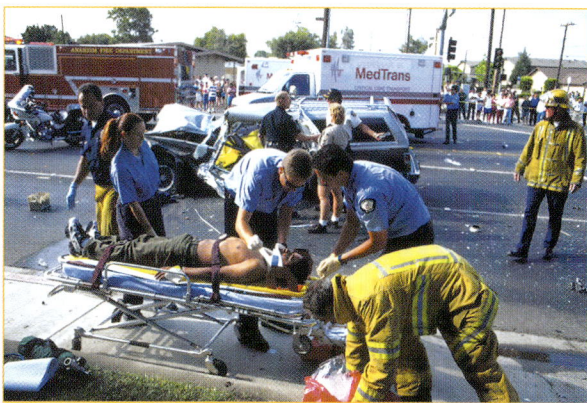

Figure 35-2 The scene of a crash should be marked properly, and traffic should be diverted so that responders have enough room to work.

clearly in charge. The team leader's assessment of the patient and the situation will dictate the way in which medical care, packaging, and transport will proceed. Customarily, the crew chief, who typically is clearly indicated on the shift schedule, is responsible for this role. If not, a team leader must be identified and agreed to before you arrive at the scene.

In some areas, there might not be enough personnel to staff multiple units. In these areas, you and your team may have two roles. However, one person must still be in charge of the overall rescue operation. If there is no identifiable leadership at the scene, the rescue effort and patient care will suffer. Leaders should be identified as part of a larger incident command system. They should be medically trained and qualified to judge the priorities of patient care, and they must also be experienced in extrication.

Scene Size-up

You must always be prepared, mentally and physically, for any incident that requires rescue or extrication. The most important part of this preparation is thinking about your safety and the safety of your team. Safety begins with the proper mind-set and the proper protective equipment.

When you arrive, you should position the unit in a safe location that does not add a hazard to the scene. Before proceeding, make sure that the scene is properly marked and that either the road is closed or traffic flow is controlled safely around the scene **Figure 35-2**. One of the important responsibilities of scene size-up is to determine what, if any, additional resources will be needed. These resources may include additional EMS units and personnel. If you are first on the scene, you may need to initiate a rescue response or call for law enforcement or specialized crews, such as HazMat or utility departments.

The equipment that you use and the gear that you wear will depend on the situation **Figure 35-3**. However, the importance of wearing blood- and fluid-impermeable gloves at all times during patient contact cannot be emphasized enough. If you will be involved with extrication, you should wear a pair of leather gloves over your disposable gloves to protect you from injury in handling ropes, tools, broken glass, hot or cold objects, or sharp metal.

Remember, you should not attempt to gain access to the patient or enter the vehicle until you are sure that the vehicle is stable and that any hazards have been identified and either properly controlled or eliminated.

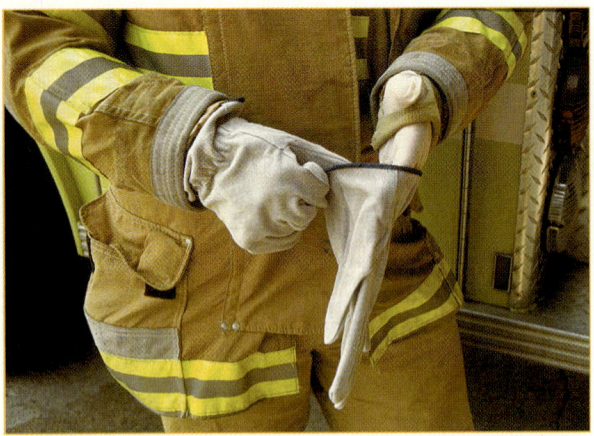

Figure 35-3 Proper protective equipment varies depending on the situation.

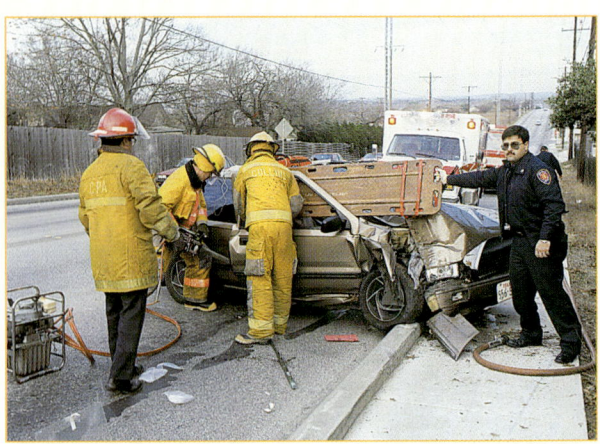

Figure 35-5 Use a long backboard or blanket to protect the patient and any rescuers who are providing care.

When there is a rescue leader present, you will only be authorized to enter when these considerations have been met.

Patient and Bystander Safety

While you are gaining access to the patient and during extrication, you must make sure that the patient remains safe. Always talk to the patient and describe what you are going to do before you do it and as you are doing it, even if you think the patient is unconscious Figure 35-4 . In many instances, you or your partner may be providing cervical spine immobilization or other care during extrication. EMS personnel should wear proper protective gear while in the working area. The patient and the EMS personnel should be covered with a heavy, nonflammable blanket to protect them against flying glass or other objects. A backboard may also be used as a protective shield Figure 35-5 . Try to keep heat, noise, and force to a minimum. Use only what is necessary to extricate the patient safely.

Bystanders and family members can be hazards themselves. If they are allowed to get too close, they are at risk of injury and may also interfere with the overall management of the incident. For these reasons, the rescue group will set up a danger zone that is off-limits to bystanders Figure 35-6 . A danger zone (hot zone)

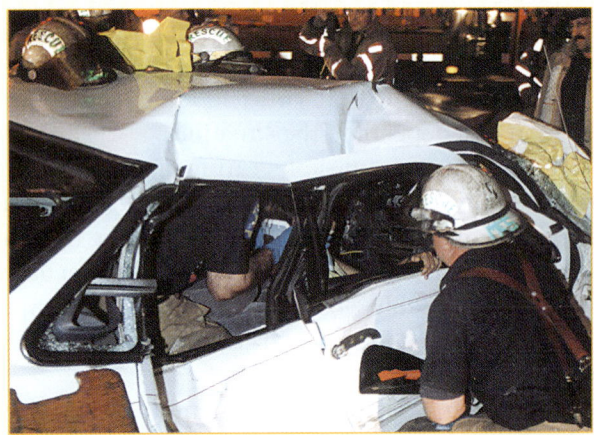

Figure 35-4 Always explain to the patient why you are there and what you are doing.

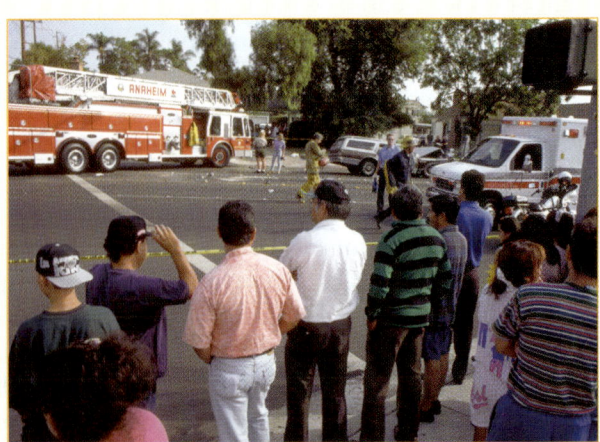

Figure 35-6 A danger zone should be established to prevent bystanders from entering the area around an incident.

Gaining Access to the Patient

The exact way you gain access to or reach the patient(s) depends on the situation. It is up to you to identify the safest, most efficient way to gain access. Darkness, uneven terrain, tall grass, shrubbery, or wreckage may make patients hard to find Figure 35-8 ▶. Multiple vehicles with multiple patients may be involved. If this is the case, you should locate and rapidly triage each patient to determine who needs urgent care. This step is important before you proceed with any treatment and patient packaging. Be sure to take these factors into account in your scene size-up. Remember that scene size-up is a continuing process, because the situation often changes. As a result, you may need to change your plans for gaining access and providing treatment.

To determine the exact location and position of the patient, you and your team should consider the following questions:

- Is the patient in a vehicle or in some other structure?
- Is the vehicle or structure severely damaged?
- What hazards exist that pose risk to the patient and rescuers?
- In what position is the vehicle? On what type of surface? Is the vehicle stable or is it apt to roll or tip?

You must also take into account the patient's injuries and their severity. You may have to change your course of action as you learn more about the patient's condition. Do not try to access the patient until you are sure that the vehicle is stable and that hazards have been identified and deemed safe. Hazards might include electrical or gas lines.

What should you do if you have to remove a patient quickly because the environment is threatening or you need to perform CPR? CPR is not effective when the patient is in a sitting position or lying on the soft seat

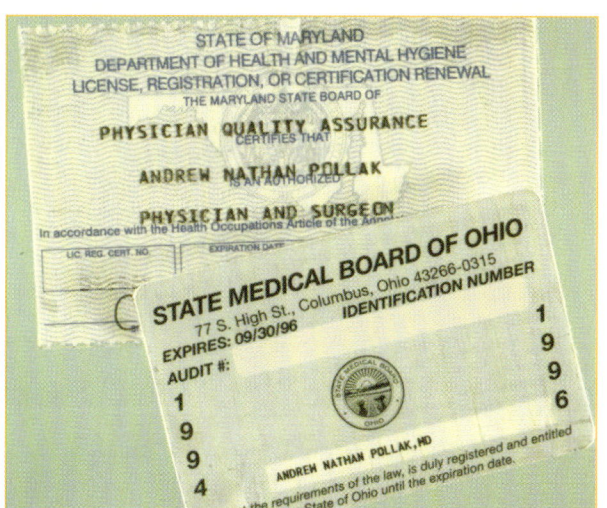

Figure 35-7 Many physicians carry a wallet-sized copy of their medical license.

is an area where individuals can be exposed to sharp metal edges, broken glass, toxic substances, lethal rays, or ignition or explosion of hazardous materials. You should help to set up and enforce this zone. If you arrive before the rescue group, you should coordinate crowd control with law enforcement officials.

Occasionally, a bystander may prove difficult to manage. This situation is especially challenging when the bystander claims to have medical credentials. Your EMS service should have a protocol for dealing with this situation. Many states provide physicians with wallet-sized copies of their medical license to use as identification Figure 35-7 ▲. However, not all physicians have training in emergency medical care. If this situation occurs, inform medical control immediately. Communication between medical control and the physician at the scene may eliminate some of the problems. You may also assign such individuals duties that will allow them to become involved in a small way. This will reduce the risk of a possible confrontation.

You are the Provider Part 2

The power company has shut off the power and has removed the power lines from the car. As the rescue team prepares for extrication, your partner enters the back of the vehicle through a broken window and manually controls the driver's cervical spine.

3. What information will be important to the continuing scene size-up?

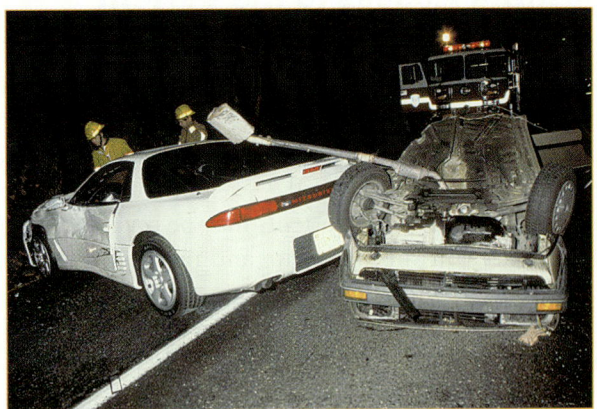

Figure 35-8 The exact way to gain access depends on many factors, including the terrain, the way in which the vehicle is situated, and the weather.

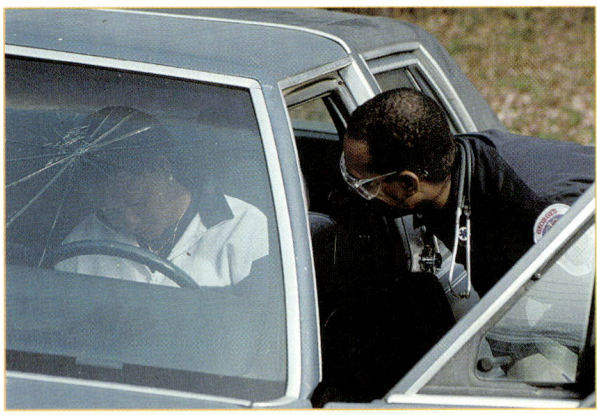

Figure 35-9 Get to the patient as quickly and simply as possible by opening the door without using tools or breaking any glass.

of a vehicle. In these instances, you and your team may have to use the rapid extrication technique to move a patient from a sitting position inside a vehicle to a supine position on a long backboard. A team of EMT-Is who are experienced in using this technique should be able to rapidly remove a patient who is not entrapped, keeping in mind the patient's condition and the group's safety. Use the rapid extrication technique only as a last resort.

Simple Access

Your first step is <u>simple access</u>, trying to get to the patient as quickly and simply as possible without using any tools or breaking any glass. Automobiles are built for easy entry and exit; however, it may be necessary to use tools or other forcible entry methods. Whenever possible, you should first try to unlock the doors (or ask the patient to unlock them) or roll down the windows. Try to open every door using the door handles to gain access before breaking any windows or using other methods of forced entry (Figure 35-9 ▶). Enter through the doors when there is no danger to the patient. The rescue group should provide the entrance you need to gain access to the patient.

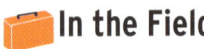

In the Field

Remember: Try before you pry!

Complex Access

<u>Complex access</u> requires the use of special tools and special training and includes breaking windows or other forcible entry. Most of these skills are too advanced for the EMT-I course and are not covered in this text. Extrication courses may be taken separately.

Patient Care During Entrapment and Extrication

Providing medical care to a patient who is trapped in a vehicle is principally the same as that for any other patient. Unless there is an immediate threat of fire, explosion, or other danger, once entrance and access to the patient have been provided, you should perform an initial assessment and provide care before further extrication begins, as follows:

1. Provide manual stabilization to protect the cervical spine, as needed.
2. Open the airway.
3. Provide high-flow oxygen.
4. Assist or provide for adequate ventilation.
5. Control any significant external bleeding.
6. Treat all critical injuries.

Preparation for Removal

As a part of your assessment, you should participate in the preparation for removal. Determine how urgently the patient must be extricated, where you should be positioned to best protect the patient during extrication, and, once the patient has been freed, how you will best move the patient from within the vehicle onto the long backboard and onto the stretcher. Carefully examine the exposed area of the limb or other part of the patient that is trapped to determine the extent of injury and whether there is a possibility of hidden bleeding. If possible, you should also evaluate sensation in the trapped area so that you will know whether increased pain indicates that an object is pressing on or impaled in the patient during extrication.

During this time, the rescue group is assessing exactly how the patient is trapped and determining the safest, easiest way to extricate him or her. Your input is essential so that the patient's injuries are considered as the rescue group plans a move that protects the patient from further harm. Once the plan has been devised and everyone understands what will be done, you should determine how best to protect the patient. Often, you or another EMT-I will be placed in the vehicle alongside the patient to monitor his or her condition and well-being as the vehicle is being forcibly cut, bent, or disassembled. Be sure to wear proper protective clothing.

Naturally, your safety and that of the patient are paramount during this process. Both you and the patient should be covered by a thick, fire-resistant canvas or blanket for protection from broken glass, flying particles, tools, or other hazards during any cutting or forceful extrication maneuvers. Extrication is often extremely noisy. You must be sure that you can communicate effectively with both the patient and the rescue group so that you can instantly let the rescuers know if it is necessary that they stop.

Once the patient has been freed, rapidly assess any previously inaccessible body parts, and reassess the patient. Make sure that the spine is manually immobilized, and apply a cervical collar if this was not previously done. Reevaluate whether the patient needs to be immediately removed by using manual immobilization and the rapid extrication technique, or whether the patient's condition and the scene allow for immobilization using an extrication vest or short backboard before he or she is moved further. In most cases, it is impractical and difficult to properly apply extremity splints within the vehicle. Extremity injuries can generally be rapidly supported and immobilized while the patient is being removed by securing an injured arm to the body and, if a leg is injured, securing one leg to the other. This will be adequate until the patient is secured to the backboard or time allows for more detailed assessment and splinting of each injury.

Removal

Moving the patient in one fast, continuous step increases the risk of harm and confusion. To ensure that each EMT-I can be positioned so that he or she can lift and carry properly at all times, move the patient in a series of smooth, slow, controlled steps, with stops designed between them to allow for the repositioning and adjustments that are needed. Plan the exact steps and pathway that you will follow in moving the patient from sitting in the vehicle to lying supine on the backboard and prepared ambulance cot. Choose a path that requires the least manipulation of the patient or equipment. Make sure that sufficient personnel are available. Once you are sure that everyone understands the steps and is ready, you can move the patient safely. Make sure that you move the patient as a unit, resisting the temptation to move the immobilization device instead. While moving the patient, continue to protect him or her from any hazards.

Once the patient has been placed on the stretcher, continue with any additional assessment and treatment that was deferred. If it is extremely cold or hot, raining or snowing, you should load the stretcher and patient into the climate-controlled ambulance before continuing assessment and treatment. If the patient's condition requires that transport be initiated without further delay, you should provide only the additional care that is essential or necessary to package the patient. Leave the remaining steps to be performed while you are en route to the hospital.

EMT-I Safety

A vehicle crash scene can present many of the hazards to rescuer and patient safety that you will encounter in emergency responses: fuel spills that pose fire and explosion risks, downed electrical lines, broken glass and torn metal, and exposure to potentially infectious body fluids. Your safety at every type of emergency scene begins with, and depends on, an initial scene size-up that leads to decisions about what kind of personal protective equipment to use and whether to call for additional or specialized assistance.

Specialized Rescue Situations

On most calls, you can drive the ambulance to within a short distance of the patient's location and, with either simple or complex access, you can reach and treat the patient. However, in some situations, the patient can be reached only by teams that are trained in making special technical rescues. Specialized skills of these teams include the following:

- Technical rope rescue (low- and high-angle rescue)

- Mountain, rock, and ice-climbing rescue
- Cross-field and trail rescue (park rangers)
- Water and small craft rescue
- White-water rescue
- Dive rescue (SCUBA)
- Cave rescue
- Mine rescue
- Confined space rescue
- Ski slope and cross-country or trail snow rescue (ski patrol)
- Search and rescue (SAR)
- Tactical response and rescue

The EMT-I and Technical Rescue Situations

Technical rescue situations may contain hidden dangers, and special technical skills are needed for personnel to safely enter and move around. It is not safe to include any personnel who do not have the necessary special training and experience in such a rescue. A technical rescue group is made up of individuals from one or more departments in a region who are trained and on call for certain types of technical rescue. Many members of a technical rescue group are also trained as first responders, EMT-Bs, or EMT-Is so that they can provide the necessary immediate care when they can safely reach the patient. Even when the technical rescue group includes a paramedic or physician, generally nothing but essential simple care is provided until the rescuers can bring the patient to the nearest point where a safe, stable setting exists.

If a technical rescue group is necessary but is not present when you arrive, you should immediately check with the incident commander to make sure that the group has been summoned and is en route to your location. The incident commander is the individual who has overall command of the scene in the field **Figure 35-10**. If no incident commander is present, follow local guidelines. (Chapter 36 discusses Incident Command in more detail.)

When you arrive at a scene where a technical rescue is already in progress, you will usually be met by a member of the rescue group and directed or led to the actual rescue site. If the rescue scene is some distance from the road, you may need to leave the ambulance on the road. The use of the ambulance stretcher is impractical in these situations; you should instead bring a long backboard and/or basket stretcher or similar rescue stretcher to carry the patient back to the waiting ambulance. Be sure that you take all of the carry-in kits and other equipment you may need to treat and immobilize the patient at the actual rescue operation site.

When you arrive at the rescue operation site, identify the stable location to which the rescue group will bring the patient, and set up your equipment there. As soon as the rescue group has brought the patient to this staging area, you should perform a rapid assessment and, after providing the treatment indicated, package the patient without delay. Although you and the other EMT-Is who responded with the ambulance will assume the primary responsibility for the patient's care at this

---

You are the Provider   Part 3

You determine that the driver is pinned in the car by the dashboard. He is unconscious, in obvious respiratory distress, and has a large bleeding laceration to his forehead. As your partner maintains manual cervical spine stabilization, you quickly perform an initial assessment.

Initial Assessment	Recording Time: 1 Minute After Patient Contact
Appearance	Unconscious, obvious respiratory distress
Level of consciousness	Unconscious and unresponsive
Airway	Open and clear
Breathing	Slow and shallow
Circulation	Radial pulse, rapid and weak; skin, cool and moist; bleeding from the forehead

4. How will you manage this patient until he can be freed from the wreckage?
5. How can your partner and the patient be protected during the extrication process?
6. What technique should you use to remove this patient from the vehicle?

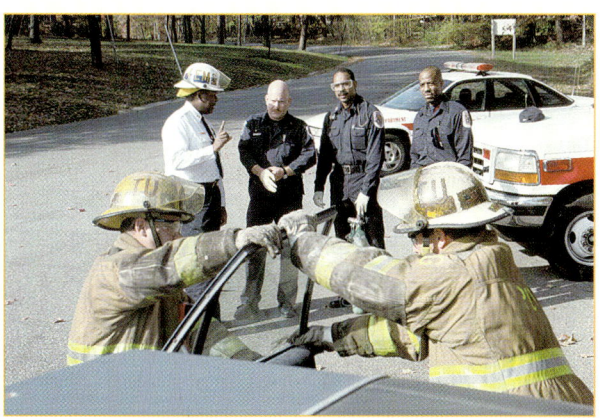

Figure 35-10 The incident commander is the individual who has overall command of the scene.

point, it usually requires a cooperative effort by both the rescue group and EMS personnel to carry the patient to the waiting ambulance. Consider using air medical transport if the patient will need to be carried and/or transported an extensive distance.

Search and Rescue

When someone is lost in the outdoors and a search effort is initiated, an ambulance is usually summoned to the search base. Each search team will be organized to include a member who is trained at either the first responder, EMT-B, or EMT-I level, carrying the essential equipment to provide simple immediate care. Your role, and that of the other EMT-Is who arrived with the ambulance, is to stand by at the search base until the lost person or people have been found.

As soon as you arrive at the scene and have been briefed on the situation, you should isolate and prepare the equipment you will need to carry in to the patient's location so that no time is lost once the patient has been found or if a member of the search team becomes injured. The prepared carry-in equipment, including a long backboard and other equipment you will need to immobilize the patient, should be left in the back of the ambulance so that it is protected from the weather. In addition, if the ambulance should need to be relocated, the equipment will not need to be reloaded or possibly be left behind. You will usually be given a portable radio that is tuned to the search frequency so that you can monitor the progress of the search and communicate with and be contacted by those in charge of the search operation.

Sometimes, you may be asked to stay with relatives of the lost individual who are at the scene. Find out from relatives whether the lost person has any medical history that may need to be addressed, and pass this information on to those who are in charge of the search. Unless you have been instructed otherwise, only incident command should communicate any news or progress of the search to the family. For this reason, you must be sure that your radio is set at a discreet volume.

Once the lost person has been found, you will be guided by search personnel to that location or a pre-arranged intersecting point where the patient will be carried to decrease the amount of time you need to reach the patient and begin treatment. You should be sure that the carry-in equipment is evenly distributed among personnel and that the pace is such that all can stay together easily. Sometimes, the time and effort that are needed to reach and carry out the patient can be decreased by relocating the ambulance or, if available, by using a four-wheel drive or all-terrain vehicle. As with other technical rescues, although the ambulance crew will assume the responsibility for patient care once they are at the patient's side, a cooperative effort of both EMS and the search team is necessary to safely carry the patient to the base and waiting ambulance.

Tactical Situations

If you are called to a scene where a <u>tactical situation</u> is taking place, such as an armed hostage situation, presence of a sniper, or exchange of shots, and the threat of violence remains, you should turn off the lights and sirens as you come close to the scene. In such situations, you should request direction from the incident commander or another appropriate authority in control of the scene. When you arrive at the outer perimeter barrier line that the police have established, you should ask a police officer to notify the incident commander of your arrival and for an officer to guide you to the shielded, safe staging area that has been selected for the ambulance and for care of the wounded and injured.

For your safety, you should exit the ambulance, stay low, and remain near the side of the vehicle unless you are directed to another place of safety. Do not turn on the vehicle's outside speakers, and turn down the volume of any radios that you are carrying. No matter how tempting it is to look, be sure that you do not look around the corner of any building or around the sides or over the top of any structure that may be serving to shield you. If it is dark outside, turn off the headlights and all clearance lights, and do not display any other light that might be reflected and serve to highlight your general location.

As in other technical rescue situations, your role, and that of the other EMT-Is, is to stand by at the staging area and treat and package injured patients after the SWAT team or other law enforcement officers have evacuated them to your shielded, safe location. When you are ready to transport a patient, you should ask a law enforcement officer to notify the incident commander. You should leave only after the incident commander has verified that it is safe for the ambulance to move. Be sure that you follow the specific route that is indicated by the incident commander or a law enforcement officer assigned to guide you. You should proceed slowly for a good distance from the incident perimeter before using your emergency lights and siren.

Structure Fires

In most areas, an ambulance is dispatched with the fire department apparatus to any structure fire, whether or not any injuries are reported. A fire in a house, apartment building, office, school, plant, warehouse, or other building is considered a <u>structure fire</u>. When responding to a major fire scene, you should determine whether, because of the fire, any special route will be necessary. Once you arrive at the scene, you should ask the incident commander where the ambulance should be parked.

> ### EMT-I Safety
>
> Physical dangers such as fire, infectious disease, and electricity are not the only risks to your safety on emergency responses. Some calls involve the possibility of deliberate violence against rescuers. Formal tactical situations are the obvious examples, but "simple" calls involving assaults, possible alcohol or drug use, and domestic disputes can be just as dangerous. Your training, your attitude when responding to calls, and your routine daily procedures should all take these risks into account.

It is essential that the ambulance be parked far enough away from the fire to be safe from the fire itself or a collapsing building. You must also ensure that the ambulance will not block or hinder other arriving equipment or become blocked in by other equipment or hose lines. However, you must also make sure that the ambulance will be close enough to be visible and that patients can be brought to it easily. The fire officer who is the incident commander will decide where this location should be.

Your next step is to determine whether there are any injured patients at the scene or whether you have been called to stand by. A number of ambulances may be dispatched to a major fire to ensure that one or more units will always remain immediately available at the scene if others leave to transport the injured.

As with other technical rescue situations, search and rescue in a burning building requires special training and equipment. Search and rescue is performed by teams of fire fighters wearing full turnout gear and self-contained breathing apparatus (SCBA), and carrying tools and fully charged hose lines. These teams will bring patients out of the burning building to the area where the ambulance is standing by. Therefore, unless otherwise ordered, you should always stay with the ambulance. Do not wander off even after the fire is basically out, in case a fire fighter becomes injured during salvage and overhaul. The ambulance should leave the scene only if transporting a patient or if the incident commander has released it.

Sometimes, the scene at a crash or fire is further complicated by the presence of hazardous materials. A <u>hazardous material</u> is any substance that is toxic, poisonous, radioactive, flammable, or explosive and can cause injury or death with exposure. In addition to posing a threat to you and others at the immediate scene, hazardous materials may pose a threat to a much larger area and population. Whenever there is a possibility that a hazardous material is involved, you will have to follow a number of additional special procedures. (Chapter 36 covers the specifics of hazardous material procedures.)

You are the Provider — Summary

1. What functions does the EMS team perform at the scene of an incident?

First and foremost, the safety and well-being of all EMS personnel must be ensured. Then, the next priority is to gain access to the patient in order to assess him or her and provide immediate life-saving treatment. As with the patient in this incident, initial assessment and management may have to occur simultaneously with extrication operations.

2. What is the connection between good communication, an accurate scene size-up, and the overall safety of the operation?

Good communication is absolutely essential to any multi-tiered rescue operation. Communication ensures team coordination and facilitates independent actions toward a common goal. An accurate scene size-up (and communication of the scene size-up) ensures that hazards are identified and addressed and that each team begins the rescue operation with a clear understanding of the "big picture."

3. What information will be important to the continuing scene size-up?

Recall that the scene size-up is an ongoing process for all who are involved in the rescue operation; it is the responsibility of each team member. A previously safe scene can become hazardous with alarming unpredictability. Remain aware of the environment in which you are functioning and be alert for the development of new hazards (ie, fire, gas leakage, etc).

4. How will you manage this patient until he can be freed from the wreckage?

Your partner is already providing manual cervical spine stabilization. Additionally, this patient will need ventilatory support because of his slow, shallow breathing; however, this may not be possible due to his position in the vehicle. Administer 100% supplemental oxygen until he is freed. You must also control the bleeding from the laceration to his forehead.

5. How can your partner and the patient be protected during the extrication process?

Your partner should be wearing heavy protective gloves over his rubber gloves. Additionally, he should be wearing a protective helmet and faceshield to protect him from flying debris. Both your partner and the patient should be covered with a heavy blanket to protect them from flying metal, glass, or other debris.

6. What technique should you use to remove this patient from the vehicle?

Once the patient has been freed from the wreckage, he should be removed with the rapid extrication technique. His critical condition clearly negates the use of a short extrication device, which is time-consuming to apply.

Prep Kit

Ready For Review

- During all phases of rescue, your primary concern is safety, and your primary role is to provide emergency medical care and prevent further injury to the patient.
- When there are not enough personnel for both an EMS team and a rescue team, you and your team may have to act as rescuers as well.
- Safety during rescue or extrication begins with the proper mind-set and the proper protective equipment.
- During scene size-up, you should identify the safest, most efficient way to access the patient. Try to get to the patient as simply and quickly as possible without using any tools or breaking any glass. Make sure that you and the patient are protected with a fireproof blanket.
- Unless there is immediate danger, perform an initial assessment of a patient while he or she is still in the vehicle. Immobilize the cervical spine before moving the patient from the vehicle.
- If a special rescue team is needed, inform the dispatcher.
- When a scene calls for a search or for specialized rescue, you may have to call for a technical rescue group, or you may find one already at work when you arrive. Your interaction and cooperation with this group, and with an incident commander when one has been designated, are important to a smooth rescue.
- You will be involved to some degree in the logistics of vehicle staging and patient movement, as well as patient care.
- Tactical situations are best directly handled by teams with specialized training. Your role will often largely consist of remaining out of danger, cooperating with the incident commander, or with police or other specialized personnel if incident command is not in effect, and remaining ready to care for any patients that are brought to you.

Technology

- Interactivities
- Vocabulary Explorer
- Anatomy Review
- Web Links
- Online Review Manual

Vital Vocabulary

access The ability to gain entry to an enclosed area and reach a patient.

complex access Complicated entry that requires special tools and training and includes breaking windows or using other force.

danger zone (hot zone) An area where individuals can be exposed to sharp metal edges, broken glass, toxic substances, lethal rays, or ignition or explosion of hazardous materials.

entrapment To be caught (trapped) within a vehicle, room, or other confined space with no way out, or to have a limb or other body part trapped.

extrication Removal of a patient from entrapment or a dangerous situation or position, such as removal from a wrecked vehicle, industrial accident, or building collapse.

hazardous material Any substance that is toxic, poisonous, radioactive, flammable, or explosive and causes injury or death with exposure.

incident commander The individual who has overall command of the scene in the field.

simple access Access that is easily achieved without the use of tools or force.

structure fire A fire in a house, apartment building, office, school, plant, warehouse, or other building.

tactical situation A hostage, robbery, or other situation in which armed conflict is threatened or shots have been fired and the threat of violence remains.

technical rescue situation A rescue that requires special technical skills and equipment in one of many specialized rescue areas, such as technical rope rescue, cave rescue, and dive rescue.

technical rescue group A team of individuals from one or more departments in a region that is trained and on call for certain types of technical rescue.

Assessment in Action

You are dispatched to a motor vehicle crash. On arrival you find a midsize car wedged under a fuel tanker and a church van overturned in a ditch.

Gasoline is leaking from the tanker, approximately 5' from the car, and flowing into the ditch. The occupant of the car is trapped. The status of the occupants of the van is unknown.

1. The group responsible for gaining access to the patient is:
   A. law enforcement personnel.
   B. fire fighters.
   C. EMS personnel.
   D. rescue personnel.

2. Your initial safety considerations will include:
   A. ensuring stability of the vehicle.
   B. removing bystanders from the danger zone.
   C. flushing the gasoline from the area.
   D. covering the occupant of the car with a blanket.

3. Before beginning treatment of the occupant of the car, you should do all of the following EXCEPT:
   A. locate and triage the patients.
   B. render the scene safe.
   C. free the patient from the car.
   D. request additional assistance if needed.

The fire department has plugged the leaking tanker and you have learned that the only occupant of the van is free from the vehicle and being treated by another ambulance crew. You can turn your attention to your only patient—the driver of the car.

4. When assessing the occupant of the car you should:
   A. assess the patient's protection needs prior to extrication.
   B. wait until the victim is free before assessing the patient.
   C. assess only the entrapped areas prior to extrication.
   D. assess only the areas of complaint prior to extrication.

5. Communication during this call will include all of the following EXCEPT:
   A. informing the patient about what is happening around them.
   B. informing the rescue team about the patient's condition.
   C. informing your partner about the patient's condition.
   D. informing the patient about his or her condition.

6. Care you will provide during extrication from the car will include all of the following EXCEPT:
   A. high-flow oxygen unless absolutely necessary.
   B. spinal immobilization.
   C. covering the patient with a nonflammable blanket.
   D. monitoring the patient's condition.

7. During the extrication process, you should occasionally reassess all of the following EXCEPT:
   A. changes in scene safety.
   B. changes in the patient's condition.
   C. the patient's response to treatment.
   D. the need for spinal immobilization.

8. Guidelines you will follow when removing the patient from the car include:
   A. splint fractures before movement.
   B. use one fast, continuous motion.
   C. use several slow, coordinated movements.
   D. avoid the use of a backboard.

Points to Ponder

You have arrived on the scene of a motor vehicle crash. The fire department is on the scene as well. A pick-up truck has struck a semitractor-trailer from behind. You note heavy front-end damage to the vehicle and the lone occupant is entrapped. During the extrication process, you are in the vehicle with the patient maintaining spinal immobilization. As the rescue team is gaining access to the patient, a window is broken and shattered glass strikes you and your patient. The patient receives cuts and you sustain eye injuries.

What went wrong? How could you have prevented these injuries?

Issue: Protecting Yourself From Dangers at Motor Vehicle Crash Scenes

Special Operations

1999 Objectives

There are no 1999 objectives for this chapter.

1985 Objectives

S1.6.66 Demonstrate the use of self-protection equipment such as air pack (breathing apparatus), etc. (p 1470-1471)

Additional Objectives*

Cognitive

1. Explain the EMT-I's role during a call involving hazardous materials. (p 1465)
2. Describe what the EMT-I should do if there is reason to believe that there is a hazard at the scene. (p 1465)
3. Describe the actions that an EMT-I should take to ensure bystander safety. (p 1468)
4. State the role the EMT-I should perform until appropriately trained personnel arrive at the scene of a hazardous materials situation. (p 1468)
5. Break down the steps to approaching a hazardous situation. (p 1465)
6. Discuss the various environmental hazards that affect EMS. (p 1464)
7. Describe the criteria for a multiple-casualty situation. (p 1473)
8. Evaluate the role of the EMT-I in the multiple-casualty situation. (p 1473)
9. Summarize the components of basic triage. (p 1473)
10. Define the role of the EMT-I in a disaster operation. (p 1477)
11. Describe basic concepts of incident management. (p 1462)
12. Explain the methods for preventing contamination of self, equipment, and facilities. (p 1470)

Affective

13. Discuss the psychological impact of wanting to act but recognizing that a scene is not safe to enter. (p 1465)

Psychomotor

14. Given a scenario of a mass-casualty incident, perform triage. (p 1473, 1476)

*These are noncurriculum objectives.

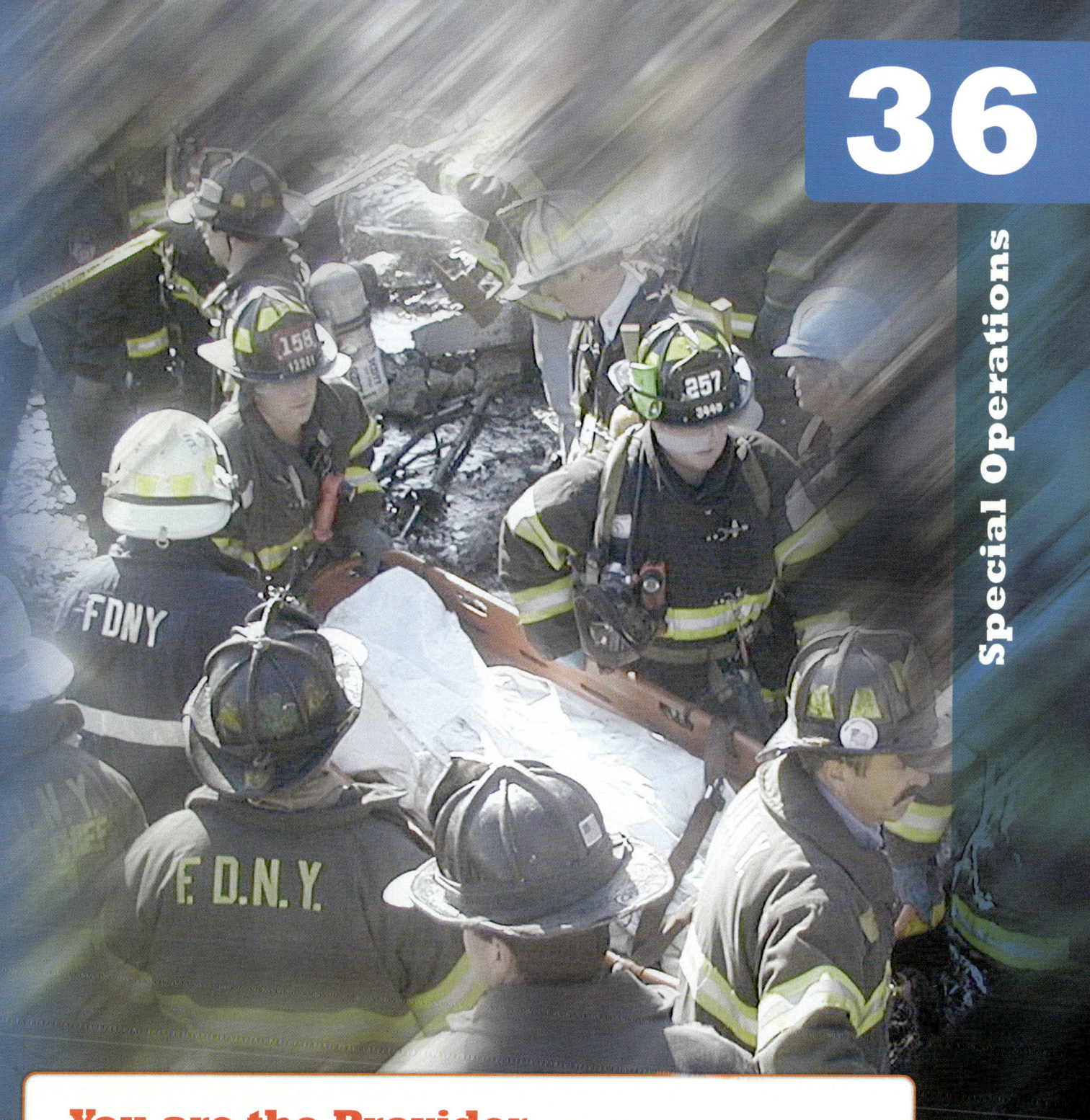

36

Special Operations

You are the Provider

Your rescue squad has been dispatched to a local manufacturing plant. Dispatch advises you that the caller stated that "a couple of employees have passed out and many more are complaining of dizziness and nausea." This chapter will help you to deal with those special operations situations encountered by the EMT-I, in addition to answering the following questions.

1. What is the incident command system (ICS)?
2. Why is the ICS helpful to all emergency responders?

Special Operations

The first section of this chapter will introduce you to incident command systems. The purpose of this section is to give you an idea of what happens during complex incidents. The role of the EMT-I within the system is explained.

The next section describes your responsibilities at a hazardous materials incident. When you are responding to this type of incident, you cannot rush in to provide patient care. Rather, you must cooperate with the incident command system, taking time to accurately assess the scene by identifying the size of the hazard area, finding a safe location to which patients can be removed, and taking self-protective measures. Safety is your primary consideration. If a hazardous materials incident is not carefully handled, many people, including rescue personnel, can become patients or casualties.

The final section describes the several roles of the EMT-I at mass-casualty incidents. Again under the incident command system, EMS personnel will have one of several roles identified to manage a large number of patients at a single event. The usual EMS response of triaging three or four patients will be difficult when there are 25 or more casualties. To ensure that every patient receives appropriate care and transportation to a hospital consistent with the severity of his or her condition, a more organized operation is required with three major responsibilities assigned: triage, treatment, and transportation.

Technology

www.EMSzone.com/EMTI

- Interactivities
- Vocabulary Explorer
- Anatomy Review
- Web Links
- Online Review Manual

Incident Command Systems

In recent years, a number of leadership and command systems have been developed to improve the on-scene management of emergency situations. The fire service has taken the lead in developing these programs to help control, direct, and coordinate emergency responders and resources. These programs are called incident command systems. They have been adapted and used by many EMS organizations to better organize their own operations. The incident command system is designed for use in daily operations. However, it is most effective when used to organize large numbers of personnel at complex incidents such as hazardous materials spills and mass-casualty incidents.

Components and Structure of an Incident Command System

At a large fire, a hazardous materials incident, or a mass-casualty incident, fire, rescue, HazMat, police, and EMS units from many different areas usually will become involved in some way. To ensure clear lines of responsibility and authority, a preestablished system is needed to identify who is in charge of different activities and who reports to whom. Even on a call with only one patient and no need for any other services, the implementation of an incident command system is helpful to identify the roles and responsibilities of each crew member, particularly if the event begins to escalate.

The incident command system is structured such that there is a single authority with overall responsibility to manage the incident. This person is identified as the incident commander. The incident commander usually remains at a command post, the designated field command center. A field command center is typically a vehicle or building at the scene where the incident commander establishes an "office." From here, the commander oversees and coordinates the activities of the various groups and leaders.

Functions normally centered at the command post include information, safety, and liaison with other agencies and groups who are responding. In a typical incident command system operation, all information to the public and the news media originates at the command post. The incident commander will usually appoint a safety officer who will circulate among responding personnel. It is essential that every EMT-I understand that any order or directive issued by a safety officer has the full authority of the incident commander and must be immediately followed. Many times EMT-Is cannot see a hazard or problem they are walking into, and the safety officer is responsible for protecting all personnel and any victims of the incident. Finally, an officer may be named by the incident commander to coordinate incoming fire, police, and EMS units.

In the initial response, the incident commander may assume direct control over the groups and task forces being set up. In this circumstance, a medical group supervisor may be named to coordinate all EMS activity, or a rescue group supervisor may be appointed to deal with people entrapped in the wreckage. In extended operations that may go on for hours, days, or longer, the typical incident command structure may have multiple sectors including operations, planning, logistics, and finance. Figure 36-1 shows a sample incident command system organization chart that includes these sectors. Each of these sections will have a single officer acting as the person in charge, the sector commander. Not all positions are used at every incident. The incident commander will select the individual positions and teams, and will choose which to use depending on the nature of the incident.

Major incidents often require another level of management, known as unified command. With unified command, the incident commander is joined at the command post by one officer who is in charge of all fire operations, one who is in charge of all rescue or HazMat operations, one who is in charge of all EMS operations, and one who is in charge of all law enforcement. This group, under the direction of the incident commander, directs the overall operations at the scene. Because the different public safety officers are stationed at the command post, they can be easily found and can collectively advise the incident commander of changes and problems that are communicated to them. The incident commander can also involve them in making the necessary decisions and in rapidly conveying orders to those under their command. In addition to unified command, this system ensures that the actions of each different type of responder are properly coordinated.

How these systems work together depends on the nature of the event. For example, with a major airplane crash, the leading agency is typically the fire department. In this situation, EMS is usually one aspect of the overall fire incident command system. Within their own system, EMS personnel establish and carry out their tasks. However, ultimate control of the incident will rest with the fire commander. Other situations, such as widespread injuries at a rock concert, are primarily civil events. Law enforcement would take the lead, establishing an incident command plan. Fire and EMS would follow the law enforcement commander's decision. EMS is seldom the lead agency.

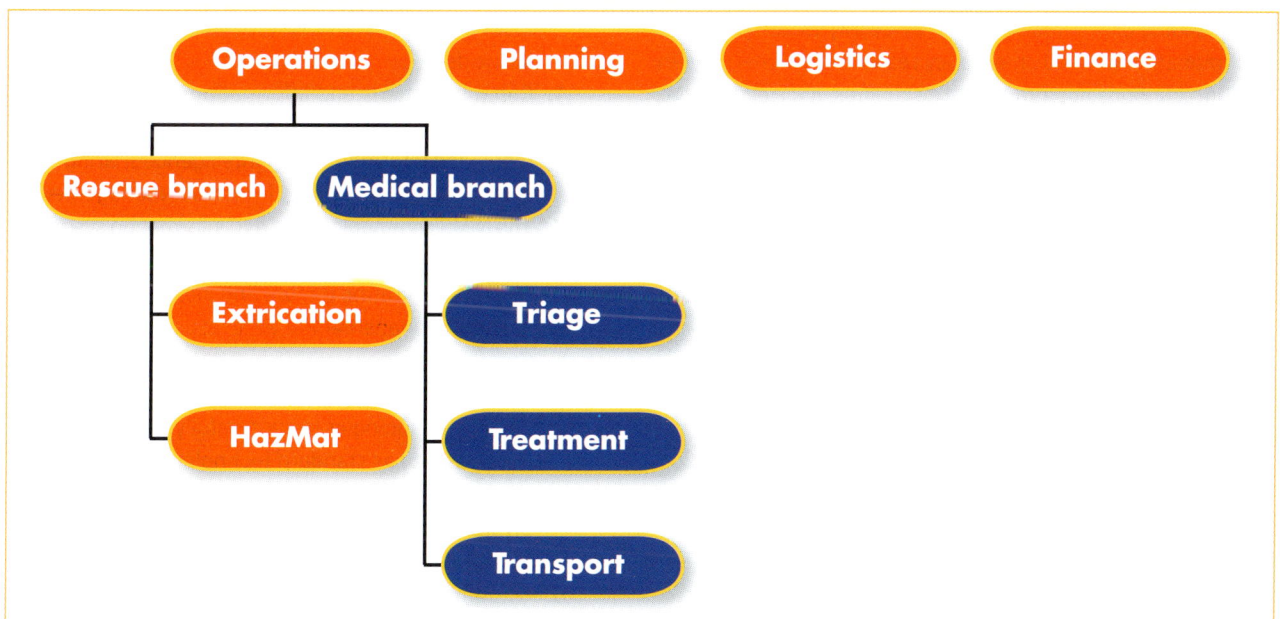

Figure 36-1 Incident command structure. Not all positions will be filled in every incident. However, the incident commander is responsible for all activity until subordinates are appointed to assist in managing the incident.

© National Wildlife Coordinating Group

EMT-I Tips

National Incident Management System

In 2003, President Bush directed the Secretary of Homeland Security to develop and administer a National Incident Management System (NIMS). This system provides a consistent nationwide template to enable federal, state, and local governments and private-sector and nongovernmental organizations to work together effectively and efficiently to prepare for, prevent, respond to, and recover from domestic incidents, regardless of cause, size, or complexity, including acts of catastrophic terrorism.

Since the September 11, 2001 attacks, much has been done to improve prevention, preparedness, response, recovery, and mitigation capabilities and coordination processes across the country. A comprehensive national approach to incident management, applicable at all jurisdictional levels and across functional disciplines would further improve the effectiveness of emergency response providers and incident management organizations across a full spectrum of potential incidents and hazard scenarios. Such an approach would also improve coordination and cooperation between public and private entities in a variety of domestic incident management activities. Incidents can include:

- Acts of terrorism
- Wildland and urban fires
- Floods
- Hazardous materials spills
- Nuclear accidents
- Aircraft accidents
- Earthquakes
- Hurricanes
- Tornadoes
- Typhoons
- War-related disasters

Building on the foundation provided by existing incident management and emergency response systems used by jurisdictions and functional disciplines at all levels, NIMS integrates the best practices that have proven effective over the years into a comprehensive framework for use by incident management organizations in an all-hazards context nationwide. To provide for interoperability and compatibility among federal, state, and local capabilities, the NIMS will include a core set of concepts, principles, terminology, and technologies covering:

- The incident command system
- Multiagency coordination systems
- Unified command
- Training
- Identification and management of resources
- Qualifications and certification
- Collection, tracking, and reporting of incident information and incident resources

While most incidents are generally handled on a daily basis by a single jurisdiction at the local level, there are important instances in which successful domestic incident management operations depend on the involvement of multiple jurisdictions, functional agencies, and emergency responder disciplines. These instances require effective and efficient coordination across this broad spectrum of organizations and activities. The NIMS uses a systems approach to integrate the best of existing processes and methods into a unified national framework for incident management. The framework forms the basis for interoperability and compatibility that will, in turn, enable a diverse set of public and private organizations to conduct well-integrated and effective incident management operations.

The NIMS is comprised of several components that work together as a system to provide a national framework for preparing for, preventing, responding to, and recovering from domestic incidents. These components include:

1. Command and Management—The NIMS standardizes incident management for all hazards and across all levels of government. The NIMS standard incident command structures are based on three key constructs: incident command system; multiagency coordination systems; and public information systems.
2. Preparedness—The NIMS establishes specific measures and capabilities that jurisdictions and agencies should develop and incorporate into an overall system to enhance operational preparedness for incident management on a steady-state basis on an all-hazards context.
3. Resource Management—The NIMS defines standardized mechanisms to describe, inventory, track, and dispatch resources before, during, and after an incident; it also defines standard procedures to recover equipment once it is no longer needed for an incident.
4. Communications and Information Management—Effective communications, information management, and information and intelligence sharing are critical aspects of domestic incident management. The NIMS communications and information systems enable the essential functions needed to provide a common operating picture and interoperability for incident management at all levels.
5. Supporting Technologies—The NIMS promotes national standards and interoperability for supporting technologies to successfully implement the NIMS, as well as standard technologies for specific professional disciplines or incident types. It provides an architecture for science and technology support to incident management.
6. Ongoing Management and Maintenance—The Department of Homeland Security will establish a multijurisdictional, multidisciplinary NIMS Integration Center. This Center will provide strategic direction for, and oversight of, the NIMS, supporting both routine maintenance and continuous improvement of the system over the long term.

Protection Level. Protection levels indicate the amount and type of protective gear that you need to prevent injury from a particular substance. The four recognized protection levels, A, B, C, and D, are as follows (Figure 36-8 ▼):

- **Level A**, the most hazardous, requires fully encapsulated, chemical-resistant protective clothing that provides full body protection, as well as SCBA and special, sealed equipment.
- **Level B** requires nonencapsulated protective clothing, or clothing that is designed to protect against a particular hazard. Usually, this clothing is made of material that will let only limited amounts of moisture and vapor pass through (nonpermeable). Level B also requires breathing devices that contain their own air supply, such as SCBA, and eye protection.
- **Level C**, like Level B, requires the use of nonpermeable clothing and eye protection. In addition, face masks that filter all inhaled outside air must be used.
- **Level D** requires a work uniform, such as coveralls, that affords minimal protection.

All levels of protection require the use of gloves. Two pairs of rubber gloves are needed for protection in case one pair must be removed because of heavy contamination.

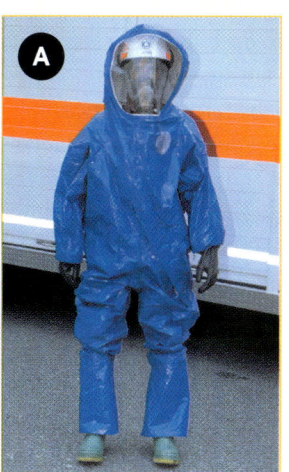 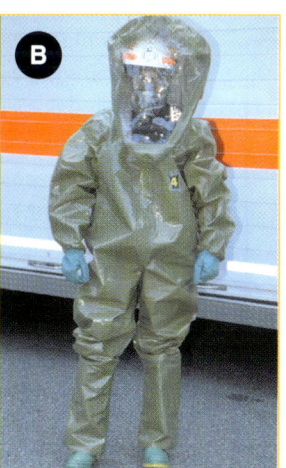 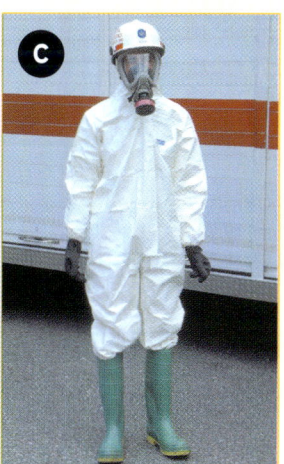 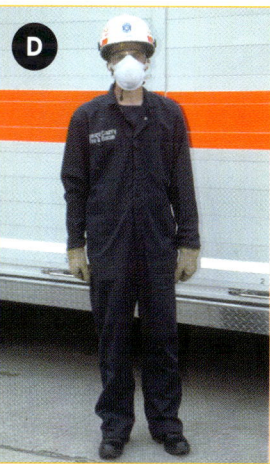

Figure 36-8 Four levels of protection. **A.** Level A protection. **B.** Level B protection. **C.** Level C protection. **D.** Level D protection. Most serious injuries and deaths from hazardous materials result from airway and breathing problems.

them again of the incomplete decontamination, obtains directions before the patient is unloaded and brought in. If there are enough ambulances at a hazardous materials scene, one may be isolated and used only to transport such patients. Remember, the ambulance needs to be decontaminated before transporting another patient.

Resources

Every ambulance, as well as the dispatch center, should have a copy of a current *Emergency Response Guidebook*, prepared by Transport Canada, the US Department of Transportation, and the Secretariat of Communications and Transportation of Mexico (Figure 36-9 ▶). This publication lists most hazardous materials. For each one, it describes the proper initial emergency action to control the scene and provide emergency medical care. Some state and local government agencies may also have information about hazardous materials that are commonly found in their areas. Be sure to keep these publications up to date and close at hand on the unit.

Another valuable resource is the Chemical Transportation Emergency Center (CHEMTREC), located in Washington, DC. CHEMTREC was established by the Chemical Manufacturers Association to assist emergency personnel in identifying and handling hazardous materials transport incidents. The center operates 24 hours a day, 7 days a week. Its toll-free number is 1-800-424-9300 from anywhere within the United States or Canada.

CHEMTREC provides information, warnings, and guidance for proper emergency management and treatment. However, it cannot identify an unknown substance. You must provide CHEMTREC with the correct DOT identification number, the chemical name, or the product name of the material.

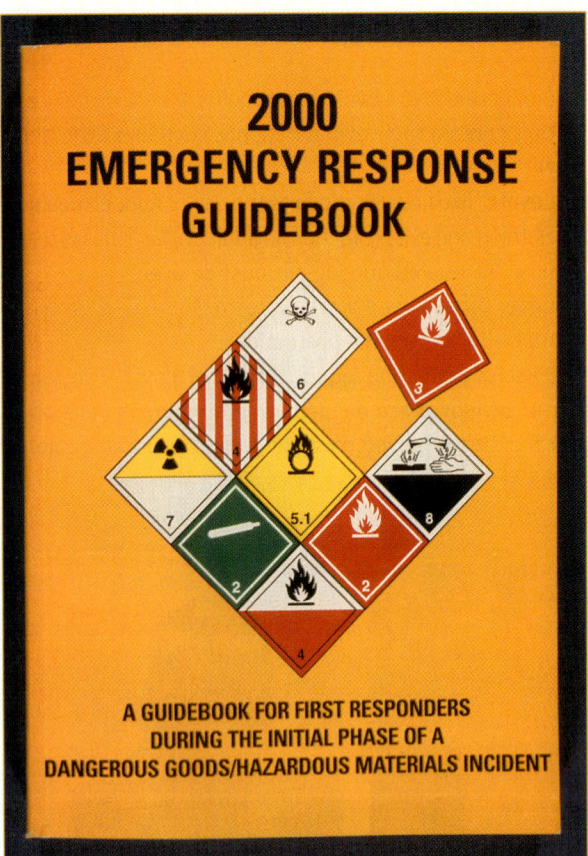

Figure 36-9 The *2000 Emergency Response Guidebook*.

If you are interested in learning more about hazardous materials incidents and rescue requirements, you can refer to the following:

- National Fire Protection Association (NFPA) standard #479
- OSHA standard #1910.120
- Federal Emergency Management Agency (FEMA) guidelines for coping with hazardous materials incidents
- EPA protective clothing

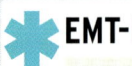

EMT-I Tips

The terminology used to describe an incident with multiple patients varies in different communities. Many communities use the term *multiple-casualty situation* to describe an emergency that involves more than one patient, but use the term *mass-casualty incident* to describe larger scale events, such as those with more than 20 patients. In this text, the term *mass-casualty incident* is used to describe any call that involves more than one patient or a situation that overwhelms your available resources.

You are the Provider — Part 3

Fire Department personnel on scene have removed ten victims to a triage area in a designated safe zone. You have been assigned to triage. As you assess your first patient, you notice the following:

Initial Assessment	Recording Time: Zero Minutes
Appearance	In respiratory distress
Level of consciousness	Responsive verbally
Airway	Open and clear
Breathing	Respiratory rate, rapid and shallow
Circulation	Skin, pale and diaphoretic; radial pulses, increased and regular

5. What is the color-coding priority system used when triaging patients in a mass-casualty incident?
6. What are the key components at a mass-casualty incident?

Mass-Casualty Incidents

In this text, a mass-casualty incident refers to any call that involves more than one patient, as well as any situation that places such a great demand on available equipment or personnel that the system is stretched to its limit or beyond. Airplane, bus, or railroad crashes, and earthquakes are obvious examples of mass-casualty incidents. However, other causes of these incidents are far more common than such disasters and are usually much smaller in scope.

Ask yourself the following questions:
- How many seriously injured patients can you care for effectively and transport in your ambulance? One? Two?
- What happens when you have three patients to deal with?
- What do you do when two cars crash head-on, resulting in eight critically injured patients, and you only have three ambulances available?

Obviously, you and your team cannot treat and transport all injured patients at the same time. At a mass-casualty incident, you will often experience a demand for equipment and personnel. For example, you may realize that there may be 15 or more minutes to wait before the next ambulance will arrive. Should you stay at the scene, placing the patients who are ready to go at some risk? Or should you leave with the patients who are loaded, leaving those at the scene without sufficient resources to manage all their needs?

If there are more patients at the scene than you can transport in your ambulance, call for back up ambulances and other mutual aid resources to assist Figure 36-10. While this may cause some delay in initiating treatment to all patients, this will not adversely affect patient care if the EMS resources on scene begin to work with the most severely injured first. Always follow local protocol.

Triage

Triage is essential at all mass-casualty incidents. Triage is the sorting of two or more patients based on the severity of their conditions to establish priorities for care based on available resources Figure 36-11.

In a smaller scale mass-casualty incident, the first provider on scene with the highest level of training usually begins the triage process. When back-up ambulances and crews are readily available, patients are ranked in order of severity. The patient with the most severe injuries is given priority attention. After counting the number of patients and notifying the dispatcher of addi-

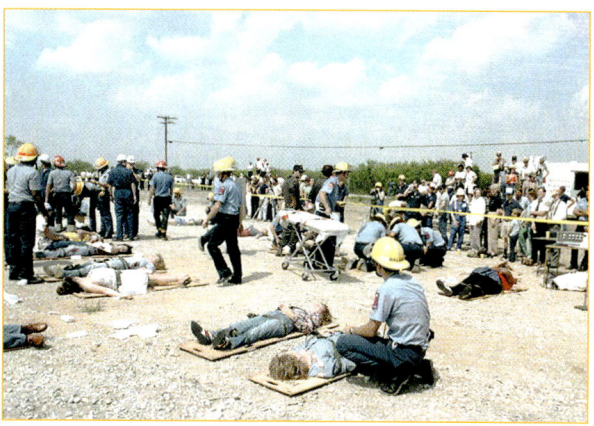

Figure 36-10 Mass-casualty incidents require additional ambulances and EMS providers from the immediate region.

tional help that is needed, initial assessment of all patients begins. As personnel arrive, the EMT-I should assign crews and equipment to priority patients first.

Triage at a large-scale mass-casualty incident should be done in several steps. The following triage steps are accepted by the majority of larger scale mass-casualty operations:
- Life-saving care rapidly administered to those in need
- Color coding to indicate priority for treatment and transportation at the scene Table 36-2. Red-tagged patients are the first priority, yellow-tagged patients are the second priority, and those tagged green or black are the lowest priority.

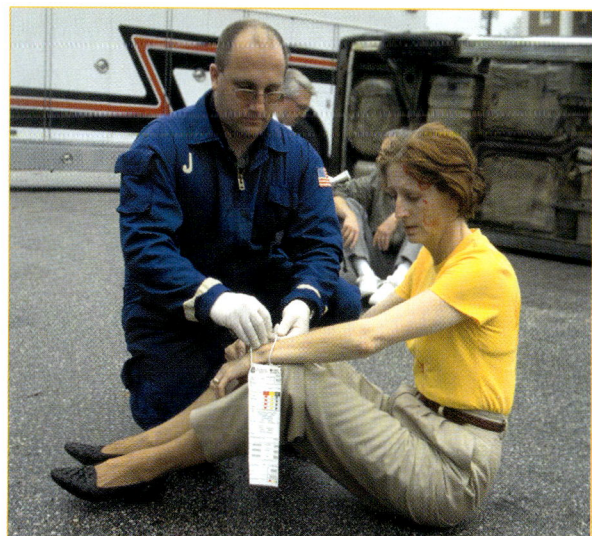

Figure 36-11 Triage is an essential component of operations at a mass-casualty incident.

TABLE 36-2	Triage Priorities
Triage Category	**Typical Injuries**
First Priority (Red) Patients who need immediate care and transport. Treat these patients first, and transport as soon as possible.	■ Airway and breathing difficulties. ■ Uncontrolled or severe bleeding ■ Decreased level of consciousness ■ Severe medical problems ■ Shock (hypoperfusion) ■ Severe burns
Second Priority (Yellow) Patients whose treatment and transportation can be temporarily delayed	■ Burns without airway problems ■ Major or multiple bone or joint injuries ■ Back injuries with or without spinal cord damage
Third Priority (Green) Patients whose treatment and transportation can be delayed until last	■ Minor fractures ■ Minor soft-tissue injuries
Fourth Priority (Black) Patients who are already dead or have little chance for survival. If resources are limited, treat salvageable patients before these patients.	■ Obvious death ■ Obviously nonsurvivable injury, such as major open brain trauma ■ Full cardiac arrest

- Rapid removal of red-tagged patients for field treatment and transportation as ambulances are available.
- Use of a separate treatment area to care for red-tagged patients if transport is not immediately available. Yellow-tagged patients can also be monitored and cared for in the treatment area while waiting for transportation.
- When there are more patients waiting for transport than there are ambulances, the Transportation Sector Officer decides which patient is the next to be loaded.
- Specialized transportation resources (air ambulance, paramedic ambulances, etc) require separate decisions when these resources are available but limited.

Triage Priorities

Patients should be color coded early to visually identify the severity of the condition and to eliminate the need for repeated patient assessments to be performed by each EMT-I who comes along later.

Patients who are tagged red should later be reassessed in the treatment area to determine who should receive limited resources such as paramedic assessment and care. The sorting of multiple red-tagged patients in the treatment area who need to be seen immediately by paramedics will depend on the number of paramedics available at that time. The order in which the patients will be transported is determined after the initial triage and treatment is completed.

If patients are entrapped, extrication is required. If circumstances such as heavy smoke or a potential hazardous materials exposure exist, triage will be difficult if not impossible. The immediate concern will be the removal of the patients to a safe area for triage to be done later. The triage area is the name usually given to such a collecting area for patients to be initially triaged and color coded. For patients located

> **Terminology Tips**
>
> *Disaster*—Any incident that overwhelms your resources.
> *Mass-casualty incident*—Any incident involving multiple patients.

in nonhazardous areas, this initial triage can begin right away.

Incident Command

To be effective, the various decision points for triage must be linked into the incident command system. The command structure must be established early and expanded as needed and as resources become available over time. Incident command systems may vary in different communities. When an EMT-I responds to another community as back up for a mass-casualty incident, he or she must follow the directions and orders given.

Table 36-3 shows the important components of an incident command system in a mass-casualty incident. As an example of how responsibilities may be assigned at a major EMS incident, consider the following typical assignments:

- **Command center.** This is typically a vehicle or building at the scene where the EMS commander establishes an "office." From here, the commander oversees and coordinates the activities of the various groups and leaders.
- **Staging area.** This is a holding area for arriving ambulances and crews until they can be assigned a particular task.
- **Extrication area.** This is where patients are disentangled and removed from a hazardous environment, allowing them to be moved to the triage area.
- **Triage area.** The triage area is a sorting point, run by a triage officer, where each patient is assessed and tagged, using color-coded tags or tape Figure 36-12, according to their injuries. These triaged patients are then directed to specific locations in the treatment area(s), according to their assigned priority.
- **Treatment area.** This is where a more thorough assessment is made and on-scene treatment is begun while transport is being arranged. The treatment area is organized and managed under the authority of the treatment officer. Patients are given care under the standards of the EMS system in the treatment area before being transported. This means that all fractures should be splinted, and all care normally rendered after a focused assessment should be accomplished before the patient is released for transportation.
- **Supply area.** This is an area in which to assemble extra equipment and supplies, such as blankets, oxygen cylinders, bandages, and backboards, for dispersal to other areas as needed.
- **Transportation area.** This is where ambulances and crews are organized to transport patients from the treatment sector to area hospitals. The transportation area is managed by the transportation officer, who will assign patients to waiting ambulances.
- **Rehabilitation area.** This area provides protection and treatment to firefighters and other personnel working at the emergency scene. As workers enter and leave the scene, they are medically monitored and provided any needed care. This helps to ensure the safety and health of emergency workers who could become injured or ill while on the job.

When you respond to a mass-casualty incident, you will be assigned to a specified area and its designated officer. Report at once to this officer for your assignment

TABLE 36-3 Key Components at a Mass-Casualty Incident

- Incident commander, command post, and incident command system
- On-site communications system
- Adequate supply of long backboards, straps, or ties
- Extrication/retrieval team
- Triage officer and designated triage area
- Staffed patient collection area
- Staffed patient treatment area
- Supply location adjacent to the treatment area
- Transportation officer and transport area
- Staging area to hold resources until they are needed
- Fire and law enforcement personnel
- A secure perimeter

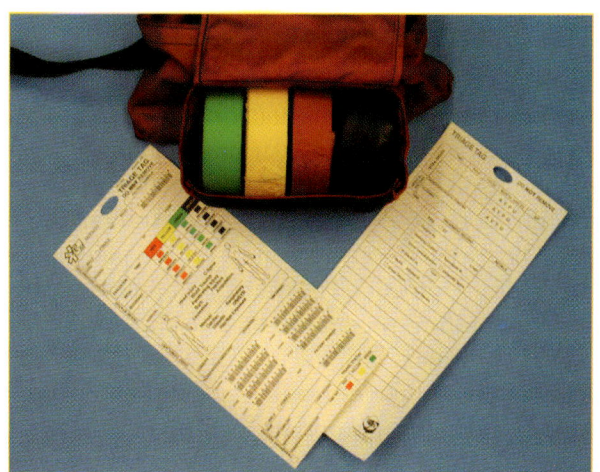

Figure 36-12 Triage tag showing front and back.

> ### ✳ EMT-I Tips
>
> **Special Triage Situations**
>
> Patients who have been contaminated by radiation or other hazardous materials are placed in a separate category of triage. This is the highest and most urgent category of all. Contaminated patients must be moved away from all other patients. They must not be allowed to contaminate other patients, EMS personnel, ambulances, or hospitals.
>
> Certain large urban areas that offer regionalized care use another concept of triage. Single patients with specific medical problems, such as burns, trauma, cardiac, or neonatal, are triaged to specialized regional centers for treatment. Making the decision to transport a patient to a special treatment center is difficult. The decision is based on many factors, including (but not limited to) the following:
>
> - The specific illness or injury
> - The severity of the illness or injury
> - The availability of local resources at the time of the event
> - Local rules and protocols
>
> These decisions are often made only after online communication with medical control.
>
> If there are special treatment centers in your area, you must know the specific triage protocols that apply. Also note that in the event of a mass-casualty incident, these protocols might not be used. For example, a school bus crash in which all 30 or 40 patients are children can overwhelm a pediatric hospital. Similarly, 10 burn patients from a petroleum plant fire could immobilize a burn center. In these cases, good triage and communication with medical control are essential in providing each patient with the best available treatment.
>
> Most urban areas have regional trauma care centers. Severe, life-threatening injuries should be treated in facilities that are prepared to deal immediately and completely with the problem. Ideally, severely injured patients should be identified in the field and sent to a designated Level I trauma center.
>
> It is not enough to know the triage techniques that your EMS system uses to identify patients for transport to specialized treatment facilities. As with the other skills you are learning, you must practice these techniques as well. Your EMS system should conduct disaster drills yearly, preferably with the participation of local hospitals and other public safety and rescue units. Disaster plans must be developed and practiced in advance of need. The mass confusion of a disaster site is no time to experiment with organization.

When you have finished your assigned task, report back to that same officer for another assignment. If your duties are complete, you may be reassigned.

Triage Procedures

If medical control is not willing or able to determine the appropriate destination hospital for each patient, a rotation system can be used to distribute patients properly to each hospital on the basis of hospital capacity and capabilities. Of course, any designated trauma centers should be used to receive the most critical patients, following local protocols. The transport officer is responsible for sending the ambulance to the appropriate hospital or the next hospital in turn. This rotation must occasionally be altered to allow specific patients to be taken to the most appropriate facility, such as a pediatric center, or to another hospital because a hospital has notified the field that it needs to be skipped for one rotation.

Normally, no more than two patients are placed in the same ambulance. However, with severe weather, a patient who has been tagged green may be seated in an ambulance next to the driver to move the patient to a comfortable, safe indoor holding area at the hospital.

As the patients are loaded into the ambulance, the transport officer logs each patient's mass-casualty tag number, each patient's overall condition, and the hospital to which they will be taken. As the ambulance leaves the scene, the transport officer radios the receiving hospital and briefly describes the patients, the unit transporting them, and the time they left the scene. To minimize radio traffic during such incidents, personnel on individual ambulances do not usually use their radios except to obtain advice from medical control or to notify the transport officer that they are leaving the hospital and returning to the field.

After giving a verbal report to hospital staff and transferring the patients, the ambulance returns to the staging area without further delay, helping to keep a continuous flow of ambulances moving between the mass-casualty incident site and the hospital. Equipment that is collected at the hospital or additional supplies that are needed in the field are brought to the staging area.

If additional ambulances are needed, the transport officer radios the command center, which then directs the resources from the staging area. If none are available at the staging area, the EMS chief notifies the dispatcher to obtain them elsewhere. To prevent a lack of ambulances, request extra ambulances as early as possible in a triage situation.

After all the first-priority (red-tagged) patients have been transported, the second-priority (yellow-tagged) patients are transported, followed by the third-priority (green-tagged) patients. After all patients have been transported, several units usually stay at the incident site to protect the other responders who will remain in case of injury. Often, ambulances will still be needed to transfer patients from the facility to which they were initially brought for stabilization to another, more appropriate facility.

Treatment and triage continue until all patients have been treated and transported. After the mass-casualty incident has ended, all personnel who were involved should be debriefed and evaluated to determine whether they need counseling. Mass-casualty incidents require regional preplanning and periodic simulation drills in which the fire, rescue, EMS, and police units are all involved. These drills usually include a large number of mock victims who are triaged and treated from the onset of the incident to delivery and re-triage at the hospital.

The success of any incident command system depends on all personnel performing their assigned tasks and working within the system. An EMT-I who is assigned to perform triage and decides instead to transport patients from the scene, bypasses the triage, treatment, and transport areas. As a result, those patients who were not yet triaged would not receive the care they need. Always remember that the cost of "doing your own thing" may include the loss of lives.

Disaster Management

A <u>disaster</u> is a widespread event that disrupts functions and resources of a community and threatens lives and property. Many disasters may not involve personal injuries. Droughts causing widespread crop damage are an example. On the other hand, many disasters such as floods, fires, and hurricanes also result in widespread injuries.

The role of the EMT-I in a disaster is to respond when requested and to report to the incident command system for assigned roles. One such role might be to record baseline vital signs and assessment of other response personnel before they enter the area. Later, the EMT-I may provide medical care and support to those who become exhausted or injured and return to the rehabilitation area.

You are the Provider   Part 4

Triage of all patients has been completed and you are now preparing to transport a patient with the following information and who has been triaged as a "red" priority.

Vital Signs	Recording Time: 4 Minutes After Patient Contact
Respirations	32 breaths/min, shallow
Pulse	132 beats/min, regular
Skin	Pale and diaphoretic
Blood pressure	88/62 mm Hg
SaO_2	95% with assisted ventilation and 100% oxygen

7. When you consult with medical control, what factors are used to determine where to transport victims of a mass-casualty incident?

Weapons of Mass Destruction

The intent of terrorism is to create chaos. To be prepared for a terrorist event, community leaders, including fire, police, and EMS officials, need to take appropriate actions to reduce the risks created by terrorism (see Chapter 37).

Six principles outline the role of the EMT-I at an incident involving a weapon of mass destruction:

1. **Carry out frequently used procedures and techniques in an emergency.** Appropriate responses to an incident involving a weapon of mass destruction must be familiar and uncomplicated.
2. **Identify an incident involving a weapon of mass destruction in one of two ways: sudden onset or delayed onset.** An incident of sudden onset can be identified almost immediately, such as a bomb blast. An incident with delayed onset can take hours or even days to appear, such as bizarre medical symptoms after exposure to some biological and chemical agents.
3. **Treat an event that is potentially or actually caused by a weapon of mass destruction as a HazMat situation.** EMS personnel should not enter the area until properly trained and equipped personnel identify the agent involved. EMS personnel should decide whether the known number of patients will require a mass-casualty response. If so, a command structure can be established immediately.
4. **Control the convergence of people.** Although public safety personnel, including EMT-Is, will tend to want to rush into the incident to help, all incidents involving a suspected weapon of mass destruction must be carefully assessed by specially trained and equipped personnel before others can enter. EMS and all safety personnel should keep all others from converging into the area where patients are located.
5. **Treat the event as a crime scene once the incident has been identified as being caused by a weapon of mass destruction.** This approach will preserve evidence and assist in later prosecution. Local and state police and the Federal Bureau of Investigation should be notified.
6. **Turn victims into patients.** People who plan and execute acts of terrorism want to create victims. Appropriate responses by EMS personnel and others can enable the treatment of these patients through local resources.

When all of these steps have been taken, the risk to public safety personnel and others is greatly reduced, which, in turn, helps those in the community return to a normal state in a shorter time.

In a disaster with an overwhelming number of casualties, area hospitals may decide that they cannot treat all patients at their facility. In this case, they may mobilize medical and nursing teams with equipment. Using a facility such as a warehouse near the disaster scene, they will set up a casualty collection area. The EMT-I would then be requested to transport patients to this alternative facility instead of to the local emergency department. Once at the **casualty collection area**, triage can be performed, medical care provided, and patients transported to the hospital on a priority basis.

If a casualty collection area is established, it will be coordinated through the incident command system in the same way as all other branches and areas of the operation. This is usually done only in a major disaster such as an earthquake when transportation to a hospital facility is impossible or has prolonged delays. It may take several hours to establish a casualty collection area. This delay can limit the number of events where such an area is an effective method for handling the incident.

Clandestine Drug Laboratories

As the war against drugs intensifies, more illegal drug manufacturing laboratories are established within the United States. The efforts of law enforcement agencies to limit illegal drug trafficking from other countries have forced many dealers and users to produce dangerous substances in clandestine labs. The volatile nature and toxic effects of the chemicals involved, as well as the unpredictable responses of drug users, increases the physical danger for emergency services personnel who may not realize the incident involves an illicit drug operation.

Several substances are abused for their mind-altering effects. Cocaine is made from coca plant, which is grown throughout South America. The opium poppy is grown widely in Asia and is used to make both morphine and heroin. Marijuana is grown throughout the world, including within the United States. Other substances are synthesized, including lysergic acid diethylamide (LSD), phencyclidine (PCP), and gamma-hydroxybutyrate (GHB), and manufactured in clandestine labs. Today, the most popular manufactured substance is methamphetamine, known on the street as "meth," "speed," or "crank."

Location of Illegal Drug Laboratories

Clandestine drug laboratories are found in every geographic and socioeconomic area. They can be found in cheap inner-city hotels, in expensive suburban homes, and in small trailer camps throughout rural America. Labs are found in vehicles such as buses, trucks, and motor homes Figure 36-13.

Recognizing Illegal Drug Laboratories

In general, there are two ways to produce methamphetamine. The first starts with a chemical known as phenyl-2-propanone (P-2-P). This method requires fairly sophisticated equipment and takes 24 to 36 hours to complete the chemical process that produces the drug. The second method is preferred not only because it is simpler, but also because it produces a drug that is two to three times more potent. In this method, ephedrine or pseudoephedrine is used as the basis for production.

The quality and quantity of equipment varies greatly. A basic laboratory may mix the compounds in buckets Figure 36-14, but there are also elaborate laboratories that use sophisticated glassware, heating mantles, and vacuum equipment. Newer labs are virtually disposable. All of the necessary ingredients Figure 36-15 for producing methamphetamine can be purchased at any discount department store and recipes are available over the Internet. Table 36-4 lists the materials common to methamphetamine labs.

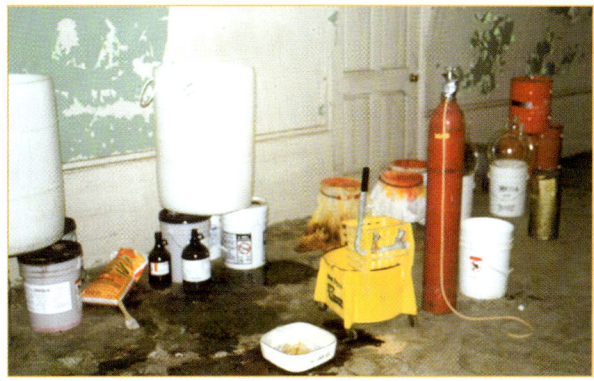

Figure 36-14 A lab capable of producing large quantities of methamphetamine.

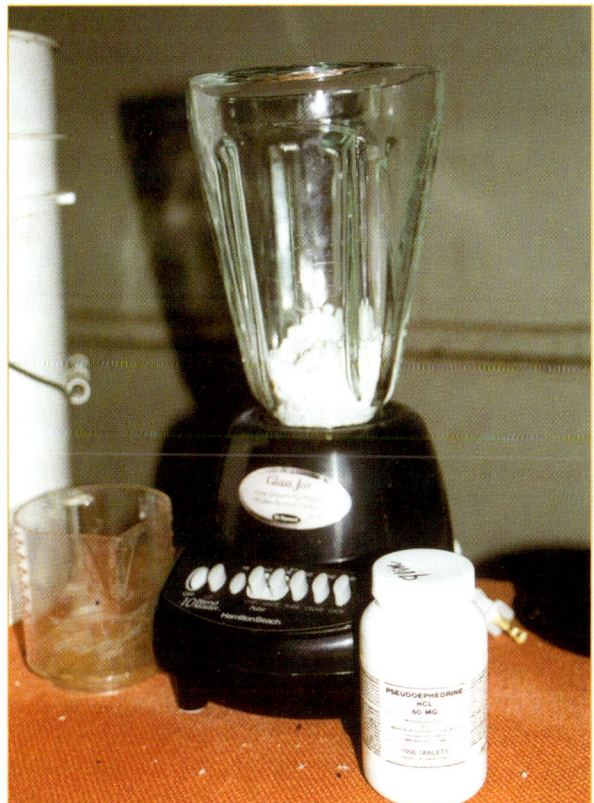

Figure 36-15 Ephedrine and pseudoephedrine tablets, available at any pharmacy, are ground in household blender as the first step in "meth" production.

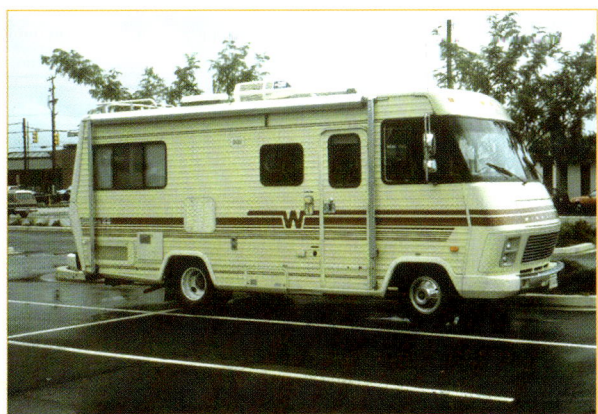

Figure 36-13 Motor homes are often used as mobile cooking labs. From the outside, this vehicle appears to be an ordinary motor home.

TABLE 36-4 Materials Common to Methamphetamine Labs

Product	Chemical	Hazard
Aluminum foil	Aluminum	Nonhazardous
Camera batteries	Lithium	Water reactive
Charcoal lighter fluid	Petroleum	Flammable
Denatured alcohol	Alcohol	Flammable
Epsom salts	Magnesium sulfate	Nonhazardous
Gasoline	Petroleum	Flammable
Heet	Methyl alcohol	Flammable
Iodine crystals	Iodine	Irritant
7% Tincture of iodine	Iodine	Irritant
Kerosene	Petroleum	Flammable
Lacquer thinner	Petroleum	Flammable
Mineral spirits	Petroleum	Flammable
Muriatic acid	Hydrochloric acid	Corrosive acid
Red Devil Lye	Sulfuric acid	Corrosive base
Roto Rooter	Sulfuric acid	Corrosive acid
Starting fluid	Ethyl ether	Flammable
Striker plates (fuses)	Phosphorus	Flammable
Table salt	Sodium chloride	Nonhazardous
Cold medications (over the counter)	Ephedrine and pseudoephedrine	Nonhazardous

Product	Use	
Coffee filter, cheesecloth, napkins	Separate liquid from solids	
Pots, pans, pressure cooker	Cooking	
Iced tea jars, sports jars	Separating layers of liquids	

Fire and EMS personnel may be exposed to the dangers of an illegal drug lab if unsuspecting neighbors request the fire department to investigate unusual odors near their home. The odors produced during the drug production process in a P-2-P lab can be mistaken for the smell of dried cat urine, cat litter, or rotten garbage. Many chemicals are used during the mixing process, including ether, which has a distinctive smell that many people recognize and report when calling for assistance.

Because of the highly flammable properties of many of the chemicals stored in an illegal drug lab, the response to a building or vehicle fire may turn into an anything-but-normal situation. Also, because many illegal drug makers are also users, you may discover an illegal drug lab whenever you respond to a reported overdose. Buildings that contain an illegal drug lab often have windows covered with black plastic, cardboard, or paint. When you enter a building or vehicle to treat an overdose victim, look for glassware and other fundamental items that you might find in a high-school chemistry laboratory.

People who work in illegal drug labs may request medical assistance if they develop symptoms of exposure to toxic, corrosive, explosive, or flammable materials. A list of chemicals that you may encounter is included in Table 36-4.

Hazards Associated With Clandestine Drug Labs

Every lab has a different configuration. Although there are no books of plans for constructing the perfect lab at the local bookstore, with the advent of the Internet, many plans are just a few keystrokes away. Recipes for drugs are usually handed down from one operator to another, or found on web sites.

Everything associated with a clandestine drug lab is hazardous! Be careful where you walk and avoid touching anything except the patient. An action as simple as shutting off the tap-water supply to a cooling condenser can cause an explosion. Turning off the heat during a heat-induced chemical reaction is even more hazardous. Many chemical reactions must be shut down in stages, and only the operator may understand the shut-down process. The operator may not even be present. Because some cooking processes take as long as 72 hours to complete, and are hazardous as well, some operators will mix the ingredients and leave the area as soon as cooking begins.

To protect the operation, operators set booby traps. Outside mechanisms include fragmentation and incendiary devices (hand grenades and claymore mines) (Figure 36-16 ▶), animal traps, and impaling stakes. Inside traps include vicious dogs, poisonous snakes, fishhooks hung at eye level, explosives connected to heating elements and electrical switches, and weapons such as crossbows and spear guns that discharge when the trigger mechanism is disturbed. Investigators have even found videotape cassettes containing plastic explosives and designed to detonate when placed in a video player.

Contact explosives are another danger you may face in an illegal drug lab. These devices are made by combining potassium chlorate or red phosphorous with another chemical that becomes unstable when it dries. The chemicals are rolled into a ball of aluminum foil and placed throughout the laboratory. If the ball is disturbed, it will explode (Figure 36-17 ▶).

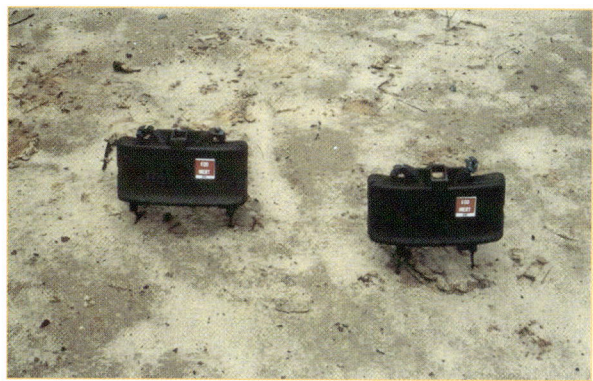

Figure 36-16 Claymore mines have been used as perimeter defense around the outside of labs.

If possible, do not touch or move anything that you did not bring with you into the area. Never disturb a suspected booby trap! Mark the location and notify the incident commander of the device. Do not use a portable radio to notify the incident commander; a radio transmission may activate an explosive device. Go to the command post and tell the commander in person.

Emergency Scene Operations

All personnel and equipment used at the scene of an illegal drug lab will be contaminated. After the area has been identified as a clandestine lab, establish a preliminary hazardous materials hot zone. Include the lab and the surrounding area as well as all personnel and equipment that came in contact with the lab (Figure 36-18 ▶). If equipment has been removed from

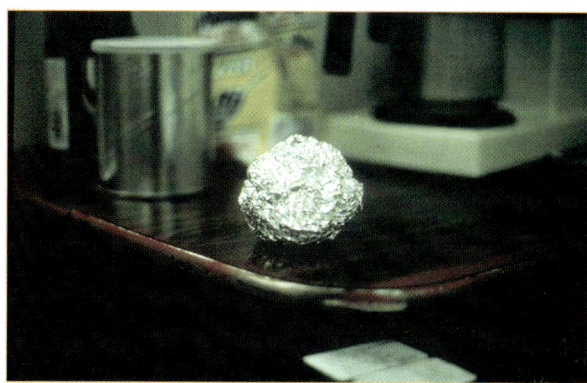

Figure 36-17 Upon exploding, this chemical booby trap can destroy a person's hand.

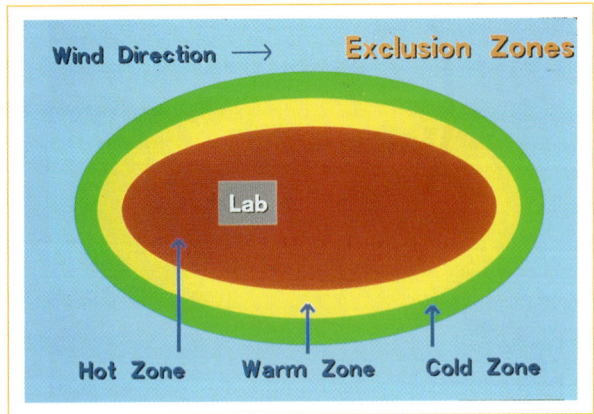

Figure 36-18 Establish safety zones for a hazardous materials response.

the lab and placed on a vehicle, include the vehicle in the hot zone. When the hazardous materials response team arrives on the scene, it will determine the final boundaries of the hot zone.

After you are clear of the building or vehicle containing the lab, notify your dispatcher that you are at the scene of an illegal drug lab, and request that the following agencies be notified to respond to the scene:

- Local law enforcement
- Drug Enforcement Administration
- Environmental Protection Agency
- Hazardous materials response team
- Additional EMS unit (ALS preferred)
- Bomb squad
- Local health department
- EMS supervisor
- Fire department

EMS Operations

If you discover an illegal drug lab during an emergency medical call, leave the lab immediately. Take the patient with you if you can do so without exposing yourself and your team to additional hazardous materials. If the patient is stable, remain in the preliminary hot zone until the hazardous materials response team arrives on the scene. If your unit is outside the hot zone, do not return to it unless you need specific equipment for patient treatment. You, your partner, your patient, and all equipment carried into the lab are considered contaminated until cleared by the hazardous materials response team. Everyone and everything must be decontaminated before leaving the hot zone.

The hazardous materials response team will set up and carry out decontamination procedures on all personnel and equipment leaving the hot zone. The decontamination stations are in a warm zone, which is adjacent to the hot zone. Access to the warm zone is limited to personnel directly involved in the incident.

If the patient's condition requires immediate transport to a hospital, notify the medical facility of the circumstances. Explain that you have been exposed to unknown hazardous materials and that you and the patient have not been decontaminated. Request that the hazardous materials response team be sent to the hospital to carry out decontamination procedures there. All hospital personnel and equipment that come into contact with you, the patient, or your equipment must be included in the decontamination procedure.

Fire Suppression Operations

If you respond to a fire that is in or around a suspected drug lab, you must wear full protective clothing, including a self-contained breathing apparatus. Use higher levels of protective clothing, such as encapsulated suits, if chemicals are involved in the fire.

Establish a hot zone as soon as possible. Again, access to the hot zone is limited to personnel directly involved in fire suppression. Personnel from other agencies that will handle the chemicals, protect the environment, and collect evidence are not allowed past the warm zone until after the fire is out or the fire ground commander specifically authorizes their presence.

Identify the warm zone as soon as the decontamination stations are erected. Back-up personnel should move charged hose lines into the warm zone in anticipation of a rapid escalation of the fire. Back up should be properly positioned, fully bunkered, and ready to advance into the hot zone.

The area within the boundary of the fire line or crime scene tape and outside of the warm zone should be established as a cold zone. This controlled area is off-limits to the general public. The incident command post is located in this area. Protective clothing is not required, and the area may be used as a staging ground for additional personnel and equipment.

If the structure or vehicle containing a known lab is burning when you arrive, protect the exposures and let it burn. Attempting to control the fire may prove deadly to the fire attack teams. Remember, the runoff of contaminated water produced by suppression efforts may cause widespread ecological damage.

If an initial fire attack is in progress when the location is identified as a drug lab, withdraw the attack teams and shift from offensive to defensive operations.

In all incidents involving drug labs, evacuate the structures on every side of the incident. When a fire or chemical spill is involved, consider evacuating people downwind from the incident.

Positive Pressure Ventilation

Never enter a known drug lab until the hazardous materials response team ventilates the area and declares it safe. All personnel responding to emergency medical situations, fire operations, chemical spills, and law enforcement activities should remain outside and upwind from the location.

Many of the chemicals used in clandestine drug labs are explosive if the proper air-to-product ratio is attained. Because this ratio will occur at some point during the ventilation process, all possible ignition sources must be eliminated.

If mechanical ventilation of the structure or vehicle is required, positive pressure ventilation should be used. All mechanical and power equipment remain outside of the area being ventilated, which further reduces the number of ignition sources during the ventilation process **Figure 36-19** .

Check with the DEA's on-scene chemist or site safety officer before turning off any utilities. Do not continue the operation until the DEA chemist arrives on the scene. After you receive permission from the chemist, secure all electric power from remote locations to prevent unwanted sparks or arcing **Figure 36-20** .

To extinguish pilot lights on stoves, heaters, and furnaces, shut off all natural and low pressure gas valves from outside the building. Do not shut off the gas if the DEA chemist believes that it is not safe to remove the heat from a chemical reaction in progress. It may be necessary to withdraw all personnel to the cold zone and wait until the process is complete.

Monitoring Personnel Working in the Hot Zone

An ALS unit (BLS unit if ALS is not available) should be assigned to all clandestine drug lab operations to monitor everyone working in the hot zone. The unit establishes a monitoring station in the warm zone. All personnel leaving the hot zone report to the monitoring station for medical evaluation after decontamination.

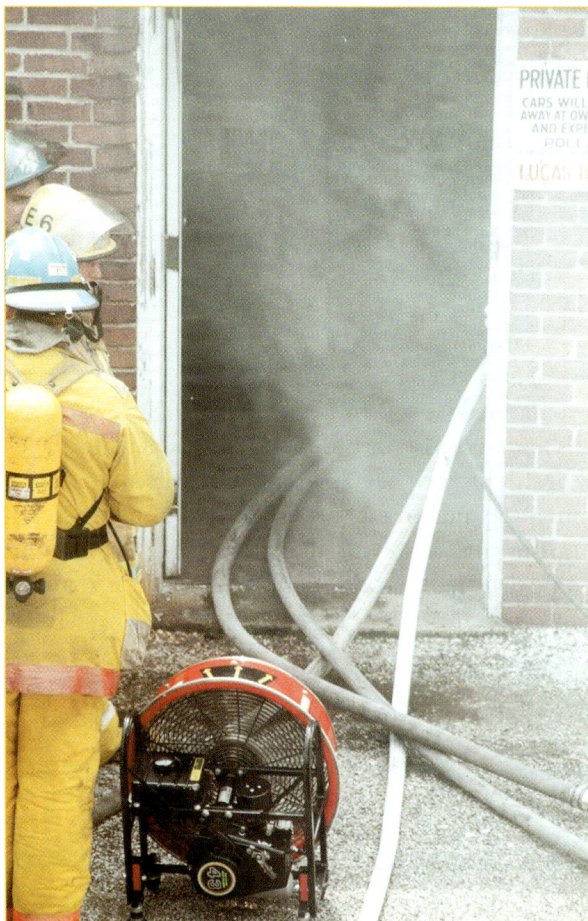

Figure 36-19 Positive-pressure ventilation is the only acceptable method of mechanical ventilation to use in drug lab operations.

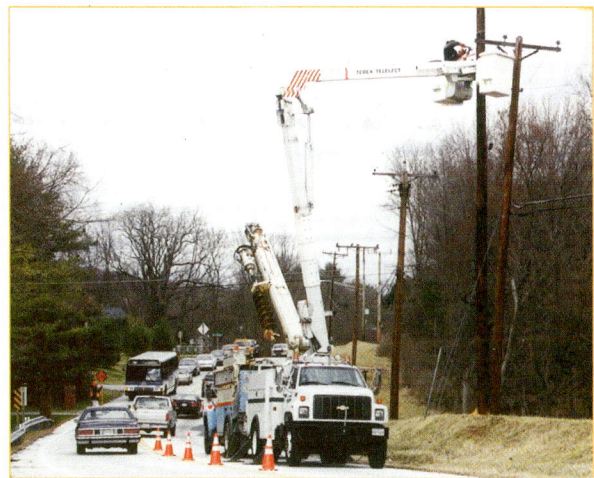

Figure 36-20 Trained personnel secure electric power to the suspected drug lab from a remote location.

Provide medical attention to anyone who develops any of the following symptoms associated with exposure to toxic chemicals:

- Nausea
- Vomiting
- Sharp headache
- Reddened face
- Burning sensation in the nose, throat, or lungs
- Drowsiness
- Numb lips
- Tingling teeth
- Unfocused eyes

Chemicals used in labs can be absorbed into the walls and floors of the building. This can create a potential health hazard that lasts days or weeks after a lab was dismantled and all chemicals and equipment removed from the site. The DEA posts warning signs on clandestine drug laboratories that have been seized and dismantled Figure 36-21 .

Interacting With a Methamphetamine User

Methamphetamine is a powerful central nervous system stimulant that can be injected, snorted, smoked, or swallowed. Because the drug produces a sense of euphoria, increased alertness, and energy, it is popular with students, truck drivers and other professions that require long hours of work. Higher doses and chronic use of the drug will produce irritability and paranoia. If a patient is suspected of using meth, you should stand approximately 7′ to 10′ away from the individual and keep your hands visible at all times, with feet shoulder-width apart and knees slightly bent. If you move closer, the paranoid user may feel threatened and attempt an attack. You should also avoid shining lights into the eyes of a suspected meth user because this may also result in a violent attack. Speak slowly in a low-pitched voice. Any movement you make should also be slow and deliberate.

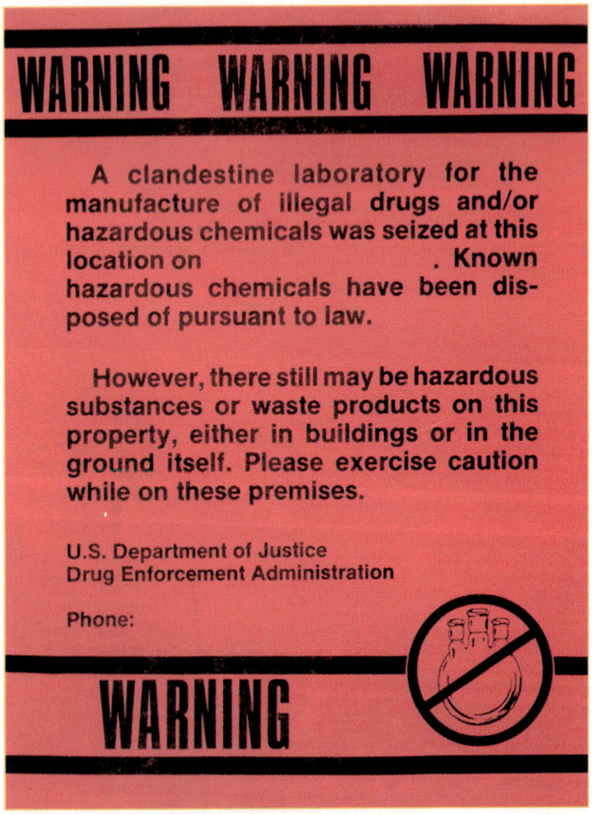

EMT-I Tips

Clandestine drug labs are extremely dangerous. Do not enter known labs until they have been secured by law enforcement personnel. All personnel and agencies responding to an incident at an illegal drug lab need an immediate plan of action. Liquid propane gas cylinders routinely used with home barbecues are now being used to hold anhydrous ammonia, a necessary chemical in the production of methamphetamine. Responders should be aware that anhydrous ammonia will react with the brass fittings of the cylinder. The reaction will cause a blue tinge on the valve and will result in failure of the container.

- The time to plan for multiagency operations is not when a clandestine drug lab is discovered—it is now!
- A drug lab is a crime scene—preserve the evidence!
- Limit overhaul to extinguishing serious hot spots that may reignite or ignite residue vapors.

Figure 36-21 Whenever you see this sign, treat the area as if the laboratory were still operating.

You are the Provider · Summary

1. What is the incident command system (ICS)?

The ICS was developed by the fire service to help control, direct, and coordinate emergency responders and resources. The system has been adapted and used by many EMS organizations to better organize their own operations.

2. Why is the ICS helpful to all emergency responders?

Even on a call with only one patient and no need for any other services, the implementation of an ICS is helpful to identify the roles and responsibilities of each crew member, particularly if the event begins to escalate.

The structure of the ICS enables a single authority to have overall responsibility to manage the incident.

3. What is the first step the EMT-I should take when arriving at a possible HazMat scene?

You must first step back and assess the situation. This can be very stressful, particularly if you can see a patient. However, rushing into a HazMat incident can have catastrophic results.

4. What two issues do you need to address at a HazMat incident?

- Any trauma that has resulted from other related mechanisms, such as vehicle collision, fire, or explosion
- The injury and harm that have resulted from exposure to the toxic hazardous substance

5. What is the color-coding priority system used when triaging patients in a mass-casualty incident?

Color coding to indicate priority for treatment and transportation at the scene is as follows: red-tagged patients are the first priority, yellow-tagged patients are the second priority, and patients tagged green or black are the lowest priority.

6. What are the key components at a mass-casualty incident?

- Incident commander, command post, and incident command system
- Onsite communications system
- Adequate supply of long backboards, straps, or ties
- Extrication/retrieval team
- Triage officer and designated triage area
- Staffed patient collection area
- Staffed patient treatment area
- Supply location adjacent to the treatment area
- Transportation officer and transport area
- Staging area to hold resources until they are needed
- Fire and law enforcement personnel
- A secure perimeter

7. When you consult with medical control, what factors are used to determine where to transport victims of a mass-casualty incident?

Making the decision to transport a patient to a special treatment center is difficult. The decision is based on many factors, including (but not limited to) the following:

- The specific illness or injury
- The severity of the illness or injury
- The availability of local resources at the time of the event
- Local rules and protocols

These decisions are often made only after online communication with medical control.

Section 8 Operations

Prep Kit

Ready for Review

- At a hazardous materials incident, safety—of you and your team, the patient, and the public—is your most important concern.
- If you arrive first, assess the situation, taking care to protect yourself, and then call for a trained HazMat team.
- The most important step in such an incident is to identify the substances involved. Do not enter the hazard zone; your job is to provide supportive care once the patient can be safely moved out of the area.
- Hazardous materials are classified according to five toxicity levels.
- Four protection levels are indicated for the amount and type of protective gear you need. Levels indicate the amount and type of protective gear that you need to prevent injury from a particular substance.
- Most serious injuries and deaths from hazardous materials incidents result from airway and breathing problems.
- Patients' injuries should be treated in the same way that you would treat any injury.
- Resources for HazMat incidents include the *Emergency Response Guidebook* and The Chemical Transportation Emergency Center (CHEMTREC). CHEMTREC is open 24 hours a day to help you identify and handle hazardous materials transport incidents.
- Incident command systems allow for coordination of police, fire, and EMS activities in an emergency situation. In major incidents, there is usually a unified command, with a single command post where decisions are made by agency leaders.
- If your unit arrives first at an incident that will involve more than one unit or agency, command should be established. Otherwise, you should report to the command post for assignment.
- You may be assigned to one of the following sectors: staging, extrication, triage, treatment, supply, transportation, or rehabilitation.
- In a mass-casualty incident, the most highly trained medical person on the scene directs triage. This means assigning treatment and transport priorities according to the severity and survivability of patients' injuries.
- There are four triage levels, each with a separate treatment area. Highest priority is given to patients whose injuries are critical but probably survivable with prompt treatment.
- The cardinal rule of triage is to do the greatest good for the greatest number. Treatment and triage continue until all patients have been transported.
- In urban areas with special treatment centers, special protocols are used to triage patients with specific injuries to the appropriate centers.
- Communication with medical control is essential for good triage.
- Disasters are widespread events that can threaten lives and property, and sometimes can cause personal injuries.
- The incident command system is used for disasters just as for other types of mass-casualty incidents. However, if the number of patients overwhelms the area's hospitals, an alternate facility and casualty collection area can be set up for triage and treatment.

Technology

- Interactivities
- Vocabulary Explorer
- Anatomy Review
- Web Links
- Online Review Manual

Vital Vocabulary

casualty collection area An area set up by physicians, nurses, and other hospital staff near a major disaster scene, where patients can receive further triage and medical care.

Chemical Transportation Emergency Center (CHEMTREC) An agency that assists emergency personnel in identifying and handling hazardous materials transport incidents.

command post The designated field command center where the incident commander and support personnel are located.

danger zone An area where individuals can be exposed to toxic substances, lethal rays, or ignition or explosion of hazardous materials.

decontamination The process of removing or neutralizing and properly disposing of hazardous materials from equipment, patients, and rescue personnel.

decontamination area The designated area in a hazardous materials incident where all patients and rescuers must be decontaminated before going to another area.

disaster A widespread event that disrupts community resources and functions, in turn threatening public safety, citizens' lives, and property.

hazardous material Any substance that is toxic, poisonous, radioactive, flammable, or explosive and causes injury or death with exposure.

hazardous materials incident An incident in which a hazardous material is no longer properly contained and isolated.

incident commander The individual who has overall command of the scene in the field.

incident command system An organizational system to help control, direct, and coordinate emergency responders and resources; known more generally as an incident management system (IMS).

mass-casualty incident An emergency situation involving more than one patient, and which can place such great demand on equipment or personnel that the system is stretched to its limit or beyond.

protection level A measure of the amount and type of protective equipment that an individual needs to avoid injury during contact with a hazardous material.

rehabilitation area This area provides protection and treatment to firefighters and other personnel working at an emergency. Here, workers are medically monitored and receive any needed care as they enter and leave the scene.

sector commander The individual delegated to oversee and coordinate activity in an incident command sector; works under the incident commander.

toxicity level A measure of the risk that a hazardous material poses to the health of an individual who comes into contact with it.

transportation area The area in a mass-casualty incident where ambulances and crews are organized to transport patients from the treatment area to receiving hospitals.

transportation officer The individual in charge of the transportation sector in a mass-casualty incident, who assigns patients from the treatment area to awaiting ambulances in the transportation area.

treatment area Location in a mass-casualty incident where patients are brought after being triaged and assigned a priority, where they are reassessed, treated, and monitored until transport to the hospital.

treatment officer The individual, usually a physician, who is in charge of and directs EMS personnel at the treatment area in a mass-casualty incident.

triage The process of sorting patients based on the severity of injury and medical need, to establish treatment and transportation priorities.

triage area Designated area in a mass-casualty incident where the triage officer is located and patients are initially triaged before being taken to the treatment center.

triage officer The individual in charge of the incident command triage sector, who directs the sorting of patients into triage categories in a mass-casualty incident.

Assessment in Action

You are the senior EMT-I on duty at a small, rural EMS unit. You are the only ambulance in service for a 20-mile radius. You are dispatched to a motor vehicle crash on the freeway. You are the first unit to arrive on the scene.

On arrival you see that an SUV has rear-ended a tanker truck. Fluid is leaking from the tanker. The roadway is completely blocked, and the occupants of several vehicles stopped by the wreckage are trying to help the victims.

1. You should immediately do all of the following EXCEPT:
   A. notify dispatch and other responding units of the situation.
   B. advise the people from the other vehicles to leave the area.
   C. attempt to visualize the truck's placard from your location.
   D. back out of the situation.

2. According to the ICS, the person who is initially in command is:
   A. the fire chief.
   B. the EMS chief.
   C. you.
   D. your partner.

3. Additional clues that may have indicated the presence of a hazardous material spill include all of the following EXCEPT:
   A. involvement of a tanker truck.
   B. "Please Drive Carefully" placard.
   C. visible cloud emanating from the substance.
   D. strong odor in the area.

Additional units have arrived. The HazMat team has designated the danger zone, decontamination area, and triage areas and has established a unified command system. Three injured patients have been identified: the driver and passenger of the SUV and the driver of the tanker truck. The driver of the SUV was unrestrained and experienced head and chest injuries in the collision. He is having difficulty breathing and is showing signs of shock. His passenger was restrained and sustained minor cuts and bruises. The tanker truck driver slipped and fell while getting out of his truck. He hit his head on the pavement, but is conscious and alert and has no complaints. All three patients are contaminated. You also notice that several of the people who tried to help are coughing and vomiting.

4. The patients would be categorized as follows:
   A. both drivers are yellow; passenger is green.
   B. the SUV driver is yellow; truck driver and passenger are green.
   C. the SUV driver is red; truck driver is yellow; passenger is green.
   D. the SUV driver is red; passenger is yellow; truck driver is green.

5. Advantages of the unified command system include:
   A. operations officers move about the incident and have more contact with rescuers.
   B. operations officers report to the incident commander hourly for updates on the rescue.
   C. multiple operations officers replace the single incident commander.
   D. operations officers function as advisors to the incident commander.

6. The decontamination area:
   A. is the exit point of the danger zone.
   B. poses no threat to emergency workers.
   C. is staffed by EMS personnel.
   D. is located in the treatment area.

7. Triage guidelines that you will use during this incident include all of the following EXCEPT:
   A. color-coding patients to indicate their treatment and transport priority.
   B. providing in-depth care prior to transport.
   C. transporting the most critical patients first.
   D. coordinating rescue efforts based on patient needs.

8. Activities that should occur in the treatment area include all of the following EXCEPT:
   A. reassessing patients.
   B. managing the ABCs.
   C. preparing patients for transport.
   D. determining who is to be transported next.

9. When treating and transporting the driver of the SUV, you should do all of the following EXCEPT:
   A. thoroughly decontaminate him prior to transport.
   B. notify the receiving facility of the situation.
   C. wear additional PPE.
   D. remove unnecessary equipment from the ambulance.

10. General guidelines for transporting patients from a mass-casualty incident include all of the following EXCEPT:
    A. transporting patients to the hospital indicated by the transportation officer.
    B. giving a brief radio report to the receiving facility.
    C. promptly returning to the staging area.
    D. transporting red-tagged patients before yellow-tagged patients.

Points to Ponder

You are dispatched to an industrial plant for an explosion. You are the first unit to arrive on the scene. You observe several people on the ground near the building, which is on fire. You report your findings to dispatch and then you and your partner approach the victims to assess injuries. As you are about 10′ from the victims, you become very dizzy and unable to breathe. You collapse to the ground and stop breathing.

What should you have done differently?

Issues: Understanding Scene Safety, Considering Environmental Risks, Thinking Before You Act

Response to Terrorism and Weapons of Mass Destruction

1999 Objectives
There are no 1999 objectives for this chapter.

1985 Objectives
There are no 1985 objectives for this chapter.

Additional Objectives*

Cognitive

1. Define international and domestic terrorism. (p 1492)
2. List the different terrorist agenda categories. (p 1492)
3. Describe the threat levels (or colors) used by the Department of Homeland Security (DHS) to notify responders of the potential for a terrorist attack:
   - SEVERE (RED)
   - HIGH (ORANGE)
   - ELEVATED (YELLOW)
   - GUARDED (BLUE)
   - LOW (GREEN) (p 1495)
4. On the basis of DHS threat levels, discuss what actions EMT-Is should take during the course of their work to heighten their ability to respond to and survive a terrorist attack. (p 1494)
5. Recognize the hallmarks of a terrorist event. (p 1494)
6. List potential terrorist targets and their vulnerability. (p 1494)
7. Discuss these key principles to assuring responder safety at the scene of a terrorist event:
   - Establishing scene safety
   - Approaching the scene
   - Protective measures
   - Establishing a safety zone
   - Ongoing reevaluation of scene safety
   - Awareness of secondary devices (p 1496)
8. Discuss the following critical actions that the EMT-I must perform to operate on the scene following a terrorist attack:
   - Notification
   - Establish command
   - Patient management (p 1496)
9. Describe and list the four weapons of mass destruction (WMD). (p 1493)
10. Describe historical events dealing with WMD. (p 1492)
11. List nuclear/chemical/biological/explosive agents that may be used by a terrorist. (p 1494)
12. Describe the routes of exposure for chemical agents. (p 1498)
13. Describe the routes of exposure for biological agents. (p 1506)
14. Describe the routes of exposure for nuclear/radiological dispersal devices (RDD). (p 1513)
15. Discuss the clinical manifestations of exposure to the various WMD agents. (p 1498)
16. Describe the treatment to be rendered to a victim of a nuclear/chemical/biological/explosive attack. (p 1499)

Affective

17. Discuss the "new age" terrorist's trend towards apocalyptic violence and indiscriminate death. (p 1493)
18. Explain the rationale behind **NOT** entering the WMD scene or being **UNABLE** to treat contaminated victims, and the possible impact on the EMT-I. (p 1496)

Psychomotor

19. Demonstrate the patient assessment skills to assist the victim of a nuclear/chemical/biological/explosive agent. (p 1499)
20. Demonstrate the use of the nerve agent antidote (MARK 1) auto-injector kit. (p 1501)
21. Given a scenario of a terrorist event, establish scene safety and begin patient management. (p 1496)

*All of these objectives are noncurriculum objectives.

37

Response to Terrorism and Weapons of Mass Destruction

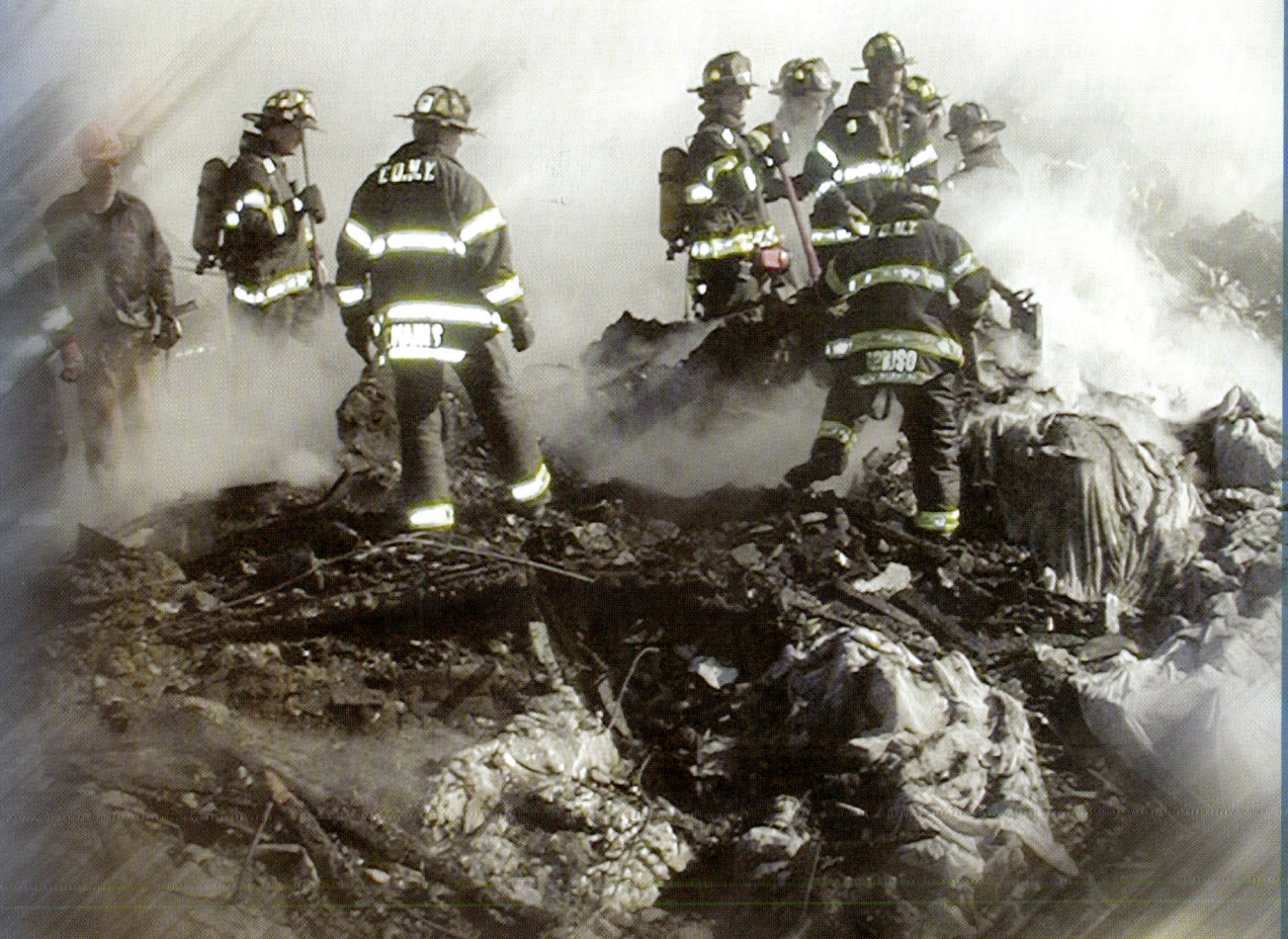

You are the Provider

You are a member of a small combination department located in a rural area. Every year, tens of thousands of people from all over the country migrate to your town to enjoy a very popular music festival. You are asked to attend the festivities to assist attendants should the need arise. You've participated in this standby of the event for the past 5 years without major incident. Today will be different.

1. Why is this event at particular risk for a terrorist attack?
2. What other factors will play a significant role should an attack occur?
3. What can agencies large and small do to prepare for mass-casualty incidents and/or terrorism?

Introduction

As a result of the increase in terrorist activity, it is possible that you may witness a terrorist event during your career. International terrorists as well as domestic groups have increased their targeting of civilian populations with acts of terror. The question is not will terrorists strike again, but rather when and where they will strike. The EMT-I must be mentally and physically prepared for the possibility of a terrorist event.

The use of weapons of mass destruction (WMD) or mass casualty further complicates the management of the terrorist incident and places the EMT-I in greater danger. Although it is difficult to plan and anticipate a response to many terrorist events, there are several key principles that apply to every response. This chapter describes how you can prepare to respond to these events by discussing types of terrorist events, personnel safety, and patient management. You will learn the signs, symptoms, and treatment of patients who have been exposed to nuclear, chemical, or biological agents or an explosive attack. At the end of this chapter, you will be able to answer the following key questions:

- What are your initial actions?
- Who should you notify, and what should you tell them?
- What type of additional resources might you require?
- How should you proceed to address the needs of the victims?
- How do you ensure your own and your partner's safety, as well as the safety of the victims?
- What is the clinical presentation of a victim exposed to a WMD?
- How are WMD patients to be assessed and treated?
- How do you avoid becoming contaminated or cross-contaminated with a WMD agent?

What Is Terrorism?

No one is quite sure who the first terrorist was, but terrorist forces have been at work since early civilizations. Today, terrorists pose a threat to nations and cultures everywhere. International terrorism has brought a new fear into the lives of many American citizens.

Modern-day terrorism is common in the Middle East, where terrorist groups have frequently attacked civilian populations. In Ireland terrorist groups have attacked the civilian population for decades under the guise of religious freedom. In Colombia, political terrorist groups target oil resources as a means to instill fear.

In the United States, domestic terrorists have struck multiple times within the last decade. The Centennial Park bombing during the 1996 Summer Olympics and the destruction of the Alfred P. Murrah Federal Building in Oklahoma City in 1995 are examples. Terrorist organizations are generally categorized. Only a small percentage of groups actually turn toward terrorism as a means to achieve their goals, such as the following:

1. **Violent religious groups/doomsday cults.** These include groups such as Aum Shinrikyo, who carried out chemical and biological attacks in Tokyo in 1994 and 1995. Some of these groups may participate in apocalyptic violence (Figure 37-1).

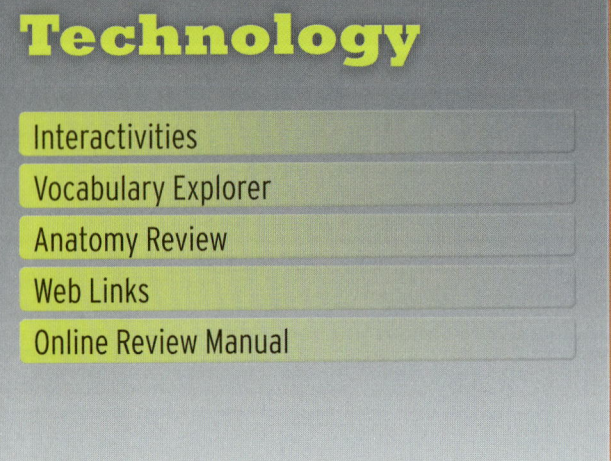

Technology
- Interactivities
- Vocabulary Explorer
- Anatomy Review
- Web Links
- Online Review Manual

www.EMSzone.com/EMTI

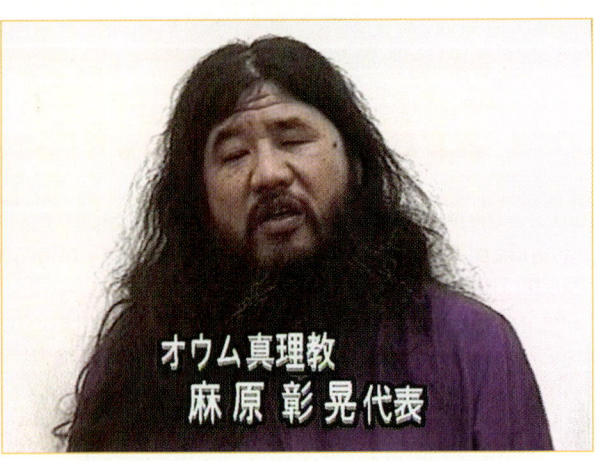

Figure 37-1 Asahara Shoko, the founder of Aum Shinrikyo.

devastating results. Terrorists who acted alone carried out all of the Atlanta abortion clinic attacks, the 1996 Summer Olympics attack, and the Oklahoma City bombing.

Weapons of Mass Destruction

What Are WMDs?

A weapon of mass destruction (WMD) or weapon of mass casualty (WMC) is any agent designed to bring about mass death, casualties, and/or massive damage to property and infrastructure (bridges, tunnels, airports, and seaports). These instruments of death and destruction include nuclear, chemical, biological, and explosive weapons. To date, the preferred WMD for terrorists has been explosive devices. Terrorist groups have favored tactics that use car or truck bombs or pedestrian suicide bombers. Many previous terrorist attempts to use either chemical or biological weapons to their full capacity have been unsuccessful. Nonetheless, as an EMT-I you should understand the destructive potential of these weapons.

As discussed earlier, the motives and tactics of the new-age terrorist groups have begun to change. As with the doomsday cults, many terrorist groups participate in apocalyptic, indiscriminate killing. This doctrine of total carnage would make the use of WMDs highly desirable. WMDs are easy to obtain or create and are specifically geared toward killing large numbers of people. Had the proper techniques been used during the 1995 attack on the Tokyo subway, there may have been tens of thousands of casualties. With the fall of the former Soviet Union, the technology and expertise to produce WMDs may be available to terrorist groups with sufficient funding. Moreover, the technical recipes for making nuclear, biological, chemical (NBC) weapons and explosive devices can be found readily on the Internet; in fact, they have even been published on terrorist group websites.

Chemical Warfare/Terrorism

Chemical agents are man-made substances that can have devastating effects on living organisms. They can be produced in liquid, powder, or vapor form, depending on the desired route of exposure and dissemination technique. Developed during World War I, these agents have been implicated in thousands of deaths since being intro-

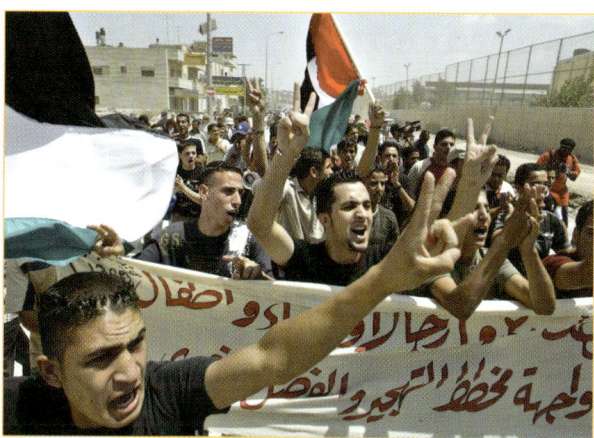

Figure 37-2 Palestinian extremist political groups have been associated with terrorism.

2. **Extremist political groups.** They may include violent separatist groups and those who seek political, religious, economic, and social freedom, such as many Middle Eastern groups **Figure 37-2**.
3. **Technology terrorists.** Those who would attack a population's technological infrastructure as a means to draw attention to their cause, such as cyber-terrorists.
4. **Single-issue groups.** These include anti-abortion, animal rights, anarchist, racist, or even eco-terrorists who threaten or use violence as a means to protect the environment **Figure 37-3**.

Most terrorist attacks require the coordination of multiple terrorists or "actors" working together. However, in a few instances, a single terrorist has struck with

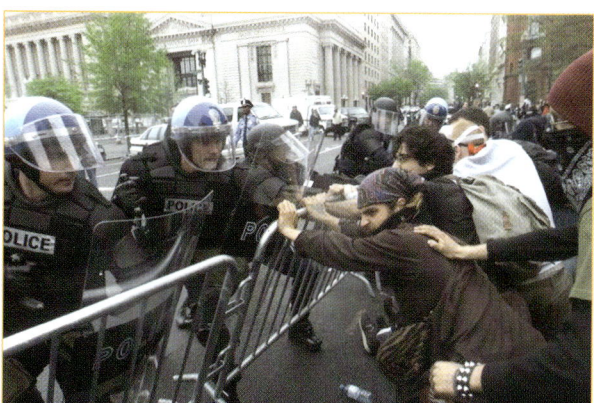

Figure 37-3 Demonstrators being held back by police near the World Bank in Washington, DC.

duced on the battlefield, and since then have been used to terrorize civilian populations. These agents consist of:

- Vesicants (blister agents)
- Respiratory agents (choking agents)
- Nerve agents
- Metabolic agents (blood agents)

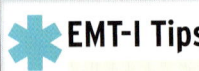

EMT-I Tips

Chemical warfare may be in the form of liquid, powder, or vapor.

Biological Terrorism/Warfare

Biological agents are organisms that cause disease. They are generally found in nature; for terrorist use, however, they are cultivated, synthesized, and mutated in a laboratory. The <u>weaponization</u> of biological agents is performed to artificially maximize the target population's exposure to the germ, thereby exposing the greatest number of people and achieving the desired result.

The primary types of biological agents that you may come into contact with during a biological event include:

- Viruses
- Bacteria
- Toxins

Nuclear/Radiological Terrorism

There have been only two publicly known incidents involving the use of a nuclear device. During World War II, Hiroshima and Nagasaki were devastated when they were targeted with nuclear bombs. The awesome destructive power demonstrated by the attack ended World War II and has served as a deterrent to nuclear war.

There are also nations that hold close ties with terrorist groups (known as <u>state-sponsored terrorism</u>) and have obtained some degree of nuclear capability.

It is also possible for a terrorist to secure radioactive materials or waste to perpetrate an act of terror. Such materials are far easier for the determined terrorist to acquire and would require less expertise to use. The difficulties in developing a nuclear weapon are well-documented. Radioactive materials, however, such as those in radiological dispersal devices (RDDs), also known as "dirty bombs," can cause widespread panic and civil disturbances. More on these devices will be covered later in this chapter.

EMT-I Response to Terrorism

Recognizing a Terrorist Event (Indicators)

Most acts of terror are <u>covert</u>, which means that the public safety community generally has no prior knowledge of the time, location, or nature of the attack. This element of surprise makes responding to an event more complex. You must constantly be aware of your surroundings and understand the possible risks for terrorism associated with certain locations, at certain times. It is therefore important that you know the current threat level issued by the federal government through the Department of Homeland Security (DHS).

The Homeland Security Advisory System alerts responders to the potential for an attack, although the specifics of the current threat will not be given. On the basis of the current threat level, the EMT-I should take appropriate actions and precautions while continuing to perform daily duties and responding to calls. The system of colors is used to inform the public safety community of the climate of terrorism (derived from intelligence gathering and the amount of terrorist communication) and to heighten the awareness of the potential for a terrorist attack. The system is designed to save lives, including yours.

The DHS has not issued specific recommendations for EMS personnel to follow in response to the alert system. Follow your local protocols, policies, and procedures.

It is your responsibility to make sure you know the advisory level at the start of your workday. Daily newspapers, television news programs, and multiple websites (including the DHS website) all give up-to-date information on the threat level. Many EMS organizations are starting to display the advisory system on boards where they can be seen once staff arrives for a shift.

Understanding and being aware of the current threat is only the beginning of responding safely to calls. Once you are on duty, you must be able to make appropriate decisions regarding the potential for a terrorist event. In determining the potential for a terrorist attack, on every call you should observe the following:

- **Type of location.** Is the location a monument, infrastructure, government building, or a specific type of location such as a church or synagogue? Is there a large gathering? Is there a special event taking place?
- **Type of call.** Is there a report of an explosion or suspicious device nearby? Does the call come

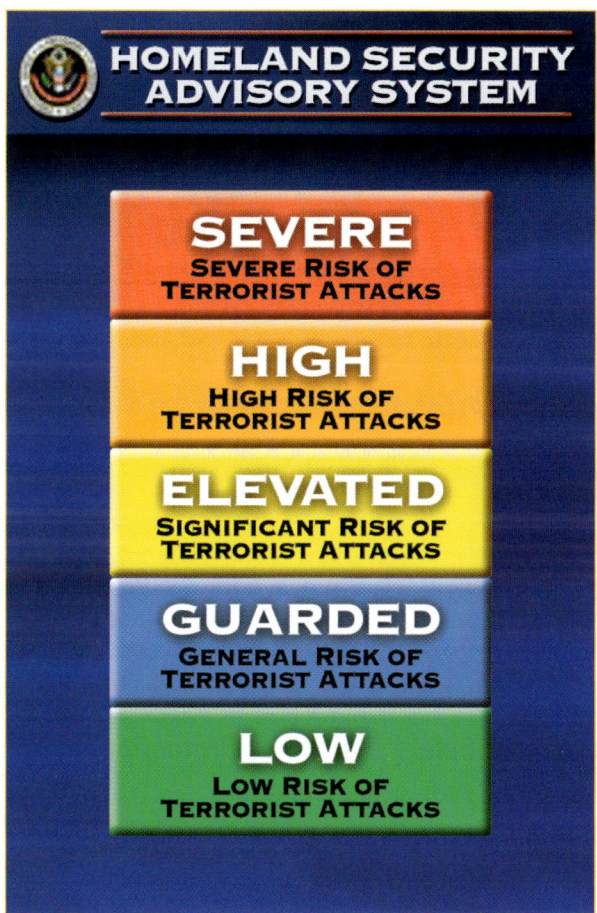

Figure 37-4 Homeland Security Advisory System.

> **EMT-I Safety**
>
> The Department of Homeland Security Advisory System is posted daily to heighten awareness of the current terrorist threat Figure 37-4.
> SEVERE (RED): Severe risk of terrorist attacks
> HIGH (ORANGE): High risk of terrorist attacks
> ELEVATED (YELLOW): Significant risk of terrorist attacks
> GUARDED (BLUE): General risk of terrorist attack
> LOW (GREEN): Low risk of terrorist attacks

into dispatch as someone having unexplained coughing and difficulty breathing? Are there reports of people fleeing the scene?

- **Number of patients.** Are there multiple victims with similar signs and symptoms? This is probably the single most important clue that a terrorist attack or an incident involving a WMD has occurred.
- **Victims' statements.** This is probably the second best indication of a terrorist or WMD event. Are the victims fleeing the scene giving statements such as, "Everyone is passing out," "There was a loud explosion," or "There are a lot of people shaking on the ground." If so, something is occurring that you do not want to rush into, even if it is determined not to be a terrorist event.
- **Preincident indicators.** Is the terror alert level high (orange) or severe (red)? Has there been a recent increase in violent political activism? Are you aware of any credible threats made against the location, gathering, or occasion?

Response Actions

Once you suspect that a terrorist event has occurred or WMDs have been used, there are certain actions to take to ensure that you will be safe and be in the proper position to help the community.

You are the Provider — Part 2

You and your partner are enjoying the music and interacting with passersby when you see, hear, and feel a significant explosion in the middle of the large crowd of spectators. A state of chaos ensues instantly as people are screaming and running in all directions.

4. What are your next actions?
5. How does the incident command system play a vital role in mass-casualty incidents?

EMT-I Tips

One of the easiest ways to distinguish between a nonterrorist mass-casualty event and a terrorist event is that the intentional use of a WMD affects multiple persons. These casualties will generally exhibit the same signs and symptoms. It is highly unlikely for more than one person to experience a seizure at any given time. It is not uncommon to find multiple patients complaining of difficulty breathing at the scene of a fire. However, the same report in the subway at rush hour, when no smell of smoke has been reported, is certainly cause for suspicion. In these situations, you must use good judgment and resist the urge to "rush in and help," especially when there are multiple victims from an unknown cause.

Scene Safety

Make sure that the scene is safe. If you have **any** doubt that it may not be safe, **do not enter**. When dealing with a WMD scene, it is safe to assume that you will not be able to enter where the event has occurred. Nor do you want to. The best location for staging is upwind and uphill from the incident. Wait for assistance from those who are trained in assessing and managing WMD scenes (Figure 37-5 ▼). Also remember:

- Failure to park your vehicle at a safe location can place you and your partner in danger (Figure 37-6 ▶).

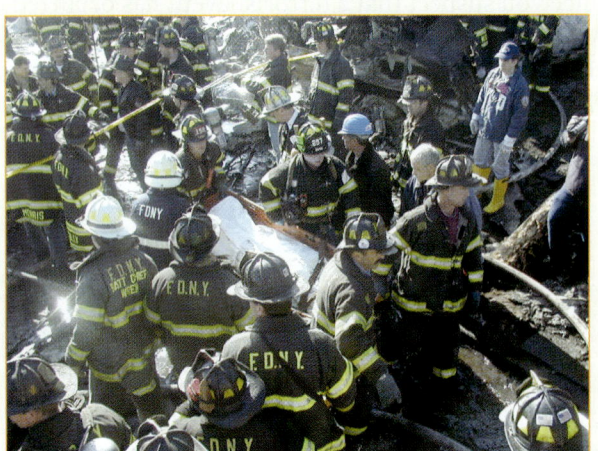

Figure 37-5 Improper staging of a mass-casualty scene could lead to injury or even death of EMS personnel. Wait for assistance from persons who are trained in assessing and managing such scenes.

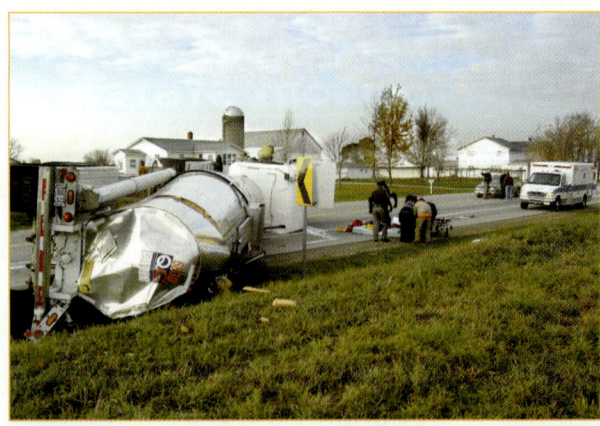

Figure 37-6 Park your vehicle at a safe location.

- If your vehicle is blocked in by other emergency vehicles or damaged by a secondary device (or event), you will be unable to provide victims with transportation (Figure 37-7 ▶) or escape yourself.

Responder Safety (Personnel Protection)

The best form of protection from a WMD agent is preventing yourself from coming into contact with the agent. The greatest threats facing an EMT-I in a WMD attack are contamination and **cross-contamination.** Contamination with an agent occurs when you have direct contact with the WMD or are exposed to it. Cross-contamination occurs when you come into contact with a contaminated person who has not yet been decontaminated.

Notification Procedures

When you suspect a terrorist or WMD event has taken place, notify the dispatcher, providing that communications function properly. Vital information needs to be communicated effectively if you are to receive the appropriate assistance (see Chapter 11 for information on effective communication). Inform dispatch of the nature of the event, any additional resources that may be required, the estimated number of patients, and the upwind route of approach or optimal route of approach.

It is extremely important to establish a staging area, where other units will converge. Be mindful of access and exit routes when you direct units to respond to a location. It is unwise to have units respond to the front entrance of a hotel or apartment building that has had an explosion (see Chapter 33 on vehicle positioning). Last, trained responders in the proper protective equipment are the only persons equipped to handle the WMD

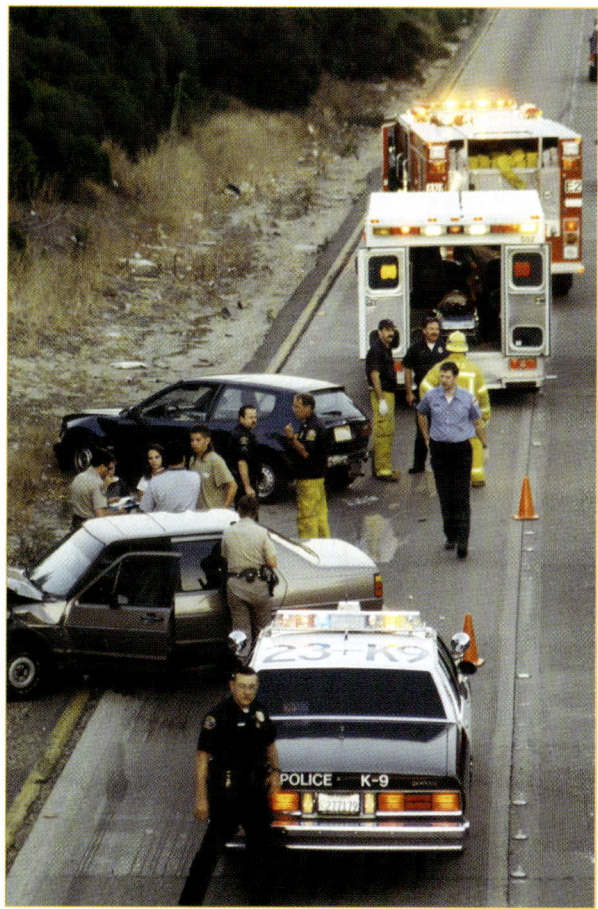

Figure 37-7 Make sure that your vehicle is not blocked in by other emergency vehicles. Parking in a way that prevents you from being able to leave the scene could become especially dangerous if a secondary device is used.

incident. These specialized units, traditionally hazardous materials (HazMat) teams, must be requested as early as possible due to the time required to assemble and dispatch the team and their equipment. Many jurisdictions share HazMat teams, and the team may have to travel a long distance to reach the location of the event. It is always better to be safe than sorry; call the team early and the outcome of the call will be more favorable.

Keep in mind that there may be more than one type of device or agent present.

Establishing Command

The first arriving provider on the scene must begin to sort out the chaos and define his or her responsibilities under the Incident Command System (ICS). As the first person on scene, the EMT-I may need to establish command until additional personnel arrive. Depending on the circumstances, you and other EMT-Is may function as med-

 Weapons of Mass Destruction

On September 11th, 2001, communications were severely affected by the collapse of the World Trade Center. The primary repeater was situated atop one of the towers. Additionally, excess radio traffic made transmitting and receiving messages extremely difficult. Not only was radio communications affected, but also most cellular phones and radio and television stations were disabled. The lesson learned is to have multiple backups to your ability to communicate with your dispatcher. In the event of a terrorist or WMD event, refrain from using the radio unless you have something important to transmit. If you do transmit, gather your thoughts and speak in as calm a tone as possible, avoiding unnecessary chatter. Remember, while you are transmitting, others may be unable to call for help.

ical branch officers, triage officers, treatment officers, transportation or logistic officers, or staff. If the ICS is already in place, you should immediately seek out the medical staging officer to receive your assignment.

Secondary Device or Event (Reassessing Scene Safety)

Terrorists have been known to plant additional explosives that are set to explode after the initial bomb. This type of <u>secondary device</u> is intended primarily to injure responders, and to secure media coverage, because the media generally arrives on scene just after the initial response. Do not rely on others to secure your safety. It is every EMT-I's responsibility to constantly assess and reassess the scene for safety. It is easy to overlook a suspicious package lying on the floor while you are treating casualties. **Stay alert.** Something as subtle as a change in the wind direction during a gas attack or an increase in the number of contaminated patients can place you in danger. Never become so involved with the tasks that you are performing that you do not look around and make sure that the scene remains safe.

 EMT-I Tips

Secondary devices may include various types of electronic equipment such as cell phones or pagers that are detonated when "answered."

> **EMT-I Tips**
>
> You are of no help to the public if you become a patient. More importantly, once you become a victim of the event, you place an additional burden on your fellow responders, who must treat you. Assess the scene and resist the urge to run in and help (do not develop tunnel vision). You may place your life and your partner in danger. Remember . . . **Don't become a victim.**

Chemical Agents

Chemical agents are liquids or gases that are dispersed to kill or injure. Modern-day chemicals were first developed during WWI and WWII. During the Cold War, many of these agents were perfected and stockpiled. While the United States has long renounced the use of chemical weapons, many nations still develop and stockpile them. These agents are deadly and pose a threat if acquired by terrorists.

Chemical weapons have several classifications. The properties or characteristics of an agent can be described as liquid, gas, or solid material. Persistency and volatility are terms used to describe how long the agent will stay on a surface before it evaporates. Persistent or nonvolatile agents can remain on a surface for long periods of time, usually longer than 24 hours. Nonpersistent or volatile agents evaporate relatively fast when left on a surface in the optimal temperature range. An agent that is described as highly persistent (such as VX, a nerve agent) can remain in the environment for weeks to months, whereas an agent that is highly volatile (such as sarin, also a nerve agent) will turn from liquid to gas (evaporate) within seconds to minutes.

Route of exposure is a term used to describe how the agent most effectively enters the body. Chemical agents can have either a vapor or contact hazard. Agents with a vapor hazard enter the body through the respiratory tract in the form of vapors. Agents with a contact hazard (skin hazard) give off very little vapor or no vapors and enter the body through the skin.

Vesicants (Blister Agents)

The primary route of exposure of blister agents, or vesicants, is the skin (contact); however, if vesicants are left on the skin or clothing long enough, they produce vapors that can enter the respiratory tract. Vesicants cause burn-like blisters to form on the victim's skin as well as in the respiratory tract. The vesicant agents consist of sulfur mustard (H), Lewisite (L), and phosgene oxime (CX) (the symbols H, L, and CX are military designations for these chemicals). The vesicants usually cause the most damage to damp or moist areas of the body, such as the armpits, groin, and respiratory tract. Signs of vesicant exposure on the skin include:

- Skin irritation, burning, and reddening
- Immediate intense skin pain (with L and CX)
- Formation of large blisters
- Gray discoloration of skin (a sign of permanent damage seen with L and CX)
- Swollen and closed or irritated eyes
- Permanent eye injury (including blindness)

If vapors were inhaled, the patient may experience the following:

- Hoarseness and stridor
- Severe cough
- Hemoptysis (coughing up of blood)
- Severe dyspnea

Sulfur mustard (agent H) is a brownish, yellowish oily substance that is generally considered very persist-

---

You are the Provider — Part 3

You can't believe what you are seeing and are stunned briefly. You take a deep breath to regain your composure and focus on the tasks at hand. You immediately notify dispatch of the explosion and request all available resources. Because you are unsure of exactly what occurred, you choose to refrain from entering the immediate area.

6. What are some reasons you should not rush into the area of explosion?
7. What else should you immediately do besides notifying the dispatch center?

ent. When released, mustard has the distinct smell of garlic or mustard and is quickly absorbed into the skin and/or mucous membranes. As the agent is absorbed into the skin, it begins an irreversible process of damage to the cells. Absorption through the skin or mucous membranes usually occurs within seconds, and damage to the underlying cells takes place within 1 to 2 minutes.

Mustard is considered a mutagen, which means that it mutates, damages, and changes the structures of cells. Eventually, cellular death will occur. On the surface, the patient will generally not produce any signs or symptoms until 4 to 6 hours after exposure (depending on concentration and amount of exposure) Figure 37-8.

The patient will develop a progressive reddening of the affected area, which will gradually develop into large blisters. These blisters are very similar in shape and appearance to those associated with thermal second-degree burns. The fluid within the blisters does not contain any of the agent; however, the skin covering the area is considered to be contaminated until decontamination by trained personnel has been performed.

Mustard also attacks vulnerable cells within the bone marrow and depletes the body's ability to produce white blood cells. As with burns, the primary complication associated with vesicant blisters is secondary infection. If the patient does survive the initial direct injury from the agent, the depletion of the white blood cells leaves the patient with a decreased resistance to infections. Although sulfur mustard is regarded as persistent, it does release enough vapors when dispersed to be inhaled. This creates upper and lower airway compromise. The result is damage and swelling of the airways. The airway compromise makes the patient's condition far more serious.

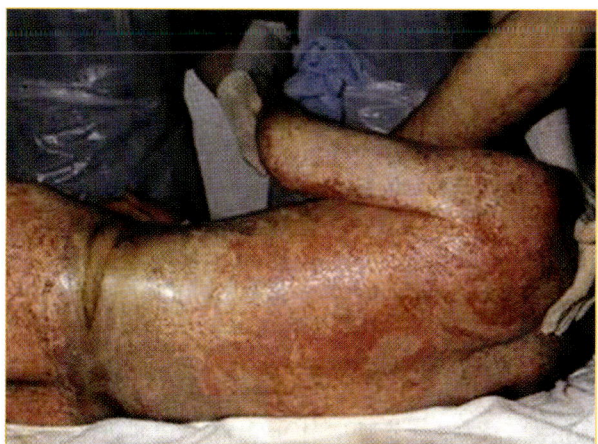

Figure 37-8 Skin damage resulting from exposure to sulfur mustard (agent H).

Lewisite (L) and phosgene oxime (CX) produce blister wounds very similar to mustard. They are highly volatile and have a rapid onset of symptoms, as opposed to the delayed onset seen with mustard. These agents produce immediate intense pain and discomfort when contact is made. The patient may have a grayish discoloration at the contaminated site. While tissue damage also occurs with exposure to these agents, they do not cause the secondary cellular injury that is associated with mustard.

Vesicant Agent Treatment

There are no antidotes for mustard or CX exposure. BAL (British Anti-Lewisite) is the antidote for agent L; however, it is not carried by civilian EMS. The EMT-I must ensure that the patient has been decontaminated before ABCs are initiated. The patient may require prompt airway support if any agent has been inhaled, but this should not occur until after decontamination. Gain IV access and initiate transport as soon as possible. Generally, burn centers are best equipped to handle the wounds and subsequent infections produced by vesicants. Follow your local protocols when deciding what facility to transport the patient to.

Place the patient on the cardiac monitor, consider early intubation if needed, and consider administering analgesics for pain according to local protocols.

Pulmonary Agents (Choking Agents)

The pulmonary agents are gases that cause immediate harm to persons exposed to them. The primary route of exposure for these agents is through the respiratory tract, which makes them an inhalation or vapor hazard. Once inside the lungs, they damage the lung tissue and fluid leaks into the lungs. Pulmonary edema develops in the patient, resulting in difficulty breathing due to the inability for air exchange. These agents produce respiratory-related symptoms such as dyspnea, tachypnea, and pulmonary edema. This class of chemical agents consists of chlorine (CL) and phosgene.

Chlorine (CL) was the first chemical agent ever used in warfare. It has a distinct odor of bleach and creates a green haze when released as a gas. Initially it produces upper airway irritation and a choking sensation. The patient may later experience:

- Shortness of breath
- Chest tightness
- Hoarseness and stridor due to upper airway constriction
- Gasping and coughing

With serious exposures, patients may develop pulmonary edema, complete airway constriction, and death. The fumes from a mixture of household bleach and ammonia create an acid gas that produces similar effects. Each year, such mixtures overcome hundreds of people when they try to mix household cleaners.

Phosgene should not be confused with phosgene oxime, a blistering agent, or vesicant. Not only has phosgene been produced for chemical warfare, but it is a product of combustion that might be produced in a fire at a textile factory or house, or from metalwork or burning Freon (a liquid chemical used in refrigeration). Therefore, you may encounter a victim of exposure to this gas during the course of a normal call or at a fire scene. Phosgene is a very potent agent that has a delayed onset of symptoms, usually hours. Unlike bleach, when phosgene enters the body, it generally does not produce severe irritation, which would possibly cause the victim to leave the area or hold his or her breath. In fact, the odor produced by the chemical is similar to that of freshly mown grass or hay. The result is that much more of the gas is allowed to enter the body unnoticed. The initial symptoms of a mild exposure may include:

- Nausea
- Chest tightness
- Severe cough
- Dyspnea upon exertion

The victim of a severe exposure may present with dyspnea at rest, and excessive pulmonary edema (the patient will actually expel large amounts of pulmonary edema from his or her lungs). The pulmonary edema that is seen with a severe exposure produces such large amounts of fluid from the lungs that the patient may actually become hypovolemic and subsequently hypotensive.

Pulmonary Agent Treatment

The best initial treatment for any pulmonary agent is to remove the patient from the contaminated atmosphere. This should be done by trained personnel in the proper PPE. Aggressive management of the ABCs should be initiated, paying particular attention to oxygenation, ventilation, and suctioning if required. **Do not allow the patient to be active, as this will worsen the condition much faster**. There are no antidotes to counteract the pulmonary agents. Performing the ABCs, gaining IV access, allowing the patient to rest in a position of comfort with the head elevated, and initiating rapid transport are the primary goals for prehospital emergency care.

Place the patient on a cardiac monitor and consider early intubation if needed to maintain the airway.

Nerve Agents

The nerve agents are among the most deadly chemicals developed. Designed to kill large numbers of people with small quantities, nerve agents can cause cardiac arrest within seconds to minutes of exposure. Nerve agents, discovered while in search of a superior pesticide, are a class of chemical called organophosphates, which are found in household bug sprays, agricultural pesticides, and some industrial chemicals, at far lower strengths than in nerve agents. Organophosphates block an essential enzyme in the parasympathetic nervous system, which cause the body's organs to become over stimulated and burn out.

G agents came from the early nerve agents, the G series, which were developed by German scientists (hence the G) in the period after WWI and into WWII. There are three G series agents, which are all designed with the same basic chemical structure with slight variations to produce different properties. The two variations of these agents are lethality and volatility. The following G agents are listed from high volatility to low volatility:

- Sarin (GB): Highly volatile colorless and odorless liquid. Turns from liquid to gas within seconds to minutes at room temperature. Highly lethal, with an LD_{50} of 1,700 mg/70 kg (about 1 drop, depending on the purity). The LD_{50} is the amount that will kill 50% of people who are exposed to this level. Sarin is primarily a vapor hazard, with the respiratory tract as the main route of entry. This agent is especially dangerous in enclosed environments such as office buildings, shopping malls, or subway cars. When this agent comes into contact with skin, it is quickly absorbed and evaporates. When sarin is on clothing, it has the effect of off-gassing, which means that the vapors are continuously released over a period of time (like perfume). This renders the victim as well as the victim's clothing contaminated.
- Soman (GD): Twice as persistent as sarin and five times as lethal. It has a fruity odor as a result of the type of alcohol used in the agent and generally has no color. This agent is both a contact and inhalation hazard that can enter the body through skin absorption and through the respiratory tract. A unique additive in GD causes it to bind to the cells that it attacks faster than any other agent. This irreversible binding is called aging, which makes it more difficult to treat patients who have been exposed.

- **Tabun (GA)**: Approximately half as lethal as sarin and 36 times more persistent; under the proper conditions it will remain for several days. It also has a fruity smell and an appearance similar to sarin. The components used to manufacture GA are easy to acquire and the agent is easy to manufacture, which make it unique. GA is both a contact and inhalation hazard that can enter the body through skin absorption as well as through the respiratory tract.
- **V agent (VX)**: Clear oily agent that has no odor and looks like baby oil. V agent was developed by the British after WWII and has similar chemical properties to the G series agents. The difference is that VX is over 100 times more lethal than sarin and is extremely persistent Figure 37-9 . In fact, VX is so persistent that given the proper conditions it will remain relatively unchanged for weeks to months. These properties make VX primarily a contact hazard, because it lets off very little vapor. It is easily absorbed into the skin, and the oily residue that remains on the skin's surface is extremely difficult to decontaminate.

Nerve agents all produce similar symptoms, but have varying routes of entry. Nerve agents differ slightly in lethal concentration or dose and also differ in their volatility. Some agents are designed to become a gas quickly (nonpersistent or highly volatile), while others remain liquid for a period of time (persistent or nonvolatile). These agents have been used successfully in warfare and to date represent the only type of chemical agent that has been used successfully in a terrorist act. Once the agent has entered the body through skin contact or through the respiratory system, the patient will begin to exhibit a pattern of predictable symptoms. Like all chemical agents, the severity of the symptoms will depend on the route of exposure and the amount of agent to which the patient was exposed. The resulting symptoms are described in Table 37-1 using the military mnemonic SLUDGEM and the medical mnemonic DUMBELS. SLUDGEM/DUMBELS mnemonics are used to describe the symptoms of nerve agent exposure. The medical mnemonic is more useful to the EMT-I because it lists the more dangerous symptoms associated with exposure to nerve agents.

There are only a handful of medical conditions that are associated with the bilateral pinpoint constricted pupils (miosis) seen with nerve agent exposure. Conditions such as a cerebrovascular accident, direct light to both eyes, and a drug overdose all can cause bilateral constricted pupils. You should therefore assess the patient for all the SLUDGEM/DUMBELS signs and symptoms to determine whether the patient has been exposed to a nerve agent.

Miosis is the most common symptom of nerve agent exposure and can remain for days to weeks. This symptom, along with the others listed in Table 37-1, will help you recognize exposure to a nerve agent early. The seizures that are associated with nerve agent exposure are unlike those found in patients with a history of seizures. The patient will continue to seize until death or until treatment is given with a nerve agent antidote (MARK 1 or NAAK).

Nerve Agent Treatment (MARK 1/NAAK)

Fatalities from severe exposure occur as a result of respiratory complications, which lead to respiratory arrest. Once the patient has been decontaminated, the EMT-I should be prepared to treat these patients aggressively, if they are to be saved. You can greatly increase the patient's chances of survival simply by providing airway and ventilatory support. As with all emergencies, securing the ABCs is the best and most important treatment that you can provide. Often patients exposed to these agents will begin seizing and will not stop. These patients will require administration of nerve agent antidote kits in addition to support of the ABCs.

Fortunately, there is an antidote for nerve agent exposure. MARK 1 kits, also known as Nerve Agent Antidote Kits (NAAK), contain two autoinjector medications: atropine and 2-PAM chloride (pralidoxime chloride). In some regions, the EMT-I may carry MARK 1 kits on the unit and will be called upon to administer one or both of the antidotes. These medications are delivered using the same technique as the Epi-Pen autoinjector; however, multiple doses may need to be administered.

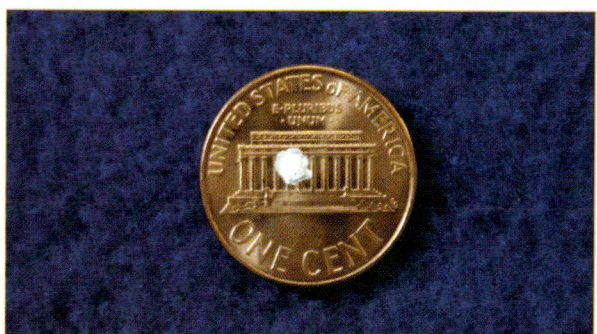

Figure 37-9 VX penny. VX is the most toxic chemical ever produced. The dot on the penny demonstrates the amount needed to achieve the lethal dose. Only a fraction of a drop is needed to kill.

TABLE 37-1	Symptoms of Persons Exposed to Nerve Agents
Military Mnemonic: SLUDGEM	**Medical Mnemonic: DUMBELS**
Salivation, **S**weating	**D**iarrhea
Lacrimation (excessive tearing)	**U**rination
Urination	**M**iosis (pinpoint pupils)
Defecation, **D**rooling, **D**iarrhea	**B**radycardia, **B**ronchospasm (spasm of the bronchioles)
Gastric upset and cramps	**E**mesis (vomiting)
Emesis (vomiting)	**L**acrimation (excessive tearing)
Muscle twitching	**S**eizures, **S**alivation, **S**weating

Atropine is used to block the nerve agent from affecting the parasympathetic nervous system. However, since the nerve agent may remain in the body for long periods of time, 2-PAM Cl is used to eliminate the agent from the body. Many of the symptoms described in the DUMBELS mnemonic will be reversed with the use of atropine; however, many doses may need to be administered to see these results. If your service carries a nerve agent antidote, please refer to your local protocols for dose and usage information.

Table 37-2 ▼ has been provided for quick reference and comparison of the nerve agents.

Industrial Chemicals/Insecticides

As previously mentioned, the basic chemical ingredient in nerve agents is organophosphate. This is a common chemical that is used in lesser concentrations for insecticides. While industrial chemicals do not possess sufficient lethality to be effective WMDs, they are easy to acquire, inexpensive, and would have similar effects as the nerve agents. Crop-duster planes could be used to disseminate these chemicals. You should be cautious when responding to calls where insecticide equipment is stored and used, such as a farm or supply store that sells these products. The symptoms and medical management of victims of organophosphate insecticide poisoning are identical to those of the nerve agents.

Metabolic Agents (Cyanides)

Hydrogen cyanide (AC) and cyanogen chloride (CK) are both agents that affect the body's ability to use oxygen. Cyanide is a colorless gas that has an odor similar to almonds. The effects of the cyanides begin on the cellular level and are very rapidly seen at the organ

TABLE 37-2	The Nerve Agents					
Name	Code Name	Odor	Special Features	Onset of Symptoms	Volatility	Route of Exposure
Tabun	GA	Fruity	Easy to manufacture	Immediate	Low	Both contact and vapor hazard
Sarin	GB	None (if pure) or strong	Nerve gas; will off-gas while on victim's clothing	Immediate	High	Primarily respiratory vapor hazard; extremely lethal if skin contact is made
Soman	GD	Fruity	Ages rapidly, making it difficult to treat	Immediate	Moderate	Contact with skin; minimal vapor hazard
V agent	VX	None	Most lethal chemical agent; difficult to decontaminate	Immediate	Very low	Contact with skin; no vapor hazard (unless aerosolized)

EMT-I Safety

On March 20th, 1995, members of a Japanese cult released sarin (GB) in the Tokyo subway. The first arriving medical responders were met with chaos as hundreds and then thousands of people fled the subway system Figure 37-10 ▶. Many were contaminated and showing signs and symptoms of nerve agent exposure. In the end, more than 5,000 people sought medical care for exposure to sarin, and 12 people had died. None of the EMS personnel wore protective clothing and most became cross-contaminated. Remember, you can avoid becoming exposed. Don't become a victim.

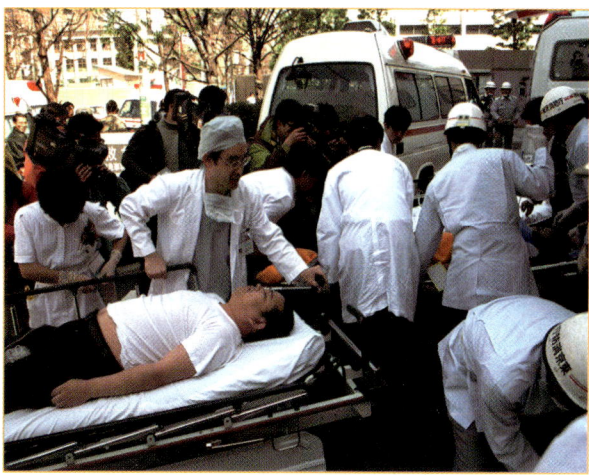

Figure 37-10 Medical professionals responding to an attack in 1995, where cult members released sarin in the Tokyo subway.

system level. Besides the nerve agents, metabolic agents are the only chemical weapons known to kill within seconds to minutes. Unlike nerve agents, however, these deadly gases are commonly found in many industrial settings. Cyanides are produced in massive quantities throughout the United States every year for industrial uses such as gold and silver mining, photography, lethal injections, and plastics processing. They are often present in fires associated with textile or plastic factories. In fact, cyanide is naturally found in the pits of many fruits in very low doses. There is very little difference in the symptoms found between AC and CK. In low doses, these chemicals are associated with dizziness, light-headedness, headache, and vomiting. Higher doses will produce symptoms that include:

- Shortness of breath and gasping respirations
- Tachypnea
- Flushed skin color
- Tachycardia
- Altered mental status
- Seizures
- Coma
- Apnea
- Cardiac arrest

The symptoms associated with the inhalation of a large amount of cyanide will all appear within several minutes. Death is likely unless the patient is treated promptly.

Cyanide Agent Treatment. Cyanide binds with the body's cells, preventing oxygen from being used. Several medications act as antidotes, but most services do not carry them. Once trained personnel in the proper PPE have removed the patient from the source of exposure, even if there is no liquid contamination, all of the patient's clothes must be removed to prevent off-gassing in the ambulance. Trained and protected personnel must decontaminate any patients who may have been exposed to liquid contamination before an EMT-I can initiate treatment. Then you should support the patient's ABCs and gain IV access. Mild effects of cyanide exposure will generally resolve by simply removing the victim from the source of contamination and administering supplemental oxygen. Severe exposure, however, will require aggressive oxygenation and perhaps ventilation with supplemental oxygen. **Always use a BVM device or oxygen-powered ventilator device to ventilate a victim of a metabolic agent.** The agent can easily be passed on from the patient to the EMT-I through mouth to mouth or mouth-to-mask ventilations. If no antidote is available, initiate transport immediately.

Place the patient on the cardiac monitor and consider early intubation to maintain the airway.

Table 37-3 ▶ summarizes the chemical agents. The odors of the particular chemicals are provided for informational purposes only. The sense of smell is a poor tool to use to determine whether there is a chemical agent present. Many persons are unable to smell the agents, and the odor could be derived from another source. This information is useful to you if you receive reports from victims claiming to smell of bleach or garlic, for example. You should never enter a potentially hazardous area and "smell" to determine if there is a chemical agent present.

> **EMT-I Safety**
>
> Always make sure that your patients have been thoroughly decontaminated by trained personnel before you come into contact with them. Chemical agents are primarily a vapor hazard, and all of the patient's clothing must still be removed to prevent off-gassing. Finally, never perform mouth-to-mouth or mouth-to-mask ventilation on a victim of a chemical agent. Many of the vapors may linger in the patient's airway and cross-contamination may occur.

Biological Agents

Biological agents pose many difficult issues when used as a WMD. Biological agents can be almost completely undetectable. Also, most of the diseases caused by these agents will be similar to other minor illnesses commonly seen by EMS providers.

Biological agents are grouped as viruses, bacterium, or neurotoxins and may be spread in various ways. **Dissemination** is the means by which a terrorist will spread the agent—for example, poisoning the water supply or aerosolizing the agent into the air or ventilation system of a building. A **disease vector** is an animal that spreads disease, once infected, to another animal. For example, the plague can be spread by infected rats, smallpox by infected persons, and West Nile virus by infected mosquitoes. How easily the disease is able to spread from one human to another human is called **communicability**. Some diseases, such as those caused by the human immunodeficiency virus, are difficult to spread by routine contact. Therefore, communicability is considered low. In other instances when communicability is high, such as with smallpox, the person is considered **contagious**. Typically, routine BSI precautions are enough to prevent contamination from contagious biological organisms.

Incubation describes the period of time between exposure to the agent and when symptoms begin.

TABLE 37-3 Chemical Agents

Class	Military Designations	Odor	Lethality	Onset of Symptoms	Volatility	Primary Route of Exposure
Nerve agents	Tabun (GA) Sarin (GB) Soman (GD) VX	Fruity or none	Most lethal chemical agents; can kill within minutes; effects are reversible with antidotes	Immediate	Moderate (GB, GD) Very high (GB) Low (VX)	GA—both GB—vapor hazard GD—both VX—contact hazard
Vesicants	Mustard (H Lewisite (L) Phosgene oxime (CX)	Garlic (H) Geranium (L)	Causes large blisters to form on victims; may severely damage upper airway if vapors are inhaled; severe intense pain and grayish skin discoloration (L and CX)	Delayed (H) Immediate (L, CX)	Very low (H, L) Moderate (CX)	Primarily contact with some vapor hazard
Pulmonary agents	Chlorine (CL) Phosgene (CG)	Bleach (CL) Cut grass (CG)	Causes irritation choking (CL); severe pulmonary edema (CG)	Immediate (CL) Delayed (CG)	Very high	Vapor hazard
Cyanide agents	Hydrogen cyanide (AC) Cyanogen chloride (CK)	Almonds (AC) Irritating (CK)	Highly lethal chemical gases; can kill within minutes; effects are reversible with antidotes	Immediate	Very high	Vapor hazard

The incubation period is especially important for the EMT-I to understand. Although your patient may not exhibit signs or symptoms, he or she may be contagious.

EMT-Is need to be aware of when they should suspect the use of biological agents. If the agent is in the form of a powder, such as in the October 2001 attacks involving anthrax powder mailed in letters, the incident must be handled by HazMat specialists. Patients who have come into direct contact with the agent need to be decontaminated before any EMS contact or treatment is initiated.

Viruses

Viruses are germs that require a living host to multiply and survive. A virus is a simple organism and cannot thrive outside of a host (living body). Once in the body, the virus will invade healthy cells and replicate itself to spread through the host. As the virus spreads, so does the disease that it carries. Viruses survive by moving from one host to another by using its transport system—vectors.

Viral agents that may be used during a biological terrorist release pose an extraordinary problem for health care providers, especially those in EMS. Although some viral agents do have vaccines, there is no treatment for a viral infection. Because of this characteristic, the following viruses have been used as terrorist agents.

Smallpox

Smallpox is a highly contagious disease. All forms of BSI precautions must be used to prevent cross-contamination to health care providers. Simply by wearing examination gloves, a HEPA-filtered respirator, and eye protection, you will greatly reduce your risk of contamination. The last natural case of smallpox in the world was seen in 1977. Before the rash and blisters show, the illness will start with a high fever and body aches and headaches. The fever is usually in the range of 101° to 104°F.

An easy and quick way to differentiate the smallpox rash from other skin disorders is to observe the size, shape, and location of the lesions. In smallpox, all the lesions are identical in their development. In other skin disorders, the lesions will be in various stages of healing and development. Smallpox blisters also begin on the face and extremities and eventually move toward the chest and abdomen. The disease is in its most contagious phase when the blisters begin to form (Figure 37-11). Unprotected contact with these blisters will promote transmission of the disease. There is a vaccine to prevent smallpox; however, it has been linked to medical complications and in very rare cases death (Table 37-4).

Viral Hemorrhagic Fevers

Viral hemorrhagic fevers (VHF) consist of a group of diseases that include the Ebola, Rift Valley, and Yellow Fever viruses, among others. This group of viruses causes the blood in the body to seep out from the tissues and blood vessels (Figure 37-12). Initially, the patient will have flu-like symptoms, progressing to more serious symptoms such as internal and external hemorrhaging. Outbreaks are not uncommon in Africa and South America. Outbreaks in the United States, however, are extremely rare. All BSI precautions must be taken when treating illnesses of this nature. Mor-

You are the Provider   Part 4

You evaluate the area from a distance using binoculars. The entire department has been activated along with three other mutual aid agencies. State resources have also been requested and you have directed the walking wounded to a safe triage area via your ambulance's loudspeaker. Information from local law enforcement indicates this was a backpack bomb filled with shrapnel. No signs of alternate chemical or biological agents exist. You then direct personnel (after addressing safety issues) to begin triage and treatment of patients.

8. Why is it important to direct the walking wounded to another location?
9. Where should you create a staging area for responding personnel and apparatus?

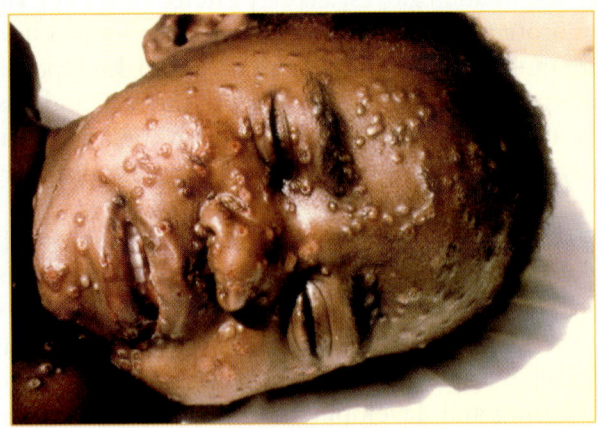

Figure 37-11 In smallpox, all the lesions are identical in their development. In other skin disorders, the lesions will be in various stages of healing and development.

tality rates can range from 5% to 90%, depending on the strain of virus, the victim's age and health condition, and the availability of a modern health care system (Table 37-5).

Bacteria

Unlike viruses, <u>bacteria</u> do not require a host to multiply and live. Bacteria are much more complex and larger than viruses and can grow up to 100 times larger than the largest virus. Bacteria contain all the cellular structures of a normal cell and are completely self-sufficient. Most importantly, bacterial infections can be fought with antibiotics.

Most bacterial infections will generally begin with flu-like symptoms, which make it quite difficult to identify whether the cause is a biological attack or a natural epidemic. Biological agents have been developed and used for centuries during times of war.

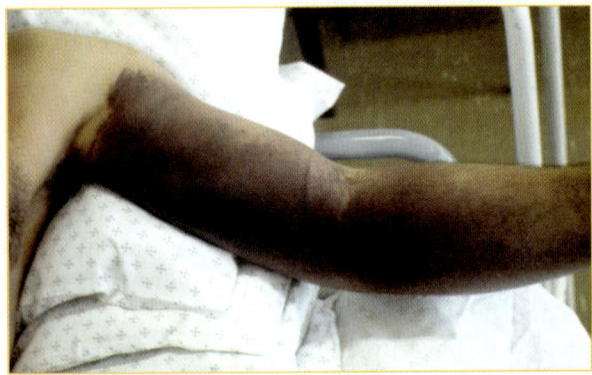

Figure 37-12 Viral hemorrhagic fevers cause the blood vessels and tissues to seep blood. The end result is ecchymosis, hemoptysis, and blood in the patient's stool. Notice the severe discoloration in this patient with Crimean Congo hemorrhagic fever, indicating internal bleeding.

> **EMT-I Tips**
>
> Because humans are acceptable hosts and vectors for many viruses and bacteria, it is important for the EMT-I to use BSI precautions at all times. If you fail to use BSI precautions you may not only become a host for a virus, but you may spread it as well. Remember, a virus moves from person to person to survive, and many infectious diseases present like common colds.

TABLE 37-4	Characteristics of Smallpox
Dissemination	Aerosolized for warfare or terrorist uses
Communicability	High from infected individuals or items (such as blankets used by infected patients). Person-to-person transmission is possible.
Route of entry	Through inhalation of coughed droplets or direct skin contact with blisters
Signs and symptoms	Severe fever, malaise, body and headaches, small blisters on the skin, bleeding of the skin and mucous membranes. Incubation period is 10 to 12 days and the duration of the illness is approximately 4 weeks.
Medical management	BSI. There is no specific treatment for smallpox. Patients should be provided supportive care (ABCs).

Inhalation and Cutaneous Anthrax (*Bacillus anthracis*)

Anthrax is a deadly bacterium that lays dormant in a spore (protective shell). When exposed to the optimal temperature and moisture, the germ will be released from the spore. The routes of entry for anthrax are inhalation, cutaneous, or gastrointestinal (from consuming food that contains spores) (Figure 37-13 ▶). The inhalational form or pulmonary anthrax is the most deadly and often presents as a severe cold. Pulmonary anthrax infections are associated with a 90% death rate if untreated. Antibiotics can be used to treat anthrax successfully. There is also a vaccine to prevent anthrax infections (Table 37-6 ▶).

Plague (Bubonic/Pneumonic)

Of all the infectious diseases known to humans, none has killed as many as the plague. The 14th century plague that ravaged Asia, the Middle East, and finally Europe (the Black Death) killed an estimated 33 to 42 million people. Later on, in the early 19th century, almost 20 million in India and China perished due to plague. The plague's natural vectors are infected rodents and fleas. When a person is either bit by an infected flea or comes into contact with an infected rodent (or the waste of the rodent), the person can contract bubonic plague.

Bubonic plague infects the lymphatic system (a passive circulatory system in the body that bathes the tissues in lymph and works with the immune system). When this occurs, the patient's lymph nodes (area of the lymphatic system where infection-fighting cells are housed) become infected and grow. The glands of the

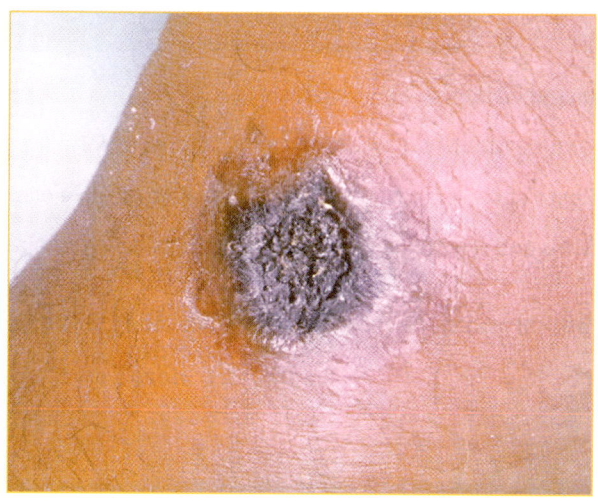

Figure 37-13 Cutaneous anthrax.

nodes will grow large (up to the size of a tennis ball) and round, forming buboes (Figure 37-14 ▶). If left untreated, the infection may spread through the body, leading to sepsis and possibly death. This form of plague is not contagious and is not likely to be seen in a bioterrorist incident.

Pneumonic plague is a lung infection, also known as plague pneumonia, that results from inhalation of plague bacteria. This form of the disease is contagious and has a much higher death rate than the bubonic form. This form of plague (aerosolized) therefore would be easier to disseminate and has a higher mortality (Table 37-7 ▶).

TABLE 37-5	Characteristics of Viral Hemorrhagic Fevers
Dissemination	Direct contact with an infected person's body fluids. It can also be aerosolized for use in an attack.
Communicability	Moderate from person to person, or contaminated items
Route of entry	Direct contact with an infected person's body fluids
Signs and symptoms	Sudden onset of fever, weakness, muscle pain, headache, and sore throat. All of these symptoms are followed by vomiting and as the virus runs it course, internal and external bleeding.
Medical management	BSI. There is no specific treatment for viral hemorrhagic fever. Patients should be provided supportive care (ABCs) and treatment for shock and hypotension, if present.

TABLE 37-6	Characteristics of Anthrax
Dissemination	Aerosol
Communicability	Only in the cutaneous form (rare)
Route of entry	Through inhalation of spore or skin contact with spore or direct contact with skin wound (cutaneous)
Signs and symptoms	Flu-like symptoms, fever, respiratory distress with tachycardia, shock, pulmonary edema and respiratory failure after 3-5 days of flu-like symptoms
Medical management	Pulmonary/Inhalation: BSI, oxygen, ventilatory support if in pulmonary edema or respiratory failure and transport. Cutaneous: BSI, apply dry sterile dressing to prevent accidental contact with wound and fluids.

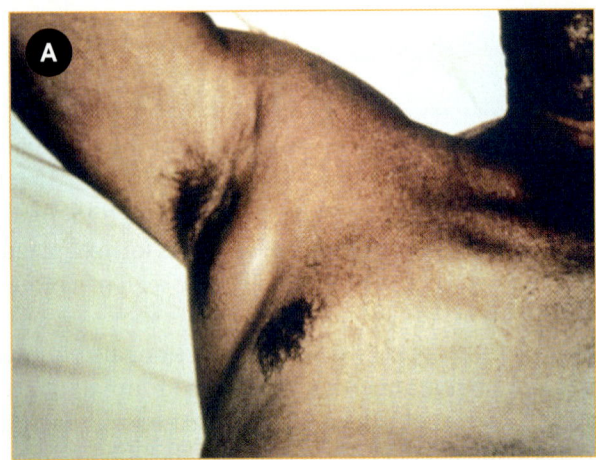

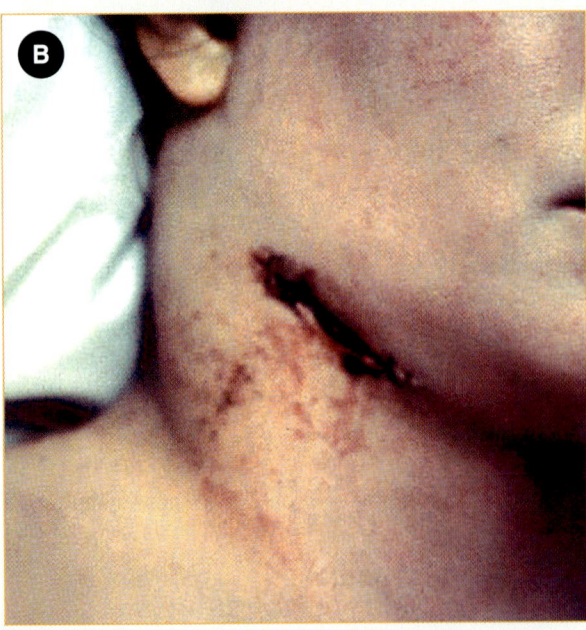

Figure 37-14 A. Plague buboe at lymph node under arm. B. Plague buboe at lymph node on neck.

Neurotoxins

Neurotoxins are the most deadly substances known to humans. The strongest neurotoxin is 15,000 times more lethal than VX and 100,000 times more lethal than sarin. These toxins are produced from plants, marine animals, molds, and bacteria. The route of entry for these toxins is through ingestion, inhalation from aerosols, or injection. Unlike viruses and bacteria, neurotoxins are not contagious and have a faster onset of symptoms. Although these biological toxins have immense destructive potential, they have not been used successfully as a WMD.

Botulinum Toxin

The most potent neurotoxin is botulinum, which is produced by bacteria. When introduced into the body, this neurotoxin affects the nervous system's ability to function. Voluntary muscle control will diminish as the toxin spreads. Eventually the toxin will cause muscle paralysis that begins at the head and face and travels downward throughout the body. The patient's accessory muscles and diaphragm will become paralyzed, and the patient will go into respiratory arrest (Table 37-8 ▶).

Ricin

While not as deadly as botulinum, ricin is still five times more lethal than VX. This toxin is derived from mash that is left from the castor bean (Figure 37-15 ▶). When introduced into the body, ricin causes pulmonary edema and respiratory and circulatory failure leading to death (Table 37-9 ▶).

(Table 37-10 ▶) summarizes the biological agents.

TABLE 37-7 Characteristics of Plague

Dissemination	Aerosol
Communicability	Bubonic: low, only from contact with fluid in a buboe Pneumonic: high, from person to person
Route of entry	Ingestion, inhalation, or cutaneous
Signs and symptoms	Fever, headache, muscle pain and tenderness, pneumonia, shortness of breath, extreme lymph node pain and enlargement (bubonic)
Medical management	BSI, ABCs, provide oxygen, and transport

TABLE 37-8 Characteristics of Botulinum Toxin

Dissemination	Aerosol or food supply sabotage or injection
Communicability	None
Route of entry	Ingestion or gastrointestinal
Signs and symptoms	Dry mouth, intestinal obstruction, urinary retention, constipation, nausea and vomiting, abnormal pupil dilation, blurred vision, double vision, drooping eyelids, difficulty swallowing, difficulty speaking, and respiratory failure due to paralysis
Medical management	ABCs, provide oxygen, and transport. Ventilatory support may be needed due to paralysis of the respiratory muscles. A vaccine is available.

Other EMT-I Roles During a Biological Event

Syndromic Surveillance

Syndromic surveillance is the monitoring, usually by local or state health departments, of patients presenting to emergency departments and alternative care facilities, the recording of EMS call volume, and monitoring the use of over-the-counter medications. Patients with signs and symptoms that resemble influenza are particularly important. Local and state health departments monitor for an unusual influx of patients with these symptoms in hopes of catching an outbreak early. The EMS role in syndromic surveillance is a small one, yet valuable in the overall tracking of a biological terrorist event or infectious disease outbreak. Quality assurance and dispatch operations need to be aware of an unusual number of calls from patients with "unexplainable flu" coming from a particular region or community.

Points of Distribution (Strategic National Stockpile)

Points of distribution (PODs) are strategically placed facilities that have been preestablished for the mass distribution of antibiotics, antidotes, vaccinations, with

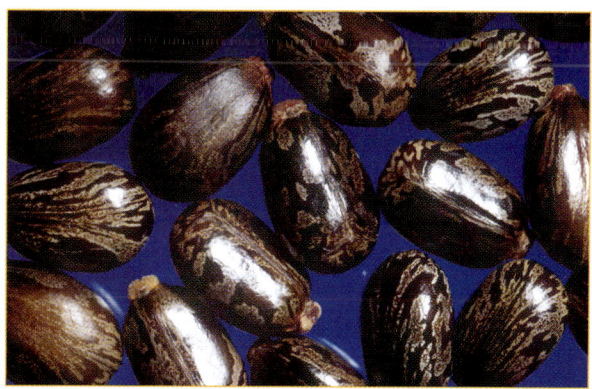

Figure 37-15 These seemingly harmless castor beans contain the key ingredient for ricin, one of the most potent toxins known to humans.

TABLE 37-9	Characteristics of Ricin
Dissemination	Aerosol or contamination of a food or water supply by sabotage
Communicability	None
Route of entry	Inhalation, ingestion, injection
Signs and symptoms	Inhaled: Cough, difficulty breathing, chest tightness, nausea, muscle aches, pulmonary edema, and hypoxia Ingested: Nausea and vomiting, internal bleeding, and death Injection: No signs except swelling at the injection site and death
Medical management	ABCs. No treatment or vaccine exists.

TABLE 37-10 Biological Agents

Disease	Transmission Person to Person	Incubation Period	Duration of Illness	Lethality (approximate case fatality rates)
Inhalation anthrax	No	1-6 d	3-5 d (usually fatal if untreated)	High
Pneumonic plague	High	2-3 d	1-6 d (usually fatal)	High unless treated within 12-24 h
Smallpox	High	7-17 d (average 12 d)	4 wk	High to moderate
Viral hemorrhagic fevers	Moderate	4-21 d	Death between 7-16 d	High to moderate, depending on type of VHF
Botulism	No	1-5 d	Death in 24-72 h; lasts months if patient does not die	High without respiratory support
Ricin	No	18-24 h	Days—death within 10-12 d for ingestion	High

You are the Provider — Part 5

Because you requested all available resources early on, established incident command, and did not become part of the problem by allowing your emotions to control your actions, the situation was well handled. It was later found out that this backpack bomb was detonated via cellular phone by a disturbed individual with no ties to domestic or foreign terrorists.

10. If this event involved the use of organophosphates, how would it affect this scenario?
11. What would likely be an issue with organophosphate poisoning?

other medications and supplies. These medications may be delivered in large containers known as "push packs" by the Centers for Disease Control and Prevention National Pharmaceutical Stockpile Figure 37-16. These containers have a delivery time of 12 hours anywhere in the country and contain antibiotics, chemical antidotes, antitoxins, life-support medications, IV administration supplies, airway maintenance supplies, and medical/surgical items. In some regions, local and state municipalities have started to stockpile their own supplies to reduce the time delay.

EMT-Is and paramedics may be called on to assist in the delivery of the medications to the public (depending on local emergency management planning). The EMT-I's role may include triage, treatment of seriously ill patients, and patient transport to the hospital. Most plans for PODs include at least one ambulance on standby for the transport of seriously ill patients.

Radiological/Nuclear Devices

What Is Radiation?

Ionizing radiation is energy that is emitted in the form of rays, or particles. This energy can be found in radioactive material, such as rocks and metals. Radioactive material is any material that emits radiation. This material is unstable, and attempts to stabilize itself by changing its structure is a natural process called decay. As the substance decays, it gives off radiation, until it stabilizes. The process of radioactive decay can take from as little as minutes to billions of years; meanwhile, the substance remains radioactive.

The energy that is emitted from a strong radiological source can be either alpha, beta, gamma (x-rays), or neutron radiation. Alpha is the least harmful penetrating type of radiation and cannot travel fast or through most objects. In fact, a sheet of paper or the body's skin easily stops it. Beta radiation is slightly more penetrating than alpha, and requires a layer of clothing to stop it. Gamma or x-rays are far faster and stronger than alpha and beta rays. These rays easily penetrate through the human body and require either several inches of lead or concrete to prevent penetration. Neutron energy is the fastest moving and most powerful form of radiation. Neutrons easily penetrate through lead and require several feet of concrete to stop them Figure 37-17.

Sources of Radiological Material

There are thousands of radioactive materials found on the earth. These materials are generally used for purposes that benefit humankind, such as medicine, killing germs in food (irradiating), and construction work. Once radiological material has been used for its purpose, the material remaining is called radiological waste. Radiological waste remains radioactive, but has no more usefulness. These materials can be found at:

- Hospitals
- Colleges and universities
- Chemical and industrial sites

Not all radioactive material is tightly guarded, and the waste is often not guarded. This makes the use of radioactive material and substances appealing to terrorists.

Radiological Dispersal Devices (RDD)

A radiological dispersal device (RDD) is any container that is designed to disperse radioactive material. This would generally require the use of a bomb, hence the nickname "dirty bomb." A dirty bomb would carry the potential to injure victims with not only the radioactive material but the explosive material used to deliver it. Just the thought of an RDD creates fear in a population, and so the ultimate goal of the terrorist—fear—is accom-

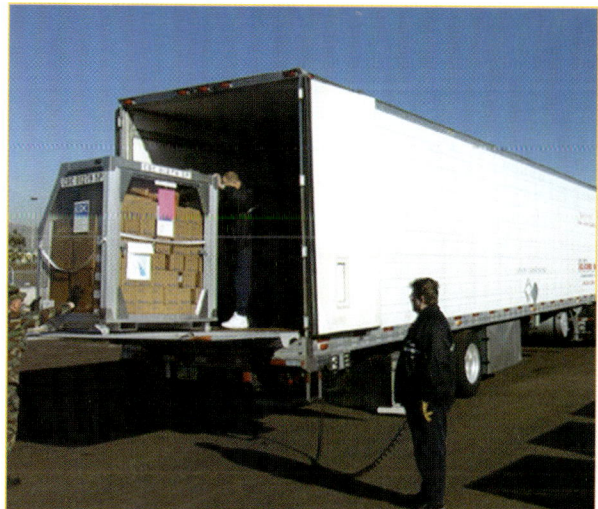

Figure 37-16 The Centers for Disease Control and Prevention Strategic National Stockpile can deliver one of many push packs to any location in the country within 12 hours of an emergency.

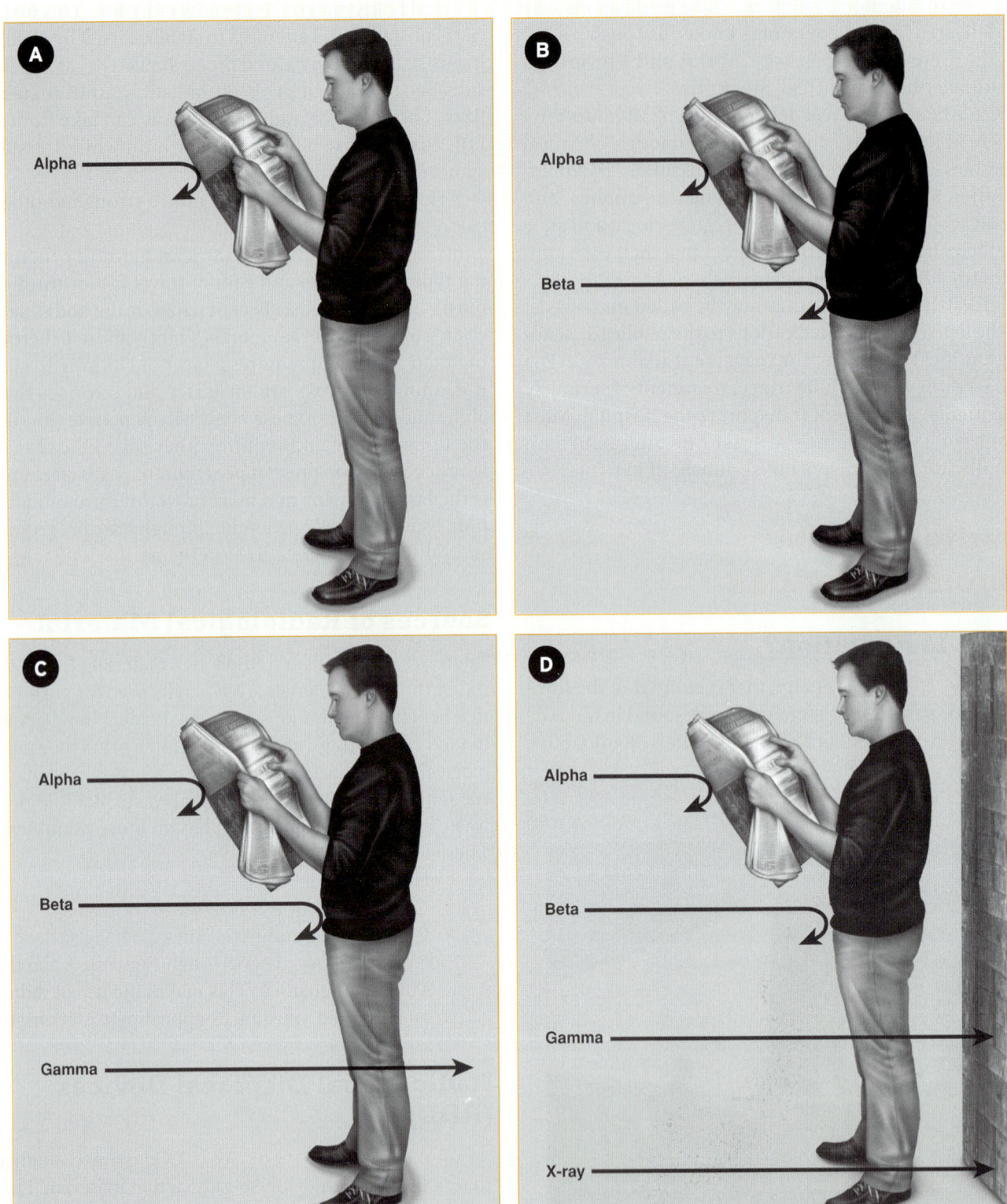

Figure 37-17 The penetrating potential of four different types of radiation. **A.** Alpha. **B.** Beta. **C.** Gamma. **D.** X-ray.

plished. In reality, however, the destructive capability of a dirty bomb is limited to the explosives that are attached to it. Therefore, if the explosive is sufficient to kill 10 persons without radioactive material, it will also kill 10 persons with the radioactive material added. There may be long-term injuries and illness associated with the use of an RDD, yet not much more than the bomb by itself would create. In short, the dirty bomb is an ineffective WMD.

Nuclear Energy

Nuclear energy is artificially made by altering (splitting) radioactive atoms. The result is an immense amount of energy that usually takes the form of heat. Nuclear material is used in medicine, weapons, naval vessels, and power plants. Nuclear material gives off all forms of radiation, including neutrons (the most deadly type). Like radioactive material, when nuclear material is no longer useful, it becomes waste that is still radioactive.

Nuclear Weapons

The destructive energy of a nuclear explosion is unlike any other weapon in the world. That is why nuclear weapons are kept only in secure facilities throughout the world. There are nations that have ties to terrorists and that have actively attempted to build nuclear weapons. Yet the ability of these nations to deliver a nuclear weapon, such as a missile or bomb, is as of yet, incomplete. There is also the deterrent of complete mutual annihilation. Therefore, the likelihood of a nuclear attack is extremely remote.

Unfortunately, however, due to the collapse of the former Soviet Union, the whereabouts of many small nuclear devices is unknown. These small suitcase-sized nuclear weapons are called Special Atomic Demolition Munitions (SADM). The SADM, or "suit-case nuke," was designed to destroy individual targets, such as important buildings, bridges, tunnels, or large ships. The estimate is that perhaps as many as 80 are missing as of 1998. No other information or updates on the whereabouts of these devices have been made public.

Symptomology

The effects of radiation exposure will vary depending on the amount of radiation that a person receives and the route of entry. Radiation can be introduced into the body by all routes of entry as well as through the body (irradiation). The patient can inhale radioactive dust from nuclear fallout or from a dirty bomb, or have radioactive liquid absorbed into the body through the skin. Once in the body, the radiation source will irradiate the person from within rather than from an external source (such as x-ray equipment). Some common signs of acute radiation sickness are listed in Table 37-11. Additional injuries will occur with a nuclear blast such as thermal and blast trauma, trauma from flying objects, and eye injuries.

Medical Management

Being exposed to a radiation source does not make a patient contaminated or radioactive. However, when patients have a radioactive source on their body (such as debris from a dirty bomb), they are contaminated and must be initially cared for by a HazMat responder. Once the patient is decontaminated and there is no threat to you, you may begin treatment with the ABCs and treat the patient for any burns or trauma.

Protective Measures

There are no suits or protective gear designed to completely shield from radiation. Those who work in high-risk areas do wear some protection (lead-lined suits); however this equipment is not available to the EMT-I. The best way to protect yourself from the effects of radiation is to use time, distance, and shielding from the source.

- **Time.** Radiation has a cumulative effect on the body. The less time that you are exposed to the

TABLE 37-11 Common Signs of Acute Radiation Sickness

Low exposure	Nausea, vomiting, and diarrhea
Moderate exposure	First-degree burns, hair loss, depletion of the immune system (death of white blood cells), and cancer
Severe exposure	Second- and third-degree burns, cancer, and death

source, the fewer effects there will be. If you realize that the patient is near a radiation source, leave the area immediately.

- **Distance.** Radiation is limited as to how far it can travel. Depending on the type of radiation, often moving only a few feet is enough to remove you from immediate danger. Alpha radiation cannot travel more than a few inches. You should take this into account when responding to a nuclear or radiological incident and make certain that responders are stationed far enough from the incident.
- **Shielding.** As discussed earlier, the path of all radiation can be stopped by a specific object. It will be impossible for you to recognize the type of radiation being emitted, or even from which direction it is coming. Therefore, you should always assume that you are dealing with the strongest form of radiation and use concrete shielding (such as buildings or walls) between yourself and the incident. The importance of shielding cannot be overemphasized. In one atomic test, a car was parked on the side of a house, opposite the direction of the oncoming blast. The house was completely destroyed, yet the car that was directly next to it sustained almost no damage.

You are the Provider — Summary

1. Why is this event at particular risk for a terrorist attack?

Large gatherings can pose unique security challenges and can be tempting targets for terrorist attacks. Any gathering, location, or event that can produce great loss of life or property can be potential terrorist targets.

2. What other factors will play a significant role should an attack occur?

This scenario involves an immediate challenge in regards to local resources. This department's resources will be overwhelmed easily. Also, a rural area implies time to receive additional resources and increased transport times to hospitals when compared with urban areas.

3. What can agencies large and small do to prepare for mass-casualty incidents and/or terrorism?

To prepare for situations such as these, your agency must identify its strengths and weaknesses and create standard operating guidelines that clearly outline actions for personnel. Using local, state, and national resources by establishing mutual aid agreements and dispatch guidelines will minimize confusion and delayed response. Training with other agencies on a consistent and frequent basis will also aid in the effective handling of terrorist attacks. Proper attitude is essential regardless of agency size or location.

4. What are your next actions?

You must immediately notify the dispatch center of what just occurred. Provide a size-up of the event from a safe distance and request all available local and statewide resources as needed.

5. How does the incident command system play a vital role in mass-casualty incidents?

Whether you are an EMT-I for a fire department or work with a private ambulance service, you must have a fundamental understanding of the incident command system. Large incidents require activation and utilization of adequate numbers of personnel and equipment. This requires an organized effort and a common language among responders. You must also be prepared to assume command until the arrival of a higher ranking officer. The actions you take in the first few moments can create an atmosphere of continued chaos or a scene that is being brought under control in a systematic fashion. An event like this will require a unified command or one that involves cooperation between various jurisdictions and organizations.

6. What are some reasons you should not rush into the area of explosion?

You do not know the nature of the explosion. It may be a conventional bomb or one that also contains chemical or biological agents. Also, secondary devices can be planted to explode later to eliminate as many first responders as possible. Making the choice to evaluate the situation from a safe distance will be one of your most difficult experiences whether you're a seasoned provider or not. Your natural reaction will be to want to immediately assist the victims. However, you must control your emotions and maintain your focus. This is where training becomes an invaluable tool in conditioning your brain to react appropriately.

You are the Provider continued

7. What else should you immediately do besides notifying the dispatch center?

You must establish yourself as the incident commander and an incident command post (so that responders know your location). If you do not practice this on a consistent basis, you will feel very uncomfortable should the need arise (especially in a mass-casualty incident). Your agency should have practice drills on MCIs and all personnel with and without rank should be required to practice establishing an incident command.

8. Why is it important to direct the walking wounded to another location?

Wounded persons walking through the scene cause further confusion. Directing the walking wounded to a different location will allow you to initially triage these individuals and obtain an idea of the total number of patients.

9. Where should you create a staging area for responding personnel and apparatus?

You should direct responding units to an area that is out of the way and is uphill and upwind from the area of explosion. It is important that the apparatus be accessible but out of the way.

10. If this event involved the use of organophosphates, how would it affect this scenario?

You must take time to identify the agent and address decontamination issues. After these issues are addressed, you must ensure all responders understand the agent, how to avoid contamination and cross-contamination, and how to treat victims.

11. What would likely be an issue with organophosphate poisoning?

Obtaining enough MARK 1 kits (especially enough atropine) will be an issue. Patients will likely require multiple doses of atropine and it is unlikely that a small, rural department would carry an adequate amount. Until the additional resources are acquired, the EMT-I should provide supportive measures and aggressive airway management when warranted.

Summary

Prep Kit

Ready for Review

- As a result of the increase in terrorist activity, it is possible that the EMT-I could witness a terrorist event. You must be mentally and physically prepared for the possibility of a terrorist event.
- The use of weapons of mass destruction or mass casualty further complicates the management of the terrorist incident. Be aware of your surroundings at all times. The best form of protection from a WMD agent is to avoid contact with the agent.
- Types of groups that tend to use terrorism include violent religious groups/doomsday cults, extremist political groups, technology terrorists, and single-issue groups.
- A WMD is any agent designed to bring about mass death, casualties, and/or massive damage to property and infrastructure (bridges, tunnels, airports, and seaports). These can be nuclear, chemical, biological, and explosive weapons.
- Chemical agents are man-made substances that can have devastating effects on living organisms. They can be produced in liquid, powder, or vapor form, depending on the desired route of exposure and dissemination technique. These agents consist of vesicants, respiratory, nerve, and metabolic agents.
- Biological agents are organisms that cause disease. They are generally found in nature and can be weaponized to maximize the number of people exposed to the germ. These types of agents include viruses, bacteria, and toxins.
- Nuclear or radiological weapons can create a massive amount of destruction. This type of weapon includes radiological dispersal devices (RDDs), also known as dirty bombs.
- Be aware of the current threat level issued by the federal government through the Department of Homeland Security (DHS). This threat level can be severe, high, elevated, guarded, or low.
- On the basis of the current threat level, take appropriate actions and precautions. Be aware of established policies that your organization may have regarding the current threat level.
- Indicators that may give you clues as to whether the emergency is the result of a WMD attack include the type of location, type of call, number of patients, victims' statements, and preincident indicators.
- If you suspect that a terrorist or WMD event has occurred, make sure that the scene is safe. If you have **any** doubt that it may not be safe, **do not enter**. Wait for assistance.
- Notification of the dispatcher is essential. Inform dispatch of the nature of the event, any additional resources that may be required, the estimated number of patients, and the upwind route of approach or optimal route of approach.
- Establish a staging area, where other units will converge. Be mindful of access and exit routes.
- The first arriving provider on the scene must begin to sort out the chaos and define his or her responsibilities under the Incident Command System (ICS).
- If the ICS is already in place, the EMT-I should immediately seek out the medical staging officer to receive his or her assignment.
- Terrorists may set secondary devices to explode after the initial bomb, to injure responders and secure media coverage. Constantly assess and reassess the scene for safety.
- Persistent or nonvolatile agents can remain on a surface for long periods of time. A highly persistent agent can remain in the environment for weeks to months.
- Nonpersistent or volatile agents evaporate relatively fast when left on a surface in the optimal temperature range. A highly volatile agent will turn from liquid to gas (evaporate) within minutes to seconds.
- Route of exposure is how the agent most effectively enters the body.
- A vesicant is an agent that enters through the skin and causes burn-like blisters on the victim's skin, as well as in the respiratory tract.

Technology

Interactivities

Vocabulary Explorer

Anatomy Review

Web Links

Online Review Manual

Prep Kit continued...

- Vesicant agent treatment includes decontamination first, then the ABCs.
- Place the patient who has been exposed to a vesicant agent on the cardiac monitor, consider early intubation if needed, and consider analgesics for pain according to local protocols.
- Pulmonary agents are gases that cause immediate harm by damaging the lung tissue.
- Pulmonary agent treatment is to remove the patient from the contaminated atmosphere. This should be done by trained personnel in the proper PPE. Then begin aggressive management of the ABCs and gain IV access. **Do not allow the patient to be active**.
- Place the patient who has been exposed to a pulmonary agent on a cardiac monitor and consider early intubation if needed to maintain the airway.
- Nerve agents are among the most deadly chemicals developed and can cause cardiac arrest within seconds to minutes of exposure.
- Securing the ABCs is the best and most important treatment that the EMT-I can render for patients exposed to nerve agents. Patients who will not stop seizing will require administration of nerve agent antidote kits in addition to support of the ABCs.
- Metabolic agents, or cyanides, affect the body's ability to utilize oxygen and are commonly found in many industrial settings.
- Before treatment begins, the patient exposed to a metabolic agent must be removed from the source of exposure by trained personnel in the proper PPE, all of the patient's clothes must be removed, and the patient must be decontaminated. Then support the patient's ABCs and gain IV access.
- Place the patient who has been exposed to a metabolic agent on the cardiac monitor and consider early intubation to maintain the airway.
- Biological agents include viruses such as smallpox and viral hemorrhagic fevers; bacteria such as anthrax and plague; and neurotoxins such as botulinum toxin and ricin.
- EMTs and paramedics may be called upon to assist in the delivery of medications to the public. The EMT-I's role may include triage, treatment of seriously ill patients, and patient transport to the hospital.
- Ionizing radiation is energy that can enter the human body and cause damage.
- Treatment for radiation exposure should begin with making sure that the patient is not contaminated. If the patient is contaminated, he or she must be initially cared for by a HazMat responder.
- There are no suits or protective gear designed to completely shield from radiation. Protect yourself by leaving an area where a radiation source is present, staying as far away as possible, and using concrete shielding when possible.

Vital Vocabulary

alpha Type of energy that is emitted from a strong radiological source; it is the least harmful penetrating type of radiation and cannot travel fast or through most objects.

anthrax A deadly bacterium (*Bacillus anthracis*) that lays dormant in a spore (protective shell); the germ is released from the spore when exposed to the optimal temperature and moisture. The route of entry is inhalation, cutaneous, or gastrointestinal (from consuming food that contains spores).

bacteria Microorganisms that reproduce by binary fission. These single-cell creatures reproduce rapidly. Some can form spores (encysted variants) when environmental conditions are harsh.

beta Type of energy that is emitted from a strong radiological source; is slightly more penetrating than alpha, and requires a layer of clothing to stop it.

botulinum Produced by bacteria, this is a very potent neurotoxin. When introduced into the body, this neurotoxin affects the nervous system's ability to function and causes botulism.

buboes Enlarged lymph nodes (up to the size of tennis balls) that are characteristic of people infected with the bubonic plague.

bubonic plague An epidemic that spread throughout Europe in the Middle Ages, causing over 25 million deaths transmitted by infected fleas and characterized by acute malaise, fever, and the formation of tender, enlarged, inflamed lymph nodes that appear as lesions, called buboes; also called the Black Death.

chlorine (CL) The first chemical agent ever used in warfare. It has a distinct odor of bleach and creates a green haze when released as a gas. Initially it produces upper airway irritation and a choking sensation.

communicability Describes how easily a disease spreads from one human to another human.

contact hazard (skin hazard) A hazardous agent that gives off very little or no vapors; the skin is the primary route for this type of chemical to enter the body.

contagious A person infected with a disease that is highly communicable.

covert Act in which the public safety community generally has no prior knowledge of the time, location, or nature of the attack.

cross-contamination Contamination that occurs when a person is contaminated by an agent as a result of coming into contact with another contaminated person.

cyanide Agent that affects the body's ability to use oxygen. It is a colorless gas that has an odor similar to almonds. The effects begin on the cellular level and are very rapidly seen at the organ system level.

decay A natural process in which a material that is unstable attempts to stabilize itself by changing its structure.

dirty bomb Name given to a bomb that is used as a radiological dispersal device (RDD).

disease vector An animal that spreads a disease, once infected, to another animal.

dissemination The means by which a terrorist will spread a disease, for example, by poisoning of the water supply, or aerosolizing the agent into the air or ventilation system of a building.

domestic terrorists Native citizens that carry out acts of terrorism against their own country.

G agents Early nerve agents, the G series, which were developed by German scientists (hence the G) in the period after WWI and into WWII. There are three G series agents: sarin, soman, and tabun.

gamma (x-rays) Type of energy that is emitted from a strong radiological source that is far faster and stronger than alpha and beta rays. These rays easily penetrate through the human body and require either several inches of lead or concrete to prevent penetration.

incubation Describes the period of time between exposure to a disease and the time when symptoms begin.

international terrorism Terrorism that is carried out by those not of the host's country; also known as cross-border terrorism.

ionizing radiation Energy that is emitted in the form of rays, or particles.

LD_{50} The amount of an agent or substance that will kill 50% of people who are exposed to this level.

Lewisite (L) A blistering agent that has a rapid onset of symptoms and produces immediate intense pain and discomfort on contact.

lymph nodes Area of the lymphatic system where infection-fighting cells are housed.

lymphatic system A passive circulatory system that transports a plasma-like liquid called lymph, a thin fluid that bathes the tissues of the body.

MARK 1 A nerve agent antidote kit containing two autoinjector medications, atropine and 2-PAM chloride (pralidoxime chloride); also known as a Nerve Agent Antidote Kit (NAAK).

miosis Bilateral pinpoint constricted pupils.

mucous membranes The lining of body cavities and passages that communicate directly or indirectly with the environment outside the body.

mutagen Substance that mutates, damages, and changes the structures of DNA in the body's cells.

NAAK A nerve agent antidote kit containing two autoinjector medications, atropine and 2-PAM chloride (pralidoxime chloride); also known as a MARK 1 kit.

nerve agents A class of chemical called organophosphates; they function by blocking an essential enzyme in the nervous system, which causes the body's organs to become overstimulated and burn out.

neurotoxins Biological agents that are the most deadly substances known to humans; they include botulinum toxin and ricin.

neutron radiation Type of energy that is emitted from a strong radiological source; neutron energy is the fastest moving and most powerful form of radiation. Neutrons easily penetrate through lead and require several feet of concrete to stop them.

off-gassing The emitting of an agent after exposure, for example from a person's clothes that have been exposed to the agent.

persistency Term used to describe how long a chemical agent will stay on a surface before it evaporates.

phosgene A pulmonary agent that is a product of combustion, such as might be produced in a fire at a textile factory or house, or from metalwork or burning

Prep Kit continued...

Freon. Phosgene is a very potent agent that has a delayed onset of symptoms, usually hours.

phosgene oxime (CX) A blistering agent that has a rapid onset of symptoms and produces immediate intense pain and discomfort on contact.

pneumonic plague A lung infection, also known as plague pneumonia, that is the result of inhalation of plague bacteria.

points of distribution (PODs) Strategically placed facilities that have been preestablished for the mass distribution of antibiotics, antidotes, vaccinations, with other medications and supplies.

radioactive material Any material that emits radiation.

radiological dispersal device (RDD) Any container that is designed to disperse radioactive material.

ricin Neurotoxin derived from mash that is left from the castor bean. When introduced into the body, ricin causes pulmonary edema and respiratory and circulatory failure, leading to death.

route of exposure Manner by which a toxic substance enters the body.

sarin (GB) A nerve agent that is one of the G agents; is a highly volatile colorless and odorless liquid that turns from liquid to gas within seconds to minutes at room temperature.

secondary device Additional explosives used by terrorists, which are set to explode after the initial bomb.

smallpox A highly contagious viral disease; it is most contagious when blisters begin to form.

soman (GD) A nerve agent that is one of the G agents. It is twice as persistent as sarin and five times as lethal; it has a fruity odor, as a result of the type of alcohol used in the agent, and is both a contact and inhalation hazard that can enter the body through skin absorption and the respiratory tract.

Special Atomic Demolition Munitions (SADM) Small suitcase-sized nuclear weapons that were designed to destroy individual targets, such as important buildings, bridges, tunnels, or large ships.

state-sponsored terrorism Terrorism that is funded and/or supported by nations that hold close ties with terrorist groups.

sulfur mustard (agent H) A vesicant; it is a brownish-yellowish oily substance that is generally considered very persistent. It has the distinct smell of garlic or mustard and, when released, it is quickly absorbed into the skin and/or mucous membranes and begins an irreversible process of damaging the cells.

syndromic surveillance The monitoring, usually by local or state health departments, of patients presenting to emergency departments and alternative care facilities, the recording of EMS call volume, and the use of over-the-counter medications.

tabun (GA) A nerve agent that is one of the G agents. This agent is 36 times more persistent than sarin and approximately half as lethal; it has a fruity smell and is unique because the components used to manufacture the agent are easy to acquire and the agent is easy to manufacture.

V agent (VX) One of the G agents; it is a clear oily agent that has no odor and looks like baby oil. VX is over 100 times more lethal than sarin and is extremely persistent.

vapor hazard An agent that enters the body through the respiratory tract.

vesicants Blister agents; the primary route of entry for vesicants is through the skin.

viral hemorrhagic fevers (VHF) A group of diseases that include the ebola, Rift Valley, and yellow fever viruses among others. This group of viruses causes the blood in the body to seep out from the tissues and blood vessels.

viruses Germs that require a living host to multiply and survive.

volatility Term used to describe how long a chemical agent will stay on a surface before it evaporates.

weapon of mass casualty (WMC) Any agent designed to bring about mass death, casualties, and/or massive damage to property and infrastructure (bridges, tunnels, airports, and seaports); also known as a weapon of mass destruction (WMD).

weapon of mass destruction (WMD) Any agent designed to bring about mass death, casualties, and/or massive damage to property and infrastructure (bridges, tunnels, airports, and seaports); also known as a weapon of mass casualty (WMC).

weaponization The creation of a weapon from a biological agent generally found in nature and that causes disease; the agent is cultivated, synthesized, and/or mutated to maximize the target population's exposure to the germ.

www.EMSzone.com/EMT

Assessment in Action

It is the Fourth of July and your department is gearing up for the city's celebration. You are expecting thousands of people to travel to the city to watch the fireworks. At about 5 pm you are dispatched to a truck stop on the outskirts of the city for an ill person.

Bystanders state that they observed the patient get out of his vehicle and collapse. You find the male patient laying on the ground, barely conscious, actively coughing and having severe respiratory distress. You attempt to gain information from four other men in the vehicle, only to find that all of them are displaying the same signs and symptoms.

1. You should immediately do all of the following EXCEPT:
   A. notify dispatch of the situation and request assistance.
   B. wear contact and respiratory PPE.
   C. remove the victims from the vehicle.
   D. isolate bystanders at a safe distance.

2. Indicators that you may be dealing with a weapon of mass destruction include all of the following EXCEPT:
   A. the upcoming festival and resulting crowds.
   B. the similarity of symptoms.
   C. the presence of multiple patients.
   D. the ethnicity of the patients.

3. Law enforcement has secured the area and the hazardous materials team is inspecting the vehicle. They find several pipe bombs in the trunk, as well as containers of an unknown substance. On the basis of this information, you should:
   A. suspect some form of contagious disease is involved.
   B. secure the pipe bombs in an isolated area.
   C. reassess scene safety.
   D. radio the hospital with this information.

4. On the basis of the patient's symptoms, you should suspect:
   A. Ebola.
   B. ricin.
   C. sarin.
   D. agent H.

5. The agent you suspect is classified as a:
   A. nerve agent.
   B. bacterial agent.
   C. blister agent.
   D. neurotoxin.

6. In treating these patients, your greatest risk of contamination will be from contact with:
   A. the patients.
   B. body fluids.
   C. the substance itself.
   D. the cough secretions.

7. Your treatment will include all of the following EXCEPT:
   A. supporting the ABCs.
   B. administering the MARK 1 antidote.
   C. administering oxygen.
   D. providing rapid transport.

8. You should expect the patient's condition to:
   A. improve with oxygen therapy.
   B. improve with administration of atropine.
   C. deteriorate to respiratory/circulatory failure.
   D. deteriorate to paralysis.

Points to Ponder

It has been a year since you responded to a mass-casualty incident that resulted in the deaths of hundreds of people, including some of your coworkers. The incident was the result of a terrorist attack. Ever since that night you have suffered from nightmares and have begun drinking heavily. You recently separated from your spouse because "she doesn't understand." You have been depressed and have not felt as passionate about your job as you used to. Over the last couple of months you have been considering suicide.

What should you do?

Issues: Understanding the Help That Is Available to You, Strength in Asking for Help

www.EMSzone.com/EMT

Enrichment

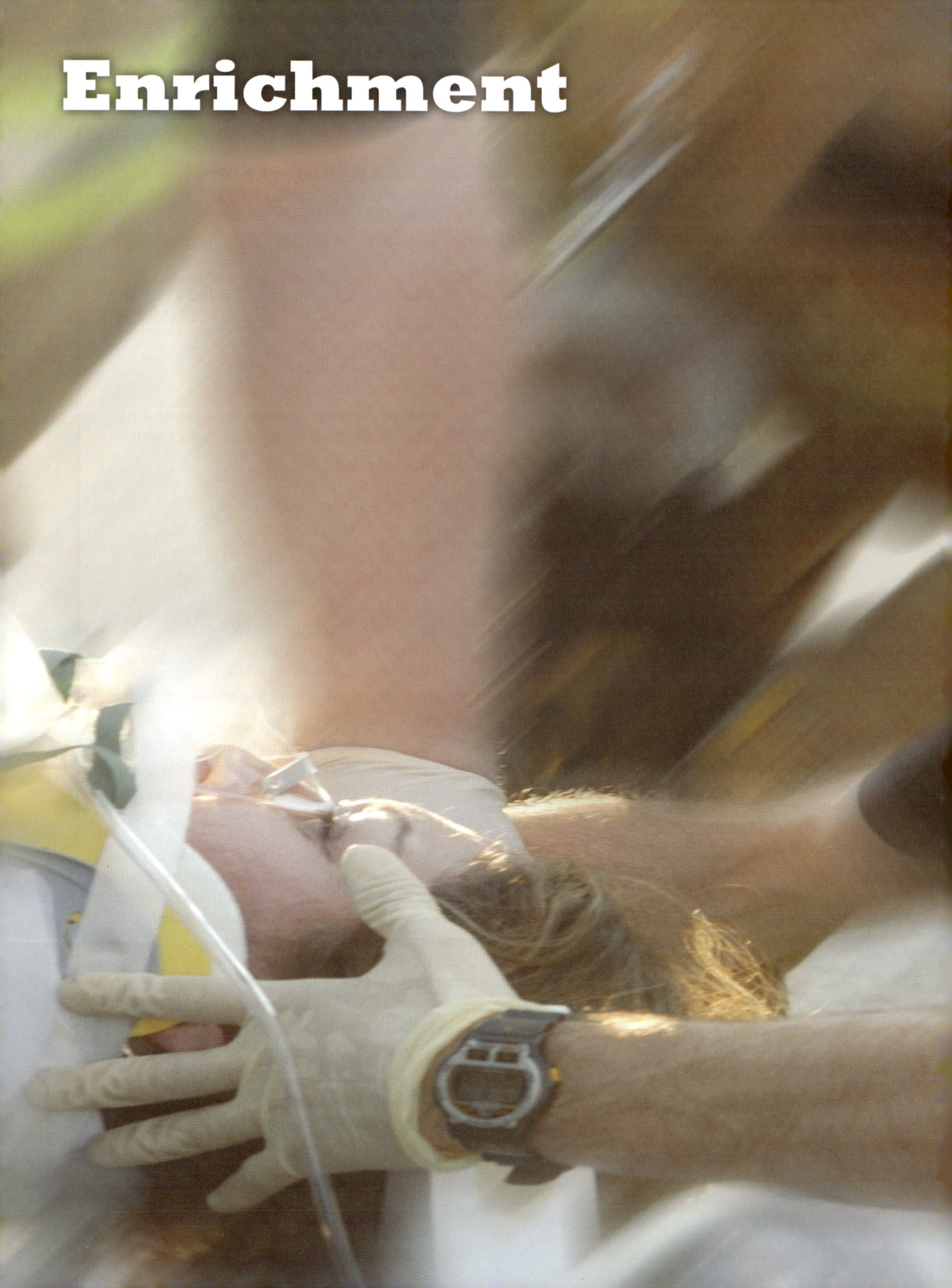

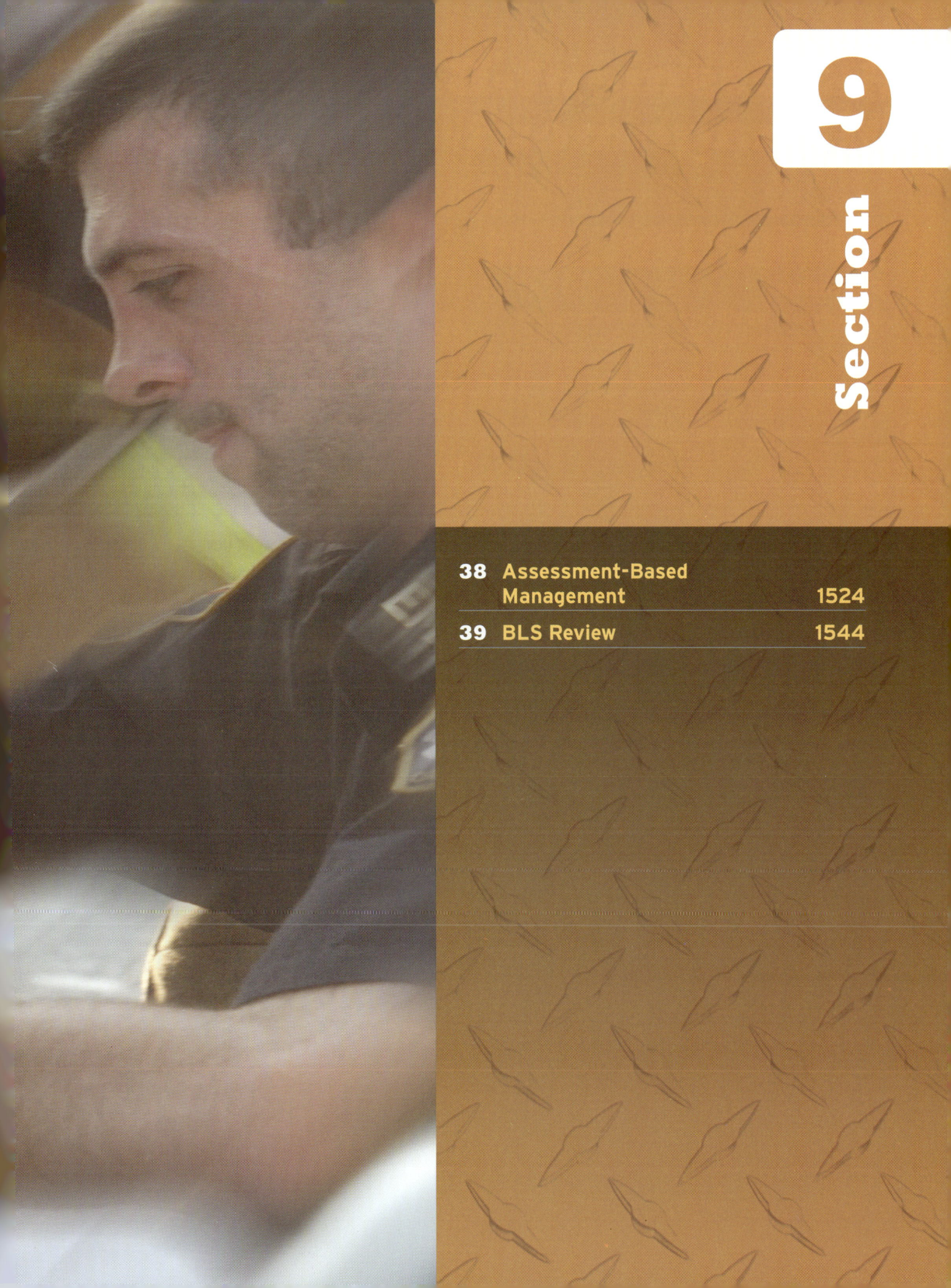

Section 9

- **38** Assessment-Based Management — 1524
- **39** BLS Review — 1544

Assessment-Based Management

1999 Objectives

Cognitive

7-1.1 Explain how effective assessment is critical to clinical decision making. (p 1528)
7-1.2 Explain how the EMT-Intermediate's attitude affects assessment and decision making. (p 1532)
7-1.3 Explain how uncooperative patients affect assessment and decision making. (p 1532)
7-1.4 Explain strategies to prevent labeling and tunnel vision. (p 1529, 1533)
7-1.5 Develop strategies to decrease environmental distractions. (p 1533)
7-1.6 Describe how manpower considerations and staffing configurations affect assessment and decision making. (p 1533)
7-1.7 Synthesize concepts of scene management and choreography to simulated emergency calls. (p 1533)
7-1.8 Explain the roles of the team leader and the patient care person. (p 1529)
7-1.9 List and explain the rationale for carrying the essential patient care items. (p 1531)
7-1.10 When given a simulated call, list the appropriate equipment to be taken to the patient. (p 1531)
7-1.11 Explain the general approach to the emergency patient. (p 1533)
7-1.12 Describe how to effectively communicate patient information face to face, over the telephone, by radio, and in writing. (p 1534)
7-1.13 Explain the general approach, patient assessment, and management priorities for patients who complain of chest pain. (p 1537)
7-1.14 Explain the general approach, patient assessment, and management priorities for medical and traumatic cardiac arrest patients. (p 1537)
7-1.15 Explain the general approach, patient assessment, and management priorities for patients who complain of acute abdominal pain. (p 1537)
7-1.16 Explain the general approach, patient assessment, and management priorities for patients who complain of GI bleeding. (p 1537)
7-1.17 Explain the general approach, patient assessment, and management priorities for altered mental status patients. (p 1537)
7-1.18 Explain the general approach, patient assessment, and management priorities for patients who complain of dyspnea. (p 1537)
7-1.19 Explain the general approach, patient assessment, and management priorities for trauma or multi trauma patients. (p 1537)
7-1.20 Explain the general approach, patient assessment, and management priorities for a patient who is having an allergic reaction. (p 1537)
7-1.21 Explain the general approach, patient assessment, and management priorities for pediatric patients. (p 1537)

Affective

7-1.22 Appreciate the use of scenarios to develop high-level clinical decision-making skills. (p 1536)
7-1.23 Advocate and practice the process of complete patient assessment on all patients. (p 1533)
7-1.24 Value the importance of presenting the patient accurately and clearly. (p 1534)

Psychomotor

7-1.25 While serving as team leader, choreograph the EMS response team, perform a patient assessment, provide local/regionally appropriate treatment, present cases verbally and in writing given a moulaged and programmed simulated patient. (p 1536)

7-1.26 While serving as team leader, assess a programmed patient or mannequin, make decisions relative to interventions and transportation, provide the interventions, patient packaging and transportation, work as a team and practice various roles for the following common emergencies:
  a. Chest pain
  b. Cardiac arrest
     - Traumatic arrest
     - Medical arrest
  c. Acute abdominal pain
  d. GI bleeding
     - Lower GI bleeding
     - Upper GI bleeding
  e. Altered mental status
  f. Dyspnea
  g. Syncope
  h. Trauma
     - Isolated extremity fracture (tibia/fibula or radius/ulna)
     - Femur fracture
     - Spine injury (no neurologic deficit, with neurologic deficit)
     - Multiple trauma—blunt
     - Penetrating trauma
     - Impaled object
     - Elderly fall
     - Athletic injury
     - Head injury (concussion, subdural/epidural)
  i. Allergic reactions/bites/envenomation
     - Local allergic reaction
     - Systemic allergic reaction
  j. Pediatric
     - Respiratory distress
     - Fever
     - Seizures (p 1537)

1985 Objectives

There are no 1985 objectives for this chapter.

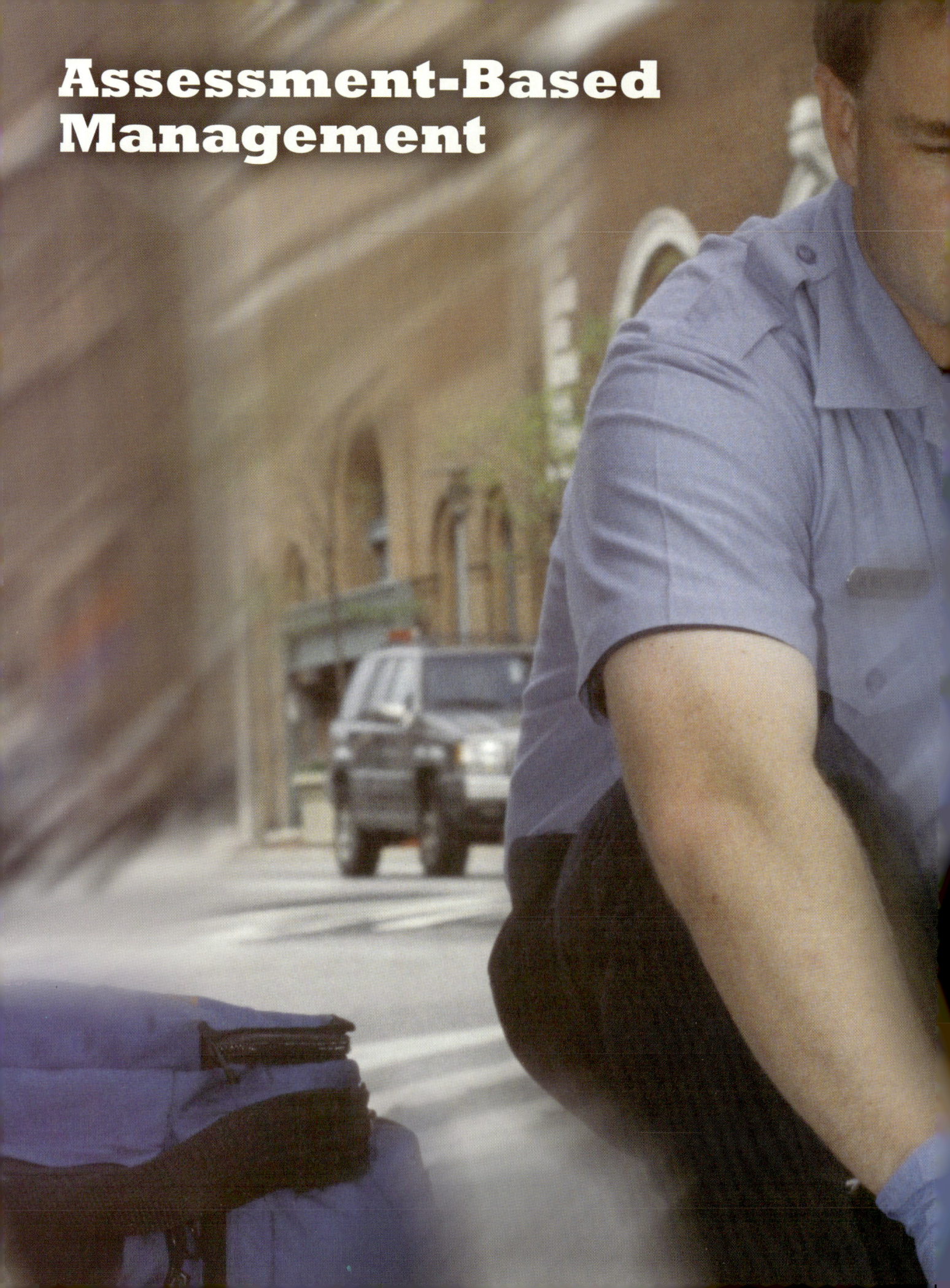

Assessment-Based Management

38

Assessment-Based Management

You are the Provider

At 1:30 AM, you and your partner are dispatched to the intersection of Harvey Shaw and Loney Road for a possible one-car motor vehicle crash. While en route to the location, you receive an update from the dispatcher. The 9-1-1 call was placed by a motorist who was flagged down by a man standing in the road. The man stated to the motorist that he'd been involved in an accident. Road conditions are wet (it started raining 15 minutes prior to the dispatch); the current temperature is 65°F with a slight breeze at 5 to 10 mph.

1. What are some considerations to be made about the time and weather conditions?
2. What is the danger of common dispatches such as this one?

Assessment-Based Management

As an EMT-I you will be called on in numerous situations to provide care for patients who may be unable to answer questions for themselves. Your assessment and reasoning skills may be all that is standing between the patient and morbidity or mortality. You must be able to accurately assess not only the patient but the scene as well. This includes drawing clues from the surrounding environment, whether it is the damage to a vehicle at a crash scene or the medications found on the night stand in the patient's home (Figure 38-1). Regardless of the type of call, you must evaluate the scene, the patient's condition, and make the appropriate choices for patient care and transportation.

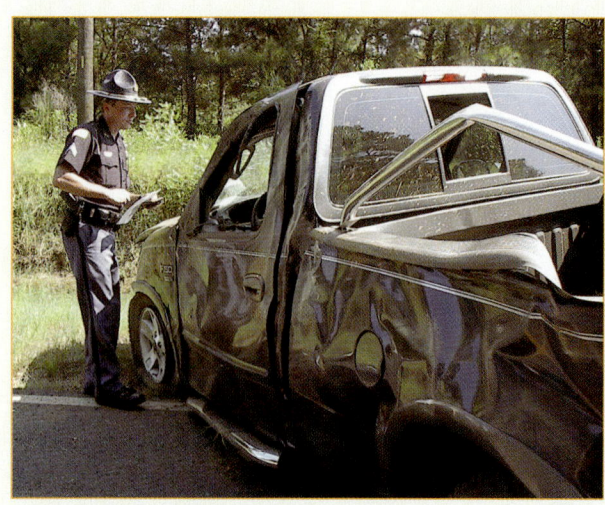

Figure 38-1 Making a sketch of the surrounding environment may help you assess the scene.

Effective Patient Assessment

In any given situation, assessment is the foundation of patient care. In order to provide the best possible care, you must gather and evaluate as much information as possible about the patient and the environment. Furthermore, you must synthesize this information, meaning the information must be processed or formed into a hypothesis for determining what is wrong and what is the best route to take for treatment. Assessment must be thorough in order to provide the best care possible.

Gathering Information

Accurate information is critical to decision making. You must work in the capacity of a medical detective and put together the clues that you find. This includes those clues garnered from the scene and from the patient.

> 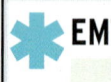 **EMT-I Tips**
>
> If you can't see it, you can't treat it! Do not forget to expose the patient.

The Importance of History

The patient's history plays a large role in medical diagnosis; oftentimes, 80% of the diagnosis is attributed to the patient's history. Medical conditions or the medication taken for those conditions may interfere with or mask signs and symptoms of the current problem. In order to be effective in gathering information you must have a good understanding of various disease processes. By applying what you know about a particular illness and maintaining a high index of suspicion, you can question a patient or family member and obtain more information. Your knowledge will help guide you in asking appropriate questions (Figure 38-2). Even though the patient may have an extensive history, make sure you are focused toward the systems associated with the current complaint and any associated problems.

Technology

- Interactivities
- Vocabulary Explorer
- Anatomy Review
- Web Links
- Online Review Manual

www.EMSzone.com/EMTI

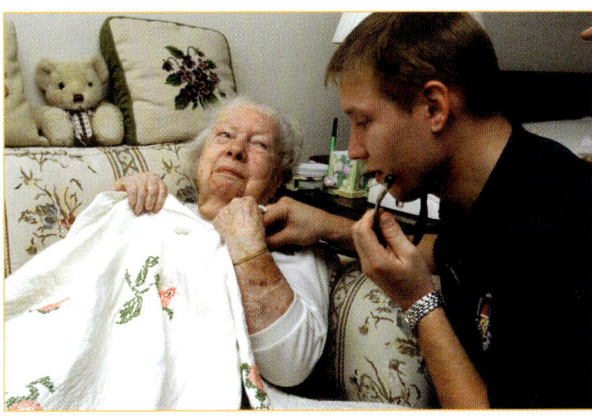

Figure 38-2 Use your knowledge of disease processes to guide patient questioning.

Physical Assessment

The physical exam is yet another tool for gaining vital information. Unfortunately, it is often overlooked or performed in a hasty manner. The effectiveness of the assessment may also be compromised by some field situations. Due to scene hazards there may not be enough time to complete a thorough assessment. The patient's condition may also hamper evaluation efforts. If the patient is apneic and pulseless, your treatment should be centered on basic life support. Another problem frequently encountered is a result of tunnel vision. Even though you should focus on the systems associated with the complaint, you must also be aware of the potential for other injuries or other systems that may be affected.

Recognizing Patterns and Obtaining a Field Impression

As you gather information from the environment, history, and patient status, that information should be compared with what you know about similar conditions. Combined with the information you obtain in your assessment, your knowledge and training will improve your chances of conducting an accurate assessment and making sound decisions.

When you are assessing a patient, look for patterns. For example, if you arrive on scene to find a combative patient exhibiting bizarre behavior and no one around that knows the patient, your examination may point you in the right direction. You note that the patient is extremely diaphoretic and on further examination you find a prescription bottle in his pocket for Glucophage (a commonly prescribed diabetic medication). All of these things should lead you to check the patient's glucose level for hypoglycemia.

The field impression that you arrive at is essentially your working diagnosis. This is formed based on pattern recognition, your knowledge of various medical conditions, and your instinct based on experience. From this impression you will formulate a plan of action. This includes what should be done to stabilize the patient on scene and what should be done en route. The patient's condition and the environment may also dictate what you can or cannot do on scene.

> **In the Field**
>
> Experience is the key to expanding your knowledge base.

BLS/ALS Treatment

Your service will have standing orders or protocols to dictate interventions that may be performed without consulting on-line medical control. In order to choose the appropriate protocol to use, you must first have a correct impression of the patient. You should also know when and how to apply those protocols to each patient as well as when to deviate from them. Not every patient presents in the same manner that you learned from your textbook. You must learn how to adapt your treatment for the problem presented. For example, you may have a trauma patient for whom you cannot apply a cervical collar because of his or her size or shape. In this case you could improvise by using towels or other material to brace the head 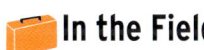.

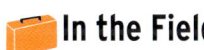

Figure 38-3 Use towels to fill voids and support the head of a patient whose body shape does not align with the straight, flat shape of a backboard, for example, older patients who are kyphotic.

Choreographing Assessment and Management

The number of responders on scene often makes effective assessment challenging. In any given situation there are multiple levels of responders ranging from laypersons and first responders to ALS providers. Often there are too many people attempting to acquire a history at the same time and creating nothing but confusion. It is even worse when the responders are at the same level and there is no clear direction for what role each provider should assume.

Members of the EMS team need to have a preplan for determining roles. If providers are trained to the same level, this may be accomplished by alternating who will serve as the lead medic on each call, or it may be that one provider is stronger in a particular area, such as pediatric care. By designating roles, confusion on scene is minimized. An EMT-I working without a paramedic partner must assume an ALS role and should have a plan for handling such situations.

When there are two EMT-Is working together, there should be a preplan, with one EMT-I designated as team leader and one EMT-I designated for patient care; however, this plan needs to be flexible, because field situations are dynamic and continuously change. Regular partners tend to develop their own plan based on their experience together. There also needs to be a universally understood plan that allows for the participation of others. Having a basic "game plan" in advance prevents chaos when you are on scene.

Team Leader

The team leader generally manages patient care throughout the call. This provider establishes contact and a dialogue with the patient and obtains the patient's history. The team leader performs the physical exam and then gives a report over the radio while en route to the hospital to the nurse or physician responsible for the patient's care at the receiving facility. Once patient care has been transferred, the team leader completes the written documentation.

The team leader tries to maintain the overall patient care and provides leadership to the team by designating tasks and coordinating transportation. During the resuscitative phase of the initial assessment, the team leader also designates who will perform critical interventions and actively participates in patient care. In a mass-casualty situation, the team leader acts as the initial EMS command. On calls that involve ACLS intervention, the team leader reads the ECG, relays information on the radio, gives the orders for appropriate drug intervention, controls the drug box, and keeps notes on drug administration and effects.

Patient Care Person(s)

The patient care person or persons provide scene cover, assisting the team leader as indicated, for example by gathering scene information (such as damage to a vehicle at a motor vehicle crash or medications belonging to the patient), talking to relatives and bystanders, and obtaining the patient's vital signs. Other roles of the patient care person involve those interventions requested

You are the Provider — Part 2

You arrive to find a county sheriff interviewing a man on the side of the road. You see no vehicle on the roadway or any indications of an accident (ie, skid marks or debris). As you approach the patient and officer, your partner begins a survey of the surrounding area using a spotlight from the ambulance.

3. Why is it helpful to split up your crew in this situation?
4. What are other issues you should consider on the scene of vehicle accidents?

by the team leader. These may include such procedures as attaching monitor leads, oxygen administration, venous access, medication administration, and gathering equipment for patient packaging in preparation for transport. In a mass-casualty situation the patient care person acts as the triage group leader. He or she may also be called on to administer drugs, monitor ET or Combitube placement, and monitor BCLS during ACLS.

The Right Stuff

The right stuff means carrying the right equipment to the patient's side. As an EMT-I you should always be prepared for the worst and hope for the best. For some patients, assessment and management are simultaneous. You may be required to control bleeding or initiate BCLS as a part of your initial assessment. Not having the right equipment compromises patient care and may cause chaos. Table 38-1 lists the essential items that should be carried to the patient's side to manage the ABCDEs. A notepad and pen or pencil are also necessary equipment.

> **EMT-I Tips**
>
> Don't forget your cardiac monitor as a part of your essential equipment!

Optional "Take In" Equipment

Drug therapy and venous access supplies need to be in portable containers too. Even though these may not be required for every patient, they should be available if needed. How supplies are carried may vary based on the type of response vehicle and how the system is designed. Some EMT-Is work on regular ambulances where others may work on nontransporting vehicles.

Particular equipment and supplies that are carried to the patient's side may depend on local protocols, but is usually dictated by the nature of the patient's problem. Standing orders allow for flexibility based on the presenting situation. Other factors that affect equipment carried to the patient include the number of EMT-I responders and the difficulty in accessing the patient.

Because venous access is required to administer most emergency drugs, venous access supplies should be carried with the drug box Figure 38-4. The drug box itself should contain those drugs allowed by local protocols for prehospital use.

TABLE 38-1	EMT-I Management of ABCDEs
Airway control	■ Oral airways
	■ Nasal airways
	■ Suction (electric or manual)
	■ Rigid Yankauer and flexible suction catheters
	■ Laryngoscopes and blades
	■ Endotracheal tubes, stylets, syringes, tape
Breathing	■ Mouth-powered ventilation devices (pocket mask)
	■ Manual ventilation bag-valve-mask
	■ Spare masks
	■ Oxygen tank and regulator
	■ Oxygen masks, cannulas, and extension tubing
	■ Occlusive dressings
	■ Large-bore IV catheter for thoracic decompression
Circulation	■ Dressings
	■ Bandages and tape
	■ Infection control supplies: gloves, eye shields
	■ Sphygmomanometer, stethoscope
Disability and dysrhythmia	■ Rigid collars
	■ Flashlight
	■ AED
	■ Cardiac monitor/defibrillator
Exposure	■ Scissors
	■ Space blanket or something to cover the patient

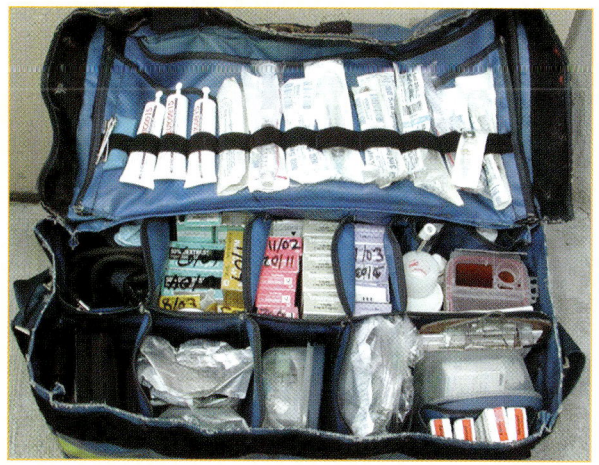

Figure 38-4 An ALS drug box.

Aspects of Assessment and Decision Making

As an EMT-I you must ensure that your attitude is nonjudgmental. When you approach a patient with preconceived notions it may "short circuit" your information gathering and lead to insufficient information to recognize patterns. For example, you arrive on scene to find a "regular" who smells strongly of alcohol and is exhibiting bizarre behavior. He has a small abrasion on his left temple and tries to tell you that his head hurts. You have picked this patient up on numerous occasions and he is always drunk. You sit him on the bench seat and transport him to the triage area of the emergency department. Upon arrival at the emergency department several hours later you find that the patient you brought in earlier is deeply comatose. A computed tomographic (CT) scan of the brain has revealed a subdural hematoma. The outlook for the patient is poor. A more thorough examination would have revealed unequal pupils and other signs of a possible head injury. Patients depend on us for medical assessment and management, not determination of social standing or "likeability."

 EMT-I Tips

Do not go into a situation with preconceived notions, which may cloud your ability to adequately assess and treat your patient.

Uncooperative Patients

It is easy to assume that a patient is intoxicated, especially if you have encountered this patient on numerous occasions; however, in *all* uncooperative, restless, belligerent patients you must consider the following as possible causes:

- Hypoxia
- Hypovolemia
- Hypoglycemia
- Head injury

Distracting Injuries

Make sure that you are not distracted by obvious injuries that may look bad, but in reality, may divert your attention away from more serious problems. Angulated fractures

You are the Provider — Part 3

The officer explains that he arrived only moments before you. He hasn't seen the vehicle yet and was in the process of obtaining information from the accident victim as you arrived. The patient hands the officer his ID, and you begin speaking with him. The patient tells you, "I'm fine. I'm not sure what happened, but I'm okay. You can go." Your partner informs you that he found the vehicle. It rolled multiple times after leaving the roadway and there is significant damage to the driver's side compartment.

Initial Assessment	Recording Time: 1 Minute After Patient Contact
Level of consciousness	Alert but appears slightly confused
Airway	Open and clear
Breathing	Respirations appear increased
Circulation	Patient will not allow you to assess his pulse; no gross bleeding noted

5. What questions should you ask this patient?
6. If the patient continues to refuse care, should you release him?

> **In the Field**
>
> "Labels" applied by responders sometimes set an inappropriate tone, are distracting, and cause biased assessment.
> - Just another drunk
> - Frequent flyer
>
> Tunnel vision causes distraction.
> - Locking on to a particular obvious injury can result in making a field impression too early.
> - "Gut instinct" sometimes causes a rush to judgment too early.

draw attention, but unless they are bleeding profusely, they are likely not going to result in death. The most obvious problems are often the least life-threatening.

The Environment, Patient Compliance, and Manpower Considerations

The environment in which you are working can be very distracting and can take your attention away from your patient care duties due to scene chaos, violent or dangerous situations, crowds of bystanders or responders, or noise levels. Moving the patient into the controlled environment of the ambulance as quickly as possible will minimize distractions.

In order to gain a sufficient history and provide the most appropriate care, the patient must have confidence in his or her rescuers. This means breaking down cultural or ethnic barriers by treating every patient with respect and courtesy. Always treat the patient as if he or she were a member of your own family.

When considering the manpower available in treating a patient, you must organize your help to avoid confusion. A single EMT-I can gather information and provide treatment sequentially. When there are two EMT-Is present, one can gather information while the second provides the treatment. With the introduction of more personnel, chaos may ensue. It is impossible to get an accurate history by "committee."

General Approach

A calm, orderly demeanor is essential. You are a professional. Your "bedside" manner is also important in making the patient feel comfortable and confident in your abilities. The patient may not be able to rate your medical performance, but he or she can rate your people skills and service.

Before entering a scene you should have a "preplan" to prevent confusion and improve the accuracy of the assessment. One team member should talk to the patient. He or she should establish a rapport by asking appropriate questions and listening actively and carefully to the patient's responses. Take notes when you obtain a history to ensure its accuracy and also to prevent asking the same questions repeatedly.

Carry in all of the essential equipment to maintain order. The patient will lose confidence if you have to run back and forth to the ambulance to obtain necessary equipment. You should also be ready to provide resuscitative care if needed.

Use the initial scene size-up to gather clues and help formulate an impression. In trauma situations, look for any hazards, the mechanism of injury, and the number of patients. Take care to avoid tunnel vision.

The Initial Assessment

The initial assessment sets the tone for the patient encounter. For a patient who is in critical condition, the resuscitative approach is best. As you assess the ABCs, perform any interventions that are necessary. This may include manually opening the airway, suctioning the airway, or initiating CPR. Immediate intervention is required for any patient with a life-threatening problem such as:

- Cardiac/respiratory arrest
- Respiratory distress/failure
- Unstable dysrhythmias
- Seizures
- Coma/altered mental status
- Shock/hypotension
- Major trauma
- Possible cervical spine injury

Acquire more history and details immediately after resuscitation. Do not delay care to talk with family members or bystanders.

For patients who are not in critical condition, a more contemplative approach to treatment may be taken. Because an immediate intervention is not needed, you can generally obtain a complete history and physical examination and then provide any necessary care.

Immediate evacuation to the ambulance may be required if the patient needs lifesaving interventions that cannot be provided by the EMT-I, the scene is unsafe, or the scene is too unstable or chaotic to allow for an

> **EMT-I Tips**
>
> To find something, you must suspect it!
> - During the initial assessment you must actively look for life-threatening problems
> - Be systematic
> - Rapidly determine the chief complaint
> - Assess the degree of distress
> - Obtain baseline vital signs early
> - Focus on the relevant history and physical findings

effective and accurate assessment. Remember that the inside of the ambulance provides a controlled environment that is not available on scene.

The Role of Experience

The greater the knowledge you possess regarding what you are looking for, the more productive the line of questioning will be. Experience also assists in developing the ability of "multi-tasking" or being able to ask questions and do other things while listening to the answer. Until you gain experience, you should concentrate on asking questions and just listening to the answers. Your partner should perform any necessary tasks while you are obtaining the history. If your attention is diverted, you may miss important clues.

The patient's ability to describe symptoms and the EMT-I's ability to listen has a great effect on the assessment. Pain severity is not necessarily in direct proportion to the life-threat potential. The location of pain and its source do not always correlate well either, especially if it is visceral pain. Your role as an EMT-I is to rapidly assess and treat for the worst-case scenario.

Transferring the Patient

Effective communication and transfer of patient information are vital to both prehospital and inhospital care. The way the patient is presented or transferred is often a weak link in care. Even though you may perform ALS interventions on few patients, every patient encounter requires accurate patient presentation and information exchange. This presentation may be accomplished face to face, over the telephone, over the radio, and in writing.

Effective presentation and communications skills are essential to establishing trust and credibility at receiving facilities Figure 38-5 ▶. A good assessment and a good presentation go hand in hand. As discussed previously, you cannot treat or report that which is not found. Good presentations suggest effective patient

---

You are the Provider — Part 4

You express your concern for the patient's well-being, and he agrees to further care and transport. You apply full cervical spine precautions from a standing position and find no deficits before or after immobilization. You obtain the following vital signs:

Vital Signs	Recording Time: 6 Minutes After Patient Contact
Level of consciousness	Alert and oriented to person, place, and time
Respirations	28 breaths/min, adequate depth
Pulse	90 beats/min, strong and regular
Blood pressure	140/80 mm Hg
SaO_2	97% on supplemental oxygen

7. Sometimes what you don't find is as important as what you do find. What is this called? What examples of this are presented in the scenario?
8. What does this mechanism of injury tell you about the forces that were placed on the patient during the crash?

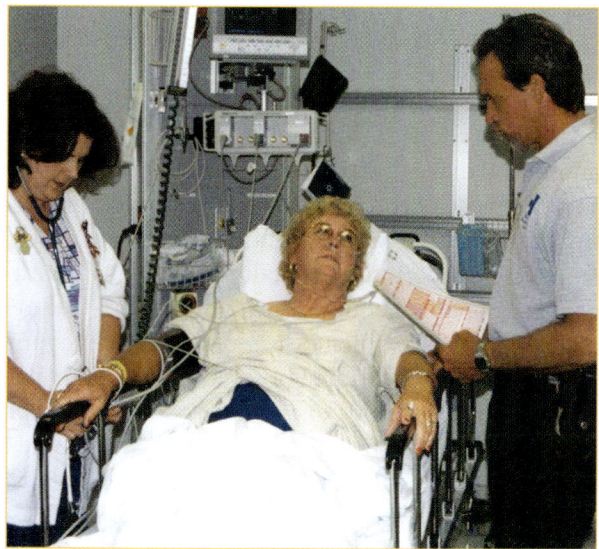

Figure 38-5 When presenting a patient to the hospital, good communication skills are essential.

assessment and care. Poor presentation suggests poor assessment and care. Other health care providers are not interested in listening to rambling, disjointed presentations covering irrelevant information. Most health care providers are used to listening to either the SOAP format, CHART format (both discussed in Chapter 11), or some close variation of it. This provides for a more organized and concise report.

Aside from damaging credibility, poor presentation can also compromise patient care. As extensions of the physician's authority, EMT-Is must contact their supervising physician for orders at one time or another. For that physician to have the confidence to give orders, the patient's needs and status must be communicated effectively. Table 38-2 ▼ lists guidelines for effective presentations.

When you are giving a report, start with the end in mind. Know what discrete areas of information will be asked for and be sure to obtain the right information. Until you become experienced and the format is committed to memory, it is a good idea to use a preprinted card or sheet to organize information and take notes during the work-up. Use the form to organize thoughts and assessment findings before making the presentation. As you gain experience, you will find the method that works best for you and with practice, the flow of the report will become second nature. Table 38-3 ▼ is a sample format that can be used for patient presentation.

The key to developing proficiency is repetition and understanding the format. Use a small pre-printed form. Eventually you will depend on the form less and less. Practice presenting on simulated and real patients. Remember, practice makes perfect. Listen to other providers' radio reports and formulate your style based on what you find to be effective.

Drills for Common Prehospital Complaints

Upon successful completion of your EMT-I course and "boards," whether you take the National Registry of Emergency Medical Technicians exam or a state-approved exam, you will be what is known as an entry-level provider. In order to develop your skill level and knowledge base, scenario-based practice and review needs to be conducted for complaints commonly encountered in the field.

TABLE 38-2　Effective Presentations

- Are very concise, usually lasting less than 1 minute
- Are usually free of extensive medical jargon
- Follow the same basic information pattern
- Generally follow the SOAP format, CHART format, or some close variation of it
- Include pertinent findings and **pertinent negatives** (expected findings given the patient's condition, but which are absent)

TABLE 38-3　Areas of an Ideal Presentation

- Patient identification, age, sex, and degree of distress
- Chief complaint
  - Why were you called?
- Present illness/injury
  - Pertinent details about the present problem
  - Pertinent negatives
- Past medical history
  - Allergies, medications, and pertinent medical history
- Physical findings
  - Vital signs
  - Pertinent positive findings
  - Pertinent negative findings
- Assessment
  - Your impression
- Plan
  - What has been done
  - Orders requested

The goal of practice sessions should be to choreograph the EMS response team. This allows for practice of assessment and decision-making on cases you are likely to encounter in the prehospital arena. It also allows for practice in providing interventions based on your assessment and treatment modalities included in your local or regional treatment protocols. You should practice presenting cases verbally and in writing.

Along with practice sessions, there should also be laboratory-based simulations. These simulations require the EMT-I student to assess a programmed patient or manikin and make decisions relative to interventions and transportation. The manikins allow for actual interventions, and scenarios should continue with patient packaging and transportation. By taking scenarios from the beginning of patient contact through transferal of care at the emergency department, the student must encounter each phase of a call. Students should work together as a team and practice various roles. Table 38-4 lists common complaints that may be encountered and should be used in practice sessions.

> **In the Field**
>
> EMT-Is should practice their interventions with practice sessions along with more formal simulated scenarios. With enough practice, dealing with an emergency situation will be second nature.

You are the Provider — Part 5

En route to the hospital, the patient now complains of neck and abdominal pain. During your reassessment (now in a well-lit environment) you notice some redness and discoloration across his abdomen, apparently from the seatbelt. You have time to start one large-bore IV prior to calling your radio report to the hospital.

Reassessment	Recording Time: 10 Minutes After Patient Contact
Level of consciousness	Alert and oriented to person, place, and time
Respirations	28 breaths/min, adequate depth
Pulse	100 beats/min, strong and regular
Blood pressure	130/88 mm Hg
SaO_2	98% on supplemental oxygen

9. Beyond his injuries, what else could be a factor given the weather conditions?
10. What could be causing his abdominal pain, and can you provide analgesics for his discomfort?

TABLE 38-4 Simulated Patient Presentations

Patient Presentation	Scenarios
Chest pain	<ul><li>Stable—no dysrhythmias</li><li>Cardiogenic shock/hypotension</li><li>Stable bradycardia *(1999)*</li><li>Unstable bradycardia (hypotension/chest pain) *(1999)*</li><li>Stable narrow complex tachycardia *(1999)*</li><li>Unstable narrow complex tachycardia *(1999)*</li><li>Stable wide complex tachycardia *(1999)*</li><li>Unstable wide complex tachycardia *(1999)*</li><li>Ventricular ectopy (ie, PVCs)</li></ul>
Cardiac arrest	<ul><li>Traumatic arrest</li><li>Medical arrest</li><li>Ventricular fibrillation *(1999)*</li><li>Ventricular tachycardia *(1999)*</li><li>Asystole *(1999)*</li><li>Pulseless electrical activity</li><li>Termination of resuscitation</li><li>No resuscitation indicated</li></ul>
Abdominal pain / GI bleeding	<ul><li>Acute abdominal pain</li><li>Upper GI bleeding</li><li>Lower GI bleeding</li></ul>
Altered mental status	<ul><li>Alcohol overdose</li><li>Drug ingestion/overdose</li><li>Seizure</li><li>Hypoglycemia</li><li>Stroke</li><li>Head injury</li></ul>
Dyspnea	<ul><li>Asthma/acute bronchospasm</li><li>Acute pulmonary edema/left-sided heart failure</li><li>Hyperventilation syndrome</li><li>Smoke/toxic inhalation</li></ul>
Syncope	<ul><li>Dehydration</li><li>Stroke</li><li>Hypoglycemia</li><li>Cardiac problems</li></ul>
Trauma	<ul><li>Isolated extremity fracture (tibia/fibula or radius/ulna)</li><li>Femur fracture (hip, midshaft, supracondylar)</li><li>Spinal injuries</li><li>Multiple trauma</li><li>Blunt trauma</li><li>Penetrating trauma</li><li>Impaled object</li><li>Elderly fall</li><li>Athletic injury</li><li>Head injury</li></ul>
Allergic reactions/bites/envenomation	<ul><li>Medication reactions</li><li>Insect stings</li><li>Animal/human bites</li></ul>
Pediatric	<ul><li>Respiratory distress/failure/arrest</li><li>Shock</li><li>Cardiopulmonary failure/arrest</li><li>Major trauma</li><li>Fever</li><li>Seizures</li></ul>

You are the Provider

1. What are some considerations to be made about the time and weather conditions?

This time of the evening can immediately raise the red flag of suspicion regarding the use of alcohol or drugs. If you believe your patient is under the influence, this is significant as it can not only impair judgment but also decrease awareness of injuries and pain. Driver fatigue and weather conditions could also be contributing factors precipitating the crash. The timing of the rain is important to note as roadways become slick at the beginning of rainstorms when the oil and other contaminants on the road surfaces are not yet washed away.

2. What is the danger of common dispatches such as this one?

Complacency can set in for responders who are dispatched to similar situations, patients, or facilities on a daily basis. Don't fall into the trap of assuming what is wrong. Each response is different. In this case, until you have assessed the patient, the scene, and the vehicle, do not assume to know whether he is uninjured, even though he is ambulatory and has no immediate complaints.

3. Why is it helpful to split up your crew in this situation?

You can expedite the gathering of information by splitting your crew. While one of you is assessing the patient, the other provider can be assessing the scene. Sometimes the condition of the patient standing in front of you would not concern you until you have viewed the damage to the vehicle. You must assess both the patient, the mechanism of injury, and the scene as a whole to get an accurate picture of the potential trauma involved.

4. What are other issues you should consider on the scene of vehicle accidents?

On every scene, you must ensure the safety of yourself and your crew first. Accident scenes can present many safety hazards. Preventing further accidents from incoming vehicles is of high concern. Until police officers are available to implement traffic control, responders should consider appropriate vehicle placement to enhance visibility and protection for both providers and patients. Other safety issues include vehicle stability; airbag deployment (for those not yet activated); use of Jaws of Life and potential for electrocution (cutting through the posts of hybrid vehicles); glass, metal, and other sharp objects causing injury to responders/patients; potential for fire; vehicle fluids containment; and requesting adequate resources for multiple patients. These are only some of the considerations that must be made when dealing with vehicle crashes.

5. What questions should you ask this patient?

You want to know whether he was wearing his seatbelt, lost consciousness, hit his head, has head/neck/back pain or numbness/tingling of his extremities, the speed he was traveling, what occurred before, during, and after the accident, if there were other passengers in the vehicle, and his medical history, including any medications or allergies.

Summary

6. If the patient continues to refuse care, should you release him?

You cannot release this patient if he is confused. A patient must be alert and oriented to person, place, time, and event; otherwise you cannot ask him to sign a refusal form. Even if a person continues to refuse care and is fully alert, you must explain the potential consequences of not accepting evaluation, care, and transport to a hospital. This explanation is not meant to scare a patient into changing his or her mind, but is a truthful explanation of potential conditions that could develop or what could happen as a result of denying care. Refusals should be signed by an objective party (ie, a police officer, family member, or bystander) as well as by you, your partner, and the patient. Attention to the details during documentation of a refusal can avoid successful litigation against you and your department. Be honest and speak clearly, avoiding technical language during your explanation. Oftentimes, if you lay out the potential injuries/consequences of refusal (when you think it's warranted), the patient will concede.

7. Sometimes what you don't find is as important as what you do find. What is this called? What examples of this are presented in the scenario?

These findings are referred to as pertinent negatives. In this situation, the lack of parasthesias/paralysis points to an intact spinal cord. Given the mechanism of injury, however, you would still suspect spinal fractures and initiate full spinal precautions. Failure to assess or document prior to patient movement, extrication, or immobilization techniques could make it difficult to differentiate between whether your care caused an exacerbation of injuries or whether the deficits were present prior to your treatment. Unfortunately, this is a common error in assessment and documentation of patients who have been in motor vehicle crashes.

8. What does this mechanism of injury tell you about the forces that were placed on the patient during the crash?

Although many rollovers do not produce significant injuries, rollovers contain almost all of the forces seen in other collisions. Therefore, you must be suspicious that significant injuries exist for victims of a rollover crash.

9. Beyond his injuries, what else could be a factor given the weather conditions?

Hypothermia can occur even in moderate temperatures. In this case, the temperature is 65°F and it is raining. Rain and wind can cause loss of body heat very quickly, and if other factors are present, such as alcohol, this can make the patient even more susceptible to hypothermia.

10. What could be causing his abdominal pain, and can you provide analgesics for his discomfort?

A variety of internal abdominal organs could have been injured during his crash. Improperly worn seatbelts can cause injuries. Contacting the interior of the vehicle (steering wheel) can cause injuries as well.

Unfortunately, because of the difficulty in pinpointing the cause of pain, you cannot provide pain management. In this case, administering pain medications could cloud a diagnosis and delay life-saving care in the hospital.

Prep Kit

Ready for Review

- Your job as an EMT-I will focus on assessments of the scene and the patient and providing appropriate care and transportation based on these findings.
- The care that you provide is only as good as the assessment you perform.
- Gathering an accurate history is crucial to decision making.
- Complete a thorough physical exam if the patient's status will allow and using this information along with the history, formulate a strategy of care based on your field impression.
- Do not let tunnel vision or attitude cloud your assessment.
- Assessment and management should be choreographed in advance to reduce chaos on scene. Establish a game plan for a team leader and patient care personnel.
- Make sure you have the right equipment at the patient's side to prevent the need for multiple trips to the ambulance, which could waste valuable time in an emergency situation.
- Your approach to the patient should be professional in appearance. This helps to instill confidence in the patient and family members present. Gather an accurate history and carefully and frequently takes notes to avoid repetitive questioning.

Technology

Interactivities

Vocabulary Explorer

Anatomy Review

Web Links

Online Review Manual

- The patient's status should dictate your order of care. For a patient in critical condition, care should be interspersed with assessment; for a patient who is not in critical condition, a history and assessment can be obtained prior to treatment.
- Experience is the key to being able to multitask. This allows you to talk with the patient while performing other procedures such as taking vital signs or starting an IV.
- Effective presentation and communications skills are essential to establishing trust and credibility. A good assessment and a good presentation go hand in hand.
- Review and practice assessment and treatment of common complaints to gain proficiency.

Vital Vocabulary

field impression Working diagnosis arrived at based on pattern recognition and experience.

pertinent negatives Expected findings given the patient's condition but which are absent.

Assessment in Action

You respond to a local gas station where the police have called for your assistance. During a traffic stop they found a 67-year-old man, alone in his vehicle, disoriented and confused. They believe he may be intoxicated.

As you approach the car, you note that the patient appears pale and diaphoretic. You introduce yourself and your partner. The patient looks at you but is unable to respond. You decide to move him into the ambulance for treatment rather than trying to work in his car. He is uncooperative and slightly combative. With the help of the officers, you get him in the ambulance and begin your assessment. Your partner finds the following vital signs: blood pressure, 96/60 mm Hg; heart rate, 56 beats/min and irregular; and respirations, 22 breaths/min. While placing him on oxygen you note that his pupils are slightly dilated. His level of consciousness continues to decline. You begin transport.

The scene does not suggest any trauma but you do a quick head to toe assessment. There are no obvious injuries found that would cause the decreased level of consciousness. You place him on the ECG and find a sinus rhythm with frequent premature ventricular contractions. You prepare to start an IV but take a blood sample first to check his blood glucose level. It is 36 mg/dL. Realizing that you have found the most likely cause of the problem, you finish placing the IV line and administer $D_{50}W$ per protocol.

Minutes later, George, as he introduced himself, is sitting up on the cot. He is alert and well oriented. His skin is now pink, warm, and dry, and the premature ventricular contractions on the monitor have resolved.

His vital signs are now: blood pressure, 124/76 mm Hg; heart rate, 72 beats/min; and respirations, 18 breaths/min. As you continue to the hospital, he tells you that he took his insulin this morning and planned to eat breakfast at a nearby restaurant but he needed to run a few errands first.

Shortly after arriving at the hospital, the emergency room staff brings the patient a breakfast tray. When he finished eating, he was reevaluated and discharged.

1. A possible cause of uncooperative, restless, or belligerent behavior is:
    A. hypoxia.
    B. head injury.
    C. hypoglycemia.
    D. all of the above.

2. Another name for your working diagnosis is:
    A. general impression.
    B. index of suspicion.
    C. field impression.
    D. mechanism of injury.

3. Given a patient's condition, findings that are expected but absent are documented as:
    A. absent findings.
    B. pertinent negatives.
    C. nonessential.
    D. not documented or reported.

4. Your radio report should contain all of the following EXCEPT:

   A. the patient's name.
   B. the chief complaint.
   C. physical findings.
   D. your impression.

5. Your patient's blood glucose level was initially 36 mg/dL. You know that a normal reading would be:

   A. 40.
   B. 60.
   C. 100.
   D. 200.

Points to Ponder

You respond to a local shopping mall for a geriatric patient who fell on the escalator. As you leave your ambulance, you take your stretcher, a backboard, your jump kit, the ECG monitor, and portable O_2. On approaching the patient, you note that a large crowd has gathered at the foot of the escalator. Making your way through, you find a frail woman supine on the floor. Her daughter introduces herself and tells you that her mother, Mrs. Harris, lost her balance and fell backwards.

You introduce yourself to the patient and she responds appropriately. You have a mall security officer hold her cervical spine in place while you begin your assessment. Because there does not appear to be any life-threatening injuries, your partner obtains a SAMPLE history from the daughter. The security officer tells you that the patient must be moved so the escalator can be restarted.

You do a rapid trauma assessment. Your findings include a hematoma above the right eye, minor skin tears on the right arm, and obvious deformity to the right hip. With the assistance of the security officer and your partner, the patient is placed on the backboard and started on oxygen therapy. You move to the more controlled setting of your ambulance. Vital signs include a blood pressure of 146/88 mm Hg, a heart rate of 106 beats/min, and respirations of 20 breaths/min. You obtain an ECG and start an IV of normal saline. The patient tolerates the transport well and is admitted to the hospital for repair of her fractured hip.

Issues: Understanding the Need to Develop Roles in Patient Care, Understanding the Need to Carry the Right Equipment to the Patient's Side, Understanding the Need to Move to the Ambulance When the Environment Is Distracting or Chaotic

BLS Review

1999 Objectives

There are no 1999 objectives for this chapter.

1985 Objectives

1.6.62 Demonstrate effective cardiopulmonary resuscitation. (p 1549)

*****S1.9.24** Demonstrate on an adult mannequin, the techniques for single and two-person CPR according to American Heart Association standards. (p 1567)

*****S1.9.25** Demonstrate on an infant mannequin, the technique for infant CPR according to American Heart Association standards. (p 1572)

*Indicates optional.

Additional Objectives†

Cognitive

1. Identify the need for basic life support, including the urgency surrounding its rapid application. (p 1546, 1549)
2. List the EMT-I's responsibilities in beginning and terminating CPR. (p 1549)
3. Describe the proper way to position an adult patient to receive basic life support. (p 1551)
4. Describe the proper way to position an infant and child to receive basic life support. (p 1551)
5. Describe the three techniques for opening the airway in infants, children, and adults. (p 1551)
6. List the steps in providing artificial ventilation in infants, children, and adults. (p 1560)
7. Describe how gastric distention occurs. (p 1562)
8. Define the recovery position. (p 1563)
9. Describe infectious disease issues related to rescue breathing. (p 1560)
10. List the steps in providing chest compressions in an adult. (p 1564)
11. List the steps in providing chest compressions in an infant and child. (p 1571)
12. List the steps in providing one-rescuer CPR in an infant, child, and adult. (p 1567)
13. List the steps in providing two-rescuer CPR in an infant, child, and adult. (p 1567)
14. Distinguish foreign body airway obstruction from other conditions that cause respiratory failure. (p 1554, 1558)
15. Distinguish a complete airway obstruction from a partial airway obstruction. (p 1554, 1557)
16. Describe the steps in removing a foreign body obstruction in an infant, child, and adult. (p 1555)

Affective

17. Recognize and respect the feelings of the patient and family during basic life support. (p 1550)
18. Explain the urgency surrounding the rapid initiation of basic life support measures. (p 1546)
19. Explain the EMT-I's responsibilities in starting and terminating CPR. (p 1549)
20. Explain the rationale for removing a foreign body obstruction. (p 1554)

Psychomotor

21. Demonstrate how to position the patient to open the airway. (p 1551)
22. Demonstrate how to perform the head tilt-chin lift maneuver in infants, children, and adults. (p 1552)
23. Demonstrate how to perform the jaw-thrust and modified jaw-thrust maneuvers in infants, children, and adults. (p 1554)
24. Demonstrate how to place a patient in the recovery position. (p 1563)
25. Demonstrate how to perform chest compressions in an adult. (p 1564)
26. Demonstrate how to perform chest compressions in an infant and child. (p 1571)
27. Demonstrate how to perform one-rescuer CPR in an infant, child, and adult. (p 1567)
28. Demonstrate how to perform two-rescuer CPR in an infant, child, and adult. (p 1567)
29. Demonstrate how to remove a foreign body obstruction in an infant, child, and adult. (p 1555, 1558)

†All of these objectives are noncurriculum objectives.

39
BLS Review

You are the Provider

You and your partner are dispatched to 1300 Blossom Lane for an unconscious male, unknown cause. A few minutes later, the dispatcher informs you that "CPR is in progress."

1. Given the initial nature of the call, what would be a good idea?
2. After the dispatcher notifies you that CPR is in progress, what should you do to prepare?

BLS Review

The principles of basic life support were introduced in 1960. Since that time, the specific techniques have been reviewed and revised every 5 to 6 years. The updated guidelines are published in *JAMA*. The most recent revision occurred as a result of the 2005 Conference on Cardiopulmonary Resuscitation and Emergency Cardiac Care. The guidelines in this chapter follow those proposed at the 2005 conference. Note that the 1994 EMT-Basic National Standard Curriculum requires basic life support (BLS) as a prerequisite to the EMT-I course; it is presented here as a review.

This chapter begins with a definition and general discussion of BLS. The next sections describe methods for opening and maintaining an airway, providing artificial ventilation to a person who is not breathing, providing artificial circulation to a person with no pulse, and removing a foreign body airway obstruction. Each of these sections is followed by a review of the changes in technique that are necessary to treat infants and children. A discussion of the methods of preventing the transmission of infectious diseases during CPR is provided in Chapter 2.

Elements of BLS

Basic life support (BLS) is noninvasive (not involving penetration of the body, such as with surgery or a hypodermic needle) emergency lifesaving care that is used to treat medical conditions, including airway obstruction, respiratory arrest, and cardiac arrest. This care focuses on what is often termed the ABCs: airway (obstruction), breathing (respiratory arrest), and circulation (cardiac arrest or severe bleeding) (Figure 39-1). BLS follows a specific sequence for adults and for infants and children (Table 39-1). Ideally, only seconds should pass between the time you recognize that a patient needs BLS and the start of treatment. Remember, brain cells die every second that they are deprived of oxygen. Permanent brain damage may occur if the brain is without oxygen for 4 to 6 minutes. After 6 minutes without oxygen, some brain damage is almost certain (Figure 39-2).

If a patient is not breathing well or at all, you may simply need to open the airway. Very often, this will help the patient breathe normally again. However, if the patient has no pulse, you must combine artificial ventilation with artificial circulation. If breathing stops before the heart stops, the patient will have enough oxygen in the lungs to stay alive for several minutes. But when a patient goes into cardiac arrest first, the heart and brain stop receiving oxygen immediately.

Cardiopulmonary resuscitation (CPR) is used to establish artificial ventilation and circulation in a patient who is not breathing and has no pulse. The steps for CPR include the following:

1. Opening the airway
2. Restoring breathing by means of rescue breathing (mouth-to-mouth ventilation, mouth-to-nose ventilation, or using mechanical devices)
3. Restoring circulation by means of chest compressions to circulate blood through the body

To maximize survival, you must be able to easily identify a patient who is in respiratory and/or cardiac arrest and begin treatment with BLS measures immediately (Figure 39-3).

> **EMT-I Safety**
>
> While your chances of contracting a disease during CPR training or actual CPR on a patient are very low, common sense and OSHA (Occupational Safety and Health Administration) guidelines both demand that you take reasonable precautions to prevent unnecessary exposure to infectious disease. Using standard precautions makes the risk *extremely* low; then you don't have to be anxious about practicing and performing the skill.

Technology

- Interactivities
- Vocabulary Explorer
- Anatomy Review
- Web Links
- Online Review Manual

www.EMSzone.com/EMTI

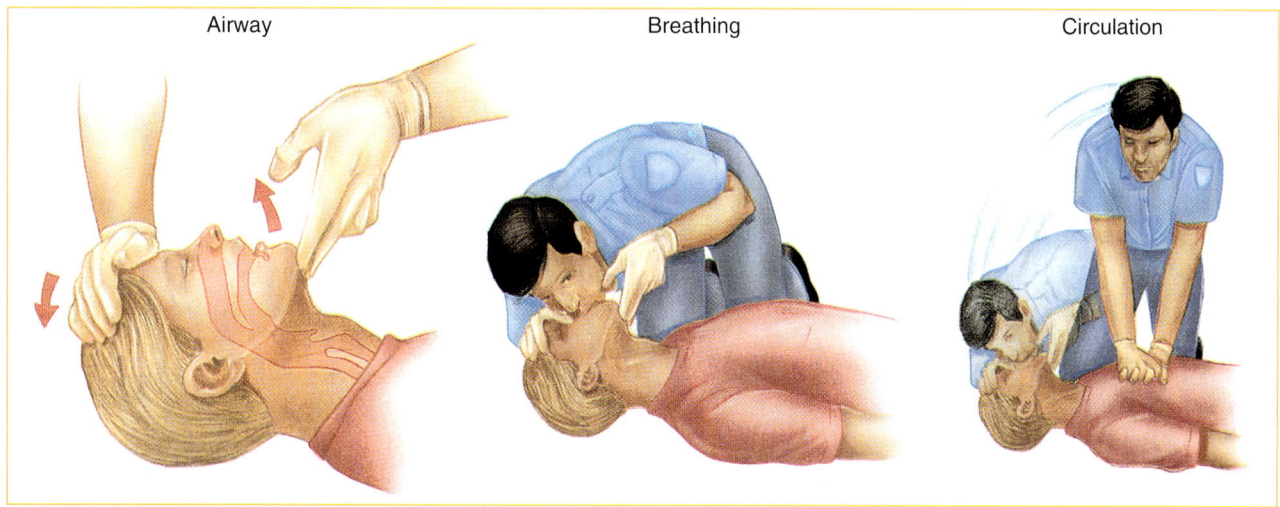

Figure 39-1 The ABCs of basic life support are airway, breathing, and circulation.

TABLE 39-1 Review of Pediatric BLS Procedures

Procedure	Infants (younger than 1 y)	Children (1 y to onset of puberty)[1]
Airway	Head tilt–chin lift; jaw thrust if spinal injury is suspected	Head tilt–chin lift; jaw thrust if spinal injury is suspected
Breathing		
Initial breaths	2 breaths with duration of 1 second each with enough volume to produce chest rise	2 breaths with duration of 1 second each with enough volume to produce chest rise
Subsequent breaths	1 breath every 3 to 5 seconds; 12 to 20 breaths/min	1 breath every 3 to 5 seconds; 12 to 20 breaths/min
Circulation		
Pulse check	Brachial artery	Carotid or femoral artery
Compression area	Just below the nipple line	In the center of the chest, in between the nipples
Compression width	2 fingers or 2-thumb hands-encircling technique	Heel of one or both hands
Compression depth	$1/3$ to $1/2$ the depth of the chest	$1/3$ to $1/2$ the depth of the chest
Compression rate	100/min	100/min
Ratio of compressions to ventilations	30:2 (one rescuer); 15:2 (two rescuers)[2]	30:2 (one rescuer); 15:2 (two rescuers)[2]
Foreign body obstruction	Conscious: back slaps and chest thrusts Unconscious: CPR	Conscious: abdominal thrusts Unconscious: CPR

[1] Onset of puberty is approximately 12-14 years of age, as defined by secondary characteristics (eg, breast development in girls and armpit hair in boys).
[2] Pause compressions to deliver ventilations.

You are the Provider — Part 2

Five minutes later, you arrive at the scene to find a hysterical woman standing at the front door. She tells you that her husband is in the back bedroom, and he's not breathing. As you enter the bedroom, you see an elderly male who is lying in bed. A dog is in the bed next to him, growling and barking at you.

3. What is your first priority?
4. What information do you need to obtain from the patient's wife?

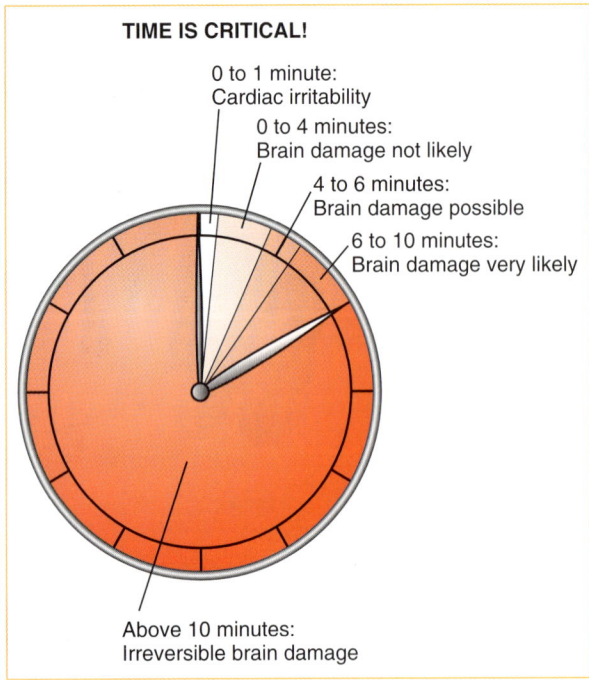

Figure 39-2 Time is critical for patients who are not breathing. If the brain is deprived of oxygen for 4 to 6 minutes, brain damage is likely to occur.

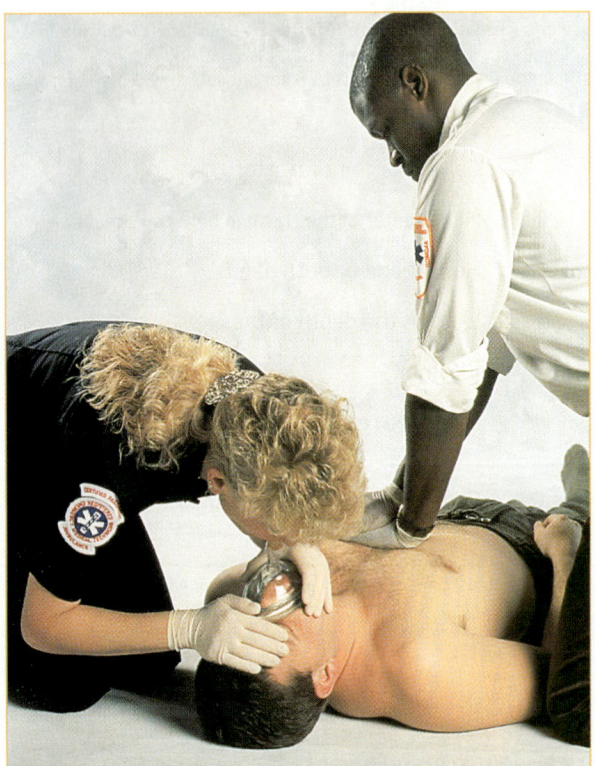

Figure 39-3 You must quickly identify patients in respiratory and/or cardiac arrest so that BLS measures can begin immediately.

Rescue breathing can be given by one or two EMT-Is or EMT-Bs, by first responders, or by trained bystanders. It does not require any equipment; however, you should use a barrier device when performing rescue breathing. Rescue breathing delivers exhaled gas from you to the patient. This gas contains 16% oxygen, which is sufficient to maintain the patient's life. Once you determine that the patient needs BLS, you should begin rescue breathing immediately, along with efforts to support the circulation and correct cardiac problems.

BLS differs from <u>advanced life support (ALS)</u>, which involves advanced lifesaving procedures, such as cardiac monitoring, administration of intravenous fluids and medications, and the use of advanced airway adjuncts. However, when done correctly, BLS can maintain life for a short time until ALS measures can be started. In some cases, such as choking, near drowning, or lightning injuries, early BLS measures may be all that is needed to restore a patient's pulse and breathing. Of course, these patients also require transport to the hospital for evaluation.

BLS measures are only as effective as the person who is performing them. Your skills will be very good immediately after training. However, as time goes on, your skills will deteriorate unless you practice them regularly.

Automated External Defibrillation

Most out-of-hospital cardiac arrests occur as the result of a sudden cardiac rhythm disturbance (dysrhythmia), such as ventricular fibrillation (V-fib) or pulseless ventricular tachycardia (V-tach). According to the American Heart Association, early defibrillation is the link in the chain of survival that is most likely to improve survival rates. For each minute the patient remains in V-fib or pulseless V-tach, there is a 7% to 10% smaller chance of survival.

The automated external defibrillator (AED) should be attached to any adult nontraumatic cardiac arrest patient as soon as possible; defibrillation, if indicated, must be performed without delay. The AED is not indicated for children less than 1 year of age, regardless of the cause of their cardiac arrest.

The AED's simple design makes it easy for EMT-Is, EMT-Bs, first responders, and laypersons to use; very little training is required.

If you witness the patient's cardiac arrest, begin CPR and apply the AED as soon as it is available. However, if the patient's cardiac arrest was not witnessed by you, especially if the call-to-arrival interval is greater than 5 minutes, the American Heart Association recommends that you perform 5 cycles (about 2 minutes) of CPR before applying the AED. The rationale for this is that the heart is more likely to respond to defibrillation within the first few minutes of the onset of ventricular fibrillation. If the arrest interval is prolonged, however, metabolic waste products accumulate within the heart, energy stores are rapidly depleted, and the chance of successful defibrillation is reduced. Therefore, a 2-minute period of CPR before applying the AED in patients with prolonged (> 5 minutes) cardiac arrest can "prime the pump," thus restoring oxygen to the heart, removing metabolic waste products, and increasing the chance of successful defibrillation.

AEDs can safely be used in patients older than 1 year of age. If using the AED on a child between 1 and 8 years of age, you should use pediatric-sized pads and a dose-attenuating system (energy reducer). However, if these are unavailable, you should use an adult AED. Refer to Chapter 20 for complete information regarding the AED, including proper use, safety considerations, and the AED algorithm.

Assessing the Need for BLS

As always, begin by surveying the scene. Is it safe? How many patients are there? What is your initial impression of the patients? Are there bystanders who may have information? Do you suspect trauma? If you were dispatched to the scene, does the dispatch information match what you are seeing?

Because of the urgent need to start CPR in a pulseless, nonbreathing patient, you must complete an initial assessment as soon as possible, evaluating the patient's ABCs. The first step is determining unresponsiveness Figure 39-4. Clearly, a patient who is conscious does not need CPR; a person who is unresponsive may need CPR, depending on further assessment findings.

You may also suspect the presence of a cervical spine injury. If so, you must protect the spinal cord from further injury as you perform CPR. If there is even a remote possibility of this type of injury, you should begin taking appropriate precautions during the initial assessment.

The basic principles of BLS are the same for infants, children, and adults. For the purposes of BLS, anyone younger than 1 year is considered an infant. A child is between 1 year of age and the onset of puberty (12 to 14 years of age). Adulthood is from onset of puberty and older. Children vary in size. Some small children may best be treated as infants and some larger children as adults. There are two basic differences in providing CPR for infants, children, and adults. The first is that the emergencies in which infants and children require CPR have different underlying causes. The second is that there are anatomic differences among adults, children, and infants. These differences include smaller airways in infants and children than in adults.

Although cardiac arrest in adults usually occurs before respiratory arrest, the reverse is true in infants and children. In most cases, cardiac arrest in children results from respiratory arrest. If untreated, respiratory arrest will quickly lead to cardiac arrest and death. Respiratory arrest in infants and children has a variety of causes, including aspiration of foreign bodies into the airway, such as parts of hot dogs, peanuts, candy, or small toys; airway infections, such as croup and epiglottitis; near-drowning incidents or electrocution; and sudden infant death syndrome (also known as SIDS).

When to Start and Stop BLS

As an EMT-I, it is your responsibility to start CPR in virtually all patients who are in cardiac arrest. There are only two general exceptions to the rule.

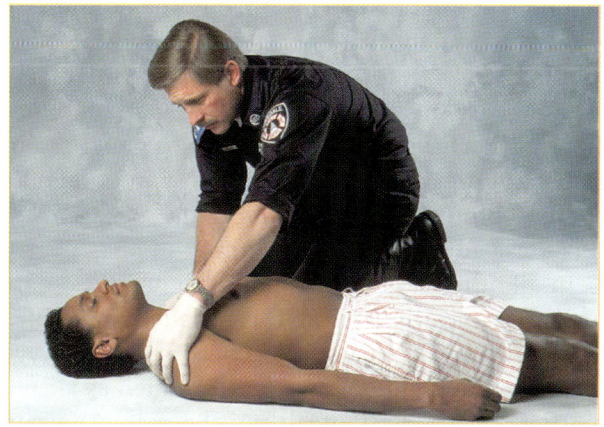

Figure 39-4 Assess airway, breathing, and circulation in an unconscious patient by first attempting to rouse the patient.

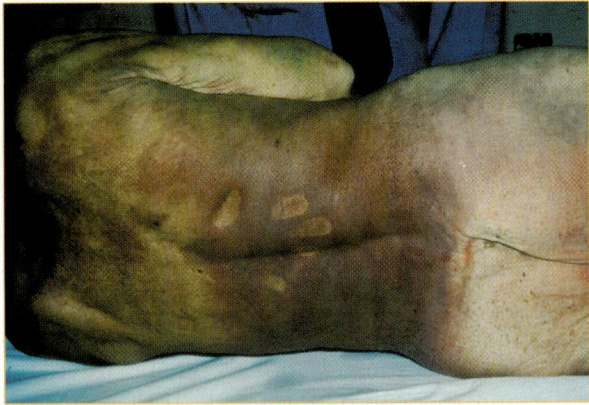

Figure 39-5 Dependent lividity is an obvious sign of death, caused by blood settling to the areas of the body not in firm contact with the ground. The lividity in this figure is seen as purple discoloration of the back, except in areas that are in firm contact with the ground (scapula and buttock).

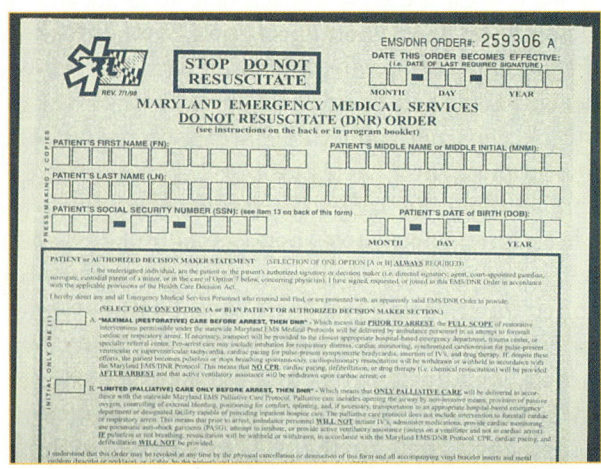

Figure 39-6 You should not start CPR if the patient and his or her physician have previously agreed on DNR or no-CPR orders. Learn your local protocols for treating terminally ill patients.

Documentation Tips

Correct handling of situations when you choose not to start CPR on a patient in cardiac arrest begins with compliance with protocols and ends with detailed documentation. In particular, record physical exam signs that led to your decision, and make reference to the protocol that states these signs as a reason not to start. If extenuating circumstances such as entrapment physically prevent resuscitation attempts, record the conditions thoroughly. These decisions occasionally give rise to questions that can often be put to rest immediately by reference to a well-written report.

First, you should not start CPR if the patient has obvious signs of death. Signs of obvious death include an absence of a pulse and breathing, along with any one of the following:

- Rigor mortis, or stiffening of the body after death
- Dependent lividity (livor mortis), a discoloration of the skin due to pooling of blood **Figure 39-5**
- Putrefaction or decomposition of the body
- Evidence of a nonsurvivable injury, such as decapitation, dismemberment, or burned beyond recognition.

Rigor mortis and dependent lividity develop after a patient has been dead for a long period.

Second, you should not start CPR if the patient and his or her physician have previously agreed on DNR (do not resuscitate) or no-CPR orders **Figure 39-6**. This may apply only to situations in which the patient is known to be in the terminal stage of an incurable disease. In this situation, CPR serves only to prolong the patient's death. However, this can be a complicated issue. Advance directives, such as living wills, may express the patient's wishes; however, these documents may not be readily producible by the patient's family or caregiver. In such cases, the safest course is to assume that an emergency exists and begin CPR under the rule of implied consent and contact medical control for further guidance. Conversely, if a valid DNR document or living will is produced, resuscitative efforts may be withheld. Learn your local protocols and the standards in your system for treating terminally ill patients. Some EMS systems have computer notes on patients who are preregistered with the system. These notes usually specify the amount and extent of treatment that are desired. Other states have specific EMS DNR forms that allow EMS providers to withhold care in situations where the patient, family, and physician have agreed in advance that such a course is most appropriate. It is critical that you understand your local protocols and are aware of the specific restrictions these advance directives imply.

In all other cases, you should begin CPR on anyone who is in cardiac arrest. It is usually impossible to know how long the patient has been without oxygen to the brain and vital organs. Factors such as air temperature and the basic health of the patient's tissues and organs can affect their ability to survive. There-

> **Pediatric Needs**
>
> Opening the airway in an infant or child is done by using the same techniques that are used for an adult. However, because a child's neck is so flexible, the head tilt–chin lift maneuver should be modified so that as you tilt the head back, you are moving it only into the neutral position or a slightly extended position (Figure 39-7). You may also use the jaw-thrust maneuver. In fact, this is the best method to use if you suspect a spinal injury in a child. If a second rescuer is present, he or she should immobilize the child's cervical spine.

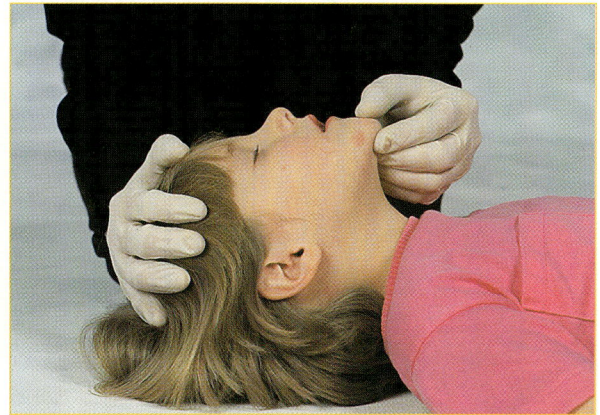

Figure 39-7 The head tilt–chin lift maneuver on a child is slightly modified in that as you tilt the head back, you move it only into the neutral position or a slightly extended position.

fore, most legal advisers recommend that, when in doubt, you should always give too much care rather than too little. You should always start CPR if any doubt exists.

You are not responsible for making the decision to stop CPR. Once you begin CPR in the field, you must continue until one of the following events occurs:

- S The patient **starts** breathing and has a pulse.
- T The patient is **transferred** to another person who is trained in BLS, to ALS-trained personnel, or to another emergency medical responder.
- O You are **out** of strength or too tired to continue.
- P A **physician** who is present or providing online medical direction assumes responsibility for the patient and gives direction to discontinue CPR.

"Out of strength" does not mean merely weary; it means no longer physically able to perform CPR. In short, CPR should always be continued until the patient's care is transferred to a physician or higher medical authority in the field. In some cases, your medical director or a designated medical control physician may order you to stop CPR on the basis of the patient's condition.

Every EMS system should have clear standing orders or protocols that provide guidelines for starting and stopping CPR. Your medical director and your system's legal adviser should agree on these protocols, which should be closely administered and reviewed by your medical director.

Positioning the Patient

The next step in providing CPR is to position the patient to ensure that the airway is open. For CPR to be effective, the patient must be lying supine on a firm surface, with enough clear space around the patient for two rescuers to perform CPR. You will need to reposition any patient who is "crumpled up" or lying face down. The few seconds that you spend to position the patient properly will greatly improve the delivery and effectiveness of CPR.

Follow the steps in (Skill Drill 39-1) to reposition an unconscious adult patient for airway management:

1. **Kneel beside the patient.** You and your partner must be far enough away so that the patient, when rolled toward you, does not come to rest in your lap (**Step 1**).
2. First EMT-I: **Place your hands** behind the patient's back, head, and neck to protect the cervical spine if you suspect spinal injury. Second EMT-I: Place your hands on the distant shoulder and the hip (**Step 2**).
3. Second EMT-I: **Turn the patient toward you** by pulling on the distant shoulder and the hip. First EMT-I: Control the head and neck so that they move as a unit with the rest of the torso. This single motion will allow the head, neck, and back to stay in the same vertical plane and will minimize aggravation of any spinal injury (**Step 3**).
4. First EMT-I: **Place the patient in a supine position,** with the legs straight and both arms at the sides (**Step 4**).

Skill Drill 39-1: Positioning the Patient

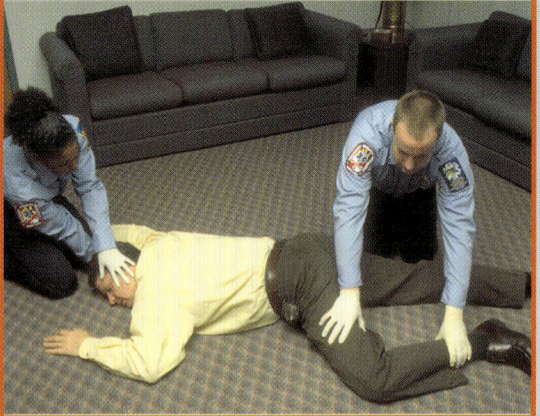

1 Kneel beside the patient, leaving room to roll the patient toward you.

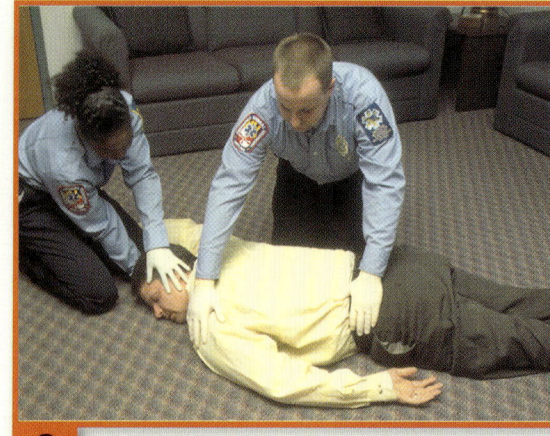

2 Grasp the patient, stabilizing the cervical spine if needed.

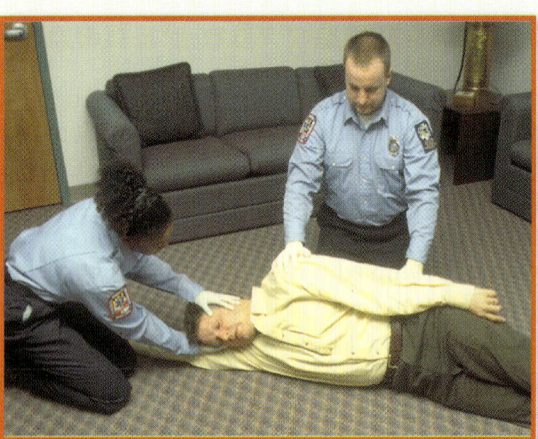

3 Move the head and neck as a unit with the torso as your partner pulls on the distant shoulder and hip.

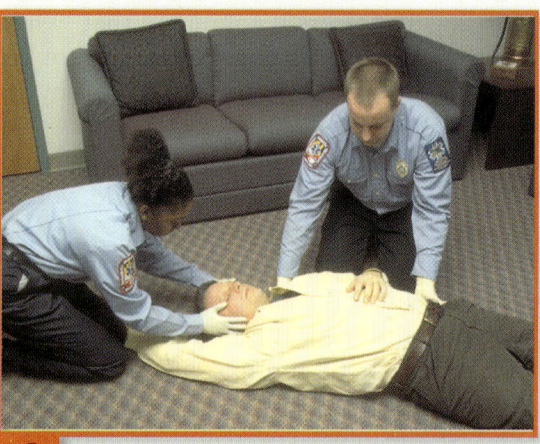

4 Move the patient to a supine position with legs straight and arms at the sides.

If possible, log roll the patient onto a long backboard as you are positioning him or her for CPR. This device will provide support during transport and emergency department care. Once the patient is properly positioned, you can easily assess airway, breathing, circulation, and the need for defibrillation and start CPR if necessary.

Opening the Airway in Adults

Without an open airway, rescue breathing will not be effective. There are two techniques for opening the airway in adults: the head tilt–chin lift maneuver and the jaw-thrust maneuver.

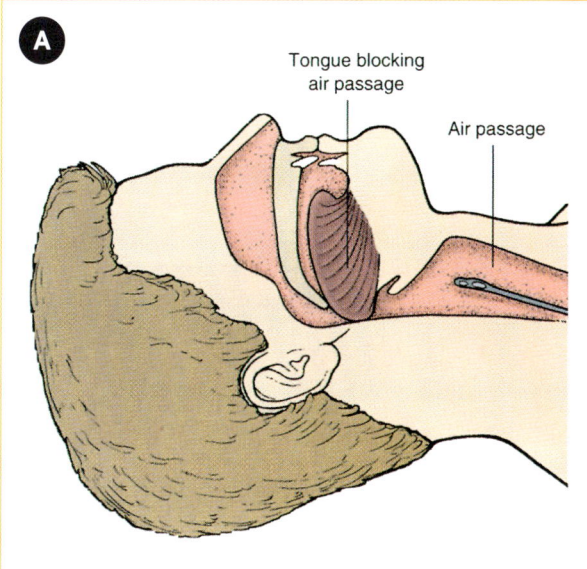

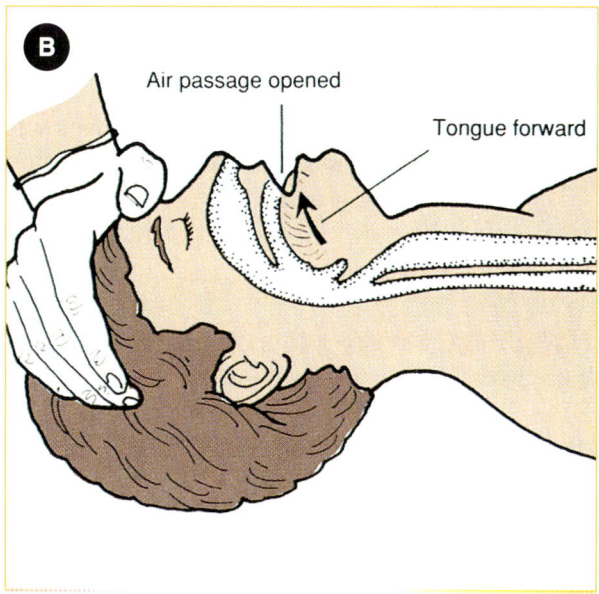

Figure 39-8 **A.** Relaxation of the tongue back into the throat causes airway obstruction. **B.** The head tilt–chin lift maneuver combines two movements of opening the airway.

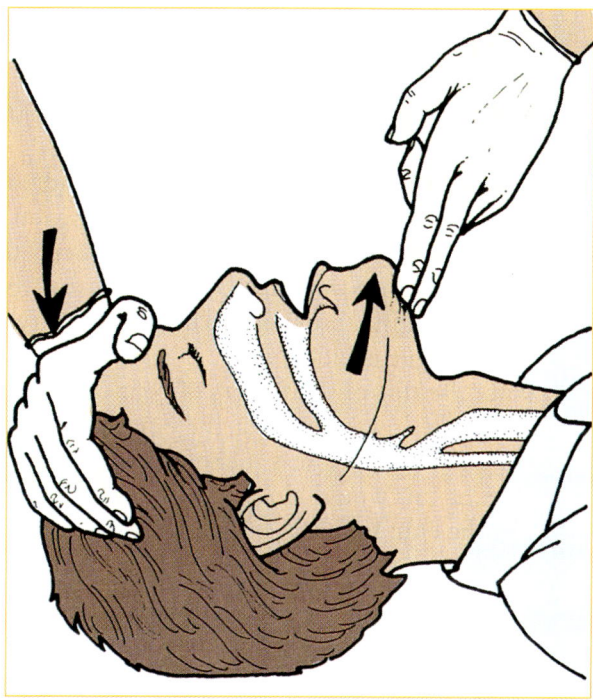

Figure 39-9 To perform the head tilt–chin lift maneuver, place one hand on the patient's forehead, and apply firm backward pressure with your palm to tilt the head back. Next, place the tips of the fingers of your other hand under the lower jaw near the bony part of the chin. Lift the chin forward, bringing the entire lower jaw with it, helping to tilt the head back.

Head Tilt–Chin Lift Maneuver

Opening the airway to relieve an obstruction caused by relaxation of the tongue can often be accomplished quickly and easily with the head tilt–chin lift maneuver Figure 39-8. In patients who have not sustained trauma, this simple maneuver is sometimes all that is required for the patient to resume breathing. If the patient has any foreign material or vomitus in the mouth, you should quickly remove it. Wipe out any liquid materials from the mouth with a piece of cloth held by your index and middle fingers; use your hooked

You are the Provider Part 3

You confirm that the patient is unresponsive, and you and your partner move the man down to the floor. As you open his airway, copious amounts of vomitus come from his mouth. While you are managing his airway, your partner checks for a carotid pulse and finds none.

5. Why should you move the patient, and what should you do if you cannot?
6. What should you do to manage his airway, and what should be the next step your partner performs?

index finger to remove any solid material. You should perform the head tilt–chin lift maneuver in an adult in the following way Figure 39-9:

1. **Make sure the patient is supine.** Kneel close beside the patient.
2. **Place one hand on the patient's forehead**, and apply firm backward pressure with your palm to tilt the patient's head back. This extension of the neck will move the tongue forward, away from the back of the throat, and will clear the airway if the tongue is blocking it.
3. **Place the tips of the fingers** of your other hand under the lower jaw near the bony part of the chin. Do not compress the soft tissue under the chin, as this would block the airway.
4. **Lift the chin forward**, bringing the entire lower jaw with it, helping to tilt the head back. Do not use your thumb to lift the chin. Lift so that the teeth are nearly brought together, but avoid closing the mouth completely.

The chin lift has the added advantage of holding loose dentures in place, making obstruction by the lips less likely. Performing ventilation is much easier when dentures are in place. However, dentures that do not stay in place should be removed. Partial dentures (plates) may come loose as a result of an accident or as you are providing care, so check these periodically.

Jaw-Thrust Maneuver

The head tilt–chin lift maneuver is effective for opening the airway in most patients. In cases of suspected spinal injury, you want to minimize movement of the patient's neck. In this case, perform a jaw-thrust maneuver. To perform a jaw-thrust maneuver, place your fingers behind the angles of the patient's lower jaw and then move the jaw forward. Keep the head in a neutral position as you move the jaw forward and open the mouth. If the patient's mouth remains closed, you can use your thumbs to pull the patient's lower lip down, to allow breathing. You can also easily apply a face mask or other barrier device with both hands while performing the jaw thrust.

Perform the jaw-thrust maneuver as follows Figure 39-10:

1. **Kneel above the patient's head.** Place your index or middle finger behind the angle of the patient's lower jaw on both sides, and forcefully move the jaw forward without manipulating the patient's neck.

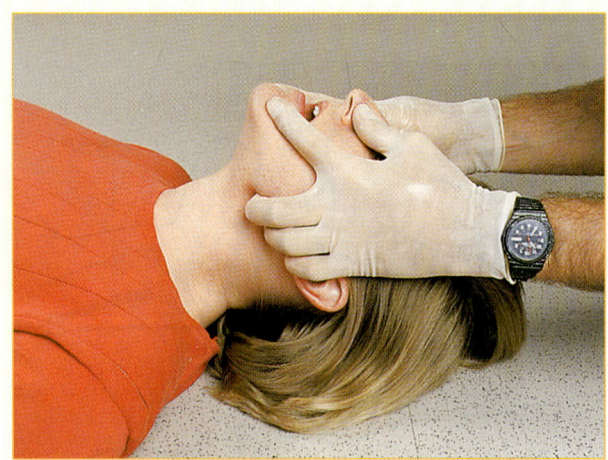

Figure 39-10 To perform the jaw-thrust maneuver, maintain the head in neutral alignment and use your index and long fingers to thrust the jaw forward.

2. **Use your thumbs to open the mouth** to allow breathing.
3. **The nose can be sealed with your cheek** when providing rescue breathing using the jaw-thrust maneuver.

Foreign Body Airway Obstruction in Adults

Airway obstruction may be caused by many things, including relaxation of the throat muscles in an unconscious patient, vomited or regurgitated stomach contents, a blood clot, damaged tissue after an injury, dentures, or a foreign body in the airway. Occasionally, a large foreign body will be aspirated and block the upper airway.

Large objects that cannot be removed from the airway with suction, such as loose dentures, large pieces of vomited food, or blood clots, should be swept forward and out with your gloved index finger. Suctioning can then be used as needed to keep the airway clear of thinner secretions, such as blood, vomitus, and mucus.

Recognizing Foreign Body Obstruction

Sudden airway obstruction by a foreign body in an adult usually occurs during a meal. In a child, it usually occurs during mealtime or at play. Children commonly choke on peanuts, large bits of hot dog, or small toys. If the foreign body is not removed quickly, the lungs will use up their oxygen supply; unconsciousness and death will follow. Your treatment will be based on the cause of the obstruction. Therefore, you must learn to tell the difference between airway problems caused by a foreign body obstruction and those due to respiratory failure or arrest.

Conscious Patients

Sudden airway obstruction is usually easy to recognize in someone who is eating or has just finished eating. The person is suddenly unable to speak or cough, grasps his or her throat, turns cyanotic, and makes exaggerated efforts to breathe. Either air is not moving into and out of the airway or the air movement is so slight that it is not detectable. At first, the patient will be conscious and able to clearly indicate the nature of the problem. Ask the patient, "Are you choking?" The patient will usually answer by nodding yes. Alternatively, he or she may use the universal sign to indicate airway blockage (Figure 39-11 ▶).

Unconscious Patients

When you encounter an unconscious patient, your first step is to determine whether he or she is breathing and has a pulse. The unconsciousness may be due to airway obstruction, cardiac arrest, or a number of other problems. Remember that you must first clear the patient's airway before addressing other problems, such as cardiac arrest. You must first ensure an open and unobstructed airway before checking for a pulse.

You should suspect an airway obstruction if the standard maneuvers to open the airway and ventilate the lungs are not effective. If you feel resistance when ventilating the patient or pressure builds up in your mouth, the patient probably has some type of obstruction.

Removing a Foreign Body Obstruction in Patients Over 1 Year of Age

The manual maneuver recommended for removing a foreign body airway obstruction in the conscious adult and child is the abdominal-thrust maneuver (the Heimlich maneuver). This technique creates an artificial cough by causing a sudden increase in intrathoracic pressure when thrusts are applied to the subdiaphragmatic region; it is a very effective method for removing a foreign body that is obstructing the airway.

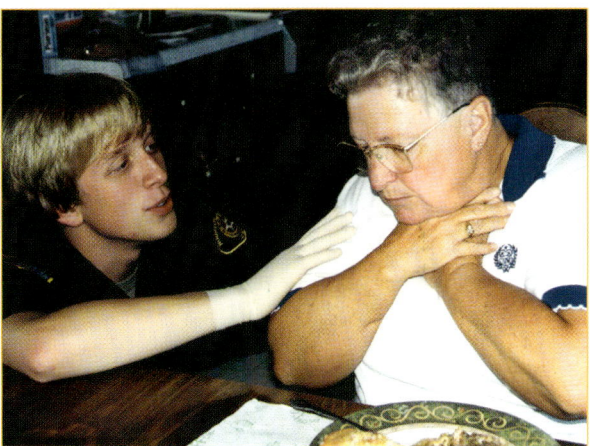

Figure 39-11 Hands at the throat are the universal sign to indicate choking.

Conscious Patients

Abdominal-thrust Maneuver

The abdominal-thrust maneuver, also called the Heimlich maneuver, is the preferred way to dislodge and force food or other material from the throat of a choking victim. Residual air, which is always present in the lungs, is compressed upward and used to expel the object. In conscious patients with a complete airway obstruction, you should repeat abdominal thrusts until the foreign body is expelled or the patient becomes unconscious. Each thrust should be deliberate, with the intent of relieving the obstruction.

To perform abdominal thrusts on the conscious adult (Figure 39-12 ▶), use the following technique:

1. **Stand behind the patient**, and wrap your arms around his or her waist.
2. **Make a fist with one hand**; grasp the fist with the other hand. Place the thumb side of the fist against the patient's abdomen, just above the umbilicus and well below the xiphoid.
3. **Press your fist into the patient's abdomen** with a quick inward and upward thrust.
4. **Continue abdominal thrusts** until the object is expelled from the airway or the patient becomes unconscious.

Chest Thrusts

You can perform the abdominal-thrust maneuver safely on all adults and children. However, you should preferentially use chest thrusts for women in advanced stages of pregnancy and patients who are very obese.

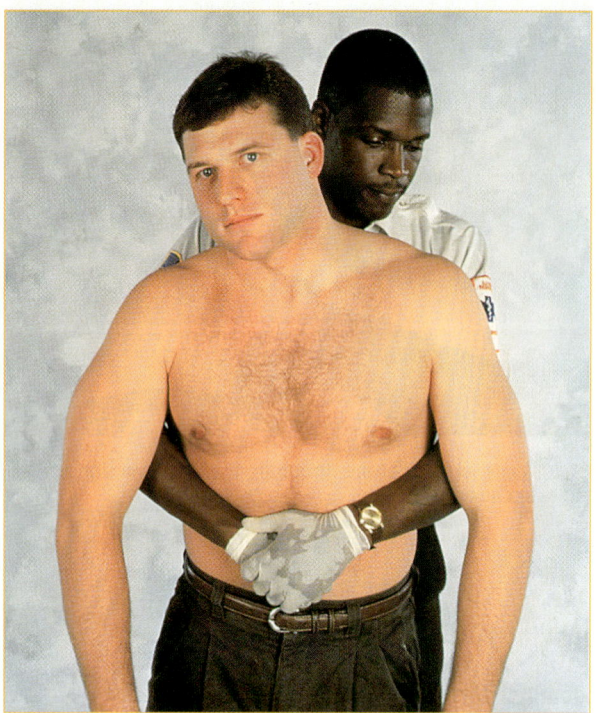

Figure 39-12 The abdominal-thrust maneuver in a conscious adult patient. Stand behind the patient, and wrap your arms around his or her waist. Press your fists into the patient's abdomen, and deliver quick inward and upward thrusts.

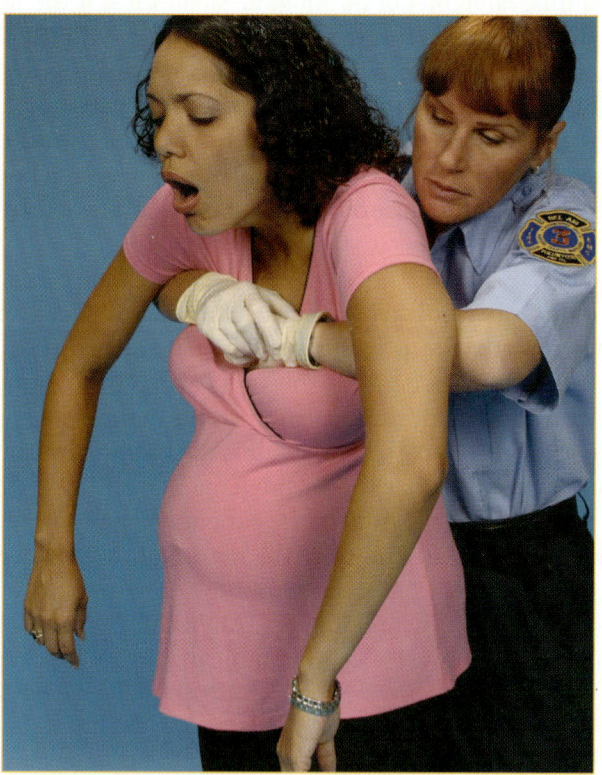

Figure 39-13 Removal of foreign body obstruction in the conscious adult patient using chest thrusts. Stand behind the patient and wrap your arms around the patient's chest. Place the thumb side of one fist against the chest while holding your fist with the other hand. Press your fists into the patient's chest with backwards thrusts.

To perform chest thrusts on the conscious adult, use the following technique (Figure 39-13 ▶):

1. **Stand behind the patient with your arms** directly under the patient's armpits, and wrap your arms around the patient's chest.
2. **Make a fist with one hand**; grasp the fist with the other hand. Place the thumb side of the fist against the patient's sternum, avoiding the xiphoid process and the edges of the rib cage.
3. **Press your fist into the patient's chest** with backward thrusts until the object is expelled or the patient becomes unconscious.

If the patient becomes unconscious, you should begin CPR (Figure 39-14 ▶).

Unconscious Patients

The patient with an airway obstruction may become unconscious and require additional care. Knowing that this patient had an obstruction will prompt the EMT-I to open the airway and look inside before completing the additional steps of resuscitation.

When a choking victim is found unconscious, it is unlikely that the EMT-I will know what caused the problem. Begin the steps of CPR by determining unresponsiveness, opening the airway, and attempting ventilation. If the first ventilation does not produce visible chest rise, reposition the head and reattempt to ventilate (Figure 39-15 ▶). If both breaths fail to produce visible chest rise, perform 30 chest compressions and then open the airway and look in the mouth. If an object is visible, attempt to remove it. *Never perform blind finger sweeps on any patient; doing so may push the obstruction further into the airway.* After opening the airway and looking inside the mouth, reattempt to ventilate the patient. Continue performing chest compressions, opening the airway and looking inside the mouth, and attempting to ventilate until the airway is clear or you reach definitive care.

Mild Airway Obstruction

Patients with a mild (partial) airway obstruction are able to exchange adequate amounts of air, but still have signs of respiratory distress. Breathing may be noisy; however, the patient usually has a strong, effective cough. Leave these patients alone! Your main concern is to pre-

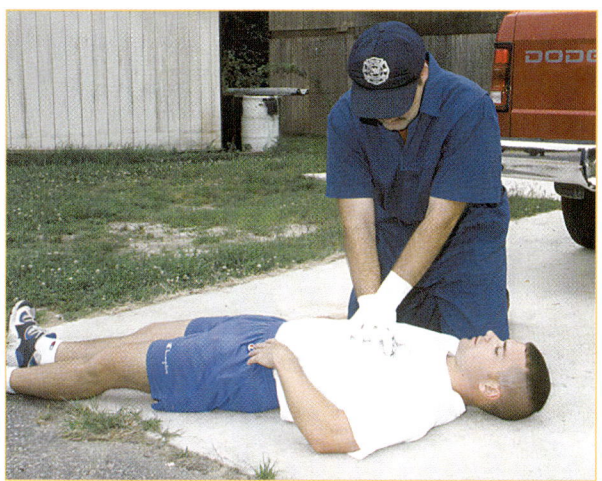

Figure 39-14 Perform chest compressions (CPR) on an unconscious patient with a severe airway obstruction.

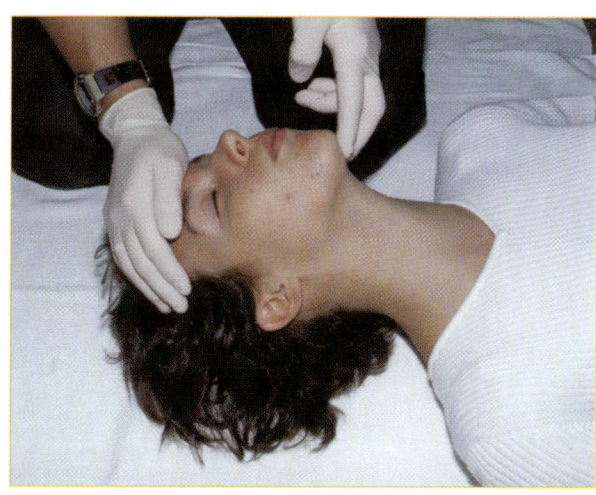

Figure 39-15 The head tilt-chin lift maneuver is a simple technique for opening the airway in a patient without a suspected cervical spine injury.

vent a mild airway obstruction from becoming a severe airway obstruction. The abdominal thrust is not indicated in patients with a mild airway obstruction.

For the patient with a mild airway obstruction, you should first encourage him or her to cough or to continue coughing if they are already doing so. Do not interfere with the patient's own attempts to expel the foreign body. Instead, give 100% oxygen with a nonrebreathing mask and provide prompt transport to the hospital. Closely monitor the patient and observe for signs of a severe airway obstruction (weak or absent cough, decreasing level of consciousness, cyanosis).

Foreign Body Obstruction in Infants and Children

Airway obstruction is a common problem in infants and children and usually is caused by a foreign body or an infection, such as croup or epiglottitis, resulting in swelling and narrowing of the airway. You should try to identify the cause of the obstruction as soon as possible. In patients who have signs and symptoms of an airway infection, you should not waste time trying to dislodge a foreign body. The child needs 100% oxygen with a nonrebreathing mask and immediate transport to the emergency department.

A previously healthy child who is eating or playing with small toys or an infant who is crawling about the house and who suddenly has difficulty breathing has probably aspirated a foreign body. As in adults, foreign bodies may cause a mild or severe airway obstruction.

With a mild airway obstruction, the patient can cough forcefully, although there may be wheezing between coughs. As long as the patient can breathe, cough, or talk, you should not interfere with his or her own attempts to expel the foreign body. As with the adult, encourage the child to continue coughing. Administer 100% oxygen with a nonrebreathing mask (if tolerated) and provide transport to the hospital.

You should intervene only if signs of a severe airway obstruction develop, such as a weak, ineffective cough, cyanosis, absent air movement, or a decreasing level of consciousness. If this occurs, stand or kneel behind the child and provide abdominal thrusts until the object is expelled or the child becomes unconscious (Figure 39-16 ▶).

Removing a Foreign Body Airway Obstruction

Conscious Infants

The abdominal-thrust maneuver might injure the liver or other abdominal organs in an infant. Therefore, use the following technique to remove a foreign body in an infant (Figure 39-17 ▶):

1. **Place one hand on the infant's back and neck** and the other on his or her chest, jaws, and face, holding the jaw firmly to support the head at a

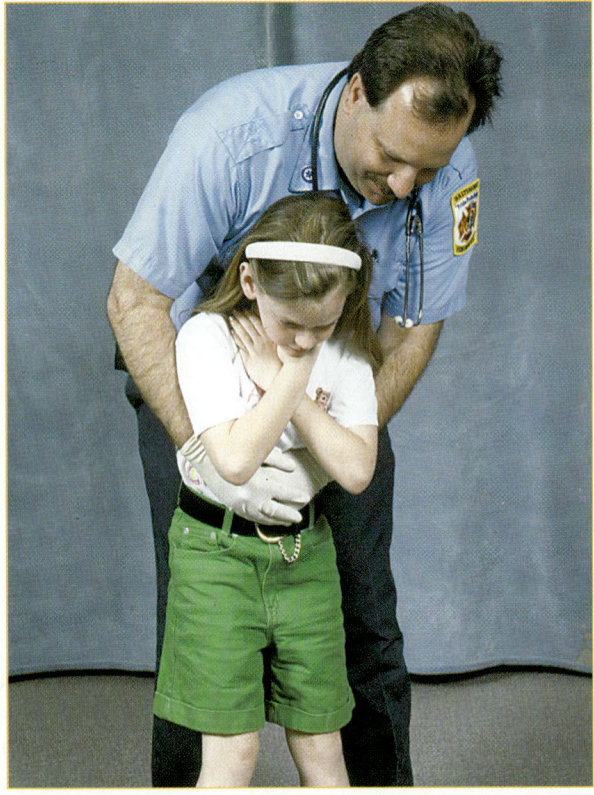

Figure 39-16 Stand behind the child, place your arms around the armpits, and wrap your arms around the patient's abdomen and chest. Press your fists into the patient's abdomen, and provide quick, upward thrusts.

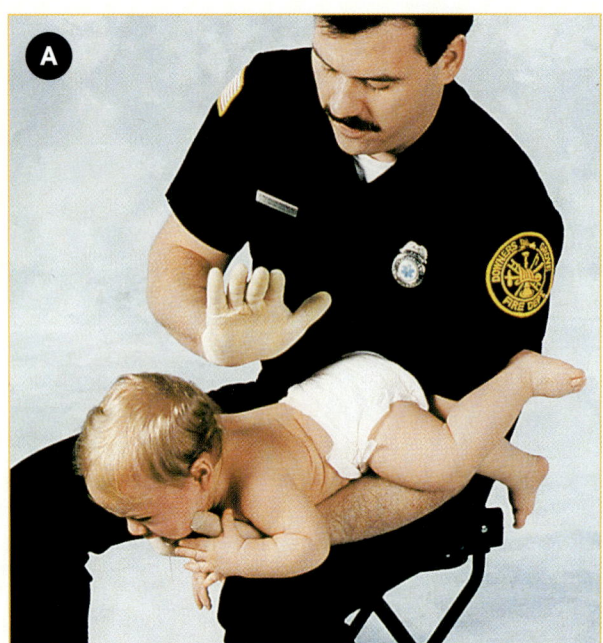

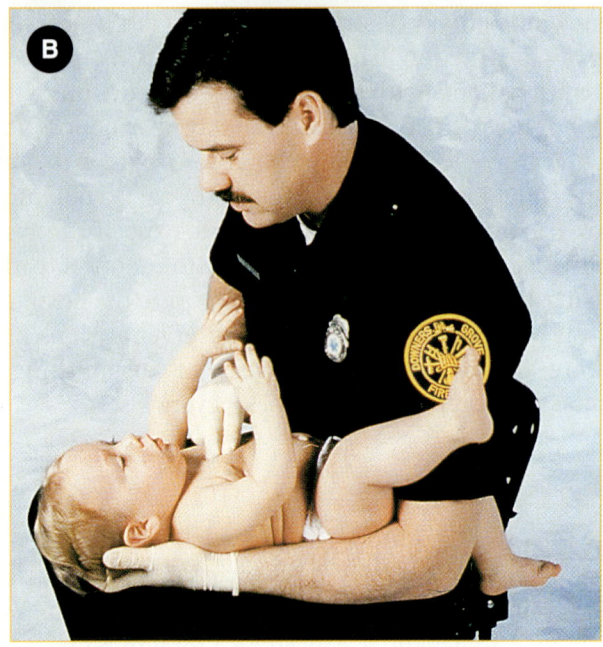

Figure 39-17 A. Deliver five quick back slaps between the shoulder blades, using the heel of your hand. **B.** Give five quick chest thrusts on the sternum at a slightly slower rate than you would give for CPR.

level lower than the trunk. This sandwiches the infant between your hands and arms. Your forearm should rest on your thigh to support the infant.
2. **Deliver five quick back slaps** between the shoulder blades, using the heel of your hand.
3. Next, **turn the infant face up**, making sure that you support the head and neck. Hold the infant in a supine position on your thigh, with the head slightly lower than the trunk.
4. **Give five quick chest thrusts on the sternum** in the same manner as for CPR, except at a slightly slower rate. If the infant is large or your hands are small, you might need to place the infant on your lap to deliver the chest thrusts.

Unconscious Infants

Begin CPR with one extra step: Look inside the airway each time before ventilating and remove the object if seen.

Rescue Breathing in Adults

Once you open the airway, check for breathing by placing your ear about 1″ above the patient's nose and mouth; listen carefully for sounds of breathing. Turn your head so that you can watch for movement of the patient's chest and abdomen **Figure 39-18**. This is called the look, listen, and feel technique. You know that the patient is

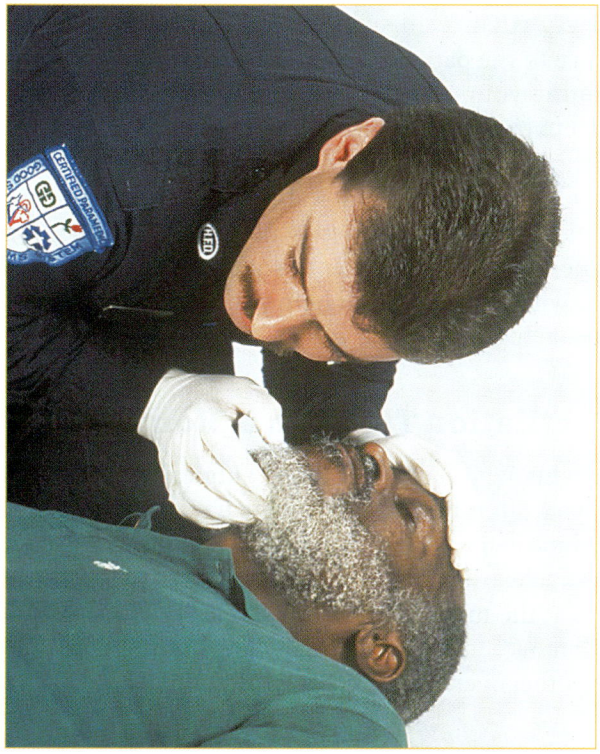

Figure 39-18 Look, listen, and feel for signs of breathing.

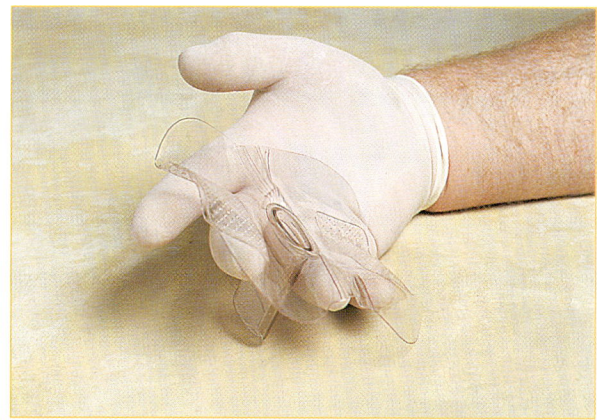

Figure 39-19 A barrier device is used in performing ventilation, because it prevents exposure to saliva, blood, and vomitus.

breathing if you see the chest and abdomen rise and fall and, more important, if you feel and hear air move during exhalation. With airway obstruction, there may be no movement of air, even though the chest and abdomen rise and fall as the patient tries to breathe. You may also have difficulty seeing movement of the chest and abdomen if the patient is fully clothed. Finally, you may see very little or no chest movement at all in some patients, particularly those with chronic lung disease. Therefore, if you do not feel any air movement as you look, listen, and feel, you must begin artificial ventilation. This evaluation should take at least 5 seconds but no more than 10 seconds.

A lack of oxygen in the blood, combined with too much carbon dioxide, is lethal. To correct this condition, you must provide slow, deliberate ventilations that last 1 second. This gentle, slow method of ventilating the patient minimizes the amount of air that is forced into the stomach.

Ventilation

Ventilations are now done routinely with barrier devices, such as masks. These devices feature a plastic barrier that covers the patient's mouth and nose and a one-way valve to prevent exposure to secretions and exhaled contaminants Figure 39-19 ▲ . Such devices also provide good infection control. Providing ventilation without a barrier device should be performed only in extreme conditions. The EMT-B should use devices that supply supplemental oxygen when possible. Devices that have an oxygen reservoir will provide higher percentages of oxygen to the patient. Regardless of whether you are ventilating the patient with or without supplemental oxygen, you should observe the chest for good rise to assess the effectiveness of your ventilation.

You should perform rescue breathing with a simple barrier device in an adult in the following way Figure 39-20 ▼ :

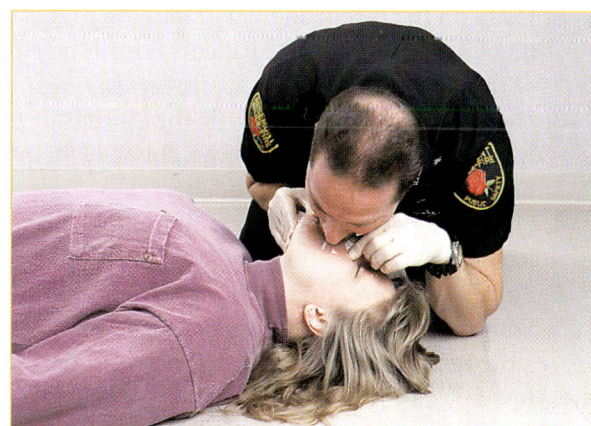

Figure 39-20 To perform ventilation, ensure that you make a tight seal with your mouth around the barrier device, and then give two slow rescue breaths, each lasting 1 second.

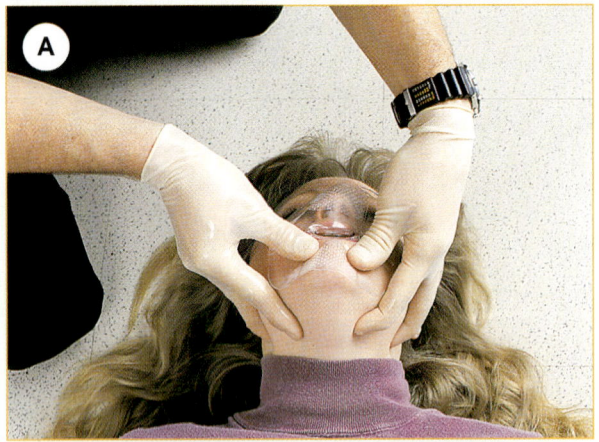
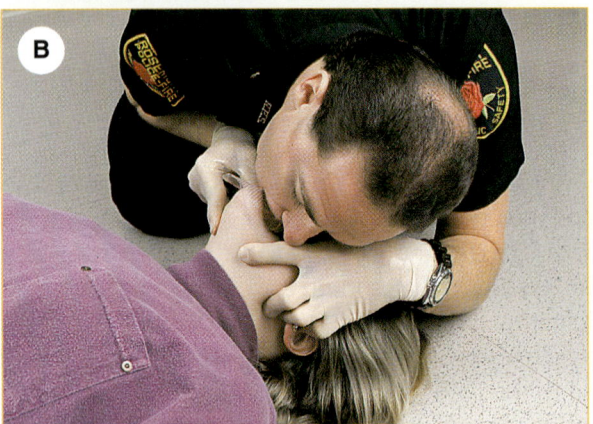

Figure 39-21 A. If you use the jaw-thrust maneuver to open the airway, keep the patient's mouth open with both thumbs as you move from above the patient's head to the side. **B.** Seal the nose by placing your cheek against the patient's nostrils.

If you use the jaw-thrust maneuver to open the airway (that is, in suspected neck injury), you must move to the patient's side to provide ventilation. Positioning yourself at the patient's head is necessary to effectively stabilize the patient's head and provide ventilation at the same time. Keep the patient's mouth open with both thumbs, and seal the nose by placing your cheek against the patient's nostrils Figure 39-21. Note that this maneuver is somewhat difficult; practice with a manikin will help you gain familiarity with this technique.

Ventilation Through a Stoma

Patients who have undergone surgical removal of the larynx often have a permanent tracheal stoma at the midline in the neck. A stoma is an opening that connects the trachea directly to the skin Figure 39-22. Because it is at the midline, the stoma is the only opening that will move air into the patient's lungs; you should ignore any other openings. Patients with a stoma should be ven-

1. **Open the airway** with the head tilt–chin lift maneuver (nontrauma patient).
2. **Press on the forehead** to maintain the backward tilt of the head. Pinch the patient's nostrils together with your thumb and index finger.
3. **Depress the lower lip** with the thumb of the hand that is lifting the chin. This will help to keep the patient's mouth open.
4. **Open the patient's mouth widely**, and place the barrier device over the patient's mouth and nose.
5. **Take a deep breath**, then make a tight seal with your mouth around the barrier device. Give two slow rescue breaths, each lasting 1 second followed by 10 to 12 breaths/min.
6. **Remove your mouth**, and allow the patient to exhale passively. Turn your head slightly to watch for movement of the patient's chest.

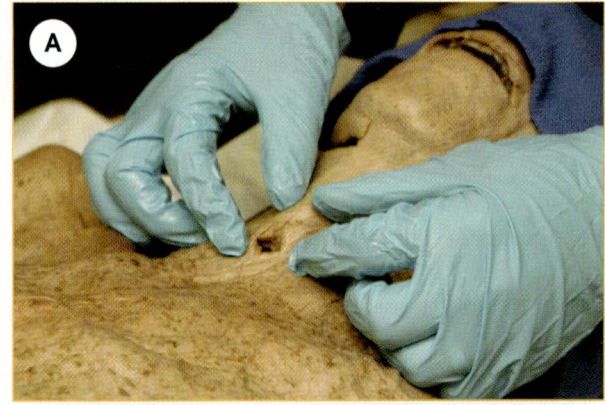
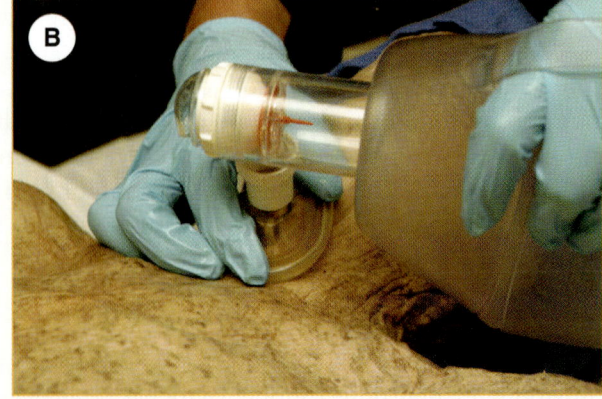

Figure 39-22 A. A stoma is an opening that connects the trachea directly to the skin. **B.** Use a BVM or pocket mask device to ventilate a patient with a stoma.

tilated with a BVM or pocket mask device, as described in Chapter 9.

Gastric Distention

Artificial ventilation may result in the stomach becoming filled with air, a condition called <u>gastric distention</u>. Although it occurs more easily in children, it also happens frequently in adults. Gastric distention is likely to occur if you blow too fast as you ventilate, if you give too much air, or if the patient's airway is not opened adequately. Therefore, it is important for you to give slow, gentle breaths. Such breaths are also more effective in ventilating the lungs. Serious inflation of the stomach is dangerous because it can cause the patient to vomit during CPR. It can also reduce lung volume by elevating the diaphragm.

If massive gastric distention interferes with adequate ventilation, you should contact medical control. Check the airway again, and reposition the patient's head, watch for rise and fall of the chest, and avoid giving forceful breaths. Medical control may order you to turn the patient on his or her side and provide gentle manual pressure to the abdomen to expel air from the stomach. Have suction readily available, and be prepared for copious amounts of vomitus. If gastric distention interferes with your ability to perform adequate artificial ventilation, it must be managed.

Recovery Position

The <u>recovery position</u> helps to maintain a clear airway in a patient with a decreased level of consciousness who has not had traumatic injuries and is breathing adequately on his or her own Figure 39-23. It also allows vomitus to drain from the mouth. Roll the patient onto his or her side so that the head, shoulders, and torso move as a unit, without twisting. Then place the patient's hands under his or her cheek. Never place a patient who

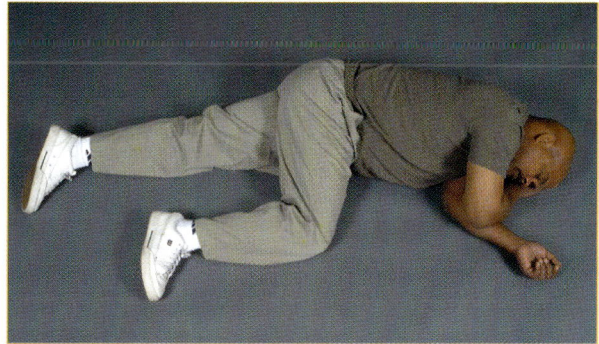

Figure 39-23 The recovery position is used to maintain an open airway in an adequately breathing patient with a decreased level of consciousness who has had no traumatic injuries. It allows vomitus, blood, and any other secretions to drain from the mouth.

> ### ▲ Pediatric Needs
>
> Children who are in respiratory distress are often struggling to breathe. As a result, they usually position themselves in a way that keeps the airway open enough for air to move. Let them stay in that position as long as breathing remains adequate. If you and your partner arrive at the scene and find that the infant or child is not breathing or has cyanosis, immediate management (that is, rescue breathing, supplemental oxygen) must be implemented. Consider requesting additional assistance, if available.
>
> For infants, the preferred technique of rescue breathing is mouth-to-nose-and-mouth ventilation. With this technique, a seal must be made over the mouth and nose. Various masks and other barrier devices are recommended for this technique. If the patient is a large child for whom a tight seal cannot be made over both mouth and nose, you should provide mouth-to-mouth ventilation as you would for an adult.
>
> Once you have made an airtight seal over the mouth, give two gentle breaths each lasting 1 second. These initial breaths will help you assess for airway obstruction and expand the lungs. Because the lungs of infants and children are much smaller than those of adults, you do not need to blow in a great amount of air. Limit the amount of air to that needed to cause the chest to rise.
>
> Remember, too, that a child's airway is smaller than that of an adult. Therefore, there is greater resistance to airflow. As a result, you will need to use a bit more ventilatory pressure to inflate the lungs. You know you are giving the correct amount of air volume as soon as you see the chest rise. Infants and children should be ventilated once every 3 to 5 seconds, or 12 to 20 times per minute.
>
> If air enters freely with your initial breaths and the chest rises, the airway is clear. You should then check the pulse. If air does not enter freely, you should check the airway for obstruction. Reposition the patient's head to open the airway, and attempt to give another breath. If air still does not enter freely, you must then take steps to relieve the obstruction.

has a suspected head or spinal injury in the recovery position because maintenance of spinal alignment in this position is not possible and further spinal injury could result.

Adult CPR

Once you have arrived at the scene and determined that the patient is unresponsive and not breathing, you must position the patient and begin rescue breathing. After you begin rescue breathing, you must assess the patient's circulation.

Cardiac arrest is determined by the absence of a palpable pulse at the carotid artery. Feel for the carotid artery by locating the larynx at the front of the neck and then sliding two fingers toward one side. The pulse is felt in the groove between the larynx and the sternocleidomastoid muscle, with the pulp of the index and long fingers held side by side (Figure 39-24 ▼). Light pressure is sufficient to palpate the pulse. Check the pulse for at least 5 seconds but no longer than 10 seconds; if a pulse cannot be felt, begin CPR.

External Chest Compression

You can provide CPR by applying rhythmic pressure and relaxation to the lower half of the sternum. The heart is located slightly to the left of the middle of the chest between the sternum and the spine

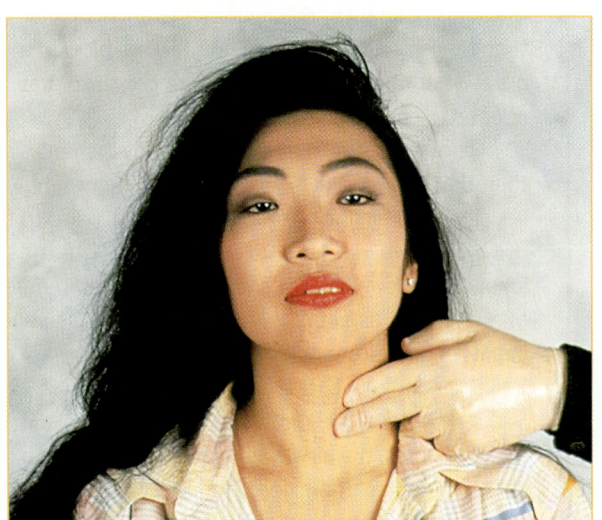

Figure 39-24 Feel for the carotid artery by locating the larynx, then sliding two fingers toward one side. You can feel the pulse in the groove between the larynx and sternocleidomastoid muscle.

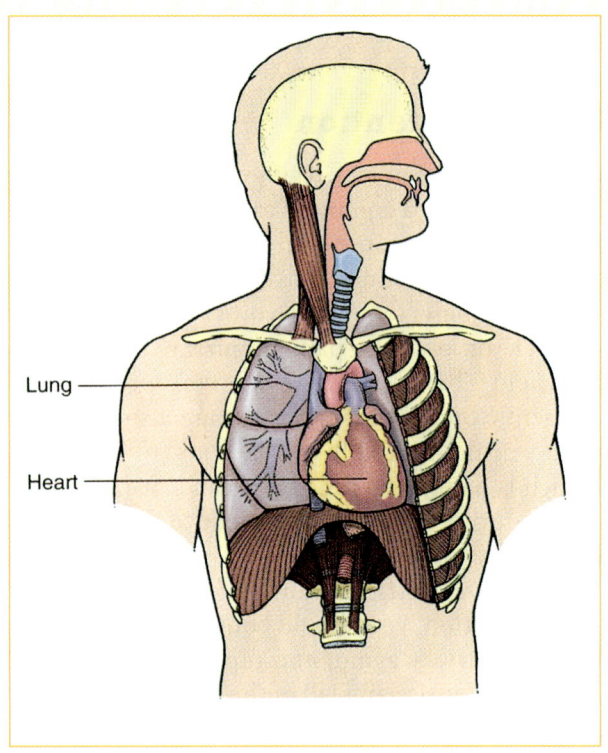

Figure 39-25 The heart lies slightly to the left of the middle of the chest between the sternum and spine.

(Figure 39-25 ▲). The blood that circulates through the lungs by chest compressions is likely to receive adequate oxygen to maintain life when accompanied by artificial ventilation. However, keep in mind that, at its best, external chest compression provides only one third of the blood that is normally pumped by the heart, so it is very important to do it properly.

The patient must be placed on a firm, flat surface, in a supine position. The head should not be elevated at a level above the heart because this will further reduce blood flow to the brain. The surface can be the ground, the floor, or a backboard on a stretcher. You cannot perform chest compressions adequately on a bed; therefore, a patient who is in bed should be moved to the floor or have a board placed under the back. Remember, too, that external chest compressions must always be accompanied by artificial ventilation.

Proper Hand Position

Correct hand position is established by placing the heel of one hand on the sternum (center of the chest) between the patient's nipples (lower half of the sternum). Follow the steps in (Skill Drill 39-2 ▶):

1. **Place the heel of one hand** on the sternum between the nipples (**Step 1**).

Skill Drill 39-2: Performing Chest Compressions

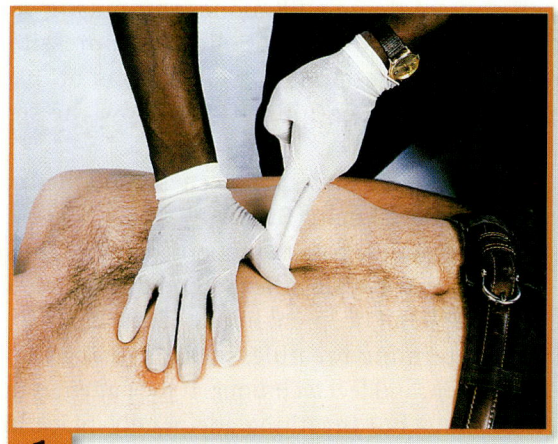

1 Place the heel of one hand on the sternum between the nipples.

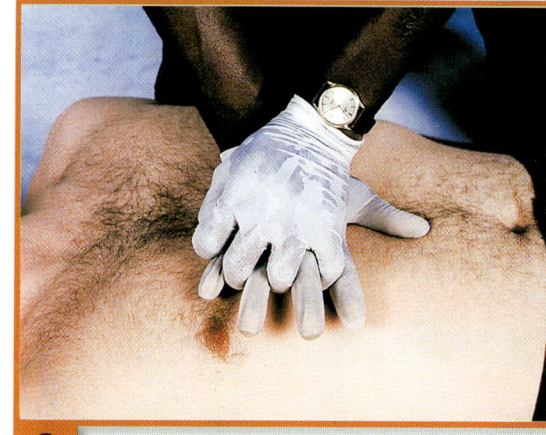

2 Place the heel of your other hand over the first hand.

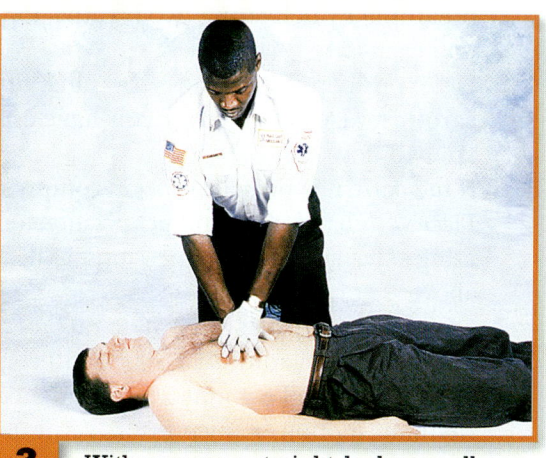

3 With your arms straight, lock your elbows, and position your shoulders directly over your hands. Depress the sternum 1½" to 2", using a direct downward movement.

2. **Place the heel of your other hand** over the first hand (**Step 2**).
3. **With your arms straight,** lock your elbows, and position your shoulders directly over your hands. Depress the sternum 1½" to 2", using direct downward movement and then rising gently upward. It is important that you allow the chest to return to its normal position. Your technique may be improved or made more comfortable if you interlock the fingers of your lower hand with the fingers of your upper hand; either way, your fingers should be kept off the patient's chest (**Step 3**).

Proper Compression Technique

Complications from chest compressions are rare but can include fractured ribs, a lacerated liver, or a fractured sternum. Although these injuries cannot be entirely avoided, you can minimize the chance that they will occur if you use good, smooth technique and proper hand placement.

Proper compressions begin by locking your elbows, with your arms straight, and positioning your shoulders directly over your hand so that the thrust of each compression is straight down on the sternum **Figure 39-26**. Depress the sternum 1½" to 2" in an adult, avoiding a rocking motion and rising gently

One-Rescuer Adult CPR

When you are doing CPR alone, you must give both artificial ventilations and chest compressions in a ratio of compressions to ventilations of 30:2. To perform one-rescuer adult CPR, follow the steps in Skill Drill 39-3:

1. **Determine unresponsiveness**, and then call for additional help (**Step 1**).
2. Position the patient properly (supine), and **open the airway** using the method that matches your suspicion of spinal injury (**Step 2**).
3. **Determine breathlessness** by using the look, listen, and feel technique. If the patient is unconscious but breathing adequately, place him or her in the recovery position, and maintain the open airway (**Step 3**).
4. If the patient is not breathing, begin **rescue breathing** by delivering two breaths, for 1 second each (**Step 4**).
5. **Determine pulselessness** by checking the carotid pulse (**Step 5**). If you have an AED, apply it now.
6. If the patient is pulseless, begin compressions. Place your hands in the proper position for delivering external chest compressions, as described above.
7. Give 30 compressions at a rate of about 100/min for an adult. Each set of 30 compressions should take about 20 seconds. Using a rhythmic motion, apply pressure vertically from your shoulders down through both arms to depress the sternum $1\frac{1}{2}''$ to $2''$ in the adult, then rise up gently and fully. Count the compressions aloud (**Step 6**).
8. **Open the airway**, and then give two ventilations, each lasting 1 second.

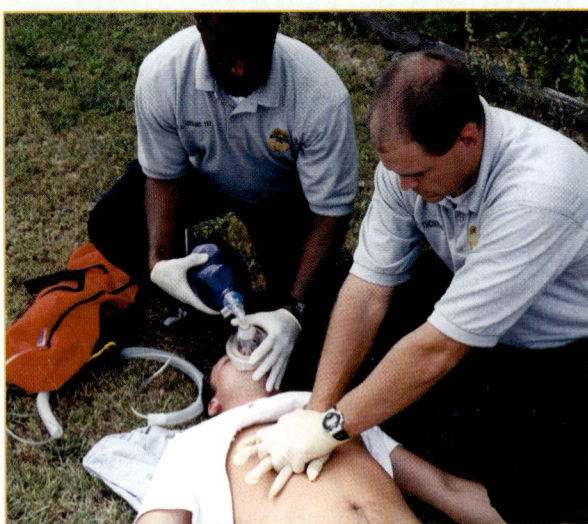

Figure 39-26 When performing CPR, be sure that your arms are in a locked position for adequate compressions, and maintain a good seal with the BVM device.

upward. This motion allows pressure to be delivered vertically down from your shoulders. Vertical downward pressure produces a compression that must be followed immediately by an equal period of relaxation. The ratio of time devoted to compression versus relaxation should be 1:1.

The actual motions must be smooth, rhythmic, and uninterrupted (Figure 39-27A). Short, jabbing compressions are not effective in producing artificial blood flow. Do not remove the heel of your hand from the patient's chest during relaxation, but make sure that you completely release pressure on the sternum so that it can return to its normal resting position between compressions (Figure 39-27B).

You are the Provider — Part 4

Your partner applies an AED, and shocks the patient one time. You and your partner then begin immediate CPR. You secure the airway according to local protocols and provide artificial respirations via a BVM device attached to high-flow oxygen while your partner performs chest compressions.

7. For adult CPR, what is the appropriate rate and depth of compressions, and how can you help your partner in determining if the compressions are adequate?
8. If family members ask if the patient will be okay, what should you say?

EMT-I Tips

Performing CPR in the field is a different experience than practicing in the classroom and requires special preparations. You and your partner should drill in advance on how you will make the best use of your skills, equipment, and personnel available to assist. Besides improving patient care, practicing how to deploy equipment, assign roles, and move patients with fire crews who may respond to help you is also an excellent way to develop good working relations.

Geriatric Needs

Proper hand position and depth of compression, always important, take on added priority in older patients who are likely to have brittle bones and chest cartilage. There is no guarantee against causing injury to these tissues, and you must compress adequately to provide adequate perfusion of vital organs. Paying particular attention to your compression technique, however, will help reduce avoidable injuries.

9. Locate the proper position, and **begin another cycle** of chest compressions. Perform five cycles of compressions and ventilations.
10. **After five cycles** of compressions and ventilations, stop CPR and check for the return of a carotid pulse. If there is no change, resume CPR.

If the patient has a pulse, check for breathing. If the patient is not breathing or is breathing inadequately, provide rescue breathing. If the patient has a pulse, is breathing adequately, but remains unresponsive, place the patient in the recovery position and closely monitor the patient.

Two-Rescuer Adult CPR

You and your team should be able to perform both one-rescuer and two-rescuer CPR with ease. Two-rescuer CPR is always the first choice because it is less tiring for the rescuers and facilitates effective chest compressions. Once one-rescuer CPR is in progress, a second rescuer can be added very easily. He or she should enter the procedure after a cycle of 30 compressions and two ventilations. You should use airway adjuncts, such as mouth-to-mask ventilations, whenever possible. To perform two-rescuer adult CPR, follow the steps in Skill Drill 39-4 ▶:

1. Moving to the head, **establish unresponsiveness** as your partner moves to the patient's side to be ready to deliver chest compressions (**Step 1**).
2. Position the patient to **open the airway** (**Step 2**).
3. **Check for breathing** by using the look, listen, and feel technique. If the patient is unconscious but breathing adequately, place him or her in the recovery position, and maintain the open airway (**Step 3**).
4. **If the patient is not breathing, begin rescue breathing** by delivering two breaths, for 1 second each (**Step 4**).

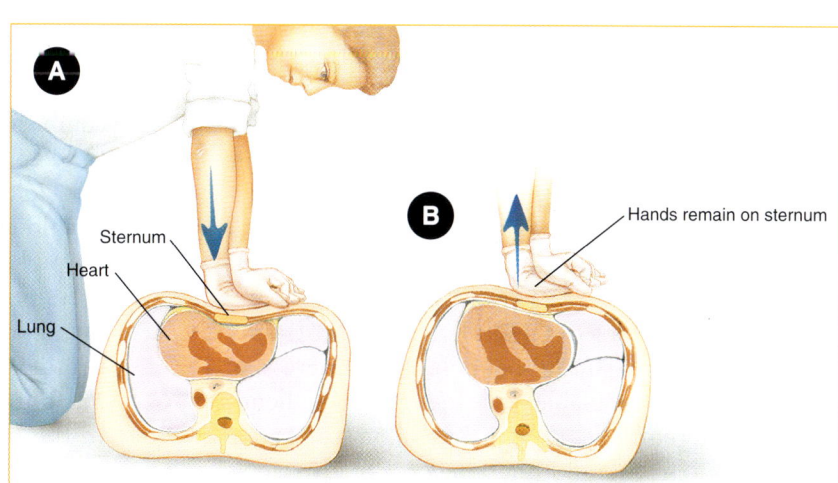

Figure 39-27 **A.** Compression and relaxation should be rhythmic and of equal duration. **B.** Pressure on the sternum must be released so that it can return to its normal resting position between compressions. However, do not remove the heel of your hand from the sternum.

Performing One-Rescuer Adult CPR

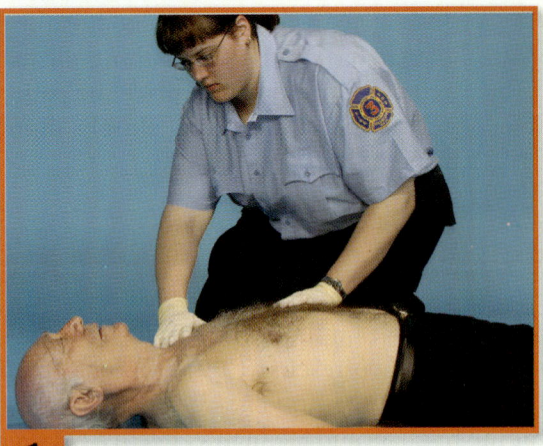

1 Establish unresponsiveness, and call for help.

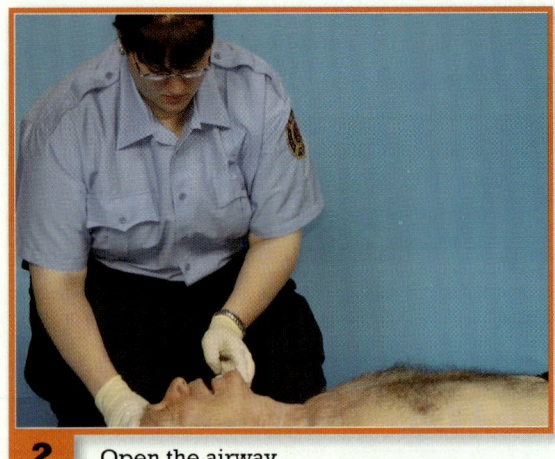

2 Open the airway.

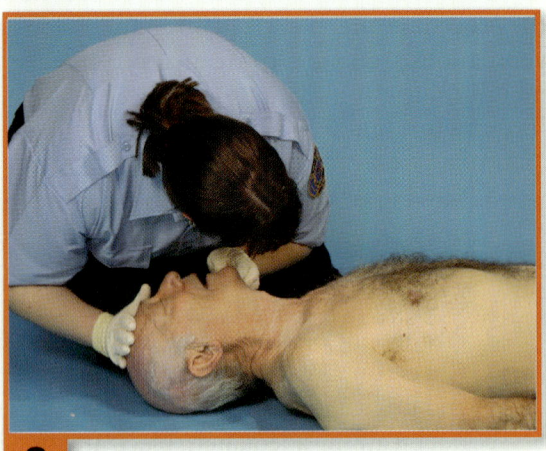

3 Look, listen, and feel for breathing. If the patient is breathing adequately, place in the recovery position and monitor.

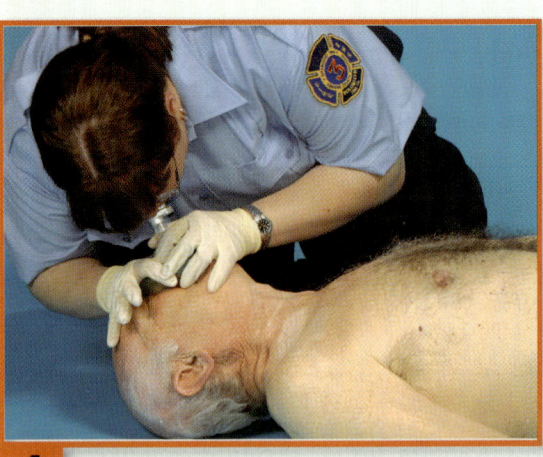

4 If not breathing, give two breaths of 1 second each.

5. **Determine pulselessness** by checking the carotid pulse (**Step 5**). If the patient has no pulse and an AED is available, apply it now.
6. **Begin chest compressions** at a compression to ventilation ratio of 30:2 (**Step 6**). Once the airway is secured (intubated) rescuers should no longer deliver cycles of CPR. Chest compressions should be delivered continuously (100/min) and rescue breaths delivered at a rate of 8 to 10 breaths/min.
7. **After five cycles of CPR**, the rescuer providing compressions should be replaced. If there is a third rescuer available, have them position themselves at the chest opposite the compressor. Make the switch when both rescuers are ready, keeping the switch time to as little as possible (no more than 5 to 10 seconds). If only two rescuers are available, make the switch mid-cycle during compressions to allow less delay during the switch to ventilations.
8. **Check for a pulse every 2 minutes.** Pulse checks should last no more than 10 seconds. If there is no pulse, continue CPR beginning with compressions. If the patient has a pulse, check for breathing. If the patient is not breathing, provide ventilations. If the patient has a pulse, is breathing, but remains unresponsive, place the patient in the recovery position and closely monitor the patient.

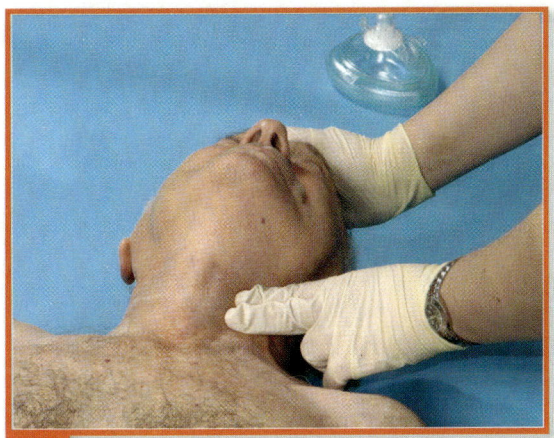

5 Check for carotid pulse.

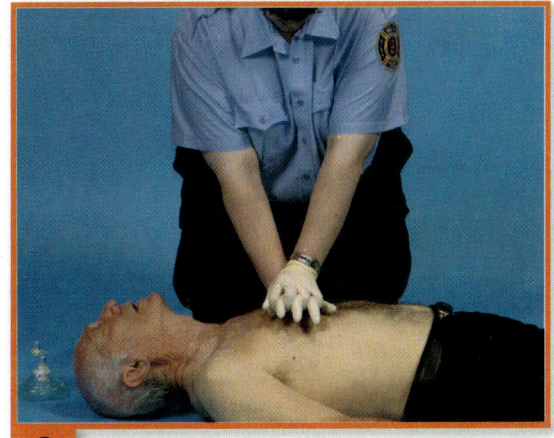

6 If no pulse is found, apply your AED. If there is no AED, place your hands in the proper position for chest compressons.

Give 30 compressions at about 100/min.

Open the airway, and give two ventilations of 1 second each.

Perform five cycles of chest compressions and ventilations.

Stop CPR, and check for return of the carotid pulse.

Depending on the patient's condition, continue CPR, continue rescue breathing only, or place the patient in the recovery position and monitor breathing and pulse.

Switching Positions

Switching rescuers during CPR is beneficial to the quality of CPR administered to the patient. After 2 minutes of CPR, the rescuer providing compressions will begin to tire and compression quality will begin to suffer. It is therefore recommended to switch the rescuer doing compressions every 2 minutes. If there are only two rescuers, the rescuers will switch positions. If additional rescuers are available, rotating the rescuer providing compressions every 2 minutes is required. During switches, every effort should be made to minimize the time that no compressions are being administered. This should be approximately 5 seconds but no more than 10 seconds of a break in between the compression cycle.

The switch can be accomplished by the two rescuers knowing what each other will do. Rescuer one will begin another cycle of 30 compressions while rescuer two moves to the opposite side of the chest and moves into position to begin compressions. During the cycle, rescuer one will stop compressing and rescuer two will begin, continuing until 30 compressions have completed. Rescuer one will then deliver two ventilations and the CPR cycles will continue as needed.

Skill Drill 39-4

Performing Two-Rescuer Adult CPR

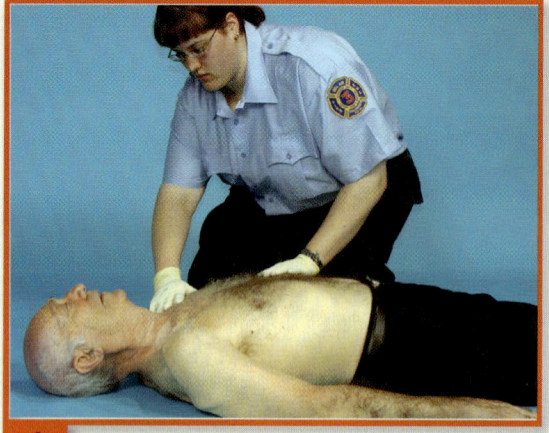

1 Establish unresponsiveness and take positions.

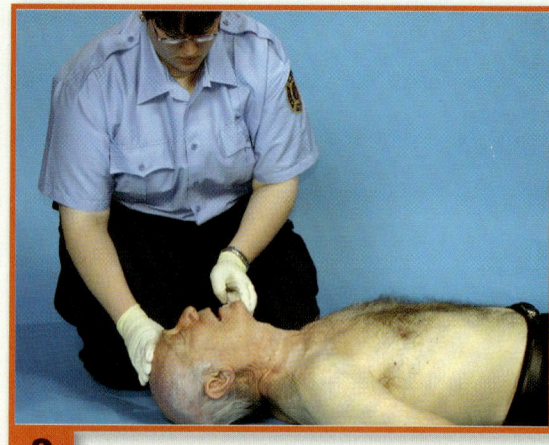

2 Open the airway.

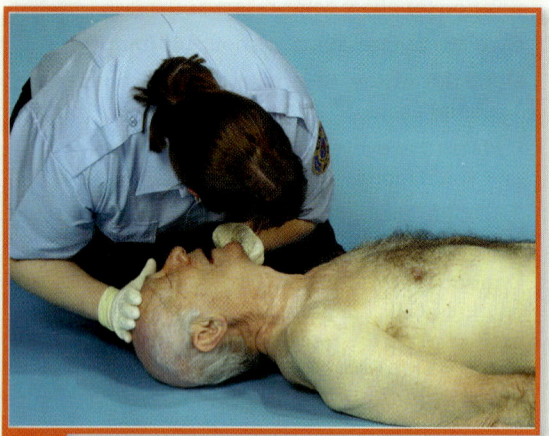

3 Look, listen, and feel for breathing. If the patient is breathing adequately, place in the recovery position and monitor.

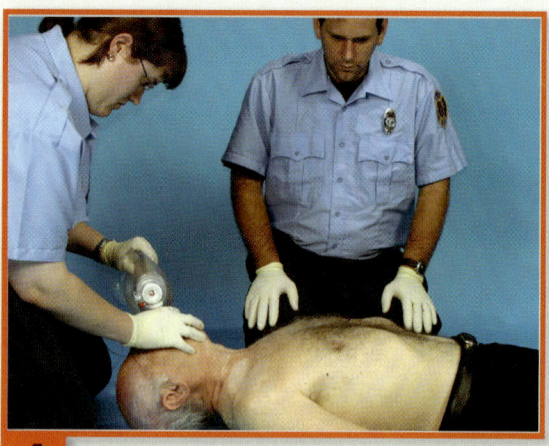

4 If the patient is not breathing, give two breaths of 1 second each.

You are the Provider — Part 5

Volunteer fire fighters now arrive to assist you. They place the patient onto a backboard (to facilitate moving him) and transfer him to the gurney. You continue CPR en route to the hospital without any changes in the patient's condition. Although a pulse is regained in the emergency department, the patient later dies.

9. What are important considerations to make involving the needs of both responders and the patient's family?
10. What should be done after every major call such as this one?

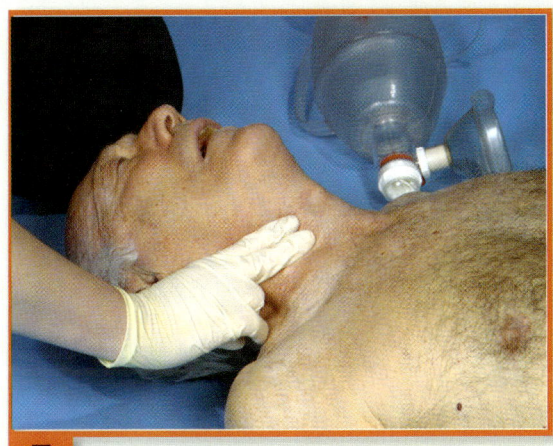

5 Check for a carotid pulse. If no pulse is felt in 10 seconds, begin CPR.

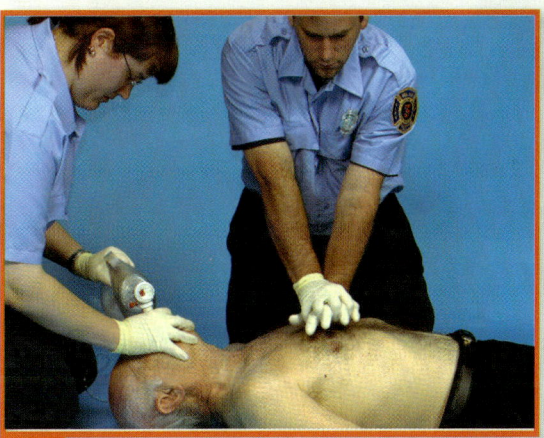

6 If there is no pulse but an AED is available, apply it now. If no AED is available, begin chest compressions at about 100/min (30 compressions to two ventilations).

After every five cycles, switch rescuer positions in order to minimize fatigue. Keep switch time to 5 to 10 seconds.

Depending on patient condition, continue CPR, continue ventilations only, or place in recovery position.

Infant and Child CPR

In most instances, cardiac arrest in infants and children follows respiratory arrest, which triggers hypoxia and ischemia of the heart. Children consume oxygen two to three times as rapidly as adults. Therefore, you must first focus on opening an airway and providing artificial ventilation. Often, this will be enough to allow the child to resume spontaneous breathing and, thus, prevent cardiac arrest.

Once the airway is open and you have delivered two breaths, you need to assess circulation. As with an adult, you should first check for a palpable pulse in a large central artery. Absence of a palpable pulse in a major central artery means that you must begin external chest compressions. You can usually palpate the carotid pulse in children older than 1 year, but it is difficult in infants, who have short and often fat necks. Therefore, in infants, palpate the brachial artery, which is located on the inner side of the arm, midway between the elbow and shoulder. Place your thumb on the outer surface of the arm between the elbow and shoulder. Then place the tips of your index and long fingers on the inside of the biceps, and press lightly toward the bone (**Figure 39-28** ▶).

External Chest Compression

Most BLS techniques are the same for infants, small children, larger children, and adults. As with an adult, an infant or child must be lying on a hard surface for the best results. If you are holding an infant, the hard surface can be your forearm, with your palm supporting

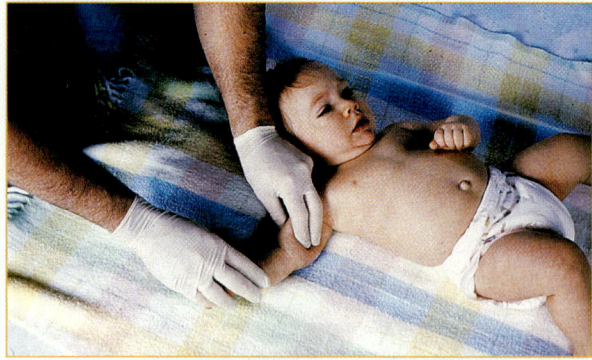

Figure 39-28 To assess circulation in an infant, palpate the brachial artery on the inner side of the arm, midway between the elbow and shoulder.

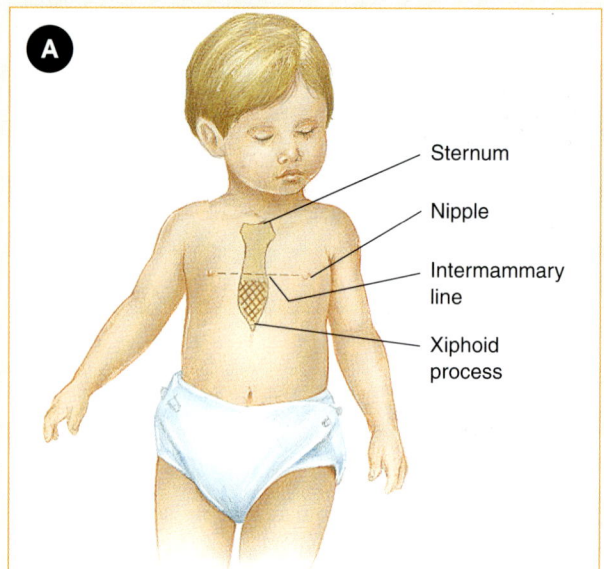

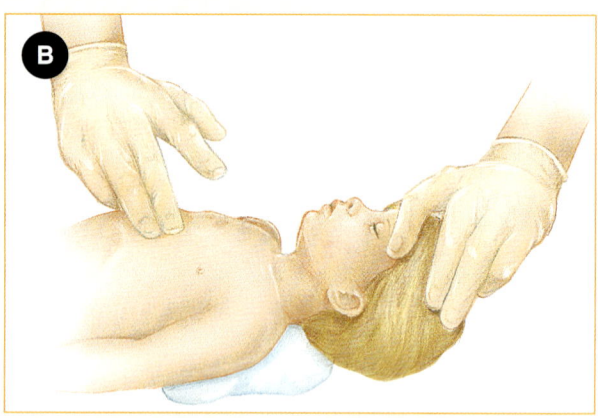

Figure 39-29 A. The proper location for chest compressions in an infant is in the midline, 1 fingerbreadth below an imaginary line drawn between the nipples at the sternum. **B.** With two fingers, compress the sternum approximately one third to one half the depth of the infant's chest. Perform compressions at a rate of approximately 100/min.

the infant's head. In this way, the infant's shoulders are elevated, and the head is slightly tilted back in a position that will keep the airway open. However, you must ensure that the infant's head is not higher than the rest of the body. The technique for chest compressions in infants and children differs because of a number of anatomic differences, including the position of the heart, the size of the chest, and the fragile organs of a child. The liver is relatively large, immediately under the right side of the diaphragm, and very fragile, especially in infants. The spleen, on the left, is much smaller and much more fragile in children than in adults. These organs are easily injured if you are not careful in performing chest compressions, so be sure that your hand position is correct before you begin.

Proper Hand Position and Compression Technique

The chest of an infant or child is smaller and more pliable than that of an adult; therefore, you should only use two fingers to compress the chest. In children, especially those older than 8 years of age, you can use the heel of one or both hands to compress the chest.

Infant CPR

In an infant, there are two methods for performing chest compressions: the two-finger technique and the two thumb–encircling hands technique.

The two-finger technique is the preferred method for performing chest compressions if you are by yourself. Place two fingers of one hand over the lower half of the sternum, approximately 1 fingerbreadth below an imaginary line located between the nipples (Figure 39-29A ▶). Compress the sternum approximately one third to one half the depth of the infant's chest. With two fingers, perform compressions at a rate of at least 100/min (Figure 39-29B ▲). Finger position is important in order to avoid compressing the xiphoid process.

The two thumb–encircling hands technique is the preferred method for performing two-rescuer infant CPR, when physically feasible (Figure 39-30 ▶). Place both thumbs side by side over the lower half of the infant's sternum, approximately 1 fingerbreadth below an imaginary line located between the nipples. Ensure that the thumbs do not compress on or near the xiphoid process. In very small infants, you may need to overlap your thumbs. Encircle the infant's chest and support the infant's back with the fingers of both hands. With your hands encircling the chest, use both thumbs to depress the sternum approximately one third to one half the

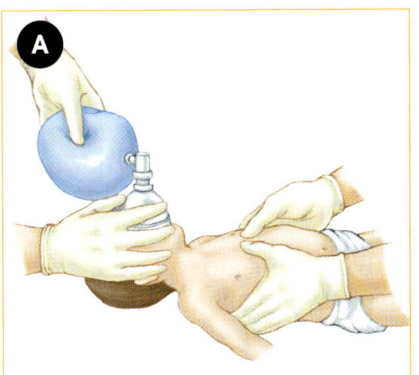 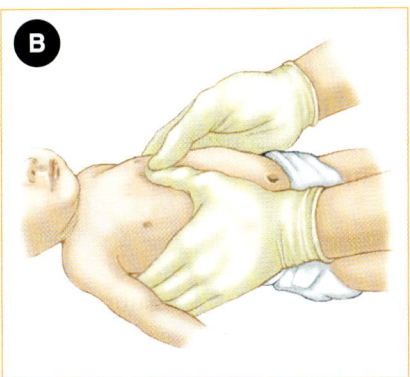 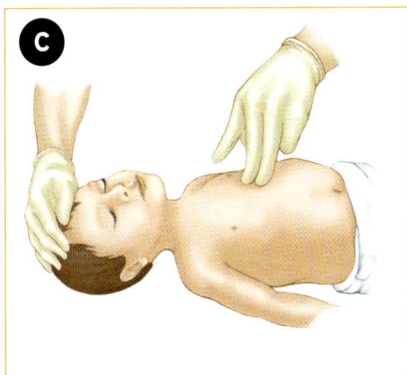

Figure 39-30 A. Place both thumbs side by side over the lower half of the infant's sternum, approximately 1 fingerbreadth below an imaginary line located between the nipples. **B.** In very small infants, you may need to overlap your thumbs. **C.** In larger infants, you may use the two-finger technique.

depth of the infant's chest. Perform compressions at a rate of at least 100/min. After 15 compressions, pause briefly for the second rescuer to deliver two ventilations. Compressions and ventilations should be coordinated to avoid simultaneous delivery and ensure adequate ventilation and chest expansion, especially when the infant's airway has not been definitively protected (intubated).

After each compression, release pressure from the sternum without removing your fingers (or thumbs) from the patient's chest. Use smooth, rhythmic motions to deliver compressions, as with adult CPR.

When performing one-rescuer CPR on an infant on a hard surface (for example, the ground, a table), make sure that the hand closest to the head remains on the infant's forehead during chest compressions. Your other hand may remain on the chest as you give rescue breathing. If the chest does not rise, remove the hand that is on the patient's chest, and reposition the airway using the appropriate maneuver. Then relocate the proper anatomic landmark and return the compression hand to the chest.

Child CPR

For a child older than 1 year, the way in which you deliver chest compressions differs. You will need to use more force with a child than with an infant, compressing the sternum with the heel of one or both hands to a depth that is approximately one third to one half the depth of the child's chest. Perform compressions at a rate of about 100/min. Your other hand (if only using one hand to compress the chest) should be used to maintain the child's head position so that you can provide rescue breathing without repositioning the head 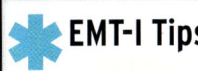. Compressions should be delivered in

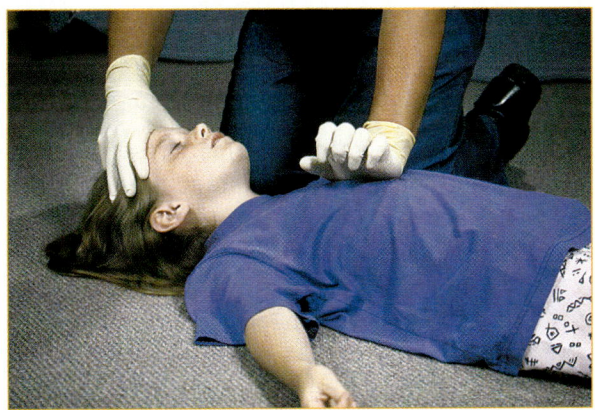

Figure 39-31 When performing chest compressions on a child, use the heel of one hand to compress the sternum to a depth that is approximately one third to one half the depth of the child's chest. Perform compressions at a rate of about 100/min. If you are using only one hand to compress the chest, the other hand should remain on the child's head to maintain an open airway.

a smooth, rhythmic manner in which the chest returns to its resting position after each compression.

As with an adult, external chest compressions on a child or infant must be coordinated with ventilations. The ratio of compression to ventilation for children is 30:2 for one-rescuer and 15:2 for two-rescuer CPR.

Reassess the child after five cycles (about 2 minutes) of CPR and every 2 minutes thereafter. Pulse checks, which should take at least 5 seconds but no more than

> **EMT-I Tips**
>
> Integrate the AED into the CPR sequence for children over 1 year of age.

10 seconds, should be done at the carotid or femoral artery. If no pulse is felt after 10 seconds, continue CPR.

Switching rescuer positions is the same for children as is it for adults, after every 5 cycles (about 2 minutes) of CPR. The best time to switch positions is when you reassess the child for breathing and circulation.

Interrupting CPR

CPR is an important holding action that provides minimal circulation and ventilation until the patient can receive definitive care in the form of defibrillation or further care at the hospital. No matter how well it is performed, however, CPR is rarely enough to save a patient's life.

Try not to interrupt CPR for more than a few seconds, except when it is absolutely necessary. For example, if you have to move a patient up or down stairs, you should continue CPR until you arrive at the head or foot of the stairs, interrupt CPR at an agreed-upon signal, and move quickly to the next level where you can resume CPR. Do not move the patient until all transport arrangements are made so that your interruptions of CPR can be kept to a minimum.

You are the Provider Summary

1. Given the initial nature of the call, what would be a good idea?

Immediately requesting more resources is always a good idea whenever the nature of the call sounds serious. Ideally, ALS should be simultaneously dispatched, but if paramedics are not available in your area, request extra hands to assist with patient transfer, equipment retrieval, etc. Use available resources, including fire fighters or other trained personnel.

2. After the dispatcher notifies you that CPR is in progress, what should you do to prepare?

Beyond the memorization of protocols, before you arrive on scene you should review who will perform which functions. This avoids confusion on the scene and decreases the overall time to administer necessary therapies. It is also beneficial to notify the receiving hospital and/or medical control of the nature of the dispatch. Most hospitals appreciate being notified to enable the emergency department staff to prepare.

3. What is your first priority?

The safety of you and your crew is always the first priority. The presence of this animal constitutes a safety risk. You must ask the wife to remove the pet and put it in another area of the house for your protection and to prevent the interference of patient care procedures. After you address this safety issue, you must determine the patient's level of consciousness.

4. What information would you like to obtain from the patient's wife?

Some examples of questions include the following. Did she witness her husband's loss of consciousness? If not, when was the last time she saw her husband alert? Was he complaining of anything before he lost consciousness? What is his medical background and does he take any medications? Does he have a DNR? (Most family members will immediately inform you if there is a do not resuscitate order but may not be able to produce the paperwork. This can put you in a very tough predicament, but be prepared for this situation as it can be common.) Did she perform CPR?

5. Why should you move the patient, and what should you do if you cannot?

In order to effectively execute CPR (adequately compressing the heart between the sternum and spine), it must be performed on a hard surface. If the patient is too large or you cannot move him for some other reason, you must place a hard surface (such as a CPR board or similar item) underneath his torso. If CPR was done prior to your arrival with the patient on a soft surface, this will be important to know and document.

You are the Provider continued

Summary

6. What do you do to manage his airway, and what should be the next step your partner performs?

You cannot perform artificial respirations with his airway full of emesis. Therefore, you must aggressively clear his airway (preferably using a portable electric suction unit). You then need to secure his airway according to your local protocols. The EMT-I scope of practice includes the use of PtLs, Combitubes, or LMAs. Some EMT-Is may intubate while others may not. At a minimum, an oral airway must be inserted to prevent the tongue from obstructing the airway, and cricoid pressure may then be applied to prevent or reduce aspiration. Regurgitation can be minimized by performing correct ventilations—not forcing air into the lungs either too much or too fast (air will follow the path of least resistance). Your partner should assess the patient for the presence of a pulse. If the patient has no pulse, the AED should be applied as quickly as possible.

7. For adult CPR, what is the appropriate rate and depth of compressions, and how can you help your partner in determining if the compressions are adequate?

Adult compressions should be at a rate of 100 times per minute at a depth of $1\frac{1}{2}''$ to $2''$. During CPR, you can assist your partner by feeling for a carotid pulse as each compression is performed. Depth of compressions can then be adjusted accordingly.

8. If family members ask if the patient will be okay, what should you say?

You should never lie or mislead the patient's friends or family members. Explain that you are doing all that you can for him, but that he is not breathing, his heart is not beating, and it is very serious. Giving them false hope will only make the situation more difficult should the patient not survive, and they will likely resent you for it.

9. What are important considerations to make involving the needs of responders and family?

Unfortunately, not every call results in a happy ending. For each minute that passes the patient's chances of survival decrease by 7 to 10%. When you factor in whether or not this was a witnessed/recognized arrest and the time it takes to access 9-1-1, to obtain the necessary information, to dispatch appropriate resources, and travel time, it's easy to understand why the national average for survival of sudden cardiac arrest in the prehospital setting is only about 5%. Early defibrillation is the key to patient survival. This is why public access defibrillation makes such a tremendous impact. Whenever possible, you should assist family members in their time of need. This can be as simple as offering to call friends or clergy members to help them, or answering their questions in an open and honest way. You should offer critical incident stress debriefing (CISD) for family members or bystanders who performed CPR. Don't leave them to deal with their feelings alone. Also, if there were new rescuers involved in helping or if there were unusual circumstances surrounding the call likely to bother seasoned providers, make sure that they receive CISD. Performing CPR for the first time as a new rescuer can be traumatic, especially if that patient does not survive.

10. What should be done after every major call such as this one?

Even seasoned providers can use constructive criticism to improve their skills and techniques. Every significant call should undergo a formal review for quality improvement or assurance. These reviews should involve all members on the call and other department personnel who did not respond but can benefit from reviewing the information. This should be performed in conjunction with the EMS coordinator and the program medical director. Reviewing calls is not about finding or placing blame, but about learning and striving to improve.

Prep Kit

Ready for Review

- Basic life support (BLS), such as CPR, is a noninvasive series of emergency lifesaving procedures that are carried out in order to treat airway obstruction, respiratory arrest, and cardiac arrest. Commonly known as cardiopulmonary resuscitation (CPR), it is a method of providing artificial ventilation and circulation.

- The effectiveness of BLS depends on prompt recognition of respiratory and/or cardiac arrest and the immediate initiation of treatment. You are expected to be able to recognize cardiac or respiratory arrest without difficulty and to quickly institute proper BLS measures.

- BLS can be given by one or two EMT-Is or EMT-Bs, by first responders, or by alert, well-trained bystanders. It does not require any equipment; however, a barrier device should be used to perform rescue breathing.

- The basic principles of BLS are the same for infants, children, and adults. According to the American Heart Association (AHA), anyone younger than 1 year is considered an infant. A child is between 1 year of age and puberty (12 to 14 years of age). Adulthood is from onset of puberty and older.

- Several methods exist for opening the airway and providing rescue breathing. Each has specific applications for conscious or unconscious patients, with or without head or spinal injury. The head tilt–chin lift maneuver is effective for opening the airway of most patients. However, for patients who have suspected spinal injury, the jaw-thrust maneuver is indicated.

- Rescue breathing is done routinely with a barrier device, such as a mask, to provide infection control.

- Sometimes, rescue breathing causes excess air to be forced into the stomach. The resulting condition is called gastric distention. A patient with gastric distention may vomit during CPR. If this condition develops, you should continue to provide slow rescue breaths; however, if gastric distention is interfering with your ability to perform effective ventilation, medical control may order you to turn the patient on his or her side and apply gentle pressure to the abdomen to relieve the gastric distention. Be sure to have suction immediately available.

- If a patient begins breathing following rescue breathing, you should place the patient in the recovery position. This position helps to maintain a clear airway in a patient with a decreased level of consciousness who has not had traumatic injuries and is breathing adequately on his or her own.

- After you begin rescue breathing, you must assess the patient's circulation. If the patient has no pulse, you must provide artificial circulation by performing chest compressions at the rate and depth appropriate for the patient's age.

- If an AED is available, immediately attach it to the patient and provide defibrillation as indicated. The AED is indicated for patients in nontraumatic cardiac arrest who are over the age of 1 year. If using an AED on a child between 1 and 8 years of age, if available, you should use pediatric-sized pads and a dose-attenuating system (energy reducer).

- Remember that the patient must be on a firm, flat surface for chest compressions to be effective. Proper hand position and proper compression technique are essential for artificial circulation to be effective.

- CPR can be done with one or two rescuers. Two-rescuer CPR is always the first choice. When a rescuer is doing adult CPR alone or with another rescuer, the ratio of compressions to ventilations is 30:2.

- In infants and children, the ratio of compressions to ventilations is 30:2 if one rescuer is present and 15:2 if two rescuers are present. For one-rescuer infant CPR, compress the chest with the two-finger technique; the two thumb-encircling hands tech-

Technology

- Interactivities
- Vocabulary Explorer
- Anatomy Review
- Web Links
- Online Review Manual

www.EMSzone.com/EMTI

nique should be used for two-rescuer infant CPR. For child CPR, compress the chest with the heel of one or both hands, depending on the child's size. In infants and children, the chest should be compressed one-third to one-half the depth of the chest at a rate of 100/min.

- Remember that you should try not to interrupt CPR for more than a few seconds, except when it is absolutely necessary.
- Specific techniques must be used for removing foreign bodies that obstruct the airway. Obstruction may be caused by many things, including relaxation of the tongue in an unconscious patient (most common), vomited or regurgitated stomach contents, a blood clot, damaged tissue after an injury, dentures, or a foreign body in the airway. Recognition of the obstruction and prompt intervention are critical.
- The manual maneuvers recommended for removing a foreign body airway obstruction are the abdominal-thrust maneuver (Heimlich maneuver) and chest thrusts.
- In infants and children, the cause of airway obstruction may be infectious. Therefore, you should try to identify the cause of the obstruction as soon as possible. Infants and children with such infections need immediate transport to the hospital and will not benefit from attempts to relieve a foreign body airway obstruction.

Vital Vocabulary

abdominal-thrust maneuver The preferred method to dislodge and force food or other material from the throat of a choking victim; also called the Heimlich maneuver.

advanced life support (ALS) Advanced lifesaving procedures, such as cardiac monitoring, administration of intravenous fluids and medications, and use of advanced airway adjuncts.

basic life support (BLS) Noninvasive emergency lifesaving care that is used to treat airway obstruction, respiratory arrest, or cardiac arrest. Although the term "BLS" represents a wide variety of procedures performed by the EMT-I, in this chapter, it is used synonymously with CPR.

cardiopulmonary resuscitation (CPR) The combination of rescue breathing and chest compressions used to establish adequate ventilation and circulation in a patient who is not breathing and has no pulse.

gastric distention A condition in which air fills the stomach as a result of high volume and pressure or airway obstruction during artificial ventilation.

head tilt–chin lift maneuver A technique to open the airway that combines tilting back the forehead and lifting the chin.

jaw-thrust maneuver A technique to open the airway by placing the fingers behind the angles of the patient's lower jaw and forcefully moving the jaw forward; can be performed with or without head tilt.

recovery position A position that helps to maintain a clear airway in a patient with a decreased level of consciousness who has had no traumatic injuries and is breathing adequately on his or her own.

Assessment in Action

You are awakened one morning to the sound of pounding on your door. It is your neighbor's daughter. She screams for help. When you open the door she tells you that she can't wake her father up. She thinks he is dead.

You grab your kit and rush over to the house. In the bedroom you find your neighbor lying prone beside the bed. You roll him over and shout his name. He is unresponsive; 9-1-1 has already been called.

You open his airway and look, listen, and feel for breathing. There is none. With your pocket mask in place you give two breaths. You check for a pulse and it too is absent. You begin chest compressions. After five cycles of CPR you reassess and find there are still no signs of life. You continue CPR. Soon, your coworkers arrive in the ambulance. You continue CPR while they attach the AED to your neighbor. After assessment, no shock is advised. One of your coworkers takes over compressions for you and you continue to ventilate. As soon as possible, the other crewmembers move the patient to the ambulance and transport. You stay behind and comfort the daughter. Later, you drive her to the hospital where her father was taken. You learn they were unable to resuscitate him.

1. What is the correct rate of compressions for this patient?
   - A. >100
   - B. 100
   - C. 80
   - D. 60

2. There was no evidence of trauma noted in this case, so the airway should have been opened by what method?
   - A. Jaw thrust
   - B. Head tilt–chin lift
   - C. Keeping the head neutral and using the jaw lift
   - D. Head tilt–jaw thrust

3. CPR must be initiated unless:
   - A. the patient is cold to the touch.
   - B. the patient's family says not to start.
   - C. rigor mortis is present.
   - D. there is no lividity.

4. Once started, you must continue CPR unless:
   - A. there is no breathing.
   - B. the patient is transferred to another trained person.
   - C. you feel like there is no longer any hope.
   - D. the patient's family requests that you stop.

5. You know that starting CPR as quickly as possible after the collapse is important because damage to brain tissue from lack of oxygen may occur within:
   - A. 4–6 minutes.
   - B. 6–8 minutes.
   - C. 8–10 minutes.
   - D. 30 minutes.

6. The ratio of your initial compressions to ventilations on this patient were:
   - A. 2:30.
   - B. 1:5.
   - C. 2:5.
   - D. 30:2.

Points to Ponder

While treating your child to an ice cream sundae at the local diner, you hear someone scream for help. You turn around in time to see a 6-year-old boy clutching his hands to his throat. He is cyanotic and not making any sounds or coughs. You run up behind him and ask, "Are you choking?" He nods. You tell him you are going to help and move behind him. You get down on your knees and wrap your arms around his torso. You make a fist and place it between his umbilicus and xiphoid. You make several attempts to dislodge the object by abdominal thrusts. Soon, a small piece off of a toy pops out of his mouth. He is awake and breathing easier but now has some coughing. You tell his mother that he should still be evaluated by a doctor to be sure the toy did not do any internal damage. The ambulance crew arrives and you tell your buddies what happened. They congratulate you on a job well done and move the boy to the ambulance.

Issues: Recognizing the Need for Abdominal Thrusts in the Choking Patient, Recognizing the Signs of Choking, Realizing the Need for Further Evaluation

Index

NOTE: Page numbers with *f* indicates figures, and *t* indicates tables.

A

Abandonment, 53–54, 82
Abbreviations.
    medical, 104, 105–10*t*
    uncertainty about, 602
ABCDEs, 1531*t*
ABCs, 508–14, 1547*f*
Abdomen.
    anatomy of, 143–45, 143–45*f*, 744–45, 1088*f*
    child's, 1240
    injuries, 688, 688*f*, 745–51, 746–50*f*, 1316
    management of injuries, 751
    nontraumatic emergencies, 1084
    physical examination, 543, 545*f*, 548–49, 746–47
    rapid trauma assessment, 520, 522*f*, 524
    venous circulation system, 194–95
Abdominal aorta, 192–93, 193*f*
Abdominal pain, 527–28, 535, 746, 1159, 1350
Abdominal quadrants, 123, 123*f*, 144, 144*f*, 745, 745*f*
Abdominal (muscular) walls, 143, 143*f*
Abdominal-thrust maneuver, 1255–56, 1255–56*f*.
    for children, 1254–55, 1255*f*
Abduction, definition of, 126
Aberrancy, 956–57, 956–57*f*, 959*f*
Abnormalities, history of, 536
Abortion, 1153, 1158, 1175
Abrasions, 681, 682*f*
Absence seizures, 1064
Absent breath sounds, 1247*t*
Absent rhythms, 1297–99
Absorption, of drugs, 257, 257*t*
Abuse
    child, 1242, 1321, 1321*t*, 1324, 1324*f*
    older, 1360–62, 1362*t*
    reporting, 89
    substance, 43–44, 1035, 1035*t*, 1041
Acceleration, vehicle, 1387
Acceptance, grief and, 29
Access ports, 297
Accessory muscles, 511, 1247
Acetaminophen poisoning, 1048
Acetylcholine, 172, 250
Acid-base balance, 378–83.
Acidosis.
    bicarbonate and, 287
    diabetic, 988
    metabolic, 380, 381–82, 988
    in newborns, 1206
    respiratory, 380–81, 719
Acidotic blood, 213
Acids/acidity, 213, 378, 701*t*
Acrocyanosis, 1214, 1246
Action, medication, 244.
Action potentials, 166, 895*f*
Activated charcoal, 262–63
    indications/contraindications for, 245
    poisonings and, 1038, 1038*f*, 1040–41
Active listening, 507
Active transport, 126, 127*f*, 128, 288
Activities of daily living (ADLs), 1133, 1341
Acuity
    levels of, 558–59
    spectrum of, 561
Acute abdomen.
    causes, 1088–91, 1089*t*
    emergency medical care, 1091–92
    older patients, 1358–59
    physiology, 1084
    signs and symptoms, 1084–88, 1085–86*f*
Acute myocardial infarction (AMI), 899–900, 899*f*, 901–12, 903–4*f*, 906*f*, 909*t*, 910–12*f*
Adam's apple, 138, 369
Addiction, 1041
Adduction, 126
Adenosine (Adenocard), 265*t*, 1282*t*
Adenosine triphosphate (ATP), 128, 130, 287, 288
Adipose tissue, 129
Administration, of drugs, 244*t*, 254–55
Administration sets, for drugs, 297–98, 297–98*f*, 318
Administrative laws, 81
Adolescents, 1154, 1154*f*, 1237–38, 1238*f*.
Adrenal glands, 171, 177–78, 177*f*, 178*f*, 248
Adrenaline, 177
Adrenergic nervous system, 249, 249*t*
Adsorption, of drugs, 262–63
Advance directives, 86–87, 1346–48
Advanced cardiac life support (ACLS), 723
Advanced life support (ALS), 10, 1529, 1529*f*, 1548
Adventitious (breath) sounds, 521
Adverse effects, of drugs, 244*t*, 259
    unpredictable, 261*t*
AEIOU-TIPS assessment, 1066, 1301
Aerobic metabolism, 129
Afterload, 187, 895, 906
Agonal respirations (breathing), 377*t*, 1285
Agonists, 250, 251, 259
Air ambulances, 1395–97, 1395–97*f*
Air embolus/embolism, 317, 1123
Air exchange, good or poor, 391
Air splints, 653–54, 654*f*, 816–18, 817–18*f*
Air trapping, 547.
Airbags, 625–26, 628*f*, 633–34, 748–49, 748*f*, 1312, 1312*f*
Airborne diseases, transmission and precautions, 45, 46*t*
Airway.
    acid-base balance and, 378–83
    anatomy, 368–71, 850*f*
    axes, 441*f*
    child's, 1238–39, 1239*f*
Airway adjuncts, 402–5, 402–6*f*, 405*t*
    pediatric, 1259–63, 1260*t*, 1261–62*f*
Airway assessment, 376–78, 509.
    children, 1246–47, 1246–47*f*
    responsive patients, 510–11
    unresponsive patients, 384–85, 384*f*, 511
Airway management.
    allergic reactions and, 1011
    diabetes and, 998
    equipment, 1377
    esophageal obturator airways, 461–63, 461*f*, 462*f*
    extubation, 451, 453, 454–55*f*
    head injuries, 783–84, 784*f*
    head tilt–chin maneuver, 385, 385*f*, 385*t*, 386*f*, 1551–53, 1553*f*
    jaw-thrust maneuver, 386–87, 387*t*, 388*f*, 1553–54, 1554*f*
    jaw-thrust maneuver with head tilt, 387
    laryngeal mask airways, 463–66, 464–66*f*, 468–69*f*
    pediatric, 1252–63, 1313–14, 1319, 1319*f*
    recovery position for, 123, 383, 383*f*, 1300*f*
    spinal injuries and, 769, 769*f*
    suctioning, 397–98, 399*f*, 399*t*
    supplemental oxygen, 406–13, 407–9*f*, 408*t*, 411–14*f*
    tongue–jaw lift maneuver, 388, 390*f*
    tracheal stoma, 466–67, 470–71*f*, 471–72, 473*f*
    tracheostomy, 466–67
    tracheostomy tubes, 466–67, 467*f*, 474*f*
Airway obstructions, 388–89, 625*t*, 863–64, 864*f*
    causes, 389–91, 392*t*
    in children, 394*f*, 396, 1252–58, 1253–58*f*, 1291
    emergency care, 392, 393–97*f*, 396–97
    recognition of, 391–92, 391*f*
Alcohol poisoning, 1041–42
Alcoholic ketoacidosis, 382
Alcoholism, diabetes *versus*, 998
Alert patients, responsiveness and, 509
Algorithms, patient care, 559
Alkalis, 701*t*
Alkalosis
    bicarbonate and, 287
    respiratory, 719
Alkalotic blood, 213
Allergens, 860, 1007, 1007*t*
Allergic reactions, 263, 316–17, 1006–16, 1010*t*, 1022.
Alpha cells, 176, 177*f*
Alpha effects, 186, 186*f*, 660, 661*t*, 892, 893*f*
Alpha radiation, 1511, 1512*f*
Alpha receptors, 172, 186, 186*f*, 249*t*
Altered levels of consciousness, 1301–2
Altered mental status, 509, 1060, 1066*f*, 1134.
    assessment, 529, 1066, 1073–74
    breathing difficulty and, 869*t*
    diabetics and, 995, 998
    hypoglycemia and, 1066–67, 1067*f*
    older patients, 1350, 1360
Alveolar air, 371
Alveolar ducts, 202
Alveoli, 201*f*, 202, 203*f*, 206*f*
Alveolocapillary membrane, 202
Alzheimer's disease, 1346
Ambient temperature, 1111
Ambulance calls, 1375, 1376–82*f*, 1376–84, 1376*t*
Ambulance drivers, 15, 1384–91
    characteristics, 1385
    chassis set and, 1387
    controlled acceleration, 1387
    controlled braking, 1388
    emergency vehicle control, 1386–87
    laws and regulations for, 1389–90
    road positioning and cornering, 1387, 1387*f*
    safe driving practices, 1385–86
    safety guidelines, 1391, 1391*t*
    speeding, 1386
    steering techniques, 1387
    vehicle size and distance judgment by, 1387
    weather conditions, 1388–89, 1388*f*
Ambulances, 1374
    cleaning, 47–48, 54–55, 58
    daily inspections, 1383
    design, 1374, 1375*f*, 1375*t*
    escorts for, 1390
    intersections hazards, 1390
    maintenance, 1395
    medical equipment and supplies, 1377–83, 1377*t*, 1378–82*f*, 1379–81*t*, 1383*t*
    personnel, 1383
    right-of-way privileges, 1390
    safety precautions, 1384
    warning lights and siren, 1390
American Standard System, 409
Americans With Disabilities Act (ADA) of 1990, 9, 54
Ammonia inhalants, contraindications for, 509

Amnesia, 779
Amniotic sac, 1172, 1184
Amphetamines, 1045–46, 1046t
Ampules, 340, 341, 341f, 342f
Amputations, 682–83, 690, 690f, 831
Anabolism, cellular, 128
Anaerobic metabolism, 129, 660–61
AnaKit, 1012f, 1014–15, 1014–15f
Anaphylaxis/anaphylactic shock, 316, 664, 861, 1006, 1007, 1010
 in children, 1295
 management, 1012–16, 1013–15f, 1013t
Anatomic movements, 123, 125–26
Anatomic planes, 120–21, 120–21f
Anatomic position, 119–20, 119f, 123
Anemia, 179, 1246
Aneurysms, 1090, 1345
Anger, 28, 30
Angina pectoris, 900–901
Angiocaths, 302
Angioedema, 1011, 1295
Angle of Louis, 141, 141f
Anions, 287, 293
Ankles, 151–52, 152f, 839, 839f.
Anorexia, 1085
Anoxia, 376
Antacids, metabolic alkalosis and, 382–83, 382f
Antagonists, 250, 251, 259
Antecubital areas, for IV administration, 300
Anterior pituitary lobe, 174, 175
Anterior plane, 120
Anterior (body) position or location, 121
Anthrax, 1507, 1507f, 1508t
Antiadrenergic agents, 249
Antiarrhythmics, chest injuries and, 723
Antibodies, 179
Anticholinergic agents, 1047–48
Anticoagulants, 304, 649–50, 651
Antidiuretic hormone (ADH), 175, 212, 212t, 213f, 288
Antidotes, 1036
Antigens, 179
Antihistamines, 1295
Antivenins, 1017
Anus, 1151, 1152f, 1170f
Anxiety, 30, 869t
Aorta, 141, 142, 183, 189–90, 886
 abdominal, 192–93, 193f
 dissection and rupture, 733, 736t
 thoracic, 192
Aortic arch, 189–90, 898
Aortic pulsations, 524
Aortic valve, 182, 548, 885
Apex position or location, 122
Apgar scores, 1210, 1210t
Aphasia, 1068
Apical pulse, 1212, 1212f, 1249
Apnea, 377t, 1211, 1257
Apothecary system, 331
Apparent life-threatening events (ALTEs), 1308–9
Appendicitis, 1085
Appendicular skeleton, 133, 145–46f, 145–48, 148f
Appendix, 144, 144f, 209
Arachnoid, 165, 165f
Arrhythmias, cardiac, 902, 903f, 951–52, 951f
Arterial ruptures, 1062
Arteries, 188, 189–93, 190f, 191f, 193f, 896.
 bleeding from, 649, 650f
 cannulation with IV catheter in, 302–3
 recognizing injury to, 625t
Arterioles, 188
Arteriosclerosis, 897–98, 1345
Articular cartilage, 802

Asbestosis, 205
Ascending aorta, 189–90, 898
Ascending fibers, 166
Ascending reticular activating system, 165
Ascites, 548
Aseptic technique, 304, 304f, 335
Asphyxia, traumatic, 734–35, 737t
Aspiration, 391, 523
Aspirin
 metabolic acidosis and, 382
 poisoning, 1048
Assault, definition of, 84–85.
Assays, of drugs, 246
Assessment-based management, 561–63, 1528
 distracting injuries, 1532–33
 drills for common complaints, 1535–36
 environment, 1533
 equipment and supplies, 1531, 1531f
 general approach, 1533–34
 manpower for, 1533
 nonjudgmental attitude for, 1532
 patient assessment, 1528–29, 1529f
 patient transfer, 1534–35, 1535f, 1535t
 simulated patient presentations, 1537t
 team coordination, 1530–31
 uncooperative patients, 1532
Asthma, 205, 860, 860f, 861, 1288–90
 acute, bronchospasm and, 204, 1289f
Asynchronous CPR, 1567
Asynchronous depolarization, 956
Asystole, 903, 903f, 947, 969t, 970–71, 972t, 1297
Ataxia, 287
Atelectasis, 370
Atherosclerosis, 897–98, 899–900, 899–900f, 1062–63, 1063f, 1345, 1345f
Atlas (C1), 139–40
Atrial fibrillation, 944, 944f, 970t
Atrial flutter, 943, 943f, 970t
Atrioventricular (AV) node, 184, 185f, 888, 888f, 889–90, 890f
Atrioventricular valves, 182, 885
Atrium/atria, 182, 885
Atropine sulfate, 266–67f, 1282t
Auscultation, 521, 521f, 523–24
Auto-injectors, 1012–13f, 1013–14
Automated external defibrillators (AEDs), 11, 916–19, 916f, 1380, 1381f.
 aftercare, 919, 921
 algorithm, 922f
 CPR and, 918–19, 920–21f, 1573
 maintenance, 923, 924f, 925
 medical direction and, 925
 operational tips, 919
 safety considerations, 913, 923
Automatic implantable cardiac defibrillators (AICD), 913–14, 914f
Automatic transport ventilators (ATVs), 422, 422f
Automaticity, of cardiac cells, 185, 891
Autonomic nervous systems (ANS), 161, 171–72, 247, 248f, 249, 661, 765
Autonomic receptors, 893f
AVPU scale, 509, 782, 1073–74, 1244, 1244t
Avulsions, 681, 682–83, 683f
Axial skeleton, 133
Axillary lines, 122
Axillary nerves, 169
Axillary veins, 194

B
Back.
 assessment, 747
 detailed physical exam, 543, 545f, 550

 rapid trauma assessment, 520, 522f, 524–25
Backboards, 1413, 1413f, 1436–37.
 for children, 791, 791f
 lifting, 1408–14, 1409–11f, 1436f
 long, 772–73f, 787–88, 787f
 short, 785, 787f
Bacteria, 1506–7, 1507f
Bad news, communication of, 31
Bag-valve-mask devices. see BVM devices
Ball-and-socket joints, 146, 147f, 156, 158f
Bandages.
 for soft-tissue injuries, 707–8
Barbiturates, 1043, 1043t
Bargaining, grief and, 28
Baroreceptors, 185, 891
Barotrauma, 1212, 1240
Barrier devices, 49–50, 414, 1560–61f
Base station radios, 580–81, 581f, 584
Bases, 213, 378, 701t
Basic life support (BLS), 11, 1529, 1529f
 ABCs, 1547f
 adult CPR, 1564, 1564–66f, 1566
 assessing need for, 1549, 1549f
 automated external defibrillation, 1548–49
 description, 1546, 1548
 foreign body airway obstructions, 1255–56, 1255–57f
 foreign body airway obstructions in children, 1558–59f, 1558–60
 interrupting CPR, 1574
 one-rescuer adult CPR, 1567
 one-rescuer CPR, 1567, 1568–69f
 opening airway, 1551–54, 1551f, 1553–54f
 partial airway obstructions, 1257–58
 pediatric CPR, 1570–73, 1571–73f
 pediatric procedures, 1547t
 rescue breathing in adults, 1560–63, 1560–63f
 starting and stopping, 1549–51
 two-rescuer CPR, 1567, 1569, 1570–71f
Basket stretchers, 1437, 1437f
Battery, definition of, 84–85
Battle's sign, 542, 544f, 546, 777, 779f
Behavior, 1132
Behavioral crisis, 1133
Behavioral emergencies, 66–67, 1132–33
 assessment, 1134–38, 1136t
 management, 1139
 medicolegal considerations, 1133, 1140–42
 pathology, 1134
 safe approach to, 1134, 1135t
 suicide, 1138–39, 1138t
Bends, 1124
Benzodiazepines, 1043, 1043t
Beta agonists, 861
Beta cells, 176, 177f
Beta effects, 186–87, 186f, 660, 661t, 892, 893f
Beta radiation, 1511, 1512f
Beta receptors, 172, 186f, 249t
Beta-blocker class, of medications, 249, 250
Bicarbonate, 287, 379
Biceps muscle, 149f, 160f
Bilateral body structures, 122, 726
Bilateral breath sounds, 377
Bioassays, of drugs, 246
Bioavailability, drug absorption and, 257t
Biological death, 27
Biological terrorism/warfare, 1494, 1504–9, 1506–9f, 1506–10t, 1511
Biological transmission of disease, 46t
Biotransformation, of drugs, 258
Black lung disease, 205
Black widow spiders, 1017, 1017f
Bladder, urinary, 145f, 209–10

Blanching, 1261
Blast injuries, 638, 720
Bleeding.
  in brain, 658, 659f, 779–80, 780f, 1069, 1069f, 1075f
  controlling external, 651–53, 652–53f
  external, 512–13
  facial injuries, 430, 430f
  hidden, 625t
  safety concerns, 647, 647f
  vaginal, 1158–59
Blood, 885.
  components of, 178–81, 179f
  drawing, 304–5
Blood clotting, 180–81, 649–51
Blood pressure, 197–98
  chest injuries and, 721, 723
  in children, 1241, 1250, 1250f
  cuffs, 303, 528f, 656, 657f, 1250f
  perfusion and, 659–60
  shock and, 663
  systolic readings, 526t
Blood vessels, 896–900, 897–900f.
  penetrating wounds to, 733–34, 736t
Blow-by technique, 1263–64, 1264f
Blowout fractures, 136, 137f
Blunt trauma, 622–23
  abdominal, 745, 745f, 747–48
  chest, 720, 722
  mechanism of injury, 499–500, 499f
  rib fractures, 723
  sternal fracture, 725
  vehicular collisions, 623–26
Body armor, 65, 66
Body language, 595, 595f
Body substance isolation (BSI), 45–47, 49, 497, 497f
  airway suctioning and, 402
  altered mental status with diabetics and, 995
  artificial ventilation and, 414
  biological terrorism/warfare, 1506
  burns and, 695, 696f
  childbirth and/or neonatal resuscitation, 1180, 1207
  closed injuries and, 681
  hemorrhage and, 651
  intubation and, 440, 441
  medication administration and, 338, 345, 349, 351
  meningitis and, 1304
  open wounds and, 684–85
  patient assessment and, 512
Body surface area, in children, 1240
Body temperature, 131–32.
  assessment of, 513, 1104f
  core, 1103, 1104t
Bolus, 349
Bone(s), 129.
  anatomy of, 152–56, 154–57f
  focused assessment of pain in, 528, 535
Botulinum toxin, 1508, 1509f
Bourdon-gauge flowmeters, 409–10, 409f
Bradycardias, 902, 903f, 1122
  in children, 1241, 1248, 1297
  management, 970–71, 971t
  in newborns, 1206, 1212
  rates, 937
Bradypnea, 380, 721, 1247
Brain
  anatomy of, 162, 191f, 194f, 762, 763f, 1060, 1061f
  disorders, 1061–67
  emergency medical care, 1074–76, 1075f, 1075t

injuries, 625t, 779–80, 1314–15
  organic syndrome, 1134
  signs and symptoms of disorders, 1068–69, 1069f
Brain attacks, 1062.
Brain stem, 162, 162f, 163–64, 164f, 762, 763f, 1061f
Breach of duty, 53–54, 81–82
Breath odors, 542, 544f, 546
Breath sounds.
  absent, 1247t
  bilateral, 377
  detailed physical exam, 542–43, 545f, 547–48
  focused trauma assessment, 521, 521f, 522f, 523–24
  obstructive airway disease and, 859–60
Breath-holding syncope, 1124–25
Breathing.
  assessment, 511–12, 625t
  determining quality of, 525t
  difficult, 869t
  inadequate, 869t
  pediatric assessment, 1244, 1245, 1247
  pediatric management, 1319–20, 1320f
  pursed-lip, 874
  rescue, 1560–62, 1560–63f
Breech presentation, 1189, 1189f, 1191
Bronchioles, 202, 370, 1289f
Bronchiolitis, 1290
Bronchitis, 855t
  chronic, 205, 858–62
Bronchoconstriction, 547
Bronchodilator, 205, 1017
Bronchospasm, 204, 523, 1288–91, 1289f
Bronchovesicular sounds, 547
Brown recluse spiders, 1018, 1018f
Bruising.
  child abuse and, 1324
  fractures and, 806, 806f
Bruit (heart sound), 184, 887
BSI precautions. see Body substance isolation
Buboes, 1507, 1508f
Bubonic plague, 1507
Buccal medications, 255t, 352
Buffer(s), 213, 287, 378–79
Buffer systems, 213–14
Bulb syringe, 1210f, 1259f
Bundle branch blocks (BBBs), 963–64f, 963–65
Bundle of His, 184, 185f, 888, 888f, 890, 890f
Burnout, stress and, 38
Burns, 678, 679.
  chemical, 699–700, 699–701f, 701t, 702
  in children, 695, 695t, 1240, 1316–18, 1317f, 1318t, 1324
  classification, 692t, 693–94, 693f, 694, 694f
  electrical, 702–5, 702f, 704–5f
  emergency medical care, 695, 696f, 697–98
  in infants, 695, 695t
  inhalation, 698–99
  management, 692
  mechanism of injury, 694
  pathophysiology, 691
  signs and symptoms, 694–95
BURP maneuver, 444, 444f
Burping, occlusive dressings, 737
Butterfly catheters, 301, 301f, 302, 302t
BVM (bag-valve-mask) devices, 50, 414–15
  chemical terrorism/warfare, 1503
  for children, 419, 1264–65, 1265f, 1266f
  direct laryngoscopy and, 449
  neonatal- or infant-sized, 1211f
  one-person, 415–17, 416f, 417f
  stoma ventilation with, 471, 471f

three-person, 418, 420
two-person, 417–18, 419f

C

Calcium, 287
Cannulation, 300, 312
Capillaries, 188, 896
  bleeding from, 649, 650f
  perfusion decreases and, 660–61
Capillary beds, 289
Capillary refill, 513
  in children, 1248, 1249f
  musculoskeletal injuries and, 810f, 811
Capnographers, 447
Capnography, 548
Capnometers, 447
Carbon dioxide
  in blood, 373
  end-tidal detection of, 448–49, 448f, 460, 1217f, 1269, 1269f
  partial pressure ($PaCO_2$), 206, 373, 375
  retention, 853
Carbon monoxide poisoning, 1045
Cardiac arrest, 902, 915.
  AED and, 916–19, 920–22f, 921, 923, 924f, 925
  resuscitation termination, 915–16
  during transport, 922–23
Cardiac cycle, 187–88, 895–96
Cardiac muscle, 130, 130f, 160, 800, 800f, 801
Cardiac output, 187, 895–96
Cardiac tamponade, 546, 885f, 1298
Cardiogenic shock, 664, 666, 666t, 903–4, 904f, 1296
Cardiopulmonary resuscitation (CPR)
  for adults, 1564f
  AED and, 918–19, 920–21f
  asynchronous, 1567
  definition, 1546
  external chest compression, 1565–66f, 1566
  interrupting, 1574
  one-rescuer, 1567, 1568–69f
  orders against, 1550, 1550f
  pediatric, 1274–75, 1275–76f, 1551f, 1570–73, 1571–73f
  positioning for, 1551, 1552f
  two-rescuer, 1567, 1569, 1570–71f
Cardiovascular emergencies, 884
  acute myocardial infarction, 901–12, 903–4f, 906f, 909t, 910–12f
  assessment, 907–12
  cardiac arrest, 915–25
  cardiac surgery, 912–13, 913f
  chest pain and stroke, 967, 969, 969t
  in children, 915
  ECG monitoring, 925–65
  electrical interventions, 965, 966f, 967
  risk and prevention strategies, 884t
Cardiovascular system, 188–95, 898f.
  aging effects, 923, 1344–45
  anatomy and physiology, 884–88, 885–87f
  cardiac cycle, 898–99
  child's, 1241
  detailed physical exam, 550–51
  electrical properties, 888–98
  hypothermia and, 1107
  physiology, 196–98
Carotid arteries, 135, 138, 139f
Carpopedal spasms, 287, 865–66
Carriers, infectious disease, 55
Carrying. see Lifting; Moves, patient
Cartilage, 129, 134, 152
Casualty collection area, 1478

Index

Catabolism, cellular, 128
Catheter shear
   IV administration and, 317
Catheters, IV
   for children, 318, 1276–77, 1277f
   choices, 301–2f, 301–3, 302t
   contaminated, 302
   feed troubles, 296
   for geriatric patients, 319
   insertion of, 303–4, 303–4f
   troubleshooting, 318
Cations, 287, 293
Caudad (body) position or location, 120, 121
Cell membrane, 126, 126f
Cells, 118, 286–92
Cellular ischemia, 660–61
Cellular perfusion, 287
Cellular respiration, 128–29, 129f, 130
Cellular telephones, 13, 582, 583–84, 583f, 585t, 1497
Centers for Disease Control and Prevention (CDC), 46, 51, 53
   WMD medications and supplies, 1511, 1511f
Central cyanosis, 1213–14, 1214f, 1285.
Central nervous system (CNS), 161, 162–66, 248f
   anatomy and physiology, 762, 763–65f, 764–65
   depressed function, 380
   injuries, 765
Central pulses, 1248
Cephalad position or location, 120–21
Cerebellum, 162, 162f, 164f, 165, 762, 763f, 1061f
Cerebral arteries, 191
Cerebral edema, 781
Cerebral embolism, 1062
Cerebral perfusion, 381
Cerebrospinal fluid (CSF), 165
   halo test for, 166, 546, 658, 659f
   infectious agents in, 169
   leakage of, 135, 166, 764, 781, 1273
Cerebrospinal fluid rhinorrhea, 1273
Cerebrovascular accidents, 506, 1061, 1062.
Cerebrum, 162, 162f, 163f, 762, 763f, 1061f
Certification
   continuing education, 19
   EMT-I, 8–9
   instructors, 17
   state standards, 80
Cervical (spine immobilization) collar, 785, 785–87f
   for infants and children, 792, 792f
   rapid trauma assessment and, 520, 521, 522f
Cervical (lymph) nodes, 200
Cervical spine, 138, 139–40, 140f
   detailed physical exam, 543, 546
   rapid trauma assessment, 520–21
   stabilization, 770–71, 770f
Cervical vertebrae, 138–40, 139f, 140f
Chairs, patient transfer. *see* Stair chair, wheeled
Channels, radio, 580
CHART format, 606t, 1535
Chassis set, 1387
Chemical burns, 699–700, 699–701f, 701t, 702
Chemical names, for drugs, 245
Chemical Transportation Emergency Center (CHEMTREC), 1471–72
Chemical warfare/terrorism, 1493–94, 1498–1504, 1504t
Chemicals, allergic reactions to, 1007
Chemoreceptors, 185, 374–75, 718, 891–92
Chest.
   barrel-shaped, 869t

child's, 1239–40
   detailed physical exam, 542, 545f, 546–48
   rapid trauma assessment, 520, 521, 522f, 523–24
Chest compressions, 1565–66f, 1566.
   for infants, 1212, 1213f, 1275f, 1571–72, 1572f
Chest injuries/wounds, 719–23.
   children, 1316
   closed, 719, 719f, 720
   and impaled objects, 690
   open, 686–87, 688f, 719–20, 719f
   sucking, 686, 687f, 727, 727f
Chest pain/discomfort
   angina pectoris, 900–901
   documentation, 902
   focused assessment of, 527, 535
   management, 967, 969, 969t
   older patients, 1349–50
   other possible causes, 901t
   pleuritic, 862
   treating conscious patient, 910–11f
Chest thrusts, 1256–57, 1256–57f.
Chest wall injuries, 723–25
Cheyne-Stokes respirations, 377t
Chief complaint, 501, 531, 531f
   focused assessment, 526–29, 535–36
Child abuse, 1242, 1321, 1324, 1324f
CHILD ABUSE mnemonic, 1321t
Child safety seats, 634, 1312, 1312f
Childbirth, 1168, 1204–5.
   breech presentation, 1189, 1189f, 1191
   cord presentation, 1190–91, 1190f
   delivery, 1182–84, 1182f, 1184–85f, 1186–89, 1188f
   field preparation, 1182, 1182f
   limb presentation, 1189–90, 1190f
   postdelivery care, 1186–88
   preparing for delivery, 1180–82
   prolapsed uterus and, 1191
   reporting, 89
   supplies, 1380f, 1380t
Children.
   abdominal injuries, 1316
   abuse of, 1242, 1321, 1321t, 1324, 1324f
   airbags and, 627
   airway adjuncts for, 1259–63, 1260t, 1261–62f
   airway anatomy, 371, 1238–39, 1239f
   airway diseases, lower, 1288–91
   airway diseases, upper, 1286–88, 1287f
   airway management, 1252–63, 1313–14, 1319, 1319f
   airway positioning, 1252, 1253f, 1551
   altered level of consciousness, 1301–2
   altered mental status in, 1076
   anatomical differences, 1310–11, 1311f
   anatomy, 1238–42, 1239f
   artificial ventilation for, 419
   assessment, 1242, 1243f, 1244–48
   brain injuries, 1314–15
   burns, 695, 1316–18, 1317f
   cardiac dysrhythmias, 1296–99
   cardiovascular emergencies, 915
   caring for, 1236t
   chest injuries, 1316
   circulation, 1273–84
   communication with, 597–98, 598f, 1284, 1284f
   CPR in, 972t, 1274–75, 1275–76f, 1570–73, 1571–73f
   critically ill, 32
   death of, 32–33, 1307–10, 1309t, 1310t
   defibrillation, 1280–81, 1282–83f, 1282t, 1283

   dehydration, 1304–5, 1305f, 1305t
   diabetic, 991
   drowning or near drowning, 1318
   electrical burns and, 702, 702f
   emergency medical care, 1318–21
   endotracheal intubation, 439, 453–57, 458–60f, 460, 1266–69, 1267f, 1269–71f, 1272
   endotracheal tube selection, 456t, 1267t
   epiphyseal (growth plate) injuries, 805, 805f, 830, 831f
   extremities injuries, 1316
   falls and, 635
   fever, 1303
   fluid resuscitation/management, 1279, 1314
   focused history and physical exam, 1251–52
   foreign body airway obstructions, 394f, 396, 1252–58, 1253–58f, 1291, 1558–59f, 1558–60
   fractures, 829
   gastric decompression, 1272–73, 1272–73f, 1272t
   growth and development, 1235–38, 1236–38f
   head injuries, 1315–16, 1315f
   helmet removal, 791, 791f
   hyperglycemia, 1306–7, 1307t
   hypoglycemia, 1305–6, 1306t
   illness and injury prevention, 1234–35
   immobilizing, 791–92, 791–92f, 1314, 1320–21, 1322–23f
   injury patterns, 1311–13
   intraosseous infusion, 310–11f, 1278–79, 1280–81f
   IV administration, 318–19, 1276–77, 1277–78f
   medical emergencies, 1234, 1284–1309
   medication dosages for, 251, 334, 335
   medications for resuscitation, 1280, 1282t
   meningitis, 1303–4
   mental status assessment, 506f, 508
   motor vehicle collisions with, 1312–13, 1313f
   oropharyngeal (oral) airways for, 405
   oxygenation, 1263–64, 1263–64f
   physiology, 1238–42
   poisoning, 1048–49, 1049t, 1302–3, 1302f, 1302t
   psychological differences, 1312
   pulse rates in, 512, 512t
   rescue breathing, 1562
   respiratory compromise, 1285–86, 1286f
   respiratory system of, 207, 207f
   seizures, 1299–1301, 1299t, 1300f
   shock, 1291–96
   significant mechanism of injury for, 518
   sports injuries, 1313
   suctioning, 1258–59
   sudden infant death syndrome, 1307–9
   transport decision, 1250, 1284
   trauma emergencies, 1234, 1310–25
   unique needs, 1234
   ventilation, 1264–66, 1319–20, 1320f
   vital functions, 1246–48
   vital signs, 1248–50, 1249f, 1249t
   weight estimations, 1279
Chloride, 287
Chlorine (CL), 1499–1500, 1504t
Choking, 391, 391f, 1555f
Choking agents, 1499–1500
Cholecystitis, 1084, 1085, 1085f
Cholinergic agents, 1048
Chronic bronchitis, 205, 858–62

Chronic obstructive pulmonary disease (COPD), 206, 381, 850, 858–62
Chronotropic state, 185, 185t, 660, 891, 892t
Cilia, 1169
Cincinnati Stroke Scale, 549, 550t, 1071, 1071t
Circulation, 1248f.
    assessment, 512–13
    blood, 188, 189f
    detailed physical exam, 543
    diabetes and, 996f
    general scheme of, 896–97, 896–97f
    head injuries and, 784
    to the heart, 183f, 188–89, 897, 898f
    musculoskeletal injuries and, 809
    pediatric, 1273–84
    pediatric assessment, 1246, 1246f, 1248
    placenta-fetal, 1172f
    pulmonary, 183f, 189, 192f, 898
    rapid trauma assessment of, 524
    restoring, 513–14
    return of spontaneous, 915
    systemic arterial, 189–93, 190f, 898
    systemic venous, 190f, 194–95
Circulatory overload, 317
Circulatory system, definition of, 187
Circumflex coronary arteries, 189, 897
Civil (tort) law, 81
Clavicles, 141, 141f, 143, 145–46, 145–46f
    injuries, 824–26, 825–26f
Cleaning, 47–48, 54–55, 58, 1395
Clinical death, 27
Clinical decision making, 557
    assessment-based management, 561–63, 563t
    critical thinking and, 559–61
    patient acuity and, 558–59
    prehospital environment and, 557–58
    protocols, standing orders, and algorithms for, 559
    six R's of, 563–64
Clonic phase, of seizures, 1064
Closed injuries
    abdominal, 745, 745f
    chest, 719
    fractures, 804
    head, 781
    soft-tissue, 679, 680–81, 680f
Clothing, protective, 63–65
Coagulation, 512–13
Coefficient of friction, 1385–86
Cold exposure, 63, 1103–10, 1104t, 1105–6f, 1108–9f, 1118
Colloid solutions, 295–96
Color.
    in newborns, 1213
    shock and, 669
    skin, 513
Coma.
    diabetic, 991
    hyperosmolar hyperglycemic nonketotic, 128, 989
Combitube (multilumen airway), 430, 431f, 433, 434–35f, 435, 436t.
    endotracheal intubation versus, 467t
Command post, 1462
Comminuted fractures, 805, 805f
Common law, 81
Communicability, 1504
Communicable diseases, 45–51, 46t, 52t, 1546
Communications, 580.
    with children, 597–98, 598f
    coordinating patient moves, 1414–15
    with older patients, 596t, 597f, 1353–54, 1353–54f
    with hearing-impaired patients, 598
    local dispatch components, 584–85
    with non-English-speaking patients, 600
    with other health care professionals, 593–94, 593–94f
    with patients, 507, 508f, 594–600, 595f
    phases of EMS event, 591t
    radio, 586–93, 592t
    systems and equipment, 580–84, 591–93
    verbal, 593–600
    WMD scenes, 1496–97
    written, 600–606, 607t
Compartment syndrome, 681, 809
Compensated (early) shock, 661–62, 1292, 1359
Competency, 86.
Complaint(s)
    chief, 501, 526–29, 531, 531f, 535–36
    drills for responding to, 1535–36
    patient's, 507
Complete airway obstruction, 391, 1254–56
Complex access, 1450
Compression, for closed injuries, 681
Compression injuries, 680–81, 680f, 767
Computers
    communications using, 585t
    for reporting, 602
Concealment, 66
Concentration gradient, 126–27, 287–88
Concentrations, of drugs, 332
Concept formation, 559–60
Concussions, 779
Conduction, definition of, 1102
Conduction system, 184–87, 185f, 888, 888f
Conductivity, of cardiac cells, 185, 891
Confidentiality, 88, 602
Congested breath sounds, 547
Congestive heart failure (CHF), 905–6, 906f
Conjunctiva, 513, 542, 544f
Connecting nerves, 764, 765f
Connective tissues, 129, 152
Consent
    advance directives, 86–87, 1346–48
    behavioral emergencies and, 1141
    definition of, 82–83
    expressed, 83
    forcible restraint, 84
    implied, 83
    mentally incompetent adults, 84
    minors and, 83
    pregnant teens and, 1154
    refusal of care, 85, 87, 604, 605f
Constricting band, 303, 307f, 318
Contact hazards, 1498
Contagious diseases, 45, 1504
Contaminated stick, 302
Contamination.
    hazardous substance, 1039
    infectious disease, 55, 681, 685
    WMD scenes, 1496, 1513
Continuing education, 19, 1235
Continuous quality improvement (CQI), 14
Continuum of care, 17
Contractility, of heart, 186, 892
Contraindications, for medications, 244–45, 244t
Contralateral body structures, 122, 123, 726
Controlled substances, classifications of, 262
Contusions, 680, 680f, 779
Convection, definition of, 1102
Copperheads, 1019, 1019f, 1020–21, 1020f
Coral snakes, 1019, 1019f, 1022
Core temperature, 1103, 1104t
Coronary arteries, 188–89, 190f
Coronary artery disease (CAD), 898
Corticosteroids, 175, 204, 871

Costal arch, 141, 142, 142f, 143, 145
Cottonmouth (snake), 1019f, 1020–21, 1020f
Coughs/coughing, 207, 377, 869t, 1304
Coup-countrecoup injuries, 624
Cover, for violent situations, 66
CPR board, 1379, 1379f
Crackles (breath sounds), 521, 547
Cranial nerves, 170–71, 170f, 248f, 550
Cranial (body) position or location, 120–21
Cranial vault, 132
Cranium, 134, 135f
Crenation, definition of, 127
Crepitus, 138, 520, 521, 806
Cribriform plate, 135
Cricoid cartilage, 138, 139f
Cricoid pressure, 420, 422–23, 423t
    for children, 1265–66, 1267f
Cricothyroid membrane, 138, 139f
Crime scenes, 89, 90
Criminal actions.
    gun shot wounds, 501, 501f, 683–84, 684f
    sexual assault, 1159–60
Criminal law, 81
Critical incident stress debriefing (CISD), 40–41
Critical incident stress management (CISM), 35–36
Critical thinking, 559–60, 561
Cross-contamination, 1496
Croup, 523, 856f, 856t, 1286–87, 1287f, 1288
Crowing (breath sounds), 523, 547, 869t
Crowning, 1179
Crushing injuries
    closed, 680–81, 680f
    open, 684, 684f
Crystalloid solutions, 294
Cullen's sign, 548
Cultural diversity, 41–42
Cumulative effect, of drugs, 261t
Cyanides, 1502–4, 1504t
Cyanosis, 513, 869t, 1246.
    central, 1213–14, 1214f, 1285
Cytotoxins, definition of, 1018

D

D_5W (5% dextrose in water), 293, 294
$D_{50}W$ (50% dextrose), 262, 267t, 294, 996, 997f
Dalton's law, 373–74
Damages, determination of, 81–82
Danger zones (hot zones), 1448–49, 1448f, 1467
Data interpretation, 560
DCAP-BTLS assessments
    abdominal injuries, 747
    chest wall, 546–47
    detailed physical exam, 543
    flail chest, 724
    musculoskeletal trauma, 809
    open soft-tissue injuries, 685
    spinal injuries, 768
    trauma patients, 520
    of unresponsive patients, 537
Dead space, 371
Death
    of children, 32–33, 1307–10, 1309t, 1310t
    definitive signs, 26–27, 28t
    fetal, 1222
    grieving process, 28–29, 29t
    local regulations, 34
    obvious signs of, 1549–50
    in older people, 1342, 1342t
    physical signs, 27
    presumptive signs, 27, 27t

Index

pronouncement of, 90
sudden, 902–3
from vehicular collisions, 625
Decay, 1511
Deceleration injuries, 627
Deceleration, vehicle, 1387
Decerebrate posturing, 782
Decision-making styles, 562, 563t
Decompensated (late) shock, 662–63, 1292, 1359
Decompression sickness, 1124
Decompression, tension pneumothorax, 727–29, 730f
Decontamination, 1377, 1469, 1504.
Decontamination area, 1468–69
Decorticate posturing, 782
Dedicated lines, radio, 581
Defamation, definition of, 88
Defibrillation, 903, 917–18, 965, 966f.
  pediatric, 1280–81, 1282–83f, 1282t, 1283
Deformities, 805, 805f, 815
Dehydration, 291–92, 292f, 1238, 1304–5, 1305f, 1305t
Delirium, 1360
Delirium tremens (DTs), 1042
Dementia, 1360
Denial, 28
Dental appliances, 428–29, 1552–53
Dependency, 30–31
Dependent lividity, 27, 1307–8, 1550f
Dependent living, 1342
Depolarization, 288, 892–93, 894f, 931f
Depression, 28, 30, 1133
Dermis, 132, 133f, 678, 679f
Designated officers, 57–58
Detailed physical exam, 541–43, 544–45f, 546–51
Dextrose, see D_5W and $D_{50}W$
Diabetes
  complications, 996–98
  definition of, 986
  emergencies, 990–92, 990f, 990t
  emergency medical care, 992–96, 994f, 997f
  gestational, 1177
  glucose, insulin and, 987–88, 987f, 989f
  hyperglycemia and, 989
  types, 986–87
Diabetic coma, 991
Diabetic ketoacidosis, 988, 990–92, 1306, 1307t
Diamond carry, 1409–10f, 1411–12
Diaphoresis, 721
Diaphoretic skin, 508
Diaphragm, 141, 142, 142f, 734, 737t
Diarrhea, older patients, 1351–52
Diastole, 197, 895
Diet, stress and, 38–39
Differential diagnosis, 557
Diffuse pain, 532, 533f
Diffusion, 126, 127f, 288, 896, 896f
  drug absorption and, 257t
  in respiration, 372, 851–52
  vascular, 188, 188f
Digestion, 207
Digestive system, 207–9
Digital communication equipment, 582–83
Dimensional analysis, 312
Direct carry methods, 1427–28, 1429f
Direct contact, of communicable diseases, 46, 46t
Direct ground lift, 1426–27, 1427f
Direct laryngoscopy. see Laryngoscopy, direct
Direct transmission of disease, 45, 46t
Directional terms, 119f, 122–23, 122t

Dirty bombs, 1511, 1513
Disasters, 1474, 1477–78
Disease vectors, 1504
Disinfection, 1395
Dislocations, 802–3, 803f, 807, 807f
  elbow, 829, 829f
  finger joint, 831, 831f
  hip, 834, 834f, 835f
  knee, 836–37
  patella, 838, 838f
  shoulder, 826–27, 826–27f
Disoriented patients, 529
Dispatch, 13, 586–88, 1384, 1384f.
  ambulance arrival at scene, 1391
  local communications components, 584–85
  required reporting, 591
  WMD scenes and, 1496–97
Displaced fractures, 805
Dissociate/dissociation, 378
Distal position or location, 119f, 121
Distributive shock, 664, 666, 666t, 1294–95
Diving emergencies, 1122–24
Diving reflex, 1122
Dizziness, 528, 535, 536, 651, 1350
DNR (do not resuscitate) orders, 27, 86–87, 1346–48, 1550, 1550f
Doctor's orders, 312, 590
Documentation, 580, 600–607.
  accuracy, 89
  acute abdomen, 1087
  AED, 924f
  ambulance inspections, 1383
  behavioral emergencies, 1133, 1140
  BLS decisions, 1549
  burn patterns, 694
  chest discomfort, 902
  childbirth, 1187
  daily ambulance inspections, 1383
  data collection, 606
  disease exposure, 58
  elder abuse, 1362
  endotracheal intubation in children, 1272
  errors in, 604, 604f, 606
  form types, 602
  general considerations, 603
  gunshot wounds, 684
  hypothermia, 1105
  inhaler treatments, 336
  insect bites and stings, 1017, 1018
  IV therapy, 313
  mechanism of trauma injury, 626
  medication administration, 263–64, 335
  minimum data set, 600, 601f
  motor vehicle crash, 749
  narrative writing systems, 604, 606, 606t, 607t
  obstetric, 1153, 1181
  occlusive chest wound dressings, 737
  of pain, 535
  patient assessment, 528–29, 536
  poisonings, 1040
  prehospital care reports, 600–601, 602t
  refusal of care, 85, 604, 605f
  respiratory emergencies, 871
  restraints, 1142
  seizure patterns, 1065, 1301
  sexual assault, 1160
  shock progression, 663
  special situations, 606
  spinal injuries, 768
  splinting, 814
  thoroughness of, 89, 561
  triage tag, 1475f
  unresponsive patients, 538–39
  vital signs, 1249

Dog bites and rabies, 1024, 1024f
Dorsal position or location, 120, 121, 122
Dorsalis pedis arteries, 193, 194f
Doses/dosages, medication, 244, 244t, 331–34
Draw sheet transfer method, 1428, 1429f
Dressings
  control of bleeding, 651, 652f
  flutter valve for chest wounds, 687, 687f
  occlusive, 687
  soft-tissue injuries, 707–8
Drills
  common complaints, 1535–36
  CPR, 1568
Drip chamber, 298
Drip rates, 312–13
Drip sets, 297–98
Dromotropic state, 185, 185t, 660, 891, 892t
Drowning or near drowning, 1117–20, 1121–22f, 1122, 1125, 1318
Drug abuse. see Substance abuse
Drug concentrations, 331, 332
Drug laboratories, clandestine, 1478–84
  emergency scene, 1481–82, 1482f
  fire suppression, 1482–83
  hazards, 1481, 1481f
  hot zone personnel monitoring, 1483–84, 1484f
  materials common to, 1480t
  positive pressure ventilation, 1483, 1483f
Drug overdose signs and symptoms, 1035t
Drug reconstitution, 340–41
Drug-related injuries, reporting, 89
Drugs. see Medications
DUMBELS assessment, 1048, 1501, 1502t
Duplex communication systems, 584, 585t
Duty to act, 53–54, 81
Dysarthria, 1068
Dysphasia, 695
Dyspnea, 376.
  burns and, 695
  chest injuries/wounds and, 721, 722
  definition of, 850
  diseases associated with, 855–56t
  focused assessment, 527, 535
  nocturnal, 861
  older patients, 1349, 1359t
  paroxysmal nocturnal, 861, 912
  two- to three-word, 510–11, 861, 869t
Dysrhythmias, 380, 902, 903f, 1296–99
Dysuria, 549

E

E (enhanced) 9-1-1 calls, 584–85
Ears
  aging effects, 1344
  anatomy of, 134, 135
  bleeding from, 653, 658, 659f
  detailed physical exam, 542, 544f
  protection, 65
Ecchymosis, 524, 680, 779, 806.
Eclampsia, 1176
Ectopic pregnancy, 1089–90, 1158, 1175–76
Edema, 290–91, 542
  cerebral, 781
  peripheral, diabetes and, 996f
  pulmonary, 373, 856–58, 857f
Education, 7–8
  continuing, 19, 1235
  EMT-I instructors, 17
Efficacy, of drugs, 259
Ejection fraction, 187, 896
Elbows, 149f, 829, 829f
Elder abuse, 1360–62, 1362t
Electrical burns, 702, 702f

history, 703
  management, 704, 705f
  mechanism of injury, 703
  pathophysiology, 703
  safety, 703–4, 705
Electrical hazards, 61
Electrical potential, 892, 894f
Electrocardiograms (ECGs), 884
  arrhythmias versus events, 951–52
  artifacts, 937–38, 938f
  basic components, 926–27, 926f
  interpretation points, 938–40
  lead placement for, 925–26, 926f
  monitoring using paddles, 927f
  rates, 936–37, 936–37f
  recording paper, 933–34, 933f
  tools, 934–36, 934–36f
  wave nomenclature, 927–33, 928–33f
Electrolytes, 126, 286–88, 892, 1112
Elevation, for injuries, 669, 681
Embolus, 864, 1063f
Embryo, 1171
Emergency, definition of, 79
Emergency Medical Act of 1973, 10
Emergency medical care, 78
Emergency Medical Dispatch (EMD), 13
Emergency medical services (EMS) system.
  components, 12–17
  description, 6–7
  history, 9–10
  regulation, 15
Emergency medical technician-basic (EMT-B), 6, 11
Emergency medical technician-intermediate (EMT-I)
  course description, 6–7
  levels of training, 10–12
  medications approved for administration by, 262
  postexposure management, 57–58
  protective clothing, 63–65
  roles and responsibilities, 18–19, 18t
  training requirements, 7–8
  well-being of, 24
Emergency medical technician-paramedic (EMT-P), 6, 12
Emergency moves, 1419–21, 1420–22f
Emesis (vomiting), 1041, 1084–85, 1351–52
Emotions, 26, 1325
Emphysema, 205, 858–62
  subcutaneous, 520–21, 723, 862
Emulsions, definition of, 252
Endocrine system, 173–78
Endometrium, 1151, 1169
End-organ perfusion, 1248
Endotracheal intubation, 438–39, 438f, 438t, 467t.
  chest injuries and, 723
  for children, 1266–69, 1267f, 1269–71f, 1272
  for neonatal resuscitation, 1208
  for newborns, 1216–17, 1216t
  pediatric, 453–57, 458–60f, 460
  tracheobronchial suctioning, 451
Endotracheal (ET) route, for drug administration, 254, 255
Endotracheal tubes, 369, 439f
  for newborns, 1216, 1216t
  pediatric, 456t, 1267f, 1267t
  securing with commercial device, 452f
End-tidal carbon dioxide detection, 448–49, 448f
  for newborns, 1217f
  pediatric, 460, 1269, 1269f
Energy, trauma and, 620–21, 622

Enteral medications, 337–40
Enteral route, for drug administration, 254, 255, 255t
Entrance wounds, 501, 501f, 683–84, 704
Entrapment, 1446
Envenomations, 1007.
  marine animals, 1025–26, 1025f, 1026t
Environmental emergencies, 1102
  cold exposure, 1102–10
  diving, 1122–24
  drowning and near drowning, 1117–20, 1121–22f, 1122
  heat exposure, 1111–16
  lightening injuries, 1116–17
  risk factors, 1102t
  water hazards, 1124–25
Epicardium, 182, 885
Epidermis, 132, 133f, 678, 679f
Epidural bleeding, 779–80, 780f, 1069
Epiglottis, 202, 202f
Epiglottitis, 523, 855–56t, 855f, 1286, 1287–88, 1287f
Epileptic seizures, 1064, 1299
Epinephrine, 187, 249, 268–69t
  administration of, 251–52, 262, 861, 1012–15f, 1012–16
  alpha and beta effects of, 661t, 892
  for children, 1282t
  low blood volume and, 198
  for newborn resuscitation, 1218, 1218t
  production of, 177
  side effects of, 245
  sodium/potassium pump and, 287
EpiPen auto-injectors, 1012f
Epiphyseal fractures, 805, 805f, 830, 831f
Epiphyseal plate, 1240
Epiphyses, 155
Epistaxis, 653, 658
Epithelial tissue, 129
Equipment.
  ambulance, 1377–83, 1377t, 1378–82f, 1379–81t
  communications, 580–84, 591–93
  EMT-I, 15
  extrication, 1383, 1383t
  neonatal resuscitation, 1207–8, 1207t
  patient transfer, 1381–82, 1381f, 1430–38
  sterile obstetric kit, 1181, 1181f
Errors, reporting, 604, 604f, 606
Eschar, 691
Escherichia coli (E. coli), 57
Escorts for ambulances, 1390
Esophageal gastric tube airways (EGTAs), 462–63, 462f
  endotracheal intubation versus, 467t
Esophageal intubation, 457
Esophageal obturator airways (EOAs), 461–63, 461f, 462f
  endotracheal intubation versus, 467t
Esophageal varices, 548
Esophagus, 138, 142, 208, 734, 737t
Estrogen, 178, 1169
Ethics, 18–19
  considerations, 78
  duty to act, 53–54, 81
  responsibilities, 87–88, 87t
Evaporation, 1102–3
Evisceration, abdominal, 688, 688f, 750–51, 750f
Excitability, of cardiac cells, 185, 891
Excretion, pharmacokinetics and, 258
Exercise, stress and, 39
Exhalation, 371
Exit wounds, 501, 501f, 683–84, 684f, 704, 704f

Exocrine glands, 173
Expiration, 372, 851
Expiration dates, medication, 263, 264
Expiratory reserve volume, 371
Exposure.
  to communicable diseases, 46
Exposure control plan, 51, 51t, 57–58
Expressed consent, 83
Extension (movement), 125, 156
Extensor posturing, 782
External auditory meatus, 135
External jugular IVs, 311–12, 312f
External nares, 202
External occipital protuberance, 136
External rotation, definition of, 125
Extracellular fluid (ECF), 212, 289
Extremities.
  child's, 1240
  pediatric injuries, 1316
  physical exam, 543, 545f, 549–50
Extremity lift, 1427, 1428f
Extrication, 1446–54
  equipment, 1383, 1383t
  patient care during, 1450–54
  triage, 1449–50
Extubation, 451, 453, 454–55f
Eye contact, 507, 594, 595f, 598f, 1136f
  pediatric assessment and, 1245, 1245f
Eyes.
  aging effects, 1343
  blunt trauma, 136, 137f
  chemical burns of, 699, 699f, 700, 701f, 702, 1039–40, 1040f
  detailed physical exam, 542, 544f
  protection, 49, 51, 65
Eyes-forward position, 770

F

Face, 134
  bones, 136
  detailed physical exam, 542, 544f, 546
  impaled objects in, 690
  injuries, 430, 430f
Face mask, simple, 413
Facial nerve, 135
Facilitated diffusion, 126, 127f, 128
Facilitating behaviors, 562
Facsimile systems, 585t
FACTS (about seizures), 1064
Fahrenheit scale, 331
Fainting. see Syncopal episodes
Fallopian tubes, 211f, 212, 1151, 1152f, 1169, 1171
Falls, 635–36, 635f
  blunt trauma and, 623
  mechanism of injury, 501
  older patients, 1351, 1351f, 1356–58
False labor, 1179
Family
  balancing work, health, and, 39–40
  dealing with grief, 29
  death of a child, 32–33, 1309–10, 1309t, 1310t
  notification of, 32
  pediatric patients and, 1242, 1284
  SIDS and, 1308
Fascia, 138, 314
Fasttrach laryngeal mask airway (LMA), 466f
Fear
  in critically ill and injured patients, 30
  separation anxiety, 1242, 1284
Febrile seizures, 1065, 1300, 1300f
Federal Communications Commission (FCC), 586
Feedback inhibition, 174

Feet.
    anatomy of, 151–52, 152f
    injuries, 839–40, 840f
Female genitalia injuries, 754–55
Female reproductive system, 210, 211f, 212, 751, 752f
    anatomy, 1151–52, 1152f, 1168–70, 1168–70f
    gestation, 1171–72
    physiology, 1152–53
Femoral arteries, 193
Femoral head, 149, 149f
Femoral nerves, 169–70
Femoral veins, 195, 197f
Femur, 149, 151f, 832
    fractures, 834–36, 835f
Fertilization, 1169f, 1171f
Fetal alcohol syndrome, 1221
Fetal death, 1222
Fetal distress, 1205–6
Fetal transition, 1204–5
Fetus, 1171–72
Fever.
    children, 1303
    older patients, 1350
Fibrin, 180
Fibula, 150, 838–39, 838f
Fick Principle, 852
Field impression, 557, 1529
Fight or flight response, 161, 248
Filtration, 257t, 288
Fire ants, 1009, 1009f
Fire scene hazards, 62
First responders, 11
First-degree burns, 693–94, 693f
First-responder vehicles, 1374
Flail chest, 521, 724–25, 724f, 725f, 735t
Flash chamber, 304
Flat bones, 155, 155f
Flexible stretchers, 1435–36, 1435f
Flexion (movement), 123, 125, 156
Flexor posturing, 782
Flexor reflex, 166
Floating ribs, 142
Flow-restricted, oxygen-powered ventilation devices (FROPVDs), 420–21, 421f, 421t, 423
Fluid balance, 212, 212t, 290–91.
    daily, 290t
    principles, 291–96
Fluid compartments, 287, 289–90
Fluids, 212
    composition, 292
    movement of, 287–88, 295f
Flutter valve, for chest wound dressing, 687, 687f, 729
Focal pain, 532, 533f
Focused history and physical exam
    behavioral emergencies, 1138
    children, 1251–52
    medical patients, 531–36, 531t
    older patients, 1352–55
    respiratory emergency, 868–70
    seizures, 1073
    strokes, 1070–71
    trauma patients with no significant MOI, 526–29
    trauma patients with significant MOI, 517–20, 518t
Fontanelles, 134, 1238
Food, allergic reactions to, 1007
Food and Drug Administration (FDA), U.S., 245, 247
Food poisoning, 1049–50, 1050t
Foramen magnum, 134, 136, 138, 140

Foramen ovale, 182, 885
Forced expiratory vital capacity (FEVI), 204
Forcible restraint, 84
Foreign body airway obstructions, 390
    in children, 1252–58, 1253–58f, 1291, 1558–59f, 1558–60
    emergency care for, 392, 393–97f, 396–97, 1255–56, 1255–57f
Fossa ovalis, 182, 885
4H and 4T mnemonic, 1298
Four-person log roll, 771, 772–73f
Fowler's position, 123
Fractures, 803–6f, 804–7
    blowout, 136, 137f
    child abuse and, 1324
    cribriform plate, 135
    definition of, 802
    femur, 834–36, 835f
    fibula, 838–39, 838f
    forearm, 830, 830f
    humerus, 827, 828f, 828t
    knee, 837
    larynx, 391
    older patients and, 155
    olecranon process, 829
    pelvis, 753, 753f, 831–34, 833f
    range of motion and, 125
    skull, 658, 777, 779f
    spine, 840, 840f
    sternum, 725, 735t
    tibia, 838–39, 838f
    wrist, 125
Fraternal twins, 1220–21
French catheters, 398, 400, 400f
Friction, 1385–86
Frontal (vehicular) collisions, 623, 625–29, 628–29f, 628t
Frontal lobe, 162, 163f
Frontal plane, 120, 120f, 121
Frostbite, 513, 1108–9f, 1108–10
Frostnip, 1108–9
Full-thickness burns, 693–94, 693f
Functional disorders, 1134
Functional reserve (residual) capacity, 371, 1240
Fundus, 1151, 1169
Furosemide, 269–70t

G

G agents, 1500–1502
Gag reflex, 377, 402
Gallbladder, 209.
Gamma (x-rays) radiation, 1511, 1512f
Gangrene, 1109, 1109f
Gas cylinders, 410, 411f
Gases for inhalation, 254
Gastric decompression, 423
    in children, 1272–73, 1272–73f
    manual, 424f
Gastric distention, 423, 1272, 1563–64
Gastric tubes, 423–24
    for children, 1272t
    dental appliances and, 428–29
    nasogastric, 424–25, 425f, 425t, 426–27f, 1272
    orogastric, 427–28, 428–30f, 430t, 1272
Gastrointestinal tract
    abdominal pain, 1088–89
    aging effects, 1346
Gauge, of needles, 340
Gels, drug administration in, 253, 253f
General adaptation syndrome, 35, 35t
General impressions, 505, 506f, 868
Generic drug names, 245

Genitourinary system, 209–10, 210f, 751–55
Geriatric patients
    abuse, 1360–62, 1362t
    acute abdomen, 1089, 1358–59
    altered mental status, 1073, 1360
    assessment, 1338–42, 1348–55
    behavioral emergencies, 1137, 1140
    with burns, 692
    cardiovascular emergencies, 923, 1358
    communicable diseases and, 57
    communication with, 596–97, 596t, 597f, 1353–54, 1353–54f
    CPR and, 1568
    falls and, 635
    fractures and, 155
    heat or cold effects on, 1116
    hemorrhage and, 651
    hip fractures, 834–35
    medications for, 254
    physiologic changes for, 1342–44f, 1342–46, 1345f
    poisonings, 1049
    respiratory system, 86
    trauma, 1356–58
    turgor assessment in, 546
    undiagnosed diabetes in, 995
Gestation, 1171–72
Gestational diabetes, 1177
Gestational period, 1221
Glands, 129, 173
Glasgow Coma Scale (GCS), 526, 782, 783f, 1071, 1071t
    pediatric, 1244–45
Glenoid fossa, 145, 145f, 146, 846
Glossopharyngeal nerves, 171
Glottic opening, 369, 443–44, 445, 447, 464
Glottis, 202
Gloves, protective
    firefighting, 64, 64f
    infection control, 47–49
    IV insertion and, 303
    removal, 47–48
Glucagon, 176, 987
Glucocorticoids, 178
Gluconeogenesis, 176, 988
Glucose
    for children, 1282t
    diabetes and, 986, 987–88
Glucose, oral
    EMT-I administration of, 262, 993–96, 994f
    packaging of, 993f
    substitute for, 994
Glycogen, 176
Glycogenolysis, 176, 987
Glycolysis, 987
Golden Hour, 517, 517f, 618, 812
Good air exchange, 391
Good Samaritan laws, 85–86
Gowns, protective, 49, 51
Gravida, definition of, 1153, 1172, 1181
Greenstick fractures, 805, 805f, 1240
Grey-Turner's sign, 548
Grieving, 28–29, 29t
Growth hormone (GH), 175
Growth plate, 1240.
    fractures, 805, 805f, 830, 831f
Grunting, breathing difficulty and, 1247t
Gtt measurement, 298
Guarding, 549, 747, 806, 1086
Guide dogs, 599, 599f
Guilt, 31
Gum bougie, 444
Gunshot wounds, 501, 501f, 683–84, 684f
Gynecologic emergencies, 1151
    assessment, 1154–56

ectopic pregnancy, 1158
history of, 1154–55
management, 1156–57
obstetric history, 1154–55
pelvic inflammatory disease, 1157–58
physical exam, 1156
ruptured ovarian cyst, 1158
sexual assault, 1159–60
traumatic abdominal pain, 1159
vaginal bleeding, 1158–59

H

Hair follicles, 133, 133f
Hairline fractures, 804–5
Half-life, of drugs, 244t, 259
Hallucinogens, 1046–47, 1046t
Halo test, 166, 546, 658, 659f
Hands.
    anatomy, 148, 148f
    injuries, 830–31, 831f
    splinting, 832f
Handwashing, 47
Hantavirus, 57
Hard palate, 136
Hare traction splint, 819–22, 820–21f
Haversian systems, 156, 157f
Hay fever, 861–62
Hazardous materials, 1454, 1465.
    protection levels, 1471, 1471f
    scene management, 60–61, 61f
    toxicity levels, 61t, 1470
    warning placards, 1467–68f, 1467–69
Hazardous materials incidents, 1465–72
    patient care at, 1469–71
    resources, 1471–72
Head.
    arterial circulation system, 190–91, 191f
    child's, 1238
    emergency medical care, 783–84
    injuries, 762, 775, 781–84, 1315–16, 1315f
    injury complications, 781
    physical exam, 542, 543, 544f, 546
    rapid trauma assessment of, 520–21, 522f
    skin color and elevation of, 669
    venous circulation system, 194, 194f, 195f
Head bobbing, 1247
Head tilt–chin maneuver, 385, 385f, 385t, 386f, 1246, 1246f, 1551–53, 1551f, 1553f
Health Insurance Portability and Accountability Act (HIPAA) of 1996, 88
Hearing-impaired patients, 598, 1344
Heart, 181–88, 884–85.
    anatomy, 181–82
    blood flow within, 182–84, 183f, 885–88, 886f
    cardiac cycle, 187–88, 898–99
    electrical properties, 184–87, 888–98
    pacemaker function, 888
    pacemaker settings, 888–89, 889f
    recognizing injury to, 625t
    regulation of, 891–92, 892t
    sounds, 184f, 548, 887f
    valves, 182, 885
Heart attack. *see* Myocardial infarction
Heart blocks, 949–51, 949–51f
    nomenclature, 950
Heart rate.
    breathing difficulty and, 869t
    low blood volume and, 198
Heat cramps, 382, 1111–12, 1112f
Heat exhaustion, 1111, 1113, 1114f
Heat exposure, 1111–16

Heatstroke, 1111, 1115, 1115f
Heimlich maneuver, 392, 396, 396f
    for children, 1254–55, 1255f
Helicopters, 1396–97, 1396–97f
Helmets, 61, 61f, 64, 64f
    removal of, 788–89, 788–91f, 791
Hematemesis, 1041, 1359
Hematochezia, 651
Hematomas, 316, 316f, 680, 680f, 779–80, 780f
Hematuria, 651, 753, 833
Hemiparesis, 1066
Hemoglobin, 179
Hemophilia, 650–51
Hemopneumothorax, 723, 731
Hemoptysis, 721–22
Hemorrhage, 646.
    assessment, 651
    brain, 780
    intracerebral, 1069
    management, 651–53, 652–53f
    PASGs for, 654, 655f, 656
    physiologic response to, 649–51, 650f
    shock and, 666, 667f, 668
    significance of, 648–49, 649f
    stages of, 650t
    subarachnoid, 166
    tourniquets for, 656, 657f, 658
Hemorrhagic strokes, 1062
Hemostasis, 180–81, 180f, 649
Hemostats, 654
Hemothorax, 686, 688f, 723, 730–31, 731f, 736t
HEPA respirators, 49–50, 51
Heparin, 180
Hepatic portal system, 195, 196f
Hepatitis, 54–55t, 55–56
Hepatomegaly, 1296
Hering-Breuer reflex, 372
Hernias, 1090–91, 1220
Hidden injuries, 518
High-level disinfection, 1395
Highway Safety Act of 1966, 10
Hinge joints, 146, 147f, 150, 156, 158f, 802
Hips.
    dislocation, 834, 834f, 835f
    fractures, 150, 150f
Histamines, 180, 1006, 1011, 1289
History of illness, 535, 537–38, 909t, 1528, 1529f
HIV infection, 50, 52, 54–55
Hollow organs, abdominal, 744, 744f, 1088f
Homeland Security Advisory System, 1494, 1495f
Homeostasis, 118–19, 126, 286, 291
Hormones, 173, 173f, 249, 986.
Hospitals
    communicating with, 588–91, 588f
    EMS medical directors of, 13–14
    mass-casualty incidents, 1478
    working with staff, 16
Hostility, 28, 30
Hosts, disease, 45
Hot lines, 581
Human bites, 1024–25, 1024f
Human body.
    abdomen, 143–45, 143–45f
    acid-base balance, 213–14
    appendicular skeleton, 145–46f, 145–48, 148f
    blood components, 178–81
    bones, 152–56, 154–56f
    cartilage, tendons, and ligaments, 152, 153t
    cellular transport mechanisms, 126–27f, 126–29, 129f

    circulation physiology, 196–98
    digestive system, 207–9
    endocrine system, 173–78
    female reproductive system, 210, 211f, 212, 751, 752f, 1151–53, 1152f, 1168–70f, 1168–72
    fluids, 212, 212t
    genital system, 210
    heart, 181–86f, 181–88
    integumentary system, 130–33, 131f, 133f
    joints, 147f, 156, 157f, 158
    lower extremities, 149–52, 149–52f
    lymphatic system, 198, 199f, 200–201, 201f
    male reproductive system, 210, 211f, 751, 752f
    musculoskeletal system, 158–60, 159–60f
    neck, 138, 139f
    nervous system, 160–72
    pelvic girdle, 148–49
    respiratory system, 201–3f, 201–7, 205–7f
    skeletal system, 133–34, 134f
    skull, 134–37f, 134–38
    spine, 139–41, 140f
    terminology, 119–26
    thorax, 141–42f, 141–43
    tissues, 129–30, 130f, 131f
    urinary system, 209–10, 210f
    vascular system, 188–95, 188–96f
Humerus, 146, 154f, 156f, 826, 827, 828f, 828t.
Hydrophilic layer, of cells, 286
Hydrophobic layer, of cells, 286
Hydroplaning, 1388
Hyoid bone, 137
Hyperbaric chambers, 1124, 1124f
Hypercalcemia, 287
Hyperextension, 125, 629
Hyperflexion, 125, 629
Hyperglycemia, 988, 990–92, 1306–7, 1307t
    treatment for hypoglycemia *versus*, 993, 1307
Hyperglycemic hyperosmolar nonketotic coma (HHNC), 128, 989
Hyperkalemia, 287, 1298
Hyperosmolar hyperglycemic nonketotic coma (HHNC), 128
Hypersensitivity, 1006
Hypertension, 906–7, 1069, 1176
Hyperthermia, 1102, 1111
Hypertonic solutions, 289, 294, 295f
Hyperventilation, 373, 377t, 865
Hyperventilation syndrome, 865–66
Hyphema, 546
Hypnotic agents, 1041.
Hypocalcemia, 287
Hypoglycemia, 987, 990–92, 1305–6, 1306t
    altered mental status and, 1066–67, 1067f
    strokes *versus*, 1069
    treatment for hyperglycemia *versus*, 993, 1307
Hypokalemia, 287, 1298
Hypoperfusion, 382
Hypotension, postural, 292
Hypothalamohypophyseal portal system, 174
Hypothalamus, 174
Hypothermia, 513, 665, 1103–7, 1104t, 1105–6f
    burns and, 697
    in children, 1298
    definition of, 1102
    neonatal, 1209, 1220
    in older patients, 1355
Hypotonic solutions, 289, 293–94, 295f
Hypovolemia
    in children, 1298
    relative, 1294
Hypovolemic shock, 663–64, 1294

definition of, 649
differential diagnosis of, 666, 666t
open soft-tissue injuries and, 685
peritonitis and, 1085
signs and symptoms, 648
signs and treatment of newborn, 1217
Hypoxemia, 376, 1298
Hypoxia, 376, 852, 854, 1241, 1357
Hypoxic drive, 207, 375, 853

I

Iatrogenic responses, to drugs, 259
Ice, 681
   amputated parts and, 690
ICES (mnemonic), 681
Identical twins, 1220–21
Idiosyncratic reactions, to drugs, 245
Ileum, 144, 145
Ileus, 1084
Iliac crest, 123, 543, 545f
Illness and injury prevention, 59, 1234–35
Immersion foot, 1108–9
Immobilization.
   children, 791–92, 791–92f, 1314, 1320–21, 1322f
   devices, 784–85, 785–86f, 787–88, 1436–37, 1436f
   infants, 792, 792f, 1323f
   spinal, 520–21, 522f, 774
   spinal-injured sitting patients, 773–74, 776–77f
   spinal-injured standing patients, 774, 778f
Immune system, 1346
Immunity
   communicable disease, 52–53, 52t
   legal, 85–86
Immunizations, 52–53
Impaled objects, 689–90, 689f, 722
Implied consent, 83, 1141
Implosion effect, pulmonary contusion and, 731
Incarcerated hernias, 1091
Incident command systems, 1462–63, 1463f, 1464
   WMD scenes, 1497
Incident commander, 1452, 1462
Incontinence, 1065
Incubation, 1504–5
Index of suspicion, 558, 618
Indications, for medications, 244, 244t, 245
Indirect contact, of communicable diseases, 46, 46t
Industrial chemicals, 1502–4
Infants, 1236f
   burns, 695
   car restraints, 633f
   caring for, 1236t
   chest compressions for, 1212, 1213f, 1275f, 1571–72, 1572f
   CPR, 1570–73, 1571–73f
   definition of, 1204, 1236
   foreign body airway obstructions, 395f, 396, 1256–57, 1258f
   immobilizing, 792, 792f
   mechanism of injury, 518
   pulse rates in, 512, 512t, 1571f
   rescue breathing, 1562
Infarcted cells, 1061
Infection control, 47–49, 58, 1395
Infections, 45
Infectious diseases, 45, 89–90, 854, 855–56t.
   virulence, 56
Inferior position or location, 119f, 121, 122
Inferior vena cava, 182, 885, 899

Infiltration, IV administration and, 314
Informed consent, 83
Ingestion, 1037–38, 1037f
Inguinal ligament, 145
Inguinal (lymph) nodes, 200
Inhalants, abused, 1044–45
Inhalation, 370
   for drug administration, 254, 256t, 336, 337f
   medications, 871–74, 872t, 1017
   poisons, 1037–38f, 1038–39
Inhalation burns, 698–99
Inhalers
   prescribed, 871–74
Inhibiting factors, 174
Initial assessments, 505, 505t.
   ABCs, 508–14
   assessment-based management, 1533–34
   behavioral emergencies, 1137–38
   breathing, 867–68
   children, 1243f, 1244
   general impressions, 505, 506f, 868
   older patients, 1348–49
   seizures, 1072
   strokes, 1069–70
Inotropic state, 185, 185t, 660, 891, 892t
Insect bites and stings, 1017–18, 1017–18f, 1023, 1023f
   allergic reactions to, 1007, 1008–10
Insecticides, 1502–4
Inspections
   AED, 923, 924f
   ambulance, 1383
Inspiration, 372, 851
Inspiratory reserve volume, 371
Insulin, 176, 345, 986, 987–88, 987f
Insulin shock, 990–92
Integumentary system, 130–33, 131f, 133f
Intercostal spaces, 143
Intermittent sites (INTs), 306
International terrorism, 1492
Internodal pathways, 889, 889f
Interpreters, 600
Interstitial fluid, 212, 287, 289, 289f
Interventions for illness, 534
Intervertebral disks, 766
Intracellular fluid (ICF), 212, 289
Intracellular fluid compartments, 289–90, 289f
Intracranial pressure, 1238
Intradermal medications, 256t
Intralingual medications, 256t
Intramuscular (IM) injections, 251, 255, 256t, 328f, 347–48f, 349
Intraosseous (IO) infusion, 255, 256t, 309–11, 351–52, 353f
   pediatric, 310–11f, 1278–79, 1280–81f
Intraosseous needles, 1278f
Intrapericardial pressure, 732
Intrathecal medications, 256t
Intravascular fluid, 212, 287, 289, 289f
Intravenous (IV) injections, 251, 255, 256t, 349–51, 350f, 1217
Intravenous (IV) solutions, 293–97, 297f, 318, 1107
Intravenous (IV) techniques, 296, 307–8f
   administration sets, 297–98, 297–98f
   assembling equipment, 296, 296t
   blood pressure level and, 1016
   catheter feed troubles, 296
   catheters, 301–2f, 301–3
   determining viability, 315f
   dimensional analysis, 312
   discontinuing the line, 306, 306f
   drip rates, 312–13
   drops per minute, 313
   external jugular, 311–12, 312f

geriatric considerations, 319
intraosseous lines, 309–11
local reactions, 313–14, 316
pediatric considerations, 318–19, 1276–77, 1277–78f
possible complications, 313–14, 316–17
saline locks, 306, 309
securing the line, 305–6, 305f
site choices, 298, 300–301, 300–301f
solution choices, 294, 297, 297f
spiking the bag, 299f
systemic complications, 313, 316–17
troubleshooting, 318
Intrinsicoid deflection, 930, 930f
Involuntary activities, 765
Involuntary muscles, 130, 160, 801
Involuntary nerves, 248f, 765
Iodine, 304
Ionic concentration, 294
Ionizing radiation, 1511
Ions, 286, 378, 892.
Irreversible shock, 663
Ischemia, 455, 660–61, 899
Ischemic cells, 1062
Ischemic strokes, 1062–63
Islets of Langerhans, 176, 177f, 987
Isoelectric line, 926
Isotonic solutions, 289, 293, 295f

J

J point, 931f
Jamshedi needle, 309, 1278
Jaundice, 513
Jaw, pain in, 138
Jaw-thrust maneuver, 386-87, 387t, 388f, 1247f, 1553-54, 1554f
   with head tilt, 387
   rescue breathing and, 1562f
   spinal injuries and, 769, 769f
Jellyfish, 1026–27, 1026t
Joint capsules, 156, 157f
Joints, 147f, 156, 157f, 158, 802, 802f.
   locked, fractures and, 807
   pain assessment, 528, 535
Jugular foramen, 136
Jugular notch, 141, 141f, 143
Jugular vein distention (JVD), 311, 542, 548
Jugular veins, 194, 542, 545f
Jump kits, 1381, 1381f, 1381t
Junctional rhythms, 944–45
JVD (jugular vein distention), 311, 542, 548

K

Kendrick splint, 819
Ketoacidosis, 377t
   alcoholic, 382
   diabetic, 988, 990–92, 1306, 1307t
Ketones, 382
Kidneys
   aging effects, 1345
   as buffer component, 379
   filtration by, 288
   injuries, 751–53
   renin-angiotensin system and, 212
   soft-tissue injuries and, 681, 682f
Kilograms, conversion from pounds, 330–31
Kinetic energy (KE), 621–22
Knees.
   anatomy, 150–51, 151f
   dislocation, 836–37
   fractures, 837
   ligament injuries, 836
   splinting, 837, 837f

Krebs cycle, 129
Kussmaul respirations, 377t, 988
KVO (keep vein open), 313
Kyphosis, 1346

L

Labia, 1151, 1152f, 1170, 1170f
Lacerations, 681, 682f
    scalp, 775, 775f
Lactated Ringer's (LR) solution, 293, 294
Lactic acidosis, 382
LAF (left anterior fascicle), 891, 891f
Language problems, 600
Lap (seat) belts, 519, 633
Large intestine, 209
Laryngeal mask airways (LMAs), 463–66, 464–66f, 467t, 468–69f
Laryngeal spasm and edema, 390–91
Laryngectomy, 471
Laryngoscope blades
    for newborns, 1216
    tongue and, 442–43, 443f
Laryngoscopy, direct, 438, 1257–58, 1258–59f
Laryngospasm, 438t, 1118
    croup and, 1286, 1288
    epiglottitis and, 1286, 1288
    esophageal airways and, 462
    extubation and, 453
Larynx, 201f, 202, 202f, 369–70
    anatomy, 138
    fractured, 391
Lasix, 269–70t
Lateral (vehicular) collisions, 623, 630–31, 631f
Lateral (body) location, 119f, 120, 121, 726
Lateral recumbent position, 123, 124f
LD$_{50}$, 1500
LEAN mnemonic, 255
Left (directional term), 119f, 122
Legal issues, 79, 80–81.
    immunity, 85–86
Legislative laws, 81
Legs, 150.
Length-based resuscitation tape, 1260t
Leukocytes, 179
Leukotrienes, 1006
Levels of consciousness, 782, 1104t, 1113.
    altered, in children, 1301–2
    consent and, 83
Lewisite (L), 1499, 1504t
Liability insurance, 86
Libel, definition of, 88
Licensure, 80
Lidocaine, 270–71t, 1282t
Lifting.
    body mechanics for, 1404–6, 1406–8f, 1408
    directions and commands, 1414–15
    guidelines, 1415–16
Ligaments, 152, 156, 802
    IV administration and damage to, 316
    knee injuries, 836
    skeleton and, 134
Lightening, 61–62, 1116–17
Limb presentation, 1189–90, 1190f
Limbic system, 164, 164f
Liquids, drug administration in, 251–52
Liver, 208
Lobes, of brain, 162
LOC. see Levels of consciousness
Locked joints, 807
Log roll, 1429, 1429f, 1431f
    four-person, 771, 772–73f
Lost person search, 1453

Lower airway, 202–4.
    pediatric diseases, 1288–91
Lower extremities
    anatomy of, 149–52, 149–52f
    arterial circulation system, 193, 193f, 194f
    rapid trauma assessment of, 520, 522f, 524
    venous circulation system, 195, 197f
LPF (left posterior fascicle), 891, 891f
Lumbar spine, 139, 140f, 840, 840f
Lumbar vertebrae, 142, 142f
Lumbosacral plexus, 168, 169–70
Lumen, 899, 899f
Lung compliance, 392
Lungs, 202–3.
    anatomy and function, 851–52f, 851–54
    child's, 1239–40
    gas exchange in, 205f, 851f
    hemothorax, 686, 688f, 723, 730–31, 731f
    open pneumothorax, 726–27
    pneumothorax, 686, 688f, 723
    pulmonary contusions, 731–32
    respiratory volumes and, 370–71
    simple pneumothorax, 725–26, 725f
    spontaneous pneumothorax, 725–26
    tension pneumothorax, 723, 727–29, 730f
Lymphatic system, 198, 199f, 200–201, 201f, 1507
Lymphocytes, 179, 180
Lysis, 127, 289

M

Macrodrip sets, 298, 319
Magill forceps, 397, 397f, 1257–58, 1258–59f
Male genitalia injuries, 754
Male reproductive system, 210, 211f, 751, 752f
Mammary glands, 1170, 1170f
Mandible, 136, 137, 542, 544f
Manubrium, 141, 547
Marijuana, 1046
Marine animals, injuries from, 1025–26, 1025f, 1026t
MARK 1, 1501–2
Masks, protective, 49–50, 51
Mass-casualty incidents, 502, 503f, 1472, 1473–77, 1473f, 1475t
MAST (military antishock trousers), 654, 818
Mastoid process, 134–35, 135f
Maxillae, 136, 542, 544f
MDI (metered-dose inhaler) medications, 252, 252f.
Mechanism of action, 244t, 246
Mechanism of injury (MOI).
    burns, 694
    documentation, 749
    electrical burns, 703
    insignificant, 526–29
    musculoskeletal, 804, 804f
    patient assessment, 499–500f, 499–501
    reconsideration, 518, 518t
    significant, 518, 520, 529
    trauma profiles, 623
    vehicular collisions, 625, 625t
Meconium, 1179–80, 1184, 1186, 1219
Meconium aspirators, 1219, 1220f
MED channels, 584
Medial (body) position or location, 120, 121, 121f
Median plane, 120
Mediastinum, 181, 884, 1240
Medical ambiguity, 559
Medical asepsis, 335
Medical control, 14.
    abnormal or complicated childbirth and, 1189

    communicating with, 588–91, 589f
Medical directors, EMS, 13–14, 78, 925
Medical equipment, 1377–82
Medical examiner cases, 28
Medical history. see History of illness
Medical identification insignia, 91
Medical patients.
    focused history and physical exam, 531–36
Medical Practices Act, 80
Medical terminology, 98
    abbreviations, 104, 105–10t
    prefixes, 99–100t
    root words, 101–2, 102–4t
    suffixes, 101, 101t
Medical waste disposal, 58–59
Medication administration, 328
    apothecary system, 331
    calculating doses, 331–33
    calculating infusion doses and rates, 333–34
    Celsius scale, 331
    converting pounds to kilograms, 330–31
    by EMT-I, 247, 247t
    enteral, 254, 255, 255t, 337–40
    Fahrenheit scale, 331
    inhalation, 336, 337f
    intramuscular, 328f, 347–48f, 349
    intraosseus, 351–52, 353f
    intravenous bolus, 349–51, 350–51f
    local medical direction on, 334–35
    metric system and, 328–29, 329t
    oral, 337–38, 337–38f
    parenteral, 256t, 340–41, 341–43f, 343
    pediatric, 334, 335
    principles, 335
    rectal, 338–40, 339f
    routes, 254–55
    safety, 338, 341
    steps in, 263–64
    subcutaneous, 343, 345–46f, 347
    sublingual, 352, 352f, 354f
    volume conversion, 329, 330
    weight conversion, 329–30
    weight-based doses, 333
Medications.
    allergic reactions, 1007
    for ambulance, 1380, 1380t
    classifications, 244t, 246
    documenting, 263–64
    drug interaction factors, 260–62
    drug profile components, 244t
    forms, 250–54
    mechanism of action, 244–45, 255–56
    names, 245–46
    neonatal resuscitation, 1208
    newborn resuscitation and, 1217–19, 1218t
    older patients, 1345, 1354–55, 1355f
    pharmacodynamics, 259, 260t
    pharmacokinetics, 257–58, 257t
    properties, 250, 349
    respiratory rates and, 375–76
    standardization, 246
    storage and security of, 262
    unpredictable adverse effects to, 261t
    volume to be administered, 332
Medicolegal considerations, 83–84, 1133, 1140–42
Medullary canal/cavity, 155, 1278
Melena, 651, 1359
Menarche, 1154, 1169
Meninges, 162f, 165, 762, 764
Meningitis, 56, 165, 764, 1303–4
Menopause, 1154, 1169
Menstrual cycle, 1169, 1169f, 1172
Menstruation, 1154, 1169

Mental capacity. *see* Competency
Mental conditioning, 562
Mental disorders, 1133–34
Mental status.
    assessment, 506f, 508–9
    in critically ill and injured patients, 31
    detailed physical exam of, 551
    rapid trauma assessment of, 520, 522f
Mentally incompetent adults, 84
Mesentery, definition of, 630
Metabolic acidosis, 380, 381–82, 988
Metabolic agents, 1502–4
Metabolic alkalosis, 380, 382–83
Metabolic seizures, 1065
Metabolism
    cellular, 128, 130, 131
    decreased perfusion and, 660–61
    pediatric *versus* adult, 1241
    respiratory rates and, 376
    water, electrolytes and, 287
Metered-dose inhalers (MDIs), 252, 252f, 336, 336f, 872f
    administration of, 262, 873–74, 873f
    for children, 1289–90, 1290f
Methamphetamines, 1045–46.
Metric system, 328–29, 329t
Microdrip sets, 298, 318
Midaxillary line, 121, 121f, 122
Midclavicular lines, 121, 121f
Midline, 119f, 120, 121
Military antishock trousers (MAST), 654, 818
Minors, consent and, 83
Minute volume, 371, 1285
Mitochondrion, 129
Mitral valve, 181, 548, 885
Mix-o-Vials, 343, 343f
Mobile radios, 581–82, 581f
MONA (medications for chest pain), 908
Motor nerves, 168, 524, 764, 809, 810–11f, 811–12
Motor vehicle crashes (MVCs), 623–26.
    ambulances, 1386, 1390
    with children, 1312–13, 1313f
    flail chest, 724–25
    frontal, 625–29
    lateral, 630–31, 631f
    mechanism of injury, 500–501, 500f
    motorcycle, 634
    pedestrians and, 635
    rear-end, 630, 630f
    rollover, 631–32, 632f
    rotational, 632–33
Motorcycle collisions, 634
Mouth
    bleeding from, 658
    digestion and, 208
    physical exam, 542, 544f, 546
Mouth-to-mask ventilation, 414–15
Mouth-to-mouth ventilation, 50, 414–15
Mouth-to-nose ventilation, 414–15
Mouth-to-stoma ventilation, 467, 470–71f
Moves, patient, 1438.
    directions and commands, 1414–15
    emergency, 1419–21, 1420–22f
    equipment, 1381–82, 1381f, 1430–38
    general considerations, 1419
    guidelines, 1415–16
    nonurgent, 1426–30
    safe reaching and pulling for, 1417–19, 1417–20f
    transfer, 1427–30, 1429–31f
    urgent, 1421–26, 1424–25f
Mucous membranes, 133, 678–79, 869t, 1499
Multilumen airways, 430–37, 431–36f, 436t
Multiple-casualty incidents (MCIs), 606, 1472.

Multiplex communication systems, 584, 585t
Murmur, heart, 184, 887
Muscles, 130, 130f, 134, 800–801
Musculocutaneous nerve, 169
Musculoskeletal injuries, 802–8.
    assessment, 808–9, 809–10f, 810–11
    emergency medical care, 812–24
    grading system, 812t
    mechanism of injury, 804, 804f
    transportation, 824
Musculoskeletal system, 158–60
    aging effects, 1346
    anatomy and physiology, 800–802
Mycobacterium tuberculosis, 56–57, 58
Myocardial contusion, 733, 736f
Myocardial infarction, 182, 506, 1358, 1359t
    acute, 899–900, 899f, 901–12
Myocardial injuries, 732–33, 732f, 733
Myocardium, 181, 884

N

NAAK, 1501–2
Naloxone hydrochloride, 272t, 1218–19, 1218t, 1282t
Narcotics, 1042–43, 1042t
Narrative reports, 602
Nasal cannulas, 412–13, 413f, 415, 1263
Nasal cavity, 135, 137, 201, 201f, 202
Nasal flaring, 511, 1247
Nasal septum, 137, 202
Nasogastric route, for drug administration, 255t
Nasogastric (NG) tubes, 423, 424–25, 425–27f, 425t, 1272–73, 1272t
Nasopharyngeal airways, 405, 405f, 406f, 407t, 1260–63, 1262f
Nasopharynx, 201, 368–69
National Highway Traffic Safety Administration (NHTSA), 10
National Incident Management System (NIMS), 1464
National Poison Control Center, 1036
National Registry of Emergency Medical Technicians (NREMT), 7, 8, 10–11
Nature of the illness (NOI), 501–2
Near drowning, 1117
Nebulizers, 336, 336f, 337f, 413, 1289, 1290f
Neck
    anatomy, 138, 139f, 190–91, 191f, 194, 195f
    physical exam, 542, 543, 544–45f, 546
    positions in supine position, 125f
    rapid trauma assessment, 520–21, 522f
    soft-tissue injuries, 690, 690f, 691f
Necrosis, 899
Needle decompression, tension pneumothorax, 727–29, 730f
Needles
    contaminated, 302
    disposal, 50, 246, 308f
    sizes and parts, 340, 340f
Negative feedback, 174
Neglect, child abuse and, 1324
Negligence
    determination of, 81–82
    presumptive, 79
Neisseria meningitidis, 1304
Nematocysts, 1026–27
Neonatal emergencies, 1204
    addicted mothers, 1221
    anticipating resuscitation, 1206–7
    diaphragmatic hernia, 1220
    fetal death, 1222
    fetal distress, 1205–6

    hypothermia, 1220
    meconium staining and aspiration, 1219–20
    newborn bradycardia, 1206
    pathophysiology, 1204–5
    premature births, 1221–22, 1221f
    risk factors, 1206–7, 1206t
    twins, 1220–21
Neonatal resuscitation
    advanced life support equipment, 1207–8
    advanced life support interventions, 1214–19
    Apgar scores, 1210, 1210t
    assessment, 1208, 1208t
    basic equipment, 1207, 1207t
    bradycardia, 1212
    cyanosis, 1213–14, 1214f
    depressed newborn, 1208–10, 1208–10f
    respiratory distress, 1211–12, 1211f
Neonates, 1204, 1236
Nerve agents, 1500–1502, 1501f, 1502t
Nerve fibers, 161
Nerve tissue, 130
Nerves, 161, 316, 374, 809
Nervous systems, 160–72.
    aging effects, 1345–46
    child's, 1241
Neural permeability, 378
Neural transmissions, 378
Neurogenic shock, 664, 1295
Neurologic emergencies, 1060.
Neurons, 130, 131, 131f
Neurotoxins, 1018, 1508
Neurotransmitters, 161, 161f, 172
Neutral position, 1268, 1320, 1322–23f
Neutron radiation, 1511
Neutrophils, 179–80, 180f
Newborns, 1204, 1236.
Newton's laws, 620–21, 622
Nitroglycerin (NTG), 244, 246, 251f, 272–73t, 912f
    administration of, 262, 352f, 908–11, 913
    erectile dysfunction medications and, 254
Nocturnal dyspnea, 861
Nondisplaced fractures, 804–5
Nonprogressive shock, 661–62
Nonrebreathing masks, 412, 412f, 1263, 1263f, 1264, 1320f
Nonsteroidal anti-inflammatory drugs (NSAIDs), 155
Norepinephrine, 172, 187, 249
    alpha and beta effects of, 661t, 892
    low blood volume and, 198
    production of, 177
Normal saline solution, 293, 294
Nose, 137.
    bleeding from, 653, 658
Nuchal rigidity, 1304
Nuclear/radiological terrorism, 1494, 1511, 1512f, 1513–14, 1513t
Nutrition, stress and, 36–39

O

Obstetric emergencies, 1168, 1189–91.
    prior to delivery, 1175–79
Obstetric kits, 1181, 1181f
Obstructive shock, 666, 666t
Obturators, 461
Occipital condyles, 135–36
Occipital lobe, 162, 163f
Occiput, 1238
Occlusion, 314, 315f, 899, 899f
Occlusive dressings, 687, 737
Occult injuries, 518

Occupational Safety and Health Administration (OSHA), 45–46, 51, 53
Off-gassing, 1500
Official drug names, 245
Olecranon process fracture, 829
Olfactory bulb, 135
Olfactory nerve, 171
Ongoing assessments, 553–55, 553f, 553t, 1252
Onset of illness, 532
Oocytes, 1151, 1168
Open injuries
 abdominal, 745–46, 745f
 chest, 686–87, 688f, 719–20, 719f
 fractures, 804, 807, 807f
 head, 782
 soft-tissue, 679, 681–85, 682–84f
Operations.
 air medical, 1395–97
 delivery phase, 1393, 1393f
 dispatch phase, 1384, 1384f
 en route to scene, 1384–91, 1385f, 1387–88f
 en route to station, 1394, 1394f
 postrun phase, 1394–95
 scene arrival, 1391–92, 1391f
 transfer phase, 1392–93, 1393f
 transport phase, 1393
Opiates (opioids), 1042–43, 1042t
OPQRST assessment, 868–70, 909t, 1349–50
OPQRST-I assessment, 532–34
Opsites, 305
Oral administration, of drugs, 255t, 337–38, 337–38f
Oral glucose, 253, 993–96, 994f
Organ collisions, 624, 629, 631
Organ(s), definition of, 118
Organ donors, 90–91
Organ systems, definition of, 118
Organic brain syndrome (OBS), 1134
Organisms, definition of, 118
Orientation tests, 509
Orogastric (OG) tubes, 423, 427–28, 428–30f, 430t
 for children, 1272–73, 1272t
 for newborns, 1214–16, 1215f
Oropharyngeal (oral) airways, 402–4, 402–5f, 1211, 1259–60, 1261f
Oropharynx
 in child with respiratory distress, 1288
 digestion and, 208, 369
Orotracheal intubation, 440–49, 441–47f, 449–50f, 449t, 451.
 end-tidal carbon dioxide detection, 448–49, 448f
 equipment preparation for, 440t
Orthostatic tilt test, 662
Osmolarity, 293, 294
Osmosis, 127, 257t, 288–89, 288f
Osmotic pressure, definition of, 127, 288
Osteocytes, 154, 154f
Osteomyelitis, 1279
Osteoporosis, 804, 1358
Ovaries, 178, 1151–52, 1152f, 1168
 abdominal pain and, 1089–90
 ruptured cysts, 1158
Overdoses, 1035t
Overhydration, 292
Over-the-counter (OTC) medications, 245
Over-the-needle catheters, 301, 301f, 302, 302t
Ovulation, 1168
Ovum, 1168
Oxidative phosphorylation, 129
Oxygen.
 administration of, 254, 262
 cellular metabolism and, 130
 chest injuries and, 722
 for children, 1263–64, 1263–64f
 decreased blood concentrations of, 373–74
 delivery devices, 412–13, 412–13f
 hazards of, 411
 IV solutions and, 295
Oxygen cylinders, 407–8, 407f, 408t, 1378, 1378f
 flowmeters, 409–10, 409f
 liquid, 408
 operating procedures, 410, 411f
 pin-indexing system, 408–9, 408f
 regulators, 409
 safety considerations, 408
Oxygen humidifiers, 413, 414f

P

P waves, 928, 928f
Pacemakers, 912–14, 913f
Paging, communications, 586
 WMD scenes, 1497
Pain.
 abdominal, 527–28, 535, 746
 in critically ill and injured patients, 30
 documentation, 535
 fractures and, 807
 in older patients, 1351, 1355
 quality of, 532, 533f
 responsiveness to, 509, 510f
 spinal injuries, 768
Palmar method, for burn estimates, 694
Palmar surface, 122
Palpation, 512, 1087–88, 1088f
Pancreas, 176–77, 177f, 208
Pancreatitis, 1086
Panic, drowning and, 1118f
Paper bag effect (syndrome), 629, 726
Papillary muscles, 181, 885
Para, definition of, 1153, 1172, 1181
Paradoxical motion, 521, 724
Paralysis, 718f, 768, 769f
Paramedic assistance
 abnormal or complicated childbirth and, 1189
Parasympathetic nervous system, 172, 248, 250
Parasympatholytics, 250
Parasympathomimetics, 250
Parathyroid glands, 176
Parathyroid hormone, 176
Parenteral medications, 254, 255, 256t, 340
 equipment, 340, 340f
 packaging, 340–41, 341–43f, 343
Parietal layer, 182, 885
Parietal lobe, 162, 163f
Parietal peritoneum, 1084
Parietal pleura, 203, 203f
Parking, ambulance, 1391–92, 1392f
Parkinson's disease, 1346
Parkland formula, 697
Paroxysmal nocturnal dyspnea, 861, 912
Partial agonists, definition of, 251
Partial airway obstruction, 391, 1254, 1254f, 1257–58
Partial pressure
 of carbon dioxide ($PaCO_2$), 206, 373, 375
 Dalton's law of, 373–74
 of oxygen (PaO_2), 206, 373, 375
Partial rebreathing masks, 413
Partial-thickness burns, 693–94, 693f
Patches, for drug administration, 253
Patellae, 150, 157f, 838, 838f.
Patency, 511
Pathogens, definition of, 45
Pathologic fractures, 805, 805f
Pathophysiology, definition of, 118
Patient(s).
 carrying, 1408–14, 1409–10f, 1409t
 communicating with, 507, 508f, 594–600, 595f
 critically ill or injured, 30–32
 dealing with grief, 29
 lifting and moving, 1404–43
 prehospital, 558–59
 quoting, for reports, 603
 uncooperative, 1532
Patient assessment, 495.
 ABCs approach to, 508
 airway, 509–11
 breathing, 511–12
 circulation, 512–14
 clinical decision making, 557
 determining reason for EMS call, 498–99
 external bleeding, 512–13
 identifying priority patients, 514–15, 515f
 initial assessment, 505
 mechanism of injury, 499–500f, 499–501
 medical or trauma, 506–8
 mental status, 506f, 508–9
 nature of the illness, 501–2
 pediatric, 1243f
 prehospital environment, 557–58, 558f
 scene size-up, 497, 497t
 triage, 502, 503f
Patient assessment flowchart, 494, 556
 detailed physical exam, 540
 initial assessment, 504
 medical, focused history and physical exam, 530
 ongoing assessment, 552
 scene size-up, 496
 trauma, focused history and physical exam, 516
Patient care person(s), 1530–31
Pedal edema, 542, 905
Pedestrians, vehicular collisions with, 635
Pediatric assessment triangle (PAT), 1244–45f, 1244–46
Pediatric patients. see Children; Infants
Peer diffusing, 36
Pelvic inflammatory disease (PID), 1089, 1157–58
Pelvis
 anatomy, 143, 145, 148–49, 149f
 circulation system, 193, 193f, 194–95
 fractures, 753, 753f, 831–34, 833f
 physical exam, 543, 545f, 549
 rapid trauma assessment, 520, 522f, 524
Penetrating trauma, 622–23
 abdominal, 745–46, 745f, 749, 749f
 chest, 719–20, 722
 great vessels, 733–34
 gunshots, 501, 501f, 683–84, 684f
 mechanism of injury, 500, 500f
 pathophysiology, 636–38, 636t, 637f
 soft-tissue, 681, 683–84, 683f
Per os (PO), 255t
Per rectum (PR), 255t
Percussion, 547–48
Percutaneous drug administration, 340
Perfusion, 197–98, 198f, 851–52, 853, 896
 cellular, 287
 compensation for decreased, 660–61
 end-organ, 1248
 patient assessment, 508
 physiology and, 646–48, 646f
 shock and, 659–60
Pericardial fluid, 182, 885

Pericardial sac, 181, 182f, 884, 885f
Pericardial tamponade, 732–33, 732f, 736t
Pericardiocentesis, 1298
Pericarditis, 187
Pericardium, 181, 732, 884
Perinatal period, 1236
Perineum, 1151, 1152f, 1170, 1170f, 1184f
Periorbital ecchymosis, 777, 779f
Peripheral cyanosis, 1214
Peripheral nerves, 130, 248f
Peripheral nervous systems (PNS), 161, 168–71, 762, 763f, 764–65
Peristalsis, 209, 1084
Peritoneal cavity, 744
Peritoneum, 1084
Peritonitis, 744, 1084–85, 1179
Persistency, of chemical agents, 1498
Personal protection, 44–45, 497–98, 498f
Personal protective equipment (PPE), 48–49, 50–51, 497, 497f, 1382.
Pertinent negatives, 602, 1535t
Petechiae, 542
pH, 206, 213, 214t
    arterial, 719
    chloride regulation of, 287
    definition of, 378
    drug absorption and, 257t
    respiratory rates and, 375
Phagocytosis, 127f, 128, 180
Phalanges, 148, 148f
Pharmacodynamics, 255, 259, 260t
Pharmacokinetics, 244t, 255, 257–58, 257t
Pharmacology, 244.
Pharyngeotracheal Lumen Airway (PtL), 430, 431–33f, 432–33, 436t, 467t.
Pharynx, 201, 201f, 368–69
Phlebitis, 314
Phosgene, 1500, 1504t
Phosgene oxime (CX), 1499, 1500, 1504t
Phospholipid bilayer, 286, 286f
Phosphorus, 287
Phrenic nerve, 169, 169f
Physical exam, 1529.
    detailed, 541–51
    gynecological emergencies, 1154
Physicians.
    emergency department, 15
    identification at scene, 1449, 1449f
Physiology, definition of, 118
Pia mater, 165, 165f
Piercing spikes, 297
    dual, 298f
"Piggyback" administration, 297f
Pin-indexing system, 408–9, 408f
Pit vipers, 1020–21, 1020f
Pitting edema, 542, 549
Pituitary gland, 174
Placenta abruptio, 1159, 1178, 1178f
Placenta previa, 1158–59, 1177–78, 1177f
Plague, 1507, 1509t
Planes, anatomic, 120–21, 120–21f
Plantar surface, 122
Plants
    allergic reactions to, 1007
    poisoning by, 1050, 1051–52f, 1053
    toxic, 1050t
Plasma, 178, 212
Platelets, 179f, 180, 180f
Platinum Ten Minutes, 517, 517f
Pleura, 203, 203f
Pleural cavity, 203
Pleural effusions, 863, 863f
Pleural friction rubs, 524, 547
Pleural space, 203
Pleurisy (pleuritic pain), 524, 721

Pleuritic chest pain, 862
Pneumatic antishock garments (PASGs), 653, 818
    applying, 654, 655f, 656
    pelvic fractures and, 833–34, 833f
    shock and, 668
Pneumonia, 855t, 863, 1290–91
Pneumonic plague, 1507
Pneumothorax, 373, 686, 688f, 723, 862f
    definition of, 862, 1123
    open, 726–27, 736t
    simple, 725–26, 725f, 735t
    spontaneous, 725–26, 862
    tension, 723, 727–29, 730f, 736t
Pocket masks, 50, 51, 414–15
Point of maximal impulse (PMI), 548
Point tenderness
    fractures and, 806, 806f
Points of distribution (PODs), 1505, 1507
Poisonings, 1034–35
    in children, 1048–49, 1049t, 1302–3, 1302f, 1302t
    documentation, 1040
    emergency medical care, 1040–41
    food, 1049–50, 1050t
    plants, 1050, 1051–52f, 1053
    substance abuse and, 1035–37
Poisons.
    absorbed, 1037f, 1039–40
    geography-specific, 1041
    ingested, 1037–38, 1037f
    inhaled, 1037–38f, 1038–39
    injected, 1037f, 1039, 1039f
    routes of administration, 1037, 1037f
Polarized state, 892
Polymorphic rhythms, 948
Polyphagia, 988
Polypharmacy, 262, 1354
Polyuria, 292, 988
Pons, 164, 164f, 165
Poor air exchange, 391
Popliteal arteries, 193, 194f
Popliteal veins, 195, 197f
Portable radios, 581–82, 582f
Portable stretchers, 1435, 1435f
Portal venous system, 1217
Portuguese man-of war, 1026–27, 1026t
Position of function, 831
Positive feedback, 174
Posterior plane, 120
Posterior position or location, 121
Posterior tibial arteries, 193, 194f
Postganglionic neurons, 172
Postictal state, 1064, 1066, 1069, 1072, 1072f, 1299, 1300f
Postsynaptic terminals, 161
Posttraumatic stress disorder (PTSD), 35
Postural hypotension, 292
Posturing, 782, 1301, 1302f
Potential energy, 622
Potentiation, as drug response, 261t
Pounds, conversion to kilograms, 330–31
Power grips, 1408, 1408f
Power lifts, 1406, 1407f
Power lines, 61
P-P interval, 933, 933f
P-R interval, 929, 929f
P-R segment, 929, 929f
Preeclampsia, 1176
Prefilled syringes, 340, 343, 343f
Prefixes, medical, 99–100t
Pregnancy.
    anatomic structures during, 1172f
    consent issues for teens, 1154
    drug therapy and, 247

    ectopic, 1089–90, 1175–76
    normal maternal changes, 1173–75
    stages of labor, 1179–80
    supine hypotensive syndrome, 755, 1177
    trimesters, 1173, 1173f
Prehospital care reports (PCRs), 600–601, 602t
Preload, of heart, 188, 906
Premature complexes, 951, 951f
Premature newborns, 1221–22, 1221f
Premature rupture of membranes, 1172
Preschool-age children, 1237, 1237f
Prescription medications, 245
Presentation, 1189
Pressure dressings, 651, 652f
Pressure points, 652, 653f
Pressure sores, 1343f
Pressure, thinking under, 561–62
Pressure-compensated flowmeters, 409, 409f
Presumptive negligence, 79
Primary apnea, 1211
Primary injury prevention, 59
Primary service areas (PSAs), 13
Professionalism
    caring for children, 1236t
    communicating with patients, 31–33
    EMT-I, 18–19
    radio communications, 588–89
    standards of care and, 79–80
Progesterone, 178, 1169
Prolapsed umbilical cord, 1189, 1190–91, 1190f
Pronator drift, 549–50
Prone position, 123, 124f
Prostaglandins, 173
Prostate gland, 210, 211f
Protection levels, 1471, 1471f
Protocols, 78, 559
Provoking/palliating factors of illness, 532
Proximal position or location, 119f, 121
Proximate cause, 54, 81–82
Psychiatric medications, 1044, 1044t
Psychogenic factors, 1137
Pubic symphysis, 143, 145, 833, 833f
Public safety agencies, 16
Pulling, safety guidelines, 1417–19, 1417–20f
Pulmonary agents, 1499–1500
Pulmonary artery, 142
Pulmonary circulation, 183f, 189, 192f, 898
Pulmonary contusion, 731–32, 736t
Pulmonary edema, 373, 906
    acute, 854, 856–58, 857f
Pulmonary function tests, 204
Pulmonary thromboembolism, 864–65, 865f
Pulmonary veins, 182
Pulmonic valves, 181, 548, 883
Pulse oximetry, 372, 373, 447, 548
    carbon monoxide and, 1045
    children and, 1251, 1252f
    preoxygenation for intubation and, 441
Pulse pressure, 661–62
Pulse rates
    average, by age, 525t
    normal infants and children, 512t
Pulseless electrical activity (PEA), 970–71, 972t, 1298
Pulseless ventricular tachycardia (V-tach), 971, 972t, 1298–99
Pulses, 196–98, 197f.
    apical, 1212, 1212f, 1249
    assessment of, 512
    carotid, 1564f
    central, 1248
    fractures and, 806f
    musculoskeletal injuries and, 809, 810–11f, 811–12

Pupil size, 527t, 783
    changes in children, 1301, 1302f
    head injury and, 782, 782f
Purkinje system, 891, 892f
Pursed-lip breathing, 874
Putrefaction, 28
P-wave axis, 953

Q

Q waves, 930, 930f
QRS complex, 928f, 929–30, 930f
Q-T interval, 931–32, 932f
Quadrants, abdominal, 123, 123f, 144, 144f, 745, 745f
Quality control, 14

R

R' waves, 928, 928f
Rabies, 1024
Raccoon eyes, 546, 777, 779f.
Radial arteries, 196
Radial head fracture, 829
Radial nerves, 169, 169f
Radiating pain or discomfort, 532–33, 533f
Radiation, definition of, 1103
Radiation exposure, 705–6, 706t, 707
Radiation sickness, 1513t
Radio communications, 586–88f, 586–93, 592t
Radioactive material, 1507
Radiological dispersal devices (RDDs), 1511, 1513
Radiological/nuclear terrorism. see Nuclear/radiological terrorism
Radios
    base station, 580–81, 581f
    maintenance, 591–93
    mobile and portable, 581–82, 581–82f
    repeaters for, 582, 582f
Radius, 125, 146, 829
Rales (breath sounds), 521, 547, 859, 1279
Range of motion (ROM), 123–24, 125f
Rape. see Sexual assault
Rapid extrication technique, 1421–26, 1421t, 1424–25f
Rapid medical assessment, 537, 538–39f
Rapid trauma assessment, 520–21, 522–23f, 523–26, 525t, 526t
Rapport, 594
Rattlesnakes, 1019, 1019f, 1020–21, 1020f
Raynaud's syndrome, 549
Reaching, safety guidelines, 1417–19, 1417–20f
Reactive airway disease (RAD), 1289–90
Rear-end (vehicular) collisions, 623, 630, 630f
Receptors, 172
Reciprocity, 8
Record keeping, 88–89.
Recovery position, 123, 383, 383f, 1300f, 1564, 1564h
Rectal administration, of drugs, 338–40, 339f
Rectum, 209
Red blood cells, 178, 179, 179f, 180f
Red Blood Gives Life (mnemonic), 304
Reduction, of dislocation, 807
Referred pain or discomfort, 533, 1084
Reflexes
    diving, 1122
    flexor, 166
    gag, 377, 402
    Hering-Breuer, 372
    spinal reflex arcs and, 166, 167f
Refusal of care, 85, 87, 604, 605f
Regional anatomy, 119

Rehabilitation areas, 1475
Relative hypovolemia, 1294
Relaxation, stress and, 39
Religion, respect for, 34
Renal pelvis, 209
Renal system. see Kidneys
Repeaters, base station, 582, 582f, 584
Repolarization, 893, 894f, 931f
Reporting requirements, 89–90, 591.
Reproduction, 175, 178.
Residual volume, 204, 371
Respiration, 851
    cellular, 128–29, 129f, 130
    definition of, 1103
    as gas exchange, 372–73, 852f
    pattern changes, 377t
    ventilation versus, 853
Respirators, 49–50, 51
Respiratory acidosis, 380–81, 719
Respiratory alkalosis, 380, 381
Respiratory arrest, 1285–86
Respiratory bronchioles, 202
Respiratory center, 205
Respiratory distress, 1285, 1286f
Respiratory emergencies, 850–51.
    acute pulmonary edema, 854, 856–57, 857f
    airway obstructions, 858–62, 859–60f, 863–64, 864f
    emergency care, 866–71
    focused history and physical exam, 868–70
    general impression, 868
    hyperventilation syndrome, 865–66
    infections, 854, 855–56t
    management, 870–71
    medications, 273–77t
    pediatric, 874, 1285–86, 1286f
    pleural effusions, 863, 863f
    pneumonia, 863
    positioning, 872
    prescribed inhalers, 871–74
    pulmonary thromboembolism, 864–65, 865f
    reassessment, 874
    signs and symptoms, 868, 869t
    spontaneous pneumothorax, 862, 862f
Respiratory failure, 1285
Respiratory rates, 374–76
    breathing difficulty and, 869t
    normal, 376t, 525t
Respiratory syncytial virus (RSV), 1290
Respiratory system, 201–3f, 205–7f
    aging effects, 1344, 1345f
    anatomy and function, 851–54
    as buffer component, 379
    in children, 207, 207f, 1240
    chronic obstructive pulmonary disease, 206
    detailed physical exam, 543, 548
    lower airway, 202–4
    physiology, 204–5, 205–6f, 207
    upper airway, 201–2
Responsiveness, evaluation of, 509, 531, 531t
Restraints
    behavioral emergencies, 1141–42, 1141–42f
    forcible, 84
    vehicle safety, 633–34, 633f
Resuscitation.
    termination of, 915–16
Retractions, chest, 521, 1245, 1245f, 1247
Retroperitoneal organs, 144, 145, 1088
Retroperitoneal space, 832
Retroperitoneum, 176
Return of spontaneous circulation (ROSC), 915
Reverse triage, 1117
Rhonchi (breath sounds), 521, 523, 547, 859

Ribs, 141, 141f, 143, 717f
    detailed physical exam, 542, 545f
    fractures, 723–24, 735t
Ricin, 1508, 1509f
Right (directional term), 119f, 122
Rights of medication administration, six, 335
Rigor mortis, 27–28, 1307–8
Rollover (vehicular) collisions, 623, 631–32, 632f
Root words, medical, 101–2, 102–4t
Rotation, 125–26
Rotational (vehicular) collisions, 623, 632–33
Route of exposure, 1498
R-R interval, 932–33, 933f
Rule of nines, 694, 694f
Rule of palms, 694

S

S' waves, 928, 928f
Sacrum, 139, 140f, 143, 143f
Saddle joints, 147f, 148
Safety.
    AED shock, 918, 923
    ambulance crashes, 1385
    behavioral emergencies, 1134, 1135t
    bleeding patients and, 647, 647f
    BLS treatment, 1546
    clandestine drug laboratories, 1484
    cold exposure, 1110
    compressed gas cylinders, 408
    coughs and, 207
    electrical burns and, 703–4
    head, spine injuries and, 783
    heat exposure, 1111
    IV solutions, 293, 293f
    lifting and moving patients, 1406
    medication administration, 338, 341
    nuclear/radiological terrorism, 1513–14
    seizures and, 1065
    stress and, 36
    water rescue, 1119, 1120f, 1122f
    WMD scenes, 1496, 1496–97f, 1498
Safety and operations equipment, 1382.
Sager splint, 819, 822–23f, 822–24
Sagittal plane, 120, 120f
Sagittal suture, 134
Saline locks, 306, 309, 309f, 351
Saline solutions, normal, 293, 294
Salivary glands, 208
SAM splints, 830f
SAMPLE history
    description, 525–26
    focused assessment and, 528
    gynecologic emergencies, 1153
    for medical patients, 534–35
    rapid trauma assessment and, 520, 522f
    for unresponsive patients, 537–38
Saphenous veins, 195, 197f
Sarin (GB), 1500–1501, 1503, 1503f, 1504t
SARS (severe acute respiratory syndrome), 57, 856t
Scalp, 132
    lacerations, 775, 775f
Scanners, 584
Scapulae, 141, 141f, 145, 145f, 146f
    injuries, 825–26, 825–26f
Scene safety
    assessment, 497–98, 498f
    fires, 62
    hazardous materials, 60–61, 1467
    lightening, 61–62
    making unsafe scene safe, 498
    personal protection and, 44–45
    physical dangers, 1454
    power lines, 61

vehicular collisions, 1451
visibility, 44–45
WMD scenes, 1496, 1496f
Scene size-up, 497, 497t.
    arrival, 1391–92, 1391f
    extrication, 1447–48, 1447–48f
    older patients, 1348
    pediatric emergency, 1242, 1243f
    respiratory emergencies, 867–68
School-age children, 1237, 1237f
Sciatic nerves, 170, 170f, 834
Sclera, 513, 542, 544f
Sclerosis, 301
Scoop stretchers, 1429–30, 1430f, 1437, 1437f
Scope of practice, 78
Scorpion stings, 1022–23, 1022f
Scuba gear, 1122, 1122f
Sea anemones, 1026–27, 1026t
Seatbelts
    abdominal injuries and, 748–49, 748f
    vehicular collisions and, 518–19, 519f, 626–27
Sebaceous glands, 132
Secondary apnea, 1211
Secondary devices, 1497
Secondary injury prevention, 59
Second-degree burns, 693–94, 693f
Sector commander, 1463
Sedative-hypnotic drugs, 1043, 1043t
Sedatives, 1041
Seizures, 1064
    assessment, 1072–73, 1072f
    causes, 1064–65, 1064t, 1299t
    in children, 1299–1301, 1300f
    description of, 1060
    diabetic, 997–98
    eclampsia, 1176
    emergency medical care, 1075–76
    older patients and, 1073
    patterns of, 1066
    postictal state, 1066
Selective permeability, 126, 126f, 286
Sellick maneuver, 369, 422–23, 423t, 444, 444f
Semi-Fowler's position, 123, 124f, 376, 511, 1182
Sensitization, 664
Sensory nerves, 168, 248f, 524, 764
    musculoskeletal injuries and, 809, 810–11f, 811–12
Separation anxiety, 1242, 1284
Sepsis, 548, 1294–95.
Septic shock, 664, 1294–95
Septum, 1262
Serous pericardium, 181, 884–85
Serum osmolality, 128
Severe acute respiratory syndrome (SARS), 57, 856t
Severity of illness, 533–34
Severity of injury, 812
Sexual abuse, 1324–25
Sexual assault, 1159–60
Sexual harassment, 42–43
Sexually transmitted diseases, 1154
Shaken baby syndrome, 1324
Sharps disposal, 50, 246, 308f
Shock.
    in children, 1291–96
    definition, 646, 647
    differential diagnosis of, 666, 666t
    etiologies, 663–65, 665f, 1294–96
    facial skin color and head elevation, 669
    hemorrhage and, 649
    indicators, 662
    management, 666, 667f, 668–69, 1292–94, 1293f

    pathophysiology, 659–60
    pharmacologic interventions, 668–69
    stages, 661–63, 662t, 664, 1292
Shock position, 123
Shoulder, 146, 826–27, 826–27f.
Shoulder (seat) belts, 519
Shoulder restraints, 633
Side effects, of drugs, 244t, 245, 259
Sign language, 598, 599f
Simple access, 1450, 1450f
Simplex communication systems, 584, 585t
Sinoatrial (SA) node, 184, 185f, 888–89f, 889
Sinuses, 137, 138
Sitting patients, immobilizing spinal-injured, 773–74, 776–77f
Situational awareness, 562–63
Six R's of clinical decision making, 563–64
Skeletal muscle, 130, 130f, 158–59, 159f, 800–801, 800–801f
Skeletal system, 766–67
Skeleton, 133–34, 134f, 801–2, 802f.
Skilled care facilities, 1356
Skin
    anatomy, 132–33, 133f, 678–79, 679f
    assessment, 513, 513f, 526t
    child's, 1240
    contact hazards, 1498
    functions, 130–32, 679
    hypothermia and, 1106
    in older people, 1343
    shock and color of, 669
Skin protection, 65
Skull, 134–37f, 134–38, 766, 766f
    base, 135–36, 136f
    floor, 135, 135f
    fractures, 658, 777, 779f
    hyoid bone, 137
    mandible, 137
    nose, 137
    orbits, 136
    temporomandibular joint, 137
Slander, definition of, 88
Slings, 825–26, 826f, 830f
SLUDGEM assessment, 1501, 1502t
Small intestine, 209
Smallpox, 1505, 1506t
Smell
    aging effects, 1344
    chemical agent identification, 1503–4
Smoke, inhalation burns and, 698–99
Smooth muscle, 130, 130f, 159f, 160, 800, 800f, 801, 801f
Snake bites, 1018–22, 1019–20f
Sniffing position, 376, 441–42, 442f, 1246
SOAP format, 606t, 1535
Sodium, 287, 293
Sodium/potassium (Na$^+$/K$^+$) pump, 287, 892, 894f
Soft-tissue injuries, 678.
    abdominal, 688, 688f
    amputations, 690, 690f
    chest, 686–87, 687f, 688f
    closed, 680–81, 680f
    controlling bleeding from, 686f
    impaled objects, 689–90, 689f
    neck, 690, 690f
    open, 681–85, 682–84f
    radiation exposure, 705–7, 706t
    types, 679
Solid organs, abdominal, 744, 745f, 1088f
Solids, drug administration in, 250–51
Solutes, 126, 292
Solutions, 251, 292
Solvents, 292
Soman (GD), 1500–1501, 1504t

Somatic nervous system, 765
Spalding effect, 731
Special Atomic Demolition Munitions (SADM), 1513
Sperm, 1171
Sphincters, capillary, 661
Spider bites, 1017–18, 1017–18f
Spinal column, 140f, 143, 766–67, 766f
Spinal cord, 165f, 166, 166f, 762, 1061f.
    injuries, 718f, 765
    nerve tracts, 167f
Spinal immobilization, 520–21, 522f.
Spinal nerves, 165f, 168, 168f, 248f
Spinal shock, 664–65, 665f
Spine
    anatomy, 139–41, 139f, 140f
    fractures, 840, 840f
    immobilization devices, 784–85, 785–86f, 787–88
    injuries, 762, 767–77, 768–70f
    recognizing injury to, 625t
    submersion incident injuries, 1120, 1121f
    transport with injured, 771, 772–73f, 773–74
Spleen, 143f, 200
Splinting, 814f
    documentation, 814
    feet, 840, 840f
    general principles, 814
    hand and wrist, 832f
    hazards of improper, 824
    in-line traction, 814–15, 815f
    knees, 837, 837f
    musculoskeletal injuries, 813–24
    supplies, 1379f, 1379t
Splints, 813–14
    bleeding control using, 653–54, 653f
    formable, 816–18, 817–19f
    padded board, 830f
    rigid, 815, 816f
    for soft-tissue injuries, 681, 685, 686f
    traction, 819–24, 820–23f
Spontaneous pneumothorax, 725–26, 862
Sprains, 152, 153t, 803, 807–8, 808f, 829
ST segment, 930–31
Stab wounds, 501
Stair chair, wheeled, 1413, 1413f, 1415–16, 1416f, 1431f, 1437–38, 1438f
Stairs, carrying patient on, 1411–12, 1412f
Standards of care, 78–81
Standing orders, 78, 559, 592
Standing patients, immobilizing spinal-injured, 774, 778f
Starling's Law of the Heart, 187, 896
Status asthmaticus, 860, 1290
Status epilepticus (seizures), 1064, 1299
Stenosis, tracheal stoma, 472
Sterile dressings, 707, 707f
Sterilization, 1395
Sternal fracture, 725, 735t
Sternal rub, contraindications, 509
Sternocleidomastoid muscles, 138, 139f
Sternum, 138, 141, 141f, 142, 143, 145f
Steroid hormones, 173f, 871
Stimulants, 1045–46, 1046t
Stoma, tracheal, 466–67
    suctioning, 471–72, 473f
    ventilation by BVM to, 471, 471f, 1561–62, 1562f
    ventilation by mouth to, 467, 470–71f
Stomach, 208
STOP (mnemonic), 1550
Strains, 152, 153t, 803
Strangulated hernias, 1091
Stress, 33–34

critical incident debriefing, 40–41
  management, 37–40, 38t
  nutrition and, 36–37, 38–39
  warning signs, 34–36, 38t
Stridor, 523, 547, 856t, 869t, 1011, 1247t
Stroke volume, 187, 895
Strokes, 506, 1060, 1061–62
  assessment, 1069–72, 1070f
  emergency medical care, 1074–75
  hemorrhagic, 1062
  ischemic, 1062–63
  management, 967, 969, 969t
  older patients and, 1073
  signs and symptoms, 1068–69
  transient ischemic attacks, 1063–64
Structure fires, 1454
Subarachnoid hemorrhage, 166
Subcutaneous emphysema, 520–21, 723, 862
Subcutaneous (SC) injections, 251, 255, 256t, 343, 345–46f, 347
Subcutaneous tissue, 133, 133f, 679f
Subdural bleeding, 779–80, 780f, 1069, 1069f
Sublingual (SL) medications, 251, 255t, 352, 352f, 354f
Submersion injuries, children, 1318
Substance abuse, 43–44, 1035, 1035t, 1041.
Sucking chest wounds, 686, 687f, 727, 727f
Suction catheters, 398, 400f, 1210f, 1259f
Suctioning, 397–98
  in children, 1258–59
  equipment for, 398, 399f, 399t, 1378
  neonatal resuscitation, 1209
  stoma, 471–72, 473f
  techniques, 398, 400–401, 401f
  time limits, 402
  tracheobronchial, 451
Sudden infant death syndrome (SIDS), 1307–9
Suffixes, medical, 101, 101t
Suicides, 1138–39, 1138t
Sulfur mustard (agent H), 1498–99, 1499f, 1504t
Superficial (directional term), 122
Superficial burns, 693–94, 693f
Superior (body) position or location, 119f, 120–21, 122
Superior vena cava, 182, 885, 899
Supination (movement), 125
Supine hypotensive syndrome, 755, 1177
Supine position, 123, 124f, 125f
Suppositories, 251
Supraglottic inhalation injury, 698
Supraventricular rhythms, 940–44, 940–44f
Supraventricular tachycardia (SVT), 970t, 1296
Surfactant, 370, 1173
Suspensions, 252
Sutures, in skull, 134, 134f
Swathe, 846
Sweat glands, 132, 133f
Swelling, fractures and, 806, 806f
Sympathetic nervous system (SNS), 562
Sympathetic pathway, 171, 247–48, 660
Sympatholytics, 249
Sympathomimetics, 249, 1045–46, 1046t
Synapses, 161
Synchronized cardioversion, 967, 1283, 1296
Syncopal episodes, 317, 506, 1073
Syncope, 913, 1073, 1358, 1359t
  breath-holding, 1124–25
  hemorrhage and, 651
Syndromic surveillance, 1509
Synergism, as drug response, 261t
Synovial fluid, 152
Syringes, 340, 340f, 341f
  prefilled, 340, 343, 343f

Systemic circulation, 189, 189f, 898
Systemic complications, IV administration and, 313, 316–17
Systole, 187, 895

T

T waves, 931, 931f, 932f
Tabun (GA), 1501, 1504t
Tachycardias, 292, 862, 902, 903f, 969–70, 970t
Tachypnea, 292, 721, 862, 866t, 1245, 1246, 1247
Tactical situations, 1453–54
Tactile stimulation, 1210
Tamponade. *see* Cardiac tamponade; Pericardial tamponade
T-bone (vehicular) collisions, 623
Technical rescue groups, 1451–53
Technical rescue situations, 1451–53
Teens, 1154, 1154f, 1237–38, 1238f.
Telemetry, 582–83
Temperature. *see* Body temperature
Temporal lobe, 162, 163f
Temporomandibular joint (TMJ), 137
Tendons, 134, 152, 156, 316, 801
Tension pneumothorax, 546, 723, 727–29, 730f, 736t, 1298
Tenting, 1251, 1305f
Teratogens/teratogenic drugs, 247, 1172
Term, in pregnancy, 1173
Terrorism, 1492–93
  biological agents, 1504–9, 1506–9f, 1506–10t, 1511
  chemical agents, 1498–1504, 1504f
  EMT-I response to, 1494–97
  nuclear/radiological devices, 1511, 1512f, 1513–14, 1513t
  WMDs and, 1493–94
Tertiary injury prevention, 59
Testes, 178
Testicles, 210
Therapeutic effect, 259
Thermogenesis, 1102
Thermolysis, 1111
Third spacing, 294
Third-degree burns, 693–94, 693f
Thoracic aorta, 192
Thoracic cage, 141, 142f
Thoracic duct, 198
Thoracic injuries, 716.
  diaphragmatic, 734
  esophageal, 734
  flail chest, 724–25, 724f, 725f
  hemothorax, 686, 688f, 723, 730–31, 731f
  management, 722–23, 735–37t
  myocardial, 732–33, 732f
  pathophysiology, 720–22
  pulmonary contusion, 731–32
  rib fractures, 723–24
  sternal fracture, 725
  tracheobronchial, 734
  traumatic asphyxia, 734–35
  vascular, 733–34
Thoracic spine, 139, 140f
Thorax.
  anatomy, 141–42f, 141–43, 181f, 716–17f, 716–18
  physiology, 718–19
  venous circulation, 194
Thromboembolism, 1298
Thrombus, 1062
Thyroid cartilage, 138, 139f
Thyroid gland, 175, 176f
Thyroid-stimulating hormone (TSH), 175

Tibia, 150, 838–39, 838f
Tibial arteries, 193, 194f
Tibial nerves, 169, 170
Tibial veins, 195, 197f
Tick bites, 1023, 1023f
Tidal volume, 204, 371, 1263
Tiered response systems, 587
Tissues, definition of, 118
TMJ syndrome, 138
Toddlers, 1236–37, 1237f.
Toes, burns of, 695
Tolerance, drug, 261t, 1041
Tongue
  airway obstruction, 389–90, 864f, 1553f
  head tilt–chin maneuver and, 385, 385f, 386f
  laryngoscope blade and, 442–43, 443f
Tongue–jaw lift maneuver, 388, 390f, 1254, 1255f
Tonic phase, of seizures, 1064
Tonic-clonic seizures, 1300
Tonicity, 288–89, 288f
Tonsil tips, 398, 400t
Tonsils, 200–201, 201f
Topical medications, 252
Topographic anatomy, 119
Torso, 123, 143
Tourniquets, 656, 657f, 658
Toxicity levels, 1470
Toxins, 1018, 1040, 1298.
Tp waves, 928–29, 929f
Trachea, 138, 139f, 201f, 202, 203f
Tracheobronchial injuries, 734, 737t
Tracheobronchial suctioning, 451
Tracheostomy, 466–67
Tracheostomy tubes, 466–67, 467f, 474f
Track marks, 301
Traction, in-line, 814–15, 815f
Traction splints, 819
  Hare, 819–22, 820–21f
  Sager, 822–23f, 822–24
Trade names, for drugs, 245
Traffic control, 1392
Tragus, 1261
Transcutaneous medications, 252–53, 253f, 256t
Transcutaneous pacing (TCP), 967, 968f
Transdermal medications, 252–53
Transfers, patient, 1392–93, 1393f
  assessment-based management, 1534–35, 1535f, 1535t
  equipment, 1381–82, 1381f
Transient ischemic attacks (TIAs), 1063–64, 1073
Transition phase, 1250
Transmission, disease, 45
Transport, 1393
  of children, 1250
  interfacility, 16
  musculoskeletal injuries, 824
  patient assessment and, 526, 528, 536, 555
  specialty centers, 15–16
  spinal-injured sitting patients, 773–74, 776–77f
  spinal-injured standing patients, 774, 778f
  spinal-injured supine patients, 771, 772–73f, 773
  stroke patients, 1072, 1072f
  of unresponsive patients, 538
Transportation area, 1475
Transportation officer, 1475
Transverse plane, 120, 120f, 121, 121f
Trauma.
  blast injuries, 638
  blunt, 622–33

energy and, 620–22
falls, 635–36, 635f
focused assessment, 526–29
gynecologic emergencies, 1159
history and physical exam, 517–20
kinematics, 618
mechanism of injury profiles and, 623, 625t
older patients, 1351
patients with no significant MOI, 526–29
patients with significant MOI, 520, 529
pediatric, 1234, 1310–25
penetrating, 622–23, 636–38, 636t, 637f
rapid assessment, 520–21, 522–23f, 523–26, 525t, 526t
recognizing developing problems, 625t
transport considerations, 619–20
Trauma centers, 619, 619t
Treatment area, 1468
Treatment officer, 1475
Treatment, refusal of, 85, 87, 604, 605f
Trendelenburg's position, 123, 124f
Trending, definition of, 525
Triage
 incident command, 1475–76
 mass-casualty incidents, 502, 503f, 1473–75, 1473f, 1475f
 priorities, 1474–75, 1474t
 procedures, 1476–77
 reverse, 1117
 special situations, 1476
Triage area, 1475
Triage officer, 1475
Tricuspid valve, 182, 548, 885
Trimesters, 1173, 1173f
Tripod position, 1285
True vocal cords, 202, 202f
Trunking, 581
Tubal pregnancy, 1175–76
Tuberculosis, 56–57, 524, 855
Tubules, 288
Turgor, 546–47, 1305f
Turnout gear, 63–64, 63f
Twins, 1220–21
Two- to three-word dyspnea, 510–11, 861, 869t
Type I diabetes, 986–87
Type II diabetes, 987

U

U wave, 932, 932f
UHF (ultra high frequency), 581
Ulcers, 1088
Ulna, 146, 829.
Ulnar nerves, 169, 169f
Umbilical cord, 1172
 around neck, 1186
 prolapsed, 1189, 1190–91, 1190f
Umbilical medications, 256t
Umbilical vein catheterization, 1207
Uncertain situations, response to, 34
Unconscious or unresponsive patients, 509.
 airway assessment, 391–92, 392f
 altered mental status and, 1066, 1066f
 diabetic, 992–93
 evaluation, 536–39, 536f, 538–39f
 foreign body airway obstructions, 392, 393–95f, 1254–56, 1255–57f, 1554–55
 positioning for airway assessment, 384–85, 384f
 rapid trauma assessment, 529
Unidentified complaints, assessment of, 529
Unilateral body structures, 122–23, 726

Universal precautions, 46, 46t
Upper extremities, 146, 148f
 circulation, 191, 194, 195f
 rapid trauma assessment of, 520, 522f, 524
Ureters, 145f, 209–10, 211f
Urethra, 210, 1151, 1152f, 1170f
Urinary bladder, 145f, 209–10, 753–54
Urinary system, 209–10, 210f, 746, 746f, 1088–89
Urticaria, 548, 1006, 1006f
Uterine rupture, 1179
Uterus, 1089–90, 1151, 1152f, 1169, 1191

V

V agent (VX), 1501, 1501f, 1504t
Vacuum mattresses, 1358, 1358f
Vacuum splints, 818, 819f
Vagina, 211f, 212, 1151, 1152f, 1170
Vapor hazards, 1498
Varicose veins, IV administration and, 319, 319f
Vascular injuries, 733–34
Vasoconstriction, 1345
Vasodilation, 1359t
Vasogenic shock, 664
Vasovagal reactions, 317
Vector-borne disease transmission, 45, 46t
Vehicle assessment, 499–500f, 623
Vehicle restraints, 633–34, 633f
Vehicle-borne disease transmission, 45, 46t
Veins, 188, 194–95, 625t, 896, 899
 bleeding from, 649, 650f
 IV administration and, 314, 316
Ventilation, 204, 372–73, 718–19, 851.
 assisted and artificial, 414
 automatic transport ventilators, 422, 422t
 barrier devices and, 1560–61, 1560–61f
 BVM to stoma, 471, 471f
 for children, 419, 1264–66
 cricoid pressure for, 420, 422–23, 423t, 1265–66, 1267f
 dental appliances and, 428–29
 devices, 1377–78
 facial bleeding and, 430, 430f
 flow-restricted, oxygen-powered devices, 420–21, 421f, 421t, 423
 mouth-to-stoma, 467, 470–71f
 multilumen airways, 430–37, 431–36f, 436t
 one-person BVM, 415–17, 416f, 417f
 rates, 415
 respiration versus, 853
 three-person BVM, 418, 420
 two-person BVM, 417–18, 419f
Ventral (body) position or location, 120, 121, 122
Ventricles, 182, 885
Ventricular fibrillation (V-fib), 902–3, 903f, 949, 949f, 971, 972t, 1106, 1298–99
Ventricular rhythms, 945
Ventricular tachycardia (V-tach), 546, 902, 903f, 947–48, 947f, 960, 1296–97
 management, 971t
 pulseless, 971, 972t, 1298–99
Verbal communications, 593–600
Verbal stimuli, responsiveness to, 509
Vertebrae, 138–41, 139–40f, 142, 142f
Vertebral canal, 166
Vertebral column, 139–41, 139f, 140f
Vesicants, 1498–99, 1499f
Vesicular sounds, 547
Vestibular folds, 202, 202f
Vestibule, 1151, 1152f, 1170, 1170f
VHF (very high frequency), 581

Violent behaviors, 1065, 1141–43.
Violent situations, 65–66
Viral hemorrhagic fevers, 1505–6, 1506f, 1507t
Virulence, infectious disease, 56
Viruses, 1505–6, 1506f, 1506t
Visually-impaired patients, 598–99, 1343
Vital capacity, 204
Vital signs
 by age, 1249t
 baseline, 525–26, 528, 536, 537, 551
 dehydration and, 1305t
 focused assessment, 528, 536
 medication administration and, 263
 pediatric, 1248–50, 1249f
 physical exam, 551
 progression of shock, 663
 rapid medical assessment, 537
 rapid trauma assessment, 520, 525–26
VITAMINS C & D mnemonic, 1350
Vocal cords, 202f
Volatility, of chemical agents, 1498
Volume
 conversion to metric units, 329, 330
 of medication to be administered, 332–33
Voluntary activities, 765
Voluntary muscles, 130, 158, 800–801, 800–801f
Voluntary nerves, 248f, 765
Volutrol IV sets, 318, 319f, 1277, 1279
Vomiting (emesis), 1041, 1084–85, 1351–52
Vomitus, bagging of, 1037, 1038

W

Warning placards, hazardous materials, 1467–68f, 1467–69
Water hazards, 1124–25
Water rescue safety, 1119, 1120f, 1122f
Weaponization, 1494
Weapons of mass destruction (WMD), 1047, 1478, 1493–94.
Weather and road conditions, 1388–89, 1388f
Weight
 conversion to metric units, 329–30
 distribution of, 1408–14
 estimates for children, 1279
 lifting and carrying, 1415–16
West Nile virus, 57
Wet breath sounds, 547
Wheals, 1009, 1009f
Wheeled ambulance stretchers, 1112–13, 1413f, 1430–35, 1432–34f, 1435t
Wheezing, 523, 547, 859, 860, 861, 869t, 1006, 1011, 1247t
Whistle-tip catheters, 398, 400, 400f
White blood cells, 178, 179–80, 179f
Whooping cough, 57
Wound care supplies, 1379, 1379f
Wrists, 125, 146, 148, 830–31, 831f, 832f.
Written communications, 600–606, 604f, 607t

X

Xiphoid process, 141, 141f, 143, 1274
X-rays, 1511, 1512f

Z

Zone of injury, 803–4, 803f
Zygomas, 542, 544f
Zygomatic arch, 136, 137f
Zygotes, 1171

Credits

Section 1
Opener © Tom Carter/PhotoEdit

Chapter 1
Opener © Mark Ide; 1-1 © Linda Gheen; 1-3 © Shout Pictures/Custom Medical Stock Photo

Chapter 2
2-1 © Luis Santana/911 Pictures; 2-2 © Stephane Brunet/911 Pictures; 2-3 © Spencer Grant, Liaison International; 2-5 © Craig Jackson/In the Dark Photography; 2-7 Courtesy of U.S. Department of Agriculture and U.S. Department of Health and Human Services; 2-8 © Digital Vision; 2-12 © Mark Ide; 2-13 © Bill Aron/PhotoEdit; 2-15 © Craig Jackson/In the Dark Photography; 2-25 © U.S. Department of Transportation; 2-26 and 2-32 © Linda Gheen

Chapter 3
Opener © Bill Aron/PhotoEdit; 3-1 and 3-3 © Craig Jackson/In the Dark Photography; 3-4 © Mark & Audrey Gibson, Gibson Stock Photography; 3-5 © Lawrence Porter/911 Pictures; 3-6 © Linda Gheen; 3-9 © EyeWire, Inc.

Chapter 4
Opener © Michael Heller/911 Pictures

Chapter 5
5-11 A and B: © John D. Cunningham/Visuals Unlimited; C: © R. Calentine/Visuals Unlimited; 5-12 A: © David M. Phillips/Visuals Unlimited; 5-113 B: © Chet Childs/Custom Medical Stock Photo; 5-114 (photo) © Art Siegel, University of Pennsylvania

Section 2
Opener © Craig Jackson/In the Dark Photography

Chapter 7
Opener © Mark Ide

Chapter 8
Opener © Craig Jackson/In the Dark Photography; 8-1 © Michael Heller/911 Pictures; 8-6 and 8-15 Used with permission of the American Academy of Pediatrics, *Pediatric Education for Prehospital Professionals*, © American Academy of Pediatrics, 2000

Section 3
Opener © Spencer Grant/PhotoEdit

Chapter 9
9-25 © Eddie Sperling; 9-52 Used with permission of the American Academy of Pediatrics, *Pediatric Education for Prehospital Professionals*, © American Academy of Pediatrics, 2000

Section 4
Opener © Tom Carter/PhotoEdit

Chapter 10
10-02 © Tony Freeman/PhotoEdit; 10-8 A. © Charles Stewart & Associates; B. © D. Willoughby/Custom Medical Stock Photography; 10-9 © Linda Gheen; 10-15 © Jones & Bartlett Publishers. Photographed by Scarlett Stoppa; 10-26 © Craig Jackson/In the Dark Photography; 10-27 © Michael Heller/911 Pictures

Chapter 11
Opener © Craig Jackson/In the Dark Photography; 11-6 Courtesy of National Academies of Emergency Dispatch

Section 5
Opener © Pete Fisher/911 Pictures

Chapter 12
Opener © Pete Fisher/911 Pictures; 12-8 and 12-9 Courtesy of the Maryland Institute of Emergency Medical Services Systems; 12-15 © D. Willoughby/Custom Medical Stock Photo

Chapter 13
Opener © James Shaffer/PhotoEdit; 13-2 © Craig Jackson/In the Dark Photography

Chapter 14
Opener © Charles Stewart & Associates; 14-2 © Jones & Bartlett Publishers. Photographed by Kimberly Potvin; 14-7 © Michael English, MD/Custom Medical Stock Photo; 14-11 © Custom Medical Stock Photo; 14-15 © Charles Stewart & Associates; 14-25 A: © St. Stephen's Hospital/Photo Researchers, Inc. B: © Charles Stewart & Associates

Chapter 15
Opener © Mark Ide; 15-4 © Charles Stewart & Associates

Chapter 16
Opener © John Meyer/Custom Medical Stock Photo; 16-5 © Custom Medical Stock Photo; 16-6 © Michael English, MD/Custom Medical Stock Photo; 16-15 © Kirk Sides/On Scene Photography

Chapter 17
Opener © Linda Gheen; 17-16 © Tony Freeman/PhotoEdit; Used with permission of the American Academy of Pediatrics, *Pediatric Education for Prehospital Professionals*, 17-28 © American Academy of Pediatrics, 2000

Chapter 18
Opener © Craig Jackson/In the Dark Photography; 18-15 Courtesy of the Maryland Institute of Emergency Medical Services Systems; 18-16 and 18-17 © Custom Medical Stock Photo; 18-18 © Steve Skjold/PhotoEdit; 18-22 © K. Shea/Custom Medical Stock Photo; 18-27 © Shout Pictures/Custom Medical Stock Photo; 18-35 Used with permission of the American Academy of Pediatrics, *Pediatric Education for Prehospital Professionals*, © American Academy of Pediatrics, 2000; 18-41 Courtesy of the Maryland Institute of Emergency Medical Services Systems; 18-46 © Science Photo Library/Photo Researchers

Section 6
Opener © Michael Newman/PhotoEdit

Chapter 19
Opener © Tom Carter/911 Pictures

Chapter 20
Opener © Craig Jackson/In the Dark Photography; 20-34 Reproduced with permission. Adapted from CPR for Family and Friends, © 2000, American Heart Association

Chapter 21
Opener © Craig Jackson/In the Dark Photography; 22-1 © Custom Medical Stock Photo

Chapter 22
Opener © Craig Jackson/In the Dark Photography; 22-2 A (photo): © AbleStock; 22-4 © Craig Jackson/In the Dark Photography; 22-6 © Andrea Randolph; 22-10 A: ©AbleStock; 22-16 Courtesy of the Moose Jaw Police Service; 22-18 B: © AbleStock

Chapter 23
Opener © Keith Hawkins/FocusGroup/PictureQuest; 23-1 A: © Mark Clarke/Photo Researchers, Inc. B: PhotoEdit, C: Eyewire Images, D: Courtesy of George Roarty/VDEM; 23-3 © Neil Schneider/911 Pictures; 23-4 © AbleStock

Chapter 24
Opener © Craig Jackson/In the Dark Photography; 24-1 Graphic World/Nadine Sokol; 24-5 © Michael Heller/911 Pictures; 24-6 © Michael Heller/911 Pictures

Chapter 25
Opener © Craig Jackson/In the Dark Photography

Chapter 26
Opener © Linda Gheen; 26-8 Courtesy of the Maryland Institute of Emergency Medical Services Systems; 26-12 © Mark Ide

Chapter 27
27-1 © Craig Jackson/In the Dark Photography; 27-2 © Mark Ide

Section 7
Opener Courtesy of the Maryland Institute of Emergency Medical Services Systems

Chapter 29
29-10 © Lennart Nilsson, *A Child is Born*; 29-19 Used with permission of the American Academy of Pediatrics, *Pediatric Education for Prehospital Professionals*, © American Academy of Pediatrics, 2000

Chapter 30
Opener © Michael Heller/911 Pictures; 30-4 Courtesy of David Burchfield, MD; 30-6 Used with permission of the American Academy of Pediatrics, *Pediatric Education for Prehospital Professionals*, © American Academy of Pediatrics, 2000; 30-7 Courtesy of Ron Dieckmann, MD; 30-9 Courtesy of Neotech Products, Inc.

Chapter 31
Opener © Craig Jackson/In the Dark Photography; 31-1 © Linda Gheen; 31-9 Courtesy of National EMSC Slide Set; 31-10 Courtesy of Dena Brownstein, MD; 31-11 and 31-12 Courtesy of National EMSC Slide Set; 31-13, 31-14, 31-20, 31-27, 31-38, 31-39, 31-41, 31-42, 31-43, 31-44, 31-45, and 31-51 Used with permission of the American Academy of Pediatrics, *Pediatric Education for Prehospital Professionals*, © American Academy of Pediatrics, 2000; 31-57 © Ron Dieckmann, MD

Chapter 32
Opener © Mark & Audrey Gibson/Gibson Stock Photography; 32-3 © Photodisc; 32-4 © Charles Stewart & Associates; 32-10 © Craig Jackson/In the Dark Photography

Section 8
Opener Courtesy of the Maryland Institute of Emergency Medical Services Systems

Chapter 33
Opener © Mark & Audrey Gibson, Gibson Stock Photography; 33-1 and Courtesy of American Emergency Vehicles; 33-16 © Mike Bucy/FireShots; 33-18 © Ken Sherman; 33-21 © Michael Heller/911 Pictures; 33-25 Courtesy of the Maryland Institute of Emergency Medical Services Systems

Chapter 34
Opener © Mark & Audrey Gibson, Gibson Stock Photography

Chapter 35
Opener © Steve Townsend/Code 3 Images; 35-1 © Spencer Grant/PhotoEdit; 35-2 © Tony Freeman/PhotoEdit/PictureQuest; 35-4 © Craig Jackson/In the Dark Photography; 35-6 © Tony Freeman/PhotoEdit; 35-8 Courtesy of the Maryland Institute of Emergency Medical Services Systems

Chapter 36
Opener © Steve Spak/911 Pictures; 36-1 Courtesy of the National Wildfire Coordinating Group; 36-5 and 36-6 © U.S. Department of Transportation; 36-7 © Chris Mickal/911 Pictures; 36-10 © Linda Gheen; 36-19 Courtesy of Craig C. Schleunes

Chapter 37
Opener © Steve Spak/911 Pictures; 37-1 © NHK/AP Photo; 37-2 © Oded Balilty/AP Photo; 37-3 © Rick Bowmer/AP Photo; 37-5 © Steve Spak/911 Pictures; 37-6 © Dennis MacDonald/PhotoEdit; 37-7 © Spencer Grant/PhotoEdit; 37-8 Courtesy of Dr. Saeed Keshavarz/RCCI, Research Center of Chemical Injuries/IRAN; 37-9 © Jones and Bartlett Publishers. Photographed by Kimberly Potvin; 37-10 © Chiaki Tsukumo/AP Photo; 37-11 Courtesy of CDC; 37-12 Courtesy of Professor Robert Swanepoel/National Institute for Communicable Diseases; 37-13 Courtesy of James H. Steele/CDC; 37-14 A and B: Courtesy of CDC; 37-15 Courtesy of Brian Prechtel/USDA; 37-16 Courtesy of the Strategic National Stockpile/CDC

Section 9
Opener © Craig Jackson/In the Dark Photography

Chapter 38
Opener Courtesy of the Maryland Institute of Emergency Medical Services Systems

Chapter 39
Opener © Craig Jackson/In the Dark Photography

Unless otherwise indicated, photographs have been supplied by the Maryland Institute of Emergency Medical Services Systems. Photographs have also been supplied by the Academy of Orthopaedic Surgeons, Rhonda Beck and Jones and Bartlett Publishers. Illustrations were created by Imagineering and Rolin Graphics.

Notes

Notes